BNF
47

MARCH 2004

BNF.org

D1386474

BRITISH
NATIONAL
FORMULARY

•

British Medical Association

**Royal Pharmaceutical Society
of Great Britain**

Published by the British Medical Association
Tavistock Square, London WC1H 9JP, UK
and the **Royal Pharmaceutical Society of Great Britain**
1 Lambeth High Street, London, SE1 7JN, UK
© 2004 British Medical Association and the Royal Pharmaceutical Society of Great Britain

ISBN: 0 85369 584 9 (Royal Pharmaceutical Society of Great Britain)

ISSN: 0260-535X

Printed in Germany by Clausen & Bosse, CPI Books, Leck

A catalogue record for this book is available from the British Library.

Copies may be obtained through any bookseller or direct from:

Pharmaceutical Press
  PO Box 151
  Wallingford
  Oxon OX10 8QU
  UK
  Tel: +44 (0) 1491 829 272
  Fax: +44 (0) 1491 829 292
  E-mail: rpsgb@cabi.org
  www.pharmpress.com

The Pharmaceutical Press also supplies the BNF in digital formats suitable for standalone use or for small networks, for use over an intranet and for use on a personal digital assistant (PDA).

NHS Responseline
General practitioners and community pharmacies in **England** can telephone the NHS Responseline for enquiries concerning the direct mailing of the *British National Formulary*
Tel: 08701 555 455

For a list of changes to approved names of drugs, see p. x

Contents

Preface

The BNF is a joint publication of the British Medical Association and the Royal Pharmaceutical Society of Great Britain. It is published under the authority of a Joint Formulary Committee which comprises representatives of the two professional bodies and of the UK Health Departments. The BNF aims to provide prescribers, pharmacists and other healthcare professionals with sound up-to-date information about the use of medicines.

The BNF includes key information on the selection, prescribing, dispensing and administration of medicines. Drugs that are generally prescribed in the UK are covered and those considered less suitable for prescribing are clearly identified. Little or no information is included on medicines that are promoted for purchase by the public.

Basic information about drugs is drawn from the manufacturers' product literature, from medical and pharmaceutical literature, from regulatory and professional authorities, and from the data used for pricing prescriptions. Advice on the therapeutic use of medicines and on the choice of drugs is constructed from clinical literature and reflects, wherever possible, an evaluation of the evidence. The advice also takes account of authoritative national guidelines. In addition, the Joint Formulary Committee receives expert clinical advice on all therapeutic areas in tune with current best evidence; this ensures that the BNF's recommendations are relevant to practice. Many individuals and organisations contribute towards the preparation of each edition of the BNF.

The BNF is designed as a digest for rapid reference and it may not always include all the information necessary for prescribing and dispensing. Also, less detail is given on areas such as obstetrics, malignant disease, and anaesthesia since it is expected that those undertaking treatment will have specialist knowledge and access to specialist literature. The BNF should be interpreted in light of professional knowledge and supplemented as necessary by specialised publications and by reference to the manufacturers' product literature. Information is also available from medicines information services (see inside front cover).

Biannual publication allows the BNF to reflect promptly changes in product availability as well as emerging safety concerns and shifts in clinical practice. The more important changes for this edition are listed on p. viii. The current edition must **always** be used for making clinical decisions.

The BNF on the internet (BNF.org) includes additional information of relevance to healthcare professionals dealing with medicines. Other digital versions of the BNF—including intranet versions—are produced in parallel with the paper version.

> The BNF welcomes comments from healthcare professionals; such comments help to ensure that the BNF remains relevant to practice. Comments and constructive criticism should be sent to:
> Executive Editor, British National Formulary,
> c/o Royal Pharmaceutical Society of Great Britain,
> 1 Lambeth High Street, London SE1 7JN.
> Email: editor@bnf.org

Acknowledgements

The Joint Formulary Committee is grateful to individuals and organisations that have provided advice and information to the BNF.

The principal contributors for this edition were:

I.H. Ahmed-Jushuf, S.P. Allison, M. Badminton, T.P. Baglin, P.R.J. Barnes, D.N. Bateman, R.H. Behrens, D. Bowsher, M.J. Brodie, R.J. Buckley, I.F. Burgess, D.J. Burn, A.J. Camm, R. Dinwiddie, P.N. Durrington, A.J. Duxbury, T.S.J. Elliott, B.G. Gazzard, A.H. Ghodse, N.J.L. Gittoes, P.J. Goadsby, E.C. Gordon-Smith, I.A. Greer, J. Guillebaud, C.H. Hawkes, C.J. Hawkey, S.H.D. Jackson, J.R. Kirwan, P.G. Kopelman, L. Lane, M.J.S. Langman, T.H. Lee, L. Luzzatto, K.E.L. McColl, G.M. Mead, E. Miller, J.M. Neuberger, J. Nooney, D.J. Nutt, D.J. Oliver, L.P. Ormerod, P.A. Poole-Wilson, D.J. Rowbotham, P.C. Rubin, R.S. Sawers, A.E. Tattersfield, S. Thomas, D.G. Waller, D.A. Warrell, A. Wilcock.

Members of the British Association of Dermatologists Therapy Guidelines and Audit Subcommittee, A. Anstey, A.S. Highet, J. McLelland, R.H. Meyrick-Thomas, A.D. Ormerod, C.H. Smith, J.C. Sterling, and D. White (Secretariat) have provided valuable advice.

The Joint British Societies' Coronary Risk Prediction Charts have been reproduced with the kind permission of P.N. Durrington who has also provided the BNF with access to the computer program for assessing coronary and stroke risk.

Correspondents in the pharmaceutical industry have provided information on new products and commented on products in the BNF. The Prescription Pricing Authority has supplied the prices of products in the BNF.

Numerous doctors, pharmacists, nurses and others have sent comments and suggestions.

The BNF has valuable access to the *Martindale* data banks by courtesy of S. Sweetman and staff.

C.L. Iskander provided considerable assistance during the production of this edition of the BNF.

Additional checks on the BNF data were undertaken by A. Breewood and M. Davis.

E.I. Connor and K.A. Parsons have assisted with the development of the electronic BNF and publishing software. Xpage and CSW Informatics Ltd have provided technical assistance with the editorial database and typesetting software.

Joint Formulary Committee 2003–2004

Chairman
Martin J. Kendall
MB, ChB, MD, FRCP

Deputy Chairman
Nicholas L. Wood
BPharm, FRPharmS

Committee Members
Nigel S. Baber
BSc, MB, FRCP, FRCP(Ed), FFPH, DipClinPharmacol

Alison Blenkinsopp
PhD, BPharm, FRPharmS

Peter Clappison
MB, ChB, MRCGP

Michael J. Goodman
MA, BM, BCh, DPhil, FRCP

Margaret L. Hewetson
BPharm, DipHospPharm, MRPharmS

Frank P. Marsh
MA, MB, BChir, FRCP

Roopendra K. Prasad
MB BS, MS, FRCS, FRCGP

Ewen Sim
BSc, MB, ChB, DipHlthMgmt

James Smith
BPharm, PhD, FRPharmS, MCPP, MIInfSc

Joint Secretaries
Vivienne H. Nathanson
MB, BS

Philip E. Green
BSc, MSc, LLM, MRPharmS

Executive Secretary
Tracy L. South
BTEC

Editorial Staff

Executive Editor
Dinesh K. Mehta
BPharm, MSc, FRPharmS

Senior Assistant Editor
John Martin
BPharm, PhD, MRPharmS

Assistant Editors
Bryony Jordan
BSc, DipPharmPract, MRPharmS

Colin R. Macfarlane
BPharm, MSc, MRPharmS

Rachel S. M. Ryan
BPharm, MRPharmS

Shama M. S. Wagle
BPharm, DipPharmPract, MRPharmS

Staff Editors
Fauziah T. Hashmi
BSc, MSc, MRPharmS

Sangeeta Kakar
BSc, MRPharmS

Maria Kouimtzi
BPharm, PhD, MRPharmS

Dawud Masieh
BPharm, MRPharmS

Vinaya K. Sharma
BPharm, MSc, MRPharmS

Mark C. Stuart
BPharm, DipCDDS, DipBotMed, MRPharmS

Rob Ticehurst
BSc, MRPharmS

Editorial Assistant
Gerard P. Gallagher

Head of Publishing Services
John Wilson

Director of Publications
Charles Fry

How to use the BNF

Notes on conditions, drugs and preparations

The main text consists of classified notes on clinical conditions, drugs and preparations. These notes are divided into 15 chapters, each of which is related to a particular system of the body or to an aspect of medical care. Each chapter is then divided into sections which begin with appropriate *notes for prescribers*. These notes are intended to provide information to doctors, pharmacists, nurses, and other healthcare professionals to facilitate the selection of suitable treatment. The notes are followed by details of relevant drugs and preparations.

Guidance on prescribing

This part includes information on prescription writing, controlled drugs and dependence, prescribing for children and the elderly, and prescribing in palliative care. Advice is given on the reporting of adverse reactions.

DRUG NAME ▭●

Indications: details of uses and indications

Cautions: details of precautions required (with cross-references to appropriate Appendixes) and also any monitoring required

COUNSELLING. Verbal explanation to the patient of specific details of the drug treatment (e.g. posture when taking a medicine)

Contra-indications: details of any contra-indications to use of drug

Side-effects: details of common and more serious side-effects

Dose: dose and frequency of administration (max. dose); CHILD and ELDERLY details of dose for specific age group

By alternative route, dose and frequency

* **Approved Name** (Non-proprietary) PoM ●
Pharmaceutical form, colour, coating, active ingredient and amount in dosage form, net price, pack size = basic NHS price. Label: (as in Appendix 9)

Proprietary Name® (Manufacturer) PoM NHS ●

Pharmaceutical form, sugar-free, active ingredient mg/mL, net price, pack size = basic NHS price. Label: (as in Appendix 9)

Excipients: includes clinically important excipients or electrolytes
* exceptions to the prescribing status indicated by a footnote.
Note. Specific notes about the product e.g. handling

Preparations

Preparations usually follow immediately after the drug which is their main ingredient.

Preparations are included under a non-proprietary title, if they are marketed under such a title, if they are not otherwise prescribable under the NHS, or if they may be prepared extemporaneously.

If proprietary preparations are of a distinctive colour this is stated.

In the case of compound preparations the indications, cautions, contra-indications, side-effects, and interactions of all constituents should be taken into account for prescribing.

Emergency treatment of poisoning

This chapter provides information on the management of acute poisoning when first seen in the home, although aspects of hospital-based treatment are mentioned.

Appendixes and indexes

The appendixes include information on interactions, liver disease, renal impairment, pregnancy, breast-feeding, intravenous additives, borderline substances, wound management products, and cautionary and advisory labels for dispensed medicines. They are designed for use in association with the main body of the text.

The Dental Practitioners' List and the Nurse Prescribers' List are also included in this section. The indexes consist of the Index of Manufacturers and the Main Index.

Drugs

Drugs appear under pharmacopoeial or other non-proprietary titles. When there is an *appropriate current monograph* (Medicines Act 1968, Section 65) preference is given to a name at the head of that monograph; otherwise a British Approved Name (BAN), if available, is used (see also p. x).

The symbol ▭ is used to denote those preparations that are considered by the Joint Formulary Committee to be less suitable for prescribing. Although such preparations may not be considered as drugs of first choice, their use may be justifiable in certain circumstances.

Prescription-only medicines PoM

This symbol has been placed against those preparations that are available only on a prescription given by an appropriate practitioner. For more detailed information see *Medicines, Ethics and Practice*, No. 27, London, Pharmaceutical Press, 2003 (and subsequent editions as available).

The symbol CD indicates that the preparation is subject to the prescription requirements of the Misuse of Drugs Act. For regulations governing prescriptions for such preparations see pages 7–9.

Preparations not available for NHS prescription NHS

This symbol has been placed against those preparations included in the BNF that are not prescribable under the NHS. Those prescribable only for specific disorders have a footnote specifying the condition(s) for which the preparation remains available. Some preparations which are not *prescribable* by brand name under the NHS may nevertheless be *dispensed* using the brand name providing that the prescription shows an appropriate non-proprietary name.

Prices

Prices have been calculated from the basic cost used in pricing NHS prescriptions dispensed in October 2003 or later, see p. vii for further details.

Patient Packs

On January 1 1994, Directive 92/27/EEC came into force, giving the requirements for the labelling of medicines and outlining the format and content of patient information leaflets to be supplied with every medicine. The directive also requires the use of Recommended International Non-proprietary Names for drugs (see p. x).

All medicines have approved labelling and patient information leaflets; anyone who supplies a medicine is responsible for providing the relevant information to the patient (see also Appendix 9).

Many medicines are available in manufacturers' original packs complete with patient information leaflets. Where patient packs are available, the BNF shows the number of dose units in the packs. In particular clinical circumstances, where patient packs need to be split or medicines are provided in bulk dispensing packs, manufacturers will provide additional supplies of patient information leaflets on request.

During the revision of each edition of the BNF careful note is taken of the information that appears on the patient information leaflets. Where it is considered appropriate to alert a prescriber to some specific limitation appearing on the patient information leaflet (for example, in relation to pregnancy) this advice now appears in the BNF.

The patient information leaflet also includes details of all inactive ingredients in the medicine. A list of common E numbers and the inactive ingredients to which they correspond is now therefore included in the BNF (see inside back cover).

PACT and SPA

PACT (Prescribing Analyses and Cost) and SPA (Scottish Prescribing Analysis) provide prescribers with information about their prescribing.

The *PACT Standard Report*, or in Scotland SPA *Level 1 Report*, is sent to all general practitioners on a quarterly basis. The PACT Standard Report contains an analysis of the practitioner's prescribing and the practice prescribing over the last 3 months, and gives comparisons with the local Primary Care Trust equivalent practice and with a national equivalent. The report also contains details of the practice prescribing for a specific topic; a different topic is chosen each quarter.

The *PACT Catalogue*, or in Scotland SPA *Level 2 Report*, provides a full inventory of the prescriptions issued by a prescriber. The PACT catalogue is available on request for periods between 1 and 24 months. To allow the prescriber to target specific areas of prescribing, a Catalogue may be requested to cover individual preparations, BNF sections, or combinations of BNF chapters.

PACT is also available electronically (ePACT.net). This system gives users on-line access through NHSnet to the 3 years' prescribing data held on the Prescription Pricing Authority's database; tools for analysing the data are also provided.

Prices in the BNF

Basic **net prices** are given in the BNF to provide an indication of relative cost. Where there is a choice of suitable preparations for a particular disease or condition the relative cost may be used in making a selection. Cost-effective prescribing must, however, take into account other factors (such as dose frequency and duration of treatment) that affect the total cost. The use of more expensive drugs is justified if it will result in better treatment of the patient or a reduction of the length of an illness or the time spent in hospital.

Prices have generally been calculated from the net cost used in pricing NHS prescriptions dispensed in October 2003, but where available later prices have been included; unless an original pack is available these prices are based on the largest pack size of the preparation in use in community pharmacies. The price for an extemporaneously prepared preparation has been omitted where the net cost of the ingredients used to make it would give a misleadingly low impression of the final price. In Appendix 8 prices stated are per dressing or bandage.

The unit of 20 is still sometimes used as a basis for comparison, but where suitable original packs or patient packs are available these are priced instead.

Gross prices vary as follows:

1. Costs to the NHS are greater than the net prices quoted and include professional fees and overhead allowances;
2. Private prescription charges are calculated on a separate basis;
3. Over-the-counter sales are at retail price, as opposed to basic net price, and include VAT.

> **BNF prices are NOT, therefore, suitable for quoting to patients seeking private prescriptions or contemplating over-the-counter purchases.**

A fuller explanation of costs to the NHS may be obtained from the Drug Tariff.

It should be noted that separate Drug Tariffs are applicable to England and Wales, Scotland, and Northern Ireland. Prices in the different tariffs may vary.

Changes for this edition

Significant changes

The BNF is revised twice yearly and numerous changes are made between issues. All copies of BNF No. 46 (September 2003) should therefore be withdrawn and replaced by BNF No. 47 (March 2004). Significant changes have been made in the following sections for BNF No. 47:

Adverse reactions to drugs [new text on side-effects], Guidance on prescribing

Emergency treatment of poisoning [updated advice on management of poisoning by ibuprofen, tricyclic antidepressants, phenothiazines, cocaine, noxious gases, and paraquat; new advice on poisoning by calcium-channel blockers, and methanol], Emergency treatment of poisoning

Infliximab for Crohn's disease [NICE guidance], section 1.5

Drug treatment of hypertension [revised text], section 2.5

Appropriate use of long-acting beta$_2$ agonists in asthma [important warnings about salmeterol and formoterol], section 3.1.1.1

Adrenal crisis in children with excessive doses of inhaled corticosteroids [important warning], section 3.2

Selective serotonin re-uptake inhibitors not to be used in those under 18 years [updated CSM advice], section 4.3.3

Antibacterial treatment of meningitis [revised text], Table 1, section 5.1

Antibacterial treatment of uncomplicated gonorrhoea [revised text], Table 1, section 5.1

Antibacterial treatment of osteomyelitis and septic arthritis [revised text], Table 1, section 5.1

Prevention of infection in urological procedures [new text], Table 2, section 5.1

Treatment of chronic hepatitis C [revised text], section 5.3

Oseltamivir, zanamivir, and amantadine for prophylaxis of influenza [NICE guidance], section 5.3

Specific recommendations for malaria prophylaxis [updated advice], section 5.4.1

Pioglitazone and rosiglitazone for type 2 diabetes mellitus [updated NICE guidance], section 6.1.2.3

Use of HRT for prevention of osteoporosis in women over 50 years of age [CSM safety update], section 6.4.1

Somatropin for adults with growth hormone deficiency [NICE guidance], section 6.5.1

Danazol for the management of endometriosis and benign fibrocystic breast disease [revised text], section 6.7.2

Liposomal doxorubicin side-effects [revised text], section 8.1.2

Imatinib for chronic myeloid leukaemia [NICE guidance], section 8.1.5

Rituximab for aggressive non-Hodgkin's lymphoma [NICE guidance], section 8.2.3

Bicalutamide no longer used for localised prostate cancer [CSM advice], section 8.3.4

Use of hydroxycarbamide for sickle-cell disease [new text], section 9.1.3

Drugs used in autoimmune thrombocytopenic purpura [revised text], section 9.1.4

Drugs used in neutropenia [reorganised text], section 9.1.6

Fluoride [revised text], section 9.5.3

Zinc [revised text], section 9.5.4

Doxycycline mouthwash for severe recurrent aphthous ulceration [new text], section 12.3.1

Immunisation schedule [MMR vaccine replaces Rubella vaccine (for non-immune women of child-bearing age)], section 14.1

Post-immunisation pyrexia in infants [revised text], section 14.1

Diphtheria vaccines [revised text], section 14.4

Influenza vaccine for children [revised text], section 14.4

Measles, Mumps and Rubella vaccine [revised text], section 14.4

Pneumococcal vaccine [revised text], section 14.4

Varicella-zoster vaccine [revised text], section 14.4

Tick-borne encephalitis vaccine [new text], section 14.4

Anti-D (Rh$_0$) immunoglobulin and MMR vaccine in postpartum women [revised text], section 14.5

International travel, tetanus booster [new text], section 14.6

NOTE. In view of changes in the plans for market withdrawal, information on primidone has been reinstated in BNF 47.

Dose changes

Changes in dose statements introduced into BNF No. 47:

Aspirin (antiplatelet), p. 118
Basiliximab, p. 425
Candesartan, p. 95
Colistin, p. 280
Copegus®, p. 311
Dexamethasone, p. 349
Diazepam [rectal solution], p. 236
Fluoxetine, p. 194
Full Marks® lotion, p. 572
Hypnomidate, p. 602
Levonorgestrel, p. 393
Meloxicam, p. 484
Midazolam [for induction of anaesthesia], p. 607
Pioglitazone, p. 337
Premarin® vaginal cream, p. 384
Rocuronium bromide, p. 611
Somatuline® LA, p. 437
Sodium nitrite, p. 27
Sumatriptan [nasal spray], p. 223
WHO formulation of rehydration salts, p. 450
Zeffix®, p. 302

Classification changes

Classification changes have been made in the following sections for BNF No. 47:

Section 1.1.1 Antacids and simeticone [title change]
Section 1.1.1 Antacid preparations containing simeticone [subtitle change]
Section 1.1.1 Simeticone alone [subtitle change]
Section 1.5 Cytokine inhibitors [new subsection]
Section 10.1.3 Cytokine inhibitors [new subsection]
Section A8.2.10 Multi-layer compression bandaging kits [subtitle removed]

Discontinued preparations

Preparations discontinued during the compilation of BNF No. 47:

AC Vax®
Adgyn Estro®
Adgyn Combi®
Adgyn Medro®
Adsorbed Diphtheria [low dose] Vaccine for Adults and Adolescents
Akineton®
Alphosyl®
Alupent® tablets
Alyrane®
Aminoplex® products
Aramine®
Atrovent® *Autohaler*®
Atrovent® *Forte* aerosol inhalation
Brasivol® *Paste No.2*
Calsynar®
Clinomel® products
Compound Thymol Glycerin, BP 1988
Cymevene® capsules
Debrisoquine
Dermestril®
Dermestril Septem®
Doloxene®
Eurax® dermatological bath oil
Estrapak®
Feldene® suppositories
Flagyl Compak®
Fucidin® gel
Gammabulin®
Haemaccel®
Hepanutrin®
Inderetic®
Inderex®
Indocid®
Indocid-R®
Jectofer®
KabiMix® products
Kefadol®
Kefzol®
Kerlone®
Medicoal®
Minihep®

Monozide® *10*
Nivaquine® injection
Oxivent®
Profasi®
Retrovir® tablets
Rubella vaccine, live
Quinoderm® lotio-gel
Sevredol® oral solution
Ster-Zac Powder®
Streflam®
Tavegil® elixir
Terra-Cortril Nystatin®
Zaditen® capsules

New preparations included in this edition

Preparations included in the relevant sections of BNF No. 47:

Anzemet®, p. 205
Avandamet®, p. 338
Busilvex®, p. 410
Cetraben®, p. 540
Duac® *Once Daily*, p. 556
Emtriva®, p. 302
Enbrel®, p. 495
Foresteo®, p. 369
FSME-IMMUN®, p. 593
Fuzeon®, p. 307
Humira®, p. 495
Kineret®, p. 495
Minijet® *Morphine Sulphate*, p. 214
Morphgesic® *SR*, p. 214
Niaspan®, p. 129
OliClinomel N4-550E, N4-720E, N6-900E, N7-1000, p. 459
Remicade®, p. 496
Stalevo®, p. 241
StructoKabiven® *Electrolyte-Free*, p. 459
Subcuvia®, p. 595
Telfast® *30*, p. 152
Zibor®, p. 113

Late additions

Gliadel® (Link) PoM
Implant, carmustine 7.7 mg, net price = £687.50. BNF section 8.1.1
For treatment of recurrent glioblastoma multiforme as an adjunct to surgery

Gonapeptyl® **Depot** (Ferring) PoM
Injection, powder for reconstitution, triptorelin (as acetate), net price 3.75-mg prefilled syringe = £105.05 (with prefilled syringe of solvent). BNF section 8.3.4.2
For the treatment of advanced prostate cancer (section 8.3.4.2); reduction in size of uterine fibroids, endometriosis, precocious puberty (section 6.7.2)

Name changes

European Law requires use of the Recommended International Non-proprietary Name (rINN) for medicinal substances. In most cases the British Approved Name (BAN) and rINN were identical. Where the two differed, the BAN was modified to accord with the rINN.

The following list shows those substances for which the former BAN has been modified to accord with the rINN. The MHRA has proposed a timetable for effecting the change from former BANs to the new names. Former BANs have been retained as synonyms in the BNF.

ADRENALINE AND NORADRENALINE. Adrenaline and noradrenaline are the terms used in the titles of monographs in the European Pharmacopoeia and are thus the official names in the member states. For these substances, BP 2003 shows the European Pharmacopoeia names and the rINNs at the head of the monographs; the BNF has adopted a similar style.

Former BAN	New BAN
adrenaline	*see above*
amethocaine	tetracaine
aminacrine	aminoacridine
amoxycillin	amoxicillin
amphetamine	amfetamine
amylobarbitone	amobarbital
amylobarbitone sodium	amobarbital sodium
beclomethasone	beclometasone
bendrofluazide	bendroflumethiazide
benorylate	benorilate
benzhexol	trihexyphenidyl
benzphetamine	benzfetamine
benztropine	benzatropine
busulphan	busulfan
butobarbitone	butobarbital
carticaine	articaine
cephalexin	cefalexin
cephradine	cefradine
chloral betaine	cloral betaine
chlorbutol	chlorobutanol
chlormethiazole	clomethiazole
chlorpheniramine	chlorphenamine
chlorthalidone	chlortalidone
cholecalciferol	colecalciferol
cholestyramine	colestyramine
clomiphene	clomifene
colistin sulphomethate sodium	colistimethate sodium
corticotrophin	corticotropin
cyclosporin	ciclosporin
cysteamine	mercaptamine
danthron	dantron
desoxymethasone	desoximetasone
dexamphetamine	dexamfetamine
dibromopropamidine	dibrompropamidine
dicyclomine	dicycloverine
dienoestrol	dienestrol
dimethicone(s)	dimeticone

Former BAN	New BAN
dimethyl sulphoxide	dimethyl sulfoxide
dothiepin	dosulepin
doxycycline hydrochloride (hemihydrate hemiethanolate)	doxycycline hyclate
eformoterol	formoterol
ethamsylate	etamsylate
ethinyloestradiol	ethinylestradiol
ethynodiol	etynodiol
flumethasone	flumetasone
flupenthixol	flupentixol
flurandrenolone	fludroxycortide
frusemide	furosemide
gestronol	gestonorone
guaiphenesin	guaifenesin
hexachlorophane	hexachlorophene
hexamine hippurate	methenamine hippurate
hydroxyurea	hydroxycarbamide
indomethacin	indometacin
lignocaine	lidocaine
lysuride	lisuride
methotrimeprazine	levomepromazine
methyl cysteine	mecysteine
methylene blue	methylthioninium chloride
mitozantrone	mitoxantrone
mustine	chlormethine
nicoumalone	acenocoumarol
noradrenaline	*see above*
oestradiol	estradiol
oestriol	estriol
oestrone	estrone
oxpentifylline	pentoxifylline
phenobarbitone	phenobarbital
pipothiazine	pipotiazine
polyhexanide	polihexanide
potassium clorazepate	dipotassium clorazepate
pramoxine	pramocaine
procaine penicillin	procaine benzylpenicillin
prothionamide	protionamide
quinalbarbitone	secobarbital
riboflavine	riboflavin
salcatonin	calcitonin (salmon)
sodium calciumedetate	sodium calcium edetate
sodium cromoglycate	sodium cromoglicate
sodium ironedetate	sodium feredetate
sodium picosulphate	sodium picosulfate
sorbitan monostearate	sorbitan stearate
stibocaptate	sodium stibocaptate
stilboestrol	diethylstilbestrol
sulphacetamide	sulfacetamide
sulphadiazine	sulfadiazine
sulphamethoxazole	sulfamethoxazole
sulphapyridine	sulfapyridine
sulphasalazine	sulfasalazine
sulphathiazole	sulfathiazole
sulphinpyrazone	sulfinpyrazone
tetracosactrin	tetracosactide
thiabendazole	tiabendazole
thioguanine	tioguanine
thiopentone	thiopental
thymoxamine	moxisylyte
thyroxine sodium	levothyroxine sodium
tribavirin	ribavirin
trimeprazine	alimemazine
urofollitrophin	urofollitropin

Guidance on prescribing
General guidance

Medicines should be prescribed only when they are necessary, and in all cases the benefit of administering the medicine should be considered in relation to the risk involved. This is particularly important during pregnancy where the risk to both mother and fetus must be considered (for further details see Prescribing in Pregnancy, Appendix 4).

It is important to discuss treatment options carefully with the patient to ensure that the patient is content to take the medicine as prescribed (see also Taking Medicines to Best Effect, below). In particular, the patient should be helped to distinguish the side-effects of prescribed drugs from the effects of the medical disorder. Where the beneficial effects of the medicine are likely to be delayed, the patient should be advised of this.

TAKING MEDICINES TO BEST EFFECT. Difficulties in compliance with drug treatment occur regardless of age. Factors contributing to poor compliance with prescribed medicines include:

- Prescription not collected or not dispensed
- Purpose of medicine not clear
- Perceived lack of efficacy
- Real or perceived side-effects
- Instructions for administration not clear
- Physical difficulty in taking medicines (e.g. with swallowing the medicine, with handling small tablets, or with opening medicine containers)
- Unattractive formulation (e.g. unpleasant taste)
- Complicated regimen

The prescriber and the patient should agree on the health outcomes that the patient desires and on the strategy for achieving them ('concordance'). Further information on concordance is available on the Internet (www.medicines-partnership.org).

Taking the time to explain to the patient (and relatives) the rationale and the potential adverse effects of treatment may improve compliance. Reinforcement and elaboration of the physician's instructions by the pharmacist also helps. Advising the patient of the possibility of alternative treatments may encourage the patient to seek advice rather than merely abandon unacceptable treatment.

Simplifying the drug regimen may help; the need for frequent administration may reduce compliance although there appears to be little difference in compliance between once-daily and twice-daily administration. Combination products reduce the number of drugs taken but this may be at the expense of the ability to titrate individual doses.

COMPLEMENTARY MEDICINE. An increasing amount of information on complementary ('alternative') medicine is becoming available. However, the BNF's scope is restricted to the discussion of conventional medicines but reference is made to complementary treatments if they affect conventional therapy (e.g. interactions with St John's wort—see Appendix 1). Further information on herbal medicines is available at www.mhra.gov.uk

ABBREVIATION OF TITLES. In general, titles of drugs and preparations should be written *in full*. Unofficial abbreviations should not be used as they may be misinterpreted; obsolete titles, such as Mist. Expect. should not be used.

NON-PROPRIETARY TITLES. Where non-proprietary ('generic') titles are given, they should be used in prescribing. This will enable any suitable product to be dispensed, thereby saving delay to the patient and sometimes expense to the health service. The only exception is where bioavailability problems are so important that the patient should always receive the same brand; in such cases, the brand name or the manufacturer should be stated. Non-proprietary titles should **not** be invented for the purposes of prescribing generically since this can lead to confusion, particularly in the case of compound and modified-release preparations.

Titles used as headings for monographs may be used freely in the United Kingdom but in other countries may be subject to restriction.

Many of the non-proprietary titles used in this book are titles of monographs in the European Pharmacopoeia, British Pharmacopoeia or British Pharmaceutical Codex 1973. In such cases the preparations must comply with the standard (if any) in the appropriate publication, as required by the Medicines Act (Section 65).

PROPRIETARY TITLES. Names followed by the symbol® are or have been used as proprietary names in the United Kingdom. These names may in general be applied only to products supplied by the owners of the trade marks.

MARKETING AUTHORISATION AND BNF ADVICE. In general the *doses, indications, cautions, contra-indications and side-effects* in the BNF reflect those in the manufacturers' data sheets or Summaries of Product Characteristics (SPCs) which, in turn, reflect those in the corresponding Marketing Authorisations (formerly known as Product Licences). Where an unlicensed drug is included in the BNF, this is indicated in brackets after the entry. Where the BNF suggests a use (or route) that is outside the licensed indication of a product ('off-label' use), this too is indicated. Unlicensed use of medicines becomes necessary if the clinical need cannot be met by licensed medicines; such use should be supported by appropriate evidence and experience. When a preparation is available from more than one manufacturer, the BNF reflects advice that is the most clinically relevant regardless of any variation in the marketing authorisations.

The doses stated in the BNF are intended for general guidance and represent, unless otherwise stated, the usual range of doses that are generally regarded as being suitable for adults.

> Prescribing medicines outside the recommendations of their Marketing Authorisation alters (and probably increases) the doctor's professional responsibility.

ORAL SYRINGES. An **oral syringe** is supplied when oral liquid medicines are prescribed in doses other than multiples of 5 mL. The oral syringe is marked in 0.5-mL divisions from 1 to 5 mL to measure doses of less than 5 mL. It is provided with an adaptor and an instruction leaflet. The *5-mL spoon* is used for doses of 5 mL (or multiples thereof).

STRENGTHS AND QUANTITIES. The strength or quantity to be contained in capsules, lozenges, tablets, etc. should be stated by the prescriber.

If a pharmacist receives an incomplete prescription for a systemically administered preparation[1] and considers it would not be appropriate for the patient to return to the doctor, the following procedures will apply:

(a) an attempt must always be made to contact the prescriber to ascertain the intention;

(b) if the attempt is successful the pharmacist must, where practicable, subsequently arrange for details of quantity, strength where applicable, and dosage to be inserted by the prescriber on the incomplete form;

(c) where, although the prescriber has been contacted, it has not proved possible to obtain the written intention regarding an incomplete prescription, the pharmacist may endorse the form 'p.c.' (prescriber contacted) and add details of the quantity and strength where applicable of the preparation supplied, and of the dose indicated. The endorsement should be initialled and dated by the pharmacist;

(d) where the prescriber cannot be contacted and the pharmacist has sufficient information to make a professional judgment the preparation may be dispensed. If the quantity is missing the pharmacist may supply sufficient to complete up to 5 days' treatment; except that where a combination pack (i.e. a proprietary pack containing more than one medicinal product) or oral contraceptive is prescribed by name only, the smallest pack shall be dispensed. In all cases the prescription must be endorsed 'p.n.c.' (prescriber not contacted) the quantity, the dose, and the strength (where applicable) of the preparation supplied must be indicated, and the endorsement must be initialled and dated;

(e) if the pharmacist has any doubt about exercising discretion, an incomplete prescription must be referred back to the prescriber.

EXCIPIENTS. Oral liquid preparations that do not contain *fructose, glucose* or *sucrose* are described as 'sugar-free' in the BNF. Preparations containing hydrogenated glucose syrup, mannitol, maltitol, sorbitol or xylitol are also marked 'sugar-free' since there is evidence that they do not cause dental caries. Patients receiving medicines containing cariogenic sugars should be advised of appropriate dental hygiene measures to prevent caries.

Where information on the presence of *aspartame, gluten, tartrazine, arachis (peanut) oil* or *sesame oil* is available, this is indicated in the BNF against the relevant preparation.

Information is provided on *selected excipients* in skin preparations (see section 13.1.3) and on *selected*

preservatives and *excipients* in eye drops and injections. Pressurised metered aerosols containing *chlorofluorocarbons* (CFCs) have also been identified throughout the BNF (see section 3.1.1.1).

The presence of *benzyl alcohol* and *polyoxyl castor oil* (polyethoxylated castor oil) in injections is indicated in the BNF. Benzyl alcohol has been associated with a fatal toxic syndrome in premature infants, and parenteral preparations containing the preservative should not be used in neonates. Polyoxyl castor oils, used as vehicles in intravenous injections, have been associated with severe anaphylactoid reactions.

The presence of *propylene glycol* in oral or parenteral medicines is indicated in the BNF; it can cause adverse effects if it's elimination is impaired, e.g. in renal failure, in neonates and young children, and in slow metabolisers of the substance. It may interact with disulfiram and metronidazole.

> In the absence of information on excipients in the BNF and in the product literature, contact the manufacturer (see Index of Manufacturers) if it is essential to check details.

EXTEMPORANEOUS PREPARATION. A product should be dispensed extemporaneously only when no product with a marketing authorisation is available.

The BP direction that a preparation must be *freshly prepared* indicates that it must be made not more than 24 hours before it is issued for use. The direction that a preparation should be *recently prepared* indicates that deterioration is likely if the preparation is stored for longer than about 4 weeks at 15–25° C.

The term **water** used without qualification means either potable water freshly drawn direct from the public supply and suitable for drinking or freshly boiled and cooled purified water. The latter should be used if the public supply is from a local storage tank or if the potable water is unsuitable for a particular preparation (Water for injections, section 9.2.2).

DRUGS AND DRIVING. Prescribers should advise patients if treatment is likely to affect their ability to drive motor vehicles. This applies especially to drugs with sedative effects; patients should be warned that these effects are increased by alcohol. General information about a patient's fitness to drive is available from the Driver and Vehicle Licensing Agency at www.dvla.gov.uk (see also Appendix 9).

PATENTS. In the BNF certain drugs have been included notwithstanding the existence of actual or potential patent rights. In so far as such substances are protected by Letters Patent, their inclusion in this Formulary neither conveys, nor implies, licence to manufacture.

HEALTH AND SAFETY. When handling chemical or biological materials particular attention should be given to the possibility of allergy, fire, explosion, radiation, or poisoning. Substances, including corticosteroids, some antimicrobials, phenothiazines, and many cytotoxics, are irritant or very potent and should be handled with caution. Contact with the skin and inhalation of dust should be avoided.

---

1. With the exception of temazepam, an incomplete prescription is **not** acceptable for controlled drugs in schedules 2 and 3 of the Misuse of Drugs Regulations 2001

SAFETY IN THE HOME. Patients must be warned to keep all medicines out of the reach of children. All solid dose and all oral and external liquid preparations must be dispensed in a reclosable *child-resistant container* unless:

- the medicine is in an original pack or patient pack such as to make this inadvisable;
- the patient will have difficulty in opening a child-resistant container;
- a specific request is made that the product shall not be dispensed in a child-resistant container;
- no suitable child-resistant container exists for a particular liquid preparation.

All patients should be advised to dispose of *unwanted medicines* by returning them to a supplier for destruction.

NAME OF MEDICINE. The name of the medicine should appear on the label unless the prescriber indicates otherwise.

1. Subject to the conditions of paragraphs 4 and 6 below, the name of the prescribed medicine is stated on the label unless the prescriber deletes the letters 'NP' which appear on NHS prescription forms.
2. The strength is also stated on the label in the case of tablets, capsules, and similar preparations that are available in different strengths.
3. If it is the wish of the prescriber that a description such as 'The Sedative Tablets' should appear on the label, the prescriber should write the desired description on the prescription form.
4. The arrangement will extend to approved names, proprietary names or titles given in the BP, BPC, BNF, DPF, or NPF. The arrangement does not apply when a prescription is written so that several ingredients are given.
5. The name written on the label is that used by the prescriber on the prescription.
6. If more than one item is prescribed on one form and the prescriber does not delete the letters 'NP', each dispensed medicine is named on the label, subject to the conditions given above in paragraph 4. If the prescriber wants only selected items on such a prescription to be so labelled this should be indicated by deleting the letters 'NP' on the form and writing 'NP' alongside the medicines to be labelled.
7. When a prescription is written other than on an NHS prescription form the name of the prescribed preparation will be stated on the label of the dispensed medicine unless the prescriber indicates otherwise.
8. The Council of the Royal Pharmaceutical Society advises that the labels of dispensed medicines should indicate the total quantity of the product dispensed in the container to which the label refers. This requirement applies equally to solid, liquid, internal, and external preparations. If a product is dispensed in more than one container, the reference should be to the amount in each container.

Non-proprietary names of **compound preparations** which appear in the BNF are those that have been compiled by the British Pharmacopoeia Commission or another recognised body; whenever possible they reflect the names of the active ingredients.

Prescribers should avoid creating their own compound names for the purposes of generic prescribing; such names do not have an approved definition and can be misinterpreted.

Special care should be taken to avoid errors when prescribing compound preparations; in particular the hyphen in the prefix 'co-' should be retained.

Special care should also be taken to avoid creating generic names for **modified-release** preparations where the use of these names could lead to confusion between formulations with different lengths of action.

SECURITY AND VALIDITY OF PRESCRIPTIONS. The Councils of the British Medical Association and the Royal Pharmaceutical Society have issued a joint statement on the security and validity of prescriptions.

In particular, prescription forms should:

- not be left unattended at reception desks;
- not be left in a car where they may be visible; and
- when not in use, be kept in a locked drawer within the surgery and at home.

Where there is any doubt about the authenticity of a prescription, the pharmacist should contact the prescriber. If this is done by telephone, the number should be obtained from the directory rather than relying on the information on the prescription form, which may be false.

PATIENT GROUP DIRECTION (PGD). In most cases, the most appropriate clinical care will be provided on an individual basis by a prescriber to a specific individual patient. However, a Patient Group Direction for supply and administration of medicines by other healthcare professionals can be used where it would benefit patient care without compromising safety.

A Patient Group Direction is a written direction relating to supply and administration (or administration only) of a prescription-only medicine by certain classes of healthcare professionals; the Direction is signed by a doctor (or dentist), and by a pharmacist. Further information on Patient Group Directions is available in Health Service Circular HSC 2000/026 (England), HDL (2001) 7 (Scotland), and WHC (2000) 116 (Wales).

Prescription writing

Shared care. In its guidelines on responsibility for prescribing (circular EL (91) 127) between hospitals and general practitioners, the Department of Health has advised that legal responsibility for prescribing lies with the doctor who signs the prescription.

Prescriptions[1] should be written legibly in ink or otherwise so as to be indelible[2], should be dated, should state the full name and address of the patient, and should be signed in ink by the prescriber[3]. The age and the date of birth of the patient should preferably be stated, and it is a legal requirement in the case of prescription-only medicines to state the age for children under 12 years.

The following should be noted:

(a) The unnecessary use of decimal points should be avoided, e.g. 3 mg, not 3.0 mg.
   Quantities of 1 gram or more should be written as 1 g etc.
   Quantities less than 1 gram should be written in milligrams, e.g. 500 mg, not 0.5 g.
   Quantities less than 1 mg should be written in micrograms, e.g. 100 micrograms, not 0.1 mg.
   When decimals are unavoidable a zero should be written in front of the decimal point where there is no other figure, e.g. 0.5 mL, not .5 mL.
   Use of the decimal point is acceptable to express a range, e.g. 0.5 to 1 g.

(b) 'Micrograms' and 'nanograms' should **not** be abbreviated. Similarly 'units' should **not** be abbreviated.

(c) The term 'millilitre' (ml or mL)[4] is used in medicine and pharmacy, and cubic centimetre, c.c., or cm^3 should not be used.

(d) Dose and dose frequency should be stated; in the case of preparations to be taken 'as required' a **minimum dose interval** should be specified.
   When doses other than multiples of 5 mL are prescribed for *oral liquid preparations* the dose-volume will be provided by means of an **oral syringe**, see p. 2 (except for preparations intended to be measured with a pipette).
   Suitable quantities:
   Elixirs, Linctuses, and Paediatric Mixtures (5-mL dose), 50, 100, or 150 mL
   Adult Mixtures (10-mL dose), 200 or 300 mL
   Ear Drops, Eye drops, and Nasal Drops, 10 mL (or the manufacturer's pack)
   Eye Lotions, Gargles, and Mouthwashes, 200 mL

(e) For suitable quantities of dermatological preparations, see section 13.1.2.

(f) The names of drugs and preparations should be written clearly and **not** abbreviated, using approved titles **only** (see also advice in box on p. 3 to **avoid** creating generic titles for modified-release preparations).

(g) The symbol 'NP' on NHS forms should be deleted if it is required that the name of the preparation should not appear on the label. For full details see p. 3.

(h) The quantity to be supplied may be stated by indicating the number of days of treatment required in the box provided on NHS forms. In most cases the exact amount will be supplied. This does not apply to items directed to be used as required—if the dose and frequency are not given the quantity to be supplied needs to be stated.
   When several items are ordered on one form the box can be marked with the number of days of treatment provided the quantity is added for any item for which the amount cannot be calculated.

(i) Although directions should preferably be in **English without abbreviation**, it is recognised that some Latin abbreviations are used (for details see Inside Back Cover).

(j) A prescription for a preparation that has been withdrawn or needs to be specially imported for a named patient should be handwritten. The name of the preparation should be endorsed with the prescriber's signature and the letters 'WD' (withdrawn or specially-imported drug); there may be considerable delay in obtaining a withdrawn medicine.

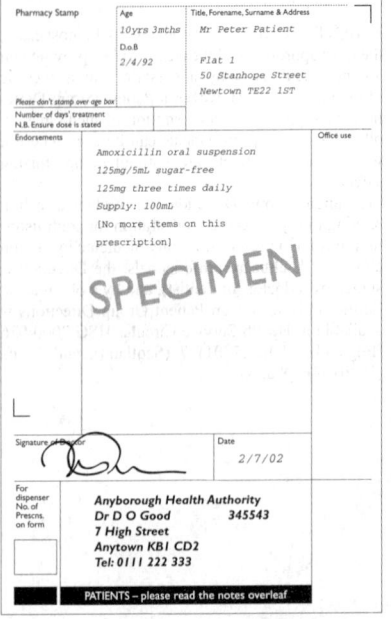

1. The above recommendations are acceptable for **prescription-only medicines** (▣ PoM ▣). For items marked ▣ CD ▣ see also Controlled Drugs and Drug Dependence p. 7.

2. It is permissible to issue carbon copies of NHS prescriptions as long as they are signed in ink.

3. Computer-generated facsimile signatures do not meet the legal requirement.

4. The use of capital 'L' in mL is a printing convention throughout the BNF; both 'mL' and 'ml' are recognised SI abbreviations.

Computer-issued prescriptions

For computer-issued prescriptions the following recommendations of the Joint Computing Group of the General Practitioners Committee and the Royal College of General Practitioners should also be noted:

1. The computer must print out the date,[1] the patient's surname, one forename, other initials, and address, and may also print out the patient's title and date of birth. The age of children under 12 years and of adults over 60 years must be printed in the box available; the age of children under 5 years should be printed in years and months. A facility may also exist to print out the age of patients between 12 and 60 years.

2. The doctor's name must be printed at the bottom of the prescription form; this will be the name of the doctor responsible for the prescription (who will normally sign it). The doctor's surgery address, reference number, and Primary Care Trust (PCT)[2] are also necessary. In addition, the surgery telephone number should be printed.

3. When prescriptions are to be signed by general practitioner registrars, assistants, locums, or deputising doctors, the name of the doctor printed at the bottom of the form must still be that of the responsible principal.

4. Names of medicines must come from a dictionary held in the computer memory, to provide a check on the spelling and to ensure that the name is written in full. The computer can be programmed to recognise both the non-proprietary and the proprietary name of a particular drug and to print out the preferred choice, but must not print out both names. For medicines not in the dictionary, separate checks are required—the user must be warned that no check was possible and the entire prescription must be entered in the lexicon.

5. The dictionary may contain information on the usual doses, formulations, and pack sizes to produce standard predetermined prescriptions for common preparations, and to provide a check on the validity of an individual prescription on entry.

6. The prescription must be printed in English without abbreviation; information may be entered or stored in abbreviated form. The dose must be in numbers, the frequency in words, and the quantity in numbers in brackets, thus: 40 mg four times daily (112). It must also be possible to prescribe by indicating the length of treatment required, see (h) above.

7. The BNF recommendations should be followed as in (a), (b), (c), (d), and (e) above.

8. Checks may be incorporated to ensure that all the information required for dispensing a particular drug has been filled in. For instructions such as 'as directed' and 'when required', the maximum daily dose should normally be specified.

9. Numbers and codes used in the system for organising and retrieving data must never appear on the form.

10. Supplementary warnings or advice should be written in full, should not interfere with the clarity of the prescription itself, and should be in line with any warnings or advice in the BNF; numerical codes should not be used.

11. A mechanism (such as printing a series of non-specific characters) should be incorporated to cancel out unused space, or wording such as 'no more items on this prescription' may be added after the last item. Otherwise the doctor should delete the space manually.

12. To avoid forgery the computer may print on the form the number of items to be dispensed (somewhere separate from the box for the pharmacist). The number of items per form need be limited only by the ability of the printer to produce clear and well-demarcated instructions with sufficient space for each item and a spacer line before each fresh item.

13. Handwritten alterations should only be made in exceptional circumstances—it is preferable to print out a new prescription. Any alterations must be made in the doctor's own handwriting and countersigned; computer records should be updated to fully reflect any alteration. Prescriptions for drugs used for contraceptive purposes (but which are not promoted as contraceptives) may need to be marked in handwriting with the symbol ♀ (or endorsed in another way to indicate that the item is prescribed for contraceptive purposes).

14. Prescriptions for controlled drugs must not be printed from the computer. Blank forms may be computer-printed with the doctor's name, surgery address and telephone number, reference number and Primary Care Trust (PCT)[2]; the remaining details must be handwritten.[3]

15. The strip of paper on the side of the FP10[4](Comp) may be used for various purposes but care should be taken to avoid including confidential information. It may be advisable for the patient's name to appear at the top, but this should be preceded by 'confidential'.

16. In rural dispensing practices prescription requests (or details of medicines dispensed) will normally be entered in one surgery. The prescriptions (or dispensed medicines) may then need to be delivered to another surgery or location; if possible the computer should hold up to 10 alternatives.

17. Prescription forms that are reprinted or issued as a duplicate should be labelled clearly as such.

---

1. The exemption for own handwriting regulations for phenobarbital does not apply to the date; a computer-generated date need not be deleted but the date must also be added by the prescriber.

2. Health Board in Scotland.

3. Except in the case of phenobarbital (but see also footnote 1) or where the prescriber has been exempted from handwriting requirements, for details see Controlled Drugs and Drug Dependence p. 7

4. GP10 in Scotland, WP10 (Comp) in Wales

Emergency supply of medicines

For details of emergency supply at the request of a doctor, see *Medicines, Ethics and Practice*, No. 27, London, Pharmaceutical Press, 2003 (and subsequent editions).

Pharmacists are sometimes called upon by members of the public to make an emergency supply of medicines. The Medicines (Products Other Than Veterinary Drugs) (Prescription Only) Order 1983, as amended, allows exemptions from the Prescription Only requirements for emergency supply to be made by a person lawfully conducting a retail pharmacy business provided:

(a) that the pharmacist has interviewed the person requesting the prescription-only medicine and is satisfied:
   (i) that there is immediate need for the prescription-only medicine and that it is impracticable in the circumstances to obtain a prescription without undue delay;
   (ii) that treatment with the prescription-only medicine has on a previous occasion been prescribed by a doctor[1], a supplementary prescriber, a district nurse or health visitor prescriber or an extended formulary nurse prescriber for the person requesting it;
   (iii) as to the dose which it would be appropriate for the person to take;
(b) that no greater quantity shall be supplied than will provide 5 days' treatment except when the prescription-only medicine is:
   (i) insulin, an ointment or, cream, or a preparation for the relief of asthma in an aerosol dispenser when the smallest pack can be supplied;
   (ii) an oral contraceptive when a full cycle may be supplied;
   (iii) an antibiotic in liquid form for oral administration when the smallest quantity that will provide a full course of treatment can be supplied;
(c) that an entry shall be made in the prescription book stating:
   (i) the date of supply;
   (ii) the name, quantity and, where appropriate, the pharmaceutical form and strength;
   (iii) the name and address of the patient;
   (iv) the nature of the emergency;
(d) that the container or package must be labelled to show:
   (i) the date of supply;
   (ii) the name, quantity and, where appropriate, the pharmaceutical form and strength;
   (iii) the name of the patient;
   (iv) the name and address of the pharmacy;
   (v) the words 'Emergency supply';
   (vi) the words 'Keep out of the reach of children' (or similar warning).
(e) that the prescription-only medicine is not a substance specifically excluded from the emergency supply provision, and does not contain a Controlled Drug specified in schedules 1, 2, or 3 to the Misuse of Drugs Regulations 2001 except for phenobarbital or phenobarbital sodium for the treatment of epilepsy: for details see *Medicines, Ethics and Practice*, No. 27, London, Pharmaceutical Press, 2003 (and subsequent editions as available).

Royal Pharmaceutical Society's Guidelines

1. The pharmacist should consider the medical consequences of *not* supplying.
2. If the patient is not known to the pharmacist, the patient's identity should be established by way of appropriate documentation.
3. It may occasionally be desirable to contact the prescriber, e.g. when the medicine requested has a potential for misuse or the prescriber is not known to the pharmacist.
4. Care should be taken to ask whether the patient's doctor has stopped the treatment, or whether the patient is taking any other medication.
5. Except for conditions which may occur infrequently (e.g. hay fever, asthma attack or migraine), a supply should not be made if the item requested was last prescribed more than 6 months ago.
6. Consideration should be given to supplying less than 5 days' quantity if this is justified.
7. Where a prescription is to be provided later, a record of emergency supply as required by law must still be made. It is good practice to add to the record the date on which the prescription is received. Payment for the medicine supplied is not a legal requirement, but may help to minimise the abuse of the emergency supply exemption. If an NHS prescription is to be provided, a refundable charge may be made.

---

1. The doctor must be a UK-registered doctor.

Controlled drugs and drug dependence

PRESCRIPTIONS. Preparations which are subject to the prescription requirements of the Misuse of Drugs Regulations 2001, i.e. preparations specified in schedules 2 and 3, are distinguished throughout the BNF by the symbol CD (Controlled Drugs). The principal legal requirements relating to medical prescriptions are listed below.

Prescriptions ordering Controlled Drugs subject to prescription requirements must be *signed* and *dated*[1] by the prescriber and specify the prescriber's *address*. The prescription must always state *in the prescriber's own handwriting*[2] in ink or otherwise so as to be indelible:

- The name and address of the patient;
- In the case of a preparation, the form[3] and where appropriate the strength[4] of the preparation;
- The total quantity of the preparation, or the number of dose units, *in both words and figures;*[5]
- The dose;[6]
- The words 'for dental treatment only' if issued by a dentist.

A prescription may order a Controlled Drug to be dispensed by instalments; the amount of the instalments and the intervals to be observed must be specified.[7,8] Prescriptions ordering 'repeats' on the same form are **not** permitted. A prescription is valid for 13 weeks from the date stated thereon.

It is an offence for a prescriber to issue an incomplete prescription and a pharmacist is **not** allowed to dispense a Controlled Drug unless all

---

1. A computer-generated date is **not** acceptable; however, the prescriber may use a date stamp.

2. Does not apply to prescriptions for temazepam. Otherwise applies unless the prescriber has been specifically exempted from this requirement or unless the prescription contains no controlled drug other than phenobarbital or phenobarbital sodium or a preparation containing either of these; the exemption does **not** apply to the date—a computer-generated date need not be deleted but the date must also be added by the prescriber.

3. The dosage form (e.g. tablets) must be included on a Controlled Drugs prescription irrespective of whether it is implicit in the proprietary name (e.g. *MST Continus*) or of whether only one form is available.

4. When more than one strength of a preparation exists the strength required must be specified.

5. Does not apply to prescriptions for temazepam.

6. The instruction 'one as directed' constitutes a dose but 'as directed' does not.

7. A total of 14 days' treatment by instalment of any drug listed in Schedule 2 of the Misuse of Drugs Regulations may be prescribed in England and Scotland. In *England*, form FP10MDA-SS (blue) or occasionally form FP10MDA (blue) should be used; in hospital, form FP10HP(AD) is being replaced by form FP10MDA-SS. In *Scotland* forms HBP(A) (hospital-based prescribers) or GP10 (general practitioners) should be used. In *Wales* a total of 14 days treatment by instalment of any drug listed in Schedules 2–5 of the Misuse of Drugs Regulations may be prescribed. In Wales form WP10(MDA) or form WP10HP(AD) for hospital prescribers should be used when available; in the meantime existing stocks of FP10(MDA) for general practice prescribers, or FP10HP(AD) for hospital prescribers should continue to be used.

8. Buprenorphine (schedule 3) may be prescribed by instalment in England on form FP10MDA-SS (or on form FP10MDA)

---

the information required by law is given on the prescription. Failure to comply with the regulations concerning the writing of prescriptions will result in inconvenience to patients and delay in supplying the necessary medicine.

DEPENDENCE AND MISUSE. The most serious drugs of addiction are **cocaine, diamorphine** (heroin), **morphine,** and the **synthetic opioids**. For arrangements for prescribing of diamorphine, dipipanone or cocaine for addicts, see p. 9.

Despite marked reduction in the prescribing of **amphetamines** there is concern that abuse of illicit amfetamine and related compounds is widespread.

Owing to problems of abuse, **flunitrazepam** and **temazepam** are subject to additional controlled drug requirements (but temazepam remains exempt from the additional prescribing requirements).

The principal **barbiturates** are now Controlled Drugs, but phenobarbital (phenobarbitone) and phenobarbital sodium (phenobarbitone sodium) or a preparation containing either of these are exempt from the handwriting requirement but must fulfil all other controlled drug prescription requirements (**important:** the own handwriting exemption does **not** apply to the date; a computer-generated date need not be deleted but the date must also be added by the prescriber). Moreover, for the treatment of epilepsy phenobarbital and phenobarbital sodium are available under the emergency supply regulations (p. 6).

Cannabis (Indian hemp) has no approved medicinal use and cannot be prescribed by doctors. Its use is illegal but has become widespread. Cannabis is a mild hallucinogen seldom accompanied by a desire to increase the dose; withdrawal symptoms are unusual. **Lysergide** (lysergic acid diethylamide, LSD) is a

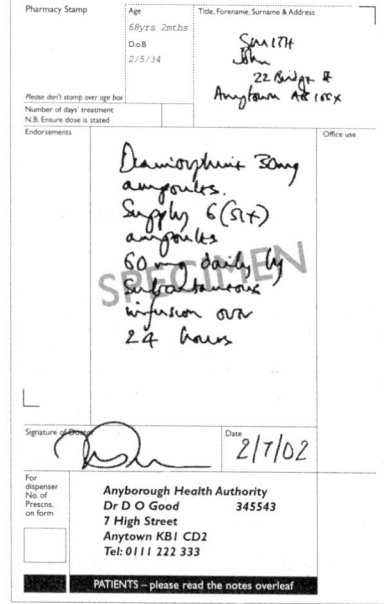

much more potent hallucinogen; its use can lead to severe psychotic states in which life may be at risk.

PRESCRIBING DRUGS LIKELY TO CAUSE DEPENDENCE OR MISUSE. The prescriber has three main responsibilities:

- To avoid creating dependence by introducing drugs to patients without sufficient reason. In this context, the proper use of the morphine-like drugs is well understood. The dangers of other controlled drugs are less clear because recognition of dependence is not easy and its effects, and those of withdrawal, are less obvious. Perhaps the most notable result of uninhibited prescribing is that a very large number of patients in the country take tablets which do them neither much good nor much harm, but are committed to them indefinitely because they cannot readily be stopped.
- To see that the patient does not gradually increase the dose of a drug, given for good medical reasons, to the point where dependence becomes more likely. This tendency is seen especially with hypnotics and anxiolytics (for CSM advice see section 4.1). The prescriber should keep a close eye on the amount prescribed to prevent patients from accumulating stocks that would enable them to arrange their own dosage or even that of their families and friends. A minimal amount should be prescribed in the first instance, or when seeing a new patient for the first time.
- To avoid being used as an unwitting source of supply for addicts. Methods include visiting more than one doctor, fabricating stories, and forging prescriptions.

Patients under temporary care should be given only small supplies of drugs unless they present an unequivocal letter from their own doctors. Doctors should also remember that their own patients may be doing a collecting round with other doctors, especially in hospitals. It is sensible to decrease dosages steadily or to issue weekly or even daily prescriptions for small amounts if it is apparent that dependence is occurring.

The stealing and misuse of prescription forms could be minimised by the following precautions:

(a) do not leave unattended if called away from the consulting room or at reception desks; do not leave in a car where they may be visible; when not in use, keep in a locked drawer within the surgery and at home;
(b) draw a diagonal line across the blank part of the form under the prescription;
(c) write the quantity in words and figures when prescribing drugs prone to abuse; this is obligatory for controlled drugs (see Prescriptions, above);
(d) alterations are best avoided but if any are made they should be clear and unambiguous; add initials against altered items;
(e) if prescriptions are left for collection they should be left in a safe place in a sealed envelope.

TRAVELLING ABROAD. Prescribed drugs listed in schedule 4 Part II (CD Anab) [only when in the form of a medicinal product and for administration by a person to himself] and schedule 5 of the Misuse of Drugs Regulations 2001 are not subject to import or export licensing, but doctors are advised that patients intending to carry schedule 2, 3 and 4 Part I (CD Benz) and Part II (CD Anab) drugs abroad may require an export licence (subject to the above exemption for schedule 4 Part II). This is dependent upon the amount of drug to be exported and further details may be obtained from the Home Office by telephoning (020) 7273 3806. Applications for licences should be sent to the Home Office, Drugs Branch, Queen Anne's Gate, London SW1H 9AT.

There is no standard application form but applications must be supported by a letter from a doctor giving details of:

- the patient's name and current address;
- the quantities of drugs to be carried;
- the strength and form in which the drugs will be dispensed;
- the dates of travel to and from the United Kingdom.

Ten days should be allowed for processing the application.

Individual doctors who wish to take Controlled Drugs abroad while accompanying patients may similarly be issued with licences. Licences are not normally issued to doctors who wish to take Controlled Drugs abroad solely in case a family emergency should arise.

These import/export licences for named individuals do not have any legal status outside the UK and are only issued to comply with the Misuse of Drugs Act and facilitate passage through UK Customs and Excise control. For clearance in the country to be visited it would be necessary to approach that country's consulate in the UK.

Misuse of Drugs Act

The Misuse of Drugs Act, 1971 prohibits certain activities in relation to 'Controlled Drugs', in particular their manufacture, supply, and possession. The penalties applicable to offences involving the different drugs are graded broadly according to the *harmfulness attributable to a drug when it is misused* and for this purpose the drugs are defined in the following three classes:

Class A includes: alfentanil, cocaine, diamorphine (heroin), dipipanone, lysergide (LSD), methadone, methylenedioxymethamfetamine (MDMA, 'ecstasy'), morphine, opium, pethidine, phencyclidine, remifentanil, and class B substances when prepared for injection

Class B includes: oral amphetamines, barbiturates, codeine, ethylmorphine, glutethimide, pentazocine, phenmetrazine, and pholcodine

Class C includes: certain drugs related to the amphetamines such as benzfetamine and chlorphentermine, buprenorphine, cannabis, cannabis resin, diethylpropion, mazindol, meprobamate, pemoline, pipradrol, most benzodiazepines, zolpidem, androgenic and anabolic steroids, clenbuterol, chorionic gonadotrophin (HCG), non-human chorionic gonadotrophin, somatotropin, somatrem, and somatropin

The Misuse of Drugs Regulations 2001 define the classes of person who are authorised to supply and possess controlled drugs while acting in their professional capacities and lay down the conditions under which these activities may be carried out. In the regulations drugs are divided into five schedules each specifying the requirements governing such activities as import, export, production, supply, possession, prescribing, and record keeping which apply to them.

Schedule 1 includes drugs such as cannabis and lysergide which are not used medicinally. Possession and supply are prohibited except in accordance with Home Office authority.

Schedule 2 includes drugs such as diamorphine (heroin), morphine, remifentanil, pethidine, secobarbital, glutethimide, amfetamine, and cocaine and are subject to the full controlled drug requirements relating to prescriptions, safe custody (except for secobarbital), the need to keep registers, etc. (unless exempted in schedule 5).

Schedule 3 includes the barbiturates (except secobarbital, now schedule 2), buprenorphine, diethylpropion, flunitrazepam, mazindol, meprobamate, pentazocine, phentermine, and temazepam. They are subject to the special prescription requirements (except for phenobarbital and temazepam, see p. 7) but not to the safe custody requirements (except for buprenorphine, diethylpropion, flunitrazepam, and temazepam) nor to the need to keep registers (although there are requirements for the retention of invoices for 2 years).

Schedule 4 includes in Part I benzodiazepines (except flunitrazepam and temazepam which are in schedule 3) and zolpidem, which are subject to minimal control. Part II includes androgenic and anabolic steroids, clenbuterol, chorionic gonadotrophin (HCG), non-human chorionic gonadotrophin, somatotropin, somatrem, and somatropin. Controlled drug prescription requirements do not apply and Schedule 4 Controlled Drugs are not subject to safe custody requirements.

Schedule 5 includes those preparations which, because of their strength, are exempt from virtually all Controlled Drug requirements other than retention of invoices for two years.

Notification of drug misusers

Doctors are expected to report on a standard form cases of drug misuse to their regional or national drug misuse database or centre—see below for contact telephone numbers. The National Drugs Treatment Monitoring System was introduced in England in April 2001; regional centres replace the Regional Drug Misuse Databases. A similar system has been introduced in Wales.

A report (notification) to their regional or national drug misuse database or centre should be made when a patient starts treatment for drug misuse. In England and Wales further information is collected in Spring, including whether or not patients are continuing to receive treatment. All types of problem drug misuse should be reported including opioid, benzodiazepine, and CNS stimulant.

The regional or national drug misuse database or centres are now the only national and local source of epidemiological data on people presenting with problem drug misuse; they provide valuable information to those working with drug misusers and those planning services for them. The databases cannot, however be used as a check on multiple prescribing for drug addicts because the data are anonymised.

Enquiries about the regional or national drug misuse database or centres (including requests for supplies of notification forms) can be made by contacting one of the centres listed below:

ENGLAND

Eastern and South East (West)
Tel: (01865) 226 734
Fax: (01865) 226 652

London and South East (East)
Tel: (020) 7972 2324
Fax: (020) 7972 2248

North West
Mersey
Tel: (0151) 231 4486
Fax: (0151) 231 4320

Northern Western
Tel: (0161) 772 3782
Fax: (0161) 772 3445

Northern and Yorkshire
Tel: (0113) 295 1337
Fax: (0113) 295 1310

South Western
Tel: (0117) 918 6880
Fax: (0117) 918 6883

Trent
Tel: (0116) 225 6360
Fax: (0116) 225 6370

West Midlands
Tel: (0121) 415 8556
Fax: (0121) 414 8197

SCOTLAND
Tel: (0131) 551 8715
Fax: (0131) 551 1392

WALES
Tel: (02920) 502 639
Fax: (02920) 502 504

In **Northern Ireland**, the Misuse of Drugs (Notification of and Supply to Addicts) (Northern Ireland) Regulations 1973 require doctors to send particulars of persons whom they consider to be addicted to certain controlled drugs to the Chief Medical Officer of the Department of Health and Social Services. The Northern Ireland contacts are:

Medical contact:

Dr Ian McMaster
C3 Castle Buildings
Belfast BT4 3PP
Tel: (028) 9052 2421
Fax: (028) 9052 0781

Administrative contact:

Health Promotion Branch
C4.22 Castle Building
Belfast BT4 3PP
Tel: (028) 9052 0532

Prescribing of diamorphine (heroin), dipipanone, and cocaine for addicts

The Misuse of Drugs (Supply to Addicts) Regulations 1997 require that only medical practitioners who hold a special licence issued by the Home Secretary may prescribe, administer or supply diamorphine, dipipanone[1] (*Diconal*®) or cocaine in the treatment of drug addiction; other practitioners must refer any addict who requires these drugs to a treatment centre. Whenever possible the addict will be introduced by a member of staff from the treatment centre to a pharmacist whose agreement has been obtained and whose pharmacy is conveniently sited for the patient. Prescriptions for weekly supplies will be sent to the pharmacy by post and will be dispensed on a daily basis as indicated by the doctor. If any alterations of the arrangements are requested by the addict, the portion of the prescription affected must be represcribed and not merely altered. *General practitioners and other doctors may still prescribe diamorphine, dipipanone, and cocaine for patients (including addicts) for relief of pain due to organic disease or injury without a special licence.*

For guidance on prescription writing, see p. 7.

---

1. Dipipanone in *Diconal*® tablets has been much misused by opioid addicts in recent years. Doctors and others should be suspicious of people who ask for the tablets, especially if temporary residents.

Adverse reactions to drugs

Any drug may produce unwanted or unexpected adverse reactions. Detection and recording of these is of vital importance. Doctors, dentists, coroners, pharmacists and nurses are urged to help by reporting suspected adverse reactions on yellow cards to:

Medicines and Healthcare products Regulatory Agency (formerly MCA)
CSM
Freepost
London SW8 5BR
Tel: (0800 731 6789)

Suspected adverse reactions to *any* therapeutic agent should be reported, including drugs *(self-medication* as well as those *prescribed)*, blood products, vaccines, radiographic contrast media and herbal products. Prepaid Yellow Cards for reporting are available from the above address and are also bound in this book (inside back cover). For on-line reporting, consult the Medicines and Healthcare products Regulatory Agency (MHRA) website: medicines.mhra.gov.uk.

A 24-hour Freefone service is available to all parts of the UK for advice and information on suspected adverse drug reactions; contact the National Yellow Card Information Service at the MHRA (formerly MCA) on 0800 731 6789. Outside office hours a telephone-answering machine will take messages.

The following regional centres also collect data:

CSM Mersey
Freepost
Liverpool L3 3AB
Tel: (0151) 794 8206

CSM Wales
Freepost
Cardiff CF4 1ZZ
Tel: (029) 2074 4181
(direct line)

CSM Northern & Yorkshire
Freepost 1085
Newcastle upon Tyne
NE1 1BR
Tel: (0191) 232 1525
(direct line)

CSM West Midlands
Freepost SW2991
Birmingham B18 7BR
Tel: (0121) 507 5672

CSM Scotland
CARDS
Freepost NAT3271
Edinburgh EH16 4BR
Tel: (0131) 242 2919

The MHRA's Adverse Drug Reactions On-line Information Tracking (ADROIT) facilitates the monitoring of adverse drug reactions.

More detailed information on reporting and a list of products currently under intensive monitoring can be found on the CSM homepage:
(medicines.mhra.gov.uk).

PRESCRIPTION-EVENT MONITORING. In addition to the CSM's Yellow Card scheme, an independent scheme monitors the safety of new medicines using a different approach. The Drug Safety Research Unit identifies patients who have been prescribed selected new medicines and collects data on clinical events in these patients. The data are submitted on a voluntary basis by general practitioners on green forms. More information about the scheme and the Unit's educational material is available from www.dsru.org.

NEWER DRUGS AND VACCINES. Only limited information is available from clinical trials on the safety of new medicines. Further understanding about the safety of medicines depends on the availability of information from routine clinical practice.

The black triangle symbol (▼) identifies newly licensed medicines that are monitored intensively by the MHRA/CSM. Such medicines include those that have been licensed for administration by a new route or drug delivery system, or for significant new indications which may alter the established risks and benefits of that drug. There is no standard time for which products retain a black triangle; safety data are usually reviewed after 2 years.

Spontaneous reporting is particularly valuable for recognising possible new hazards rapidly. For medicines showing the black triangle symbol, the MHRA/CSM asks that **all** suspected reactions (including those considered not to be serious) are reported through the Yellow Card scheme. An adverse reaction should be reported even if it is not certain that the drug has caused it, or if the reaction is well recognised, or if other drugs have been given at the same time.

ESTABLISHED DRUGS AND VACCINES. Doctors, dentists, coroners, pharmacists and nurses are asked to report *all* serious suspected reactions, including those that are fatal, life-threatening, disabling, incapacitating, or which result in or prolong hospitalisation; they should be reported even if the effect is well recognised. Examples include anaphylaxis, blood disorders, endocrine disturbances, effects on fertility, haemorrhage from any site, renal impairment, jaundice, ophthalmic disorders, severe CNS effects, severe skin reactions, reactions in pregnant women, and any drug interactions. Reports of serious adverse reactions are required to enable comparison with other drugs of a similar class. Reports of overdoses (deliberate or accidental) can complicate the assessment of adverse drug reactions, but provides important information on the potential toxicity of drugs.

For established drugs there is no need to report well-known, relatively minor side-effects, such as dry mouth with tricyclic antidepressants or constipation with opioids.

ADVERSE REACTIONS TO MEDICAL DEVICES. Suspected adverse reactions to medical devices including dental or surgical materials, intra-uterine devices and contact lens fluids should be reported. Information on reporting these can be found at: devices.mhra.gov.uk

SIDE-EFFECTS IN THE BNF. The BNF includes clinically relevant side-effects for most drugs; an exhaustive list is not included for drugs that are used by specialists (e.g. cytotoxics and drugs used in anaesthesia). Side-effects in the manufacturers' literature whose causality has not been established may be omitted from the BNF.

Side-effects are generally listed in order of frequency and arranged broadly by body systems. Occasionally a rare side-effect might be listed first if it is considered to be particularly important because of its seriousness.

In the product literature the frequency of side-effects is generally described as follows:

Very common	greater than 1 in 10
Common	1 in 100 to 1 in 10
Uncommon	1 in 1000 to 1 in 100
Rare	1 in 10 000 to 1 in 1000
Very rare	less than 1 in 10 000

Special problems

Delayed drug effects. Some reactions (e.g. cancers, chloroquine retinopathy, and retroperitoneal fibrosis) may become manifest months or years after exposure. Any suspicion of such an association should be reported.

The elderly. Particular vigilance is required to identify adverse reactions in the elderly.

Congenital abnormalities. When an infant is born with a congenital abnormality or there is a malformed aborted fetus doctors are asked to consider whether this might be an adverse reaction to a drug and to report all drugs (including self-medication) taken during pregnancy.

Children. Particular vigilance is required to identify and report adverse reactions in children, including those resulting from the unlicensed use of medicines; **all** suspected reactions should be reported (see below).

Prevention of adverse reactions

Adverse reactions may be prevented as follows:

1. Never use any drug unless there is a good indication. If the patient is pregnant do not use a drug unless the need for it is imperative.
2. Allergy and idiosyncrasy are important causes of adverse drug reactions. Ask if the patient had previous reactions.
3. Ask if the patient is already taking other drugs *including self-medication drugs*; interactions may occur.

4. Age and hepatic or renal disease may alter the metabolism or excretion of drugs, so that much smaller doses may be needed. Genetic factors may also be responsible for variations in metabolism, notably of isoniazid and the tricyclic antidepressants.
5. Prescribe as few drugs as possible and give very clear instructions to the elderly or any patient likely to misunderstand complicated instructions.
6. When possible use a familiar drug. With a new drug be particularly alert for adverse reactions or unexpected events.
7. If serious adverse reactions are liable to occur warn the patient.

Defective medicines

During the manufacture or distribution of a medicine an error or accident may occur whereby the finished product does not conform to its specification. While such a defect may impair the therapeutic effect of the product and could adversely affect the health of a patient, it should **not** be confused with an Adverse Drug Reaction where the product conforms to its specification.

The Defective Medicines Report Centre assists with the investigation of problems arising from licensed medicinal products thought to be defective and co-ordinates any necessary protective action. Reports on suspect defective medicinal products should include the brand or the non-proprietary name, the name of the manufacturer or supplier, the strength and dosage form of the product, the product licence number, the batch number or numbers of the product, the nature of the defect, and an account of any action already taken in consequence. The Centre can be contacted at:

The Defective Medicines Report Centre
Medicines and Healthcare products Regulatory Agency
Room 1801, Market Towers
1 Nine Elms Lane
London SW8 5NQ
(020) 7273 0574 (weekdays 9.00 am–5.00 pm)
or (020) 7210 3000 or 5371 (any other time)

Prescribing for children

Children, and particularly neonates, differ from adults in their response to drugs. Special care is needed in the neonatal period (first 30 days of life) and doses should always be calculated with care. At this age, the risk of toxicity is increased by inefficient renal filtration, relative enzyme deficiencies, differing target organ sensitivity, and inadequate detoxifying systems causing delayed excretion.

Whenever possible painful intramuscular injections should be **avoided** in children.

Where possible, medicines for children should be prescribed within the terms of the product licence (marketing authorisation). However, many children may require medicines not specifically licensed for paediatric use.

Although medicines cannot be promoted outside the limits of the licence, the Medicines Act does not prohibit the use of unlicensed medicines. It is recognised that the informed use of unlicensed medicines or of licensed medicines for unlicensed applications ('off-label' use) is often necessary in paediatric practice.

ADVERSE DRUG REACTIONS IN CHILDREN. The reporting of all suspected adverse drug reactions in children is **strongly encouraged** through the Yellow Card scheme (see p. 10) even if the intensive monitoring symbol (▼) has been removed, because experience in children may still be limited.

The identification and reporting of adverse reactions to drugs in children is particularly important because:

- the action of the drug and its pharmacokinetics in children (especially in the very young) may be different from that in adults
- drugs are not extensively tested in children
- many drugs are not specifically licensed for use in children and are used 'off-label'
- suitable formulations may not be available to allow precise dosing in children
- the nature and course of illnesses and adverse drug reactions may differ between adults and children.

PRESCRIPTION WRITING. Prescriptions should be written according to the guidelines in Prescription Writing (p. 4) Inclusion of age is a legal requirement in the case of prescription-only medicines for children under 12 years of age, but it is preferable to state the age for **all** prescriptions for children.

It is particularly important to state the strengths of capsules or tablets. Although liquid preparations are particularly suitable for children, they may contain sugar which encourages dental decay. Sugar-free medicines are preferred for long-term treatment.

Many children are able to swallow tablets or capsules and may prefer a solid dose form; involving the child and parents in choosing the formulation is helpful.

When a prescription for a liquid oral preparation is written and the dose ordered is smaller than 5 mL an **oral syringe** will be supplied (for details, see p. 2) . Parents should be advised not to add any medicines to the infant's feed, since the drug may interact with the milk or other liquid in it; moreover the ingested dosage may be reduced if the child does not drink all the contents.

Parents must be warned to keep **all** medicines out of reach of children, see Safety in the Home, p. 3

Rare paediatric conditions

Information on substances such as *biotin* and *sodium benzoate* used in rare metabolic conditions can be obtained from:

Alder Hey Children's Hospital
Drug Information Centre
Liverpool L12 2AP
Tel: (0151) 252 5381

Great Ormond Street Hospital for Children
Pharmacy
Great Ormond St
London WC1N 3JH
Tel: (020) 7405 9200

Dosage in Children

Children's doses in the BNF are stated in the individual drug entries as far as possible, except where paediatric use is not recommended, information is not available, or there are special hazards.

Doses are generally based on body-weight (in kilograms) or the following age ranges:

first month (neonate)
up to 1 year (infant)
1–5 years
6–12 years

Unless the age is specified, the term 'child' in the BNF includes persons aged 12 years and younger.

DOSE CALCULATION. Children's doses may be calculated from adult doses by using age, body-weight, or body-surface area, or by a combination of these factors. The most reliable methods are those based on body-surface area.

Body-weight may be used to calculate doses expressed in mg/kg. Young children may require a higher dose per kilogram than adults because of their higher metabolic rates. Other problems need to be considered. For example, calculation by body-weight in the obese child may result in much higher doses being administered than necessary; in such cases, dose should be calculated from an ideal weight, related to height and age.

Body-surface area (BSA) estimates are more accurate for calculation of paediatric doses than body-weight since many physiological phenomena correlate better to body-surface area. The average body-surface area of a 70-kilogram human is about 1.8 m^2. Thus, to calculate the dose for a child the following formula may be used:

Approximate dose for patient =

$$\frac{\text{surface area of patient } (\text{m}^2)}{1.8} \times \text{adult dose}$$

More precise body-surface values may be calculated from height and weight by means of a nomogram (e.g. J. Insley, *A Paediatric Vade-Mecum*, 13th Edition, London, Arnold, 1996); see also inside back cover.

Where the dose for children is not stated, prescribers should seek advice from a drug information centre or refer to a current edition of a specialist text on the use of medicines in children.

DOSE FREQUENCY. Antibacterials are generally given at regular intervals throughout the day. Some flexibility should be allowed in children to avoid waking them during the night. For example, the night-time dose may be given at the parent's bedtime.

Where new or potentially toxic drugs are used, the manufacturers' recommended doses should be carefully followed.

Prescribing in palliative care

Palliative care is the active total care of patients whose disease is not responsive to curative treatment. Control of pain, of other symptoms, and of psychological, social and spiritual problems, is paramount to provide the best quality of life for patients and their families. Careful assessment of symptoms and needs of the patient should be undertaken by a multidisciplinary team.

Specialist palliative care is available in most areas as day hospice care, home care teams (often known as Macmillan teams), in-patient hospice care, and hospital teams. Many acute hospitals and teaching centres now have consultative, hospital-based teams.

Hospice care of terminally ill patients has shown the importance of symptom control and psychosocial support of the patient and family. Families should be included in the care of the patient if they wish.

Many patients wish to remain at home with their families. Although some families may at first be afraid of caring for the patient at home, support can be provided by community nursing services, social services, voluntary agencies and hospices together with the general practitioner. The family may be reassured by the knowledge that the patient will be admitted to a hospital or hospice if the family cannot cope.

DRUG TREATMENT. The number of drugs should be as few as possible, for even the taking of medicine may be an effort. Oral medication is usually satisfactory unless there is severe nausea and vomiting, dysphagia, weakness, or coma, in which case parenteral medication may be necessary.

Pain

Analgesics are more effective in preventing pain than in the relief of established pain; it is important that they are given regularly.

The non-opioid analgesics **paracetamol** or an **NSAID** (section 10.1.1) given regularly will often make the use of opioids unnecessary. The NSAID may also control the pain of *bone secondaries*; if necessary, flurbiprofen or indometacin can be given rectally. Radiotherapy, bisphosphonates (section 6.6.2) and radioactive isotopes of **strontium** (*Metastron®* available from Amersham) may also be useful for pain due to bone metastases.

An opioid such as **codeine** or **dextropropoxyphene**, alone or in combination with a non-opioid analgesic at adequate dosage, may be helpful in the control of moderate pain if non-opioids alone are not sufficient. Alternatively, **tramadol** can be considered for mderate pain. If these preparations are not controlling the pain, **morphine** is the most useful opioid analgesic. Alternatives to morphine include **hydromorphone**, **methadone**, **oxycodone** (section 4.7.2) and transdermal **fentanyl** (see below and section 4.7.2); these drugs are best initiated by those with experience in palliative care. Initiation of an opioid analgesic should not be delayed by concern over a theoretical likelihood of psychological dependence (addiction).

Equivalent single doses of strong analgesics
These equivalences are intended **only** as an approximate guide; patients should be carefully monitored after **any** change in medication and dose titration may be required

Analgesic	Dose
Morphine salts (oral)	10 mg
Diamorphine hydrochloride (intramuscular)	3 mg
Hydromorphone hydrochloride	1.3 mg
Oxycodone (oral)	5 mg

ORAL ROUTE. Morphine is given *by mouth* as an oral solution or as standard ('immediate release') tablets regularly every 4 hours, the initial dose depending largely on the patient's previous treatment. A dose of 5–10 mg is enough to replace a weaker analgesic (such as paracetamol or co-proxamol), but 10–20 mg or more is required to replace a strong one (comparable to morphine itself). If the first dose of morphine is no more effective than the previous analgesic, the next dose should be increased by 50%, the aim being to choose the lowest dose which prevents pain. The dose should be adjusted with careful assessment of the pain and the use of adjuvant analgesics (such as NSAIDs) should also be considered. Although morphine in a dose of 5–20 mg is usually adequate there should be no hesitation in increasing it stepwise according to response to 100 mg or occasionally up to 500 mg or higher if necessary. It may be possible to omit the overnight dose if double the usual dose is given at bedtime.

If pain occurs between regular doses of morphine ('breakthrough pain'), an additional dose ('rescue dose') should be given. An additional dose should also be given 30 minutes before an activity that causes pain (e.g. wound dressing). Fentanyl lozenges are also licensed for breakthrough pain.

When the pain is controlled and the patient's 24–hour morphine requirement is established, the daily dose can be given as a single dose or in 2 divided doses as a *modified-release preparation*.

Preparations suitable for twice daily administration include *MST Continus®* tablets or suspension, and *Zomorph®* capsules. Preparations that allow administration of the total daily morphine requirement as a single dose include *MXL®* capsules. *Morcap SR®* capsules may be given either twice daily or as a single daily dose.

The starting dose of modified-release preparations designed for twice daily administration is usually 10–20 mg every 12 hours if no other analgesic (or only paracetamol) has been taken previously, but to replace a weaker opioid analgesic (such as co-proxamol) the starting dose is usually 20–30 mg every 12 hours. Increments should be made to the dose, not to the frequency of administration, which should remain at every 12 hours.

The effective dose of modified-release preparations can alternatively be determined by giving the oral solution of morphine every 4 hours in increasing doses until the pain has been controlled, and then transferring the patient to the same total 24-hour dose of morphine given as the modified-release preparation (divided into two portions for 12-hourly administration). The first dose of the modified-release preparation is given 4 hours after the last dose of the oral solution.[1]

Morphine, as oral solution or standard formulation tablets, should be prescribed for breakthrough pain; the dose should be about one-sixth of the total daily dose of oral morphine repeated every 4 hours if necessary (review pain management if analgesic required more frequently).

PARENTERAL ROUTE. If the patient becomes unable to swallow, the equivalent intramuscular dose of morphine is half the oral solution dose; in the case of the modified-release tablets it is half the total 24-hour dose (which is then divided into 6 portions to be given every 4 hours). **Diamorphine** is preferred for injection because, being more soluble, it can be given in a smaller volume. The equivalent intramuscular (or subcutaneous) is approximately a third of the oral dose of morphine. *Subcutaneous infusion* of diamorphine via syringe driver can be useful (for details, see p. 15).

If the patient can resume taking medicines by mouth, then oral morphine may be substituted for subcutaneous infusion of diamorphine; see table of equivalent doses of morphine (p. 17) for equivalences between the two opioids.

RECTAL ROUTE. Morphine is also available for *rectal administration* as suppositories; alternatively **oxycodone** suppositories can be obtained on special order.

TRANSDERMAL ROUTE. Transdermal preparations of fentanyl are available (section 4.7.2). Careful conversion from oral morphine to transdermal fentanyl is necessary. The following 24-hour doses of morphine are considered to be equivalent to the fentanyl patches shown:

Morphine salt 90 mg daily ≡ fentanyl '25' patch
Morphine salt 180 mg daily ≡ fentanyl '50' patch
Morphine salt 270 mg daily ≡ fentanyl '75' patch
Morphine salt 360 mg daily ≡ fentanyl '100' patch

Morphine (as oral solution or standard formulation tablets) is given for breakthrough pain.

GASTRO-INTESTINAL PAIN. The pain of *bowel colic* may be reduced by loperamide 2–4 mg 4 times daily. Hyoscine hydrobromide may also be helpful, given sublingually at a dose of 300 micrograms 3 times daily as *Kwells*® (Roche Consumer Health) tablets. For the dose by subcutaneous infusion using a syringe driver, see p. 16).

Gastric distension pain due to pressure on the stomach may be helped by a preparation incorporating an antacid with an antiflatulent (section 1.1.1) and by domperidone 10 mg 3 times daily before meals.

MUSCLE SPASM. The pain of muscle spasm can be helped by a muscle relaxant such as diazepam 5–10 mg daily or baclofen 5–10 mg 3 times daily.

NEUROPATHIC PAIN. Patients with neuropathic pain (section 4.7.3) may benefit from a trial of a tricyclic antidepressant for several weeks. An anticonvulsant may be added or substituted if pain persists; gabapentin is licensed for neuropathic pain (section 4.8.1).

Pain due to nerve compression may be reduced by a corticosteroid such as dexamethasone 8 mg daily, which reduces oedema around the tumour, thus reducing compression.

Nerve blocks may be considered when pain is localised to a specific area. **Transcutaneous electrical nerve stimulation** (TENS) may also help.

Miscellaneous conditions

Non-licensed indications or routes. Several recommendations in this section involve non-licensed indications or routes.

RAISED INTRACRANIAL PRESSURE. Headache due to raised intracranial pressure often responds to a high dose of a corticosteroid, such as dexamethasone 16 mg daily for 4 to 5 days, subsequently reduced to 4–6 mg daily if possible; dexamethasone should be given before 6 p.m. to reduce the risk of insomnia.

INTRACTABLE COUGH. Intractable cough may be relieved by moist inhalations or by regular administration of oral morphine in an initial dose of 5 mg every 4 hours. Methadone linctus should be avoided because it has a long duration of action and tends to accumulate.

DYSPNOEA. Breathlessness at rest may be relieved by regular oral morphine in carefully titrated doses, starting at 5 mg every 4 hours. Diazepam 5–10 mg daily may be helpful for dyspnoea associated with anxiety. A corticosteroid, such as dexamethasone 4–8 mg daily, may also be helpful if there is bronchospasm or partial obstruction.

EXCESSIVE RESPIRATORY SECRETION. Excessive respiratory secretion (death rattle) may be reduced by subcutaneous injection of hyoscine hydrobromide 400–600 micrograms every 4 to 8 hours; care must however be taken to avoid the discomfort of dry mouth. Alternatively glycopyrronium may be given by subcutaneous or intramuscular injection in a dose of 200 micrograms every 4 hours. For the dose by subcutaneous infusion using a syringe driver, see p. 16.

RESTLESSNESS AND CONFUSION. Restlessness and confusion may require treatment with haloperidol 1–3 mg by mouth every 8 hours. Chlorpromazine 25–50 mg by mouth every 8 hours is an alternative, but causes more sedation. Levomepromazine (methotrimeprazine) is also used occasionally for restlessness. For the dose by subcutaneous infusion using a syringe driver, see p. 16.

HICCUP. Hiccup due to gastric distension may be helped by a preparation incorporating an antacid with an antiflatulent (section 1.1). If this fails, metoclopramide 10 mg every 6 to 8 hours by mouth or by subcutaneous or intramuscular injection can be added; if this also fails baclofen 5 mg twice daily, or nifedipine 10 mg three times daily, or chlorpromazine 10–25 mg every 6 to 8 hours can be tried.

ANOREXIA. Anorexia may be helped by prednisolone 15–30 mg daily or dexamethasone 2–4 mg daily.

---

1. Studies have indicated that administration of the last dose of the *oral solution* with the first dose of the *modified-release tablets* is not necessary.

CONSTIPATION. Constipation is a very common cause of distress and is almost invariable after administration of an opioid. It should be prevented if possible by the regular administration of laxatives; a faecal softener with a peristaltic stimulant (e.g. co-danthramer), or lactulose solution with a senna preparation should be used (section 1.6.2 and section 1.6.3).

FUNGATING GROWTH. Fungating growth may be treated by regular dressing and oral administration of metronidazole; topical application of metronidazole is also used.

CAPILLARY BLEEDING. Capillary bleeding may be reduced by applying gauze soaked in adrenaline (epinephrine) solution 1 mg/mL (1 in 1000).

DRY MOUTH. Dry mouth may be relieved by good mouth care and measures such as the sucking of ice or pineapple chunks or the use of artificial saliva (section 12.3.5); dry mouth associated with candidiasis can be treated by oral preparations of nystatin or miconazole (section 12.3.2); alternatively, fluconazole can be given by mouth (section 5.2). Dry mouth may be caused by certain medication including opioids, antimuscarinic drugs (e.g. hyoscine), antidepressants and some anti-emetics; if possible, an alternative preparation should be considered.

PRURITUS. Pruritus, even when associated with obstructive jaundice, often responds to simple measures such as application of emollients (section 13.2.1). In the case of obstructive jaundice, further measures include administration of colestyramine (section 1.9.2).

CONVULSIONS. Patients with cerebral tumours or uraemia may be susceptible to convulsions. Prophylactic treatment with phenytoin or carbamazepine (section 4.8.1) should be considered. When oral medication is no longer possible, diazepam as suppositories 10–20 mg every 4 to 8 hours, or phenobarbital by injection 50–200 mg twice daily is continued as prophylaxis. For the use of midazolam by subcutaneous infusion using a syringe driver, see below.

DYSPHAGIA. A corticosteroid such as dexamethasone 8 mg daily may help, temporarily, if there is an obstruction due to tumour. See also under Dry Mouth.

NAUSEA AND VOMITING. Nausea and vomiting are common in patients with advanced cancer. Ideally, the cause should be determined before treatment with an anti-emetic (section 4.6) is started.
  Nausea and vomiting may occur with opioid therapy particularly in the initial stages but can be prevented by giving an anti-emetic such as haloperidol or metoclopramide. An anti-emetic is usually necessary only for the first 4 or 5 days and therefore combined preparations containing an opioid with an anti-emetic are not recommended because they lead to unnecessary anti-emetic therapy (and associated side-effects when used long-term).
  Metoclopramide has a prokinetic action and is used in a dose of 10 mg 3 times daily by mouth for nausea and vomiting associated with gastritis, gastric stasis, and functional bowel obstruction. Drugs with antimuscarinic effects antagonise prokinetic drugs and,

where possible, should not therefore be used concurrently.
  Haloperidol is used in a dose of 1.5 mg daily (or twice daily if nausea continues) by mouth for most chemical causes of vomiting (e.g. hypercalcaemia, renal failure).
  Cyclizine is given in a dose of 50 mg up to 3 times daily by mouth. It is used for nausea and vomiting due to mechanical bowel obstruction, raised intracranial pressure, and motion sickness.
  Anti-emetic therapy should be reviewed every 24 hours; it may be necessary to substitute the anti-emetic or to add another one.
  Levomepromazine (methotrimeprazine) may be used if first-line anti-emetics are inadequate; it is given by mouth in a dose of 6–25 mg daily [6-mg tablets available on named-patient basis]. Dexamethasone 8–16 mg daily by mouth may be used as an adjunct.
  For the administration of anti-emetics by subcutaneous infusion using a syringe driver, see below.
  For the treatment of nausea and vomiting associated with cancer chemotherapy, see section 8.1.

INSOMNIA. Patients with advanced cancer may not sleep because of discomfort, cramps, night sweats, joint stiffness, or fear. There should be appropriate treatment of these problems before hypnotics are used. Benzodiazepines, such as temazepam, may be useful (section 4.1.1).

HYPERCALCAEMIA. See section 9.5.1.2.

Syringe drivers

Although drugs can usually be administered *by mouth* to control the symptoms of advanced cancer, the parenteral route may sometimes be necessary. If the parenteral route is necessary, repeated administration of *intramuscular injections* can be difficult in a cachectic patient. This has led to the use of a portable syringe driver to give a *continuous subcutaneous infusion*, which can provide good control of symptoms with little discomfort or inconvenience to the patient.

> **Syringe driver rate settings.** Staff using syringe drivers should be **adequately trained** and different rate settings should be **clearly identified** and **differentiated**; incorrect use of syringe drivers is a common cause of drug errors.

Indications for the **parenteral route** are:

- the patient is unable to take medicines by mouth owing to *nausea and vomiting, dysphagia, severe weakness,* or *coma;*
- there is *malignant bowel obstruction* in patients for whom further surgery is inappropriate (avoiding the need for an intravenous infusion or for insertion of a nasogastric tube);
- occasionally when the patient *does not wish* to take regular medication by mouth.

NAUSEA AND VOMITING. Haloperidol is given in a *subcutaneous infusion dose* of 2.5–10 mg/24 hours.
  Levomepromazine (methotrimeprazine) causes sedation in about 50% of patients; it is given in a *subcutaneous infusion dose* of 25–200 mg/24 hours, although lower doses of 5–25 mg/24 hours may be effective with less sedation.

Cyclizine is particularly liable to precipitate if mixed with diamorphine or other drugs (see under Mixing and Compatibility, below); it is given in a *subcutaneous infusion dose* of 150 mg/24 hours.

Metoclopramide may cause skin reactions; it is given in a *subcutaneous infusion dose* of 30–100 mg/24 hours.

Octreotide (section 8.3.4.3), which stimulates water and electrolyte absorption and inhibits water secretion in the small bowel, can be used by subcutaneous infusion, in a dose of 300–600 micrograms/24 hours to reduce intestinal secretions and vomiting.

BOWEL COLIC AND EXCESSIVE RESPIRATORY SECRETIONS. Hyoscine hydrobromide effectively reduces respiratory secretions and is sedative (but occasionally causes paradoxical agitation); it is given in a *subcutaneous infusion dose* of 0.6–2.4 mg/24 hours.

Hyoscine butylbromide is effective in bowel colic, is less sedative than hyoscine hydrobromide, but is not always adequate for the control of respiratory secretions; it is given in a *subcutaneous infusion dose* of 20–60 mg/24 hours (**important:** this dose of *hyoscine butylbromide* must not be confused with the much lower dose of *hyoscine hydrobromide*, above).

Glycopyrronium 0.6–1.2 mg/24 hours may also be used.

RESTLESSNESS AND CONFUSION. Haloperidol has little sedative effect; it is given in a *subcutaneous infusion dose* of 5–15 mg/24 hours.

Levomepromazine (methotrimeprazine) has a sedative effect; it is given in a *subcutaneous infusion dose* of 50–200 mg/24 hours.

Midazolam is a sedative and an antiepileptic, and is therefore suitable for a very restless patient; it is given in a *subcutaneous infusion dose* of 20–100 mg/24 hours.

CONVULSIONS. If a patient has previously been receiving an antiepileptic *or* has a primary or secondary cerebral tumour *or* is at risk of convulsion (e.g. owing to uraemia) antiepileptic medication should not be stopped. Midazolam is the benzodiazepine antiepileptic of choice for *continuous subcutaneous infusion*, and it is given initially in a dose of 20–40 mg/24 hours.

PAIN CONTROL. Diamorphine is the preferred opioid since its high solubility permits a large dose to be given in a small volume (see under Mixing and Compatibility, below). The table below gives the approximate doses of *morphine by mouth* (as oral solution or standard formulation tablets or as modified-release tablets) equivalent to *diamorphine by injection* (intramuscularly or by subcutaneous infusion).

MIXING AND COMPATIBILITY. The general principle that injections should be given into separate sites (and should not be mixed) does not apply to the use of syringe drivers in palliative care. Provided that there is evidence of compatibility, selected injections can be mixed in syringe drivers. Not all types of medication can be used in a subcutaneous infusion. In particular, chlorpromazine, prochlorperazine and diazepam are **contra-indicated** as they cause skin reactions at the injection site; to a lesser extent cyclizine and levomepromazine (methotrimeprazine) may also sometimes cause local irritation.

In theory injections dissolved in water for injections are more likely to be associated with pain (possibly owing to their hypotonicity). The use of physiological saline (sodium chloride 0.9%) however increases the likelihood of precipitation when more than one drug is used; moreover subcutaneous infusion rates are so slow (0.1–0.3 mL/hour) that pain is not usually a problem when water is used as a diluent.

Diamorphine can be given by subcutaneous infusion in a strength of up to 250 mg/mL; up to a strength of 40 mg/mL either *water for injections* or *physiological saline* (sodium chloride 0.9%) is a suitable diluent—above that strength only *water for injections* is used (to avoid precipitation).

The following can be mixed with *diamorphine*:

Cyclizine[1]	Hyoscine hydrobromide
Dexamethasone[2]	Levomepromazine
Haloperidol[3]	Metoclopramide[4]
Hyoscine butylbromide	Midazolam

Subcutaneous infusion solution should be monitored regularly both to check for precipitation (and discoloration) and to ensure that the infusion is running at the correct rate

PROBLEMS ENCOUNTERED WITH SYRINGE DRIVERS. The following are problems that may be encountered with syringe drivers and the action that should be taken:

- if the subcutaneous infusion runs *too quickly* check the rate setting and the calculation;
- if the subcutaneous infusion runs *too slowly* check the start button, the battery, the syringe driver, the cannula, and make sure that the injection site is not inflamed;
- if there is an *injection site reaction* make sure that the site does not need to be changed—firmness or swelling at the site of injection is not in itself an indication for change, but pain or obvious inflammation is.

---

1. Cyclizine may precipitate at concentrations above 10mg/mL *or* in the presence of physiological saline *or* as the concentration of diamorphine relative to cyclizine increases; mixtures of diamorphine and cyclizine are also liable to precipitate after 24 hours.

2. Special care is needed to avoid precipitation of dexamethasone when preparing.

3. Mixtures of haloperidol and diamorphine are liable to precipitate after 24 hours if haloperidol concentration is above 2mg/mL.

4. Under some conditions metoclopramide may become discoloured; such solutions should be discarded.

Equivalent doses of morphine sulphate by mouth (as oral solution or standard tablets or as modified-release tablets) or of diamorphine hydrochloride by intramuscular injection or by subcutaneous infusion

These equivalences are approximate only and may need to be adjusted according to response

ORAL MORPHINE		PARENTERAL DIAMORPHINE	
Morphine sulphate oral solution or standard tablets	Morphine sulphate modified-release tablets	Diamorphine hydrochloride by intramuscular injection	Diamorphine hydrochloride by subcutaneous infusion
every 4 hours	every 12 hours	every 4 hours	every 24 hours
5 mg	20 mg	2.5 mg	15 mg
10 mg	30 mg	5 mg	20 mg
15 mg	50 mg	5 mg	30 mg
20 mg	60 mg	7.5 mg	45 mg
30 mg	90 mg	10 mg	60 mg
40 mg	120 mg	15 mg	90 mg
60 mg	180 mg	20 mg	120 mg
80 mg	240 mg	30 mg	180 mg
100 mg	300 mg	40 mg	240 mg
130 mg	400 mg	50 mg	300 mg
160 mg	500 mg	60 mg	360 mg
200 mg	600 mg	70 mg	400 mg

If breakthrough pain occurs give a subcutaneous (preferable) or intramuscular injection of diamorphine equivalent to one-sixth of the total 24-hour subcutaneous infusion dose. It is kinder to give an intermittent bolus injection *subcutaneously*—absorption is smoother so that the risk of adverse effects at peak absorption is avoided (an even better method is to use a subcutaneous butterfly needle).

To minimise the risk of infection no individual subcutaneous infusion solution should be used for longer than 24 hours.

Prescribing for the elderly

Old people, especially the very old, require special care and consideration from prescribers. *Medicines for Older People*, a component document of the National Service Framework for Older People,[1] describes how to maximise the benefits of medicines and how to avoid excessive, inappropriate, or inadequate consumption of medicines by older people.

APPROPRIATE PRESCRIBING. Elderly patients often receive multiple drugs for their multiple diseases. This greatly increases the risk of drug interactions as well as adverse reactions, and may affect compliance (see Taking medicines to best effect under General guidance). The balance of benefit and harm of some medicines may be altered in the elderly. Therefore, elderly patients' medicines should be reviewed regularly and medicines which are not of benefit should be stopped. In some cases prophylactic drugs may be inappropriate if they are likely to complicate existing treatment or introduce unnecessary side-effects, especially in elderly patients with poor prognosis or with poor overall health. However, elderly patients should not be denied medicines which may help them, such as anticoagulants or antiplatelet drugs for atrial fibrillation, antihypertensives, statins, and drugs for osteoporosis.

FORM OF MEDICINE. Frail elderly patients may have difficulty swallowing tablets; if left in the mouth, ulceration may develop. They should always be encouraged to take their tablets or capsules with enough fluid, and whilst in an upright position to

1. Department of Health. National Service Framework for Older People. London: Department of Health, March 2001

avoid the possibility of oesophageal ulceration. It may be helpful to discuss with the patient the possibility of taking the drug as a liquid if available.

MANIFESTATIONS OF AGEING. In the very old, manifestations of normal ageing may be mistaken for disease and lead to inappropriate prescribing. In addition, age-related muscle weakness and difficulty in maintaining balance should not be confused with neurological disease. Disorders such as lightheadedness not associated with postural or postprandial hypotension are unlikely to be helped by drugs.

SELF-MEDICATION. Just as in a younger patient self-medication with over-the-counter products or with drugs prescribed for a previous illness (or even for another person) may be an added complication. Discussion with both the patient and relatives as well as a home visit may be needed to establish exactly what is being taken.

SENSITIVITY. The ageing nervous system shows increased *susceptibility* to many commonly used drugs, such as opioid analgesics, benzodiazepines, antipsychotics, and antiparkinsonian drugs, all of which must be used with caution. Similarly, other organs may also be more susceptible to the effects of drugs such as antihypertensives and NSAIDs.

Pharmacokinetics

The most important effect of age is reduction in renal clearance. Many aged patients thus *excrete drugs slowly*, and are *highly susceptible to nephrotoxic drugs*. Acute illness may lead to rapid reduction in renal clearance, especially if accompanied by dehydration. Hence, a patient stabilised on a drug with a narrow margin between the therapeutic and the toxic dose (e.g. digoxin) may rapidly develop adverse effects in the aftermath of a myocardial infarction or a respiratory-tract infection. The metabolism of some drugs may be reduced in the elderly.

Pharmacokinetic changes may markedly increase the tissue concentration of a drug in the elderly, especially in debilitated patients.

Adverse reactions

Adverse reactions often present in the elderly in a vague and non-specific fashion. *Confusion* is often the presenting symptom (caused by almost any of the commonly used drugs). Other common manifestations are *constipation* (with antimuscarinics and many tranquillisers) and postural *hypotension* and *falls* (with diuretics and many psychotropics).

HYPNOTICS. Many hypnotics with long half-lives have serious hangover effects of drowsiness, unsteady gait, and even slurred speech and confusion. Those with short half-lives should be used but they too can present problems (section 4.1.1). Short courses of hypnotics are occasionally useful for helping a patient through an acute illness or some other crisis but every effort must be made to avoid dependence. Benzodiazepines impair balance, which may result in falls.

DIURETICS. Diuretics are overprescribed in old age and should **not** be used on a long-term basis to treat simple gravitational oedema which will usually respond to increased movement, raising the legs, and support stockings. A few days of diuretic treatment may speed the clearing of the oedema but it should rarely need continued drug therapy.

NSAIDs. Bleeding associated with *aspirin* and *other NSAIDs* is more common in the elderly who are more likely to have a fatal or serious outcome. NSAIDs are also a special hazard in patients with cardiac disease or renal impairment which may again place older patients at particular risk.

Owing to the *increased susceptibilty of the elderly* to the *side-effects of NSAIDs* the following recommendations are made:

- for *osteoarthritis, soft-tissue lesions* and *back pain* first try measures such as weight reduction (if obese), warmth, exercise and use of a walking stick;
- for *osteoarthritis, soft-tissue lesions, back pain* and *pain in rheumatoid arthritis*, paracetamol should be used first and can often provide adequate pain relief;
- alternatively, a low-dose NSAID (e.g. ibuprofen up to 1.2 g daily may be given;
- for pain relief when either drug is inadequate, paracetamol in a full dose plus a low-dose NSAID may be given;
- if necessary, the NSAID dose can be increased or an opioid analgesic given with paracetamol;
- do not give two NSAIDs at the same time.

For advice on prophylaxis of NSAID-induced peptic ulcers if continued NSAID treatment is necessary, see section 1.3.

OTHER DRUGS. Other drugs which commonly cause adverse reactions are *antiparkinsonian drugs, antihypertensives, psychotropics*, and *digoxin*. The usual maintenance dose of digoxin in very old patients is 125 micrograms daily (62.5 micrograms in those with renal disease); lower doses are often inadequate but toxicity is common in those given 250 micrograms daily.

Drug-induced blood disorders are much more common in the elderly. Therefore drugs with a tendency to cause bone marrow depression (e.g. *co-trimoxazole, mianserin*) should be avoided unless there is no acceptable alternative.

The elderly generally require a lower maintenance dose of *warfarin* than younger adults; once again, the outcome of bleeding tends to be more serious.

Guidelines

First always question whether a drug is indicated at all.

LIMIT RANGE. It is a sensible policy to prescribe from a limited range of drugs and to be thoroughly familiar with their effects in the elderly.

REDUCE DOSE. Dosage should generally be substantially lower than for younger patients and it is common to start with about 50% of the adult dose. Some drugs (e.g. long-acting antidiabetic drugs such as glibenclamide and chlorpropamide) should be avoided altogether.

REVIEW REGULARLY. Review repeat prescriptions regularly. In many patients it may be possible to stop some drugs, provided that clinical progress is monitored. It may be necessary to reduce the dose of some drugs as renal function declines.

SIMPLIFY REGIMENS. Elderly patients benefit from simple treatment regimens. Only drugs with a clear indication should be prescribed and whenever possible given once or twice daily. In particular, regimens which call for a confusing array of dosage intervals should be avoided.

EXPLAIN CLEARLY. Write full instructions on every prescription (*including* repeat prescriptions) so that containers can be properly labelled with full directions. Avoid imprecisions like 'as directed'. Child-resistant containers may be unsuitable.

REPEATS AND DISPOSAL. Instruct patients what to do when drugs run out, and also how to dispose of any that are no longer necessary. Try to prescribe matching quantities.

If these guidelines are followed most elderly people will cope adequately with their own medicines. If not then it is essential to enrol the help of a third party, usually a relative or a friend.

Drugs and sport

uk sport
sporting excellence

Drug-Free Sport Advice Card
January 2004

Prohibited Classes of Substances and Prohibited Methods
and Examples of Permitted Substances in Sport

If in doubt - check it out

If the substance you're searching for is not on this card, check UK Sport's Drug Information
Database to find the status of your medication or substance at www.uksport.gov.uk/did

Examples of Permitted Substances

Anti-allergic	acrivastine, brompheniramine, cetirizine, chlorpheniramine, desloratadine, loratadine, mizolastine, terfenadine
Anti-bacterial	all antibiotics are PERMITTED
Anti-diarrhoeal	atropine, diphenoxylate, loperamide, and products containing electrolytes
Anti-fungal	amphotericin, clotrimazole, fluconazole, miconazole, nystatin, terbinafine
Anti-viral	aciclovir, idoxuridine, penciclovir
Asthma	sodium cromoglicate and theophylline are permitted. Beclometasone, fluticasone, formoterol, salbutamol (below 1000ng/mL), salmeterol and terbutaline are permitted when administered by inhalation only and with the submission of a Therapeutic Use Exemption (TUE)* form (see overleaf)
Cough/Cold	non-sedative antihistamines, codeine, dextromethorphan, guaiphenesin, oxymetazoline, paracetamol, phenylephrine, phenylpropanolamine, pholcodine, pseudoephedrine, steam and menthol inhalations, terfenadine and xylometazoline
Ear/Nose	ear and nasal drops or sprays containing docusate sodium, tramazoline. Preparations containing glucocorticosteroids such as beclometasone, betamethasone, dexamethasone, fluticasone, and hydrocortisone are permitted with the submission of a TUE* form (see overleaf)
Eye	eye drops or creams containing antazoline, sodium cromoglicate, chloramphenicol. Those containing glucocorticosteroids such as betamethasone, dexamethasone, fluorometholone and hydrocortisone
Hayfever	acetate are permitted with the submission of a TUE* form (see overleaf) all antihistamines (see anti-allergic), phenylephrine, pseudoephedrine, sodium cromoglicate and xylometazoline. Nasal sprays containing a glucocorticosteroid such as beclometasone are permitted with the submission of a TUE* form (see overleaf)
Haemorrhoids	preparations containing benzocaine, cinchocaine and lidocaine
Local anaesthetics	are permitted (except for cocaine)
Oral contraceptives	those containing one or more of the following: desogestrel, drospirenone, ethinylestradiol, etynodiol diacetate, gestodene, levonorgestrel, mestranol, norethisterone, norgestimate
Pain/inflammation	all non-steroidal anti-inflammatory drugs (NSAIDs), aspirin, caffeine, codeine, dextropropoxyphene, diclofenac, dihydrocodeine, ibuprofen, paracetamol, tramadol
Vomiting/nausea	cinnarizine, cyclizine, domperidone, hyoscine, meclozine, metoclopramide, prochlorperazine, promethazine

WARNING: Many prescription and over-the-counter medicines and substances contain prohibited substances. Inform your doctor and pharmacist of your need to take only those substances that are permitted. Consider giving your doctor and pharmacist a copy of this advice card and the link to the D.I.D at www.uksport.gov.uk/did

SUPPLEMENTS: Some vitamin, herbal and nutritional supplements may contain prohibited substances. Use of these products is at your own risk. Visit UK Sport's website at www.uksport.gov.uk for more information on the reasons why athletes are at risk if using supplements in sport.

Use caution when travelling abroad as ingredients may differ in other countries.

USEFUL CONTACTS:
UK Sport Drug Information Database (DID):   www.uksport.gov.uk/did
UK Sport Drug Information Line: +44 (0)800 528 0004
Drug-Free Sport email address: drug-free@uksport.gov.uk

Add your own useful numbers:

_____

_____

NOTE: The information on this card is based on the World Anti-Doping Code list of prohibited substances and methods effective from January 1 2004. You have been provided with examples only of permitted and prohibited substances. Check UK Sport's website for the latest information regarding this list at www.uksport.gov.uk

Version 3 January 2004

Classes of Prohibited Substances and Methods with examples

Stimulants including their optical D- and L- isomers (in competition): e.g. amfetamine, bromantan, cathine, cocaine, ephedrine, fenproporex, mefenorex, methamfetamine, methylephedrine, methylphenidate, modafinil, phenmetrazine and other related substances

Narcotics (in competition): buprenorphine, dextromoramide, diamorphine (heroin), hydromorphone, methadone, morphine, oxycodone, oxymorphone, pentazocine and pethidine

Cannabinoids (in competition): hashish and marijuana are prohibited

Anabolic Agents (in and out-of-competition): e.g. androstadienone, androstenedione, bolasterone, clenbuterol, DHEA, methandienone, nandrolone, norbolethone, 19 nor-steroids, stanozolol, testosterone, trenbolone and other related substances

Peptide Hormones (in and out-of-competition): including their mimetics, analogues and releasing factors, chorionic gonadotrophin and pituitary and synthetic gonadotrophins are prohibited in males only. Corticotrophins, erythropoietin (EPO), growth hormone (hGH), insulin-like growth factor (IGF-1) and insulin (for insulin dependent diabetics a TUE* form is required (see below))

Beta-2 Agonists (in and out-of-competition): All beta-2 agonists are prohibited except for formoterol, salbutamol (below 1000ng/mL), salmeterol, terbutaline which are permitted by inhalation only when a TUE* has been granted (see below)

Anti-oestrogenic agents (in and out-of-competition): e.g. clomiphene, cyclofenil, tamoxifen, anastrozole, letrozole, exemestane and related substances are prohibited in males only

Masking Agents (in and out-of-competition): e.g. epitestosterone, plasma expanders (e.g.hydroxyethyl starch), probenecid and diuretics including amiloride, bendrofluazide, furosemide, hydrochlorothiazide, mannitol (prohibited by intravenous injection) and triamterene

Glucocorticosteroids (in competition): Prohibited when administered orally, rectally, or by intravenous or intramuscular injection. All other routes of administration require the submission of a TUE* form (see below).

WARNING TO ATHLETES: Strict liability means that you are responsible for any prohibited substance found in your system. The presence of a prohibited substance constitutes a doping violation, whether or not the substance was taken in or out of competition. Be aware when taking medication that substances do take time to pass through the system.

Classes of Prohibited Methods with examples:

Enhancement of Oxygen Transfer: blood doping and the use of products that enhance the uptake, transport, or delivery of oxygen and other methods

Pharmacological, Chemical or Physical Manipulation: substances or methods including masking agents which alter the validity of a sample

Gene Doping: non-therapeutic use of genes, genetic elements and/or cells that have the capacity to enhance athletic performance.

Classes of prohibited substances in specific sports:

Alcohol (Each sport has a different doping violation threshold. See the January 2004 prohibited list for more details)
Alcohol is prohibited in competition only in aeronautics, archery, automobile, billiards, boules, football, gymnastics, karate, modern pentathlon, motor cycling, roller sports, skiing, triathlon and wrestling

Beta-blockers (in competition): including but not limited to acebutolol, atenolol, carvedilol, oxprenolol, propranolol are prohibited in the following sports, aeronautic, archery (also prohibited out of competition), automobile, billiards, bobsleigh, boules, bridge, chess, curling, diving, football, freestyle snowboard, gymnastics, motorcycling, modern pentathlon, nine-pin bowling, sailing (race helms only), shooting (also prohibited out of competition), ski jumping, synchronised swimming and wrestling

Diuretics (prohibited in all sports in and out of competition): Diuretics are prohibited in all sports however, a TUE* will not be granted for diuretics for athletes competing in these sports: body-building, boxing, judo, karate, powerlifting, rowing (light weight), ski jumping, taekwondo, weightlifting, wrestling, wushu (see below). Contact your governing body for anti-doping regulations.

*Therapeutic Use Exemptions (TUE)
Athletes who have been invited to participate in the UK's registered testing pool are required to submit a Therapeutic Use Exemption (TUE) for the use of a prohibited substance for a medical condition. Athletes in the registered testing pool will be able to access the TUE application form via the Drug-Free Sport registration programme.

Beware of medications to treat the following conditions that may contain prohibited substances, for example:

Asthma	sympathomimetics e.g. ephedrine, fenoterol, isoprenaline and rimiterol
Cough/Cold	sympathomimetics/stimulants e.g. ephedrine and amfetamine related substances
Diarrhoea	strong opioids e.g. morphine
Hayfever	strong opioids e.g. morphine
Haemorrhoids	suppositories containing glucocorticosteroids
Pain/inflammation	strong opioids e.g. morphine

It is the responsibility of the athlete to check the status of all medications and substances

Supplies of this card are available from: UK Sport, Ethics & Anti-Doping, 40 Bernard Street, London WC1N 1ST.

A similar card detailing classes of drugs and doping methods prohibited in football is available from the Football Association.

General Medical Council's advice. Doctors who prescribe or collude in the provision of drugs or treatment with the intention of improperly enhancing an individual's performance in sport would be contravening the GMC's guidance, and such actions would usually raise a question of a doctor's continued registration. This does not preclude the provision of any care or treatment where the doctor's intention is to protect or improve the patient's health.

Emergency treatment of poisoning

These notes provide only an overview and it is strongly recommended that either a **poisons information centre** or **TOXBASE** (see below) be consulted in cases where there is doubt about the degree of risk or about appropriate management.

HOSPITAL ADMISSION. All patients who show features of poisoning should generally be admitted to hospital. Patients who have taken poisons with delayed actions should also be admitted, even if they appear well. Delayed-action poisons include aspirin, iron, paracetamol, tricyclic antidepressants, co-phenotrope (diphenoxylate with atropine, *Lomotil*®), and paraquat; the effects of modified-release preparations are also delayed. A note of all relevant information including what treatment has been given should accompany the patient to hospital.

TOXBASE

TOXBASE, the primary clinical toxicology database of the National Poisons Information Service, is available on the Internet to registered users (www.spib.axl.co.uk). It provides information about routine diagnosis, treatment and management of patients exposed to drugs, household products, and industrial and agricultural chemicals. **Important:** for specialised information telephone a Poisons Information Centre.

TICTAC

TICTAC is a computer-aided tablet and capsule identification system. It is available to authorised users including Regional Medicines Information Centres (see inside front cover) and Poisons Information Centres.

Poisons information centres (consult day and night)

The following single number for the UK National Poisons Information Service directs the caller to the local poisons information centre:
Tel: (0870) 600 6266

NOTE. Some centres also advise on laboratory analytical services which may be of help in the diagnosis and management of a small number of cases. For advice on snake bites see p. 29.

> The **poisons information centres** (see above) will provide advice on all aspects of poisoning day and night

General care

It is often impossible to establish with certainty the identity of the poison and the size of the dose. Fortunately this is not usually important because only a few poisons (such as opioids, paracetamol, and iron) have specific antidotes; few patients require active removal of the poison. In most patients, treatment is directed at managing symptoms as they arise. Nevertheless, knowledge of the type and timing of poisoning can help in anticipating the course of events. All relevant information should be sought from the poisoned individual and from carers or parents. However, such information should be interpreted with care because it may not be complete or entirely reliable. Sometimes symptoms arise from other illnesses and patients should be assessed carefully. Accidents may involve a number of domestic and industrial products (the contents of which are not generally known). A **poisons information centre** should be consulted where there is doubt about any aspect of suspected poisoning.

Respiration

Respiration is often impaired in unconscious patients. An obstructed airway requires immediate attention. In the absence of trauma, the airway should be opened with simple measures such as chin lift or jaw thrust. An oropharyngeal or nasopharyngeal airway may be useful in patients with reduced consciousness to prevent obstruction, provided ventilation is adequate. Intubation and ventilation should be considered in patients whose airway cannot be protected or who have inadequate ventilation because of respiratory acidosis; such patients should be monitored in a critical care area.

Most poisons that impair consciousness also depress respiration. Assisted ventilation by mouth-to-mouth or *Ambu-bag* inflation may be needed. Oxygen is not a substitute for adequate ventilation, though it should be given in the highest concentration possible in poisoning with carbon monoxide and irritant gases.

Respiratory stimulants do not help and should be avoided.

Blood pressure

Hypotension is common in severe poisoning with central nervous system depressants. A systolic blood pressure of less than 70 mmHg may lead to irreversible brain damage or renal tubular necrosis. Hypotension should be corrected initially by tilting down the head of the bed and administration of either sodium chloride intravenous infusion or a colloidal infusion. Vasoconstrictor sympathomimetics (section 2.7.2) are rarely required and their use may be discussed with a poisons information centre.

Fluid depletion without hypotension is common after prolonged coma and after aspirin poisoning due to vomiting, sweating, and hyperpnoea.

Hypertension, often transient, occurs less frequently than hypotension in poisoning; it may be associated with sympathomimetic drugs such as amphetamines, phencyclidine, and cocaine.

Heart

Cardiac conduction defects and arrhythmias may occur in acute poisoning, notably with tricyclic antidepressants, some antipsychotics, some antihistamines, and co-proxamol. Arrhythmias often respond to correction of underlying hypoxia, acidosis, or other biochemical abnormalities. Ventricular arrhythmias that have been confirmed by ECG and which are causing serious hypotension may require treatment. If the QT interval is prolonged, specialist advice should be sought because the use of some anti-arrhythmic drugs may be inappropriate. Supraventricular arrhythmias are seldom life-threatening and drug treatment is best withheld until the patient reaches hospital.

Body temperature

Hypothermia may develop in patients of any age who have been deeply unconscious for some hours particularly following overdose with barbiturates or phenothiazines. It may be missed unless core temperature is measured using a low-reading rectal thermometer or by some other means. Hypothermia is best treated by wrapping the patient (e.g. in a 'space blanket') to conserve body heat.

Hyperthermia can develop in patients taking CNS stimulants; children and the elderly are also at risk when taking drugs with antimuscarinic properties at therapeutic doses. It is initially managed by removing all unnecessary clothing and using a fan. Sponging with tepid water will promote evaporation; iced water should **not** be used.

Both hypothermia and hyperthermia require urgent hospitalisation for assessment and supportive treatment.

Convulsions

Single short-lived convulsions do not require treatment. If convulsions are protracted or recur frequently, lorazepam 4 mg or diazepam (preferably as emulsion) up to 10 mg should be given by slow intravenous injection into a large vein; the benzodiazepines should not be given intramuscularly.

Removal and elimination

Removal from the gastro-intestinal tract

Gastric lavage is rarely required and should be considered only if a life-threatening amount of a drug has been ingested within the preceding hour. It should be carried out only if the airway can be protected adequately. Gastric lavage is contra-indicated if a corrosive substance or a petroleum distillate has been ingested but it may occasionally be considered in patients who have ingested drugs that are not absorbed by charcoal, such as iron or lithium. Induction of *emesis* (e.g. with ipecacuanha) is **not** recommended because there is no evidence that it affects absorption and it may increase the risk of aspiration.

Whole bowel irrigation (by means of a bowel cleansing solution) has been used in poisoning with certain modified-release or enteric-coated formula-

tions, in severe poisoning with iron and lithium salts, and if illicit drugs are carried in the gastro-intestinal tract ('body-packing'). However, it is not clear that the procedure improves outcome and advice should be sought from a poisons information centre.

Prevention of absorption

Given by mouth, **activated charcoal** can bind many poisons in the gastro-intestinal system, thereby *reducing their absorption*. The **sooner** it is given the **more effective** it is, but it may still be effective up to 1 hour after ingestion of the poison—longer in the case of modified-release preparations or of drugs with antimuscarinic (anticholinergic) properties. It is relatively safe and is particularly useful for the prevention of absorption of poisons which are toxic in small amounts, e.g. antidepressants.

For the use of charcoal in active elimination techniques, see below.

CHARCOAL, ACTIVATED

Indications: adsorption of poisons in the gastro-intestinal system; see also active elimination techniques, below

Cautions: drowsy or comatose patient (risk of aspiration); reduced gastro-intestinal motility (risk of obstruction); not for poisoning with petroleum distillates, corrosive substances, alcohols, clofenotane (dicophane, DDT), malathion, and metal salts including iron and lithium salts

Side-effects: black stools

Dose: see under preparations below

Actidose-Aqua® Advance (Cambridge)
Oral suspension, activated charcoal, net price 50-g pack (240 mL) = £12.50
NOTE. The brand name *Actidose-Aqua®* was formerly used
Dose: reduction of absorption, 50–100 g; INFANT under 1 year 1 g/kg (approx. 5 mL/kg), CHILD 1–12 years 25–50 g
Active elimination (see below for ADULT dose); INFANT under 1 year, 1 g/kg (approx. 5 mL/kg) every 4–6 hours; CHILD 1–12 years, 25–50 g every 4–6 hours

Carbomix® (Meadow)
Powder, activated charcoal, net price 25-g pack = £8.50, 50-g pack = £11.90
Dose: reduction of absorption, 50 g, repeated if necessary; CHILD under 12 years 25 g (50 g in severe poisoning)
Active elimination, see below

Charcodote® (PLIVA)
Oral suspension, activated charcoal, net price 50-g pack = £12.50
Dose: reduction of absorption, 50 g; CHILD under 12 years 25 g (50 g in severe poisoning)
Active elimination, see below

Active elimination techniques

Repeated doses of **activated charcoal** by mouth *enhance the elimination* of some drugs after they have been absorbed; repeated doses are given after overdosage with:

Barbiturates	Quinine
Carbamazepine	Theophylline
Dapsone	

The usual adult dose of activated charcoal is 50 g initially then 50 g every 4 hours. Vomiting should be treated (e.g. with an anti-emetic drug) since it may reduce the efficacy of charcoal treatment. In cases of intolerance, the dose may be reduced and the frequency increased (e.g. 25 g every 2 hours *or* 12.5 g every hour) but this may compromise efficacy.

Other techniques intended to enhance the elimination of poisons after absorption are only practicable in hospital and are only suitable for a small number of severely poisoned patients. Moreover, they only apply to a limited number of poisons. Examples include:

- Haemodialysis for salicylates, phenobarbital, methyl alcohol (methanol), ethylene glycol, and lithium
- Haemoperfusion for medium- and short-acting barbiturates, chloral hydrate, meprobamate, and theophylline.

Alkalinisation of the urine increases elimination of salicylates, but forced alkaline diuresis is no longer recommended.

Specific drugs

Alcohol

Acute intoxication with alcohol (ethanol) is common in adults but also occurs in children. The features include ataxia, dysarthria, nystagmus, and drowsiness, which may progress to coma, with hypotension and acidosis. Aspiration of vomit is a special hazard and hypoglycaemia may occur in children and some adults. Patients are managed supportively with particular attention to maintaining a clear airway and measures to reduce the risk of aspiration of gastric contents. The blood glucose is measured and glucose given if indicated.

> The **poisons information centres** (see p. 20) will provide advice on all aspects of poisoning day and night

Analgesics (non-opioid)

ASPIRIN. The chief features of salicylate poisoning are hyperventilation, tinnitus, deafness, vasodilatation, and sweating. Coma is uncommon but indicates very severe poisoning. The associated acid-base disturbances are complex.

Treatment must be in hospital where plasma salicylate, pH, and electrolytes can be measured. Fluid losses are replaced and sodium bicarbonate (1.26%) given to enhance urinary salicylate excretion when the plasma-salicylate concentration is greater than:
500 mg/litre (3.6 mmol/litre) in adults *or*
350 mg/litre (2.5 mmol/litre) in children.
Haemodialysis is the treatment of choice for severe salicylate poisoning and should be given serious consideration when the plasma-salicylate concentration is greater than 700 mg/litre (5.1 mmol/litre) or in the presence of severe metabolic acidosis.

NSAIDS. Mefenamic acid has important consequences in overdosage because it can cause convulsions, which if prolonged or recurrent, require treatment with intravenous lorazepam or diazepam.

Ibuprofen may cause nausea, vomiting, and tinnitus, but more serious toxicity is very uncommon. Activated charcoal followed by symptomatic mea-

sures are indicated if more than 400 mg/kg has been ingested within the preceding hour, followed by symptomatic measures.

PARACETAMOL. As little as 10–15 g (20–30 tablets) or 150 mg/kg of paracetamol taken within 24 hours may cause severe hepatocellular necrosis and, less frequently, renal tubular necrosis. Nausea and vomiting, the only early features of poisoning, usually settle within 24 hours. Persistence beyond this time, often associated with the onset of right subcostal pain and tenderness, usually indicates development of hepatic necrosis. Liver damage is maximal 3–4 days after ingestion and may lead to encephalopathy, haemorrhage, hypoglycaemia, cerebral oedema, and death.

Therefore, despite a lack of significant early symptoms, patients who have taken an overdose of paracetamol should be transferred to hospital urgently.

Administration of activated charcoal should be considered if paracetamol in excess of 150 mg/kg or 12 g **whichever is the smaller**, is thought to have been ingested within the previous hour.

Antidotes such as **acetylcysteine** and **methionine** protect the liver if given within 10–12 hours of ingestion; acetylcysteine is effective up to and possibly beyond 24 hours.

Patients at risk of liver damage and therefore requiring treatment can be identified from a single measurement of the plasma-paracetamol concentration, related to the time from ingestion, provided this time interval is not less than 4 hours; earlier samples may be misleading. The concentration is plotted on a paracetamol treatment graph of a reference line ('normal treatment line') joining plots of 200 mg/litre (1.32 mmol/litre) at 4 hours and 6.25 mg/litre (0.04 mmol/litre) at 24 hours (see p. 23). Those whose plasma-paracetamol concentration is above the *normal treatment line* are treated with acetylcysteine by intravenous infusion (or, if acetylcysteine is not available, with methionine by mouth, provided the overdose has been taken **within 10–12 hours** *and* the patient is not vomiting). Patients on enzyme-inducing drugs (e.g. carbamazepine, phenobarbital, phenytoin, primidone, rifampicin, alcohol, and St John's wort) or who are malnourished (e.g. in anorexia, in alcoholism, or those who are HIV-positive) may develop toxicity at **lower** plasma-paracetamol concentrations and should be treated if concentrations are above the *high-risk treatment line* (which joins plots that are at 50% of the plasma-paracetamol concentrations of the normal treatment line).

The prognostic accuracy after 15 hours is uncertain but a plasma-paracetamol concentration above the relevant treatment line should be regarded as carrying a serious risk of liver damage.

Plasma-paracetamol concentration may be difficult to interpret when paracetamol has been ingested over several hours. If there is doubt about timing or the need for treatment then the patient should be treated with an antidote.

In remote areas methionine (2.5 g) should be given by mouth since it is seldom practicable to give acetylcysteine outside hospital. Once the patient reaches hospital the need to continue treatment with the antidote will be assessed from the plasma-paracetamol concentration (related to the time from ingestion).

See also Co-proxamol, under Analgesics (opioid).

Time (hours)

Patients whose plasma-paracetamol concentrations are above the **normal treatment line** should be treated with acetylcysteine by intravenous infusion (or with methionine by mouth, provided the overdose has been taken **within 10–12 hours** and the patient is not vomiting). Patients on enzyme-inducing drugs (e.g. carbamazepine, phenobarbital, phenytoin, primidone, rifampicin, alcohol, and St John's wort) or who are malnourished (e.g. in anorexia, in alcoholism, or those who are HIV-positive) should be treated if their plasma-paracetamol concentrations are above the **high-risk treatment line**. The prognostic accuracy after 15 hours is uncertain but a plasma-paracetamol concentration above the relevant treatment line should be regarded as carrying a serious risk of liver damage.

Graph reproduced courtesy of University of Wales College of Medicine Therapeutics and Toxicology Centre

ACETYLCYSTEINE

Indications: paracetamol overdosage, see notes above

Cautions: asthma

Side-effects: rashes, anaphylaxis

Dose: *by intravenous infusion*, in glucose intravenous infusion 5%, initially 150 mg/kg in 200 mL over 15 minutes, followed by 50 mg/kg in 500 mL over 4 hours, then 100 mg/kg in 1000 mL over 16 hours

NOTE. Manufacturer also recommends other infusion fluids, but glucose is preferable

Parvolex® (Celltech) **PoM**
Injection, acetylcysteine 200 mg/mL, net price 10-mL amp = £2.65

METHIONINE

Indications: paracetamol overdosage, see notes above

Cautions: hepatic impairment (Appendix 2)

Side-effects: nausea, vomiting, drowsiness, irritability

Dose: ADULT and CHILD over 6 years initially 2.5 g, followed by 3 further doses of 2.5 g every 4 hours, CHILD under 6 years initially 1 g, followed by 3 further doses of 1 g every 4 hours

Methionine (Non-proprietary)
Tablets, DL-methionine 250 mg, net price 200-tab pack = £66.05
Available from Celltech

Analgesics (opioid)

Opioids (narcotic analgesics) cause varying degrees of coma, respiratory depression, and pinpoint pupils. The specific antidote **naloxone** is indicated if there is coma or bradypnoea. Since naloxone has a shorter duration of action than many opioids, close monitoring and repeated injections are necessary according to the respiratory rate and depth of coma. Alternatively, it may be given by continuous intravenous infusion, the rate of administration being adjusted according to response and based on close monitoring of vital signs. The effects of some opioids, such as buprenorphine, are only partially reversed by naloxone. Dextropropoxyphene and methadone have very long durations of action; patients may need to be monitored for long periods following large overdoses.

CO-PROXAMOL. A combination of dextropropoxyphene and paracetamol (co-proxamol) is frequently taken in overdosage and is the most frequent prescription product to cause death. The initial features are those of acute opioid overdosage with coma, respiratory depression, and pinpoint pupils. Patients may die of acute cardiovascular collapse before reaching hospital (particularly if alcohol has also been consumed) unless adequately resuscitated.
  Naloxone reverses the opioid effects of dextropropoxyphene; the long duration of action of dextropropoxyphene calls for prolonged monitoring and further doses of naloxone may be required . Norpropoxyphene, a metabolite of dextropropoxyphene, also has cardiotoxic effects which may require treatment with **sodium bicarbonate**, or **magnesium sulphate**, or both; arrhythmias may occur for up to 12 hours. Paracetamol hepatotoxicity may develop later and should be anticipated and treated as indicated above.

NALOXONE HYDROCHLORIDE

Indications: overdosage with opioids; postoperative respiratory depression (section 15.1.7)
Cautions: physical dependence on opioids; cardiac irritability; naloxone is short-acting, see notes above
Dose: *by intravenous injection,* 0.8–2 mg repeated at intervals of 2–3 minutes to a max. of 10 mg if respiratory function does not improve (then question diagnosis); CHILD 10 micrograms/kg; subsequent dose of 100 micrograms/kg if no response
By subcutaneous or intramuscular injection, as intravenous injection but only if intravenous route not feasible (onset of action slower)
By continuous intravenous infusion using an infusion pump, 10 mg diluted in 50 mL intravenous infusion solution at a rate adjusted according to the response
IMPORTANT. Doses used in acute opioid overdosage may not be appropriate for the management of opioid-induced respiratory depression and sedation in those receiving palliative care and in chronic opioid use, see also section 15.1.7 for management of postoperative respiratory depression

Naloxone (Non-proprietary) PoM
Injection, naloxone hydrochloride 400 micrograms/ mL, net price 1-mL amp = £6.92; 1 mg/mL, 2-mL prefilled syringe = £6.30
Available from Antigen, Aurum, Mayne

Minijet® Naloxone (Celltech) PoM
Injection, naloxone hydrochloride 400 micrograms/ mL, net price 1-mL disposable syringe = £5.57; 2-mL disposable syringe = £10.71

Narcan® (Bristol-Myers Squibb) PoM
Injection, naloxone hydrochloride 400 micrograms/ mL, net price 1-mL amp = £4.54

Neonatal preparations —section 15.1.7

Antidepressants

Tricyclic and related antidepressants cause dry mouth, coma of varying degree, hypotension, hypothermia, hyperreflexia, extensor plantar responses, convulsions, respiratory failure, cardiac conduction defects, and arrhythmias. Dilated pupils and urinary retention also occur. Metabolic acidosis may complicate severe poisoning; delirium with confusion, agitation, and visual and auditory hallucinations, is common during recovery.
  Symptomatic treatment and activated charcoal by mouth may reasonably be given before transfer but hospital admission is strongly advised, and supportive measures to ensure a clear airway and adequate ventilation during transfer are mandatory. Intravenous diazepam (preferably in emulsion form) may be required for control of convulsions. Although arrhythmias are worrying, some will respond to correction of hypoxia and acidosis. The use of anti-arrhythmic drugs is best avoided but intravenous infusion of sodium bicarbonate can arrest arrythmias or prevent them in those with an extended QRS duration. Diazepam given by mouth is usually adequate to sedate delirious patients but large doses may be required.

Antimalarials

Overdosage with chloroquine and hydroxychloroquine is extremely hazardous and difficult to treat. Urgent advice from a poisons information centre is essential. Life-threatening features include arrhythmias (which can have a very rapid onset) and convulsions (which can be intractable). Quinine overdosage is also a severe hazard and calls for urgent advice from a poisons information centre.

Beta-blockers

Therapeutic overdosages with beta-blockers may cause lightheadedness, dizziness, and possibly syncope as a result of bradycardia and hypotension; heart failure may be precipitated or exacerbated. These complications are most likely in patients with conduction system disorders or impaired myocardial function. Bradycardia is the most common arrhythmia caused by beta-blockers, but sotalol may induce ventricular tachyarrhythmias (sometimes of the torsades de pointes type). The effects of massive overdosage may vary from one beta-blocker to another; propranolol overdosage in particular may cause coma and convulsions.
  Acute massive overdosage must be managed in hospital and expert advice should be obtained. Maintenance of a clear airway and adequate ventilation is mandatory. An intravenous injection of atropine is required to treat bradycardia and hypotension

(3 mg for an adult, 40 micrograms/kg for a child). Cardiogenic shock unresponsive to atropine is probably best treated with an intravenous injection of glucagon 2–10 mg (CHILD 50–150 micrograms/kg) [unlicensed indication and dose] in glucose 5% (with precautions to protect the airway in case of vomiting) followed by an intravenous infusion of 50 micrograms/kg/hour. If glucagon is not available, intravenous isoprenaline [special order only] is an alternative. A cardiac pacemaker may be used to increase the heart rate.

Calcium-channel blockers

Features of calcium-channel blocker poisoning include nausea, vomiting, dizziness, agitation, confusion, and coma in severe poisoning. Metabolic acidosis and hyperglycaemia may occur. Verapamil and diltiazem have a profound cardiac depressant effect causing hypotension and arrhythmias including complete heart block and asystole. The dihydropyridine calcium-channel blockers cause severe hypotension secondary to profound peripheral vasodilatation.

Activated charcoal is given if the patient presents within 1 hour of overdosage with a calcium-channel blocker; repeated doses of activated charcoal are considered if a modified-release preparation is involved. In patients with significant features of poisoning, calcium chloride or calcium gluconate (section 9.5.1.1) is given by injection; atropine is given to correct symptomatic bradycardia. For the management of hypotension, the choice of inotropic sympathomimetic depends on whether hypotension is secondary to vasodilation or to myocardial depression and advice should be sought from a poisons information centre.

> The **poisons information centres** (see p. 20) will provide advice on all aspects of poisoning day and night

Hypnotics and anxiolytics

BARBITURATES. These cause drowsiness, coma, respiratory depression, hypotension, and hypothermia. The duration and depth of cerebral depression vary greatly with the drug, the dose, and the tolerance of the patient. The severity of poisoning is often greater with a large dose of barbiturate hypnotics than with the longer-acting phenobarbital. The majority of patients survive with supportive measures alone. Repeated doses of activated charcoal (see Active Elimination Techniques, above) may be used for barbiturate poisoning. Charcoal haemoperfusion is the treatment of choice for the small minority of patients with very severe barbiturate poisoning who fail to improve, or who deteriorate despite good supportive care.

BENZODIAZEPINES. Benzodiazepines taken alone cause drowsiness, ataxia, dysarthria, and occasionally minor and short-lived depression of consciousness. They potentiate the effects of other central nervous system depressants taken concomitantly. Use of the benzodiazepine antagonist flumazenil can be hazardous, particularly in mixed overdoses involving tricyclic antidepressants or in benzodiazepine-dependent patients. Flumazenil should be used on **expert advice** only.

Iron salts

Iron poisoning is commonest in childhood and is usually accidental. The symptoms are nausea, vomiting, abdominal pain, diarrhoea, haematemesis, and rectal bleeding. Hypotension, coma, and hepatocellular necrosis occur later. Mortality is reduced with intensive and specific therapy with **desferrioxamine**, which chelates iron. The stomach should be emptied by gastric lavage (with a wide-bore tube) within 1 hour of ingesting a significant quantity of iron or if radiography reveals tablets in the stomach; whole bowel irrigation may be considered in severe poisoning but advice should be sought from a poisons information centre. The serum-iron concentration is measured as an emergency and intravenous desferrioxamine given to chelate absorbed iron in excess of the expected iron binding capacity. In **severe toxicity** intravenous desferrioxamine should be given *immediately* without waiting for the result of the serum-iron measurement (contact a poisons information centre for advice).

DESFERRIOXAMINE MESILATE
(Deferoxamine Mesilate)
Indications: iron poisoning; chronic iron overload (section 9.1.3)
Cautions: section 9.1.3
Side-effects: section 9.1.3
Dose: *by continuous intravenous infusion*, ADULT and CHILD up to 15 mg/kg/hour; max. 80 mg/kg in 24 hours (in severe cases, higher doses on advice from a poisons information centre)

■ Preparations
Section 9.1.3

Lithium

Most cases of lithium intoxication occur as a complication of long-term therapy and are caused by reduced excretion of the drug due to a variety of factors including dehydration, deterioration of renal function, infections, and co-administration of diuretics or NSAIDs (or other drugs that interact). Acute deliberate overdoses may also occur with delayed onset of symptoms (12 hours or more) due to slow entry of lithium into the tissues and continuing absorption from modified-release formulations.

The early clinical features are non-specific and may include apathy and restlessness which could be confused with mental changes due to the patient's depressive illness. Vomiting, diarrhoea, ataxia, weakness, dysarthria, muscle twitching, and tremor may follow. Severe poisoning is associated with convulsions, coma, renal failure, electrolyte imbalance, dehydration, and hypotension.

Therapeutic lithium concentrations are within the range of 0.4–1.0 mmol/litre; concentrations in excess of 2.0 mmol/litre are usually associated with serious toxicity and such cases may need treatment with haemodialysis (if there is renal failure). In acute overdosage much higher serum concentrations may be present without features of toxicity and all that is usually necessary is to take measures to increase urine production (e.g. by ensuring adequate fluid intake; but avoid diuretics). Otherwise treatment is supportive with special regard to electrolyte balance, renal function, and control of convulsions. Whole bowel irrigation should be considered for significant ingestion, but advice should be sought from a poisons information centre.

Phenothiazines and related drugs

Phenothiazines cause less depression of consciousness and respiration than other sedatives. Hypotension, hypothermia, sinus tachycardia, and arrhythmias (particularly with thioridazine) may complicate poisoning. Dystonic reactions can occur with therapeutic doses, (particularly with prochlorperazine and trifluoperazine) and convulsions may occur in severe cases. Arrhythmias may respond to correction of hypoxia, acidosis and other biochemical abnormalities but specialist advice should be sought if arrhythmias result from a prolonged QT interval; the use of some anti-arrhythmic drugs may worsen such arrhythmias. Dystonic reactions are rapidly abolished by injection of drugs such as benzatropine or diazepam (section 4.8.2, emulsion preferred).

Stimulants

AMPHETAMINES. These cause wakefulness, excessive activity, paranoia, hallucinations, and hypertension followed by exhaustion, convulsions, hyperthermia, and coma. The early stages can be controlled by diazepam or lorazepam; advice should be sought from a poisons information centre on the management of hypertension. Later, tepid sponging, anticonvulsants, and artificial respiration may be needed.

COCAINE. Cocaine stimulates the central nervous system, causing agitation, dilated pupils, tachycardia, hypertension, hallucinations, hyperthermia, hypertonia, and hyperreflexia; cardiac effects include chest pain, myocardial infarction, and arrhythmias.
Initial treatment of cocaine poisoning involves intravenous administration of diazepam to control agitation and cooling measures for hyperthermia (see Body temperature, p. 21); hypertension and cardiac effects require specific treatment and expert advice should be sought.

ECSTASY. Ecstasy (methylenedioxymethamfetamine, MDMA) may cause severe reactions, even at doses that were previously tolerated. The most serious effects are delirium, coma, convulsions, ventricular arrhythmias, hyperpyrexia, rhabdomyolysis, acute renal failure, acute hepatitis, disseminated intravascular coagulation, adult respiratory distress syndrome, hyperreflexia, hypotension and intracerebral haemorrhage; hyponatraemia has also been associated with ecstasy use.
Treatment is supportive, with diazepam to control severe agitation or persistent convulsions and close monitoring including ECG. Self-induced water intoxication should be considered in patients with ecstasy poisoning.

Theophylline

Theophylline and related drugs are often prescribed as modified-release formulations and toxicity may therefore be delayed. They cause vomiting (which may be severe and intractable), agitation, restlessness, dilated pupils, sinus tachycardia, and hyperglycaemia. More serious effects are haematemesis, convulsions, and supraventricular and ventricular arrhythmias. Profound **hypokalaemia** may develop rapidly.
The stomach should be emptied if the patient presents within 2 hours. Elimination of theophylline is enhanced by repeated doses of activated charcoal by mouth (see also under Active Elimination Techniques). Hypokalaemia is corrected by intravenous infusion of potassium chloride and may be so severe as to require 60 mmol/hour (high doses under ECG monitoring). Convulsions should be controlled by intravenous administration of diazepam (emulsion preferred). Sedation with diazepam may be necessary in agitated patients.
Provided the patient does **not** suffer from asthma, **propranolol** (section 2.4) may be administered intravenously to reverse extreme tachycardia, hypokalaemia, and hyperglycaemia.

Other poisons

Consult either a poisons information centre day and night or TOXBASE, see p. 20.

> The **poisons information centres** (see p. 20) will provide advice on all aspects of poisoning day and night

Cyanides

Cyanide antidotes include dicobalt edetate, given alone, and sodium nitrite followed by sodium thiosulphate. These antidotes are held for emergency use in hospitals as well as in centres where cyanide poisoning is a risk such as factories and laboratories. Hydroxocobalamin is an alternative antidote but its use should ideally be discussed with a poisons information centre; the usual dose is hydroxocobalamin 70 mg/kg by intravenous infusion (repeated once or twice according to severity). *Cyanokit®*, which provides hydroxocobalamin 2.5 g/bottle, is available but it is not licensed for use in the UK.

DICOBALT EDETATE

Indications: acute poisoning with cyanides
Cautions: owing to toxicity to be used only when patient tending to lose, or has lost, consciousness; not to be used as a precautionary measure
Side-effects: hypotension, tachycardia, and vomiting
Dose: *by intravenous injection*, ADULT 300 mg over 1 minute (5 minutes if condition less serious) followed immediately by 50 mL of glucose intravenous infusion 50%; if response inadequate a second dose of both may be given; if no response after further 5 minutes a third dose of both may be given; CHILD consult a poisons information centre

Dicobalt Edetate (Cambridge) PoM
Injection, dicobalt edetate 15 mg/mL, net price 20-mL (300-mg) amp = £9.80

SODIUM NITRITE

Indications: poisoning with cyanides (used in conjunction with sodium thiosulphate)
Side-effects: flushing and headache due to vasodilatation
Dose: see under preparation below

Sodium Nitrite Injection PoM
Injection, sodium nitrite 3% (30 mg/mL) in water for injections
Dose: 10 mL (CHILD 0.13–0.33 mL/kg) *by intravenous injection* over 5–20 minutes, followed by sodium thiosulphate injection 50% 25 mL (CHILD 0.8 mL/kg), *by intravenous injection* over 10 minutes
'Special-order' [unlicensed] product: contact Martindale, or regional hospital manufacturing unit

SODIUM THIOSULPHATE

Indications: poisoning with cyanides (used in conjunction with sodium nitrite)

Sodium Thiosulphate Injection PoM
Injection, sodium thiosulphate 50% (500 mg/mL) in water for injections
Dose: see above under Sodium Nitrite Injection
'Special-order' [unlicensed] product: contact Martindale, or regional hospital manufacturing unit

Ethylene glycol and methanol

Ethanol (by mouth or by intravenous infusion) is used for the treatment of ethylene glycol or methanol (methyl alcohol) poisoning. Fomepizole (*Antizol*, available on named-patient basis from poisons information centres or from IDIS) has also been used for the treatment of ethylene glycol or methanol poisoning. Advice on the treatment of ethylene glycol or methanol poisoning should be obtained from a poisons information centre.

Heavy metals

Heavy metal antidotes include dimercaprol, penicillamine, and sodium calcium edetate. Other antidotes for heavy metal poisoning include succimer (DMSA) and unithiol (DMPS) [both unlicensed]; their use may be valuable in certain cases and the advice of a poisons information centre should be sought.

DIMERCAPROL

(BAL)
Indications: poisoning by antimony, arsenic, bismuth, gold, mercury, possibly thallium; adjunct (with sodium calcium edetate) in lead poisoning
Cautions: hypertension, renal impairment (discontinue or use with extreme caution if impairment develops during treatment; elderly, pregnancy and breast-feeding; **interactions:** Appendix 1 (dimercaprol)
Contra-indications: not indicated for iron, cadmium, or selenium poisoning; severe hepatic impairment (unless due to arsenic poisoning)
Side-effects: hypertension, tachycardia, malaise, nausea, vomiting, salivation, lacrimation, sweat-

ing, burning sensation (mouth, throat, and eyes), feeling of constriction of throat and chest, headache, muscle spasm, abdominal pain, tingling of extremities; pyrexia in children; local pain and abscess at injection site
Dose: *by intramuscular injection*, ADULT and CHILD 2.5–3 mg/kg every 4 hours for 2 days, 2–4 times on the third day, then 1–2 times daily for 10 days or until recovery

Dimercaprol (Sovereign) PoM
Injection, dimercaprol 50 mg/mL. Net price 2-mL amp = £42.73
NOTE. Contains arachis (peanut) oil as solvent

PENICILLAMINE

Indications: lead poisoning
Cautions: see section 10.1.3
Contra-indications: see section 10.1.3
Side-effects: see section 10.1.3
Dose: 1–2 g daily in divided doses before food until urinary lead is stabilised at less than 500 micrograms/day; CHILD 20 mg/kg daily

■ Preparations
Section 10.1.3

SODIUM CALCIUM EDETATE

(Sodium Calciumedetate)
Indications: poisoning by heavy metals, especially lead
Cautions: renal impairment
Side-effects: nausea, diarrhoea, abdominal pain, pain at site of injection, thrombophlebitis if given too rapidly, renal damage particularly in overdosage; hypotension, lacrimation, myalgia, nasal congestion, sneezing, malaise, thirst, fever, chills, headache also reported
Dose: *by intravenous infusion*, ADULT and CHILD up to 40 mg/kg twice daily for up to 5 days, repeated if necessary after 48 hours

Ledclair® (Durbin) PoM
Injection, sodium calcium edetate 200 mg/mL, net price 5-mL amp = £7.29

Noxious gases

CARBON MONOXIDE. Carbon monoxide poisoning is usually due to inhalation of smoke, car exhaust, or fumes caused by blocked flues or incomplete combustion of fuel gases in confined spaces. Its toxic effects are entirely due to hypoxia.

Immediate treatment of carbon monoxide poisoning is essential. The person should be removed into the fresh air, the airway cleared, and **oxygen** 100% administered as soon as available. Artificial respiration should be given as necessary and continued until adequate spontaneous breathing starts, or stopped only after persistent and efficient treatment of cardiac arrest has failed. The patient should be admitted to hospital because complications may arise after a delay of hours or days. Cerebral oedema should be anticipated in severe poisoning and is treated with an intravenous infusion of mannitol (section 2.2.5). Referral for hyperbaric oxygen treatment should be discussed with the poisons information services if the victim is or has been unconscious, or has a blood carboxyhaemoglobin concentration of more than 20%, or is pregnant.

CS SPRAY. CS spray, which is used for riot control, irritates the eyes (hence 'tear gas') and the respiratory tract; symptoms normally settle spontaneously within 15 minutes. If symptoms persist, the patient should be removed to a well-ventilated area, and the exposed skin washed with soap and water after removal of contaminated clothing. Contact lenses should be removed and hard ones washed (soft ones should be discarded). Eye symptoms should be treated by irrigating the eyes with physiological saline (or water if saline not available) and advice sought from an ophthalmologist. Patients with features of severe poisoning, particularly respiratory complications, should be admitted to hospital for symptomatic treatment.

SULPHUR DIOXIDE, CHLORINE, PHOSGENE, AMMONIA. All of these gases can cause upper respiratory tract and conjunctival irritation. Pulmonary oedema, with severe breathlessness and cyanosis may develop suddenly up to 36 hours after exposure. Death may occur. Patients are kept under observation and those who develop pulmonary oedema are given oxygen. Assisted ventilation may be necessary in the most serious cases.

NERVE AGENTS. Treatment of nerve agent poisoning is similar to organophosphorus insecticide poisoning (see below), but advice should be sought from a poisons information centre. The risk of cross-contamination is significant; adequate decontamination and protective clothing for healthcare personnel are essential. In emergencies involving the release of nerve agents, kits ('NAAS pods') which contain **pralidoxime mesilate** may be obtained through the Ambulance Service from the National Blood Service (or the Welsh Blood Service in South Wales or designated hospital pharmacies in Northern Ireland and Scotland—see TOXBASE for list of designated centres). If the patient does not respond to atropine and pralidoxime it may be appropriate to use **obidoxime**, but advice should be sought from a poisons information centre. In the very rare circumstances where the nerve agent is tabun (GA), obidoxime will also be supplied as part of the pod.

Pesticides

PARAQUAT. Concentrated liquid paraquat preparations (e.g. *Gramoxone®*), available to farmers and horticulturists, contain 10–20% paraquat and are extremely toxic. Granular preparations, for garden use, contain only 2.5% paraquat and have caused few deaths.

Paraquat has local and systemic effects. Splashes in the eyes irritate and ulcerate the cornea and conjunctiva. Copious washing of the eye should aid healing but it may be a long process. Skin irritation, blistering, and ulceration can occur from prolonged contact both with the concentrated and dilute forms. Inhalation of spray, mist, or dust containing paraquat may cause nose bleeding and sore throat but not systemic toxicity.

Ingestion of concentrated paraquat solutions is followed by nausea, vomiting, and diarrhoea. Painful ulceration of the tongue, lips, and fauces may appear after 36 to 48 hours together with renal failure. Some days later there may be dyspnoea with pulmonary fibrosis due to proliferative alveolitis and bronchiolitis.

Treatment should be started immediately. The single most useful measure is oral administration of **activated charcoal**. Vomiting may preclude the use of activated charcoal and an anti-emetic may be required. Gastric lavage is of doubtful value. Intravenous fluids and analgesics are given as necessary. Oxygen therapy should be avoided in the early stages of management since this may exacerbate damage to the lungs, but oxygen may be required in the late stages to palliate symptoms. Measures to enhance elimination of absorbed paraquat are probably valueless but should be discussed with the poisons information centres who will also give guidance on predicting the likely outcome from plasma concentrations. Paraquat absorption can be confirmed by a simple qualitative urine test.

ORGANOPHOSPHORUS INSECTICIDES. Organophosphorus insecticides are usually supplied as powders or dissolved in organic solvents. All are absorbed through the bronchi and intact skin as well as through the gut and inhibit cholinesterase activity thereby prolonging and intensifying the effects of acetylcholine. Toxicity between different compounds varies considerably, and onset may be delayed after skin exposure.

Anxiety, restlessness, dizziness, headache, miosis, nausea, hypersalivation, vomiting, abdominal colic, diarrhoea, bradycardia, and sweating are common. Muscle weakness and fasciculation may develop and progress to generalised flaccid paralysis including the ocular and respiratory muscles. Convulsions, coma, pulmonary oedema with copious bronchial secretions, hypoxia, and arrhythmias occur in severe cases. Hyperglycaemia and glycosuria without ketonuria may also be present.

Further absorption should be prevented by moving the patient to fresh air, removing soiled clothing, and washing contaminated skin. In severe poisoning it is vital to ensure a clear airway, frequent removal of bronchial secretions, and adequate ventilation and oxygenation; gastric lavage may be considered provided that the airway is protected. **Atropine** will reverse the muscarinic effects of acetylcholine and is given in a dose of 2 mg (20 micrograms/kg in a child) as atropine sulphate (intramuscularly or intravenously according to the severity of poisoning) every 5 to 10 minutes until the skin becomes flushed and dry, the pupils dilate, and tachycardia develops.

Pralidoxime mesilate (P2S), a cholinesterase reactivator, is used, as an adjunct to atropine, in moderate or severe poisoning but it is effective only if given within 24 hours. It produces muscle improvement within 30 minutes but further doses may be required; an intravenous infusion may be required in severe cases. Pralidoxime mesilate may be obtained from designated centres, the names of which are held by the poisons information centres (see p. 20).

PRALIDOXIME MESILATE

(P2S)

Indications: adjunct to atropine in the treatment of poisoning by organophosphorus insecticide or nerve agent

Cautions: renal impairment, myasthenia gravis

Contra-indications: poisoning due to carbamates and to organophosphorus compounds without anticholinesterase activity

Side-effects: drowsiness, dizziness, disturbances of vision, nausea, tachycardia, headache, hyperventilation, and muscular weakness

Dose: *by slow intravenous injection* (diluted to 10–15 mL with water for injections) over 5–10 minutes, initially 30 mg/kg followed by 1–2 further doses if necessary *or by intravenous infusion*, 8 mg/kg/hour; usual max. 12 g in 24 hours

CHILD 20–60 mg/kg as required depending on severity of poisoning and response

NOTE. Pralidoxime mesilate doses in BNF may differ from those in product literature

Pralidoxime Mesilate [PoM]

Injection, pralidoxime mesilate 200 mg/mL
Available as 5-mL amps (from designated centres for organophosphorus insecticide poisoning or from the National Blood Service and the Welsh Blood Service for nerve agent poisoning—see TOXBASE for list of designated centres)

> The **poisons information centres** (see p. 20) will provide advice on all aspects of poisoning day and night

---

Snake bites and animal stings

SNAKE BITES. Envenoming from snake bite is uncommon in the UK. Many exotic snakes are kept, some illegally, but the only indigenous venomous snake is the adder (*Vipera berus*). The bite may cause local and systemic effects. Local effects include pain, swelling, bruising, and tender enlargement of regional lymph nodes. Systemic effects include early anaphylactoid symptoms (transient hypotension with syncope, angioedema, urticaria, abdominal colic, diarrhoea, and vomiting), with later persistent or recurrent hypotension, ECG abnormalities, spontaneous systemic bleeding, coagulopathy, adult respiratory distress syndrome, and acute renal failure. Fatal envenoming is rare but the potential for severe envenoming must not be underestimated.

Early anaphylactoid symptoms should be treated with **adrenaline (epinephrine)** (section 3.4.3). Indications for antivenom treatment include systemic envenoming, especially hypotension (see above), ECG abnormalities, vomiting, haemostatic abnormalities, and marked local envenoming such that after bites on the hand or foot, swelling extends beyond the wrist or ankle within 4 hours of the bite. For both **adults** and **children**, the contents of one vial (10 mL) of **European viper venom antiserum** (available from Farillon) is given *by intravenous injection* over 10–15 minutes or *by intravenous infusion* over 30 minutes after diluting in sodium chloride intravenous infusion 0.9% (use 5 mL diluent/kg body-weight). The **same dose** should be used for **adults** and **children**. The dose can be repeated in 1–2 hours if symptoms of **systemic envenoming** persist. Adrenaline (epinephrine) injection must be immediately to hand for treatment of anaphylactic reactions to the antivenom (for the management of anaphylaxis see section 3.4.3).

Antivenom is available for certain foreign snakes, spiders and scorpions. For information on identification, management, and supply, telephone:

Oxford	(01865) 220 968
or	(01865) 221 332
or	(01865) 741 166
Liverpool	(0151) 708 9393
Liverpool (Royal Liverpool University Hospital)	
(emergency supply only)	(0151) 706 2000
London (emergency supply only)	(020) 7771 5394

INSECT STINGS. Stings from ants, wasps, hornets, and bees cause local pain and swelling but seldom cause severe direct toxicity unless many stings are inflicted at the same time. If the sting is in the mouth or on the tongue local swelling may threaten the upper airway. The stings from these insects are usually treated by cleaning the area. Bee stings should be removed as quickly as possible. Anaphylactic reactions require immediate treatment with intramuscular **adrenaline (epinephrine)**; self-administered intramuscular adrenaline (e.g. *EpiPen*®) is the best first-aid treatment for patients with severe hypersensitivity. An inhaled bronchodilator should be used for asthmatic reactions. For the management of anaphylaxis, see section 3.4.3. A short course of an **oral antihistamine** or a **topical corticosteroid** may help to reduce inflammation and relieve itching.

MARINE STINGS. The severe pain of weeverfish (*Trachinus vipera*) stings can be relieved by immersing the stung area in uncomfortably hot, but not scalding, water (not more than 45° C). People stung by jellyfish and Portugese man-o'-war around the UK coast should be removed from the sea as soon as possible. Adherent tentacles should be lifted off carefully (wearing gloves or using tweezers) or washed off with seawater. Alcoholic solutions including suntan lotions should **not** be applied because they may cause further discharge of stinging hairs. Ice packs will reduce pain and a slurry of baking soda (sodium bicarbonate), but not vinegar, may be useful for treating stings from UK species.

1: Gastro-intestinal system

1.1 Dyspepsia and gastro-oesophageal reflux disease

Dyspepsia

Dyspepsia covers pain, fullness, early satiety, bloating, or nausea. It can occur with gastric and duodenal ulceration (section 1.3) and gastric cancer but most commonly it is of uncertain origin.

Helicobacter pylori infection may be present in patients with dyspepsia. *H. pylori* eradication therapy (section 1.3) should be considered for dyspepsia if it is ulcer-like. However, most individuals with functional (investigated, non-ulcer) dyspepsia do not benefit symptomatically from *H. pylori* eradication. Urgent investigation is required if the dyspepsia is accompanied by 'alarm symptoms' (e.g. bleeding, dysphagia, recurrent vomiting, and weight loss).

Gastro-oesophageal reflux disease

Gastro-oesophageal reflux disease (including non-erosive gastro-oesophageal reflux and erosive oesophagitis) is characterised by symptoms which include heartburn, acid regurgitation, and sometimes, difficulty in swallowing (dysphagia); oesophageal inflammation (oesophagitis), ulceration, and stricture formation may occur and there is an association with asthma.

The management of gastro-oesophageal reflux disease includes drug treatment, lifestyle changes and, in some cases, surgery. Initial treatment is guided by the severity of symptoms and treatment is then adjusted according to response. The extent of healing depends on the severity of the disease, the treatment chosen, and the duration of therapy.

For *mild symptoms* of gastro-oesophageal reflux disease, initial management may include the use of **antacids** and **alginates**. Alginate-containing antacids form a 'raft' that floats on the surface of the stomach contents to reduce reflux and protect the oesophageal mucosa. **Histamine H_2-receptor antagonists** (section 1.3.1) suppress acid secretion and they may relieve symptoms and permit reduction in antacid consumption. For refractory cases, a course of a **proton pump inhibitor** (section 1.3.5) may be considered (as described for severe symptoms, below).

For *severe symptoms* of gastro-oesophageal reflux disease or for patients with a proven or severe pathology (e.g. *oesophagitis, oesophageal ulceration, oesophagopharyngeal reflux, Barrett's oesophagus*), initial management involves the use of a **proton pump inhibitor** (section 1.3.5); patients need to be reassessed if symptoms persist despite 4–6 weeks of treatment with a proton pump inhibitor.

When symptoms abate, treatment is titrated down to a level which maintains remission (e.g. by reducing the dose of the proton pump inhibitor or by giving it intermittently, or by substituting treatment with a histamine H_2-receptor antagonist). However, for endoscopically confirmed *erosive, ulcerative,* or *stricturing* disease, treatment with a proton pump inhibitor usually needs to be maintained at the minimum effective dose.

A prokinetic drug such as **metoclopramide** (section 4.6) may improve gastro-oesophageal sphincter function and accelerate gastric emptying.

Patients with gastro-oesophageal reflux disease need to be advised about lifestyle changes (avoidance of excess alcohol and of aggravating foods such as fats); other measures include weight reduction, smoking cessation, and raising the head of the bed.

CHILDREN. Gastro-oesophageal reflux disease is common in infancy but most symptoms resolve between 12 and 18 months of age. Mild or moderate reflux without complications can be managed initially by changes in posture and thickening of liquid feeds (see Appendix 7 for suitable products) followed if necessary by treatment with an alginate-containing product (low sodium and low aluminium content for infants). For older children, life-style changes similar to those for adults (see above) may be helpful followed if necessary by treatment with an alginate-containing product.

Children who do not respond to these measures or who have problems such as respiratory disorders or suspected oesophagitis need to be referred to hospital; an H_2-receptor antagonist such as cimetidine (section 1.3.1) may be needed to reduce acid secretion. If the oesophagitis is resistant to H_2-receptor blockade, the proton pump inhibitor omeprazole (section 1.3.5) can be tried.

1.1.1   Antacids and simeticone

Antacids (usually containing aluminium or magnesium compounds) can often relieve symptoms in *ulcer dyspepsia* and in *non-erosive gastro-oesophageal reflux* (see also section 1.1); they are also sometimes used in functional (non-ulcer) dyspepsia but the evidence of benefit is uncertain. Antacids are best given when symptoms occur or are expected, usually between meals and at bedtime, 4 or more times daily; additional doses may be required up to once an hour. Conventional doses e.g. 10 mL 3 or 4 times daily of liquid magnesium–aluminium antacids promote ulcer healing, but less well than antisecretory drugs (section 1.3); proof of a relationship between healing and neutralising capacity is lacking. Liquid preparations are more effective than solids.

Aluminium- and **magnesium-containing** antacids (e.g. aluminium hydroxide, and magnesium carbonate, hydroxide and trisilicate), being relatively insoluble in water, are long-acting if retained in the stomach. They are suitable for most antacid purposes. Magnesium-containing antacids tend to be laxative whereas aluminium-containing antacids may be constipating; antacids containing both magnesium and aluminium may reduce these colonic side-effects. Aluminium accumulation does not appear to be a risk if renal function is normal (see also Appendix 3).

The acid-neutralising capacity of preparations that contain more than one antacid may be the same as simpler preparations. Complexes such as **hydrotalcite** confer no special advantage.

Sodium bicarbonate has been used in the relief of dyspepsia. Some individuals may still use sodium bicarbonate, but it has largely fallen from use as an antacid. However, it retains a place in the management of urinary-tract disorders (section 7.4.3) and acidosis (section 9.2.1.3 and section 9.2.2). Sodium bicarbonate should be avoided in patients on salt-restricted diets.

Bismuth-containing antacids (unless chelates) are not recommended because absorbed bismuth can be neurotoxic, causing encephalopathy; they tend to be constipating. **Calcium-containing** antacids can induce rebound acid secretion: with modest doses the clinical significance is doubtful, but prolonged high doses also cause hypercalcaemia and alkalosis, and can precipitate the milk-alkali syndrome.

Simeticone (activated dimeticone) is added to an antacid as an antifoaming agent to relieve flatulence. These preparations may be useful for the relief of hiccup in palliative care. **Alginates** added as protectants against gastro-oesophageal reflux disease (section 1.1) may be useful. The amount of additional ingredient or antacid in individual preparations varies widely, as does their sodium content, so that preparations may not be freely interchangeable

For **preparations** on sale to the public (not prescribable on the NHS), see p. 34.

See also section 1.3 for drugs used in the treatment of peptic ulceration.

INTERACTIONS. Antacids should preferably not be taken at the same time as other drugs since they may impair absorption. Antacids may also damage enteric coatings designed to prevent dissolution in the stomach. See also **Appendix 1** (antacids, calcium salts).

> **Low Na^+.** The words low Na^+ added after some preparations indicate a sodium content of less than 1 mmol per tablet or 10-mL dose.

Aluminium- and magnesium-containing antacids

ALUMINIUM HYDROXIDE

Indications: dyspepsia; hyperphosphataemia (section 9.5.2.2)

Cautions: see notes above; **interactions:** Appendix 1 (antacids)

Contra-indications: hypophosphataemia; porphyria (section 9.8.2)

Side-effects: see notes above

■ Aluminium-only preparations

Aluminium Hydroxide (Non-proprietary)
Tablets, dried aluminium hydroxide 500 mg. Net price 20 = 28p
Dose: 1–2 tablets chewed 4 times daily and at bedtime or as required

Oral suspension, about 4% w/w Al_2O_3 in water, with a peppermint flavour. Net price 200 mL = 41p
Dose: antacid, 5–10 mL 4 times daily between meals and at bedtime or as required; CHILD 6–12 years, up to 5 mL 3 times daily
NOTE. The brand name *Aludrox®* NHS (Pfizer Consumer) is used for aluminium hydroxide mixture; net price 200 mL = £1.42. *Aludrox®* NHS tablets also contain magnesium.

Alu-Cap® (3M)
Capsules, green/red, dried aluminium hydroxide 475 mg (low Na^+). Net price 120-cap pack = £4.03
Dose: antacid, 1 capsule 4 times daily and at bedtime; CHILD not recommended for antacid therapy

■ Co-magaldrox
Co-magaldrox is a mixture of aluminium hydroxide and magnesium hydroxide; the proportions are expressed in the form x/y where x and y are the strengths in milligrams per unit dose of magnesium hydroxide and aluminium hydroxide respectively

Maalox® (Rhône-Poulenc Rorer)
Suspension, sugar-free, co-magaldrox 195/220 (magnesium hydroxide 195 mg, dried aluminium hydroxide 220 mg/5 mL (low Na^+)). Net price 500 mL = £2.38
Dose: 10–20 mL 20–60 minutes after meals and at bedtime or when required; CHILD under 14 years not recommended

Mucogel® (Forest)
Suspension, sugar-free, co-magaldrox 195/220 (magnesium hydroxide 195 mg, dried aluminium hydroxide 220 mg/5 mL (low Na^+)). Net price 500 mL = £1.82
Dose: 10–20 mL 3 times daily, 20–60 minutes after meals, and at bedtime or when required; CHILD under 12 years not recommended

MAGNESIUM CARBONATE

Indications: dyspepsia
Cautions: renal impairment; see also notes above; **interactions:** Appendix 1 (antacids)
Contra-indications: hypophosphataemia
Side-effects: diarrhoea; belching due to liberated carbon dioxide

Aromatic Magnesium Carbonate Mixture, BP
(Aromatic Magnesium Carbonate Oral Suspension)
Oral suspension, light magnesium carbonate 3%, sodium bicarbonate 5%, in a suitable vehicle containing aromatic cardamom tincture. Contains about 6 mmol Na^+/10 mL. Net price 200 mL = 60p
Dose: 10 mL 3 times daily in water
For **preparations** also containing aluminium, see above and section 1.1.2.

MAGNESIUM TRISILICATE

Indications: dyspepsia
Cautions: see under Magnesium Carbonate
Contra-indications: see under Magnesium Carbonate
Side-effects: diarrhoea; silica-based renal stones reported on long-term treatment

Magnesium Trisilicate Tablets, Compound, BP
Tablets, magnesium trisilicate 250 mg, dried aluminium hydroxide 120 mg
Dose: 1–2 tablets chewed when required

Magnesium Trisilicate Mixture, BP
(Magnesium Trisilicate Oral Suspension)
Oral suspension, 5% each of magnesium trisilicate, light magnesium carbonate, and sodium bicarbonate in a suitable vehicle with a peppermint flavour. Contains about 6 mmol Na^+/10 mL
Dose: 10 mL 3 times daily in water
For **preparations** also containing aluminium, see above and section 1.1.2.

Aluminium-magnesium complexes

HYDROTALCITE
Aluminium magnesium carbonate hydroxide hydrate

Indications: dyspepsia
Cautions: see notes above; **interactions:** Appendix 1 (antacids)
Side-effects: see notes above

Hydrotalcite (Peckforton)
Suspension, hydrotalcite 500 mg/5 mL (low Na^+). Net price 500-mL pack = £1.96
Dose: 10 mL between meals and at bedtime; CHILD under 6 years not recommended, 6–12 years 5 mL
NOTE. The brand name *Altacite®* NHS is used for hydrotalcite suspension; for *Altacite Plus®* suspension, see below

Antacid preparations containing simeticone

Altacite Plus® (Peckforton)
Suspension, sugar-free, co-simalcite 125/500 (simeticone 125 mg, hydrotalcite 500 mg)/5 mL (low Na^+). Net price 500 mL = £1.96
Dose: 10 mL between meals and at bedtime when required; CHILD 8–12 years 5 mL
Tablets NHS, see p. 34

Asilone® (Thornton & Ross)
Suspension, sugar-free, dried aluminium hydroxide 420 mg, simeticone 135 mg, light magnesium oxide 70 mg/5 mL (low Na^+). Net price 500 mL = £1.95
Dose: 5–10 mL after meals and at bedtime or when required up to 4 times daily; CHILD under 12 years not recommended
Tablets NHS, see p. 34
Liquid NHS, see p. 34

Maalox Plus® (Rhône-Poulenc Rorer)
Suspension, sugar-free, dried aluminium hydroxide 220 mg, simeticone 25 mg, magnesium hydroxide 195 mg/5 mL (low Na^+). Net price 500 mL = £2.38
Dose: 5–10 mL 4 times daily (after meals and at bedtime or when required); CHILD under 5 years 5 mL 3 times daily, over 5 years appropriate proportion of adult dose
Tablets NHS, see p. 34

Simeticone alone

Simeticone (activated dimeticone) is an antifoaming agent. It is licensed for infantile colic but evidence of benefit is uncertain.

Dentinox® (DDD) ▰

Colic drops (= emulsion), simeticone 21 mg/2.5-mL dose. Net price 100 mL = £1.40

Dose: gripes, colic or wind pains, INFANT 2.5 mL with or after each feed (max. 6 doses in 24 hours); may be added to bottle feed

NOTE. The brand name *Dentinox®* is also used for other preparations including teething gel

Infacol® (Forest) ▰

Liquid, sugar-free, simeticone 40 mg/mL (low Na⁺). Net price 50 mL = £1.97. Counselling, use of dropper

Dose: gripes, colic or wind pains, INFANT 0.5–1 mL before feeds

Woodward's Colic Drops® (SSL) ▰

Oral drops, simeticone 20 mg/0.3-mL dose, net price 30 mL = £1.78

Dose: gripes, colic or wind pains, CHILD under 2 years 0.3–0.6 mL 4 times daily before feeds

---

1.1.2   Compound alginates and proprietary indigestion preparations

Alginate-containing antacids form a 'raft' that floats on the surface of the stomach contents to reduce reflux and protect the oesophageal mucosa; they are used in the management of mild symptoms of gastro-oesophageal reflux disease.

Indigestion preparations on sale to the public include antacids with other ingredients such as alginates, simeticone, and peppermint oil.

Compound alginate preparations

Algicon® (Rhône-Poulenc Rorer)

Tablets, aluminium hydroxide-magnesium carbonate co-gel 360 mg, magnesium alginate 500 mg, heavy magnesium carbonate 320 mg, potassium bicarbonate 100 mg, sucrose 1.5 g (low Na⁺). Net price 60-tab pack = £2.64

Cautions: diabetes mellitus (high sugar content)

Dose: 1–2 tablets chewed 4 times daily (after meals and at bedtime); CHILD under 12 years not recommended

Suspension, yellow, aluminium hydroxide-magnesium carbonate co-gel 140 mg, magnesium alginate 250 mg, magnesium carbonate 175 mg, potassium bicarbonate 50 mg/5 mL (low Na⁺). Net price 500 mL (lemon- or mint-flavoured) = £3.07

Dose: 10–20 mL 4 times daily (after meals and at bedtime); CHILD under 12 years not recommended

Gastrocote® (Thornton & Ross)

Tablets, alginic acid 200 mg, dried aluminium hydroxide 80 mg, magnesium trisilicate 40 mg, sodium bicarbonate 70 mg. Contains about 1 mmol Na⁺/tablet. Net price 100-tab pack = £3.51

Cautions: diabetes mellitus (high sugar content)

Dose: 1–2 tablets chewed 4 times daily (after meals and at bedtime); CHILD under 6 years not recommended

Liquid, sugar-free, peach-coloured, dried aluminium hydroxide 80 mg, magnesium trisilicate 40 mg, sodium alginate 220 mg, sodium bicarbonate 70 mg/5 mL. Contains 1.8 mmol Na⁺/5 mL. Net price 500 mL = £2.67

Dose: 5–15 mL 4 times daily (after meals and at bedtime)

Gaviscon® (R&C)

Tablets, sugar-free, alginic acid 500 mg, dried aluminium hydroxide 100 mg, magnesium trisilicate 25 mg, sodium bicarbonate 170 mg. Contains 2 mmol Na⁺/tablet. Net price 60-tab pack (peppermint- or lemon-flavoured) = £2.25

Dose: 1–2 tablets chewed after meals and at bedtime, followed by water; CHILD 2–6 years 1 tablet (on doctor's advice only) and 6–12 years 1 tablet

Liquid, sugar-free, sodium alginate 250 mg, sodium bicarbonate 133.5 mg, calcium carbonate 80 mg/ 5 mL. Contains about 3 mmol Na⁺/5 mL. Net price 500 mL (aniseed- or peppermint-flavour) = £2.70

Dose: 10–20 mL after meals and at bedtime; CHILD 2–6 years (on doctor's advice only) and 6–12 years 5–10 mL

Gaviscon 250® ▰, *Gaviscon 500® Tablets*, and *Gaviscon® Liquid Sachets*, see p. 34

Gaviscon® Advance (R&C)

Suspension, sugar-free, sodium alginate 500 mg, potassium bicarbonate 100 mg/5 mL. Contains 2.3 mmol Na⁺, 1 mmol K⁺/5 mL. Net price 500 mL (aniseed- or peppermint-flavour) = £5.40

Dose: ADULT and CHILD over 12 years, 5–10 mL after meals and at bedtime

Gaviscon® Infant (R&C)

Oral powder, sugar-free, sodium alginate 225 mg, magnesium alginate 87.5 mg, with colloidal silica and mannitol/dose (half dual-sachet). Contains 0.92 mmol Na⁺/dose. Net price 15 dual-sachets (30 doses) = £2.46

Dose: INFANT under 4.5 kg 1 dose (half dual-sachet) mixed with feeds (or water in breast-fed infants) when required; over 4.5 kg 2 doses (1 dual-sachet); CHILD 2 doses (1 dual-sachet) in water after each meal

NOTE. Not to be used in premature infants, or where excessive water loss likely (e.g. fever, diarrhoea, vomiting, high room temperature), or if intestinal obstruction. Not to be used with other preparations containing thickening agents

IMPORTANT. Each half of the dual-sachet is identified as 'one dose'. To avoid errors prescribe as 'dual-sachet' with directions in terms of 'dose'

Peptac® (IVAX)

Suspension, sugar-free, sodium bicarbonate 133.5 mg, sodium alginate 250 mg, calcium carbonate 80 mg/5 mL. Contains 3.1 mmol Na⁺/5mL. Net price 500 mL (aniseed-flavoured) = £2.16

Dose: 10–20 mL after meals and at bedtime; CHILD 6–12 years 5–10 mL

Rennie® Duo (Roche Consumer Health)

Suspension, sugar-free, calcium carbonate 600 mg, magnesium carbonate 70 mg, sodium alginate 150 mg/5 mL. Contains 2.6 mmol Na+/5 mL. Net price 500 mL (mint flavour) = £2.67

Dose: ADULT and CHILD over 12 years, 10 mL after meals and at bedtime; an additional 10 mL may be taken between doses for heartburn if necessary, max. 80 mL daily

Excipients: include propylene glycol

Rennie® ▰ and *Rennie Deflatine®*, see p. 34

Topal® (Ceuta)

Tablets, alginic acid 200 mg, dried aluminium hydroxide 30 mg, light magnesium carbonate 40 mg with lactose 220 mg, sucrose 880 mg, sodium bicarbonate 40 mg (low Na⁺). Net price 42-tab pack = £1.67

Cautions: diabetes mellitus (high sugar content)

Dose: 1–3 tablets chewed 4 times daily (after meals and at bedtime); CHILD half adult dose

Indigestion preparations

Indigestion **preparations** on sale to the public (may not be prescribable on the NHS) include:

Actal® (alexitol = aluminium), **Actonorm Gel**® (aluminium, magnesium, peppermint oil, simeticone), **Actonorm Powder**® (section 1.2), **Altacite**® (hydrotalcite = aluminium, magnesium), **Aludrox Liquid**® (aluminium), **Aludrox Tablets**® (aluminium, magnesium), **Andrews Antacid**® (calcium, magnesium), **APP**® (section 1.2), **Asilone Antacid Liquid**® (aluminium, magnesium, simeticone), **Asilone Antacid Tablets**® (aluminium, simeticone), **Asilone Heartburn Liquid**® (sodium alginate, aluminium, magnesium, sodium bicarbonate), **Asilone Heartburn Tablets**® (alginic acid, aluminium, magnesium, sodium bicarbonate), **Asilone Windcheaters**® **Capsules** (simeticone)

Barum Antacid® (calcium), **Birley**® (aluminium, magnesium), **Bismag**® (magnesium, sodium bicarbonate), **Bisma-Rex**® (bismuth, calcium, magnesium, peppermint oil), **Bisodol Heartburn Relief Tablets**® (alginic acid, magaldrate, sodium bicarbonate), **Bisodol Indigestion Relief Powder**® (magnesium, sodium bicarbonate), **Bisodol Indigestion Relief Tablets**® and **Bisodol Extra Strong Mint Tablets**® (calcium, magnesium, sodium bicarbonate), **Bisodol Wind Relief Tablets**® (calcium, magnesium, simeticone, sodium bicarbonate), **Boots Heartburn Relief**® (sodium alginate, calcium, sodium bicarbonate), **Boots Indigestion Tablets**® (calcium, magnesium, sodium bicarbonate), **Boots Gripe Mixture 1 Month Plus**® (sodium bicarbonate)

Carbellon® (magnesium, charcoal, peppermint oil)

De Witt's Antacid Powder® (calcium, magnesium, sodium bicarbonate, light kaolin, peppermint oil), **De Witt's Antacid Tablets**® (calcium, magnesium, peppermint oil), **Dijex**® (aluminium, magnesium), **Dynese**® (magaldrate = aluminium, magnesium)

Eno® (sodium bicarbonate, sodium carbonate), **Entrotabs**® (aluminium, attapulgite, pectin)

Gaviscon 250® **Tablets** (alginic acid, aluminium, magnesium, sodium bicarbonate; **Gaviscon**® and **Gaviscon 500**® **Tablets** are prescribable), **Gaviscon**® **Liquid Sachets** (sodium alginate, calcium, sodium bicarbonate), **Gelusil**® (aluminium, magnesium)

Maalox Plus Tablets® (aluminium, magnesium, simeticone), **Maclean**® (aluminium, calcium, magnesium), **Magnatol**® (alexitol, magnesium, potassium bicarbonate, xanthan gum), **Moorland**® (aluminium, bismuth, calcium, magnesium, light kaolin)

Nulacin® (calcium, magnesium, peppermint oil; *contains* gluten)

Opas® (calcium, magnesium, sodium bicarbonate), **Original Andrews Salts**® (citric acid, magnesium, sodium bicarbonate)

Pepto-Bismol® (bismuth), **Phillips' Milk of Magnesia**® (magnesium), **Premiums**® (aluminium, calcium, magnesium, peppermint oil)

Rap-eze® (calcium), **Remegel**®, **Remegel Alpine Mint with Lemon**® and **Remegel Freshmint**® (calcium), **Remegel Wind Relief**® (calcium, simeticone), **Rennie**® (calcium, magnesium), **Rennie Deflatine**® (calcium, magnesium, simeticone), **Roter**® (bismuth, frangula, magnesium, sodium bicarbonate)

Setlers Antacid® (calcium), **Setlers Heartburn and Indigestion Liquid**® (calcium, sodium alginate, sodium bicarbonate), **Simeco**® (aluminium, magnesium, simeticone), **Sovol**® (aluminium, magnesium, simeticone)

Tums® (calcium)

Wind-eze® (simeticone)

1.2 Antispasmodics and other drugs altering gut motility

Drugs in this section include antimuscarinic compounds and drugs believed to be direct relaxants of intestinal smooth muscle. The smooth muscle relaxant properties of antimuscarinic and other antispasmodic drugs may be useful in *irritable bowel syndrome* and in *diverticular disease*.

The dopamine-receptor antagonists metoclopramide and domperidone (section 4.6) stimulate transit in the gut.

Antimuscarinics

Antimuscarinics (formerly termed 'anticholinergics') reduce intestinal motility. They are used for the management of *irritable bowel syndrome* and *diverticular disease*. However, the evidence of their value in irritable bowel syndrome has not been established and response varies. Other indications of antimuscarinic drugs include arrhythmias (section 2.3.1), asthma and airways disease (section 3.1.2), motion sickness (section 4.6), parkinsonism (section 4.9.2), urinary incontinence (section 7.4.2), mydriasis and cycloplegia (section 11.5), premedication (section 15.1.3) and as an antidote to organophosphorus poisoning (p. 28).

Antimuscarinics that are used for gastro-intestinal smooth muscle spasm include the tertiary amines **atropine sulphate** and **dicycloverine hydrochloride** (dicyclomine hydrochloride) and the quaternary ammonium compounds **propantheline bromide** and **hyoscine butylbromide**. The quaternary ammonium compounds are less lipid soluble than atropine and so may be less likely to cross the blood-brain barrier; they are also less well absorbed.

Dicycloverine hydrochloride has a much less marked antimuscarinic action than atropine and may also have some direct action on smooth muscle. Hyoscine butylbromide is advocated as a gastro-intestinal antispasmodic, but it is poorly absorbed; the injection is useful in endoscopy and radiology. Atropine and the belladonna alkaloids are outmoded treatments, any clinical virtues being outweighed by atropinic side-effects.

CAUTIONS. Antimuscarinics should be used with caution (due to increased risk of side-effects) in Down's syndrome, in children and in the elderly; they should also be used with caution in gastro-oesophageal reflux disease, diarrhoea, ulcerative colitis, acute myocardial infarction, hypertension, conditions characterised by tachycardia (including hyperthyroidism, cardiac insufficiency, cardiac surgery), pyrexia, pregnancy and breast-feeding. **Interactions:** Appendix 1 (antimuscarinics).

CONTRA-INDICATIONS. Antimuscarinics are contra-indicated in angle-closure glaucoma, myasthenia gravis (but may be used to decrease muscarinic side-effects of anticholinesterases—section 10.2.1), paralytic ileus, pyloric stenosis and prostatic enlargement.

SIDE-EFFECTS. Side-effects of antimuscarinics include constipation, transient bradycardia (followed by tachycardia, palpitations and arrhythmias), reduced bronchial secretions, urinary urgency and retention, dilatation of the pupils with loss of accommodation, photophobia, dry mouth, flushing and dryness of the skin. Side-effects that occur occasionally include confusion (particularly in the elderly), nausea, vomiting and giddiness.

ATROPINE SULPHATE ▰

Indications: symptomatic relief of gastro-intestinal disorders characterised by smooth muscle spasm; mydriasis and cycloplegia (section 11.5); pre-medication (section 15.1.3); see also notes above
Cautions: see notes above
Contra-indications: see notes above
Side-effects: see notes above

Atropine (Non-proprietary) PoM
Tablets, atropine sulphate 600 micrograms. Net price 28-tab pack = £6.60
Available from CP
Dose: 0.6–1.2 mg at night

■ Preparations on sale to the public
Preparations on sale to the public (not prescribable on the NHS) containing atropine or related compounds include:
Actonorm Powder® (atropine, aluminium, calcium, magnesium, sodium bicarbonate, peppermint oil), **APP**® (homatropine, aluminium, bismuth, calcium, magnesium)

DICYCLOVERINE HYDROCHLORIDE
(Dicyclomine hydrochloride)
Indications: symptomatic relief of gastro-intestinal disorders characterised by smooth muscle spasm
Cautions: see notes above
Contra-indications: see notes above; infants under 6 months
Side-effects: see notes above
Dose: 10–20 mg 3 times daily; CHILD 6–24 months 5–10 mg up to 3–4 times daily, 15 minutes before feeds, 2–12 years 10 mg 3 times daily

[1]**Merbentyl**® (Florizel) PoM
Tablets, dicycloverine hydrochloride 10 mg, net price 20 = £1.08; 20 mg (*Merbentyl 20*®), 84-tab pack = £9.11
Syrup, dicycloverine hydrochloride 10 mg/5 mL, net price 120 mL = £1.98

1. Dicycloverine hydrochloride can be sold to the public provided that max. single dose is 10 mg and max. daily dose is 60 mg

■ Compound preparations
Kolanticon® (Peckforton)
Gel, sugar-free, dicycloverine hydrochloride 2.5 mg, dried aluminium hydroxide 200 mg, light magnesium oxide 100 mg, simeticone 20 mg/5 mL, net price 200 mL = £1.69, 500 mL = £1.85
Dose: 10–20 mL every 4 hours when required

HYOSCINE BUTYLBROMIDE
Indications: symptomatic relief of gastro-intestinal or genito-urinary disorders characterised by smooth muscle spasm
Cautions: see notes above
Contra-indications: see notes above; avoid in porphyria (section 9.8.2)
Side-effects: see notes above

Dose: *by mouth* (but poorly absorbed, see notes above), 20 mg 4 times daily; CHILD 6–12 years, 10 mg 3 times daily
Irritable bowel syndrome, 10 mg 3 times daily, increased if required up to 20 mg 4 times daily
By intramuscular or intravenous injection, acute spasm and spasm in diagnostic procedures, 20 mg repeated after 30 minutes if necessary (may be repeated more frequently in endoscopy); CHILD not recommended

Buscopan® (Boehringer Ingelheim) PoM
[1]*Tablets*, coated, hyoscine butylbromide 10 mg. Net price 56-tab pack = £2.59
Injection, hyoscine butylbromide 20 mg/mL. Net price 1-mL amp = 20p

1. Hyoscine butylbromide can be sold to the public provided single dose does not exceed 20 mg, daily dose does not exceed 80 mg, and pack does not contain a total of more than 240 mg.

PROPANTHELINE BROMIDE
Indications: symptomatic relief of gastro-intestinal disorders characterised by smooth muscle spasm; urinary frequency (section 7.4.2); gustatory sweating (section 6.1.5)
Cautions: see notes above
Contra-indications: see notes above
Side-effects: see notes above
Dose: 15 mg 3 times daily at least 1 hour before meals and 30 mg at night, max. 120 mg daily; CHILD not recommended

Pro-Banthine® (Hansam) PoM
Tablets, pink, s/c, propantheline bromide 15 mg, net price 112-tab pack = £15.32. Label: 23

Other antispasmodics

Alverine, **mebeverine**, and **peppermint oil** are believed to be direct relaxants of intestinal smooth muscle and may relieve pain in *irritable bowel syndrome* and *diverticular disease*. They have no serious adverse effects but, like all antispasmodics, should be avoided in paralytic ileus. Peppermint oil occasionally causes heartburn.

ALVERINE CITRATE
Indications: adjunct in gastro-intestinal disorders characterised by smooth muscle spasm; dys-menorrhoea
Cautions: pregnancy and breast-feeding
Contra-indications: paralytic ileus; when combined with sterculia, intestinal obstruction, faecal impaction, colonic atony
Side-effects: nausea, headache, pruritus, rash and dizziness reported
Dose: 60–120 mg 1–3 times daily; CHILD under 12 years not recommended

Spasmonal® (Norgine)
Capsules, alverine citrate 60 mg (blue/grey), net price 100-cap pack = £11.69; 120 mg (*Spasmonal® Forte*, blue/grey), 60-cap pack = £13.50
NOTE. A proprietary brand of alverine citrate 60 mg (*Relaxyl*®) is on sale to the public for irritable bowel syndrome

■ Compound preparations

Spasmonal Fibre® (Norgine)
Granules, beige, coated, sterculia 62%, alverine citrate 0.5%. Net price 500 g = £13.70. Label: 25, 27, counselling, see below
Dose: irritable bowel syndrome, 1–2 heaped 5-mL spoonfuls swallowed without chewing with water once or twice daily after meals; CHILD not recommended
COUNSELLING. Preparations that swell in contact with liquid should always be carefully swallowed with water and should not be taken immediately before going to bed

MEBEVERINE HYDROCHLORIDE

Indications: adjunct in gastro-intestinal disorders characterised by smooth muscle spasm
Cautions: pregnancy and breast-feeding; avoid in porphyria (section 9.8.2.)
Contra-indications: paralytic ileus
Side-effects: rarely allergic reactions (including rash, urticaria, angioedema)
Dose: ADULT and CHILD over 10 years 135–150 mg 3 times daily preferably 20 minutes before meals

[1]**Mebeverine Hydrochloride** (Non-proprietary)
PoM
Tablets, mebeverine hydrochloride 135 mg, net price 20 = £1.55
Available from Alpharma, APS, Arrow, Generics, Hillcross, IVAX

1. Mebeverine hydrochloride can be sold to the public for symptomatic relief of irritable bowel syndrome provided that max. single dose is 135 mg and max. daily dose is 405 mg; for uses other than symptomatic relief of irritable bowel syndrome provided that max. single dose is 100 mg and max. daily dose is 300 mg; proprietary brands on sale to the public include *Colofac 100®*, *Colofac IBS®* (135 mg), *Equilon®* (135 mg), *IBS Relief®*

Colofac® (Solvay) PoM
Tablets, s/c, mebeverine hydrochloride 135 mg. Net price 20 = £1.67
Liquid, yellow, sugar-free, mebeverine hydrochloride 50 mg (as embonate)/5 mL. Net price 300 mL = £3.50

■ Modified release

Colofac® MR (Solvay) PoM
Capsules, m/r, mebeverine hydrochloride 200 mg, net price 60-cap pack = £7.41. Label: 25
Dose: irritable bowel syndrome, 1 capsule twice daily preferably 20 minutes before meals; CHILD not recommended

■ Compound preparations

[1]**Fybogel® Mebeverine** (R&C) PoM
Granules, buff, effervescent, ispaghula husk 3.5 g, mebeverine hydrochloride 135 mg/sachet. Contains 7 mmol K+/sachet (caution in renal impairment). Net price 60 sachets = £15.00. Label: 13, 22, counselling, see below
Dose: irritable bowel syndrome, ADULT, 1 sachet in water, morning and evening 30 minutes before food; an additional sachet may also be taken before the midday meal if necessary; CHILD not recommended
COUNSELLING. Preparations that swell in contact with liquid should always be carefully swallowed with water and should not be taken immediately before going to bed

1. 10-sachet pack can be sold to the public

PEPPERMINT OIL

Indications: relief of abdominal colic and distension, particularly in irritable bowel syndrome
Cautions: rarely sensitivity to menthol

Side-effects: heartburn, perianal irritation; rarely, allergic reactions (including rash, headache, bradycardia, muscle tremor, ataxia)
LOCAL IRRITATION. Capsules should not be broken or chewed because peppermint oil may irritate mouth or oesophagus

Colpermin® (Pharmacia)
Capsules, m/r, e/c, light blue/dark blue, blue band, peppermint oil 0.2 mL. Net price 100-cap pack = £10.96. Label: 5, 22, 25
Excipients: include arachis (peanut) oil
Dose: 1–2 capsules, swallowed whole with water, 3 times daily for up to 2–3 months if necessary; CHILD under 15 years not recommended

Mintec® (Shire)
Capsules, e/c, green/ivory, peppermint oil 0.2 mL. Net price 84-cap pack = £7.04. Label: 5, 22, 25
Dose: 1–2 capsules swallowed whole with water, 3 times daily before meals for up to 2–3 months if necessary; CHILD not recommended

Motility stimulants

Metoclopramide and **domperidone** (section 4.6) are dopamine antagonists which stimulate gastric emptying and small intestinal transit, and enhance the strength of oesophageal sphincter contraction. They are used in some patients with *non-ulcer dyspepsia*. Metoclopramide is also used to speed the transit of barium during intestinal follow-through examination, and as accessory treatment for *gastro-oesophageal reflux disease*. Metoclopramide and domperidone are useful in non-specific and in cytotoxic-induced nausea and vomiting. Metoclopramide and occasionally domperidone may induce an acute dystonic reaction, particularly in young women and children—for further details of this and other side-effects, see section 4.6.

1.3   Ulcer-healing drugs

Peptic ulceration commonly involves the stomach, duodenum, and lower oesophagus; after gastric surgery it involves the gastro-enterostomy stoma.
Healing can be promoted by general measures, stopping smoking and taking antacids and by antisecretory drug treatment, but relapse is common when treatment ceases. Nearly all duodenal ulcers and most gastric ulcers not associated with NSAIDs are caused by *Helicobacter pylori*.
The management of *H. pylori* infection and of NSAID-associated ulcers is discussed below.

Helicobacter pylori infection
Long-term healing of gastric and duodenal ulcers can be achieved rapidly by eradicating *Helicobacter pylori*; it is recommended that the presence of *H. pylori* is confirmed before starting eradication treatment. Acid inhibition combined with antibacterial treatment is highly effective in the eradication of *H. pylori*; reinfection is rare. Antibiotic-induced colitis is an uncommon risk.

One-week triple-therapy regimens that comprise a proton pump inhibitor, amoxicillin, and either clarithromycin or metronidazole, eradicate *H. pylori* in over 90% of cases. There is normally no need to continue antisecretory treatment (with a proton pump inhibitor or H$_2$-receptor antagonist) unless the ulcer is complicated by haemorrhage or perforation. Resistance to clarithromycin or to metronidazole is much more common than to amoxicillin and can develop during treatment. A regimen containing amoxicillin and clarithromycin is therefore recommended for initial therapy and one containing amoxicillin and metronidazole for eradication failure. Ranitidine bismuth citrate may be substituted for a proton pump inhibitor. Other regimens, including those combining clarithromycin and metronidazole are best used in specialist settings. Treatment failure usually indicates antibacterial resistance or poor compliance.

Two-week triple-therapy regimens offer the possibility of higher eradication rates compared to one-week regimens, but adverse effects are common and poor compliance is likely to offset any possible gain.

Two-week dual-therapy regimens using a proton pump inhibitor and a single antibacterial are licensed, but produce low rates of *H. pylori* eradication and are **not** recommended.

A two-week regimen using tripotassium dicitrato-bismuthate *plus* a proton pump inhibitor *plus* two antibacterials may have a role in the treatment of resistant cases after confirmation of the presence of *H. pylori*.

Tinidazole or tetracycline are also used occasionally for *H. pylori* eradication; they should be used in combination with antisecretory drugs and other antibacterials.

There is insufficient evidence to support eradication therapy in patients infected with *H. pylori* who continue to take NSAIDs.

Test for *Helicobacter pylori*

^{13}C-Urea breath test kits are available for the diagnosis of gastro-duodenal infection with *Helicobacter pylori*. The test involves collection of breath samples before and after ingestion of an oral solution of ^{13}C-urea; the samples are sent for analysis by an appropriate laboratory. The test should not be performed within 4 weeks of treatment with an antibacterial or within 2 weeks of treatment with an antisecretory drug.

diabact UBT® (MDE) PoM
Tablets, ^{13}C-urea 50 mg, net price 1 kit (including 1 tablet, 4 breath-sample containers, straws) = £12.75 (analysis included), 10-kit pack (hosp. only) = £89.50 (analysis included)

Helicobacter Test Hp-Plus® (Espire) PoM
Soluble tablets, ^{13}C-urea 100 mg, net price 1 kit (including 4 breath-sample containers, straws, citric acid test meal) = £19.75 (analysis included)

Helicobacter Test INFAI® (Infai) PoM
Oral powder, ^{13}C-urea 75 mg for dissolving in water, net price 1 kit (including 4 breath-sample containers, straws) = £21.01 (analysis included)

Pylobactell® (Torbet) PoM
Soluble tablets, ^{13}C-urea 100 mg, net price 1 kit (including 6 breath-sample containers, 30-mL mixing and administration vial, straws) = £20.75 (analysis included)

NSAID-associated ulcers

Gastro-intestinal bleeding and ulceration can occur with NSAID use (section 10.1.1). Wherever possible, NSAIDs should be **withdrawn** if an ulcer occurs.

Recommended regimens for *Helicobacter pylori* eradication

Acid suppressant	Antibacterial			Price for 7–day course
	Amoxicillin	Clarithromycin	Metronidazole	
Esomeprazole	1 g twice daily	500 mg twice daily	—	£34.24
20 mg twice daily	—	500 mg twice daily	400 mg twice daily	£33.36
Lansoprazole	1 g twice daily	500 mg twice daily	—	£36.87
30 mg twice daily	1 g twice daily	—	400 mg twice daily	£13.88
	—	500 mg twice daily	400 mg twice daily	£35.99
Omeprazole	1 g twice daily	500 mg twice daily	—	£31.36
20 mg twice daily	500 mg 3 times daily	—	400 mg 3 times daily	£9.77
	—	500 mg twice daily	400 mg twice daily	£30.49
Pantoprazole	1 g twice daily	500 mg twice daily	—	£36.82
40 mg twice daily	—	500 mg twice daily	400 mg twice daily	£35.94
Rabeprazole	1 g twice daily	500 mg twice daily	—	£36.37
20 mg twice daily	—	500 mg twice daily	400 mg twice daily	£35.49
Ranitidine bismuth	1 g twice daily	500 mg twice daily	—	£37.99
citrate	1 g twice daily	—	400 mg twice daily	£15.00
400 mg twice daily	—	500 mg twice daily	400 mg twice daily	£37.11

Regimens that include amoxicillin with either clarithromycin or metronidazole are suitable for use in the community. Regimens that combine clarithromycin with metronidazole are best used in specialist settings (see also notes above)

In those at risk of ulceration a proton pump inhibitor or misoprostol may be considered for protection against NSAID-associated gastric and duodenal ulcers; colic and diarrhoea may limit the dose of misoprostol. An H$_2$-receptor antagonist may be effective for protection against NSAID-associated duodenal ulcers only.

NSAID use and *H. pylori* infection are independent risk factors for gastro-intestinal bleeding and ulceration. In patients already on an NSAID, eradication of *H. pylori* is not recommended because it is unlikely to reduce the risk of NSAID-induced bleeding or ulceration. However, in patients about to start long-term NSAID treatment who are *H. pylori* positive and have dyspepsia or a history of gastric or duodenal ulcer, eradication of *H. pylori* may reduce the overall risk of ulceration.

If the *NSAID can be discontinued* in a patient who has developed an ulcer, a proton pump inhibitor usually produces the most rapid healing, but the ulcer can be treated with an H$_2$-receptor antagonist or misoprostol.

If *NSAID treatment needs to continue*, the following options are suitable (see also NICE guidance, section 1.3.5 and section 10.1.1):

- Treat ulcer with a proton pump inhibitor and on healing continue the proton pump inhibitor (dose not normally reduced because asymptomatic ulcer deterioration may occur);
- Treat ulcer with a proton pump inhibitor and on healing switch to misoprostol for maintenance therapy (colic and diarrhoea may limit the dose of misoprostol);
- Treat ulcer with a proton pump inhibitor and switch NSAID to a cyclo-oxygenase-2 selective inhibitor.

1.3.1   H$_2$-receptor antagonists

All H$_2$-receptor antagonists heal *gastric and duodenal ulcers* by reducing gastric acid output as a result of histamine H$_2$-receptor blockade; they can also be expected to relieve *gastro-oesophageal reflux disease* (section 1.1). High doses of H$_2$-receptor antagonists have been used in the *Zollinger–Ellison syndrome*, but a proton pump inhibitor may now be preferred.

Maintenance treatment with low doses has largely been replaced in *Helicobacter pylori* positive patients by eradication regimens (section 1.3). Maintenance treatment may occasionally be used for those with frequent severe recurrences and for the elderly who suffer ulcer complications.

Treatment of *undiagnosed dyspepsia* with H$_2$-receptor antagonists may be acceptable in younger patients but care is required in older people because of the possibility of gastric cancer in these patients.

H$_2$-receptor antagonist therapy can promote healing of *NSAID-associated ulcers* (particularly duodenal) (section 1.3).

Treatment has not been shown to be beneficial in haematemesis and melaena, but prophylactic use reduces the frequency of bleeding from *gastroduodenal erosions in hepatic coma*, and possibly in other conditions requiring intensive care. Treatment also

reduces the risk of *acid aspiration* in obstetric patients at delivery (Mendelson's syndrome).

CAUTIONS. H$_2$-receptor antagonists should be used with caution in hepatic impairment (Appendix 2), in renal impairment (Appendix 3), pregnancy (Appendix 4), and in breast-feeding (Appendix 5). H$_2$-receptor antagonists might mask symptoms of gastric cancer; particular care is required in those whose symptoms change and in those who are middle-aged or over.

SIDE-EFFECTS. Side-effects of the H$_2$-receptor antagonists include diarrhoea and other gastro-intestinal disturbances, altered liver function tests (rarely liver damage), headache, dizziness, rash, and tiredness. Rare side-effects include acute pancreatitis, bradycardia, AV block, confusion, depression, and hallucinations particularly in the elderly or the very ill, hypersensitivity reactions (including fever, arthralgia, myalgia, anaphylaxis), blood disorders (including agranulocytosis, leucopenia, pancytopenia, thrombocytopenia), and skin reactions (including erythema multiforme and toxic epidermal necrolysis). There have been occasional reports of gynaecomastia and impotence.

INTERACTIONS. Cimetidine retards oxidative hepatic drug metabolism by binding to microsomal cytochrome P450. It should be avoided in patients stabilised on warfarin, phenytoin, and theophylline (or aminophylline), but other interactions (see **Appendix 1**) may be of less clinical relevance. Famotidine, nizatidine, and ranitidine do not share the drug metabolism inhibitory properties of cimetidine.

CIMETIDINE

Indications: benign gastric and duodenal ulceration, stomal ulcer, reflux oesophagitis, Zollinger–Ellison syndrome, other conditions where gastric acid reduction is beneficial (see notes above and section 1.9.4)

Cautions: see notes above; also preferably avoid intravenous injection (use intravenous infusion) particularly in high dosage and in cardiovascular impairment (risk of arrhythmias); **interactions:** Appendix 1 (histamine H$_2$-antagonists) and notes above

Side-effects: see notes above; also alopecia; very rarely tachycardia, interstitial nephritis

Dose: *by mouth*, 400 mg twice daily (with breakfast and at night) *or* 800 mg at night (benign gastric and duodenal ulceration) for at least 4 weeks (6 weeks in gastric ulceration, 8 weeks in NSAID-associated ulceration); when necessary the dose may be increased to 400 mg 4 times daily; INFANT under 1 year 20 mg/kg daily in divided doses has been used; CHILD over 1 year 25–30 mg/kg daily in divided doses

Maintenance, 400 mg at night *or* 400 mg morning and night

Reflux oesophagitis, 400 mg 4 times daily for 4–8 weeks

Zollinger–Ellison syndrome (but see notes above), 400 mg 4 times daily or occasionally more (max. 2.4 g daily)

Prophylaxis of stress ulceration, 200–400 mg every 4–6 hours

Gastric acid reduction (prophylaxis of acid aspiration; do not use syrup), obstetrics 400 mg at start of labour, then up to 400 mg every 4 hours if required (max. 2.4 g daily); surgical procedures 400 mg 90–120 minutes before induction of general anaesthesia

Short-bowel syndrome, 400 mg twice daily (with breakfast and at bedtime) adjusted according to response

To reduce degradation of pancreatic enzyme supplements, 0.8–1.6 g daily in 4 divided doses 1–1½ hours before meals

By intramuscular injection, 200 mg every 4–6 hours

By slow intravenous injection (but see Cautions above) over at least 5 minutes, 200 mg; may be repeated every 4–6 hours; if larger dose needed or if cardiovascular impairment, dilute and give injection over at least 10 minutes (infusion preferable); max. 2.4 g daily

By intravenous infusion, 200–400 mg (may be repeated every 4–6 hours) *or by continuous intravenous infusion* usually at a rate of 50–100 mg/hour over 24 hours, max. 2.4 g daily; INFANT under 1 year, *by slow intravenous injection or by intravenous infusion,* 20 mg/kg daily in divided doses has been used; CHILD over 1 year, 25–30 mg/kg daily in divided doses

[1]**Cimetidine** (Non-proprietary) PoM

Tablets, cimetidine 200 mg, net price 60-tab pack = £2.72; 400 mg, 60-tab pack = £5.58; 800 mg, 30-tab pack = £5.72

Available from Alpharma, APS, Ashbourne (*Peptimax*®), Berk (*Ultec*®), BHR (*Phimetin*®), CP, Dexcel Pharma, Eastern (*Zita*®), Hillcross, IVAX, Kent, Opus (*Acitak*®), Sovereign

Oral solution, cimetidine 200 mg/5 mL, net price 300 mL = £14.04

Available from Rosemont (sugar-free)

1. Cimetidine can be sold to the public for adults and children over 16 years (provided packs do not contain more than 2 weeks' supply) for the short-term symptomatic relief of heartburn, dyspepsia, and hyperacidity (max. single dose 200 mg, max. daily dose 800 mg), and for the prophylactic management of nocturnal heartburn (single night-time dose 100 mg); a proprietary brand (*Tagamet 100*® containing cimetidine 100 mg) is on sale to the public

Dyspamet® (Goldshield) PoM

Suspension, sugar-free, cimetidine 200 mg/5 mL. Contains sorbitol 2.79 g/5 mL. Net price 600 mL = £24.08

Tagamet® (GSK) PoM

Tablets, all green, f/c, cimetidine 200 mg, net price 120-tab pack = £19.58; 400 mg, 60-tab pack = £22.62; 800 mg, 30-tab pack = £22.62

Syrup, orange, cimetidine 200 mg/5 mL. Net price 600 mL = £28.49

Injection, cimetidine 100 mg/mL. Net price 2-mL amp = 36p

FAMOTIDINE

Indications: see under Dose

Cautions: see notes above; **interactions:** Appendix 1 (histamine H$_2$-antagonists) and notes above

Side-effects: see notes above; also very rarely anxiety, anorexia, dry mouth, cholestatic jaundice

Dose: benign gastric and duodenal ulceration, treatment, 40 mg at night for 4–8 weeks; maintenance (duodenal ulceration), 20 mg at night; CHILD not recommended

Reflux oesophagitis, 20–40 mg twice daily for 6–12 weeks; maintenance, 20 mg twice daily

Zollinger–Ellison syndrome (but see notes above), 20 mg every 6 hours (higher dose in those who have previously been receiving another H$_2$-antagonist); up to 800 mg daily in divided doses has been used

[1]**Famotidine** (Non-proprietary) PoM

Tablets, famotidine 20 mg, net price 28-tab pack = £12.40; 40 mg, 28-tab pack = £23.12

Available from APS, Arrow, Generics, Niche, Sandoz

1. Famotidine can be sold to the public for adults and children over 16 years (provided packs do not contain more than 2 weeks' supply) for the short-term symptomatic relief of heartburn, dyspepsia, and hyperacidity, and for the prevention of these symptoms when associated with consumption of food or drink including when they cause sleep disturbance (max. single dose 10 mg, max. daily dose 20 mg); proprietary brands (*Boots Excess Acid Control*®, *Pepcid*® *AC*, *Pepcid*®*AC Chewable* all containing famotidine 10 mg) are on sale to the public; a combination of famotidine and antacids (*Pepcidtwo*®) is also available for sale to the public

Pepcid® (MSD) PoM

Tablets, f/c, famotidine 20 mg (beige), net price 28-tab pack = £13.37; 40 mg (brown), 28-tab pack = £25.40

NIZATIDINE

Indications: see under Dose

Cautions: see notes above; also avoid rapid intravenous injection (risk of arrhythmias and postural hypotension); **interactions:** Appendix 1 (histamine H$_2$-antagonists) and notes above

Side-effects: see notes above; also sweating; rarely hyperuricaemia

Dose: *by mouth,* benign gastric, duodenal or NSAID-associated ulceration, treatment, 300 mg in the evening *or* 150 mg twice daily for 4–8 weeks; maintenance, 150 mg at night; CHILD not recommended

Gastro-oesophageal reflux disease, 150–300 mg twice daily for up to 12 weeks

By intravenous infusion, for short-term use in peptic ulcer hospital inpatients as alternative to oral route, *by intermittent intravenous infusion* over 15 minutes, 100 mg 3 times daily, *or by continuous intravenous infusion,* 10 mg/hour; max. 480 mg daily; CHILD not recommended

[1]**Nizatidine** (Non-proprietary) PoM

Capsules, nizatidine 150 mg, net price 30-cap pack = £6.81; 300 mg, 30-cap pack = £13.70

Available from APS, Generics, Niche

1. Nizatidine can be sold to the public for the prevention and treatment of symptoms of food-related heartburn and meal-induced indigestion in adults and children over 16 years; max. single dose 75 mg, max. daily dose 150 mg for max. 14 days

Axid® (Lilly) PoM

Capsules, nizatidine 150 mg (pale yellow/dark yellow), net price 28-cap pack (hosp. only) = £6.87, 30-cap pack = £8.27; 300 mg (pale yellow/brown), 30-cap pack = £16.40

Injection, nizatidine 25 mg/mL. For dilution and use as an intravenous infusion. Net price 4-mL amp = £1.14

RANITIDINE

Indications: see under Dose, other conditions where reduction of gastric acidity is beneficial (see notes above and section 1.9.4)

Cautions: see notes above; also avoid in porphyria (section 9.8.2); **interactions:** Appendix 1 (histamine H_2-antagonists) and notes above

Side-effects: see notes above; also rarely tachycardia, agitation, visual disturbances, alopecia; very rarely interstitial nephritis

Dose: *by mouth*, 150 mg twice daily *or* 300 mg at night (benign gastric and duodenal ulceration) for 4 to 8 weeks, up to 6 weeks in chronic episodic dyspepsia, and up to 8 weeks in NSAID-associated ulceration (in duodenal ulcer 300 mg can be given twice daily for 4 weeks to achieve a higher healing rate); maintenance, 150 mg at night; CHILD (peptic ulcer) 2–4 mg/kg twice daily, max. 300 mg daily

Duodenal ulceration associated with *H. pylori* (but see p. 37 for recommended regimens), ranitidine 300 mg daily in 1–2 divided doses (plus amoxicillin 750 mg 3 times daily and metronidazole 500 mg 3 times daily) for 2 weeks; ranitidine treatment continued for a further 2 weeks

Prophylaxis of NSAID-induced duodenal ulcer, 150 mg twice daily

Reflux oesophagitis, 150 mg twice daily *or* 300 mg at night for up to 8 weeks, or if necessary 12 weeks (moderate to severe, 600 mg daily in 2–4 divided doses for up to 12 weeks); long-term treatment of healed oesophagitis, 150 mg twice daily

Zollinger–Ellison syndrome (but see notes above), 150 mg 3 times daily; doses up to 6 g daily in divided doses have been used

Gastric acid reduction (prophylaxis of acid aspiration) in obstetrics, *by mouth*, 150 mg at onset of labour, then every 6 hours; surgical procedures, *by intramuscular or slow intravenous injection*, 50 mg 45–60 minutes before induction of anaesthesia (intravenous injection diluted to 20 mL and given over at least 2 minutes), or *by mouth*, 150 mg 2 hours before induction of anaesthesia, and also, when possible on the preceding evening

By intramuscular injection, 50 mg every 6–8 hours

By slow intravenous injection, 50 mg diluted to 20 mL and given over at least 2 minutes; may be repeated every 6–8 hours

By intravenous infusion, 25 mg/hour for 2 hours; may be repeated every 6–8 hours

Prophylaxis of stress ulceration, initial *slow intravenous injection* of 50 mg (as above) then *continuous infusion*, 125–250 micrograms/kg per hour (may be followed by 150 mg twice daily *by mouth* when oral feeding commences)

¹**Ranitidine** (Non-proprietary) PoM
Tablets, ranitidine (as hydrochloride) 150 mg, net price 60-tab pack = £8.16; 300 mg, 30-tab pack = £8.16
Available from Alpharma, APS, Ashbourne (*Zaedoc®*), Berk (*Rantec®*), CP, Generics, Genus, Goldshield, Hillcross, IVAX, PLIVA, Ranbaxy, Sovereign, Sterwin, Tillomed (*Ranitic®*)
Effervescent tablets, ranitidine (as hydrochloride) 150 mg, net price 60-tab pack = £26.05; 300 mg, 30-tab pack = £25.12. Label: 13
Excipients: may include sodium (check with supplier)
Available from Alpharma, Ratiopharm, Sandoz

Oral solution, ranitidine (as hydrochloride) 75 mg/5 mL, net price 300 mL = £22.32
Available from Rosemont (sugar-free, contains alcohol 8%)

1. Ranitidine can be sold to the public for adults and children over 16 years (provided packs do not contain more than 2 weeks' supply) for the short-term symptomatic relief of heartburn, dyspepsia, and hyperacidity, and for the prevention of these symptoms when associated with consumption of food or drink (max. single dose 75 mg, max. daily dose 300 mg); proprietary brands (*Gavilast-P®*, *Zantac® 75*, *Ranzac®* containing ranitidine (as hydrochloride) 75 mg) are on sale to the public

Zantac® (GSK) PoM
Tablets, f/c, ranitidine (as hydrochloride) 150 mg, net price 60-tab pack = £19.52; 300 mg, 30-tab pack = £19.20
Effervescent tablets, pale yellow, ranitidine (as hydrochloride) 150 mg (contains 14.3 mmol Na^+/tablet), net price 60-tab pack = £27.89; 300 mg (contains 20.8 mmol Na^+/tablet), 30-tab pack = £27.43. Label: 13
Excipients: include aspartame (section 9.4.1)
Syrup, sugar-free, ranitidine (as hydrochloride) 75 mg/5 mL. Net price 300 mL = £22.32
Excipients: include alcohol 8%
Injection, ranitidine (as hydrochloride) 25 mg/mL. Net price 2-mL amp = 64p

RANITIDINE BISMUTH CITRATE

(Ranitidine bismutrex)

Indications: see under Dose

Cautions: see notes above; see also under Tripotassium Dicitratobismuthate; **interactions:** Appendix 1 (histamine H_2-antagonists) and notes above

Contra-indications: moderate to severe renal impairment; pregnancy (Appendix 4); breast-feeding (Appendix 5); porphyria (section 9.8.2)

Side-effects: see notes above; may darken tongue or blacken faeces; rarely tachycardia, agitation, visual disturbances, erythema multiforme, alopecia

Dose: 400 mg twice daily, preferably with food, for 8 weeks in benign gastric ulceration or 4–8 weeks in duodenal ulceration; CHILD not recommended

Eradication of *Helicobacter pylori*, see eradication regimens on p. 37; ranitidine bismuth citrate treatment may be continued for a total of 4 weeks; long-term (maintenance) treatment not recommended (max. total of 16 weeks treatment in any 1 year); CHILD not recommended

COUNSELLING. May darken tongue and blacken faeces

Pylorid® (GSK) PoM
Tablets, blue, f/c, ranitidine bismuth citrate 400 mg. Net price 14-tab pack = £13.00; Counselling (discoloration of tongue and faeces)

1.3.2 Selective antimuscarinics

Pirenzepine is a selective antimuscarinic drug which was used for the treatment of gastric and duodenal ulcers. It has been discontinued.

1.3.3 Chelates and complexes

Tripotassium dicitratobismuthate is a bismuth chelate effective in healing gastric and duodenal ulcers, but not on its own in maintaining remission. For the role of tripotassium dicitratobismuthate in a *Helicobacter pylori* eradication regimen for those who have not responded to first-line regimens, see section 1.3.

The bismuth content of tripotassium dicitratobismuthate is low but absorption has been reported; encephalopathy (described with older high-dose bismuth preparations) has not been reported.

Ranitidine bismuth citrate (section 1.3.1) is used in the management of gastric and duodenal ulcers, and in combination with two antibacterials for the eradication of *H. pylori* (section 1.3).

Sucralfate may act by protecting the mucosa from acid-pepsin attack in gastric and duodenal ulcers. It is a complex of aluminium hydroxide and sulphated sucrose but has minimal antacid properties. It should be used with caution in patients under intensive care (**important:** reports of bezoar formation, see CSM advice below)

TRIPOTASSIUM DICITRATOBISMUTHATE

Indications: benign gastric and duodenal ulceration; see also *Helicobacter pylori* infection, section 1.3

Cautions: see notes above; **interactions:** Appendix 1 (tripotassium dicitratobismuthate)

Contra-indications: renal impairment, pregnancy

Side-effects: may darken tongue and blacken faeces; nausea and vomiting reported

De-Noltab® (Yamanouchi)
Tablets, f/c, tripotassium dicitratobismuthate 120 mg. Net price 112-tab pack = £7.11. Counselling, see below
Dose: 2 tablets twice daily *or* 1 tablet 4 times daily; taken for 28 days followed by further 28 days if necessary; maintenance not indicated but course may be repeated after interval of 1 month; CHILD not recommended
COUNSELLING. Each dose to be swallowed with half a glass of water; twice daily dosage to be taken 30 minutes before breakfast and main evening meal; four times daily dosage to be taken as follows: one dose 30 minutes before breakfast, midday meal and main evening meal, and one dose 2 hours after main evening meal; milk should not be drunk by itself during treatment but small quantities may be taken in tea or coffee or on cereal; antacids should not be taken half an hour before or after a dose; may darken tongue and blacken faeces

SUCRALFATE

Indications: see under Dose

Cautions: renal impairment (avoid if severe, see Appendix 3); pregnancy and breast-feeding; administration of sucralfate and enteral feeds should be separated by 1 hour; **interactions:** Appendix 1 (sucralfate)
BEZOAR FORMATION. Following reports of bezoar formation associated with sucralfate, the **CSM** has advised caution in seriously ill patients, especially those receiving concomitant enteral feeds or those with predisposing conditions such as delayed gastric emptying

Side-effects: constipation, diarrhoea, nausea, indigestion, gastric discomfort, dry mouth, rash,
hypersensitivity reactions, back pain, dizziness, headache, vertigo and drowsiness, bezoar formation (see above)

Dose: benign gastric and duodenal ulceration and chronic gastritis, 2 g twice daily (on rising and at bedtime) *or* 1 g 4 times daily 1 hour before meals and at bedtime, taken for 4–6 weeks or in resistant cases up to 12 weeks; max. 8 g daily
Prophylaxis of stress ulceration, 1 g 6 times daily (max. 8 g daily)
CHILD not recommended

Sucralfate (Non-proprietary) PoM
Tablets, sucralfate 1 g. Net price 112-tab pack = £9.80. Label: 5
Available from Hillcross

Antepsin® (Chugai) PoM
Tablets, scored, sucralfate 1 g, net price 100-tab pack = £8.75. Label: 5
COUNSELLING. Tablets may be dispersed in water
Suspension, sucralfate, 1 g/5 mL, net price 250 mL (aniseed- and caramel-flavoured) = £4.37. Label: 5

1.3.4 Prostaglandin analogues

Misoprostol, a synthetic prostaglandin analogue has antisecretory and protective properties, promoting healing of *gastric and duodenal ulcers*. It can prevent NSAID-associated ulcers, its use being most appropriate for the frail or very elderly from whom NSAIDs cannot be withdrawn.

For comment on the use of misoprostol to induce abortion or labour [unlicensed indications], see section 7.1.1.

MISOPROSTOL

Indications: see notes above and under Dose

Cautions: conditions where hypotension might precipitate severe complications (e.g. cerebrovascular disease, cardiovascular disease)

Contra-indications: pregnancy or planning pregnancy (increases uterine tone)—**important:** women of childbearing age, see also below, and breast-feeding
WOMEN OF CHILDBEARING AGE. Manufacturer advises that misoprostol should not be used in women of childbearing age unless the patient requires non-steroidal anti-inflammatory (NSAID) therapy and is at high risk of complications from NSAID-induced ulceration. In such patients it is advised that misoprostol should only be used if the patient takes *effective contraceptive measures* and has been advised of the *risks of taking misoprostol if pregnant*.

Side-effects: diarrhoea (may occasionally be severe and require withdrawal, reduced by giving single doses not exceeding 200 micrograms and by avoiding magnesium-containing antacids); also reported: abdominal pain, dyspepsia, flatulence, nausea and vomiting, abnormal vaginal bleeding (including intermenstrual bleeding, menorrhagia, and postmenopausal bleeding), rashes, dizziness

Dose: benign gastric and duodenal ulceration and NSAID-associated ulceration, 800 micrograms daily (in 2–4 divided doses) with breakfast (or main meals) and at bedtime; treatment should be continued for at least 4 weeks and may be continued for up to 8 weeks if required
Prophylaxis of NSAID-induced gastric and duo-

denal ulcer, 200 micrograms 2–4 times daily taken with the NSAID

CHILD not recommended

Cytotec® (Pharmacia) [PoM]
Tablets, scored, misoprostol 200 micrograms, net price 60-tab pack = £10.03, 140-tab pack = £23.40. Label: 21

▪ With diclofenac or naproxen
Section 10.1.1

1.3.5 Proton pump inhibitors

The proton pump inhibitors **omeprazole**, **esomeprazole**, **lansoprazole**, **pantoprazole** and **rabeprazole** inhibit gastric acid by blocking the hydrogen-potassium adenosine triphosphatase enzyme system (the 'proton pump') of the gastric parietal cell. Proton pump inhibitors are effective short-term treatments for *gastric and duodenal ulcers*; they are also used in combination with antibacterials for the eradication of *Helicobacter pylori* (see p. 37 for specific regimens). An initial short course of a proton pump inhibitor is the treatment of choice in *gastro-oesophageal reflux disease* with severe symptoms; patients with endoscopically confirmed *erosive, ulcerative*, or *stricturing oesophagitis* usually need to be maintained on a proton pump inhibitor (section 1.1).

Proton pump inhibitors are also used in the prevention and treatment of NSAID-associated ulcers (see p. 37 and guidance issued by NICE, below). In patients who need to continue NSAID treatment after an ulcer has healed, the dose of proton pump inhibitor should normally not be reduced because asymptomatic ulcer deterioration may occur.

Omeprazole is effective in the treatment of the *Zollinger-Ellison syndrome* (including cases resistant to other treatment); lansoprazole is also indicated for this condition.

CAUTIONS. Proton pump inhibitors should be used with caution in patients with liver disease (Appendix 2), in pregnancy (Appendix 4) and in breast-feeding. Proton pump inhibitors may mask symptoms of gastric cancer; particular care is required in those whose symptoms change and in those over 45 years of age; the presence of gastric malignancy should be excluded before treatment.

SIDE-EFFECTS. Side-effects of the proton pump inhibitors include dry mouth, gastro-intestinal disturbances (including diarrhoea, nausea and vomiting, constipation, flatulence, abdominal pain), liver dysfunction, taste disturbance, hypersensitivity reactions (including rash, urticaria, angioedema, bronchospasm, anaphylaxis), peripheral oedema, depression, dizziness, drowsiness, headache, insomnia, fever, haematological changes (including agranulocytosis, leucocytosis, leucopenia, pancytopenia, thrombocytopenia), interstitial nephritis, muscle and joint pain, blurred vision, photosensitivity, pruritus, severe skin reactions (including Stevens-Johnson syndrome, toxic epidermal necrolysis, bullous eruption), sweating, malaise. Proton pump inhibitors decrease gastric acidity and may increase the risk of gastro-intestinal infections.

> **NICE advice (proton pump inhibitors).** NICE has provided guidance (July 2000) on the use of proton pump inhibitors for the following indications:
>
> - Gastro-oesophageal reflux disease—use only for severe symptoms (reduce dose when symptoms abate) and in disease complicated by stricture, ulceration, or haemorrhage (full dose should be maintained);
> - NSAID-associated ulceration in patients who need to continue NSAID treatment—on healing of the ulcer a lower dose of proton pump inhibitor may be used [but see notes above].

ESOMEPRAZOLE

Indications: see under Dose
Cautions: see notes above; renal impairment (Appendix 3); **interactions:** Appendix 1 (proton pump inhibitors)
Side-effects: see notes above; also reported, dermatitis
Dose: duodenal ulcer associated with *Helicobacter pylori*, see eradication regimens on p. 37

Gastro-oesophageal reflux disease, 40 mg once daily for 4 weeks, followed by a further 4 weeks if not fully healed or symptoms persist; maintenance 20 mg daily; symptomatic treatment in the absence of oesophagitis, 20 mg daily for up to 4 weeks, followed by 20 mg daily when required

CHILD not recommended

COUNSELLING. Swallow whole *or* disperse in water

Nexium® (AstraZeneca) [PoM]
Tablets, f/c, esomeprazole (as magnesium trihydrate) 20 mg (light pink), net price 28-tab pack = £18.50 (also 7-tab pack, hosp. only); 40 mg (pink), 28-tab pack = £28.56 (also 7-tab pack, hosp. only). Counselling, administration

LANSOPRAZOLE

Indications: see under Dose
Cautions: see notes above; **interactions:** Appendix 1 (proton pump inhibitors)
Side-effects: see notes above; also reported, alopecia, paraesthesia, bruising, purpura, petechiae, fatigue, vertigo, hallucinations, confusion; rarely gynaecomastia, impotence
Dose: benign gastric ulcer, 30 mg daily in the morning for 8 weeks

Duodenal ulcer, 30 mg daily in the morning for 4 weeks; maintenance 15 mg daily

NSAID-associated duodenal or gastric ulcer, 15–30 mg once daily for 4 weeks, followed by a further 4 weeks if not fully healed; prophylaxis, 15–30 mg once daily

Duodenal ulcer associated with *Helicobacter pylori*, see eradication regimens on p. 37

Zollinger-Ellison syndrome (and other hypersecretory conditions), initially 60 mg once daily adjusted according to response; daily doses of 120 mg or more given in two divided doses

Gastro-oesophageal reflux disease, 30 mg daily in the morning for 4 weeks, followed by a further 4 weeks if not fully healed; maintenance 15–30 mg daily

Acid-related dyspepsia, 15–30 mg daily in the morning for 2–4 weeks

CHILD not recommended

Zoton® (Wyeth) PoM
Capsules, enclosing e/c granules, lansoprazole 15 mg (yellow), net price 28-cap pack = £12.98, 56-cap pack = £25.96; 30 mg (lilac/purple), 14-cap pack = £11.88, 28-cap pack = £23.75, 56-cap pack = £47.50 (also 7-cap pack, hosp. only). Label: 5, 25
FasTab® (= orodispersible tablet), lansoprazole 15 mg, net price 28-tab pack = £11.68; 30 mg, 7-tab pack = £5.35, 14-tab pack = £10.69, 28-tab pack = £21.38. Label: 5, counselling, administration
Excipients: include aspartame (section 9.4.1)
COUNSELLING. Tablets should be placed on the tongue, allowed to disperse and swallowed, or may be swallowed whole with a glass of water; tablets should not be crushed or chewed.
Suspension, pink, powder for reconstitution, lansoprazole 30 mg/sachet (strawberry flavour), net price 28-sachet pack = £34.14. Label: 5, 13

■ With antibacterials
For additional cautions, contra-indications and side-effects see Amoxicillin (section 5.1.1), Clarithromycin (section 5.1.5), and Metronidazole (section 5.1.11)

HeliClear® (Wyeth) PoM
Triple pack, lansoprazole capsules 30 mg (*Zoton*®), amoxicillin (as trihydrate) capsules 500 mg, clarithromycin tablets 500 mg (*Klaricid*®). Net price 7-day pack (14 × lansoprazole caps, 28 × amoxicillin caps, 14 × clarithromycin tabs) = £36.82. Label: 5, 9, 25
Dose: eradication of *Helicobacter pylori* in patients with duodenal ulcer, lansoprazole 30 mg twice daily, clarithromycin 500 mg twice daily, and amoxicillin 1 g twice daily for 7–14 days; CHILD not recommended

HeliMet® (Wyeth) PoM
Triple pack, lansoprazole capsules 30 mg (*Zoton*®), clarithromycin tablets 500 mg (*Klaricid*®), metronidazole tablets 400 mg, net price 7-day pack (14 × lansoprazole caps, 14 × clarithromycin tabs, 14 × metronidazole tabs) = £35.42. Label: 4, 5, 9, 25, 27
Dose: eradication of *Helicobacter pylori* in patients with duodenal ulcer, lansoprazole 30 mg twice daily, clarithromycin 500 mg twice daily, and metronidazole 400 mg twice daily for 7 days; CHILD not recommended

---

OMEPRAZOLE

Indications: see under Dose
Cautions: see notes above; **interactions:** Appendix 1 (proton pump inhibitors)
Side-effects: see notes above; also reported, paraesthesia, vertigo, alopecia, gynaecomastia, rarely impotence, stomatitis, encephalopathy in severe liver disease; hyponatraemia; reversible confusion, agitation, and hallucinations in the severely ill; visual impairment reported with high-dose injection
Dose: *by mouth*, benign gastric and duodenal ulcers, 20 mg once daily for 4 weeks in duodenal ulceration or 8 weeks in gastric ulceration; in severe or recurrent cases increase to 40 mg daily; maintenance for recurrent duodenal ulcer, 20 mg once daily; prevention of relapse in duodenal ulcer, 10 mg daily increasing to 20 mg once daily if symptoms return
NSAID-associated duodenal or gastric ulcer and gastroduodenal erosions, 20 mg once daily for 4 weeks, followed by a further 4 weeks if not fully healed; prophylaxis in patients with a history of

NSAID-associated duodenal or gastric ulcers, gastroduodenal lesions, or dyspeptic symptoms who require continued NSAID treatment, 20 mg once daily
Duodenal ulcer associated with *Helicobacter pylori*, see eradication regimens on p. 37
Benign gastric ulcer associated with *H. pylori*, omeprazole 40 mg daily in 1–2 divided doses (plus amoxicillin 0.75–1 g twice daily) for 2 weeks
Zollinger–Ellison syndrome, initially 60 mg once daily; usual range 20–120 mg daily (above 80 mg in 2 divided doses)
Gastric acid reduction during general anaesthesia (prophylaxis of acid aspiration), 40 mg on the preceding evening then 40 mg 2–6 hours before surgery
Gastro-oesophageal reflux disease, 20 mg once daily for 4 weeks, followed by a further 4–8 weeks if not fully healed; 40 mg once daily has been given for 8 weeks in gastro-oesophageal reflux disease refractory to other treatment; maintenance 20 mg once daily
Acid reflux disease (long-term management), 10 mg daily increasing to 20 mg once daily if symptoms return
Acid-related dyspepsia, 10–20 mg once daily for 2–4 weeks according to response
CHILD over 2 years, severe ulcerating reflux oesophagitis, 0.7–1.4 mg/kg daily for 4–12 weeks; max. 40 mg daily (to be initiated by hospital paediatrician)
By intravenous injection over 5 minutes or by intravenous infusion, gastric acid reduction during anaesthesia (prophylaxis of acid aspiration), 40 mg completed 1 hour before surgery
Benign gastric ulcer, duodenal ulcer and gastro-oesophageal reflux, 40 mg once daily until oral administration possible
CHILD not recommended
COUNSELLING. Swallow whole, *or* disperse *MUPS*® tablets in water, *or* mix capsule contents or *MUPS*® tablets with fruit juice or yoghurt

Omeprazole (Non-proprietary) PoM
Capsules, enclosing e/c granules, omeprazole 10 mg, net price 28-cap pack = £11.40; 20 mg, 28-cap pack = £12.75; 40 mg, 7-cap pack = £10.05. Label: 5, counselling, administration
Available from Alpharma, APS, Generics, Kent, PLIVA, Ratiopharm
Tablets, e/c, omeprazole 10 mg, net price 28-tab pack = £11.40; 20 mg, 28-tab pack = £12.75; 40 mg, 7-tab pack = £10.05. Label: 25
Available from Alpharma, Dexcel

Losec® (AstraZeneca) PoM
MUPS® (multiple-unit pellet system = dispersible tablets), f/c, omeprazole 10 mg (light pink), net price 28-tab pack = £19.34; 20 mg (pink), 28-tab pack = £29.22; 40 mg (red-brown), 7-tab pack = £14.61. Counselling, administration
Capsules, enclosing e/c granules, omeprazole 10 mg (pink), net price 28-cap pack = £19.34; 20 mg (pink/brown), 28-cap pack = £29.22; 40 mg (brown), 7-cap pack = £14.61. Counselling, administration
Intravenous infusion ▼, powder for reconstitution, omeprazole (as sodium salt), net price 40-mg vial = £5.21

Injection ▼, powder for reconstitution, omeprazole (as sodium salt), net price 40-mg vial (with solvent) = £5.21

PANTOPRAZOLE

Indications: see under Dose

Cautions: see notes above; also renal impairment (Appendix 3); **interactions:** Appendix 1 (proton pump inhibitors)

Side-effects: see notes above; also reported, raised triglycerides

Dose: *by mouth,* benign gastric ulcer, 40 mg daily in the morning for 4 weeks, continued for further 4 weeks if not fully healed

Gastro-oesophageal reflux disease, 20–40 mg daily in the morning for 4 weeks, continued for further 4 weeks if not fully healed; maintenance 20 mg daily, increased to 40 mg daily if symptoms return

Duodenal ulcer, 40 mg daily in the morning for 2 weeks, continued for further 2 weeks if not fully healed

Duodenal ulcer associated with *Helicobacter pylori,* see eradication regimens on p. 37

Prophylaxis of NSAID-associated gastric or duodenal ulcer in patients with an increased risk of gastroduodenal complications who require continued NSAID treatment, 20 mg daily

Zollinger–Ellison syndrome (and other hypersecretory conditions), initially 80 mg once daily adjusted according to response (ELDERLY max. 40 mg daily); daily doses above 80 mg given in 2 divided doses

CHILD not recommended

By intravenous injection over at least 2 minutes *or by intravenous infusion,* duodenal ulcer, gastric ulcer, and gastro-oesophageal reflux, 40 mg daily until oral administration can be resumed

Zollinger–Ellison syndrome (and other hypersecretory conditions), initially 80 mg (160 mg if rapid acid control required) then 80 mg once daily adjusted according to response; daily doses above 80 mg given in 2 divided doses

CHILD not recommended

Protium® (Altana) [PoM]
Tablets, yellow, e/c, pantoprazole (as sodium sesquihydrate) 20 mg, net price 28-tab pack = £12.88; 40 mg, 28-tab pack = £23.65. Label: 25
Injection, powder for reconstitution, pantoprazole (as sodium sesquihydrate), net price 40-mg vial = £5.71

RABEPRAZOLE SODIUM

Indications: see under Dose

Cautions: see notes above; **interactions:** Appendix 1 (proton pump inhibitors)

Side-effects: see notes above; also reported, cough, pharyngitis, rhinitis, asthenia, influenza-like syndrome; less commonly chest pain, sinusitis, nervousness; rarely stomatitis, encephalopathy in severe liver disease, anorexia, weight gain

Dose: benign gastric ulcer, 20 mg daily in the morning for 6 weeks, followed by a further 6 weeks if not fully healed

Duodenal ulcer, 20 mg daily in the morning for 4 weeks, followed by a further 4 weeks if not fully healed

Gastro-oesophageal reflux disease, 10–20 mg daily in the morning for 4–8 weeks; maintenance 10–20 mg daily

Duodenal and benign gastric ulcer associated with *Helicobacter pylori,* see eradication regimens on p. 37

CHILD not recommended

Pariet® (Janssen-Cilag, Eisai) [PoM]
Tablets, e/c, rabeprazole sodium 10 mg (pink), net price 28-tab pack = £12.43; 20 mg (yellow), 28-tab pack = £22.75. Label: 25

1.3.6 Other ulcer-healing drugs

Carbenoxolone is a synthetic derivative of glycyrrhizinic acid (a constituent of liquorice).

The only oral preparation of carbenoxolone remaining on the UK market is in the form of a combination with antacids for *oesophageal ulceration and inflammation.*

Side-effects of carbenoxolone (commonly sodium and water retention and occasionally hypokalaemia) may cause or exacerbate hypertension, oedema, cardiac failure, and muscle weakness. For these reasons other drugs are preferred; if used, regular monitoring of weight, blood pressure, and electrolytes is advisable during treatment. Carbenoxolone may act by protecting the mucosal barrier from acid–pepsin attack and increasing mucosal mucin production.

CARBENOXOLONE SODIUM ▱

Indications: oesophageal inflammation and ulceration

Cautions: cardiac disease, hypertension, hepatic and renal disease (see contra-indications); elderly (see under preparation); not recommended in children; see also notes above; **interactions:** Appendix 1 (carbenoxolone)

Contra-indications: hypokalaemia, cardiac failure and in those receiving cardiac glycosides (unless electrolyte levels monitored weekly and measures taken to avoid hypokalaemia); hepatic and renal impairment (see Appendixes 2 and 3); pregnancy

Side-effects: sodium and water retention (provoking hypertension and cardiac failure), hypokalaemia (leading to impaired neuromuscular function and muscle damage and to renal damage if prolonged)

Dose: see under preparations

■ Compound preparation

Pyrogastrone® (Sanofi-Synthelabo) [PoM] ▱
Tablets, chewable, carbenoxolone sodium 20 mg, alginic acid 600 mg, dried aluminium hydroxide 240 mg, magnesium trisilicate 60 mg, sodium bicarbonate 210 mg (Na^+ 3 mmol/tablet). Net price 100-tab pack = £24.85. Label: 21, 24
Dose: for oesophageal inflammation and ulceration, 1 tablet, chewed, 3 times daily after meals, and 2 at night, for 6–12 weeks; not recommended for children or for adults over 75 years

1.4   Acute diarrhoea

1.4.1   Adsorbents and bulk-forming drugs
1.4.2   Antimotility drugs

The priority in acute diarrhoea, as in gastro-enteritis, is the prevention or reversal of fluid and electrolyte depletion. This is particularly important in infants and in frail and elderly patients. For details of **oral rehydration preparations**, see section 9.2.1.2. Severe dehydration requires immediate admission to hospital and urgent replacement of fluid and electrolytes.

Antimotility drugs (section 1.4.2) relieve symptoms of acute diarrhoea. They are used in the management of uncomplicated acute diarrhoea in adults; fluid and electrolyte replacement may be necessary in case of dehydration. However, antimotility drugs are **not** recommended for acute diarrhoea in young children.

Antispasmodics (section 1.2) are occasionally of value in treating abdominal cramp associated with diarrhoea but they should **not** be used for primary treatment. Antispasmodics and antiemetics should be **avoided** in young children with gastro-enteritis since they are rarely effective and have troublesome side-effects.

Antibacterial drugs are generally unnecessary in simple gastro-enteritis because the complaint will usually resolve quickly without such treatment, and infective diarrhoeas in the UK often have a viral cause. Systemic bacterial infection does, however, need appropriate systemic treatment; for drugs used in campylobacter enteritis, shigellosis, and salmonellosis, see section 5.1, table 1. **Ciprofloxacin** is occasionally used for prophylaxis against travellers' diarrhoea, but routine use is **not** recommended. Lactobacillus preparations have not been shown to be effective.

Colestyramine (cholestyramine, section 1.9.2) and **aluminium hydroxide mixture** (section 1.1.1), bind unabsorbed bile salts and provide symptomatic relief of diarrhoea following ileal disease or resection.

1.4.1   Adsorbents and bulk-forming drugs

Adsorbents such as kaolin are **not** recommended for *acute diarrhoeas*. Bulk-forming drugs, such as ispaghula, methylcellulose, and sterculia (section 1.6.1) are useful in controlling faecal consistency in ileostomy and colostomy, and in controlling diarrhoea associated with diverticular disease.

KAOLIN, LIGHT

Indications: diarrhoea but see notes above
Cautions: interactions: Appendix 1 (kaolin)

Kaolin Mixture, BP
(Kaolin Oral Suspension)
Oral suspension, light kaolin or light kaolin (natural) 20%, light magnesium carbonate 5%, sodium bicarbonate 5% in a suitable vehicle with a peppermint flavour.
Dose: 10–20 mL every 4 hours
NOTE. Kaolin-containing preparations on sale to the public include *KLN*®

1.4.2   Antimotility drugs

Antimotility drugs have a role in the management of uncomplicated *acute diarrhoea* in adults but not in young children; see also section 1.4. However, in the case of dehydration, fluid and electrolyte replacement (section 9.2.1.2) are of primary importance.

For comments on their role in *chronic diarrhoeas* see section 1.5.

CODEINE PHOSPHATE

Indications: see notes above; cough suppression (section 3.9.1); pain (section 4.7.2)
Cautions: see section 4.7.2; also not recommended for children; tolerance and dependence may occur with prolonged use; **interactions:** Appendix 1 (opioid analgesics)
Contra-indications: see section 4.7.2; also conditions where inhibition of peristalsis should be avoided, where abdominal distension develops, or in acute diarrhoeal conditions such as acute ulcerative colitis or antibiotic-associated colitis
Side-effects: see section 4.7.2
Dose: see preparations

Codeine Phosphate (Non-proprietary) PoM
Tablets, codeine phosphate 15 mg, net price 28 = £1.03; 30 mg, 28 = £1.45; 60 mg, 28 = £2.60. Label: 2
Dose: acute diarrhoea, 30 mg 3–4 times daily (range 15–60 mg); CHILD not recommended
NOTE. Travellers needing to take codeine phosphate tablets abroad may require a doctor's letter explaining why they are necessary.

Kaodene® (Sovereign) NHS
Suspension, codeine phosphate 5 mg, light kaolin 1.5 g/5 mL. Net price 250 mL = £2.06
Dose: 20 mL 3–4 times daily; CHILD under 5 years not recommended, over 5 years 10 mL but see cautions and notes above

CO-PHENOTROPE

A mixture of diphenoxylate hydrochloride and atropine sulphate in the mass proportions 100 parts to 1 part respectively
Indications: adjunct to rehydration in acute diarrhoea (but see notes above); chronic mild ulcerative colitis
Cautions: see under Codeine Phosphate; also young children are particularly susceptible to **overdosage** and symptoms may be delayed and observation is needed for at least 48 hours after ingestion; presence of subclinical doses of atropine may give rise to atropine side-effects in susceptible individuals or in overdosage; **interactions:** Appendix 1 (opioid analgesics)
Contra-indications: see under Codeine Phosphate
Side-effects: see under Codeine Phosphate, section 4.7.2
Dose: see preparation

Lomotil® (Goldshield) PoM
Tablets, co-phenotrope 2.5/0.025 (diphenoxylate hydrochloride 2.5 mg, atropine sulphate 25 micrograms), net price 20 = £1.63
Dose: initially 4 tablets, followed by 2 tablets every 6 hours until diarrhoea controlled; CHILD under 4 years not recommended, 4–8 years 1 tablet 3 times daily, 9–12 years 1 tablet 4 times daily, 13–16 years 2 tablets 3 times daily, but see also notes above

LOPERAMIDE HYDROCHLORIDE

Indications: symptomatic treatment of acute diarrhoea; adjunct to rehydration in acute diarrhoea in adults and children over 4 years (but see notes above); chronic diarrhoea in adults only

Cautions: see notes above; also liver disease; pregnancy (Appendix 4); **interactions:** Appendix 1 (loperamide)

Contra-indications: conditions where inhibition of peristalsis should be avoided, where abdominal distension develops, or in conditions such as active ulcerative colitis or antibiotic-associated colitis

Side-effects: abdominal cramps, dizziness, drowsiness, and skin reactions, including urticaria reported; paralytic ileus and abdominal bloating also reported

Dose: acute diarrhoea, 4 mg initially followed by 2 mg after each loose stool for up to 5 days; usual dose 6–8 mg daily; max. 16 mg daily; CHILD under 4 years not recommended, 4–8 years 1 mg 3–4 times daily for up to *3 days only*, 9–12 years 2 mg 4 times daily for up to 5 days

Chronic diarrhoea in adults, initially, 4–8 mg daily in divided doses, subsequently adjusted according to response and given in 2 divided doses for maintenance; max. 16 mg daily

[1]**Loperamide** (Non-proprietary) [PoM]
Capsules, loperamide hydrochloride 2 mg. Net price 30-cap pack = £1.98
Available from Alpharma, APS, Berk (*Diocaps*®), Generics, Hillcross, IVAX, Tillomed (*Norimode*®)

[1]**Imodium**® (Janssen-Cilag) [PoM]
Capsules, green/grey, loperamide hydrochloride 2 mg. Net price 30 = £1.22
Syrup, red, sugar-free, loperamide hydrochloride 1 mg/5 mL. Net price 100 mL = £1.05

■ Compound preparations

Imodium® Plus (Janssen-Cilag)
Tablets (chewable), scored, loperamide hydrochloride 2 mg, simeticone 125 mg, net price 6-tab pack = £1.97, 18-tab pack = £4.54. Label: 24
Dose: acute diarrhoea with abdominal colic, initially 2 tablets (ADOLESCENT 12–18 years 1 tablet) then 1 tablet after each loose stool; max. 4 tablets daily for up to 2 days; CHILD not recommended

MORPHINE

Indications: see notes above

Cautions: see notes above and under Codeine Phosphate (section 4.7.2)

Contra-indications: see notes above and under Codeine Phosphate

Side-effects: see notes above and under Codeine Phosphate (section 4.7.2); sedation and the risk of dependence are greater

Dose: see preparation

Kaolin and Morphine Mixture, BP ▱
(Kaolin and Morphine Oral Suspension)
Oral suspension, light kaolin or light kaolin (natural) 20%, sodium bicarbonate 5%, and

chloroform and morphine tincture 4% in a suitable vehicle. Contains anhydrous morphine 550–800 micrograms/10 mL.
Dose: 10 mL every 4 hours in water

■ Preparations on sale to the public
Preparations on sale to the public containing morphine include:
Diocalm® (attapulgite, morphine)
Enterosan® (belladonna, morphine, kaolin)
Opazimes® (belladonna, morphine, aluminium, kaolin)

1.5 Chronic bowel disorders

Once tumours are ruled out individual symptoms of chronic bowel disorders need specific treatment including dietary manipulation as well as drug treatment and the maintenance of a liberal fluid intake.

Irritable bowel syndrome

Irritable bowel syndrome can present with pain, constipation, or diarrhoea. In some patients there may be important psychological aggravating factors which respond to reassurance. A laxative (section 1.6) may be needed to relieve constipation. Antimotility drugs such as loperamide (section 1.4.2) may relieve diarrhoea and antispasmodic drugs (section 1.2) may relieve pain. Opioids with a central action such as codeine are better avoided because of the risk of dependence.

Malabsorption syndromes

Individual conditions need specific management and also general nutritional consideration. Thus coeliac disease (gluten enteropathy) usually needs a gluten-free diet (Appendix 7) and pancreatic insufficiency needs pancreatin supplements (section 1.9.4).

Inflammatory bowel disease

The chronic inflammatory bowel diseases include *ulcerative colitis* and *Crohn's disease*. Effective management calls for drug therapy, attention to nutrition, and in severe or chronic active disease, surgery.

Aminosalicylates (balsalazide, mesalazine, olsalazine, and sulfasalazine), and **corticosteroids** (hydrocortisone, budesonide, and prednisolone) form the basis of drug treatment.

TREATMENT OF ACUTE ULCERATIVE COLITIS AND CROHN'S DISEASE. Acute mild to moderate disease affecting the rectum (proctitis) or the rectosigmoid (distal colitis) is treated initially with local application of a corticosteroid or an aminosalicylate; foam preparations and suppositories are especially useful where patients have difficulty retaining liquid enemas.

Diffuse inflammatory bowel disease or disease that does not respond to local therapy requires oral treatment; mild disease affecting the colon may be treated with an aminosalicylate alone but refractory or moderate disease usually requires adjunctive use of an oral corticosteroid such as **prednisolone** for 4–8 weeks. Modified-release **budesonide** is licensed for Crohn's disease affecting the ileum and the

---

1. Loperamide can be sold to the public, for adults and children over 12 years, provided it is licensed and labelled for the treatment of acute diarrhoea; proprietary brands including *Arret*® capsules [NHS], *Boots Diareze*® capsules, *Diasorb*® capsules, *Diocalm Ultra*® capsules [NHS] and *Imodium*® [NHS] (8- and 12-cap packs), *Imodium*® liquid and *Normaloe*® tablets are on sale to the public

ascending colon; it causes fewer systemic side-effects than oral prednisolone but may be less effective.

Severe inflammatory bowel disease calls for hospital admission and treatment with intravenous corticosteroid; other therapy may include intravenous fluid and electrolyte replacement, blood transfusion, and possibly parenteral nutrition and antibiotics. Specialist supervision is required for patients who fail to respond adequately to these measures. Patients with ulcerative colitis may benefit from a short course of ciclosporin (section 8.2.2) [unlicensed indication]. Patients with unresponsive or chronically active Crohn's disease may benefit from azathioprine, mercaptopurine (see below), or once-weekly methotrexate (section 8.1.3) [all unlicensed indications].

Infliximab (*Remicade*®, Schering-Plough) is licensed for the treatment of severe active Crohn's disease in patients whose condition has not responded adequately to treatment with a corticosteroid and a conventional immunosuppressant or who are intolerant of them. Infliximab is also licensed for the treatment of refractory fistulas of Crohn's disease.

> **NICE guidance (infliximab for Crohn's disease).** NICE has recommended (April 2002) that infliximab is used only for the treatment of severe active Crohn's disease (with or without fistulae) when treatment with immunomodulating drugs and corticosteroids has failed or is not tolerated and when surgery is inappropriate. Treatment may be repeated if the condition responded to the initial course but relapsed subsequently. Infliximab should be prescribed only by a gastroenterologist.

Metronidazole (section 5.1.11) may be beneficial for the treatment of active Crohn's disease with perianal involvement, possibly through its antibacterial activity. Metronidazole in doses of 0.6–1.5 g daily in divided doses has been used; it is usually given for a month but no longer than 3 months because of concerns about developing peripheral neuropathy. Other antibacterials should be given if specifically indicated (e.g. sepsis associated with fistulas and perianal disease) and for managing bacterial overgrowth in the small bowel.

MAINTENANCE OF REMISSION OF ACUTE ULCERATIVE COLITIS AND CROHN'S DISEASE. **Aminosalicylates** are of great value in the maintenance of remission of ulcerative colitis. They are of less value in the maintenance of remission of Crohn's disease; an oral formulation of mesalazine is licensed for the long-term management of ileal disease. Corticosteroids are **not** suitable for maintenance treatment because of side-effects. In resistant or frequently relapsing cases either **azathioprine** (section 8.2.1), 2–2.5 mg/kg daily [unlicensed indication] or **mercaptopurine** (section 8.1.3), 1–1.5 mg/kg daily [unlicensed indication], given under close supervision may be helpful.

ADJUNCTIVE TREATMENT OF INFLAMMATORY BOWEL DISEASE. Due attention should be paid to diet; high-fibre or low-residue diets should be used as appropriate. Irritable bowel syndrome during remission of ulcerative colitis calls for avoidance of a high-fibre diet and possible treatment with an antispasmodic (section 1.2).

Antimotility drugs such as codeine and loperamide, and antispasmodic drugs may precipitate paralytic ileus and megacolon in active ulcerative colitis; treatment of the inflammation is more logical. Laxatives may be required in proctitis. Diarrhoea resulting from the loss of bile-salt absorption (e.g. in terminal ileal disease or bowel resection) may improve with **colestyramine** (section 1.9.2), which binds bile salts.

Antibiotic-associated colitis

Antibiotic-associated colitis (pseudomembranous colitis) is caused by colonisation of the colon with *Clostridium difficile* which may follow antibiotic therapy. It is usually of acute onset, but may run a chronic course; it is a particular hazard of clindamycin but few antibiotics are free of this side-effect. Oral **vancomycin** (see section 5.1.7) or **metronidazole** (see section 5.1.11) are used as specific treatment; vancomycin may be preferred for very sick patients.

Diverticular disease

Diverticular disease is treated with a high-fibre diet, **bran supplements**, and **bulk-forming drugs**. **Antispasmodics** may provide symptomatic relief when colic is a problem (section 1.2). **Antibacterials** are used only when the diverticula in the intestinal wall become infected (specialist referral). **Antimotility** drugs which slow intestinal motility, e.g. codeine, diphenoxylate, and loperamide could possibly exacerbate the symptoms of diverticular disease and are **contra-indicated**.

Aminosalicylates

Sulfasalazine is a combination of 5-aminosalicylic acid ('5-ASA') and sulfapyridine; sulfapyridine acts only as a carrier to the colonic site of action but still causes side-effects. In the newer aminosalicylates, **mesalazine** (5-aminosalicylic acid), **balsalazide** (a prodrug of 5-aminosalicylic acid) and **olsalazine** (a dimer of 5-aminosalicylic acid which cleaves in the lower bowel), the sulphonamide-related side-effects of sulfasalazine are avoided, but 5-aminosalicylic acid alone can still cause side-effects including blood disorders (see recommendation below) and lupoid phenomenon also seen with sulfasalazine.

CAUTIONS. Aminosalicylates should be used with caution in renal impairment (Appendix 3), during pregnancy (Appendix 4) and breast-feeding (Appendix 5); blood disorders can occur (see recommendation below).

> **Blood disorders**
> It is recommended that patients receiving aminosalicylates should be advised to report any unexplained bleeding, bruising, purpura, sore throat, fever or malaise that occurs during treatment. A blood count should be performed and the drug stopped immediately if there is suspicion of a blood dyscrasia.

CONTRA-INDICATIONS. Aminosalicylates should be avoided in salicylate hypersensitivity.

SIDE-EFFECTS. Side-effects of the aminosalicylates include diarrhoea, nausea, vomiting, abdominal pain, exacerbation of symptoms of colitis, headache, hypersensitivity reactions (including rash, urticaria); side-effects that occur rarely include acute pancreatitis, hepatitis, myocarditis, pericarditis, lung complications (including eosinophilia, fibrosing alveolitis), peripheral neuropathy, blood disorders (including agranulocytosis, aplastic anaemia, leucopenia, methaemoglobinaemia, neutropenia, thrombocytopenia—see also recommendation above), renal dysfunction (interstitial nephritis, nephrotic syndrome), myalgia, arthralgia, skin reactions (including lupus erythematosus-like syndrome, Stevens-Johnson syndrome), alopecia.

BALSALAZIDE SODIUM

Indications: treatment of mild to moderate ulcerative colitis and maintenance of remission
Cautions: see notes above; also history of asthma; **interactions:** Appendix 1 (aminosalicylates)
BLOOD DISORDERS. See recommendation above
Contra-indications: see notes above; also severe hepatic impairment
Side-effects: see notes above; also cholelithiasis
Dose: acute attack, 2.25 g 3 times daily until remission occurs or for up to max. 12 weeks
Maintenance, 1.5 g twice daily, adjusted according to response (max. 6 g daily)
CHILD not recommended

Colazide® (Shire) [PoM]
Capsules, beige, balsalazide sodium 750 mg. Net price 130-cap pack = £39.00. Label: 21, 25, counselling, blood disorder symptoms (see recommendation above)

MESALAZINE

Indications: treatment of mild to moderate ulcerative colitis and maintenance of remission; see also under preparations
Cautions: see notes above; elderly; with oral preparations, test renal function initially and every 3 months for first year then every 6 months for next 4 years and annually thereafter (risk of serious renal toxicity); **interactions:** Appendix 1 (aminosalicylates)
BLOOD DISORDERS. See recommendation above
Contra-indications: see notes above; also severe hepatic impairment; blood clotting abnormalities
Side-effects: see notes above
Dose: see under preparations, below
NOTE. The delivery characteristics of enteric-coated mesalazine preparations may vary; these preparations should not be considered interchangeable

Asacol® (Procter & Gamble Pharm.) [PoM]
Foam enema, mesalazine 1 g/metered application, net price 14-application cannister with disposable applicators and plastic bags = £37.82. Counselling, blood disorder symptoms (see recommendation above)
Dose: acute attack affecting the rectosigmoid region, 1 metered application (mesalazine 1 g) into the rectum daily for 4–6 weeks; acute attack affecting the descending colon, 2 metered applications (mesalazine 2 g) once daily for 4–6 weeks; CHILD not recommended

Suppositories, mesalazine 250 mg, net price 20-suppos pack = £6.83; 500 mg, 10 = £6.83. Counselling, blood disorder symptoms (see recommendation above)
Dose: 3–6 suppositories of 250 mg (max. 3 suppositories of 500 mg) daily in divided doses, with last dose at bedtime; CHILD not recommended

Asacol® MR (Procter & Gamble Pharm.) [PoM]
Tablets, red, e/c, mesalazine 400 mg, net price 90-tab pack = £31.22, 120-tab pack = £41.62. Label: 5, 25, counselling, blood disorder symptoms (see recommendation above)
Dose: ulcerative colitis, acute attack, 6 tablets daily in divided doses; maintenance of remission of ulcerative colitis and Crohn's ileo-colitis, 3–6 tablets daily in divided doses; CHILD not recommended
NOTE. Preparations that lower stool pH (e.g. lactulose) may prevent release of mesalazine

Ipocol® (Sandoz) [PoM]
Tablets, e/c, mesalazine 400 mg, net price 120-tab pack = £41.62. Label: 5, 25, counselling, blood disorder symptoms (see recommendation above)
Dose: acute attack, 6 tablets daily in divided doses; maintenance of remission, 3–6 tablets daily in divided doses; CHILD not recommended
NOTE. Preparations that lower stool pH (e.g. lactulose) may prevent release of mesalazine

Mesren MR® (IVAX) [PoM]
Tablets, red-brown, e/c, mesalazine 400 mg, net price 90-tab pack = £31.22, 120-tab pack = £41.62. Label: 5, 25, counselling, blood disorder symptoms (see recommendation above)
Dose: acute attack, 6 tablets daily in divided doses; maintenance of remission, 3–6 tablets daily in divided doses; CHILD not recommended
NOTE. Preparations that lower stool pH (e.g. lactulose) may prevent release of mesalazine

Pentasa® (Ferring) [PoM]
Slow Release tablets, m/r, scored, mesalazine 500 mg (grey), net price 100-tab pack = £25.82. Counselling, administration, see dose, blood disorder symptoms (see recommendation above)
Dose: acute attack, up to 4 g daily in 2–3 divided doses; maintenance, 1.5 g daily in 2–3 divided doses; tablets may be dispersed in water, but should not be chewed; CHILD under 15 years not recommended
Prolonged Release granules, m/r, pale brown, mesalazine 1 g/sachet, net price 50-sachet pack = £31.60. Counselling, administration, see dose, blood disorder symptoms (see recommendation above)
Dose: acute attack, up to 4 g daily in 2–4 divided doses; maintenance, 2 g daily in 2 divided doses; granules should be placed on tongue and washed down with water or orange juice without chewing; CHILD under 12 years not recommended
Retention enema, mesalazine 1 g in 100-mL pack. Net price 7 enemas = £19.45. Counselling, blood disorder symptoms (see recommendation above)
Dose: 1 enema at bedtime; CHILD not recommended
Suppositories, mesalazine 1 g. Net price 28-suppos pack = £44.68. Counselling, blood disorder symptoms (see recommendation above)
Dose: ulcerative proctitis, acute attack, 1 suppository daily for 2–4 weeks; maintenance, 1 suppository daily; CHILD under 15 years not recommended

Salofalk® (Provalis) [PoM]
Tablets, e/c, yellow, mesalazine 250 mg. Net price 100-tab pack = £18.41. Label: 5, 25, counselling,

blood disorder symptoms (see recommendation above)

Dose: acute attack, 6 tablets daily in 3 divided doses; maintenance 3–6 tablets daily in divided doses; CHILD not recommended

Granules, m/r, grey, mesalazine 500 mg/sachet, net price 100-sachet pack = £31.00; 1 g/sachet, 50-sachet pack = £31.00. Counselling, administration, see dose, blood disorder symptoms (see recommendation above)
Excipients: include aspartame (section 9.4.1)

Dose: acute attack, 0.5–1 g 3 times daily; maintenance, 500 mg 3 times daily; CHILD over 6 years, body-weight under 40 kg half adult dose, body-weight over 40 kg, adult dose; granules should be placed on tongue and washed down with water without chewing
NOTE. Preparations that lower stool pH (e.g. lactulose) may prevent release of mesalazine

Suppositories, mesalazine 500 mg. Net price 30-suppos pack = £16.75. Counselling, blood disorder symptoms (see recommendation above)

Dose: acute attack, 1–2 suppositories 2–3 times daily adjusted according to response; CHILD not recommended

Enema, mesalazine 2 g in 59-mL pack. Net price 7 enemas = £32.95. Counselling, blood disorder symptoms (see recommendation above)

Dose: acute attack *or* maintenance, 1 enema daily at bedtime; CHILD not recommended

Rectal foam, mesalazine 1 g/metered application, net price 14-application cannister with disposable applicators and plastic bags = £32.95. Counselling, blood disorder symptoms (see recommendation above)

Dose: mild ulcerative colitis affecting sigmoid colon and rectum, 2 metered applications (mesalazine 2 g) into the rectum at bedtime increased if necessary to 2 metered applications (mesalazine 2 g) twice daily; CHILD not recommended

---

OLSALAZINE SODIUM

Indications: treatment of mild ulcerative colitis and maintenance of remission

Cautions: see notes above; **interactions:** Appendix 1 (aminosalicylates)
BLOOD DISORDERS. See recommendation above

Contra-indications: see notes above

Side-effects: see notes above; also watery diarrhoea

Dose: acute attack, 1 g daily in divided doses after meals increased if necessary over 1 week to max. 3 g daily (max. single dose 1 g)
Maintenance, 500 mg twice daily after meals; CHILD not recommended

Dipentum® (Celltech) [PoM]
Capsules, brown, olsalazine sodium 250 mg. Net price 112-cap pack = £27.42. Label: 21, counselling, blood disorder symptoms (see recommendation above)
Tablets, yellow, scored, olsalazine sodium 500 mg. Net price 60-tab pack = £29.38. Label: 21, counselling, blood disorder symptoms (see recommendation above)

SULFASALAZINE
(Sulphasalazine)

Indications: treatment of mild to moderate and severe ulcerative colitis and maintenance of remission; active Crohn's disease; rheumatoid arthritis (section 10.1.3)

Cautions: see notes above; also history of allergy; hepatic and renal impairment; G6PD deficiency (section 9.1.5); slow acetylator status; risk of haematological and hepatic toxicity (differential white cell, red cell and platelet counts initially and at monthly intervals for first 3 months, liver function tests at monthly intervals for first 3 months); kidney function tests at regular intervals; upper gastro-intestinal side-effects common over 4 g daily; porphyria (section 9.8.2); **interactions:** Appendix 1 (aminosalicylates)
BLOOD DISORDERS. See recommendation above

Contra-indications: see notes above; also sulphonamide hypersensitivity; CHILD under 2 years of age

Side-effects: see notes above; also loss of appetite; fever; blood disorders (including Heinz body anaemia, megaloblastic anaemia); hypersensitivity reactions (including exfoliative dermatitis, epidermal necrolysis, pruritus, photosensitisation, anaphylaxis, serum sickness); ocular complications (including periorbital oedema); stomatitis, parotitis; ataxia, aseptic meningitis, vertigo, tinnitus, insomnia, depression, hallucinations; kidney reactions (including proteinuria, crystalluria, haematuria); oligospermia; urine may be coloured orange; some soft contact lenses may be stained

Dose: *by mouth*, acute attack 1–2 g 4 times daily (but see **cautions**) until remission occurs (if necessary corticosteroids may also be given), reducing to a maintenance dose of 500 mg 4 times daily; CHILD over 2 years, acute attack 40–60 mg/kg daily, maintenance dose 20–30 mg/kg daily

By rectum, in suppositories, alone or in conjunction with oral treatment 0.5–1 g morning and night after a bowel movement. As an enema, 3 g at night, retained for at least 1 hour

Sulfasalazine (Non-proprietary) [PoM]
Tablets, sulfasalazine 500 mg. Net price 112 = £7.71. Label: 14, counselling, blood disorder symptoms (see recommendation above), contact lenses may be stained
Available from Generics, Hillcross
Tablets, e/c, sulfasalazine 500 mg. Net price 112-tab pack = £8.43. Label: 5, 14, 25, counselling, blood disorder symptoms (see recommendation above), contact lenses may be stained
Available from Alpharma (*Sulazine EC*®)

Salazopyrin® (Pharmacia) [PoM]
Tablets, yellow, scored, sulfasalazine 500 mg. Net price 112-tab pack = £6.97. Label: 14, counselling, blood disorder symptoms (see recommendation above), contact lenses may be stained
EN-Tabs® (= tablets e/c), yellow, f/c, sulfasalazine 500 mg. Net price 112-tab pack = £8.43. Label: 5, 14, 25, counselling, blood disorder symptoms (see recommendation above), contact lenses may be stained
Suspension, yellow, sulfasalazine 250 mg/5 mL. Net price 500 mL = £18.84. Label: 14, counselling, blood disorder symptoms (see recommendation above), contact lenses may be stained
Suppositories, yellow, sulfasalazine 500 mg. Net price 10 = £3.30. Label: 14, counselling, blood disorder symptoms (see recommendation above), contact lenses may be stained
Retention enema, sulfasalazine 3 g in 100-mL single-dose disposable packs fitted with a nozzle. Net price 7× 100 mL = £11.87. Label: 14,

counselling, blood disorder symptoms (see recommendation above), contact lenses may be stained

Corticosteroids

BUDESONIDE

Indications: see preparations
Cautions: see section 6.3.2
Contra-indications: see section 6.3.2
Side-effects: see section 6.3.2
Dose: see preparations

Budenofalk® (Provalis) PoM
Capsules, pink, enclosing e/c pellets, budesonide 3 mg, net price 100-cap pack = £81.20. Label: 5, 10, steroid card, 22, 25
Dose: mild to moderate Crohn's disease affecting the ileum or ascending colon, 3 mg 3 times daily for up to 8 weeks; reduce dose for the last 2 weeks of treatment. See also section 6.3.2
CHILD not recommended

Entocort® (AstraZeneca) PoM
CR Capsules, grey/pink, enclosing e/c, m/r granules, budesonide 3 mg, net price 100-cap pack = £99.00. Label: 5, 10, steroid card, 22, 25
NOTE. Dispense in original container (contains dessicant)
Dose: mild to moderate Crohn's disease affecting the ileum or ascending colon, 9 mg once daily in the morning before breakfast for up to 8 weeks; reduce dose for the last 2–4 weeks of treatment. See also section 6.3.2
CHILD not recommended
Enema, budesonide 2 mg/100 mL when dispersible tablet reconstituted in isotonic saline vehicle, net price pack of 7 dispersible tablets and bottles of vehicle = £33.00
Dose: ulcerative colitis involving rectal and rectosigmoid disease, 1 enema at bedtime for 4 weeks; CHILD not recommended

HYDROCORTISONE

Indications: ulcerative colitis, proctitis, proctosigmoiditis
Cautions: see section 6.3.2; systemic absorption may occur; prolonged use should be avoided
Contra-indications: use of enemas and rectal foams in obstruction, bowel perforation, and extensive fistulas; untreated infection
Side-effects: see section 6.3.2; local irritation
Dose: rectal, see preparations

Colifoam® (Meda) PoM
Foam in aerosol pack, hydrocortisone acetate 10%, net price 14-application cannister with applicator = £7.46
Dose: initially 1 metered application (125 mg hydrocortisone acetate) inserted into the rectum once or twice daily for 2–3 weeks, then once on alternate days

PREDNISOLONE

Indications: ulcerative colitis, and Crohn's disease; other indications, see section 6.3.2, see also preparations
Cautions: see under Hydrocortisone and section 6.3.2
Contra-indications: see under Hydrocortisone and section 6.3.2
Side-effects: see under Hydrocortisone and section 6.3.2

Dose: *by mouth*, initially 20–40 mg daily in single or divided doses, until remission occurs, followed by reducing doses
By rectum, see under preparations

■ Oral preparations
Section 6.3.2

■ Rectal preparations
Predenema® (Forest) PoM
Retention enema, prednisolone 20 mg (as sodium metasulphobenzoate) in 100-mL single-dose disposable pack. Net price 1 (standard tube) = 76p, 1 (long tube) = £1.29
Dose: ulcerative colitis, initially 1 enema at bedtime for 2–4 weeks, continued if good response; CHILD not recommended

Predfoam® (Forest) PoM
Foam in aerosol pack, prednisolone 20 mg (as metasulphobenzoate sodium)/metered application, net price 14-application cannister with disposable applicators = £6.74
Dose: proctitis and distal ulcerative colitis, 1 metered application (20 mg prednisolone) inserted into the rectum once or twice daily for 2 weeks, continued for further 2 weeks if good response; CHILD not recommended

Predsol® (Celltech) PoM
Retention enema, prednisolone 20 mg (as sodium phosphate) in 100-mL single-dose disposable packs fitted with a nozzle. Net price 7 = £6.39
Dose: rectal and rectosigmoidal ulcerative colitis and Crohn's disease, initially 1 enema at bedtime for 2–4 weeks, continued if good response; CHILD not recommended
Suppositories, prednisolone 5 mg (as sodium phosphate). Net price 10 = £1.23
Dose: ADULT and CHILD proctitis and rectal complications of Crohn's disease, 1 suppository inserted night and morning after a bowel movement

Cytokine inhibitors

Infliximab is a monoclonal antibody which inhibits the pro-inflammatory cytokine, tumour necrosis factor α. It should be used by specialists where adequate resuscitation facilities are available.

INFLIXIMAB

Indications: see under Inflammatory Bowel Disease above; ankylosing spondylitis, rhematoid arthritis (section 10.1.3)
Cautions: see section 10.1.3
HYPERSENSITIVITY REACTIONS. Risk of delayed hypersensitivity if drug-free interval exceeds 16 weeks
Contra-indications: see section 10.1.3
Side-effects: see section 10.1.3
Dose: *by intravenous infusion*, severe active Crohn's disease, ADULT and ADOLESCENT over 17 years, initially 5 mg/kg, then if the condition responds within 2 weeks of initial dose, either 5 mg/kg 2 weeks and 6 weeks after initial dose, then 5 mg/kg every 8 weeks *or* after initial dose, further dose of 5 mg/kg if signs and symptoms recur
Fistulating Crohn's disease, ADULT and ADOLESCENT over 17 years, initially 5 mg/kg, then 5 mg/kg 2 weeks and 6 weeks after initial dose, then if condition has responded, consult literature for guidance on further doses

■ Preparations
Section 10.1.3

Food allergy

Allergy with classical symptoms of vomiting, colic and diarrhoea caused by specific foods such as shellfish should be managed by strict avoidance. The condition should be distinguished from symptoms of occasional food intolerance in those with irritable bowel syndrome. **Sodium cromoglicate** (sodium cromoglycate) may be helpful as an adjunct to dietary avoidance.

SODIUM CROMOGLICATE
(Sodium cromoglycate)

Indications: food allergy (in conjunction with dietary restriction); asthma (section 3.3); allergic conjunctivitis (section 11.4.2); allergic rhinitis (section 12.2.1)

Side-effects: occasional nausea, rashes, and joint pain

Dose: 200 mg 4 times daily before meals; CHILD 2–14 years 100 mg; capsules may be swallowed whole or the contents dissolved in hot water and diluted with cold water before taking. May be increased if necessary after 2–3 weeks to a max. of 40 mg/kg daily and then reduced according to the response

Nalcrom® (Pantheon) [PoM]
Capsules, sodium cromoglicate 100 mg. Net price 100-cap pack = £66.85. Label: 22, counselling, see dose above

1.6   Laxatives

1.6.1   Bulk-forming laxatives
1.6.2   Stimulant laxatives
1.6.3   Faecal softeners
1.6.4   Osmotic laxatives
1.6.5   Bowel cleansing solutions

Before prescribing laxatives it is important to be sure that the patient *is* constipated and that the constipation is *not* secondary to an underlying undiagnosed complaint.

It is also important for those who complain of constipation to understand that bowel habit can vary considerably in frequency without doing harm. Some people tend to consider themselves constipated if they do not have a bowel movement each day. A useful definition of constipation is the passage of hard stools less frequently than the patient's own normal pattern and this can be explained to the patient.

Misconceptions about bowel habits have led to excessive laxative use. Abuse may lead to hypokalaemia and an atonic non-functioning colon.

Thus, laxatives should generally be **avoided** except where straining will exacerbate a condition (such as angina) or increase the risk of rectal bleeding as in haemorrhoids. Laxatives are also of value in *drug-induced constipation*, for the expulsion of *parasites* after anthelmintic treatment, and to clear the alimentary tract before *surgery and radiological procedures*. Prolonged treatment of constipation is seldom necessary except occasionally in the elderly.

CHILDREN. The use of laxatives in children should be discouraged unless prescribed by a doctor. Infrequent defaecation may be normal in breast-fed babies or in response to poor intake of fluid or fibre. Delays of greater than 3 days between stools may increase the likelihood of pain on passing hard stools leading to anal fissure, anal spasm and eventually to a learned response to avoid defaecation.

If increased fluid and fibre intake is insufficient, an osmotic laxative such as lactulose or a bulk-forming laxative such as methylcellulose may be effective; methylcellulose is given in a dose of 0.5–1 g twice daily for a child over 7 years [unlicensed use]—an appropriate formulation for a younger child is not readily available. If there is evidence of minor faecal retention, the addition of a stimulant laxative such as senna may overcome withholding but may lead to colic or, in the presence of faecal impaction in the rectum, an increase of faecal overflow. Referral to hospital may be needed unless the child evacuates the impacted mass spontaneously. In hospital, enemas or suppositories may clear the mass but their use is frequently distressing for the child and may lead to a persistence of withholding. Enemas may be administered under heavy sedation in hospital or alternatively a bowel cleansing solution (section 1.6.5) may be tried. In severe cases or where the child is afraid, a manual evacuation under anaesthetic may be appropriate.

Long-term use of stimulant laxatives such as senna or sodium picosulfate (sodium picosulphate, section 1.6.2) is essential to prevent recurrence of the faecal impaction. Parents should be encouraged to use them regularly for many months; intermittent use may provoke a series of relapses.

> The laxatives that follow have been divided into 5 main groups (sections 1.6.1–1.6.5). This simple classification disguises the fact that some laxatives have a complex action.

1.6.1   Bulk-forming laxatives

Bulk-forming laxatives relieve constipation by increasing faecal mass which stimulates peristalsis; patients should be advised that the full effect may take some days to develop.

Bulk-forming laxatives are of particular value in those with small hard stools, but should not be required unless fibre cannot be increased in the diet. A balanced diet, including adequate fluid intake and fibre is of value in preventing constipation.

Bulk-forming laxatives are useful in the management of patients with *colostomy, ileostomy, haemorrhoids, anal fissure, chronic diarrhoea associated with diverticular disease, irritable bowel syndrome*, and as adjuncts in *ulcerative colitis* (section 1.5). Adequate fluid intake must be maintained to avoid intestinal obstruction. Unprocessed wheat **bran**, taken with food or fruit juice, is a most effective bulk-forming preparation. Finely ground bran, though more palatable, has poorer water-retaining properties, but can be taken as bran bread or biscuits in appropriately increased quantities. Oat bran is also used.

Methylcellulose, **ispaghula**, and **sterculia** are useful in patients who cannot tolerate bran. Methylcellulose also acts as a faecal softener.

ISPAGHULA HUSK

Indications: see notes above; hypercholesterolaemia (section 2.12)

Cautions: adequate fluid intake should be maintained to avoid intestinal obstruction—it may be necessary to supervise elderly or debilitated patients or those with intestinal narrowing or decreased motility

Contra-indications: difficulty in swallowing, intestinal obstruction, colonic atony, faecal impaction

Side-effects: flatulence, abdominal distension, gastro-intestinal obstruction or impaction; hypersensitivity reported

Dose: see preparations below

COUNSELLING. Preparations that swell in contact with liquid should always be carefully swallowed with water and should not be taken immediately before going to bed

Fybogel® (R&C)
Granules, buff, effervescent, sugar- and gluten-free, ispaghula husk 3.5 g/sachet (low Na⁺), net price 30 sachets (plain, lemon, or orange flavour) = £2.12, 150 g (orange flavour) = £3.44. Label: 13, counselling, see above
Excipients: include aspartame 16 mg/sachet (see section 9.4.1)
Dose: 1 sachet or 2 level 5-mL spoonfuls in water twice daily preferably after meals; CHILD (but see section 1.6) 6–12 years ½–1 level 5-mL spoonful (children under 6 years on doctor's advice only)

Isogel® (Pfizer Consumer)
Granules, brown, sugar- and gluten-free, ispaghula husk 90%. Net price 200 g = £2.59. Label: 13, counselling, see above
Dose: constipation, 2 teaspoonfuls in water once or twice daily, preferably at mealtimes; CHILD (but see section 1.6) 1 teaspoonful
Diarrhoea (section 1.4.1), 1 teaspoonful 3 times daily

Ispagel Orange® (Richmond)
Granules, beige, effervescent, sugar- and gluten-free, ispaghula husk 3.5 g/sachet, net price 30 sachets = £2.10. Label: 13, counselling, see above
Excipients: include aspartame (section 9.4.1)
Dose: 1 sachet in water 1–3 times daily; CHILD (but see section 1.6) 6–12 years ½ adult dose (children under 6 years on doctor's advice only)

Konsyl® (Eastern)
Powder, sugar- and gluten-free, ispaghula husk (micronised) 6 g/sachet, net price 30-sachet pack = £3.99. Label: 13, counselling, see above
Dose: 1 sachet in water 1–3 times daily before or after meals; CHILD (but see section 1.6) over 6 years, ½ adult dose or less (children under 6 years on doctor's advice only)
Diarrhoea (section 1.4.1), 1 sachet in water 3 times daily

Regulan® (Procter & Gamble)
Powder, beige, sugar- and gluten-free, ispaghula husk 3.4 g/5.85-g sachet (orange or lemon/lime flavour). Net price 30 sachets = £2.12. Label: 13, counselling, see above
Excipients: include aspartame (section 9.4.1)
Dose: 1 sachet in 150 mL water 1–3 times daily; CHILD (but see section 1.6) 6–12 years 2.5–5 mL

METHYLCELLULOSE

Indications: see notes above and section 1.6 [unlicensed dose in children]; adjunct in obesity (but see section 4.5.1)

Cautions: see under Ispaghula Husk

Contra-indications: see under Ispaghula Husk; also infective bowel disease

Side-effects: see under Ispaghula Husk

Dose: see preparations below

COUNSELLING. Preparations that swell in contact with liquid should always be carefully swallowed with water and should not be taken immediately before going to bed

Celevac® (Shire)
Tablets, pink, scored, methylcellulose '450' 500 mg. Net price 112-tab pack = £2.69. Counselling, see above and dose
Dose: constipation and diarrhoea, 3–6 tablets twice daily. In constipation the dose should be taken with at least 300 mL liquid. In diarrhoea, ileostomy, and colostomy control, minimise liquid intake for 30 minutes before and after dose
Adjunct in obesity (but see section 4.5.1), 3 tablets with at least 300 mL warm liquid 30 minutes before food or when hungry

STERCULIA

Indications: see notes above

Cautions: see under Ispaghula Husk

Contra-indications: see under Ispaghula Husk

Side-effects: see under Ispaghula Husk

Dose: see under preparations below

COUNSELLING. Preparations that swell in contact with liquid should always be carefully swallowed with water and should not be taken immediately before going to bed

Normacol® (Norgine)
Granules, coated, gluten-free, sterculia 62%. Net price 500 g = £6.05; 60 × 7-g sachets = £5.11. Label: 25, 27, counselling, see above
Dose: 1–2 heaped 5-mL spoonfuls, or the contents of 1–2 sachets, washed down without chewing with plenty of liquid once or twice daily after meals; CHILD (but see section 1.6) 6–12 years half adult dose

Normacol Plus® (Norgine)
Granules, brown, coated, gluten-free, sterculia 62%, frangula (standardised) 8%. Net price 500 g = £6.50; 60 × 7 g sachets = £5.45. Label: 25, 27, counselling, see above
Dose: constipation and after haemorrhoidectomy, 1–2 heaped 5-mL spoonfuls or the contents of 1–2 sachets washed down without chewing with plenty of liquid once or twice daily after meals

1.6.2 Stimulant laxatives

Stimulant laxatives include **bisacodyl** and members of the **anthraquinone** group, **senna** and **dantron** (danthron). The indications for dantron are limited (see below) by its potential carcinogenicity (based on *rodent* carcinogenicity studies) and evidence of genotoxicity. Powerful stimulants such as **cascara** (an anthraquinone) and **castor oil** are obsolete. **Docusate** sodium probably acts both as a stimulant and as a softening agent.

Stimulant laxatives increase intestinal motility and often cause abdominal cramp; they should be avoided in intestinal obstruction. Prolonged use of stimulant laxatives can precipitate the onset of an atonic non-functioning colon and hypokalaemia; however, prolonged use may be justifiable in some circumstances (see section 1.6 for the use of stimulant laxatives in children).

Glycerol suppositories act as a rectal stimulant by virtue of the mildly irritant action of glycerol.

The **parasympathomimetics** bethanechol, distigmine, neostigmine, and pyridostigmine (see section 7.4.1 and section 10.2.1) enhance parasympathetic activity in the gut and increase intestinal motility. They are rarely used for their gastro-intestinal effects. Organic obstruction of the gut must first be excluded and they should not be used shortly after bowel anastomosis.

BISACODYL

Indications: see under Dose; tablets act in 10–12 hours; suppositories act in 20–60 minutes

Cautions: see notes above

Contra-indications: see notes above

Side-effects: see notes above; tablets, griping; suppositories, local irritation

Dose: constipation, *by mouth*, 5–10 mg at night; occasionally necessary to increase to 15–20 mg; CHILD (but see section 1.6) under 10 years 5 mg
By rectum in suppositories, 10 mg in the morning; CHILD (but see section 1.6) under 10 years 5 mg

Before radiological procedures and surgery, *by mouth*, 10 mg at bedtime for 2 days before examination and, if necessary, *by rectum* in suppositories, 10 mg 1 hour before examination; CHILD half adult dose

Bisacodyl (Non-proprietary)
Tablets, e/c, bisacodyl 5 mg. Net price 20 = 59p. Label: 5, 25
Suppositories, bisacodyl 10 mg. Net price 12 = 77p
Paediatric suppositories, bisacodyl 5 mg. Net price 5 = 89p
NOTE. The brand name *Dulco-lax®* [NHS] (Boehringer Ingelheim) is used for bisacodyl tablets, net price 10-tab pack = 71p; suppositories (10 mg), 10 = £1.48; paediatric suppositories (5 mg), 5 = 89p
The brand names *Dulco-lax® Liquid* and *Dulco-lax Perles®* are used for sodium picosulfate preparations

---

DANTRON
(Danthron)

Indications: only for constipation in terminally ill patients of all ages

Cautions: see notes above; avoid prolonged contact with skin (as in incontinent patients)—risk of irritation and excoriation; avoid in pregnancy and breast-feeding; *rodent* studies indicate potential carcinogenic risk

Contra-indications: see notes above

Side-effects: see notes above; urine may be coloured red

Dose: see under preparations

■ With poloxamer '188' (as co-danthramer)
NOTE. Co-danthramer suspension 5 mL = one co-danthramer capsule, **but** strong co-danthramer suspension 5 mL = two strong co-danthramer capsules

Co-danthramer (Non-proprietary) [PoM]
Capsules, co-danthramer 25/200 (dantron 25 mg, poloxamer '188' 200 mg). Net price 60-cap pack = £12.86. Label: 14, (urine red)
Dose: 1–2 capsules at bedtime; CHILD 1 capsule at bedtime (restricted indications, see notes above)
Available from Napp
Strong capsules, co-danthramer 37.5/500 (dantron 37.5 mg, poloxamer '188' 500 mg). Net price 60-cap pack = £15.55. Label: 14, (urine red)
Dose: 1–2 capsules at bedtime (restricted indications, see notes above); CHILD under 12 years not recommended
Available from Napp

Suspension, co-danthramer 25/200 in 5 mL (dantron 25 mg, poloxamer '188' 200 mg/5 mL). Net price 300 mL = £11.27, 1 litre = £37.57. Label: 14, (urine red)
Dose: 5–10 mL at night; CHILD 2.5–5 mL (restricted indications, see notes above)
Available from Hillcross, Napp (*Codalax®* [NHS]), Sovereign (*Danlax®*)
Strong suspension, co-danthramer 75/1000 in 5 mL (dantron 75 mg, poloxamer '188' 1 g/5 mL). Net price 300 mL = £30.13. Label: 14, (urine red)
Dose: 5 mL at night (restricted indications, see notes above); CHILD under 12 years not recommended
Available from Hillcross, Napp (*Codalax Forte®* [NHS])

■ With docusate sodium (as co-danthrusate)
Co-danthrusate (Non-proprietary) [PoM]
Capsules, co-danthrusate 50/60 (dantron 50 mg, docusate sodium 60 mg). Net price 63-cap pack = £13.46. Label: 14, (urine red)
Dose: 1–3 capsules, usually at night; CHILD 6–12 years 1 capsule (restricted indications, see notes above)
Available from APS, Celltech (*Normax®* [NHS]), Galen (*Capsuvac®*), Hillcross, IVAX, Sterwin
Suspension, yellow, co-danthrusate 50/60 (dantron 50 mg, docusate sodium 60 mg/5 mL). Net price 200 mL = £8.75. Label: 14, (urine red)
Dose: 5–15 mL at night; CHILD 6–12 years 5 mL at night (restricted indications, see notes above)
Available from Celltech (*Normax®*)

DOCUSATE SODIUM
(Dioctyl sodium sulphosuccinate)

Indications: constipation (oral preparations act within 1–2 days); adjunct in abdominal radiological procedures

Cautions: see notes above; do not give with liquid paraffin; rectal preparations not indicated if haemorrhoids or anal fissure

Contra-indications: see notes above

Side-effects: see notes above

Dose: *by mouth*, chronic constipation, up to 500 mg daily in divided doses; CHILD (but see section 1.6) over 6 months 12.5 mg 3 times daily, 2–12 years 12.5–25 mg 3 times daily (use paediatric oral solution only)
With barium meal, 400 mg

Dioctyl® (Schwarz)
Capsules, yellow/white, docusate sodium 100 mg, net price 30-cap pack = £2.40, 100-cap pack = £8.00

Docusol® (Typharm)
Adult oral solution, sugar-free, docusate sodium 50 mg/5 mL, net price 300 mL = £2.48
Paediatric oral solution, sugar-free, docusate sodium 12.5 mg/5 mL, net price 300 mL = £1.63

■ Rectal preparations
Fletchers' Enemette® (Forest)
Enema, docusate sodium 90 mg, glycerol 3.78 g/5 mL with macrogol and sorbic acid. Net price 5-mL unit = 31p
Dose: ADULT and CHILD (but see section 1.6) over 3 years, 5-mL unit when required

Norgalax Micro-enema® (Norgine)
Enema, docusate sodium 120 mg in 10-g single-dose disposable packs. Net price 10-g unit = 64p
Dose: ADULT and CHILD (but see section 1.6) over 12 years, 10-g unit

GLYCEROL

(Glycerin)
Indications: constipation
Dose: see below

Glycerol Suppositories, BP
(Glycerin Suppositories)
Suppositories, gelatin 140 mg, glycerol 700 mg, purified water to 1 g. Net price 12 = 81p (infant), 82p (child), 74p (adult)
Dose: 1 suppository moistened with water before use. The usual sizes are for *infants* small (1-g mould), *children* medium (2-g mould), *adults* large (4-g mould)

SENNA

Indications: constipation; acts in 8–12 hours
Cautions: see notes above
Contra-indications: see notes above
Side-effects: see notes above
Dose: see under preparations

Senna (Non-proprietary)
Tablets, total sennosides (calculated as sennoside B) 7.5 mg. Net price 20 = 29p
Dose: 2–4 tablets, usually at night; initial dose should be low then gradually increased; CHILD (but see section 1.6) over 6 years, half adult dose in the morning (on doctor's advice only)
NOTE. Lower dose on packs on sale to the public
Available from Alpharma, APS, R&C (*Senokot®* NHS)

Manevac® (Galen)
Granules, coated, senna fruit 12.4%, ispaghula 54.2%, net price 400 g = £7.49, 56 × 4-g sachets = £3.80. Label: 25, 27, counselling, see Ispaghula Husk
Dose: 1–2 level 5-mL spoonfuls (or sachets) with water or warm drink after supper and, if necessary, before breakfast *or* every 6 hours in resistant cases for 1–3 days; CHILD (but see section 1.6) 5–12 years 1 level 5-mL spoonful (or sachet) daily
NOTE. One level 5-mL spoonful is equivalent to one 4-g sachet
COUNSELLING. Preparations that swell in contact with liquid should always be carefully swallowed with water and should not be taken immediately before going to bed

Senokot® (R&C)
Tablets NHS, see above
Granules, brown, total sennosides (calculated as sennoside B) 15 mg/5 mL or 5.5 mg/g (one 5-mL spoonful = 2.7 g). Net price 100 g = £2.99
Dose: 5–10 mL, usually at bedtime; CHILD (but see section 1.6) over 6 years 2.5–5 mL in the morning
NOTE. Lower dose on packs on sale to the public
Syrup, brown, total sennosides (calculated as sennoside B) 7.5 mg/5 mL. Net price 100 mL = £2.27
Dose: 10–20 mL, usually at bedtime; CHILD (but see section 1.6) 2–6 years 2.5–5 mL in the morning (doctor's advice only), over 6 years 5–10 mL
NOTE. Lower dose on packs on sale to the public; the brand name *Senokot®* is also used for glycerol suppositories

SODIUM PICOSULFATE

(Sodium picosulphate)
Indications: constipation; bowel evacuation before abdominal radiological and endoscopic procedures on the colon, and surgery (section 1.6.5); acts within 6–12 hours
Cautions: see notes above
Contra-indications: see notes above
Side-effects: see notes above
Dose: 5–10 mg at night; CHILD (but section 1.6) under 4 years 250 micrograms/kg, 4–10 years 2.5–5 mg at night, over 10 years 5–10 mg at night

Sodium Picosulfate (Non-proprietary)
Elixir, sodium picosulfate 5 mg/5 mL, net price 100 mL = £1.85
NOTE. The brand names *Laxoberal®* NHS and *Dulco-lax® Liquid* (both Boehringer Ingelheim) are used for sodium picosulfate elixir 5 mg/5 mL

Dulco-lax® (Boehringer Ingelheim)
Perles® (= capsules), sodium picosulfate 2.5 mg, net price 50-cap pack = £2.73
NOTE. The brand name *Dulco-lax®* is also used for bisacodyl tablets and suppositories

■ Bowel cleansing solutions
Section 1.6.5

Other stimulant laxatives

Unstandardised preparations of cascara, frangula, rhubarb, and senna should be **avoided** as their laxative action is unpredictable. Aloes, colocynth, and jalap should be **avoided** as they have a drastic purgative action.

■ Preparations on sale to the public
Stimulant laxative preparations on sale to the public (not prescribable on the NHS) together with their significant ingredients:
Boots Compound Laxative Syrup of Figs® (fig, senna),
  Boots Senna Tablets® (senna)
Califig® (fig, senna), **Calsalettes®** (aloin)
Ex-lax Senna® (senna)
Fam-Lax Senna® (Irish moss, rhubarb, senna)
Jackson's Herbal Laxative® (cascara, rhubarb, senna)
Juno Junipah Salts® (juniper berry oil, sodium bicarbonate, sodium phosphate, sodium sulphate)
Nylax with Senna® (senna)
Potter's Cleansing Herb® (aloes, cascara, senna)

1.6.3   Faecal softeners

Liquid paraffin, the classical lubricant, has disadvantages (see below). Bulk laxatives (section 1.6.1) and non-ionic surfactant 'wetting' agents e.g. docusate sodium (section 1.6.2) also have softening properties. Such drugs are useful for oral administration in the management of haemorrhoids and anal fissure; glycerol suppositories (section 1.6.2) are useful for rectal use.

Enemas containing **arachis oil** (ground-nut oil, peanut oil) lubricate and soften impacted faeces and promote a bowel movement.

ARACHIS OIL

Indications: see notes above
Dose: see below

Fletchers' Arachis Oil Retention Enema®
(Forest)
Enema, arachis (peanut) oil in 130-mL single-dose disposable packs. Net price 130 mL = £1.02
Dose: to soften impacted faeces, 130 mL; the enema should be warmed before use; CHILD (but see section 1.6) under 3 years not recommended; over 3 years reduce adult dose in proportion to body-weight (medical supervision only)

LIQUID PARAFFIN ▱

Indications: constipation

Cautions: CSM recommends avoid prolonged use, and has contra-indicated in children less than 3 years of age

Side-effects: anal seepage of paraffin and consequent anal irritation after prolonged use, granulomatous reactions caused by absorption of small quantities of liquid paraffin (especially from the emulsion), lipoid pneumonia, and interference with the absorption of fat-soluble vitamins

Dose: see under preparation

Liquid Paraffin Oral Emulsion, BP ▱

Oral emulsion, liquid paraffin 5 mL, vanillin 5 mg, chloroform 0.025 mL, benzoic acid solution 0.2 mL, methylcellulose-20 200 mg, saccharin sodium 500 micrograms, water to 10 mL
Dose: 10–30 mL at night when required
COUNSELLING. Should not be taken immediately before going to bed

---

1.6.4   Osmotic laxatives

Osmotic laxatives increase the amount of water in the large bowel, either by drawing fluid from the body into the bowel or by retaining the fluid they were administered with.

Saline purgatives such as **magnesium hydroxide** are commonly abused but are satisfactory for occasional use; adequate fluid intake should be maintained. **Magnesium salts** are useful where rapid bowel evacuation is required. **Sodium salts** should be avoided as they may give rise to sodium and water retention in susceptible individuals. **Phosphate enemas** are useful in bowel clearance before radiology, endoscopy, and surgery.

Lactulose is a semi-synthetic disaccharide which is not absorbed from the gastro-intestinal tract. It produces an osmotic diarrhoea of low faecal pH, and discourages the proliferation of ammonia-producing organisms. It is therefore useful in the treatment of *hepatic encephalopathy*.

Macrogols are inert polymers of ethylene glycol which sequester fluid in the bowel; giving fluid with macrogols may reduce the dehydrating effect sometimes seen with osmotic laxatives.

LACTULOSE

Indications: constipation (may take up to 48 hours to act), hepatic encephalopathy (portal systemic encephalopathy)

Cautions: lactose intolerance

Contra-indications: galactosaemia, intestinal obstruction

Side-effects: flatulence, cramps, and abdominal discomfort

Dose: see under preparations below

Lactulose (Non-proprietary)

Solution, lactulose 3.1–3.7 g/5 mL with other ketoses. Net price 500-mL pack = £2.43
Dose: constipation, initially 15 mL twice daily, adjusted according to patient's needs; CHILD (but see section 1.6) under 1 year 2.5 mL twice daily, 1–5 years 5 mL twice

daily, 5–10 years 10 mL twice daily
Hepatic encephalopathy, 30–50 mL 3 times daily, subsequently adjusted to produce 2–3 soft stools daily
Available from Alpharma, APS, Arrow, CP, Hillcross, Intrapharm (*Lactugal*®), IVAX, Novartis Consumer Health (*Regulose*®), Sandoz, Solvay (*Duphalac*® ▱NHS▱)
NOTE. A proprietary brand of lactulose 3.3 g/5 mL (*Regulose*®) is on sale to the public

---

MACROGOLS

(Polyethylene glycols)

Indications: see preparation below

Cautions: pregnancy and breast-feeding; discontinue if symptoms of fluid and electrolyte disturbance

Contra-indications: intestinal perforation or obstruction, paralytic ileus, severe inflammatory conditions of the intestinal tract (such as Crohn's disease, ulcerative colitis, and toxic megacolon)

Side-effects: abdominal distension and pain, nausea

Dose: see preparation below

Idrolax® (Schwarz)

Oral powder, macrogol '4000' (polyethylene glycol '4000') 10 g/sachet, net price 20-sachet pack (orange-grapefruit flavour) = £4.90. Label: 13
Dose: constipation, 1–2 sachets as a single dose preferably in the morning; content of each sachet dissolved in a glass of water; CHILD over 8 years, as adult dose for max. 3 months

Movicol® (Norgine)

Oral powder, macrogol '3350' (polyethylene glycol '3350') 13.125 g, sodium bicarbonate 178.5 mg, sodium chloride 350.7 mg, potassium chloride 46.6 mg/sachet, net price 20-sachet pack (lime and lemon flavour) = £4.98, 30-sachet pack = £7.47. Label: 13
Cautions: patients with impaired cardiovascular function should not take more than 2 sachets in any 1 hour
Dose: chronic constipation, 1–3 sachets daily in divided doses usually for up to 2 weeks; content of each sachet dissolved in half a glass (approx. 125 mL) of water; maintenance, 1–2 sachets daily; CHILD not recommended
Faecal impaction, 8 sachets daily dissolved in 1 litre water and drunk within 6 hours, usually for max. 3 days; CHILD not recommended.
After reconstitution the solution should be kept in a refrigerator and discarded if unused after 6 hours

Movicol-Half® (Norgine)

Oral powder, macrogol '3350' (polyethylene glycol '3350') 6.563 g, sodium bicarbonate 89.3 mg, sodium chloride 175.4 mg, potassium chloride 23.3 mg/sachet, net price 20-sachet pack (lime and lemon flavour) = £2.99, 30-sachet pack = £4.48. Label: 13
Cautions: patients with impaired cardiovascular function should not take more than 4 sachets in any 1 hour
Dose: chronic constipation, 2–6 sachets daily in divided doses usually for up to 2 weeks; content of each sachet dissolved in quarter of a glass (approx. 62.5 mL) of water; maintenance, 2–4 sachets daily; CHILD not recommended
Faecal impaction, 16 sachets daily dissolved in 1 litre water and drunk within 6 hours, usually for max. 3 days; CHILD 2–11 years, consult product literature
After reconstitution the solution should be kept in a refrigerator and discarded if unused after 24 hours

---

MAGNESIUM SALTS

Indications: see under preparations below

Cautions: renal impairment (risk of magnesium accumulation); hepatic impairment (see Appendix

2); elderly and debilitated; see also notes above;
interactions: Appendix 1 (antacids)
Contra-indications: acute gastro-intestinal conditions
Side-effects: colic
Dose: see under preparations below

■ Magnesium hydroxide

Magnesium Hydroxide Mixture, BP
(Cream of Magnesia)
Aqueous suspension containing about 8% hydrated
magnesium oxide. Do not store in cold place
Dose: constipation, 25–50 mL when required

■ Magnesium hydroxide with liquid paraffin

**Liquid Paraffin and Magnesium Hydroxide Oral
Emulsion, BP** ☐◢
Oral emulsion, 25% liquid paraffin in aqueous
suspension containing 6% hydrated magnesium
oxide
Dose: constipation, 5–20 mL when required
NOTE. Liquid paraffin and magnesium hydroxide preparations
on sale to the public include: *Milpar®* [NHS]

■ Magnesium sulphate

Magnesium Sulphate
Label: 13, 23
Dose: rapid bowel evacuation (acts in 2–4 hours) 5–10 g
in a glass of water preferably before breakfast
NOTE. Magnesium sulphate is on sale to the public as
Epsom Salts

■ Bowel cleansing solutions
Section 1.6.5

PHOSPHATES (RECTAL)

Indications: rectal use in constipation; bowel
evacuation before abdominal radiological procedures,
endoscopy, and surgery
Cautions: elderly and debilitated; see also notes
above
Contra-indications: acute gastro-intestinal conditions
Side-effects: local irritation
Dose: see under preparations

Carbalax® (Forest)
Suppositories, sodium acid phosphate (anhydrous)
1.3 g, sodium bicarbonate 1.08 g, net price 12 =
£2.14
Dose: constipation, 1 suppository, inserted 30 minutes
before evacuation required; moisten with water before
use; CHILD under 12 years not recommended

Fleet® Ready-to-use Enema (De Witt)
Enema, sodium acid phosphate 21.4 g, sodium
phosphate 9.4 g/118 mL. Net price single-dose
pack (standard tube) = 46p
Dose: ADULT and CHILD (but see section 1.6) over 12
years, 118 mL; CHILD 3–12 years, on doctor's advice only
(under 3 years not recommended)

Fletchers' Phosphate Enema® (Forest)
Enema, sodium acid phosphate 12.8 g, sodium
phosphate 10.24 g, purified water, freshly boiled
and cooled, to 128 mL (corresponds to Phosphates
Enema Formula B). Net price 128 mL with
standard tube = 44p, with long rectal tube = 61p
Dose: 128 mL; CHILD (but see section 1.6) over 3 years,
reduced according to body weight (under 3 years not
recommended)

SODIUM CITRATE (RECTAL)

Indications: rectal use in constipation
Cautions: elderly and debilitated; see also notes
above
Contra-indications: acute gastro-intestinal conditions
Dose: see under preparations

Micolette Micro-enema® (Dexcel)
Enema, sodium citrate 450 mg, sodium lauryl
sulphoacetate 45 mg, glycerol 625 mg, together
with citric acid, potassium sorbate, and sorbitol in a
viscous solution, in 5-mL single-dose disposable
packs with nozzle. Net price 5 mL = 31p
Dose: ADULT and CHILD over 3 years, 5–10 mL (but see
section 1.6)

Micralax Micro-enema® (Celltech)
Enema, sodium citrate 450 mg, sodium alkylsulphoacetate
45 mg, sorbic acid 5 mg, together with
glycerol and sorbitol in a viscous solution in 5-mL
single-dose disposable packs with nozzle. Net
price 5 mL = 33p
Dose: ADULT and CHILD over 3 years, 5 mL (but see
section 1.6)

Relaxit Micro-enema® (Crawford)
Enema, sodium citrate 450 mg, sodium lauryl
sulphate 75 mg, sorbic acid 5 mg, together with
glycerol and sorbitol in a viscous solution in 5-mL
single-dose disposable packs with nozzle. Net
price 5 mL = 32p
Dose: ADULT and CHILD (but see section 1.6) 5 mL (insert
only half nozzle length in child under 3 years)

1.6.5   Bowel cleansing solutions

Bowel cleansing solutions are used before colonic
surgery, colonoscopy, or radiological examination to
ensure the bowel is free of solid contents. They are
not treatments for constipation.

BOWEL CLEANSING SOLUTIONS

Indications: see above
Cautions: pregnancy; renal impairment (avoid if
severe—Appendix 3); heart disease; ulcerative
colitis; diabetes mellitus; reflux oesophagitis;
impaired gag reflex; unconscious or semiconscious
or possibility of regurgitation or aspiration
Contra-indications: gastro-intestinal obstruction,
gastric retention, gastro-intestinal ulceration, perforated
bowel, congestive cardiac failure; toxic
colitis, toxic megacolon or ileus
Side-effects: nausea and bloating; less frequently
abdominal cramps (usually transient—reduced by
taking more slowly); vomiting
Dose: see under preparations

Citramag® (Sanochemia)
Powder, effervescent, magnesium carbonate
11.57 g, anhydrous citric acid 17.79 g/sachet, net
price 10-sachet pack (lemon and lime flavour) =
£14.90. Label: 10, patient information leaflet, 13,
counselling, see below
Dose: bowel evacuation for surgery, colonoscopy or
radiological examination, on day before procedure, 1
sachet at 8 a.m. and 1 sachet between 2 and 4 p.m.; CHILD

5–9 years one-third adult dose; over 10 years and frail ELDERLY one-half adult dose
COUNSELLING. The patient information leaflet advises that hot water (200 mL) is needed to make the solution and provides guidance on the timing and procedure for reconstitution; it also mentions need for high fluid, low residue diet beforehand (according to hospital advice), and explains that only clear fluids can be taken after *Citramag*® until procedure completed

Fleet Phospho-soda® (De Witt)
Oral solution, sugar-free, sodium dihydrogen phosphate dihydrate 24.4 g, disodium phosphate dodecahydrate 10.8 g/45 mL. Net price 2 × 45-mL bottles = £4.79. Label: 10, patient information leaflet, counselling
Dose: 45 mL diluted with half a glass (120 mL) of cold water, followed by one full glass (240 mL) of cold water
Timing of doses is dependent on the time of the procedure
For morning procedure, first dose should be taken at 7 a.m. and second at 7 p.m. on day before the procedure
For afternoon procedure, first dose should be taken at 7 p.m. on day before and second dose at 7 a.m. on day of the procedure
Solid food must not be taken during dosing period; clear liquids or water should be substituted for meals
CHILD and ADOLESCENT under 15 years not recommended

Klean-Prep® (Norgine)
Oral powder, macrogol '3350' (polyethylene glycol '3350') 59 g, anhydrous sodium sulphate 5.685 g, sodium bicarbonate 1.685 g, sodium chloride 1.465 g, potassium chloride 743 mg/sachet, net price 4 sachets = £9.20. Label: 10, patient information leaflet, counselling
Excipients: include aspartame (section 9.4.1)
Four sachets when reconstituted with water to 4 litres provides an iso-osmotic solution for bowel cleansing before surgery, colonoscopy or radiological procedures
Dose: a glass (approx. 250 mL) of reconstituted solution every 10–15 minutes, or by nasogastric tube 20–30 mL/minute, until 4 litres have been consumed or watery stools are free of solid matter; CHILD not recommended
The solution from all 4 sachets should be drunk within 4–6 hours (250 mL drunk rapidly every 10–15 minutes); flavouring such as clear fruit cordials may be added if required; to facilitate gastric emptying domperidone or metoclopramide may be given 30 minutes before starting. Alternatively the administration may be divided into two, e.g. taking the solutions from 2 sachets on the evening before examination and the remaining 2 on the morning of the examination
After reconstitution the solution should be kept in a refrigerator and discarded if unused after 24 hours
NOTE. Allergic reactions reported

Picolax® (Nordic)
Oral powder, sugar-free, sodium picosulfate 10 mg/sachet, with magnesium citrate (for bowel evacuation before radiological procedure, endoscopy, and surgery), net price 2-sachet pack = £3.95. Label: 10, patient information leaflet, 13, counselling, see below
Dose: ADULT and CHILD over 9 years, 1 sachet in water in morning (before 8 a.m.) and a second in afternoon (between 2 and 4 p.m.) of day preceding procedure; CHILD 1–2 years quarter sachet morning and afternoon, 2–4 years half sachet morning and afternoon, 4–9 years 1 sachet morning and half sachet afternoon
Acts within 3 hours of first dose
NOTE. Low residue diet recommended for 2 days before procedure and copious intake of water or other clear fluids recommended during treatment
COUNSELLING. Patients should be warned that heat is generated on addition to water; for this reason the powder

should be added initially to 30 mL (2 tablespoonfuls) of water; after 5 minutes (when reaction complete) the solution should be further diluted to 150 mL (approx. half a glass)

1.7 Local preparations for anal and rectal disorders

1.7.1   Soothing haemorrhoidal preparations
1.7.2   Compound haemorrhoidal preparations with corticosteroids
1.7.3   Rectal sclerosants

Anal and perianal pruritus, soreness, and excoriation are best treated by application of bland ointments and suppositories (section 1.7.1). These conditions occur commonly in patients suffering from haemorrhoids, fistulas, and proctitis. Careful local toilet with attention to any minor faecal soiling, adjustment of the diet to avoid hard stools, the use of bulk-forming materials such as bran (section 1.6.1) and a high residue diet are helpful. In proctitis these measures may supplement treatment with corticosteroids or sulfasalazine (see section 1.5).

When necessary topical preparations containing **local anaesthetics** (section 1.7.1) or **corticosteroids** (section 1.7.2) are used provided perianal thrush has been excluded. Perianal thrush is best treated with **nystatin** by mouth and by local application (see section 5.2, section 7.2.2, and section 13.10.2).

The management of *anal fissures* requires stool softening by increasing dietary fibre in the form of bran or by using a bulk-forming laxative. Short-term use of local anaesthetic preparations may help (section 1.7.1). If these measures are inadequate, the patient should be referred for specialist treatment in hospital; surgery or the use of a topical nitrate (e.g. glyceryl trinitrate 0.2–0.3% ointment) may be considered [unlicensed indication].

1.7.1 Soothing haemorrhoidal preparations

Soothing preparations containing mild astringents such as bismuth subgallate, zinc oxide, and hamamelis may give symptomatic relief in haemorrhoids. Many proprietary preparations also contain lubricants, vasoconstrictors, or mild antiseptics.

Local anaesthetics are used to relieve pain associated with *haemorrhoids*, and *pruritus ani* but good evidence is lacking. Lidocaine (lignocaine) ointment (section 15.2) is used before emptying the bowel to relieve pain associated with *anal fissure*. Alternative local anaesthetics include tetracaine (amethocaine), cinchocaine, and pramocaine (pramoxine), but they are more irritant. Local anaesthetic ointments can be absorbed through the rectal mucosa therefore excessive application should be **avoided**, particularly in infants and children. They should be used for short periods only (no longer than a few days) since they may cause sensitisation of the anal skin.

■ Preparations on sale to the public

Soothing haemorrhoidal preparations on sale to the public together with their significant ingredients include:

Anacal® (heparinoid, laureth '9'), **Anodesyn**® (allantoin, lidocaine (lignocaine)), **Anusol**® **cream** (bismuth oxide, Peru balsam, zinc oxide), **Anusol**® **ointment** and **suppositories** (bismuth oxide, bismuth subgallate, Peru balsam, zinc oxide)

Boots Haemorrhoid Ointment® (lidocaine (lignocaine), zinc oxide), **Boots Suppositories for Haemorrhoids**® (benzyl alcohol, glycol monosalicylate, methyl salicylate, zinc oxide)

Germoloids® (lidocaine (lignocaine), zinc oxide)

Hemocane® (benzoic acid, bismuth oxide, cinnamic acid, lidocaine (lignocaine), zinc oxide)

Lanacane® **cream** (benzocaine, chlorothymol)

Nupercainal® (cinchocaine)

Preparation H® **gel** (hamamelis water), **Preparation H**® **ointment and suppositories** (shark liver oil, yeast cell extract)

1.7.2 Compound haemorrhoidal preparations with corticosteroids

Corticosteroids are often combined with local anaesthetics and soothing agents in preparations for haemorrhoids. They are suitable for occasional short-term use after exclusion of infections, such as herpes simplex; prolonged use can cause atrophy of the anal skin. See section 13.4 for general comments on topical corticosteroids and section 1.7.1 for comment on local anaesthetics.

CHILDREN. Haemorrhoids in children are rare. Treatment is usually symptomatic and the use of a locally applied cream is appropriate for short periods; however, local anaesthetics can cause stinging initially and this may aggravate the child's fear of defaecation.

Anugesic-HC® (Pfizer) PoM

Cream, benzyl benzoate 1.2%, bismuth oxide 0.875%, hydrocortisone acetate 0.5%, Peru balsam 1.85%, pramocaine hydrochloride 1%, zinc oxide 12.35%. Net price 30 g (with rectal nozzle) = £3.71

Dose: apply night and morning and after a bowel movement; do not use for longer than 7 days; CHILD not recommended

Suppositories, buff, benzyl benzoate 33 mg, bismuth oxide 24 mg, bismuth subgallate 59 mg, hydrocortisone acetate 5 mg, Peru balsam 49 mg, pramocaine hydrochloride 27 mg, zinc oxide 296 mg, net price 12 = £2.69

Dose: insert 1 suppository night and morning and after a bowel movement; do not use for longer than 7 days; CHILD not recommended

Anusol-HC® (Kestrel) PoM

Ointment, benzyl benzoate 1.25%, bismuth oxide 0.875%, bismuth subgallate 2.25%, hydrocortisone acetate 0.25%, Peru balsam 1.875%, zinc oxide 10.75%. Net price 30 g (with rectal nozzle) = £3.19

Dose: apply night and morning and after a bowel movement; do not use for longer than 7 days; CHILD not recommended

NOTE. A proprietary brand (*Anusol Plus HC*® ointment) is on sale to the public

Suppositories, benzyl benzoate 33 mg, bismuth oxide 24 mg, bismuth subgallate 59 mg, hydrocortisone acetate 10 mg, Peru balsam 49 mg, zinc oxide 296 mg. Net price 12 = £2.24

Dose: insert 1 suppository night and morning and after a bowel movement; do not use for longer than 7 days; CHILD not recommended

NOTE. A proprietary brand (*Anusol Plus HC*® suppositories) is on sale to the public

Perinal® (Dermal)

Spray application, hydrocortisone 0.2%, lidocaine hydrochloride (lignocaine hydrochloride) 1%. Net price 30-mL pack = £6.87

Dose: spray twice over the affected area up to 3 times daily; do not use for longer than 1–2 weeks; CHILD under 14 years not recommended

NOTE. Also available as *Germoloids*® HC (Bayer Consumer Care)

Proctofoam HC® (Meda) PoM

Foam in aerosol pack, hydrocortisone acetate 1%, pramocaine hydrochloride 1%. Net price 21.2-g pack (approx. 40 applications) with applicator = £5.06

Dose: haemorrhoids and proctitis, 1 applicatorful (4–6 mg hydrocortisone acetate, 4–6 mg pramocaine hydrochloride) by rectum 2–3 times daily and after a bowel movement (max. 4 times daily); do not use for longer than 7 days; CHILD not recommended

Proctosedyl® (Aventis Pharma) PoM

Ointment, cinchocaine (dibucaine) hydrochloride 0.5%, hydrocortisone 0.5%. Net price 30 g = £7.13 (with cannula)

Dose: apply morning and night and after a bowel movement, externally or by rectum; do not use for longer than 7 days

Suppositories, cinchocaine (dibucaine) hydrochloride 5 mg, hydrocortisone 5 mg. Net price 12 = £3.22

Dose: insert 1 suppository night and morning and after a bowel movement; do not use for longer than 7 days

Scheriproct® (Schering Health) PoM

Ointment, cinchocaine (dibucaine) hydrochloride 0.5%, prednisolone hexanoate 0.19%. Net price 30 g = £3.53

Dose: apply twice daily for 5–7 days (3–4 times daily on 1st day if necessary), then once daily for a few days after symptoms have cleared

Suppositories, cinchocaine (dibucaine) hydrochloride 1 mg, prednisolone hexanoate 1.3 mg. Net price 12 = £1.66

Dose: insert 1 suppository daily after a bowel movement, for 5–7 days (in severe cases initially 2–3 times daily)

Ultraproct® (Meadow) PoM

Ointment, cinchocaine (dibucaine) hydrochloride 0.5%, fluocortolone caproate 0.095%, fluocortolone pivalate 0.092%, net price 30 g (with rectal nozzle) = £4.57

Dose: apply twice daily for 5–7 days (3–4 times daily on 1st day if necessary), then once daily for a few days after symptoms have cleared

Suppositories, cinchocaine (dibucaine) hydrochloride 1 mg, fluocortolone caproate 630 micrograms, fluocortolone pivalate 610 micrograms, net price 12 = £2.15

Dose: insert 1 suppository daily after a bowel movement, for 5–7 days (in severe cases initially 2–3 times daily) then 1 suppository every other day for 1 week

Uniroid-HC® (Chemidex) PoM

Ointment, cinchocaine (dibucaine) hydrochloride 0.5%, hydrocortisone 0.5%. Net price 30 g (with applicator) = £4.23

Dose: apply twice daily and after a bowel movement, externally or by rectum; do not use for longer than 7 days; CHILD under 12 years not recommended

Suppositories, cinchocaine (dibucaine) hydrochloride 5 mg, hydrocortisone 5 mg. Net price 12 = £1.91

Dose: insert 1 suppository twice daily and after a bowel movement; do not use for longer than 7 days; CHILD under 12 years not recommended

Xyloproct® (AstraZeneca) PoM

Ointment (water-miscible), aluminium acetate 3.5%, hydrocortisone acetate 0.275%, lidocaine (lignocaine) 5%, zinc oxide 18%, net price 20 g (with applicator) = £2.26

Dose: apply several times daily; short-term use only

1.7.3 Rectal sclerosants

Oily phenol injection is used to inject haemorrhoids particularly when unprolapsed.

PHENOL

Indications: see notes above
Side-effects: irritation, tissue necrosis

Oily Phenol Injection, BP PoM

phenol 5% in a suitable fixed oil. Net price 5-mL amp = £5.12

Dose: 2–3 mL into the submucosal layer at the base of the pile; several injections may be given at different sites, max. total injected 10 mL at any one time
Available from Celltech

1.8 Stoma care

Prescribing for patients with stoma calls for special care. The following is a brief account of some of the main points to be borne in mind.

Enteric-coated and *modified-release* preparations are **unsuitable**, particularly in patients with ileostomies, as there may not be sufficient release of the active ingredient.

Laxatives. Enemas and washouts should **not** be prescribed for patients with ileostomies as they may cause rapid and severe dehydration.

Colostomy patients may suffer from constipation and whenever possible should be treated by increasing fluid intake or dietary fibre. **Bulk-forming drugs** (section 1.6.1) should be tried. If they are insufficient, as small a dose as possible of senna (section 1.6.2) should be used.

Antidiarrhoeals. Drugs such as **loperamide**, **codeine phosphate**, or **co-phenotrope** (diphenoxylate with atropine) are effective. Bulk-forming drugs (section 1.6.1) may be tried but it is often difficult to adjust the dose appropriately.

Antibacterials should **not** be given for an episode of acute diarrhoea.

Antacids. The tendency to diarrhoea from magnesium salts or constipation from aluminium salts may be increased in these patients.

Diuretics should be used with caution in patients with ileostomies as they may become excessively dehydrated and potassium depletion may easily occur. It is usually advisable to use a **potassium-sparing** diuretic (see section 2.2.3).

Digoxin. Patients with a stoma are particularly susceptible to hypokalaemia if on digoxin therapy and potassium supplements or a potassium-sparing diuretic may be advisable (for comment see section 9.2.1.1).

Potassium supplements. Liquid formulations are preferred to modified-release formulations (see above).

Analgesics. Opioid analgesics (see section 4.7.2) may cause troublesome constipation in colostomy patients. When a non-opioid analgesic is required **paracetamol** is usually suitable but anti-inflammatory analgesics may cause gastric irritation and bleeding.

Iron preparations may cause loose stools and sore skin in these patients. If this is troublesome and if iron is definitely indicated an intramuscular iron preparation (see section 9.1.1.2) should be used. Modified-release preparations should be **avoided** for the reasons given above.

Patients are usually given advice about the use of *cleansing agents, protective creams, lotions, deodorants,* and *sealants* whilst in hospital, either by the surgeon or by the health authority stoma care nurses. Voluntary organisations offer help and support to patients with stoma.

1.9 Drugs affecting intestinal secretions

1.9.1	Drugs affecting biliary composition and flow
1.9.2	Bile acid sequestrants
1.9.3	Aprotinin
1.9.4	Pancreatin

1.9.1 Drugs affecting biliary composition and flow

The use of laparoscopic cholecystectomy and of endoscopic biliary techniques has limited the place of the bile acid **ursodeoxycholic acid** in gallstone disease. Ursodeoxycholic acid is suitable for patients with unimpaired gall bladder function, small or medium-sized radiolucent stones, and whose mild symptoms are not amenable to other treatment; it should be used cautiously in those with liver disease (but see below). Patients should be given dietary advice (including avoidance of excessive cholesterol and calories) and they require radiological monitoring. Long-term prophylaxis may be needed after complete dissolution of the gallstones has been confirmed because they may recur in up to 25% of patients within one year of stopping treatment.

Ursodeoxycholic acid is also used in primary biliary cirrhosis; liver tests improve in most patients but the effect on overall survival is uncertain. Ursodeoxycholic acid has also been tried in primary sclerosing cholangitis [unlicensed indication].

URSODEOXYCHOLIC ACID

Indications: see under Dose and under preparations

Cautions: see notes above; **interactions:** Appendix 1 (ursodeoxycholic acid)

Contra-indications: radio-opaque stones, pregnancy (Appendix 4), non-functioning gall bladder, inflammatory diseases and other conditions of the small intestine, colon and liver which interfere with entero-hepatic circulation of bile salts

Side-effects: nausea, vomiting, diarrhoea; gallstone calcification; pruritus

Dose: dissolution of gallstones, 8–12 mg/kg daily as a single dose at bedtime *or* in two divided doses, for up to 2 years; treatment is continued for 3–4 months after stones dissolve

Primary biliary cirrhosis, see under *Ursofalk®*

Ursodeoxycholic Acid (Non-proprietary) PoM
Tablets, ursodeoxycholic acid 150 mg, net price 60-tab pack = £18.56. Label: 21
Available from Hillcross
Capsules, ursodeoxycholic acid 250 mg, net price 60-cap pack = £35.15. Label: 21
Available from Hillcross

Destolit® (Norgine) PoM
Tablets, scored, ursodeoxycholic acid 150 mg, net price 60-tab pack = £19.77. Label: 21

Urdox® (CP) PoM
Tablets, f/c, ursodeoxycholic acid 300 mg, net price 60-tab pack = £30.24. Label: 21

Ursofalk® (Provalis) PoM
Capsules, ursodeoxycholic acid 250 mg. Net price 60 = £32.95. Label: 21
Suspension, sugar-free, ursodeoxycholic acid 250 mg/5 mL, net price 250 mL = £30.20. Label: 21
Dose: primary biliary cirrhosis, 10–15 mg/kg daily in 2–4 divided doses
Dissolution of gallstones, see Dose, above

Ursogal® (Galen) PoM
Tablets, scored, ursodeoxycholic acid 150 mg, net price 60-tab pack = £17.05. Label: 21
Capsules, ursodeoxycholic acid 250 mg, net price 60-cap pack = £30.50. Label: 21

Other preparations for biliary disorders

A **terpene** mixture (*Rowachol®*) raises biliary cholesterol solubility. It is not considered to be a useful adjunct.

Rowachol® (Rowa) PoM ◼
Capsules, green, e/c, borneol 5 mg, camphene 5 mg, cineole 2 mg, menthol 32 mg, menthone 6 mg, pinene 17 mg in olive oil. Net price 50-cap pack = £7.35. Label: 22
Dose: 1–2 capsules 3 times daily before food (but see notes above)
Interactions: Appendix 1 (*Rowachol®*)

1.9.2 Bile acid sequestrants

Colestyramine (cholestyramine) is an anion-exchange resin that is not absorbed from the gastro-intestinal tract. It relieves diarrhoea and pruritus by forming an insoluble complex with bile acids in the intestine. Colestyramine can interfere with the

absorption of a number of drugs. Colestyramine is also used in hypercholesterolaemia (section 2.12).

COLESTYRAMINE
(Cholestyramine)

Indications: pruritus associated with partial biliary obstruction and primary biliary cirrhosis; diarrhoea associated with Crohn's disease, ileal resection, vagotomy, diabetic vagal neuropathy, and radiation; hypercholesterolaemia (section 2.12)

Cautions: see section 2.12

Contra-indications: see section 2.12

Side-effects: see section 2.12

Dose: pruritus, 4–8 g daily in water (or other suitable liquid)
Diarrhoea, after initial introduction over 3–4 week period, 12–24 g daily mixed with water (or other suitable liquid) in 1–4 divided doses, then adjusted as required; max. 36 g daily
CHILD 6–12 years, consult product literature
COUNSELLING. Other drugs should be taken at least 1 hour before or 4–6 hours after colestyramine to reduce possible interference with absorption

◼ Preparations
Section 2.12

1.9.3 Aprotinin

Section 2.11.

1.9.4 Pancreatin

Supplements of pancreatin are given by mouth to compensate for reduced or absent exocrine secretion in cystic fibrosis, and following pancreatectomy, total gastrectomy, or chronic pancreatitis. They assist the digestion of starch, fat, and protein.

Pancreatin is inactivated by gastric acid therefore pancreatin preparations are best taken with food (or immediately before or after food). Gastric acid secretion may be reduced by giving cimetidine or ranitidine an hour beforehand (section 1.3). Concurrent use of antacids also reduces gastric acidity. Enteric-coated preparations deliver a higher enzyme concentration in the duodenum (provided the capsule contents are swallowed whole without chewing). Higher-strength versions are now also available (**important:** see CSM advice below).

Since pancreatin is also inactivated by heat, excessive heat should be avoided if preparations are mixed with liquids or food; the resulting mixtures should not be kept for more than one hour.

Dosage is adjusted according to size, number, and consistency of stools, so that the patient thrives; extra allowance may be needed if snacks are taken between meals.

Pancreatin can irritate the perioral skin and buccal mucosa if retained in the mouth, and excessive doses can cause perianal irritation. The most frequent side-effects are gastro-intestinal, including nausea, vomiting, and abdominal discomfort; hyperuricaemia and hyperuricosuria have been associated with very high doses. Hypersensitivity reactions occur occasionally and may affect those handling the powder.

PANCREATIN

NOTE. The pancreatin preparations which follow are all of porcine origin

Indications: see also above

Cautions: see also above and (for higher-strength preparations) see below

Side-effects: see also above and (for higher-strength preparations) see below

Dose: see preparations

Creon® 10 000 (Solvay)
Capsules, brown/clear, enclosing buff-coloured e/c granules of pancreatin, providing: protease 600 units, lipase 10 000 units, amylase 8000 units. Net price 100-cap pack = £16.66. Counselling, see dose
Dose: ADULT and CHILD initially 1–2 capsules with meals either taken whole or contents mixed with fluid or soft food (then swallowed immediately without chewing)

Nutrizym GR® (Merck)
Capsules, green/orange, enclosing e/c pellets of pancreatin, providing minimum of: protease 650 units, lipase 10 000 units, amylase 10 000 units. Net price 100 = £14.47. Counselling, see dose
Dose: ADULT and CHILD 1–2 capsules with meals swallowed whole or contents sprinkled on soft food (then swallowed immediately without chewing); higher doses may be required according to response

Nutrizym 10® (Merck)
Capsules, red/yellow, enclosing e/c minitablets of pancreatin providing minimum of: protease 500 units, lipase 10 000 units, amylase 9000 units. Net price 100 = £14.47. Counselling, see dose
Dose: ADULT and CHILD 1–2 capsules with meals and 1 capsule with snacks, swallowed whole or contents taken with water or sprinkled on soft food (then swallowed immediately without chewing); higher doses may be required according to response

Pancrease® (Janssen-Cilag)
Capsules, enclosing e/c beads of pancrelipase USP, providing minimum of: protease 330 units, lipase 5000 units, amylase 2900 units. Net price 100 = £17.07. Counselling, see dose
Dose: ADULT and CHILD 1–2 (occasionally 3) capsules during each meal and 1 capsule with snacks swallowed whole or contents sprinkled on liquid or soft food (then swallowed immediately without chewing); higher doses may be required according to response

Pancrex® (Paines & Byrne)
Granules, pancreatin, providing minimum of: protease 300 units, lipase 5000 units, amylase 4000 units/g. Net price 300 g = £20.39. Label: 25, counselling, see dose
Dose: ADULT and CHILD 5–10 g just before meals washed down or mixed with liquid

Pancrex V® (Paines & Byrne)
Capsules, pancreatin, providing minimum of: protease 430 units, lipase 8000 units, amylase 9000 units. Net price 300-cap pack = £15.80. Counselling, see dose
Dose: ADULT and CHILD over 1 year 2–6 capsules with meals, swallowed whole or sprinkled on food; CHILD up to 1 year 1–2 capsules mixed with feeds
Capsules '125', pancreatin, providing minimum of: protease 160 units, lipase 2950 units, amylase 3300 units. Net price 300-cap pack = £9.72. Counselling, see dose
Dose: NEONATE 1–2 capsules with feeds

Tablets, e/c, s/c, pancreatin, providing minimum of: protease 110 units, lipase 1900 units, amylase 1700 units. Net price 300-tab pack = £4.51. Label: 5, 25, counselling, see dose
Dose: ADULT and CHILD 5–15 tablets before meals
Tablets forte, e/c, s/c, pancreatin, providing minimum of: protease 330 units, lipase 5600 units, amylase 5000 units. Net price 300-tab pack = £13.74. Label: 5, 25, counselling, see dose
Dose: ADULT and CHILD 6–10 tablets before meals
Powder, pancreatin, providing minimum of: protease 1400 units, lipase 25 000 units, amylase 30 000 units/g. Net price 300 g = £24.28. Counselling, see dose
Dose: ADULT and CHILD 0.5–2 g with meals washed down or mixed with liquid; NEONATE 250–500 mg with each feed

■ **Higher-strength preparations**

The **CSM** has advised of data associating the high-strength pancreatin preparations *Nutrizym 22®* and *Pancreatin HL®* with the development of large bowel strictures (fibrosing colonopathy) in children with cystic fibrosis aged between 2 and 13 years. No association was found with *Creon® 25 000*. The following was recommended:

- *Pancrease HL®*, *Nutrizym 22®*, *Panzytrat® 25 000* [now discontinued] should not be used in children aged 15 years or less with cystic fibrosis;

- the total dose of pancreatic enzyme supplements used in patients with cystic fibrosis should not usually exceed 10 000 units of lipase per kg body-weight daily;

- if a patient on any pancreatin preparation develops new abdominal symptoms (or any change in existing abdominal symptoms) the patient should be reviewed to exclude the possibility of colonic damage.

Possible risk factors are gender (boys at greater risk than girls), more severe cystic fibrosis, and concomitant use of laxatives. The peak age for developing fibrosing colonopathy is between 2 and 8 years.

COUNSELLING. It is important to ensure adequate hydration at all times in patients receiving higher-strength pancreatin preparations.

Creon® 25 000 (Solvay) PoM
Capsules, orange/clear, enclosing brown-coloured e/c pellets of pancreatin, providing: protease (total) 1000 units, lipase 25 000 units, amylase 18 000 units, net price 100-cap pack = £39.00. Counselling, see above and under dose
Dose: ADULT and CHILD initially 1 capsule with meals either taken whole or contents mixed with fluid or soft food (then swallowed immediately without chewing)

Creon® 40 000 (Solvay) ▼ PoM
Capsules, brown/clear, enclosing brown-coloured e/c granules of pancreatin, providing: protease (total) 1600 units, lipase 40 000 units, amylase 25 000 units, net price 100-cap pack = £60.00. Counselling, see above and under dose
Dose: ADULT and CHILD initially 1–2 capsules with meals either taken whole or contents mixed with fluid or soft food (then swallowed immediately without chewing)

Nutrizym 22® (Merck) PoM
Capsules, red/yellow, enclosing e/c minitablets of pancreatin, providing minimum of: protease 1100 units, lipase 22 000 units, amylase

19 800 units. Net price 100-cap pack = £33.33.
Counselling, see above and under dose

Dose: 1–2 capsules with meals and 1 capsule with snacks,
swallowed whole or contents taken with water or
sprinkled on soft food (then swallowed immediately
without chewing)

CHILD under 15 years not recommended

Pancrease HL® (Janssen-Cilag) PoM

Capsules, enclosing light brown e/c minitablets of
pancreatin, providing minimum of: protease
1250 units, lipase 25 000 units, amylase
22 500 units. Net price 100 = £36.18. Counselling,
see above and under dose

Dose: 1–2 capsules during each meal and 1 capsule with
snacks swallowed whole or contents sprinkled on liquid
or soft food (then swallowed immediately without
chewing)

CHILD under 15 years not recommended

2: Cardiovascular system

2.1   Positive inotropic drugs

2.1.1   Cardiac glycosides
2.1.2   Phosphodiesterase inhibitors

Positive inotropic drugs increase the force of contraction of the myocardium; for sympathomimetics with inotropic activity see section 2.7.1.

2.1.1   Cardiac glycosides

Cardiac glycosides increase the force of myocardial contraction and reduce conductivity within the atrioventricular (AV) node. Digoxin is the most commonly used cardiac glycoside.

Cardiac glycosides are most useful in the treatment of supraventricular tachycardias, especially for controlling ventricular response in persistent atrial fibrillation (section 2.3.1). For reference to the role of digoxin in heart failure, see section 2.5.5.

For management of atrial fibrillation the maintenance dose of the cardiac glycoside can usually be determined by the ventricular rate at rest which should not be allowed to fall below 60 beats per minute except in special circumstances, e.g. with the concomitant administration of a beta-blocker.

Digoxin is now rarely used for rapid control of heart rate (see section 2.3 for the management of supraventricular arrhythmias). Even with intravenous administration, response may take many hours; persistence of tachycardia is therefore not an indication for exceeding the recommended dose. The intramuscular route is **not** recommended.

In patients with mild heart failure a loading dose is not required, and a satisfactory plasma-digoxin concentration can be achieved over a period of about a week, using a dose of digoxin 125 to 250 micrograms twice a day which is then reduced.

Digoxin has a long half-life and maintenance doses need to be given only once daily (although higher doses may be divided to avoid nausea). **Digitoxin** also has a long half-life and maintenance doses need to be given only once daily or on alternate days. Renal function is the most important determinant of digoxin dosage, whereas elimination of digitoxin depends on metabolism by the liver.

Unwanted effects depend both on the concentration of the cardiac glycoside in the plasma and on the sensitivity of the conducting system or of the myocardium, which is often increased in heart disease. Thus plasma concentration alone cannot indicate toxicity reliably but the likelihood of toxicity increases progressively through the range 1.5 to 3 micrograms/litre for digoxin. Cardiac glycosides should be used with special care in the elderly who may be particularly susceptible to digitalis toxicity.

Regular monitoring of plasma-digoxin concentration during maintenance treatment is not necessary unless problems occur. Care should be taken to avoid hypokalaemia if a diuretic is used with a cardiac glycoside because hypokalaemia predisposes the patient to digitalis toxicity. Hypokalaemia is managed by giving a potassium-sparing diuretic or, if necessary, potassium supplements (or foods rich in potassium).

Toxicity can often be managed by discontinuing digoxin and correcting hypokalaemia if appropriate; serious manifestations require urgent specialist management. **Digoxin-specific antibody fragments** are available for reversal of life-threatening overdosage (see below).

CHILDREN. The dose is based on body-weight; they require a relatively larger dose of digoxin than adults.

DIGOXIN

Indications: heart failure, supraventricular arrhythmias (particularly atrial fibrillation)

Cautions: recent infarction; sick sinus syndrome; thyroid disease; reduce dose in the elderly and in renal impairment; avoid hypokalaemia; avoid rapid intravenous administration (nausea and risk of arrhythmias); pregnancy (see also Appendix 4); **interactions:** Appendix 1 (cardiac glycosides)

Contra-indications: intermittent complete heart block, second degree AV block; supraventricular arrhythmias caused by Wolff-Parkinson-White syndrome; hypertrophic obstructive cardiomyopathy (unless concomitant atrial fibrillation and heart failure — but with caution)

Side-effects: usually associated with excessive dosage, include: anorexia, nausea, vomiting, diarrhoea, abdominal pain; visual disturbances, headache, fatigue, drowsiness, confusion, delirium, hallucinations, depression; arrhythmias, heart block; rarely rash, intestinal ischaemia; gynaecomastia on long-term use; thrombocytopenia reported; see also notes above

Dose: *by mouth*, rapid digitalisation, 1–1.5 mg in divided doses over 24 hours; less urgent digitalisation, 250–500 micrograms daily (higher dose may be divided)

Maintenance, 62.5–500 micrograms daily (higher dose may be divided) according to renal function and, in atrial fibrillation, on heart-rate response; usual range, 125–250 micrograms daily (lower dose may be appropriate in elderly)

Emergency loading dose *by intravenous infusion*, 0.75–1 mg over at least 2 hours (see also Cautions) then maintenance dose *by mouth* on the following day

NOTE. The above doses may need to be reduced if digoxin (or another cardiac glycoside) has been given in the preceding 2 weeks. Digoxin doses in the BNF may differ from those in product literature. For plasma concentration monitoring, blood should ideally be taken at least 6 hours after a dose

Digoxin (Non-proprietary) PoM
Tablets, digoxin 62.5 micrograms, net price 20 = 55p; 125 micrograms, 20 = 43p; 250 micrograms, 20 = 43p
Injection, digoxin 250 micrograms/mL, net price 2-mL amp = 70p
Available from Antigen
Paediatric injection, digoxin 100 micrograms/mL (hosp. only, available from BCM Specials)

Lanoxin® (GSK) PoM
Tablets, digoxin 125 micrograms, net price 20 = 32p; 250 micrograms (scored), 20 = 35p
Injection, digoxin 250 micrograms/mL. Net price 2-mL amp = 71p

Lanoxin-PG® (GSK) PoM
Tablets, blue, digoxin 62.5 micrograms. Net price 20 = 35p
Elixir, yellow, digoxin 50 micrograms/mL. Do not dilute, measure with pipette. Net price 60 mL = £5.75. Counselling, use of pipette

DIGITOXIN

Indications: heart failure, supraventricular arrhythmias (particularly atrial fibrillation)
Cautions: see under Digoxin but not necessary to reduce dose in mild to moderate renal impairment
Contra-indications: see under Digoxin
Side-effects: see under Digoxin
Dose: maintenance, 100 micrograms daily *or* on alternate days; may be increased to 200 micrograms daily if necessary

Digitoxin (Non-proprietary) PoM
Tablets, digitoxin 100 micrograms, net price 20 = £2.66

Digoxin-specific antibody

Digoxin-specific antibody fragments are indicated for the treatment of known or strongly suspected digoxin or digitoxin overdosage, where measures beyond the withdrawal of the cardiac glycoside and correction of any electrolyte abnormality are felt to be necessary (see also notes above).

Digibind® (GSK) PoM
Injection, powder for preparation of infusion, digoxin-specific antibody fragments (F(ab)) 38 mg. Net price per vial = £101.04 (hosp. and poisons centres only)
Dose: consult product literature

2.1.2 Phosphodiesterase inhibitors

Enoximone and **milrinone** are selective phosphodiesterase inhibitors which exert most of their effect on the myocardium. Sustained haemodynamic benefit has been observed after administration, but there is no evidence of any beneficial effect on survival.

ENOXIMONE

Indications: congestive heart failure where cardiac output reduced and filling pressures increased

Cautions: heart failure associated with hypertrophic cardiomyopathy, stenotic or obstructive valvular disease or other outlet obstruction; monitor blood pressure, heart rate, ECG, central venous pressure, fluid and electrolyte status, renal function, platelet count, hepatic enzymes; renal impairment (Appendix 3); avoid extravasation; pregnancy and breast-feeding

Side-effects: ectopic beats; less frequently ventricular tachycardia or supraventricular arrhythmias (more likely in patients with pre-existing arrhythmias); hypotension; also headache, insomnia, nausea and vomiting, diarrhoea; occasionally, chills, oliguria, fever, urinary retention; upper and lower limb pain

Dose: *by slow intravenous injection* (rate not exceeding 12.5 mg/minute), diluted before use, initially 0.5–1 mg/kg, then 500 micrograms/kg every 30 minutes until satisfactory response or total of 3 mg/kg given; maintenance, initial dose of up to 3 mg/kg may be repeated every 3–6 hours as required

By intravenous infusion, initially 90 micrograms/kg/minute over 10–30 minutes, followed by continuous or intermittent infusion of 5–20 micrograms/kg/minute

Total dose over 24 hours should not usually exceed 24 mg/kg

Perfan® (Myogen) ▭PoM▭
Injection, enoximone 5 mg/mL. For dilution before use. Net price 20-mL amp = £15.02
Excipients: include alcohol, propylene glycol
NOTE. Plastic apparatus should be used; crystal formation if glass used

MILRINONE

Indications: short-term treatment of severe congestive heart failure unresponsive to conventional maintenance therapy (not immediately after myocardial infarction); acute heart failure, including low output states, following heart surgery

Cautions: see under Enoximone; also correct hypokalaemia, monitor renal function

Side-effects: see under Enoximone; also chest pain, tremor, bronchospasm, anaphylaxis and rash reported

Dose: *by intravenous injection* over 10 minutes, diluted before use, 50 micrograms/kg followed by *intravenous infusion* at a rate of 375–750 nanograms/kg/minute, usually for up to 12 hours following surgery or for 48–72 hours in congestive heart failure; max. daily dose 1.13 mg/kg

Primacor® (Sanofi-Synthelabo) ▭PoM▭
Injection, milrinone (as lactate) 1 mg/mL. For dilution before use. Net price 10-mL amp = £16.61

2.2   Diuretics

2.2.1	Thiazides and related diuretics
2.2.2	Loop diuretics
2.2.3	Potassium-sparing diuretics
2.2.4	Potassium-sparing diuretics with other diuretics
2.2.5	Osmotic diuretics
2.2.6	Mercurial diuretics
2.2.7	Carbonic anhydrase inhibitors
2.2.8	Diuretics with potassium

Thiazides (section 2.2.1) are used to relieve oedema due to chronic heart failure (section 2.5.5) and, in lower doses, to reduce blood pressure.

Loop diuretics (section 2.2.2) are used in pulmonary oedema due to left ventricular failure and in patients with chronic heart failure (section 2.5.5).

Combination diuretic therapy may be effective in patients with oedema resistant to treatment with one diuretic. Vigorous diuresis, particularly with loop diuretics, may induce acute hypotension; rapid reduction of plasma volume should be avoided.

ELDERLY. Lower initial doses of diuretics should be used in the elderly because they are particularly susceptible to the side-effects. The dose should then be adjusted according to renal function. Diuretics should not be used continuously on a long-term basis to treat simple gravitational oedema (which will usually respond to increased movement, raising the legs, and support stockings).

POTASSIUM LOSS. Hypokalaemia may occur with both thiazide and loop diuretics. The risk of hypokalaemia depends on the duration of action as well as the potency and is thus greater with thiazides than with an equipotent dose of a loop diuretic.

Hypokalaemia is dangerous in severe coronary artery disease and in patients also being treated with cardiac glycosides. Often the use of potassium-sparing diuretics (section 2.2.3) avoids the need to take potassium supplements.

In hepatic failure hypokalaemia caused by diuretics can precipitate encephalopathy, particularly in alcoholic cirrhosis; diuretics may also increase the risk of hypomagnesaemia in alcoholic cirrhosis, leading to arrhythmias.

Potassium supplements are seldom necessary when thiazides are used in the routine treatment of hypertension (see also section 9.2.1.1).

2.2.1   Thiazides and related diuretics

Thiazides and related compounds are moderately potent diuretics; they inhibit sodium reabsorption at the beginning of the distal convoluted tubule. They act within 1 to 2 hours of oral administration and most have a duration of action of 12 to 24 hours; they are usually administered early in the day so that the diuresis does not interfere with sleep.

In the management of *hypertension* a low dose of a thiazide, e.g. bendroflumethiazide (bendrofluazide) 2.5 mg daily, produces a maximal or near-maximal blood pressure lowering effect, with very little biochemical disturbance. Higher doses cause more marked changes in plasma potassium, uric acid, glucose, and lipids, with no advantage in blood pressure control, and should not be used. For reference to the use of thiazides in chronic heart failure see section 2.5.5.

Bendroflumethiazide (bendrofluazide) is widely used for mild or moderate heart failure and for hypertension—alone in the treatment of mild hypertension or with other drugs in more severe hypertension.

Chlortalidone (chlorthalidone), a thiazide-related compound, has a longer duration of action than the thiazides and may be given on alternate days to control oedema. It is also useful if acute retention is liable to be precipitated by a more rapid diuresis or if patients dislike the altered pattern of micturition promoted by other diuretics.

Other thiazide diuretics (including benzthiazide, clopamide, cyclopenthiazide, hydrochlorothiazide and hydroflumethiazide) do not offer any significant advantage over bendroflumethiazide and chlortalidone.

Metolazone is particularly effective when combined with a loop diuretic (even in renal failure); profound diuresis may occur and the patient should therefore be monitored carefully.

Xipamide and **indapamide** are chemically related to chlortalidone. Indapamide is claimed to lower blood pressure with less metabolic disturbance, particularly less aggravation of diabetes mellitus.

BENDROFLUMETHIAZIDE
(Bendrofluazide)

Indications: oedema, hypertension (see also notes above)

Cautions: may cause hypokalaemia, aggravates diabetes and gout; may exacerbate systemic lupus erythematosus; elderly; pregnancy (Appendix 4) and breast-feeding; hepatic and renal impairment (avoid if severe, see Appendixes 2 and 3); see also notes above; porphyria (section 9.8.2); **interactions:** Appendix 1 (diuretics)

Contra-indications: refractory hypokalaemia, hyponatraemia, hypercalcaemia; severe renal and hepatic impairment; symptomatic hyperuricaemia; Addison's disease

Side-effects: postural hypotension and mild gastrointestinal effects; impotence (reversible on withdrawal of treatment); hypokalaemia (see also notes above), hypomagnesaemia, hyponatraemia, hypercalcaemia, hypochloraemic alkalosis, hyperuricaemia, gout, hyperglycaemia, and altered plasma lipid concentration; less commonly rashes, photosensitivity; blood disorders (including neutropenia and thrombocytopenia—when given in late pregnancy neonatal thrombocytopenia has been reported); pancreatitis, intrahepatic cholestasis, and hypersensitivity reactions (including pneumonitis, pulmonary oedema, severe skin reactions) also reported

Dose: oedema, initially 5–10 mg in the morning, daily *or* on alternate days; maintenance 5–10 mg 1–3 times weekly

Hypertension, 2.5 mg in the morning; higher doses rarely necessary (see notes above)

Bendroflumethiazide (Non-proprietary) PoM
Tablets, bendroflumethiazide 2.5 mg, net price 20 = 53p; 5 mg, 20 = 52p
Available from Alpharma, APS, Generics, Goldshield (*Neo-NaClex®*, 5 mg only), Hillcross, IVAX, Sovereign (*Aprinox®*)

CHLORTALIDONE
(Chlorthalidone)

Indications: ascites due to cirrhosis in stable patients (under close supervision), oedema due to nephrotic syndrome, hypertension (see also notes above), mild to moderate chronic heart failure; diabetes insipidus (see section 6.5.2)

Cautions: see under Bendroflumethiazide

Contra-indications: see under Bendroflumethiazide

Side-effects: see under Bendroflumethiazide

Dose: oedema, up to 50 mg daily for limited period
Hypertension, 25 mg in the morning, increased to 50 mg if necessary (but see notes above)
Heart failure, 25–50 mg in the morning, increased if necessary to 100–200 mg daily

Hygroton® (Alliance) PoM
Tablets, yellow, scored, chlortalidone 50 mg, net price 28-tab pack = £1.68

CYCLOPENTHIAZIDE

Indications: oedema, hypertension (see also notes above)

Cautions: see under Bendroflumethiazide

Contra-indications: see under Bendroflumethiazide

Side-effects: see under Bendroflumethiazide

Dose: heart failure, 250–500 micrograms daily in the morning increased if necessary to 1 mg daily (reduce to lowest effective dose for maintenance)
Hypertension, initially 250 micrograms daily in the morning, increased if necessary to 500 micrograms daily (but see notes above)
Oedema, up to 500 micrograms daily for a short period

Navidrex® (Goldshield) PoM
Tablets, scored, cyclopenthiazide 500 micrograms. Net price 28-tab pack = £1.27
Excipients: include gluten

INDAPAMIDE

Indications: essential hypertension

Cautions: renal impairment (stop if deterioration); monitor plasma potassium and urate concentrations in elderly, hyperaldosteronism, gout, or with concomitant cardiac glycosides; hyperparathyroidism (discontinue if hypercalcaemia); pregnancy and breast-feeding; **interactions:** Appendix 1 (diuretics)

Contra-indications: severe hepatic impairment

Side-effects: hypokalaemia, headache, dizziness, fatigue, muscular cramps, nausea, anorexia, diarrhoea, constipation, dyspepsia, rashes (erythema multiforme, epidermal necrolysis reported); rarely postural hypotension, palpitations, increase in liver enzymes, blood disorders (including thrombocytopenia), hyponatraemia, metabolic alkalosis, hyperglycaemia, increased plasma urate concentrations, paraesthesia, photosensitivity, impotence, renal impairment, reversible acute myopia; diuresis with doses above 2.5 mg daily

Dose: 2.5 mg in the morning

Indapamide (Non-proprietary) [PoM]
Tablets, s/c, indapamide 2.5 mg, net price 28-tab
pack = £2.82, 56-tab pack = £5.10
Available from Alpharma, APS, Ashbourne (*Nindaxa
2.5®*), Hillcross, IVAX, Niche, Sterwin

Natrilix® (Servier) [PoM]
Tablets, f/c, indapamide 2.5 mg. Net price 30-tab
pack = £4.27, 60-tab pack = £8.45

▪ Modified release
Natrilix SR® (Servier) [PoM]
Tablets, m/r, indapamide 1.5 mg. Net price 30-tab
pack = £4.79. Label: 25
Dose: hypertension, 1 tablet daily, preferably in the
morning

METOLAZONE
Indications: oedema, hypertension (see also notes
above)
Cautions: see under Bendroflumethiazide; also
profound diuresis on concomitant administration
with furosemide (monitor patient carefully)
Contra-indications: see under Bendroflumethiazide
Side-effects: see under Bendroflumethiazide
Dose: oedema, 5–10 mg in the morning, increased if
necessary to 20 mg daily in resistant oedema, max.
80 mg daily
Hypertension, initially 5 mg in the morning; maintenance 5 mg on alternate days

Metenix 5® (Borg) [PoM]
Tablets, blue, metolazone 5 mg. Net price 100-tab
pack = £20.37

XIPAMIDE
Indications: oedema, hypertension (see also notes
above)
Cautions: see under Bendroflumethiazide
Contra-indications: see under Bendroflumethiazide
Side-effects: gastro-intestinal disturbances; mild
dizziness; hypokalaemia, more rarely other
electrolyte disturbances such as hyponatraemia
Dose: oedema, initially 40 mg in the morning,
increased to 80 mg in resistant cases; maintenance
20 mg in the morning
Hypertension, 20 mg in the morning

Diurexan® (Viatris) [PoM]
Tablets, scored, xipamide 20 mg. Net price 140-tab
pack = £20.92

2.2.2 Loop diuretics

Loop diuretics are used in pulmonary oedema due to
left ventricular failure; intravenous administration
produces relief of breathlessness and reduces pre-
load sooner than would be expected from the time of
onset of diuresis. Loop diuretics are also used in
patients with chronic heart failure. Diuretic-resistant
oedema (except lymphoedema and oedema due to
peripheral venous stasis or calcium-channel blockers) can be treated with a loop diuretic combined
with a thiazide or related diuretic (e.g. bendroflumethiazide 5–10 mg daily or metolazone 5–20 mg
daily).

A loop diuretic is sometimes used to lower blood
pressure especially in hypertension resistant to
thiazide therapy.
Loop diuretics inhibit reabsorption from the
ascending limb of the loop of Henlé in the renal
tubule and are powerful diuretics. Hypokalaemia
may develop, and care is needed to avoid hypotension. If there is an enlarged prostate, urinary
retention may occur; this is less likely if small doses
and less potent diuretics are used initially.
Furosemide (frusemide) and **bumetanide** are
similar in activity; both act within 1 hour of oral
administration and diuresis is complete within 6
hours so that, if necessary, they can be given twice in
one day without interfering with sleep. Following
intravenous administration they have a peak effect
within 30 minutes. The diuresis associated with these
drugs is dose related. In patients with impaired renal
function very large doses may occasionally be
needed; in such doses both drugs can cause deafness
and bumetanide can cause myalgia.
Torasemide has properties similar to those of
furosemide and bumetanide, and is indicated for
oedema and for hypertension.

FUROSEMIDE
(Frusemide)
Indications: oedema (see notes above), oliguria due
to renal failure
Cautions: pregnancy and breast-feeding; hypotension; correct hypovolaemia before using in
oliguria; liver failure, prostatic enlargement; porphyria (section 9.8.2); although manufacturer
advises that rate of intravenous administration
should not exceed 4 mg/minute, single doses of
up to 80 mg may be administered more rapidly;
interactions: Appendix 1 (diuretics)
Contra-indications: precomatose states associated
with liver cirrhosis; renal failure with anuria
Side-effects: hyponatraemia, hypokalaemia, and
hypomagnesaemia (see also section 2.2), hypochloraemic alkalosis, increased calcium excretion,
hypotension; less commonly nausea, gastro-intestinal disturbances, hyperuricaemia and gout;
hyperglycaemia (less common than with thiazides); temporary increase in plasma cholesterol
and triglyceride concentrations; rarely rashes,
photosensitivity and bone marrow depression
(withdraw treatment), pancreatitis (with large parenteral doses), tinnitus and deafness (usually with
large parenteral doses and rapid administration and
in renal impairment)
Dose: *by mouth*, oedema, initially 40 mg in the
morning; maintenance 20–40 mg daily, increased
in resistant oedema to 80 mg daily or more; CHILD
1–3 mg/kg daily, max. 40 mg daily
Oliguria, initially 250 mg daily; if necessary larger
doses, increasing in steps of 250 mg, may be given
every 4–6 hours to a max. of a single dose of 2 g
(rarely used)
*By intramuscular injection or slow intravenous
injection* (see Cautions, above), initially 20–
50 mg; CHILD 0.5–1.5 mg/kg to a max. daily dose
of 20 mg
By intravenous infusion (by syringe pump if necessary), in oliguria, initially 250 mg over 1 hour (rate
not exceeding 4 mg/minute), if satisfactory urine
output not obtained in the subsequent hour further
500 mg over 2 hours, then if no satisfactory

response within subsequent hour, further 1 g over 4 hours, if no response obtained dialysis probably required; effective dose (up to 1 g) can be repeated every 24 hours

Furosemide (Non-proprietary) PoM
Tablets, furosemide 20 mg, net price 20 = 46p; 40 mg, 28-tab pack = 78p; 500 mg, 20 = £6.44
Various strengths available from Alpharma, APS, Ashbourne (*Froop®*), CP (including *Rusyde®*), Generics, Hillcross, IVAX, Sovereign
Oral solution, sugar-free, furosemide, net price 4 mg/mL, 150 mL = £12.84; 8 mg/mL, 150 mL = £16.57; 10 mg/mL, 150 mL = £17.91
Available from Rosemont (*Frusol®*)
Injection, furosemide 10 mg/mL, net price 2-mL amp = 55p
Available from Antigen, Celltech, Phoenix (all as 5-mL amp)

Lasix® (Celltech) PoM
Tablets, all scored, furosemide 20 mg, net price 28-tab pack = £1.57; 40 mg, 28-tab pack = £2.27; 500 mg (yellow), 20 = £21.74
Paediatric liquid, sugar-free, furosemide 1 mg/mL when reconstituted with purified water, freshly boiled and cooled, net price 150 mL = £3.68
Injection, furosemide 10 mg/mL, net price 2-mL amp = 84p
NOTE. Large volume furosemide injections available from Antigen, Celltech (*Minijet®*)

BUMETANIDE

Indications: oedema (see notes above), oliguria due to renal failure
Cautions: see under Furosemide (but has been used in porphyria, see section 9.8.2)
Contra-indications: see under Furosemide
Side-effects: see under Furosemide; also myalgia
Dose: *by mouth*, 1 mg in the morning, repeated after 6–8 hours if necessary; severe cases, increased up to 5 mg or more daily
ELDERLY, 500 micrograms daily may be sufficient
By intravenous injection, 1–2 mg, repeated after 20 minutes; when *intramuscular injection* considered necessary, 1 mg initially then adjusted according to response
By intravenous infusion, 2–5 mg over 30–60 minutes

Bumetanide (Non-proprietary) PoM
Tablets, bumetanide 1 mg, net price 28-tab pack = £1.69; 5 mg, 28-tab pack = £11.14
Available from Alpharma, APS, CP, Generics, Hillcross, IVAX
Liquid, bumetanide 1 mg/5 mL, net price 150 mL = £9.51
Available from Leo
Injection, bumetanide 500 micrograms/mL, net price 4-mL amp = £1.79
Available from Leo

Burinex® (Leo) PoM
Tablets, both scored, bumetanide 1 mg, net price 28-tab pack = £1.64; 5 mg, 28 = £10.45

TORASEMIDE

Indications: oedema (see notes above), hypertension
Cautions: see under Furosemide
Contra-indications: see under Furosemide; pregnancy and breast-feeding
Side-effects: see under Furosemide; also dry mouth; rarely limb paraesthesia

Dose: oedema, 5 mg once daily, preferably in the morning, increased if required to 20 mg once daily; usual max. 40 mg daily
Hypertension, 2.5 mg daily, increased if necessary to 5 mg once daily

Torasemide (Non-proprietary) PoM
Tablets, torasemide 5 mg, net price 28-tab pack = £5.94; 10 mg, 28-tab pack = £8.74
Available from PLIVA

Torem® (Roche) PoM
Tablets, torasemide 2.5 mg, net price 28-tab pack = £4.06; 5 mg (scored), 28-tab pack = £5.95; 10 mg (scored), 28-tab pack = £8.75

2.2.3   Potassium-sparing diuretics

Amiloride and **triamterene** on their own are weak diuretics. They cause retention of potassium and are therefore used as a more effective alternative to giving potassium supplements with thiazide or loop diuretics. (See section 2.2.4 for compound preparations with thiazides or loop diuretics.)

Spironolactone is also a potassium-sparing diuretic, and potentiates thiazide or loop diuretics by antagonising aldosterone. It is of value in the treatment of the oedema of cirrhosis of the liver. Low doses of spironolactone are beneficial in severe heart failure, see section 2.5.5.

Spironolactone is also used in primary hyperaldosteronism (Conn's syndrome). It is given before surgery or if surgery is not appropriate, in the lowest effective dose for maintenance.

Potassium supplements must **not** be given with potassium-sparing diuretics. It is also important to bear in mind that administration of a potassium-sparing diuretic to a patient receiving an ACE inhibitor can cause severe hyperkalaemia.

AMILORIDE HYDROCHLORIDE

Indications: oedema, potassium conservation with thiazide and loop diuretics
Cautions: pregnancy and breast-feeding; monitor in renal impairment (avoid if moderate to severe, see also Appendix 3); diabetes mellitus; elderly; **interactions:** Appendix 1 (diuretics)
Contra-indications: hyperkalaemia, renal failure
Side-effects: include gastro-intestinal disturbances, dry mouth, rashes, confusion, postural hypotension, hyperkalaemia, hyponatraemia
Dose: used alone, initially 10 mg daily *or* 5 mg twice daily, adjusted according to response; max. 20 mg daily
With other diuretics, congestive heart failure and hypertension, initially 5–10 mg daily; cirrhosis with ascites, initially 5 mg daily

Amiloride (Non-proprietary) PoM
Tablets, amiloride hydrochloride 5 mg, net price 20 = £1.08
Available from Alpharma, APS, CP, Hillcross, IVAX
Oral solution, sugar-free, amiloride hydrochloride 5 mg/5 mL, net price 150 mL = £39.73
Available from Rosemont (*Amilamont®*)

■ Compound preparations with thiazide or loop diuretics
See section 2.2.4

TRIAMTERENE

Indications: oedema, potassium conservation with thiazide and loop diuretics

Cautions: see under Amiloride Hydrochloride; may cause blue fluorescence of urine

Contra-indications: see under Amiloride Hydrochloride

Side-effects: include gastro-intestinal disturbances, dry mouth, rashes; slight decrease in blood pressure, hyperkalaemia, hyponatraemia; photosensitivity and blood disorders also reported; triamterene found in kidney stones

Dose: initially 150–250 mg daily, reducing to alternate days after 1 week; taken in divided doses after breakfast and lunch; lower initial dose when given with other diuretics

COUNSELLING. Urine may look slightly blue in some lights

Dytac® (Goldshield) PoM

Capsules, maroon, triamterene 50 mg. Net price 30-cap pack = £17.35 Label: 14, (see above), 21

■ Compound preparations with thiazides or loop diuretics

See section 2.2.4

Aldosterone antagonists

SPIRONOLACTONE

Indications: oedema and ascites in cirrhosis of the liver, malignant ascites, nephrotic syndrome, congestive heart failure (section 2.5.5); primary hyperaldosteronism

Cautions: potential metabolic products carcinogenic in *rodents*; elderly; hepatic impairment; renal impairment (avoid if moderate to severe; Appendix 3); monitor electrolytes (discontinue if hyperkalaemia); porphyria (section 9.8.2); **interactions:** Appendix 1 (diuretics)

Contra-indications: hyperkalaemia, hyponatraemia; pregnancy and breast-feeding; Addison's disease

Side-effects: gastro-intestinal disturbances; impotence, gynaecomastia; menstrual irregularities; lethargy, headache, confusion; rashes; hyperkalaemia (discontinue); hyponatraemia; hepatotoxicity, osteomalacia, and blood disorders reported

Dose: 100–200 mg daily, increased to 400 mg if required; CHILD initially 3 mg/kg daily in divided doses

Heart failure, see section 2.5.5

Spironolactone (Non-proprietary) PoM

Tablets, spironolactone 25 mg, net price 20 = £1.50; 50 mg, 20 = £3.21; 100 mg, 20 = £3.31

Available from Alpharma, APS, Ashbourne (*Spirospare®*), Hillcross, IVAX

Oral suspensions, sugar-free, spironolactone 5 mg/5 mL, 10 mg/5 mL, 25 mg/5 mL, 50 mg/5 mL and 100 mg/5 mL available from Rosemont (special order)

Aldactone® (Searle) PoM

Tablets, all f/c, spironolactone 25 mg (buff), net price 100-tab pack = £8.89; 50 mg (off-white), 100-tab pack = £17.78; 100 mg (buff), 28-tab pack = £9.96

■ With thiazides or loop diuretics

See section 2.2.4

2.2.4 Potassium-sparing diuretics with other diuretics

Although it is preferable to prescribe thiazides (section 2.2.1) and potassium-sparing diuretics (section 2.2.3) separately, the use of fixed combinations may be justified if compliance is a problem. Potassium-sparing diuretics are not usually necessary in the routine treatment of hypertension, unless hypokalaemia develops. For **interactions**, see Appendix 1 (diuretics).

■ Amiloride with thiazides

Co-amilozide (Non-proprietary) PoM

Tablets, co-amilozide 2.5/25 (amiloride hydrochloride 2.5 mg, hydrochlorothiazide 25 mg), net price 28-tab pack = £1.85

Available from CP, Bristol-Myers Squibb (*Moduret 25®*)

Dose: hypertension, initially 1 tablet daily, increased if necessary to max. 2 tablets daily

Congestive heart failure, initially 1 tablet daily, increased if necessary to max. 4 tablets daily

Oedema and ascites in cirrhosis of the liver, initially 2 tablets daily, increased if necessary to max. 4 tablets daily; reduce for maintenance if possible

Tablets, co-amilozide 5/50 (amiloride hydrochloride 5 mg, hydrochlorothiazide 50 mg), net price 28 = £1.99

Available from Alpharma, APS, CP, Bristol-Myers Squibb (*Moduretic®*), Hillcross, IVAX (*Amil-Co®*)

Dose: hypertension, initially ½ tablet daily, increased if necessary to max. 1 tablet daily

Congestive heart failure, initially ½ tablet daily, increased if necessary to max. 1 tablet daily

Oedema and ascites in cirrhosis of the liver, initially 1 tablet daily, increased if necessary to max. 2 tablets daily; reduce for maintenance if possible

Navispare® (Novartis) PoM

Tablets, f/c, orange, amiloride hydrochloride 2.5 mg, cyclopenthiazide 250 micrograms. Net price 28-tab pack = £2.25

Excipients: include gluten

Dose: hypertension, 1–2 tablets in the morning

■ Amiloride with loop diuretics

Co-amilofruse (Non-proprietary) PoM

Tablets, co-amilofruse 2.5/20 (amiloride hydrochloride 2.5 mg, furosemide 20 mg). Net price 28-tab pack = £4.42, 56-tab pack = £3.12

Available from Alpharma, CP, Helios (*Frumil LS®*), Sandoz

Dose: oedema, 1 tablet in the morning

Tablets, co-amilofruse 5/40 (amiloride hydrochloride 5 mg, furosemide 40 mg). Net price 28-tab pack = £2.58

Available from Alpharma, APS, Ashbourne (*Froop-Co®*), Borg (*Lasoride®*), CP, Helios (*Frumil®*), Hillcross, IVAX (*Fru-Co®*), Sandoz, Sovereign

Dose: oedema, 1–2 tablets in the morning

Tablets, co-amilofruse 10/80 (amiloride hydrochloride 10 mg, furosemide 80 mg). Net price 28-tab pack = £7.46, 56-tab pack = £21.56

Available from CP (*Aridil®*), Helios (*Frumil Forte®*)

Dose: oedema, 1 tablet in the morning

Burinex A® (Leo) [PoM]
Tablets, ivory, scored, amiloride hydrochloride
5 mg, bumetanide 1 mg. Net price 28-tab pack =
£3.06
Dose: oedema, 1–2 tablets daily

■ Triamterene with thiazides
COUNSELLING. Urine may look slightly blue in some lights
Co-triamterzide (Non-proprietary) [PoM]
Tablets, co-triamterzide 50/25 (triamterene 50 mg,
hydrochlorothiazide 25 mg), net price 30-tab pack
= £1.75. Label: 14, (see above), 21
Dose: hypertension, 1 tablet daily after breakfast,
increased if necessary, max. 4 daily
Oedema, 2 tablets daily (1 after breakfast and 1 after
midday meal) increased to 3 daily if necessary (2 after
breakfast and 1 after midday meal); usual maintenance in
oedema, 1 daily or 2 on alternate days; max. 4 daily
Available from Ashbourne (*TriamaxCo*®), IVAX (*Triam-
Co*®)

Dyazide® (Goldshield) [PoM]
Tablets, peach, scored, co-triamterzide 50/25
(triamterene 50 mg, hydrochlorothiazide 25 mg).
Net price 30-tab pack = £1.75. Label: 14, (see
above), 21
Dose: hypertension, 1 tablet daily after breakfast,
increased if necessary, max. 4 daily
Oedema, 2 tablets daily (1 after breakfast and 1 after
midday meal) increased to 3 daily if necessary (2 after
breakfast and 1 after midday meal); usual maintenance in
oedema, 1 daily or 2 on alternate days; max. 4 daily

Dytide® (Goldshield) [PoM]
Capsules, clear/maroon, triamterene 50 mg, benzthiazide 25 mg. Net price 30-cap pack = £17.35.
Label: 14, (see above), 21
Dose: oedema, initially 3 capsules daily (2 after breakfast
and 1 after midday meal) for 1 week then 1 or 2 on
alternate days

Kalspare® (PLIVA) [PoM]
Tablets, orange, f/c, scored, triamterene 50 mg,
chlortalidone 50 mg. Net price 28-tab pack = £3.05.
Label: 14, (see above), 21
Dose: hypertension, oedema, 1–2 tablets in the morning

■ Triamterene with loop diuretics
COUNSELLING. Urine may look slightly blue in some lights
Frusene® (Orion) [PoM]
Tablets, yellow, scored, triamterene 50 mg, furose-
mide 40 mg. Net price 56-tab pack = £4.54.
Label: 14, (see above), 21
Dose: oedema, ½–2 tablets daily in the morning

■ Spironolactone with thiazides
Co-flumactone (Non-proprietary) [PoM] ▱
Tablets, co-flumactone 25/25 (hydroflumethiazide
25 mg, spironolactone 25 mg). Net price 100-tab
pack = £20.23
Available from Searle (*Aldactide 25*®)
Dose: congestive heart failure, initially 4 tablets daily;
range 1–8 daily (but not recommended because spironolactone generally given in lower dose)
Tablets, co-flumactone 50/50 (hydroflumethiazide
50 mg, spironolactone 50 mg). Net price 28-tab
pack = £10.70
Available from Searle (*Aldactide 50*®)
Dose: congestive heart failure, initially 2 tablets daily;
range 1–4 daily (but not recommended because spironolactone generally given in lower dose)

■ Spironolactone with loop diuretics
Lasilactone® (Borg) [PoM]
Capsules, blue/white, spironolactone 50 mg, furo-
semide 20 mg. Net price 28-cap pack = £8.91
Dose: resistant oedema, 1–4 capsules daily

2.2.5   Osmotic diuretics

Osmotic diuretics are rarely used in heart failure as
they may acutely expand the blood volume. **Mannitol** is used in cerebral oedema—a typical dose is 1 g/
kg as a 20% solution given by rapid intravenous
infusion.

MANNITOL

Indications: see notes above; glaucoma (section
11.6)
Cautions: extravasation causes inflammation and
thrombophlebitis
Contra-indications: congestive cardiac failure,
pulmonary oedema
Side-effects: chills, fever
Dose: *by intravenous infusion*, diuresis, 50–200 g
over 24 hours, preceded by a test dose of 200 mg/
kg by slow intravenous injection
Cerebral oedema, see notes above

Mannitol (Non-proprietary) [PoM]
Intravenous infusion, mannitol 10% and 20%
Available from Baxter

2.2.6   Mercurial diuretics

Mercurial diuretics are effective but are now almost
never used because of their nephrotoxicity.

2.2.7   Carbonic anhydrase inhibitors

The carbonic anhydrase inhibitor **acetazolamide** is a
weak diuretic and is little used for its diuretic effect.
It is used for prophylaxis against mountain sickness
[unlicensed indication] but is not a substitute for
acclimatisation.
   Acetazolamide and eye drops of dorzolamide and
brinzolamide inhibit the formation of aqueous
humour and are used in glaucoma (section 11.6).

2.2.8   Diuretics with potassium

Many patients on diuretics do not need potassium
supplements (section 9.2.1.1). For many of those
who do, the amount of potassium in combined
preparations may not be enough, and for this reason
their use is to be discouraged.
   Diuretics with potassium and potassium-sparing
diuretics should **not** usually be given together.
COUNSELLING. Modified-release potassium tablets should
be swallowed whole with plenty of fluid during meals while
sitting or standing

Burinex K® (Leo) [PoM] ▱
Tablets, bumetanide 500 micrograms, potassium
7.7 mmol for modified release. Net price 20 = 80p.
Label: 25, 27, counselling, see above

Centyl K® (Leo) PoM ◾️◤
Tablets, green, s/c, bendroflumethiazide 2.5 mg, potassium 7.7 mmol for modified release, net price 56-tab pack = £7.50. Label: 25, 27, counselling, see above

Lasikal® (Borg) PoM ◾️◤
Tablets, white/yellow, f/c, furosemide 20 mg, potassium 10 mmol for modified release. Net price 100-tab pack = £15.21. Label: 25, 27, counselling, see above

Neo-NaClex-K® (Goldshield) PoM ◾️◤
Tablets, pink/white, f/c, bendroflumethiazide 2.5 mg, potassium 8.4 mmol for modified release. Net price 20 = £1.59. Label: 25, 27, counselling, see above

2.3   Anti-arrhythmic drugs

2.3.1   Management of arrhythmias
2.3.2   Drugs for arrhythmias

2.3.1   Management of arrhythmias

Management of an arrhythmia requires precise diagnosis of the type of arrhythmia, and electro-cardiography is essential; underlying causes such as heart failure require appropriate treatment.

ECTOPIC BEATS. If spontaneous with a normal heart, ectopic beats rarely require treatment beyond reassurance. If they are particularly troublesome, beta-blockers are sometimes effective and may be safer than other suppressant drugs.

ATRIAL FIBRILLATION. The ventricular rate in atrial fibrillation can be controlled with a beta-blocker, or diltiazem [unlicensed indication], or verapamil. Digoxin is usually effective for controlling the rate at rest; it is also appropriate if atrial fibrillation is accompanied by congestive heart failure. If the rate at rest or during exercise cannot be controlled, diltiazem or verapamil may be combined with digoxin, but care is required if the ventricular function is diminished. In some cases, e.g. acute atrial fibrillation or paroxysmal atrial fibrillation, diltiazem or verapamil or a beta-blocker may be more effective than digoxin (see also Paroxysmal Supraventricular Tachycardia and Supraventricular Arrhythmias below). Anticoagulants are indicated especially in valvular or myocardial disease, and in the elderly; in the very elderly the overall benefit and risk needs careful assessment. Younger patients with lone atrial fibrillation in the absence of heart disease probably do not need anticoagulation. Aspirin is less effective than warfarin at preventing emboli but may be appropriate if there are no other risk factors for stroke; aspirin 75 mg may be used.

ATRIAL FLUTTER. The ventricular rate at rest can sometimes be controlled with digoxin. Reversion to sinus rhythm (if indicated) may be achieved by appropriately synchronised d.c. shock. Alternatively, amiodarone may be used to restore sinus rhythm, and amiodarone or sotalol to maintain it. If the arrhythmia is long-standing a period of treatment with anticoagulants should be considered before cardioversion to avoid the complication of emboli.

PAROXYSMAL SUPRAVENTRICULAR TACHYCARDIA. In most patients this remits spontaneously or can be returned to sinus rhythm by reflex vagal stimulation with respiratory manoeuvres, prompt squatting, or pressure over one carotid sinus (**important:** pressure over carotid sinus should be restricted to monitored patients—it can be dangerous in recent ischaemia, digitalis toxicity, or the elderly).

If vagal stimulation fails, intravenous administration of adenosine is usually the treatment of choice. Intravenous administration of verapamil is useful for patients without myocardial or valvular disease (**important:** never in patients recently treated with beta-blockers, see p. 106). For arrhythmias that are poorly tolerated, synchronised d.c. shock usually provides rapid relief.

In cases of paroxysmal supraventricular tachycardia with block, digitalis toxicity should be suspected. In addition to stopping administration of the cardiac glycoside and giving potassium supplements, intravenous administration of a beta-blocker may be useful. Specific digoxin antibody is available if the toxicity is considered life-threatening (section 2.1.1).

ARRHYTHMIAS AFTER MYOCARDIAL INFARCTION. In patients with a paroxysmal tachycardia or rapid irregularity of the pulse it is best not to administer an antiarrhythmic until an ECG record has been obtained. Bradycardia, particularly if complicated by hypotension, should be treated with atropine sulphate, given intravenously in a dose of 0.3–1 mg. If the initial dose is effective it may be repeated if necessary.

VENTRICULAR TACHYCARDIA. Drug treatment is used both for the treatment of ventricular tachycardia and for prophylaxis of recurrent attacks that merit suppression. Ventricular tachycardia requires treatment most commonly in the acute stage of myocardial infarction, but the likelihood of this and other life-threatening arrhythmias diminishes sharply over the first 24 hours after the attack, especially in patients without heart failure or shock. Lidocaine (lignocaine) is the preferred drug for emergency use. Other drugs are best administered under specialist supervision. Very rapid ventricular tachycardia causes profound circulatory collapse and should be treated urgently with d.c. shock.

Torsades de pointes is a special form of ventricular tachycardia which tends to occur in the presence of a long QT interval (usually drug induced, but other factors including hypokalaemia, severe bradycardia, and genetic predisposition may also be implicated). The episodes are usually self-limiting, but are frequently recurrent and may cause impairment (or loss) of consciousness. If not controlled, the arrhythmia may progress to ventricular fibrillation. Intravenous infusion of magnesium sulphate (section 9.5.1.3) is usually effective. A beta-blocker (but not sotalol) and atrial (or ventricular) pacing may be considered. Anti-arrhythmics (including lidocaine) may further prolong the QT interval, thus worsening the condition.

2.3.2 Drugs for arrhythmias

Anti-arrhythmic drugs can be classified clinically into those that act on supraventricular arrhythmias (e.g. verapamil), those that act on both supraventricular and ventricular arrhythmias (e.g. disopyramide), and those that act on ventricular arrhythmias (e.g. lidocaine (lignocaine)).

They can also be classified according to their effects on the electrical behaviour of myocardial cells during activity:

Class Ia, b, c: membrane stabilising drugs (e.g. quinidine, lidocaine, flecainide respectively)
Class II: beta-blockers
Class III: amiodarone, bretylium, and sotalol (also Class II)
Class IV: calcium-channel blockers (includes verapamil but not dihydropyridines)

This latter classification (the Vaughan Williams classification) is of less clinical significance.

CAUTIONS. The negative inotropic effects of anti-arrhythmic drugs tend to be additive. Therefore special care should be taken if two or more are used, especially if myocardial function is impaired. Most or all drugs that are effective in countering arrhythmias can also provoke them in some circumstances; moreover, hypokalaemia enhances the arrhythmogenic (pro-arrhythmic) effect of many drugs.

Supraventricular arrhythmias

Adenosine is usually the treatment of choice for terminating paroxysmal supraventricular tachycardia. As it has a very short duration of action (half-life only about 8 to 10 seconds, but prolonged in those taking dipyridamole), most side-effects are short lived. Unlike verapamil, adenosine may be used after a beta-blocker. Verapamil may be preferable to adenosine in asthma.

Oral administration of a **cardiac glycoside** (such as digoxin, section 2.1.1) slows the ventricular response in cases of atrial fibrillation and atrial flutter. However, intravenous infusion of digoxin is rarely effective for rapid control of ventricular rate. Cardiac glycosides are contra-indicated in supraventricular arrhythmias associated with Wolff-Parkinson-White syndrome.

Verapamil (section 2.6.2) is usually effective for supraventricular tachycardias. An initial intravenous dose (**important**: serious beta-blocker interaction hazard, see p. 106) may be followed by oral treatment; hypotension may occur with larger doses. It should not be used for tachyarrhythmias where the QRS complex is wide (i.e. broad complex) unless a supraventricular origin has been established beyond reasonable doubt. It is also contra-indicated in atrial fibrillation with pre-excitation (e.g. Wolff-Parkinson-White syndrome). It should not be used in children with arrhythmias without specialist advice; some supraventricular arrhythmias in childhood can be accelerated by verapamil with dangerous consequences.

Intravenous administration of a **beta-blocker** (section 2.4) such as esmolol or propranolol, can achieve rapid control of the ventricular rate.

Drugs for both supraventricular and ventricular arrhythmias include **amiodarone**, **beta-blockers**, **disopyramide**, **flecainide**, **procainamide**, **propafenone** and **quinidine**, see below under Supraventricular and Ventricular Arrhythmias.

ADENOSINE

Indications: rapid reversion to sinus rhythm of paroxysmal supraventricular tachycardias, including those associated with accessory pathways (e.g. Wolff-Parkinson-White syndrome); aid to diagnosis of broad or narrow complex supraventricular tachycardias

Cautions: atrial fibrillation or flutter with accessory pathway (conduction down anomalous pathway may increase); heart transplant (see below); **interactions:** Appendix 1 (adenosine)

Contra-indications: second- or third-degree AV block and sick sinus syndrome (unless pacemaker fitted); asthma

Side-effects: include transient facial flush, chest pain, dyspnoea, bronchospasm, choking sensation, nausea, light-headedness; severe bradycardia reported (requiring temporary pacing); ECG may show transient rhythm disturbances

Dose: *by rapid intravenous injection* into central or large peripheral vein, 3 mg over 2 seconds with cardiac monitoring; if necessary followed by 6 mg after 1–2 minutes, and then by 12 mg after a further 1–2 minutes; increments should not be given if high level AV block develops at any particular dose

NOTE. 3-mg dose ineffective in a number of patients, therefore higher initial dose sometimes used but patients with *heart transplant* are **very sensitive** to effects of adenosine, and should **not** receive higher initial dose. Also if essential to give with dipyridamole reduce initial dose to 0.5–1 mg

Adenocor® (Sanofi-Synthelabo) [PoM]
Injection, adenosine 3 mg/mL in physiological saline. Net price 2-mL vial = £4.45 (hosp. only)
NOTE. Intravenous infusion of adenosine (*Adenoscan*®, Sanofi Winthrop) may be used in conjunction with radionuclide myocardial perfusion imaging in patients who cannot exercise adequately or for whom exercise is inappropriate—consult product literature

Supraventricular and ventricular arrhythmias

Amiodarone is used in the treatment of arrhythmias particularly when other drugs are ineffective or contra-indicated. It may be used for paroxysmal supraventricular, nodal and ventricular tachycardias, atrial fibrillation and flutter, and ventricular fibrillation. It should be initiated only under hospital or specialist supervision. Amiodarone may be given by intravenous infusion as well as by mouth, and has the advantage of causing little or no myocardial depression. Unlike oral amiodarone, intravenous amiodarone may act relatively rapidly.

Intravenous injection of amiodarone may be used in cardiopulmonary resuscitation for ventricular fibrillation or pulseless tachycardia unresponsive to other interventions (section 2.7.3).

Amiodarone has a very long half-life (extending to several weeks) and only needs to be given once daily (but high doses may cause nausea unless divided). Many weeks or months may be required to achieve steady-state plasma-amiodarone concentration; this is particularly important when drug interactions are likely (see also Appendix 1).

Most patients taking amiodarone develop corneal microdeposits (reversible on withdrawal of treatment); these rarely interfere with vision, but drivers may be dazzled by headlights at night. Because of the possibility of phototoxic reactions, patients should be advised to shield the skin from light and to use a wide-spectrum sunscreen (section 13.8.1) to protect against both long ultraviolet and visible light.

Amiodarone contains iodine and can cause disorders of thyroid function; both hypothyroidism and hyperthyroidism may occur. Clinical assessment alone is unreliable, and laboratory tests should be performed before treatment and every 6 months. Thyroxine (T4) may be raised in the absence of hyperthyroidism; therefore tri-iodothyronine (T3), T4, and thyroid-stimulating hormone (thyrotrophin, TSH) should all be measured. A raised T3 and T4 with a very low or undetectable TSH concentration suggests the development of thyrotoxicosis. The thyrotoxicosis may be very refractory, and amiodarone should usually be withdrawn at least temporarily to help achieve control; treatment with carbimazole may be required. Hypothyroidism can be treated with replacement therapy without withdrawing amiodarone if it is essential.

Pneumonitis should always be suspected if new or progressive shortness of breath or cough develops in a patient taking amiodarone. Fresh neurological symptoms should raise the possibility of peripheral neuropathy.

Amiodarone is also associated with hepatotoxicity and treatment should be discontinued if severe liver function abnormalities or clinical signs of liver disease develop.

Beta-blockers act as anti-arrhythmic drugs principally by attenuating the effects of the sympathetic system on automaticity and conductivity within the heart, for details see section 2.4. For special reference to the role of **sotalol** in ventricular arrhythmias, see also p. 78.

Disopyramide may be given by intravenous injection to control arrhythmias after myocardial infarction (including those not responding to lidocaine (lignocaine)), but it impairs cardiac contractility. Oral administration of disopyramide is useful but it has an antimuscarinic effect which limits its use in patients with glaucoma or prostatic hypertrophy.

Flecainide belongs to the same general class as lidocaine. It may be of value in serious symptomatic ventricular arrhythmias. It may also be indicated for junctional re-entry tachycardias and for paroxysmal atrial fibrillation. As with quinidine it may precipitate serious arrhythmias in a small minority of patients (including those with otherwise normal hearts).

Procainamide is given by intravenous injection to control ventricular arrhythmias.

Propafenone is used for the prophylaxis and treatment of ventricular arrhythmias and also for some supraventricular arrhythmias. It has complex mechanisms of action, including weak beta-blocking activity (therefore caution is needed in obstructive airways disease—contra-indicated if severe).

Quinidine may be effective in suppressing supraventricular and ventricular arrhythmias. It may itself precipitate rhythm disorders, and is best used on

specialist advice; it can cause hypersensitivity reactions and gastro-intestinal upsets.

Drugs for supraventricular arrhythmias include **adenosine**, **cardiac glycosides** and **verapamil**, see above under Supraventricular Arrhythmias. Drugs for ventricular arrhythmias include **bretylium**, **lidocaine**, **mexiletine**, and **phenytoin**, see below under Ventricular Arrhythmias.

AMIODARONE HYDROCHLORIDE

Indications: see notes above (should be initiated in hospital or under specialist supervision)

Cautions: liver-function and thyroid-function tests required before treatment and then every 6 months (see notes above for tests of thyroid function); chest x-ray required before treatment; heart failure; renal impairment; elderly; severe bradycardia and conduction disturbances in excessive dosage; intravenous use may cause moderate and transient fall in blood pressure (circulatory collapse precipitated by rapid administration or overdosage); porphyria (section 9.8.2); **interactions:** Appendix 1 (amiodarone)

Contra-indications: sinus bradycardia, sino-atrial heart block; unless pacemaker fitted avoid in severe conduction disturbances or sinus node disease; history of thyroid dysfunction; pregnancy and breast-feeding (see also Appendixes 4 and 5); iodine sensitivity; avoid *intravenous use* in severe respiratory failure, circulatory collapse (except in cardiac arrest, see section 2.7.3), severe arterial hypotension; avoid bolus injection in congestive heart failure or cardiomyopathy; avoid injections containing benzyl alcohol in neonates

Side-effects: reversible corneal microdeposits (sometimes with night glare), rarely impaired vision due to optic neuritis; peripheral neuropathy and myopathy (usually reversible on withdrawal); bradycardia and conduction disturbances (see Cautions); phototoxicity and rarely persistent slate-grey skin discoloration (see also notes); hypothyroidism, hyperthyroidism, diffuse pulmonary alveolitis, pneumonitis, and fibrosis; raised serum transaminases (may require dose reduction or withdrawal if accompanied by acute liver disorders); jaundice, hepatitis and cirrhosis reported; rarely nausea, vomiting, metallic taste, tremor, hot flushes, sweating, nightmares, vertigo, headache, sleeplessness, fatigue, alopecia, paraesthesia, benign raised intracranial pressure, impotence, epididymo-orchitis; ataxia, rashes (including exfoliative dermatitis); hypersensitivity including vasculitis, renal involvement and thrombocytopenia; haemolytic or aplastic anaemia; anaphylaxis on rapid injection, also bronchospasm or apnoea in respiratory failure

Dose: *by mouth*, 200 mg 3 times daily for 1 week reduced to 200 mg twice daily for a further week; maintenance, usually 200 mg daily or the minimum required to control the arrhythmia

By intravenous infusion via caval catheter, initially 5 mg/kg over 20–120 minutes with ECG monitoring; subsequent infusion given if necessary according to response up to max. 1.2 g in 24 hours

Ventricular fibrillation or pulseless ventricular tachycardia, *by intravenous injection* over at least 3 minutes, 300 mg (section 2.7.3)

Amiodarone (Non-proprietary) PoM
Tablets, amiodarone hydrochloride 100 mg, net price 28-tab pack = £4.28; 200 mg, 28-tab pack = £6.45. Label: 11
Available from Alpharma, APS, Generics, Hillcross, IVAX, Lexon (*Amyben*®), Sterwin
Injection, amiodarone hydrochloride 30 mg/mL, net price 10-mL prefilled syringe = £10.25
Excipients: may include benzyl alcohol (avoid in neonates, see Excipients, p. 2)
Available from Aurum
Sterile concentrate, amiodarone hydrochloride 50 mg/mL, net price 3-mL amp= £1.43, 6-mL amp = £2.86. For dilution and use as an infusion
Excipients: may include benzyl alcohol (avoid in neonates, see Excipients, p. 2)
Available from Mayne

Cordarone X® (Sanofi-Synthelabo) PoM
Tablets, both scored, amiodarone hydrochloride 100 mg, net price 28-tab pack = £4.78; 200 mg, 28-tab pack = £7.82. Label: 11
Sterile concentrate, amiodarone hydrochloride 50 mg/mL. Net price 3-mL amp = £1.43. For dilution and use as an infusion
Excipients: include benzyl alcohol (avoid in neonates, see Excipients, p. 2)

DISOPYRAMIDE

Indications: ventricular arrhythmias, especially after myocardial infarction; supraventricular arrhythmias
Cautions: discontinue if hypotension, hypoglycaemia, ventricular tachycardia, ventricular fibrillation or torsades de pointes develop; atrial flutter or tachycardia with partial block, bundle branch block, heart failure (avoid if severe); prostatic enlargement; glaucoma; hepatic and renal impairment (see Appendixes 2 and 3); pregnancy and breast-feeding (see Appendixes 4 and 5); **interactions:** Appendix 1 (disopyramide)
Contra-indications: second-and third-degree heart block and sinus node dysfunction (unless pacemaker fitted); cardiogenic shock; severe uncompensated heart failure
Side-effects: ventricular tachycardia, ventricular fibrillation or torsades de pointes (usually associated with prolongation of QRS complex or QT interval—see Cautions above), myocardial depression, hypotension, AV block; antimuscarinic effects include dry mouth, blurred vision, urinary retention; gastro-intestinal irritation; psychosis, cholestatic jaundice, hypoglycaemia also reported (see Cautions above)
Dose: *by mouth*, 300–800 mg daily in divided doses
By slow intravenous injection, 2 mg/kg over at least 5 minutes to a max. of 150 mg, with ECG monitoring, followed immediately *either* by 200 mg *by mouth*, then 200 mg every 8 hours for 24 hours *or* 400 micrograms/kg/hour *by intravenous infusion*; max. 300 mg in first hour and 800 mg daily

Disopyramide (Non-proprietary) PoM
Capsules, disopyramide (as phosphate) 100 mg, net price 20 = £3.76; 150 mg, 20 = £4.99
Available from Hillcross, IVAX (100 mg)

Rythmodan® (Borg) PoM
Capsules, disopyramide 100 mg (green/beige), net price 84-cap pack = £15.82; 150 mg, 84-cap pack = £20.99
Injection, disopyramide (as phosphate) 10 mg/mL, net price 5-mL amp = £2.92

■ Modified release
Isomide® **CR** (Tillomed) PoM
Capsules, m/r, disopyramide (as phosphate) 250 mg, net price 56-cap pack = £31.00. Label: 25
Dose: 250 mg every 12 hours

Rythmodan Retard® (Borg) PoM
Tablets, m/r, scored, f/c, disopyramide (as phosphate) 250 mg. Net price 56-tab pack = £31.02. Label: 25
Dose: 250–375 mg every 12 hours

FLECAINIDE ACETATE

Indications: *Tablets and injection:* AV nodal reciprocating tachycardia, arrhythmias associated with Wolff-Parkinson-White syndrome and similar conditions with accessory pathways; paroxysmal atrial fibrillation in patients with disabling symptoms (arrhythmias of recent onset will respond more readily)
Tablets only: symptomatic sustained ventricular tachycardia, premature ventricular contractions and/or non-sustained ventricular tachycardia causing disabling symptoms in patients resistant to or intolerant of other therapy
Injection only: ventricular tachyarrhythmias resistant to other treatment
Cautions: patients with pacemakers (especially those who may be pacemaker dependent because stimulation threshold may rise appreciably; avoid in sinus node dysfunction, atrial conduction defects, second-degree or greater AV block, bundle branch block or distal block unless pacing rescue available; atrial fibrillation following heart surgery; elderly (accumulation may occur); hepatic impairment (Appendix 2); renal impairment (monitor plasma-flecainide concentration, see also Appendix 3); pregnancy (Appendix 4) and breast-feeding (Appendix 5); **interactions:** Appendix 1 (flecainide)
Contra-indications: heart failure; history of myocardial infarction and either asymptomatic ventricular ectopics or asymptomatic non-sustained ventricular tachycardia; long-standing atrial fibrillation where no attempt has been made to convert to sinus rhythm; haemodynamically significant valvular heart disease
Side-effects: nausea, vomiting; pro-arrhythmic effects; dyspnoea; visual disturbances; less commonly gastro-intestinal disturbances, jaundice, hepatic dysfunction, AV block, heart failure, myocardial infarction, hypotension, pneumonitis, hallucinations, depression, convulsions, peripheral neuropathy, paraesthesia, ataxia, dyskinesia, hypoaesthesia, tinnitus, vertigo, reduction in red blood cells, in white blood cells and in platelets, corneal deposits, rashes, alopecia, sweating, urticaria, photosensitivity, increased antinuclear antibodies
Dose: *by mouth* (initiated under direction of hospital consultant), ventricular arrhythmias, initially 100 mg twice daily (max. 400 mg daily usually reserved for rapid control or in heavily built patients), reduced after 3–5 days if possible
Supraventricular arrhythmias, 50 mg twice daily, increased if required to max. 300 mg daily
By slow intravenous injection (in hospital), 2 mg/kg over 10–30 minutes, max. 150 mg, with ECG monitoring; followed if required by *infusion* at a

rate of 1.5 mg/kg/hour for 1 hour, subsequently reduced to 100–250 micrograms/kg/hour for up to 24 hours; max. cumulative dose in first 24 hours, 600 mg; transfer to *oral* treatment, as above
NOTE. Plasma-flecainide concentration for optimum response 0.2–1 mg/litre

Flecainide (Non-proprietary) [PoM]
Tablets, flecainide acetate 50 mg, net price 60-tab pack = £15.55; 100 mg, 60-tab pack = £22.21
Available from Alpharma, APS, Generics, Sterwin

Tambocor® (3M) [PoM]
Tablets, flecainide acetate 50 mg, net price 60-tab pack = £15.55; 100 mg (scored), 60-tab pack = £22.21
Injection, flecainide acetate 10 mg/mL. Net price 15-mL amp = £4.73

PROCAINAMIDE HYDROCHLORIDE

Indications: ventricular arrhythmias, especially after myocardial infarction; atrial tachycardia
Cautions: elderly; hepatic and renal impairment; asthma; myasthenia gravis; pregnancy; **interactions:** Appendix 1 (procainamide)
Contra-indications: heart block, heart failure, hypotension; systemic lupus erythematosus; not indicated for torsades de pointes (can exacerbate); breast-feeding
Side-effects: nausea, diarrhoea, rashes, fever, myocardial depression, heart failure, lupus erythematosus-like syndrome, agranulocytosis after prolonged treatment; psychosis and angioedema also reported
Dose: *by slow intravenous injection*, rate not exceeding 50 mg/minute, 100 mg with ECG monitoring, repeated at 5-minute intervals until arrhythmia controlled; max. 1 g
By intravenous infusion, 500–600 mg over 25–30 minutes with ECG monitoring, followed by maintenance at rate of 2–6 mg/minute, then if necessary oral treatment as above, starting 3–4 hours after infusion
NOTE. Serum procainamide concentration for optimum response 3–10 mg/litre

Pronestyl® (Squibb) [PoM]
Injection, procainamide hydrochloride 100 mg/mL. Net price 10-mL vial = £1.90

PROPAFENONE HYDROCHLORIDE

Indications: ventricular arrhythmias; paroxysmal supraventricular tachyarrhythmias which include paroxysmal atrial flutter or fibrillation and paroxysmal re-entrant tachycardias involving the AV node or accessory pathway, where standard therapy ineffective or contra-indicated
Cautions: heart failure; hepatic and renal impairment; elderly; pacemaker patients; pregnancy and breast-feeding (see Appendixes 4 and 5); great caution in obstructive airways disease owing to beta-blocking activity (contra-indicated if severe); **interactions:** Appendix 1 (propafenone)
Contra-indications: uncontrolled congestive heart failure, cardiogenic shock (except arrhythmia induced), severe bradycardia, electrolyte disturbances, severe obstructive pulmonary disease, marked hypotension; myasthenia gravis; unless adequately paced avoid in sinus node dysfunction, atrial conduction defects, second degree or greater AV block, bundle branch block or distal block

Side-effects: antimuscarinic effects including constipation, blurred vision, and dry mouth; dizziness, nausea and vomiting, fatigue, bitter taste, diarrhoea, headache, and allergic skin reactions reported; postural hypotension, particularly in elderly; bradycardia, sino-atrial, atrioventricular, or intraventricular blocks; arrhythmogenic (pro-arrhythmic) effect; rarely hypersensitivity reactions (cholestasis, blood disorders, lupus syndrome), seizures; myoclonus also reported
Dose: 70 kg and over, initially 150 mg 3 times daily after food under direct hospital supervision with ECG monitoring and blood pressure control (if QRS interval prolonged by more than 20%, reduce dose or discontinue until ECG returns to normal limits); may be increased at intervals of at least 3 days to 300 mg twice daily and, if necessary, to max. 300 mg 3 times daily; under 70 kg, reduce dose
ELDERLY may respond to lower doses

Arythmol® (Abbott) [PoM]
Tablets, both f/c, propafenone hydrochloride 150 mg, net price 90-tab pack = £21.43; 300 mg (scored), 60-tab pack = £21.43. Label: 21, 25

QUINIDINE

Indications: suppression of supraventricular tachycardias and ventricular arrhythmias (see notes above)
Cautions: 200-mg test dose to detect hypersensitivity reactions; extreme care in uncompensated heart failure, myocarditis, severe myocardial damage and in myasthenia gravis; **interactions:** Appendix 1 (quinidine)
Contra-indications: heart block
Side-effects: see under Procainamide Hydrochloride; also ventricular arrhythmias, thrombocytopenia, haemolytic anaemia; rarely granulomatous hepatitis; also cinchonism (see Quinine, section 5.4.1)
Dose: *by mouth*, quinidine sulphate 200–400 mg 3–4 times daily
NOTE. Quinidine sulphate 200 mg = quinidine bisulphate 250 mg

Quinidine Sulphate (Non-proprietary) [PoM]
Tablets, quinidine sulphate 200 mg, net price 100-tab pack = £32.95
Available from Regent

■ Modified release
Kinidin Durules® (AstraZeneca) [PoM]
Tablets, m/r, f/c, quinidine bisulphate 250 mg. Net price 100-tab pack = £11.05. Label: 25
Dose: 500 mg every 12 hours, adjusted as required

Ventricular arrhythmias

Bretylium is only used as an anti-arrhythmic drug in resuscitation. It is given both intramuscularly and intravenously but can cause severe hypotension, particularly after intravenous administration; nausea and vomiting can occur with either route. The intravenous route should only be used in emergency when there is doubt about absorption because of inadequate circulation.

Lidocaine (lignocaine) is relatively safe when used by slow intravenous injection and should be considered first for emergency use. Though effective in suppressing ventricular tachycardia and reducing the risk of ventricular fibrillation following myocardial infarction, it has not been shown to reduce mortality when used prophylactically in this condition. In patients with cardiac or hepatic failure doses may need to be reduced to avoid convulsions, depression of the central nervous system, or depression of the cardiovascular system.

Mexiletine may be given as a slow intravenous injection if lidocaine is ineffective; it has a similar action. Adverse cardiovascular and central nervous system effects may limit the dose tolerated; nausea and vomiting may prevent an effective dose being given by mouth.

Moracizine (*Ethmozine®*, Shire) is available on a named-patient basis for the prophylaxis and treatment of serious and life-threatening ventricular arrhythmias for patients already stabilised on moracizine.

Phenytoin (section 4.8.2) by slow intravenous injection was formerly used in ventricular arrhythmias particularly those caused by cardiac glycosides, but this use is now obsolete.

Drugs for both supraventricular and ventricular arrhythmias include **amiodarone**, **beta-blockers**, **disopyramide**, **flecainide**, **procainamide**, **propafenone** and **quinidine**, see above under Supraventricular and Ventricular Arrhythmias.

BRETYLIUM TOSILATE

Indications: ventricular arrhythmias resistant to other treatment

Cautions: do not give noradrenaline (norepinephrine) or other sympathomimetic amines; may exacerbate ventricular arrhythmias due to cardiac glycosides; **interactions:** Appendix 1 (adrenergic neurone blockers)

Contra-indications: phaeochromocytoma

Side-effects: hypotension, nausea and vomiting; tissue necrosis reported after intramuscular injection (rotate sites)

Dose: *by slow intravenous injection*, 5–10 mg/kg over 8–10 minutes (preferably 15–30 minutes) with blood pressure and ECG monitoring; may be repeated after 1–2 hours to a total dosage of 30 mg/kg (intravenous dose being diluted to 10 mg/mL in glucose 5% or sodium chloride intravenous infusion)

Maintenance 5–10 mg/kg *by intramuscular injection*, *by intravenous infusion* (over 15–30 minutes) every 6–8 hours, *or* 1–2 mg/minute *by continuous intravenous infusion*

Minijet® Bretylium Tosylate (Celltech) PoM
Injection, bretylium tosilate 50 mg/mL, net price 10-mL disposable syringe = £23.66

LIDOCAINE HYDROCHLORIDE

(Lignocaine hydrochloride)

Indications: ventricular arrhythmias, especially after myocardial infarction

Cautions: lower doses in congestive cardiac failure, in hepatic failure, and following cardiac surgery; elderly; **interactions:** Appendix 1 (lidocaine)

Contra-indications: sino-atrial disorders, all grades of atrioventricular block, severe myocardial depression; porphyria (see section 9.8.2)

Side-effects: dizziness, paraesthesia, or drowsiness (particularly if injection too rapid); other CNS effects include confusion, respiratory depression and convulsions; hypotension and bradycardia (may lead to cardiac arrest); hypersensitivity reported

Dose: *by intravenous injection*, in patients without gross circulatory impairment, 100 mg as a bolus over a few minutes (50 mg in lighter patients or those whose circulation is severely impaired), followed immediately by *infusion* of 4 mg/minute for 30 minutes, 2 mg/minute for 2 hours, then 1 mg/minute; reduce concentration further if infusion continued beyond 24 hours (ECG monitoring and specialist advice for infusion)

IMPORTANT. Following intravenous injection lidocaine has a short duration of action (lasting for 15–20 minutes). If an *intravenous infusion* is not immediately available the initial *intravenous injection* of 50–100 mg can be repeated if necessary once or twice at intervals of not less than 10 minutes

Lidocaine (Non-proprietary) PoM
Injection 2%, lidocaine hydrochloride 20 mg/mL, net price 2-mL amp = 28p; 5-mL amp = 25p; 10-mL amp = 60p; 20-mL amp = 61p
Available from Braun
Infusion, lidocaine hydrochloride 0.1% (1 mg/mL) and 0.2% (2 mg/mL) in glucose intravenous infusion 5%. 500-mL containers
Available from Baxter

Minijet® Lignocaine (Celltech) PoM
Injection, lidocaine hydrochloride 1% (10 mg/mL), net price 10-mL disposable syringe = £4.40; 2% (20 mg/mL), 5-mL disposable syringe = £4.30

MEXILETINE HYDROCHLORIDE

Indications: ventricular arrhythmias, especially after myocardial infarction

Cautions: hepatic impairment; close monitoring on initiation of therapy (including ECG, blood pressure, etc.); **interactions:** Appendix 1 (mexiletine)

Contra-indications: bradycardia, cardiogenic shock; high degree AV block (unless pacemaker fitted)

Side-effects: nausea, vomiting, constipation; bradycardia, hypotension, atrial fibrillation, palpitations, conduction defects, exacerbation of arrhythmias, torsades de pointes; drowsiness, confusion, convulsions, psychiatric disorders, dysarthria, ataxia, paraesthesia, nystagmus, tremor; jaundice, hepatitis, and blood disorders reported; see also notes above

Dose: *by mouth*, initial dose 400 mg (may be increased to 600 mg if opioid analgesics also given), followed after 2 hours by 200–250 mg 3–4 times daily

By intravenous injection, 100–250 mg at a rate of 25 mg/minute with ECG monitoring followed by *infusion* of 250 mg as a 0.1% solution over 1 hour, 125 mg/hour for 2 hours, then 500 micrograms/minute

Mexitil® (Boehringer Ingelheim) PoM
Capsules, mexiletine hydrochloride 50 mg (purple/red), net price 100-cap pack = £4.95; 200 mg (red), 100-cap pack = £11.87
Injection, mexiletine hydrochloride 25 mg/mL. Net price 10-mL amp = £1.49

2.4 Beta-adrenoceptor blocking drugs

Beta-adrenoceptor blocking drugs (beta-blockers) block the beta-adrenoreceptors in the heart, peripheral vasculature, bronchi, pancreas, and liver.

Many beta-blockers are now available and in general they are all equally effective. There are, however, differences between them which may affect choice in treating particular diseases or individual patients; esmolol and sotalol are used for the management of arrhythmia only (see below).

Intrinsic sympathomimetic activity (ISA, partial agonist activity) represents the capacity of beta-blockers to stimulate as well as to block adrenergic receptors. **Oxprenolol, pindolol, acebutolol** and **celiprolol** have intrinsic sympathomimetic activity; they tend to cause less bradycardia than the other beta-blockers and may also cause less coldness of the extremities.

Some beta-blockers are lipid soluble and some are water soluble. **Atenolol, celiprolol, nadolol**, and **sotalol** are the most water-soluble; they are less likely to enter the brain, and may therefore cause less sleep disturbance and nightmares. Water-soluble beta-blockers are excreted by the kidneys; they accumulate in renal impairment and dosage reduction is therefore often necessary.

Beta-blockers with a relatively short duration of action have to be given two or three times daily. Many of these are, however, available in modified-release formulations so that administration once daily is adequate for hypertension. For angina twice-daily treatment may sometimes be needed even with a modified-release formulation. Some beta-blockers such as atenolol, bisoprolol, carvedilol, celiprolol, and nadolol have an intrinsically longer duration of action and need to be given only once daily.

Beta-blockers slow the heart and can depress the myocardium; they are contra-indicated in patients with second- or third-degree heart block. Beta-blockers should also be avoided in patients with worsening unstable heart failure; care is required when initiating a beta-blocker in those with stable heart failure (see also section 2.5.5). **Sotalol** may prolong the QT interval, and it occasionally causes life-threatening ventricular arrhythmias (**important:** particular care is required to avoid hypokalaemia in patients taking sotalol).

Labetalol, celiprolol, carvedilol and **nebivolol** are beta-blockers which have, in addition, an arteriolar vasodilating action, by diverse mechanisms, and thus lower peripheral resistance. There is no evidence that these drugs have important advantages over other beta-blockers in the treatment of hypertension.

Beta-blockers may precipitate asthma and this effect can be dangerous. Beta-blockers should be **avoided** in patients with a history of asthma or bronchospasm; if there is no alternative, a cardioselective beta-blocker may be used with extreme caution under specialist supervision. **Atenolol, bisoprolol, metoprolol, nebivolol** and (to a lesser extent) **acebutolol**, have less effect on the beta$_2$ (bronchial) receptors and are, therefore, relatively *cardioselective*, but they are **not** *cardiospecific*. They have a lesser effect on airways resistance but are **not** free of this side-effect.

Beta-blockers are also associated with fatigue, coldness of the extremities (may be less common with those with ISA, see above), and sleep disturbances with nightmares (may be less common with the water-soluble ones, see above).

Beta-blockers are not contra-indicated in diabetes; however they can lead to a small deterioration of glucose tolerance and interfere with metabolic and autonomic responses to hypoglycaemia. Cardioselective beta-blockers (see above) may be preferable and beta-blockers should be avoided altogether in those with frequent episodes of hypoglycaemia.

HYPERTENSION. Beta-blockers are effective antihypertensives but their mode of action is not understood; they reduce cardiac output, alter baroceptor reflex sensitivity, and block peripheral adrenoceptors. Some beta-blockers depress plasma renin secretion. It is possible that a central effect may also explain their mode of action. Blood pressure can usually be controlled with relatively few side-effects. In general the dose of beta-blocker does not have to be high; for example **atenolol** is given in a dose of 50 mg daily and it is usually not necessary to increase the dose to 100 mg.

Combined thiazide and beta-blocker preparations may help compliance but combined preparations should only be used when blood pressure is not adequately controlled by a thiazide or a beta-blocker alone. Beta-blockers reduce, but do not abolish, the tendency for diuretics to cause hypokalaemia.

Beta-blockers can be used to control the pulse rate in patients with *phaeochromocytoma* (section 2.5.4). However, they should never be used alone as beta-blockade without concurrent alpha-blockade may lead to a hypertensive crisis. For this reason phenoxybenzamine should always be used together with the beta-blocker.

ANGINA. By reducing cardiac work beta-blockers improve exercise tolerance and relieve symptoms in patients with *angina* (for further details on the management of stable and unstable angina see section 2.6). As with hypertension there is no good evidence of the superiority of any one drug, although occasionally a patient will respond better to one beta-blocker than to another. There is some evidence that sudden withdrawal may cause an exacerbation of angina and therefore gradual reduction of dose is preferable when beta-blockers are to be stopped. There is a risk of precipitating heart failure when beta-blockers and verapamil are used together in established ischaemic heart disease (**important**: see p. 106).

MYOCARDIAL INFARCTION. For advice on the management of myocardial infarction see section 2.10.1.

Several studies have shown that some beta-blockers can reduce the recurrence rate of *myocardial infarction*. However, uncontrolled heart failure, hypotension, bradyarrhythmias, and obstructive airways disease render beta-blockers unsuitable in some patients following a myocardial infarction. **Atenolol** and **metoprolol** may reduce early mortality after intravenous and subsequent oral administration in the acute phase, while **acebutolol, metoprolol, propranolol**, and **timolol** have protective value when started in the early convalescent phase. The evidence relating to other beta-blockers is less convincing; some have not been tested in trials of secondary protection. It is also not known whether the protective effect of beta-blockers continues after 2–3 years; it is possible that sudden cessation may cause a rebound worsening of myocardial ischaemia.

ARRHYTHMIAS. Beta-blockers act as *anti-arrhythmic drugs* principally by attenuating the effects of the sympathetic system on automaticity and conductivity within the heart. They may be used in conjunction with digoxin to control the ventricular response in atrial fibrillation, especially in patients with thyrotoxicosis. Beta-blockers are also useful in the management of supraventricular tachycardias, and are used to control those following myocardial infarction, see above.

Esmolol is a relatively cardioselective beta-blocker with a very short duration of action, used intravenously for the short-term treatment of supraventricular arrhythmias, sinus tachycardia, or hypertension, particularly in the peri-operative period. It may also be used in other situations, such as acute myocardial infarction, where sustained beta blockade might be hazardous.

Sotalol, a non-cardioselective beta-blocker with additional class III anti-arrhythmic activity, is used for prophylaxis in paroxysmal supraventricular arrhythmias. It also suppresses ventricular ectopic beats and non-sustained ventricular tachycardia. It has been shown to be more effective than lidocaine (lignocaine) in the termination of spontaneous sustained ventricular tachycardia due to coronary disease or cardiomyopathy. However, it may induce torsades de pointes in susceptible patients.

HEART FAILURE. Beta-blockers may produce benefit in heart failure by blocking sympathetic activity. **Bisoprolol** and **carvedilol** reduce mortality in any grade of stable heart failure. Treatment should be initiated by those experienced in the management of heart failure (see section 2.5.5 for details on heart failure).

THYROTOXICOSIS. Beta-blockers are used in preoperative preparation for thyroidectomy. Administration of propranolol can reverse clinical symptoms of *thyrotoxicosis* within 4 days. Routine tests of increased thyroid function remain unaltered. The thyroid gland is rendered less vascular thus making surgery easier (section 6.2.2).

OTHER USES. Beta-blockers have been used to alleviate some symptoms of *anxiety*; probably patients with palpitations, tremor, and tachycardia respond best (see also section 4.1.2 and section 4.9.3). Beta-blockers are also used in the *prophylaxis of migraine* (section 4.7.4.2). Betaxolol, carteolol, levobunolol, metipranolol and timolol are used topically in *glaucoma* (section 11.6).

PROPRANOLOL HYDROCHLORIDE

Indications: see under Dose

Cautions: pregnancy and breast-feeding (see also Appendixes 4 and 5); avoid abrupt withdrawal especially in angina; first-degree AV block; reduce oral dose of propranolol in liver disease; portal hypertension (risk of deterioration in liver function); renal impairment (Appendix 3); diabetes; history of obstructive airways disease (introduce cautiously and monitor lung function—see also

Bronchospasm below); myasthenia gravis; history of hypersensitivity—may increase sensitivity to allergens and result in more serious hypersensitivity response, also may reduce response to adrenaline (epinephrine) (see also section 3.4.3); see also notes above; **interactions:** Appendix 1 (beta-blockers), **important:** verapamil interaction, see also p. 106

Contra-indications: asthma (**important:** see Bronchospasm below), uncontrolled heart failure, Prinzmetal's angina, marked bradycardia, hypotension, sick sinus syndrome, second- or third-degree AV block, cardiogenic shock, metabolic acidosis, severe peripheral arterial disease; phaeochromocytoma (apart from specific use with alpha-blockers, see also notes above)

BRONCHOSPASM. The CSM has advised that beta-blockers, including those considered to be cardioselective, should not be given to patients with a history of asthma or bronchospasm. However, in rare situations where there is no alternative a cardioselective beta-blocker is given to these patients with extreme caution and under specialist supervision

Side-effects: bradycardia, heart failure, hypotension, conduction disorders, bronchospasm, peripheral vasoconstriction (including exacerbation of intermittent claudication and Raynaud's phenomenon), gastro-intestinal disturbances, fatigue, sleep disturbances; rare reports of rashes and dry eyes (reversible on withdrawal), sexual dysfunction, and exacerbation of psoriasis; see also notes above; **overdosage:** see Emergency Treatment of Poisoning, p. 24

Dose: *by mouth*, hypertension, initially 80 mg twice daily, increased at weekly intervals as required; maintenance 160–320 mg daily

Portal hypertension, initially 40 mg twice daily, increased to 80 mg twice daily according to heart-rate; max. 160 mg twice daily

Phaeochromocytoma (only with an alpha-blocker), 60 mg daily for 3 days before surgery *or* 30 mg daily in patients unsuitable for surgery

Angina, initially 40 mg 2–3 times daily; maintenance 120–240 mg daily

Arrhythmias, hypertrophic obstructive cardiomyopathy, anxiety tachycardia, and thyrotoxicosis (adjunct), 10–40 mg 3–4 times daily

Anxiety with symptoms such as palpitations, sweating, tremor, 40 mg once daily, increased to 40 mg 3 times daily if necessary

Prophylaxis after myocardial infarction, 40 mg 4 times daily for 2–3 days, then 80 mg twice daily, beginning 5 to 21 days after infarction

Migraine prophylaxis and essential tremor, initially 40 mg 2–3 times daily; maintenance 80–160 mg daily

By intravenous injection, arrhythmias and thyrotoxic crisis, 1 mg over 1 minute; if necessary repeat at 2-minute intervals; max. 10 mg (5 mg in anaesthesia)

NOTE. Excessive bradycardia can be countered with intravenous injection of atropine sulphate 0.6–2.4 mg in divided doses of 600 micrograms; for **overdosage** see Emergency Treatment of Poisoning, p. 24

Propranolol (Non-proprietary) PoM
Tablets, propranolol hydrochloride 10 mg, net price 20 = 42p; 40 mg, 20 = 46p; 80 mg, 20 = 34p; 160 mg, 20 = 85p. Label: 8

Available from Alpharma, APS, DDSA (*Angilol®*), Hillcross

Oral solution, propranolol hydrochloride 5 mg/
5 mL, net price 150 mL = £13.30; 10 mg/5 mL,
150 mL = £17.50; 50 mg/5 mL, 150 mL = £21.25
Available from Rosemont (*Syprol*®)

Inderal® (AstraZeneca) PoM
Tablets, all pink, f/c, propranolol hydrochloride
10 mg, net price 100-tab pack = 89p; 40 mg, 100-
tab pack = £2.40; 80 mg, 60-tab pack = £2.35.
Label: 8
Injection, propranolol hydrochloride 1 mg/mL, net
price 1-mL amp = 21p

■ Modified release

Half-Inderal LA® (AstraZeneca) PoM
Capsules, m/r, lavender/pink, propranolol hydro-
chloride 80 mg. Net price 28-cap pack = £5.40.
Label: 8, 25
NOTE. Modified-release capsules containing propranolol
hydrochloride 80 mg also available from APS, Sandoz
(*Bedranol SR*)®, Tillomed (*Half Beta Prograne*®)

Inderal-LA® (AstraZeneca) PoM
Capsules, m/r, lavender/pink, propranolol hydro-
chloride 160 mg. Net price 28-cap pack = £6.67.
Label: 8, 25
NOTE. Modified-release capsules containing propranolol
hydrochloride 160 mg also available from APS, Hillcross,
Opus (*Lopranol LA*®), Sandoz (*Bedranol SR*®), Tillomed
(*Beta Prograne*®)

ACEBUTOLOL

Indications: see under Dose
Cautions: see under Propranolol Hydrochloride
Contra-indications: see under Propranolol Hydro-
chloride
Side-effects: see under Propranolol Hydrochloride
Dose: hypertension, initially 400 mg once daily *or*
200 mg twice daily, increased after 2 weeks to
400 mg twice daily if necessary
Angina, initially 400 mg once daily *or* 200 mg twice
daily; 300 mg 3 times daily in severe angina; up to
1.2 g daily has been used
Arrhythmias, 0.4–1.2 g daily in 2–3 divided doses

Sectral® (Akita) PoM
Capsules, acebutolol (as hydrochloride) 100 mg
(buff/white), net price 84-cap pack = £16.10;
200 mg (buff/pink), 56-cap pack = £20.63. Label: 8
Tablets, f/c, acebutolol 400 mg (as hydrochloride).
Net price 28-tab pack = £20.02. Label: 8

■ With diuretic

Secadrex® (Akita) PoM
Tablets, f/c, acebutolol 200 mg (as hydrochloride),
hydrochlorothiazide 12.5 mg. Net price 28-tab
pack = £18.91. Label: 8
Dose: hypertension, 1 tablet daily, increased to 2 daily as
a single dose if necessary

ATENOLOL

Indications: see under Dose
Cautions: see under Propranolol Hydrochloride;
reduce dose in renal impairment
Contra-indications: see under Propranolol Hydro-
chloride
Side-effects: see under Propranolol Hydrochloride
Dose: *by mouth,*
Hypertension, 50 mg daily (higher doses rarely
necessary)
Angina, 100 mg daily in 1 or 2 doses
Arrhythmias, 50–100 mg daily

By intravenous injection, arrhythmias, 2.5 mg at a
rate of 1 mg/minute, repeated at 5-minute intervals
to a max. of 10 mg
NOTE. Excessive bradycardia can be countered with
intravenous injection of atropine sulphate 0.6–2.4 mg in
divided doses of 600 micrograms; for **overdosage** see
Emergency Treatment of Poisoning, p. 24
By intravenous infusion, arrhythmias, 150 micr-
ograms/kg over 20 minutes, repeated every 12
hours if required
Early intervention within 12 hours of myocardial
infarction (section 2.10.1), *by intravenous injection* over 5 minutes, 5 mg, then *by mouth,* 50 mg
after 15 minutes, 50 mg after 12 hours, then
100 mg daily

Atenolol (Non-proprietary) PoM
Tablets, atenolol 25 mg, net price 28-tab pack = 76p;
50 mg, 28-tab pack = 86p; 100 mg, 28-tab pack =
£1.01. Label: 8
Various strengths available from Alpharma, APS, Ashbourne (*Atenix*®), CP, Hillcross, IVAX, Sterwin, Tillomed

Tenormin® (AstraZeneca) PoM
'25' *tablets*, f/c, atenolol 25 mg. Net price 28-tab
pack = £4.41. Label: 8
LS tablets, orange, f/c, scored, atenolol 50 mg. Net
price 28-tab pack = £5.11. Label: 8
Tablets, orange, f/c, scored, atenolol 100 mg. Net
price 28-tab pack = £6.50. Label: 8
Syrup, sugar-free, atenolol 25 mg/5mL. Net price
300 mL = £8.55. Label: 8
Injection, atenolol 500 micrograms/mL. Net price
10-mL amp = 96p (hosp. only)

■ With diuretic

Co-tenidone (Non-proprietary) PoM
Tablets, co-tenidone 50/12.5 (atenolol 50 mg,
chlortalidone 12.5 mg), net price 28-tab pack =
£2.71; co-tenidone 100/25 (atenolol 100 mg,
chlortalidone 25 mg), 28-tab pack = £3.83. Label: 8
Available from Alpharma, APS, Ashbourne (*AtenixCo*®),
Berk (*Tenchlor*®), CP (*Totaretic*®), Hillcross, IVAX
Dose: hypertension, 1 tablet daily (but see also under
Dose above)

Kalten® (AstraZeneca) PoM
Capsules, red/ivory, co-amilozide 50 mg, co-amilozide
2.5/25 (anhydrous amiloride hydrochloride
2.5 mg, hydrochlorothiazide 25 mg). Net price 28-
cap pack = £8.39. Label: 8
Dose: hypertension, 1 capsule daily

Tenoret 50® (AstraZeneca) PoM
Tablets, brown, f/c, co-tenidone 50/12.5 (atenolol
50 mg, chlortalidone 12.5 mg). Net price 28-tab
pack = £5.70. Label: 8
Dose: hypertension, 1 tablet daily

Tenoretic® (AstraZeneca) PoM
Tablets, brown, f/c, co-tenidone 100/25 (atenolol
100 mg, chlortalidone 25 mg). Net price 28-tab
pack = £8.12. Label: 8
Dose: hypertension, 1 tablet daily (but see also under
Dose above)

■ With calcium-channel blocker
NOTE. Only indicated when calcium-channel blocker or
beta-blocker alone proves inadequate

Beta-Adalat® (Bayer) PoM
Capsules, reddish-brown, atenolol 50 mg, nifedipine 20 mg (m/r). Net price 28-cap pack =
£10.41. Label: 8, 25
Dose: hypertension, 1 capsule daily, increased if necessary to twice daily; elderly, 1 daily
Angina, 1 capsule twice daily

Tenif® (AstraZeneca) PoM
Capsules, reddish-brown, atenolol 50 mg, nifedipine 20 mg (m/r). Net price 28-cap pack = £10.63. Label: 8, 25
Dose: hypertension, 1 capsule daily, increased if necessary to twice daily; elderly, 1 daily
Angina, 1 capsule twice daily

BISOPROLOL FUMARATE

Indications: see under Dose
Cautions: see under Propranolol Hydrochloride; reduce dose in hepatic (Appendix 2) and renal impairment (Appendix 3); in heart failure monitor clinical status for 4 hours after initiation (with low dose) and ensure heart failure not worsening before increasing each dose; psoriasis
Contra-indications: see under Propranolol Hydrochloride; also acute or decompensated heart failure requiring intravenous inotropes; sino-atrial block
Side-effects: see under Propranolol Hydrochloride
Dose: hypertension and angina, usually 10 mg once daily (5 mg may be adequate in some patients); max. 20 mg daily
Adjunct in stable moderate to severe heart failure (section 2.5.5), initially 1.25 mg once daily (in the morning) for 1 week then, if well tolerated, increased to 2.5 mg once daily for 1 week, then 3.75 mg once daily for 1 week, then 5 mg once daily for 4 weeks, then 7.5 mg once daily for 4 weeks, then 10 mg once daily; max. 10 mg daily

Bisoprolol Fumarate (Non-proprietary) PoM
Tablets, bisoprolol fumarate 5 mg, net price 28-tab pack = £7.49; 10 mg, 28-tab pack = £8.63. Label: 8
Available from Alpharma, APS, Ashbourne (*Bipranix*®), Generics, Goldshield (*Soloc*®), Lexon (*Vivacor*®), Niche, PLIVA

Cardicor® (Merck) ▼ PoM
Tablets, f/c, bisoprolol fumarate 1.25 mg, net price 28-tab pack = £8.56; 2.5 mg (scored), 28-tab pack = £8.56; 3.75 mg (scored, white-yellow), 28-tab pack = £8.56; 5 mg (scored, light yellow), 28-tab pack = £8.56; 7.5 mg (scored, yellow), 28-tab pack = £9.09; 10 mg (scored, orange), 28-tab pack = £9.61. Label: 8

Emcor® (Merck) PoM
LS Tablets, yellow, f/c, scored, bisoprolol fumarate 5 mg. Net price 28-tab pack = £8.56. Label: 8
Tablets, orange, f/c, scored, bisoprolol fumarate 10 mg. Net price 28-tab pack = £9.61. Label: 8

Monocor® (Lederle) PoM
Tablets, both f/c, bisoprolol fumarate 5 mg (pink), net price 28-tab pack = £8.56; 10 mg, 28-tab pack £9.61. Label: 8

CARVEDILOL

Indications: hypertension; angina; adjunct to diuretics, digoxin, or ACE inhibitors in symptomatic chronic heart failure
Cautions: see under Propranolol Hydrochloride; before increasing dose ensure renal function and heart failure not deteriorating; severe heart failure, avoid in acute or decompensated heart failure requiring intravenous inotropes
Contra-indications: see under Propranolol Hydrochloride; severe chronic heart failure; hepatic impairment (Appendix 2)
Side-effects: postural hypotension, dizziness, headache, fatigue, gastro-intestinal disturbances, brady-

cardia; occasionally diminished peripheral circulation, peripheral oedema and painful extremities, dry mouth, dry eyes, eye irritation or disturbed vision, impotence, disturbances of micturition, influenza-like symptoms; rarely angina, AV block, exacerbation of intermittent claudication or Raynaud's phenomenon; allergic skin reactions, exacerbation of psoriasis, nasal stuffiness, wheezing, depressed mood, sleep disturbances, paraesthesia, heart failure, changes in liver enzymes, thrombocytopenia, leucopenia also reported
Dose: hypertension, initially 12.5 mg once daily, increased after 2 days to usual dose of 25 mg once daily; if necessary may be further increased at intervals of at least 2 weeks to max. 50 mg daily in single or divided doses; ELDERLY initial dose of 12.5 mg daily may provide satisfactory control
Angina, initially 12.5 mg twice daily, increased after 2 days to 25 mg twice daily
Adjunct in heart failure (section 2.5.5) initially 3.125 mg twice daily (with food), dose increased at intervals of at least 2 weeks to 6.25 mg twice daily, then to 12.5 mg twice daily, then to 25 mg twice daily; increase to highest dose tolerated, max. 25 mg twice daily in patients with severe heart failure or body-weight less than 85 kg and 50 mg twice daily in patients over 85 kg

Eucardic® (Roche) ▼ PoM
Tablets, all scored, carvedilol 3.125 mg (pink), net price 28-tab pack = £8.14; 6.25 mg (yellow), 28-tab pack = £9.04; 12.5 mg (peach), 28-tab pack = £10.05; 25 mg, 28-tab pack = £12.56. Label: 8

CELIPROLOL HYDROCHLORIDE

Indications: mild to moderate hypertension
Cautions: see under Propranolol Hydrochloride
Contra-indications: see under Propranolol Hydrochloride; also avoid in severe renal impairment
Side-effects: headache, dizziness, fatigue, nausea and somnolence; also bradycardia, bronchospasm; depression and pneumonitis reported rarely
Dose: 200 mg once daily in the morning, increased to 400 mg once daily if necessary

Celiprolol (Non-proprietary) PoM
Tablets, celiprolol hydrochloride 200 mg, net price 28-tab pack = £14.61; 400 mg, 28-tab pack = £33.09. Label: 8, 22
Available from APS, Generics, IVAX, Sovereign

Celectol® (Pantheon) PoM
Tablets, both f/c, scored, celiprolol hydrochloride 200 mg (yellow), net price 28-tab pack = £17.19; 400 mg, 28-tab pack = £34.38. Label: 8, 22

ESMOLOL HYDROCHLORIDE

Indications: short-term treatment of supraventricular arrhythmias (including atrial fibrillation, atrial flutter, sinus tachycardia); tachycardia and hypertension in peri-operative period
Cautions: see under Propranolol Hydrochloride; renal impairment
Contra-indications: see under Propranolol Hydrochloride
Side-effects: see under Propranolol Hydrochloride
Dose: *by intravenous infusion*, usually within range 50–200 micrograms/kg/minute (consult product literature for details of dose titration and doses during peri-operative period)

Brevibloc® (Baxter) [PoM]
Injection, esmolol hydrochloride 10 mg/mL, net price 10-mL vial = £6.49, 250-mL infusion bag = £74.75
Injection concentrate, esmolol hydrochloride 250 mg/mL (for dilution before infusion), 10-mL amp = £72.49

LABETALOL HYDROCHLORIDE

Indications: hypertension (including hypertension in pregnancy, hypertension with angina, and hypertension following acute myocardial infarction); hypertensive crisis (but see section 2.5); controlled hypotension in anaesthesia

Cautions: see under Propranolol Hydrochloride; interferes with laboratory tests for catecholamines; liver damage (see below)

LIVER DAMAGE. Severe hepatocellular damage reported after both short-term and long-term treatment. Appropriate laboratory testing needed at first symptom of liver dysfunction and if laboratory evidence of damage (or if jaundice) labetalol should be stopped and not restarted

Contra-indications: see under Propranolol Hydrochloride

Side-effects: postural hypotension (avoid upright position during and for 3 hours after intravenous administration), tiredness, weakness, headache, rashes, scalp tingling, difficulty in micturition, epigastric pain, nausea, vomiting; liver damage (see above); rarely lichenoid rash

Dose: *by mouth*, initially 100 mg (50 mg in elderly) twice daily with food, increased at intervals of 14 days to usual dose of 200 mg twice daily; up to 800 mg daily in 2 divided doses (3–4 divided doses if higher); max. 2.4 g daily
By intravenous injection, 50 mg over at least 1 minute, repeated after 5 minutes if necessary; max. 200 mg

NOTE. Excessive bradycardia can be countered with intravenous injection of atropine sulphate 0.6–2.4 mg in divided doses of 600 micrograms; for **overdosage** see Emergency Treatment of Poisoning, p. 24

By intravenous infusion, 2 mg/minute until satisfactory response then discontinue; usual total dose 50–200 mg, (**not** recommended for phaeochromocytoma, see under Phaeochromocytoma, section 2.5.4)
Hypertension of pregnancy, 20 mg/hour, doubled every 30 minutes; usual max. 160 mg/hour
Hypertension following myocardial infarction, 15 mg/hour, gradually increased to max. 120 mg/hour

Labetalol Hydrochloride (Non-proprietary) [PoM]
Tablets, all f/c, labetalol hydrochloride 100 mg, net price 20 = £1.69; 200 mg, 20 = £2.29; 400 mg, 20 = £3.97. Label: 8, 21
Available from Alpharma, Hillcross, Ivax

Trandate® (Celltech) [PoM]
Tablets, all orange, f/c, labetalol hydrochloride 50 mg, net price 56-tab pack = £5.05; 100 mg, 56-tab pack = £5.56; 200 mg, 56-tab pack = £9.02; 400 mg, 56-tab pack = £12.56. Label: 8, 21
Injection, labetalol hydrochloride 5 mg/mL. Net price 20-mL amp = £2.83

METOPROLOL TARTRATE

Indications: see under Dose
Cautions: see under Propranolol Hydrochloride; reduce dose in hepatic impairment

Contra-indications: see under Propranolol Hydrochloride
Side-effects: see under Propranolol Hydrochloride
Dose: *by mouth*, hypertension, initially 100 mg daily, maintenance 100–200 mg daily in 1–2 doses
Angina, 50–100 mg 2–3 times daily
Arrhythmias, usually 50 mg 2–3 times daily; up to 300 mg daily in divided doses if necessary
Migraine prophylaxis, 100–200 mg daily in divided doses
Hyperthyroidism (adjunct), 50 mg 4 times daily
By intravenous injection, arrhythmias, up to 5 mg at rate 1–2 mg/minute, repeated after 5 minutes if necessary, total dose 10–15 mg

NOTE. Excessive bradycardia can be countered with intravenous injection of atropine sulphate 0.6–2.4 mg in divided doses of 600 micrograms; for **overdosage** see Emergency Treatment of Poisoning, p. 24

In surgery, 2–4 mg *by slow intravenous injection* at induction or to control arrhythmias developing during anaesthesia; 2-mg doses may be repeated to a max. of 10 mg
Early intervention within 12 hours of infarction, 5 mg *by intravenous injection* every 2 minutes to a max. of 15 mg, followed after 15 minutes by 50 mg *by mouth* every 6 hours for 48 hours; maintenance 200 mg daily in divided doses

Metoprolol Tartrate (Non-proprietary) [PoM]
Tablets, metoprolol tartrate 50 mg, net price 20 = 63p; 100 mg, 20 = £1.15. Label: 8
Available from Alpharma, APS, Hillcross, IVAX

Betaloc® (AstraZeneca) [PoM]
Tablets, both scored, metoprolol tartrate 50 mg, net price 100-tab pack = £3.30; 100 mg, 100-tab pack = £6.13. Label: 8
Injection, metoprolol tartrate 1 mg/mL. Net price 5-mL amp = 42p

Lopresor® (Novartis) [PoM]
Tablets, both f/c, scored, metoprolol tartrate 50 mg (pink), net price 56-tab pack = £2.57; 100 mg (blue), 56-tab pack = £6.68. Label: 8

■ Modified release
Betaloc-SA® (AstraZeneca) [PoM]
Durules® (= tablets, m/r), metoprolol tartrate 200 mg, net price 28-tab pack = £4.56. Label: 8, 25
Dose: hypertension, angina, 200 mg daily in the morning, increased to 400 mg daily if necessary; migraine prophylaxis, 200 mg daily

Lopresor SR® (Novartis) [PoM]
Tablets, m/r, yellow, f/c, metoprolol tartrate 200 mg, net price 28-tab pack = £9.80. Label: 8, 25
Dose: hypertension, 200 mg daily; angina, 200–400 mg daily; migraine prophylaxis, 200 mg daily

■ With diuretic
Co-Betaloc® (Searle) [PoM]
Tablets, scored, metoprolol tartrate 100 mg, hydrochlorothiazide 12.5 mg, net price 28-tab pack = £5.59. Label: 8
Dose: hypertension, 1–3 tablets daily in single or divided doses

Co-Betaloc SA® (Searle) [PoM]
Tablets, yellow, f/c, metoprolol tartrate (m/r) 200 mg, hydrochlorothiazide 25 mg, net price 28-tab pack = £6.89. Label: 8, 25
Dose: hypertension, 1 tablet daily

NADOLOL

Indications: see under Dose
Cautions: see under Propranolol Hydrochloride; reduce dose in renal impairment
Contra-indications: see under Propranolol Hydrochloride
Side-effects: see under Propranolol Hydrochloride
Dose: hypertension, 80 mg daily, increased at weekly intervals if required; max. 240 mg daily
Angina, 40 mg daily, increased at weekly intervals if required; usual max. 160 mg daily
Arrhythmias, initially 40 mg daily, increased to 160 mg if required; reduce to 40 mg if bradycardia occurs
Migraine prophylaxis, initially 40 mg daily, increased by 40 mg at weekly intervals; usual maintenance dose 80–160 mg daily
Thyrotoxicosis (adjunct), 80–160 mg daily

Corgard® (Sanofi-Synthelabo) PoM
Tablets, blue, scored, nadolol 80 mg, net price 28-tab pack = £5.20. Label: 8

■ With diuretic
Corgaretic® (Sanofi-Synthelabo) PoM
Tablets, scored, nadolol 40 mg, bendroflumethiazide 5 mg (*Corgaretic 40*®), net price 28-tab pack = £5.92. Label: 8
Dose: hypertension, 1–2 tablets daily

NEBIVOLOL

Indications: essential hypertension
Cautions: see under Propranolol Hydrochloride; reduce dose in renal impairment (Appendix 3); elderly
Contra-indications: see under Propranolol Hydrochloride; hepatic impairment
Side-effects: see under Propranolol Hydrochloride; oedema, headache, depression, visual disturbances, paraesthesia, impotence
Dose: 5 mg daily; ELDERLY initially 2.5 mg daily, increased if necessary to 5 mg daily

Nebilet® (Menarini) PoM
Tablets, scored, nebivolol (as hydrochloride) 5 mg, net price 28-tab pack = £9.80

OXPRENOLOL HYDROCHLORIDE

Indications: see under Dose
Cautions: see under Propranolol Hydrochloride
Contra-indications: see under Propranolol Hydrochloride
Side-effects: see under Propranolol Hydrochloride
Dose: hypertension, 80–160 mg daily in 2–3 divided doses, increased as required; max. 320 mg daily
Angina, 80–160 mg daily in 2–3 divided doses; max. 320 mg daily
Arrhythmias, 40–240 mg daily in 2–3 divided doses; max. 240 mg daily
Anxiety symptoms (short-term use), 40–80 mg daily in 1–2 divided doses

Oxprenolol (Non-proprietary) PoM
Tablets, all coated, oxprenolol hydrochloride 20 mg, net price 20 = 55p; 40 mg, 20 = £1.11; 80 mg, 20 = £2.21; 160 mg, 20 = £2.36. Label: 8
Available from Hillcross, IVAX

Trasicor® (Novartis) PoM
Tablets, all f/c, oxprenolol hydrochloride 20 mg (contain gluten), net price 56-tab pack = £1.55; 40 mg (contain gluten), 56-tab pack = £3.11; 80 mg (yellow), 56-tab pack = £6.20. Label: 8

■ Modified release
Slow-Trasicor® (Novartis) PoM
Tablets, m/r, f/c, oxprenolol hydrochloride 160 mg. Net price 28-tab pack = £6.63. Label: 8, 25
Dose: hypertension, angina, initially 160 mg once daily; if necessary may be increased to max. 320 mg daily
NOTE. Modified-release tablets containing oxprenolol hydrochloride 160 mg also available from IVAX

■ With diuretic
Trasidrex® (Novartis) PoM
Tablets, red, s/c, co-prenozide 160/0.25 (oxprenolol hydrochloride 160 mg (m/r), cyclopenthiazide 250 micrograms). Net price 28-tab pack = £8.88. Label: 8, 25
Dose: hypertension, 1 tablet daily, increased if necessary to 2 daily as a single dose

PINDOLOL

Indications: see under Dose
Cautions: see under Propranolol Hydrochloride; reduce dose in renal impairment
Contra-indications: see under Propranolol Hydrochloride
Side-effects: see under Propranolol Hydrochloride
Dose: hypertension, initially 5 mg 2–3 times daily *or* 15 mg once daily, increased as required at weekly intervals; usual maintenance 15–30 mg daily; max. 45 mg daily
Angina, 2.5–5 mg up to 3 times daily

Visken® (Novartis) PoM
Tablets, both scored, pindolol 5 mg, net price 56-tab pack = £4.88; 15 mg, 28-tab pack = £7.33. Label: 8

■ With diuretic
Viskaldix® (Novartis) PoM
Tablets, scored, pindolol 10 mg, clopamide 5 mg. Net price 28-tab pack = £6.70. Label: 8
Dose: hypertension, 1 tablet daily in the morning, increased if necessary to 2 daily; max. 3 daily

SOTALOL HYDROCHLORIDE

Indications: *Tablets and injection:* life-threatening arrhythmias including ventricular tachyarrhythmias, symptomatic non-sustained ventricular tachyarrhythmias
Tablets only: prophylaxis of paroxysmal atrial tachycardia or fibrillation, paroxysmal AV re-entrant tachycardias (both nodal and involving accessory pathways), paroxysmal supraventricular tachycardia after cardiac surgery, maintenance of sinus rhythm following cardioversion of atrial fibrillation or flutter
Injection only: electrophysiological study of inducible ventricular and supraventricular arrhythmias; temporary substitution for tablets
CSM advice. The use of sotalol should be limited to the treatment of ventricular arrhythmias or prophylaxis of supraventricular arrhythmias (see above). It should no longer be used for angina, hypertension, thyrotoxicosis or for secondary prevention after myocardial infarction; when stopping sotalol for these indications, the dose should be reduced gradually

Cautions: see under Propranolol Hydrochloride; reduce dose in renal impairment (avoid if severe); correct hypokalaemia, hypomagnesaemia, or other electrolyte disturbances; severe or prolonged diarrhoea; **interactions:** Appendix 1 (beta-blockers), **important:** verapamil interaction see also p. 106

Contra-indications: see under Propranolol Hydrochloride; congenital or acquired long QT syndrome; torsades de pointes; renal failure

Side-effects: see under Propranolol Hydrochloride; arrhythmogenic (pro-arrhythmic) effect (torsades de pointes—increased risk in women)

Dose: *by mouth* with ECG monitoring and measurement of corrected QT interval, arrhythmias, initially 80 mg daily in 1–2 divided doses increased gradually at intervals of 2–3 days to usual dose of 160–320 mg daily in 2 divided doses; higher doses of 480–640 mg daily for life-threatening ventricular arrhythmias under specialist supervision

By intravenous injection over 10 minutes, acute arrhythmias, 20–120 mg with ECG monitoring, repeated if necessary with 6-hour intervals between injections

Diagnostic use, see product literature

NOTE. Excessive bradycardia can be countered with intravenous injection of atropine sulphate 0.6–2.4 mg in divided doses of 600 micrograms; for **overdosage** see Emergency Treatment of Poisoning, p. 24

Sotalol (Non-proprietary) PoM
Tablet, sotalol hydrochloride 40 mg, net price 20 = 79p; 80 mg, 28-tab pack = £1.65; 160 mg, 28-tab pack = £6.13. Label: 8
Available from Generics, Hillcross, Taro, Tillomed

Beta-Cardone® (Celltech) PoM
Tablets, all scored, sotalol hydrochloride 40 mg (green), net price 56-tab pack = £2.22; 80 mg (pink), 56-tab pack = £3.29; 200 mg, 28-tab pack = £4.15. Label: 8

Sotacor® (Bristol-Myers Squibb) PoM
Tablets, sotalol hydrochloride 80 mg, net price 28-tab pack = £3.49; 160 mg, 28-tab pack = £6.89. Label: 8
Injection, sotalol hydrochloride 10 mg/mL. Net price 4-mL amp = £1.76

TIMOLOL MALEATE

Indications: see under Dose; glaucoma (section 11.6)

Cautions: see under Propranolol Hydrochloride

Contra-indications: see under Propranolol Hydrochloride

Side-effects: see under Propranolol Hydrochloride

Dose: hypertension, initially 5 mg twice daily *or* 10 mg once daily; gradually increased if necessary to max. 60 mg daily (given in divided doses above 20 mg daily)

Angina, initially 5 mg 2–3 times daily, usual maintenance 35–45 mg daily (range 15–45 mg daily)

Prophylaxis after myocardial infarction, initially 5 mg twice daily, increased after 2 days to 10 mg twice daily, starting 7 to 28 days after infarction

Migraine prophylaxis, 10–20 mg once daily

Betim® (ICN) PoM
Tablets, scored, timolol maleate 10 mg. Net price 30-tab pack = £2.45. Label: 8

■ With diuretic
Moducren® (MSD) PoM
Tablets, blue, scored, timolol maleate 10 mg, co-amilozide 2.5/25 (amiloride hydrochloride 2.5 mg, hydrochlorothiazide 25 mg). Net price 28-tab pack = £8.00. Label: 8
Dose: hypertension, 1–2 tablets daily as a single dose

Prestim® (ICN) PoM
Tablets, scored, timolol maleate 10 mg, bendroflumethiazide 2.5 mg. Net price 30-tab pack = £4.11. Label: 8
Dose: hypertension, 1–2 tablets daily; max. 4 daily

2.5 Drugs affecting the renin-angiotensin system and some other antihypertensive drugs

2.5.1	Vasodilator antihypertensive drugs
2.5.2	Centrally acting antihypertensive drugs
2.5.3	Adrenergic neurone blocking drugs
2.5.4	Alpha-adrenoceptor blocking drugs
2.5.5	Drugs affecting the renin-angiotensin system
2.5.6	Ganglion-blocking drugs
2.5.7	Tyrosine hydroxylase inhibitors

Lowering raised blood pressure decreases the frequency of stroke, coronary events, heart failure, and renal failure. Advice on antihypertensive therapy in this section reflects the recommendations of the British Hypertension Society (Guidelines for management of hypertension: report of the third working party of the British Hypertension Society. *J Hum Hypertens* 1999; **13:** 569–92).

Possible causes of hypertension (e.g. renal disease, endocrine causes), contributory factors, risk factors, and the presence of any complications of hypertension, such as left ventricular hypertrophy, should be established. Patients should be given advice on lifestyle changes to reduce blood pressure or cardiovascular risk; these include smoking cessation, weight reduction, reduction of excessive intake of alcohol, reduction of dietary salt, reduction of total and saturated fat, increasing exercise, and increasing fruit and vegetable intake.

THRESHOLDS AND TARGETS FOR TREATMENT. The following thresholds for treatment are recommended:

- Accelerated (malignant) hypertension (with papilloedema or fundal haemorrhages and exudates) *or* impending cardiovascular complications, admit for **immediate treatment**;
- Where the initial blood pressure is systolic ≥ 220 mmHg *or* diastolic ≥ 120 mmHg, **treat immediately**;
- Where the initial blood pressure is systolic 200–219 mmHg *or* diastolic 110–119 mmHg, confirm over 1–2 weeks then **treat** if these values are sustained;
- Where the initial blood pressure is systolic 160–199 mmHg *or* diastolic 100–109 mmHg, *and* the patient has cardiovascular complications, end-organ damage (e.g. left ventricular hyper-

trophy, renal impairment) or diabetes mellitus (type 1 or 2), confirm over 3–4 weeks then **treat** if these values are sustained;
- Where the initial blood pressure is systolic 160–199 mmHg *or* diastolic 100–109 mmHg, but the patient has *no* cardiovascular complications, end-organ damage or diabetes, advise lifestyle changes, reassess weekly initially and **treat** if these values are sustained on repeat measurements over 4–12 weeks;
- Where the initial blood pressure is systolic 140–159 mmHg *or* diastolic 90–99 mmHg *and* the patient has cardiovascular complications, end-organ damage or diabetes, confirm within 4–12 weeks and **treat** if these values are sustained;
- Where the initial blood pressure is systolic 140–159 mmHg *or* diastolic 90–99 mmHg and *no* cardiovascular complications, end-organ damage or diabetes, advise lifestyle changes and **reassess** monthly; if mild hypertension persists, **treat** if coronary heart disease risk[1] is $\geq 15\%$ over 10 years.

An optimal target systolic blood pressure < 140 mmHg *and* diastolic blood pressure < 85 mmHg is suggested.[2]

DRUG TREATMENT OF HYPERTENSION. No consistent or important differences have been found between the major classes of antihypertensive drugs in terms of antihypertensive efficacy, side-effects or changes to quality of life (but there are differences in response related to age and ethnic group). The choice of antihypertensive drug will depend on the relevant indications or contra-indications for the individual patient; *some* indications and contra-indications for various antihypertensive drugs are shown below (see also under individual drug entries for details):

- **Thiazides** (section 2.2.1)—particularly indicated for hypertension in the elderly (see below); a contra-indication is gout;
- **Beta-blockers** (section 2.4)—indications include myocardial infarction, angina; compelling contra-indications include asthma, heart block;
- **ACE inhibitors** (section 2.5.5.1)—indications include heart failure, left ventricular dysfunction and diabetic nephropathy; contra-indications include renovascular disease (but see section 2.5.5.1) and pregnancy;
- **Angiotensin-II receptor antagonists** (section 2.5.5.2) are alternatives for those who cannot tolerate ACE inhibitors because of persistent dry cough, but they have the same contra-indications as ACE inhibitors;
- **Calcium-channel blockers**. There are important differences between calcium-channel blockers (section 2.6.2). **Dihydropyridine calcium-channel blockers** are valuable in isolated

systolic hypertension in the elderly when a low-dose thiazide is contra-indicated or not tolerated (see below). **'Rate-limiting' calcium-channel blockers** (e.g. diltiazem, verapamil) may be valuable in angina; contra-indications include heart failure and heart block;
- **Alpha-blockers** (section 2.5.4)—a possible indication is prostatism; a contra-indication is urinary incontinence.

A single antihypertensive drug is often not adequate and other antihypertensive drugs are usually added in a step-wise manner until control is achieved. Unless it is necessary to lower the blood pressure urgently, an interval of at least 4 weeks should be allowed to determine response. Where two antihypertensive drugs are needed, an ACE inhibitor *or* an angiotensin-II receptor antagonist *or* a beta-blocker may be combined with *either* a thiazide *or* a calcium-channel blocker. In patients with **primary hyperaldosteronism**, spironolactone (section 2.2.3) is effective.

Response to drug treatment for hypertension may be affected by the patient's age and ethnic background. A beta-blocker or an ACE inhibitor may be the most appropriate initial drug in younger Caucasians; Afro-Caribbean patients respond less well to these drugs and a thiazide or a calcium-channel blocker may be chosen for initial treatment.

OTHER MEASURES TO REDUCE CARDIOVASCULAR RISK. **Aspirin** (section 2.9) in a dose of 75 mg daily reduces the risk of cardiovascular events and myocardial infarction; however, concerns about an increased risk of bleeding need to be considered. Unless it is contra-indicated, aspirin is recommended for *secondary prevention* in patients with cardiovascular complications (myocardial infarction, angina, non-haemorrhagic cerebrovascular disease, peripheral vascular disease, or atherosclerotic renovascular disease), and for *primary prevention* in patients aged over 50 years with controlled blood pressure (systolic pressure < 150 mmHg and diastolic pressure < 90 mmHg) who have end-organ damage, type 2 diabetes, or a coronary heart disease risk[1] $\geq 15\%$ over 10 years.

A **statin** can be of benefit in those at high risk of coronary heart disease and stroke and in those with hypercholesterolaemia (see section 2.12 for details).

HYPERTENSION IN THE ELDERLY. Benefit from antihypertensive therapy is evident up to at least 85 years of age, but it is probably inappropriate to apply a strict age limit when deciding on drug therapy. Elderly individuals who have a good outlook for longevity should have their blood pressure lowered if they are hypertensive. The thresholds for treatment are diastolic pressure averaging ≥ 90 mmHg *or* systolic pressure averaging ≥ 160 mmHg over 3 to 6 months' observation (despite appropriate non-drug treatment). A low dose of a thiazide is the clear drug of first choice, with addition of a beta-blocker when necessary.

ISOLATED SYSTOLIC HYPERTENSION. Isolated systolic hypertension (systolic pressure ≥ 160 mmHg, diastolic pressure < 90 mmHg) is associated with an increased risk of stroke and coronary events, particularly in those aged over 60 years. Systolic blood pressure averaging 160 mmHg or higher over 3 to 6 months (despite appropriate non-drug treat-

---

1. Coronary heart disease risk may be formally estimated using the Joint British Societies' 'Cardiac Risk Assessor' computer program or chart (British Cardiac Society, British Hyperlipidaemia Association, British Hypertension Society. *Heart* 1998; **80** (suppl 2): S1–29)

See inside back cover

2. A lower target for blood pressure should be considered for the secondary prevention of stroke, and for patients with diabetes and renal disease

ment) should be lowered in those over 60 years, even if diastolic hypertension is absent. Treatment with a low dose of a thiazide, with addition of a beta-blocker when necessary is effective; a long-acting dihydropyridine calcium-channel blocker is recommended when a thiazide is contra-indicated or not tolerated. Patients with severe postural hypotension should not receive blood pressure lowering drugs.

Isolated systolic hypertension in younger patients is uncommon but treatment may be indicated in those with a threshold systolic pressure of 160 mmHg or less if at increased risk of coronary heart disease, see above).

HYPERTENSION IN DIABETES. Hypertension is common in type 2 (non-insulin-dependent) diabetes and treatment prevents both macrovascular and microvascular complications. Systolic blood pressure $\geq$ 140 mmHg *or* diastolic pressure $\geq$ 90 mmHg should be lowered to a target systolic blood pressure < 140 mmHg and a diastolic pressure < 80 mmHg. Low-dose thiazides, beta-blockers, ACE inhibitors and dihydropyridine calcium-channel blockers have all shown benefit in type 2 diabetes.

In type 1 (insulin-dependent) diabetes, hypertension usually indicates the presence of diabetic nephropathy and ACE inhibitors and angiotensin-II receptor antagonists have a specific role in this condition (section 6.1.5). The threshold for treatment of hypertension in type 1 diabetes is the same as that for type 2 diabetes, and the target for patients without nephropathy is a systolic blood pressure < 140 mmHg and a diastolic pressure < 80 mmHg; if nephropathy is present the target is a systolic blood pressure < 130 mmHg and a diastolic pressure < 80 mmHg, or even lower if proteinuria exceeds 1 g in 24 hours.

HYPERTENSION IN RENAL DISEASE. The threshold for antihypertensive treatment in patients with renal impairment or persistent proteinuria is a systolic blood pressure $\geq$ 140 mmHg *or* a diastolic blood pressure $\geq$ 90 mmHg. Optimal blood pressure is a systolic blood pressure < 130 mmHg and a diastolic pressure < 85 mmHg, or lower if proteinuria exceeds 1 g in 24 hours. Thiazides may be ineffective and high doses of loop diuretics may be required. Specific cautions apply to the use of ACE inhibitors in renal impairment, see section 2.5.5.1.

HYPERTENSION IN PREGNANCY. High blood pressure in pregnancy may usually be due to pre-existing essential hypertension or to pre-eclampsia. Methyldopa (section 2.5.2) is safe in pregnancy. Beta-blockers are effective and safe in the third trimester. Modified-release preparations of nifedipine [unlicensed] are also used for hypertension in pregnancy. Intravenous administration of labetalol (section 2.4) can be used to control hypertensive crises; alternatively hydralazine (section 2.5.1) may be used by the intravenous route. For use of magnesium sulphate in eclampsia, see section 9.5.1.3.

ACCELERATED OR VERY SEVERE HYPERTENSION. Accelerated (or malignant) hypertension or very severe hypertension (e.g. diastolic blood pressure > 140 mmHg) requires urgent treatment in hospital, but it is not an indication for parenteral antihypertensive therapy. Normally treatment should be by

mouth with a beta-blocker (atenolol or labetalol) or a long-acting calcium-channel blocker (e.g. amlodipine or modified-release nifedipine). Within the first 24 hours the diastolic blood pressure should be reduced to 100–110 mmHg. Over the next 2 or 3 days blood pressure should be normalised by using beta-blockers, calcium-channel blockers, diuretics, vasodilators, or ACE inhibitors. Very rapid reduction in blood pressure can reduce organ perfusion leading to cerebral infarction and blindness, deterioration in renal function, and myocardial ischaemia. Parenteral antihypertensive drugs are rarely necessary; sodium nitroprusside by infusion is the drug of choice on the rare occasions when parenteral treatment is necessary.

For advice on short-term management of hypertensive episodes in phaeochromocytoma, see under Phaeochromocytoma, section 2.5.4.

2.5.1 Vasodilator antihypertensive drugs

These are potent drugs, especially when used in combination with a beta-blocker and a thiazide. **Important:** for a warning on the hazards of a very rapid fall in blood pressure, see section 2.5.

Diazoxide has been used by intravenous injection in hypertensive emergencies.

Hydralazine given by mouth is a useful adjunct to other treatment, but when used alone causes tachycardia and fluid retention. Side-effects can be few if the dose is kept below 100 mg daily, but systemic lupus erythematosus should be suspected if there is unexplained weight loss, arthritis, or any other unexplained ill health.

Sodium nitroprusside is given by intravenous infusion to control severe hypertensive crises on the rare occasions when parenteral treatment is necessary.

Minoxidil should be reserved for the treatment of severe hypertension resistant to other drugs. Vasodilatation is accompanied by increased cardiac output and tachycardia and the patients develop fluid retention. For this reason the addition of a beta-blocker and a diuretic (usually furosemide, in high dosage) are mandatory. Hypertrichosis is troublesome and renders this drug unsuitable for women.

Prazosin, doxazosin, and terazosin (section 2.5.4) have alpha-blocking and vasodilator properties.

Bosentan is licensed for the treatment of pulmonary arterial hypertension.

BOSENTAN

Indications: pulmonary arterial hypertension

Cautions: not to be initiated if systemic systolic blood pressure is below 85 mmHg; monitor liver function before and during treatment (reduce dose or suspend treatement if liver enzymes raised significantly) — discontinue if symptoms of liver impairment; monitor haemoglobin; **interactions:** Appendix 1 (bosentan)

Contra-indications: hepatic impairment (Appendix 2); **avoid** pregnancy **during** and for **3 months after** treatment; breast feeding

Side-effects: dyspepsia, flushing, hypotension, palpitations, fatigue, oedema, anaemia, pruritus, nasopharyngitis, hepatic impairment (see Cautions above)

Dose: initially 62.5 mg twice daily increased after 4 weeks to 125 mg twice daily; max. 250 mg twice daily

Tracleer® (Actelion) ▼ PoM
Tablets, f/c, orange, bosentan (as monohydrate) 62.5 mg, net price 56-tab pack = £1615.00; 125 mg, 56-tab pack = £1615.00

DIAZOXIDE

Indications: severe hypertension associated with renal disease (but see section 2.5); hypoglycaemia (section 6.1.4)

Cautions: ischaemic heart disease, pregnancy, labour, impaired renal function; **interactions:** Appendix 1 (diazoxide)

Side-effects: tachycardia, hyperglycaemia, sodium and water retention

Dose: *by rapid intravenous injection* (less than 30 seconds), 1–3 mg/kg to max. single dose of 150 mg (see below); may be repeated after 5–15 minutes if required
NOTE. Single doses of 300 mg have been associated with angina and with myocardial and cerebral infarction

Eudemine® (Goldshield) PoM [▬]
Injection, diazoxide 15 mg/mL. Net price 20-mL amp = £30.00

HYDRALAZINE HYDROCHLORIDE

Indications: moderate to severe hypertension (adjunct); heart failure (with long-acting nitrate, but see section 2.5.5); hypertensive crisis (including during pregnancy) (but see section 2.5)

Cautions: hepatic impairment (Appendix 2), renal impairment (Appendix 3); coronary artery disease (may provoke angina, avoid after myocardial infarction until stabilised), cerebrovascular disease; occasionally blood pressure reduction too rapid even with low parenteral doses; pregnancy (Appendix 4), breast-feeding; manufacturer advises test for antinuclear factor and for proteinuria every 6 months and check acetylator status before increasing dose above 100 mg daily, but evidence of clinical value unsatisfactory; **interactions:** Appendix 1 (hydralazine)

Contra-indications: idiopathic systemic lupus erythematosus, severe tachycardia, high output heart failure, myocardial insufficiency due to mechanical obstruction, cor pulmonale, dissecting aortic aneurysm; porphyria (section 9.8.2)

Side-effects: tachycardia, palpitations, flushing, hypotension, fluid retention, gastro-intestinal disturbances; headache, dizziness; systemic lupus erythematosus-like syndrome after long-term therapy with over 100 mg daily (or less in women and in slow acetylator individuals) (see also notes above); rarely rashes, fever, peripheral neuritis, polyneuritis, paraesthesia, arthralgia, myalgia, increased lacrimation, nasal congestion, dyspnoea, agitation, anxiety, anorexia; blood disorders (including leucopenia, thrombocytopenia, haemolytic anaemia), abnormal liver function, jaundice, raised plasma creatinine, proteinuria and haematuria reported

Dose: *by mouth*, hypertension, 25 mg twice daily, increased to usual max. 50 mg twice daily (see notes above)

Heart failure (initiated in hospital) 25 mg 3–4 times daily, increased every 2 days if necessary; usual maintenance dose 50–75 mg 4 times daily

By slow intravenous injection, hypertension with renal complications and hypertensive crisis, 5–10 mg diluted with 10 mL sodium chloride 0.9%; may be repeated after 20–30 minutes (see Cautions)

By intravenous infusion, hypertension with renal complications and hypertensive crisis, initially 200–300 micrograms/minute; maintenance usually 50–150 micrograms/minute

Hydralazine (Non-proprietary) PoM
Tablets, hydralazine hydrochloride 25 mg, net price 20 = 54p; 50 mg, 20 = £1.06

Apresoline® (Sovereign) PoM
Tablets, yellow, s/c, hydralazine hydrochloride 25 mg, net price 84-tab pack = £2.35
Excipients: include gluten
Injection, powder for reconstitution, hydralazine hydrochloride. Net price 20-mg amp = £1.54

MINOXIDIL

Indications: severe hypertension, in addition to a diuretic and a beta-blocker

Cautions: see notes above; angina; after myocardial infarction (until stabilised); lower doses in dialysis patients; pregnancy; porphyria (section 9.8.2); **interactions:** Appendix 1 (minoxidil)

Contra-indications: phaeochromocytoma

Side-effects: sodium and water retention; weight gain, peripheral oedema, tachycardia, hypertrichosis; reversible rise in creatinine and blood urea nitrogen; occasionally, gastro-intestinal disturbances, breast tenderness, rashes

Dose: initially 5 mg (elderly, 2.5 mg) daily, in 1–2 doses, increased by 5–10 mg every 3 or more days; max. usually 50 mg daily

Loniten® (Pharmacia) PoM
Tablets, all scored, minoxidil 2.5 mg, net price 60-tab pack = £8.88; 5 mg, 60-tab pack = £15.83; 10 mg, 60-tab pack = £30.68

SODIUM NITROPRUSSIDE

Indications: hypertensive crisis (but see section 2.5); controlled hypotension in anaesthesia; acute or chronic heart failure

Cautions: hypothyroidism, renal impairment, hyponatraemia, ischaemic heart disease, impaired cerebral circulation, elderly; hypothermia; monitor blood pressure and blood-cyanide concentration and if treatment exceeds 3 days, also blood-thiocyanate concentration; avoid sudden withdrawal—terminate infusion over 15–30 minutes; pregnancy and breast-feeding; **interactions:** Appendix 1 (nitroprusside)

Contra-indications: severe hepatic impairment; severe vitamin B_{12} deficiency; Leber's optic atrophy; compensatory hypertension

Side-effects: associated with over rapid reduction in blood pressure (reduce infusion rate): headache, dizziness, nausea, retching, abdominal pain, perspiration, palpitations, apprehension, retrosternal discomfort; occasionally reduced platelet count, acute transient phlebitis
CYANIDE. Side-effects caused by excessive plasma concentration of the cyanide metabolite include tachycardia,

sweating, hyperventilation, arrhythmias, marked metabolic acidosis (discontinue and give antidote, see p. 26)

Dose: hypertensive crisis, *by intravenous infusion*, initially 0.5–1.5 micrograms/kg/minute, then increased in steps of 500 nanograms/kg/minute every 5 minutes within range 0.5–8 micrograms/kg/minute (lower doses in patients already receiving other antihypertensives); stop if response unsatisfactory with max. dose in 10 minutes

NOTE. Lower initial dose of 300 nanograms/kg/minute has been used

Maintenance of blood pressure at 30–40% lower than pretreatment diastolic blood pressure, 20–400 micrograms/minute (lower doses for patients being treated with other antihypertensives)

Controlled hypotension in surgery, *by intravenous infusion*, max. 1.5 micrograms/kg/minute

Heart failure, *by intravenous infusion*, initially 10–15 micrograms/minute, increased every 5–10 minutes as necessary; usual range 10–200 micrograms/minute normally for max. 3 days

Sodium Nitroprusside (Non-proprietary) PoM
Intravenous infusion, powder for reconstitution, sodium nitroprusside 10 mg/mL. For dilution and use as an infusion, net price 5-mL vial = £6.64
Available from Faulding DBL

2.5.2 Centrally acting antihypertensive drugs

Methyldopa is a centrally acting antihypertensive; it may be used for the management of hypertension in pregnancy. Side-effects are minimised if the daily dose is kept below 1 g.

Clonidine has the disadvantage that sudden withdrawal may cause a hypertensive crisis. Reserpine and rauwolfia are no longer used in Britain.

Moxonidine, a centrally acting drug, is licensed for mild to moderate essential hypertension. It may have a role when thiazides, beta-blockers, ACE inhibitors and calcium-channel blockers are not appropriate or have failed to control blood pressure.

CLONIDINE HYDROCHLORIDE

Indications: hypertension; migraine (section 4.7.4.2); menopausal flushing (section 6.4.1.1)

Cautions: must be withdrawn gradually to avoid hypertensive crisis; Raynaud's syndrome or other occlusive peripheral vascular disease; history of depression; avoid in porphyria (section 9.8.2); **interactions:** Appendix 1 (clonidine)
DRIVING. Drowsiness may affect performance of skilled tasks (e.g. driving); effects of alcohol may be enhanced

Side-effects: dry mouth, sedation, depression, fluid retention, bradycardia, Raynaud's phenomenon, headache, dizziness, euphoria, nocturnal unrest, rash, nausea, constipation, rarely impotence

Dose: *by mouth*, 50–100 micrograms 3 times daily, increased every second or third day; usual max. dose 1.2 mg daily
By slow intravenous injection, 150–300 micrograms; max. 750 micrograms in 24 hours

Catapres® (Boehringer Ingelheim) PoM
Tablets, both scored, clonidine hydrochloride 100 micrograms, net price 100-tab pack = £5.60; 300 micrograms, 100-tab pack = £13.04. Label: 3, 8

Injection, clonidine hydrochloride 150 micrograms/mL. Net price 1-mL amp = 29p

Dixarit® PoM
(migraine), section 4.7.4.2

METHYLDOPA

Indications: hypertension

Cautions: history of liver impairment (Appendix 2); renal impairment (Appendix 3); blood counts and liver-function tests advised; history of depression; positive direct Coombs' test in up to 20% of patients (may affect blood cross-matching); interference with laboratory tests; **interactions:** Appendix 1 (methyldopa)
DRIVING. Drowsiness may affect performance of skilled tasks (e.g. driving); effects of alcohol may be enhanced

Contra-indications: depression, active liver disease, phaeochromocytoma; porphyria (section 9.8.2)

Side-effects: gastro-intestinal disturbances, dry mouth, stomatitis, sialadenitis; bradycardia, exacerbation of angina, postural hypotension, oedema; sedation, headache, dizziness, asthenia, myalgia, arthralgia, paraesthesia, nightmares, mild psychosis, depression, impaired mental acuity, parkinsonism, Bell's palsy; abnormal liver function tests, hepatitis, jaundice; pancreatitis; haemolytic anaemia; bone-marrow depression, leucopenia, thrombocytopenia, eosinophilia; hypersensitivity reactions including lupus erythematosus-like syndrome, drug fever, myocarditis, pericarditis; rashes (including toxic epidermal necrolysis); nasal congestion, failure of ejaculation, impotence, decreased libido, gynaecomastia, hyperprolactinaemia, amenorrhoea

Dose: initially 250 mg 2–3 times daily, increased gradually at intervals of 2 or more days, max. 3 g daily; ELDERLY initially 125 mg twice daily, increased gradually, max. 2 g daily

Methyldopa (Non-proprietary) PoM
Tablets, coated, methyldopa (anhydrous) 125 mg, net price 20 = 57p; 250 mg, 20 = 60p; 500 mg, 20 = £1.23. Label: 3, 8
Available from Alpharma, CP, Hillcross, IVAX, Sovereign

Aldomet® (MSD) PoM
Tablets, all yellow, f/c, methyldopa (anhydrous) 250 mg, net price 20 = 63p; 500 mg, 20 = £1.27. Label: 3, 8

MOXONIDINE

Indications: mild to moderate essential hypertension

Cautions: renal impairment (see Appendix 3); avoid abrupt withdrawal (if concomitant treatment with beta-blocker has to be stopped, discontinue beta-blocker first, then moxonidine after few days); **interactions:** see Appendix 1 (moxonidine)

Contra-indications: history of angioedema; conduction disorders (sick sinus syndrome, sino-atrial block, second- or third-degree AV block); bradycardia; life-threatening arrhythmia; severe heart failure; severe coronary artery disease, unstable angina; severe liver disease or severe renal impairment; also on theoretical grounds: Raynaud's syndrome, intermittent claudication, epilepsy, depression, Parkinson's disease, glaucoma; pregnancy and breast-feeding

Side-effects: dry mouth; headache, fatigue, dizziness, nausea, sleep disturbance (rarely sedation), asthenia, vasodilatation; rarely skin reactions

Dose: 200 micrograms once daily in the morning, increased if necessary after 3 weeks to 400 micrograms daily in 1–2 divided doses; max. 600 micrograms daily in 2 divided doses (max. single dose 400 micrograms)

Physiotens® (Solvay) [PoM]
Tablets, f/c, moxonidine 200 micrograms (pink), net price 28-tab pack = £10.45; 300 micrograms (red), 28-tab pack = £12.35; 400 micrograms (red), 28-tab pack = £14.26. Label: 3

2.5.3 Adrenergic neurone blocking drugs

Adrenergic neurone blocking drugs prevent the release of noradrenaline from postganglionic adrenergic neurones. These drugs do not control supine blood pressure and may cause postural hypotension. For this reason they have largely fallen from use, but may be necessary with other therapy in resistant hypertension.

Guanethidine, which also depletes the nerve endings of noradrenaline, is licensed for the rapid control of blood pressure.

Bretylium (section 2.3.2) is licensed for ventricular arrhythmias.

GUANETHIDINE MONOSULPHATE

Indications: hypertensive crisis (but see section 2.5)

Cautions: renal impairment (avoid if creatinine clearance < 40 mL/minute; Appendix 3); coronary or cerebral arteriosclerosis, asthma, history of peptic ulceration; pregnancy; **interactions:** Appendix 1 (adrenergic neurone blockers)

Contra-indications: phaeochromocytoma, heart failure

Side-effects: postural hypotension, failure of ejaculation, fluid retention, nasal congestion, headache, diarrhoea, drowsiness

Dose: *by intramuscular injection*, 10–20 mg, repeated after 3 hours if required

Ismelin® (Sovereign) [PoM]
Injection, guanethidine monosulphate 10 mg/mL. Net price 1-mL amp = £1.56

2.5.4 Alpha-adrenoceptor blocking drugs

Prazosin has post-synaptic alpha-blocking and vasodilator properties and rarely causes tachycardia. It may, however, cause a rapid reduction in blood pressure after the first dose and should be introduced with caution. **Doxazosin, indoramin**, and **terazosin** have properties similar to those of prazosin.

Alpha-blockers may be used with other antihypertensive drugs in the treatment of hypertension.

PROSTATIC HYPERPLASIA. Alfuzosin, doxazosin, indoramin, prazosin, tamsulosin and terazosin are indicated for benign prostatic hyperplasia (section 7.4.1).

DOXAZOSIN

Indications: hypertension; benign prostatic hyperplasia (section 7.4.1)

Cautions: care with initial dose (postural hypotension); hepatic impairment (Appendix 2); susceptibility to heart failure; pregnancy (Appendix 4) and breast-feeding (Appendix 5); **interactions:** Appendix 1 (alpha-blockers)

Side-effects: postural hypotension; dizziness, vertigo, headache, fatigue, asthenia, oedema, somnolence, nausea, rhinitis; less frequently abdominal discomfort, diarrhoea, vomiting, agitation, tremor, rash, pruritus; rarely blurred vision, epistaxis, haematuria, thrombocytopenia, purpura, leucopenia, hepatitis, jaundice, cholestasis, and urinary incontinence; isolated cases of priapism and impotence reported

Dose: hypertension, 1 mg daily, increased after 1–2 weeks to 2 mg once daily, and thereafter to 4 mg once daily, if necessary; max. 16 mg daily

Doxazosin (Non-proprietary) [PoM]
Tablets, doxazosin (as mesilate) 1 mg, net price 28-tab pack = £8.17; 2 mg, 28-tab pack = £10.48; 4 mg, 28-tab pack = £12.34
Available from APS, Discovery (*Doxadura*®), Generics, Sterwin

Cardura® (Pfizer) [PoM]
Tablets, doxazosin (as mesilate) 1 mg, net price 28-tab pack = £10.56; 2 mg, 28-tab pack = £14.08

■ Modified-release

Cardura® **XL** (Pfizer) [PoM]
Tablets, m/r, doxazosin (as mesilate) 4 mg, net price 28-tab pack = £14.08; 8 mg, 28-tab pack = £28.16. Label: 25
Dose: 4 mg once daily, increased to 8 mg once daily after 4 weeks if necessary

INDORAMIN

Indications: hypertension; benign prostatic hyperplasia (section 7.4.1)

Cautions: avoid alcohol (enhances rate and extent of absorption); control incipient heart failure with diuretics and digoxin; hepatic or renal impairment; elderly patients; Parkinson's disease; epilepsy (convulsions in *animal* studies); history of depression; **interactions:** Appendix 1 (alpha-blockers)
DRIVING. Drowsiness may affect performance of skilled tasks (e.g. driving); effects of alcohol may be enhanced

Contra-indications: established heart failure; patients receiving MAOIs

Side-effects: sedation; also dizziness, depression, failure of ejaculation, dry mouth, nasal congestion, extrapyramidal effects, weight gain

Dose: hypertension, initially 25 mg twice daily, increased by 25–50 mg daily at intervals of 2 weeks; max. daily dose 200 mg in 2–3 divided doses

Baratol® (Shire) [PoM]
Tablets, blue, f/c, indoramin (as hydrochloride) 25 mg, net price 84-tab pack = £9.00. Label: 2

■ Prostatic hyperplasia

Doralese® [PoM] see section 7.4.1

PRAZOSIN

Indications: see under Dose

Cautions: first dose may cause collapse due to hypotension (therefore should be taken on retiring to bed); elderly; renal impairment (Appendix 3); hepatic impairment (Appendix 2); pregnancy and breast-feeding; **interactions:** Appendix 1 (alpha-blockers)

Contra-indications: not recommended for congestive heart failure due to mechanical obstruction (e.g. aortic stenosis)

Side-effects: postural hypotension, drowsiness, weakness, dizziness, headache, lack of energy, nausea, palpitations; urinary frequency, incontinence and priapism reported

Dose: hypertension, 500 micrograms 2–3 times daily, the initial dose on retiring to bed at night (to avoid collapse, see Cautions); increased to 1 mg 2–3 times daily after 3–7 days; further increased if necessary to max. 20 mg daily

Congestive heart failure (but see section 2.5.5), 500 micrograms 2–4 times daily (initial dose at bedtime, see above), increasing to 4 mg daily in divided doses; maintenance 4–20 mg daily (but rarely used)

Raynaud's syndrome (but efficacy not established, see section 2.6.4.1), initially 500 micrograms twice daily (initial dose at bedtime, see above); maintenance 1–2 mg twice daily

Benign prostatic hyperplasia, section 7.4.1

Prazosin (Non-proprietary) ▣PoM▣
Tablets, prazosin (as hydrochloride) 500 micrograms, net price 56-tab pack = £2.51; 1 mg, 56-tab pack = £3.23; 2 mg, 56-tab pack = £4.39; 5 mg, 56-tab pack = £8.75. Label: 3, counselling, see dose above
Available from APS, Hillcross, IVAX, Kent (*Kentovase*®)

Hypovase® (Pfizer) ▣PoM▣
Tablets, prazosin (as hydrochloride) 500 micrograms, net price 56-tab pack = £2.51; 1 mg (orange, scored), 56-tab pack = £3.23; 2 mg (scored), 56-tab pack = £4.39; starter pack of 8 × 500-microgram tabs with 32 × 1-mg tabs = £3.02. Label: 3, counselling, see dose above

TERAZOSIN

Indications: mild to moderate hypertension; benign prostatic hyperplasia (section 7.4.1)

Cautions: first dose may cause collapse due to hypotension (within 30–90 minutes, therefore should be taken on retiring to bed) (may also occur with rapid dose increase); **interactions:** Appendix 1 (alpha-blockers)

Side-effects: dizziness, lack of energy, peripheral oedema; urinary frequency and priapism reported

Dose: hypertension, 1 mg at bedtime (compliance with bedtime dose important, see Cautions); dose doubled after 7 days if necessary; usual maintenance dose 2–10 mg once daily; more than 20 mg daily rarely improves efficacy

Terazosin (Non-proprietary) ▣PoM▣
Tablets, terazosin (as hydrochloride) 2 mg, net price 28-tab pack = £7.75; 5 mg, 28-tab pack = £12.58; 10 mg, 28-tab pack = £25.73
Available from Alpharma, APS, Generics, Ratiopharm

Hytrin® (Abbott) ▣PoM▣
Tablets, terazosin (as hydrochloride) 2 mg (yellow), net price 28-tab pack = £8.07; 5 mg (tan), 28-tab pack = £13.07; 10 mg (blue), 28-tab pack = £26.59; starter pack of 7 × 1-mg tabs with 21 × 2-mg tabs = £13.00. Label: 3, counselling, see dose above

Phaeochromocytoma

Long-term management of phaeochromocytoma involves surgery. Alpha-blockers are used in the short-term management of hypertensive episodes in phaeochromocytoma. Once alpha blockade is established, tachycardia can be controlled by the cautious addition of a beta-blocker (section 2.4); a cardioselective beta-blocker is preferred.

Phenoxybenzamine, a powerful alpha-blocker, is effective in the management of phaeochromocytoma but it has many side-effects. **Phentolamine** is a short-acting alpha-blocker used mainly during surgery of phaeochromocytoma; its use for the diagnosis of phaeochromocytoma has been superseded by measurement of catecholamines in blood and urine.

PHENOXYBENZAMINE HYDROCHLORIDE

Indications: hypertensive episodes in phaeochromocytoma

Cautions: elderly; congestive heart failure; severe heart disease (see also Contra-indications); cerebrovascular disease (avoid if history of cerebrovascular accident); renal impairment; carcinogenic in *animals*; pregnancy; avoid in porphyria (section 9.8.2); avoid infusion in hypovolaemia; avoid extravasation (irritant to tissues)

Contra-indications: history of cerebrovascular accident; during recovery period after myocardial infarction (usually 3–4 weeks)

Side-effects: postural hypotension with dizziness and marked compensatory tachycardia, lassitude, nasal congestion, miosis, inhibition of ejaculation; rarely gastro-intestinal disturbances; decreased sweating and dry mouth after intravenous infusion; idiosyncratic profound hypotension within few minutes of starting infusion

Dose: see under preparations

Phenoxybenzamine (Goldshield) ▣PoM▣
Injection concentrate, phenoxybenzamine hydrochloride 50 mg/mL. To be diluted before use. Net price 3 × 2-mL amp = £94.88 (hosp. only)
Dose: by *intravenous infusion* (preferably through large vein), adjunct in severe shock (but rarely used) and phaeochromocytoma, 1 mg/kg daily over at least 2 hours; do not repeat within 24 hours (intensive care facilities needed)
CAUTION. Owing to risk of contact sensitisation healthcare professionals should avoid contamination of hands

Dibenyline® (Goldshield) ▣PoM▣
Capsules, red/white, phenoxybenzamine hydrochloride 10 mg. Net price 30-cap pack = £10.84
Dose: phaeochromocytoma, 10 mg daily, increased by 10 mg daily; usual dose 1–2 mg/kg daily in 2 divided doses

PHENTOLAMINE MESILATE

Indications: hypertensive episodes due to phaeochromocytoma e.g. during surgery; diagnosis of phaeochromocytoma

Cautions: monitor blood pressure (avoid in hypotension), heart rate; renal impairment; gastritis, peptic ulcer; elderly; pregnancy and breast-feeding; **interactions:** Appendix 1 (alpha-blockers)

ASTHMA. Presence of sulphites in ampoules may (especially in patients with asthma) lead to hypersensitivity (with bronchospasm and shock)

Contra-indications: hypotension; history of myocardial infarction; coronary insufficiency, angina, or other evidence of coronary artery disease

Side-effects: postural hypotension, tachycardia, dizziness, flushing; nausea and vomiting, diarrhoea, nasal congestion; also acute or prolonged hypotension, angina, chest pain, arrhythmias

Dose: hypertensive episodes, *by intravenous injection*, 2–5 mg repeated if necessary

Diagnosis of phaeochromocytoma, consult product literature

Rogitine® (Alliance) [PoM]
Injection, phentolamine mesilate 10 mg/mL. Net price 1-mL amp = £1.70

2.5.5 Drugs affecting the renin-angiotensin system

2.5.5.1 Angiotensin-converting enzyme inhibitors

2.5.5.2 Angiotensin-II receptor antagonists

Heart failure

The treatment of chronic heart failure aims to relieve symptoms, improve exercise tolerance, reduce the incidence of acute exacerbations and reduce mortality. An **ACE inhibitor** given at an adequate dose[1] generally achieves these aims; a diuretic is also necessary in most patients to reduce symptoms of fluid overload. Digoxin improves symptoms and exercise tolerance and reduces hospitalisation due to acute exacerbations but it does not reduce mortality. Drug treatment of chronic systolic heart failure is covered below; optimal management of diastolic heart failure is less certain but digoxin should probably be avoided.

An ACE inhibitor (section 2.5.5.1) is generally advised for patients with asymptomatic left ventricular dysfunction or symptomatic heart failure.

Patients with fluid overload should also receive either a loop or a thiazide diuretic (with salt or fluid restriction where appropriate). A **thiazide diuretic** (section 2.2.1) may be of benefit in patients with mild heart failure and good renal function; however, thiazide diuretics are ineffective in patients with poor renal function (estimated creatinine clearance less than 30 mL/minute, see Appendix 3) and a **loop diuretic** (section 2.2.2) is preferred. If diuresis with a single diuretic is insufficient, a combination of a loop diuretic and a thiazide diuretic may be tried; addition of metolazone (section 2.2.1) may also be considered but the resulting diuresis may be profound and care is

needed to avoid potentially dangerous electrolyte disturbances.

The aldosterone antagonist **spironolactone** (section 2.2.3) may be considered for patients with severe heart failure who are already receiving an ACE inhibitor and a diuretic; low doses of spironolactone (usually 25 mg) daily have been shown to reduce symptoms and mortality in these patients. Close monitoring of serum creatinine and potassium is necessary with any change in treatment or in the patient's clinical condition.

The **beta-blockers** bisoprolol and carvedilol (section 2.4) are of value in any grade of stable heart failure and left-ventricular systolic dysfunction. Beta-blocker treatment should be started by those experienced in the management of heart failure, at a very low dose and titrated very slowly over a period of weeks or months. Symptoms may deteriorate initially, calling for adjustment of concomitant therapy.

Digoxin (section 2.1) is given to patients with atrial fibrillation and also to those in sinus rhythm who remain symptomatic despite treatment with an ACE inhibitor, a diuretic, and a beta-blocker.

Patients who cannot tolerate ACE inhibitors or in whom they are contra-indicated may be given **isosorbide dinitrate** (section 2.6.1) with **hydralazine** (section 2.5.1), but this combination may be poorly tolerated. **Angiotensin-II receptor antagonists** (section 2.5.5.2), although not licensed for heart failure, may be useful alternatives for patients who, because of symptoms such as cough, cannot tolerate ACE inhibitors.

2.5.5.1 Angiotensin-converting enzyme inhibitors

Angiotensin-converting enzyme inhibitors (ACE inhibitors) inhibit the conversion of angiotensin I to angiotensin II. They are effective antihypertensives and generally well tolerated. The main indications of ACE inhibitors are shown below.

HEART FAILURE. ACE inhibitors have a valuable role in all grades of heart failure, usually combined with a diuretic (section 2.5.5). Potassium supplements and potassium-sparing diuretics should be discontinued before introducing an ACE inhibitor because of the risk of hyperkalaemia. However, a low dose of spironolactone may be beneficial in severe heart failure (section 2.5.5) and can be used with an ACE inhibitor provided serum potassium is monitored carefully. Profound first-dose hypotension may occur when ACE inhibitors are introduced to patients with heart failure who are already taking a high dose of a loop diuretic (e.g. furosemide 80 mg or more). Temporary withdrawal of the loop diuretic reduces the risk, but may cause severe rebound pulmonary oedema. Therefore, for patients on high doses of loop diuretics, the ACE inhibitor may need to be initiated under specialist supervision, see below. An ACE inhibitor can be initiated in the community in patients who are receiving a low dose of a diuretic or who are not otherwise at risk of serious hypotension; nevertheless, care is required and a very low dose of the ACE inhibitor is given initially.

---

1. For heart failure the dose of the ACE inhibitor is titrated to a 'target' dose (or to the maximum tolerated dose if lower). Target doses of some ACE inhibitors may exceed licensed ones, e.g. captopril (target dose 50 mg three times daily), enalapril (10–20 mg twice daily), lisinopril (30–35 mg daily), ramipril (5 mg twice daily), trandolapril (4 mg daily [unlicensed indication])

HYPERTENSION. ACE inhibitors should be considered for hypertension when thiazides and beta-blockers are contra-indicated, not tolerated, or fail to control blood pressure; they are particularly indicated for hypertension in insulin-dependent diabetics with nephropathy (see also section 6.1.5). ACE inhibitors may cause very rapid falls of blood pressure in some patients particularly in those receiving diuretic therapy (see Cautions, below); the first dose should preferably be given at bedtime.

DIABETIC NEPHROPATHY. For comment on the role of ACE inhibitors in the management of diabetic nephropathy, see section 6.1.5.

PROPHYLAXIS OF CARDIOVASCULAR EVENTS. ACE inhibitors are used in the early and long-term management of patients who have had a myocardial infarction, see section 2.10.1. An ACE inhibitor may also have a role in preventing cardiovascular events and stroke in those at risk because of stable coronary heart disease.

INITIATION UNDER SPECIALIST SUPERVISION. ACE inhibitors should be initiated under specialist supervision and with careful clinical monitoring in those with severe heart failure or in those:

- receiving multiple or high-dose diuretic therapy (e.g. more than 80 mg of furosemide daily or its equivalent);
- with hypovolaemia;
- with hyponatraemia (plasma-sodium concentration below 130 mmol/litre);
- with pre-existing hypotension (systolic blood pressure below 90 mmHg);
- with unstable heart failure;
- with renal impairment (plasma-creatinine concentration above 150 micromol/litre);
- receiving high-dose vasodilator therapy;
- aged 70 years or more.

RENAL EFFECTS. In patients with severe bilateral renal artery stenosis (or severe stenosis of the artery supplying a single functioning kidney), ACE inhibitors reduce or abolish glomerular filtration and are likely to cause severe and progressive renal failure. They are thus contra-indicated in patients known to have these forms of critical renovascular disease.

ACE inhibitor treatment is unlikely to have an adverse effect on overall renal function in patients with severe unilateral renal artery stenosis and a normal contralateral kidney, but glomerular filtration is likely to be reduced (or even abolished) in the affected kidney and the long-term consequences are unknown.

In general, ACE inhibitors are therefore best avoided in patients with known or suspected renovascular disease, unless the blood pressure cannot be controlled by other drugs. If they are used in these circumstances renal function needs to be monitored.

ACE inhibitors should also be used with particular caution in patients who may have undiagnosed and clinically silent renovascular disease. This includes patients with peripheral vascular disease or those with severe generalised atherosclerosis.

Renal function and electrolytes should be checked before starting ACE inhibitors and monitored during treatment (more frequently if features mentioned above present). Although ACE inhibitors now have a specialised role in some forms of renal disease they also occasionally cause impairment of renal function which may progress and become severe in other circumstances (at particular risk are the elderly).

Concomitant treatment with NSAIDs increases the risk of renal damage, and potassium-sparing diuretics (or potassium-containing salt substitutes) increase the risk of hyperkalaemia.

CAUTIONS. ACE inhibitors need to be initiated with care in patients receiving diuretics (**important:** see Concomitant diuretics, below); first doses may cause hypotension especially in patients taking high doses of diuretics, on a low-sodium diet, on dialysis, dehydrated or with heart failure (see above). They should also be used with caution in peripheral vascular disease or generalised atherosclerosis owing to risk of clinically silent renovascular disease (see also above). Renal function should be monitored before and during treatment, and the dose reduced in renal impairment (see also above and Appendix 3). The risk of agranulocytosis is possibly increased in collagen vascular disease (blood counts recommended). ACE inhibitors should be used with care in patients with severe or symptomatic aortic stenosis (risk of hypotension). They should be used with care (or avoided) in those with a history of idiopathic or hereditary angioedema. Use ACE inhibitors with caution in breast-feeding (see Appendix 5). **Interactions:** Appendix 1 (ACE inhibitors)

ANAPHYLACTOID REACTIONS. To prevent anaphylactoid reactions, ACE inhibitors should be avoided during dialysis with high-flux polyacrylonitrile membranes and during low-density lipoprotein apheresis with dextran sulphate; they should also be withheld before desensitisation with wasp or bee venom

Concomitant diuretics. ACE inhibitors can cause a very rapid fall in blood pressure in volume-depleted patients; treatment should therefore be initiated with very low doses. If the dose of diuretic is greater than 80 mg furosemide or equivalent, the ACE inhibitor should be initiated under close supervision and in some patients the diuretic dose may need to be reduced or the diuretic discontinued at least 24 hours beforehand. If high-dose diuretic therapy cannot be stopped, close observation is recommended after administration of the first dose of ACE inhibitor, for at least 2 hours or until the blood pressure has stabilised.

CONTRA-INDICATIONS. ACE inhibitors are contra-indicated in patients with hypersensitivity to ACE inhibitors (including angioedema) and in known or suspected renovascular disease (see also above). ACE inhibitors should not be used in pregnancy (Appendix 4).

SIDE-EFFECTS. ACE inhibitors can cause profound hypotension (see Cautions) and renal impairment (see Renal effects above), and a persistent dry cough. They may also cause angioedema (onset may be delayed), rash (which may be associated with pruritus and urticaria), pancreatitis and upper respiratory-tract symptoms such as sinusitis, rhinitis and sore throat. Gastro-intestinal effects reported with ACE inhibitors include nausea, vomiting, dyspepsia, diarrhoea and constipation. Altered liver function tests, cholestatic jaundice and hepatitis have been reported. Blood disorders including thrombocytopenia, leucopenia, neutropenia and haemolytic anaemia have also been reported. Other reported side-effects include headache, dizziness, fatigue, malaise, taste disturbance, paraesthesia, bronchospasm, fever, serositis, vasculitis, myalgia, arthralgia, positive anti-nuclear antibody, raised erythrocyte sedimentation rate, eosinophilia, leucocytosis and photosensitivity.

COMBINATION PRODUCTS. A number of products incorporating an ACE inhibitor with a thiazide diuretic are now available for the treatment of hypertension. Use of these combination products should be reserved for patients whose blood pressure has not responded to a thiazide diuretic or an ACE inhibitor alone.

Products combining an ACE inhibitor with a calcium-channel blocker are also available for the management of hypertension. Use of such a combination is rarely justified; the range of adverse effects may be increased considerably. A combination product should be considered only for those patients who have been stabilised on the individual components in the same proportions.

CAPTOPRIL

Indications: mild to moderate essential hypertension alone or with thiazide therapy and severe hypertension resistant to other treatment; congestive heart failure (adjunct—see section 2.5.5); following myocardial infarction, see dose; diabetic nephropathy (microalbuminuria greater than 30 mg/day) in insulin-dependent diabetes

Cautions: see notes above

Contra-indications: see notes above; porphyria (section 9.8.2)

Side-effects: see notes above; tachycardia, serum sickness, weight loss, stomatitis, maculopapular rash, photosensitivity, flushing and acidosis

Dose: hypertension, used alone, initially 12.5 mg twice daily; if used in addition to diuretic (see notes above), or in elderly, initially 6.25 mg twice daily (first dose at bedtime); usual maintenance dose 25 mg twice daily; max. 50 mg twice daily (rarely 3 times daily in severe hypertension)

Heart failure (adjunct), initially 6.25–12.5 mg under close medical supervision (see notes above); usual maintenance dose 25 mg 2–3 times daily (but see section 2.5.5); usual max. 150 mg daily

Prophylaxis after infarction in clinically stable patients with asymptomatic or symptomatic left ventricular dysfunction (radionuclide ventriculography or echocardiography undertaken before initiation), initially 6.25 mg, starting as early as 3 days after infarction, then increased over several weeks to 150 mg daily (if tolerated) in divided doses

Diabetic nephropathy, 75–100 mg daily in divided doses; if further blood pressure reduction required, other antihypertensives may be used in conjunction with captopril; in severe renal impairment, initially 12.5 mg twice daily (if concomitant diuretic therapy required, loop diuretic rather than thiazide should be chosen)

Captopril (Non-proprietary) [PoM]
Tablets, captopril 12.5 mg, net price 56-tab pack = £2.24; 25 mg, 56-tab pack = £3.22; 50 mg, 56-tab pack = £4.09
Available from Alpharma, Berk (*Kaplon*®), CP, Generics, Goldshield (*Ecopace*®), Hillcross, IVAX (*Tensopril*®), Sandoz, Sovereign, Sterwin, Tillomed

Capoten® (Squibb) [PoM]
Tablets, captopril 12.5 mg (scored), net price 56-tab pack = £10.56; 25 mg, 56-tab pack = £12.03, 84-tab

pack = £18.05; 50 mg (scored), 56-tab pack = £20.50, 84-tab pack = £30.75 (also available as *Acepril*®)

■ With diuretic
NOTE. For mild to moderate hypertension in patients stabilised on the individual components in the same proportions

Co-zidocapt (Non-proprietary) [PoM]
Tablets, co-zidocapt 12.5/25 (hydrochlorothiazide 12.5 mg, captopril 25 mg), net price 28-tab pack = £11.25
Available from IVAX (*Capto-co*®), Ratiopharm
Tablets, co-zidocapt 25/50 (hydrochlorothiazide 25 mg, captopril 50 mg), net price 28-tab pack = £10.60
Available from IVAX (*Capto-co*®), Ratiopharm

Capozide® (Squibb) [PoM]
LS tablets, scored, co-zidocapt 12.5/25 (hydrochlorothiazide 12.5 mg, captopril 25 mg). Net price 28-tab pack = £11.25
Tablets, scored, co-zidocapt 25/50 (hydrochlorothiazide 25 mg, captopril 50 mg). Net price 28-tab pack = £14.14 (also available as *Acezide*®)

CILAZAPRIL

Indications: essential hypertension; congestive heart failure (adjunct—see section 2.5.5)

Cautions: see notes above; severe hepatic impairment (Appendix 2)

Contra-indications: see notes above; ascites

Side-effects: see notes above; dyspnoea and bronchitis

Dose: hypertension, initially 1 mg once daily (reduced to 500 micrograms daily in those receiving a diuretic, in the elderly, and in renal impairment), then adjusted according to response; usual maintenance dose 2.5–5 mg once daily; max. 5 mg daily

Heart failure (adjunct), initially 500 micrograms once daily under close medical supervision (see notes above), increased to 1 mg once daily; usual maintenance dose 1–2.5 mg daily; max. 5 mg daily

Vascace® (Roche) [PoM]
Tablets, f/c, cilazapril 500 micrograms (white), net price 28-tab pack = £3.92; 1 mg (yellow), 28-tab pack = £6.46; 2.5 mg (pink), 28-tab pack = £8.21; 5 mg (brown), 28-tab pack = £14.28

ENALAPRIL MALEATE

Indications: essential and renovascular hypertension (but see notes above); congestive heart failure (adjunct—see section 2.5.5); prevention of symptomatic heart failure and prevention of coronary ischaemic events in patients with left ventricular dysfunction

Cautions: see notes above

Contra-indications: see notes above

Side-effects: see notes above; also palpitations, arrhythmias, angina, chest pain, Raynaud's syndrome, syncope, cerebrovascular accident, myocardial infarction; anorexia, ileus, stomatitis, hepatic failure; dermatological side-effects including erythema multiforme, Stevens-Johnson syndrome, toxic epidermal necrolysis, exfoliative dermatitis and pemphigus; confusion, depression, nervousness, asthenia, drowsiness, insomnia, dream abnormalities, blurred vision, tinnitus, sweating, flushing, impotence, alopecia, dyspnoea, asthma, pulmonary infiltrates and muscle cramps

Dose: hypertension, used alone, initially 5 mg once daily; if used in addition to diuretic (see notes above), in elderly patients, or in renal impairment, initially 2.5 mg daily; usual maintenance dose 10–20 mg once daily; in severe hypertension may be increased to max. 40 mg once daily

Heart failure (adjunct), asymptomatic left ventricular dysfunction, initially 2.5 mg daily under close medical supervision (see notes above); usual maintenance dose 20 mg daily in 1–2 divided doses (but see section 2.5.5)

Enalapril Maleate (Non-proprietary) PoM
Tablets, enalapril maleate 2.5 mg, net price 28-tab pack = £2.46; 5 mg, 28-tab pack = £3.59; 10 mg, 28-tab pack = £4.96; 20 mg, 28-tab pack = £5.93
Available from Alpharma, APS (*Enacard®*), Dexcel, IVAX, Opus (*Pralenal®*), PLIVA (*Ednyt®*), Sterwin

Innovace® (MSD) PoM
Tablets, enalapril maleate 2.5 mg, net price 28-tab pack = £5.35; 5 mg (scored), 28-tab pack = £7.51; 10 mg (red), 28-tab pack = £10.53; 20 mg (peach), 28-tab pack = £12.51

■ **With diuretic**
NOTE. For mild to moderate hypertension in patients stabilised on the individual components in the same proportions

Innozide® (MSD) PoM
Tablets, yellow, scored, enalapril maleate 20 mg, hydrochlorothiazide 12.5 mg. Net price 28-tab pack = £13.90

FOSINOPRIL

Indications: hypertension; congestive heart failure (adjunct—see section 2.5.5)
Cautions: see notes above
Contra-indications: see notes above
Side-effects: see notes above; chest pain and musculoskeletal pain
Dose: hypertension, initially 10 mg daily, increased if necessary after 4 weeks; usual dose range 10–40 mg (doses over 40 mg not shown to increase efficacy); if used in addition to diuretic see notes above

Heart failure (adjunct), initially 10 mg daily under close medical supervision (see notes above); if initial dose well tolerated, may be increased to up to 40 mg once daily

Staril® (Squibb) PoM
Tablets, fosinopril sodium 10 mg, net price 28-tab pack = £12.04; 20 mg, 28-tab pack = £13.00

IMIDAPRIL HYDROCHLORIDE

Indications: essential hypertension
Cautions: see notes above
Contra-indications: see notes above
Side-effects: see notes above; dry mouth, glossitis, abdominal pain, ileus; bronchitis, dyspnoea; sleep disturbances, depression, confusion, blurred vision, tinnitus, impotence
Dose: initially 5 mg daily before food; if used in addition to diuretic (see notes above), in elderly, in patients with heart failure, angina or cerebrovascular disease, or in renal or hepatic impairment, initially 2.5 mg daily; if necessary increase dose at intervals of at least 3 weeks; usual maintenance

dose 10 mg once daily; max. 20 mg daily (elderly, 10 mg daily)

Tanatril (Trinity) PoM
Tablets, scored, imidapril hydrochloride 5 mg, net price 28-tab pack = £5.65; 10 mg, 28-tab pack = £6.39; 20 mg, 28-tab pack = £7.67

LISINOPRIL

Indications: essential and renovascular hypertension (but see notes above); congestive heart failure (adjunct—see section 2.5.5); following myocardial infarction in haemodynamically stable patients; diabetic nephropathy in normotensive insulin-dependent and hypertensive non-insulin-dependent diabetes mellitus
Cautions: see notes above
Contra-indications: see notes above
Side-effects: see notes above; tachycardia, cerebrovascular accident, myocardial infarction; dry mouth, blurred vision, confusion, mood changes, asthenia, sweating, impotence and alopecia
Dose: hypertension, initially 2.5 mg daily; usual maintenance dose 10–20 mg daily; max. 40 mg daily; if used in addition to diuretic see notes above

Heart failure (adjunct), initially 2.5 mg daily under close medical supervision (see notes above); usual maintenance dose 5–20 mg daily (but see section 2.5.5)

Prophylaxis after myocardial infarction, systolic blood pressure over 120 mmHg, 5 mg within 24 hours, followed by further 5 mg 24 hours later, then 10 mg after a further 24 hours, and continuing with 10 mg once daily for 6 weeks (or continued if heart failure); systolic blood pressure 100–120 mmHg, initially 2.5 mg, increasing to maintenance dose of 5 mg once daily
NOTE. Should not be started after myocardial infarction if systolic blood pressure less than 100 mmHg; temporarily reduce maintenance dose to 5 mg and if necessary 2.5 mg daily if systolic blood pressure 100 mmHg or less during treatment; withdraw if prolonged hypotension occurs (systolic blood pressure less than 90 mmHg for more than 1 hour)

Diabetic nephropathy, initially 2.5 mg daily adjusted to achieve a sitting diastolic blood pressure below 75 mmHg in normotensive insulin-dependent diabetes and below 90 mmHg in hypertensive non-insulin dependent diabetes; usual dose range 10–20 mg daily

Lisinopril (Non-proprietary) PoM
Tablets, lisinopril (as dihydrate) 2.5 mg, net price 28-tab pack = £5.14; 5 mg, 28-tab pack = £6.49; 10 mg, 28-tab pack = £8.23; 20 mg, 28-tab pack = £9.36
Available from APS, Generics, Sandoz

Carace® (Bristol-Myers Squibb) PoM
Tablets, lisinopril 2.5 mg (blue), net price 28-tab pack = £7.30; 5 mg (scored), 28-tab pack= £9.15; 10 mg (yellow, scored), 28-tab pack= £11.30; 20 mg (orange, scored), 28-tab pack = £12.78

Zestril® (AstraZeneca) PoM
Tablets, lisinopril (as dihydrate) 2.5 mg, net price 28-tab pack = £6.26; 5 mg (pink, scored), 28-tab pack = £7.86; 10 mg (pink), 28-tab pack = £9.70; 20 mg (pink), 28-tab pack = £10.97

■ **With diuretic**

NOTE. For mild to moderate hypertension in patients stabilised on the individual components in the same proportions

Carace Plus® (Bristol-Myers Squibb) PoM

Carace 10 Plus tablets, blue, lisinopril 10 mg, hydrochlorothiazide 12.5 mg. Net price 28-tab pack = £11.30

Carace 20 Plus tablets, yellow, scored, lisinopril 20 mg, hydrochlorothiazide 12.5 mg. Net price 28-tab pack = £12.78

Zestoretic® (AstraZeneca) PoM

Zestoretic 10 tablets, peach, lisinopril (as dihydrate) 10 mg, hydrochlorothiazide 12.5 mg. Net price 28-tab pack = £13.01

Zestoretic 20 tablets, lisinopril (as dihydrate) 20 mg, hydrochlorothiazide 12.5 mg. Net price 28-tab pack = £14.72

MOEXIPRIL HYDROCHLORIDE

Indications: essential hypertension

Cautions: see notes above

Contra-indications: see notes above

Side-effects: see notes above; arrhythmias, angina, chest pain, syncope, cerebrovascular accident, myocardial infarction; appetite and weight changes; dry mouth, photosensitivity, flushing, nervousness, mood changes, anxiety, drowsiness, sleep disturbance, tinnitus, influenza-like syndrome, sweating and dyspnoea

Dose: used alone, initially 7.5 mg once daily; if used in addition to diuretic (see notes above), with nifedipine, in elderly, in renal or hepatic impairment, initially 3.75 mg once daily; usual range 15–30 mg once daily; doses above 30 mg daily not shown to increase efficacy

Perdix® (Schwarz) PoM

Tablets, f/c, both pink, scored, moexipril hydrochloride 7.5 mg, net price 28-tab pack = £8.12; 15 mg, 28-tab pack = £9.36

PERINDOPRIL

Indications: essential and renovascular hypertension (but see notes above); congestive heart failure (adjunct—see section 2.5.5)

Cautions: see notes above

Contra-indications: see notes above

Side-effects: see notes above; asthenia, flushing, mood and sleep disturbances

Dose: hypertension, initially 2 mg daily (before food); usual maintenance dose 4 mg once daily; max. 8 mg daily; if used in addition to diuretic see notes above

Heart failure (adjunct), initial dose 2 mg in the morning under close medical supervision (see notes above); usual maintenance 4 mg once daily (before food)

Coversyl® (Servier) PoM

Tablets, perindopril erbumine (= tert-butylamine) 2 mg (white), net price 30-tab pack = £10.68; 4 mg (light green, scored), 30-tab pack = £10.68; 8 mg (green), 30-tab pack = £14.97

■ **With diuretic**

NOTE. For hypertension not adequately controlled by perindopril alone

Coversyl® Plus (Servier) ▼ PoM

Tablets, perindopril erbumine (= tert-butylamine) 4 mg, indapamide 1.25 mg, net price 30-tab pack = £14.97

QUINAPRIL

Indications: essential hypertension; congestive heart failure (adjunct—see section 2.5.5)

Cautions: see notes above

Contra-indications: see notes above

Side-effects: see notes above; asthenia, chest pain, oedema, flatulence, nervousness, depression, insomnia, blurred vision, impotence, back pain and myalgia

Dose: hypertension, initially 10 mg once daily; with a diuretic, in elderly, or in renal impairment initially 2.5 mg daily; usual maintenance dose 20–40 mg daily in single or 2 divided doses; up to 80 mg daily has been given

Heart failure (adjunct), initial dose 2.5 mg under close medical supervision (see notes above); usual maintenance 10–20 mg daily in single or 2 divided doses; up to 40 mg daily has been given

Accupro® (Parke-Davis) PoM

Tablets, all brown, f/c, quinapril (as hydrochloride) 5 mg, net price 28-tab pack = £7.17; 10 mg, 28-tab pack = £7.17; 20 mg, 28-tab pack = £8.99; 40 mg, 28-tab pack = £9.75

■ **With diuretic**

NOTE. For hypertension in patients stabilised on the individual components in the same proportions

Accuretic® (Parke-Davis) PoM

Tablets, pink, f/c, scored, quinapril (as hydrochloride) 10 mg, hydrochlorothiazide 12.5 mg. Net price 28-tab pack = £11.75

RAMIPRIL

Indications: mild to moderate hypertension; congestive heart failure (adjunct—see section 2.5.5); following myocardial infarction in patients with clinical evidence of heart failure; susceptible patients over 55 years, prevention of myocardial infarction, stroke, cardiovascular death or need of revascularisation procedures (consult product literature)

Cautions: see notes above

Contra-indications: see notes above

Side-effects: see notes above; arrhythmias, angina, chest pain, syncope, cerebrovascular accident, myocardial infarction, loss of appetite, stomatitis, dry mouth, skin reactions including erythema multiforme and pemphigoid exanthema; precipitation or exacerbation of Raynaud's syndrome; conjunctivitis, onycholysis, confusion, nervousness, depression, anxiety, impotence, decreased libido, alopecia, bronchitis and muscle cramps

Dose: hypertension, initially 1.25 mg once daily, increased at intervals of 1–2 weeks; usual range 2.5–5 mg once daily; max. 10 mg once daily; if used in addition to diuretic see notes above

Heart failure (adjunct), initially 1.25 mg once daily under close medical supervision (see notes above), increased if necessary at intervals of 1–2 weeks; max. 10 mg daily (daily doses of 2.5 mg or more may be taken in 1–2 divided doses) (see also section 2.5.5)

Prophylaxis after myocardial infarction (started in hospital 3 to 10 days after infarction), initially 2.5 mg twice daily, increased after 2 days to 5 mg twice daily; maintenance 2.5–5 mg twice daily NOTE. If initial 2.5-mg dose not tolerated, give 1.25 mg twice daily for 2 days before increasing to 2.5 mg twice daily, then 5 mg twice daily; withdraw if 2.5 mg twice daily not tolerated

Prophylaxis of cardiovascular events or stroke, initially 2.5 mg once daily, increased after 1 week to 5 mg once daily, then increased after a further 3 weeks to 10 mg once daily

Tritace® (Aventis Pharma) PoM
Tablets, all scored, ramipril 1.25 mg (white), net price 28-tab pack = £5.30; 2.5 mg (yellow), 28-tab pack = £7.51; 5 mg (red), 28-tab pack = £10.46; 10 mg (white), 28-tab pack = £14.24
Titration pack, capsules, 35-day starter pack of ramipril 7 x 2.5 mg with 21 x 5 mg and 7 x 10 mg, net price = £13.00

■ **With calcium-channel blocker**
NOTE. For hypertension in patients stabilised on the individual components in the same proportions, but combination with calcium-channel blocker not first-line treatment. For cautions, contra-indications and side-effects of felodipine, see section 2.6.2
Triapin® (Aventis Pharma) ▼ PoM ▭
Triapin® *tablets*, f/c, brown, ramipril 5 mg, felodipine 5 mg (m/r), net price 28-tab pack = £24.46. Label: 25
Triapin mite® *tablets*, f/c, orange, ramipril 2.5 mg, felodipine 2.5 mg (m/r), net price 28-tab pack = £19.37. Label: 25

TRANDOLAPRIL

Indications: mild to moderate hypertension; following myocardial infarction in patients with left ventricular dysfunction; heart failure [unlicensed] see section 2.5.5
Cautions: see notes above
Contra-indications: see notes above
Side-effects: see notes above; tachycardia, arrhythmias, angina, transient ischaemic attacks, cerebral haemorrhage, myocardial infarction; ileus, dry mouth; skin reactions including Stevens-Johnson syndrome, toxic epidermal necrolysis, psoriasis-like efflorescence; asthenia, alopecia, dyspnoea and bronchitis
Dose: hypertension, initially 500 micrograms once daily, increased at intervals of 2–4 weeks; usual range 1–2 mg once daily; max. 4 mg daily; if used in addition to diuretic see notes above
Prophylaxis after myocardial infarction (starting as early as 3 days after infarction), initially 500 micrograms daily, gradually increased to max. 4 mg once daily
NOTE. If symptomatic hypotension develops during titration, do not increase dose further; if possible, reduce dose of any adjunctive treatment and if this is not effective or feasible, reduce dose of trandolapril

Gopten® (Abbott) PoM
Capsules, trandolapril 500 micrograms (red/yellow), net price 14-cap pack = £2.65; 1 mg (red/orange), 28-cap pack = £12.28; 2 mg (red/red), 28-cap pack = £8.39

Odrik® (Hoechst Marion Roussel) PoM
Capsules, trandolapril 500 micrograms (red/yellow), net price 28-cap pack = £8.19; 1 mg (red/orange), 28-cap pack = £10.34; 2 mg (red/red), 28-cap pack = £12.29

■ **With calcium-channel blocker**
NOTE. For hypertension in patients stabilised on the individual components in the same proportions, but combination with calcium-channel blocker not first-line treatment. For cautions, contra-indications and side-effects of verapamil, see section 2.6.2
Tarka® (Abbott) ▼ PoM ▭
Capsules, pink, trandolapril 2 mg, verapamil hydrochloride 180 mg (m/r). Net price 28 cap-pack = £17.85. Label: 25

2.5.5.2 Angiotensin-II receptor antagonists

Candesartan, **irbesartan**, **losartan**, and **valsartan** are specific angiotensin-II receptor antagonists with many properties similar to those of the ACE inhibitors; **eprosartan**, **olmesartan**, and **telmisartan** have been introduced more recently. However, unlike ACE inhibitors, they do not inhibit the breakdown of bradykinin and other kinins, and thus do not appear to cause the persistent dry cough which commonly complicates ACE inhibitor therapy. They are therefore a useful alternative for patients who have to discontinue an ACE inhibitor because of persistent cough.

An angiotensin-II receptor antagonist may be used as an alternative to an ACE inhibitor in the management of heart failure [unlicensed indication](section 2.5.5) or diabetic nephropathy (section 6.1.5).

CAUTIONS. Angiotensin-II receptor antagonists should be used with caution in renal artery stenosis (see also Renal Effects under ACE Inhibitors, section 2.5.5.1). Monitoring of plasma-potassium concentration is advised, particularly in the elderly and in patients with renal impairment; lower initial doses may be appropriate in these patients. Angiotensin-II receptor antagonists should be used with caution in aortic or mitral valve stenosis and in obstructive hypertrophic cardiomyopathy. **Interactions:** Appendix 1 (as for ACE inhibitors).

CONTRA-INDICATIONS. Angiotensin-II receptor antagonists, like the ACE inhibitors, should be avoided in pregnancy (see also Appendix 4).

SIDE-EFFECTS. Side-effects are usually mild. Symptomatic hypotension including dizziness may occur, particularly in patients with intravascular volume depletion (e.g. those taking high-dose diuretics). Hyperkalaemia occurs occasionally; angioedema has also been reported with some angiotensin-II receptor antagonists.

CANDESARTAN CILEXETIL

Indications: hypertension (see also notes above)
Cautions: see notes above; hepatic and renal impairment (Appendixes 2 and 3)
Contra-indications: see notes above; breast-feeding (Appendix 5), cholestasis
Side-effects: see notes above; also upper respiratory-tract and influenza-like symptoms including rhinitis and pharyngitis; abdominal pain, back

pain, arthralgia, myalgia, nausea, headache, peripheral oedema, rash also reported; rarely urticaria, pruritus, blood disorders reported

Dose: initially 8 mg (hepatic impairment 2 mg, renal impairment or intravascular volume depletion 4 mg) once daily adjusted according to response; usual maintenance dose 8 mg once daily; max. 16 mg once daily

Amias® (AstraZeneca, Takeda) PoM
Tablets, candesartan cilexetil 2 mg, net price 7-tab pack = £2.99; 4 mg (scored), 7-tab pack = £3.24, 28-tab pack = £12.95; 8 mg (pink, scored), 28-tab pack = £14.95; 16 mg (pink, scored), 28-tab pack = £17.75

EPROSARTAN

Indications: hypertension (see also notes above)
Cautions: see notes above; also renal impairment (Appendix 3); breast-feeding (Appendix 5)
Contra-indications: see notes above; also severe hepatic impairment (Appendix 2)
Side-effects: see notes above; also flatulence, arthralgia, rhinitis; hypertriglyceridaemia, rarely anaemia
Dose: 600 mg once daily (elderly over 75 years, mild to moderate hepatic impairment, renal impairment, initially 300 mg once daily); if necessary increased after 2–3 weeks to 800 mg once daily

Teveten® (Solvay) PoM
Tablets, f/c, eprosartan (as mesilate) 300 mg, net price 28-tab pack = £12.50; 400 mg, 56-tab pack = £16.96; 600 mg, 28-tab pack = £14.75. Label: 21

IRBESARTAN

Indications: hypertension; renal disease in hypertensive type 2 diabetes mellitus (see also notes above)
Cautions: see notes above
Contra-indications: see notes above; breast-feeding (Appendix 5)
Side-effects: see notes above; nausea, vomiting, fatigue, musculoskeletal pain; less commonly diarrhoea, dyspepsia, flushing, tachycardia, cough; rarely rash, urticaria; very rarely tinnitus
Dose: hypertension, initially 150 mg once daily, increased if necessary to 300 mg once daily. Renal disease in hypertensive type 2 diabetes mellitus, initially 150 mg once daily, increased according to response to 300 mg once daily (in haemodialysis or in elderly over 75 years, initial dose of 75 mg once daily may be used)

Aprovel® (Bristol-Myers Squibb, Sanofi-Synthelabo) PoM
Tablets, irbesartan 75 mg, net price 28-tab pack = £14.80; 150 mg, 28-tab pack = £16.45; 300 mg, 28-tab pack = £22.21

■ With diuretic
NOTE. For hypertension not adequately controlled on individual components
CoAprovel® (Bristol-Myers Squibb, Sanofi-Synthelabo) PoM
Tablets, both peach, irbesartan 150 mg, hydrochlorothiazide 12.5 mg, net price 28-tab pack = £16.45; irbesartan 300 mg, hydrochlorothiazide 12.5 mg, 28-tab pack = £22.21

LOSARTAN POTASSIUM

Indications: hypertension; diabetic nephropathy in type 2 diabetes mellitus (see also notes above)
Cautions: see notes above; hepatic and renal impairment (Appendixes 2 and 3)
Contra-indications: see notes above; breast-feeding (Appendix 5)
Side-effects: see notes above; diarrhoea, taste disturbance, cough, myalgia, migraine, urticaria, pruritus, rash; rarely hepatitis, anaemia (in severe renal disease or following renal transplant), vasculitis (including Henoch-Schönlein purpura)
Dose: usually 50 mg once daily (elderly over 75 years, moderate to severe renal impairment, intravascular volume depletion, initially 25 mg once daily); if necessary increased after several weeks to 100 mg once daily

Cozaar® (MSD) PoM
Tablets, f/c, losartan potassium 25 mg (Half Strength), net price 7-tab pack = £4.31; 50 mg (scored), 28-tab pack = £17.23; 100 mg, 28-tab pack = £22.00

■ With diuretic
NOTE. For hypertension not adequately controlled on individual components
Cozaar-Comp® (MSD) PoM
Tablets, f/c, yellow, losartan potassium 50 mg, hydrochlorothiazide 12.5 mg. Net price 28-tab pack = £17.23

OLMESARTAN MEDOXOMIL

Indications: hypertension (see also notes above)
Cautions: see notes above
Contra-indications: hepatic impairment; moderate to severe renal impairment (Appendix 3); biliary obstruction; breast-feeding (Appendix 5)
Side-effects: see notes above; also abdominal pain, diarrhoea, dyspepsia, nausea, influenza-like symptoms, cough, pharyngitis, rhinitis, haematuria, urinary-tract infection, peripheral oedema, arthritis, musculoskeletal pain; less commonly angina, vertigo, rash
Dose: initially 10 mg once daily; if necessary increased to 20 mg once daily; max. 40 mg daily (ELDERLY max. 20 mg daily)

Olmetec® (Sankyo) ▼ PoM
Tablets, olmesartan medoxomil 10 mg, net price 28-tab pack = £11.75; 20 mg, 28-tab pack = £14.10; 40 mg, 28-tab pack = £18.00

TELMISARTAN

Indications: hypertension (see also notes above)
Cautions: see notes above; hepatic impairment—avoid if severe (Appendix 2); active gastric or duodenal ulceration or other gastro-intestinal disease (increased risk of gastro-intestinal bleeding)
Contra-indications: see notes above; also severe renal impairment; biliary obstruction; breast-feeding
Side-effects: see notes above; gastro-intestinal disturbances (rarely gastro-intestinal bleeding), pharyngitis, back pain, myalgia; rarely decrease in haemoglobin, increase in uric acid, urticaria
Dose: usually 40 mg once daily, increased if necessary to max. 80 mg once daily

Micardis® (Boehringer Ingelheim) PoM
Tablets, telmisartan 20 mg, net price 28-tab pack = £12.60; 40 mg, 28-tab pack = £12.60; 80 mg, 28-tab pack = £15.75

■ With diuretic
NOTE. For patients with hypertension not adequately controlled by telmisartan alone
Micardis Plus® (Boehringer Ingelheim) ▼ PoM
Tablets 40/12.5, red/white, telmisartan 40 mg, hydrochlorothiazide 12.5 mg, net price 28-tab pack = £12.60
Tablets 80/12.5, red/white, telmisartan 80 mg, hydrochlorothiazide 12.5 mg, net price 28-tab pack = £15.75

VALSARTAN
Indications: hypertension (see also notes above)
Cautions: see notes above; mild to moderate hepatic impairment (Appendix 2) and renal impairment (Appendix 3)
Contra-indications: see notes above; severe hepatic impairment (Appendix 2), cirrhosis, biliary obstruction, breast-feeding (Appendix 5)
Side-effects: see notes above; fatigue, rarely diarrhoea, headache, epistaxis; thrombocytopenia, arthralgia, myalgia, taste disturbance, neutropenia reported
Dose: usually 80 mg once daily (elderly over 75 years, mild to moderate hepatic impairment, moderate to severe renal impairment, intravascular volume depletion, initially 40 mg once daily); if necessary increased after at least 4 weeks to 160 mg daily (80 mg daily in hepatic impairment)

Diovan® (Novartis) PoM
Capsules, valsartan 40 mg (grey), net price 7-cap pack = £3.35; 80 mg (grey/pink), 7-cap pack = £3.94 (hosp. only), 28-cap pack = £15.75; 160 mg (dark grey/pink), 7-cap pack = £4.92 (hosp. only), 28-cap pack = £19.69

2.5.6 Ganglion-blocking drugs

TRIMETAPHAN CAMSILATE
Indications: controlled hypotension in surgery
Cautions: hepatic or renal impairment, diabetes mellitus, elderly, cerebral or coronary vascular disease, adrenal insufficiency, Addison's disease, CNS degenerative disease; **interactions:** Appendix 1 (trimetaphan)
Contra-indications: severe arteriosclerosis, severe cardiac disease, pyloric stenosis, pregnancy
Side-effects: tachycardia and respiratory depression (particularly with muscle relaxants); constipation, increased intra-ocular pressure, pupillary dilatation
Dose: *by intravenous infusion*, 3–4 mg/minute initially, then adjusted according to response

Trimetaphan Camsilate (Cambridge) PoM
Injection, trimetaphan camsilate 50 mg/mL. Net price 5-mL amp = £17.42. For dilution and use as an infusion

2.5.7 Tyrosine hydroxylase inhibitors

Metirosine (*Demser*®, MSD, available on named-patient basis) inhibits the enzyme tyrosine hydroxylase, and hence the synthesis of catecholamines. It is used in the pre-operative management of phaeochromocytoma, and long term in patients unsuitable for surgery; an alpha-adrenoceptor blocking drug (e.g. phenoxybenzamine, section 2.5.4) may also be required. Metirosine should **not** be used to treat essential hypertension.

2.6 Nitrates, calcium-channel blockers, and potassium-channel activators

2.6.1	Nitrates
2.6.2	Calcium-channel blockers
2.6.3	Potassium-channel activators
2.6.4	Peripheral and cerebral vasodilators

Nitrates, calcium-channel blockers and potassium-channel activators have a vasodilating effect. Vasodilators are known to act in heart failure either by arteriolar dilatation which reduces both peripheral vascular resistance and left ventricular pressure at systole and results in improved cardiac output, *or* venous dilatation which results in dilatation of capacitance vessels, increase of venous pooling, and diminution of venous return to the heart (decreasing left ventricular end-diastolic pressure).

Angina
Stable angina usually results from atherosclerotic plaques in the coronary arteries, whereas *unstable angina* is usually due to plaque rupture and may occur either in patients with a history of stable angina or in those with previously silent coronary artery disease. It is important to distinguish unstable from stable angina; unstable angina is usually characterised by new onset severe angina or sudden worsening of previously stable angina.

STABLE ANGINA. Acute attacks of stable angina should be managed with sublingual **glyceryl trinitrate**. If attacks occur more than twice a week, regular drug therapy is required and should be introduced in a stepwise manner according to response. **Aspirin** (section 2.9) should be given to patients with angina; a dose of 75 mg daily is suitable. Revascularisation procedures may also be appropriate.

Patients with mild or moderate stable angina who do not have left ventricular dysfunction, may be managed effectively with sublingual glyceryl trinitrate and regular administration of a **beta-blocker** (section 2.4). If necessary a long-acting **dihydropyridine calcium-channel blocker** (section 2.6.2) and then a **long-acting nitrate** (section 2.6.1) may be added. For those without left ventricular dysfunction and in whom beta-blockers are inappropriate, **diltiazem** or **verapamil** may be given (section 2.6.2) and a long-acting nitrate (section 2.6.1) may be added if symptom control is not adequate. For those intolerant of standard treatment, or where standard treatment has failed, nicorandil may be tried.

For patients with left ventricular dysfunction a long-acting nitrate (section 2.6.1) should be used and a long-acting dihydropyridine calcium-channel blocker (section 2.6.2) may be added if necessary.

A **statin** (section 2.12) should be prescribed for those with an elevated plasma-cholesterol concentration.

UNSTABLE ANGINA. Patients with unstable angina should be admitted to hospital. The aims of management of unstable angina are to provide supportive care and pain relief during the acute attack and to prevent myocardial infarction and death.

Initial management. **Aspirin** (chewed or dispersed in water) is given for its antiplatelet effect at a dose of 300 mg (section 2.9). If aspirin is given before arrival at hospital, a note saying that it has been given should be sent with the patient.

Heparin (section 2.8.1) or the low molecular weight heparins **dalteparin** or **enoxaparin** (section 2.8.1) should also be given.

Nitrates (section 2.6.1) are used to relieve ischaemic pain. If sublingual glyceryl trinitrate is not effective, intravenous or buccal glyceryl trinitrate or intravenous isosorbide dinitrate is given.

Patients without contra-indications should receive intravenous or oral **beta-blockers** (section 2.4). In patients without left ventricular dysfunction and in whom beta-blockers are inappropriate, **diltiazem** or **verapamil** may be given (section 2.6.2).

The glycoprotein IIb/IIIa inhibitors **eptifibatide** and **tirofiban** (section 2.9) are recommended (with aspirin and heparin) for unstable angina in patients with a high risk of developing myocardial infarction. **Abciximab**, eptifibatide or tirofiban may also be used with aspirin and heparin in patients undergoing percutaneous coronary intervention, to reduce the immediate risk of vascular occlusion.

Revascularisation procedures are often appropriate for patients with unstable angina.

Long-term management. The importance of life-style changes, especially stopping smoking, should be emphasised. Patients should receive low-dose **aspirin** indefinitely—a dose of 75 mg daily is suitable. A **statin** (section 2.12) should also be prescribed. The need for long-term angina treatment or for coronary angiography should be assessed. If there is continuing ischaemia, standard angina treatment should be continued; if not, antianginal treatment may be withdrawn cautiously at least 2 months after the acute attack.

2.6.1   Nitrates

Nitrates have a useful role in *angina* (for details on the management of stable angina, see section 2.6). Although they are potent coronary vasodilators, their principal benefit follows from a reduction in venous return which reduces left ventricular work. Unwanted effects such as flushing, headache, and postural hypotension may limit therapy, especially when angina is severe or when patients are unusually sensitive to the effects of nitrates.

Sublingual **glyceryl trinitrate** is one of the most effective drugs for providing rapid symptomatic relief of angina, but its effect lasts only for 20 to 30 minutes; the 300-microgram tablet is often appropriate when glyceryl trinitrate is first used. The *aerosol spray* provides an alternative method of rapid relief of symptoms for those who find difficulty in dissolving sublingual preparations. Duration of action may be prolonged by *modified-release* and *transdermal* preparations (but tolerance may develop, see below).

Isosorbide dinitrate is active *sublingually* and is a more stable preparation for those who only require nitrates infrequently. It is also effective by mouth for prophylaxis; although the effect is slower in onset, it may persist for several hours. Duration of action of up to 12 hours is claimed for *modified-release* preparations. The activity of isosorbide dinitrate may depend on the production of active metabolites, the most important of which is isosorbide mononitrate. **Isosorbide mononitrate** itself is also licensed for angina prophylaxis; modified-release formulations (for once daily administration) are available.

Glyceryl trinitrate or isosorbide dinitrate may be tried by *intravenous injection* when the sublingual form is ineffective in patients with chest pain due to myocardial infarction or severe ischaemia. Intravenous injections are also useful in the treatment of acute left ventricular failure.

TOLERANCE. Many patients on long-acting or transdermal nitrates rapidly develop tolerance (with reduced therapeutic effects). Reduction of blood-nitrate concentrations to low levels for 4 to 8 hours each day usually maintains effectiveness in such patients. If tolerance is suspected during the use of transdermal patches they should be left off for several consecutive hours in each 24 hours; in the case of modified-release tablets of isosorbide dinitrate (and conventional formulations of isosorbide mononitrate), the second of the two daily doses can be given after about 8 hours rather than after 12 hours. Conventional formulations of isosorbide mononitrate should not usually be given more than twice daily unless small doses are used; modified-release formulations of isosorbide mononitrate should only be given once daily, and used in this way do not produce tolerance.

GLYCERYL TRINITRATE

Indications: prophylaxis and treatment of angina; left ventricular failure

Cautions: severe hepatic or renal impairment; hypothyroidism, malnutrition, or hypothermia; head trauma, cerebral haemorrhage; recent history of myocardial infarction; metal-containing transdermal systems should be removed before cardioversion or diathermy; tolerance (see notes above); **interactions:** Appendix 1 (glyceryl trinitrate)

Contra-indications: hypersensitivity to nitrates; hypotensive conditions and hypovolaemia; hypertrophic obstructive cardiomyopathy, aortic stenosis, cardiac tamponade, constrictive pericarditis, mitral stenosis; marked anaemia, closed-angle glaucoma

Side-effects: throbbing headache, flushing, dizziness, postural hypotension, tachycardia (but paradoxical bradycardia has occurred)

INJECTION. Specific side-effects following injection (particularly if given too rapidly) include severe hypotension, nausea and retching, diaphoresis, apprehension, restlessness, muscle twitching, retrosternal discomfort, palpitations, abdominal pain, syncope; prolonged administration has been associated with methaemoglobinaemia

Dose: *sublingually*, 0.3–1 mg, repeated as required

By mouth, see under preparations

By intravenous infusion, 10–200 micrograms/minute

■ Short-acting tablets and sprays

Glyceryl Trinitrate (Non-proprietary)
Sublingual tablets, glyceryl trinitrate 300 micrograms, net price 100 = £2.91; 500 micrograms, 100 = £1.06; 600 micrograms, 100 = £2.31. Label: 16

NOTE. Glyceryl trinitrate tablets should be supplied in glass containers of not more than 100 tablets, closed with a foil-lined cap, and containing no cotton wool wadding; they should be discarded after 8 weeks in use

Aerosol spray, glyceryl trinitrate 400 micrograms/metered dose. Net price 200-dose unit = £3.13

Dose: treatment or prophylaxis of angina, spray 1–2 doses under tongue and then close mouth

Available from Alpharma

Coro-Nitro Pump Spray® (Roche)
Aerosol spray, glyceryl trinitrate 400 micrograms/metered dose. Net price 200-dose unit = £3.13

Dose: treatment or prophylaxis of angina, spray 1–2 doses under tongue and then close mouth

Glytrin Spray® (Sanofi-Synthelabo)
Aerosol spray, glyceryl trinitrate 400 micrograms/metered dose. Net price 200-dose unit = £3.49

Dose: treatment or prophylaxis of angina, spray 1–2 doses under tongue and then close mouth

Caution: flammable

GTN 300 mcg (Martindale)
Sublingual tablets, glyceryl trinitrate 300 micrograms. Net price 100 = £2.91. Label: 16

Nitrolingual Pumpspray® (Merck)
Aerosol spray, glyceryl trinitrate 400 micrograms/metered dose. Net price 200-dose unit = £3.65; *Duo Pack* (250-dose unit and 75-dose unit) = £4.98

Dose: treatment or prophylaxis of angina, spray 1–2 doses under tongue and then close mouth

Nitromin® (Servier)
Aerosol spray, glyceryl trinitrate 400 micrograms/metered dose, net price 180-dose unit = £2.63, 200-dose unit = £2.82

Dose: treatment or prophylaxis of angina, spray 1–2 doses under tongue and then close mouth

■ Longer-acting tablets

Suscard® (Forest)
Buccal tablets, m/r, glyceryl trinitrate 2 mg, net price 100-tab pack = £13.55; 3 mg, 100-tab pack = £19.56; 5 mg, 100-tab pack = £26.63. Counselling, see below

Dose: treatment of angina, 2 mg as required (1 mg in sensitive patients), increased to 3 mg if necessary; prophylaxis 1–3 mg 3 times daily; 5 mg in severe angina

Unstable angina (adjunct), up to 5 mg with ECG monitoring

Congestive heart failure, 5 mg 3 times daily, increased to 10 mg 3 times daily in severe cases

Acute heart failure, 5 mg repeated until symptoms abate

COUNSELLING. Tablets have rapid onset of effect; they are placed between upper lip and gum, and left to dissolve; vary site to reduce risk of dental caries

Sustac® (Forest)
Tablets, m/r, all pink, glyceryl trinitrate 2.6 mg, net price 90-tab pack = £5.12; 6.4 mg, 90-tab pack = £7.38; 10 mg, 60-tab pack = £6.85. Label: 25

Dose: prophylaxis of angina, 2.6–12.8 mg 3 times daily *or* 10 mg 2–3 times daily

■ Parenteral preparations

NOTE. Glass or polyethylene apparatus is preferable; loss of potency will occur if PVC is used

Glyceryl Trinitrate (Non-proprietary) PoM
Injection, glyceryl trinitrate 5 mg/mL. To be diluted before use. Net price 5-mL amp = £6.49; 10-mL amp = £12.98

Available from Faulding DBL

Nitrocine® (Schwarz) PoM
Injection, glyceryl trinitrate 1 mg/mL. To be diluted before use or given undiluted with syringe pump. Net price 10-mL amp = £7.90; 50-mL bottle = £18.51

Nitronal® (Merck) PoM
Injection, glyceryl trinitrate 1 mg/mL. To be diluted before use or given undiluted with syringe pump. Net price 5-mL vial = £2.06; 50-mL vial = £16.85

■ Transdermal preparations

Deponit® (Schwarz)
Patches, self-adhesive, transparent, glyceryl trinitrate, *'5' patch* (releasing approx. 5 mg/24 hours when in contact with skin), net price 28 = £17.16; *'10' patch* (releasing approx.10 mg/24 hours), 28 = £18.89

Dose: prophylaxis of angina, apply one '5' or one '10' patch to lateral chest wall, upper arm, or shoulder; replace every 24 hours, siting replacement patch on different area; see also notes above

Minitran® (3M)
Patches, self-adhesive, transparent, glyceryl trinitrate, *'5' patch* (releasing approx. 5 mg/24 hours when in contact with skin), net price 30 = £12.49; *'10' patch* (releasing approx. 10 mg/24 hours), 30 = £13.84; *'15' patch* (releasing approx. 15 mg/24 hours), 30 = £15.26

Dose: prophylaxis of angina, apply one '5' patch to chest or upper arm; replace every 24 hours, siting replacement patch on different area; adjust dose according to response; see also notes above

Maintenance of venous patency ('5' patch only), consult product literature

Nitro-Dur® (Schering-Plough)
Patches, self-adhesive, buff, glyceryl trinitrate, *'0.2 mg/h' patch* (releasing approx. 5 mg/24 hours when in contact with skin), net price 28 = £11.84; *'0.4 mg/h' patch* (releasing approx. 10 mg/24 hours), 28 = £13.10; *'0.6 mg/h' patch* (releasing approx.15 mg/24 hours), 28 = £14.42

Dose: prophylaxis of angina, apply one '0.2 mg/h' patch to chest or outer upper arm; replace every 24 hours, siting replacement patch on different area; adjust dose according to response; see also notes above

Percutol® (PLIVA)
Ointment, glyceryl trinitrate 2%. Net price 60 g = £10.49. Counselling, see administration below

Excipients: include wool fat

Dose: prophylaxis of angina, usual dose 1–2 inches of ointment measured on to *Applirule*®, and applied (usually

to chest, arm, or thigh) without rubbing in and secured with surgical tape, every 3–4 hours as required; to determine dose, ½ inch on first day then increased by ½ inch/day until headache occurs, then reduced by ½ inch
NOTE. Approx. 800 micrograms/hour absorbed from 1 inch of ointment

Transiderm-Nitro® (Novartis)
Patches, self-adhesive, pink, glyceryl trinitrate, '5' patch (releasing approx. 5 mg/24 hours when in contact with skin), net price 28 = £21.31; '10' patch (releasing approx. 10 mg/24 hours), 28 = £23.43
Dose: prophylaxis of angina, apply one '5' or one '10' patch to lateral chest wall; replace every 24 hours, siting replacement patch on different area; max. two '10' patches daily; see also notes above
Prophylaxis of phlebitis and extravasation ('5' patch only), consult product literature

Trintek® (Goldshield)
Patches, self-adhesive, glyceryl trinitrate, '5' patch (releasing approx. 5 mg/24 hours when in contact with skin), net price 30 = £11.84; '10' patch (releasing approx. 10 mg/24 hours), net price 30 = £13.10; '15' patch (releasing approx. 15 mg/24 hours), net price 30 = £14.42
Dose: prophylaxis of angina, apply one '5' patch to lateral chest wall; replace every 24 hours, siting replacement patch on different area; adjust dose according to response, max one '15' patch daily; see also notes above

ISOSORBIDE DINITRATE

Indications: prophylaxis and treatment of angina; left ventricular failure
Cautions: see under Glyceryl Trinitrate
Contra-indications: see under Glyceryl Trinitrate
Side-effects: see under Glyceryl Trinitrate
Dose: *By mouth,* daily in divided doses, angina 30–120 mg, left ventricular failure 40–160 mg, up to 240 mg if required
By intravenous infusion, 2–10 mg/hour; higher doses up to 20 mg/hour may be required

■ Short-acting tablets and sprays
Isosorbide Dinitrate (Non-proprietary)
Tablets, isosorbide dinitrate 10 mg, net price 20 = 39p; 20 mg, 20 = 66p
Available from Alpharma, Hillcross, IVAX

Angitak® (Eastern)
Aerosol spray, isosorbide dinitrate 1.25 mg/metered dose, net price 200-dose unit = £3.95
Dose: treatment or prophylaxis of angina, spray 1–3 doses under tongue whilst holding breath; allow 30 second interval between each dose

■ Modified-release preparations
Cedocard Retard® (Pharmacia)
Retard-20 tablets, m/r, yellow, scored, isosorbide dinitrate 20 mg. Net price 60-tab pack = £6.85. Label: 25
Dose: prophylaxis of angina, 1 tablet every 12 hours
Retard-40 tablets, m/r, orange-red, scored, isosorbide dinitrate 40 mg. Net price 60-tab pack = £13.31. Label: 25
Dose: prophylaxis of angina, 1–2 tablets every 12 hours

Isoket Retard® (Schwarz)
Retard-20 tablets, m/r, scored, isosorbide dinitrate 20 mg. Net price 56-tab pack = £3.47. Label: 25
Retard-40 tablets, m/r, scored, isosorbide dinitrate 40 mg. Net price 56-tab pack = £8.55. Label: 25
Dose: prophylaxis of angina, 20–40 mg every 12 hours

■ Parenteral preparations
Isoket® (Schwarz) [PoM]
Injection 0.05%, isosorbide dinitrate 500 micrograms/mL. To be diluted before use or given undiluted with syringe pump. Net price 50-mL bottle = £9.61
Injection 0.1%, isosorbide dinitrate 1 mg/mL. To be diluted before use. Net price 10-mL amp = £3.62; 50-mL bottle = £17.96; 100-mL bottle = £25.98
NOTE. Glass or polyethylene infusion apparatus is preferable; loss of potency if PVC used

ISOSORBIDE MONONITRATE

Indications: prophylaxis of angina; adjunct in congestive heart failure
Cautions: see under Glyceryl Trinitrate
Contra-indications: see under Glyceryl Trinitrate
Side-effects: see under Glyceryl Trinitrate
Dose: initially 20 mg 2–3 times daily *or* 40 mg twice daily (10 mg twice daily in those who have not previously received nitrates); up to 120 mg daily in divided doses if required

Isosorbide Mononitrate (Non-proprietary)
Tablets, isosorbide mononitrate 10 mg, net price 56 = £1.13; 20 mg, 56 = £2.10; 40 mg, 56 = £3.59. Label: 25
Various strengths available from Alpharma, APS, Berk (*Dynamin®*), Hillcross, IVAX, Opus (*Angeze®*), PLIVA

Elantan® (Schwarz)
Elantan 10 tablets, scored, isosorbide mononitrate 10 mg. Net price 56 = £3.56; 84 = £5.34. Label: 25
Elantan 20 tablets [PoM], scored, isosorbide mononitrate 20 mg. Net price 56 = £4.64; 84 = £6.59. Label: 25
Elantan 40 tablets [PoM], scored, isosorbide mononitrate 40 mg. Net price 56 = £7.56; 84 = £11.35. Label: 25

Ismo® (Roche)
Ismo 10 tablets, isosorbide mononitrate 10 mg. Net price 60-tab pack = £3.24. Label: 25
Ismo 20 tablets, scored, isosorbide mononitrate 20 mg. Net price 60-tab pack = £4.75. Label: 25
Ismo 40 tablets, scored, isosorbide mononitrate 40 mg. Net price 60-tab pack = £7.80. Label: 25

Isotrate® (Bioglan)
Tablets, isosorbide mononitrate 20 mg. Net price 60-tab pack = £7.09. Label: 25

Monit® (Sanofi-Synthelabo)
LS Tablets, isosorbide mononitrate 10 mg. Net price 56-tab pack = £3.22. Label: 25

■ Modified release
Chemydur® 60XL (Sovereign) [PoM]
Tablets, m/r, scored, ivory, isosorbide mononitrate 60 mg, net price 28-tab pack = £15.83. Label: 25
Dose: prophylaxis of angina, 1 tablet in the morning (half a tablet for 2–4 days to minimise possibility of headache), increased if necessary to 2 tablets

Elantan LA® (Schwarz)
Elantan LA 25 capsules, m/r, brown/white, enclosing white micropellets, isosorbide mononitrate 25 mg. Net price 28-cap pack = £6.69. Label: 25
Dose: prophylaxis of angina, 1 capsule in the morning, increased if necessary to 2 capsules
Elantan LA 50 capsules, m/r, brown/pink, enclosing white micropellets, isosorbide mononitrate 50 mg. Net price 28-cap pack = £10.79. Label: 25
Dose: prophylaxis of angina, 1 capsule daily in the morning, increased if necessary to 2 capsules

Imdur® (AstraZeneca)
Durules® (= tablets m/r), yellow, f/c, scored, isosorbide mononitrate 60 mg. Net price 28-tab pack = £11.14. Label: 25
Dose: prophylaxis of angina, 1 tablet in the morning (half a tablet if headache occurs), increased to 2 tablets in the morning if required

Isib 60XL® (Ashbourne)
Tablets, m/r, scored, ivory, isosorbide mononitrate 60 mg. Net price 28-tab pack = £9.47. Label: 25
Dose: prophylaxis of angina, 1 tablet in the morning (half a tablet for 2–4 days if headache occurs), increased if necessary to 2 tablets

Ismo Retard® (Roche)
Tablets, m/r, s/c, isosorbide mononitrate 40 mg, net price 30-tab pack= £10.48. Label: 25
Dose: prophylaxis of angina, 1 tablet daily in morning

Isodur® (Galen)
Isodur 25XL capsules, m/r, brown/white, isosorbide mononitrate 25 mg, net price 28-cap pack = £6.05. Label: 25
Isodur 50XL capsules, m/r, brown/pink, isosorbide mononitrate 50 mg, net price 28-cap pack = £9.75. Label: 25
Dose: prophylaxis of angina, 25–50 mg daily in the morning, increased if necessary to 50–100 mg once daily

Isotard® (Strakan)
Isotard 25XL tablets, m/r, ivory, isosorbide mononitrate 25 mg, net price 28-tab pack = £6.60. Label: 25
Isotard 40XL tablets, m/r, ivory, isosorbide mononitrate 40 mg, net price 28-tab pack = £7.88. Label: 25
Isotard 50XL tablets, m/r, ivory, isosorbide mononitrate 50 mg, net price 28-tab pack = £7.95. Label: 25
Isotard 60XL tablets, m/r, ivory, isosorbide mononitrate 60 mg, net price 28-tab pack = £7.95. Label: 25
Dose: prophylaxis of angina, 25–60 mg daily in the morning (if headache occurs with 60-mg tablet, half a 60-mg tablet may be given for 2–4 days), increased if necessary to 50–120 mg daily

¹**MCR-50**® (Pharmacia)
Capsules, m/r, containing white micropellets, isosorbide mononitrate 50 mg. Net price 28-cap pack = £13.22. Label: 25
Dose: prophylaxis of angina, 1 capsule in the morning, increased to 2 capsules if required
1. Full product name Mono Cedocard Retard-50®

Modisal XL® (Sandoz)
Tablets, m/r, ivory, isosorbide mononitrate 60 mg. Net price 28-tab pack = £15.97. Label: 25
Dose: prophylaxis of angina, 1 tablet daily in the morning (half a tablet for first 2–4 days to minimise possibility of headache), increased if necessary to 2 tablets once daily

Monit SR® (Sanofi-Synthelabo)
Tablets, m/r, s/c, isosorbide mononitrate 40 mg. Net price 28-tab pack = £9.78. Label: 25
Dose: prophylaxis of angina, 1 tablet daily in morning

Monit XL® (Sterwin)
Tablets, m/r, f/c, scored, orange, isosorbide mononitrate 60 mg, net price 28-tab pack = £11.14. Label: 25
Dose: prophylaxis of angina, 1 tablet in the morning (half a tablet if headache occurs), increased to 2 tablets in the morning if required

Monomax® (Trinity) PoM
Monomax® *SR, capsules,* m/r, isosorbide mononitrate 40 mg, net price 28-cap pack = £8.31; 60 mg, 28-cap pack = £9.03. Label: 25
Dose: prophylaxis of angina, 40–60 mg daily in the morning, increased if necessary to 120 mg daily
NOTE. Also available as *Angeze SR*® (Opus)
Monomax® *XL tablets,* m/r, isosorbide mononitrate 60 mg, net price 28-tab pack = £7.99. Label: 25
Dose: prophylaxis of angina, 1 tablet in the morning (half a tablet for first 2–4 days to minimise possibility of headache), increased if necessary to 2 tablets

Monosorb XL 60® (Dexcel) PoM
Tablets, m/r, f/c, isosorbide mononitrate 60 mg. Net price 28-tab pack = £16.70. Label: 25
Dose: prophylaxis of angina, 1 tablet daily in the morning (half a tablet for first 2–4 days to minimise possibility of headache), increased if necessary to 2 tablets
NOTE. Also available as *Trangina*® *XL* (Alpharma) and as *Xismox*® *XL 60* (Genus)

■ With aspirin
NOTE. For prophylaxis of angina and secondary prevention of myocardial infarction; for cautions, contra-indications and side-effects of aspirin see section 2.9

Imazin® **XL** (Napp)
Tablets, aspirin 75 mg, isosorbide mononitrate 60 mg (m/r), net price 28-tab pack = £10.76. Label: 25, 32
Dose: 1 tablet in the morning, increased to 2 tablets if required
Forte tablets, aspirin 150 mg, isosorbide mononitrate 60 mg (m/r), net price 28-tab pack = £10.76. Label: 25, 32
Dose: 1 tablet in the morning

2.6.2 Calcium-channel blockers

Calcium-channel blockers (less correctly called 'calcium-antagonists') interfere with the inward displacement of calcium ions through the slow channels of active cell membranes. They influence the myocardial cells, the cells within the specialised conducting system of the heart, and the cells of vascular smooth muscle. Thus, myocardial contractility may be reduced, the formation and propagation of electrical impulses within the heart may be depressed, and coronary or systemic vascular tone may be diminished.

Calcium-channel blockers differ in their predilection for the various possible sites of action and, therefore, their therapeutic effects are disparate, with much greater variation than those of beta-blockers. There are important differences between verapamil, diltiazem, and the dihydropyridine calcium-channel blockers (amlodipine, felodipine, isradipine, lacidipine, lercanidipine, nicardipine, nifedipine, nimodipine, and nisoldipine). Verapamil and diltiazem should usually be **avoided** in *heart failure* because they may further depress cardiac function and cause clinically significant deterioration.

Verapamil is used for the treatment of *angina* (section 2.6), *hypertension*, and *arrhythmias* (section 2.3.2). It is a highly negatively inotropic calcium channel-blocker and it reduces cardiac output, slows the heart rate, and may impair atrioventricular conduction. It may precipitate heart failure, exacerbate conduction disorders, and cause hypotension at high doses and should **not** be used with beta-blockers (see p. 106). Constipation is the most common side-effect.

Nifedipine relaxes vascular smooth muscle and dilates coronary and peripheral arteries. It has more influence on vessels and less on the myocardium than does verapamil, and unlike verapamil has no anti-arrhythmic activity. It rarely precipitates heart failure because any negative inotropic effect is offset by a reduction in left ventricular work. Short-acting formulations of nifedipine are not recommended for angina or long-term management of hypertension; their use may be associated with large variations in blood pressure and reflex tachycardia. **Nicardipine** has similar effects to those of nifedipine and may produce less reduction of myocardial contractility. **Amlodipine** and **felodipine** also resemble nifedipine and nicardipine in their effects and do not reduce myocardial contractility and they do not produce clinical deterioration in heart failure. They have a longer duration of action and can be given once daily. Nifedipine, nicardipine, amlodipine, and felodipine are used for the treatment of angina (section 2.6) or hypertension. All are valuable in forms of *angina associated with coronary vasospasm.* Side-effects associated with vasodilatation such as flushing and headache (which become less obtrusive after a few days), and ankle swelling (which may respond only partially to diuretics) are common.

Isradipine, **lacidipine**, **lercanidipine** and **nisoldipine** have similar effects to those of nifedipine and nicardipine; isradipine, lacidipine, and lercanidipine are only indicated for *hypertension* whereas nisoldipine is indicated for angina and hypertension.

Nimodipine is related to nifedipine but the smooth muscle relaxant effect preferentially acts on cerebral arteries. Its use is confined to prevention of *vascular spasm following aneurysmal subarachnoid haemorrhage.*

Diltiazem is effective in most forms of *angina* (section 2.6); the longer-acting formulation is also used for *hypertension.* It may be used in patients for whom beta-blockers are contra-indicated or ineffective. It has a less negative inotropic effect than verapamil and significant myocardial depression occurs rarely. Nevertheless because of the risk of bradycardia it should be used with caution in association with beta-blockers.

UNSTABLE ANGINA. Calcium-channel blockers do not reduce the risk of myocardial infarction in unstable angina. The use of diltiazem or verapamil should be reserved for patients resistant to treatment with beta-blockers.

WITHDRAWAL. There is some evidence that sudden withdrawal of calcium-channel blockers may be associated with an exacerbation of angina.

AMLODIPINE BESILATE

Indications: hypertension, prophylaxis of angina

Cautions: hepatic impairment; **interactions:** Appendix 1 (calcium-channel blockers)

Contra-indications: cardiogenic shock, unstable angina, significant aortic stenosis; pregnancy and breast-feeding

Side-effects: headache, oedema, fatigue, nausea, flushing, dizziness, gum hyperplasia, rashes (including rarely pruritus and very rarely erythema multiforme); rarely gastro-intestinal disturbances, dry mouth, sweating, palpitations, dyspnoea, drowsiness, mood changes, myalgia, arthralgia, asthenia, peripheral neuropathy, impotence, increased urinary frequency, visual disturbances; also reported, jaundice, pancreatitis, hyperglycaemia, thrombocytopenia, vasculitis, angioedema, alopecia, gynaecomastia

Dose: hypertension or angina, initially 5 mg once daily; max. 10 mg once daily

Istin® (Pfizer) PoM
Tablets, amlodipine (as besilate) 5 mg. Net price 28-tab pack = £13.04; 10 mg, 28-tab pack = £19.47

DILTIAZEM HYDROCHLORIDE

Indications: prophylaxis and treatment of angina; hypertension

Cautions: reduce dose in hepatic and renal impairment; heart failure or significantly impaired left ventricular function, bradycardia (avoid if severe), first degree AV block, or prolonged PR interval; **interactions:** Appendix 1 (calcium-channel blockers)

Contra-indications: severe bradycardia, left ventricular failure with pulmonary congestion, second- or third-degree AV block (unless pacemaker fitted), sick sinus syndrome; pregnancy and breast-feeding (see Appendixes 4 and 5)

Side-effects: bradycardia, sino-atrial block, AV block, palpitations, dizziness, hypotension, malaise, asthenia, headache, hot flushes, gastrointestinal disturbances, oedema (notably of ankles); rarely rashes (including erythema multiforme and exfoliative dermatitis), photosensitivity; hepatitis, gynaecomastia, gum hyperplasia, extrapyramidal symptoms, depression reported

Dose: angina, 60 mg 3 times daily (elderly initially twice daily); increased if necessary to 360 mg daily
Longer-acting formulations, see under preparations below

■ Standard formulations
NOTE. These formulations are licensed as generics and there is no requirement for brand name dispensing. Although their means of formulation has called for the strict designation 'modified-release' their duration of action corresponds to that of tablets requiring administration 3 times daily

Diltiazem (Non-proprietary) PoM
Tablets, m/r (but see note above), diltiazem hydrochloride 60 mg. Net price 100 = £5.25. Label: 25
Available from Alpharma, APS, Ashbourne (*Angiozem*®), Hillcross, IVAX, Niche, Opus (*Optil*®), Sterwin

Tildiem® (Sanofi-Synthelabo) PoM
Tablets, m/r (but see note above), off-white, diltiazem hydrochloride 60 mg. Net price 90-tab pack = £8.28. Label: 25

■ Longer-acting formulations
NOTE. Different versions of modified-release preparations may not have the same clinical effect. To avoid confusion between these different formulations of diltiazem, prescribers should specify the brand to be dispensed

Adizem-SR® (Napp) PoM
Capsules, m/r, diltiazem hydrochloride 90 mg (white), net price 56-cap pack = £10.56; 120 mg (brown/white), 56-cap pack = £11.74; 180 mg (brown/white), 56-cap pack = £17.60. Label: 25

Tablets, m/r, f/c, scored, diltiazem hydrochloride 120 mg. Net price 56-tab pack = £17.32. Label: 25
Dose: mild to moderate hypertension, usually 120 mg twice daily (dose form not appropriate for initial dose titration)
Angina, initially 90 mg twice daily (elderly, dose form not appropriate for initial dose titration); increased to 180 mg twice daily if required

Adizem-XL® (Napp) PoM
Capsules, m/r, diltiazem hydrochloride 120 mg (pink/blue), net price 28-cap pack = £10.24; 180 mg (dark pink/blue), 28-cap pack = £11.61; 200 mg (brown), 28-cap pack = £11.61; 240 mg (red/blue), 28-cap pack = £12.90; 300 mg (maroon/blue), 28-cap pack = £10.24. Label: 25
Dose: angina and mild to moderate hypertension, initially 240 mg once daily, increased if necessary to 300 mg once daily; in elderly and in hepatic or renal impairment, initially 120 mg daily

Angitil SR® (Trinity) PoM
Capsules, m/r, diltiazem hydrochloride 90 mg (white), net price 56-cap pack = £8.45; 120 mg (brown), 56-cap pack = £9.39; 180 mg (brown), 56-cap pack = £14.08. Label: 25
Dose: angina and mild to moderate hypertension, initially 90 mg twice daily; increased if necessary to 120 mg or 180 mg twice daily
NOTE. Also available as *Disogram*® *SR* (Ranbaxy)

Angitil XL® (Trinity) PoM
Capsules, m/r, diltiazem hydrochloride 240 mg (white), net price 28-cap pack = £10.15; 300 mg (yellow), 28-cap pack = £9.22. Label: 25
Dose: angina and mild to moderate hypertension, initially 240 mg once daily (elderly and in hepatic and renal impairment, dose form not appropriate for initial dose titration); increased if necessary to 300 mg once daily
NOTE. Also available as *Disogram*® *SR* (Ranbaxy)

Calcicard CR® (IVAX) PoM
Tablets, m/r, both f/c, diltiazem hydrochloride 90 mg, net price 56-tab pack = £6.33; 120 mg, 56-tab pack = £7.04. Label: 25
Dose: mild to moderate hypertension, initially 90 mg or 120 mg twice daily; up to 360 mg daily may be required; ELDERLY and in hepatic and renal impairment, initially 120 mg once daily; up to 240 mg daily may be required
Angina, initially 90 mg or 120 mg twice daily; up to 480 mg daily in divided doses may be required; ELDERLY and in hepatic and renal impairment, dose form not appropriate for initial dose titration; up to 240 mg daily may be required
NOTE. Also available as *Angiozem CR*® (Ashbourne)

Dilcardia SR® (Generics) PoM
Capsules, m/r, diltiazem hydrochloride 60 mg (pink/white), net price 56-cap pack = £8.13; 90 mg (pink/yellow), 56-cap pack = £10.33; 120 mg (pink/orange), 56-cap pack = £11.49. Label: 25
Dose: angina and mild to moderate hypertension, initially 90 mg twice daily; increased if necessary to 180 mg twice daily; ELDERLY and in hepatic and renal impairment, initially 60 mg twice daily, max. 90 mg twice daily

Dilzem SR® (Elan) PoM
Capsules, m/r, beige, diltiazem hydrochloride 60 mg, net price 56-cap pack = £8.32; 90 mg, 56-cap pack = £11.23; 120 mg, 56-cap pack = £12.47. Label: 25
Dose: angina and mild to moderate hypertension, initially 90 mg twice daily (elderly 60 mg twice daily); up to 180 mg twice daily may be required

Dilzem XL® (Elan) PoM
Capsules, m/r, diltiazem hydrochloride 120 mg, net price 28-cap pack = £8.32; 180 mg, 28-cap pack = £11.40; 240 mg, 28-cap pack = £11.70. Label: 25
Dose: angina and mild to moderate hypertension, initially 180 mg once daily (elderly and in hepatic and renal impairment, 120 mg once daily); if necessary may be increased to 360 mg once daily

Slozem® (Merck) PoM
Capsules, m/r, diltiazem hydrochloride 120 mg (pink/clear), net price 28-cap pack = £7.00; 180 mg (pink/clear), 28-cap pack = £7.80; 240 mg (red/clear), 28-cap pack = £8.20; 300 mg (red/white), 28-cap pack = £8.50. Label: 25
Dose: angina and mild to moderate hypertension, initially 240 mg once daily (elderly and in hepatic and renal impairment, 120 mg once daily); if necessary may be increased to 360 mg once daily

Tildiem LA® (Sanofi-Synthelabo) PoM
Capsules, m/r, diltiazem hydrochloride 200 mg (pink/grey, containing white pellets), net price 28-cap pack = £11.61; 300 mg (white/yellow, containing white pellets), 28-cap pack = £12.80. Label: 25
Dose: angina and mild to moderate hypertension, initially 200 mg once daily before or with food, increased if necessary to 300–400 mg daily, max. 500 mg daily; ELDERLY and in hepatic or renal impairment, initially 200 mg daily, increased if necessary to 300 mg daily

Tildiem Retard® (Sanofi-Synthelabo) PoM
Tablets, m/r, diltiazem hydrochloride 90 mg, net price 56-tab pack = £9.95; 120 mg, 56-tab pack = £11.06. Label: 25
COUNSELLING. Tablet membrane may pass through gastro-intestinal tract unchanged, but being porous has no effect on efficacy
Dose: mild to moderate hypertension, initially 90 mg or 120 mg twice daily; increased if necessary to 360 mg daily in divided doses; ELDERLY and in hepatic or renal impairment, initially 120 mg once daily; increased if necessary to 120 mg twice daily
Angina, initially 90 mg or 120 mg twice daily; increased if necessary to 480 mg daily in divided doses; ELDERLY and in hepatic or renal impairment, dose form not appropriate for initial titration; up to 120 mg twice daily may be required

Viazem XL® (Genus) PoM
Capsules, m/r, diltiazem hydrochloride 120 mg (lavender), net price 28-cap pack = £6.95; 180 mg (white/blue-green), 28-cap pack = £7.75; 240 mg (blue-green/lavender), 28-cap pack = £8.15; 300 mg (white/lavender), 28-cap pack = £8.45; 360 mg (blue-green), 28-cap pack = £14.95. Label: 25
Dose: angina and mild to moderate hypertension, initially 180 mg once daily, adjusted according to response to 240 mg once daily; max. 360 mg once daily; ELDERLY and in hepatic or renal impairment, initially 120 mg once daily, adjusted according to response

Zemtard® (Galen) PoM
Zemtard 120XL capsules, m/r, brown/orange, diltiazem hydrochloride 120 mg, net price 28-cap pack = £7.65. Label: 25
Zemtard 180XL capsules, m/r, grey/pink, diltiazem hydrochloride 180 mg, net price 28-cap pack = £7.80. Label: 25
Zemtard 240XL capsules, m/r, blue, diltiazem hydrochloride 240 mg, net price 28-cap pack = £8.20. Label: 25

Zemtard 300XL capsules, m/r, white/blue, diltiazem hydrochloride 300 mg, net price 28-cap pack = £8.50. Label: 25

Dose: angina and mild to moderate hypertension, 180–300 mg once daily, increased if necessary to 360 mg once daily in hypertension and to 480 mg once daily in angina; ELDERLY and in hepatic or renal impairment, initially 120 mg once daily

FELODIPINE

Indications: hypertension, prophylaxis of angina

Cautions: withdraw if ischaemic pain occurs or existing pain worsens shortly after initiating treatment or if cardiogenic shock develops; severe left ventricular dysfunction; hepatic impairment; breast-feeding; avoid grapefruit juice (may affect metabolism); **interactions:** Appendix 1 (calcium-channel blockers)

Contra-indications: pregnancy; unstable angina, uncontrolled heart failure; significant aortic stenosis; within 1 month of myocardial infarction

Side-effects: flushing, headache, palpitations, dizziness, fatigue, gravitational oedema; rarely rash, pruritus, cutaneous vasculitis, gum hyperplasia, urinary frequency, impotence, fever

Dose: hypertension, initially 5 mg (elderly 2.5 mg) daily in the morning; usual maintenance 5–10 mg once daily; doses above 20 mg daily rarely needed
Angina, initially 5 mg daily in the morning, increased if necessary to 10 mg once daily

Felodipine (Non-proprietary) PoM
Tablets, m/r felodipine 5 mg, net price 30-tab pack = £7.95; 10 mg, 28-tab pack = £10.91, 30-tab pack = £9.95. Label: 25
Available from Generics (*Felogen XL®*), Genus (*Felotens XL®*)

Plendil® (AstraZeneca) PoM
Tablets, m/r, f/c, felodipine 2.5 mg (yellow), net price 28-tab pack = £6.70; 5 mg (pink), 28-tab pack = £8.93; 10 mg (brown), 28-tab pack = £12.01. Label: 25

ISRADIPINE

Indications: hypertension

Cautions: tight aortic stenosis; sick sinus syndrome (if pacemaker not fitted); reduce dose in hepatic or renal impairment; pregnancy (may prolong labour); avoid grapefruit juice (may affect metabolism); **interactions:** Appendix 1 (calcium-channel blockers)

Side-effects: headache, flushing, dizziness, tachycardia and palpitations, localised peripheral oedema; hypotension uncommon; rarely weight gain, fatigue, abdominal discomfort, rashes

Dose: 2.5 mg twice daily (1.25 mg twice daily in elderly, hepatic or renal impairment); increased if necessary after 3–4 weeks to 5 mg twice daily (exceptionally up to 10 mg twice daily); maintenance 2.5 or 5 mg once daily may be sufficient

Prescal® (Novartis) PoM
Tablets, yellow, scored, isradipine 2.5 mg. Net price 56-tab pack = £15.04

LACIDIPINE

Indications: hypertension

Cautions: cardiac conduction abnormalities; poor cardiac reserve; hepatic impairment; withdraw if ischaemic pain occurs shortly after initiating treatment or if cardiogenic shock develops; avoid grapefruit juice (may affect metabolism); **interactions:** Appendix 1 (calcium-channel blockers)

Contra-indications: aortic stenosis; pregnancy and breast-feeding; avoid within 1 month of myocardial infarction

Side-effects: headache, flushing, oedema, dizziness, palpitations; also asthenia, rash (including pruritus and erythema), gastro-intestinal disturbances, gum hyperplasia, muscle cramps, polyuria, chest pain (see Cautions); mood disturbances

Dose: initially 2 mg as a single daily dose, preferably in the morning; increased after 3–4 weeks to 4 mg daily, then if necessary to 6 mg daily

Motens® (Boehringer Ingelheim) PoM
Tablets, both f/c, lacidipine 2 mg, net price 28-tab pack = £10.23; 4 mg (scored), 28-tab pack = £15.30

LERCANIDIPINE HYDROCHLORIDE

Indications: mild to moderate hypertension

Cautions: hepatic and renal impairment (Appendixes 2 and 3); left ventricular dysfunction; sick sinus syndrome (if pacemaker not fitted); avoid grapefruit juice (may affect metabolism); **interactions:** Appendix 1 (calcium-channel blockers)

Contra-indications: aortic stenosis; unstable angina, uncontrolled heart failure; within 1 month of myocardial infarction; pregnancy and breast-feeding

Side-effects: flushing, peripheral oedema, palpitations, tachycardia, headache, dizziness, asthenia; also gastro-intestinal disturbances, hypotension, drowsiness, myalgia, polyuria, rash

Dose: initially 10 mg once daily; increased, if necessary, after at least 2 weeks to 20 mg daily

Zanidip® (Napp) PoM
Tablets, yellow, f/c, lercanidipine hydrochloride 10 mg, net price 28-tab pack = £6.24. Label: 22

NICARDIPINE HYDROCHLORIDE

Indications: prophylaxis of angina; mild to moderate hypertension

Cautions: withdraw if ischaemic pain occurs or existing pain worsens within 30 minutes of initiating treatment or increasing dose; congestive heart failure or significantly impaired left ventricular function; elderly; hepatic or renal impairment; avoid grapefruit juice (may affect metabolism); **interactions:** Appendix 1 (calcium-channel blockers)

Contra-indications: cardiogenic shock; advanced aortic stenosis; unstable or acute attacks of angina; pregnancy and breast-feeding; avoid within 1 month of myocardial infarction

Side-effects: dizziness, headache, peripheral oedema, flushing, palpitations, nausea; also gastro-intestinal disturbances, drowsiness, insomnia, tinnitus, hypotension, rashes, dyspnoea, paraesthesia, frequency of micturition; thrombocytopenia, depression and impotence reported

Dose: initially 20 mg 3 times daily, increased, after at least three days, to 30 mg 3 times daily (usual range 60–120 mg daily)

Nicardipine (Non-proprietary) [PoM]
Capsules, nicardipine hydrochloride 20 mg, net price 56-cap pack = £8.36; 30 mg, 56-cap pack = £9.72
Available from Generics

Cardene® (Yamanouchi) [PoM]
Capsules, nicardipine hydrochloride 20 mg (blue/white), net price 56-cap pack = £9.22; 30 mg (blue/pale blue), 56-cap pack = £10.70

■ Modified release

Cardene SR® (Yamanouchi) [PoM]
Capsules, m/r, nicardipine hydrochloride 30 mg, net price 56-cap pack = £10.98; 45 mg (blue), 56-cap pack = £15.98. Label: 25
Dose: mild to moderate hypertension, initially 30 mg twice daily; usual effective dose 45 mg twice daily (range 30–60 mg twice daily)

NIFEDIPINE

Indications: prophylaxis of angina; hypertension; Raynaud's phenomenon
Cautions: withdraw if ischaemic pain occurs or existing pain worsens shortly after initiating treatment; poor cardiac reserve; heart failure or significantly impaired left ventricular function (heart failure deterioration observed); severe hypotension; reduce dose in hepatic impairment; diabetes mellitus; may inhibit labour; pregnancy (Appendix 4); breast-feeding (Appendix 5); avoid grapefruit juice (may affect metabolism); **interactions:** Appendix 1 (calcium-channel blockers)
Contra-indications: cardiogenic shock; advanced aortic stenosis; within 1 month of myocardial infarction; unstable or acute attacks of angina; porphyria (section 9.8.2)
Side-effects: headache, flushing, dizziness, lethargy; tachycardia, palpitations; short-acting preparations may induce an exaggerated fall in blood pressure and reflex tachycardia which may lead to myocardial or cerebrovascular ischaemia; gravitational oedema, rash (erythema multiforme reported), pruritus, urticaria, nausea, constipation or diarrhoea, increased frequency of micturition, eye pain, visual disturbances, gum hyperplasia, paraesthesia, myalgia, tremor, impotence, gynaecomastia; depression, telangiectasia, cholestasis, jaundice reported
Dose: see preparations below

Nifedipine (Non-proprietary) [PoM]
Capsules, nifedipine 5 mg, net price 84-cap pack = £3.49; 10 mg, 84-cap pack = £4.47
Dose: angina prophylaxis (but not recommended, see notes above) and Raynaud's phenomenon, initially 5 mg 3 times daily, adjusted according to response to 20 mg 3 times daily
Hypertension, not recommended therefore no dose stated
Available from Alpharma, APS, CP, Hillcross, IVAX

Adalat® (Bayer) [PoM]
Capsules, both orange, nifedipine 5 mg, net price 90-cap pack = £6.08; 10 mg, 90-cap pack = £7.74
Dose: angina prophylaxis (but not recommended, see notes above) and Raynaud's phenomenon, initially 5 mg 3 times daily, adjusted according to response to 20 mg 3 times daily
Hypertension, not recommended therefore no dose stated

■ Modified release
NOTE. Different versions of modified-release preparations may not have the same clinical effect. To avoid confusion between these different formulations of nifedipine, prescribers should specify the brand to be dispensed. Modified-release formulations may not be suitable for dose titration in hepatic disease

Adalat® LA (Bayer) [PoM]
LA 20 tablets, m/r, pink, nifedipine 20 mg, net price 28-tab pack = £8.15. Label: 25
LA 30 tablets, m/r, pink, nifedipine 30 mg, net price 28-tab pack = £9.89. Label: 25
LA 60 tablets, m/r, pink, nifedipine 60 mg, net price 28-tab pack = £15.40. Label: 25
COUNSELLING. Tablet membrane may pass through gastro-intestinal tract unchanged, but being porous has no effect on efficacy
Dose: hypertension, 20–30 mg once daily, increased if necessary; max. 90 mg once daily
Angina prophylaxis, 30 mg once daily, increased if necessary; max. 90 mg once daily
Caution: dose form not appropriate for use in hepatic impairment or where there is a history of oesophageal or gastro-intestinal obstruction, decreased lumen diameter of the gastro-intestinal tract, or inflammatory bowel disease (including Crohn's disease)

Adalat® Retard (Bayer) [PoM]
Retard 10 tablets, m/r, pink, nifedipine 10 mg. Net price 56-tab pack = £8.50. Label: 25
Retard 20 tablets, m/r, pink, nifedipine 20 mg. Net price 56-tab pack = £10.20. Label: 25
Dose: hypertension and angina prophylaxis, 10 mg twice daily, adjusted according to response to 40 mg twice daily

Adipine® MR (Trinity) [PoM]
Tablets, m/r, nifedipine 10 mg (apricot), net price 56-tab pack = £6.62; 20 mg (pink), 56-tab pack = £8.26. Label: 21, 25
Dose: hypertension and angina prophylaxis, 20 mg twice daily after food (initial titration 10 mg twice daily); max. 40 mg twice daily

Cardilate MR® (IVAX) [PoM]
Tablets, m/r, nifedipine 10 mg (pink), net price 56-tab pack = £4.97; 20 mg (brown), net price 100-tab pack = £16.62. Label: 25
Dose: hypertension and angina prophylaxis, 20 mg twice daily (initial titration 10 mg twice daily); max. 80 mg daily

Coracten SR® (Celltech) [PoM]
Capsules, m/r, nifedipine 10 mg (grey/pink, enclosing yellow pellets), net price 60-cap pack = £6.25; 20 mg (pink/brown, enclosing yellow pellets), 60-cap pack = £8.67. Label: 25
Dose: hypertension and angina prophylaxis, one 20-mg capsule every 12 hours, adjusted within range 10–40 mg every 12 hours

Coracten XL® (Celltech) [PoM]
Capsules, m/r, nifedipine 30 mg (brown), net price 28-cap pack = £6.73; 60 mg (orange), 28-cap pack = £10.01. Label: 25
Dose: hypertension and angina prophylaxis, 30 mg once daily, increased if necessary; max. 90 mg once daily

Coroday MR® (Generics) [PoM]
Tablets, m/r, red, nifedipine 20 mg, net price 56-tab pack = £9.94. Label: 25
Dose: hypertension and angina prophylaxis, 20 mg every 12 hours, increased if necessary to 40 mg every 12 hours

Fortipine LA 40® (Goldshield) [PoM]
Tablets, m/r, red, nifedipine 40 mg, net price 30-tab pack = £8.00. Label: 21, 25
Dose: hypertension and angina prophylaxis, 40 mg once daily, increased if necessary to 80 mg daily in 1–2 divided doses

Hypolar® Retard 20 (Sandoz) PoM
Tablets, m/r, red, f/c, nifedipine 20 mg. Net price 56-tab pack = £10.12. Label: 25
Dose: hypertension and angina prophylaxis, 20 mg twice daily, increased if necessary to 40 mg twice daily

Nifedipress® MR (Dexcel) PoM
Tablets, m/r, pink, nifedipine 10 mg, net price 56-tab pack = £9.93. Label: 25
Dose: hypertension and angina prophylaxis, initially 10 mg twice daily adjusted according to response to 40 mg twice daily

Nifopress® Retard (Goldshield) PoM
Tablets, m/r, pink, nifedipine 20 mg, net price 112-tab pack = £10.80. Label: 21, 25
Dose: mild to moderate hypertension, angina prophylaxis and Raynaud's phenomenon, usually 20 mg twice daily, adjusted according to response to 40 mg twice daily

Slofedipine® (Sterwin) PoM
Tablets, m/r, pink, nifedipine 20 mg, net price 56-tab pack = £10.32. Label: 25
Dose: hypertension and angina prophylaxis, initially 20 mg twice daily adjusted according to response to 40 mg twice daily

Slofedipine XL® (Sterwin) PoM
Tablets, m/r, brown, nifedipine 30 mg, net price 28-tab pack = £9.89; 60 mg, 28-tab pack = £14.71. Label: 25
Dose: hypertension and angina prophylaxis, 30 mg once daily, increased if necessary to 90 mg once daily
Caution: dose form not appropriate for use in hepatic impairment or where there is a history of oesophageal or gastro-intestinal obstruction, decreased lumen diameter of the gastro-intestinal tract, or inflammatory bowel disease (including Crohn's disease)

Tensipine MR® (Genus) PoM
Tablets, m/r, both pink, nifedipine 10 mg, net price 56-tab pack = £4.65; 20 mg, 56-tab pack = £5.99. Label: 21, 25
Dose: hypertension and angina prophylaxis, initially 10 mg twice daily adjusted according to response to 40 mg twice daily

■ With atenolol
Section 2.4

NIMODIPINE

Indications: prevention and treatment of ischaemic neurological deficits following aneurysmal subarachnoid haemorrhage
Cautions: cerebral oedema or severely raised intracranial pressure; hypotension; avoid concomitant administration of nimodipine tablets and infusion, other calcium-channel blockers, or beta-blockers; renal impairment or concomitant nephrotoxic drugs; hepatic impairment (Appendix 2); pregnancy; avoid grapefruit juice (may affect metabolism); **interactions:** Appendix 1 (calcium-channel blockers, alcohol (infusion only))
Contra-indications: within 1 month of myocardial infarction; unstable angina
Side-effects: hypotension, variation in heart-rate, flushing, headache, gastro-intestinal disorders, nausea, sweating and feeling of warmth; thrombocytopenia and ileus reported
Dose: prevention, *by mouth*, 60 mg every 4 hours, starting within 4 days of aneurysmal subarachnoid haemorrhage and continued for 21 days
Treatment, *by intravenous infusion* via central catheter, initially 1 mg/hour (up to 500 micr-ograms/hour if body-weight less than 70 kg or if blood pressure unstable), increased after 2 hours to 2 mg/hour if no severe fall in blood pressure; continue for at least 5 days (max. 14 days); if surgical intervention during treatment, continue for at least 5 days after surgery; max. total duration of nimodipine use 21 days

Nimotop® (Bayer) PoM
Tablets, yellow, f/c, nimodipine 30 mg. Net price 100-tab pack = £38.85
Intravenous infusion, nimodipine 200 micrograms/mL; also contains ethanol 20% and macrogol '400' 17%. Net price 50-mL vial (with polyethylene infusion catheter) = £13.24
NOTE. Polyethylene, polypropylene or glass apparatus should be used; PVC should be avoided

NISOLDIPINE

Indications: prophylaxis of angina, mild to moderate hypertension
Cautions: elderly; hypotension; avoid grapefruit juice (may affect metabolism); **interactions:** Appendix 1 (calcium-channel blockers)
Contra-indications: cardiogenic shock, aortic stenosis, unstable or acute attacks of angina; within 1 week of myocardial infarction; hepatic impairment (dose form not appropriate); pregnancy and breast-feeding
Side-effects: gravitational oedema, headache, flushing, tachycardia, palpitations; dizziness, asthenia, gastro-intestinal disturbances (including nausea, constipation); less frequently paraesthesia, myalgia, tremor, hypotension, weakness, dyspnoea, allergic skin reactions, increased frequency of micturition; rarely exacerbation of angina, visual disturbances, gynaecomastia, gum hyperplasia
Dose: initially 10 mg daily, preferably before breakfast; if necessary increase at intervals of at least 1 week (usual maintenance in angina 20–40 mg once daily); max. 40 mg daily

Syscor MR® (Forest) PoM
Tablets, m/r, all f/c, yellow, nisoldipine 10 mg, net price 28-tab pack = £9.36; 20 mg, 28-tab pack = £13.10; 30 mg, 28-tab pack = £16.85. Label: 22, 25

VERAPAMIL HYDROCHLORIDE

Indications: see under Dose and preparations
Cautions: first-degree AV block; acute phase of myocardial infarction (avoid if bradycardia, hypotension, left ventricular failure); patients taking beta-blockers (**important:** see below); hepatic impairment (Appendix 2); children, specialist advice only (section 2.3.2); pregnancy (Appendix 4) and breast-feeding (Appendix 5); avoid grapefruit juice (may affect metabolism); **interactions:** Appendix 1 (calcium-channel blockers)
VERAPAMIL AND BETA-BLOCKERS. **Verapamil** injection should not be given to patients recently treated with beta-blockers because of the risk of hypotension and asystole. The suggestion that when verapamil injection has been given first, an interval of 30 minutes before giving a beta-blocker is sufficient has not been confirmed. It may also be hazardous to give verapamil and a beta-blocker together by mouth (should only be contemplated if myocardial function well preserved).
Contra-indications: hypotension, bradycardia, second- and third-degree AV block, sick sinus syndrome, cardiogenic shock, sino-atrial block;

history of heart failure or significantly impaired left ventricular function, even if controlled by therapy; atrial flutter or fibrillation complicating Wolff-Parkinson-White syndrome; porphyria (section 9.8.2)

Side-effects: constipation; less commonly nausea, vomiting, flushing, headache, dizziness, fatigue, ankle oedema; rarely allergic reactions (erythema, pruritus, urticaria, angioedema, Stevens-Johnson syndrome); myalgia, arthralgia, paraesthesia, erythromelalgia; increased prolactin concentration; rarely gynaecomastia and gingival hyperplasia after long-term treatment; after intravenous administration or high doses, hypotension, heart failure, bradycardia, heart block, and asystole

Dose: *by mouth,* supraventricular arrhythmias (but see also Contra-indications), 40–120 mg 3 times daily

Angina, 80–120 mg 3 times daily

Hypertension, 240–480 mg daily in 2–3 divided doses

By slow intravenous injection over 2 minutes (3 minutes in elderly), 5–10 mg (preferably with ECG monitoring); in paroxysmal tachyarrhythmias a further 5 mg after 5–10 minutes if required

Verapamil (Non-proprietary) PoM
Tablets, coated, verapamil hydrochloride 40 mg, net price 20 = 38p; 80 mg, 20 = 50p; 120 mg, 20 = 72p; 160 mg, 20 = £1.71
Various strengths available from Alpharma, APS, Generics, Hillcross, IVAX
Oral solution, verapamil hydrochloride 40 mg/ 5 mL, net price 150 mL = £39.25
Available from Rosemont (*Zolvera*®)

Cordilox® (IVAX) PoM
Tablets, all yellow, f/c, verapamil hydrochloride 40 mg, net price 84-tab pack = £1.50; 80 mg, 84-tab pack = £2.05; 120 mg, 28-tab pack = £1.15; 160 mg, 56-tab pack = £2.80
Injection, verapamil hydrochloride 2.5 mg/mL, net price 2-mL amp = £1.11

Securon® (Abbott) PoM
Tablets, f/c, verapamil hydrochloride 40 mg, net price 100 = £4.57; 120 mg (scored), 60-tab pack = £7.67
Injection, verapamil hydrochloride 2.5 mg/mL. Net price 2-mL amp = £1.08

■ Modified release
Half Securon SR® (Abbott) PoM
Tablets, m/r, f/c, verapamil hydrochloride 120 mg. Net price 28-tab pack = £7.50. Label: 25
Dose: see *Securon SR*®

Securon SR® (Abbott) PoM
Tablets, m/r, pale green, f/c, scored, verapamil hydrochloride 240 mg. Net price 28-tab pack = £10.64. Label: 25
Dose: hypertension, 240 mg daily (new patients initially 120 mg), increased if necessary to max. 480 mg daily (doses above 240 mg daily as 2 divided doses)
Angina, 240 mg twice daily (may sometimes be reduced to once daily)
Prophylaxis after myocardial infarction where betablockers not appropriate (started at least 1 week after infarction), 360 mg daily in divided doses, given as 240 mg in the morning and 120 mg in the evening *or* 120 mg 3 times daily

Univer® (Elan) PoM
Capsules, m/r, verapamil hydrochloride 120 mg (yellow/dark blue), net price 28-cap pack = £7.51; 180 mg (yellow), 56-cap pack = £18.15; 240 mg (yellow/dark blue), 28-cap pack = £12.24.
Label: 25
Dose: hypertension, 240 mg daily, max. 480 mg daily (new patients, initial dose 120 mg); angina, 360 mg daily, max. 480 mg daily

Verapress MR® (Dexcel) PoM
Tablets, m/r, pale green, f/c, verapamil hydrochloride 240 mg. Net price 28-tab pack = £10.64.
Label: 25
Dose: hypertension, 1 tablet daily, increased to twice daily if necessary; angina, 1 tablet twice daily (may sometimes be reduced to once daily)
NOTE. Also available as *Cordilox*® *MR* (IVAX)

Vertab® **SR 240** (Trinity) PoM
Tablets, m/r, pale green, f/c, scored, verapamil hydrochloride 240 mg, net price 28-tab pack = £8.63. Label: 25
Dose: mild to moderate hypertension, 240 mg daily, increased to twice daily if necessary; angina, 240 mg twice daily (may sometimes be reduced to once daily)

2.6.3 Potassium-channel activators

Nicorandil, a potassium-channel activator with a nitrate component, has both arterial and venous vasodilating properties and is licensed for the prevention and long-term treatment of angina (section 2.6). Nicorandil has similar efficacy to other antianginal drugs in controlling symptoms; it may produce additional symptomatic benefit in combination with other antianginal drugs [unlicensed indication].

NICORANDIL

Indications: prophylaxis and treatment of angina
Cautions: hypovolaemia; low systolic blood pressure; acute pulmonary oedema; acute myocardial infarction with acute left ventricular failure and low filling pressures; pregnancy and breast-feeding; **interactions:** Appendix 1 (nicorandil)
DRIVING. Patients should be warned not to drive or operate machinery until it is established that their performance is unimpaired
Contra-indications: cardiogenic shock; left ventricular failure with low filling pressures; hypotension
Side-effects: headache (especially on initiation, usually transitory); cutaneous vasodilatation with flushing; nausea, vomiting, dizziness, weakness also reported; rarely oral ulceration and myalgia; at high dosage, reduction in blood pressure and/or increase in heart rate; angioedema, hepatic dysfunction also reported
Dose: initially 10 mg twice daily (if susceptible to headache 5 mg twice daily); usual dose 10–20 mg twice daily; up to 30 mg twice daily may be used

Ikorel® (Rhône-Poulenc Rorer) PoM
Tablets, both scored, nicorandil 10 mg, net price 60-tab pack = £8.16; 20 mg, 60-tab pack = £15.54

2.6.4 Peripheral and cerebral vasodilators

2.6.4.1 Peripheral vasodilators and related drugs
2.6.4.2 Cerebral vasodilators

2.6.4.1 Peripheral vasodilators and related drugs

Most serious peripheral vascular disorders, such as *intermittent claudication*, are due to occlusion of vessels, either by spasm or sclerotic plaques. Lifestyle changes including smoking cessation and exercise training are the most important measures in the conservative management of intermittent claudication. Low-dose aspirin (75 mg daily) should be given as long-term prophylaxis against cardiovascular events and a statin (section 2.12) should be considered if serum total cholesterol is raised. **Naftidrofuryl** 200 mg 3 times daily may alleviate symptoms and improve pain-free walking distance in moderate disease, but it is not known whether naftidrofuryl has any effect on the outcome of the disease. Patients receiving naftidrofuryl should be assessed for improvement after 3–6 months. **Cilostazol** is licensed for use in intermittent claudication to improve walking distance in patients without peripheral tissue necrosis and who do not have pain at rest. Inositol nicotinate, pentoxifylline (oxpentifylline) and cinnarizine are not established as being effective.

Management of *Raynaud's syndrome* includes avoidance of exposure to cold and stopping smoking. More severe symptoms may require vasodilator treatment, which is most often successful in primary Raynaud's syndrome. **Nifedipine** (section 2.6.2) is useful for reducing the frequency and severity of vasospastic attacks. Alternatively, **naftidrofuryl** may produce symptomatic improvement; **inositol nicotinate** (a nicotinic acid derivative) may also be considered. Cinnarizine, pentoxifylline, prazosin and moxisylyte (thymoxamine) are not established as being effective.

Vasodilator therapy is not established as being effective for *chilblains* (section 13.14).

CILOSTAZOL

Indications: intermittent claudication in patients without rest pain and no peripheral tissue necrosis
Cautions: atrial or ventricular ectopy, atrial fibrillation, atrial flutter; diabetes mellitus (higher risk of intra-ocular bleeding); **interactions:** Appendix 1 (cilostazol)
Contra-indications: predisposition to bleeding (e.g. active peptic ulcer, haemorrhagic stroke in previous 6 months, surgery in previous 3 months, proliferative diabetic retinopathy, poorly controlled hypertension); history of ventricular tachycardia, of ventricular fibrillation and of multifocal ventricular ectopics, prolongation of QT interval; congestive heart failure; moderate or severe hepatic impairment (Appendix 2), renal impairment (Appendix 3); pregnancy (Appendix 4) and breast-feeding (Appendix 5)

Side-effects: diarrhoea, abnormal stools, and headache are very common; nausea, vomiting, dyspepsia, flatulence, abdominal pain; tachycardia, palpitation, angina, arrhythmia, chest pain; rhinitis; dizziness; ecchymosis; rash, pruritus; oedema, asthenia; less commonly, gastritis, myocardial infarction, congestive heart failure, postural hypotension, insomnia, anxiety, abnormal dreams, dyspnoea, pneumonia, cough, hypersensitivity reactions, diabetes mellitus, anaemia, haemorrhage, thrombocythaemia, myalgia, renal impairment
Dose: 100 mg twice daily (30 minutes before or 2 hours after food)

Pletal (Otsuka) ▼ PoM
Tablets, cilostazol 100 mg, net price 56-tab pack = £35.31

CINNARIZINE

Indications: peripheral vascular disease, Raynaud's syndrome
Cautions: see section 4.6
Contra-indications: see section 4.6
Side-effects: see section 4.6
Dose: initially, 75 mg 3 times daily; maintenance, 75 mg 2–3 times daily

Stugeron Forte® (Janssen-Cilag)
Capsules, orange/ivory, cinnarizine 75 mg. Net price 100-cap pack = £5.50. Label: 2

Stugeron®
See section 4.6

MOXISYLYTE

(Thymoxamine)
Indications: primary Raynaud's syndrome (short-term treatment)
Cautions: diabetes mellitus
Contra-indications: active liver disease
Side-effects: nausea, diarrhoea, flushing, headache, dizziness; hepatic reactions including cholestatic jaundice and hepatitis reported to CSM
Dose: initially 40 mg 4 times daily, increased to 80 mg 4 times daily if poor initial response; discontinue after 2 weeks if no response

Opilon® (Hansam) PoM
Tablets, yellow, f/c, moxisylyte 40 mg (as hydrochloride). Net price 112-tab pack = £79.98. Label: 21

NAFTIDROFURYL OXALATE

Indications: see under Dose
Side-effects: nausea, epigastric pain, rash, hepatitis, hepatic failure
Dose: peripheral vascular disease (see notes above), 100–200 mg 3 times daily; cerebral vascular disease, 100 mg 3 times daily

Naftidrofuryl (Non-proprietary) PoM
Capsules, naftidrofuryl oxalate 100 mg. Net price 84-cap pack = £7.63. Label: 25, 27
Available from Alpharma

Praxilene® (Merck) PoM
Capsules, pink, naftidrofuryl oxalate 100 mg. Net price 84-cap pack = £8.60. Label: 25, 27

NICOTINIC ACID DERIVATIVES

Indications: peripheral vascular disease; hyperlipidaemia (section 2.12)
Side-effects: flushing, dizziness, nausea, vomiting, hypotension (more frequent with nicotinic acid than derivatives); occasional diabetogenic effect reported with nicotinic acid and nicotinyl alcohol; rarely associated with nodular changes to liver (monitor on prolonged high dosage)

Hexopal® (Sanofi-Synthelabo)
Tablets, scored, inositol nicotinate 500 mg. Net price 20 = £4.10
Dose: 1 g 3 times daily, increased to 4 g daily if required
Tablets forte, scored, inositol nicotinate 750 mg. Net price 112-tab pack = £34.02
Dose: 1.5 g twice daily

PENTOXIFYLLINE
(Oxpentifylline)
Indications: peripheral vascular disease; venous leg ulcers [unlicensed indication] (Appendix A8.2.5)
Cautions: hypotension, coronary artery disease; renal impairment (Appendix 3), severe hepatic impairment; avoid in porphyria (section 9.8.2); **interactions:** Appendix 1 (pentoxifylline)
Contra-indications: cerebral haemorrhage, extensive retinal haemorrhage, acute myocardial infarction; pregnancy and breast-feeding
Side-effects: gastro-intestinal disturbances, dizziness, agitation, sleep disturbances, headache; rarely flushing, tachycardia, angina, hypotension, thrombocytopenia, intrahepatic cholestasis, hypersensitivity reactions including rash, pruritus and bronchospasm
Dose: 400 mg 2–3 times daily

Trental® (Aventis Pharma) PoM
Tablets, m/r, pink, s/c, pentoxifylline 400 mg. Net price 90-tab pack = £23.81. Label: 21, 25

Other preparations used in peripheral vascular disease

Rutosides (oxerutins, *Paroven*®) are not vasodilators and are not generally regarded as effective preparations as capillary sealants or for the treatment of cramps; side-effects include headache, flushing, rashes, mild gastro-intestinal disturbances.

Paroven® (Novartis Consumer Health)
Capsules, yellow, oxerutins 250 mg. Net price 120-cap pack = £13.05
Dose: relief of symptoms of oedema associated with chronic venous insufficiency, 500 mg twice daily

2.6.4.2 Cerebral vasodilators

The cerebral vasodilator **co-dergocrine** is claimed to improve mental function. Some improvements in performance of psychological tests have been reported but it has not been shown clinically to be of much benefit in dementia. For other drugs used in dementia, see section 4.11.

CO-DERGOCRINE MESILATE

A mixture in equal proportions of dihydroergocornine mesilate, dihydroergocristine mesilate, and (in the ratio 2 : 1) α- and β-dihydroergocryptine mesilates

Indications: adjunct in elderly patients with mild to moderate dementia
Cautions: severe bradycardia
Side-effects: gastro-intestinal disturbances, flushing, headache, rash, nasal congestion; dizziness and postural hypotension in hypertensive patients
Dose: 1.5 mg 3 times daily before meals *or* 4.5 mg once daily before a meal

Hydergine® (Novartis) PoM
Tablets, co-dergocrine mesilate 1.5 mg (scored), net price 100-tab pack = £12.94. Label: 22

2.7 Sympathomimetics

2.7.1 Inotropic sympathomimetics
2.7.2 Vasoconstrictor sympathomimetics
2.7.3 Cardiopulmonary resuscitation

The properties of sympathomimetics vary according to whether they act on alpha or on beta adrenergic receptors. Adrenaline (epinephrine) (section 2.7.3) acts on both alpha and beta receptors and increases both heart rate and contractility (beta$_1$ effects); it can cause peripheral vasodilation (a beta$_2$ effect) or vasoconstriction (an alpha effect).

2.7.1 Inotropic sympathomimetics

The cardiac stimulants **dobutamine** and **dopamine** act on beta$_1$ receptors in cardiac muscle, and increase contractility with little effect on rate.

Dopexamine acts on beta$_2$ receptors in cardiac muscle to produce its positive inotropic effect; and on peripheral dopamine receptors to increase renal perfusion; it is reported not to induce vasoconstriction.

Isoprenaline injection is available on special order only.

SHOCK. Shock is a medical emergency associated with a high mortality. The underlying causes of shock such as haemorrhage, sepsis or myocardial insufficiency should be corrected. The profound hypotension of shock must be treated promptly to prevent tissue hypoxia and organ failure. Volume replacement is essential to correct the hypovolaemia associated with haemorrhage and sepsis but may be detrimental in cardiogenic shock. Depending on haemodynamic status, cardiac output may be improved by the use of sympathomimetic inotropes such as adrenaline (epinephrine), dobutamine or dopamine (see notes above). In septic shock, when fluid replacement and inotropic support fail to maintain blood pressure, the vasoconstrictor noradrenaline (norepinephrine) (section 2.7.2) may be considered. In cardiogenic shock peripheral resistance is frequently high and to raise it further may worsen myocardial performance and exacerbate tissue ischaemia.

The use of sympathomimetic inotropes and vasoconstrictors should preferably be confined to the intensive care setting and undertaken with invasive haemodynamic monitoring.

For advice on the management of anaphylactic shock, see section 3.4.3.

DOBUTAMINE

Indications: inotropic support in infarction, cardiac surgery, cardiomyopathies, septic shock, and cardiogenic shock

Cautions: severe hypotension complicating cardiogenic shock; **interactions:** Appendix 1 (sympathomimetics)

Side-effects: tachycardia and marked increase in systolic blood pressure indicate overdosage

Dose: *by intravenous infusion*, 2.5–10 micrograms/kg/minute, adjusted according to response

Dobutrex® (Lilly) [PoM]
Strong sterile solution, dobutamine (as hydrochloride) 12.5 mg/mL. For dilution and use as an intravenous infusion. Net price 20-mL amp = £8.35
NOTE. Strong sterile solution containing dobutamine (as hydrochloride) 12.5 mg/mL also available in 20-mL amps from Phoenix

Posiject® (Boehringer Ingelheim) [PoM]
Strong sterile solution, dobutamine (as hydrochloride) 50 mg/mL. For dilution and use as an intravenous infusion. Net price 5-mL amp = £3.85

DOPAMINE HYDROCHLORIDE

Indications: cardiogenic shock in infarction or cardiac surgery

Cautions: correct hypovolaemia; low dose in shock due to acute myocardial infarction—see notes above; **interactions:** Appendix 1 (sympathomimetics)

Contra-indications: tachyarrhythmia, phaeochromocytoma

Side-effects: nausea and vomiting, peripheral vasoconstriction, hypotension, hypertension, tachycardia

Dose: *by intravenous infusion*, 2–5 micrograms/kg/minute initially (see notes above)

Dopamine (Non-proprietary) [PoM]
Sterile concentrate, dopamine hydrochloride 40 mg/mL, net price 5-mL amp = £3.88; 160 mg/mL, net price 5-mL amp = £14.75. For dilution and use as an intravenous infusion
Available from Antigen, Faulding DBL
Intravenous infusion, dopamine hydrochloride 1.6 mg/mL in glucose 5% intravenous infusion, net price 250-mL container (400 mg) = £11.69; 3.2 mg/mL, 250-mL container (800 mg) = £22.93 (both hosp. only)
Available from Abbott

Select-A-Jet® Dopamine (Celltech) [PoM]
Strong sterile solution, dopamine hydrochloride 40 mg/mL. Net price 5-mL vial = £4.55; 10-mL vial = £7.32. For dilution and use as an intravenous infusion

DOPEXAMINE HYDROCHLORIDE

Indications: inotropic support and vasodilator in exacerbations of chronic heart failure and in heart failure associated with cardiac surgery

Cautions: myocardial infarction, recent angina, hypokalaemia, hyperglycaemia; correct hypovolaemia before starting, monitor blood pressure, pulse, plasma potassium, blood glucose; avoid abrupt withdrawal; **interactions:** Appendix 1 (sympathomimetics)

Contra-indications: left ventricular outlet obstruction such as hypertrophic cardiomyopathy or aortic stenosis; phaeochromocytoma, thrombocytopenia

Side-effects: tachycardia, other arrhythmias; also reported: nausea, vomiting, anginal pain, tremor, headache

Dose: *by intravenous infusion* into central or large peripheral vein, 500 nanograms/kg/minute, may be increased to 1 microgram/kg/minute and further increased up to 6 micrograms/kg/minute in increments of 0.5–1 microgram/kg/minute at intervals of not less than 15 minutes

Dopacard® (Elan) [PoM]
Strong sterile solution, dopexamine hydrochloride 10 mg/mL (1%). For dilution and use as an intravenous infusion. Net price 5-mL amp = £21.00
NOTE. Contact with metal in infusion apparatus should be minimised

2.7.2   Vasoconstrictor sympathomimetics

Vasoconstrictor sympathomimetics raise blood pressure transiently by acting on alpha-adrenergic receptors to constrict peripheral vessels. They are sometimes used as an emergency method of elevating blood pressure where other measures have failed (see also section 2.7.1).

The danger of vasoconstrictors is that although they raise blood pressure they do so at the expense of perfusion of vital organs such as the kidney.

Spinal and epidural anaesthesia may result in sympathetic block with resultant hypotension. Management may include intravenous fluids (which are usually given prophylactically), oxygen, elevation of the legs, and injection of a pressor drug such as ephedrine or methoxamine. As well as constricting peripheral vessels **ephedrine** also accelerates the heart rate (by acting on beta receptors). Use is made of this dual action of ephedrine to manage associated bradycardia (although intravenous injection of atropine sulphate 400 to 600 micrograms may also be required if bradycardia persists).

EPHEDRINE HYDROCHLORIDE

Indications: see under Dose

Cautions: hyperthyroidism, diabetes mellitus, ischaemic heart disease, hypertension, angle-closure glaucoma, elderly, pregnancy (Appendix 4); may cause acute urine retention in prostatic hypertrophy; **interactions:** Appendix 1 (sympathomimetics)

Contra-indications: breast-feeding (Appendix 5)

Side-effects: nausea, vomiting, anorexia; tachycardia (sometimes bradycardia), arrhythmias, anginal pain, vasoconstriction with hypertension, vasodilation with hypotension, dizziness and flushing; dyspnoea; headache, anxiety, restlessness, confusion, psychoses, insomnia, tremor; difficulty in micturition, urine retention; sweating, hypersalivation; changes in blood-glucose concentration

Dose: reversal of hypotension from spinal or epidural anaesthesia, *by slow intravenous injection* of a solution containing ephedrine hydrochloride 3 mg/mL, 3–6 mg (max. 9 mg) repeated every 3–4 minutes to max. 30 mg

Ephedrine Hydrochloride (Non-proprietary) PoM
Injection, ephedrine hydrochloride 3 mg/mL, net price 10-mL amp = £2.70; 30 mg/mL, net price 1-mL amp = £1.40
Available from Auden McKenzie, Aurum

METARAMINOL

Indications: acute hypotension (see notes above)
Cautions: see under Noradrenaline Acid Tartrate; longer duration of action than noradrenaline (norepinephrine), see below; cirrhosis
HYPERTENSIVE RESPONSE. Metaraminol has a longer duration of action than noradrenaline, and an excessive vasopressor response may cause a prolonged rise in blood pressure
Contra-indications: see under Noradrenaline Acid Tartrate
Side-effects: see under Noradrenaline Acid Tartrate; tachycardia; fatal ventricular arrhythmia reported in Laennec's cirrhosis
Dose: *by intravenous infusion*, 15–100 mg, adjusted according to response
In emergency, *by intravenous injection*, 0.5–5 mg then *by intravenous infusion*, 15–100 mg, adjusted according to response

Metaraminol (Non-proprietary) PoM
Injection, metaraminol 10 mg (as tartrate)/mL.
NOTE. May be difficult to obtain

NORADRENALINE ACID TARTRATE/ NOREPINEPHRINE BITARTRATE

Indications: see under dose
Cautions: coronary, mesenteric, or peripheral vascular thrombosis; following myocardial infarction, Prinzmetal's variant angina, hyperthyroidism, diabetes mellitus; hypoxia or hypercapnia; uncorrected hypovolaemia; elderly; extravasation at injection site may cause necrosis; **interactions:** Appendix 1 (sympathomimetics)
Contra-indications: hypertension (monitor blood pressure and rate of flow frequently), pregnancy
Side-effects: hypertension, headache, bradycardia, arrhythmias, peripheral ischaemia
Dose: acute hypotension, *by intravenous infusion*, via central venous catheter, of a solution containing noradrenaline acid tartrate 80 micrograms/mL (equivalent to noradrenaline base 40 micrograms/mL) at an initial rate of 0.16–0.33 mL/minute, adjusted according to response
Cardiac arrest, *by rapid intravenous or intracardiac injection*, 0.5–0.75 mL of a solution containing noradrenaline acid tartrate 200 micrograms/mL (equivalent to noradrenaline base 100 micrograms/mL)

Noradrenaline/Norepinephrine (Non-proprietary) PoM
Injection, noradrenaline acid tartrate 2 mg/mL (equivalent to noradrenaline base 1 mg/mL). For dilution before use. Net price 2-mL amp = £1.01, 20-mL amp = £6.35
Available from Abbott

PHENYLEPHRINE HYDROCHLORIDE

Indications: acute hypotension (see notes above)
Cautions: see under Noradrenaline Acid Tartrate; longer duration of action than noradrenaline (norepinephrine), see below; coronary disease
HYPERTENSIVE RESPONSE. Phenylephrine has a longer duration of action than noradrenaline, and an excessive vasopressor response may cause a prolonged rise in blood pressure
Contra-indications: see under Noradrenaline Acid Tartrate; severe hyperthyroidism
Side-effects: see under Noradrenaline Acid Tartrate; tachycardia or reflex bradycardia
Dose: *by subcutaneous or intramuscular injection*, 2–5 mg, followed if necessary by further doses of 1–10 mg
By slow intravenous injection of a 1 mg/mL solution, 100–500 micrograms repeated as necessary after at least 15 minutes
By intravenous infusion, initial rate up to 180 micrograms/minute reduced to 30–60 micrograms/minute according to response

Phenylephrine (Sovereign) PoM
Injection, phenylephrine hydrochloride 10 mg/mL (1%). Net price 1-mL amp = £5.00

2.7.3 Cardiopulmonary resuscitation

The algorithm for cardiopulmonary resuscitation (see inside back cover) reflects the most recent recommendations of the Resuscitation Council (UK). In cardiac arrest **adrenaline (epinephrine)** 1 in 10 000 (100 micrograms/mL) is recommended in a dose of 10 mL by intravenous injection, preferably through a central line. If injected through a peripheral line, the drug must be flushed with at least 20 mL sodium chloride 0.9% injection (to aid entry into the central circulation). Intravenous injection of **amiodarone** 300 mg (from a prefilled syringe *or* diluted in glucose intravenous infusion 5%) should be considered after adrenaline to treat ventricular fibrillation or pulseless ventricular tachycardia in cardiac arrest refractory to defibrillation. **Atropine** 3 mg by intravenous injection (section 15.1.3) as a single dose is also used in cardiopulmonary resuscitation to block vagal activity.

For the management of acute anaphylaxis see section 3.4.3.

ADRENALINE/EPINEPHRINE

Indications: see notes above
Cautions: heart disease, diabetes mellitus, hyperthyroidism, hypertension, arrhythmias, cerebrovascular disease, angle-closure glaucoma, avoid during second stage of labour; **interactions:** Appendix 1 (sympathomimetics)
Side-effects: anxiety, tremor, tachycardia, headache, cold extremities; in overdosage arrhythmias, cerebral haemorrhage, pulmonary oedema; nausea, vomiting, sweating, weakness, dizziness and hyperglycaemia also reported
Dose: see notes above

Adrenaline/Epinephrine 1 in 10 000, Dilute
(Non-proprietary) PoM
Injection, adrenaline (as acid tartrate) 100 micrograms/mL. 10-mL amp.
Available from Aurum, Martindale (special order); also from Aurum (1-mL and 10-mL prefilled syringe), Celltech (*Minijet® Adrenaline* 3- and 10-mL disposable syringes)

2.8　Anticoagulants and protamine

2.8.1　Parenteral anticoagulants
2.8.2　Oral anticoagulants
2.8.3　Protamine sulphate

The main use of anticoagulants is to prevent thrombus formation or extension of an existing thrombus in the slower-moving venous side of the circulation, where the thrombus consists of a fibrin web enmeshed with platelets and red cells. They are therefore widely used in the prevention and treatment of *deep-vein thrombosis in the legs*.

Anticoagulants are of less use in preventing thrombus formation in arteries, for in faster-flowing vessels thrombi are composed mainly of platelets with little fibrin. They are used to prevent thrombi forming on *prosthetic heart valves*.

2.8.1　Parenteral anticoagulants

Heparin

Heparin initiates anticoagulation rapidly but has a short duration of action. It is now often referred to as being **standard** or **unfractionated heparin** to distinguish it from the **low molecular weight heparins** (see p. 113), which have a longer duration of action. For patients at high risk of bleeding, heparin is more suitable than low molecular weight heparin because its effect can be terminated rapidly by stopping the infusion.

TREATMENT. For the initial treatment of *deep-vein thrombosis and pulmonary embolism* heparin is given as an *intravenous loading dose*, followed by *continuous intravenous infusion* (using an infusion pump) or by *intermittent subcutaneous injection*; the use of *intermittent intravenous injection* is no longer recommended. Alternatively, a low molecular weight heparin is given for initial treatment of deep vein thrombosis and pulmonary embolism. An oral anticoagulant (usually warfarin, section 2.8.2) is started at the same time as the heparin (the heparin needs to be continued for at least 5 days and until the INR has been in the therapeutic range for 2 consecutive days). Laboratory monitoring is essential—preferably on a daily basis, determination of the activated partial thromboplastin time (APTT) being the most widely used technique. Heparin is also used in regimens for the management of *myocardial infarction* (see also section 2.10.1), the management of *unstable angina* (section 2.6), and the management of *acute peripheral arterial occlusion*.

PROPHYLAXIS. In patients undergoing *general surgery*, low-dose heparin by subcutaneous injection is widely advocated to *prevent postoperative deep-vein thrombosis and pulmonary embolism* in 'high risk' patients (i.e. those with obesity, malignant disease, history of deep-vein thrombosis or pulmonary embolism, patients over 40 years, or those with an established thrombophilic disorder or who are undergoing large or complicated surgical procedures); laboratory monitoring is not required with this *standard prophylactic regimen*.

To combat the increased risk in *major orthopaedic surgery* an *adjusted dose regimen* may be used (with monitoring) or *low molecular weight heparin* (see p. 113), or aspirin, or in patients at high risk of thromboembolism, warfarin may be selected.

EXTRACORPOREAL CIRCUITS. Heparin is also used in the maintenance of extracorporeal circuits in *cardiopulmonary bypass* and *haemodialysis*.

HAEMORRHAGE. If haemorrhage occurs it is usually sufficient to withdraw heparin, but if rapid reversal of the effects of heparin is required, protamine sulphate (section 2.8.3) is a specific antidote (but only partially reverses the effects of low molecular weight heparins).

HEPARIN

Indications: see under Dose

Cautions: hepatic and renal impairment (Appendix 2 and Appendix 3); pregnancy; hypersensitivity to low molecular weight heparins; **interactions:** Appendix 1 (heparin)

THROMBOCYTOPENIA. Clinically important thrombocytopenia is immune-mediated, and does not usually develop until after 6 to 10 days; it may be complicated by thrombosis. Platelet counts are recommended for patients receiving heparin (including low molecular weight heparins) for longer than 5 days (heparin should be stopped immediately, and not repeated, in those who develop thrombocytopenia or a 50% reduction of platelet count). Patients requiring continued anticoagulation should preferably be given lepirudin or a heparinoid such as danaparoid

HYPERKALAEMIA. Inhibition of aldosterone secretion by heparin (including low molecular weight heparins) may result in hyperkalaemia; patients with diabetes mellitus, chronic renal failure, acidosis, raised plasma potassium or those taking potassium-sparing drugs seem to be more susceptible. The risk appears to increase with duration of therapy and the CSM has recommended that plasma potassium should be measured in patients at risk before starting heparin and monitored regularly thereafter, particularly if heparin is to be continued for more than 7 days

Contra-indications: haemophilia and other haemorrhagic disorders, thrombocytopenia (including history of heparin-induced thrombocytopenia), peptic ulcer, recent cerebral haemorrhage, severe hypertension, severe liver disease (including oesophageal varices), after major trauma or recent surgery to eye or nervous system; spinal or epidural anaesthesia with treatment doses of heparin; hypersensitivity to heparin

Side-effects: haemorrhage (see notes above), skin necrosis, thrombocytopenia (see Cautions), hyperkalaemia (see Cautions), hypersensitivity reactions (including urticaria, angioedema, and anaphylaxis); osteoporosis after prolonged use (and rarely alopecia)

Dose: treatment of deep-vein thrombosis and pulmonary embolism, *by intravenous injection*, loading dose of 5000 units (10 000 units in severe pulmonary embolism) followed by continuous *infusion* of 15–25 units/kg/hour *or* treatment of deep-vein thrombosis, *by subcutaneous injection* of 15 000 units every 12 hours (laboratory monitoring essential—preferably on a daily basis, and dose adjusted accordingly)

SMALL ADULT OR CHILD, lower loading dose *then*, 15–25 units/kg/hour *by intravenous infusion, or* 250 units/kg every 12 hours *by subcutaneous injection*

Unstable angina, acute peripheral arterial occlusion, as intravenous regimen for deep-vein thrombosis and pulmonary embolism, above

Prophylaxis in orthopaedic surgery, see notes above

Prophylaxis in general surgery (see notes above), *by subcutaneous injection*, 5000 units 2 hours before surgery, then every 8–12 hours for 7 days or until patient is ambulant (monitoring not needed); during pregnancy (with monitoring), 5000–10 000 units every 12 hours (**important:** not intended to cover prevention of prosthetic heart valve thrombosis in pregnancy which calls for separate specialist management)

MYOCARDIAL INFARCTION. For the prevention of *coronary re-occlusion after thrombolysis* heparin is used in a variety of regimens according to locally agreed protocols. For the prevention of *mural thrombosis* heparin is considered effective when given *by subcutaneous injection* of 12 500 units every 12 hours for at least 10 days.

Prevention of clotting in extracorporeal circuits, consult product literature

> *Note.* Doses above reflect the guidelines of the British Society for Haematology; for doses of the low molecular weight heparins, see below

Heparin (Non-proprietary) PoM
Injection, heparin sodium 1000 units/mL, net price 1-mL amp = 19p, 5-mL amp = 52p, 5-mL vial = 46p, 10-mL amp = 69p, 20-mL amp = £1.24; 5000 units/mL, 1-mL amp = 36p, 5-mL amp = £1.00, 5-mL vial = 92p; 25 000 units/mL, 1-mL amp = £1.01, 5-mL vial = £3.68

Calciparine® (Sanofi-Synthelabo) PoM
Injection (subcutaneous only), heparin calcium 25 000 units/mL. Net price 0.2-mL syringe = 65p; 0.5-mL syringe = £1.46

Monoparin® (CP) PoM
Injection, heparin sodium (mucous) 1000 units/mL, net price 1-mL amp = 19p; 5-mL amp = 52p; 10-mL amp = 69p; 20-mL amp = £1.24; 5000 units/mL, 1-mL amp = 36p; 5-mL amp = £1.00; 25 000 units/mL, 0.2-mL amp = 46p, 1-mL amp = £1.01

Monoparin Calcium® (CP) PoM
Injection, heparin calcium 25 000 units/mL. Net price 0.2-mL amp = 48p

Multiparin® (CP) PoM
Injection, heparin sodium (mucous) 1000 units/mL, net price 5-mL vial = 47p; 5000 units/mL, 5-mL vial = 92p; 25 000 units/mL, 5-mL vial = £3.68

Low molecular weight heparins

Bemiparin, **certoparin**, **dalteparin**, **enoxaparin**, **reviparin**, and **tinzaparin** are low molecular weight heparins. Low molecular weight heparins are as effective and as safe as unfractionated heparin in the prevention of venous thrombo-embolism; in orthopaedic practice they are probably more effective. They have a longer duration of action than unfractionated heparin; *once-daily subcutaneous* dosage means that they are convenient to use. The standard prophylactic regimen does not require monitoring.

Some low molecular weight heparins are also used in the treatment of deep-vein thrombosis, pulmonary embolism, unstable coronary artery disease (section 2.6) and for the prevention of clotting in extracorporeal circuits.

HAEMORRHAGE. See under Heparin.

BEMIPARIN SODIUM

Indications: see notes above and under preparations
Cautions: see under Heparin
Contra-indications: see under Heparin
Side-effects: see under Heparin
Dose: see under preparations below

Zibor® (Amdipharm) ▼ PoM
Injection, bemiparin sodium 12 500 units/mL, net price 0.2-mL (2500-unit) prefilled syringe = £3.39; 17 500 units/mL, 0.2-mL (3500-unit) prefilled syringe = £4.50
Dose: prophylaxis of deep-vein thrombosis, *by subcutaneous injection*, moderate risk, 2500 units 2 hours before or 6 hours after surgery then 2500 units every 24 hours for 7–10 days; high risk, 3500 units 2 hours before or 6 hours after surgery then 3500 units every 24 hours for 7–10 days
   Prevention of clotting in extracorporeal circuits, consult product literature

Injection, bemiparin sodium 25 000 units/mL, net price 0.2-mL (5000-unit) prefilled syringe = £6.96, 0.3-mL (7500-unit) prefilled syringe = £8.63, 0.4-mL (10 000-unit) prefilled syringe = £12.60
Dose: treatment of deep-vein thrombosis (with or without pulmonary embolism), *by subcutaneous injection*, 115 units/kg every 24 hours for 5–9 days (and until adequate oral anticoagulation established)

CERTOPARIN SODIUM

Indications: see notes above and under preparations
Cautions: see under Heparin
Contra-indications: see under Heparin
Side-effects: see under Heparin
Dose: see under preparation below

Alphaparin® (Grifols) PoM
Injection, certoparin sodium 3000 units/0.3-mL syringe, net price 1 syringe = £2.87
Dose: prophylaxis of deep-vein thrombosis, *by subcutaneous injection*, 3000 units 1–2 hours before surgery, then 3000 units every 24 hours for 7–10 days (or until the patient is mobile)

DALTEPARIN SODIUM

Indications: see notes above and under preparations
Cautions: see under Heparin
Contra-indications: see under Heparin
Side-effects: see under Heparin
Dose: see under preparations below

Fragmin® (Pharmacia) PoM
Injection (single-dose syringe), dalteparin sodium 12 500 units/mL, net price 0.2-mL (2500-unit) syringe = £1.86; 25 000 units/mL, 0.2-mL (5000-unit) syringe = £2.82, 0.3-mL (7500-unit) syringe =

£4.23, 0.4-mL (10 000-unit) syringe = £5.65, 0.5-mL (12 500-unit) syringe = £7.06, 0.6-mL (15 000-unit) syringe = £8.47, 0.72-mL (18 000-unit) syringe = £10.16

Dose: prophylaxis of deep-vein thrombosis, *by subcutaneous injection*, moderate risk, 2500 units 1–2 hours before surgery then 2500 units every 24 hours for 5–7 days or longer; high risk, 2500 units 1–2 hours before surgery, then 2500 units 8–12 hours later (*or* 5000 units on the evening before surgery, then 5000 units on the following evening), then 5000 units every 24 hours for 5–7 days or longer (5 weeks in hip replacement)

Treatment of deep-vein thrombosis and of pulmonary embolism, *by subcutaneous injection*, as a single daily dose, ADULT body-weight under 46 kg, 7500 units daily; body-weight 46–56 kg, 10 000 units daily; body-weight 57–68 kg, 12 500 units daily; body-weight 69–82 kg, 15 000 units daily; body-weight 83 kg and over, 18 000 units daily, with oral anticoagulant treatment until prothrombin complex concentration in therapeutic range (usually for at least 5 days); monitoring of anti-factor Xa not usually required; for patients at increased risk of haemorrhage, see below

Injection, dalteparin sodium 2500 units/mL (for subcutaneous or intravenous use), net price 4-mL (10 000-unit) amp = £5.12; 10 000-units/mL (for subcutaneous or intravenous use), 1-mL (10 000-unit) amp = £5.12; 25 000 units/mL (for subcutaneous use only), 4-mL (100 000-unit) vial = £48.66

Dose: treatment of deep-vein thrombosis and of pulmonary embolism, *by subcutaneous injection*, 200 units/kg (max. 18 000 units) as a single daily dose (*or* 100 units/kg twice daily if increased risk of haemorrhage) with oral anticoagulant treatment until prothrombin complex concentration in therapeutic range (usually for at least 5 days)

NOTE. For monitoring, blood should be taken 3–4 hours after a dose (recommended plasma concentration of anti-Factor Xa 0.5–1 unit/mL); monitoring not required for once-daily treatment regimen and not generally necessary for twice-daily regimen

Unstable coronary artery disease, *by subcutaneous injection,* 120 units/kg every 12 hours (max. 10 000 units twice daily) for 5–8 days

Prevention of clotting in extracorporeal circuits, consult product literature

Injection (graduated syringe), dalteparin sodium 10 000 units/mL, net price 1-mL (10 000-unit) syringe = £5.65

Dose: unstable coronary artery disease (including non-ST-segment-elevation myocardial infarction), *by subcutaneous injection*, 120 units/kg every 12 hours (max. 10 000 units twice daily) for up to 8 days; beyond 8 days (if awaiting angiography or revascularisation) women body-weight less than 80 kg and men less than 70 kg, 5000 units every 12 hours, women body-weight greater than 80 kg and men greater than 70 kg, 7500 units every 12 hours, until day of procedure (max. 45 days)

ENOXAPARIN SODIUM

Indications: see notes above and under preparations
Cautions: see under Heparin
Contra-indications: see under Heparin
Side-effects: see under Heparin
Dose: see under preparation below

Clexane® (Rhône-Poulenc Rorer) PoM
Injection, enoxaparin sodium 100 mg/mL, net price 0.2-mL syringe (20 mg, 2000 units) = £3.39, 0.4-mL syringe (40 mg, 4000 units) = £4.52, 0.6-mL syringe (60 mg, 6000 units) = £5.11, 0.8-mL syringe (80 mg, 8000 units) = £5.81, 1-mL syringe (100 mg, 10 000 units) = £7.19; 150 mg/mL (*Clexane*® *Forte*), 0.8-mL syringe (120 mg,

12 000 units) = £10.51, 1-mL syringe (150 mg, 15 000 units) = £11.94

Dose: prophylaxis of deep-vein thrombosis especially in surgical patients, *by subcutaneous injection, moderate risk*, 20 mg (2000 units) approx. 2 hours before surgery then 20 mg (2000 units) every 24 hours for 7–10 days; *high risk* (e.g. orthopaedic surgery), 40 mg (4000 units) 12 hours before surgery then 40 mg (4000 units) every 24 hours for 7–10 days

Prophylaxis of deep-vein thrombosis in medical patients, *by subcutaneous injection*, 40 mg (4000 units) every 24 hours for at least 6 days until patient ambulant (max. 14 days)

Treatment of deep-vein thrombosis or pulmonary embolism, *by subcutaneous injection*, 1.5 mg/kg (150 units/kg) every 24 hours, usually for at least 5 days (and until adequate oral anticoagulation established)

Unstable angina and non-ST-segment-elevation myocardial infarction, *by subcutaneous injection*, 1 mg/kg (100 units/kg) every 12 hours usually for 2–8 days (minimum 2 days)

Prevention of clotting in extracorporeal circuits, consult product literature

REVIPARIN SODIUM

Indications: see notes above and under preparation
Cautions: see under Heparin; platelet count recommended before treatment, on days 1 and 4 of treatment then twice weekly for first 3 weeks of treatment
Contra-indications: see under Heparin
Side-effects: see under Heparin
Dose: see under preparation below

Clivarine® (ICN) ▼ PoM
Injection, reviparin sodium 1432 units/0.25-mL syringe, net price 1 syringe = £3.63
Dose: prophylaxis of deep-vein thrombosis, *by subcutaneous injection*, 1432 units 2 hours before surgery, then 1432 units every 24 hours for 7 days (or until patient is mobile)

TINZAPARIN SODIUM

Indications: see notes above and under preparations
Cautions: see under Heparin
Contra-indications: see under Heparin
Side-effects: see under Heparin
Dose: see under preparations below

Innohep® (Leo) PoM
Injection, tinzaparin sodium 10 000 units/mL, net price 2500-unit (0.25-mL) syringe = £2.13, 3500-unit (0.35-mL) syringe = £2.98, 4500-unit (0.45-mL) syringe = £3.83, 20 000-unit (2-mL) vial = £11.36

Dose: prophylaxis of deep-vein thrombosis, *by subcutaneous injection*, general surgery, 3500 units 2 hours before surgery, then 3500 units every 24 hours for 7–10 days; orthopaedic surgery (high risk), 50 units/kg 2 hours before surgery, then 50 units/kg every 24 hours for 7–10 days *or* 4500 units 12 hours before surgery, then 4500 units every 24 hours for 7–10 days

Prevention of clotting in extracorporeal circuits, consult product literature

Injection, tinzaparin sodium 20 000 units/mL, net price 0.5-mL (10 000-unit) syringe = £9.65, 0.7-mL (14 000-unit) syringe = £13.51, 0.9-mL (18 000-unit) syringe = £17.37, 2-mL (40 000-unit) vial = £36.77

Dose: treatment of deep-vein thrombosis and of pulmonary embolism, *by subcutaneous injection*, 175 units/kg once daily for at least 6 days (and until adequate oral anticoagulation established)

NOTE. This treatment regimen does not require antic-oagulation monitoring

ASTHMA. Presence of sulphites in formulation may (especially in patients with asthma) lead to hypersensi-tivity (with bronchospasm and shock)

Heparinoids

Danaparoid (available on a named-patient basis from Durbin (*Organan*®) is a heparinoid used for prophylaxis of deep-vein thrombosis in patients undergoing general or orthopaedic surgery. Provid-ing there is no evidence of cross-reactivity, it also has a role in patients who develop thrombocytopenia in association with heparin.

Hirudins

Lepirudin, a recombinant hirudin, is licensed for anticoagulation in patients with Type II (immune) heparin-induced thrombocytopenia who require par-enteral antithrombotic treatment. The dose of lepir-udin is adjusted according to activated partial thromboplastin time (APTT).

LEPIRUDIN

Indications: thromboembolic disease requiring par-enteral anticoagulation in patients with heparin-induced thrombocytopenia type II

Cautions: renal impairment (Appendix 3); hepatic impairment (Appendix 2); recent bleeding or risk of bleeding including recent puncture of large vessels, organ biopsy, recent major surgery, stroke, haemorrhagic diathesis, severe uncontrolled hypertension, bacterial endocarditis; determine activated partial thromboplastin time 4 hours after start of treatment (or after infusion rate altered) and at least once daily thereafter

Contra-indications: pregnancy and breast-feeding

Side-effects: bleeding manifestations; reduced hae-moglobin concentration without obvious source of bleeding; fever, hypersensitivity reactions (includ-ing rash); injection site reactions

Dose: initially *by slow intravenous injection* (of 5 mg/mL solution), 400 micrograms/kg followed by *continuous intravenous infusion* of 150 micr-ograms/kg/hour (max. 16.5 mg/hour), adjusted according to activated partial thromboplastin time, for 2–10 days (longer if necessary)

Refludan® (Pharmion) PoM
Injection, powder for reconstitution, lepirudin. Net price 50-mg vial = £52.30

Heparin flushes

For maintaining patency of peripheral venous cathe-ters, sodium chloride injection 0.9% is as effective as heparin flushes.

Heparin Sodium (Non-proprietary) PoM
Solution, heparin sodium 10 units/mL, net price 5-mL amp = 25p; 100 units/mL, 2-mL amp = 28p
To maintain patency of catheters, cannulas etc. 10–200 units flushed through every 4–8 hours. Not for therapeutic use
Available from Leo

Canusal® (CP) PoM
Solution, heparin sodium 100 units/mL. Net price 2-mL amp = 27p
To maintain patency of catheters, cannulas, etc., 200 units flushed through every 4 hours or as required. Not for therapeutic use

Hepsal® (CP) PoM
Solution, heparin sodium 10 units/mL. Net price 5-mL amp = 25p
To maintain patency of catheters, cannulas, etc., 50 units flushed through every 4 hours or as required. Not for therapeutic use

Epoprostenol

Epoprostenol (prostacyclin) can be given to inhibit platelet aggregation during renal dialysis either alone or with heparin. It is also licensed for the treatment of primary pulmonary hypertension resistant to other treatment, usually with oral anticoagulation. Since its half-life is only about 3 minutes it must be given by continuous intravenous infusion. It is a potent vasodilator and therefore its side-effects include flushing, headache, and hypotension.

EPOPROSTENOL

Indications: see notes above

Cautions: anticoagulant monitoring required when given with heparin; haemorrhagic diathesis; dose titration for pulmonary hypertension should be in hospital (risk of pulmonary oedema); pregnancy (Appendix 4) and breast-feeding (Appendix 5)

Contra-indications: severe left ventricular dys-function

Side-effects: see notes above; also bradycardia, tachycardia, pallor, sweating with higher doses; gastro-intestinal disturbances; lassitude, anxiety, agitation; dry mouth, jaw pain, chest pain; also reported, hyperglycaemia and injection-site reac-tions

Dose: see product literature

Flolan® (GSK) PoM
Infusion, powder for reconstitution, epoprostenol (as sodium salt). Net price 500-microgram vial (with diluent) = £69.43; 1.5-mg vial (with diluent) = £139.86

Fondaparinux

Fondaparinux sodium is a synthetic pentasacchar-ide that inhibits activated factor X. It has been introduced recently for prophylaxis of venous thromboembolism in those undergoing major ortho-paedic surgery of the legs.

FONDAPARINUX SODIUM

Indications: see notes above

Cautions: hepatic impairment; renal impairment (Appendix 3); bleeding disorders, active gastro-intestinal ulcer disease; recent intra-cranial haemorrhage; brain, spinal, or ophthalmic surgery; spinal or epidural anaesthesia (risk of spinal haematoma); pregnancy (Appendix 4); breast-feeding (Appendix 5)

THROMBOCYTOPENIA. Platelet counts recommended at baseline and at end of treatment, especially when considering follow-up therapy with heparin or a low molecular weight heparin

Contra-indications: severe renal impairement; active bleeding; bacterial endocarditis

Side-effects: haemorrhage (see notes above); anaemia, thrombocytopenia, purpura; oedema; liver enzyme changes; less frequently nausea, vomiting, abdominal pain, dyspepsia, gastritis, constipation, diarrhoea, hypotension, vertigo, headache, rash, pruritus, injection site reactions

Dose: see under preparation below

Arixtra® (Sanofi-Synthelabo) ▼ PoM

Injection, fondaparinux sodium 5 mg/mL, net price 0.5-mL (2.5 mg) prefilled syringe = £7.17

Dose: by subcutaneous injection, 2.5 mg 6 hours after surgery then 2.5 mg daily for 5–9 days, CHILD under 17 years not recommended

2.8.2   Oral anticoagulants

Oral anticoagulants antagonise the effects of vitamin K, and take at least 48 to 72 hours for the anticoagulant effect to develop fully; if an immediate effect is required, heparin must be given concomitantly.

USES. The main indication for an oral anticoagulant is *deep-vein thrombosis.* Patients with *pulmonary embolism* should also be treated, as should those with *atrial fibrillation who are at risk of embolisation* (see also section 2.3.1), and those with *mechanical prosthetic heart valves* (to prevent emboli developing on the valves); an antiplatelet drug may also be useful in these patients.

Warfarin is the drug of choice; **acenocoumarol** (nicoumalone) and **phenindione** are seldom required.

Oral anticoagulants should not be used in cerebral artery thrombosis or peripheral artery occlusion as first-line therapy; aspirin (section 2.9) is more appropriate for reduction of risk in transient ischaemic attacks.

DOSE. Whenever possible, the base-line prothrombin time should be determined but the initial dose should not be delayed whilst awaiting the result.

The usual adult induction dose of warfarin is 10 mg[1] daily for 2 days (higher doses no longer recommended). The subsequent maintenance dose depends upon the prothrombin time, reported as INR (international normalised ratio). The daily maintenance dose of warfarin is usually 3 to 9 mg (taken at the **same time** each day). The indications and target INRs[2] currently recommended by the British Society for Haematology[3] are:

- INR 2–2.5 for prophylaxis of deep-vein thrombosis including surgery on high-risk patients;

- INR 2.5 for treatment of deep-vein thrombosis and pulmonary embolism (or for recurrence in patients no longer receiving warfarin), atrial fibrillation, cardioversion, dilated cardiomyopathy, mural thrombus following myocardial infarction, and rheumatic mitral valve disease;

- INR 3.5 for recurrent deep-vein thrombosis and pulmonary embolism (in patients currently receiving warfarin with INR above 2) and mechanical prosthetic heart valves.

MONITORING. It is essential that the INR be determined daily or on alternate days in early days of treatment, *then* at longer intervals (depending on response[4]) *then* up to every 12 weeks.

HAEMORRHAGE. The main adverse effect of all oral anticoagulants is haemorrhage. Checking the INR and omitting doses when appropriate is essential; if the anticoagulant is stopped but not reversed, the INR should be measured 2–3 days later to ensure that it is falling. The following recommendations of the British Society for Haematology are based on the result of the INR and whether there is major or minor bleeding; the recommendations apply to patients taking warfarin:

- Major bleeding—stop warfarin; give phytomenadione (vitamin K_1) 5 mg by slow intravenous injection; give prothrombin complex concentrate (factors II, VII, IX and X) 50 units/kg *or* (if no concentrate available) fresh frozen plasma 15 mL/kg

- INR > 8.0, no bleeding or minor bleeding—stop warfarin, restart when INR < 5.0; if there are other risk factors for bleeding give phytomenadione (vitamin K_1) 0.5 mg by slow intravenous injection or 5 mg by mouth (for partial reversal of anticoagulation give smaller oral doses of phytomenadione e.g. 0.5–2.5 mg using the intravenous preparation orally); repeat dose of phytomenadione if INR still too high after 24 hours

- INR 6.0–8.0, no bleeding or minor bleeding—stop warfarin, restart when INR < 5.0

- INR < 6.0 but more than 0.5 units above target value—reduce dose or stop warfarin, restart when INR < 5.0

- Unexpected bleeding at therapeutic levels—always investigate possibility of underlying cause e.g. unsuspected renal or gastro-intestinal tract pathology

PREGNANCY. Oral anticoagulants are teratogenic and should not be given in the first trimester of pregnancy. Women at risk of pregnancy should be warned of this danger since stopping warfarin before the sixth week of gestation may largely avoid the risk of fetal abnormality. Oral anticoagulants cross the placenta with risk of placental or fetal haemorrhage, especially during the last few weeks of pregnancy and at delivery. Therefore, if at all possible, oral anticoagulants should be avoided in pregnancy, especially in the first and third trimesters. Difficult decisions may

---

1. First dose less than 10 mg if base-line prothrombin time prolonged, if liver-function tests abnormal, or if patient in cardiac failure, on parenteral feeding, less than average body weight, elderly, or receiving other drugs known to potentiate oral anticoagulants.

2. An INR which is within 0.5 units of the target value is generally satisfactory; larger deviations require dosage adjustment. Target values (rather than ranges) are now recommended (except for prophylaxis of deep-vein thrombosis where a range is still recommended).

3. Guidelines on Oral Anticoagulation: third edition. *Br J Haematol* 1998; **101**: 374–87

4. Change in patient's clinical condition, particularly associated with liver disease, intercurrent illness, or drug administration, necessitates more frequent testing. See also **interactions,** Appendix 1 (warfarin). Major changes in diet (especially involving salads and vegetables) and in alcohol consumption may also affect warfarin control.

have to be made, particularly in women with prosthetic heart valves or with a history of recurrent venous thrombosis or pulmonary embolism.

TREATMENT BOOKLETS. Anticoagulant treatment booklets should be issued to patients, and are available for distribution to local healthcare professionals from Health Authorities and also from:

England and Wales:
Astron
The Causeway
Oldham Broadway
Business Park
Chadderton
Oldham OL9 9XD
(0161) 683 2376

Scotland:
Banner Business Supplies
20 South Gyle Crescent
Edinburgh EH12 9EB
(0131) 479 3279

Northern Ireland:
Central Services Agency
25 Adelaide St
Belfast BT2 8FH
(028) 9053 5652

These booklets include advice for patients on anticoagulant treatment.

WARFARIN SODIUM

Indications: prophylaxis of embolisation in rheumatic heart disease and atrial fibrillation; prophylaxis after insertion of prosthetic heart valve; prophylaxis and treatment of venous thrombosis and pulmonary embolism; transient ischaemic attacks

Cautions: hepatic or renal disease (Appendixes 2 and 3), recent surgery; breast-feeding (Appendix 5); **interactions:** Appendix 1 (warfarin)

Contra-indications: pregnancy (see notes above), peptic ulcer, severe hypertension, bacterial endocarditis

Side-effects: haemorrhage—see notes above for British Society for Haematology recommendations; other side-effects reported include hypersensitivity, rash, alopecia, diarrhoea, unexplained drop in haematocrit, 'purple toes', skin necrosis, jaundice, hepatic dysfunction; also nausea, vomiting, and pancreatitis

Dose: see notes above

Warfarin (Non-proprietary) PoM
Tablets, warfarin sodium 0.5 mg (white), net price 28-tab pack = £1.00; 1 mg (brown), 20 = 99p; 3 mg (blue), 20 = £1.11; 5 mg (pink), 20 = £1.21.
Label: 10, anticoagulant card
Available from Alpharma, APS, Generics, Goldshield (*Marevan*®), Hillcross, IVAX, Taro

ACENOCOUMAROL

(Nicoumalone)
Indications: see under Warfarin Sodium
Cautions: see under Warfarin Sodium
Contra-indications: see under Warfarin Sodium
Side-effects: see under Warfarin Sodium
Dose: 8–12 mg on 1st day; 4–8 mg on 2nd day; maintenance dose usually 1–8 mg daily

Sinthrome® (Alliance) PoM
Tablets, acenocoumarol 1 mg. Net price 20 = 95p.
Label: 10, anticoagulant card

PHENINDIONE

Indications: prophylaxis of embolisation in rheumatic heart disease and atrial fibrillation; prophylaxis after insertion of prosthetic heart valve;

prophylaxis and treatment of venous thrombosis and pulmonary embolism

Cautions: see under Warfarin Sodium; **interactions:** Appendix 1 (phenindione)

Contra-indications: see under Warfarin Sodium; avoid breast-feeding

Side-effects: see under Warfarin Sodium; also hypersensitivity reactions including rashes, exfoliative dermatitis, exanthema, fever, leucopenia, agranulocytosis, eosinophilia, diarrhoea, renal and hepatic damage; urine coloured pink or orange

Dose: 200 mg on day 1; 100 mg on day 2; maintenance dose usually 50–150 mg daily

Phenindione (Non-proprietary) PoM
Tablets, phenindione 10 mg, net price 100 = £6.80; 25 mg, 100 = £9.50; 50 mg, 100 = £12.10.
Label: 10, anticoagulant card, 14, (urine pink or orange)
Available from Goldshield

2.8.3 Protamine sulphate

Although protamine sulphate is used to counteract overdosage with heparin, if used in excess it has an anticoagulant effect.

PROTAMINE SULPHATE

(Protamine Sulfate)
Indications: see above
Cautions: see above; also if increased risk of allergic reaction to protamine (includes previous treatment with protamine or protamine insulin, allergy to fish, men who are infertile or who have had a vasectomy)
Side-effects: nausea, vomiting, lassitude, flushing, hypotension, bradycardia, dyspnoea; hypersensitivity reactions (including angioedema, anaphylaxis) reported
Dose: *by intravenous injection* over approx. 10 minutes, 1 mg neutralises 80–100 units heparin when given within 15 minutes of heparin; if longer time, less protamine required as heparin rapidly excreted; max. 50 mg

Protamine Sulphate (Non-proprietary) PoM
Injection, protamine sulphate 10 mg/mL, net price 5-mL amp = £1.14, 10-mL amp = £3.30
Available from Celltech, Sovereign

Prosulf® (CP) PoM
Injection,, protamine sulphate 10 mg/mL. Net price 5-mL amp = 96p (glass), £1.20 (polypropylene)

2.9 Antiplatelet drugs

Antiplatelet drugs decrease platelet aggregation and may inhibit thrombus formation in the arterial circulation, where anticoagulants have little effect.

A low dose of **aspirin** is used for the *secondary prevention* of thrombotic cerebrovascular or cardiovascular disease. A single dose of aspirin 150–300 mg is given as soon as possible after an ischaemic event, preferably dispersed in water or chewed. The initial dose is followed by maintenance treatment with aspirin 75 mg daily.

A low dose of aspirin is also of benefit in the *primary prevention* of vascular events when the estimated 10-year coronary heart disease risk is 15% or greater and provided that blood pressure is controlled (section 2.5).

A low dose of aspirin (75 mg daily) is also given following coronary bypass surgery. For details on the use of aspirin in atrial fibrillation see section 2.3.1, for stable angina see section 2.6 and for intermittent claudication see section 2.6.4.1.

Clopidogrel is licensed for the prevention of ischaemic events in patients with a history of symptomatic ischaemic disease. Clopidogrel, in combination with low-dose aspirin, is also licensed for acute coronary syndrome without ST-segment elevation; in these circumstances the combination is given for at least 1 month but usually no longer than 9–12 months. However, long-term routine use of clopidogrel with aspirin increases the risk of bleeding and the evidence of benefit of such use is not compelling.

Dipyridamole is used by mouth as an adjunct to oral anticoagulation for prophylaxis of thromboembolism associated with prosthetic heart valves. Modified-release preparations are licensed for secondary prevention of ischaemic stroke and transient ischaemic attacks. Dipyridamole is also used in combination with low-dose aspirin; evidence of long-term benefit has not been established.

GLYCOPROTEIN IIb/IIIa INHIBITORS. Glycoprotein IIb/IIIa inhibitors prevent platelet aggregation by blocking the binding of fibrinogen to receptors on platelets. **Abciximab** is a monoclonal antibody which binds to glycoprotein IIb/IIIa receptors and to other related sites; it is licensed as an adjunct to heparin and aspirin for the prevention of ischaemic complications in high-risk patients undergoing percutaneous transluminal coronary intervention. Abciximab should be used once only. **Eptifibatide** and **tirofiban** also inhibit glycoprotein IIb/IIIa receptors; they are licensed for use with heparin and aspirin to prevent early myocardial infarction in patients with unstable angina (section 2.6) or non-ST-segment-elevation myocardial infarction. Abciximab, eptifibatide and tirofiban should be used by specialists only.

For use of epoprostenol, see section 2.8.1.

> **NICE guidance (glycoprotein IIb/IIIa inhibitors for acute coronary syndromes).** NICE has recommended (September 2002) that a glycoprotein IIb/IIIa inhibitor (abciximab, eptifibatide, and tirofiban) should be considered in the management of unstable angina or non-ST-segment-elevation myocardial infarction.
>
> A glycoprotein IIb/IIIa inhibitor is recommended for patients at high risk of myocardial infarction or death when early percutaneous coronary intervention is desirable but does not occur immediately; either eptifibatide or tirofiban is recommended in addition to other appropriate drug treatment.
>
> A glycoprotein IIb/IIIa inhibitor is recommended as an adjunct to percutaneous coronary intervention:
>
> - when early percutaneous coronary intervention is indicated but it is delayed;
> - in patients with diabetes;
> - if the procedure is complex.
>
> NOTE. Only abciximab is licensed as an adjunct to percutaneous coronary intervention

ABCIXIMAB

Indications: prevention of ischaemic cardiac complications in patients undergoing percutaneous coronary intervention; short-term prevention of myocardial infarction in patients with unstable angina not responding to conventional treatment and who are scheduled for percutaneous coronary intervention (use under specialist supervision)

Cautions: measure baseline prothrombin time, activated partial thromboplastin time, platelet count, haemoglobin and haematocrit; monitor haemoglobin and haematocrit 12 hours and 24 hours after start of treatment and platelet count 2–4 hours and 24 hours after start of treatment; concomitant use of drugs that increase risk of bleeding; discontinue if uncontrollable serious bleeding occurs or emergency cardiac surgery needed; consult product literature for details of procedures to minimise bleeding; pregnancy (Appendix 4)

Contra-indications: active internal bleeding, major surgery, intracranial or intraspinal surgery or trauma within last 2 months, stroke within last 2 years; intracranial neoplasm, arteriovenous malformation or aneurysm, severe hypertension, haemorrhagic diathesis, thrombocytopenia, vasculitis, hypertensive or diabetic retinopathy; severe hepatic or renal impairment (Appendixes 2 and 3); breast-feeding

Side-effects: bleeding manifestations; nausea, vomiting, hypotension, bradycardia, chest pain, back pain, headache, fever, puncture site pain, thrombocytopenia; rarely cardiac tamponade, adult respiratory distress, hypersensitivity reactions

Dose: ADULT initially *by intravenous injection* over 1 minute, 250 micrograms/kg, then *by intravenous infusion*, 125 nanograms/kg/minute (max. 10 micrograms/minute); for prevention of ischaemic complications start 10–60 minutes before percutaneous coronary intervention and continue infusion for 12 hours; for unstable angina start up to 24 hours before possible percutaneous coronary intervention and continue infusion for 12 hours after intervention

ReoPro® (Lilly) PoM
Injection, abciximab 2 mg/mL, net price 5-mL vial = £280.00

ASPIRIN (antiplatelet)

(Acetylsalicylic Acid)

Indications: prophylaxis of cerebrovascular disease or myocardial infarction (see section 2.10.1 and notes above)

Cautions: asthma; uncontrolled hypertension; previous peptic ulceration (but manufacturer's package insert may advise avoidance of low-dose aspirin in history of peptic ulceration); pregnancy (but see Appendix 4); **interactions:** Appendix 1 (aspirin)

Contra-indications: children under 16 years and in breast-feeding (Reye's syndrome, section 4.7.1); active peptic ulceration; haemophilia and other bleeding disorders

Side-effects: bronchospasm; gastro-intestinal haemorrhage (occasionally major), also other haemorrhage (e.g. subconjunctival)

Dose: see notes above

[1]**Aspirin** (Non-proprietary) [PoM]
Dispersible tablets, aspirin 75 mg, net price 20 = 13p; 300 mg, see section 4.7.1. Label: 13, 21, 32
Tablets, e/c, aspirin 75 mg, net price 56-tab pack = £3.03; 300 mg, see section 4.7.1. Label: 5, 25, 32
Available from Dexcel (*Micropirin*®), Genus (*Gencardia*®), Sandoz

Angettes 75® (Bristol-Myers Squibb)
Tablets, aspirin 75 mg. Net price 28-tab pack = 94p. Label: 32

Caprin® (Sinclair) [PoM]
Tablets, e/c, pink, aspirin 75 mg, net price 56-tab pack = £3.08; 300 mg, see section 4.7.1. Label: 5, 25, 32

Nu-Seals® **Aspirin** (Alliance) [PoM]
Tablets, e/c, aspirin 75 mg, net price 56-tab pack = £3.09; 300 mg, see section 4.7.1. Label: 5, 25, 32
NOTE. Tablets may be chewed at diagnosis for rapid absorption

■ With isosorbide mononitrate
Section 2.6.1

CLOPIDOGREL

Indications: prevention of atherosclerotic events in peripheral arterial disease, or within 35 days of myocardial infarction, or within 6 months of ischaemic stroke, or (given with aspirin—see notes above) in acute coronary syndrome without ST-segment-elevation

Cautions: avoid for first few days after myocardial infarction and for 7 days after ischaemic stroke; patients at risk of increased bleeding from trauma, surgery or other pathological conditions; discontinue 7 days before elective surgery if antiplatelet effect not desirable; liver impairment (Appendix 2), renal impairment; pregnancy (Appendix 4); **interactions:** Appendix 1 (clopidogrel)

Contra-indications: active bleeding, breast-feeding

Side-effects: dyspepsia, abdominal pain, diarrhoea; bleeding disorders (including gastro-intestinal and intracranial); less commonly nausea, vomiting, gastritis, flatulence, constipation, gastric and duodenal ulcers, headache, dizziness, paraesthesia, vertigo, leucopenia, decreased platelets (very rarely severe thrombocytopenia), eosinophilia, rash, pruritus; very rarely colitis, pancreatitis, hepatitis, vasculitis, confusion, hallucinations, taste disturbance, blood disorders (including thrombocytopenic purpura, agranulocytosis and pancytopenia), hypersensitivity-like reactions (including hypotension, bronchospasm, arthralgia, erythema multiforme, angioedema, fever, glomerulonephritis

Dose: 75 mg once daily
Acute coronary syndrome, initially 300 mg then 75 mg daily (with aspirin, but see notes above)

Plavix® (Bristol-Myers Squibb, Sanofi-Synthelabo) [PoM]
Tablets, pink, f/c, clopidogrel (as hydrogen sulphate) 75 mg, net price 28-tab pack = £35.31

1. Aspirin tablets 75 mg may be sold to the public in packs of up to 100 tablets; for details relating to other strengths see section 4.7.1 and *Medicines, Ethics and Practice*, No. 27, London, Pharmaceutical Press, 2003 (and subsequent editions as available)

DIPYRIDAMOLE

Indications: see notes above and under Dose

Cautions: rapidly worsening angina, aortic stenosis, recent myocardial infarction, heart failure; may exacerbate migraine; hypotension; myasthenia gravis (risk of exacerbation); **interactions:** Appendix 1 (dipyridamole)

Side-effects: gastro-intestinal effects, dizziness, myalgia, throbbing headache, hypotension, hot flushes and tachycardia; worsening symptoms of coronary heart disease; hypersensitivity reactions such as rash, urticaria, severe bronchospasm and angioedema; increased bleeding during or after surgery; thrombocytopenia reported

Dose: *by mouth*, 300–600 mg daily in 3–4 divided doses before food
Modified-release preparations, see under preparation below
By intravenous injection, diagnostic only, consult product literature

Dipyridamole (Non-proprietary) [PoM]
Tablets, coated, dipyridamole 25 mg, net price 20 = 40p; 100 mg, 20 = £1.09; 84 = £4.57. Label: 22
Available from Alpharma, Hillcross, IVAX
Oral suspension, dipyridamole 50 mg/5 mL, net price 150 mL = £34.00
Available from Rosemont (sugar-free)

Persantin® (Boehringer Ingelheim) [PoM]
Tablets, both s/c, dipyridamole 25 mg (orange), net price 84-tab pack = £1.70; 100 mg, 84-tab pack = £4.73. Label: 22
Injection, dipyridamole 5 mg/mL. Net price 2-mL amp = 11p

■ Modified release
Persantin® **Retard** (Boehringer Ingelheim) [PoM]
Capsules, m/r, red/orange containing yellow pellets, dipyridamole 200 mg. Net price 60-cap pack = £9.75. Label: 21, 25
Dose: secondary prevention of ischaemic stroke and transient ischaemic attacks (used alone or with aspirin), adjunct to oral anticoagulation for prophylaxis of thromboembolism associated with prosthetic heart valves, 200 mg twice daily preferably with food
NOTE. Dispense in original container (pack contains a desiccant) and discard any capsules remaining 6 weeks after opening

■ With aspirin
For cautions, contra-indications and side-effects of aspirin, see under Aspirin, above
Asasantin® **Retard** (Boehringer Ingelheim) [PoM]
Capsules, red/ivory, aspirin 25 mg, dipyridamole 200 mg (m/r), net price 60-cap pack = £9.75. Label: 21, 25
Dose: secondary prevention of ischaemic stroke and transient ischaemic attacks, 1 capsule twice daily
Note: Dispense in original container (pack contains a desiccant) and discard any capsules remaining 6 weeks after opening

EPTIFIBATIDE

Indications: prevention of early myocardial infarction in patients with unstable angina or non-ST-segment-elevation myocardial infarction and with last episode of chest pain within 24 hours (use under specialist supervision)

Cautions: renal impairment (Appendix 3); risk of bleeding, concomitant drugs that increase risk of bleeding—discontinue immediately if uncontrolled serious bleeding; measure baseline prothrombin time, activated partial thromboplastin time, platelet count, haemoglobin, haematocrit and serum creatinine; monitor haemoglobin, haematocrit and platelets within 6 hours after start of treatment then at least once daily; discontinue if thrombolytic therapy, intra-aortic balloon pump or emergency cardiac surgery necessary; pregnancy (Appendix 4)

Contra-indications: abnormal bleeding within 30 days, major surgery or severe trauma within 6 weeks, stroke within last 30 days or any history of haemorrhagic stroke, intracranial disease (aneurysm, neoplasm or arteriovenous malformation), severe hypertension, haemorrhagic diathesis, increased prothrombin time or INR, thrombocytopenia, significant hepatic impairment; breast-feeding

Side-effects: bleeding manifestations

Dose: initially *by intravenous injection*, 180 micrograms/kg, then *by intravenous infusion*, 2 micrograms/kg/minute for up to 72 hours (up to 96 hours if percutaneous coronary intervention during treatment)

Integrilin® (Schering-Plough) PoM
Injection, eptifibatide 2 mg/mL, net price 10-mL (20-mg) vial = £15.54
Infusion, eptifibatide 750 micrograms/mL, net price 100-mL (75-mg) vial = £48.84

TIROFIBAN

Indications: prevention of early myocardial infarction in patients with unstable angina or non-ST-segment-elevation myocardial infarction and with last episode of chest pain within 12 hours (use under specialist supervision)

Cautions: renal impairment (Appendix 3); hepatic impairment (avoid if severe; Appendix 2); major surgery or severe trauma within 3 months (avoid if within 6 weeks); traumatic or protracted cardiopulmonary resuscitation, organ biopsy or lithotripsy within last 2 weeks; risk of bleeding including active peptic ulcer within 3 months; acute pericarditis, aortic dissection, haemorrhagic retinopathy, vasculitis, haematuria, faecal occult blood; severe heart failure, cardiogenic shock, anaemia; puncture of non-compressible vessel within 24 hours; concomitant drugs that increase risk of bleeding (including within 48 hours after thrombolytic); monitor platelet count, haemoglobin and haematocrit before treatment, 2–6 hours after start of treatment and then at least once daily; discontinue if thrombolytic therapy, intra-aortic balloon pump or emergency cardiac surgery necessary; discontinue immediately if serious bleeding uncontrolled by pressure occurs; pregnancy (Appendix 4)

Contra-indications: abnormal bleeding within 30 days, stroke within 30 days or any history of haemorrhagic stroke, intracranial disease (aneurysm, neoplasm or arteriovenous malformation), severe hypertension, haemorrhagic diathesis, increased prothrombin time or INR, thrombocytopenia; breast-feeding

Side-effects: bleeding manifestations; reversible thrombocytopenia

Dose: *by intravenous infusion*, initially 400 nanograms/kg/minute for 30 minutes, then 100 nan-ograms/kg/minute for at least 48 hours (continue during and for 12–24 hours after percutaneous coronary intervention); max. duration of treatment 108 hours

Aggrastat® (MSD) PoM
Concentrate for intravenous infusion, tirofiban (as hydrochloride) 250 micrograms/mL. For dilution before use, net price 50-mL (12.5-mg) vial = £146.11
Intravenous infusion, tirofiban (as hydrochloride) 50 micrograms/mL, net price 250-mL *Intravia*® bag = £160.72

2.10   Myocardial infarction and fibrinolysis

2.10.1	Management of myocardial infarction
2.10.2	Fibrinolytic drugs

2.10.1   Management of myocardial infarction

> Local guidelines for the management of myocardial infarction should be followed where they exist

These notes give an overview of the initial and long-term management of myocardial infarction. The aims of management are to provide supportive care and pain relief, to promote revascularisation and to reduce mortality. Oxygen, diamorphine and nitrates provide initial support and pain relief; aspirin and percutaneous coronary intervention or thrombolytics promote revascularisation; long-term use of aspirin, beta-blockers, ACE inhibitors and statins help to reduce mortality further.

INITIAL MANAGEMENT. **Oxygen** (section 3.6) is administered unless the patient has severe chronic obstructive pulmonary disease.

The pain (and anxiety) of myocardial infarction is managed with slow intravenous injection of **diamorphine** (section 4.7.2); an antiemetic such as metoclopramide (or, if left ventricular function is not compromised, cyclizine) by intravenous injection should also be given (section 4.6).

Aspirin (chewed or dispersed in water) is given for its antiplatelet effect (section 2.9); a dose of 150–300 mg is suitable. If aspirin is given before arrival at hospital, a note saying that it has been given should be sent with the patient.

Patency of the occluded artery can be restored by percutaneous coronary intervention or by giving a **thrombolytic drug** (section 2.10.2), unless contra-indicated. Alteplase, reteplase and streptokinase need to be given within 12 hours of a myocardial infarction, ideally within 1 hour; use after 12 hours requires specialist advice. Tenecteplase should be given within 6 hours of a myocardial infarction. Streptokinase remains the drug of choice but antibodies appear after 4 days and streptokinase should not therefore be used again after this time. **Heparin** is used as adjunctive therapy with alteplase, reteplase, and tenecteplase to prevent re-thrombosis; heparin treatment should be continued for at least 24 hours (consult product literature).

Nitrates (section 2.6.1) are used to relieve ischaemic pain. If sublingual glyceryl trinitrate is not effective, intravenous glyceryl trinitrate or isosorbide dinitrate is given.

Early intravenous administration of some **beta-blockers** (section 2.4) has been shown to be of benefit and patients without contra-indications should receive **atenolol** by intravenous injection at a dose of 5 mg over 5 minutes, and the dose repeated once after 10–15 minutes; **metoprolol** by intravenous injection is an alternative.

ACE inhibitors (section 2.5.5.1) are also of benefit to patients who have no contra-indications; in hypertensive and normotensive patients treatment with an ACE inhibitor can be started within 24 hours of the myocardial infarction and continued for at least 5–6 weeks (see below for long-term treatment).

All patients should be closely monitored for hyperglycaemia; those with diabetes or raised blood-glucose concentration should receive **insulin**.

LONG-TERM MANAGEMENT. Long-term management involves the use of several drugs which should ideally be started before the patient is discharged from hospital.

Aspirin (section 2.9) should be given to all patients, unless contra-indicated, at a dose of 75 mg daily. **Warfarin** (with or without aspirin) may confer greater benefit than aspirin alone, but the risk of bleeding is increased.

Beta-blockers (section 2.4) should be given to all patients in whom they are not contra-indicated and continued for at least 2–3 years. Acebutolol, metoprolol, propranolol and timolol are suitable; for patients with left ventricular dysfunction, carvedilol, bisoprolol or long-acting metoprolol may be appropriate (section 2.5.5).

Although other calcium-channel blockers (section 2.6.2) have no place in routine management, **verapamil** may be useful in patients in whom beta-blockers are inappropriate.

An **ACE inhibitor** (section 2.5.5.1) should be considered for all patients, especially those with evidence of left ventricular dysfunction.

Nitrates (section 2.6.1) are used for patients with angina.

Statins are beneficial in preventing recurrent coronary events (section 2.12).

2.10.2   Fibrinolytic drugs

Fibrinolytic drugs act as thrombolytics by activating plasminogen to form plasmin, which degrades fibrin and so breaks up thrombi.

The value of thrombolytic drugs for the treatment of *myocardial infarction* has been established (section 2.10.1). **Streptokinase** and **alteplase** have been shown to reduce mortality. **Reteplase** and, more recently, **tenecteplase** are also licensed for acute myocardial infarction; they are given by intravenous injection (tenecteplase is given as a bolus injection). Thrombolytic drugs are indicated for any patient with acute myocardial infarction for whom the benefit is likely to outweigh the risk of treatment. Trials have shown that the benefit is greatest in those with ECG changes that include ST segment elevation (especially in those with anterior infarction) and in patients with bundle branch block. Patients should not be denied thrombolytic treatment on account of

age alone because mortality in this group is high and the reduction in mortality is the same as in younger patients.

Streptokinase is used in the treatment of *life-threatening venous thrombosis*, and in *pulmonary embolism*, but treatment must be started promptly.

CAUTIONS. Risk of bleeding including that from venepuncture or invasive procedures, external chest compression, pregnancy (see Appendix 4), abdominal aneurysm or conditions in which thrombolysis might give rise to embolic complications such as enlarged left atrium with atrial fibrillation (risk of dissolution of clot and subsequent embolisation), diabetic retinopathy (very small risk of retinal bleeding), recent or concurrent anticoagulant therapy.

CONTRA-INDICATIONS. Recent haemorrhage, trauma, or surgery (including dental extraction), coagulation defects, bleeding diatheses, aortic dissection, coma, history of cerebrovascular disease especially recent events or with any residual disability, recent symptoms of possible peptic ulceration, heavy vaginal bleeding, severe hypertension, active pulmonary disease with cavitation, acute pancreatitis, severe liver disease, oesophageal varices; also in the case of streptokinase, previous allergic reactions to either streptokinase or anistreplase (no longer available).

Prolonged persistence of antibodies to streptokinase and anistreplase (no longer available) may reduce the effectiveness of subsequent treatment, therefore streptokinase should not be used again beyond 4 days of first administration of either streptokinase or anistreplase.

SIDE-EFFECTS. Side-effects of thrombolytics are mainly nausea and vomiting and bleeding. When thrombolytics are used in myocardial infarction, reperfusion arrhythmias may occur. Hypotension may also occur and can usually be controlled by elevating the patient's legs, or by reducing the rate of infusion or stopping it temporarily. Back pain has been reported. Bleeding is usually limited to the site of injection, but intracerebral haemorrhage or bleeding from other sites may occur. Serious bleeding calls for discontinuation of the thrombolytic and may require administration of coagulation factors and antifibrinolytic drugs (aprotinin or tranexamic acid). Streptokinase may cause allergic reactions (including rash, flushing and uveitis) and anaphylaxis has been reported (for details of management see Allergic Emergencies, section 3.4.3). Guillain-Barré syndrome has been reported rarely after streptokinase treatment.

ALTEPLASE

(rt-PA, tissue-type plasminogen activator)

Indications: acute myocardial infarction (see notes above and section 2.10.1); pulmonary embolism; acute ischaemic stroke (treatment under specialist neurology physician **only**)

Cautions: see notes above; *in acute stroke*, monitor for intracranial haemorrhage, monitor blood pressure (antihypertensive recommended if systolic above 180 mm Hg or diastolic above 105 mmHg)

Contra-indications: see notes above; *in acute stroke*, convulsion accompanying stroke, severe stroke, history of stroke in patients with diabetes, stroke in last 3 months, hypoglycaemia, hyperglycaemia

Side-effects: see notes above; also risk of cerebral bleeding increased in acute stroke

Dose: myocardial infarction, accelerated regimen (initiated within 6 hours), 15 mg *by intravenous injection*, followed *by intravenous infusion* of 50 mg over 30 minutes, then 35 mg over 60 minutes (total dose 100 mg over 90 minutes); lower doses in patients less than 65 kg

Myocardial infarction, initiated within 6–12 hours, 10 mg *by intravenous injection*, followed *by intravenous infusion* of 50 mg over 60 minutes, then 4 *infusions* each of 10 mg over 30 minutes (total dose 100 mg over 3 hours; max. 1.5 mg/kg in patients less than 65 kg

Pulmonary embolism, 10 mg *by intravenous injection* over 1–2 minutes, followed *by intravenous infusion* of 90 mg over 2 hours; max. 1.5 mg/kg in patients less than 65 kg

Acute stroke (treatment **must** begin within 3 hours), *by intravenous administration* over 60 minutes, 900 micrograms/kg (max. 90 mg); initial 10% of dose by intravenous injection, remainder by intravenous infusion; ELDERLY over 80 years not recommended

Actilyse® (Boehringer Ingelheim) [PoM]
Injection, powder for reconstitution, alteplase 10 mg (5.8 million units)/vial, net price per vial (with diluent) = £135.00; 20 mg (11.6 million units)/vial (with diluent and transfer device) = £180.00; 50 mg (29 million units)/vial (with diluent, transfer device, and infusion bag) = £300.00

RETEPLASE

Indications: acute myocardial infarction (see notes above and section 2.10.1)
Cautions: see notes above
Contra-indications: see notes above
Side-effects: see notes above
Dose: *by intravenous injection*, 10 units over not more than 2 minutes, followed after 30 minutes by a further 10 units

Rapilysin® (Roche) [PoM]
Injection, powder for reconstitution, reteplase 10 units/vial, net price pack of 2 vials (with 2 prefilled syringes of diluent and transfer device) = £716.25

STREPTOKINASE

Indications: acute myocardial infarction (see notes above and section 2.10.1); deep-vein thrombosis, pulmonary embolism, acute arterial thromboembolism, and central retinal venous or arterial thrombosis; topical use (section 13.11.7)
Cautions: see notes above
Contra-indications: see notes above
Side-effects: see notes above
Dose: myocardial infarction, 1 500 000 units over 60 minutes

Deep-vein thrombosis, pulmonary embolism, acute arterial thromboembolism, central retinal venous or arterial thrombosis, *by intravenous infusion*, 250 000 units over 30 minutes, then 100 000 units every hour for up to 12–72 hours according to condition with monitoring of clotting parameters (consult product literature)

Streptokinase (Non-proprietary) [PoM]
Injection, powder for reconstitution, streptokinase, net price 100 000-unit vial = £10.00; 250 000-unit vial = £14.33; 750 000-unit vial = £38.20; 1.5 million-unit vial = £81.18
Available from Braun

Streptase® (Aventis Behring) [PoM]
Injection, powder for reconstitution, streptokinase, net price 250 000-unit vial = £17.11; 750 000-unit vial = £44.86; 1.5 million-unit vial = £89.72 (hosp. only)

TENECTEPLASE

Indications: acute myocardial infarction (see notes above and section 2.10.1)
Cautions: see notes above
Contra-indications: see notes above
Side-effects: see notes above; also fever
Dose: *by intravenous injection* over 10 seconds, 30–50 mg according to body-weight (500–600 micrograms/kg)—consult product literature; max. 50 mg

Metalyse® (Boehringer Ingelheim) [PoM]
Injection, powder for reconstitution, tenecteplase, net price 40-mg (8000-unit) vial = £700.00; 50-mg (10 000-unit) vial = £770.00 (both with prefilled syringe of water for injection)

2.11   Antifibrinolytic drugs and haemostatics

Fibrin dissolution can be impaired by the administration of **tranexamic acid**, which inhibits fibrinolysis. It may be useful to prevent bleeding (e.g. in prostatectomy and dental extraction in haemophilia) and can be particularly useful in menorrhagia. Tranexamic acid may also be used in hereditary angioedema, epistaxis and in thrombolytic overdose.

Desmopressin (section 6.5.2) is used in the management of mild to moderate haemophilia.

Aprotinin is a proteolytic enzyme inhibitor acting on plasmin and kallidinogenase (kallikrein). It is indicated for patients at high risk of major blood loss during and after open heart surgery with extracorporeal circulation and for patients in whom optimal blood conservation during open heart surgery is an absolute priority; it is also indicated for the treatment of life-threatening haemorrhage due to hyperplasminaemia (occasionally observed during the mobilisation and dissection of malignant tumours, in acute promyelocytic leukaemia, and following thrombolytic therapy). Aprotinin is also used in liver transplantation [unlicensed].

Etamsylate (ethamsylate) reduces capillary bleeding in the presence of a normal number of platelets. It does not act by fibrin stabilisation, but probably by correcting abnormal adhesion.

APROTININ

Indications: see notes above
Side-effects: occasionally hypersensitivity reactions and localised thrombophlebitis
Dose: *by slow intravenous injection or infusion*
Open heart surgery, loading dose, 2 000 000 units (200 mL) after induction of anaesthesia and before sternotomy—initial 50 000 units (5 mL) *by slow intravenous injection* over several minutes (to

detect allergy), remainder *by intravenous infusion* over 20 minutes; maintenance dose, *by intravenous infusion* 500 000 units (50 mL) every hour until end of operation (or early postoperative period in septic endocarditis); pump prime, 2 000 000 units (200 mL) in priming volume of extracorporeal circuit; in septic endocarditis 3 000 000 units (300 mL) added to pump prime Hyperplasminaemia, *by slow intravenous injection or by intravenous infusion*, initially 500 000–1 000 000 units (50–100 mL) at max. rate 10 mL/minute; followed if necessary by 200 000 units (20 mL) every hour until bleeding stops

Trasylol® (Bayer) PoM
Injection, aprotinin 10 000 kallikrein inactivator units/mL. Net price 50-mL vial = £20.53
NOTE. Aprotinin injection containing 10 000 kallikrein inactivator units/mL also available from Nordic

ETAMSYLATE
(Ethamsylate)
Indications: see under preparations
Contra-indications: porphyria (see section 9.8.2)
Side-effects: nausea, headache, rashes
Dose: see below

Dicynene® (Sanofi-Synthelabo) PoM
Tablets, scored, etamsylate 500 mg, net price 100-tab pack = £21.13
Dose: short-term treatment of blood loss in menorrhagia, 500 mg 4 times daily during menstruation

TRANEXAMIC ACID
Indications: see notes above
Cautions: renal impairment (avoid if severe—Appendix 3); massive haematuria (avoid if risk of ureteric obstruction); not for use in disseminated intravascular coagulation; pregnancy (Appendix 4); regular eye examinations and liver function tests in long-term treatment of hereditary angio-edema
NOTE. Requirement for regular eye examinations during long-term treatment is based on unsatisfactory evidence
Contra-indications: severe renal impairment, thromboembolic disease
Side-effects: nausea, vomiting, diarrhoea (reduce dose); disturbances in colour vision (discontinue) and thromboembolic events reported rarely; giddiness on rapid intravenous injection
Dose: *by mouth*, local fibrinolysis, 15–25 mg/kg 2–3 times daily
Menorrhagia (initiated when menstruation has started), 1 g 3 times daily for up to 4 days; max. 4 g daily
Hereditary angioedema, 1–1.5 g 2–3 times daily
By slow intravenous injection, local fibrinolysis, 0.5–1 g 3 times daily

Cyklokapron® (Pharmacia) PoM
Tablets, f/c, scored, tranexamic acid 500 mg. Net price 60-tab pack = £14.30
Injection, tranexamic acid 100 mg/mL. Net price 5-mL amp = £1.55

Blood products

ANTITHROMBIN III CONCENTRATE
Dried antithrombin III is prepared from human plasma
Indications: congenital deficiency of antithrombin III
Side-effects: nausea, flushing, headache; rarely, allergic reactions and fever
Available from BPL (Dried Antithrombin III)

DROTRECOGIN ALFA (ACTIVATED)
Recombinant activated protein C
Indications: adjunctive treatment of severe sepsis with multiple organ failure
Cautions: increased risk of bleeding, concomittant use of drugs that increase risk of bleeding; pregnancy (Appendix 4) and breast-feeding (Appendix 5); **interactions:** Appendix 1 (drotrecogin alfa)
Contra-indications: internal bleeding; intracranial neoplasm or cerebral herniation; chronic severe hepatic disease; thrombocytopenia
Side-effects: bleeding; headache; ecchymosis; pain
Available from Lilly (*Xigris*®▼)

FACTOR VIIa (RECOMBINANT)
Recombinant factor VIIa is used in patients with inhibitors to factors VIII and IX
Available from Novo Nordisk (*NovoSeven*®)

FACTOR VIII FRACTION, DRIED
(Human Antihaemophilic Fraction, Dried)
Dried factor VIII fraction is prepared from human plasma by a suitable fractionation technique
Indications: treatment and prophylaxis of haemorrhage in haemophilia A
Cautions: intravascular haemolysis after large or frequently repeated doses in patients with blood groups A, B, or AB—less likely with high potency concentrates
Side-effects: allergic reactions including chills, fever; hyperfibrinogenaemia occurred after massive doses with earlier products but less likely since fibrinogen content has now been substantially reduced
Available from Aventis Behring (*Beriate*® *P*▼, *Haemate*® P, *Monoclate-P*®), Baxter (*Hemofil M*®), BPL (*Replenate*®, *8Y*®), Grifols (*Alphanate*®, *Fanhdi*®), SNBTS (*Liberate*®, High Potency Factor VIII Concentrate)
NOTE. Preparation of recombinant human antihaemophilic factor VIII (octocog alfa) available from Aventis Behring (*Helixate*® NexGen), Baxter Bioscience (*Recombinate*®), Bayer (*Kogenate Bayer*®), Wyeth (*ReFacto*® ▼)

FACTOR VIII INHIBITOR BYPASSING FRACTION
Preparations with factor VIII inhibitor bypassing activity are prepared from human plasma
Human Factor VIII Inhibitor Bypassing Fraction (*FEIBA*, Baxter Bioscience)) is used in patients with factor VIII inhibitors
NOTE. A porcine preparation of antihaemophilic factor for patients with inhibitors to human factor VIII is available from Ipsen (*Hyate C*®)

FACTOR IX FRACTION, DRIED

Dried factor IX fraction is prepared from human plasma by a suitable fractionation technique; it may also contain clotting factors II, VII, and X

Indications: congenital factor IX deficiency (haemophilia B)

Cautions: risk of thrombosis—principally with former low purity products

Contra-indications: disseminated intravascular coagulation

Side-effects: allergic reactions, including chills, fever

Available from Aventis Behring (*Mononine*®), BPL (Dried Factor IX Fraction; *Replenine*®-*VF*), Grifols (*AlphaNine*®), SNBTS (Human Factor IX Concentrate, Heat Treated; *HT Defix*®)

NOTE. Preparation of recombinant coagulation factor IX (nonacog alfa) available from Baxter Bioscience (*Bene-FIX*® ▼)

FACTOR XIII FRACTION, DRIED
(Human Fibrin-stabilising Factor, Dried)

Indications: congenital factor XIII deficiency
Side-effects: rarely, allergic reactions and fever
Available from Aventis Behring (*Fibrogammin*® *P*)

FRESH FROZEN PLASMA

Fresh frozen plasma is prepared from the supernatant liquid obtained by centrifugation of one donation of whole blood

Indications: to replace coagulation factors or other plasma proteins where their concentration or functional activity is critically reduced, e.g. to reverse warfarin effect

Cautions: avoid in circulatory overload; need for compatibility

Side-effects: allergic reactions including chills, fever, bronchospasm; adult respiratory distress syndrome

Available from Regional Blood Transfusion Services and BPL

NOTE. A preparation of solvent/detergent treated human plasma (frozen) is available from Octapharma (*Octaplas*®)

PROTEIN C CONCENTRATE

Protein C is prepared from human plasma
Indications: congenital protein C deficiency
Cautions: hypersensitivity to heparin
Side-effects: fever, arrhythmia, bleeding and thrombosis reported; rarely allergic reactions
Available from Baxter (*Ceprotin*®▼)

2.12 Lipid-regulating drugs

Lowering the concentration of low density lipoprotein (LDL) cholesterol and raising high density lipoprotein (HDL) cholesterol reduces the progression of coronary atherosclerosis and may even induce regression.

There is evidence that lowering total cholesterol by 20–25% (or lowering the LDL-cholesterol by about 30%) is effective in both the primary and secondary prevention of clinical manifestations of coronary heart disease. Therefore, treatment with a lipid-regulating drug should be considered in patients with coronary heart disease and in those at high risk of developing it because of multiple risk factors (including smoking, hypertension, diabetes mellitus,

and a family history of premature coronary heart disease). Treatment with statins (see Statins, below) has been shown to reduce myocardial infarction, coronary deaths and overall mortality rate and they are the drugs of choice in patients with a high risk of coronary heart disease. Lipid-regulating drug therapy must be combined with advice on diet and lifestyle measures to reduce coronary risk including, if appropriate, reduction of blood pressure (section 2.5) and use of aspirin (section 2.9).

A number of conditions, some familial, are characterised by very high plasma concentrations of cholesterol, or triglycerides, or both. Statins are drugs of first choice for treating hypercholesterolaemia and fibrates for treating hypertriglyceridaemia; statins or fibrates can be used, either alone or together, to treat mixed hyperlipidaemia.

Severe hyperlipidaemia often requires a combination of lipid-regulating drugs such as a statin with ezetimibe or with a fibrate; such treatment should generally be under specialist supervision. Combinations of a statin with nicotinic acid or a fibrate carry an increased risk of side-effects (including rhabdomyolysis) and should be used with caution. In particular, concomitant administration of gemfibrozil with a statin may increase the risk of rhabdomyolysis considerably (see also below); gemfibrozil and statins should therefore **not** be used concomitantly.

Patients with hypothyroidism should receive adequate thyroid replacement therapy before assessing their requirement for lipid-regulating treatment because correction of hypothyroidism itself may resolve the lipid abnormality. Untreated hypothyroidism increases the risk of myositis with lipid-regulating drugs.

CSM advice (muscle effects). The CSM has advised that rhabdomyolysis associated with lipid-regulating drugs such as the fibrates and statins appears to be rare (approx. 1 case in every 100 000 treatment years) but may be increased in those with renal impairment and possibly in those with hypothyroidism (see also notes above). Concomitant treatment with drugs that increase plasma-statin concentration increase the risk of muscle toxicity; concomitant treatment with a fibrate and a statin may also be associated with an increased risk of serious muscle toxicity.

Anion-exchange resins

Colestyramine (cholestyramine) and **colestipol** are anion-exchange resins used in the management of hypercholesterolaemia. They act by binding bile acids, preventing their reabsorption; this promotes hepatic conversion of cholesterol into bile acids; the resultant increased LDL-receptor activity of liver cells increases the clearance of LDL-cholesterol. Thus both compounds effectively reduce LDL-cholesterol but can aggravate hypertriglyceridaemia.

CAUTIONS. Anion-exchange resins interfere with the absorption of fat-soluble vitamins; supplements of vitamins A, D and K may be required when treatment is prolonged. **Interactions:** Appendix 1 (colestyramine and colestipol).

SIDE-EFFECTS. As colestyramine and colestipol are not absorbed, gastro-intestinal side-effects predominate. Constipation is common, but diarrhoea has occurred, as have nausea, vomiting, and gastro-intestinal discomfort. Hypertriglyceridaemia may be aggravated. An increased bleeding tendency has been reported due to hypoprothrombinaemia associated with vitamin K deficiency.

COUNSELLING. Other drugs should be taken at least 1 hour (in the case of ezetimibe, at least 2 hours) before or 4–6 hours after colestyramine or colestipol to reduce possible interference with absorption.

COLESTYRAMINE
(Cholestyramine)

Indications: hyperlipidaemias, particularly type IIa, in patients who have not responded adequately to diet and other appropriate measures; primary prevention of coronary heart disease in men aged 35–59 years with primary hypercholesterolaemia who have not responded to diet and other appropriate measures; pruritus associated with partial biliary obstruction and primary biliary cirrhosis (section 1.9.2); diarrhoeal disorders (section 1.9.2)

Cautions: see notes above; pregnancy and breast-feeding

Contra-indications: complete biliary obstruction (not likely to be effective)

Side-effects: see notes above; hyperchloraemic acidosis reported on prolonged use

Dose: lipid reduction (after initial introduction over 3–4 weeks) 12–24 g daily in water (or other suitable liquid) in single or up to 4 divided doses; up to 36 g daily if necessary

Pruritus, see section 1.9.2

Diarrhoeal disorders, see section 1.9.2

CHILD 6–12 years, see product literature

Colestyramine (Non-proprietary) PoM
Powder, colestyramine (anhydrous) 4 g/sachet, net price 50-sachet pack = £17.55. Label: 13, counselling, avoid other drugs at same time (see notes above)
Excipients: include aspartame (section 9.4.1)
Available from PLIVA

Questran® (Bristol-Myers Squibb) PoM
Powder, colestyramine (anhydrous) 4 g/sachet. Net price 50-sachet pack = £17.55. Label: 13, counselling, avoid other drugs at same time (see notes above)
Excipients: include sucrose 3.79g/sachet

Questran Light® (Bristol-Myers Squibb) PoM
Powder, sugar-free, colestyramine (anhydrous) 4 g/sachet, net price 50-sachet pack = £18.43. Label: 13, counselling, avoid other drugs at same time (see notes above)
Excipients: include aspartame (section 9.4.1)

COLESTIPOL HYDROCHLORIDE

Indications: hyperlipidaemias, particularly type IIa, in patients who have not responded adequately to diet and other appropriate measures

Cautions: see notes above; pregnancy

Side-effects: see notes above

Dose: 5 g 1–2 times daily in liquid increased if necessary at intervals of 1–2 months to max. of 30 g daily (in single or 2 divided doses)

Colestid® (Pharmacia) PoM
Granules, yellow, colestipol hydrochloride 5 g/sachet. Net price 30 sachets = £15.05. Label: 13,

counselling, avoid other drugs at same time (see notes above)
Colestid Orange, granules, yellow/orange, colestipol hydrochloride 5 g/sachet, with aspartame. Net price 30 sachets = £15.05. Label: 13, counselling, avoid other drugs at same time (see notes above)

Ezetimibe

Ezetimibe inhibits the intestinal absorption of cholesterol. It is licensed as adjunctive therapy to dietary manipulation in patients with hyper-cholesterolaemia in combination with a statin or alone (if a statin is inappropriate), in patients with homozygous familial hypercholesterolaemia in combination with a statin, and in patients with homozygous familial sitosterolaemia (phytosterolaemia).

EZETIMIBE

Indications: adjunct to dietary measures and statin in primary and homozygous familial hyper-cholesterolaemia (statin omitted in primary hyper-cholesterolaemia if inappropriate or not tolerated); adjunct to dietary measures in homozygous sitos-terolaemia

Cautions: liver impairment (avoid if moderate or severe; Appendix 2); **interactions:** Appendix 1 (ezetimibe)

Contra-indications: breast-feeding (Appendix 5)

Side-effects: diarrhoea, abdominal pain, headache; angioedema and rash reported

Dose: 10 mg once daily; CHILD under 10 years not recommended

Ezetrol (MSD, Schering-Plough) ▼ PoM
Tablets, ezetimibe 10 mg, net price 28-tab pack = £26.31

Fibrates

Bezafibrate, **ciprofibrate**, **fenofibrate**, and **gem-fibrozil** act mainly by decreasing serum tri-glycerides; they have variable effects on LDL-cholesterol. Fibrates may reduce the risk of coronary heart disease events in those with low HDL-cholesterol or with raised triglycerides.

All can cause a myositis-like syndrome, especially in patients with impaired renal function. Also, combination of a fibrate with a statin increases the risk of muscle effects (especially rhabdomyolysis) and should be used with caution (see CSM advice in section 2.12).

BEZAFIBRATE

Indications: hyperlipidaemias of types IIa, IIb, III, IV and V in patients who have not responded adequately to diet and other appropriate measures

Cautions: renal impairment (Appendix 3—see also under Myotoxicity below); correct hypothyroidism before initiating treatment (see section 2.12); **interactions:** Appendix 1 (fibrates)

MYOTOXICITY. Special care needed in patients with renal disease, as progressive increases in serum creatinine concentration or failure to follow dosage guidelines may result in myotoxicity (rhabdomyolysis); discontinue if myotoxicity suspected or creatine kinase concentration increases significantly

Contra-indications: severe hepatic and renal impairment, hypoalbuminaemia, primary biliary cirrhosis, gall bladder disease, nephrotic syndrome, pregnancy and breast-feeding

Side-effects: gastro-intestinal (e.g. nausea, anorexia, gastric pain), pruritus, urticaria, raised serum creatinine (unrelated to renal impairment), impotence; also headache, dizziness, vertigo, fatigue, hair loss; myotoxicity (with myasthenia or myalgia)—special risk in renal impairment (see Cautions); also reported, anaemia, leucopenia, thrombocytopenia

Dose: see preparations below

Bezafibrate (Non-proprietary) PoM
Tablets, bezafibrate 200 mg, net price 100-tab pack = £9.76. Label: 21
Dose: 200 mg 3 times daily after food
Available from Generics, PLIVA

Bezalip® (Roche) PoM
Tablets, f/c, bezafibrate 200 mg. Net price 100-tab pack = £9.84. Label: 21
Dose: 200 mg 3 times daily with or after food

■ Modified release
Bezalip® Mono (Roche) PoM
Tablets, m/r, f/c, bezafibrate 400 mg. Net price 30-tab pack = £8.70. Label: 21, 25
Dose: 1 tablet daily after food (dose form not appropriate in renal impairment)
NOTE. Modified-release tablets containing bezafibrate 400 mg also available from Generics (*Bezagen® XL*), Link (*Zimbacol®XL*)

CIPROFIBRATE

Indications: hyperlipidaemias of types IIa, IIb, III, and IV in patients who have not responded adequately to diet

Cautions: see under Bezafibrate

Contra-indications: see under Bezafibrate

Side-effects: see under Bezafibrate

Dose: 100 mg daily

Modalim® (Sanofi-Synthelabo) PoM
Tablets, scored, ciprofibrate 100 mg. Net price 28-tab pack = £14.72

FENOFIBRATE

Indications: hyperlipidaemias of types IIa, IIb, III, IV, and V in patients who have not responded adequately to diet and other appropriate measures

Cautions: see under Bezafibrate; renal impairment (Appendix 3); liver function tests recommended every 3 months for first year (discontinue treatment if significantly raised)

Contra-indications: severe renal or hepatic impairment, existing gall bladder disease; pregnancy (Appendix 4) and breast-feeding (Appendix 5); photosensitivity to ketoprofen

Side-effects: see under Bezafibrate; also reported rash, photosensitivity, raised serum transaminases, hepatitis

Dose: see preparations below

Fenofibrate (Non-proprietary) PoM
Capsules, fenofibrate 200 mg, net price 30-cap pack = £14.75. Label: 21
Dose: 1 capsule daily (dose form not appropriate for children or in renal impairment)
Available from Genus (*Fenogal®*)

Lipantil® (Fournier) PoM
Lipantil® Micro 67 capsules, yellow, fenofibrate (micronised) 67 mg, net price 90-cap pack = £23.30. Label: 21
Dose: initially 3 capsules daily in divided doses; usual range 2–4 capsules daily; CHILD 1 capsule/20 kg daily
Lipantil® Micro 200 capsules, orange, fenofibrate (micronised) 200 mg, net price 28-cap pack = £17.95. Label: 21
Dose: initially 1 capsule daily (dose form not appropriate for children or in renal impairment)
Lipantil® Micro 267 capsules, orange/cream, fenofibrate (micronised) 267 mg, net price 28-cap pack = £21.75. Label: 21
Dose: severe hyperlipidaemia, 1 capsule daily (dose form not appropriate for children or in renal impairment)
NOTE. For an equivalent therapeutic effect, 100 mg previously available non-micronised fenofibrate ≡ 67 mg micronised fenofibrate

■ Modified release
Supralip® 160 (Fournier) PoM
Tablets, m/r, f/c, fenofibrate 160 mg, net price 28-tab pack = £14.75. Label: 21, 25
Dose: 160 mg daily (dose form not appropriate for children or in renal impairment)

GEMFIBROZIL

Indications: hyperlipidaemias of types IIa, IIb, III, IV and V in patients who have not responded adequately to diet and other appropriate measures; primary prevention of coronary heart disease in men aged 40–55 years with hyperlipidaemias that have not responded to diet and other appropriate measures

Cautions: lipid profile, blood counts, and liver-function tests before initiating long-term treatment; renal impairment (Appendix 3); preferably avoid use with statins (high risk of rhabdomyolysis); correct hypothyroidism before initiating treatment (see section 2.12); **interactions:** Appendix 1 (fibrates)

Contra-indications: alcoholism, hepatic impairment, gallstones; pregnancy and breast-feeding

Side-effects: gastro-intestinal disturbances; also rash, dermatitis, pruritus, urticaria, impotence, headache, dizziness, blurred vision, cholestatic jaundice, angioedema, laryngeal oedema, atrial fibrillation, pancreatitis, myasthenia, myopathy, rhabdomyolysis, painful extremities, myalgia accompanied by increases in creatine kinase

Dose: 1.2 g daily, usually in 2 divided doses; range 0.9–1.5 g daily

Gemfibrozil (Non-proprietary) PoM
Capsules, gemfibrozil 300 mg, net price 112-cap pack = £24.43
Available from APS
Tablets, gemfibrozil 600 mg, net price 30-tab pack = £13.90
Available from APS, IVAX

Lopid® (Pfizer) PoM
'300' capsules, white/maroon, gemfibrozil 300 mg. Net price 112-cap pack = £35.57
'600' tablets, f/c, gemfibrozil 600 mg. Net price 56-tab pack = £35.57

Statins

The statins (**atorvastatin**, **fluvastatin**, **pravastatin**, **rosuvastatin**, and **simvastatin**) competitively inhibit 3-hydroxy-3-methylglutaryl coenzyme A (HMG CoA) reductase, an enzyme involved in cholesterol synthesis, especially in the liver. They are more effective than other classes of drugs in lowering LDL-cholesterol but less effective than the fibrates in reducing triglycerides.

Statins reduce coronary events, all cardiovascular events, and total mortality. They should be considered for all patients, including the elderly, at risk of cardiovascular disease such as those with coronary heart disease (including history of angina or acute myocardial infarction), occlusive arterial disease (including peripheral vascular disease, non-haemorrhagic stroke or transient ischaemic attacks), or diabetes mellitus.

Statins are also used for the *secondary prevention* of coronary and cardiovascular events in patients with coronary heart disease (including history of angina or acute myocardial infarction), peripheral artery disease, or a history of stroke. Although statins produce these benefits irrespective of the initial cholesterol concentration, patients with a total serum-cholesterol concentration of 5 mmol/litre or greater are likely to benefit most. Statins also reduce the incidence of non-haemorrhagic stroke when used for secondary prevention in coronary heart disease.

Statins are also used in the *primary prevention* of coronary events in patients at increased risk. Risk of coronary events is not accurately predicted from cholesterol concentrations alone and methods that take into account factors such as smoking, hypertension and diabetes mellitus should be used to estimate risk. Patients at an increased risk of coronary heart disease (10-year risk of 15% or possibly less), stand to benefit from primary prevention irrespective of the cholesterol concentration. However, statins should particularly be considered for patients with a total serum-cholesterol concentration of 5 mmol/litre or greater and a coronary heart disease risk[1] of 30% or greater over 10 years, in association with lifestyle measures and other appropriate interventions.

For primary and secondary prevention of coronary heart disease, statin treatment should be adjusted to achieve a target total cholesterol concentration of less than 5 mmol/litre (or a reduction of 20–25% if that produces a lower concentration); in terms of LDL-cholesterol, the target should be below 3 mmol/litre (or a reduction of about 30% if that produces a lower concentration).

CAUTIONS. Statins should be used with caution in those with a history of liver disease or with a high alcohol intake (use should be avoided in active liver disease). Hypothyroidism should be managed adequately before starting treatment with a statin (see section 2.12). Liver-function tests should be carried out before and within 1–3 months of starting treatment and thereafter at intervals of 6 months for 1 year, unless indicated sooner by signs or symptoms suggestive of hepatotoxicity. Treatment should be discontinued if serum transaminase concentration rises to, and persists at, 3 times the upper limit of the reference range. Patients should be advised to report unexplained muscle pain (see Muscle Effects below). **Interactions:** Appendix 1 (statins).

CONTRA-INDICATIONS. Statins are contra-indicated in active liver disease (or persistently abnormal liver function tests) and in pregnancy (adequate contraception required during treatment and for 1 month afterwards) and breast-feeding (see Appendixes 4 and 5).

SIDE-EFFECTS. Reversible myositis is a rare but significant side-effect of the statins (see also Muscle Effects, p. 124 and below). The statins also cause headache, altered liver-function tests (rarely, hepatitis), paraesthesia, and gastro-intestinal effects including abdominal pain, flatulence, diarrhoea, nausea and vomiting. Rash and hypersensitivity reactions (including angioedema and anaphylaxis) have been reported rarely.

MUSCLE EFFECTS. Myalgia, myositis and myopathy have been reported with the statins; if myopathy is suspected and creatine kinase is markedly elevated (more than 5 times upper limit of normal), treatment should be discontinued; in patients at high risk of muscle effects, a statin should not be started if creatine kinase is elevated. There is an increased incidence of myopathy if the statins are given with a fibrate (see also CSM advice in section 2.12), with lipid-lowering doses of nicotinic acid, or with immunosuppressants such as ciclosporin; close monitoring of liver function and, if symptomatic, of creatine kinase is required in patients receiving these drugs. Rhabdomyolysis with acute renal impairment secondary to myoglobinuria has also been reported.

COUNSELLING. Advise patient to report promptly unexplained muscle pain, tenderness, weakness.

ATORVASTATIN

Indications: primary hypercholesterolaemia, heterozygous familial hypercholesterolaemia, homozygous familial hypercholesterolaemia or combined (mixed) hyperlipidaemia in patients who have not responded adequately to diet and other appropriate measures

Cautions: see notes above

Contra-indications: see notes above

Side-effects: see notes above; also insomnia, angioedema, anorexia, asthenia, peripheral neuropathy, alopecia, pruritus, rash, impotence, chest pain, hypoglycaemia and hyperglycaemia reported; thrombocytopenia reported rarely

Dose: primary hypercholesterolaemia and combined hyperlipidaemia, usually 10 mg once daily

Familial hypercholesterolaemia, initially 10 mg daily, increased at intervals of at least 4 weeks to 40 mg once daily; if necessary, further increased to max. 80 mg once daily (or combined with anion-exchange resin in heterozygous familial hypercholesterolaemia)

Lipitor® (Parke-Davis) PoM

Tablets, all f/c, atorvastatin (as calcium trihydrate) 10 mg, net price 28-tab pack = £18.03; 20 mg, 28-tab pack = £29.69; 40 mg 28-tab pack = £29.69; 80 mg, 28-tab pack = £29.69. Counselling, muscle effects, see notes above

---

1. Coronary heart disease risk may be formally estimated using the Joint British Societies' 'Cardiac Risk Assessor' computer program or chart (British Cardiac Society, British Hyperlipidaemia Association, British Hypertension Society. *Heart* 1998; **80** (suppl 2): S1–29)

See inside back cover

FLUVASTATIN

Indications: adjunct to diet in primary hyper-cholesterolaemia or combined (mixed) hyperlipid-aemia (types IIa and IIb) in patients who have not responded adequately to dietary control; adjunct to diet in retarding progression of coronary athero-sclerosis in primary hypercholesterolaemia and concomitant coronary heart disease; prevention of coronary events after percutaneous coronary intervention

Cautions: see notes above

Contra-indications: see notes above; also severe renal impairment

Side-effects: see notes above; also insomnia; rarely dysaesthesia and hypoesthesia

Dose: initially 20–40 mg daily in the evening, adjusted at intervals of at least 4 weeks; up to 40 mg twice daily may be required

Following percutaneous coronary intervention, 80 mg daily

Lescol® (Novartis) PoM
Capsules, fluvastatin (as sodium salt) 20 mg (brown/yellow), net price 28-cap pack = £12.72; 40 mg (brown/orange), 28-cap pack = £12.72, 56-cap pack = £25.44. Counselling, muscle effects, see notes above

■ Modified release
Lescol® XL (Novartis) PoM
Tablets, m/r, yellow, fluvastatin (as sodium salt) 80 mg, net price 28-tab pack = £16.00. Label: 25, counselling, muscle effects, see notes above
Dose: 80 mg once daily (dose form not appropriate for initial dose titration)

PRAVASTATIN SODIUM

Indications: primary hypercholesterolaemia in patients who have not responded adequately to dietary control; adjunct to diet to slow progression of coronary atherosclerosis and reduce incidence of cardiac events in patients with hypercholesterol-aemia and atherosclerotic coronary artery disease; adjunct in hypercholesterolaemia without clinically evident coronary heart disease; preven-tion of stroke, recurrent coronary events (including myocardial infarction), or need for revasculariza-tion procedure in patients with previous myo-cardial infarction or unstable angina and total serum cholesterol concentration greater than 4.8 mmol/litre (or LDL-cholesterol greater than 3.2 mmol/litre) (see also notes above)

Cautions: see notes above

Contra-indications: see notes above

Side-effects: see notes above; also chest pain, fatigue; angioedema, polyneuropathy, hepatitis and fulminant hepatic necrosis, jaundice, pancreat-itis, lupus erythematosus-like syndrome and thrombocytopenia reported rarely

Dose: usual range 10–40 mg once daily at night, adjusted at intervals of not less than 4 weeks

Lipostat® (Squibb) PoM
Tablets, all yellow, pravastatin sodium 10 mg, net price 28-tab pack = £16.18; 20 mg, 28-tab pack = £29.69; 40 mg, 28-tab pack = £29.69. Counselling, muscle effects, see notes above

ROSUVASTATIN

Indications: primary hypercholesterolaemia (type IIa including heterozygous familial hyper-cholesterolaemia), mixed dyslipidaemia (type IIb), or homozygous familial hypercholesterol-aemia in patients who have not responded ade-quately to diet and other appropriate measures

Cautions: see notes above

Contra-indications: see notes above; also renal impairment (Appendix 3)

Side-effects: see notes above; also dizziness and asthenia; proteinuria

Dose: 10 mg once daily increased if necessary after not less than 4 weeks to 20 mg once daily, further increased to 40 mg in severe hypercholesterol-aemia and high cardiovascular risk

Crestor® (AstraZeneca) ▼ PoM
Tablets, all pink, f/c, rosuvastatin (as calcium salt) 10 mg, net price 28-tab pack = £18.03; 20 mg, 28-tab pack = £29.69; 40 mg, 28-tab pack = £29.69. Counselling, muscle effects, see notes above

SIMVASTATIN

Indications: primary hypercholesterolaemia, het-erozygous familial hypercholesterolaemia, homo-zygous familial hypercholesterolaemia or com-bined (mixed) hyperlipidaemia in patients who have not responded adequately to diet and other appropriate measures; prevention of coronary events, need for revascularisation procedures, and to slow progression of coronary atherosclerosis in patients with coronary heart disease and total cholesterol concentration of 5.5 mmol/litre or greater (see also notes above)

Cautions: see notes above; severe renal impairment (Appendix 3)

Contra-indications: see notes above; also por-phyria (see section 9.8.2)

Side-effects: see notes above; also alopecia, anae-mia, dizziness, peripheral neuropathy, hepatitis, jaundice, pancreatitis

Dose: primary hypercholesterolaemia, heterozy-gous familial hypercholesterolaemia, combined hyperlipidaemia, 10 mg daily at night, adjusted at intervals of not less than 4 weeks; usual range 10–80 mg once daily at night

Homozygous familial hypercholesterolaemia, 40 mg daily at night *or* 80 mg daily in 3 divided doses (with largest dose at night)

Coronary heart disease, initially 20 mg once daily at night, adjusted at intervals of not less than 4 weeks; max. 80 mg once daily

NOTE. Max. 10 mg daily with concomitant ciclosporin, fibrate or lipid-lowering dose of nicotinic acid

Simvastatin (Non-proprietary) PoM
Tablets, simvastatin 10 mg, net price 28-tab pack = £15.18, 20 mg, 28-tab pack = £24.21; 40 mg, 28-tab pack = £26.81; 80 mg, 28-tab pack = £29.08. Counselling, muscle effects, see notes above
Available from APS (*Simzal®*), Discovery (*Simvador®*), Generics, Ratiopharm

Zocor® (MSD) PoM
Tablets, all f/c, simvastatin 10 mg (peach), net price 28-tab pack = £18.03; 20 mg (tan), 28-tab pack = £29.69; 40 mg (red), 28-tab pack = £29.69; 80 mg (red), 28-tab pack = £29.69. Counselling, muscle effects, see notes above

Nicotinic acid group

The value of **nicotinic acid** is limited by its side-effects, especially vasodilatation. In doses of 1.5 to 3 g daily it lowers both cholesterol and triglyceride concentrations by inhibiting synthesis; it also increases HDL-cholesterol. **Acipimox** seems to have fewer side-effects but may be less effective in its lipid-modulating capabilities.

ACIPIMOX

Indications: hyperlipidaemias of types IIa, IIb, and IV in patients who have not responded adequately to diet and other appropriate measures

Cautions: renal impairment (Appendix 3)

Contra-indications: peptic ulcer; pregnancy and breast-feeding

Side-effects: vasodilatation, flushing, itching, rashes, urticaria, erythema; heartburn, epigastric pain, nausea, diarrhoea, headache, malaise, dry eyes; rarely angioedema, bronchospasm, anaphylaxis

Dose: usually 500–750 mg daily in divided doses

Olbetam® (Pharmacia) PoM
Capsules, brown/pink, acipimox 250 mg. Net price 90-cap pack = £46.33. Label: 21

NICOTINIC ACID

Indications: see notes above

Cautions: diabetes mellitus, gout, liver disease, peptic ulcer; **interactions:** Appendix 1 (nicotinic acid)

Contra-indications: pregnancy, breast-feeding

Side-effects: flushing, dizziness, headache, palpitations, pruritus (prostaglandin-mediated symptoms can be reduced by low initial doses taken with meals, or by taking aspirin 75 mg 30 minutes before the dose); nausea, vomiting; rarely impaired liver function and rashes

Dose: initially 100–200 mg 3 times daily (see above), gradually increased over 2–4 weeks to 1–2 g 3 times daily

NOTE. Doses of standard-release and modified-release formulations are **not** equivalent; when switching formulation initiate treatment with low dose and increase gradually as recommended

¹**Nicotinic Acid** (Non-proprietary) PoM
Tablets, nicotinic acid 50 mg, net price 100 = £9.25. Label: 21

1. May be sold to the public unless max. daily dose exceeds 600 mg or if intended for treatment of hyperlipidaemia

■ Modified release

Niaspan® (Merck) PoM
Tablets, m/r, nicotinic acid 500 mg, net price 56-tab pack = £17.25; 750 mg, 56-tab pack = £26.25; 1 g, 56-tab pack = £29.50; 21-day starter pack of 7 × 375-mg tab with 7 × 750-mg tab and 7 × 1-g tab = £14.00. Label: 21, 25

Dose: 375 mg once daily at night for 1 week, then 500 mg once daily at night for 1 week, then 750 mg once daily at night for 1 week, then 1 g once daily at night for 4 weeks, increased if necessary in steps of 500 mg at intervals of at least 4 weeks to max. 2 g daily; usual maintenance dose 1–2 g once daily at night

Fish oils

A fish-oil preparation (*Maxepa*®), rich in **omega-3-marine triglycerides**, is useful in the treatment of severe hypertriglyceridaemia; however, it can sometimes aggravate hypercholesterolaemia.

The preparation *Omacor*®, which contains **omega-3-acid ethyl esters**, is licensed for hypertriglyceridaemia and secondary prevention after myocardial infarction.

OMEGA-3-ACID ETHYL ESTERS

Indications: adjunct in the reduction of plasma triglycerides in patients with hypertriglyceridaemia judged to be at special risk of ischaemic heart disease or pancreatitis; adjunct in secondary prevention after myocardial infarction

Cautions: haemorrhagic disorders, anticoagulant treatment

Side-effects: nausea, belching, diarrhoea, constipation; eczema and acne reported

Dose: see under preparation below

Omacor® (Solvay)
Capsules, 1 g of 90% omega-3-acid ethyl esters containing eicosapentaenoic acid 46% and docosahexaenoic acid 38%, alpha-tocopherol 4 mg, net price 28-cap pack = £13.89. Label: 21
Dose: hypertriglyceridaemia, 4 capsules daily in 1–2 divided doses with food
Secondary prevention after myocardial infarction 1 capsule daily with food

OMEGA-3-MARINE TRIGLYCERIDES

Indications: adjunct in the reduction of plasma triglycerides in patients with severe hypertriglyceridaemia judged to be at special risk of ischaemic heart disease or pancreatitis

Cautions: haemorrhagic disorders, anticoagulant treatment; aspirin-sensitive asthma; diabetes mellitus

Side-effects: occasional nausea and belching

Dose: see under preparations below

Maxepa® (Seven Seas)
Capsules, 1 g (approx. 1.1 mL) concentrated fish oils containing eicosapentaenoic acid 170 mg, docosahexaenoic acid 115 mg. Vitamin A content less than 100 units/g, vitamin D content less than 10 units/g, net price 200-cap pack = £27.28. Label: 21
Dose: 5 capsules twice daily with food
Liquid, golden-coloured, concentrated fish oils containing eicosapentaenoic acid 170 mg, docosahexaenoic acid 115 mg/g (1.1 mL). Vitamin A content less than 100 units/g, vitamin D content less than 10 units/g, net price 150 mL = £20.46. Label: 21
Dose: 5 mL twice daily with food

2.13 Local sclerosants

Ethanolamine oleate and sodium tetradecyl sulphate are used in sclerotherapy of varicose veins, and phenol is used in haemorrhoids (section 1.7.3).

ETHANOLAMINE OLEATE
(Monoethanolamine Oleate)

Indications: sclerotherapy of varicose veins

Cautions: extravasation may cause necrosis of tissues

Contra-indications: inability to walk, acute phlebitis, oral contraceptive use, obese legs

Side-effects: allergic reactions (including anaphylaxis)

Ethanolamine Oleate PoM

Injection, ethanolamine oleate 5%. Net price 5-mL amp = £2.23

Available from Celltech

Dose: by slow injection into empty isolated segment of vein, 2–5 mL divided between 3–4 sites; repeated at weekly intervals

SODIUM TETRADECYL SULPHATE

Indications: sclerotherapy of varicose veins

Cautions: see under Ethanolamine Oleate

Contra-indications: see under Ethanolamine Oleate

Side-effects: see under Ethanolamine Oleate

Fibro-Vein® (STD Pharmaceutical) PoM

Injection, sodium tetradecyl sulphate 0.2%, net price 5-mL amp = £2.34; 0.5%, 2-mL amp = £1.39; 1%, 2-mL amp = £1.50; 3%, 2-mL amp = £1.69, 5-mL vial = £3.25

Dose: by slow injection into empty isolated segment of vein, 0.1–1 mL according to site and condition being treated (consult product literature)

3: Respiratory system

3.1 Bronchodilators

3.1.1   Adrenoceptor agonists
3.1.2   Antimuscarinic bronchodilators
3.1.3   Theophylline
3.1.4   Compound bronchodilator preparations
3.1.5   Peak flow meters, inhaler devices and nebulisers

Asthma

Drugs used in the management of asthma include beta$_2$ agonists (section 3.1.1), antimuscarinic bronchodilators (section 3.1.2), theophylline (section 3.1.3), corticosteroids (section 3.2), cromoglicate and nedocromil (section 3.3.1), and leukotriene receptor antagonists (section 3.3.2).

For tables outlining the management of chronic asthma and acute severe asthma see p. 132 and p. 133.

Administration of drugs for asthma

INHALATION. This route delivers the drug directly to the airways; the dose is smaller than that for the drug given by mouth and side-effects are reduced. *Pressurised metered-dose inhalers* are an effective and convenient method of administering many drugs used for asthma. A spacer device (section 3.1.5) may improve drug delivery, particularly for young children and those who have difficulty using a pressurised metered-dose inhaler; spacers also reduce local adverse effects from inhaled corticosteroids. Breath-actuated devices including dry powder inhalers are also available.

Solutions for nebulisation are available for use in acute severe asthma. They are administered over 5–10 minutes from a nebuliser, usually driven by oxygen in hospital. Electric compressors are best suited to domiciliary use.

ORAL. The oral route is used when administration by inhalation is not possible. Systemic side-effects occur more frequently when a drug is given orally rather than by inhalation. Drugs given by mouth for the treatment of asthma include beta$_2$ agonists, corticosteroids, theophylline and leukotriene receptor antagonists.

PARENTERAL. Drugs such as beta$_2$ agonists, corticosteroids, and aminophylline may be given by injection in acute severe asthma when administration by nebulisation is inadequate or inappropriate. If the patient is being treated in the community, urgent transfer to hospital should be arranged.

Pregnancy and breast-feeding

It is particularly important that asthma should be well controlled during pregnancy; where this is achieved asthma has no important effects on pregnancy,

MANAGEMENT OF CHRONIC ASTHMA IN ADULTS AND CHILDREN

Start at step most appropriate to initial severity

Chronic asthma: adults and schoolchildren

Step 1: occasional relief bronchodilators
Inhaled short-acting beta$_2$ agonist as required (up to once daily)

NOTE. Move to step 2 if needed more than once daily (or if night-time symptoms or if lung function impaired); check compliance and inhaler technique

Step 2: regular inhaled preventer therapy
Inhaled short-acting beta$_2$ agonist as required
   plus
Regular standard-dose[1] inhaled corticosteroid (alternatives[2] are considerably less effective)

Step 3: inhaled corticosteroids + long-acting inhaled beta$_2$ agonist
Inhaled short-acting beta$_2$ agonist as required
   plus
Regular standard-dose[1] inhaled corticosteroid
   plus
Regular inhaled long-acting beta$_2$ agonist (salmeterol *or* formoterol (eformoterol)) but discontinue long-acting beta$_2$ agonist in the absence of response

If asthma not controlled
Increase dose of inhaled corticosteroid to upper end of standard dose[1]

If asthma still not controlled
Add one of
   Leukotriene receptor antagonist
   Modified-release oral theophylline
   Modified-release oral beta$_2$ agonist

Step 4: high-dose inhaled corticosteroids + regular bronchodilators
Inhaled short-acting beta$_2$ agonist as required
   with
Regular high-dose[3] inhaled corticosteroid
   plus
Inhaled long-acting beta$_2$ agonist
   plus
In adults 6-week sequential therapeutic trial of one or more of
   Leukotriene receptor antagonist
   Modified-release oral theophylline
   Modified-release oral beta$_2$ agonist

Step 5: regular corticosteroid tablets
Inhaled short-acting beta$_2$ agonist as required
   with
Regular high-dose[3] inhaled corticosteroid
   and
one or more long-acting bronchodilators (see step 4)
   plus
Regular prednisolone tablets (as single daily dose)

NOTE. In addition to regular prednisolone, continue high-dose inhaled corticosteroid (in exceptional cases may exceed licensed doses); these patients should normally be referred to an asthma clinic

Stepping down
Review treatment every 3 months; if control achieved stepwise reduction may be possible; use lowest possible dose of corticosteroid; reduce dose of *inhaled* corticosteroid slowly (consider reduction every 3 months, decreasing dose by approx. 25–50% each time) to the lowest dose which controls asthma

Chronic asthma: children under 5 years

Step 1: occasional relief bronchodilators
Short-acting beta$_2$ agonist as required (not more than once daily)

NOTE. Whenever possible inhaled (less effective and more side-effects when given by mouth); check compliance, technique and that inhaler device is appropriate

Step 2: regular preventer therapy
Inhaled short-acting beta$_2$ agonist as required
   plus
Either regular standard-dose[1] inhaled corticosteroid
Or (if inhaled corticosteroid cannot be used) leukotriene receptor antagonist

Step 3: add-on therapy

Children 2–5 years:
Inhaled short-acting beta$_2$ agonist as required
   plus
Regular inhaled corticosteroid in standard dose[1]
   plus
Leukotriene receptor antagonist

Children under 2 years:
Refer to respiratory paediatrician

Step 4: persistent poor control
Refer to respiratory paediatrician

Stepping down
Regularly review need for treatment

1. Standard-dose inhaled corticosteroids (given through metered dose inhaler) are beclometasone dipropionate or budesonide 100–400 micrograms (CHILD 100–200 micrograms) twice daily *or* fluticasone propionate 50–200 micrograms (CHILD 50–100 micrograms) twice daily; initial dose according to severity of asthma; use large-volume spacer in children under 5 years

2. Alternatives to inhaled corticosteroid are leukotriene receptor antagonist, theophylline, and in adults, regular cromoglicate, and in children, regular nedocromil

3. High-dose inhaled corticosteroids (given through metered dose inhaler) are beclometasone dipropionate or budesonide 0.8–2 mg daily (in divided doses) *or* fluticasone propionate 0.4–1 mg daily (in divided doses); CHILD 5–12 years, beclometasone dipropionate or budesonide up to 400 micrograms twice daily *or* fluticasone propionate up to 200 micrograms twice daily; use a large-volume spacer

Based on tables in: British Thoracic Society and Scottish Intercollegiate Guidelines Network. British Guideline on the Management of Asthma. *Thorax* 2003; **58** (suppl I); i1–i94. Reproduced with permission of BMJ Specialist Journals

MANAGEMENT OF ACUTE SEVERE ASTHMA IN GENERAL PRACTICE

MANAGEMENT OF ACUTE SEVERE ASTHMA IN GENERAL PRACTICE

Moderate asthma exacerbation

— Peak flow >50–75% of predicted or best
— No features of acute severe asthma
— Increasing symptoms

Treat at home but response to treatment **must** be assessed before doctor leaves

Treatment:
High-flow oxygen if available
Salbutamol or terbutaline via large-volume spacer or nebuliser
Monitor response 15–30 minutes after nebulisation
Give oral prednisolone 40–50 mg daily for at least 5 days and step up usual treatment

Follow up
Monitor symptoms and peak flow
Set up asthma action plan
Review in surgery within 48 hours
Modify treatment at review according to guidelines for chronic asthma (see Management of Chronic Asthma in Adults and Children)

Important: regard each emergency consultation as being for **acute severe asthma** until shown otherwise.

Important: failure to respond adequately **at any time** requires immediate referral to hospital.

Acute severe asthma in adults

— Cannot complete sentences in one breath
— Pulse ≥ 110 beats/minute
— Respiration ≥ 25 breaths/minute
— Peak flow 33–50% of predicted or best
Seriously consider hospital admission if more than one of above features present

Treatment:
High-flow oxygen if available
Salbutamol or terbutaline via large-volume spacer or nebuliser (oxygen driven if available)
Oral prednisolone 40–50 mg daily for at least 5 days (or i/v hydrocortisone 400 mg daily in 4 divided doses)
Monitor response 15–30 minutes after nebulisation

If any signs of acute asthma persist:
Arrange hospital admission
While awaiting ambulance repeat nebulised beta₂ agonist and give with nebulised ipratropium 500 micrograms
Alternatively if symptoms have improved, respiration and pulse settling, and peak flow >50% of predicted or best:
Step up usual treatment *and* continue prednisolone for at least 5 days

Follow up
Monitor symptoms and peak flow
Set up asthma action plan
Review in surgery within 24 hours
Modify treatment at review (see Management of Chronic Asthma)

Life-threatening asthma in adults

— Silent chest
— Cyanosis
— Feeble respiratory effort
— Bradycardia, exhaustion, arrhythmia, hypotension, confusion, or coma
— Peak flow <33% of predicted or best
— Arterial oxygen saturation <92%
Arrange **immediate** hospital admission
Treatment:
Oral prednisolone 40–50 mg daily for at least 5 days (or i/v hydrocortisone 400 mg daily in 4 divided doses) (immediately)
Oxygen-driven nebuliser in ambulance
Nebulised beta₂ agonist with nebulised ipratropium
Stay with patient until ambulance arrives

I. If nebuliser not available give 1 puff of beta₂ agonist using large-volume spacer and repeat 10–20 times

Important: patients with severe or life-threatening attacks may not be distressed and may not have all these abnormalities; the presence of any should alert doctor.

Acute episodes or exacerbations of asthma in young children

Mild/moderate episode in young children
— short-acting beta₂ agonist from metered dose inhaler *via* large-volume spacer (and face mask in very young), up to 10 puffs; alternatively give by nebuliser
— if favourable response (respiratory rate reduced, reduced use of accessory muscles, improved 'behaviour' pattern), repeat inhaled beta₂ agonist as needed

Acute asthma in children in primary care

— start short course of oral prednisolone for 3 days (under 2 years 10 mg; 2–5 years 20 mg; over 5 years 30–40 mg daily; those already on prednisolone tablets 2 mg/kg up to max. 60 mg)
— consider i/v hydrocortisone in those who are unable to retain oral prednisolone

If unresponsive or relapse within 3–4 hours:
— immediately refer to hospital
— give nebulised beta₂ agonist with nebulised ipratropium 250 micrograms every 20–30 minutes
— give high-flow oxygen *via* face mask

Signs of acute asthma in children

Acute severe asthma:
— too breathless to talk
— too breathless to feed
— respiration >50 breaths/minute (> 30/minute in children over 5 years)
— pulse >130 beats/minute (>120 beats/minute in children over 5 years)
— in younger children, use of accessory muscles of breathing
— in older children, peak flow ≤50% of predicted or best

Life-threatening features:
— cyanosis, silent chest, or poor respiratory effort
— exhaustion
— agitation, hypotension, confusion, reduced level of consciousness, or coma
— in older children, peak flow <33% of predicted or best

labour, or on the fetus. Drugs for asthma should preferably be administered by inhalation to minimise exposure of the fetus.

Severe exacerbations of asthma can have an adverse effect on pregnancy and should be treated promptly with conventional therapy, including oral or parenteral administration of a corticosteroid and nebulisation of a beta$_2$ agonist; prednisolone is the preferred corticosteroid for oral administration since very little of the drug reaches the fetus. Oxygen should be given immediately to maintain arterial oxygen saturation above 95% and prevent maternal and fetal hypoxia. Inhaled drugs, theophylline, and prednisolone can be taken as normal during breast-feeding.

Acute severe asthma

Severe asthma can be fatal and **must** be treated promptly and energetically. It is characterised by persistent dyspnoea poorly relieved by broncho-dilators, exhaustion, a high pulse rate (usually over 110/minute), and a very low peak expiratory flow. As asthma becomes more severe, wheezing may be absent. Such patients should be given **oxygen** (if available) and **salbutamol** or **terbutaline** by nebu-liser. This should be followed by a large dose of a **corticosteroid** (section 6.3.2)—for adults, predniso-lone 30–60 mg by mouth or hydrocortisone 200 mg (preferably as sodium succinate) intravenously; for children, prednisolone 1–2 mg/kg by mouth (1–4 years max. 20 mg, 5–15 years max. 40 mg) or hydrocortisone 100 mg (preferably as sodium succinate) intravenously; if vomiting occurs, the parenteral route may be preferred for the first dose. For a table outlining the management of acute severe asthma, see p. 133.

If there is little response **ipratropium** by nebuliser (section 3.1.2) should be considered. Most patients do not require and do not benefit from the addition of intravenous aminophylline or of a beta$_2$ agonist; both cause more adverse effects than nebulised beta$_2$ agonists. Nevertheless, an occasional patient who has not been taking theophylline, may benefit from a slow intravenous infusion of aminophylline. Patients with severe asthma may be helped by **magnesium sulphate** [unlicensed indication] but evidence of benefit is limited; it may be given by intravenous infusion of magnesium sulphate 1.2–2 g over 20 minutes or by nebulisation of 2.5 mL isotonic magnesium sulphate (60 mg/mL) in 2.5 mL salbut-amol nebuliser solution (1 mg/mL).

Treatment of these patients is safer in hospital where resuscitation facilities are immediately available. Treatment should **never** be delayed for investigations, patients should **never** be sedated, and the possibility of a pneumothorax should be considered.

If the patient deteriorates despite appropriate pharmacological treatment, intermittent positive pressure ventilation may be needed.

Chronic obstructive pulmonary disease

Chronic obstructive pulmonary disease (chronic bronchitis and emphysema) may be helped by an inhaled **short-acting beta$_2$ agonist** (section 3.1.1.1) used as required *or* when the airways obstruction is more severe, by a regular inhaled **antimuscarinic**

bronchodilator (section 3.1.2) *or* an inhaled **long-acting beta$_2$ agonist**. Although many patients are treated with an inhaled corticosteroid, long-term studies have shown no reduction in the decline in lung function in patients taking regular inhaled corticosteroids (section 3.2). A limited trial of high-dose inhaled corticosteroid *or* an oral cortico-steroid is recommended for patients with moderate airflow obstruction to ensure that asthma has not been overlooked.

Long-term **oxygen** therapy (section 3.6) prolongs survival in some patients with chronic obstructive pulmonary disease. For the management of infections in bronchitis see Table 1, section 5.1.

Croup

Mild croup requires no specific treatment and can be managed in the community. More severe croup calls for hospital admission; a single dose of a cortico-steroid (e.g. dexamethasone 150 micrograms/kg by mouth) may be administered before transfer to hospital. In hospital, dexamethasone 150 micr-ograms/kg (by mouth or by injection) or budesonide 2 mg (by nebulisation) will often reduce symptoms. For severe croup not effectively controlled with corticosteroid treatment, nebulised adrenaline solu-tion 1 in 1000 (1 mg/mL) may be given with close clinical monitoring in a dose of 400 micrograms/kg (max. 5 mg) repeated after 30 minutes if necessary; the effects of nebulised adrenaline last 2–3 hours.

3.1.1   Adrenoceptor agonists
(Sympathomimetics)

3.1.1.1   Selective beta$_2$ agonists
3.1.1.2   Other adrenoceptor agonists

The selective beta$_2$ agonists (selective beta$_2$-adreno-ceptor agonists, selective beta$_2$ stimulants) (section 3.1.1.1) such as salbutamol or terbutaline are the safest and most effective short-acting beta$_2$ agonists for asthma. They are recommended over the less selective beta$_2$ agonists such as orciprenaline (sec-tion 3.1.1.2), which should be avoided whenever possible.

Adrenaline (epinephrine) (which has both alpha- and beta-adrenoceptor agonist properties) is used in the emergency management of allergic and anaphy-lactic reactions (section 3.4.3).

3.1.1.1   Selective beta$_2$ agonists

Mild to moderate symptoms of asthma respond rapidly to the inhalation of a selective short-acting beta$_2$ agonist such as **salbutamol** or **terbutaline**. If beta$_2$ agonist inhalation is needed more often than once daily, prophylactic treatment should be con-sidered, using a stepped approach as outlined on p. 132.

Salmeterol and **formoterol** (eformoterol) are longer-acting beta$_2$ agonists which are administered by inhalation. They should not be used for the relief of an acute asthma attack. Salmeterol and formoterol should be added to existing corticosteroid therapy and not replace it. They can be useful in nocturnal asthma. Patients with asthma who use salmeterol must also use an inhaled corticosteroid (see Chronic

Asthma table, p. 132) because salmeterol may increase life-threatening attacks when given without an inhaled corticosteroid. Formoterol is also licensed for short-term symptom relief. Higher doses of formoterol (e.g. 24 micrograms twice daily) may be associated with an increase in severe exacerbations; lower doses are equally effective in most patients and should be tried first.

REGULAR TREATMENT. Short-acting beta$_2$ agonists should not be prescribed for use on a regular basis in patients with mild or moderate asthma since regular treatment provides no clinical benefit. However, regular use of the longer acting beta$_2$ agonists, salmeterol and formoterol, is of benefit.

Chronic Asthma table, see p. 132
Acute Severe Asthma table, see p. 133

INHALATION. *Pressurised-metered dose inhalers* are an effective and convenient method of drug administration in mild to moderate asthma. A spacer device (section 3.1.5) may improve drug delivery. At recommended inhaled doses the duration of action of salbutamol, terbutaline and fenoterol is about 3 to 5 hours and for salmeterol and formoterol 12 hours. The **dose**, the frequency, and the maximum number of inhalations in 24 hours of the beta$_2$ agonist should be **stated explicitly** to the patient. High doses of beta$_2$ agonists can be dangerous in some patients. Excessive use is usually an indication of **inadequately controlled** asthma and should be managed with a prophylactic drug such as an inhaled corticosteroid. The patient should be advised to seek medical advice when the prescribed dose of beta$_2$ agonist fails to provide the usual degree of symptomatic relief because this usually indicates a worsening of the asthma and the patient may require alternative medication (see Chronic Asthma table, p. 132).

CFC-FREE INHALERS. Chlorofluorocarbon (CFC) propellants in pressurised metered-dose inhalers are being replaced by hydrofluoroalkane (HFA) propellants. Patients receiving CFC-free inhalers should be reassured about the efficacy of the new inhalers and counselled that the aerosol may feel and taste different; any difficulty with the new inhaler should be discussed with the doctor or pharmacist.

Respirator (or nebuliser) solutions of salbutamol and terbutaline are used for the treatment of acute asthma both in hospital and in general practice. Patients with a severe attack of asthma should have oxygen if possible during nebulisation since beta$_2$ agonists can increase arterial hypoxaemia. The dose given by nebuliser is substantially higher than that given by inhaler. Patients should therefore be warned that it is dangerous to exceed the prescribed dose and they should seek medical advice if they fail to respond to the usual dose of the respirator solution. See also guidelines in section 3.1.5.

ORAL. Oral preparations of beta$_2$ agonists may be used by patients who cannot manage the inhaled route. They are sometimes used for children, but inhaled beta$_2$ agonists are more effective and have fewer side-effects; and most children can use one of the inhaler systems available. The longer-acting oral preparations including bambuterol may be of value in nocturnal asthma as an alternative to modified-release theophylline preparations (section 3.1.3) but they have a limited role and inhaled long-acting beta$_2$ agonists are usually preferred.

PARENTERAL. Salbutamol or terbutaline are given by intravenous infusion for severe asthma. Although some patients with chronic asthma are treated with a beta$_2$ agonist by subcutaneous injection on a regular basis, this route is not recommended since the evidence of benefit is uncertain and it may be difficult to withdraw such treatment once started. Patients supplied with a selective beta$_2$ agonist injection for severe attacks should be advised to attend hospital immediately after using the injection, for further assessment. Beta$_2$ agonists may also be given by intramuscular injection.

CHILDREN. Selective beta$_2$ agonists are useful even in children under the age of 18 months. They are most effective by the inhaled route; a pressurised metered-dose inhaler should be used with a spacer device in children under 5 years (see NICE guidance, section 3.1.5). A beta$_2$ agonist may also be given by mouth but administration by inhalation is preferred; a long-acting inhaled beta$_2$ agonist may be used where appropriate (see Chronic Asthma table, p. 132). In severe attacks nebulisation using a selective beta$_2$ agonist or ipratropium is advisable (see also Asthma tables, p. 132 and p. 133).

CAUTIONS. Beta$_2$ agonists should be used with caution in hyperthyroidism, cardiovascular disease, arrhythmias, susceptibility to QT-interval prolongation, and hypertension. If high doses are necessary in pregnancy or when breast-feeding, particular care should be taken. Beta$_2$ agonists should be used with caution in diabetes—monitor blood glucose (risk of ketoacidosis, especially when beta$_2$ agonist given intravenously). **Interactions:** Appendix 1 (sympathomimetics, beta$_2$)

HYPOKALAEMIA. The CSM has advised that potentially serious hypokalaemia may result from beta$_2$ agonist therapy. Particular caution is required in severe asthma, because this effect may be potentiated by concomitant treatment with theophylline and its derivatives, corticosteroids, and diuretics, and by hypoxia. Plasma-potassium concentration should therefore be monitored in severe asthma

SIDE-EFFECTS. Side-effects of the beta$_2$ agonists include fine tremor (particularly in the hands), nervous tension, headache, peripheral dilatation and palpitations. Other side-effects include tachycardia and arrhythmias and disturbances of sleep and behaviour in children. Muscle cramps and hypersensitivity reactions including paradoxical bronchospasm, urticaria, and angioedema have also been reported. Beta$_2$ agonists are associated with hypokalaemia after high doses (for CSM advice see under Cautions). Pain may occur on intramuscular injection.

SALBUTAMOL

Indications: asthma and other conditions associated with reversible airways obstruction; premature labour (section 7.1.3)

Cautions: see notes above

Side-effects: see notes above

Dose: *by mouth*, 4 mg (elderly and sensitive patients initially 2 mg) 3–4 times daily; max. single dose 8 mg (but unlikely to provide much extra benefit or to be tolerated); CHILD under 2 years 100 micrograms/kg 4 times daily [unlicensed]; 2–6 years 1–2 mg 3–4 times daily, 6–12 years 2 mg 3–4 times daily

By subcutaneous or intramuscular injection, 500 micrograms, repeated every 4 hours if necessary

By slow intravenous injection, 250 micrograms, repeated if necessary

By intravenous infusion, initially 5 micrograms/minute, adjusted according to response and heart-rate usually in range 3–20 micrograms/minute, or more if necessary; CHILD 1 month–12 years 0.1–1 microgram/kg/minute [unlicensed]

By aerosol inhalation, 100–200 micrograms (1–2 puffs); for persistent symptoms up to 3–4 times daily (but see also Chronic Asthma table); CHILD 100 micrograms (1 puff), increased to 200 micrograms (2 puffs) if necessary; for persistent symptoms up to 3–4 times daily (but see also Chronic Asthma table)

Prophylaxis in exercise-induced bronchospasm, 200 micrograms (2 puffs); CHILD 100 micrograms (1 puff), increased to 200 micrograms (2 puffs) if necessary

By inhalation of powder (for *Ventolin Accuhaler* and *Asmasal* dose see under preparation), 200–400 micrograms; for persistent symptoms up to 3–4 times daily (but see also Chronic Asthma table); CHILD 200 micrograms

Prophylaxis in exercise-induced bronchospasm (*powder*), 400 micrograms; CHILD 200 micrograms

NOTE. Bioavailability appears to be lower, so recommended doses for dry powder inhalers are twice those in a metered inhaler

By inhalation of nebulised solution, chronic bronchospasm unresponsive to conventional therapy and severe acute asthma, ADULT and CHILD over 18 months 2.5 mg, repeated up to 4 times daily; may be increased to 5 mg if necessary, but medical assessment should be considered since alternative therapy may be indicated; CHILD under 18 months, [unlicensed] (transient hypoxaemia may occur—consider supplemental oxygen), 1.25–2.5 mg up to 4 times daily but more frequent administration may be needed in severe cases

■ Oral

Salbutamol (Non-proprietary) PoM
Tablets, salbutamol (as sulphate) 2 mg, net price 20 = 59p; 4 mg, 20 = £1.09
Available from Alpharma, APS, Hillcross, IVAX
Oral solution, salbutamol (as sulphate) 2 mg/5 mL, net price 150 mL = 64p
Available from Pinewood (*Salapin*, sugar-free), Sandoz (sugar-free)

Ventmax® SR (Trinity) PoM
Capsules, m/r, salbutamol (as sulphate) 4 mg (green/grey), net price 56-cap pack = £8.57; 8 mg (white), 56-cap pack = £10.28. Label: 25
Dose: 8 mg twice daily; CHILD 3–12 years 4 mg twice daily

Ventolin® (A&H) PoM
Syrup, sugar-free, salbutamol (as sulphate) 2 mg/5 mL, net price 150 mL = 64p

Volmax® (A&H) PoM
Tablets, m/r, salbutamol (as sulphate) 4 mg, net price 56-tab pack = £10.55; 8 mg, 56-tab pack = £12.66. Label: 25
Dose: 8 mg twice daily; CHILD 3–12 years 4 mg twice daily

■ Parenteral

Salbutamol (Non-proprietary) PoM
Injection, salbutamol (as sulphate) 100 micrograms/mL, net price 50-mL vial = £5.25
Available from Aurum

Ventolin® (A&H) PoM
Injection, salbutamol (as sulphate) 500 micrograms/mL, 1-mL amp = 43p
Solution for intravenous infusion, salbutamol (as sulphate) 1 mg/mL. Dilute before use. Net price 5-mL amp = £2.78

■ Inhalation

COUNSELLING. Advise patients not to exceed prescribed dose and to follow manufacturer's directions; if a previously effective dose of inhaled salbutamol fails to provide at least 3 hours relief, a doctor's advice should be obtained as soon as possible.
Patients receiving CFC-free inhalers should be reassured about their efficacy and counselled that aerosol may feel and taste different

Salbutamol (Non-proprietary) PoM
Aerosol inhalation, salbutamol 100 micrograms/metered inhalation, net price 200-dose unit = £1.92. Counselling, dose
Available from Arrow, Generics, Hillcross
Excipients: include CFC propellants
Aerosol inhalation (CFC-free), salbutamol (as sulphate) 100 micrograms/metered inhalation, net price 200-dose unit = £1.92. Counselling, dose, change to CFC-free inhaler
Available from APS, IVAX (*Salamol®*)
Excipients: include HFA-134a (a non-CFC propellant), alcohol
NOTE. Can be supplied against a generic prescription but if CFC-free not specified will be reimbursed at price for CFC-containing inhaler
Dry powder for inhalation, salbutamol 200 micrograms/metered inhalation, net price 100-dose unit = £5.05. Counselling, dose
Available from Trinity (*Pulvinal® Salbutamol*)
Inhalation powder, hard capsule (for use with *Cyclohaler®* device), salbutamol 200 micrograms, net price 120-cap pack = £5.14; 400 micrograms, 120-cap pack = £8.69
Available from APS (*Salbutamol Cyclocaps®*)
Nebuliser solution, salbutamol (as sulphate) 1 mg/mL, net price 20 × 2.5 mL (2.5 mg) = £2.74; 2 mg/mL, 20 × 2.5 mL (5 mg) = £5.47. May be diluted with sterile sodium chloride 0.9%
Available from Galen, Generics, IVAX (*Salamol Steri-Neb®*)

Airomir® (IVAX) PoM
Aerosol inhalation, salbutamol (as sulphate) 100 micrograms/metered inhalation, net price 200-dose unit = £1.97. Counselling, dose, change to CFC-free inhaler
Excipients: include HFA-134a (a non-CFC propellant), alcohol
Also available as *Salbulin®* (3M)
NOTE. Can be supplied against a generic prescription but if 'CFC-free' not specified will be reimbursed at price for CFC-containing inhaler
Autohaler (breath-actuated aerosol inhalation), salbutamol (as sulphate) 100 micrograms/metered inhalation, net price 200-dose unit = £6.02. Counselling, dose, change to CFC-free inhaler
Excipients: include HFA-134a (a non-CFC propellant), alcohol

Asmasal Clickhaler® (Celltech) PoM
Dry powder for inhalation, salbutamol (as sulphate) 95 micrograms/metered inhalation, net price 200-dose unit = £6.32. Counselling, dose
Dose: acute bronchospasm 1–2 puffs
Persistent symptoms, 2 puffs 3–4 times daily
Prophylaxis in exercise-induced bronchospasm, 2 puffs

Salamol Easi-Breathe® (IVAX) [PoM]

CFC-Free aerosol inhalation, salbutamol 100 micrograms/metered inhalation, net price 200-dose breath-actuated unit = £6.30 Counselling, dose

Excipients: include alcohol, HFA-134a (a non-CFC propellant)

Ventodisks® (A&H) [PoM]

Dry powder for inhalation, disks containing 8 blisters of salbutamol (as sulphate) 200 micrograms/blister, 15 disks with *Diskhaler*® device = £7.50, 15-disk refill = £6.94; 400 micrograms/blister, 15 disks with *Diskhaler*® device = £12.72, 15-disk refill = £12.14. Counselling, dose

Ventolin® (A&H) [PoM]

Accuhaler® (dry powder for inhalation), disk containing 60 blisters of salbutamol (as sulphate) 200 micrograms/blister with *Accuhaler*® device, net price = £5.50. Counselling, dose

Dose: by inhalation of powder, 200 micrograms; for persistent symptoms up to 4 times daily (but see also Chronic Asthma table); CHILD 200 micrograms Prophylaxis in allergen- or exercise-induced bronchospasm, 200 micrograms

Evohaler® aerosol inhalation, salbutamol (as sulphate) 100 micrograms/metered inhalation, net price 200-dose unit = £2.30. Counselling, dose, change to CFC-free inhaler

Excipients: include HFA-134a (a non-CFC propellant)

NOTE. Can be supplied against a generic prescription but if CFC-free not specified will be reimbursed at price for CFC-containing inhaler

Nebules® (for use with nebuliser), salbutamol (as sulphate) 1 mg/mL, net price 20 × 2.5 mL (2.5 mg) = £3.40; 2 mg/mL, 20 × 2.5 mL (5 mg) = £6.92. May be diluted with sterile sodium chloride 0.9% if administration time in excess of 10 minutes is required

Respirator solution (for use with a nebuliser or ventilator), salbutamol (as sulphate) 5 mg/mL. Net price 20 mL = £2.44 (hosp. only). May be diluted with sterile sodium chloride 0.9%

■ Compound preparations

For some **compound preparations** containing salbutamol, see section 3.1.4

Chronic Asthma table, see p. 132
Acute Severe Asthma table, see p. 133

TERBUTALINE SULPHATE

Indications: asthma and other conditions associated with reversible airways obstruction; premature labour (section 7.1.3)

Cautions: see notes above

Side-effects: see notes above

Dose: *by mouth*, initially 2.5 mg 3 times daily for 1–2 weeks, then up to 5 mg 3 times daily CHILD 75 micrograms/kg 3 times daily; 7–15 years 2.5 mg 2–3 times daily

By subcutaneous, intramuscular, or slow intravenous injection, 250–500 micrograms up to 4 times daily; CHILD 2–15 years 10 micrograms/kg to a max. of 300 micrograms

By continuous intravenous infusion as a solution containing 3–5 micrograms/mL, 1.5–5 micrograms/minute for 8–10 hours; reduce dose for children

By aerosol inhalation, ADULT and CHILD 250–500 micrograms (1–2 puffs); for persistent symptoms up to 3–4 times daily (but see also Chronic Asthma table)

By inhalation of powder (*Turbohaler*®), 500 micrograms (1 inhalation); for persistent symptoms up to 4 times daily (but see also Chronic Asthma table)

By inhalation of nebulised solution, 5–10 mg 2–4 times daily; additional doses may be necessary in severe acute asthma; CHILD, up to 3 years 2 mg, 3–6 years 3 mg; 6–8 years 4 mg, over 8 years 5 mg, 2–4 times daily

■ Oral and parenteral

Bricanyl® (AstraZeneca) [PoM]

Tablets, scored, terbutaline sulphate 5 mg. Net price 20 = 82p

Syrup, sugar-free, terbutaline sulphate 1.5 mg/5 mL. Net price 300 mL = £2.60

Injection, terbutaline sulphate 500 micrograms/mL. Net price 1-mL amp = 30p; 5-mL amp = £1.40

Bricanyl SA® (AstraZeneca) [PoM]

Tablets, m/r, terbutaline sulphate 7.5 mg. Net price 20 = £1.71. Label: 25

Dose: 7.5 mg twice daily

Monovent® (Sandoz) [PoM]

Syrup, sugar-free, terbutaline sulphate 1.5 mg/5 mL. Net price 300 mL = £2.15

■ Inhalation

COUNSELLING. Advise patients not to exceed prescribed dose and to follow manufacturer's directions; if a previously effective dose of inhaled terbutaline fails to provide at least 3 hours relief, a doctor's advice should be obtained as soon as possible

Terbutaline Sulphate (Non-proprietary) [PoM]

Nebuliser solution, terbutaline sulphate 2.5 mg/mL, net price 20 × 2 mL (5 mg) = £3.67. May be diluted with sterile sodium chloride 0.9%

Available from Galen

Bricanyl® (AstraZeneca) [PoM]

Aerosol inhalation, terbutaline sulphate 250 micrograms/metered inhalation. Net price 400-dose unit = £5.84. Counselling, dose

Excipients: include CFC propellants

Turbohaler® (= dry powder inhaler), terbutaline sulphate 500 micrograms/inhalation. Net price 100-dose unit = £6.92. Counselling, dose

Respules® (= single-dose units for nebulisation), terbutaline sulphate 2.5 mg/mL. Net price 20 × 2-mL units (5-mg) = £4.04

Respirator solution (for use with a nebuliser or ventilator), terbutaline sulphate 10 mg/mL. Net price 20 mL = £2.91. Before use dilute with sterile sodium chloride 0.9%

BAMBUTEROL HYDROCHLORIDE

NOTE. Bambuterol is a pro-drug of terbutaline

Indications: asthma and other conditions associated with reversible airways obstruction

Cautions: see notes above; renal impairment (Appendix 3); avoid in cirrhosis, severe hepatic impairment; manufacturer advises avoid in pregnancy

Side-effects: see notes above

Dose: 20 mg once daily at bedtime if patient has previously tolerated beta$_2$ agonists; other patients, initially 10 mg once daily at bedtime, increased if necessary after 1–2 weeks to 20 mg once daily; CHILD not recommended

Bambec® (AstraZeneca) [PoM]
Tablets, both scored, bambuterol hydrochloride
10 mg, net price 28-tab pack = £12.05; 20 mg, 28-
tab pack = £13.14

FENOTEROL HYDROBROMIDE

Indications: reversible airways obstruction
Cautions: see notes above
Side-effects: see notes above

■ Compound preparations
For some **compound preparations** containing
fenoterol, see section 3.1.4

FORMOTEROL FUMARATE

(Eformoterol fumarate)
Indications: reversible airways obstruction (including nocturnal asthma and prevention of exercise-
induced bronchospasm) in patients requiring long-
term regular bronchodilator therapy, see also
Chronic Asthma table, p. 132; chronic obstructive
pulmonary disease
Cautions: see notes above; severe liver cirrhosis;
pregnancy (Appendix 4 and notes above); breast-
feeding (Appendix 5)
Side-effects: see notes above; oropharyngeal irritation, taste disturbances, rash, insomnia, nausea and
pruritus also reported; **important:** potential for
paradoxical bronchospasm (calling for discontinuation and alternative therapy)
Dose: see under preparations below
COUNSELLING. Advise patients not to exceed prescribed
dose, and to follow manufacturer's directions; if a
previously effective dose of inhaled formoterol fails to
provide adequate relief, a doctor's advice should be
obtained as soon as possible

Foradil® (Novartis) [PoM]
Dry powder for inhalation, formoterol fumarate
12 micrograms/capsule, net price 56-dose unit
(with inhaler device) = £24.80. Counselling, dose
Dose: by inhalation of powder, asthma, ADULT and CHILD
over 5 years, 12 micrograms twice daily, increased to
24 micrograms twice daily in more severe airways
obstruction
Chronic obstructive pulmonary disease, 12 micrograms
twice daily

Oxis® (AstraZeneca) [PoM]
Turbohaler® (= dry powder inhaler), formoterol
fumarate 6 micrograms/inhalation, net price 60-
dose unit = £24.80; 12 micrograms/inhalation, 60-
dose unit = £24.80. Counselling, dose
Dose: by inhalation of powder, asthma, 6–12 micrograms
1–2 times daily, increased to 24 micrograms twice daily in
more severe airways obstruction; for short-term symptom
relief (but not acute asthma) additional doses may be
taken to max. 72 micrograms daily (max. single dose
36 micrograms); reassess treatment if additional doses
required on more than 2 days a week
CHILD over 6 years, 12 micrograms 1–2 times daily, max.
24 micrograms daily
Prevention of exercise-induced bronchospasm ADULT and
CHILD over 6 years, 12 micrograms before exercise
Chronic obstructive pulmonary disease, 12 micrograms
1–2 times daily; max. 48 micrograms daily (max. single
dose 24 micrograms)

SALMETEROL

Indications: reversible airways obstruction (including nocturnal asthma and prevention of exercise-
induced bronchospasm) in patients requiring long-

term regular bronchodilator therapy, see also
Chronic Asthma table, p. 132; chronic obstructive
pulmonary disease
NOTE. CSM has emphasised that salmeterol is not for
immediate relief of acute attacks and that existing
corticosteroid therapy should not be reduced or withdrawn
Cautions: see notes above
Side-effects: see notes above; **important:** potential
for paradoxical bronchospasm (calling for discontinuation and alternative therapy)
Dose: *by inhalation*, asthma, 50 micrograms (2
puffs or 1 blister) twice daily; up to 100 micrograms (4 puffs or 2 blisters) twice daily in more
severe airways obstruction; CHILD over 4 years,
50 micrograms (2 puffs or 1 blister) twice daily
Chronic obstructive pulmonary disease 50 micrograms (2 puffs or 1 blister) twice daily
COUNSELLING. Advise patients that salmeterol should **not**
be used for relief of acute attacks, not to exceed
prescribed dose, and to follow manufacturer's directions;
if a previously effective dose of inhaled salmeterol fails to
provide adequate relief, a doctor's advice should be
obtained as soon as possible

Serevent® (A&H) [PoM]
Accuhaler® (dry powder for inhalation), disk
containing 60 blisters of salmeterol (as xinafoate (=
hydroxynaphthoate)) 50 micrograms/blister with
Accuhaler® device, net price = £31.46. Counselling, dose
Aerosol inhalation, salmeterol (as xinafoate
(= hydroxynaphthoate)) 25 micrograms/metered
inhalation, net price 120-dose unit = £31.46.
Counselling, dose
Excipients: include CFC propellants
Diskhaler® (dry powder for inhalation), disks
containing 4 blisters of salmeterol (as xinafoate
(= hydroxynaphthoate)) 50 micrograms/blister, net
price 15 disks with *Diskhaler®* device = £38.48, 15-
disk refill = £37.80. Counselling, dose

3.1.1.2   Other adrenoceptor agonists

Ephedrine and the partially selective beta agonist,
orciprenaline, are less suitable and less safe for use as
bronchodilators than the selective beta$_2$ agonists,
because they are more likely to cause arrhythmias
and other side-effects. They should be avoided
whenever possible.
  Adrenaline (epinephrine) injection (1 in 1000) is
used in the emergency treatment of acute allergic and
anaphylactic reactions (section 3.4.3).

EPHEDRINE HYDROCHLORIDE

Indications: reversible airways obstruction, but see
notes above
Cautions: hyperthyroidism, diabetes mellitus,
ischaemic heart disease, hypertension, renal impairment, elderly; prostatic hypertrophy (risk of acute
retention); interaction with MAOIs a disadvantage;
interactions: Appendix 1 (sympathomimetics)
Side-effects: tachycardia, anxiety, restlessness,
insomnia common; also tremor, arrhythmias, dry
mouth, cold extremities
Dose: 15–60 mg 3 times daily; CHILD up to 1 year
7.5 mg 3 times daily, 1–5 years 15 mg 3 times
daily, 6–12 years 30 mg 3 times daily

¹**Ephedrine Hydrochloride** (Non-proprietary) PoM ▨

Tablets, ephedrine hydrochloride 15 mg, net price 28 = £1.76; 30 mg, 28 = £1.70

1. For exemptions see *Medicines, Ethics and Practice*, No. 27, London, Pharmaceutical Press, 2003 (and subsequent editions as available)

■ Preparations on sale to the public

For a list of **cough and decongestant preparations on sale to the public**, including those containing ephedrine, see section 3.9.2

───

ORCIPRENALINE SULPHATE ▨

Indications: reversible airways obstruction, but see notes above

Cautions: see section 3.1.1.1 and notes above; **interactions:** Appendix 1 (sympathomimetics)

Side-effects: see section 3.1.1.1 and notes above

Dose: 20 mg 4 times daily; CHILD up to 1 year 5–10 mg 3 times daily, 1–3 years 5–10 mg 4 times daily, 3–12 years 40–60 mg daily in divided doses

Alupent® (Boehringer Ingelheim) PoM ▨

Syrup, sugar-free, orciprenaline sulphate 10 mg/ 5 mL, net price 300 mL = £2.26

───

3.1.2 Antimuscarinic bronchodilators

Ipratropium can be used to provide short-term relief in chronic asthma, but short-acting beta₂ agonists work more quickly. Ipratropium by nebulisation may be added to other standard treatment in life-threatening asthma or where acute asthma fails to improve with standard therapy (see Acute Severe Asthma table, p. 133).

Antimuscarinic bronchodilators are effective in patients with chronic obstructive pulmonary disease. The aerosol inhalation of ipratropium has a maximum effect 30–60 minutes after use; its duration of action is 3 to 6 hours and bronchodilation can usually be maintained with treatment 3 times a day.

Tiotropium, a long-acting antimuscarinic bronchodilator, is licensed for maintenance treatment of chronic obstructive pulmonary disease; it is not suitable for the relief of acute bronchospasm.

CAUTIONS. Antimuscarinic bronchodilators should be used with caution in glaucoma (see below), prostatic hyperplasia and bladder outflow obstruction, pregnancy (Appendix 4), and breast-feeding (Appendix 5); **interactions:** Appendix 1 (antimuscarinics)

GLAUCOMA. *Acute angle-closure glaucoma* reported with nebulised ipratropium, particularly when given with nebulised salbutamol (and possibly other beta₂ agonists); care needed to protect patient's eyes from nebulised drug or from drug powder

SIDE-EFFECTS. The side-effects of antimuscarinic bronchodilators include dry mouth, nausea, constipation, and headache.

IPRATROPIUM BROMIDE

Indications: reversible airways obstruction, particularly in chronic obstructive pulmonary disease

Cautions: see notes above

Side-effects: see notes above

Dose: *by aerosol inhalation*, 20–40 micrograms, in early treatment up to 80 micrograms at a time, 3–4 times daily; CHILD up to 6 years 20 micrograms 3 times daily, 6–12 years 20–40 micrograms 3 times daily

By inhalation of powder, 40 micrograms 3–4 times daily (may be doubled in less responsive patients); CHILD under 12 years, not recommended

By inhalation of nebulised solution, 100–500 micrograms up to 4 times daily; CHILD 1 month–3 years 62.5–250 micrograms up to 3 times daily [unlicensed]; 3–14 years 100–500 micrograms up to 3 times daily. Dilution of solution is adjusted according to equipment and length of administration. Because paradoxical bronchospasm has occurred, *first dose* should be inhaled under medical supervision

COUNSELLING. Advise patient not to exceed prescribed dose and to follow manufacturer's directions

Ipratropium Bromide (Non-proprietary) PoM

Nebuliser solution, ipratropium bromide 250 micrograms/mL, net price 20 × 1-mL (250-microgram) unit-dose vials = £7.26, 60 × 1-mL = £19.20; 20 × 2-mL (500-microgram) = £7.43, 60 × 2-mL = £22.50. If dilution is necessary use only sterile sodium chloride 0.9%

Available from Galen, Generics

Atrovent® (Boehringer Ingelheim) PoM

Aerocaps® (dry powder for inhalation; for use with *Atrovent Aerohaler*®), green, ipratropium bromide 40 micrograms, net price pack of 100 caps with *Aerohaler*® = £14.53; 100 caps = £10.53. Counselling, dose

Aerosol inhalation, ipratropium bromide 20 micrograms/metered inhalation, net price 200-dose unit = £4.21. Counselling, dose

Excipients: include CFC propellants

Nebuliser solution, isotonic, ipratropium bromide 250 micrograms/mL, net price 20 × 1-mL unit-dose vials = £6.48, 60 × 1-mL vials = £19.44; 20 × 2-mL vials = £7.60, 60 × 2-mL vials = £22.80. If dilution is necessary use only sterile sodium chloride 0.9%

NOTE. One *Atrovent Aerocap*® is equivalent to 2 puffs of *Atrovent*® metered aerosol inhalation *or* 1 puff of *Atrovent Forte*® metered aerosol inhalation

Ipratropium Steri-Neb® (IVAX) PoM

Nebuliser solution, isotonic, ipratropium bromide 250 micrograms/mL, net price 20 × 1-mL (250-microgram) unit-dose vials = £7.67; 20 × 2-mL (500-microgram) = £8.99. If dilution is necessary use only sterile sodium chloride 0.9%

Respontin® (A&H) PoM

Nebuliser solution, isotonic, ipratropium bromide 250 micrograms/mL, net price 20 × 1-mL (250-microgram) unit-dose vials = £5.44; 20 × 2-mL (500-microgram) = £6.40. If dilution is necessary use only sterile sodium chloride 0.9%

■ Compound ipratropium preparations

Section 3.1.4

TIOTROPIUM

Indications: maintenance treatment of chronic obstructive pulmonary disease

Cautions: see notes above; renal impairment (Appendix 3)

Side-effects: see notes above; also pharyngitis, sinusitis, candidiasis; rarely tachycardia, difficulty in micturition (urinary retention reported in elderly men with prostatic hyperplasia)

Dose: *by inhalation of powder*, 18 micrograms daily, CHILD and ADOLESCENT under 18 years, not recommended

Spiriva® (Boehringer Ingelheim) ▼ PoM
Inhalation powder, hard capsule (for use with *HandiHaler*® device), tiotropium (as tiotropium bromide monohydrate) 18 micrograms, net price 30-cap pack with *HandiHaler*® device = £37.62, 30-cap refill = £36.60

3.1.3   Theophylline

Theophylline is a bronchodilator used for reversible airways obstruction. It may have an additive effect when used in conjunction with small doses of beta$_2$ agonists; the combination may increase the risk of side-effects, including hypokalaemia (for CSM advice see p. 135).

Theophylline is metabolised in the liver; there is considerable variation in plasma-theophylline concentration particularly in smokers, in patients with hepatic impairment or heart failure, or if certain drugs are taken concurrently. The plasma-theophylline concentration is *increased* in heart failure, cirrhosis, viral infections, in the elderly, and by drugs that inhibit its metabolism. The plasma-theophylline concentration is *decreased* in smokers and in chronic alcoholism and by drugs that induce liver metabolism. For other interactions of theophylline see Appendix 1.

These differences in theophylline half-life are important because its toxic dose is close to the therapeutic dose. In most individuals a plasma-theophylline concentration of between 10–20 mg/litre is required for satisfactory bronchodilation, although a plasma-theophylline concentration of 10 mg/litre (or less) may be effective. Adverse effects can occur within the range 10–20 mg/litre and both the frequency and severity increase at concentrations above 20 mg/litre.

Theophylline is given by injection as **aminophylline**, a mixture of theophylline with ethylenediamine, which is 20 times more soluble than theophylline alone. Aminophylline injection is needed rarely for severe attacks of asthma. It must be given by **very slow** intravenous injection (over at least 20 minutes); it is too irritant for intramuscular use. Measurement of plasma theophylline concentration may be helpful, and is **essential** if aminophylline is to be given to patients who have been taking theophylline, because serious side-effects such as convulsions and arrhythmias can occasionally precede other symptoms of toxicity.

THEOPHYLLINE

Indications: reversible airways obstruction, acute severe asthma; for guidelines see also Asthma tables (p. 132 and p. 133)

Cautions: cardiac disease, hypertension, hyperthyroidism, peptic ulcer, hepatic impairment (Appendix 2), epilepsy, pregnancy and breastfeeding (Appendices 4 and 5), elderly, fever; CSM advice on hypokalaemia risk, p. 135; avoid in porphyria (section 9.8.2); **interactions:** Appendix 1 (theophylline) and notes above

Side-effects: tachycardia, palpitations, nausea and other gastro-intestinal disturbances, headache, CNS stimulation, insomnia, arrhythmias, and convulsions especially if given rapidly by intravenous injection; **overdosage:** see Emergency Treatment of Poisoning, p. 26

Dose: see below

NOTE. Plasma theophylline concentration for optimum response 10–20 mg/litre (55–110 micromol/litre); narrow margin between therapeutic and toxic dose, see also notes above

Nuelin® (3M)
Tablets, scored, theophylline 125 mg. Net price 90-tab pack = £3.29. Label: 21
Dose: 125 mg 3–4 times daily after food, increased to 250 mg if required; CHILD 7–12 years 62.5–125 mg 3–4 times daily
Liquid, brown, theophylline hydrate (as sodium glycinate) 60 mg/5 mL. Net price 300 mL = £2.93. Label: 21
Dose: 120–240 mg 3–4 times daily after food; CHILD 2–6 years 60–90 mg, 7–12 years 90–120 mg, 3–4 times daily

---

■ Modified release

NOTE. The Council of the Royal Pharmaceutical Society of Great Britain advises pharmacists that if a general practitioner prescribes a modified-release oral theophylline preparation without specifying a brand name, the pharmacist should contact the prescriber and agree the brand to be dispensed. Additionally, it is essential that a patient discharged from hospital should be maintained on the brand on which that patient was stabilised as an in-patient.

Nuelin SA® (3M)
SA tablets, m/r, theophylline 175 mg. Net price 60-tab pack = £3.43. Label: 25
Dose: 175–350 mg every 12 hours; CHILD over 6 years 175 mg every 12 hours
SA 250 tablets, m/r, scored, theophylline 250 mg. Net price 60-tab pack = £4.80. Label: 25
Dose: 250–500 mg every 12 hours; CHILD over 6 years 125–250 mg every 12 hours

Slo-Phyllin® (Merck)
Capsules, all m/r, theophylline 60 mg (white/clear, enclosing white pellets), net price 56-cap pack = £2.11; 125 mg (brown/clear, enclosing white pellets), 56-cap pack = £2.66; 250 mg (blue/clear, enclosing white pellets), 56-cap pack = £3.32. Label: 25, or counselling, see below
Dose: 250–500 mg every 12 hours; CHILD, every 12 hours, 2–6 years 60–120 mg, 7–12 years 125–250 mg
COUNSELLING. Swallow whole with fluid *or* swallow enclosed granules with soft food (e.g. yoghurt)

Uniphyllin Continus® (Napp)
Tablets, m/r, all scored, theophylline 200 mg, net price 56-tab pack = £4.12; 300 mg, 56-tab pack = £6.27; 400 mg, 56-tab pack = £7.44. Label: 25
Dose: 200 mg every 12 hours increased according to response to 400 mg every 12 hours
May be appropriate to give larger evening or morning dose to achieve optimum therapeutic effect when symptoms most severe; in patients whose night or daytime symptoms persist despite other therapy, who are not currently receiving theophylline, total daily requirement may be added as single evening or morning dose
CHILD 9 mg/kg twice daily; some children with chronic asthma may require 10–16 mg/kg every 12 hours

For a list of **cough and decongestant preparations on sale to the public**, including those containing theophylline, see section 3.9.2

AMINOPHYLLINE

NOTE. Aminophylline is a stable mixture or combination of theophylline and ethylenediamine; the ethylenediamine confers greater solubility in water

Indications: reversible airways obstruction, acute severe asthma

Cautions: see under Theophylline

Side-effects: see under Theophylline; also allergy to ethylenediamine can cause urticaria, erythema, and exfoliative dermatitis

Dose: see under preparations, below

NOTE. Plasma theophylline concentration for optimum response 10–20 mg/litre (55–110 micromol/litre); narrow margin between therapeutic and toxic dose, see also notes above

Aminophylline (Non-proprietary)

Tablets, aminophylline 100 mg, net price 20 = 77p. Label: 21

Dose: by mouth, 100–300 mg, 3–4 times daily, after food

Injection, aminophylline 25 mg/mL, net price 10-mL amp = 69p [PoM]

Available from Celltech (*Minijet®*), Phoenix

Dose: deteriorating acute severe asthma **not** previously treated with theophylline, *by slow intravenous injection* over at least 20 minutes (with close monitoring), 250–500 mg (5 mg/kg), then as for acute severe asthma; CHILD 5 mg/kg, then as for acute severe asthma

Acute severe asthma, *by intravenous infusion* (with close monitoring), 500 micrograms/kg/hour, adjusted according to plasma-theophylline concentration; CHILD 6 months–9 years 1 mg/kg/hour, 10–16 years 800 micrograms/kg/hour, adjusted according to plasma-theophylline concentration

NOTE. Patients taking oral theophylline or aminophylline should not normally receive intravenous aminophylline unless plasma-theophylline concentration is available to guide dosage

■ Modified release

NOTE. Advice about modified-release theophylline preparations on p. 140 also applies to modified-release aminophylline preparations

Phyllocontin Continus® (Napp)

Tablets, m/r, yellow, f/c, aminophylline hydrate 225 mg. Net price 56-tab pack = £3.34. Label: 25

Dose: 1 tablet twice daily initially, increased after 1 week to 2 tablets twice daily

NOTE. Modified-release tablets containing aminophylline 225 mg also available from Ashbourne (*Amnivent® 225 SR*), IVAX (*Norphyllin® SR*)

Forte tablets, m/r, yellow, f/c, aminophylline hydrate 350 mg. Net price 56-tab pack = £5.55. Label: 25

NOTE. *Forte* tablets are for smokers and other patients with decreased theophylline half-life (see notes above)

Paediatric tablets, m/r, peach, aminophylline hydrate 100 mg. Net price 56-tab pack = £2.15. Label: 25

Dose: CHILD over 3 years, 6 mg/kg twice daily initially, increased after 1 week to 12 mg/kg twice daily; some children with chronic asthma may require 13–20 mg/kg every 12 hours

3.1.4   Compound bronchodilator preparations

In general, patients are best treated with single-ingredient preparations, such as a selective beta$_2$ agonist (section 3.1.1.1) or ipratropium bromide (section 3.1.2), so that the dose of each drug can be adjusted. This flexibility is lost with combinations. However, a combination product may be appropriate for patients stabilised on individual components in the same proportion.

For **cautions, contra-indications** and **side-effects** see under individual drugs.

Combivent® (Boehringer Ingelheim) [PoM]

Aerosol inhalation, ipratropium bromide 20 micrograms, salbutamol (as sulphate) 100 micrograms/metered inhalation. Net price 200-dose unit = £6.45. Counselling, dose

Excipients: include CFC propellants

Dose: bronchospasm associated with chronic obstructive pulmonary disease, 2 puffs 4 times daily; CHILD under 12 years not recommended

Nebuliser solution, isotonic, ipratropium bromide 500 micrograms, salbutamol (as sulphate) 2.5 mg/2.5-mL vial, net price 60 unit-dose vials = £31.35

Dose: bronchospasm in chronic obstructive pulmonary disease, *by inhalation of nebulised solution*, 1 vial 3–4 times daily; CHILD under 12 years not recommended

GLAUCOMA. In addition to other potential side-effects acute angle-closure glaucoma has been reported with nebulised ipratropium—for details, see p. 139

Duovent® (Boehringer Ingelheim) [PoM]

Nebuliser solution, isotonic, fenoterol hydrobromide 1.25 mg, ipratropium bromide 500 micrograms/4-mL vial, net price 20 unit-dose vials = £11.00

Dose: acute severe asthma or acute exacerbation of chronic asthma, *by inhalation of nebulised solution*, 1 vial (4 mL); may be repeated up to max. 4 vials in 24 hours; CHILD under 14 years, not recommended

GLAUCOMA. In addition to other potential side-effects acute angle-closure glaucoma has been reported with nebulised ipratropium—for details see p. 139

3.1.5   Peak flow meters, inhaler devices and nebulisers

Peak flow meters

Measurement of peak flow is particularly helpful to patients who are 'poor perceivers' and hence slow to detect deterioration in their asthma, and for those with moderate or severe asthma. Patients must be given clear guidelines as to the action they should take if their peak flow falls below a certain level. Patients can be encouraged to adjust some of their own treatment (within specified limits) according to changes in peak flow rate.

Asmaplan® (Vitalograph)

Peak flow meter, standard (50 to 750 litres/minute), net price = £5.95, low range (25 to 280 litres /minute) = £5.95, replacement mouthpiece = 40p (for adult or child)

Ferraris Pocketpeak® (Ferraris)

Peak flow meter, standard (90–710 litres/minute), net price = £6.53, low range (40–370 litres/minute) = £6.53, replacement mouthpiece = 38p (for adult or child)

Mini-Wright® (Clement Clarke)

Peak flow meter, standard (60 to 800 litres/minute), net price = £6.86, low range (30 to 400 litres/minute) = £6.90, replacement mouthpiece = 38p (for adult or child)

Drug delivery devices

INHALER DEVICES. These include *pressurised metered-dose inhalers, breath-actuated inhalers* and *dry powder inhalers*. Many patients can be taught to use a pressurised metered-dose inhaler effectively but some patients, particularly the elderly and small children, find it difficult to use them. *Spacer devices* (see below) can help such patients because they remove the need to co-ordinate actuation with inhalation and are effective even for children under 5 years. Alternatively, breath-actuated inhalers or dry powder inhalers (which are activated by patient's inhalation) may be used but they are less suitable for young children. On changing from a pressurised metered-dose inhaler to a dry powder inhaler patients may notice a lack of sensation in the mouth and throat previously associated with each actuation. Coughing may also occur.

The patient should be instructed carefully on the use of the inhaler and it is important to check that the inhaler continues to be used correctly because inadequate inhalation technique may be mistaken for a lack of response to the drug.

NICE Guidance (inhaler devices for children with chronic asthma)
The National Institute for Clinical Excellence has advised that the child's needs, ability to develop and maintain effective technique, and likelihood of good compliance should govern the choice of inhaler and spacer device; only then should cost be considered For children aged under 5 years:

- corticosteroid and bronchodilator therapy should be routinely delivered by pressurised metered-dose inhaler and spacer device, with a facemask if necessary;

- if this is not effective, and depending on the child's condition, nebulised therapy may be considered and, in children over 3 years, a dry powder inhaler may also be considered [but see notes above];

For children aged 5–15 years:

- corticosteroid therapy should be routinely delivered by a pressurised metered-dose inhaler and spacer device

- children and their carers should be trained in the use of the chosen device; suitability of the device should be reviewed at least annually. Inhaler technique and compliance should be monitored

---

SPACER DEVICES. Spacer devices remove the need for co-ordination between actuation of a pressurised metered-dose inhaler and inhalation. The spacer device reduces the velocity of the aerosol and subsequent impaction on the oropharynx. In addition the device allows more time for evaporation of the propellant so that a larger proportion of the particles can be inhaled and deposited in the lungs. The size of the spacer is important, the larger spacers with a one-way valve (*Nebuhaler®, Volumatic®*) being most effective. Spacer devices are particularly useful for patients with poor inhalation technique, for children, for patients requiring higher doses, for nocturnal asthma, and for patients prone to candidiasis with inhaled corticosteroids. It is important to prescribe a spacer device that is compatible with the metered-dose inhaler.

USE AND CARE OF SPACER DEVICES. Patients should inhale from the spacer device as soon as possible after actuation since the drug aerosol is very short-lived; single-dose actuation is recommended. The device should be cleansed once a month by washing in mild detergent, rinsing and then allowing to dry in air (wiping should be avoided since any electrostatic charge may affect drug delivery). Spacer devices should be replaced every 6–12 months.

Able Spacer® (Clement Clarke)
Spacer device, small-volume device. For use with pressurised (aerosol) inhalers, net price standard device = £4.20; with infant, child or adult mask = £6.86

AeroChamber® Plus (3M)
Spacer device, medium-volume device. For use with *Airomir®, Atrovent®, Atrovent® Forte, Combivent®, Duovent®, Oxivent®, Salbulin®,* and *Qvar®* inhalers, net price standard device (blue) = £4.36, with mask (blue) = £7.27; infant device (orange) with mask = £4.36; child device (yellow) with mask = £7.27

Babyhaler® (A&H) NHS
Spacer device for paediatric use with *Becotide®-50* and *Ventolin®* inhalers. Net price = £11.34

E-Z Spacer® (Vitalograph) NHS
Spacer device, large-volume, collapsible device. For use with pressurised (aerosol) inhalers, price (direct from manufacturer) = £23.00

Haleraid® (A&H) NHS
Device to place over standard inhalers to aid when strength in hands is impaired (e.g. in arthritis). Available as *Haleraid®-120* for 120-dose inhalers and *Haleraid®-200* for 200-dose inhalers. Net price = 80p

Nebuhaler® (AstraZeneca)
Spacer inhaler, large-volume device. For use with *Bricanyl®* and *Pulmicort®* inhalers, net price = £4.28; with paediatric mask = £4.28

PARI Space Chamber® (Pari)
Spacer device, medium volume device. For use with a pressurised (aerosol) inhaler, net price £4.25; with mask for infant, child 1–4 years or child 4–7 years = £6.85

Pocket Chamber® (Ferraris)
Spacer device, small-volume device. For use with a pressurised (aerosol) inhaler, net price = £4.18; with infant, small, medium, or large mask = £9.75

Spinhaler® (Rhône-Poulenc Rorer)
Breath-actuated device for use with *Intal Spincaps®*. Net price = £2.08

Volumatic® (A&H)
Spacer inhaler, large-volume device. For use with *Becloforte®, Becotide®, Flixotide®, Seretide®, Serevent®,* and *Ventolin®* inhalers, net price = £2.75; with paediatric mask = £2.75

Nebulisers

In England and Wales nebulisers and compressors are not available on the NHS (but they are free of VAT); some nebulisers (but not compressors) are available on form GP10A in Scotland (for details consult Scottish Drug Tariff).

A nebuliser converts a solution of a drug into an aerosol for inhalation. It is used to deliver higher doses of drug to the airways than is usual with standard inhalers. The main indications for use of a nebuliser are:

- to deliver a beta agonist or ipratropium to a patient with an *acute exacerbation* of asthma or of airways obstruction;

- to deliver a beta agonist or ipratropium on a *regular basis* to a patient with severe asthma or reversible airways obstruction who has been shown to benefit from regular treatment with higher doses;
- to deliver *prophylactic medication* such as cromoglicate or a corticosteroid to a patient unable to use other inhalational devices (particularly a young child);
- to deliver an antibiotic (such as colistin) to a patient with chronic purulent infection (as in cystic fibrosis or bronchiectasis);
- to deliver pentamidine for the prophylaxis and treatment of pneumocystis pneumonia to a patient with AIDS.

The proportion of a nebuliser solution that reaches the lungs depends on the type of nebuliser and although it can be as high as 30% it is more frequently close to 10% and sometimes below 10%. The remaining solution is left in the nebuliser as residual volume or it is deposited in the mouthpiece and tubing. The extent to which the nebulised solution is deposited in the airways or alveoli depends on particle size. Particles with a mass median diameter of 1–5 microns are deposited in the airways and are therefore appropriate for asthma whereas a particle size of 1–2 microns is needed for alveolar deposition of pentamidine to combat pneumocystis infection. The type of nebuliser is therefore chosen according to the deposition required and according to the viscosity of the solution (antibiotic solutions usually being more viscous).

Some jet nebulisers are able to increase drug output during inspiration and hence increase efficiency.

The patient should be aware that the dose of a bronchodilator given by nebulisation is usually **much higher** than that from an aerosol inhaler; see below for British Thoracic Society guidelines.

The British Thoracic Society has advised that nebulised bronchodilators may be given to patients with chronic persistent asthma or those with sudden catastrophic severe asthma (brittle asthma). In chronic asthma, nebulised bronchodilators should only be used to relieve persistent daily wheeze (see Chronic Asthma table p. 132). The British Thoracic Society has further recommended that the use of nebulisers in chronic persistent asthma should only be considered:

- after a review of the diagnosis;
- if the airflow obstruction is significantly reversible by bronchodilators without unacceptable side-effects;
- after the patient has been using the usual hand-held inhaler correctly;
- after a larger dose of bronchodilator from a hand-held inhaler (with a spacer if necessary) has been tried for at least 2 weeks;
- if the patient is complying with the prescribed dose and frequency of anti-inflammatory treatment including regular use of high-dose inhaled corticosteroid.

Before prescribing a nebuliser, a home trial should preferably be undertaken to monitor peak flow for up to 2 weeks on standard treatment and up to 2 weeks on nebulised treatment. If prescribed, patients must:

- have clear instructions from doctor, specialist nurse or pharmacist on the use of the nebuliser and on peak-flow monitoring;
- be instructed not to treat acute attacks at home without also seeking help;
- receive an education program;
- have regular follow up including peak-flow monitoring and be seen by doctor, specialist nurse or physiotherapist.

■ Jet nebulisers

Jet nebulisers are more widely used than ultrasonic nebulisers. Most jet nebulisers require an optimum gas flow rate of 6–8 litres/minute and in hospital can be driven by piped air or oxygen. Domiciliary oxygen cylinders do not provide an adequate flow rate therefore an electrical compressor is required for domiciliary use.

For patients with *chronic obstructive pulmonary disease and hypercapnia*, oxygen can be dangerous and the nebuliser should be driven by air (see also p. 135).

> **Important:** the Department of Health has reminded users of the need to use the correct grade of tubing when connecting a nebuliser to a medical gas supply or compressor.

Medix Lifecare Nebuliser Chamber® (Medix) NHS
Jet nebuliser, disposable; for use with bronchodilators, antimuscarinics, corticosteroids, and antibiotics, replacement recommended every 2–3 months if used 4 times a day. Compatible with *AC 2000 Hi Flo*® NHS, *World Traveller Hi Flo*® NHS, and *Econoneb*® NHS, net price = £1.00

Medix Lifecare Nebuliser System® (Medix) NHS
Jet nebuliser, consisting of mouthpiece, tubing, and nebuliser chamber, net price = £2.00; mask kits with tubing and nebuliser chamber also available, net price (adult)= £2.00; (child) = £2.10

Omron CX® (Omron) NHS
Jet nebuliser, non-disposable, with *Omron VC*® nebuliser kit, net price = £56.25

PARI LC PLUS FILTER® (Pari) NHS
Jet nebuliser, closed system, non-disposable, for hospital or home use; for use with bronchodilators, antibiotics and corticosteroids; replacement recommended yearly if used 4 times a day. Compatible with *PARI Turbo BOY'N'*® NHS, *PARI Junior BOY'N'*® NHS and *PARI UNI light mobil*® NHS compressors, net price = £24.80, replacement filters 100 = £35.70

PARI LC PLUS® (Pari) NHS
Jet nebuliser, non-disposable, for hospital or home use; for use with bronchodilators, antibiotics, and corticosteroids, replacement recommended yearly if used 4 times a day. Compatible with *PARI Turbo BOY'N'*® NHS, *PARI Junior BOY'N'*® NHS, *PARI UNI light mobil*® NHS and *PARI WALK BOY*® NHS compressors, net price = £15.45

PARI BABY® (Pari) NHS
Jet nebuliser, non-disposable, for hospital or home use; for use with bronchodilators, antibiotics and corticosteroids; replacement recommended yearly if used 4 times a day. Compatible with *PARI Turbo BOY'N'*® NHS, *PARI Junior BOY'N'*® NHS, *PARI UNI light mobil*® NHS, *PARI WALK BOY*® NHS compressors. Available separately for children aged less than 1 year, 1–4 years or 4–7 years, net price (with mask and connection tube) = £31.40

Sidestream Durable® (Profile Respiratory) NHS
Jet nebuliser, non-disposable, for home use; for use with bronchodilators; yearly replacement recommended if 4 six-minute treatments used per day. Compatible with *Freeway Freedom*® NHS and *Porta-Neb*® NHS, net price year pack = £25.50 (*Porta-Neb*®), £29.00 (*Freeway Freedom*®). Disposable *Sidestream*® NHS nebuliser also available

Ventstream® (Profile Respiratory) NHS
Jet nebuliser, closed-system, for use with low flow compressors, compatible with *Porta-Neb*® NHS, and *Freeway Freedom*® NHS compressors; for use with antibiotics, bronchodilators, and corticosteroids, replacement recommended yearly if used 3 times a day, net price year pack with filter = £39.00 (*Porta-Neb*®), £41.00 (*Freeway Freedom*®)

■ **Home compressors with nebulisers**

AC 2000 HI FLO® (Medix) 〔NHS〕
Home and hospital use, containing 1 *Jet Nebuliser*® 〔NHS〕 set with mouthpiece, 1 adult and 1 child mask,1 spare inlet filter, filter spanner. Mains operated. Nebulises bronchodilators, corticosteroids, and antibiotics, net price = £117.00; carrying case available

AC 4000® (Medix) 〔NHS〕
Home and hospital use, containing 1 *Jet Nebuliser*® 〔NHS〕 set with mouthpiece, 1 adult and 1 child face mask, 1 spare inlet filter, filter spanner. Mains operated. Nebulises bronchodilators, corticosteroids, and antibiotics, net price = £80.10

Aquilon® (Henleys) 〔NHS〕
Portable, home use, with 1 adult or 1 child mask and tubing. Mains operated; for use with bronchodilators, corticosteroids and antibiotics, net price = £59.00

Econoneb® (Medix) 〔NHS〕
Home, clinic and hospital use, used with 1 *Jet Nebuliser*® 〔NHS〕 set with mouthpiece, 1 adult and 1 child mask, 1 spare inlet filter, filter spanner. Nebulises bronchodilators, corticosteroids, and antibiotics. Mains operated, net price = £99.00

Freeway Freedom® (Profile Respiratory) 〔NHS〕
Portable, containing *Sidestream Durable*® 〔NHS〕 nebuliser, 1 adult mask, 1 child mask, 1 angled mouthpiece, 1 coiled *Duratube*®, 4 inlet filters, charger and power lead, net price = £254.00; with *Ventstream*® 〔NHS〕 nebuliser, 1 straight mouthpiece, 1 coiled *Duratube*®, 4 inlet filters, 1 aerosol hose, charger and power lead, net price = £254.00

PARI Junior BOY'N'® (Pari) 〔NHS〕
Portable, for hospital or home use, containing *PARI LC PLUS Junior*® nebuliser with child mouthpiece, mask, connection tube, and mains cable. Filter replacement recommended every 12 months. Compatible with *PARI LC PLUS*® 〔NHS〕, *PARI LC PLUS Filter*® 〔NHS〕, and *PARI Baby*® 〔NHS〕 nebulisers, net price = £125.00

PARI Turbo BOY'N'® (Pari) 〔NHS〕
Portable, for hospital or home use, containing *PARI LC PLUS*® nebuliser with adult mouthpiece, mask, connection tube and mains cable. Filter replacement recommended every 12 months. Compatible with *PARI LC PLUS*® 〔NHS〕, *PARI LC PLUS FILTER*® 〔NHS〕, and *PARI BABY*® 〔NHS〕 nebulisers, net price = £115.00

PARI UNI light mobil® (Pari) 〔NHS〕
Portable, containing *PARI LC PLUS*® 〔NHS〕 nebuliser with connection tube, mains cable, car battery adaptor, and carrying case. Compatible with *PARI BABY*® 〔NHS〕, and *PARI LC PLUS FILTER*® 〔NHS〕 nebulisers. Nebulises bronchodilators, corticosteroids, and antibiotics, net price = £235.00

PARI WALK BOY® (Pari) 〔NHS〕
Portable, containing *PARI LC PLUS*® 〔NHS〕 nebuliser with connection tube, cable, rechargeable battery and carrying bag. Compatible with *PARI LC PLUS*® 〔NHS〕 and *PARI BABY*® 〔NHS〕 nebulisers, net price = £225.00; car cigarette lighter adaptor = £57.75

Porta-Neb® (Profile Respiratory) 〔NHS〕
Portable, containing *Sidestream Durable*® 〔NHS〕 nebuliser, 1 adult mask, 1 child mask, 1 angled mouthpiece, 1 coiled *Duratube*®, 4 inlet filters. Mains operated, net price = £117.50; with *Ventstream*® 〔NHS〕 nebuliser, 1 straight mouthpiece, 1 coiled *Duratube*®, 4 inlet filters, aerosol hose. Mains operated, net price = £131.00

De Vilbiss 5650® (De Vilbiss) 〔NHS〕
Home, clinic use, containing disposable nebuliser set, mouthpiece, mask, mains lead, tubing, thumb-valve. For use with bronchodilators, net price = £142.14

De Vilbiss 4650® (De Vilbiss) 〔NHS〕
Home, clinic and hospital use, with mouthpiece. Mains operated, net price = £93.95

Tourer® (Henleys) 〔NHS〕
Portable, home use. Mains/car battery operated; for use with bronchodilators, corticosteroids and antibiotics, net price = £135.00

Ultima® (Henleys) 〔NHS〕
Portable, home use. Rechargable or mains/car battery operated. Nebulises bronchodilators and corticosteroids, net price = £208.00 (includes case)

World Traveller HI FLO® (Medix) 〔NHS〕
Portable, containing 1 *Jet Nebuliser*® 〔NHS〕 set with mouthpiece, 1 adult and 1 child mask, 1 spare inlet filter, filter spanner. Battery, car, and mains operated; rechargeable battery pack available. Nebulises bronchodilators, corticosteroids, and antibiotics, net price excluding battery = £166.00; with battery = £216.00; carrying case available

■ **Compressors**

Omron CX3® (Omron) 〔NHS〕
Home and hospital use. Mains operated, net price = £48.75

System 22 CR50® (Profile Respiratory) 〔NHS〕
Home, clinic and hospital use. Mains operated, net price = £89.50. Also compatible with *Ventstream*® 〔NHS〕, and *Sidestream Durable*® 〔NHS〕

System 22 CR60® (Profile Respiratory) 〔NHS〕
Hospital use, high flow compressor. Mains operated, net price = £199.90. Also compatible with *System 22 Antibiotic Tee*® 〔NHS〕 for nebulisation of high viscosity drugs such as antibiotics

Turboneb® (Medix) 〔NHS〕
Hospital use, high flow compressor. Nebulises bronchodilators, corticosteroids, antibiotics, and pentamidine. Mains operated, net price = £125.00

■ **Ultrasonic nebulisers**
Ultrasonic nebulisers produce an aerosol by ultrasonic vibration of the drug solution and therefore do not require a gas flow

F16 Wave® (Parkside) 〔NHS〕
Portable, adjustable delivery rate. Mains/car battery operated or rechargeable battery pack (supplied), net price = £159.00

Liberty® (Medix) 〔NHS〕
Portable, home and clinic use, containing disposable mouthpiece and chamber cover. Mains and car battery operated. Nebulises bronchodilators and antibiotics, net price £124.99

Omron U1® (Omron) 〔NHS〕
Portable. Battery operated/mains adaptor, net price = £146.25

Omron NE U07® (Omron) 〔NHS〕
Portable. Mains operated or rechargeable battery pack, net price = £146.25 (mains version), rechargeable battery pack = £95.00

Ultra Neb 2000® (De Vilbiss) 〔NHS〕
Hospital, clinic and home use, delivery rate adjustable. Supplied with stand, net price = £1205.00

Nebuliser diluent

Nebulisation may be carried out using an undiluted nebuliser solution or it may require dilution beforehand. The usual diluent is sterile sodium chloride 0.9% (physiological saline).

Sodium Chloride (Non-proprietary) 〔PoM〕
Nebuliser solution, sodium chloride 0.9%, net price 20 × 2.5 mL = £5.49
Available from Galen (*Saline Steripoule*®), IVAX (*Saline Steri-Neb*®)

3.2   Corticosteroids

Corticosteroids are very effective in *asthma*; they reduce airway inflammation (and hence reduce oedema and secretion of mucus into the airway).

Patients with *chronic obstructive pulmonary disease* usually show little or no response to corticosteroids. Long-term studies have shown no reduction in the decline in lung function in chronic obstructive pulmonary disease in patients taking regular inhaled corticosteroids. Higher doses of inhaled corticosteroids may reduce symptoms and exacerbations slightly in patients with more severe chronic obstructive pulmonary disease. A trial of a corticosteroid can distinguish patients who in fact have asthma from those who have chronic obstructive pulmonary disease.

INHALATION. Inhaled corticosteroids are recommended for prophylactic treatment of asthma when patients are using a beta$_2$ agonist more than once daily (see Chronic Asthma table, p. 132). *Regular use* of inhaled corticosteroids reduces the risk of exacerbation of asthma.

Corticosteroid inhalers must be used regularly for maximum benefit; alleviation of symptoms usually occurs 3 to 7 days after initiation. **Beclometasone dipropionate** (beclomethasone dipropionate), **budesonide** and **fluticasone propionate** appear to be equally effective. Doses for CFC-free corticosteroid inhalers may be different from those that contain CFCs.

CFC-FREE INHALERS. Chlorofluorocarbon (CFC) propellants in pressurised aerosol inhalers are being replaced by hydrofluoroalkane (HFA) propellants. Patients receiving CFC-free inhalers should be reassured about the efficacy of the new inhalers and counselled that the aerosol may feel and taste different; any difficulty with the new inhaler should be discussed with the doctor or pharmacist.

If the inhaled corticosteroid causes coughing, the use of a beta$_2$ agonist beforehand may help.

Patients who have been taking long-term oral corticosteroids can often be transferred to an inhaled corticosteroid but the transfer must be slow, with gradual reduction in the dose of oral corticosteroid, and at a time when the asthma is well controlled.

High-dose inhalers are available for patients who respond only partially to standard-dose inhalers and long-acting beta$_2$ agonists or other long-acting bronchodilators (see Chronic Asthma, table, p. 132). High doses should be continued only if there is clear benefit over the lower dose. The recommended maximum doses of inhaled corticosteroids should not generally be exceeded. However, if higher doses are required (e.g. fluticasone in a dose above 500 micrograms twice daily in an adult or 200 micrograms twice daily in a child 4–16 years), then they should be initiated by specialists.

Systemic therapy may be necessary during episodes of infection or if asthma is worsening, when higher doses are needed and access of inhaled drug to small airways may be reduced; patients may need a reserve supply of tablets.

CAUTIONS OF INHALED CORTICOSTEROIDS. Caution is required in active or quiescent tuberculosis; systemic therapy may be required during periods of stress or when airways obstruction or mucus prevent drug access to smaller airways; **interactions:** Appendix 1 (corticosteroids).

PARADOXICAL BRONCHOSPASM. The potential for paradoxical bronchospasm (calling for discontinuation and alternative therapy) should be borne in mind—if mild it may be prevented by inhalation of a beta$_2$-adrenoceptor stimulant (or by transfer from an aerosol inhalation to a dry powder inhalation)

SIDE-EFFECTS OF INHALED CORTICOSTEROIDS. Inhaled corticosteroids have considerably fewer systemic effects than oral corticosteroids, but adverse effects have been reported.

Higher doses of inhaled corticosteroids have the potential to induce adrenal suppression (section 6.3.2) and patients on high doses should be given a 'steroid card'; such patients may need corticosteroid cover during an episode of stress (e.g. an operation). Inhaled corticosteroids in children have been associated with adrenal crisis and coma; excessive doses should be **avoided**, particularly of fluticasone, which should be given in a dose of 50–100 micrograms twice daily and the dose should not exceed 200 micrograms twice daily.

Bone mineral density is reduced following long-term inhalation of higher doses of corticosteroids, and this may predispose patients to osteoporosis (section 6.6). It is therefore sensible to ensure that the dose of inhaled corticosteroid is no higher than necessary to keep a patient's asthma under good control. The dose may therefore be reduced cautiously when the asthma has been well controlled for a few weeks as long as the patient knows that it is necessary to reinstate it should the asthma deteriorate or the peak flow rate fall.

In children, growth retardation associated with oral corticosteroid therapy does not seem to be a significant problem with recommended doses of inhaled therapy; although initial growth velocity may be reduced, there appears to be no effect on normal adult height. However, the CSM recommends that the height of children receiving prolonged treatment is monitored; if growth is slowed, referral to a paediatrician should be considered. Large-volume spacer devices should be used for administering inhaled corticosteroids in children under 5 years (see NICE guidance, section 3.1.5); they are also useful in older children and adults, particularly if high doses are required. Spacer devices increase airway deposition and reduce oropharyngeal deposition.

A small increased risk of glaucoma with prolonged high doses of inhaled corticosteroids has been reported; cataracts have also been reported with inhaled corticosteroids. Hoarseness and candidiasis of the mouth or throat have been reported, usually only with large doses (see also below). Hypersensitivity reactions (including rash and angioedema) have been reported rarely.

CANDIDIASIS. Candidiasis can be reduced by using spacer, see notes above, and responds to antifungal lozenges (section 12.3.2) without discontinuation of therapy—rinsing the mouth with water (or cleaning child's teeth) after inhalation of a dose may also be helpful

ORAL. Acute attacks of asthma should be treated with short courses of oral corticosteroids starting with a high dose, e.g. prednisolone 40–50 mg daily for a few days. Patients whose asthma has deteriorated rapidly usually respond quickly to corticosteroids. The dose can usually be stopped abruptly in a mild exacerbation of asthma (see also Withdrawal of Corticosteroids, section 6.3.2) but it should be reduced gradually in those with poorer asthma control, to reduce the possibility of serious relapse. For use of corticosteroids in the emergency treatment of acute severe asthma see table on p. 133.

In chronic continuing asthma, when the response to other anti-asthma drugs has been relatively small, longer term administration of oral corticosteroids may be necessary; in such cases high doses of an inhaled corticosteroid should be continued to minimise oral corticosteroid requirements. Oral corticosteroids should normally be taken as a single dose in the morning to reduce the disturbance to circadian cortisol secretion. Dosage should always be titrated to the lowest dose that controls symptoms. Regular peak flow measurements often help to optimise the dose.

Alternate-day administration has not been very successful in the management of asthma in adults because control can deteriorate during the second 24 hours. If alternate-day administration is introduced, pulmonary function should be monitored carefully over the 48 hours.

PARENTERAL. For the use of hydrocortisone injection in the emergency treatment of acute severe asthma, see Acute Severe Asthma table, p. 133.

BECLOMETASONE DIPROPIONATE

(Beclomethasone Dipropionate)

Indications: prophylaxis of asthma (see also Chronic Asthma table, p. 132)

Cautions: see notes above

Side-effects: see notes above

Dose: Standard-dose inhalers

By aerosol inhalation (for *Qvar®* dose see under preparation), 200 micrograms twice daily *or* 100 micrograms 3–4 times daily (in more severe cases initially 600–800 micrograms daily); CHILD 50–100 micrograms 2–4 times daily

By inhalation of powder (*Becodisks®*; for *Asmabec®* dose see under preparation), 400 micrograms twice daily *or* 200 micrograms 3–4 times daily; CHILD 100 micrograms 2–4 times daily *or* 200 micrograms twice daily

High-dose inhalers

By aerosol inhalation (for *Qvar®* dose see under preparation), 500 micrograms twice daily *or* 250 micrograms 4 times daily; if necessary may be increased to 500 micrograms 4 times daily; CHILD not recommended

By inhalation of powder (*Becloforte®* disks; for *Asmabec®* dose see under preparation), 400 micrograms twice daily; if necessary may be increased to 800 micrograms twice daily; CHILD not recommended

---

■ Standard-dose inhalers

Beclometasone (Non-proprietary) PoM

Aerosol inhalation, beclometasone dipropionate 50 micrograms/metered inhalation, net price 200-dose unit = £4.31; 100 micrograms/metered inhalation, 200-dose unit = £8.24; 200 micrograms/metered inhalation, 200-dose unit = £19.61.

Label: 8, counselling, dose
Available from APS, Generics, and IVAX (*Beclazone®*)
Excipients: include CFC propellants

Dry powder for inhalation, beclometasone dipropionate 100 micrograms/metered inhalation, net price 100-dose unit = £5.58; 200 micrograms/metered inhalation, 100-dose unit = £10.29.

Label: 8, counselling, dose
Available from Trinity (*Pulvinal® Beclometasone Dipropionate*)

Inhalation powder, hard capsule (for use with *Cyclohaler®* device), beclometasone dipropionate 100 micrograms, net price 120-cap pack = £9.08; 200 micrograms, 120-cap pack = £16.07. Label: 8, counselling, dose
Available from APS (*Beclometasone Cyclocaps®*)

AeroBec® (3M) PoM

AeroBec 50 Autohaler® (breath-actuated aerosol inhalation), beclometasone dipropionate 50 micrograms/metered inhalation, net price 200-dose unit = £4.34. Label: 8, counselling, dose
Excipients: include CFC propellants

AeroBec 100 Autohaler® (breath-actuated aerosol inhalation), beclometasone dipropionate 100 micrograms/metered inhalation, net price 200-dose unit = £8.24. Label: 8, counselling, dose
Excipients: include CFC propellants

Asmabec Clickhaler® (Celltech) PoM

Dry powder for inhalation, beclometasone dipropionate 50 micrograms/metered inhalation, net price 200-dose unit = £7.18; 100 micrograms/metered inhalation, 200-dose unit = £10.55.

Label: 8, counselling, dose
Dose: by inhalation of powder, 200–400 micrograms daily, in 2–4 divided doses (in more severe cases initially 0.8–1.6 mg daily, in 2–4 divided doses—see also High-dose inhalers); CHILD 50–100 micrograms 2–4 times daily

Beclazone Easi-Breathe® (IVAX) PoM

Aerosol inhalation, beclometasone dipropionate 50 micrograms/metered inhalation, net price 200-dose breath-actuated unit = £4.34; 100 micrograms/metered inhalation, 200-dose breath-actuated unit = £8.24. Label: 8, counselling, dose
Excipients: include CFC propellants

Becodisks® (A&H) PoM

Dry powder for inhalation, disks containing 8 blisters of beclometasone dipropionate 100 micrograms/blister, net price 15 disks with *Diskhaler®* device = £12.90, 15-disk refill = £12..28; 200 micrograms/blister, 15 disks with *Diskhaler®* device = £24.59, 15-disk refill = £23.96; 400 micrograms/blister, 15 disks with *Diskhaler®* device = £48.54, 15-disk refill = £47.92. Label: 8, counselling, dose

Becotide® (A&H) PoM

Becotide®-50 aerosol inhalation, beclometasone dipropionate 50 micrograms/metered inhalation. Net price 200-dose unit = £5.43. Label: 8, counselling, dose
Excipients: include CFC propellants

Becotide®-100 aerosol inhalation, beclometasone dipropionate 100 micrograms/metered inhalation. Net price 200-dose unit = £10.32. Label: 8, counselling, dose
Excipients: include CFC propellants

Becotide®-200 aerosol inhalation, beclometasone dipropionate 200 micrograms/metered inhalation. Net price 200-dose unit = £19.61. Label: 8, counselling, dose, 10 steroid card
Excipients: include CFC propellants
NOTE. *Becotide®-200* not indicated for children

Qvar® (IVAX) PoM

Qvar® 50 aerosol inhalation, beclometasone dipropionate 50 micrograms/metered inhalation, net price 200-dose unit = £7.87. Label: 8, counselling, dose

Qvar® 100 aerosol inhalation, beclometasone dipropionate 100 micrograms/metered inhalation, net price 200-dose unit = £17.21. Label: 8, counselling, dose, 10 steroid card

Qvar 50 Autohaler® (breath-actuated aerosol inhalation), beclometasone dipropionate 50 micrograms/metered inhalation, net price 200-dose unit = £7.87. Label: 8, counselling, dose

Qvar 100 Autohaler® (breath-actuated aerosol inhalation), beclometasone dipropionate 100 micrograms/metered inhalation, net price 200-dose unit = £17.21. Label: 8, counselling, dose, 10 steroid card
Excipients: include HFA-134a (a non-CFC propellant), ethanol
Dose: by aerosol inhalation, 50–200 micrograms twice daily, if necessary may be increased to max. 400 micrograms twice daily; CHILD not recommended
NOTE. When transferring a patient from a CFC-containing inhaler (asthma well controlled), initially a 100-microgram metered dose of *Qvar*® should be substituted for:

- 200–250 micrograms of beclometasone dipropionate or budesonide
- 100 micrograms of fluticasone propionate

When transferring a patient from a CFC-containing inhaler (asthma poorly controlled), initially a 100-microgram metered dose of *Qvar*® should be substituted for 100 micrograms of beclometasone dipropionate, budesonide or fluticasone propionate

■ High-dose inhalers
NOTE. High-dose inhalers not indicated for children

> Chronic Asthma table, see p. 132
> Acute Severe Asthma table, see p. 133

Beclometasone (Non-proprietary) PoM
Aerosol inhalation, beclometasone dipropionate 250 micrograms/metered inhalation, net price 200-dose unit = £17.88. Label: 8, counselling, dose, 10 steroid card
Available from APS, Generics, and IVAX (*Beclazone*®)
Excipients: include CFC propellants
Dry powder for inhalation, beclometasone dipropionate 400 micrograms/metered inhalation, net price 100-dose unit = £20.41. Label: 8, counselling, dose, 10 steroid card
Available from Trinity (*Pulvinal*® *Beclometasone Dipropionate*)
Inhalation powder, hard capsule (for use with *Cyclohaler*® device), beclometasone dipropionate 400 micrograms, net price 120-cap pack = £32.72. Label: 8, counselling, dose, 10, steroid card
Available from APS (*Beclometasone 400 Cyclocaps*®)

AeroBec Forte® (3M) PoM
Aerosol inhalation, beclometasone dipropionate 250 micrograms/metered inhalation, net price 200-inhalation breath-actuated unit (*Autohaler*®) = £18.02. Label: 8, counselling, dose, 10 steroid card
Excipients: include CFC propellants

Asmabec Clickhaler® (Celltech) PoM
Dry powder for inhalation, beclometasone dipropionate 250 micrograms/metered inhalation, net price 100-dose unit = £13.24. Label: 8, counselling, dose, 10 steroid card
Dose: by inhalation of powder, 500 micrograms twice daily *or* 250 micrograms 4 times daily; if necessary may be increased to 500 micrograms 4 times daily; CHILD not recommended

Beclazone Easi-Breathe® (IVAX) PoM
Aerosol inhalation, beclometasone dipropionate 250 micrograms/metered inhalation, net price 200-dose breath-actuated unit = £18.02. Label: 8, counselling, dose, 10 steroid card
Excipients: include CFC propellants

Becloforte® (A&H) PoM
Aerosol inhalation, beclometasone dipropionate 250 micrograms/metered inhalation. Net price 200-dose unit = £23.10. Label: 8, counselling, dose, 10 steroid card
Excipients: include CFC propellants

Qvar® (IVAX) PoM
See under Standard-dose inhalers

BUDESONIDE

Indications: prophylaxis of asthma (see also Chronic Asthma table, p. 132)
Cautions: see notes above
Side-effects: see notes above
Dose: see preparations below

Budesonide (Non-proprietary) PoM
Inhalation powder, hard capsule (for use with *Cyclohaler*® device), budesonide 200 micrograms, net price 100-cap pack = £16.65; 400 micrograms, 50-cap pack = £16.65. Label: 8, counselling, dose, 10, steroid card
Dose: 0.2–1.6 mg daily in divided doses adjusted as necessary; CHILD over 6 years 200–400 micrograms daily in divided doses adjusted as necessary (max. 800 micrograms daily)
Available from APS (*Budesonide Cyclocaps*®)

Pulmicort® (AstraZeneca) PoM
LS aerosol inhalation, budesonide 50 micrograms/metered inhalation. Net price 200-dose unit = £7.33. Label: 8, counselling, dose
Excipients: include CFC propellants
Aerosol inhalation, budesonide 200 micrograms/metered inhalation. Net price 200-dose unit with or without *NebuChamber*® = £20.90; 100-dose unit = £7.60 (hosp. only). Label: 8, counselling, dose, 10 steroid card
Excipients: include CFC propellants
Dose: by aerosol inhalation, 200 micrograms twice daily; may be reduced in well-controlled asthma to not less than 200 micrograms daily; in severe asthma dose may be increased to 1.6 mg daily; CHILD 50–400 micrograms twice daily; in severe asthma may be increased to 800 micrograms daily
Turbohaler® (= dry powder inhaler), budesonide 100 micrograms/inhalation, net price 200-dose unit = £18.50; 200 micrograms/inhalation, 100-dose unit = £18.50; 400 micrograms/inhalation, 50-dose unit = £18.50. Label: 8, counselling, dose, 10 steroid card
Dose: by inhalation of powder, when starting treatment, during periods of severe asthma, and while reducing or discontinuing oral corticosteroid, 0.2–1.6 mg daily in 2 divided doses; in less severe cases 200–400 micrograms once daily (each evening); patients already controlled on inhaled beclometasone dipropionate or budesonide administered twice daily may be transferred to once-daily dosing (each evening) at the same equivalent total daily dose (up to 800 micrograms once daily); CHILD under 12 years 200–800 micrograms daily in 2 divided doses (800 micrograms daily in severe asthma) *or* 200–400 micrograms once daily (each evening)
Respules® (= single-dose units for nebulisation), budesonide 250 micrograms/mL, net price 20 × 2-mL (500-microgram) unit = £32.00; 500 micrograms/mL, 20 × 2-mL (1-mg) unit = £44.64. May be diluted with sterile sodium chloride 0.9%. Label: 8, counselling, dose, 10 steroid card
Dose: by inhalation of nebulised suspension, when starting treatment, during periods of severe asthma, and while reducing or discontinuing oral corticosteroids, 1–2 mg twice daily (may be increased further in very severe asthma); CHILD 3 months–12 years, 0.5–1 mg twice daily Maintenance, usually half above dose
Croup, 2 mg as a single dose (*or* as two 1-mg doses separated by 30 minutes)

■ Compound preparations

Symbicort® (AstraZeneca) PoM

Symbicort 100/6 Turbohaler® (= dry powder inhaler), budesonide 80 micrograms, formoterol fumarate 4.5 micrograms/metered inhalation, net price 120-dose unit = £33.00. Label: 8, counselling, dose, 10 steroid card

NOTE. Each metered inhalation of *Symbicort® 100/6* delivers the same quantity of budesonide as a 100-microgram metered inhalation of *Pulmicort Turbohaler®* and of formoterol as a 6-microgram metered inhalation of *Oxis Turbohaler®*

Dose: by inhalation of powder, asthma, ADULT and CHILD over 12 years, 1–2 puffs twice daily, CHILD over 6 years, 2 puffs twice daily; may be reduced in well-controlled asthma to once daily

Symbicort 200/6 Turbohaler® (= dry powder inhaler), budesonide 160 micrograms, formoterol fumarate 4.5 micrograms/metered inhalation, net price 120-dose unit = £38.00. Label: 8, counselling, dose, 10 steroid card

NOTE. Each metered inhalation of *Symbicort® 200/6* delivers the same quantity of budesonide as a 200-microgram metered inhalation of *Pulmicort Turbohaler®* and of formoterol as a 6-microgram metered inhalation of *Oxis Turbohaler®*

Dose: by inhalation of powder, asthma, ADULT and CHILD over 12 years, 1–2 puffs twice daily, may be reduced in well-controlled asthma to 1–2 puffs once daily

Chronic obstructive pulmonary disease, 2 puffs twice daily; CHILD not recommended

Symbicort 400/12 Turbohaler® (= dry powder inhaler), budesonide 320 micrograms, formoterol fumarate 9 micrograms/metered inhalation, net price 60-dose unit = £38.00. Label: 8, counselling, dose, 10 steroid card

NOTE. Each metered inhalation of *Symbicort® 400/12* delivers the same quantity of budesonide as a 400-microgram metered inhalation of *Pulmicort Turbohaler®* and of formoterol as a 12-microgram metered inhalation of *Oxis Turbohaler®*

Dose: by inhalation of powder, asthma, ADULT and CHILD over 12 years, 1 puff twice daily, may be reduced in well-controlled asthma to 1 puff once daily

Chronic obstructive pulmonary disease, 1 puff twice daily; CHILD not recommended

---

FLUTICASONE PROPIONATE

Indications: prophylaxis of asthma (see also Chronic Asthma table, p. 132)

Cautions: see notes above

Side-effects: see notes above

Dose: see preparations below

Flixotide® (A&H) PoM

Accuhaler® (dry powder for inhalation), disk containing 60 blisters of fluticasone propionate 50 micrograms/blister with *Accuhaler®* device, net price = £6.86; 100 micrograms/blister with *Accuhaler®* device = £9.60; 250 micrograms/blister with *Accuhaler®* device = £22.86; 500 micrograms/blister with *Accuhaler®* device = £38.86. Label: 8, counselling, dose; 250- and 500-microgram strengths also label 10 steroid card

NOTE. *Flixotide Accuhaler®* 250 micrograms and 500 micrograms are not indicated for children

Dose: by inhalation of powder, ADULT and CHILD over 16 years, 100–250 micrograms twice daily, increased according to severity of asthma to 1 mg twice daily; CHILD 4–16 years, 50–100 micrograms twice daily adjusted as necessary; max. 200 micrograms twice daily

Aerosol inhalation, fluticasone propionate 25 micrograms/metered inhalation, net price 120-dose unit = £6.86. Label: 8, counselling, dose

Excipients: include CFC propellants

Dose: by aerosol inhalation, CHILD over 4 years, 50–100 micrograms twice daily adjusted as necessary; max. 200 micrograms twice daily

Diskhaler® (dry powder for inhalation), fluticasone propionate 50 micrograms/blister, net price 15 disks of 4 blisters with *Diskhaler®* device = £8.78, 15-disk refill = £8.21; 100 micrograms/blister, 15 disks of 4 blisters with *Diskhaler®* device = £13.67, 15-disk refill = £13.10; 250 micrograms/blister, 15 disks of 4 blisters with *Diskhaler®* device = £25.92, 15-disk refill = £25.35; 500 micrograms/blister, 15 disks of 4 blisters with *Diskhaler®* device = £43.06, 15-disk refill = £42.49. Label: 8, counselling, dose; 250- and 500-microgram strengths also label 10 steroid card

NOTE. *Flixotide Diskhaler®* 250 micrograms and 500 micrograms are not indicated for children

Dose: by inhalation of powder, ADULT and CHILD over 16 years, 100–250 micrograms twice daily, increased according to severity of asthma to 1 mg twice daily; CHILD 4–16 years, 50–100 micrograms twice daily adjusted as necessary; max. 200 micrograms twice daily

Evohaler® ▼ *aerosol inhalation*, fluticasone propionate 50 micrograms/metered inhalation, net price 120-dose unit = £5.85; 125 micrograms/metered inhalation, 120-dose unit = £22.86; 250 micrograms/metered inhalation, 120-dose unit = £38.86. Label: 8, counselling, dose, change to CFC-free inhaler; 250-microgram strength also label 10 steroid card

Excipients: include HFA-134a (a non-CFC propellant)

NOTE. *Flixotide Evohaler®* 125 micrograms and 250 micrograms not indicated for children

Dose: by aerosol inhalation, ADULT and CHILD over 16 years, 100–250 micrograms twice daily, increased according to severity of asthma to 1 mg twice daily; CHILD 4–16 years, 50–100 micrograms twice daily adjusted as necessary; max. 200 micrograms twice daily

Nebules® (= single-dose units for nebulisation) fluticasone propionate 250 micrograms/mL, net price 10 × 2-mL (500-microgram) unit = £10.04; 1 mg/mL, 10 × 2-mL (2-mg) unit = £40.16. May be diluted with sterile sodium chloride 0.9%. Label: 8, counselling, dose, 10 steroid card

Dose: by inhalation of nebulised suspension, ADULT and CHILD over 16 years, 0.5–2 mg twice daily

■ Compound preparations

Seretide® (A&H) PoM

Seretide 100 Accuhaler® (dry powder for inhalation), disk containing 60 blisters of fluticasone propionate 100 micrograms, salmeterol (as xinafoate) 50 micrograms/blister with *Accuhaler®* device, net price = £33.54. Label: 8, counselling, dose

Dose: by inhalation of powder, asthma, ADULT and CHILD over 4 years, 1 blister twice daily, reduced to 1 blister once daily if control maintained

Seretide 250 Accuhaler® (dry powder for inhalation), disk containing 60 blisters of fluticasone propionate 250 micrograms, salmeterol (as xinafoate) 50 micrograms/blister with *Accuhaler®* device, net price = £39.41. Label: 8, counselling, dose, 10 steroid card

Dose: by inhalation of powder, asthma, ADULT and CHILD over 12 years, 1 blister twice daily

Seretide 500 Accuhaler® (dry powder for inhalation), disk containing 60 blisters of fluticasone

propionate 500 micrograms, salmeterol (as xinafoate) 50 micrograms/blister with *Accuhaler*® device, net price = £44.00. Label: 8, counselling, dose, 10 steroid card
Dose: by inhalation of powder, asthma, ADULT and CHILD over 12 years, 1 blister twice daily
Chronic obstructive pulmonary disease, ADULT 1 blister twice daily

Seretide 50 Evohaler® (aerosol inhalation), flutica-sone propionate 50 micrograms, salmeterol (as xinafoate) 25 micrograms/metered inhalation, net price 120-dose unit = £19.50. Label: 8, counsel-ling, dose, change to CFC-free inhaler
Excipients: include HFA-134a (a non-CFC propellant)
Dose: by aerosol inhalation, asthma, ADULT and CHILD over 12 years, 2 puffs twice daily, reduced to 2 puffs once daily if control maintained

Seretide 125 Evohaler® (aerosol inhalation), flu-ticasone propionate 125 micrograms, salmeterol (as xinafoate) 25 micrograms/metered inhalation, net price 120-dose unit = £39.41. Label: 8, counselling, dose, change to CFC-free inhaler, 10 steroid card
Excipients: include HFA-134a (a non-CFC propellant)
Dose: by aerosol inhalation, asthma, ADULT and CHILD over 12 years, 2 puffs twice daily

Seretide 250 Evohaler® (aerosol inhalation), flu-ticasone propionate 250 micrograms, salmeterol (as xinafoate) 25 micrograms/metered inhalation, net price 120-dose unit = £66.98. Label: 8, counselling, dose, change to CFC-free inhaler, 10 steroid card
Excipients: include HFA-134a (a non-CFC propellant)
Dose: by aerosol inhalation, asthma, ADULT and CHILD over 12 years, 2 puffs twice daily

MOMETASONE FUROATE

Indications: prophylaxis of asthma (see also Chronic Asthma table, p. 132)
Cautions: see notes above
Side-effects: see notes above; also pharyngitis
Dose: *by inhalation of powder*, 200–400 micr-ograms as a single dose in the evening or in 2 divided doses; dose increased to 400 micrograms twice daily if necessary; CHILD not recommended

Asmanex® (Schering-Plough) ▼ PoM
Twisthaler (= dry powder inhaler), mometasone furoate 200 micrograms/metered inhalation, net price 30-dose unit = £16.00, 60-dose unit = £24.00; 400 micrograms/metered inhalation, 30-dose unit = £22.20, 60-dose unit = £36.75. Label: 8, counselling, dose, 10 steroid card

3.3 Cromoglicate, related therapy and leukotriene receptor antagonists

3.3.1	Cromoglicate and related therapy
3.3.2	Leukotriene receptor antagonists

3.3.1 Cromoglicate and related therapy

The mode of action of **sodium cromoglicate** and **nedocromil** is not completely understood. They may be of value in asthma with an allergic basis, but, in practice, it is difficult to predict who will benefit; they could probably be given for 4 to 6 weeks to assess response. Dose frequency is adjusted accord-ing to response but is usually 3 to 4 times a day initially; this may subsequently be reduced.

In general, *prophylaxis* with sodium cromoglicate is less effective than prophylaxis with corticosteroid inhalations (see Chronic Asthma table, p. 132). There is evidence of efficacy of nedocromil in children aged 5–12 years. Sodium cromoglicate is of no value in the treatment of acute attacks of asthma.

Sodium cromoglicate can prevent exercise-induced asthma. However, exercise-induced asthma may reflect poor overall control and the patient should be assessed.

If inhalation of the dry powder form of sodium cromoglicate causes bronchospasm a selective beta$_2$-adrenoceptor stimulant such as salbutamol or terbut-aline should be inhaled a few minutes beforehand. The nebuliser solution is an alternative means of delivery for children who cannot manage the dry powder inhaler or the aerosol.

SODIUM CROMOGLICATE

(Sodium Cromoglycate)
Indications: prophylaxis of asthma; food allergy (section 1.5); allergic conjunctivitis (section 11.4.2); allergic rhinitis (section 12.2.1)
Side-effects: coughing, transient bronchospasm, and throat irritation due to inhalation of powder (see also notes above)
Dose: *by aerosol inhalation*, ADULT and CHILD, 10 mg (2 puffs) 4 times daily, increased in severe cases or during periods of risk to 6–8 times daily; additional doses may also be taken before exercise; maintenance 5 mg (1 puff) 4 times daily
By inhalation of powder (Spincaps®), ADULT and CHILD, 20 mg 4 times daily, increased in severe cases to 8 times daily; additional doses may also be taken before exercise
By inhalation of nebulised solution, ADULT and CHILD, 20 mg 4 times daily, increased in severe cases to 6 times daily
COUNSELLING. Regular use is necessary

Sodium Cromoglicate (Non-proprietary) PoM
Aerosol inhalation, sodium cromoglicate 5 mg/metered inhalation. Net price 112-dose unit = £15.30. Label: 8
Available from IVAX (*Cromogen*®)
Excipients: include CFC propellants
Nebuliser solution, sodium cromoglicate 10 mg/mL. Net price 60 × 2-mL unit-dose vials = £11.58
Available from IVAX (*Cromogen Steri-Neb*®)

Cromogen Easi-Breathe® (IVAX) PoM
Aerosol inhalation, sodium cromoglicate 5 mg/metered inhalation. Net price 112-dose breath-actuated unit = £13.91. Label: 8
Excipients: include CFC propellants

Intal® (Rhône-Poulenc Rorer) PoM
Aerosol inhalation, sodium cromoglicate 5 mg/metered inhalation. Net price 112-dose unit = £19.09; 2 × 112-dose unit with spacer device (*Syncroner*®) = £37.98; also available with large volume spacer inhaler (*Fisonair*®), complete unit = £22.06. Label: 8
Excipients: include CFC propellants

Spincaps®, yellow/clear, sodium cromoglicate 20 mg. Net price 112-cap pack = £16.60. Label: 8
Spinhaler insufflator® (for use with *Intal Spincaps*). Net price = £1.92
Nebuliser solution sodium cromoglicate 10 mg/mL. Net price 2-mL amp = 34p. For use with power-operated nebuliser

■ Compound preparations
NOTE. The compound inhalation of sodium cromoglicate with a beta-adrenoceptor stimulant is not recommended as the inhalation is liable to be used inappropriately for relief of bronchospasm rather than for its prophylactic effect

Aerocrom® (Castlemead) [PoM] [▭]
Aerosol inhalation, sodium cromoglicate 1 mg, salbutamol (as sulphate) 100 micrograms/metered inhalation, net price 200-dose unit = £34.42; 200-dose unit with spacer device (*Syncroner*®) = £34.42. Label: 8
Excipients: include CFC propellants
Dose: by aerosol inhalation, 2 inhalations 4 times daily; CHILD, not recommended

NEDOCROMIL SODIUM

Indications: prophylaxis of asthma
Side-effects: see under Sodium Cromoglicate; also headache, nausea, vomiting, dyspepsia and abdominal pain; bitter taste (masked by mint flavour)
Dose: *by aerosol inhalation*, ADULT and CHILD over 6 years 4 mg (2 puffs) 4 times daily, when control achieved may be possible to reduce to twice daily
COUNSELLING. Regular use is necessary

Tilade® (Pantheon) [PoM]
Aerosol inhalation, mint-flavoured, nedocromil sodium 2 mg/metered inhalation. Net price 2 × 56-dose units = £42.98; 2 × 112-dose units with spacer device (*Syncroner*®) = £85.96. Label: 8
Excipients: include CFC propellants

Related therapy

Antihistamines are of no value in the treatment of bronchial asthma. **Ketotifen** is an antihistamine with an action said to resemble that of sodium cromoglicate, but it has proved disappointing.

KETOTIFEN

Indications: see notes above
Cautions: previous anti-asthmatic treatment should be continued for a minimum of 2 weeks after initiation of ketotifen treatment; pregnancy and breast-feeding (see Appendixes 4 and 5); **interactions:** Appendix 1 (antihistamines)—also, manufacturer advises avoid with oral antidiabetics (fall in thrombocyte count reported)
DRIVING. Drowsiness may affect performance of skilled tasks (e.g. driving); effects of alcohol enhanced
Side-effects: drowsiness, dry mouth, slight dizziness; CNS stimulation, weight gain also reported
Dose: 1 mg twice daily with food increased if necessary to 2 mg twice daily; initial treatment in readily sedated patients 0.5–1 mg at night; CHILD over 2 years 1 mg twice daily

Zaditen® (Novartis) [PoM]
Tablets, scored, ketotifen (as hydrogen fumarate) 1 mg. Net price 60-tab pack = £9.77. Label: 2, 8, 21
Elixir, ketotifen (as hydrogen fumarate) 1 mg/5 mL. Net price 300 mL = £11.57. Label: 2, 8, 21

The leukotriene receptor antagonists, **montelukast** and **zafirlukast**, block the effects of cysteinyl leukotrienes in the airways. They are effective in asthma when used alone or with an inhaled corticosteroid (see Chronic Asthma table, p. 132). Montelukast has not been shown to be more effective than a standard dose of inhaled corticosteroid but the two drugs appear to have an additive effect. The leukotriene receptor antagonists may be of benefit in exercise-induced asthma and in those with concomitant rhinitis but they are less effective in those with severe asthma who are also receiving high doses of other drugs.

The **CSM** has advised that leukotriene receptor antagonists should not be used to relieve an attack of acute severe asthma and that their use does not necessarily allow a reduction in existing corticosteroid treatment.

CHURG-STRAUSS SYNDROME. Churg-Strauss syndrome (characterised by a history of asthma, and often rhinitis and sinusitis, with systemic vasculitis and eosinophilia) has been associated with the use of leukotriene receptor antagonists; in many cases the reaction followed the reduction or withdrawal of oral corticosteroid therapy. The CSM has advised that in patients prescribed leukotriene receptor antagonists prescribers should be alert to the development of eosinophilia, vasculitic rash, worsening pulmonary symptoms, cardiac complications, or peripheral neuropathy.

MONTELUKAST

Indications: prophylaxis of asthma, see notes above and Chronic Asthma table, p. 132
Cautions: pregnancy (Appendix 4) and breast-feeding (Appendix 5); Churg-Strauss syndrome, see notes above; **interactions:** Appendix 1 (leukotriene antagonists)
Side-effects: gastro-intestinal disturbances, dry mouth, thirst; hypersensitivity reactions including anaphylaxis, angioedema and skin reactions; asthenia, dizziness, irritability, restlessness, headache, sleep disorders (insomnia, drowsiness, abnormal dreams, nightmares); upper respiratory-tract infection, fever; arthralgia, myalgia; palpitations, increased bleeding tendency, oedema, hallucinations, and seizures also reported
Dose: 10 mg daily at bedtime; CHILD 2–5 years 4 mg daily at bedtime, 6–14 years 5 mg daily at bedtime

Singulair® (MSD) [PoM]
Chewable tablets, both pink, cherry-flavoured, montelukast (as sodium salt) 4 mg, net price 28-tab pack = £25.69; 5 mg, 28-tab pack = £25.69. Label: 23, 24
Excipients: include aspartame equivalent to phenylalanine 674 micrograms/4-mg tablet and 842 micrograms/5-mg tablet (section 9.4.1)
Tablets, beige, f/c, montelukast (as sodium salt) 10 mg, net price 28-tab pack = £25.69

ZAFIRLUKAST

Indications: prophylaxis of asthma, see notes above and Chronic Asthma table, p. 132
Cautions: elderly, pregnancy (Appendix 4), renal

impairment (Appendix 3); Churg-Strauss syndrome, see notes above; **interactions:** Appendix 1 (leukotriene antagonists)

HEPATIC DISORDERS. Patients or their carers should be told how to recognise development of liver disorder and advised to seek medical attention if symptoms or signs such as persistent nausea, vomiting, malaise or jaundice develop

Contra-indications: hepatic impairment (Appendix 2); breast-feeding (Appendix 5)

Side-effects: gastro-intestinal disturbances; headache; rarely bleeding disorders, hypersensitivity reactions including angioedema and skin reactions, arthralgia, myalgia, lower limb oedema, raised liver enzymes, hepatitis, thrombocytopenia and very rarely agranulocytosis; also respiratory-tract infection in the elderly

Dose: 20 mg twice daily; CHILD under 12 years, not recommended

Accolate® (AstraZeneca) [PoM]
Tablets, f/c, zafirlukast 20 mg, net price 56-tab pack = £28.26. Label: 23

3.4 Antihistamines, hyposensitisation, and allergic emergencies

3.4.1 Antihistamines
3.4.2 Hyposensitisation
3.4.3 Allergic emergencies

3.4.1 Antihistamines

All antihistamines are of potential value in the treatment of nasal allergies, particularly seasonal allergic rhinitis (hay fever), and they may be of some value in vasomotor rhinitis. They reduce rhinorrhoea and sneezing but are usually less effective for nasal congestion. Antihistamines are used topically in the eye (section 11.4.2), in the nose (section 12.2.1), and on the skin (section 13.3).

Oral antihistamines are also of some value in preventing urticaria and are used to treat urticarial rashes, pruritus, and insect bites and stings; they are also used in drug allergies. Injections of chlorphenamine (chlorpheniramine) or promethazine are used as an adjunct to adrenaline (epinephrine) in the emergency treatment of anaphylaxis and angioedema (section 3.4.3). For the use of antihistamines (including cinnarizine, cyclizine, and promethazine teoclate) in nausea and vomiting, see section 4.6. Buclizine is included as an anti-emetic in a preparation for migraine (section 4.7.4.1). For reference to the use of antihistamines for occasional insomnia, see section 4.1.1.

Antihistamines differ in their duration of action and incidence of drowsiness and antimuscarinic effects. Many older antihistamines are relatively short acting but some (e.g. promethazine) act for up to 12 hours, while most of the newer non-sedating antihistamines are long acting.

All older antihistamines cause sedation but **alimemazine** (trimeprazine) and **promethazine** may be more sedating whereas **chlorphenamine** and

cyclizine (section 4.6) may be less so. This sedating activity is sometimes used to manage the pruritus associated with some allergies. There is little evidence that any one of the older, 'sedating' antihistamines is superior to another and patients vary widely in their response.

Non-sedating antihistamines such as **acrivastine**, **cetirizine**, **desloratadine** (an active metabolite of loratadine), **fexofenadine** (an active metabolite of terfenadine), **levocetirizine** (an isomer of cetirizine), **loratadine**, **mizolastine**, and **terfenadine** cause less sedation and psychomotor impairment than the older antihistamines because they penetrate the blood brain barrier only to a slight extent. Terfenadine is associated with hazardous arrhythmias.

CAUTIONS AND CONTRA-INDICATIONS. Sedating antihistamines have significant antimuscarinic activity and they should therefore be used with caution in prostatic hypertrophy, urinary retention, glaucoma and pyloroduodenal obstruction. Antihistamines should be used with caution in hepatic disease (Appendix 2) and dose reduction may be necessary in renal impairment (Appendix 3). Caution may be required in epilepsy. Children and the elderly are more susceptible to side-effects. Many antihistamines should be avoided in porphyria although some (e.g. chlorphenamine and cetirizine) are thought to be safe (section 9.8.2). **Interactions:** Appendix 1 (antihistamines); **important:** see also under Terfenadine.

SIDE-EFFECTS. Drowsiness is a significant side-effect with most of the older antihistamines although paradoxical stimulation may occur rarely, especially with high doses or in children and the elderly. Drowsiness may diminish after a few days of treatment and is considerably less of a problem with the newer antihistamines (see also notes above). Side-effects that are more common with the older antihistamines include headache, psychomotor impairment, and antimuscarinic effects such as urinary retention, dry mouth, blurred vision, and gastro-intestinal disturbances.

Other side-effects of antihistamines include palpitations and arrhythmias (**important:** see especially risks associated with *terfenadine,* below), hypotension, hypersensitivity reactions (including bronchospasm, angioedema, and anaphylaxis, rashes and photosensitivity reactions), extrapyramidal effects, dizziness, confusion, depression, sleep disturbances, tremor, convulsions, blood disorders, and liver dysfunction.

Non-sedating antihistamines

DRIVING. Although drowsiness is rare, nevertheless patients should be advised that it can occur and may affect performance of skilled tasks (e.g. driving); excess alcohol should be avoided.

ACRIVASTINE
Indications: symptomatic relief of allergy such as hay fever, urticaria
Cautions: see notes above; pregnancy (Appendix 4) and breast-feeding (Appendix 5)
Contra-indications: see notes above; also avoid in renal impairment; hypersensitivity to triprolidine

Side-effects: see notes above; incidence of sedation and antimuscarinic effects low

Dose: 8 mg 3 times daily; CHILD under 12 years, not recommended; ELDERLY not recommended

■ Preparations

Capsules can be sold to the public for the treatment of hayfever and allergic skin conditions in adults and children over 12 years provided packs do not contain over 10 days' supply (*Benadryl® Allergy Relief*)

CETIRIZINE HYDROCHLORIDE

Indications: symptomatic relief of allergy such as hay fever, urticaria

Cautions: see notes above

Contra-indications: see notes above; also pregnancy (Appendix 4) and breast-feeding (Appendix 5)

Side-effects: see notes above; incidence of sedation and antimuscarinic effects low

Dose: ADULT and CHILD over 6 years, 10 mg daily *or* 5 mg twice daily; CHILD 2–6 years, hayfever, 5 mg daily *or* 2.5 mg twice daily

Cetirizine (Non-proprietary)
Tablets, cetirizine hydrochloride 10 mg, net price 30-tab pack = £7.17. Counselling, driving
Available from Alpharma, APS (*Cetirocol®*), CP, Generics, Ratiopharm, Sandoz, Sterwin
Oral solution, cetirizine hydrochloride 5 mg/5 mL, net price 200 mL = £10.50. Counselling, driving
Available from Ratiopharm, Sandoz
Proprietary brands of cetirizine on sale to the public include *AllerTek®, Benadryl® One A Day, Piriteze® Allergy, Zirtek® Allergy, Zirtek® Allergy Relief*

DESLORATADINE

NOTE. Desloratadine is a metabolite of loratadine

Indications: symptomatic relief of allergy such as hay fever, urticaria

Cautions: see notes above

Contra-indications: see notes above; also hypersensitivity to loratadine; pregnancy (Appendix 4) and breast-feeding (Appendix 5)

Side-effects: see notes above; also fatigue; incidence of sedation and antimuscarinic effects low

Dose: ADULT and ADOLESCENT over 12 years, 5 mg daily; CHILD 2–5 years 1.25 mg daily, 6–11 years 2.5 mg daily

Neoclarityn® (Schering-Plough) ▼ PoM
Tablets, blue, f/c, desloratadine 5 mg, net price 30-tab pack = £7.57. Counselling, driving
Syrup, desloratadine 2.5 mg/5 mL, net price 100 mL (bubblegum-flavour) = £7.57. Counselling, driving

FEXOFENADINE HYDROCHLORIDE

NOTE. Fexofenadine is a metabolite of terfenadine

Indications: see under preparations below

Cautions: see notes above; also pregnancy (Appendix 4)

Contra-indications: see notes above; also breast-feeding (Appendix 5)

Side-effects: see notes above; incidence of sedation and antimuscarinic effects low

Dose: see under preparations below

Telfast® 30 (Aventis Pharma) PoM
Tablets, f/c, peach, fexofenadine hydrochloride 30 mg, net price 60-tab pack = £5.55
Dose: symptomatic relief of seasonal allergic rhinitis, CHILD 6–11 years, 30 mg twice daily; CHILD under 6 years, not recommended

Telfast® 120 (Aventis Pharma) PoM
Tablets, f/c, peach, fexofenadine hydrochloride 120 mg. Net price 30-tab pack = £7.40. Counselling, driving
Dose: symptomatic relief of seasonal allergic rhinitis, 120 mg once daily; CHILD under 12 years, not recommended

Telfast® 180 (Aventis Pharma) PoM
Tablets, f/c, peach, fexofenadine hydrochloride 180 mg. Net price 30-tab pack = £9.63. Counselling, driving
Dose: symptomatic relief of chronic idiopathic urticaria, 180 mg once daily; CHILD under 12 years, not recommended

LEVOCETIRIZINE DIHYDROCHLORIDE

NOTE. Levocetirizine is an isomer of cetirizine

Indications: symptomatic relief of allergy such as hay fever, urticaria

Cautions: see notes above; also pregnancy (Appendix 4) and breast-feeding (Appendix 5)

Contra-indications: see notes above; also severe renal impairment

Side-effects: see notes above; incidence of sedation and antimuscarinic effects low

Dose: ADULT and CHILD over 6 years, 5 mg daily

Xyzal (UCB Pharma) ▼ PoM
Tablets, f/c, levocetirizine dihydrochloride 5 mg, net price 30-tab pack = £7.45. Counselling, driving

LORATADINE

Indications: symptomatic relief of allergy such as hay fever, urticaria

Cautions: see notes above

Contra-indications: see notes above; also pregnancy (Appendix 4) and breast-feeding (Appendix 5)

Side-effects: see notes above; incidence of sedation and antimuscarinic effects low

Dose: ADULT and CHILD over 6 years 10 mg daily; CHILD 2–5 years 5 mg daily

Loratadine (Non-proprietary)
Tablets, loratadine 10 mg, net price 30-tab pack = £6.38
Syrup, loratadine 5 mg/5 mL, net price 100 mL = £5.43. Counselling, driving
Proprietary brands of loratadine on sale to the public include *Boots Hayfever and Allergy Relief All Day®*, and *Clarityn Allergy®* NHS

MIZOLASTINE

Indications: symptomatic relief of allergy such as hay fever, urticaria

Cautions: see notes above

Contra-indications: see notes above; also susceptibility to QT-interval prolongation (including cardiac disease and hypokalaemia); significant hepatic impairment; pregnancy (Appendix 4) and breast-feeding (Appendix 5)

Side-effects: see notes above; also may cause weight gain; incidence of sedation and antimuscarinic effects low

Dose: 10 mg daily; CHILD under 12 years, not recommended

Mizollen® (Schwarz) PoM
Tablets, m/r, f/c, scored, mizolastine 10 mg, net price 30-tab pack = £6.20. Label: 25, Counselling, driving

TERFENADINE

Indications: symptomatic relief of allergy such as allergic rhinitis, urticaria

Cautions: see notes above

Contra-indications: see notes above; avoid grapefruit juice (may inhibit metabolism of terfenadine); **important:** see also Arrhythmias, below; also pregnancy (Appendix 4) and breast-feeding (Appendix 5)

ARRHYTHMIAS. Rare hazardous arrhythmias are associated with terfenadine particularly in association with increased terfenadine blood concentration. Recommendations include:

- not to exceed recommended dose
- avoid in significant hepatic impairment
- avoid in hypokalaemia (or other electrolyte imbalance)
- avoid in known or suspected prolonged QT interval
- avoid concomitant administration of drugs that prolong the QT interval or inhibit the metabolism of terfenadine, or those liable to produce electrolyte imbalance or are potentially arrhythmogenic; for details, see **interactions**: Appendix 1 (antihistamines)
- discontinue if syncope occurs and evaluate for potential arrhythmias

Side-effects: see notes above; incidence of sedation and antimuscarinic effects low; erythema multiforme and galactorrhoea reported; **important:** ventricular arrhythmias (including torsades de pointes) have followed excessive dosage, see also Arrhythmias above

Dose: allergic rhinitis and conjunctivitis, ADULT and CHILD over 50 kg, 60 mg daily increased if necessary to 120 mg daily in single or 2 divided doses
Allergic skin disorders, ADULT and CHILD over 50 kg, 120 mg daily in single or 2 divided doses

Terfenadine (Non-proprietary) PoM
Tablets, terfenadine 60 mg, net price 60-tab pack = £2.44. Counselling, driving
NOTE. May be difficult to obtain

Sedating antihistamines

DRIVING. Drowsiness may affect performance of skilled tasks (e.g. driving); sedating effects enhanced by alcohol.

ALIMEMAZINE TARTRATE

(Trimeprazine tartrate)

Indications: urticaria and pruritus, premedication

Cautions: see notes above; also pregnancy (Appendix 4); see also section 4.2.1

Contra-indications: see notes above; also breast-feeding (Appendix 5); see also section 4.2.1

Side-effects: see notes above; see also section 4.2.1

Dose: 10 mg 2–3 times daily, in severe cases up to max. 100 mg daily has been used; ELDERLY 10 mg 1–2 times daily; CHILD under 2 years not recom-

mended, over 2 years 2.5–5 mg 3–4 times daily
Premedication, CHILD 2–7 years up to 2 mg/kg 1–2 hours before operation

Vallergan® (Castlemead) PoM
Tablets, blue, f/c, alimemazine tartrate 10 mg, net price 28-tab pack = £3.24. Label: 2
Syrup, straw-coloured, alimemazine tartrate 7.5 mg/5 mL, net price 100 mL = £3.70. Label: 2
Syrup forte, alimemazine tartrate 30 mg/5 mL, net price 100 mL = £5.72. Label: 2

BROMPHENIRAMINE MALEATE

Indications: symptomatic relief of allergy such as hay fever, urticaria

Cautions: see notes above; also pregnancy (Appendix 4)

Contra-indications: see notes above

Side-effects: see notes above

Dose: 4–8 mg 3–4 times daily; CHILD up to 3 years 0.4–1 mg/kg daily in 4 divided doses, 3–6 years 2 mg 3–4 times daily, 6–12 years 2–4 mg 3–4 times daily

Dimotane® (Goldshield)
Elixir, yellow-green, cola-flavoured, brompheniramine maleate 2 mg/5 mL, net price 200 mL = £1.56. Label: 2
For a list of **cough and decongestant preparations on sale to the public,** including those containing brompheniramine, see section 3.9.2.

CHLORPHENAMINE MALEATE

(Chlorpheniramine maleate)

Indications: symptomatic relief of allergy such as hay fever, urticaria; emergency treatment of anaphylactic reactions (section 3.4.3)

Cautions: see notes above; also pregnancy (Appendix 4) and breast-feeding (Appendix 5)

Contra-indications: see notes above

Side-effects: see notes above; also exfoliative dermatitis and tinnitus reported; injections may cause transient hypotension or CNS stimulation and may be irritant

Dose: *by mouth,* 4 mg every 4–6 hours, max. 24 mg daily; CHILD under 1 year not recommended, 1–2 years 1 mg twice daily; 2–5 years 1 mg every 4–6 hours, max. 6 mg daily; 6–12 years 2 mg every 4–6 hours, max. 12 mg daily
By subcutaneous or intramuscular injection, 10–20 mg, repeated if required; max. 40 mg in 24 hours
By intravenous injection over 1 minute, 10–20 mg; CHILD [unlicensed] under 1 year 250 micrograms/kg, 1–5 years 2.5–5 mg, 6–12 years 5–10 mg

Chlorphenamine (Non-proprietary)
Tablets, chlorphenamine maleate 4 mg, net price 20 = 31p. Label: 2
Oral solution, chlorphenamine maleate 2 mg/5 mL, net price 150 mL = £2.28. Label: 2
Available from Sandoz (sugar-free)
Injection PoM, chlorphenamine maleate 10 mg/mL, net price 1-mL amp = £1.62
Available from Link

Piriton® (GSK Consumer Healthcare)
Tablets, yellow, scored, chlorphenamine maleate 4 mg, net price 20 = 19p. Label: 2

Syrup, chlorphenamine maleate 2 mg/5 mL, net price 150 mL = £2.28. Label: 2

NOTE. In addition to *Piriton Allergy*® $\boxed{\text{NHS}}$, proprietary brands of chlorphenamine maleate tablets on sale to the public include *Allerief*®, *Boots Allergy Relief Antihistamine Tablets*, *Calimal*®

For a list of **cough and decongestant preparations on sale to the public**, including those containing chlorphenamine, see section 3.9.2

CLEMASTINE

Indications: symptomatic relief of allergy such as hay fever, urticaria
Cautions: see notes above; also pregnancy (Appendix 4) and breast-feeding (Appendix 5)
Contra-indications: see notes above
Side-effects: see notes above
Dose: 1 mg twice daily, increased up to 6 mg daily if required; CHILD under 1 year not recommended, 1–3 years 250–500 micrograms twice daily; 3–6 years 500 micrograms twice daily; 6–12 years 0.5–1 mg twice daily

Tavegil® (Novartis Consumer Health)
Tablets, scored, clemastine (as hydrogen fumarate) 1 mg. Net price 60-tab pack = £2.35. Label: 2

CYPROHEPTADINE HYDROCHLORIDE

Indications: symptomatic relief of allergy such as hay fever, urticaria; migraine (section 4.7.4.2)
Cautions: see notes above; also pregnancy
Contra-indications: see notes above; also breast-feeding
Side-effects: see notes above
Dose: allergy, usual dose 4 mg 3–4 times daily; usual range 4–20 mg daily, max. 32 mg daily; CHILD under 2 years not recommended, 2–6 years 2 mg 2–3 times daily, max. 12 mg daily; 7–14 years 4 mg 2–3 times daily, max. 16 mg daily
Migraine, 4 mg with a further 4 mg after 30 minutes if necessary; maintenance, 4 mg every 4–6 hours

Periactin® (MSD)
Tablets, scored, cyproheptadine hydrochloride 4 mg. Net price 30 = 86p. Label: 2

DIPHENHYDRAMINE HYDROCHLORIDE

Indications: see under Preparations
Cautions: see notes above
Contra-indications: see notes above
Side-effects: see notes above

■ Preparations
Proprietary brands of diphenhydramine hydrochloride on sale to the public to aid relief of temporary sleep disturbance in adults include:
Dreemon® (diphenhydramine hydrochloride 10 mg/5 mL, diphenhydramine hydrochloride tablets 25 mg), *Medinex*® (diphenhydramine hydrochloride 10 mg/5 mL), *Nightcalm*® (diphenhydramine hydrochloride tablets 25 mg), *Nytol*® $\boxed{\text{NHS}}$ (diphenhydramine hydrochloride tablets 25 mg and 50 mg), and *Panadol Night*® (diphenhydramine hydrochloride 25 mg and paracetamol 500 mg, for relief of temporary sleeplessness and night-time pain)

For a list of **cough and decongestant preparations on sale to the public**, including those containing diphenhydramine, see section 3.9.2

DIPHENYLPYRALINE HYDROCHLORIDE

Cautions: see notes above
Contra-indications: see notes above
Side-effects: see notes above

■ Preparations
For a list of **cough and decongestant preparations on sale to the public**, including those containing diphenylpyraline, see section 3.9.2

DOXYLAMINE

Cautions: see notes above
Contra-indications: see notes above
Side-effects: see notes above

■ Preparations
Ingredient of **cough and decongestant preparations** (section 3.9.2.) and of **compound analgesics** (section 4.7.1.) on sale to the public

HYDROXYZINE HYDROCHLORIDE

Indications: pruritus, anxiety (short-term) (section 4.1.2)
Cautions: see notes above
Contra-indications: see notes above; also pregnancy (Appendix 4) and breast-feeding (Appendix 5)
Side-effects: see notes above
Dose: pruritus, initially 25 mg at night increased if necessary to 25 mg 3–4 times daily; CHILD 6 months–6 years initially 5–15 mg daily increased if necessary to 50 mg daily in divided doses; over 6 years initially 15–25 mg daily increased if necessary to 50–100 mg daily in divided doses
Anxiety (adults only), 50–100 mg 4 times daily

Atarax® (Pfizer) $\boxed{\text{PoM}}$
Tablets, both s/c, hydroxyzine hydrochloride 10 mg (orange), net price 84-tab pack = £1.82; 25 mg (green), 28-tab pack = £1.22. Label: 2

Ucerax® (UCB Pharma) $\boxed{\text{PoM}}$
Tablets $\boxed{\text{NHS}}$, f/c, scored, hydroxyzine hydrochloride 25 mg, net price 25-tab pack = 91p. Label: 2
Syrup, hydroxyzine hydrochloride 10 mg/5 mL. Net price 200-mL pack = £1.91. Label: 2

PROMETHAZINE HYDROCHLORIDE

Indications: symptomatic relief of allergy such as hay fever, urticaria; premedication; emergency treatment of anaphylactic reactions (section 3.4.3); sedation (section 4.1.1); motion sickness (section 4.6)
Cautions: see notes above; also pregnancy (Appendix 4) and breast-feeding (Appendix 5)
Contra-indications: see notes above
Side-effects: see notes above; intramuscular injection may be painful
Dose: *by mouth*, 25 mg at night increased to 25 mg twice daily if necessary *or* 10–20 mg 2–3 times daily; CHILD under 2 years not recommended, 2–5 years 5–15 mg daily in 1–2 divided doses, 5–10 years 10–25 mg daily in 1–2 divided doses
Premedication, CHILD under 2 years not recom-

mended, 2–5 years 15–20 mg, 5–10 years 20–25 mg

By deep intramuscular injection, 25–50 mg; max. 100 mg; CHILD 5–10 years 6.25–12.5 mg

Premedication, 25–50 mg 1 hour before operation; CHILD 5–10 years, 6.25–12.5 mg

By slow intravenous injection in emergencies, 25–50 mg as a solution containing 2.5 mg/mL in water for injections; max. 100 mg

Phenergan® (Rhône-Poulenc Rorer)

Tablets, both blue, f/c, promethazine hydrochloride 10 mg, net price 56-tab pack = £1.57; 25 mg, 56-tab pack = £2.34. Label: 2

Elixir, sugar-free, golden, promethazine hydrochloride 5 mg/5 mL. Net price 100 mL = £1.49. Label: 2

Injection PoM, promethazine hydrochloride 25 mg/mL. Net price 1-mL amp = 54p

Promethazine hydrochloride injection 25 mg/mL (1-mL and 2-mL ampoules) also available from Antigen

NOTE. Proprietary brands of promethazine hydrochloride on sale to the public include *Phenergan Nightime*® (promethazine hydrochloride tablets 25 mg, for occasional insomnia in adults), *Sominex*® NHS (promethazine hydrochloride tablets 20 mg, for occasional insomnia in adults)

For a list of **cough and decongestant preparations on sale to the public**, including those containing promethazine, see section 3.9.2

TRIPROLIDINE HYDROCHLORIDE

Cautions: see notes above
Contra-indications: see notes above
Side-effects: see notes above

■ Preparations

For a list of **cough and decongestant preparations on sale to the public**, including those containing triprolidine, see section 3.9.2

3.4.2 Hyposensitisation

Except for wasp and bee sting allergy, specific hyposensitisation with allergen extract vaccines has usually shown little benefit in asthma. Hyposensitisation may be effective in allergic rhinitis if sensitisation to a particular allergen can be proven. However, the benefit of hyposensitisation needs to be balanced against the significant risk of anaphylaxis, particularly in patients with asthma (see CSM advice below).

Diagnostic skin tests are unreliable and can only be used in conjunction with a detailed history of allergen exposure.

> **CSM advice.** After re-examination of the efficacy and safety of desensitising vaccines, the CSM has concluded that they should only be used for the following indications:
>
> • Seasonal allergic hay fever (which has not responded to anti-allergy drugs) caused by pollens, using licensed products only—patients with *asthma* should not be treated with desensitising vaccines as they are more likely to develop severe adverse reactions.
>
> • Hypersensitivity to wasp and bee venoms—since reactions can be life-threatening, *asthma* is not an absolute contra-indication.

There is inadequate evidence of benefit from desensitisation to other allergens such as house dust, house dust mite, animal danders and foods and desensitisation is **not** recommended. Desensitising vaccines should be avoided in pregnant women, in children under five years old, and in those taking beta-blockers.

Bronchospasm usually develops within 1 hour and anaphylaxis within 30 minutes of injection. Therefore patients need to be monitored for 1 hour after injection. If symptoms or signs of hypersensitivity develop (e.g. rash, urticaria, bronchospasm, faintness), **even when mild**, the patient should be observed until these have **resolved completely**.

For details of the management of anaphylactic shock, see section 3.4.3.

Each set of allergen extracts usually contains vials for the administration of graded amounts of allergen to patients undergoing hyposensitisation. Maintenance sets containing vials at the highest strength are also available. Product literature must be consulted for details of allergens, vial strengths, and administration

BEE AND WASP ALLERGEN EXTRACTS

Indications: hypersensitivity to wasp or bee venom (see notes above)

Cautions: see notes above including CSM advice and consult product literature

CSM advice. The CSM has advised that facilities for cardiopulmonary resuscitation must be immediately available and patients monitored closely for one hour after each injection, for full details see above.

Contra-indications: see notes above and consult product literature

Side-effects: consult product literature

Dose: *by subcutaneous injection*, consult product literature

Pharmalgen® (ALK-Abelló) PoM

Bee venom extract (*Apis mellifera*) or wasp venom extract (*Vespula* spp.). Net price initial treatment set = £59.77 (bee), £73.28 (wasp); maintenance treatment set = £69.54 (bee), £89.45 (wasp)

GRASS AND TREE POLLEN EXTRACTS

Indications: treatment of seasonal allergic hayfever due to grass or tree pollen in patients who have failed to respond to anti-allergy drugs (see notes above)

Cautions: see notes above including CSM advice and consult product literature

CSM advice. The CSM has advised that facilities for cardiopulmonary resuscitation must be immediately available and patients must be monitored closely for one hour after each injection, for full details see above.

Contra-indications: see notes above and consult product literature

Side-effects: consult product literature

Dose: *by subcutaneous injection*, consult product literature

Pollinex® (Allergy) PoM

Grass or tree pollen extract, net price initial treatment set (3 vials) = £80.00; extension course treatment (1 vial) = £70.00

3.4.3 Allergic emergencies

Adrenaline (epinephrine) provides physiological reversal of the immediate symptoms (such as laryngeal oedema, bronchospasm, and hypotension) associated with hypersensitivity reactions such as *anaphylaxis* and *angioedema*. See below for full details of adrenaline administration and for adjunctive treatment.

Anaphylaxis

Anaphylactic shock requires prompt energetic treatment of *laryngeal oedema, bronchospasm,* and *hypotension.* Atopic individuals are particularly susceptible. Insect stings are a recognised risk (in particular wasp and bee stings). Certain foods, including eggs, fish, cow's milk protein, peanuts, and nuts may also precipitate anaphylaxis. Medicinal products particularly associated with anaphylaxis include blood products, vaccines, hyposensitising (allergen) preparations, antibiotics, aspirin and other NSAIDs, heparin, and neuromuscular blocking drugs. In the case of drugs, anaphylaxis is more likely after parenteral administration; resuscitation facilities must always be available for injections associated with special risk. Anaphylactic reactions may also be associated with *additives and excipients* in foods and medicines. Refined arachis (peanut) oil, which may be present in some medicinal products, is unlikely to cause an allergic reaction—nevertheless it is wise to check the full formula of preparations which may contain allergenic fats or oils.

First-line treatment includes securing the airway, restoration of blood pressure (laying the patient flat, raising the feet), and administration of **adrenaline** (epinephrine) injection. This is given **intramuscularly** in a dose of 500 micrograms (0.5 mL adrenaline injection 1 in 1000); a dose of 300 micrograms (0.3 mL adrenaline injection 1 in 1000) may be appropriate for *immediate self-administration*. The dose is repeated if necessary at 5-minute intervals according to blood pressure, pulse and respiratory function [important: possible need for *intravenous route* using *dilute solution*, see below]. **Oxygen** administration is also of primary importance. An antihistamine (e.g. **chlorphenamine** (chlorpheniramine), given by slow intravenous injection in a dose of 10–20 mg, see p. 153) is a useful adjunctive treatment, given after adrenaline injection and continued for 24 to 48 hours to prevent relapse. Patients receiving beta-blockers or those receiving antidepressants require special consideration (see under Adrenaline, p. 157).

Continuing deterioration requires further treatment including intravenous fluids (section 9.2.2), intravenous aminophylline (see p. 141) or a nebulised beta$_2$ agonist (such as salbutamol or terbutaline, see p. 135 and p. 137); in addition to oxygen, assisted respiration and possibly emergency tracheotomy may be necessary.

An intravenous corticosteroid e.g. **hydrocortisone** (as sodium succinate) in a dose of 100–300 mg (section 6.3.2) is of secondary value in the initial management of anaphylactic shock because the onset of action is delayed for several hours, but should be given to prevent further deterioration in severely affected patients.

When a patient is so ill that there is doubt as to the adequacy of the circulation, the initial injection of adrenaline may need to be given as a *dilute solution* by the *intravenous route*, for details of cautions, dose

and strength, see under Intravenous Adrenaline (Epinephrine), below.

Some patients with severe allergy to insect stings or foods are encouraged to carry prefilled adrenaline syringes for *self-administration* during periods of risk.

Angioedema

Angioedema is dangerous if *laryngeal oedema* is present. In this circumstance adrenaline (epinephrine) injection and oxygen should be given as described under Anaphylaxis (see above); antihistamines and corticosteroids should also be given (see again above). Tracheal intubation and other measures may be necessary.

The administration of C$_1$ esterase inhibitor (in fresh frozen plasma or in partially purified form) may terminate acute attacks of *hereditary angioedema*, but is not practical for long-term prophylaxis. **Tranexamic acid** (section 2.11) and **danazol** (section 6.7.2) [unlicensed indication] are used for long-term prophylaxis of hereditary angioedema.

Intramuscular adrenaline (epinephrine)

The *intramuscular route* is the *first choice route* for the administration of adrenaline (epinephrine) in the management of anaphylactic shock. Adrenaline has a rapid onset of action after intramuscular administration and in the shocked patient its absorption from the intramuscular site is faster and more reliable than from the subcutaneous site (the intravenous route should be reserved for extreme emergency when there is doubt about the adequacy of the circulation; for details of cautions, dose and strength see under Intravenous Adrenaline (Epinephrine), below).

Patients with severe allergy should ideally be instructed in the self-administration of adrenaline by intramuscular injection (for details see under Self-administration of Adrenaline (Epinephrine), below).

Prompt injection of adrenaline is of paramount importance. The following adrenaline doses are based on the revised recommendations of the Project Team of the Resuscitation Council (UK).

Dose of **intramuscular** injection of adrenaline (epinephrine) for anaphylactic shock. Subcutaneous injection **not** generally recommended.

Age	Dose	Volume of adrenaline 1 in 1000 (1 mg/mL)
Under 6 months	50 micrograms	0.05 mL[1]
6 months–6 years	120 micrograms	0.12 mL[1]
6–12 years	250 micrograms	0.25 mL
Adult and adolescent	500 micrograms	0.5 mL

These doses may be repeated several times if necessary at 5-minute intervals according to blood pressure, pulse and respiratory function.

1. Use suitable syringe for measuring small volume

Intravenous adrenaline (epinephrine)

Where the patient is severely ill and there is real doubt about adequacy of the circulation and absorption from the intramuscular injection site, adrenaline (epinephrine) may be given by **slow** *intravenous injection* in a dose of 500 micrograms (5 mL of the dilute 1 in 10 000 adrenaline injection) given at a rate of 100 micrograms (1 mL of the dilute 1 in 10 000 adrenaline injection) per minute, *stopping when a response has been obtained*; children can be given a dose of 10 micrograms/kg (0.1 mL/kg of the dilute 1 in 10 000 adrenaline injection) by **slow** *intravenous injection* over several minutes. Great vigilance is needed to ensure that the *correct strength* is used; anaphylactic shock kits need to make a *very clear distinction* between the 1 in 10 000 strength and the 1 in 1000 strength. It is also important that, where intramuscular injection might still succeed, time should not be wasted seeking intravenous access.

For reference to the use of the intravenous route for *cardiac resuscitation*, see section 2.7.3.

Self-administration of adrenaline (epinephrine)

Individuals at considerable risk of anaphylaxis need to carry adrenaline (epinephrine) at all times and need to be *instructed in advance* how to inject it. In addition, the packs need to be labelled so that in the case of rapid collapse someone else is able to administer the adrenaline. It is important to ensure that an adequate supply is provided to treat symptoms until medical assistance is available.

Some patients may best cope with a pre-assembled syringe fitted with a needle suitable for very rapid administration (if necessary by a bystander). *Anapen*® and *EpiPen*® consist of a fully assembled syringe and needle delivering a dose of 300 micrograms of adrenaline by *intramuscular injection*; 150-microgram versions (*Anapen*® *Junior*, *EpiPen*® *Jr*) are also available for use in children. Other products for the immediate treatment of anaphylaxis are available but are not licensed for use in the UK. *Ana-Guard*® is a prefilled syringe that delivers two 300-microgram doses of adrenaline by *subcutaneous or intramuscular injection*; it can be adjusted to administer smaller doses for children. *Ana-Kit*® includes a prefilled adrenaline syringe, chewable tablets of chlorphenamine maleate (chlorphenamine maleate) 2 mg, 2 sterile pads impregnated with 70% isopropyl alcohol, and a tourniquet. *Ana-Guard*® and *Ana-Kit*® are available on a named-patient basis from IDIS.

ADRENALINE/EPINEPHRINE

Indications: emergency treatment of acute anaphylaxis; angioedema; cardiopulmonary resuscitation (section 2.7.3)

Cautions: hyperthyroidism, diabetes mellitus, heart disease, hypertension, arrhythmias, cerebrovascular disease, angle-closure glaucoma, second stage of labour, elderly patients

INTERACTIONS: Severe anaphylaxis in patients on non-cardioselective beta-blockers may not respond to adrenaline injection calling for intravenous injection of salbutamol (see p. 135); furthermore, adrenaline may cause severe hypertension in those receiving beta-blockers. Patients on tricyclic antidepressants are considerably more susceptible to arrhythmias, calling for a much reduced dose of adrenaline. Other **interactions**, see Appendix 1 (sympathomimetics).

Side-effects: anxiety, tremor, tachycardia, arrhythmias, headache, cold extremities; also hypertension (risk of cerebral haemorrhage) and pulmonary oedema (on excessive dosage or extreme sensitivity); nausea, vomiting, sweating, weakness, dizziness and hyperglycaemia also reported

Dose: acute anaphylaxis, *by intramuscular injection* (preferably midpoint in anterolateral thigh) (*or by subcutaneous injection*) of 1 in 1000 (1 mg/mL) solution, see notes and table above

Acute anaphylaxis when there is doubt as to the adequacy of the circulation, *by slow intravenous injection* of 1 in 10 000 (100 micrograms/mL) solution (extreme caution), see notes above

IMPORTANT. Intravenous route should be used with **extreme care**, see notes above

■ Intramuscular or subcutaneous

Adrenaline/Epinephrine 1 in 1000 (Non-proprietary) PoM
Injection, adrenaline (as acid tartrate) 1 mg/mL, net price 0.5-mL amp = 50p; 1-mL amp = 42p
Available from Antigen, BCM Specials, Hillcross, Martindale, Phoenix; also available from Aurum (1-mL prefilled syringe)
Excipients: include sulphites

Minijet® **Adrenaline** (Celltech) PoM
Injection, adrenaline (as hydrochloride) 1 in 1000 (1 mg/mL). Net price 1 mL (with 25 gauge × 0.25 inch needle for subcutaneous injection) = £8.11, 1 mL (with 21 gauge × 1.5 inch needle for intramuscular injection) = £5.00 (both disposable syringes)
Excipients: include sulphites

■ Intravenous

Extreme caution, see notes above

Adrenaline/Epinephrine 1 in 10 000, Dilute (Non-proprietary) PoM
Injection, adrenaline (as acid tartrate) 100 micrograms/mL, 10-mL amp
Available from Aurum, Martindale (special order); also from Aurum (1-mL and 10-mL prefilled syringe) and Celltech (*Minijet*® *Adrenaline* 3- and 10-mL disposable syringes)
Excipients: include sulphites

■ Intramuscular injection for self-administration

Anapen® (Celltech) PoM
Anapen® *0.3 mg solution for injection* (delivering a single dose of adrenaline 300 micrograms), adrenaline 1 mg/mL (1 in 1000), net price 1.05-mL auto-injector device = £25.37
Excipients: include sulphites
NOTE. 0.75 mL of the solution remains in the auto-injector device after use
Dose: by intramuscular injection, ADULT and CHILD over 30 kg, 300 micrograms repeated after 10–15 minutes as necessary
Anapen® *Junior 0.15 mg solution for injection* (delivering a single dose of adrenaline 150 micrograms), adrenaline 500 micrograms/mL (1 in 2000), net price 1.05-mL auto-injector device = £25.37
Excipients: include sulphites
NOTE. 0.75 mL of the solution remains in the auto-injector device after use
Dose: by intramuscular injection, CHILD 15–30 kg, 150 micrograms repeated after 10–15 minutes as necessary

EpiPen® (ALK-Abelló) PoM
EpiPen® *Auto-injector 0.3 mg* (delivering a single dose of adrenaline 300 micrograms), adrenaline

1 mg/mL (1 in 1000), net price 2-mL auto-injector = £28.19

Excipients: include sulphites

NOTE. 1.7 mL of the solution remains in the *Auto-injector* after use

Dose: by intramuscular injection, ADULT and CHILD over 30 kg, 300 micrograms repeated after 15 minutes as necessary

Epipen® Jr Auto-injector 0.15 mg (delivering a single dose of adrenaline 150 micrograms), adrenaline 500 micrograms/mL (1 in 2000), net price 2-mL auto-injector = £28.19

Excipients: include sulphites

NOTE. 1.7 mL of the solution remains in the *Auto-injector* after use

Dose: by intramuscular injection, CHILD 15–30 kg, 150 micrograms (but on the basis of a dose of 10 micrograms/kg, 300 micrograms may be more appropriate for some children) repeated after 15 minutes as necessary

3.5 Respiratory stimulants and pulmonary surfactants

3.5.1 Respiratory stimulants
3.5.2 Pulmonary surfactants

3.5.1 Respiratory stimulants

Respiratory stimulants (analeptic drugs) have a limited place in the treatment of ventilatory failure in patients with chronic obstructive pulmonary disease. They are effective only when given by intravenous injection or infusion and have a short duration of action. Their use has largely been replaced by ventilatory support including nasal intermittent positive pressure ventilation. However, occasionally when ventilatory support is contra-indicated and in patients with hypercapnic respiratory failure who are becoming drowsy or comatose, respiratory stimulants in the short term may arouse patients sufficiently to co-operate and clear their secretions.

Respiratory stimulants can also be harmful in respiratory failure since they stimulate non-respiratory as well as respiratory muscles. They should only be given under **expert supervision** in hospital and must be combined with active physiotherapy. There is at present no oral respiratory stimulant available for long-term use in chronic respiratory failure.

Doxapram is given by continuous intravenous infusion. Frequent arterial blood gas and pH measurements are necessary during treatment to ensure correct dosage.

Nikethamide (now discontinued by most suppliers) is not recommended because the effective doses are close to those causing toxic effects, especially convulsions.

DOXAPRAM HYDROCHLORIDE

Indications: see under Dose

Cautions: give with oxygen in severe irreversible airways obstruction or severely decreased lung compliance (because of increased work load of breathing); give with beta₂ agonist in bronchoconstriction; hypertension (avoid if severe), impaired cardiac reserve; hepatic impairment, pregnancy (compelling reasons only); **interactions:** Appendix 1 (doxapram)

Contra-indications: severe hypertension, status asthmaticus, coronary artery disease, thyrotoxicosis, epilepsy, physical obstruction of respiratory tract

Side-effects: perineal warmth, dizziness, sweating, moderate increase in blood pressure and heart rate; side-effects reported in postoperative period (causal effect not established) include muscle fasciculation, hyperactivity, confusion, hallucinations, cough, dyspnoea, laryngospasm, bronchospasm, sinus tachycardia, bradycardia, extrasystoles, nausea, vomiting and salivation

Dose: postoperative respiratory depression, *by intravenous injection* over at least 30 seconds, 1–1.5 mg/kg repeated if necessary after intervals of 1 hour *or* alternatively *by intravenous infusion*, 2–3 mg/minute adjusted according to response; CHILD not recommended

Acute respiratory failure, *by intravenous infusion*, 1.5–4 mg/minute adjusted according to response (given concurrently with oxygen and whenever possible monitor with frequent measurement of blood gas tensions); CHILD not recommended

Dopram® (Anpharm) PoM

Injection, doxapram hydrochloride 20 mg/mL. Net price 5-mL amp = £2.04

Intravenous infusion, doxapram hydrochloride 2 mg/mL in glucose 5%. Net price 500-mL bottle = £21.33

3.5.2 Pulmonary surfactants

Pulmonary surfactants are used in the management of respiratory distress syndrome (hyaline membrane disease) in newborn and preterm infants. They may also be given prophylactically to those considered at risk of developing the syndrome.

CAUTIONS. Continuous monitoring is required to avoid hyperoxaemia (due to rapid improvement in arterial oxygen concentration).

SIDE-EFFECTS. Pulmonary haemorrhage, especially in more premature infants, is a rare complication of therapy; obstruction of the endotracheal tube by mucous secretions has also been reported.

BERACTANT

Indications: treatment of respiratory distress syndrome in neonates over 700 g; prophylaxis of respiratory distress syndrome in preterm infants

Cautions: see notes above

Side-effects: see notes above

Dose: *by endotracheal tube*, phospholipid 100 mg/kg equivalent to a volume of 4 mL/kg, preferably within 8 hours of birth; may be repeated within 48 hours at intervals of at least 6 hours for up to 4 doses

Survanta® (Abbott) PoM

Suspension, beractant (bovine lung extract) providing phospholipid 25 mg/mL, with lipids and proteins, net price 8-mL vial = £306.43

PORACTANT ALFA

Indications: treatment of respiratory distress syndrome or hyaline membrane disease in neonates over 700 g; prophylaxis of respiratory distress syndrome in preterm infants

Cautions: see notes above

Side-effects: see notes above

Dose: *by endotracheal tube*, treatment, 100–200 mg/kg; further doses of 100 mg/kg may be repeated 12 hours later and after further 12 hours if still intubated; max. total dose 300–400 mg/kg; prophylaxis, 100–200 mg/kg soon after birth (preferably within 15 minutes); further doses of 100 mg/kg may be repeated 6–12 hours later and after further 12 hours if still intubated; max. total dose 300–400 mg/kg

Curosurf® (Trinity) PoM

Suspension, poractant alfa (porcine lung phospholipid fraction) 80 mg/mL, net price 1.5-mL vial = £382.00; 3-mL vial = £764.00

3.6   Oxygen

Oxygen should be regarded as a drug. It is prescribed for hypoxaemic patients to increase alveolar oxygen tension and decrease the work of breathing necessary to maintain a given arterial oxygen tension. The concentration depends on the condition being treated; an inappropriate concentration may have serious or even lethal effects.

High concentration oxygen therapy, with concentrations of up to 60%, is safe in conditions such as pneumonia, pulmonary thromboembolism, and fibrosing alveolitis. In such conditions low arterial oxygen (P_aO_2) is usually associated with low or normal arterial carbon dioxide (P_aCO_2), therefore there is little risk of hypoventilation and carbon dioxide retention.

In acute severe asthma, the arterial carbon dioxide (P_aCO_2) is usually subnormal but as asthma deteriorates it may rise steeply (particularly in children). These patients usually require high concentrations of oxygen and if the arterial carbon dioxide (P_aCO_2) remains high despite other treatment intermittent positive pressure ventilation needs to be considered urgently. Where facilities for blood gas measurements are not immediately available, for example while transferring the patient to hospital, 35% to 50% oxygen delivered through a conventional mask is recommended.

Low concentration oxygen therapy (controlled oxygen therapy) is reserved for patients with ventilatory failure due to chronic obstructive pulmonary disease or other causes. The concentration should not exceed 28% and in some patients a concentration above 24% may be excessive. The aim is to provide the patient with enough oxygen to improve hypoxaemia but without worsening existing carbon dioxide retention and respiratory acidosis. Treatment should be initiated in hospital because repeated blood gas measurements are required to assess the correct concentration.

DOMICILIARY OXYGEN. Oxygen should only be prescribed for patients in the home after careful evaluation in hospital by respiratory experts; it should never be prescribed on a placebo basis.

Patients should be **advised of the fire risks** when receiving oxygen therapy.

AIR TRAVEL. Some patients with arterial hypoxaemia will require supplementary oxygen for air travel. The patient's requirement should be discussed with the airline before travel.

Intermittent oxygen therapy

Oxygen is occasionally prescribed for intermittent use for episodes of hypoxaemia of short duration, for example asthma. It is important, however, that the patient does not rely on oxygen instead of obtaining medical help or taking more specific treatment.

Alternatively, intermittent oxygen may be prescribed for patients with advanced irreversible respiratory disorders to increase mobility and capacity for exercise and to ease discomfort, for example in chronic obstructive pulmonary disease. Appropriate patients may be prescribed portable equipment through the hospital service, refillable from cylinders in the home.

Under the NHS oxygen may be supplied by pharmacy contractors as **oxygen cylinders**. Oxygen flow can be adjusted as the cylinders are equipped with an oxygen flow meter with 'medium' (2 litres/minute) and 'high' (4 litres/minute) settings. The Health Authorities have lists of pharmacy contractors who provide domiciliary oxygen services.

Patients are supplied with either constant or variable performance masks. The *Intersurgical 010 28%* or *Ventimask Mk IV 28%* are constant performance masks and provide a nearly constant supply of oxygen (28%) despite variations in oxygen flow rate and the patient's breathing pattern. The variable performance masks include the *Intersurgical 005 Mask* and the *Venticaire Mask*; the concentration of oxygen supplied to the patient varies with the rate of flow of oxygen and with the patient's breathing pattern. If a mask which provides 24% oxygen is required, it may be ordered from BOC Medical.

Giving oxygen by nasal cannula allows the patient to talk and eat but the concentration is not controlled and the method may not be appropriate for acute respiratory failure. When given through a nasal cannula at a rate of 1–2 litres/minute the inspiratory oxygen concentration is usually low, but it varies with ventilation and can be high if the patient is underventilating.

PORTABLE OXYGEN CYLINDERS. Medigas and BOC supply a portable oxygen cylinder called 'PD oxygen cylinder', which has the same bull-nose fitting as the normal domiciliary headsets (prescriptions must therefore specify 'PD oxygen cylinder'). The PD oxygen cylinder holds 300 litres of oxygen which will last approximately 2 hours at a standard flow rate of 2 litres/minute.

Long-term oxygen therapy

Long-term administration of oxygen (at least 15 hours daily) prolongs survival in some patients with chronic obstructive pulmonary disease.

The Royal College of Physicians has produced guidelines for oxygen therapy (*Domiciliary oxygen therapy services: Clinical guidelines and advice for prescribers*; June 1999). Assessment for long-term oxygen therapy requires measurement of arterial blood gas tensions. Measurements should be taken on 2 occasions at least 3 weeks apart to demonstrate clinical stability, and not sooner than 4 weeks after an acute exacerbation of the disease. The guidelines recommend that long-term oxygen therapy should be considered for patients with:

- chronic obstructive pulmonary disease with $P_aO_2 < 7.3$ kPa when breathing air during a period of clinical stability;
- chronic obstructive pulmonary disease with P_aO_2 7.3–8 kPa in the presence of secondary polycythaemia, nocturnal hypoxaemia, peripheral oedema or evidence of pulmonary hypertension;
- interstitial lung disease with $P_aO_2 < 8$ kPa and in patients with $P_aO_2 > 8$ kPa with disabling dyspnoea;
- cystic fibrosis when $P_aO_2 < 7.3$ kPa *or* if P_aO_2 7.3–8 kPa in the presence of secondary polycythaemia, nocturnal hypoxaemia, pulmonary hypertension or peripheral oedema;
- pulmonary hypertension, without parenchymal lung involvement when $P_aO_2 < 8$ kPa;
- neuromuscular or skeletal disorders, after specialist assessment;
- obstructive sleep apnoea despite continuous positive airways pressure therapy, after specialist assessment;
- pulmonary malignancy or other terminal disease with disabling dyspnoea;
- heart failure with daytime $P_aO_2 < 7.3$ kPa (on air) or with nocturnal hypoxaemia;
- paediatric respiratory disease, after specialist assessment.

Increased respiratory depression is seldom a problem in patients with stable respiratory failure treated with low concentrations of oxygen although it may occur during exacerbations; patients and relatives should be warned to call for medical help if drowsiness or confusion occur.

Oxygen concentrators are more economical for patients requiring oxygen for long periods, and in England and Wales are prescribable on the NHS on a regional tendering basis (see below). A concentrator is cost-effective for a patient requiring oxygen for 8 hours a day (or 21 cylinders per month). Exceptionally if a higher concentration of oxygen is required the output of 2 oxygen concentrators can be combined using a 'Y' connection.

A nasal cannula is usually preferred for long-term oxygen therapy from an oxygen concentrator. It can, however, produce dermatitis and mucosal drying in sensitive individuals. Nasal cannulas are supplied with oxygen concentrators but they are not prescribable on the NHS.

Prescribing arrangements for oxygen concentrators

Prescribe concentrator and accessories (face mask, nasal cannula, and humidifier) on form FP10 or form WP10 in Wales. Specify amount of oxygen required (hours per day) and flow rate. If required, prescribe back-up oxygen set and cylinder at same time. Inform patient that the supplier will be in contact to make arrangements and that the prescription form is

to be given to the person who installs the concentrator.

Inform supplier by telephone (see table below) that a concentrator has been prescribed. The supplier will send written confirmation of the order to the prescriber, the patient, and the Health Authority.

Follow the same procedure if a back-up oxygen set and cylinder are required later.

Health Authority regional group	Supplier
South Western London South (includes Kent, Surrey, and Sussex)	BOC Medical *to order*: Dial 0800 136 603
Eastern London North North Western and North Wales West Midlands	De Vilbiss Medequip Ltd *to order*: Dial 0800 020 202
Central and South Wales Northern Yorkshire (South and West) and Humberside	Oxygen Therapy Co Ltd *to order*: Dial 0800 373 580

In **Scotland** refer the patient for assessment by a respiratory consultant. If the need for a concentrator is confirmed the consultant will arrange for the provision of a concentrator through the Common Services Agency.

3.7 Mucolytics

Mucolytics are sometimes prescribed to facilitate expectoration by reducing sputum viscosity. Regular use of oral mucolytics may be of some benefit in patients with chronic obstructive pulmonary disease who suffer from particularly troublesome exacerbations. Steam inhalation with postural drainage, is good expectorant therapy in bronchiectasis and in some cases of chronic bronchitis.

For reference to dornase alfa, see below.

CARBOCISTEINE

Indications: reduction of sputum viscosity
Contra-indications: active peptic ulceration
Side-effects: occasional gastro-intestinal irritation, rashes
Dose: 750 mg 3 times daily initially, then 1.5 g daily in divided doses; CHILD 2–5 years 62.5–125 mg 4 times daily, 6–12 years 250 mg 3 times daily

Carbocisteine (Non-proprietary) PoM
Capsules, carbocisteine 375 mg. Net price 30-cap pack = £4.48
Available from Beacon (*Mucodyne®*)
Oral liquid, carbocisteine 125 mg/5 mL, net price 300 mL = £4.91; 250 mg/5 mL, 300 mL = £6.28
Available from Beacon (*Mucodyne® Paediatric* 125 mg/5 mL and *Mucodyne®* 250 mg/5 mL)

MECYSTEINE HYDROCHLORIDE

(Methyl Cysteine Hydrochloride)
Indications: reduction of sputum viscosity
Dose: 200 mg 4 times daily for 2 days, then 200 mg 3 times daily for 6 weeks, then 200 mg twice daily; CHILD over 5 years 100 mg 3 times daily

Visclair® (Sinclair)
Tablets, yellow, s/c, e/c, mecysteine hydrochloride
100 mg. Net price 20 = £3.66. Label: 5, 22, 25

Dornase alfa

Dornase alfa is a genetically engineered version of a naturally occurring human enzyme which cleaves extracellular deoxyribonucleic acid (DNA). It is used in cystic fibrosis and is administered by inhalation using a jet nebuliser (section 3.1.5).

DORNASE ALFA
Phosphorylated glycosylated recombinant human deoxyribonuclease 1 (rhDNase)
Indications: management of cystic fibrosis patients with a forced vital capacity (FVC) of greater than 40% of predicted to improve pulmonary function
Cautions: pregnancy (Appendix 4); breast-feeding (Appendix 5)
Side-effects: pharyngitis, voice changes, chest pain; occasionally laryngitis, rashes, urticaria, conjunctivitis
Dose: *by inhalation of nebulised solution* (by jet nebuliser), 2500 units (2.5 mg) once daily (patients over 21 years may benefit from twice daily dosage); CHILD under 5 years not recommended

Pulmozyme® (Roche) PoM
Nebuliser solution, dornase alfa 1000 units (1 mg)/mL. Net price 2.5-mL (2500 units) vial = £18.89
NOTE. For use undiluted with jet nebulisers only; ultrasonic nebulisers are unsuitable

3.8   Aromatic inhalations

Inhalations containing volatile substances such as eucalyptus oil are traditionally used and although the vapour may contain little of the additive it encourages deliberate inspiration of warm moist air which is often comforting in bronchitis; boiling water should not be used owing to the risk of scalding. Inhalations are also used for the relief of nasal obstruction in acute rhinitis or sinusitis.

CHILDREN. The use of strong aromatic decongestants (applied as rubs or to pillows) is not advised for infants under the age of 3 months. Mothers with young infants in whom nasal obstruction with mucus is a problem can readily be taught appropriate techniques of suction aspiration.

Benzoin Tincture, Compound, BP
(Friars' Balsam)
Tincture, balsamic acids approx. 4.5%. Label: 15
Dose: add one teaspoonful to a pint of hot, **not** boiling, water and inhale the vapour

Menthol and Eucalyptus Inhalation, BP 1980
Inhalation, racementhol or levomenthol 2 g, eucalyptus oil 10 mL, light magnesium carbonate 7 g, water to 100 mL
Dose: add one teaspoonful to a pint of hot, **not** boiling, water and inhale the vapour

Karvol® (Crookes) NHS
Inhalation capsules, levomenthol 35.55 mg, with chlorobutanol, pine oils, terpineol, and thymol, net price 10-cap pack = £1.44; 20-cap pack = £2.59

Inhalation solution, levomenthol 7.9%, with chlorobutanol, pine oils, terpineol, and thymol, net price 12-mL dropper bottle = £1.89
Dose: express into handkerchief or add to a pint of hot, **not** boiling, water the contents of 1 capsule or 6 drops of solution; avoid in infants under 3 months

3.9   Cough preparations

3.9.1   Cough suppressants
3.9.2   Expectorant and demulcent cough preparations

3.9.1   Cough suppressants

Cough is usually a symptom of an underlying disorder e.g. asthma (section 3.1.1), gastro-oesophageal reflux disease (section 1.1), and 'post-nasal drip'; where there is no identifiable cause, cough suppressants may be useful, for example if sleep is disturbed. They may cause sputum retention and this may be harmful in patients with chronic bronchitis and bronchiectasis.

Codeine may be effective but it is constipating and can cause dependence; **dextromethorphan** and **pholcodine** have fewer side-effects.

Sedating antihistamines, such as diphenhydramine, are used as the cough suppressant component of many compound cough preparations on sale to the public; all tend to cause drowsiness which may reflect their main mode of action.

CHILDREN. The use of cough suppressants containing codeine or similar opioid analgesics is not generally recommended in children and should be avoided altogether in those under 1 year of age.

CODEINE PHOSPHATE
Indications: dry or painful cough; diarrhoea (section 1.4.2); pain (section 4.7.2)
Cautions: asthma; hepatic and renal impairment; history of drug abuse; see also notes above and section 4.7.2; **interactions:** Appendix 1 (opioid analgesics)
Contra-indications: liver disease, ventilatory failure
Side-effects: constipation, respiratory depression in sensitive patients or if given large doses

[1]**Codeine Linctus, BP** PoM
Linctus (= oral solution), codeine phosphate 15 mg/5 mL. Net price 100 mL = 40p (diabetic, 73p)
Dose: 5–10 mL 3–4 times daily; CHILD (but not generally recommended) 5–12 years, 2.5–5 mL
Available from Alpharma, IVAX, Thornton & Ross (*Galcodine*®)
NOTE. BP directs that when Diabetic Codeine Linctus is prescribed, Codeine Linctus formulated with a vehicle appropriate for administration to diabetics, whether or not labelled 'Diabetic Codeine Linctus', shall be dispensed or supplied

1. Can be sold to the public provided the maximum single dose does not exceed 5 mL

Codeine Linctus, Paediatric, BP
Linctus (= oral solution), codeine phosphate 3 mg/
5 mL. Net price 100 mL = 21p
Dose: CHILD (but not generally recommended) 1–5 years
5 mL 3–4 times daily
Available from Thornton & Ross (*Galcodine® Paediatric*,
sugar-free)
NOTE. BP directs that Paediatric Codeine Linctus may be
prepared extemporaneously by diluting Codeine Linctus
with a suitable vehicle in accordance with the manufacturer's instructions
For a list of **cough and decongestant preparations on sale
to the public**, including those containing codeine, see
section 3.9.2

PHOLCODINE
Indications: dry or painful cough
Cautions: see under Codeine Phosphate
Contra-indications: see under Codeine Phosphate
Side-effects: see under Codeine Phosphate

Pholcodine Linctus, BP
Linctus (= oral solution), pholcodine 5 mg/5 mL in a
suitable flavoured vehicle, containing citric acid
monohydrate 1%. Net price 100 mL = 24p
Dose: 5–10 mL 3–4 times daily; CHILD (but not generally
recommended, see notes above) 5–12 years 2.5–5 mL
Available from IVAX, Ransom (*Pavacol-D®*, sugar-free),
Thornton & Ross (*Galenphol®*, sugar-free)

Pholcodine Linctus, Strong, BP
Linctus (= oral solution), pholcodine 10 mg/5 mL in
a suitable flavoured vehicle, containing citric acid
monohydrate 2%. Net price 100 mL = 33p
Dose: 5 mL 3–4 times daily
Available from IVAX, Thornton & Ross (*Galenphol®*)

Galenphol® (Thornton & Ross)
Paediatric linctus (= oral solution), orange, sugar-
free, pholcodine 2 mg/5 mL. Net price 90-mL pack
= £1.58
Dose: CHILD (but not generally recommended, see notes
above) 1–5 years 5 mL 3 times daily; 6–12 years 5–10 mL
For a list of **cough and decongestant preparations on sale
to the public**, including those containing pholcodine, see
section 3.9.2

Palliative care

Diamorphine and methadone have been used to
control distressing cough in terminal lung cancer
although morphine is now preferred (see p. 14). In
other circumstances they are contra-indicated
because they induce sputum retention and ventilatory failure as well as causing opioid dependence.
Methadone linctus should be avoided because it has
a long duration of action and tends to accumulate.

METHADONE HYDROCHLORIDE
Indications: cough in terminal disease
Cautions: see notes in section 4.7.2
Contra-indications: see notes in section 4.7.2
Side-effects: see notes in section 4.7.2; longer-
acting than morphine therefore effects may be
cumulative
Dose: see below

Methadone Linctus ▣CD▣ ◼️
Linctus (= oral solution), methadone hydrochloride
2 mg/5 mL in a suitable vehicle with a tolu flavour.
Label: 2
Dose: 2.5–5 mL every 4–6 hours, reduced to twice daily
on prolonged use

MORPHINE HYDROCHLORIDE
Indications: cough in terminal disease (see also
Prescribing in Palliative Care p. 14)
Cautions: see notes in section 4.7.2
Contra-indications: see notes in section 4.7.2
Side-effects: see notes in section 4.7.2
Dose: initially 5 mg every 4 hours

■ Preparation
Section 4.7.2

3.9.2 Expectorant and demulcent cough preparations

Expectorants are claimed to promote expulsion of
bronchial secretions but there is no evidence that any
drug can specifically facilitate expectoration. The
assumption that sub-emetic doses of expectorants,
such as ammonium chloride, ipecacuanha, and squill
promote expectoration is a myth. However, a simple
expectorant mixture may serve a useful placebo
function and has the advantage of being inexpensive.

Demulcent cough preparations contain soothing
substances such as syrup or glycerol and certainly
some patients believe that such preparations relieve a
dry irritating cough. Preparations such as **simple
linctus** have the advantage of being harmless and
inexpensive; **paediatric simple linctus** is particularly useful in children and sugar-free versions are
available.

Compound cough preparations are on sale to the
public; the rationale for some is dubious.

Ammonia and Ipecacuanha Mixture, BP
Mixture, ammonium bicarbonate 200 mg, liquorice
liquid extract 0.5 mL, ipecacuanha tincture 0.3 mL,
concentrated camphor water 0.1 mL, concentrated
anise water 0.05 mL, double-strength chloroform
water 5 mL, water to 10 mL. It should be recently
prepared
Dose: 10–20 mL 3–4 times daily

Simple Linctus, BP
Linctus (= oral solution), citric acid monohydrate
2.5% in a suitable vehicle with an anise flavour.
Net price 100 mL = 18p
Dose: 5 mL 3–4 times daily
A sugar-free version is available from Pinewood and
various wholesalers.

Simple Linctus, Paediatric, BP
Linctus (= oral solution), citric acid monohydrate
0.625% in a suitable vehicle with an anise flavour.
Net price 100 mL = 17p
Dose: CHILD 5–10 mL 3–4 times daily
A sugar-free version is available from Pinewood and
various wholesalers.

■ Preparations on sale to the public
**Systemic cough and decongestant preparations
on sale to the public**, together with their significant
ingredients.

Important: in overdose contact **Poisons Information Services** (p. 20) for full details of the
ingredients.

Adult Meltus® Expectorant with Decongestant (guai-
fenesin, pseudoephedrine, menthol), **Advil Cold and
Sinus®** (ibuprofen, pseudoephedrine)
Baby Meltus® (dilute acetic acid), **Beechams All-In-
One®** (guaifenesin, paracetamol, phenylephrine),
Beechams Flu-Plus Caplets® (paracetamol, phenyl-

ephrine), **Beechams Hot Lemon**®, **Hot Lemon and Honey**®, **Hot Blackcurrant**®, **Beechams Powders Capsules**® **with Decongestant** (paracetamol, phenylephrine), **Benadryl Plus Capsules**® (acrivastine, pseudoephedrine), **Benylin Chesty Coughs**® **Original** (diphenhydramine, menthol), **Benylin Children's Chesty Coughs**® (guaifenesin), **Benylin Children's Night Coughs**® (diphenhydramine, menthol), **Benylin Children's Dry Coughs**® (pholcodine), **Benylin Children's Coughs and Colds**® (dextromethorphan, triprolidine), **Benylin with Codeine**® (codeine, diphenhydramine, menthol), **Benylin Cough and Congestion**® (dextromethorphan, diphenhydramine, menthol, pseudoephedrine), **Benylin Dry Cough**® (dextromethorphan, diphenhydramine, menthol), **Benylin Four Flu**® (diphenhydramine, paracetamol, pseudoephedrine), **Benylin Non-drowsy for Chesty Coughs**® (guaifenesin, menthol), **Benylin Non-drowsy for Dry Coughs**® (dextromethorphan), **Benylin Day & Night Tablets**® (*day tablets*, paracetamol, pseudoephedrine, *night tablets*, paracetamol, diphenhydramine), **Boots Bronchial Cough Mixture**® (ammonium carbonate, ammonium chloride, guaifenesin), **Boots Catarrh Cough Syrup**® (codeine, creosote), **Boots Chesty Cough Syrup 1 Year Plus**® (guaifenesin), **Boots Cough and Decongestant Syrup 2 Years Plus**® (guaifenesin, pseudoephedrine), **Boots Cough Syrup 3 Months Plus**® (glycerol), **Boots Cold and Flu Relief Tablets**® (paracetamol, phenylephrine), **Boots Decongestant Tablets**® (pseudoephedrine), **Boots Decongestant Tablets with Paracetamol** ® (paracetamol, pseudoephedrine), **Boots Night Time Cough Syrup 1 Year Plus**® (diphenhydramine, pholcodine), **Buttercup Infant Cough Syrup**® (ipecacuanha,), **Buttercup Syrup**® (capsicum, squill), **Buttercup Syrup Honey and Lemon Flavour**® (ipecacuanha, menthol)
Cabdrivers® (dextromethorphan, menthol), **CAM**® (ephedrine), **Contac**® **Non Drowsy 12 Hour Relief** (pseudoephedrine), **Covonia Bronchial Balsam**® (dextromethorphan, menthol), **Covonia Mentholated Cough Mixture**® (liquorice, menthol, squill), **Covonia Night Time Formula**® (dextromethorphan, diphenhydramine)
Day Nurse® (dextromethorphan, paracetamol, phenylpropanolamine), **Dimotane Elixir**® (brompheniramine), **Dimotane Expectorant**® (brompheniramine, guaifenesin, pseudoephedrine), **Dimotane Co**® and **Dimotane Co Paediatric**® (brompheniramine, codeine, pseudoephedrine), **Dimotane Plus**® and **Dimotane Plus Paediatric**® (brompheniramine, pseudoephedrine), **Do-Do Chesteze**® (ephedrine, theophylline)
Expulin® (chlorphenamine, menthol, pholcodine, pseudoephedrine), **Expulin Children's Cough Linctus**® (chlorphenamine, menthol, pholcodine)
Famel Original® (codeine, creosote), **Franol**® and **Franol Plus**® (both ephedrine, theophylline)
Galcodine® (codeine), **Galcodine Paediatric**® (codeine), **Galenphol**® (pholcodine), **Galenphol Paediatric**® (pholcodine), **Galenphol Strong**® (pholcodine), **Galloway's**® (ipecacuanha, squill), **Galpseud**® (pseudoephedrine), **Galpseud Plus**® (chlorphenamine, pseudoephedrine)
Haymine® (chlorphenamine, ephedrine), **Hill's Balsam Adult Expectorant**® (ipecacuanha, pholcodine), **Hill's Balsam Cough Suppressant**® (pholcodine), **Histalix**® (ammonium chloride, diphenhydramine, menthol)
Jackson's All Fours® (guaifenesin), **Jackson's Bronchial Balsam**® (guaifenesin), **Jackson's Little Healers**® (ipecacuanha), **Jackson's Troublesome Coughs**® (ipecacuanha), **Junior Meltus Dry Cough**® (dextromethorphan, pseudoephedrine), **Junior Meltus Expectorant**® (guaifenesin)
Lemsip Lemcaps®, **Lemsip Flu Strength**®, **Lemsip Lemon**® or **Blackcurrant**®, **Lemsip Chesty Cough**® (guaifenesin), **Lemsip Power +**® (ibuprofen, pseudoephedrine), **Liqufruta Garlic**® (guaifenesin)
Medised® (paracetamol, promethazine), **Meltus Baby**® (dilute acetic acid), **Meltus Dry Cough**® (dextromethorphan, pseudoephedrine), **Meltus Expectorant**®,

Meltus Honey and Lemon® (guaifenesin), **Mu-Cron Tablets**® (paracetamol, phenylpropanolamine) **Multi-action Actifed Tablets**® (pseudoephedrine, triprolidine), **Multi-action Actifed Dry Coughs**® (dextromethorphan, pseudoephedrine, triprolidine), **Multi-action Actifed Syrup**® (pseudoephedrine, triprolidine), **Multi-action Actifed Chesty Coughs**® (guaifenesin, pseudoephedrine, triprolidine)
Night Nurse® (dextromethorphan, paracetamol, promethazine), **Nirolex for Chesty Coughs with Decongestant**® (guaifenesin, pseudoephedrine), **Nirolex Chesty Cough Linctus**® (guaifenesin), **Nirolex Day Cold Comfort**® (paracetamol, pholcodine, pseudoephedrine), **Nirolex Dry Cough Linctus**® (glycerol), **Nirolex for Dry Coughs with Decongestant**® (dextromethorphan, pseudoephedrine), **Nirolex for Night Time Coughs**® (diphenhydramine, pholcodine), **Non-Drowsy Sinutab**® (paracetamol, pseudoephedrine), **Non-Drowsy Sudafed Congestion Relief**® (phenylephrine), **Non-Drowsy Sudafed Co Tablets**® (paracetamol, pseudoephedrine), **Non-Drowsy Sudafed Decongestant Tablets**® (pseudoephedrine), **Non-Drowsy Sudafed Dual Relief**® (paracetamol, phenylephrine), **Non-Drowsy Sudafed Dual Relief Max**® (ibuprofen, pseudoephedrine), **Non-Drowsy Sudafed Expectorant**® (guaifenesin, pseudoephedrine), **Non-Drowsy Sudafed 12 Hour Relief**® (pseudoephedrine), **Non-Drowsy Sudafed Linctus**® (dextromethorphan, pseudoephedrine), **Non-Drowsy Sudafed Plus Tablets**® (pseudoephedrine, triprolidine), **Numark Cold Relief Powders**® (paracetamol), **Nurofen**® **Cold and Flu** (ibuprofen, pseudoephedrine), **Nurofen**® **Sinus** (ibuprofen, pseudoephedrine)
Otrivine® **Mu-Cron** (paracetamol, pseudoephedrine)
Pavacol D® (pholcodine), **Pulmo Bailly**® (codeine, guaiacol)
Robitussin Chesty Cough® (guaifenesin), **Robitussin Chesty Cough with Congestion**® (guaifenesin, pseudoephedrine), **Robitussin Dry Cough**® (dextromethorphan), **Robitussin Junior Persistant Cough**® (dextromethorphan), **Robitussin Night-Time**® (brompheniramine, codeine, pseudoephedrine)
Tixycolds® (diphenhydramine, pseudoephedrine), **Tixylix Chesty Cough**® (guaifenesin), **Tixylix Cough and Cold**® (chlorphenamine, pholcodine, pseudoephedrine), **Tixylix Daytime**® (pholcodine), **Tixylix Night-time**® (pholcodine, promethazine), **Tixyplus**® **Active Relief for Colds and Flu** (diphenhydramine, paracetamol)
Uniflu with Gregovite C® (caffeine, codeine, diphenhydramine, paracetamol, phenylephrine)
Venos for Dry Coughs®, **Venos Expectorant**® (guaifenesin), **Venos Honey and Lemon**®, **Vicks Medinite**® (dextromethorphan, doxylamine, ephedrine, paracetamol), **Vicks Vaposyrup for Tickly Coughs**® (honey, menthol), **Vicks Vaposyrup Chesty Cough**® (guaifenesin), **Vicks Vaposyrup Dry Cough**® (dextromethorphan)

3.10 Systemic nasal decongestants

Nasal decongestants for administration by mouth may not be as effective as preparations for local application (section 12.2.2) but they do not give rise to rebound nasal congestion on withdrawal. Some systemic nasal decongestants can have unwanted sympathomimetic effects. **Pseudoephedrine** is available over-the-counter; it has few sympathomimetic effects.

Systemic decongestants should be used with **caution** in diabetes, hypertension, hyperthyroidism, raised intraocular pressure, prostate hypertrophy, hepatic impairment, renal impairment, and ischaemic heart disease and **avoided** in patients taking monoamine oxidase inhibitors; **interactions:** Appendix 1 (sympathomimetics). See below for CSM advice on phenylpropanolamine.

CSM advice. The CSM has advised that evidence of a link between phenylpropanolamine and an increased risk of haemorrhagic stroke is weak and is mainly associated with indications that are not licensed in the UK. The CSM has issued a reminder that:

- the maximum daily dose of phenylpropanolamine should not exceed 100 mg;

- patients with high blood pressure, hyperthyroidism, heart disease or who are receiving MAOIs should not take products containing phenylpropanolamine;

- phenylpropanolamine may aggravate conditions such as diabetes, glaucoma or prostatic enlargement.

The main ingredients in systemic nasal decongestant preparations are shown in the list of cough and decongestant preparations on sale to the public (section 3.9.2). Many preparations also contain antihistamines, which may cause drowsiness and affect the ability to drive or operate machinery.

PSEUDOEPHEDRINE HYDROCHLORIDE

Indications: see notes above
Cautions: see notes above
Side-effects: tachycardia, anxiety, restlessness, insomnia; rarely hallucinations, rash; urinary retention also reported
Dose: see preparations below

Galpseud® (Thornton & Ross) � ━
Tablets, pseudoephedrine hydrochloride 60 mg. Net price 20 = 91p
  Dose: 1 tablet 4 times daily
Linctus, orange, sugar-free, pseudoephedrine hydrochloride 30 mg/5 mL. Net price 140 mL = 96p
  Dose: 10 mL 3 times daily; CHILD 2–6 years 2.5 mL, 6–12 years 5 mL

Sudafed® (Warner Lambert) ━
Tablets, red, f/c, pseudoephedrine hydrochloride 60 mg. Net price 20 = 96p
  Dose: 1 tablet every 4–6 hours (up to 4 times daily)
Elixir, red, pseudoephedrine hydrochloride 30 mg/5 mL. Net price 100 mL = 77p
  Dose: 10 mL every 4–6 hours (up to 4 times daily); CHILD 2–5 years 2.5 mL, 6–12 years 5 mL
NOTE. The brand name *Sudafed®* is also used for preparations containing dextromethorphan, guaifenesin, ibuprofen, paracetamol, phenylephrine, triprolidine (p. 162–3 and p. 210), oxymetazoline, and xylometazoline (p. 528)

■ Preparations on sale to the public
For a list of **cough and decongestant preparations on sale to the public**, including those containing pseudoephedrine, see p. 162–3

4: Central nervous system

4.1   Hypnotics and anxiolytics

Most anxiolytics ('sedatives') will induce sleep when given at night and most hypnotics will sedate when given during the day. Prescribing of these drugs is widespread but dependence (both physical and psychological) and tolerance occurs. This may lead to difficulty in withdrawing the drug after the patient has been taking it regularly for more than a few weeks (see Dependence and Withdrawal, below). Hypnotics and anxiolytics should therefore be reserved for short courses to alleviate acute conditions after causal factors have been established.

Benzodiazepines are the most commonly used anxiolytics and hypnotics; they act at benzodiazepine receptors which are associated with gamma-aminobutyric acid (GABA) receptors. Older drugs such as meprobamate and barbiturates (section 4.1.3) are **not** recommended—they have more side-effects and interactions than benzodiazepines and are much more dangerous in overdosage.

PARADOXICAL EFFECTS. A paradoxical increase in hostility and aggression may be reported by patients taking benzodiazepines. The effects range from talkativeness and excitement, to aggressive and antisocial acts. Adjustment of the dose (up or down) usually attenuates the impulses. Increased anxiety and perceptual disorders are other paradoxical effects. Increased hostility and aggression after barbiturates and alcohol usually indicates intoxication.

DRIVING. Hypnotics and anxiolytics may impair judgement and increase reaction time, and so affect ability to drive or operate machinery; they increase the effects of alcohol. Moreover the hangover effects of a night dose may impair driving on the following day. See also Drugs and Driving under General Guidance, p. 2.

DEPENDENCE AND WITHDRAWAL. Withdrawal of a benzodiazepine should be gradual because abrupt withdrawal may produce confusion, toxic psychosis, convulsions, or a condition resembling delirium tremens. Abrupt withdrawal of a barbiturate (section 4.1.3) is even more likely to have serious effects.

The benzodiazepine withdrawal syndrome may develop at any time up to 3 weeks after stopping a long-acting benzodiazepine, but may occur within a few hours in the case of a short-acting one. It is characterised by insomnia, anxiety, loss of appetite and of body-weight, tremor, perspiration, tinnitus, and perceptual disturbances. These symptoms may be similar to the original complaint and encourage further prescribing; some symptoms may continue for weeks or months after stopping benzodiazepines.

A benzodiazepine can be withdrawn in steps of about one-eighth (range one-tenth to one-quarter) of the daily dose every fortnight. A suggested withdrawal protocol for patients who have difficulty is as follows:

1. Transfer patient to equivalent daily dose of diazepam[1] preferably taken at night
2. Reduce diazepam dose in fortnightly steps of 2 or 2.5 mg; if withdrawal symptoms occur, maintain this dose until symptoms improve
3. Reduce dose further, if necessary in smaller fortnightly steps[2]; it is better to reduce too slowly rather than too quickly
4. Stop completely; time needed for withdrawal can vary from about 4 weeks to a year or more

Counselling may help; beta-blockers should **only** be tried if other measures fail; antidepressants should be used **only** for clinical depression or for panic disorder; **avoid** antipsychotics (which may aggravate withdrawal symptoms).

CSM advice.

1. Benzodiazepines are indicated for the short-term relief (two to four weeks only) of anxiety that is severe, disabling or subjecting the individual to unacceptable distress, occurring alone or in association with insomnia or short-term psychosomatic, organic or psychotic illness.
2. The use of benzodiazepines to treat short-term 'mild' anxiety is inappropriate and unsuitable.
3. Benzodiazepines should be used to treat insomnia only when it is severe, disabling, or subjecting the individual to extreme distress.

4.1.1 Hypnotics

Before a hypnotic is prescribed the cause of the insomnia should be established and, where possible, underlying factors should be treated. However, it should be noted that some patients have unrealistic sleep expectations, and others understate their alcohol consumption which is often the cause of the insomnia.

Transient insomnia may occur in those who normally sleep well and may be due to extraneous factors such as noise, shift work, and jet lag. If a hypnotic is indicated one that is rapidly eliminated should be chosen, and only one or two doses should be given.

Short-term insomnia is usually related to an emotional problem or serious medical illness. It may last for a few weeks and may recur; a hypnotic can be useful but should not be given for more than three weeks (preferably only one week). Intermittent use is

1. Approximate equivalent doses, diazepam 5 mg
   ≡ chlordiazepoxide 15 mg
   ≡ loprazolam 0.5–1 mg
   ≡ lorazepam 500 micrograms
   ≡ lormetazepam 0.5–1 mg
   ≡ nitrazepam 5 mg
   ≡ oxazepam 15 mg
   ≡ temazepam 10 mg

2. Steps may be adjusted according to initial dose and duration of treatment and can range from diazepam 500 micrograms (one-quarter of a 2-mg tablet) to 2.5 mg

desirable with omission of some doses. A rapidly eliminated drug is generally appropriate.

Chronic insomnia is rarely benefited by hypnotics and is more often due to mild dependence caused by injudicious prescribing. Psychiatric disorders such as anxiety, depression, and abuse of drugs and alcohol are common causes. Sleep disturbance is very common in depressive illness and early wakening is often a useful pointer. The underlying psychiatric complaint should be treated, adapting the drug regimen to alleviate insomnia. For example, amitriptyline and mirtazapine prescribed for depression, will also help to promote sleep if taken at night. Other causes of insomnia include daytime catnapping and physical causes such as pain, pruritus, and dyspnoea.

Hypnotics should **not** be prescribed indiscriminately and routine prescribing is undesirable. They should be reserved for short courses in the acutely distressed. Tolerance to their effects develops within 3 to 14 days of continuous use and long-term efficacy cannot be assured. A major drawback of long-term use is that withdrawal causes rebound insomnia and precipitates a withdrawal syndrome (section 4.1).

Where prolonged administration is unavoidable hypnotics should be discontinued as soon as feasible and the patient warned that sleep may be disturbed for a few days before normal rhythm is re-established; broken sleep with vivid dreams and increased REM (rapid eye movement) sleep may persist for several weeks.

CHILDREN. The prescribing of hypnotics to children, except for occasional use such as for night terrors and somnambulism (sleep-walking), is not justified.

ELDERLY. Hypnotics should be avoided in the elderly, who are at risk of becoming ataxic and confused and so liable to fall and injure themselves.

Benzodiazepines

Benzodiazepines used as hypnotics include **nitrazepam, flunitrazepam**, and **flurazepam** which have a prolonged action and may give rise to residual effects on the following day; repeated doses tend to be cumulative.

Loprazolam, lormetazepam, and **temazepam** act for a shorter time and they have little or no hangover effect. Withdrawal phenomena however are more common with the short-acting benzodiazepines.

If insomnia is associated with daytime anxiety then the use of a long-acting benzodiazepine anxiolytic such as **diazepam** given as a single dose at night may effectively treat both symptoms.

For general guidelines on benzodiazepine prescribing see section 4.1.2 and for benzodiazepine withdrawal see section 4.1.

NITRAZEPAM

Indications: insomnia (short-term use)

Cautions: respiratory disease, muscle weakness, history of drug or alcohol abuse, marked personality disorder, pregnancy and breast-feeding (Appendixes 4 and 5); reduce dose in elderly and debilitated, and in hepatic (avoid if severe) and renal impairment (Appendixes 2 and 3); avoid prolonged use (and abrupt withdrawal thereafter); porphyria (section 9.8.2); **interactions:** Appendix 1 (anxiolytics and hypnotics)

DRIVING. Drowsiness may persist the next day and affect performance of skilled tasks (e.g. driving); effects of alcohol enhanced

Contra-indications: respiratory depression; acute pulmonary insufficiency; severe hepatic impairment, myasthenia gravis, sleep apnoea syndrome; not for use alone to treat depression (or anxiety associated with depression) or chronic psychosis

Side-effects: drowsiness and lightheadedness the next day; confusion and ataxia (especially in the elderly); amnesia may occur; dependence; see also under Diazepam (section 4.1.2); **overdosage:** see Emergency Treatment of Poisoning, p. 25

Dose: 5–10 mg at bedtime; ELDERLY (or debilitated) 2.5–5 mg; CHILD not recommended

Nitrazepam (Non-proprietary) PoM
Tablets, nitrazepam 5 mg, net price 20 = 59p. Label: 19
Available from Alpharma, APS, CP, DDSA (*Remnos*® DHS), Generics, ICN (*Mogadon*® DHS), IVAX
Oral suspension, nitrazepam 2.5 mg/5 mL. Net price 150 mL = £5.30. Label: 19
Available from Norgine (*Somnite*® DHS)

FLUNITRAZEPAM

Indications: insomnia (short-term use)
Cautions: see under Nitrazepam
Contra-indications: see under Nitrazepam
Side-effects: see under Nitrazepam
Dose: 0.5–1 mg at bedtime; max. 2 mg; ELDERLY (or debilitated) 500 micrograms (max. 1 mg); CHILD not recommended

Rohypnol® (Roche) CD DHS
Tablets, grey-green, f/c, scored, flunitrazepam 1 mg. Net price 30-tab pack = £4.41. Label: 19
WARNING. Flunitrazepam tablets may be particularly subject to abuse

FLURAZEPAM

Indications: insomnia (short-term use)
Cautions: see under Nitrazepam
Contra-indications: see under Nitrazepam
Side-effects: see under Nitrazepam
Dose: 15–30 mg at bedtime; ELDERLY (or debilitated) 15 mg; CHILD not recommended

Dalmane® (ICN) PoM DHS
Capsules, flurazepam (as hydrochloride), 15 mg (grey/yellow), net price 30-cap pack = £5.44; 30 mg (black/grey), 30-cap pack = £6.98. Label: 19

LOPRAZOLAM

Indications: insomnia (short-term use)
Cautions: see under Nitrazepam
Contra-indications: see under Nitrazepam
Side-effects: see under Nitrazepam; shorter acting
Dose: 1 mg at bedtime, increased to 1.5 or 2 mg if required; ELDERLY (or debilitated) 0.5 or 1 mg; CHILD not recommended

Loprazolam (Non-proprietary) PoM
Tablets, loprazolam 1 mg (as mesilate). Net price 28-tab pack = £4.46. Label: 19
Available from Hoechst Marion Roussel (previously *Dormonoct*® DHS)

LORMETAZEPAM

Indications: insomnia (short-term use)
Cautions: see under Nitrazepam
Contra-indications: see under Nitrazepam
Side-effects: see under Nitrazepam; shorter acting
Dose: 0.5–1.5 mg at bedtime; ELDERLY (or debilitated) 500 micrograms; CHILD not recommended

Lormetazepam (Non-proprietary) PoM
Tablets, lormetazepam 500 micrograms, net price 28-tab pack = £3.40; 1 mg, 28-tab pack = £4.08. Label: 19
Available from Generics, Genus

TEMAZEPAM

Indications: insomnia (short-term use); see also section 15.1.4.1 for peri-operative use
Cautions: see under Nitrazepam
Contra-indications: see under Nitrazepam
Side-effects: see under Nitrazepam; shorter acting
Dose: 10–20 mg at bedtime, exceptional circumstances 30–40 mg; ELDERLY (or debilitated) 10 mg at bedtime, exceptional circumstances 20 mg; CHILD not recommended

¹**Temazepam** (Non-proprietary) CD
Tablets, temazepam 10 mg, net price 28-tab pack = 90p; 20 mg, 28-tab pack = £1.63. Label: 19
Oral solution, temazepam 10 mg/5 mL, net price 300 mL = £9.95. Label: 19
Available from Generics (sugar-free), Hillcross (sugar-free), Pharmacia (sugar-free), Rosemont (sugar-free), Sandoz

1. See p. 7 for prescribing requirements for temazepam

Zaleplon, zolpidem, and zopiclone

Zaleplon, **zolpidem** and **zopiclone** are non-benzodiazepine hypnotics, but they act at the benzodiazepine receptor. Zolpidem and zopiclone have a short duration of action; zaleplon is very short acting. All three drugs are not licensed for long-term use; dependence has been reported in a small number of patients.

ZALEPLON

Indications: insomnia (short-term use—up to 2 weeks)
Cautions: respiratory insufficiency (avoid if severe); hepatic impairment (avoid if severe; Appendix 2); history of drug or alcohol abuse; avoid prolonged use (and abrupt withdrawal thereafter); pregnancy (Appendix 4); not for use alone to treat depression
Contra-indications: sleep apnoea syndrome; myasthenia gravis; not for use alone to treat psychosis; breast-feeding
Side-effects: amnesia, paraesthesia, drowsiness, asthenia; nausea, incoordination, confusion, impaired concentration, dizziness, hallucinations, disturbances of hearing, smell, speech, and vision, photosensitivity; dependence; paradoxical effects (discontinue—see also section 4.1)
Dose: 10 mg at bedtime or after going to bed if difficulty falling asleep; ELDERLY 5 mg; CHILD under 18 years not recommended
NOTE. Patients should be advised not to take a second dose during a single night

Sonata® (Wyeth) PoM
Capsules, zaleplon 5 mg (white/light brown), net
price 14-cap pack = £3.36; 10 mg (white), 14-cap
pack = £4.04. Label: 2

ZOLPIDEM TARTRATE

Indications: insomnia (short-term use—up to 4
weeks)

Cautions: depression, history of drug or alcohol
abuse, hepatic impairment (avoid if severe; Appendix 2); renal impairment; elderly; avoid prolonged
use (and abrupt withdrawal thereafter); **interactions:** Appendix 1 (anxiolytics and hypnotics)
DRIVING. Drowsiness may persist the next day and affect
performance of skilled tasks (e.g. driving); effects of
alcohol enhanced

Contra-indications: obstructive sleep apnoea,
acute or severe respiratory depression, myasthenia
gravis, severe hepatic impairment, psychotic illness, pregnancy and breast-feeding

Side-effects: diarrhoea, nausea, vomiting, vertigo,
dizziness, headache, drowsiness, asthenia, amnesia; dependence, memory disturbances, nightmares, nocturnal restlessness, depression, confusion, perceptual disturbances or diplopia, tremor,
ataxia, falls, skin reactions, changes in libido;
paradoxical effects—see section 4.1

Dose: 10 mg at bedtime; ELDERLY (or debilitated)
5 mg; CHILD not recommended

Zolpidem (Non-proprietary) PoM
Tablets, zolpidem tartrate 5 mg, net price 28-tab
pack = £2.89; 10 mg, 28-tab pack = £4.20. Label: 19
Available from APS, Generics, Genus, Sandoz

Stilnoct® (Sanofi-Synthelabo) PoM
Tablets, both f/c, zolpidem tartrate 5 mg, net price
28-tab pack = £3.08; 10 mg, 28-tab pack = £4.48.
Label: 19

ZOPICLONE

Indications: insomnia (short-term use—up to 4
weeks)

Cautions: hepatic (avoid if severe) and renal
impairment (Appendixes 2 and 3); elderly; history
of drug abuse, psychiatric illness; avoid prolonged
use (and abrupt withdrawal thereafter); **interactions:** Appendix 1 (anxiolytics and hypnotics)
DRIVING. Drowsiness may persist the next day and affect
performance of skilled tasks (e.g. driving); effects of
alcohol enhanced

Contra-indications: myasthenia gravis, respiratory failure, severe sleep apnoea syndrome,
severe hepatic impairment; pregnancy and breast-
feeding

Side-effects: bitter or metallic taste; gastro-intestinal disturbances including nausea and vomiting,
dry mouth, aggression; irritability, confusion,
depressed mood; drowsiness, dizziness, lightheadedness, and incoordination, headache; dependence; hypersensitivity reactions reported (including urticaria and rashes); hallucinations,
nightmares, amnesia reported

Dose: 7.5 mg at bedtime; ELDERLY initially 3.75 mg
at bedtime increased if necessary; CHILD not
recommended

Zopiclone (Non-proprietary) PoM
Tablets, zopiclone 3.75 mg, net price 28-tab pack =
£3.07; 7.5 mg, 28-tab pack = £4.47. Label: 19
Available from Alpharma, APS, Arrow, CP, Dominon,
Generics, IVAX, Opus (*Zileze®*)

Zimovane® (Rhône-Poulenc Rorer) PoM
Tablets, f/c, zopiclone 3.75 mg (*Zimovane®* LS ,
blue), net price 28-tab pack = £2.94; 7.5 mg, 28-tab
pack = £4.28. Label: 19

Chloral and derivatives

Chloral hydrate and derivatives were formerly
popular hypnotics for children (but the use of
hypnotics in children is not usually justified). There
is no convincing evidence that they are particularly
useful in the elderly and their role as hypnotics is
now very limited. **Triclofos** causes fewer gastro-
intestinal disturbances than chloral hydrate.

CHLORAL HYDRATE ▱

Indications: insomnia (short-term use)

Cautions: respiratory disease, history of drug or
alcohol abuse, marked personality disorder; reduce
dose in elderly and debilitated; avoid prolonged
use (and abrupt withdrawal thereafter); avoid
contact with skin and mucous membranes; **interactions:** Appendix 1 (anxiolytics and hypnotics)
DRIVING. Drowsiness may persist the next day and affect
performance of skilled tasks (e.g. driving); effects of
alcohol enhanced

Contra-indications: cardiac disease, gastritis,
hepatic impairment, renal impairment; pregnancy
and breast-feeding; porphyria

Side-effects: gastric irritation (nausea and vomiting
reported), abdominal distention and flatulence;
also vertigo, ataxia, staggering gait, rashes, headache, light headedness, malaise, ketonuria, excitement, nightmares, delirium (especially in the
elderly), eosinophilia, reduction in white cell
count; dependence (may be associated with gastritis and renal damage) on prolonged use

Dose: insomnia, 0.5–1 g (max. 2 g) with plenty of
water at bedtime; CHILD 30–50 mg/kg up to a max.
single dose of 1 g

Chloral Mixture, BP PoM ▱
(Chloral Oral Solution)
Mixture, chloral hydrate 500 mg/5 mL in a suitable
vehicle. Extemporaneous preparations should be
recently prepared according to the following
formula: chloral hydrate 1 g, syrup 2 mL, water to
10 mL. Net price 100 mL = 44p. Label: 19, 27
Dose: 5–20 mL; CHILD 1–5 years 2.5–5 mL, 6–12 years
5–10 mL, taken well diluted with water at bedtime

Chloral Elixir, Paediatric, BP PoM ▱
(Chloral Oral Solution, Paediatric)
Elixir, chloral hydrate 4% in a suitable vehicle with
a blackcurrant flavour. Extemporaneous preparations should be recently prepared according to the
following formula: chloral hydrate 200 mg, water
0.1 mL, blackcurrant syrup 1 mL, syrup to 5 mL.
Net price 100 mL = 95p. Label: 1, 27
Dose: up to 1 year 5 mL, taken well diluted with water at
bedtime

Welldorm® (S&N Hlth.) PoM ▰

Tablets, blue-purple, f/c, cloral betaine 707 mg
(≡ chloral hydrate 414 mg). Net price 30-tab pack
= £2.43. Label: 19, 27
Dose: 1–2 tablets with water or milk at bedtime, max. 5
tablets (2 g chloral hydrate) daily

Elixir, red, chloral hydrate 143.3 mg/5 mL. Net
price 150-mL pack = £2.05. Label: 19, 27
Dose: 15–45 mL (0.4–1.3 g chloral hydrate) with water or
milk, at bedtime, max. 70 mL (2 g chloral hydrate) daily;
CHILD 1–1.75 mL/kg (30–50 mg/kg chloral hydrate),
max. 35 mL (1 g chloral hydrate) daily

TRICLOFOS SODIUM ▰

Indications: insomnia (short-term use)
Cautions: see Chloral Hydrate
Contra-indications: see Chloral Hydrate
Side-effects: see Chloral Hydrate but less gastric
irritation
Dose: see under preparation below

Triclofos Oral Solution, BP PoM ▰
(Triclofos Elixir)
Oral solution, triclofos sodium 500 mg/5 mL. Net
price 300 mL = £27.83. Label: 19
Available from Celltech
Dose: 10–20 mL (1–2 g triclofos sodium) at bedtime;
CHILD up to 1 year 25–30 mg/kg, 1–5 years 2.5–5 mL
(250–500 mg triclofos sodium), 6–12 years 5–10 mL
(0.5–1 g triclofos sodium)

Clomethiazole

Clomethiazole (chlormethiazole) may be a useful
hypnotic for elderly patients because of its freedom
from hangover but, as with all hypnotics, routine
administration is undesirable and dependence
occurs. It is licensed for use as a hypnotic only in
the elderly (and for *very short-term use* in younger
adults to attenuate alcohol withdrawal symptoms,
see section 4.10).

CLOMETHIAZOLE
(Chlormethiazole)
Indications: see under Dose; alcohol withdrawal
(section 4.10)
Cautions: cardiac and respiratory disease (confusional state may indicate hypoxia); history of drug
abuse; marked personality disorder; elderly; excessive sedation may occur (particularly with higher
doses); hepatic impairment (especially if severe
because sedation can mask hepatic coma); renal
impairment; avoid prolonged use (and abrupt
withdrawal thereafter); **interactions:** Appendix 1
(anxiolytics and hypnotics)
DRIVING. Drowsiness may persist the next day and affect
performance of skilled tasks (e.g. driving); effects of
alcohol enhanced
Contra-indications: acute pulmonary insufficiency; alcohol-dependent patients who continue
to drink
Side-effects: nasal congestion and irritation
(increased nasopharyngeal and bronchial secretions), conjunctival irritation, headache; rarely,
paradoxical excitement, confusion, dependence,
gastro-intestinal disturbances, rash, urticaria, bullous eruption, anaphylaxis, alterations in liver
enzymes

Dose: severe insomnia in the elderly (short-term
use), 1–2 capsules (*or* 5–10 mL syrup) at bedtime;
CHILD not recommended
Restlessness and agitation in the elderly, 1 capsule
(*or* 5 mL syrup) 3 times daily
Alcohol withdrawal, initially 2–4 capsules, if necessary repeated after some hours;
day 1 (first 24 hours), 9–12 capsules in 3–4 divided
doses;
day 2, 6–8 capsules in 3–4 divided doses;
day 3, 4–6 capsules in 3–4 divided doses; then
gradually reduced over days 4–6; total treatment
for not more than 9 days
NOTE. For an equivalent therapeutic effect 1 capsule ≡
5 mL syrup

Heminevrin® (AstraZeneca) PoM
Capsules, grey-brown, clomethiazole base 192 mg
in an oily basis. Net price 60-cap pack = £4.78.
Label: 19
Syrup, sugar-free, clomethiazole edisilate 250 mg/
5 mL. Net price 300-mL pack = £4.00. Label: 19

Antihistamines

Some **antihistamines** such as diphenhydramine
(section 3.4.1) and promethazine are on sale to the
public for occasional insomnia; their prolonged
duration of action may often lead to drowsiness the
following day. The sedative effect of antihistamines
may diminish after a few days of continued treatment; antihistamines are associated with headache,
psychomotor impairment and antimuscarinic effects.
Promethazine is also popular for use in children, but
the use of hypnotics in children is not usually
justified.

PROMETHAZINE HYDROCHLORIDE
▰

Indications: night sedation and insomnia (short-
term use); other indications (section 3.4.1, section
4.6)
Cautions: section 3.4.1
Contra-indications: section 3.4.1
Side-effects: section 3.4.1
Dose: *by mouth,* 25 mg at bedtime increased to
50 mg if necessary; CHILD under 2 years not
recommended, 2–5 years 15–20 mg, 5–10 years
20–25 mg, at bedtime

■ Preparations
Section 3.4.1

Alcohol

Alcohol is a poor hypnotic because its diuretic action
interferes with sleep during the latter part of the
night. With chronic use, alcohol disturbs sleep
patterns and causes insomnia; **interactions:** Appendix 1 (alcohol).

4.1.2 Anxiolytics

Benzodiazepine anxiolytics can be effective in
alleviating anxiety states. Although these drugs are
often prescribed to almost anyone with stress-related
symptoms, unhappiness, or minor physical disease,
their use in many situations is unjustified. In

particular, they are not appropriate for treating depression or chronic psychosis. In bereavement, psychological adjustment may be inhibited by benzodiazepines. In children anxiolytic treatment should be used only to relieve acute anxiety (and related insomnia) caused by fear (e.g. before surgery).

Anxiolytic treatment should be limited to the lowest possible dose for the shortest possible time (see CSM advice, section 4.1). Dependence is particularly likely in patients with a history of alcohol or drug abuse and in patients with marked personality disorders.

Anxiolytics, particularly the benzodiazepines, have been termed 'minor tranquillisers'. This term is misleading because not only do they differ markedly from the antipsychotic drugs ('major tranquillisers') but their use is by no means minor. Antipsychotics, in low doses, are also sometimes used in severe anxiety for their sedative action but long-term use should be avoided in view of a possible risk of tardive dyskinesia (section 4.2.1).

Some antidepressants (section 4.3) are licensed for use in anxiety and related disorders; see section 4.3 for a comment on their role in generalised anxiety disorder and panic disorders. The use of antihistamines (e.g. hydroxyzine, section 3.4.1) for their sedative effect in anxiety is not considered to be appropriate.

Benzodiazepines

Benzodiazepines are indicated for the *short-term relief of severe anxiety* but long-term use should be avoided (see p. 165). Diazepam, alprazolam, chlordiazepoxide, clobazam, and clorazepate have a sustained action. Shorter-acting compounds such as **lorazepam** and **oxazepam** may be preferred in patients with hepatic impairment but they carry a greater risk of withdrawal symptoms.

In *panic disorders* (with or without agoraphobia) resistant to antidepressant therapy (section 4.3), a benzodiazepine (lorazepam 3–5 mg daily or clonazepam 1–2 mg daily (section 4.8.1) [both unlicensed]) may be used; alternatively a benzodiazepine may be used as short-term adjunctive therapy at the start of antidepressant treatment to prevent the initial worsening of symptoms.

Diazepam or lorazepam are very occasionally administered intravenously for the *control of panic attacks*. This route is the most rapid but the procedure is not without risk (section 4.8.2) and should be used only when alternative measures have failed. The intramuscular route has no advantage over the oral route.

For guidelines on benzodiazepine withdrawal, see p. 165.

DIAZEPAM

Indications: short-term use in anxiety or insomnia, adjunct in acute alcohol withdrawal; status epilepticus (section 4.8.2); febrile convulsions (section 4.8.3); muscle spasm (section 10.2.2); perioperative use (section 15.1.4.1)

Cautions: respiratory disease, muscle weakness, history of drug or alcohol abuse, marked personality disorder, pregnancy and breast-feeding (Appendixes 4 and 5); reduce dose in elderly and

debilitated, and in hepatic impairment (avoid if severe, Appendix 2), renal impairment (Appendix 3); avoid prolonged use (and abrupt withdrawal thereafter); special precautions for intravenous injection (section 4.8.2); porphyria (section 9.8.2); **interactions:** Appendix 1 (anxiolytics and hypnotics)

DRIVING. Drowsiness may affect performance of skilled tasks (e.g. driving); effects of alcohol enhanced

Contra-indications: respiratory depression; acute pulmonary insufficiency; sleep apnoea syndrome; severe hepatic impairment; not for chronic psychosis; should not be used alone in depression or in anxiety with depression; avoid injections containing benzyl alcohol in neonates (see under preparations below)

Side-effects: drowsiness and lightheadedness the next day; confusion and ataxia (especially in the elderly); amnesia; dependence; paradoxical increase in aggression (see also section 4.1); muscle weakness; *occasionally:* headache, vertigo, hypotension, salivation changes, gastro-intestinal disturbances, visual disturbances, dysarthria, tremor, changes in libido, incontinence, urinary retention; blood disorders and jaundice reported; skin reactions; on intravenous injection, pain, thrombophlebitis, and rarely apnoea; **overdosage:** see Emergency Treatment of Poisoning, p. 25

Dose: *by mouth*, anxiety, 2 mg 3 times daily increased if necessary to 15–30 mg daily in divided doses; ELDERLY (or debilitated) half adult dose

Insomnia associated with anxiety, 5–15 mg at bedtime

CHILD night terrors and somnambulism, 1–5 mg at bedtime

By intramuscular injection or slow intravenous injection (into a large vein, at a rate of not more than 5 mg/minute), for severe acute anxiety, control of acute panic attacks, and acute alcohol withdrawal, 10 mg, repeated if necessary after not less than 4 hours

NOTE. Only use intramuscular route when oral and intravenous routes not possible; special precautions for intravenous injection see section 4.8.2

By intravenous infusion—section 4.8.2

By rectum as rectal solution, acute anxiety and agitation, 500 micrograms/kg repeated after 12 hours as required; ELDERLY 250 micrograms/kg; CHILD not recommended

CHILD febrile convulsions, see p. 238

By rectum as suppositories, anxiety when oral route not appropriate, 10–30 mg (higher dose divided); dose form not appropriate for less than 10 mg

Diazepam (Non-proprietary) PoM
Tablets, diazepam 2 mg, net price 20 = 38p; 5 mg, 20 = 41p; 10 mg, 20 = 60p. Label: 2 or 19
Available from Alpharma, APS, Arrow, DDSA (*Tensium®* NHS), Generics, IVAX, Ranbaxy (*Rimapam®* NHS)

Oral solution, diazepam 2 mg/5 mL, net price 100 mL = £1.45. Label: 2 or 19
Available from Alpharma, Sandoz (*Dialar®* NHS)

Strong oral solution, diazepam 5 mg/5 mL, net price 100-mL pack = £6.38. Label: 2 or 19 NHS
Available from Sandoz (*Dialar®* NHS)

Injection (solution), diazepam 5 mg/mL. Do not dilute (except for intravenous infusion). Net price 2-mL amp = 32p
Excipients: may include benzyl alcohol (avoid in neonates, see Excipients, p. 2), ethanol, propylene glycol
Available from CP, Phoenix

Injection (emulsion), diazepam 5 mg/mL. For intravenous injection or infusion. Net price 2-mL amp = 73p
Available from Alpharma (*Diazemuls*®)
Rectal tubes (= rectal solution), diazepam 2 mg/mL, net price 1.25-mL (2.5-mg) tube = 90p, 2.5-mL (5-mg) tube = £1.28; 4 mg/mL, 2.5-mL (10-mg) tube = £1.62
Available from Alpharma (*Stesolid*® 5 mg, 10 mg), CP (*Diazepam Rectubes*® 2.5 mg, 5 mg, 10 mg), Sandoz
Suppositories, diazepam 10 mg, net price 6 = £10.20. Label: 2 or 19
Available from Durbin (*Valclair*®)

ALPRAZOLAM

Indications: anxiety (short-term use)
Cautions: see under Diazepam
Contra-indications: see under Diazepam
Side-effects: see under Diazepam
Dose: 250–500 micrograms 3 times daily (elderly or debilitated 250 micrograms 2–3 times daily), increased if necessary to a total of 3 mg daily; CHILD not recommended

Xanax® (Pharmacia) PoM NHS
Tablets, both scored, alprazolam 250 micrograms, net price 60-tab pack = £2.97; 500 micrograms (pink), 60-tab pack = £5.69. Label: 2

CHLORDIAZEPOXIDE

Indications: anxiety (short-term use); adjunct in acute alcohol withdrawal (section 4.10)
Cautions: see under Diazepam
Contra-indications: see under Diazepam
Side-effects: see under Diazepam
Dose: anxiety, 10 mg 3 times daily increased if necessary to 60–100 mg daily in divided doses; ELDERLY (or debilitated) half adult dose; CHILD not recommended
NOTE. The doses stated above refer equally to chlordiazepoxide and to its hydrochloride

Chlordiazepoxide (Non-proprietary) PoM
Capsules, chlordiazepoxide hydrochloride 5 mg, net price 20 = 83p; 10 mg, 20 = £1.15. Label: 2
Various strengths available from Alpharma, DDSA (*Tropium*® NHS), Hillcross, ICN (*Librium*® NHS), Sandoz

Chlordiazepoxide Hydrochloride (Non-proprietary) PoM
Tablets, chlordiazepoxide hydrochloride 5 mg, net price 20 = 79p; 10 mg, 20 = £1.09; 25 mg, 20 = 70p. Label: 2

CLORAZEPATE DIPOTASSIUM

Indications: anxiety (short-term use)
Cautions: see under Diazepam
Contra-indications: see under Diazepam
Side-effects: see under Diazepam
Dose: 7.5–22.5 mg daily in 2–3 divided doses *or* a single dose of 15 mg at bedtime; ELDERLY (or debilitated) half adult dose; CHILD not recommended

Tranxene® (Boehringer Ingelheim) PoM NHS
Capsules, clorazepate dipotassium 7.5 mg (maroon/grey), net price 20-cap pack = £2.66; 15 mg (pink/grey), 20-cap pack = £2.78. Label: 2 or 19

LORAZEPAM

Indications: short-term use in anxiety or insomnia; status epilepticus (section 4.8.2); peri-operative (section 15.1.4.1)
Cautions: see under Diazepam; short acting; when given parenterally, facilities for managing respiratory depression with mechanical ventilation must be at hand
Contra-indications: see under Diazepam
Side-effects: see under Diazepam
Dose: *by mouth*, anxiety, 1–4 mg daily in divided doses; ELDERLY (or debilitated) half adult dose
Insomnia associated with anxiety, 1–2 mg at bedtime; CHILD not recommended
By intramuscular or slow intravenous injection (into a large vein), acute panic attacks, 25–30 micrograms/kg (usual range 1.5–2.5 mg), repeated every 6 hours if necessary; CHILD not recommended
NOTE. Only use intramuscular route when oral and intravenous routes not possible

Lorazepam (Non-proprietary) PoM
Tablets, lorazepam 1 mg, net price 20 = 89p; 2.5 mg, 20 = £1.24. Label: 2 or 19
Available from Genus, IVAX
Injection, lorazepam 4 mg/mL. Net price 1-mL amp = 40p
Excipients: include benzyl alcohol, propylene glycol (see Excipients, p. 2)
Available from Wyeth (*Ativan*®)
NOTE. For intramuscular injection it should be diluted with an equal volume of water for injections or physiological saline (but only use when oral and intravenous routes not possible)

OXAZEPAM

Indications: anxiety (short-term use)
Cautions: see under Diazepam; short acting
Contra-indications: see under Diazepam
Side-effects: see under Diazepam
Dose: anxiety, 15–30 mg (elderly or debilitated 10–20 mg) 3–4 times daily; CHILD not recommended
Insomnia associated with anxiety, 15–25 mg (max. 50 mg) at bedtime; CHILD not recommended

Oxazepam (Non-proprietary) PoM
Tablets, oxazepam 10 mg, net price 20 = 74p; 15 mg, 20 = 84p; 30 mg, 20 = 49p. Label: 2
Available from most generic manufacturers

Buspirone

Buspirone is thought to act at specific serotonin (5HT$_{1A}$) receptors. Response to treatment may take up to 2 weeks. It does not alleviate the symptoms of benzodiazepine withdrawal. Therefore a patient taking a benzodiazepine still needs to have the benzodiazepine withdrawn gradually; it is advisable to do this before starting buspirone. The dependence and abuse potential of buspirone is low; it is, however, licensed for short-term use only (but specialists occasionally use it for several months).

BUSPIRONE HYDROCHLORIDE

Indications: anxiety (short-term use)
Cautions: does not alleviate benzodiazepine withdrawal (see notes above); **interactions:** Appendix 1 (anxiolytics and hypnotics)
DRIVING. May affect performance of skilled tasks (e.g. driving); effects of alcohol may be enhanced

Contra-indications: epilepsy, severe hepatic impairment, moderate to severe renal impairment, pregnancy and breast-feeding

Side-effects: nausea, dizziness, headache, nervousness, lightheadedness, excitement; rarely tachycardia, palpitations, chest pain, drowsiness, confusion, seizures, dry mouth, fatigue, and sweating

Dose: initially 5 mg 2–3 times daily, increased as necessary every 2–3 days; usual range 15–30 mg daily in divided doses; max. 45 mg daily; CHILD not recommended

Buspirone Hydrochloride (Non-proprietary) PoM
Tablets, buspirone hydrochloride 5 mg, net price 30-tab pack = £8.42; 10 mg, 30-tab pack = £11.16.
Counselling, driving
Available from Alpharma

Buspar® (Bristol-Myers Squibb) PoM
Tablets, buspirone hydrochloride 5 mg, net price 90-tab pack = £28.08; 10 mg, 90-tab pack = £42.12.
Counselling, driving

Beta-blockers

Beta-blockers (e.g. propranolol, oxprenolol) (section 2.4) do not affect psychological symptoms, such as worry, tension, and fear, but they do reduce autonomic symptoms, such as palpitations and tremor; they do not reduce non-autonomic symptoms, such as muscle tension. Beta-blockers are therefore indicated for patients with predominantly somatic symptoms; this, in turn, may prevent the onset of worry and fear. Patients with predominantly psychological symptoms may obtain no benefit.

Meprobamate

Meprobamate is **less effective** than the benzodiazepines, more hazardous in overdosage, and can also induce dependence. It is **not** recommended.

MEPROBAMATE

Indications: short-term use in anxiety, but see notes above

Cautions: respiratory disease, muscle weakness, epilepsy (may induce seizures), history of drug or alcohol abuse, marked personality disorder, pregnancy; elderly and debilitated; hepatic and renal impairment; avoid prolonged use, abrupt withdrawal may precipitate convulsions; **interactions:** Appendix 1 (anxiolytics and hypnotics)
DRIVING. Drowsiness may affect performance of skilled tasks (e.g. driving); effects of alcohol enhanced

Contra-indications: acute pulmonary insufficiency; respiratory depression; porphyria (section 9.8.2); breast-feeding

Side-effects: see under Diazepam, but incidence greater and drowsiness most common side-effect; also gastro-intestinal disturbances, hypotension, paraesthesia, weakness, CNS effects including headache, paradoxical excitement, disturbances of vision; rarely agranulocytosis and rashes

Dose: 400 mg 3–4 times daily; elderly patients half adult dose or less; CHILD not recommended

Meprobamate (Non-proprietary) CD
Tablets, scored, meprobamate 400 mg. Net price 84-tab pack = £9.49. Label: 2
Available from Genus

4.1.3   Barbiturates

The intermediate-acting **barbiturates** have a place only in the treatment of severe intractable insomnia in patients **already taking** barbiturates; they should be avoided in the elderly. The long-acting barbiturate, phenobarbital is still sometimes of value in epilepsy (section 4.8.1) but its use as a sedative is unjustified. The very short-acting barbiturate thiopental is used in anaesthesia (section 15.1.1).

BARBITURATES

Indications: severe intractable insomnia **only** in patients already taking barbiturates; see also notes above

Cautions: avoid use where possible; dependence and tolerance readily occur; abrupt withdrawal may precipitate serious withdrawal syndrome (rebound insomnia, anxiety, tremor, dizziness, nausea, convulsions, delirium, and death); repeated doses are cumulative and may lead to excessive sedation; respiratory disease, renal disease, hepatic impairment; **interactions:** Appendix 1 (barbiturates)
DRIVING. Drowsiness may persist the next day and affect performance of skilled tasks (e.g. driving); effects of alcohol enhanced

Contra-indications: insomnia caused by pain; porphyria (section 9.8.2), pregnancy, breast-feeding; children, young adults, elderly and debilitated patients, also patients with history of drug or alcohol abuse

Side-effects: include hangover with drowsiness, dizziness, ataxia, respiratory depression, hypersensitivity reactions, headache, particularly in elderly; paradoxical excitement and confusion occasionally precede sleep; **overdosage:** see Emergency Treatment of Poisoning, p. 25

Dose: see under preparations below

Amytal® (Flynn) CD
Tablets, amobarbital (amylobarbitone) 50 mg, net price 20 = £1.84. Label: 19
Dose: 100–200 mg at bedtime (**important:** but see also contra-indications)

Sodium Amytal® (Flynn) CD
Capsules, both blue, amobarbital (amylobarbitone) sodium 60 mg, net price 20 = £3.43; 200 mg, 20 = £6.75. Label: 19
Dose: 60–200 mg at bedtime (**important:** but see also contra-indications)

Soneryl® (Concord) CD
Tablets, pink, scored, butobarbital (butobarbitone) 100 mg. Net price 56-tab pack = £10.65. Label: 19
Dose: 100–200 mg at bedtime (**important:** but see also contra-indications)

■ Preparations containing secobarbital (quinalbarbitone)
NOTE. Secobarbital (quinalbarbitone) is in schedule 2 of the Misuse of Drugs Regulations 2001; receipt and supply must therefore be recorded in the CD register.

Seconal Sodium® (Flynn) CD
Capsules, both orange, secobarbital (quinalbarbitone) sodium 50 mg, net price 20 = £5.30; 100 mg, 20 = £6.96. Label: 19
Dose: 100 mg at bedtime (**important:** but see also contra-indications)

Tuinal® (Flynn) ▢ ▭
Capsules, orange/blue, a mixture of amobarbital (amylobarbitone) sodium 50 mg, secobarbital (quinalbarbitone) sodium 50 mg. Net price 20 = £3.88. Label: 19
Dose: 1–2 capsules at bedtime (**important:** but see also contra-indications)
NOTE. Prescriptions need only specify 'Tuinal capsules'

4.2 Drugs used in psychoses and related disorders

4.2.1 Antipsychotic drugs
4.2.2 Antipsychotic depot injections
4.2.3 Antimanic drugs

Advice of Royal College of Psychiatrists on doses above BNF upper limit. Unless otherwise stated, doses in the BNF are licensed doses—any higher dose is therefore **unlicensed** (for an explanation of the significance of this, see p. 1).

1. Consider alternative approaches including adjuvant therapy and newer or atypical neuroleptics such as clozapine.
2. Bear in mind risk factors, including obesity—particular caution is indicated in older patients especially those over 70.
3. Consider potential for drug interactions—see **interactions:** Appendix 1 (antipsychotics).
4. Carry out ECG to exclude untoward abnormalities such as prolonged QT interval; repeat ECG periodically and reduce dose if prolonged QT interval or other adverse abnormality develops.
5. Increase dose slowly and not more often than once weekly.
6. Carry out regular pulse, blood pressure, and temperature checks; ensure that patient maintains adequate fluid intake.
7. Consider high-dose therapy to be for limited period and review regularly; abandon if no improvement after 3 months (return to standard dosage).

Important: When prescribing an antipsychotic for administration on an emergency basis, the intramuscular dose should be **lower** than the corresponding oral dose (owing to absence of first-pass effect), particularly if the patient is very active (increased blood flow to muscle considerably increases the rate of absorption). The prescription should specify the dose for **each route** and should **not** imply that the same dose can be given by mouth or by intramuscular injection. The dose of antipsychotic for emergency use should be reviewed at least **daily**.

4.2.1 Antipsychotic drugs

Antipsychotic drugs are also known as 'neuroleptics' and (misleadingly) as 'major tranquillisers'. Antipsychotic drugs generally tranquillise without impairing consciousness and without causing paradoxical excitement but they should not be regarded merely as tranquillisers. For conditions such as schizophrenia the tranquillising effect is of secondary importance.

In the short term they are used to quieten disturbed patients whatever the underlying psychopathology, which may be schizophrenia, brain damage, mania,

toxic delirium, or agitated depression. Antipsychotic drugs are used to alleviate severe anxiety but this too should be a short-term measure.

SCHIZOPHRENIA. Antipsychotic drugs relieve florid psychotic symptoms such as thought disorder, hallucinations, and delusions, and prevent relapse. Although they are usually less effective in apathetic withdrawn patients, they sometimes appear to have an activating influence. Patients with acute schizophrenia generally respond better than those with chronic symptoms.

Long-term treatment of a patient with a definite diagnosis of schizophrenia may be necessary even after the first episode of illness in order to prevent the manifest illness from becoming chronic. Withdrawal of drug treatment requires careful surveillance because the patient who appears well on medication may suffer a disastrous relapse if treatment is withdrawn inappropriately. In addition the need for continuation of treatment may not become immediately evident because relapse is often delayed for several weeks after cessation of treatment.

Antipsychotic drugs are considered to act by interfering with dopaminergic transmission in the brain by blocking dopamine D_2 receptors, which may give rise to the extrapyramidal effects described below, and also to hyperprolactinaemia. Antipsychotic drugs may also affect cholinergic, alpha-adrenergic, histaminergic, and serotonergic receptors.

CAUTIONS AND CONTRA-INDICATIONS. Antipsychotics should be used with **caution** in patients with hepatic impairment (Appendix 2), renal impairment (Appendix 3), cardiovascular disease, Parkinson's disease (may be exacerbated by antipsychotics), epilepsy (and conditions predisposing to epilepsy), depression, myasthenia gravis, prostatic hypertrophy, or a personal or family history of angle-closure glaucoma (avoid chlorpromazine, pericyazine and prochlorperazine in these conditions). Caution is also required in severe respiratory disease and in patients with a history of jaundice or who have blood dyscrasias (perform blood counts if unexplained infection or fever develops). Antipsychotics should be used with caution in the elderly, who are particularly susceptible to postural hypotension and to hyper- or hypothermia in very hot or cold weather. Serious consideration should be given before prescribing these drugs for elderly patients. As photosensitisation may occur with higher dosages, patients should avoid direct sunlight.

Antipsychotic drugs may be **contra-indicated** in comatose states, CNS depression, and phaeochromocytoma. Most antipsychotics are best avoided during pregnancy, unless essential (Appendix 4) and it is advisable to discontinue breast-feeding during treatment (Appendix 5); **interactions:** Appendix 1 (antipsychotics)

DRIVING. Drowsiness may affect performance of skilled tasks (e.g. driving or operating machinery), especially at start of treatment; effects of alcohol are enhanced

WITHDRAWAL. Withdrawal of antipsychotic drugs after long-term therapy should always be gradual and closely monitored to avoid the risk of acute withdrawal syndromes or rapid relapse.

SIDE-EFFECTS. Extrapyramidal symptoms are the most troublesome. They occur most frequently with the piperazine phenothiazines (fluphenazine, perphenazine, prochlorperazine, and trifluoperazine), the butyrophenones (benperidol and haloperidol), and the depot preparations. They are easy to recognise but cannot be predicted accurately because they depend on the dose, the type of drug, and on individual susceptibility.

Extrapyramidal symptoms consist of:

- *parkinsonian symptoms* (including tremor), which may occur more commonly in adults or the elderly and may appear gradually;
- *dystonia* (abnormal face and body movements) and *dyskinesia*, which occur more commonly in children or young adults and appear after only a few doses;
- *akathisia* (restlessness), which characteristically occurs after large initial doses and may resemble an exacerbation of the condition being treated; and
- *tardive dyskinesia* (rhythmic, involuntary movements of tongue, face, and jaw), which usually develops on long-term therapy or with high dosage, but it may develop on short-term treatment with low doses—short-lived tardive dyskinesia may occur after withdrawal of the drug.

Parkinsonian symptoms remit if the drug is withdrawn and may be suppressed by the administration of **antimuscarinic** drugs (section 4.9.2). However, routine administration of such drugs is not justified because not all patients are affected and because they may unmask or worsen tardive dyskinesia.

Tardive dyskinesia is of particular concern because it may be irreversible on withdrawing therapy and treatment is usually ineffective. However, some manufacturers suggest that drug withdrawal at the earliest signs of tardive dyskinesia (fine vermicular movements of the tongue) may halt its full development. Tardive dyskinesia occurs fairly frequently, especially in the elderly, and treatment must be carefully and regularly reviewed.

Hypotension and interference with temperature regulation are dose-related side-effects and are liable to cause dangerous falls and hypothermia or hyperthermia in the elderly.

Neuroleptic malignant syndrome (hyperthermia, fluctuating level of consciousness, muscular rigidity, and autonomic dysfunction with pallor, tachycardia, labile blood pressure, sweating, and urinary incontinence) is a rare but potentially fatal side-effect of some drugs. Discontinuation of the antipsychotic is essential because there is no proven effective treatment, but cooling, bromocriptine, and dantrolene have been used. The syndrome, which usually lasts for 5–7 days after drug discontinuation, may be unduly prolonged if depot preparations have been used.

Other side-effects include: drowsiness; apathy; agitation, excitement and insomnia; convulsions; dizziness; headache; confusion; gastro-intestinal disturbances; nasal congestion; antimuscarinic symptoms (such as dry mouth, constipation, difficulty with micturition, and blurred vision); cardiovascular symptoms (such as hypotension, tachycardia, and arrhythmias); ECG changes (cases of sudden death have occurred); endocrine effects such as menstrual disturbances, galactorrhoea, gynaecomastia, impotence, and weight gain; blood dyscrasias (such as agranulocytosis and leucopenia), photosensitisation, contact sensitisation and rashes, and jaundice (including cholestatic); corneal and lens opacities, and purplish pigmentation of the skin, cornea, conjunctiva, and retina.

Overdosage: for poisoning with phenothiazines and related compounds, see Emergency Treatment of Poisoning, p. 26.

CLASSIFICATION OF ANTIPSYCHOTICS. The **phenothiazine** derivatives can be divided into 3 main groups.

Group 1: chlorpromazine, levomepromazine (methotrimeprazine), and promazine, generally characterised by pronounced sedative effects and moderate antimuscarinic and extrapyramidal side-effects.

Group 2: pericyazine, pipotiazine, and thioridazine, generally characterised by moderate sedative effects, marked antimuscarinic effects, but fewer extrapyramidal side-effects than groups 1 or 3.

Group 3: fluphenazine, perphenazine, prochlorperazine, and trifluoperazine, generally characterised by fewer sedative effects, fewer antimuscarinic effects, but more pronounced extrapyramidal side-effects than groups 1 and 2.

Drugs of other chemical groups tend to resemble the phenothiazines of *group 3*. They include the **butyrophenones** (benperidol and haloperidol); **diphenylbutylpiperidines** (pimozide); **thioxanthenes** (flupentixol and zuclopenthixol); and the **substituted benzamides** (sulpiride).

For details of the newer antipsychotic drugs amisulpride, clozapine, olanzapine, quetiapine, risperidone, sertindole, and zotepine, see under Atypical Antipsychotics, p. 179.

CHOICE. As indicated above, the various drugs differ somewhat in predominant actions and side-effects. Selection is influenced by the degree of sedation required and the patient's susceptibility to extrapyramidal side-effects. However, the differences between antipsychotic drugs are less important than the great variability in patient response; moreover, tolerance to secondary effects such as sedation usually develops. The atypical antipsychotics may be appropriate if extrapyramidal side-effects are a particular concern (see under Atypical Antipsychotics, below). Clozapine is used for schizophrenia when other antipsychotics are ineffective or not tolerated.

Prescribing of more than one antipsychotic at the same time is **not** recommended; it may constitute a hazard and there is no significant evidence that side-effects are minimised.

Chlorpromazine is still widely used despite the wide range of adverse effects associated with it. It has a marked sedating effect and is useful for treating violent patients without causing stupor. Agitated states in the elderly can be controlled without confusion, a dose of 10 to 25 mg once or twice daily usually being adequate.

Flupentixol (flupenthixol) and **pimozide** (see CSM advice p. 177) are less sedating than chlorpromazine.

Sulpiride in high doses controls florid positive symptoms, but in lower doses it has an alerting effect on apathetic withdrawn schizophrenics.

Fluphenazine, haloperidol, and **trifluoperazine** are also of value but their use is limited by the high incidence of extrapyramidal symptoms. Haloperidol may be preferred for the rapid control of hyperactive psychotic states; it causes less hypotension than chlorpromazine and is therefore also popular for agitation and restlessness in the elderly, despite the high incidence of extrapyramidal side-effects.

Thioridazine is associated with rare reports of ventricular arrhythmia and it is now restricted for use as second-line treatment for schizophrenia in adults; it should be prescribed under specialist supervision only.

Promazine is not sufficiently active by mouth to be used as an antipsychotic drug; it has been used to treat agitation and restlessness in the elderly (see Other uses, below).

OTHER USES. Nausea and vomiting (section 4.6), choreas, motor tics (section 4.9.3), and intractable hiccup (see under Chlorpromazine Hydrochloride and under Haloperidol). **Benperidol** is used in deviant antisocial sexual behaviour but its value is not established; see also section 6.4.2 for the role of cyproterone acetate.

Psychomotor agitation and, in the elderly, agitation and restlessness, should be investigated for an underlying cause; they can be managed with low doses of chlorpromazine or haloperidol used for short periods. The use of promazine for agitation and restlessness in the elderly has declined. **Olanzapine** and **risperidone** may be effective for agitation and restlessness in the elderly [both unlicensed].

Equivalent doses of oral antipsychotics

These equivalences are intended **only** as an approximate guide; individual dosage instructions should **also** be checked; patients should be carefully monitored after **any** change in medication

Antipsychotic	Daily dose
Chlorpromazine	100 mg
Clozapine	50 mg
Haloperidol	2–3 mg
Pimozide	2 mg
Risperidone	0.5–1 mg
Sulpiride	200 mg
Thioridazine	100 mg
Trifluoperazine	5 mg

Important. These equivalences must **not** be extrapolated beyond the max. dose for the drug. Higher doses require careful titration in specialist units and the equivalences shown here may not be appropriate

> **Dosage.** After an initial period of stabilisation, in most patients, the long half-life of antipsychotic drugs allows the total daily oral dose to be given as a single dose. For the advice of The Royal College of Psychiatrists on doses above the BNF upper limit, see p. 173.

BENPERIDOL

Indications: control of deviant antisocial sexual behaviour (but see notes above)

Cautions: see notes above; also manufacturer advises regular blood counts and liver function tests during long-term treatment

Contra-indications: see notes above

Side-effects: see notes above

Dose: 0.25–1.5 mg daily in divided doses, adjusted according to the response; ELDERLY (or debilitated) initially half adult dose; CHILD not recommended

Benquil® (Hansam) PoM

Tablets, scored, benperidol 250 micrograms, net price 112-tab pack = £104.00. Label: 2

CHLORPROMAZINE HYDROCHLORIDE

WARNING. Owing to the risk of contact sensitisation, pharmacists, nurses, and other health workers should avoid direct contact with chlorpromazine; tablets should not be crushed and solutions should be handled with care

Indications: see under Dose; antiemetic in palliative care (section 4.6)

Cautions: see notes above; also patients should remain supine and the blood pressure monitored for 30 minutes after intramuscular injection

Contra-indications: see notes above

Side-effects: see notes above; also intramuscular injection may be painful, cause hypotension and tachycardia, and give rise to nodule formation

Dose: *by mouth*, schizophrenia and other psychoses, mania, short-term adjunctive management of severe anxiety, psychomotor agitation, excitement, and violent or dangerously impulsive behaviour initially 25 mg 3 times daily (*or* 75 mg at night), adjusted according to response, to usual maintenance dose of 75–300 mg daily (but up to 1 g daily may be required in psychoses); ELDERLY (or debilitated) third to half adult dose; CHILD (childhood schizophrenia and autism) 1–5 years 500 micrograms/kg every 4–6 hours (max. 40 mg daily); 6–12 years third to half adult dose (max. 75 mg daily)

Intractable hiccup, 25–50 mg 3–4 times daily

By deep intramuscular injection, (for relief of acute symptoms but see also Cautions and Side-effects), 25–50 mg every 6–8 hours; CHILD, 1–5 years 500 micrograms/kg every 6–8 hours (max. 40 mg daily); 6–12 years 500 micrograms/kg every 6–8 hours (max. 75 mg daily)

Induction of hypothermia (to prevent shivering), *by deep intramuscular injection*, 25–50 mg every 6–8 hours; CHILD 1–12 years, initially 0.5–1 mg/kg, followed by maintenance 500 micrograms/kg every 4–6 hours

By rectum in suppositories as chlorpromazine base 100 mg every 6–8 hours [unlicensed]

NOTE. For equivalent therapeutic effect 100 mg chlorpromazine base given *rectally* as a suppository ≡ 20–25 mg chlorpromazine hydrochloride *by intramuscular injection* ≡ 40–50 mg of chlorpromazine base or hydrochloride *by mouth*

Chlorpromazine (Non-proprietary) PoM

Tablets, coated, chlorpromazine hydrochloride 10 mg, net price 56-tab pack = 71p; 25 mg, 28-tab pack = 96p; 50 mg, 28-tab pack = 95p; 100 mg, 28-tab pack = £1.16. Label: 2, 11
Available from Antigen, APS, Arrow, DDSA (*Chloractil*®), Genus, Hillcross, IVAX

Oral solution, chlorpromazine hydrochloride 25 mg/5 mL, net price 150 mL = £1.35, 100 mg/5 mL, 150 mL = £3.76. Label: 2, 11
Available from Hillcross, Rosemont

Injection, chlorpromazine hydrochloride 25 mg/mL, net price 1-mL amp = 60p; 2-mL amp = 67p
Available from Antigen

Suppositories, chlorpromazine 100 mg. Label: 2, 11
'Special order' [unlicensed] product; contact Martindale or regional hospital manufacturing unit

Largactil® (Hawgreen) [PoM]
Tablets, all off-white, f/c, chlorpromazine hydro-chloride 10 mg. Net price 56-tab pack= 71p; 25 mg, 56-tab pack = 98p; 50 mg, 56-tab pack = £2.05; 100 mg, 56-tab pack = £3.81. Label: 2, 11
Syrup, brown, chlorpromazine hydrochloride 25 mg/5 mL. Net price 100-mL pack = £1.11. Label: 2, 11
Suspension forte, orange, sugar-free, chlorprom-azine hydrochloride 100 mg (as embonate)/5 mL. Net price 100-mL pack = £2.56. Label: 2, 11
Injection, chlorpromazine hydrochloride 25 mg/mL. Net price 2-mL amp = 67p

FLUPENTIXOL

(Flupenthixol)
Indications: schizophrenia and other psychoses, particularly with apathy and withdrawal but not mania or psychomotor hyperactivity; depression (section 4.3.4)
Cautions: see notes above; avoid in porphyria (section 9.8.2)
Contra-indications: see notes above; also excita-ble and overactive patients
Side-effects: see notes above; less sedating but extrapyramidal symptoms frequent
Dose: psychosis, initially 3–9 mg twice daily adjusted according to the response; max. 18 mg daily; ELDERLY (or debilitated) initially quarter to half adult dose; CHILD not recommended

Depixol® (Lundbeck) [PoM]
Tablets, yellow, s/c, flupentixol 3 mg (as dihy-drochloride). Net price 20 = £2.99. Label: 2
Depot injection (flupentixol decanoate): section 4.2.2

FLUPHENAZINE HYDROCHLORIDE

Indications: see under Dose
Cautions: see notes above
Contra-indications: see notes above
Side-effects: see notes above; less sedating and fewer antimuscarinic or hypotensive symptoms, but extrapyramidal symptoms, particularly dys-tonic reactions and akathisia, more frequent; sys-temic lupus erythematosus
Dose: schizophrenia and other psychoses, mania, initially 2.5–10 mg daily in 2–3 divided doses, adjusted according to response to 20 mg daily; doses above 20 mg daily (10 mg in elderly) only with special caution; CHILD not recommended
Short-term adjunctive management of severe anxiety, psychomotor agitation, excitement, and violent or dangerously impulsive behaviour, initi-ally 1 mg twice daily, increased as necessary to 2 mg twice daily; CHILD not recommended

Moditen® (Sanofi-Synthelabo) [PoM]
Tablets, all s/c, fluphenazine hydrochloride 1 mg (pink), net price 20 = £1.06; 2.5 mg (yellow), 20 = £1.33; 5 mg, 20 = £1.77. Label: 2

Modecate® [PoM] Section 4.2.2

HALOPERIDOL

Indications: see under Dose; motor tics (section 4.9.3)

Cautions: see notes above; also subarachnoid haemorrhage and metabolic disturbances such as hypokalaemia, hypocalcaemia, or hypomagnes-aemia
Contra-indications: see notes above
Side-effects: see notes above, but less sedating and fewer antimuscarinic or hypotensive symptoms; pigmentation and photosensitivity reactions rare; extrapyramidal symptoms, particularly dystonic reactions and akathisia especially in thyrotoxic patients; rarely weight loss; hypoglycaemia; inap-propriate antidiuretic hormone secretion
Dose: *by mouth*, schizophrenia and other psychoses, mania, short-term adjunctive management of psy-chomotor agitation, excitement, and violent or dangerously impulsive behaviour, initially 1.5–3 mg 2–3 times daily *or* 3–5 mg 2–3 times daily in severely affected or resistant patients; in resistant schizophrenia up to 30 mg daily may be needed; adjusted according to response to lowest effective maintenance dose (as low as 5–10 mg daily); ELDERLY (or debilitated) initially half adult dose; CHILD initially 25–50 micrograms/kg daily (in 2 divided doses) to max. 10 mg
Agitation and restlessness in the elderly, initially 0.5–1.5 mg once or twice daily
Short-term adjunctive management of severe anxiety, 500 micrograms twice daily; CHILD not recommended
Intractable hiccup, 1.5 mg 3 times daily adjusted according to response; CHILD not recommended
Nausea and vomiting, 1 mg daily (see also Pre-scribing in Palliative Care, p. 15)
By intramuscular or by intravenous injection, initi-ally 2–10 mg, then every 4–8 hours according to response to total max. 18 mg daily; severely disturbed patients may require initial dose of up to 18 mg; ELDERLY (or debilitated) initially half adult dose; CHILD not recommended
Nausea and vomiting, 0.5–2 mg

Haloperidol (Non-proprietary) [PoM]
Tablets, haloperidol 500 micrograms, net price 28-tab pack = 91p; 1.5 mg, 20 = £1.02; 5 mg, 20 = £2.41; 10 mg, 20 = £3.27; 20 mg, 20 = £8.47. Label: 2

Dozic® (Rosemont) [PoM]
Oral liquid, sugar-free, haloperidol 1 mg/mL. Net price 100-mL pack = £7.30. Label: 2

Haldol® (Janssen-Cilag) [PoM]
Tablets, both scored, haloperidol 5 mg (blue), net price 20 = £1.65; 10 mg (yellow), 20 = £3.21. Label: 2
Oral liquid, sugar-free, haloperidol 2 mg/mL. Net price 100-mL pack (with pipette) = £5.08. Label: 2
Injection, haloperidol 5 mg/mL. Net price 1-mL amp = 33p
Depot injection (haloperidol decanoate): section 4.2.2

Serenace® (IVAX) [PoM]
Capsules, green, haloperidol 500 micrograms, net price 30-cap pack = 98p. Label: 2
Tablets, haloperidol 1.5 mg, net price 30-tab pack = £1.73; 5 mg (pink), 30-tab pack = £4.90; 10 mg (pale pink), 30-tab pack = £8.81. Label: 2
Oral liquid, sugar-free, haloperidol 2 mg/mL, net price 500-mL pack = £43.83. Label: 2
Injection, haloperidol 5 mg/mL, net price 1-mL amp = 59p; 10 mg/mL, 2-mL amp = £2.03

LEVOMEPROMAZINE
(Methotrimeprazine)

Indications: see under Dose

Cautions: see notes above; patients receiving large initial doses should remain supine

ELDERLY. Risk of postural hypotension; not recommended for ambulant patients over 50 years unless risk of hypotensive reaction assessed

Contra-indications: see notes above

Side-effects: see notes above; occasionally raised erythrocyte sedimentation rate occurs

Dose: *by mouth*, schizophrenia, initially 25–50 mg daily in divided doses increased as necessary; bedpatients initially 100–200 mg daily usually in 3 divided doses, increased if necessary to 1 g daily; ELDERLY, see Cautions

Adjunctive treatment in palliative care (including management of pain and associated restlessness, distress, or vomiting), 12.5–50 mg every 4–8 hours, but see also Prescribing in Palliative Care, p. 14

By intramuscular injection or by intravenous injection (by intravenous injection after dilution with an equal volume of sodium chloride 0.9% injection), adjunct in palliative care, 12.5–25 mg (severe agitation up to 50 mg) every 6–8 hours if necessary

By continuous subcutaneous infusion, adjunct in palliative care (via syringe driver), diluted in a suitable volume of sodium chloride 0.9% injection, see Prescribing in Palliative Care, p. 15; CHILD (experience limited), 0.35–3 mg/kg daily

Nozinan® (Link) PoM

Tablets, scored, levomepromazine maleate 25 mg, net price 84-tab pack = £21.42. Label: 2

Injection, levomepromazine hydrochloride 25 mg/mL, net price 1-mL amp = £2.13

PERICYAZINE
(Periciazine)

Indications: see under Dose

Cautions: see notes above

Contra-indications: see notes above

Side-effects: see notes above; more sedating; hypotension common when treatment initiated; respiratory depression

Dose: schizophrenia and other psychoses, initially 75 mg daily in divided doses increased at weekly intervals by steps of 25 mg according to response; usual max. 300 mg daily (elderly initially 15–30 mg daily)

Short-term adjunctive management of severe anxiety, psychomotor agitation, and violent or dangerously impulsive behaviour, initially 15–30 mg (elderly 5–10 mg) daily divided into 2 doses, taking the larger dose at bedtime, adjusted according to response

CHILD (severe mental or behavioural disorders only), initially, 500 micrograms daily for 10-kg child, increased by 1 mg for each additional 5 kg to max. total daily dose of 10 mg; dose may be gradually increased according to response but maintenance should not exceed twice initial dose

INFANT under 1 year not recommended

Neulactil® (JHC) PoM

Tablets, all yellow, scored, pericyazine 2.5 mg, net price 84-tab pack = £7.69; 10 mg, 84-tab pack = £20.79. Label: 2

Syrup forte, brown, pericyazine 10 mg/5 mL. Net price 100-mL pack = £10.07. Label: 2

PERPHENAZINE

Indications: see under Dose; anti-emetic (section 4.6)

Cautions: see notes above

Contra-indications: see notes above; also agitation and restlessness in the elderly

Side-effects: see notes above; less sedating; extrapyramidal symptoms, especially dystonia, more frequent, particularly at high dosage; rarely systemic lupus erythematosus

Dose: schizophrenia and other psychoses, mania, short-term adjunctive management of anxiety, severe psychomotor agitation, excitement, and violent or dangerously impulsive behaviour, initially 4 mg 3 times daily adjusted according to the response; max. 24 mg daily; ELDERLY quarter to half adult dose (but see Cautions); CHILD under 14 years not recommended

Fentazin® (Goldshield) PoM

Tablets, both s/c, perphenazine 2 mg, net price 20 = £3.73; 4 mg, 20 = £4.39. Label: 2

PIMOZIDE

Indications: see under Dose

Cautions: see notes above

CSM WARNING. Following reports of sudden unexplained death, the CSM recommends ECG before treatment. The CSM also recommends that patients on pimozide should have an annual ECG (if the QT interval is prolonged, treatment should be reviewed and either withdrawn or dose reduced under close supervision) and that pimozide should **not** be given with other antipsychotic drugs (including depot preparations), tricyclic antidepressants or other drugs which prolong the QT interval, such as certain antimalarials, anti-arrhythmic drugs and certain antihistamines and should **not** be given with drugs which cause electrolyte disturbances (especially diuretics)

Contra-indications: see notes above; history of arrhythmias or congenital QT prolongation

Side-effects: see notes above; less sedating; serious arrhythmias reported; glycosuria and, rarely, hyponatraemia reported

Dose: schizophrenia, initially 2 mg daily, increased according to response in steps of 2–4 mg at intervals of not less than 1 week; usual dose range 2–20 mg daily; ELDERLY half usual starting dose; CHILD not recommended

Monosymptomatic hypochondriacal psychosis, paranoid psychosis, initially 4 mg daily, increased according to response in steps of 2–4 mg at intervals of not less than 1 week; max. 16 mg daily; ELDERLY half usual starting dose; CHILD not recommended

Orap® (Janssen-Cilag) PoM

Tablets, scored, green, pimozide 4 mg, net price 20 = £6.13. Label: 2

PROCHLORPERAZINE

Indications: see under Dose; anti-emetic (section 4.6)

Cautions: see notes above; also hypotension more likely after intramuscular injection

Contra-indications: see notes above; children, but see section 4.6 for use as anti-emetic

Side-effects: see notes above; less sedating; extrapyramidal symptoms, particularly dystonias, more frequent; respiratory depression may occur in susceptible patients

Dose: *by mouth*, schizophrenia and other psychoses, mania, prochlorperazine maleate or mesilate, 12.5 mg twice daily for 7 days adjusted at intervals of 4–7 days to usual dose of 75–100 mg daily according to response; CHILD not recommended

Short-term adjunctive management of severe anxiety, 15–20 mg daily in divided doses; max. 40 mg daily; CHILD not recommended

By deep intramuscular injection, psychoses, mania, prochlorperazine mesilate 12.5–25 mg 2–3 times daily; CHILD not recommended

By rectum in suppositories, psychoses, mania, the equivalent of prochlorperazine maleate 25 mg 2–3 times daily; CHILD not recommended

■ Preparations
Section 4.6

PROMAZINE HYDROCHLORIDE

Indications: see under Dose
Cautions: see notes above; also cerebral arteriosclerosis
Contra-indications: see notes above
Side-effects: see notes above; also haemolytic anaemia
Dose: *by mouth*, short-term adjunctive management of psychomotor agitation, 100–200 mg 4 times daily; CHILD not recommended
Agitation and restlessness in elderly, 25–50 mg 4 times daily
By intramuscular injection, short-term adjunctive management of psychomotor agitation, 50 mg (25 mg in elderly or debilitated), repeated if necessary after 6–8 hours; CHILD not recommended

Promazine (Non-proprietary) PoM
Tablets ▬, coated, promazine hydrochloride 25 mg, net price 20 = 50p; 50 mg, 20 = 88p. Label: 2
Available from APS
Oral solution ▬, promazine hydrochloride 25 mg/5 mL, net price 150 mL = £3.50; 50 mg/5 mL, 150 mL = £3.50. Label: 2
Available from Rosemont
Injection, promazine hydrochloride 50 mg/mL. Net price 1-mL amp = 30p
NOTE. May be difficult to obtain

SULPIRIDE

Indications: schizophrenia
Cautions: see notes above; also excited, agitated, or aggressive patients (even low doses may aggravate symptoms)
Contra-indications: see notes above; also porphyria (section 9.8.2)
Side-effects: see notes above; also hepatitis
Dose: 200–400 mg twice daily; max. 800 mg daily in predominantly negative symptoms, and 2.4 g daily in mainly positive symptoms; ELDERLY, lower initial dose, increased gradually according to response; CHILD under 14 years not recommended

Sulpiride (Non-proprietary) PoM
Tablets, sulpiride 200 mg, net price 100-tab pack = £14.98; 400 mg, 100-tab pack = £36.29. Label: 2
Available from APS, Arrow, CP, Generics, IVAX

Dolmatil® (Sanofi-Synthelabo) PoM
Tablets, both scored, sulpiride 200 mg, net price 100-tab pack = £13.85; 400 mg (f/c), 100-tab pack = £36.29. Label: 2

Sulpitil® (Pharmacia) PoM
Tablets, scored, sulpiride 200 mg. Net price 28-tab pack = £4.29; 112-tab pack = £12.85. Label: 2

Sulpor® (Rosemont) PoM
Oral solution, sugar-free, lemon- and aniseed-flavoured, sulpiride 200 mg/5 mL, net price 150 mL = £27.00. Label: 2

THIORIDAZINE

Indications: under specialist supervision, second-line treatment of schizophrenia in adults (see Contra-indications, below)
Cautions: see notes above; ECG screening and electrolyte measurement before treatment, after each dose increase and at 6-month intervals; also monitor for visual defects on prolonged use; avoid in porphyria (section 9.8.2)
Contra-indications: see under Cardiotoxicity, below; for general contra-indications see notes above
CARDIOTOXICITY. Thioridazine is associated with QT-interval prolongation and increased risk of ventricular arrhythmias. The CSM has advised that thioridazine should be restricted to second-line treatment of schizophrenia in adults under specialist supervision. Thioridazine is **contra-indicated** in patients with:

- significant cardiac disease, such as angina, bradycardia, second- or third-degree heart block, cardiac failure;
- history of ventricular arrhythmia;
- QT-interval prolongation or a family history of the condition;
- uncorrected hypokalaemia or hypomagnesaemia;
- concomitant use with other drugs known to cause QT-interval prolongation;
- reduced cytochrome P450 2D6 activity;
- concomitant use with drugs that inhibit or are metabolised by cytochrome P450 2D6.

Side-effects: see notes above; less sedating than chlorpromazine, and extrapyramidal symptoms and hypothermia rarely occur; more likely to induce hypotension and increased risk of cardiotoxicity and prolongation of QT interval (see above); pigmentary retinopathy (with reduced visual acuity, brownish colouring of vision, and impaired night vision) occurs rarely with high doses; sexual dysfunction, particularly retrograde ejaculation, may occur
Dose: 50–300 mg daily (initially in divided doses); max. 600 mg daily (in hospital patients only); CHILD not recommended

Thioridazine (Non-proprietary) PoM
Tablets, coated, thioridazine hydrochloride 25 mg, net price 20 = 35p; 50 mg, 20 = £1.14; 100 mg, 20 = £1.63. Label: 2
Available from DDSA (*Rideril*®), Hillcross, IVAX
Oral solution, thioridazine (as hydrochloride) 25 mg/5 mL. Net price 500-mL = £3.00. Label: 2
Available from Hillcross, Rosemont

Melleril® (Novartis) PoM
Tablets, all f/c, thioridazine hydrochloride 10 mg, net price 84-tab pack = £1.10; 25 mg, 84-tab pack = £1.83; 50 mg, 84-tab pack = £3.55; 100 mg, 84-tab pack = £6.86. Label: 2

Suspension 25 mg/5 mL, thioridazine 25 mg/5 mL, net price 300 mL = £2.18. Label: 2
Suspension 100 mg/5 mL, thioridazine 100 mg/5 mL, net price 300 mL = £7.85. Label: 2
NOTE. These suspensions should not be diluted but the two preparations may be mixed with each other to provide intermediate strengths
Syrup, brown, thioridazine (as hydrochloride) 25 mg/5 mL, net price 300 mL = £2.18. Label: 2

TRIFLUOPERAZINE

Indications: see under Dose; anti-emetic (section 4.6)
Cautions: see notes above
Contra-indications: see notes above
Side-effects: see notes above; extrapyramidal symptoms more frequent, especially at doses exceeding 6 mg daily; pancytopenia; thrombocytopenia; hyperpyrexia; anorexia
Dose: *by mouth* (reduce initial doses in elderly by at least half)
Schizophrenia and other psychoses, short-term adjunctive management of psychomotor agitation, excitement, and violent or dangerously impulsive behaviour, initially 5 mg twice daily, *or* 10 mg daily in modified-release form, increased by 5 mg after 1 week, then at intervals of 3 days, according to the response; CHILD up to 12 years, initially up to 5 mg daily in divided doses, adjusted according to response, age, and body-weight
Short-term adjunctive management of severe anxiety, 2–4 mg daily in divided doses *or* 2–4 mg daily in modified-release form, increased if necessary to 6 mg daily; CHILD 3–5 years up to 1 mg daily, 6–12 years up to 4 mg daily

Trifluoperazine (Non-proprietary) PoM
Tablets, coated, trifluoperazine (as hydrochloride) 1 mg, net price 20 = 57p; 5 mg, 20 = 87p. Label: 2
Available from most generic manufacturers
Oral solution, trifluoperazine (as hydrochloride) 5 mg/5 mL. Net price 200-mL = £11.07. Label: 2
Available from Rosemont (sugar-free)

Stelazine® (Goldshield) PoM
Tablets, both blue, f/c, trifluoperazine (as hydrochloride) 1 mg, net price 20 = 61p; 5 mg, 20 = 87p. Label: 2
Spansules® (= capsules m/r), all clear/yellow, enclosing dark blue, light blue, and white pellets, trifluoperazine (as hydrochloride) 2 mg, net price 60-cap pack = £4.65; 10 mg, 30-cap pack = £2.83; 15 mg, 30-cap pack = £4.27. Label: 2, 25
Syrup, yellow, sugar-free, trifluoperazine (as hydrochloride) 1 mg/5 mL. Net price 200-mL pack = £2.95. Label: 2

ZUCLOPENTHIXOL ACETATE

Indications: short-term management of acute psychosis, mania, or exacerbations of chronic psychosis
Cautions: see notes above; avoid in porphyria (section 9.8.2)
Contra-indications: see notes above
Side-effects: see notes above
Dose: *by deep intramuscular injection* into the gluteal muscle or lateral thigh, 50–150 mg (elderly 50–100 mg), if necessary re... (1 additional dose may be ... the first injection); max. cu... per course and max. 4 inject... treatment 2 weeks—if m... necessary change to an or... days after last injection, *or* to a longer acting antipsychotic depot injection given concomitantly with last injection of zuclopenthixol acetate; CHILD not recommended

Clopixol Acuphase® (Lundbeck) PoM
Injection (oily), zuclopenthixol acetate 50 mg/mL. Net price 1-mL amp = £5.20; 2-mL amp = £10.03

ZUCLOPENTHIXOL DIHYDROCHLORIDE

Indications: schizophrenia and other psychoses, particularly when associated with agitated, aggressive, or hostile behaviour
Cautions: see notes above; avoid in porphyria (section 9.8.2)
Contra-indications: see notes above; apathetic or withdrawn states
Side-effects: see notes above; urinary frequency or incontinence; weight loss (less common than weight gain)
Dose: initially 20–30 mg daily in divided doses, increasing to a max. of 150 mg daily if necessary; usual maintenance dose 20–50 mg daily; ELDERLY (or debilitated) initially quarter to half adult dose; CHILD not recommended

Clopixol® (Lundbeck) PoM
Tablets, all f/c, pink, zuclopenthixol (as dihydrochloride) 2 mg, net price 20 = 64p; 10 mg, 20 = £1.73; 25 mg, 20 = £3.47. Label: 2
Depot injection (zuclopenthixol decanoate): section 4.2.2

Atypical antipsychotics

The 'atypical antipsychotics' **amisulpride, clozapine, olanzapine, quetiapine, risperidone,** and **zotepine** may be better tolerated than other antipsychotics; extrapyramidal symptoms may be less frequent than with older antipsychotics.

Clozapine, olanzapine, quetiapine, and sertindole do not elevate the prolactin concentration to the same extent as other antipsychotics; when changing from other antipsychotics, a reduction in prolactin may increase fertility.

Clozapine is licensed for the treatment of schizophrenia only in patients unresponsive to, or intolerant of, conventional antipsychotic drugs. It can cause agranulocytosis and its use is restricted to patients registered with the Clozaril Patient Monitoring Service (see under Clozapine, below).

Sertindole has been reintroduced following an earlier suspension of the drug because of concerns about arrhythmias; its use is restricted to patients who are enrolled in clinical studies and who are intolerant of at least one other antipsychotic.

CAUTIONS AND CONTRA-INDICATIONS. While atypical antipsychotics have not generally been associated with clinically significant prolongation of the QT interval, they should be used with care if prescribed with other drugs that increase the QT interval. Atypical antipsychotics should be used with caution in patients with cardiovascular disease, or a history of epilepsy; they should be used with caution in the elderly; **interactions**: Appendix 1 (antipsychotics).

DRIVING. Atypical antipsychotics may affect performance of skilled tasks (e.g. driving); effects of alcohol are enhanced.

WITHDRAWAL. Withdrawal of antipsychotic drugs after long-term therapy should always be gradual and closely monitored to avoid the risk of acute withdrawal syndromes or rapid relapse.

SIDE-EFFECTS. Side-effects of the atypical antipsychotics include weight gain, dizziness, postural hypotension (especially during initial dose titration) which may be associated with syncope or reflex tachycardia in some patients, extrapyramidal symptoms (usually mild and transient which respond to dose reduction or to an antimuscarinic drug), and occasionally tardive dyskinesia on long-term administration (discontinue drug on appearance of early signs). Hyperglycaemia and sometimes diabetes can occur, particularly with clozapine and olanzapine; monitoring weight and plasma glucose may identify the development of hyperglycaemia. Neuroleptic malignant syndrome has been reported rarely.

AMISULPRIDE

Indications: schizophrenia

Cautions: see notes above; also renal impairment (Appendix 3); Parkinson's disease; elderly (risk of hypotension or sedation)

Contra-indications: see notes above; also pregnancy (Appendix 4) and breast-feeding (Appendix 5), phaeochromocytoma, prolactin-dependent tumours

Side-effects: see notes above; also insomnia, anxiety, agitation, drowsiness, gastro-intestinal disorders such as constipation, nausea, vomiting, and dry mouth; hyperprolactinaemia (with galactorrhoea, amenorrhoea, gynaecomastia, breast pain, sexual dysfunction), occasionally bradycardia

Dose: acute psychotic episode, 400–800 mg daily in divided doses, adjusted according to response; max. 1.2 g daily

Predominantly negative symptoms, 50–300 mg daily; CHILD under 15 years, not recommended

NOTE. Doses up to 300 mg may be administered once daily

Solian® (Sanofi-Synthelabo) PoM
Tablets, scored, amisulpride 50 mg, net price 60-tab pack = £19.74; 100 mg, 60-tab pack = £39.48; 200 mg, 60-tab pack = £66.00, 400 mg, 60-tab pack = £132.00. Label: 2
Solution, 100 mg/mL, net price 60 mL (caramel flavour) = £33.00. Label: 2

CLOZAPINE

Indications: schizophrenia (including psychosis in Parkinson's disease) in patients unresponsive to, or intolerant of, conventional antipsychotic drugs

Cautions: see notes above; monitor leucocyte and differential blood counts (see Agranulocytosis, below); taper off conventional neuroleptic before starting; hepatic impairment (Appendix 2); renal impairment (Appendix 3); prostatic hypertrophy, angle-closure glaucoma

WITHDRAWAL. On planned withdrawal reduce dose over 1–2 weeks to avoid risk of rebound psychosis. If abrupt withdrawal necessary observe patient carefully

AGRANULOCYTOSIS. Neutropenia and potentially fatal agranulocytosis reported. Leucocyte and differential blood counts must be normal before starting; monitor counts every week for 18 weeks then at least every 2 weeks and if clozapine continued and blood count stable after 1 year at least every 4 weeks (and 4 weeks after discontinuation); if leucocyte count below $3000/mm^3$ or if absolute neutrophil count below $1500/mm^3$ discontinue permanently and refer to haematologist. Avoid drugs which depress leucopoiesis; patients should report immediately symptoms of infection, especially influenza-like illness

MYOCARDITIS AND CARDIOMYOPATHY. Fatal myocarditis (most commonly in first 2 months) and cardiomyopathy reported. The CSM has advised:

- physical examination and medical history before starting clozapine;

- specialist examination if cardiac abnormalities or history of heart disease found—clozapine initiated only in absence of severe heart disease and if benefit outweighs risk;

- persistent tachycardia especially in first 2 months should prompt observation for other indicators for myocarditis or cardiomyopathy;

- if myocarditis or cardiomyopathy suspected clozapine should be stopped and patient evaluated urgently by cardiologist;

- discontinue permanently in clozapine-induced myocarditis or cardiomyopathy

GASTRO-INTESTINAL OBSTRUCTION. Reactions resembling gastro-intestinal obstruction reported. Clozapine should be used cautiously with drugs which cause constipation (e.g. antimuscarinic drugs) or in history of colonic disease or bowel surgery. Monitor for constipation and prescribe laxative if required

Contra-indications: severe cardiac disorders (e.g. myocarditis; see Myocarditis and Cardiomyopathy, above); active liver disease (Appendix 2), severe renal impairment (Appendix 3); history of neutropenia or agranulocytosis; bone-marrow disorders; paralytic ileus (see Gastro-intestinal Obstruction, above); alcoholic and toxic psychoses; history of circulatory collapse; drug intoxication; coma or severe CNS depression; uncontrolled epilepsy; pregnancy (Appendix 4) and breast-feeding (Appendix 5)

Side-effects: see notes above; also constipation (see Gastro-intestinal Obstruction, above), hypersalivation, nausea, vomiting; tachycardia, ECG changes, hypertension; drowsiness, blurred vision, headache, tremor, rigidity, extrapyramidal symptoms, convulsions, fatigue, impaired temperature regulation, fever; hepatitis, cholestatic jaundice, pancreatitis; urinary incontinence and retention; agranulocytosis (**important:** see Agranulocytosis, above), leucopenia, eosinophilia, leucocytosis; rarely dysphagia, circulatory collapse, arrhythmias, myocarditis (**important:** see Myocarditis and Cardiomyopathy, above), pericarditis, thromboembolism, confusion, delirium, restlessness, agitation, diabetes mellitus; also reported, intestinal obstruction, paralytic ileus (see Gastro-intestinal Obstruction, above), enlarged parotid gland, fulminant hepatic necrosis, thrombocytopenia, hypertriglyceridaemia, cardiomyopathy, cardiac arrest, respiratory arrest, interstitial nephritis, priapism, skin reactions

Dose: schizophrenia, ADULT over 16 years (close medical supervision on initiation—risk of collapse due to hypotension) 12.5 mg once or twice on first day then 25–50 mg on second day then increased gradually (if well tolerated) in steps of 25–50 mg daily over 14–21 days up to 300 mg daily in divided doses (larger dose at night, up to 200 mg daily may be taken as a single dose at bedtime); if necessary may be further increased in steps of 50–100 mg once (preferably) or twice weekly; usual dose 200–450 mg daily (max. 900 mg daily)

NOTE. *Restarting* after *interval of more than 2 days*, 12.5 mg once or twice on first day (but may be feasible to increase more quickly than on initiation)—extreme caution if previous respiratory or cardiac arrest with initial dosing

ELDERLY AND SPECIAL RISK GROUPS. In *elderly*, 12.5 mg once on first day—subsequent adjustments restricted to 25 mg daily

Psychosis in Parkinson's disease, ADULT over 16 years, 12.5 mg at bedtime then increased in steps of 12.5 mg up to twice weekly to 50 mg at bedtime; usual dose range 25–37.5 mg at bedtime; exceptionally, dose may be increased further in steps of 12.5 mg weekly to max. 100 mg daily in 1–2 divided doses

Clozaril® (Novartis) [PoM]
Tablets, both yellow, clozapine 25 mg (scored), net price 28-tab pack = £12.33, 84-tab pack (hosp. only) = £36.97; 100 mg, 28-tab pack = £49.28, 84-tab pack (hosp. only) = £147.84. Label: 2, 10, patient information leaflet
NOTE. Patient, prescriber, and supplying pharmacist must be registered with the Clozaril Patient Monitoring Service—takes several days to do this

OLANZAPINE

Indications: schizophrenia, treatment of moderate to severe episodes of mania

Cautions: see notes above; also pregnancy (Appendix 4), prostatic hypertrophy, paralytic ileus, hepatic impairment (Appendix 2), renal impairment (Appendix 3), diabetes mellitus (risk of exacerbation or ketoacidosis), low leucocyte or neutrophil count, bone-marrow depression, hypereosinophilic disorders, myeloproliferative disease, Parkinson's disease

Contra-indications: angle-closure glaucoma; breast-feeding

Side-effects: see notes above; also mild, transient antimuscarinic effects; drowsiness, speech difficulty, exacerbation of Parkinson's disease, akathisia, asthenia, increased appetite, raised triglyceride concentration, oedema, hyperprolactinaemia (but clinical manifestations rare), occasionally blood dyscrasias, rarely bradycardia, rash, photosensitivity, diabetes mellitus, priapism, hepatitis, pancreatitis, and elevated creatine kinase concentration

Dose: schizophrenia, combination therapy for mania, ADULT over 18 years, 10 mg daily adjusted to usual range of 5–20 mg daily; doses greater than 10 mg daily only after reassessment

Monotherapy for mania, ADULT over 18 years, 15 mg daily adjusted to usual range of 5–20 mg daily; doses greater than 15 mg only after reassessment
NOTE. When one or more factors present that might result in slower metabolism (e.g. female gender, elderly, non-smoker) consider lower initial dose and more gradual dose increase

Zyprexa® (Lilly) [PoM]
Tablets, f/c, olanzapine 2.5 mg, net price 28-tab pack = £33.29; 5 mg, 28-tab pack = £48.78; 7.5 mg, 56-tab pack = £146.34; 10 mg, 28-tab pack = £97.56, 56-tab pack = £195.11; 15 mg (blue), 28-tab pack = £146.34. Label: 2
Orodispersible tablet (*Velotab*®), olanzapine 5 mg, net price 28-tab pack = £56.10; 10 mg, 28-tab pack = £112.19; 15 mg, 28-tab pack = £168.29. Label: 2, counselling, administration
Excipients: include aspartame (section 9.4.1)
COUNSELLING. *Velotab*® may be placed on the tongue and allowed to dissolve or dispersed in water, orange juice, apple juice, milk, or coffee

QUETIAPINE

Indications: schizophrenia

Cautions: see notes above; also pregnancy, hepatic impairment (Appendix 2), renal impairment (Appendix 3), cerebrovascular disease

Contra-indications: breast-feeding (Appendix 5)

Side-effects: see notes above; also drowsiness, dyspepsia, constipation, dry mouth, mild asthenia, rhinitis, hypertension, tachycardia; anxiety, fever, myalgia, ear pain, rash; leucopenia, neutropenia and occasionally eosinophilia reported; elevated plasma-triglyceride and cholesterol concentrations, reduced plasma-thyroid hormone concentrations; possible QT interval prolongation; rarely oedema; very rarely priapism

Dose: 25 mg twice daily on day 1, 50 mg twice daily on day 2, 100 mg twice daily on day 3, 150 mg twice daily on day 4, then adjusted according to response, usual range 300–450 mg daily in 2 divided doses; max. 750 mg daily; ELDERLY initially 25 mg daily, increased in steps of 25–50 mg daily; CHILD and ADOLESCENT not recommended

Seroquel® (AstraZeneca) PoM
Tablets, f/c, quetiapine (as fumarate) 25 mg (peach), net price 60-tab pack = £28.20; 100 mg (yellow), 60-tab pack = £113.10; 150 mg (pale yellow), 60-tab pack = £113.10; 200 mg (white), 60-tab pack = £113.10; 300 mg (white), 60-tab pack = £170.00; starter pack of 6 × 25-mg tabs, 2 × 100-mg tabs, and 2 × 150-mg tabs = £10.36. Label: 2

RISPERIDONE

Indications: acute and chronic psychoses
Cautions: see notes above; Parkinson's disease; pregnancy; hepatic impairment (Appendix 2), renal impairment (Appendix 3)
Contra-indications: breast-feeding (Appendix 5)
Side-effects: see notes above; also insomnia, agitation, anxiety, headache, drowsiness, impaired concentration, fatigue, blurred vision, constipation, nausea and vomiting, dyspepsia, abdominal pain, hyperprolactinaemia (with galactorrhoea, menstrual disturbances, amenorrhoea, gynaecomastia), sexual dysfunction, priapism, urinary incontinence, tachycardia, hypertension, rash, rhinitis; cerebrovascular accidents, neutropenia and thrombocytopenia have been reported; rarely, seizures, hyponatraemia, abnormal temperature regulation, oedema
Dose: 2 mg in 1–2 divided doses on first day *then* 4 mg in 1–2 divided doses on second day (slower titration appropriate in some patients); usual dose range 4–6 mg daily; doses above 10 mg daily only if benefit considered to outweigh risk (max. 16 mg daily); ELDERLY (or in hepatic or renal impairment) initially 500 micrograms twice daily increased in steps of 500 micrograms twice daily to 1–2 mg twice daily; CHILD under 15 years not recommended

Risperdal® (Organon, Janssen-Cilag) PoM
Tablets, f/c, scored, risperidone 500 micrograms (brown-red), net price 20-tab pack = £7.67; 1 mg (white), 20-tab pack = £13.45, 60-tab pack = £40.35; 2 mg (orange), 60-tab pack = £79.56; 3 mg (yellow), 60-tab pack = £117.00; 4 mg (green), 60-tab pack = £154.44; 6 mg (yellow), 28-tab pack = £109.20. Label: 2
Orodispersible tablets (*Quicklet®*), both pink, risperidone 1 mg, net price 28-tab pack = £21.30; 2 mg, 28-tab pack = £40.14. Label: 2, counselling, administration
Excipients: include aspartame (section 9.4.1)
COUNSELLING. Tablets should be placed on the tongue, allowed to dissolve and swallowed
Liquid, risperidone 1 mg/mL, net price 100 mL = £65.00. Label: 2
NOTE. Liquid may be diluted with mineral water, orange juice or black coffee (should be taken immediately)
Depot injection: section 4.2.2

SERTINDOLE

Indications: schizophrenia, see also notes above
Cautions: see notes above; hepatic impairment (Appendix 2); diabetes; correct hypokalaemia or hypomagnesaemia before treatment; monitor ECG during treatment; monitor blood pressure during dose titration and early maintenance therapy (risk

of postural hypotension); **interactions:** Appendix 1 (antipsychotics)
Contra-indications: see notes above; pregnancy and breast-feeding, severe hepatic impairment, QT interval prolongation (ECG required before and during treatment—consult product literature); concomitant administration of drugs which prolong QT interval (see interactions); uncorrected hypokalaemia or hypomagnesaemia
Side-effects: see notes above; prolonged QT interval, peripheral oedema, dry mouth, rhinitis, nasal congestion, dyspnoea, paraesthesia, abnormal ejaculation (decreased volume); rarely seizures, hyperglycaemia
Dose: initially 4 mg daily increased in steps of 4 mg at intervals of 4–5 days to usual maintenance of 12–20 mg as a single daily dose; max. 24 mg daily; ELDERLY consider slower dose titration and lower maintenance dose; CHILD and ADOLESCENT not recommended

Serdolect® (Lundbeck) ▼ PoM
Tablets, f/c, sertindole 4 mg, 30-tab pack; 12 mg 28-tab pack; 16 mg, 28-tab pack; 20 mg 28-tab pack
Available only on named-patient basis (see notes above)

ZOTEPINE

Indications: schizophrenia
Cautions: see notes above; personal or close family history of epilepsy; withdrawal of concomitantly prescribed CNS depressants; QT interval prolongation—ECG required (before treatment and at each dose increase) in patients at risk of arrhythmias; monitor plasma electrolytes particularly before treatment and at each dose increase; hepatic impairment (Appendix 2); renal impairment (Appendix 3); prostatic hypertrophy, urinary retention, angle-closure glaucoma, paralytic ileus, pregnancy
Contra-indications: acute intoxication with CNS depressants; high doses of concomitantly prescribed antipsychotics; acute gout (avoid for 3 weeks after episode resolves), history of nephrolithiasis; breast-feeding
Side-effects: see notes above; constipation, dyspepsia, dry mouth, tachycardia, QT interval prolongation, rhinitis, agitation, anxiety, depression, asthenia, headache, EEG abnormalities, insomnia, drowsiness, hyperthermia or hypothermia, increased salivation, blood dyscrasias (including leucocytosis, leucopenia), raised erythrocyte sedimentation rate, blurred vision, sweating; less frequently anorexia, diarrhoea, nausea and vomiting, abdominal pain, hypertension, influenza-like syndrome, cough, dyspnoea, confusion, convulsions, decreased libido, speech disorder, vertigo, hyperprolactinaemia, anaemia, thrombocythaemia, increased serum creatinine, hypoglycaemia and hyperglycaemia, hyperlipidaemia, hypouricaemia, oedema, thirst, impotence, urinary incontinence, arthralgia, myalgia, conjunctivitis, acne, dry skin, rash; rarely bradycardia, epistaxis, abdominal enlargement, amnesia, ataxia, coma, delirium, hypaesthesia, myoclonus, thrombocytopenia, abnormal ejaculation, urinary retention, menstrual irregularities, myasthenia, alopecia, photosensitivity
Dose: initially 25 mg 3 times daily increased according to response at intervals of 4 days to

max. 100 mg 3 times daily; ELDERLY initially 25 mg twice daily increased according to response to max. 75 mg twice daily; CHILD and ADOLESCENT under 18 years not recommended

Zoleptil® (Orion) PoM
Tablets, s/c, zotepine 25 mg (white), net price 30-tab pack = £14.33, 90-tab pack = £42.98; 50 mg (yellow), 30-tab pack = £19.10, 90-tab pack = £57.30; 100 mg (pink), 30-tab pack = £31.52, 90-tab pack = £94.55. Label: 2

4.2.2 Antipsychotic depot injections

Long-acting depot injections are used for maintenance therapy especially when compliance with oral treatment is unreliable. However, depot injections of conventional antipsychotics may give rise to a higher incidence of extrapyramidal reactions than oral preparations; extrapyramidal reactions occur less frequently with atypical antipsychotics such as risperidone.

ADMINISTRATION. Depot antipsychotics are administered by deep intramuscular injection at intervals of 1 to 4 weeks. Patients should first be given a small test-dose as undesirable side-effects are prolonged. In general not more than 2–3 mL of oily injection should be administered at any one site; correct injection technique (including the use of z-track technique) and rotation of injection sites are essential. If the dose needs to be reduced to alleviate side-effects, it is important to recognise that the plasma-drug concentration may not fall for some time after reducing the dose, therefore it may be a month or longer before side-effects subside.

> DOSAGE. Individual responses to neuroleptic drugs are very variable and to achieve optimum effect, dosage and dosage interval must be titrated according to the patient's response. For the advice of The Royal College of Psychiatrists on doses above the BNF upper limit, see p. 173

Equivalent doses of depot antipsychotics
These equivalences are intended **only** as an approximate guide; individual dosage instructions should **also** be checked; patients should be carefully monitored after **any** change in medication

Antipsychotic	Dose (mg)	Interval
Flupentixol decanoate	40	2 weeks
Fluphenazine decanoate	25	2 weeks
Haloperidol (as decanoate)	100	4 weeks
Pipotiazine palmitate	50	4 weeks
Zuclopenthixol decanoate	200	2 weeks

IMPORTANT. These equivalences must **not** be extrapolated beyond the max. dose for the drug

CHOICE. There is no clear-cut division in the use of these drugs, but **zuclopenthixol** may be suitable for the treatment of agitated or aggressive patients whereas **flupentixol** can cause over-excitement in such patients. The incidence of extrapyramidal reactions is similar for the conventional antipsychotics.

CAUTIONS. See section 4.2.1. Treatment requires careful monitoring for optimum effect. When trans-

ferring from oral to depot therapy, dosage by mouth should be reduced gradually.

CONTRA-INDICATIONS. See section 4.2.1. Do not use in children.

SIDE-EFFECTS. See section 4.2.1. Pain may occur at injection site and occasionally erythema, swelling, and nodules. For side-effects of specific antipsychotics see under the relevant drug.

FLUPENTIXOL DECANOATE
(Flupenthixol Decanoate)
Indications: maintenance in schizophrenia and other psychoses
Cautions: see notes on p. 173 and also under Flupentixol (section 4.2.1) and notes above; an alternative antipsychotic may be necessary if symptoms such as aggression or agitation appear
Contra-indications: see notes on p. 173 and also under Flupentixol (section 4.2.1) and notes above
Side-effects: see notes on p. 174 and also under Flupentixol (section 4.2.1) and notes above, but may have a mood elevating effect
Dose: *by deep intramuscular injection* into the gluteal muscle, test dose 20 mg, then after at least 7 days 20–40 mg repeated at intervals of 2–4 weeks, adjusted according to response; max. 400 mg weekly; usual maintenance dose 50 mg every 4 weeks to 300 mg every 2 weeks; ELDERLY initially quarter to half adult dose; CHILD not recommended

Depixol® (Lundbeck) PoM
Injection (oily), flupentixol decanoate 20 mg/mL. Net price 1-mL amp = £1.63; 2-mL amp = £2.73

Depixol Conc.® (Lundbeck) PoM
Injection (oily), flupentixol decanoate 100 mg/mL. Net price 0.5-mL amp = £3.67; 1-mL amp = £6.72

Depixol Low Volume® (Lundbeck) PoM
Injection (oily), flupentixol decanoate 200 mg/mL. Net price 1-mL amp = £20.99

FLUPHENAZINE DECANOATE
Indications: maintenance in schizophrenia and other psychoses
Cautions: see notes on p. 173 and also notes above
Contra-indications: see notes on p. 173 and also notes above
Side-effects: see notes on p. 174 and also under Fluphenazine Hydrochloride (section 4.2.1) and notes above; also extrapyramidal symptoms usually appear a few hours after injection and continue for about 2 days but may be delayed
Dose: *by deep intramuscular injection* into the gluteal muscle, test dose 12.5 mg (6.25 mg in elderly), then after 4–7 days 12.5–100 mg repeated at intervals of 14–35 days, adjusted according to response; CHILD not recommended

Modecate® (Sanofi-Synthelabo) PoM
Injection (oily), fluphenazine decanoate 25 mg/mL. Net price 0.5-mL amp = £1.35, 1-mL amp = £2.35, 2-mL amp = £4.62
Excipients: include sesame oil
NOTE. Fluphenazine decanoate injection also available from Antigen, Mayne, Hillcross—some versions contain sesame oil

Modecate Concentrate® (Sanofi-Synthelabo)
PoM
Injection (oily), fluphenazine decanoate 100 mg/mL. Net price 0.5-mL amp = £4.66, 1-mL amp = £9.10
Excipients: include sesame oil
NOTE. Fluphenazine decanoate injection also available from Antigen, Mayne, Hillcross—some versions contain sesame oil

HALOPERIDOL DECANOATE

Indications: maintenance in schizophrenia and other psychoses
Cautions: see notes on p. 173 and also under Haloperidol (section 4.2.1) and notes above
Contra-indications: see notes on p. 173 and also under Haloperidol (section 4.2.1) and notes above
Side-effects: see notes on p. 174 and also under Haloperidol (section 4.2.1) and notes above
Dose: by deep intramuscular injection into the gluteal muscle, haloperidol (as decanoate), initially 50 mg every 4 weeks, if necessary increasing by 50-mg increments to 300 mg every 4 weeks; higher doses may be needed in some patients; ELDERLY, initially 12.5–25 mg every 4 weeks; CHILD not recommended
NOTE. If 2-weekly administration preferred, doses should be halved

Haldol Decanoate® (Janssen-Cilag) PoM
Injection (oily), haloperidol (as decanoate) 50 mg/mL, net price 1-mL amp = £4.35; 100 mg/mL, 1-mL amp = £5.77
Excipients: include sesame oil

PIPOTIAZINE PALMITATE

(Pipothiazine Palmitate)
Indications: maintenance in schizophrenia and other psychoses
Cautions: see notes on p. 173 and notes above
Contra-indications: see notes on p. 173 and notes above
Side-effects: see notes on p. 174 and notes above
Dose: by deep intramuscular injection into the gluteal muscle, test dose 25 mg, then a further 25–50 mg after 4–7 days, then adjusted according to response at intervals of 4 weeks; usual maintenance range 50–100 mg (max. 200 mg) every 4 weeks; ELDERLY initially 5–10 mg; CHILD not recommended

Piportil Depot® (JHC) PoM
Injection (oily), pipotiazine palmitate 50 mg/mL. Net price 1-mL amp = £11.31; 2-mL amp = £18.51
Excipients: include sesame oil

RISPERIDONE

Indications: schizophrenia and other psychoses in patients tolerant to risperidone by mouth
Cautions: see under Risperidone (section 4.2.1) and notes above
Contra-indications: see under Risperidone (section 4.2.1)
Side-effects: see under Risperidone (section 4.2.1); injection-site reactions also reported
Dose: by deep intramuscular injection into the gluteal muscle, patients taking oral risperidone up to 4 mg daily, initially 25 mg every 2 weeks; patients taking oral risperidone over 4 mg daily, initially 37.5 mg every 2 weeks; dose adjusted at intervals of at least 4 weeks in steps of 12.5 mg to

max. 50 mg (ELDERLY 25 mg) every 2 weeks; CHILD and ADOLESCENT under 18 years not recommended
NOTE. During initiation risperidone by mouth continued if necessary for max. 3 weeks; risperidone by mouth may also be used during dose adjustment of depot injection

Risperdal Consta® (Janssen-Cilag) ▼ PoM
Injection, powder for reconstitution, risperidone 25-mg vial, net price = £82.92; 37.5-mg vial = £115.84; 50-mg vial = £148.55 (all with diluent)

ZUCLOPENTHIXOL DECANOATE

Indications: maintenance in schizophrenia and other psychoses, particularly with aggression and agitation
Cautions: see notes on p. 173 and notes above; avoid in porphyria (section 9.8.2)
Contra-indications: see notes on p. 173 and notes above
Side-effects: see notes on p. 174 and notes above
Dose: by deep intramuscular injection into the gluteal muscle, test dose 100 mg, followed after at least 7 days by 200–500 mg or more, repeated at intervals of 1–4 weeks, adjusted according to response; max. 600 mg weekly; ELDERLY quarter to half usual starting dose; CHILD not recommended

Clopixol® (Lundbeck) PoM
Injection (oily), zuclopenthixol decanoate 200 mg/mL. Net price 1-mL amp = £3.39

Clopixol Conc.® (Lundbeck) PoM
Injection (oily), zuclopenthixol decanoate 500 mg/mL. Net price 1-mL amp = £8.00

4.2.3   Antimanic drugs

Drugs are used in mania both to control acute attacks and also to prevent their recurrence.

Benzodiazepines

Use of benzodiazepines (section 4.1) may be helpful in the initial stages of treatment until lithium achieves its full effect; they should not be used for long periods because of the risk of dependence.

Antipsychotic drugs

In an acute attack of mania, treatment with an antipsychotic drug (section 4.2.1) is usually required because it may take a few days for lithium to exert its antimanic effect. Lithium may be given concurrently with the antipsychotic drug, and treatment with the antipsychotic gradually tailed off as lithium becomes effective. Alternatively, lithium therapy may be commenced once the patient's mood has been stabilised with the antipsychotic. The adjunctive use of atypical antipsychotics such as olanzapine (section 4.2.1) and risperidone [unlicensed indication] with either lithium or valproic acid may also be of benefit.

High doses of haloperidol, fluphenazine, or flupentixol may be hazardous when used with lithium; irreversible toxic encephalopathy has been reported.

Carbamazepine

Carbamazepine (section 4.8.1) may be used for the prophylaxis of bipolar disorder (manic-depressive disorder) in patients unresponsive to lithium; it seems to be particularly effective in patients with rapid cycling manic-depressive illness (4 or more affective episodes per year).

Valproic acid

Valproic acid (as the semisodium salt) is licensed for the treatment of manic episodes associated with bipolar disorder. It may be useful in patients unresponsive to lithium. Sodium valproate (section 4.8.1) has also been used, but it is unlicensed for this indication.

VALPROIC ACID

Indications: treatment of manic episodes associated with bipolar disorder
Cautions: see Sodium Valproate (section 4.8.1); monitor closely if dose greater than 45 mg/kg daily
Contra-indications: see Sodium Valproate (section 4.8.1)
Side-effects: see Sodium Valproate (section 4.8.1)
Dose: initially 750 mg daily in 2–3 divided doses, increased according to response, usual dose 1–2 g daily; CHILD and ADOLESCENT under 18 years not recommended

Depakote® (Sanofi-Synthelabo) PoM
Tablets, e/c, valproic acid (as semisodium valproate) 250 mg, net price 90-tab pack = £43.19; 500 mg, 90-tab pack = £72.19. Label: 25
NOTE. Semisodium valproate comprises equimolar amounts of sodium valproate and valproic acid.

Lithium

Lithium salts are used in the prophylaxis and treatment of mania, in the prophylaxis of bipolar disorder (manic-depressive disorder) and in the prophylaxis of recurrent depression (unipolar illness or unipolar depression). Lithium is unsuitable for children.

The decision to give prophylactic lithium usually requires *specialist advice*, and must be based on careful consideration of the likelihood of recurrence in the individual patient, and the benefit weighed against the risks. In long-term use lithium has been associated with thyroid disorders and mild cognitive and memory impairment. Long-term treatment should therefore be undertaken only with careful assessment of risk and benefit, and with regular monitoring of thyroid function. The need for continued therapy should be assessed regularly and patients should be maintained on lithium after 3–5 years only if benefit persists.

SERUM CONCENTRATIONS. Lithium salts have a narrow therapeutic/toxic ratio and should therefore not be prescribed unless facilities for monitoring serum-lithium concentrations are available. There seem few if any reasons for preferring one or other of the salts of lithium available. Doses are adjusted to achieve serum-lithium concentration of 0.4–1 mmol/litre (lower end of the range for maintenance therapy and elderly patients) on samples taken 12 hours after

the preceding dose. It is important to determine the optimum range for each individual patient.

Overdosage, usually with serum-lithium concentration of over 1.5 mmol/litre, may be fatal and toxic effects include tremor, ataxia, dysarthria, nystagmus, renal impairment, and convulsions. If these potentially hazardous signs occur, treatment should be stopped, serum-lithium concentrations redetermined, and steps taken to reverse lithium toxicity. In mild cases withdrawal of lithium and administration of generous amounts of sodium and fluid will reverse the toxicity. Serum-lithium concentration in excess of 2 mmol/litre require urgent treatment as indicated under Emergency Treatment of Poisoning, p. 25.

INTERACTIONS. Lithium toxicity is made worse by sodium depletion, therefore concurrent use of diuretics (particularly thiazides) is hazardous and should be avoided. For other **interactions** with lithium, see Appendix 1 (lithium).

WITHDRAWAL. While there is no clear evidence of withdrawal or rebound psychosis, abrupt discontinuation of lithium increases the risk of relapse. If lithium is to be discontinued, the dose should be reduced gradually over a period of a few weeks and patients should be warned of possible relapse if discontinued abruptly.

> **Lithium cards.** A lithium treatment card available from pharmacies tells patients how to take lithium preparations, what to do if a dose is missed, and what side-effects to expect. It also explains why regular blood tests are important and warns that some medicines and illnesses can change serum-lithium concentration
> Cards may be obtained from NPA Services, 38–42 St. Peter's St, St. Albans, Herts AL1 3NP.

LITHIUM CARBONATE

Indications: treatment and prophylaxis of mania, bipolar disorder, and recurrent depression (see also notes above); aggressive or self-mutilating behaviour
Cautions: measure serum-lithium concentration regularly (every 3 months on stabilised regimens), measure thyroid function every 6–12 months on stabilised regimens and advise patient to seek attention if symptoms of hypothyroidism develop (women are at greater risk) e.g. lethargy, feeling cold; maintain adequate sodium and fluid intake; test renal function before initiating and if evidence of toxicity, avoid in renal impairment, cardiac disease, and conditions with sodium imbalance such as Addison's disease; reduce dose or discontinue in diarrhoea, vomiting and intercurrent infection (especially if sweating profusely); caution in pregnancy (Appendix 4), breast-feeding, elderly (reduce dose), diuretic treatment, myasthenia gravis; surgery (section 15.1); if possible avoid abrupt withdrawal (see notes above); **interactions:** Appendix 1 (lithium)
COUNSELLING. Patients should maintain an adequate fluid intake and should avoid dietary changes which might reduce or increase sodium intake; lithium treatment cards are available from pharmacies (see above)
Side-effects: gastro-intestinal disturbances, fine tremor, renal impairment (particularly impaired urinary concentration and polyuria), polydipsia, leucocytosis; also weight gain and oedema (may

respond to dose reduction); hyperparathyroidism and hypercalcaemia reported; signs of intoxication are blurred vision, increasing gastro-intestinal disturbances (anorexia, vomiting, diarrhoea), muscle weakness, increased CNS disturbances (mild drowsiness and sluggishness increasing to giddiness with ataxia, coarse tremor, lack of co-ordination, dysarthria), and require withdrawal of treatment; with severe **overdosage** (serum-lithium concentration above 2 mmol/litre) hyperreflexia and hyperextension of limbs, convulsions, toxic psychoses, syncope, renal failure, circulatory failure, coma, and occasionally, death; goitre, raised antidiuretic hormone concentration; hypothyroidism, hypokalaemia, ECG changes, exacerbation of psoriasis, and kidney changes may also occur; see also Emergency Treatment of Poisoning, p. 25

Dose: see under preparations below, adjusted to achieve a serum-lithium concentration of 0.4– 1 mmol/litre 12 hours after a dose on days 4–7 of treatment, then every week until dosage has remained constant for 4 weeks and every 3 months thereafter; doses are initially divided throughout the day, but once daily administration is preferred when serum-lithium concentration stabilised
NOTE. **Preparations vary widely in bioavailability**; changing the preparation requires the same precautions as initiation of treatment
NOTE. Lithium carbonate 200 mg ≡ lithium citrate 509 mg

Camcolit® (Norgine) PoM
Camcolit 250® tablets, f/c, scored, lithium carbonate 250 mg (Li⁺ 6.8 mmol), net price 20 = 67p. Label: 10, lithium card, counselling, see above
Camcolit 400® tablets, m/r, f/c, scored, lithium carbonate 400 mg (Li⁺ 10.8 mmol), net price 20 = 81p. Label: 10, lithium card, 25, counselling, see above
Dose: (serum monitoring, see above):
Treatment, initially 1–1.5 g daily; prophylaxis, initially 300–400 mg daily; CHILD not recommended
NOTE. *Camcolit 400®* also available as *Lithonate®* (APS)

Liskonum® (GSK) PoM
Tablets, m/r, f/c, scored, lithium carbonate 450 mg (Li⁺ 12.2 mmol), net price 60-tab pack = £3.10. Label: 10, lithium card, 25, counselling, see above
Dose: (serum monitoring, see above):
Treatment, initially 450–675 mg twice daily (elderly initially 225 mg twice daily); prophylaxis, initially 450 mg twice daily (elderly 225 mg twice daily); CHILD not recommended

Priadel® (Sanofi-Synthelabo) PoM
Tablets, m/r, both scored, lithium carbonate 200 mg (Li⁺ 5.4 mmol), 400 mg (Li⁺ 10.8 mmol), 20 = 98p. Label: 10, lithium card, 25, counselling, see above
Dose: (serum monitoring, see above):
Treatment and prophylaxis, initially 0.4–1.2 g daily as a single dose or in 2 divided doses (elderly or patients less than 50 kg, 400 mg daily); CHILD not recommended
Liquid, see under Lithium Citrate below

LITHIUM CITRATE

Indications: see under Lithium Carbonate and notes above

Cautions: see under Lithium Carbonate and notes above
COUNSELLING. Patients should maintain an adequate fluid intake and should avoid dietary changes which might reduce or increase sodium intake; lithium treatment cards are available from pharmacies (see above)

Side-effects: see under Lithium Carbonate and notes above

Dose: see under preparations below, adjusted to achieve serum-lithium concentration of 0.4– 1 mmol/litre as described under Lithium Carbonate
NOTE. **Preparations vary widely in bioavailability**; changing the preparation requires the same precautions as initiation of treatment
NOTE. Lithium carbonate 200 mg ≡ lithium citrate 509 mg

Li-Liquid® (Rosemont) PoM
Oral solution, lithium citrate 509 mg/5 mL (Li⁺ 5.4 mmol/5 mL), yellow, net price 150-mL pack = £6.16; 1.018 g/5 mL (Li⁺ 10.8 mmol/5 mL), orange, 150-mL pack = £12.32. Label: 10, lithium card, counselling, see above
Dose: (plasma monitoring, see above):
Treatment and prophylaxis, initially 1.018–3.054 g daily in 2 divided doses (elderly or patients less than 50 kg, initially 509 mg twice daily); CHILD not recommended

Priadel® (Sanofi-Synthelabo) PoM
Tablets, see under Lithium Carbonate, above
Liquid, sugar-free, lithium citrate 520 mg/5 mL (approx. Li⁺ 5.4 mmol/5 mL), net price 150-mL pack = £6.28. Label: 10, lithium card, counselling, see above
Dose: (plasma monitoring, see above):
Treatment and prophylaxis, initially 1.04–3.12 g daily in 2 divided doses (elderly or patients less than 50 kg, 520 mg twice daily); CHILD not recommended

4.3 Antidepressant drugs

4.3.1	Tricyclic and related antidepressant drugs
4.3.2	Monoamine-oxidase inhibitors
4.3.3	Selective serotonin re-uptake inhibitors
4.3.4	Other antidepressant drugs

Antidepressant drugs are effective in the treatment of major depression of moderate and severe degree including major depression associated with physical illness and that following childbirth; they are also effective for dysthymia (lower grade chronic depression). Antidepressant drugs are not generally effective in milder forms of acute depression but a trial may be considered in cases refractory to psychological treatments.

CHOICE. The major classes of antidepressants include the tricyclics and related antidepressants, the selective serotonin re-uptake inhibitors (SSRIs), and the monoamine oxidase inhibitors (MAOIs). A number of antidepressants cannot be accommodated easily into this classification; these are included in section 4.3.4.

Choice of antidepressant should be based on the individual patient's requirements, including the presence of concomitant disease, existing therapy, suicide risk, and previous response to antidepressant therapy.

Either tricyclic and related antidepressants or SSRIs are generally preferred because MAOIs may be less effective and show dangerous interactions with some foods and drugs.

Tricyclic antidepressants may be suitable for many depressed patients. If the potential side-effects of the older tricyclics are of concern, an SSRI or one of the newer classes of antidepressants may be appropriate.

Although SSRIs appear to be better tolerated than older drugs, the difference is too small to justify always choosing an SSRI as first-line treatment.

Compared to older **tricyclics** (e.g. amitriptyline), the **tricyclic-related drugs** (e.g. trazodone) have a lower incidence of antimuscarinic side-effects, such as dry mouth and constipation. The tricyclic-related drugs may also be associated with a lower risk of cardiotoxicity in overdosage, but some have additional side-effects (for further details see section 4.3.1).

The **selective serotonin re-uptake inhibitors** (SSRIs) have fewer antimuscarinic side-effects than the older tricyclics and they are also less cardiotoxic in overdosage. Therefore, although no more effective, they are preferred where there is a significant risk of deliberate overdosing or where concomitant conditions preclude the use of other antidepressants. SSRIs are also preferred to tricyclic antidepressants for depression in patients with diabetes. The SSRIs do, however, have characteristic side-effects of their own; gastro-intestinal side-effects such as nausea and vomiting are common and bleeding disorders have been reported.

For severely ill inpatients and those in whom maximising efficacy is of overriding importance, a tricyclic may be more effective than an SSRI or an MAOI. Venlafaxine, at a dose of 150 mg or greater, may also be more effective than SSRIs for major depression of at least moderate severity. Where the depression is very severe electroconvulsive therapy (ECT) may be indicated

MAOIs may be more effective than tricyclics in non-hospitalised patients with 'atypical depression'; MAOI treatment should be initiated by those experienced in its use.

Although anxiety is often present in depressive illness (and may be the presenting symptom), the use of an antipsychotic or an anxiolytic may mask the true diagnosis. Anxiolytics (section 4.1.2) or antipsychotics (section 4.2.1) should therefore be used with caution in depression but they are useful adjuncts in agitated patients.

See also section 4.2.3 for references to the management of bipolar disorders.

St John's wort (*Hypericum perforatum*) is a popular herbal remedy for treating mild depression. However, preparations of St John's wort can induce drug metabolising enzymes and a number of important drug interactions with conventional drugs have been identified, see Appendix 1 (St John's wort). The amount of active ingredient can vary between different preparations of St John's wort and switching from one to another can change the degree of enzyme induction. Furthermore, when a patient stops taking St John's wort, concentrations of interacting drugs may increase, leading to toxicity. Antidepressants should **not** be used with St John's wort because of the potential for interaction.

Hyponatraemia and antidepressant therapy. Hyponatraemia (usually in the elderly and possibly due to inappropriate secretion of antidiuretic hormone) has been associated with all types of antidepressants; however, it has been reported more frequently with SSRIs than with other antidepressants. The CSM has advised that hyponatraemia should be considered in all patients who develop drowsiness, confusion, or convulsions while taking an antidepressant.

MANAGEMENT. Patients should be reviewed every 1–2 weeks at the start of antidepressant treatment. Treatment should be continued for at least 4 weeks (6 weeks in the elderly) before considering whether to switch antidepressant due to lack of efficacy. In cases of partial response, continue for a further 2 weeks (elderly patients may take longer to respond).

Following remission, antidepressant treatment should be continued at the same dose for at least 4–6 months (about 12 months in the elderly). Patients with a history of recurrent depression should continue to receive maintenance treatment (for at least 5 years and possibly indefinitely). Lithium (section 4.2.3) is an effective second-line alternative for maintenance treatment.

Combination of two antidepressants can be dangerous and is rarely justified (except under specialist supervision).

FAILURE TO RESPOND. Failure to respond to an initial course of antidepressant, may necessitate an increase in the dose, switching to a different antidepressant class, or in patients with 'atypical' major depression, the use of an MAOI. Failure to respond to a second antidepressant may require the addition of an augmenting drug such as lithium or liothyronine (specialist use), psychotherapy, or ECT. Adjunctive therapy with lithium or an MAOI should only be initiated by doctors with special experience of these combinations.

WITHDRAWAL. Gastro-intestinal symptoms of nausea, vomiting, and anorexia, accompanied by headache, giddiness, 'chills', and insomnia, and sometimes by hypomania, panic-anxiety, and extreme motor restlessness may occur if an antidepressant (particularly an MAOI) is stopped suddenly after regular administration for 8 weeks or more. The dose should preferably be reduced gradually over about 4 weeks, or longer if withdrawal symptoms emerge (6 months in patients who have been on long-term maintenance treatment). SSRIs have been associated with a specific withdrawal syndrome (section 4.3.3).

ANXIETY. Management of *acute anxiety* generally involves the use of a benzodiazepine or buspirone (section 4.1.2). For *chronic anxiety* (of longer than 4 weeks' duration), it may be appropriate to use an antidepressant before a benzodiazepine. *Generalised anxiety disorder* which does not respond to buspirone or to a benzodiazepine is treated with an antidepressant. Antidepressants such as SSRIs and venlafaxine may be effective in specific anxiety disorders.

Compound preparations of an antidepressant and an anxiolytic are not recommended because it is not possible to adjust the dosage of the individual components separately. Whereas antidepressants are given continuously over several months, anxiolytics are prescribed on a short-term basis.

PANIC DISORDERS. Antidepressants are generally used for *panic disorders* and *phobias*; clomipramine (section 4.3.1) is licensed for *obsessional and phobic states*; paroxetine (section 4.3.3) and moclobemide (section 4.3.2) are licensed for the management of social phobia. However, in panic disorders (with or without agarophobia) resistant to antidepressant therapy, a benzodiazepine may be considered (section 4.1.2).

Tricyclic and related antidepressant drugs

This section covers tricyclic antidepressants and also 1-, 2-, and 4-ring structured drugs with broadly similar properties.

These drugs are most effective for treating moderate to severe *endogenous depression* associated with psychomotor and physiological changes such as loss of appetite and sleep disturbances; improvement in sleep is usually the first benefit of therapy. Since there may be an interval of 2 weeks before the antidepressant action takes place electroconvulsive treatment may be required in severe depression when delay is hazardous or intolerable.

Some tricyclic antidepressants are also effective in the management of *panic disorder*.

For reference to the role of some tricyclic antidepressants in some forms of *neuralgia*, see section 4.7.3, and in *nocturnal enuresis* in children, see section 7.4.2.

DOSAGE. About 10 to 20% of patients fail to respond to tricyclic and related antidepressant drugs and inadequate dosage may account for some of these failures. It is important to use doses that are sufficiently high for effective treatment but not so high as to cause toxic effects. Low doses should be used for initial treatment in the **elderly** (see under Side-effects, below).

In most patients the long half-life of tricyclic antidepressant drugs allows **once-daily** administration, usually at night; the use of modified-release preparations is therefore unnecessary.

CHOICE. Tricyclic and related antidepressant drugs can be roughly divided into those with additional sedative properties and those which are less so. Agitated and anxious patients tend to respond best to the sedative compounds whereas withdrawn and apathetic patients will often obtain most benefit from the less sedating ones. Those with **sedative** properties include amitriptyline, clomipramine, dosulepin (dothiepin), doxepin, maprotiline, mianserin, trazodone, and trimipramine. Those with **less seda-tive** properties include amoxapine, imipramine, lofepramine, and nortriptyline.

Imipramine and **amitriptyline** are well established and relatively safe and effective, but they have more marked antimuscarinic and cardiac side-effects than compounds such as **doxepin**, **mianserin**, and **trazodone**; this may be important in individual patients. **Lofepramine** also has a lower incidence of antimuscarinic and sedative side-effects and is less dangerous in overdosage; it is, however, infrequently associated with hepatic toxicity. **Amoxapine** is related to the antipsychotic loxapine and its side-effects include tardive dyskinesia.

For a comparison of tricyclic and related antidepressants with SSRIs and related antidepressants and MAOIs, see section 4.3.

SIDE-EFFECTS. *Arrhythmias* and *heart block* occasionally follow the use of tricyclic antidepressants, particularly amitriptyline, and may be a factor in the sudden death of patients with cardiac disease. They are also sometimes associated with *convulsions* (and should be prescribed with special caution in epilepsy as they lower the convulsive threshold); maprotiline has particularly been associated with convulsions. *Hepatic* and *haematological* reactions may occur and have been particularly associated with mianserin.

Other side-effects of tricyclic and related antidepressants include *drowsiness, dry mouth, blurred vision, constipation,* and *urinary retention* (all attributed to antimuscarinic activity), and sweating. The patient should be encouraged to persist with treatment as some tolerance to these side-effects seems to develop. They are reduced if low doses are given initially and then gradually increased, but this must be balanced against the need to obtain a full therapeutic effect as soon as possible. Gradual introduction of treatment is particularly important in the elderly, who, because of the hypotensive effects of these drugs, are prone to attacks of *dizziness* or even *syncope*. Another side-effect to which the elderly are particularly susceptible is *hyponatraemia* (see CSM advice on p. 187).

Neuroleptic malignant syndrome (section 4.2.1) may, very rarely, arise in the course of antidepressant treatment.

Limited quantities of tricyclic antidepressants should be prescribed at any one time because they are dangerous in overdosage. For advice on **overdosage** see Emergency Treatment of Poisoning, p. 24.

WITHDRAWAL. If possible tricyclic and related antidepressants should be withdrawn slowly (see also section 4.3).

INTERACTIONS. A tricyclic or related antidepressant (or an SSRI or related antidepressant) should not be started until 2 weeks after stopping an MAOI (3 weeks if starting clomipramine or imipramine). Conversely, an MAOI should not be started until at least 7–14 days after a tricyclic or related antidepressant (3 weeks in the case of clomipramine or imipramine) has been stopped. For guidance relating to the reversible monoamine oxidase inhibitor, moclobemide, see p. 192. For other tricyclic antidepressant **interactions**, see Appendix 1 (antidepressants, tricyclic and antidepressants, tricyclic (related)).

Tricyclic antidepressants

AMITRIPTYLINE HYDROCHLORIDE

Indications: depressive illness, particularly where sedation is required; nocturnal enuresis in children (section 7.4.2)

Cautions: cardiac disease (particularly with arrhythmias, see Contra-indications below), history of epilepsy, pregnancy and breast-feeding (Appendixes 4 and 5), elderly, hepatic impairment (avoid if severe), thyroid disease, phaeochromocytoma, history of mania, psychoses (may aggravate psychotic symptoms), angle-closure glaucoma, history of urinary retention, concurrent electroconvulsive therapy; if possible avoid abrupt withdrawal; anaesthesia (increased risk of arrhythmias and hypotension, see surgery section 15.1); porphyria (section 9.8.2); see section 7.4.2 for additional nocturnal enuresis warnings; **interactions:** Appendix 1 (antidepressants, tricyclic)

DRIVING. Drowsiness may affect performance of skilled tasks (e.g. driving); effects of alcohol enhanced

Contra-indications: recent myocardial infarction, arrhythmias (particularly heart block), not indicated in manic phase, severe liver disease

Side-effects: dry mouth, sedation, blurred vision (disturbance of accommodation, increased intra-ocular pressure), constipation, nausea, difficulty with micturition; cardiovascular side-effects (such as ECG changes, arrhythmias, postural hypotension, tachycardia, syncope, particularly with high doses); sweating, tremor, rashes and hypersensitivity reactions (including urticaria, photosensitivity), behavioural disturbances (particularly children), hypomania or mania, confusion (particularly elderly), interference with sexual function, blood sugar changes; increased appetite and weight gain (occasionally weight loss); endocrine side-effects such as testicular enlargement, gynaecomastia, galactorrhoea; also convulsions (see also Cautions), movement disorders and dyskinesias, fever, agranulocytosis, leucopenia, eosinophilia, purpura, thrombocytopenia, hyponatraemia (may be due to inappropriate antidiuretic hormone secretion) see CSM advice, p. 187, abnormal liver function tests (jaundice); for a general outline of side-effects see also notes above; **overdosage:** see Emergency Treatment of Poisoning, p. 24

Dose: depression, initially 75 mg (elderly and adolescents 30–75 mg) daily in divided doses *or* as a single dose at bedtime increased gradually as necessary to 150–200 mg; CHILD under 16 years not recommended for depression

Nocturnal enuresis, CHILD 7–10 years 10–20 mg, 11–16 years 25–50 mg at night; max. period of treatment (including gradual withdrawal) 3 months—full physical examination before further course

Amitriptyline (Non-proprietary) PoM
Tablets, coated, amitriptyline hydrochloride 10 mg, net price 20 = 56p; 25 mg, 20 = 58p; 50 mg, 20 = 86p. Label: 2
Available from Alpharma, APS
Oral solution, amitriptyline (as hydrochloride) 25 mg/5 mL, net price 200 mL = £16.53; 50 mg/5 mL, 200 mL = £18.00. Label: 2
Available from Rosemont (sugar-free)

■ Compound preparations
Triptafen® (Goldshield) PoM [▨]
Tablets, pink, s/c, amitriptyline hydrochloride 25 mg, perphenazine 2 mg. Net price 20 = £4.25. Label: 2

Triptafen-M® (Goldshield) PoM [▨]
Tablets, pink, s/c, amitriptyline hydrochloride 10 mg, perphenazine 2 mg. Net price 20 = £3.80. Label: 2

AMOXAPINE

Indications: depressive illness
Cautions: see under Amitriptyline Hydrochloride
Contra-indications: see under Amitriptyline Hydrochloride
Side-effects: see under Amitriptyline Hydrochloride; tardive dyskinesia reported; menstrual irregularities, breast enlargement, and galactorrhoea reported in women

Dose: initially 100–150 mg daily in divided doses *or* as a single dose at bedtime increased as necessary to max. 300 mg daily; ELDERLY initially 25 mg twice daily increased as necessary after 5–7 days to max. 50 mg 3 times daily; CHILD under 16 years not recommended

Asendis® (Goldshield) PoM
Tablets, amoxapine 50 mg (orange, scored), net price 84-tab pack = £16.78; 100 mg (blue, scored), 56-tab pack = £18.65. Label: 2

CLOMIPRAMINE HYDROCHLORIDE

Indications: depressive illness, phobic and obsessional states; adjunctive treatment of cataplexy associated with narcolepsy
Cautions: see under Amitriptyline Hydrochloride
Contra-indications: see under Amitriptyline Hydrochloride
Side-effects: see under Amitriptyline Hydrochloride
Dose: initially 10 mg daily, increased gradually as necessary to 30–150 mg daily in divided doses *or* as a single dose at bedtime; max. 250 mg daily; ELDERLY initially 10 mg daily increased carefully over approx. 10 days to 30–75 mg daily; CHILD not recommended

Phobic and obsessional states, initially 25 mg daily (ELDERLY 10 mg daily) increased over 2 weeks to 100–150 mg daily; CHILD not recommended

Adjunctive treatment of cataplexy associated with narcolepsy, initially 10 mg daily gradually increased until satisfactory response (range 10–75 mg daily)

Clomipramine (Non-proprietary) PoM
Capsules, clomipramine hydrochloride 10 mg, net price 28-cap pack = £1.21; 25 mg, 28-cap pack = £1.94; 50 mg, 28-cap pack = £2.42. Label: 2
Available from Alpharma, APS, Generics, Hillcross, IVAX

Anafranil® (Cephalon) PoM
Capsules, clomipramine hydrochloride 10 mg (yellow/caramel), net price 84-cap pack = £3.23; 25 mg (orange/caramel), 84-cap pack = £6.35; 50 mg (grey/caramel), 56-cap pack = £8.06. Label: 2

Anafranil SR® (Cephalon) PoM [▨]
Tablets, m/r, grey-red, f/c, clomipramine hydrochloride 75 mg. Net price 28-tab pack = £8.83. Label: 2, 25

DOSULEPIN HYDROCHLORIDE

(Dothiepin hydrochloride)
Indications: depressive illness, particularly where sedation is required
Cautions: see under Amitriptyline Hydrochloride
Contra-indications: see under Amitriptyline Hydrochloride
Side-effects: see under Amitriptyline Hydrochloride
Dose: initially 75 mg (ELDERLY 50–75 mg) daily in divided doses *or* as a single dose at bedtime, increased gradually as necessary to 150 mg daily (ELDERLY 75 mg may be sufficient); up to 225 mg daily in some circumstances (e.g. hospital use); CHILD not recommended

Dosulepin (Non-proprietary) PoM
Capsules, dosulepin hydrochloride 25 mg, net price 20 = 72p. Label: 2
Available from Alpharma, APS, Ashbourne (*Dothapax*®), Berk (*Prepadine*®), Generics, Hillcross, IVAX, Kent, Sandoz, Sanofi-Synthelabo, Sovereign, Sterwin
Tablets, dosulepin hydrochloride 75 mg, net price 28-tab pack = £2.78. Label: 2
Available from Alpharma, APS, Ashbourne (*Dothapax*®), Berk (*Prepadine*®), Generics, Hillcross, IVAX, Kent, Sandoz, Sanofi-Synthelabo, Sovereign, Sterwin

Prothiaden® (Abbott) PoM
Capsules, red/red-brown, dosulepin hydrochloride 25 mg. Net price 20 = £1.26. Label: 2
Tablets, red, s/c, dosulepin hydrochloride 75 mg. Net price 28-tab pack = £4.20. Label: 2

DOXEPIN

Indications: depressive illness, particularly where sedation is required; skin (section 13.3)
Cautions: see under Amitriptyline Hydrochloride
Contra-indications: see under Amitriptyline Hydrochloride; breast-feeding (Appendix 5)
Side-effects: see under Amitriptyline Hydrochloride
Dose: initially 75 mg daily in divided doses *or* as a single dose at bedtime, increased as necessary to max. 300 mg daily in 3 divided doses (up to 100 mg may be given as a single dose); ELDERLY initially 10–50 mg daily, range of 30–50 mg daily may be adequate; CHILD not recommended

Sinequan® (Pfizer) PoM
Capsules, doxepin (as hydrochloride) 10 mg (orange), net price 56-cap pack =£1.21; 25 mg (orange/blue), 28-cap pack= 87p; 50 mg (blue), 28-cap pack = £1.43; 75 mg (yellow/blue), 28-cap pack= £2.26. Label: 2

IMIPRAMINE HYDROCHLORIDE

Indications: depressive illness; nocturnal enuresis in children (see section 7.4.2)
Cautions: see under Amitriptyline Hydrochloride
Contra-indications: see under Amitriptyline Hydrochloride
Side-effects: see under Amitriptyline Hydrochloride, but less sedating
Dose: depression, initially up to 75 mg daily in divided doses increased gradually to 150–200 mg (up to 300 mg in hospital patients); up to 150 mg may be given as a single dose at bedtime; ELDERLY initially 10 mg daily, increased gradually to 30–50 mg daily; CHILD not recommended for depression
Nocturnal enuresis, CHILD 7 years 25 mg, 8–11 years 25–50 mg, over 11 years 50–75 mg at bedtime; max. period of treatment (including gradual withdrawal) 3 months—full physical examination before further course

Imipramine (Non-proprietary) PoM
Tablets, coated, imipramine hydrochloride 10 mg, net price 20 = 85p; 25 mg, 20 = 72p. Label: 2

Tofranil® (Novartis) PoM
Tablets, red-brown, s/c, imipramine hydrochloride 25 mg, net price 84-tab pack = £3.66. Label: 2

LOFEPRAMINE

Indications: depressive illness
Cautions: see under Amitriptyline Hydrochloride

Contra-indications: see under Amitriptyline Hydrochloride; hepatic and severe renal impairment
Side-effects: see under Amitriptyline Hydrochloride, but less sedating, lower incidence of antimuscarinic effects and less dangerous in overdosage; hepatic disorders reported
Dose: 140–210 mg daily in divided doses; ELDERLY may respond to lower doses; CHILD not recommended

Lofepramine (Non-proprietary) PoM
Tablets, lofepramine 70 mg (as hydrochloride). Net price 56-tab pack = £10.25. Label: 2
Available from Alpharma, APS, Ashbourne (*Feprapax*®), Hillcross, Sandoz, Sterwin
Oral suspension, lofepramine 70 mg/5 mL (as hydrochloride). Net price 150 mL = £23.64. Label: 2
Available from Rosemont (*Lomont*®, sugar-free)

Gamanil® (Merck) PoM
Tablets, f/c, brown-violet, lofepramine 70 mg (as hydrochloride). Net price 56-tab pack = £9.84. Label: 2

NORTRIPTYLINE

Indications: depressive illness; nocturnal enuresis in children (section 7.4.2)
Cautions: see under Amitriptyline Hydrochloride; manufacturer advises plasma-nortriptyline concentration monitoring if dose above 100 mg daily, but evidence of practical value uncertain
Contra-indications: see under Amitriptyline Hydrochloride
Side-effects: see under Amitriptyline Hydrochloride, but less sedating
Dose: depression, low dose initially increased as necessary to 75–100 mg daily in divided doses *or* as a single dose (max. 150 mg daily); ADOLESCENT and ELDERLY 30–50 mg daily in divided doses; CHILD not recommended for depression
Nocturnal enuresis, CHILD 7 years 10 mg, 8–11 years 10–20 mg, over 11 years 25–35 mg, at night; max period of treatment (including gradual withdrawal) 3 months—full physical examination and ECG before further course

Allegron® (King) PoM
Tablets, nortriptyline (as hydrochloride) 10 mg, net price 20 = £2.48; 25 mg (orange, scored), 20 = £5.04. Label: 2

■ Compound preparations

Motival® (Sanofi-Synthelabo) PoM
Tablets, pink, s/c, fluphenazine hydrochloride 500 micrograms, nortriptyline 10 mg (as hydrochloride). Net price 20 = 67p. Label: 2

TRIMIPRAMINE

Indications: depressive illness, particularly where sedation required
Cautions: see under Amitriptyline Hydrochloride
Contra-indications: see under Amitriptyline Hydrochloride
Side-effects: see under Amitriptyline Hydrochloride
Dose: initially 50–75 mg daily in divided doses *or* as a single dose at bedtime, increased as necessary to 150–300 mg daily; ELDERLY initially 10–25 mg 3 times daily, maintenance half adult dose may be sufficient; CHILD not recommended

Surmontil® (Aventis Pharma) PoM
Capsules, green/white, trimipramine 50 mg (as maleate). Net price 28-cap pack = £8.51. Label: 2
Tablets, trimipramine (as maleate) 10 mg, net price 28-tab pack = £3.84, 84-tab pack = £11.49; 25 mg, 28-tab pack = £5.06, 84-tab pack = £15.16. Label: 2

Related antidepressants

MAPROTILINE HYDROCHLORIDE
Indications: depressive illness, particularly where sedation is required
Cautions: see under Amitriptyline Hydrochloride; **interactions:** Appendix 1 (antidepressants, tricyclic (related))
Contra-indications: see under Amitriptyline Hydrochloride; history of epilepsy
Side-effects: see under Amitriptyline Hydrochloride, antimuscarinic effects may occur less frequently but rashes common and increased risk of convulsions at higher dosage
Dose: initially 25–75 mg (elderly 30 mg) daily in 3 divided doses *or* as a single dose at bedtime, increased gradually as necessary to max. 150 mg daily; CHILD not recommended

Ludiomil® (Novartis) PoM
Tablets, all f/c, maprotiline hydrochloride 25 mg (greyish-red), net price 28-tab pack = £2.53; 50 mg (light orange), 28-tab pack = £5.02; 75 mg (brownish-orange), 28-tab pack = £7.46. Label: 2
Excipients: include gluten

MIANSERIN HYDROCHLORIDE
Indications: depressive illness, particularly where sedation is required
Cautions: see under Amitriptyline Hydrochloride; **interactions:** Appendix 1 (antidepressants, tricyclic (related))
BLOOD COUNTS. A full **blood count** is recommended every 4 weeks during the first 3 months of treatment; clinical monitoring should continue subsequently and treatment should be stopped and a full blood count obtained if *fever, sore throat, stomatitis*, or other signs of infection develop.
Contra-indications: see under Amitriptyline Hydrochloride
Side-effects: see under Amitriptyline Hydrochloride, fewer and milder antimuscarinic and cardiovascular effects; leucopenia, agranulocytosis and aplastic anaemia (particularly in the elderly); jaundice; arthritis, arthralgia
Dose: initially 30–40 mg (elderly 30 mg) daily in divided doses *or* as a single dose at bedtime, increased gradually as necessary; usual dose range 30–90 mg; CHILD not recommended

Mianserin (Non-proprietary) PoM
Tablets, mianserin hydrochloride 10 mg, net price 20 = £1.93; 20 mg, 20 = £2.95; 30 mg, 20 = £2.89. Label: 2, 25
Available from Alpharma, IVAX

TRAZODONE HYDROCHLORIDE
Indications: depressive illness, particularly where sedation is required; anxiety
Cautions: see under Amitriptyline Hydrochloride; **interactions:** Appendix 1 (antidepressants, tricyclic (related))

Contra-indications: see under Amitriptyline Hydrochloride
Side-effects: see under Amitriptyline Hydrochloride but fewer antimuscarinic and cardiovascular effects; rarely priapism (discontinue immediately)
Dose: depression, initially 150 mg (elderly 100 mg) daily in divided doses after food *or* as a single dose at bedtime; may be increased to 300 mg daily; hospital patients up to max. 600 mg daily in divided doses
Anxiety, 75 mg daily, increasing if necessary to 300 mg daily
CHILD not recommended

Trazodone (Non-proprietary) PoM
Capsules, trazodone hydrochloride 50 mg, net price 84-cap pack = £17.01; 100 mg, 56-cap pack = £20.70. Label: 2, 21
Available from APS, Generics, Sterwin
Tablets, trazodone hydrochloride 150 mg, net price 28-tab pack = £12.10. Label: 2, 21
Available from APS, Generics, Sterwin

Molipaxin® (Hoechst Marion Roussel) PoM
Capsules, trazodone hydrochloride 50 mg (violet/green), net price 84-cap pack = £19.04; 100 mg (violet/fawn), 56-cap pack = £22.42. Label: 2, 21
Tablets, pink, f/c, trazodone hydrochloride 150 mg. Net price 28-tab pack = £12.78. Label: 2, 21
Liquid, sugar-free, trazodone hydrochloride 50 mg/5 mL, net price 120 mL = £8.51. Label: 2, 21

4.3.2 Monoamine-oxidase inhibitors
(MAOIs)

Monoamine-oxidase inhibitors are used much less frequently than tricyclic and related antidepressants, or SSRIs and related antidepressants because of the dangers of dietary and drug interactions and the fact that it is easier to prescribe MAOIs when tricyclic antidepressants have been unsuccessful than vice versa. **Tranylcypromine** is the most **hazardous** of the MAOIs because of its stimulant action. The drugs of choice are **phenelzine** or **isocarboxazid** which are less stimulant and therefore safer.

Phobic patients and depressed patients with atypical, hypochondriacal, or hysterical features are said to respond best to MAOIs. However, MAOIs should be tried in any patients who are refractory to treatment with other antidepressants as there is occasionally a dramatic response. Response to treatment may be delayed for 3 weeks or more and may take an additional 1 or 2 weeks to become maximal.

WITHDRAWAL. If possible MAOIs should be withdrawn slowly (see also section 4.3).

INTERACTIONS. MAOIs inhibit monoamine oxidase, thereby causing an accumulation of amine neurotransmitters. The metabolism of some amine drugs such as *indirect-acting sympathomimetics* (present in many cough and decongestant preparations, see section 3.10) is also inhibited and their pressor action may be potentiated; the pressor effect of tyramine (in some foods, such as mature cheese, pickled herring, broad bean pods, and *Bovril®*, *Oxo®*, *Marmite®* or any similar meat or yeast extract or fermented soya bean extract) may also be dangerously potentiated. These interactions may cause a dangerous rise in blood pressure. An early warning symptom may be a throbbing headache. Patients should be advised to eat only fresh foods and avoid food that is suspected of being stale or 'going off'. This is especially important with meat, fish, poultry or offal; game should be avoided. The danger of interaction persists for up to 2 weeks after treatment with MAOIs is discontinued. Patients should also avoid alcoholic drinks or de-alcoholised (low alcohol) drinks.

Other antidepressants should **not** be started for 2 weeks after treatment with MAOIs has been stopped (3 weeks if starting clomipramine or imipramine). Some psychiatrists use selected tricyclics in conjunction with MAOIs but this is hazardous, indeed potentially lethal, except in experienced hands and there is no evidence that the combination is more effective than when either constituent is used alone. The combination of tranylcypromine with clomipramine is particularly **dangerous**.

Conversely, an MAOI should not be started until at least 7–14 days after a tricyclic or related antidepressant (3 weeks in the case of clomipramine or imipramine) has been stopped.

In addition, an MAOI should not be started for at least 2 weeks after a previous MAOI has been stopped (then started at a reduced dose).

For other interactions with MAOIs including those with opioid analgesics (notably pethidine), see Appendix 1 (MAOIs). For guidance on interactions relating to the reversible monoamine oxidase inhibitor, moclobemide, see below; for guidance on interactions relating to SSRIs, see p. 193.

PHENELZINE ▰

Indications: depressive illness

Cautions: diabetes mellitus, cardiovascular disease, epilepsy, blood disorders, concurrent electroconvulsive therapy; elderly (great caution); monitor blood pressure (risk of postural hypotension and hypertensive responses—discontinue if palpitations or frequent headaches); if possible avoid abrupt withdrawal; severe hypertensive reactions to certain drugs and foods; avoid in agitated patients; porphyria (section 9.8.2); pregnancy and breast-feeding; surgery (section 15.1); **interactions:** Appendix 1 (MAOIs)

DRIVING. Drowsiness may affect performance of skilled tasks (e.g. driving)

Contra-indications: hepatic impairment or abnormal liver function tests (Appendix 2), cerebrovascular disease, phaeochromocytoma; not indicated in manic phase

Side-effects: commonly postural hypotension (especially in elderly) and dizziness; less common side-effects include drowsiness, insomnia, headache, weakness and fatigue, dry mouth, constipation and other gastro-intestinal disturbances, oedema, myoclonic movement, hyperreflexia, elevated liver enzymes; agitation and tremors, nervousness, euphoria, arrhythmias, blurred vision, nystagmus, difficulty in micturition, sweating, convulsions, rashes, purpura, leucopenia, sexual disturbances, and weight gain with inappropriate appetite may also occur; psychotic episodes with hypomanic behaviour, confusion, and hallucinations may be induced in susceptible persons; jaundice has been reported and, on rare occasions, fatal progressive hepatocellular necrosis; paraes-

thesia, peripheral neuritis, peripheral neuropathy may be due to pyridoxine deficiency; for CSM advice on possible hyponatraemia, see p. 187

Dose: 15 mg 3 times daily, increased if necessary to 4 times daily after 2 weeks (hospital patients, max. 30 mg 3 times daily), then reduced gradually to lowest possible maintenance dose (15 mg on alternate days may be adequate); CHILD not recommended

Nardil® (Hansam) PoM ▰

Tablets, orange, f/c, phenelzine (as sulphate) 15 mg, net price 20 = £3.99. Label: 3, 10, patient information leaflet

ISOCARBOXAZID ▰

Indications: depressive illness

Cautions: see under Phenelzine

Contra-indications: see under Phenelzine

Side-effects: see under Phenelzine

Dose: initially 30 mg daily in single or divided doses until improvement occurs (increased after 4 weeks if necessary to max. 60 mg daily for 4–6 weeks under close supervision), then reduced to usual maintenance dose 10–20 mg daily (but up to 40 mg daily may be required); ELDERLY 5–10 mg daily; CHILD not recommended

Isocarboxazid (Non-proprietary) PoM ▰

Tablets, pink, scored, isocarboxazid 10 mg. Net price 50 = £26.71. Label: 3, 10, patient information leaflet

Available from Cambridge

TRANYLCYPROMINE ▰

Indications: depressive illness

Cautions: see under Phenelzine

Contra-indications: see under Phenelzine; hyperthyroidism

Side-effects: see under Phenelzine; insomnia if given in evening; hypertensive crises with throbbing headache requiring discontinuation of treatment more frequent than with other MAOIs; liver damage less frequent than with phenelzine

Dose: initially 10 mg twice daily not later than 3 p.m., increasing the second daily dose to 20 mg after 1 week if necessary; doses above 30 mg daily under close supervision only; usual maintenance dose 10 mg daily; CHILD not recommended

Tranylcypromine (Non-proprietary) PoM ▰

Tablets, tranylcypromine (as sulphate) 10 mg. Net price 28-tab pack = £5.08. Label: 3, 10, patient information leaflet

Available from Goldshield

Reversible MAOIs

Moclobemide is indicated for major depression and social phobia; it is reported to act by reversible inhibition of monoamine oxidase type A (it is therefore termed a RIMA). It should be reserved as a second-line treatment.

INTERACTIONS. Moclobemide is claimed to cause less potentiation of the pressor effect of tyramine than the traditional (irreversible) MAOIs, but patients should avoid consuming large amounts of tyramine-rich food (such as mature cheese, yeast extracts and fermented soya bean products).

The risk of drug interactions is also claimed to be less but patients still need to avoid sympathomimetics such as ephedrine, pseudoephedrine, and phenylpropanolamine. In addition, moclobemide should not be given with another antidepressant. Owing to its short duration of action no treatment-free period is required after it has been stopped but it should not be started until at least a week after a tricyclic or related antidepressant or an SSRI or related antidepressant has been stopped (2 weeks in the case of paroxetine and sertraline, and at least 5 weeks in the case of fluoxetine), or for at least a week after an MAOI has been stopped. For other interactions, see Appendix 1 (moclobemide).

MOCLOBEMIDE

Indications: depressive illness; social phobia

Cautions: avoid in agitated or excited patients (or give with sedative for up to 2–3 weeks), thyrotoxicosis, hepatic impairment (Appendix 2), may provoke manic episodes in bipolar disorders, pregnancy and breast-feeding (patient information leaflet advises avoid); **interactions:** see notes above and Appendix 1 (moclobemide)

Contra-indications: acute confusional states, phaeochromocytoma

Side-effects: sleep disturbances, dizziness, gastro-intestinal disorders, headache, restlessness, agitation; paraesthesia, dry mouth, visual disturbances, oedema, skin reactions, confusional states reported; rarely raised liver enzymes, galactorrhoea; for CSM advice on possible hyponatraemia, see p. 187

Dose: depression, initially 300 mg daily usually in divided doses after food, adjusted according to response; usual range 150–600 mg daily; CHILD not recommended

Social phobia, initially 300 mg daily increased on fourth day to 600 mg daily in 2 divided doses, continued for 8–12 weeks to assess efficacy; CHILD not recommended

Moclobemide (Non-proprietary) PoM
Tablets, moclobemide 150 mg, net price 30-tab pack = £9.41; 300 mg, 30-tab pack = £14.78. Label: 10, patient information leaflet, 21
Available from APS, Generics, PLIVA, Ratiopharm, Sandoz

Manerix® (Roche) PoM
Tablets, yellow, f/c, scored, moclobemide 150 mg, net price 30-tab pack = £10.03; 300 mg, 30-tab pack = £15.04. Label: 10, patient information leaflet, 21

4.3.3 Selective serotonin re-uptake inhibitors

Citalopram, escitalopram, fluoxetine, fluvoxamine, paroxetine, and **sertraline** selectively inhibit the re-uptake of serotonin (5-hydroxytryptamine, 5-HT); they are termed selective serotonin re-uptake inhibitors (SSRIs). For a general comment on the management of depression and on the comparison between *tricyclic and related antidepressants* and the *SSRIs and related antidepressants*, see section 4.3.

CAUTIONS. SSRIs should be used with caution in patients with epilepsy (avoid if poorly controlled,

discontinue if convulsions develop), concurrent electroconvulsive therapy (prolonged seizures reported with fluoxetine), history of mania, cardiac disease, diabetes mellitus, angle-closure glaucoma, concomitant use of drugs that increase risk of bleeding, history of bleeding disorders (especially gastro-intestinal bleeding), hepatic and renal impairment (Appendixes 2 and 3), pregnancy and breast-feeding (Appendixes 4 and 5). SSRIs may also impair performance of skilled tasks (e.g. driving). Abrupt withdrawal of SSRIs should be avoided (associated with headache, nausea, paraesthesia, dizziness and anxiety); **interactions:** see below and Appendix 1 (antidepressants, SSRI).

INTERACTIONS. An SSRI or related antidepressant should not be started until 2 weeks after stopping an MAOI. Conversely, an MAOI should not be started until at least a week after an SSRI or related antidepressant has been stopped (2 weeks in the case of paroxetine and sertraline, at least 5 weeks in the case of fluoxetine). For guidance relating to the reversible monoamine oxidase inhibitor, moclobemide, see above. For other SSRI antidepressant interactions, see Appendix 1 (antidepressants, SSRI).

CONTRA-INDICATIONS. SSRIs should not be used if the patient enters a manic phase.

> **CSM advice.** The CSM has advised that the SSRIs citalopram, escitalopram, fluvoxamine, paroxetine, and sertraline, as well as venlafaxine should **not** be used in children and adolescents under 18 years to treat depressive illness. Trials in children and adolescents suggest an increase in the risk of harmful outcomes including self-harm and potentially suicidal behaviour.

SIDE-EFFECTS. SSRIs are less sedating and have fewer antimuscarinic and cardiotoxic effects than tricyclic antidepressants (section 4.3). Side-effects of the SSRIs include gastro-intestinal effects (dose–related and fairly common—include nausea, vomiting, dyspepsia, abdominal pain, diarrhoea, constipation), anorexia with weight loss (increased appetite and weight gain also reported) and hypersensitivity reactions including rash (consider discontinuation—may be sign of impending serious systemic reaction, possibly associated with vasculitis); urticaria, angioedema, anaphylaxis, arthralgia, myalgia and photosensitivity; other side-effects include dry mouth, nervousness, anxiety, headache, insomnia, tremor, dizziness, asthenia, hallucinations, drowsiness, convulsions (see Cautions above), galactorrhoea, sexual dysfunction, urinary retention, sweating, hypomania or mania (see Cautions above), movement disorders and dyskinesias, visual disturbances, hyponatraemia (may be due to inappropriate antidiuretic hormone secretion—see CSM warning, section 4.3), and cutaneous bleeding disorders including ecchymoses and purpura. Suicidal ideation has been linked with SSRIs but causality has not been established.

CITALOPRAM

Indications: depressive illness, panic disorder

Cautions: see notes above

Contra-indications: see notes above

Side-effects: see notes above; also palpitations, tachycardia, postural hypotension, coughing, yawning, confusion, impaired concentration, malaise, amnesia, migraine, paraesthesia, abnormal dreams, taste disturbance, increased salivation, rhinitis, tinnitus, polyuria, micturition disorders, euphoria

Dose: see preparations below

Citalopram (Non-proprietary) [PoM]
Tablets, citalopram (as hydrobromide) 10 mg, net price 28-tab pack = £9.64; 20 mg, 28-tab pack = £16.03; 40 mg, 28-tab pack = £27.10. Counselling, driving
Available from Generics, Niche, Sandoz, Sterwin

Cipramil® (Lundbeck) [PoM]
Tablets, f/c, citalopram (as hydrobromide) 10 mg, net price 28-tab pack = £9.64; 20 mg (scored), 28-tab pack = £16.03; 40 mg, 28-tab pack = £27.10. Counselling, driving
Dose: depressive illness, 20 mg daily as a single dose in the morning or evening increased if necessary to max. 60 mg daily (ELDERLY max. 40 mg daily); CHILD and ADOLESCENT under 18 years not recommended (see notes above)
Panic disorder, initially 10 mg daily increased to 20 mg after 7 days, usual dose 20–30 mg daily; max. 60 mg daily (ELDERLY max. 40 mg daily); CHILD not recommended
Oral drops, sugar-free, citalopram (as hydrochloride) 40 mg/mL, net price 15 mL = £21.68. Counselling, driving, administration
Dose: depressive illness, 16 mg daily as a single dose in the morning or evening increased if necessary to max. 48 mg daily (ELDERLY max. 32 mg daily); CHILD and ADOLESCENT under 18 years not recommended (see notes above)
Panic disorder, initially 8 mg daily as a single dose increased to 16 mg daily after 7 days, usual dose 16–24 mg daily; max. 48 mg daily; (ELDERLY max. 32 mg daily); CHILD and ADOLESCENT under 18 years not recommended (see notes above)
Excipients: include alcohol
NOTE. 8 mg (4 drops) Cipramil® oral drops may be considered to be equivalent in therapeutic effect to 10-mg Cipramil® tablet
Mix with water, orange juice, or apple juice before taking

ESCITALOPRAM

NOTE. Escitalopram is an isomer of citalopram
Indications: depressive illness, panic disorder
Cautions: see notes above
Contra-indications: see notes above
Side-effects: see notes above; also postural hypotension, sinusitis, yawning, pyrexia, taste disturbance reported
Dose: depressive illness, 10 mg once daily increased if necessary to max. 20 mg daily; ELDERLY initially half adult dose, lower maintenance dose may be sufficient; CHILD and ADOLESCENT under 18 years not recommended (see notes above)
Panic disorder, initially 5 mg daily increased to 10 mg daily after 7 days; max. 20 mg daily; ELDERLY lower maintenance dose may be sufficient; CHILD and ADOLESCENT under 18 years not recommended

Cipralex® (Lundbeck) ▼ [PoM]
Tablets, f/c, scored, escitalopram (as oxalate) 10 mg, net price 28-tab pack = £16.03; 20 mg, 28-tab pack = £27.10. Counselling, driving

FLUOXETINE

Indications: see under Dose
Cautions: see notes above

Contra-indications: see notes above
Side-effects: see notes above; also possible changes in blood sugar, fever, neuroleptic malignant syndrome-like event; also reported (no causal relationship established): abnormal bleeding, aplastic anaemia, cerebrovascular accident, ecchymoses, eosinophilic pneumonia, gastro-intestinal haemorrhage, haemolytic anaemia, pancreatitis, pancytopenia, thrombocytopenia, thrombocytopenic purpura, vaginal bleeding on withdrawal, violent behaviour; hair loss also reported
Dose: depressive illness, 20 mg once daily increased after 3 weeks if necessary, usual dose 20–60 mg (ELDERLY 20–40 mg) once daily; max. 80 mg (ELDERLY max. 60 mg) once daily; CHILD and ADOLESCENT under 18 years not recommended
Bulimia nervosa, 60 mg once daily; max. 80 mg once daily; CHILD and ADOLESCENT under 18 years not recommended
Obsessive-compulsive disorder, initially 20 mg once daily increased after two weeks if necessary, usual dose 20–60 mg (ELDERLY 20–40 mg) once daily; max. 80 mg (ELDERLY max. 60 mg) once daily; discontinue if no improvement within 10 weeks; CHILD and ADOLESCENT under 18 years not recommended
LONG DURATION OF ACTION. Consider the long half-life of fluoxetine when adjusting dosage (or in overdosage)

Fluoxetine (Non-proprietary) [PoM]
Capsules, fluoxetine (as hydrochloride) 20 mg, net price 30-cap pack = £4.33; 60 mg, 30-cap pack = £47.61. Counselling, driving
Available from Alpharma, APS, Arrow, CP, Generics, Genus (*Oxactin*®), IVAX, Sandoz, Sterwin
Liquid, fluoxetine (as hydrochloride) 20 mg/mL, net price 70 mL = £11.82. Counselling, driving
Available from APS

Prozac® (Dista) [PoM]
Capsules, fluoxetine (as hydrochloride) 20 mg (green/yellow), net price 30-cap pack = £14.21; 60 mg (yellow), 30-cap pack = £47.61. Counselling, driving
Liquid, fluoxetine (as hydrochloride) 20 mg/5 mL. Net price 70 mL = £13.26. Counselling, driving

FLUVOXAMINE MALEATE

Indications: depressive illness, obsessive-compulsive disorder
Cautions: see notes above
CSM ADVICE. The CSM has advised that concomitant use of fluvoxamine and theophylline or aminophylline should usually be avoided; see also **interactions:** Appendix 1 (antidepressants, SSRIs)
Contra-indications: see notes above
Side-effects: see notes above; palpitations, tachycardia (may also cause bradycardia), rarely postural hypotension, confusion, ataxia, neuroleptic malignant syndome-like event, abnormal liver function tests, usually symptomatic (discontinue treatment)
Dose: depression, initially 50–100 mg daily in the evening, increased if necessary to 300 mg daily (over 150 mg in divided doses); usual maintenance dose 100 mg daily; CHILD and ADOLESCENT under 18 years not recommended (see notes above)
Obsessive-compulsive disorder, initially 50 mg in the evening for 3–4 days, increasing if necessary to 300 mg daily (over 150 mg in divided doses); CHILD over 8 years initially 25 mg daily increased

if necessary in steps of 25 mg every 3–4 days to max. 200 mg daily in divided doses
NOTE. If no improvement in obsessive-compulsive disorder within 10 weeks, treatment should be reconsidered

Fluvoxamine (Non-proprietary) PoM
Tablets, fluvoxamine maleate 50 mg, net price 60-tab pack = £17.73; 100 mg, 30-tab pack = £18.04. Counselling, driving
Available from APS, Arrow, IVAX, Ratiopharm

Faverin® (Solvay) PoM
Tablets, f/c, scored, fluvoxamine maleate 50 mg, net price 60-tab pack = £19.00; 100 mg, 30-tab pack = £19.00. Counselling, driving

PAROXETINE

Indications: depressive illness, obsessive-compulsive disorder, panic disorder; social phobia; post-traumatic stress disorder; generalised anxiety disorder
Cautions: see notes above
IMPORTANT. During initial treatment of panic disorder, there is potential for worsening of panic symptoms
CSM ADVICE. Extrapyramidal reactions (including orofacial dystonias) and withdrawal syndrome are reported to the CSM more commonly with paroxetine than with other SSRIs
Contra-indications: see notes above
Side-effects: see notes above; postural hypotension; very rarely hepatic disorders (e.g. hepatitis)
Dose: depressive illness, post–traumatic stress disorder, usually 20 mg each morning, if necessary increased gradually in steps of 10 mg; max. 50 mg daily (ELDERLY 40 mg daily); CHILD and ADOLESCENT under 18 years not recommended (see notes above)
Obsessive-compulsive disorder, initially 20 mg each morning, if necessary increased gradually in weekly steps of 10 mg to usual dose of 40 mg daily; max. 60 mg daily (ELDERLY 40 mg daily); CHILD not recommended
Panic disorder, initially 10 mg each morning, if necessary increased gradually in weekly steps of 10 mg to usual dose of 40 mg daily; max. 50 mg daily (ELDERLY 40 mg daily); CHILD not recommended
Social phobia, initially 20 mg each morning; if no improvement after at least 2 weeks, increase in steps of 10 mg at intervals of at least 1 week; max. 50 mg daily (ELDERLY 40 mg daily); CHILD not recommended
Generalised anxiety disorder, 20 mg each morning; CHILD not recommended

Paroxetine (Non-proprietary) PoM
Tablets, paroxetine (as hydrochloride) 20 mg, net price 30-tab pack = £15.21. Label: 21, counselling, driving
Available from Alpharma, Generics, Norton

Seroxat® (GSK) PoM
Tablets, both f/c, scored, paroxetine (as hydrochloride) 20 mg, net price 30-tab pack = £17.76; 30 mg (blue), 30-tab pack = £31.16. Label: 21, counselling, driving
Liquid, orange, sugar-free, paroxetine (as hydrochloride) 10 mg/5 mL. Net price 150-mL pack = £20.77. Label: 21, counselling, driving

4.3.4 Other a...

196   4.3.4 Oth...

Cautions: ...
disorde...
conf...
d...

SERTRALINE

Indications: depressive ... sive disorder (under ... children), post-trauma...
Cautions: see notes ab...
Contra-indications: s...
Side-effects: see notes ...
sion, amnesia, aggressive behaviour, psychosis, pancreatitis, hepatitis, jaundice, liver failure, menstrual irregularities, paraesthesia; thrombocytopenia also reported (causal relationship not established)
Dose: depressive illness, initially 50 mg daily, increased if necessary by increments of 50 mg over several weeks to max. 200 mg daily; usual maintenance dose 50 mg daily; CHILD and ADOLESCENT under 18 years not recommended (see notes above)
Obsessive-compulsive disorder, ADULT and ADOLESCENT over 13 years initially 50 mg daily, increased if necessary in steps of 50 mg over several weeks; usual dose range 50–200 mg daily; CHILD 6–12 years initially 25 mg daily, increased to 50 mg daily after 1 week, further increased if necessary in steps of 50 mg at intervals of at least 1 week (max. 200 mg daily); CHILD under 6 years not recommended
Post-traumatic stress disorder, initially 25 mg daily, increased after 1 week to 50 mg daily; if response is partial and if drug tolerated, dose increased in steps of 50 mg over several weeks to max. 200 mg daily; CHILD not recommended

Lustral® (Pfizer) PoM
Tablets, both f/c, sertraline (as hydrochloride) 50 mg (scored), net price 28-tab pack = £16.20; 100 mg, 28-tab pack = £26.51. Counselling, driving

4.3.4   Other antidepressant drugs

The thioxanthene **flupentixol** (*Fluanxol*®) has antidepressant properties, and low doses (1 to 3 mg daily) are given by mouth for this purpose. Flupentixol is also used for the treatment of psychoses (section 4.2.1 and section 4.2.2)

Mirtazapine, a presynaptic α_2-antagonist, increases central noradrenergic and serotonergic neurotransmission. It has few antimuscarinic effects, but causes sedation during initial treatment.

Reboxetine, a selective inhibitor of noradrenaline re-uptake, has been introduced for the treatment of depressive illness.

Tryptophan appears to benefit some patients with resistant depression when given as adjunctive therapy but tryptophan products have been associated with the eosinophilia-myalgia syndrome; *Optimax*® (Merck) is available for patients for whom no alternative treatment is suitable.

Venlafaxine is a serotonin and noradrenaline re-uptake inhibitor (SNRI); it lacks the sedative and antimuscarinic effects of the tricyclic antidepressants.

FLUPENTIXOL

(Flupentixol)
Indications: depressive illness; psychoses (section 4.2.1)

rdiovascular disease (including cardiac , and cerebral arteriosclerosis), senile ,ional states, parkinsonism, renal and hepatic ease; avoid in excitable and overactive patients; orphyria (section 9.8.2); **interactions**: Appendix 1 (antipsychotics)

Side-effects: restlessness, insomnia; hypomania reported; rarely dizziness, tremor, visual disturbances, headache, hyperprolactinaemia, extrapyramidal symptoms

Dose: initially 1 mg (elderly 500 micrograms) in the morning, increased after 1 week to 2 mg (elderly 1 mg) if necessary; max. 3 mg (elderly 2 mg) daily, doses above 2 mg (elderly 1 mg) being divided in 2 portions, second dose not after 4 p.m. Discontinue if no response after 1 week at max. dosage; CHILD not recommended

COUNSELLING. Although drowsiness may occur, can also have an alerting effect so should not be taken in the evening

Fluanxol® (Lundbeck) PoM
Tablets, both red, s/c, flupentixol (as dihydrochloride) 500 micrograms, net price 60-tab pack = £3.10; 1 mg, 60-tab pack = £5.23. Label: 2, counselling, administration

MIRTAZAPINE

Indications: depressive illness

Cautions: epilepsy, hepatic or renal impairment, cardiac disorders, hypotension, history of urinary retention, angle-closure glaucoma, diabetes mellitus, psychoses (may aggravate psychotic symptoms), history of bipolar depression, avoid abrupt withdrawal; manufacturer advises avoid in pregnancy and in breast-feeding (Appendix 5); **interactions:** Appendix 1 (mirtazapine)

BLOOD DISORDERS. Patients should be advised to report any fever, sore throat, stomatitis or other signs of infection during treatment. Blood count should be performed and the drug stopped immediately if blood dyscrasia suspected

Side-effects: increased appetite and weight gain, oedema, sedation; less commonly dizziness, headache; rarely postural hypotension, abnormal dreams, mania, convulsions, tremor, myoclonus, paraesthesia, arthralgia, myalgia, restless legs, exanthema, reversible agranulocytosis (see Cautions above)

Dose: initially 15 mg daily at bedtime increased according to response up to 45 mg daily as a single dose at bedtime or in 2 divided doses; CHILD not recommended

Mirtazapine (Non-proprietary) PoM
Oral solution, mirtazapine 15 mg/mL, net price 66 mL = £60.00. Label: 2
Available from Rosemont

Zispin® (Organon) PoM
Tablets, scored, red/brown, mirtazapine 30 mg. Net price 28-tab pack = £22.92. Label: 2, 25
Orodispersible tablets (*Zispin SolTab®*), mirtazapine 30 mg, net price 30-tab pack = £20.63.
Label: 2, counselling, administration
Excipients: include aspartame
COUNSELLING. *Zispin SolTab®* should be placed on the tongue, allowed to disperse and swallowed

REBOXETINE

Indications: depressive illness

Cautions: severe renal impairment (Appendix 3), hepatic impairment (Appendix 2), history of cardiovascular disease and epilepsy, bipolar disorders, urinary retention, prostatic hypertrophy, glaucoma; **interactions:** Appendix 1 (reboxetine)

Contra-indications: pregnancy (Appendix 4) and breast-feeding (Appendix 5)

Side-effects: insomnia, sweating, dizziness, postural hypotension, vertigo, paraesthesia, impotence, dysuria, urinary retention (mainly in men), dry mouth, constipation, tachycardia; lowering of plasma-potassium concentration on prolonged administration in the elderly

Dose: 4 mg twice daily increased if necessary after 3–4 weeks to 10 mg daily in divided doses, max. 12 mg daily; CHILD and ELDERLY not recommended

Edronax® (Pharmacia) PoM
Tablets, scored, reboxetine (as mesilate) 4 mg. Net price 60-tab pack = £18.91. Counselling, driving

TRYPTOPHAN
(L-Tryptophan)

Indications: restricted to use by hospital specialists *only* for patients with severe and disabling depressive illness of more than 2 years continuous duration, *only* after an adequate trial of standard antidepressant drug treatment, and *only* as an adjunct to other antidepressant medication

Cautions: eosinophilia-myalgia syndrome has been reported with tryptophan-containing products therefore close and regular surveillance required; monitor eosinophil count, haematological changes and muscle symptomatology; pregnancy and breast-feeding; **interactions:** Appendix 1 (tryptophan)

Contra-indications: history of eosinophilia-myalgia syndrome following use of tryptophan

Side-effects: drowsiness, nausea, headache, lightheadedness; eosinophilia-myalgia syndrome, see Cautions

Dose: 1 g 3 times daily; max. 6 g daily; ELDERLY lower dose may be appropriate especially where renal or hepatic impairment; CHILD not recommended

Optimax® (Merck) PoM
Tablets, scored, tryptophan 500 mg. Net price 84-tab pack = £19.56. Label: 3
Important. Patient and prescriber must be registered with the *Optimax®* Information and Clinical Support (OPTICS) Unit (Tel 0845 7626902). A **safety questionnaire** is sent to the prescriber after **3** and **6 months** of treatment and **every 6 months** thereafter. The information is reviewed by the CSM—it is **important** that the questionnaires should be completed

VENLAFAXINE

Indications: depressive illness; generalised anxiety disorder

Cautions: history of myocardial infarction or unstable heart disease, blood pressure monitoring advisable if dose exceeds 200 mg daily, history of epilepsy, mania, hepatic or renal impairment (Appendixes 2 and 3), avoid abrupt withdrawal (if taken for more than 1 week withdraw over at least 1 week); glaucoma; concomitant use of drugs that increase risk of bleeding, history of bleeding disorders; **interactions:** Appendix 1 (venlafaxine)

CSM advice on the potential for harmful outcomes in children and adolescents (see p. 193)

DRIVING. May affect performance of skilled tasks (e.g. driving)

SKIN REACTIONS. Advise patients to contact doctor if rash, urticaria or related allergic reaction develops

Contra-indications: severe hepatic or renal impairment; pregnancy and breast-feeding

Side-effects: constipation, nausea; dizziness, dry mouth, insomnia, nervousness, drowsiness, asthenia, headache; sexual dysfunction; sweating; commonly anorexia, weight changes, diarrhoea, dyspepsia, vomiting, abdominal pain; hypertension, palpitation, vasodilatation, changes in serum cholesterol; chills, pyrexia, dyspnoea, yawning; abnormal dreams, agitation, anxiety, confusion, hypertonia, paraesthesia, tremor; urinary frequency, menstrual disturbances; arthralgia, myalgia; visual disturbances, mydriasis; tinnitus; pruritus, rash (see Skin Reactions above); less commonly bruxism, taste disturbances; postural hypotension, arrhythmias, syndrome of inappropriate anti-diuretic hormone secretion (see advice on Hyponatraemia, p. 187); hallucinations, myoclonus; urinary retention; bleeding disorders (including ecchymosis and rarely haemorrhage); hypersensitivity reactions including angioedema, urticaria, photosensitivity; rarely ataxia, incoordination, speech disorder, extrapyramidal effects, mania and hypomania, seizures, serotonin syndrome; galactorrhoea; thrombocytopenia; erythema multiforme, Stevens-Johnson syndrome; hepatitis reported

Dose: depression, initially 75 mg daily in 2 divided doses increased if necessary after several weeks to 150 mg daily in 2 divided doses; CHILD and ADOLESCENT under 18 years not recommended (see CSM advice, p. 193)

Severely depressed or hospitalised patients, initially 150 mg daily in 2 divided doses increased if necessary in steps of up to 75 mg every 2–3 days to max. 375 mg daily then gradually reduced; CHILD and ADOLESCENT under 18 years not recommended (see CSM advice, p. 193)

Generalised anxiety disorder, see under preparations below

Efexor® (Wyeth) PoM
Tablets, all peach, venlafaxine (as hydrochloride) 37.5 mg, net price 56-tab pack = £23.97; 50 mg, 42-tab pack = £23.97; 75 mg, 56-tab pack = £39.97. Label: 21, counselling, driving, skin reactions

■ Modified release
Efexor® XL (Wyeth) PoM
Capsules, m/r, venlafaxine (as hydrochloride) 75 mg (peach), net price 28-cap pack = £23.97, 150 mg (orange), 28-cap pack = £39.97. Label: 21, 25, counselling, driving, skin reactions
Dose: depression, 75 mg daily as a single dose, increased if necessary after at least 2 weeks to 150 mg once daily; max. 225 mg once daily; ADOLESCENT and CHILD under 18 years not recommended
Generalised anxiety disorder, 75 mg daily as a single dose; discontinue if no response after 8 weeks; ADOLESCENT and CHILD under 18 years not recommended

4.4 Central nervous system stimulants

Central nervous system stimulants include the **amphetamines** (notably dexamfetamine) **and related drugs** (e.g. methylphenidate). They have very few indications and in particular, should **not** be used to treat depression, obesity, senility, debility, or for relief of fatigue.

Caffeine is a weak stimulant present in tea and coffee. It is included in many analgesic preparations (section 4.7.1) but does not contribute to their analgesic or anti-inflammatory effect. Over-indulgence may lead to a state of anxiety.

The **amphetamines** have a limited field of usefulness and their use should be **discouraged** as they may cause dependence and psychotic states. They have **no place** in the management of **depression** or **obesity**.

Patients with *narcolepsy* may derive benefit from treatment with dexamfetamine.

Methylphenidate is used for the management of *attention deficit hyperactivity disorder* (ADHD) (see NICE guidance below); growth is not generally affected but it is advisable to monitor growth during treatment. **Dexamfetamine** (dexamphetamine) is an alternative in children who do not respond to methylphenidate. Drug treatment of attention deficit/hyperactivity disorder should be supervised by specialists.

Modafinil is used for the treatment of daytime sleepiness associated with narcolepsy or obstructive sleep apnoea syndrome; dependence with long-term use cannot be excluded and it should therefore be used with caution

NICE guidance (methylphenidate). NICE has recommended (October 2000) that methylphenidate should be used as part of a comprehensive treatment programme for children and adolescents with a diagnosis of severe attention deficit/hyperactivity disorder (ADHD). Treatment should be initiated by a specialist in ADHD but may be continued by general practitioners, under a shared-care arrangement. When a child receiving methylphenidate shows improvement and the condition appears stable, treatment can be suspended periodically in order to assess the need for continuation of therapy.

DEXAMFETAMINE SULPHATE
(Dexamphetamine sulphate)
Indications: narcolepsy, adjunct in the management of refractory hyperkinetic states in children (under specialist supervision)
Cautions: mild hypertension (contra-indicated if moderate or severe)—monitor blood pressure; history of epilepsy (discontinue if convulsions occur); tics and Tourette syndrome (use with caution)—discontinue if tics occur; monitor growth in children (see also below); avoid abrupt withdrawal; data on safety and efficacy of long-term use not complete; porphyria (see section 9.8.2); **interactions:** Appendix 1 (sympathomimetics)
SPECIAL CAUTIONS IN CHILDREN. Monitor height and weight as growth retardation may occur during prolonged therapy (drug free periods may allow catch-up in growth but withdraw slowly to avoid inducing depression or

renewed hyperactivity). In psychotic children may exacerbate behavioural disturbances and thought disorder

Contra-indications: cardiovascular disease including moderate to severe hypertension, hyper-excitability or agitated states, hyperthyroidism, history of drug or alcohol abuse, glaucoma, pregnancy and breast-feeding
DRIVING. May affect performance of skilled tasks (e.g. driving); effects of alcohol unpredictable

Side-effects: insomnia, restlessness, irritability and excitability, nervousness, night terrors, euphoria, tremor, dizziness, headache; convulsions (see also Cautions); dependence and tolerance, sometimes psychosis, anorexia, gastro-intestinal symptoms, growth retardation in children (see also under Cautions); dry mouth, sweating, tachycardia (and anginal pain), palpitations, increased blood pressure; visual disturbances; cardiomyopathy reported with chronic use; central stimulants have provoked choreoathetoid movements, tics and Tourette syndrome in predisposed individuals (see also Cautions above); **overdosage:** see Emergency Treatment of Poisoning, p. 26

Dose: narcolepsy, 10 mg (ELDERLY, 5 mg) daily in divided doses increased by 10 mg (ELDERLY, 5 mg) daily at intervals of 1 week to a max. of 60 mg daily
Hyperkinesia, CHILD over 6 years 5–10 mg daily, increased if necessary by 5 mg at intervals of 1 week to usual max. 20 mg daily (older children have received max. 40 mg daily); under 6 years not recommended

Dexedrine® (Celltech) CD
Tablets, scored, dexamfetamine sulphate 5 mg. Net price 28-tab pack = £1.92. Counselling, driving

METHYLPHENIDATE HYDROCHLORIDE

Indications: part of a comprehensive treatment programme for attention-deficit hyperactivity disorder when remedial measures alone prove insufficient (under specialist supervision)

Cautions: see under Dexamfetamine Sulphate; also manufacturer recommends periodic complete and differential blood and platelet counts; **interactions:** Appendix 1 (sympathomimetics)

Contra-indications: see under Dexamfetamine Sulphate

Side-effects: see under Dexamfetamine Sulphate; also sleep disturbances, depression, confusion, rash, pruritus, urticaria, fever, arthralgia, alopecia, exfoliative dermatitis, erythema multiforme, thrombocytopenic purpura, thrombocytopenia, leucopenia, urinary disorders, and very rarely liver damage, muscle cramps, cerebral arteritis

Dose: CHILD over 6 years, initially 5 mg 1–2 times daily, increased if necessary at weekly intervals by 5–10 mg daily to max. 60 mg daily in divided doses; discontinue if no response after 1 month, also suspend periodically to assess child's condition (usually finally discontinued during or after puberty); under 6 years not recommended
EVENING DOSE. If effect wears off in evening (with rebound hyperactivity) a dose at bedtime may be appropriate (establish need with trial bedtime dose)

Methylphenidate Hydrochloride (Non-proprietary) CD
Tablets, 5 mg, net price 30-tab pack = £2.78; 10 mg, 30-tab pack = £5.57; 20 mg, 30-tab pack = £9.98
Available from Celltech (*Equasym®*), Link (*Tranquilyn®*)

Ritalin® (Cephalon) CD
Tablets, scored, methylphenidate hydrochloride 10 mg, net price 30-tab pack = £5.57

■ Modified release

Concerta® XL (Janssen-Cilag) CD
Tablets, m/r, methylphenidate hydrochloride 18 mg (yellow), net price 30-tab pack = £27.00; 36 mg (white), 30-tab pack = £36.75. Label: 25
COUNSELLING. Tablet membrane may pass through gastro-intestinal tract unchanged
Cautions: dose form not appropriate for use in dysphagia or where gastro-intestinal lumen restricted
Dose: CHILD over 6 years, initially 18 mg once daily (in the morning), increased if necessary in weekly steps of 18 mg according to response, max. 54 mg once daily; discontinue if no response after 1 month; suspend periodically to assess condition (usually finally discontinued during or after puberty); under 6 years not recommended
NOTE. Total daily dose of 15 mg of standard-release formulation is considered equivalent to *Concerta® XL* 18 mg once daily

MODAFINIL

Indications: daytime sleepiness associated with narcolepsy or obstructive sleep apnoea syndrome

Cautions: hepatic impairment (Appendix 2); renal impairment (Appendix 3); monitor blood pressure and heart rate in hypertensive patients (but see below); possibility of dependence; **interactions:** Appendix 1 (modafinil)

Contra-indications: pregnancy and breast-feeding; moderate to severe hypertension; history of left ventricular hypertrophy or of clinically significant signs of CNS stimulant-induced mitral valve prolapse (including ischaemic ECG changes, chest pain and arrhythmias)

Side-effects: dry mouth, appetite changes, gastro-intestinal disturbances (including nausea, diarrhoea, constipation and dyspepsia), abdominal pain; tachycardia, vasodilation, chest pain; headache (uncommonly migraine), anxiety, insomnia, dizziness, depression, confusion, paraesthesia, hypertonia, asthenia; visual disturbances; less commonly, taste disturbances; hypertension, hypotension, arrhythmia, peripheral oedema; dyspnoea, rhinitis; dyskinesia, amnesia, emotional lability, abnormal dreams, agitation, tremor, vertigo, decreased libido, weight changes, hyperglycaemia; urinary frequency, menstrual disturbances; eosinophilia, leucopenia; myalgia, arthralgia; sweating, rash, pruritus, dry eye

Dose: 200–400 mg daily, *either* in 2 divided doses morning and at noon *or* as a single dose in the morning; ELDERLY initiate at 100 mg daily; CHILD not recommended

Provigil® (Cephalon) PoM
Tablets, modafinil 100 mg, net price 30-tab pack = £60.00; 200 mg, 30 tab-pack = £120.00

Cocaine

Cocaine is a drug of addiction which causes central nervous stimulation. Its clinical use is mainly as a topical local anaesthetic (section 15.2). It has been included in analgesic elixirs for the relief of pain in palliative care but this use is obsolete. For management of cocaine poisoning, see p. 26.

4.5 Drugs used in the treatment of obesity

4.5.1 Anti-obesity drugs acting on the gastro-intestinal tract

4.5.2 Centrally acting appetite suppressants

Obesity is associated with many health problems including cardiovascular disease, diabetes mellitus, gallstones and osteoarthritis. Factors that aggravate obesity may include depression, other psychosocial problems, and some drugs.

The main treatment of the obese individual is a suitable diet, carefully explained to the individual, with appropriate support and encouragement; the individual should also be advised to increase physical activity. Smoking cessation (while maintaining body weight) may be worthwhile before attempting supervised weight loss since cigarette smoking may be more harmful than obesity. Attendance at groups (e.g. 'weight-watchers') helps some individuals.

Severe obesity should be managed in an appropriate setting by staff who have been trained in the management of obesity; the individual should receive advice on diet and lifestyle modification and be monitored for changes in weight as well as in blood pressure, blood lipids and other associated conditions.

An anti-obesity drug should be considered only for those with a body mass index (BMI, individual's body-weight divided by the square of the individual's height) of 30 kg/m^2 or greater in whom at least 3 months of managed care involving supervised diet, exercise and behaviour modification fails to achieve a realistic reduction in weight. In the presence of risk factors (such as diabetes, coronary heart disease, hypertension, and obstructive sleep apnoea), it may be appropriate to prescribe a drug to individuals with a BMI of 27 kg/m^2 or greater, provided that such use is permitted by the drug's marketing authorisation. Drugs should **never** be used as the sole element of treatment. The individual should be monitored on a regular basis; drug treatment should be discontinued if weight loss is less than 5% after the first 12 weeks or if the individual regains weight at any time whilst receiving drug treatment.

Drugs specifically licensed for the treatment of obesity are **orlistat** (section 4.5.1) and **sibutramine** (section 4.5.2). There is little evidence to guide selection between the two drugs, but it may be appropriate to choose orlistat for those who have a high intake of fats whereas sibutramine may be chosen for those who cannot control their eating; the cautions, contra-indications and side-effects of the two drugs should also be considered.

Combination therapy involving more than one anti-obesity drug is **contra-indicated** until further information about efficacy and long-term safety is available.

Thyroid hormones have **no** place in the treatment of obesity except in biochemically proven hypothyroid patients. The use of diuretics, chorionic gonadotrophin, or amphetamines is **not** appropriate for weight reduction.

4.5.1 ## Anti-obesity drugs acting on the gastro-intestinal tract

Orlistat, a lipase inhibitor, reduces the absorption of dietary fat. It is used in conjunction with a mildly hypocaloric diet in individuals with a body mass index (BMI) of 30 kg/m^2 or more *or* in individuals with a BMI of 28 kg/m^2 in the presence of other risk factors such as type 2 diabetes, hypertension, or hypercholesterolaemia.

Some of the weight loss in those taking orlistat probably results from individuals reducing their fat intake to avoid severe gastro-intestinal effects including steatorrhoea. Vitamin supplementation (especially of vitamin D) may be considered if there is concern about deficiency of fat-soluble vitamins. Orlistat is not licensed for use longer than 2 years because there is insufficient experience beyond this period. However, on stopping orlistat, there may be a gradual reversal of weight loss.

> **NICE guidance (orlistat).** NICE has recommended (March 2001) that orlistat should be prescribed under the following conditions:
>
> - only for individuals who have lost at least 2.5 kg body-weight by dietary control and increased physical activity in the preceding month
> - only for individuals aged between 18 and 75 years
> - arrangements should exist for primary care staff (mostly practice nurses) supported by community dieticians to offer specific advice, support and counselling on diet, physical activity, and behavioural strategies
> - treatment should continue beyond 3 months only if weight loss is greater than 5% from start of treatment
> - treatment should continue beyond 6 months only if weight loss is greater than 10% from start of treatment
> - treatment should not usually continue beyond 1 year and never beyond 2 years [see also notes above]

The most commonly used bulk-forming drug is **methylcellulose** (section 1.6.1). It is claimed to reduce intake by producing a feeling of satiety but there is little evidence to support its use in the management of obesity.

ORLISTAT

Indications: adjunct in obesity (see notes above)

Cautions: diabetes mellitus; may impair absorption of fat-soluble vitamins; **interactions:** Appendix 1 (orlistat)

MULTIVITAMINS. If a multivitamin supplement is required, it should be taken at least 2 hours after orlistat dose or at bedtime

Contra-indications: chronic malabsorption syndrome; cholestasis; pregnancy and breast-feeding

Side-effects: liquid oily stools, faecal urgency, faecal incontinence, flatulence, less frequently abdominal and rectal pain (gastro-intestinal effects minimised by reduced fat diet); headache; menstrual irregularities; anxiety, fatigue; rarely hepatitis, hypersensitivity reactions

Dose: 120 mg taken immediately before, during, or up to 1 hour after each main meal (up to max. 360 mg daily); max. period of treatment 2 years; CHILD not recommended

NOTE. If a meal is missed or contains no fat, the dose of orlistat should be omitted

Xenical® (Roche) ▼ PoM

Capsules, turquoise, orlistat 120 mg, net price 84-cap pack = £41.16

4.5.2 Centrally acting appetite suppressants

Sibutramine inhibits the re-uptake of noradrenaline and serotonin. It is used in the adjunctive management of obesity in individuals with a body mass index (BMI) of 30 kg/m^2 or more (and no associated co-morbidity) or in individuals with a BMI of 27 kg/m^2 or more in the presence of other risk factors such as type 2 diabetes or hypercholesterolaemia. Sibutramine is not licensed for use longer than 1 year; on stopping it, there may be a reversal of weight loss.

Dexfenfluramine, fenfluramine, and phentermine have been associated with valvular heart disease and the rare but serious risk of pulmonary hypertension.

NICE guidance (sibutramine). NICE has recommended that sibutramine should be prescribed in accordance with the summary of product characteristics and under the following conditions:

- it should be prescribed only for individuals who have attempted seriously to lose weight by diet, exercise, and other behavioural modification;
- arrangements should exist for appropriate healthcare professionals to offer specific advice, support, and counselling on diet, physical activity, and behavioural strategies to those receiving sibutramine.

SIBUTRAMINE HYDROCHLORIDE

Indications: adjunct in obesity (see notes above)

Cautions: monitor blood pressure and pulse rate (every 2 weeks for first 3 months *then* monthly for 3 months *then* at least every 3 months)—discontinue if blood pressure exceeds 145/90 mmHg or if systolic or diastolic pressure raised by more than 10 mmHg or if pulse rate raised by 10 beats per minute at 2 consecutive visits; sleep apnoea syndrome (increased risk of hypertension); epilepsy; hepatic impairment (avoid if severe; Appendix 2); renal impairment (avoid if severe); open angle glaucoma, history of ocular hypertension; monitor for pulmonary hypertension; family history of motor or vocal tics, history of depression; predisposition to bleeding, concomitant use of drugs that increase risk of bleeding; **interactions:** Appendix 1 (sibutramine)

DISCONTINUATION OF TREATMENT. Discontinue treatment if:

- weight loss after 3 months less than 5% of initial body-weight;
- weight loss stabilises at less than 5% of initial body-weight;
- individuals regain 3 kg or more after previous weight loss

In individuals with co-morbid conditions, treatment should be continued only if weight loss is associated with other clinical benefits

Contra-indications: history of major eating disorders; psychiatric illness, Tourette syndrome; history of coronary artery disease, congestive heart failure, tachycardia, peripheral arterial occlusive disease, arrhythmias, and of cerebrovascular disease; uncontrolled hypertension; hyperthyroidism; prostatic hypertrophy; phaeochromocytoma; angle closure glaucoma; history of drug or alcohol abuse; pregnancy (Appendix 4); breast-feeding (Appendix 5)

Side-effects: constipation, dry mouth, nausea, taste disturbances, diarrhoea, vomiting; tachycardia, palpitations, hypertension, flushing, insomnia, lightheadedness, paraesthesia, headache, anxiety, depression, seizures; sexual dysfunction, menstrual disturbances, urinary retention; thrombocytopenia; blurred vision, seating, hypersensitivity reactions including Henoch-Shönlein purpura, rash, urticaria, angioedema and anaphylaxis; interstitial nephritis, glomerulonephritis

Dose: initially 10 mg daily in the morning, increased if weight loss less than 2 kg after 4 weeks to 15 mg daily; discontinue if weight loss less than 2 kg after 4 weeks at higher dose (see also Duration of Treatment above); max. period of treatment 1 year; CHILD, ADOLESCENT under 18 years, and ELDERLY over 65 years not recommended

Reductil® (Abbott) ▼ PoM

Capsules, sibutramine hydrochloride 10 mg (blue/yellow), net price 28-cap pack = £37.54; 15 mg (blue/white), 28-cap pack = £41.74

4.6 Drugs used in nausea and vertigo

Anti-emetics should be prescribed only when the cause of vomiting is known because otherwise they may delay diagnosis, particularly in children. Anti-emetics are unnecessary and sometimes harmful when the cause can be treated, such as in diabetic ketoacidosis, or in digoxin or antiepileptic overdose.

If anti-emetic drug treatment is indicated, the drug is chosen according to the aetiology of vomiting.

Antihistamines are effective against nausea and vomiting resulting from many underlying conditions. There is no evidence that any one antihistamine is superior to another but their duration of action and incidence of adverse effects (drowsiness and antimuscarinic effects) differ.

The **phenothiazines** are dopamine antagonists and act centrally by blocking the chemoreceptor trigger zone. They are of considerable value for the prophylaxis and treatment of nausea and vomiting associated with diffuse neoplastic disease, radiation sickness, and the emesis caused by drugs such as opioids, general anaesthetics, and cytotoxics. **Prochlorperazine**, **perphenazine**, and **trifluoperazine** are less sedating than **chlorpromazine**; severe dystonic reactions sometimes occur with phenothiazines, especially in children. Other antipsychotic drugs including **haloperidol** and **levomepromazine** (**methotrimeprazine**) (section 4.2.1) are also used for the relief of nausea. Some phenothiazines are available as rectal suppositories, which can be useful in patients with persistent vomiting or with severe nausea; prochlorperazine can also be administered as a buccal tablet which is placed between the upper lip and the gum.

Metoclopramide is an effective anti-emetic and its activity closely resembles that of the phenothiazines. Metoclopramide also acts directly on the gastro-intestinal tract and it may be superior to the pheno-thiazines for emesis associated with gastroduodenal, hepatic, and biliary disease. In postoperative nausea and vomiting, metoclopramide in a dose of 10 mg has limited efficacy. High-dose metoclopramide injection is now less commonly used for cytotoxic-induced nausea and vomiting. As with the phenothi-azines, metoclopramide can induce acute dystonic reactions involving facial and skeletal muscle spasms and oculogyric crises. These dystonic effects are more common in the young (especially girls and young women) and the very old; they usually occur shortly after starting treatment with metoclopramide and subside within 24 hours of stopping it. Injection of an antiparkinsonian drug such as procyclidine (section 4.9.2) will abort dystonic attacks.

Domperidone acts at the chemoreceptor trigger zone; it is used for the relief of nausea and vomiting, especially when associated with cytotoxic therapy. It has the advantage over metoclopramide and the phenothiazines of being less likely to cause central effects such as sedation and dystonic reactions because it does not readily cross the blood-brain barrier. In Parkinson's disease, it is used to prevent nausea and vomiting during treatment with apomor-phine and also to treat nausea caused by other dopaminergic drugs (section 4.9.1). Domperidone is also used to treat vomiting due to emergency hormonal contraception (section 7.3.1).

Granisetron, ondansetron, and **tropisetron** are specific $5HT_3$ antagonists which block $5HT_3$ recep-tors in the gastro-intestinal tract and in the CNS. They are of value in the management of nausea and vomiting in patients receiving cytotoxics and in postoperative nausea and vomiting.

Nabilone is a synthetic cannabinoid with anti-emetic properties. It may be used for nausea and vomiting caused by cytotoxic chemotherapy that is unresponsive to conventional anti-emetics. Side-effects such as drowsiness and dizziness occur frequently with standard doses.

Dexamethasone (section 6.3.2) has anti-emetic effects and it is used in vomiting associated with cancer chemotherapy. It can be used alone or with metoclopramide, prochlorperazine, lorazepam, or a $5HT_3$ antagonist (see also section 8.1).

Vomiting of pregnancy

Nausea in the first trimester of pregnancy is generally mild and does not require drug therapy. On rare occasions if vomiting is severe, short-term treatment with an antihistamine, such as **promethazine,** may be required. **Prochlorperazine** or **metoclopramide** may be considered as second-line treatments. If symptoms do not settle in 24 to 48 hours then specialist opinion should be sought. Hyperemesis gravidarum is a more serious condition, which requires intravenous fluid and electrolyte replace-ment and sometimes nutritional support. Supple-mentation with thiamine must be considered to reduce the risk of Wernicke's encephalopathy.

Postoperative nausea and vomiting

The incidence of postoperative nausea and vomiting depends on many factors including the anaesthetic used, the type and duration of surgery, and the patient's sex. The aim is to prevent postoperative nausea and vomiting from occurring. Drugs used include some **phenothiazines** (e.g. prochlorper-azine), **metoclopramide** (but 10-mg dose has lim-ited efficacy and higher parenteral doses associated with greater side-effects), **$5HT_3$ antagonists, anti-histamines** (such as cyclizine), and **dexamethasone.** A combination of two anti-emetic drugs acting at different sites may be considered in resistant post-operative nausea and vomiting.

Motion sickness

Anti-emetics should be given prophylactically for the prevention of motion sickness rather than after nausea or vomiting develop. The most effective drug for the prevention of motion sickness is **hyoscine.** A transdermal hyoscine patch provides prolonged activity but it needs to be applied several hours before travelling. The sedating antihistamines are slightly less effective against motion sickness, but are generally better tolerated than hyoscine. If a sedative effect is desired **promethazine** is useful, but generally a slightly less sedating antihistamine such as **cyclizine** or **cinnarizine** is preferred. The $5HT_3$ antagonists, domperidone, metoclopramide, and the phenothiazines (except the antihistamine phenothia-zine promethazine) are **ineffective** in motion sick-ness.

Other vestibular disorders

Management of vestibular diseases is aimed at treating the underlying cause as well as treating symptoms of the balance disturbance and associated nausea and vomiting. Vertigo and nausea associated with Ménière's disease and middle-ear surgery can be difficult to treat.

Betahistine is an analogue of histamine and is claimed to reduce endolymphatic pressure by improving the microcirculation. Betahistine is licensed for vertigo, tinnitus, and hearing loss associated with Ménière's disease.

A **diuretic** alone or combined with salt restriction may provide some benefit in vertigo associated with Ménière's disease. **Antihistamines** (such as cinnari-zine), and **phenothiazines** (such as prochlorper-azine) are effective for prophylaxis and treatment.

For advice to avoid the inappropriate prescribing of drugs (notably phenothiazines) for dizziness in the elderly, see Prescribing for the Elderly, p. 17

Cytotoxic chemotherapy

For the management of nausea and vomiting induced by cytotoxic chemotherapy, see section 8.1.

Palliative care

For the management of nausea and vomiting in palliative care, see p. 15.

Migraine

For the management of nausea and vomiting associated with migraine, see p. 224

Antihistamines

CINNARIZINE

Indications: vestibular disorders, such as vertigo, tinnitus, nausea, and vomiting in Ménière's disease; motion sickness; vascular disease (section 2.6.4)

Cautions: see under Cyclizine; risk of hypotension with high doses; avoid in porphyria (section 9.8.2)

Contra-indications: see under Cyclizine

Side-effects: see under Cyclizine; allergic skin reactions, fatigue; rarely, extrapyramidal symptoms in elderly on prolonged therapy

Dose: vestibular disorders, 30 mg 3 times daily; CHILD 5–12 years half adult dose

Motion sickness, 30 mg 2 hours before travel then 15 mg every 8 hours during journey if necessary; CHILD 5–12 years half adult dose

Cinnarizine (Non-proprietary)
Tablets, cinnarizine 15 mg. Net price 20 = £1.09. Label: 2
Available from Alpharma, APS, Ashbourne (*Cinazière®*), Generics, Hillcross, IVAX

Stugeron® (Janssen-Cilag)
Tablets, scored, cinnarizine 15 mg. Net price 20 = 75p. Label: 2

Stugeron Forte®
See section 2.6.4

CYCLIZINE

Indications: nausea, vomiting, vertigo, motion sickness, labyrinthine disorders

Cautions: see section 3.4.1; severe heart failure; may counteract haemodynamic benefits of opioids; **interactions:** Appendix 1 (antihistamines)
DRIVING. Drowsiness may affect performance of skilled tasks (e.g. driving); effects of alcohol enhanced

Contra-indications: see section 3.4.1

Side-effects: see section 3.4.1

Dose: *by mouth*, cyclizine hydrochloride 50 mg up to 3 times daily; CHILD 6–12 years 25 mg up to 3 times daily

By intramuscular or intravenous injection, cyclizine lactate 50 mg 3 times daily

Valoid® (CeNeS)
Tablets, scored, cyclizine 50 mg. Net price 20 = 95p. Label: 2
Injection PoM, cyclizine lactate 50 mg/mL. Net price 1-mL amp = 54p

MECLOZINE HYDROCHLORIDE

Indications: see under preparations

Cautions: see section 3.4.1; **interactions:** Appendix 1 (antihistamines)
DRIVING. Drowsiness may affect performance of skilled tasks (e.g. driving); effects of alcohol enhanced

Contra-indications: see section 3.4.1

Side-effects: see section 3.4.1

■ Preparations
A proprietary brand of meclozine hydrochloride tablets 12.5 mg (*Sea-legs®*) is on sale to the public for motion sickness

PROMETHAZINE HYDROCHLORIDE

Indications: nausea, vomiting, vertigo, labyrinthine disorders, motion sickness; other indications (section 3.4.1, section 4.1.1, section 15.1.4.1)

Cautions: see under Cyclizine; avoid in porphyria (section 9.8.2)

Contra-indications: see under Cyclizine

Side-effects: see under Cyclizine but more sedating; intramuscular injection may be painful

Dose: motion sickness prevention, 20–25 mg at bedtime on night before travel, repeat following morning if necessary; CHILD under 2 years not recommended, 2–5 years 5 mg at night and following morning if necessary, 5–10 years 10 mg at night and following morning if necessary

■ Preparations
Section 3.4.1

PROMETHAZINE TEOCLATE

Indications: nausea, vertigo, labyrinthine disorders, motion sickness (acts longer than the hydrochloride)

Cautions: see under Promethazine Hydrochloride

Contra-indications: see under Promethazine Hydrochloride

Side-effects: see under Promethazine Hydrochloride

Dose: 25–75 mg, max. 100 mg, daily; CHILD 5–10 years, 12.5–37.5 mg daily

Motion sickness prevention, 25 mg at bedtime on night before travel *or* 25 mg 1–2 hours before travel; CHILD 5–10 years half adult dose

Severe vomiting in pregnancy, 25 mg at bedtime, increased if necessary to max. 100 mg daily (but see also Vomiting of Pregnancy in notes above)

Avomine® (Manx)
Tablets, scored, promethazine teoclate 25 mg. Net price 10-tab pack = £1.13; 28-tab pack = £3.13. Label: 2

Phenothiazines and related drugs

CHLORPROMAZINE HYDROCHLORIDE

Indications: nausea and vomiting of terminal illness (where other drugs have failed or are not available); other indications (section 4.2.1 and section 15.1.4.1)

Cautions: see Chlorpromazine Hydrochloride, section 4.2.1

Contra-indications: see Chlorpromazine Hydrochloride, section 4.2.1

Side-effects: see Chlorpromazine Hydrochloride, section 4.2.1

Dose: *by mouth*, 10–25 mg every 4–6 hours; CHILD 500 micrograms/kg every 4–6 hours (1–5 years max. 40 mg daily, 6–12 years max. 75 mg daily)

By deep intramuscular injection initially 25 mg then 25–50 mg every 3–4 hours until vomiting stops; CHILD 500 micrograms/kg every 6–8 hours (1–5

years max. 40 mg daily, 6–12 years max. 75 mg daily)

By rectum in suppositories, chlorpromazine 100 mg every 6–8 hours [unlicensed]

■ Preparations
Section 4.2.1

PERPHENAZINE

Indications: severe nausea, vomiting (see notes above); other indications (section 4.2.1)
Cautions: see Perphenazine (section 4.2.1)
Contra-indications: see Perphenazine (section 4.2.1)
Side-effects: see Perphenazine (section 4.2.1); extrapyramidal symptoms particularly in young adults, elderly, and debilitated
Dose: 4 mg 3 times daily, adjusted according to response; max. 24 mg daily (chemotherapy-induced); ELDERLY quarter to half adult dose; CHILD under 14 years not recommended

■ Preparations
Section 4.2.1

PROCHLORPERAZINE

Indications: severe nausea, vomiting, vertigo, labyrinthine disorders (see notes above); other indications section 4.2.1
Cautions: see under Prochlorperazine (section 4.2.1); oral route only for children (avoid if under 10 kg); elderly (see notes above)
Contra-indications: see under Prochlorperazine (section 4.2.1)
Side-effects: see under Prochlorperazine (section 4.2.1); extrapyramidal symptoms, particularly in children, elderly, and debilitated
Dose: doses are expressed as prochlorperazine maleate or mesilate; 1 mg prochlorperazine maleate ≡ 1 mg prochlorperazine mesilate
By mouth, nausea and vomiting, acute attack, 20 mg initially then 10 mg after 2 hours; prevention 5–10 mg 2–3 times daily; CHILD (over 10 kg only) 250 micrograms/kg 2–3 times daily
Labyrinthine disorders, 5 mg 3 times daily, gradually increased if necessary to 30 mg daily in divided doses, then reduced after several weeks to 5–10 mg daily; CHILD not recommended
By deep intramuscular injection, nausea and vomiting, 12.5 mg when required followed if necessary after 6 hours by an oral dose, as above; CHILD not recommended
By rectum in suppositories, nausea and vomiting, 25 mg followed if necessary after 6 hours by oral dose, as above; *or* due to migraine, 5 mg 3 times daily; CHILD not recommended

Prochlorperazine (Non-proprietary) PoM
Tablets, prochlorperazine maleate 5 mg, net price 20 = £1.02. Label: 2
Available from Alpharma, APS, Ashbourne (*Prozière*®), Generics, Hillcross, IVAX

Stemetil® (Castlemead) PoM
Tablets, prochlorperazine maleate 5 mg (off-white), net price 84-tab pack = £6.65; 25 mg (scored), 56-tab pack = £11.73. Label: 2
Syrup, straw-coloured, prochlorperazine mesilate 5 mg/5 mL. Net price 100-mL pack = £3.74. Label: 2

Eff (= effervescent granules), sugar-free, prochlorperazine mesilate 5 mg/sachet. Net price 21-sachet pack = £6.95. Label: 2, 13
Injection, prochlorperazine mesilate 12.5 mg/mL. Net price 1-mL amp = 59p
Suppositories, prochlorperazine maleate (as prochlorperazine), 5 mg, net price 10 = £9.40; 25 mg, 10 = £12.32. Label: 2

■ Buccal preparation
[1]**Buccastem**® (R&C) PoM
Tablets (buccal), pale yellow, prochlorperazine maleate 3 mg. Net price 5 × 10-tab pack = £5.75. Label: 2, counselling, administration, see under Dose below
Dose: 1–2 tablets twice daily; tablets are placed high between upper lip and gum and left to dissolve; CHILD not recommended

1. Prochlorperazine maleate can be sold to the public for adults over 18 years (provided packs do not contain more than 24 mg) for the treatment of nausea and vomiting in previously diagnosed migraine only (max. daily dose 12 mg); a proprietary brand (*Buccastem*® M) is on sale to the public

TRIFLUOPERAZINE

Indications: severe nausea and vomiting (see notes above); other indications (section 4.2.1)
Cautions: see under Trifluoperazine (section 4.2.1)
Contra-indications: see under Trifluoperazine (section 4.2.1)
Side-effects: see under Trifluoperazine (section 4.2.1); extrapyramidal symptoms, particularly in children, elderly, and debilitated
Dose: 2–4 mg daily in divided doses *or* as a single dose of a modified-release preparation; max. 6 mg daily; CHILD 3–5 years up to 1 mg daily, 6–12 years up to 4 mg daily

■ Preparations
Section 4.2.1

Domperidone and metoclopramide

DOMPERIDONE

Indications: see under Dose
   CHILDREN. Use in children is restricted to nausea and vomiting following cytotoxics or radiotherapy
Cautions: pregnancy and breast-feeding; not recommended for routine prophylaxis of post-operative vomiting or for chronic administration; **interactions:** Appendix 1 (domperidone)
Side-effects: raised prolactin concentrations (possible galactorrhoea and gynaecomastia), reduced libido reported; rashes and other allergic reactions; acute dystonic reactions reported
Dose: *by mouth*, acute nausea and vomiting, (including nausea and vomiting induced by levodopa and bromocriptine), 10–20 mg every 4–8 hours, max. period of treatment 12 weeks; CHILD, nausea and vomiting following cytotoxic therapy or radiotherapy only, 200–400 micrograms/kg every 4–8 hours
Functional dyspepsia, 10–20 mg 3 times daily before food and 10–20 mg at night; max. period of treatment 12 weeks; CHILD not recommended
By rectum in suppositories, nausea and vomiting, 30–60 mg every 4–8 hours; CHILD over 2 years

(following cytotoxic therapy or radiotherapy only), body-weight 10–15 kg max. 15 mg twice daily, body-weight 15.5–25 kg max. 30 mg twice daily, body-weight 25.5–35 kg max. 30 mg 3 times daily, body-weight 35.5–45 kg max. 30 mg 4 times daily; since dose needs to be divided throughout day, suppositories may be cut in half for younger children

¹Domperidone (Non-proprietary) PoM
Tablets, 10 mg (as maleate), net price 30-tab pack = £2.51; 100-tab pack = £8.31
Available from Arrow, CP, Generics, Hillcross, Sterwin

1. Domperidone can be sold to the public (provided packs do not contain more than 200 mg) for the relief of postprandial symptoms of excessive fullness, nausea, epigastric bloating and belching occasionally accompanied by epigastric discomfort and heartburn (max. single dose 10 mg, max. daily dose 40 mg); a proprietary brand (*Motilium® 10*) is on sale to the public

Motilium® (Sanofi-Synthelabo) PoM
Tablets, f/c, domperidone 10 mg (as maleate). Net price 30-tab pack = £2.35; 100-tab pack = £7.84
Suspension, sugar-free, domperidone 5 mg/5 mL. Net price 200-mL pack = £1.80
Suppositories domperidone 30 mg. Net price 10 = £2.65

■ Compound preparations (for migraine), section 4.7.4.1

METOCLOPRAMIDE HYDROCHLORIDE

Indications: adults, nausea and vomiting, particularly in gastro-intestinal disorders (section 1.2) and treatment with cytotoxics or radiotherapy; migraine (section 4.7.4.1)
PATIENTS UNDER 20 YEARS. Use restricted to severe intractable vomiting of known cause, vomiting of radiotherapy and cytotoxics, aid to gastro-intestinal intubation, pre-medication; also, dose should be determined on the basis of body-weight

Cautions: hepatic and renal impairment; elderly, young adults, and children (measure dose accurately, preferably with a pipette); may mask underlying disorders such as cerebral irritation; epilepsy; pregnancy; porphyria (section 9.8.2); **interactions:** Appendix 1 (metoclopramide)

Contra-indications: gastro-intestinal obstruction, perforation or haemorrhage; 3–4 days after gastro-intestinal surgery; phaeochromocytoma; breast-feeding (Appendix 5)

Side-effects: extrapyramidal effects (especially in children and young adults), hyperprolactinaemia, occasionally tardive dyskinesia on prolonged administration; also reported, drowsiness, restlessness, diarrhoea, depression, neuroleptic malignant syndrome, rashes, pruritus, oedema; cardiac conduction abnormalities reported following intravenous administration; rarely methaemoglobinaemia (more severe in G6PD deficiency)

Dose: *by mouth, or by intramuscular injection or by intravenous injection* over 1–2 minutes, 10 mg (5 mg in young adults 15–19 years under 60 kg) 3 times daily; CHILD up to 1 year (up to 10 kg) 1 mg twice daily, 1–3 years (10–14 kg) 1 mg 2–3 times daily, 3–5 years (15–19 kg) 2 mg 2–3 times daily,

5–9 years (20–29 kg) 2 mg 3 times daily, 9–14 years (30 kg and over) 5 mg 3 times daily
NOTE. Daily dose of metoclopramide should not normally exceed 500 micrograms/kg, particularly for children and young adults (restricted use, see above)
For diagnostic procedures, as a single dose 5–10 minutes before examination, 10–20 mg (10 mg in young adults 15–19 years); CHILD under 3 years 1 mg, 3–9 years 2 mg, 9–14 years 5 mg

Metoclopramide (Non-proprietary) PoM
Tablets, metoclopramide hydrochloride 10 mg, net price 28-tab pack = 87p
Available from Alpharma, Antigen, APS, CP, IVAX
Oral solution, metoclopramide hydrochloride 5 mg/5 mL, net price 100-mL pack = £2.55
Available from Rosemont (sugar-free), Sandoz
Injection, metoclopramide hydrochloride 5 mg/mL, net price 2-mL amp = 28p
Available from Antigen, Phoenix

Maxolon® (Shire) PoM
Tablets, scored, metoclopramide hydrochloride 5 mg, net price 84-tab pack = £4.69; 10 mg, 84-tab pack = £5.24
Syrup, sugar-free, metoclopramide hydrochloride 5 mg/5 mL. Net price 200-mL pack = £3.83
Paediatric liquid, sugar-free, metoclopramide hydrochloride 1 mg/mL. Net price 15-mL pack with pipette = £1.51. Counselling, use of pipette
Injection, metoclopramide hydrochloride 5 mg/mL. Net price 2-mL amp = 27p

■ High-dose (with cytotoxic chemotherapy only)
Maxolon High Dose® (Shire) PoM
Injection, metoclopramide hydrochloride 5 mg/mL. Net price 20-mL amp = £2.67.
For dilution and use as an intravenous infusion in nausea and vomiting associated with cytotoxic chemotherapy only
Dose: by continuous intravenous infusion (preferred method), initially (before starting chemotherapy), 2–4 mg/kg over 15–20 minutes, then 3–5 mg/kg over 8–12 hours; max. in 24 hours, 10 mg/kg
By intermittent intravenous infusion, initially (before starting chemotherapy), up to 2 mg/kg over at least 15 minutes then up to 2 mg/kg over at least 15 minutes every 2 hours; max. in 24 hours, 10 mg/kg
NOTE. Injection of metoclopramide hydrochloride 5 mg/mL also available in 20-mL ampoules from Phoenix

■ Modified-release preparations
NOTE. All unsuitable for patients under 20 years
Gastrobid Continus® (Napp) PoM ▱
Tablets, m/r, metoclopramide hydrochloride 15 mg. Net price 56-tab pack = £10.33. Label: 25
Dose: patients over 20 years, 1 tablet twice daily

Maxolon SR® (Shire) PoM ▱
Capsules, m/r, clear, enclosing white granules, metoclopramide hydrochloride 15 mg. Net price 56-cap pack = £7.01. Label: 25
Dose: patients over 20 years, 1 capsule twice daily

■ Compound preparations (for migraine)
Section 4.7.4.1

5HT₃ antagonists

DOLASETRON MESILATE

Indications: see under Dose
Cautions: prolonged QT interval, cardiac conduction disorders, concomitant administration of

drugs that prolong QT interval, congestive cardiac failure; pregnancy and breast-feeding; **interactions:** Appendix 1 (dolasetron)
Side-effects: diarrhoea, constipation, dyspepsia, abdominal pain, flatulence, taste disturbances; tachycardia, bradycardia, ECG changes, flushing; fever, shivering; headache, sleep disorder, fatigue, dizziness, drowsiness, anorexia; hypersensitivity reactions including rash, pruritus, urticaria, angio-edema and anaphylaxis; rarely intestinal obstruction, pancreatitis, jaundice, seizures, cardiac arrhythmia, injection-site reactions; very rarely severe hypotension and bradycardia following intravenous injection
Dose: prevention of nausea and vomiting induced by cytotoxic chemotherapy, *by mouth*, 200 mg one hour before treatment *or by intravenous injection* (over 30 seconds) *or by intravenous infusion*, 100 mg 30 minutes before treatment
Prevention of delayed nausea and vomiting after chemotherapy cycle, *by mouth*, 200 mg once daily
NOTE. Dolasetron can be used for a maximum of 4 consecutive days in relation to any one chemotherapy cycle
Prevention of postoperative nausea and vomiting, *by mouth*, 50 mg before induction of anaesthesia *or by intravenous injection* (over 30 seconds) *or by intravenous infusion*, 12.5 mg at cessation of anaesthesia
Treatment of postoperative nausea and vomiting, *by intravenous injection* (over 30 seconds) *or by intravenous infusion*, 12.5 mg
CHILD not recommended

Anzemet® (Amdipharm) ▼ PoM
Tablets, f/c, pink, dolasetron mesilate 50 mg, net price 3-tab pack = £13.50; 200 mg, 3-tab pack = £42.00, 6-tab pack = £84.00
Injection, dolasetron mesilate 20 mg/mL, net price 0.625-mL (12.5-mg) amp = £4.00, 5-mL (100-mg) amp = £13.00

GRANISETRON

Indications: see under Dose
Cautions: pregnancy and breast-feeding
Side-effects: constipation, headache, rash; transient increases in liver enzymes; hypersensitivity reactions reported
Dose: nausea and vomiting induced by cytotoxic chemotherapy or radiotherapy, *by mouth*, 1–2 mg within 1 hour before start of treatment, then 2 mg daily in 1–2 divided doses during treatment; when intravenous infusion also used, max. combined total 9 mg in 24 hours; CHILD 20 micrograms/kg (max. 1 mg) within 1 hour before start of treatment, then 20 micrograms/kg (max. 1 mg) twice daily for up to 5 days during treatment
By intravenous injection (diluted in 15 mL sodium chloride 0.9% and given over not less than 30 seconds) *or by intravenous infusion* (over 5 minutes, see Appendix 6), prevention, 3 mg before start of cytotoxic therapy (up to 2 additional 3-mg doses may be given within 24 hours); treatment, as for prevention (the two additional doses must not be given less than 10 minutes apart); max. 9 mg in 24 hours; CHILD, *by intravenous infusion*, (over 5 minutes), prevention, 40 micrograms/kg (max. 3 mg) before start of cytotoxic therapy; treatment, as for prevention—one additional dose of 40 micr-

ograms/kg (max. 3 mg) may be given within 24 hours (not less than 10 minutes after initial dose)
Postoperative nausea and vomiting, *by intravenous injection* (diluted to 5 mL and given over 30 seconds), prevention, 1 mg before induction of anaesthesia; treatment, 1 mg, given as for prevention; max. 2 mg in one day; CHILD not recommended

Kytril® (Roche) PoM
Tablets, f/c, granisetron (as hydrochloride) 1 mg, net price 10-tab pack = £87.32; 2 mg, 5-tab pack = £87.32
Paediatric liquid, sugar-free, granisetron (as hydrochloride) 1 mg/5 mL, net price 30 mL = £52.39
Sterile solution, granisetron (as hydrochloride) 1 mg/mL, for dilution and use as injection or infusion, net price 1-mL amp = £11.46, 3-mL amp = £34.38

ONDANSETRON

Indications: see under Dose
Cautions: pregnancy and breast-feeding; moderate or severe hepatic impairment (max. 8 mg daily)
Side-effects: constipation; headache, sensation of warmth or flushing, hiccups; occasional alterations in liver enzymes; hypersensitivity reactions reported; occasional transient visual disturbances and dizziness following intravenous administration; involuntary movements, seizures, chest pain, arrhythmias, hypotension and bradycardia also reported; suppositories may cause rectal irritation
Dose: moderately emetogenic chemotherapy or radiotherapy, *by mouth*, 8 mg 1–2 hours before treatment *or by rectum*, 16 mg 1–2 hours before treatment *or by intramuscular injection or slow intravenous injection*, 8 mg immediately before treatment
then by mouth, 8 mg every 12 hours for up to 5 days *or by rectum*, 16 mg daily for up to 5 days
Severely emetogenic chemotherapy, *by intramuscular injection or slow intravenous injection*, 8 mg immediately before treatment, where necessary followed by 8 mg at intervals of 2–4 hours for 2 further doses (*or followed by 1 mg/hour by continuous intravenous infusion* for up to 24 hours)
then by mouth, 8 mg every 12 hours for up to 5 days *or by rectum*, 16 mg daily for up to 5 days
alternatively, by intravenous infusion over at least 15 minutes, 32 mg immediately before treatment *or by rectum*, 16 mg 1–2 hours before treatment
then by mouth, 8 mg every 12 hours for up to 5 days *or by rectum*, 16 mg daily for up to 5 days
NOTE. Efficacy may be enhanced by addition of a single dose of dexamethasone sodium phosphate 20 mg by intravenous injection
CHILD, *by slow intravenous injection or by intravenous infusion* over 15 minutes, 5 mg/m² immediately before chemotherapy then, 4 mg *by mouth* every 12 hours for up to 5 days
Prevention of postoperative nausea and vomiting, *by mouth*, 16 mg 1 hour before anaesthesia *or* 8 mg 1 hour before anaesthesia followed by 8 mg at intervals of 8 hours for 2 further doses
alternatively, by intramuscular or slow intravenous injection, 4 mg at induction of anaesthesia; CHILD over 2 years, *by slow intravenous injection*,

100 micrograms/kg (max. 4 mg) before, during, or after induction of anaesthesia

Treatment of postoperative nausea and vomiting, *by intramuscular or slow intravenous injection*, 4 mg; CHILD over 2 years, *by slow intravenous injection*, 100 micrograms/kg (max. 4 mg)

Zofran® (GSK) [PoM]
Tablets, both yellow, f/c, ondansetron (as hydrochloride) 4 mg, net price 30-tab pack = £116.03; 8 mg, 10-tab pack = £77.36
Oral lyophilisates (*Zofran Melt*®), ondansetron 4 mg, net price 10-tab pack = £38.68; 8 mg, 10-tab pack = £77.36. Counselling, administration
COUNSELLING. Tablets should be placed on the tongue, allowed to disperse and swallowed
Excipients: include aspartame (section 9.4.1)
Syrup, sugar-free, ondansetron (as hydrochloride) 4 mg/5 mL. Net price 50-mL pack = £38.68
Injection, ondansetron (as hydrochloride) 2 mg/mL, net price 2-mL amp = £6.45; 4-mL amp = £12.89
Suppositories, ondansetron 16 mg. Net price 5 = £77.35

TROPISETRON

Indications: see under Dose
Cautions: uncontrolled hypertension (has been aggravated by doses higher than recommended); cardiac conduction disorders; arrhythmias, concomitant administration of drugs that prolong QT interval; pregnancy and breast-feeding; **interactions:** Appendix 1 (tropisetron)
DRIVING. Dizziness or drowsiness may affect performance of skilled tasks (e.g. driving)
Side-effects: constipation, diarrhoea, abdominal pain; headache, dizziness, fatigue; hypersensitivity reactions reported (including facial flushing, urticaria, chest tightness, dyspnoea, bronchospasm and hypotension); collapse, syncope, bradycardia, cardiovascular collapse also reported (causal relationship not established)
Dose: prevention of nausea and vomiting induced by cytotoxic chemotherapy, *by slow intravenous injection or by intravenous infusion*, 5 mg shortly before chemotherapy, then 5 mg *by mouth* every morning at least 1 hour before food for 5 days; CHILD over 2 years, *by intravenous injection* over at least 1 minute or *by intravenous infusion*, 200 micrograms/kg (max. 5 mg) shortly before chemotherapy, then 200 micrograms/kg daily for 4 days; CHILD 25 kg and over, *by intravenous injection* over at least 1 minute or *by intravenous infusion*, 5 mg shortly before chemotherapy, then *by mouth* (preferably) or *by intravenous injection* over at least 1 minute or *by intravenous infusion*, 5 mg daily for 5 days
Postoperative nausea and vomiting, *by slow intravenous injection or by intravenous infusion*, prevention, 2 mg shortly before induction of anaesthesia; treatment, 2 mg within 2 hours of the end of anaesthesia

Navoban® (Novartis) [PoM]
Capsules, white/yellow, tropisetron (as hydrochloride) 5 mg, net price 5-cap pack = £53.86; 50-cap pack = £538.60. Label: 23
Injection, tropisetron (as hydrochloride), 1 mg/mL, net price 2-mL amp = £4.86, 5-mL amp = £12.16

Cannabinoid

NABILONE

Indications: nausea and vomiting caused by cytotoxic chemotherapy, unresponsive to conventional anti-emetics (under close observation, preferably in in-patient setting)
Cautions: history of psychiatric disorder; elderly; hypertension; heart disease; adverse effects on mental state can persist for 48–72 hours after stopping; **interactions:** Appendix 1 (nabilone)
DRIVING. Drowsiness may affect performance of skilled tasks (e.g. driving); effects of alcohol enhanced
Contra-indications: severe hepatic impairment; pregnancy and breast-feeding
Side-effects: drowsiness, vertigo, euphoria, dry mouth, ataxia, visual disturbance, concentration difficulties, sleep disturbance, dysphoria, hypotension, headache and nausea; also confusion, disorientation, hallucinations, psychosis, depression, decreased coordination, tremors, tachycardia, decreased appetite, and abdominal pain
BEHAVIOURAL EFFECTS. Patients should be made aware of possible changes of mood and other adverse behavioural effects
Dose: initially 1 mg twice daily, increased if necessary to 2 mg twice daily, throughout each cycle of cytotoxic therapy and, if necessary, for 48 hours after the last dose of each cycle; max. 6 mg daily given in 3 divided doses. The first dose should be taken the night before initiation of cytotoxic treatment and the second dose 1–3 hours before the first dose of cytotoxic drug; ADOLESCENT and CHILD under 18 years not recommended

Nabilone (Cambridge) [PoM]
Capsules, blue/white, nabilone 1 mg. Net price 20-cap pack = £114.40. Label: 2, counselling, behavioural effects

Hyoscine

HYOSCINE HYDROBROMIDE

(Scopolamine Hydrobromide)
Indications: motion sickness; premedication (section 15.1.3)
Cautions: elderly, urinary retention, cardiovascular disease, gastro-intestinal obstruction, hepatic or renal impairment; porphyria (section 9.8.2); pregnancy and breast-feeding; **interactions:** Appendix 1 (antimuscarinics)
DRIVING. Drowsiness may affect performance of skilled tasks (e.g. driving) and may persist for up to 24 hours or longer after removal of patch; effects of alcohol enhanced
Contra-indications: closed-angle glaucoma
Side-effects: drowsiness, dry mouth, dizziness, blurred vision, difficulty with micturition
Dose: motion sickness, *by mouth*, 300 micrograms 30 minutes before start of journey followed by 300 micrograms every 6 hours if required; max. 3 doses in 24 hours; CHILD 4–10 years 75–150 micrograms, over 10 years 150–300 micrograms
NOTE. Proprietary brands of hyoscine hydrobromide tablets (*Joy-rides*®, *Kwells*®) are on sale to the public for motion sickness
Injection, see section 15.1.3

Scopoderm TTS® (Novartis Consumer Health) [PoM]
Patch, self-adhesive, pink, releasing hyoscine approx. 1 mg/72 hours when in contact with skin. Net price 2 = £4.30. Label: 19, counselling, see below

Dose: motion sickness prevention, apply 1 patch to hairless area of skin behind ear 5–6 hours before journey; replace if necessary after 72 hours, siting replacement patch behind other ear; CHILD under 10 years not recommended

COUNSELLING. Explain accompanying instructions to patient and in particular emphasise advice to wash hands after handling and to wash application site after removing, and to use one patch at a time

Other drugs for Ménière's disease

Betahistine has been promoted as a specific treatment for Ménière's disease.

BETAHISTINE DIHYDROCHLORIDE

Indications: vertigo, tinnitus and hearing loss associated with Ménière's disease
Cautions: asthma, history of peptic ulcer; pregnancy and breast-feeding; **interactions:** Appendix 1 (betahistine)
Contra-indications: phaeochromocytoma
Side-effects: gastro-intestinal disturbances; headache, rashes and pruritus reported
Dose: initially 16 mg 3 times daily, preferably with food; maintenance 24–48 mg daily; CHILD not recommended

Betahistine Dihydrochloride (Non-proprietary) [PoM]
Tablets, betahistine dihydrochloride 8 mg, net price 120-tab pack = £6.63; 16 mg, 84-tab pack = £13.73. Label: 21

Serc® (Solvay) [PoM]
Tablets, betahistine dihydrochloride 8 mg (*Serc*®-8), net price 120-tab pack = £10.04; 16 mg (*Serc*®-16), 84-tab pack = £14.06. Label: 21

4.7 Analgesics

4.7.1	Non-opioid analgesics
4.7.2	Opioid analgesics
4.7.3	Neuropathic pain
4.7.4	Antimigraine drugs

The non-opioid drugs (section 4.7.1), paracetamol and aspirin (and other NSAIDs), are particularly suitable for pain in musculoskeletal conditions, whereas the opioid analgesics (section 4.7.2) are more suitable for moderate to severe pain, particularly of visceral origin.

PAIN IN PALLIATIVE CARE. For advice on pain relief in palliative care see p. 13.

PAIN IN SICKLE-CELL DISEASE. The pain of mild sickle-cell crises is managed with paracetamol, an NSAID, codeine, or dihydrocodeine. Severe crises may require the use of morphine or diamorphine; concomitant use of an NSAID may potentiate analgesia and allow lower doses of the opioid to be used. Pethidine should be avoided if possible because accumulation of a neurotoxic metabolite can precipitate seizures; the relatively short half-life of pethidine necessitates frequent injections.

DYSMENORRHOEA. Use of an oral contraceptive prevents the pain of dysmenorrhoea which is generally associated with ovulatory cycles. If treatment is necessary paracetamol or an NSAID (section 10.1.1) will generally provide adequate relief of pain. The vomiting and severe pain associated with dysmenorrhoea in women with endometriosis may call for an antiemetic (in addition to an analgesic). Antispasmodics (such as alverine citrate, section 1.2) have been advocated for dysmenorrhoea but the antispasmodic action does not generally provide significant relief.

4.7.1 Non-opioid analgesics

Aspirin is indicated for headache, transient musculoskeletal pain, dysmenorrhoea and pyrexia. In inflammatory conditions, most physicians prefer anti-inflammatory treatment with another NSAID which may be better tolerated and more convenient for the patient. Aspirin is used increasingly for its antiplatelet properties (section 2.9). Aspirin tablets or dispersible aspirin tablets are adequate for most purposes as they act rapidly.

Gastric irritation may be a problem; it is minimised by taking the dose after food. Enteric-coated preparations are available, but have a slow onset of action and are therefore unsuitable for single-dose analgesic use (though their prolonged action may be useful for night pain).

Aspirin interacts significantly with a number of other drugs and its interaction with warfarin is a **special hazard**, see **interactions:** Appendix 1 (aspirin).

Paracetamol is similar in efficacy to aspirin, but has no demonstrable anti-inflammatory activity; it is less irritant to the stomach and for that reason is now generally preferred to aspirin, particularly in the elderly. **Overdosage** with paracetamol is particularly dangerous as it may cause hepatic damage which is sometimes not apparent for 4 to 6 days (see Emergency Treatment of Poisoning, p. 22). **Benorilate** (section 10.1.1) is an aspirin–paracetamol ester.

Nefopam may have a place in the relief of persistent pain unresponsive to other non-opioid analgesics. It causes little or no respiratory depression, but sympathomimetic and antimuscarinic side-effects may be troublesome.

Non-steroidal anti-inflammatory analgesics (NSAIDs, section 10.1.1) are particularly useful for the treatment of patients with chronic disease accompanied by pain and inflammation. Some of them are also used in the short-term treatment of mild to moderate pain including transient musculoskeletal pain but paracetamol is now often preferred, particularly in the elderly (see also p. 18). They are also suitable for the relief of pain in *dysmenorrhoea* and to treat pain caused by *secondary bone tumours*, many of which produce lysis of bone and release prostaglandins (see Prescribing in Palliative Care, p. 13). NSAIDs including ketorolac are also used for peri-operative analgesia (section 15.1.4.2).

Compound analgesic preparations

Compound analgesic preparations that contain a simple analgesic (such as aspirin or paracetamol) with an opioid component reduce the scope for effective titration of the individual components in the management of pain of varying intensity.

Compound analgesic preparations containing paracetamol or aspirin with a *low dose* of an opioid analgesic (e.g. 8 mg of codeine phosphate per compound tablet) are commonly used, but the advantages have not been substantiated. The low dose of the opioid may be enough to cause opioid side-effects (in particular, constipation) and can complicate the treatment of **overdosage** (see p. 24) yet may not provide significant additional relief of pain.

A *full dose* of the opioid component (e.g. 60 mg codeine phosphate) in compound analgesic preparations effectively augments the analgesic activity but is associated with the full range of opioid side-effects (including nausea, vomiting, severe constipation, drowsiness, respiratory depression, and risk of dependence on long-term administration). For details of the **side-effects**, **cautions** and **contra-indications** of opioid analgesics, see p. 211 (**important:** the elderly are particularly susceptible to opioid side-effects and should receive lower doses).

In general, when assessing pain, it is necessary to weigh up carefully whether there is a need for a non-opioid and an opioid analgesic to be taken simultaneously.

Caffeine is a weak stimulant that is often included, in small doses, in analgesic preparations. It is claimed that the addition of caffeine may enhance the analgesic effect, but the alerting effect, mild habit-forming effect and possible provocation of headache may not always be desirable. Moreover, in excessive dosage or on withdrawal caffeine may itself induce headache.

ASPIRIN

(Acetylsalicylic Acid)

Indications: mild to moderate pain, pyrexia; see also section 10.1.1; antiplatelet (section 2.9)

Cautions: asthma, allergic disease, impaired renal or hepatic function (avoid if severe), dehydration; preferably avoid during fever or viral infection in adolescents (risk of Reye's syndrome, see below); pregnancy; elderly; G6PD-deficiency (section 9.1.5); **interactions:** Appendix 1 (aspirin)

Contra-indications: children and adolescents under 16 years and in breast-feeding (Reye's syndrome, see below); previous or active peptic ulceration, haemophilia; not for treatment of gout

HYPERSENSITIVITY. Aspirin and other NSAIDs are **contra-indicated** in patients with a history of hypersensitivity to aspirin or any other NSAID—*which includes those* in whom attacks of *asthma, angioedema, urticaria or rhinitis* have been precipitated by aspirin or any other NSAID

REYE'S SYNDROME. Owing to an association with Reye's syndrome, the CSM has advised that aspirin-containing preparations should not be given to children and adolescents under 16 years, unless specifically indicated, e.g. for Kawasaki syndrome.

Side-effects: generally mild and infrequent but high incidence of gastro-intestinal irritation with slight asymptomatic blood loss, increased bleeding time, bronchospasm and skin reactions in hypersensitive patients. Prolonged administration, see section

10.1.1. Overdosage: see Emergency Treatment of Poisoning, p. 22

Dose: 300–900 mg every 4–6 hours when necessary; max. 4 g daily; CHILD and ADOLESCENT not recommended (see Reye's syndrome above)
Rectal route, see below

Aspirin (Non-proprietary)
Tablets PoM[1], aspirin 300 mg. Net price 20 = 19p. Label: 21, 32
Tablets PoM[1], e/c, aspirin 300 mg, net price 100-tab pack = £5.78; 75 mg, see section 2.9. Label: 5, 25, 32
Available from Ashbourne, Galen
Dispersible tablets PoM[1], aspirin 300 mg, net price 20 = 22p; 75 mg, see section 2.9. Label: 13, 21, 32
NOTE. BP directs that when no strength is stated the 300-mg strength should be dispensed, and that when soluble aspirin tablets are prescribed, dispersible aspirin tablets shall be dispensed.
Suppositories, aspirin 300 mg, net price 10 = £9.59. Label: 32
Dose: 2–3 suppositories inserted every 4 hours when necessary (max. 12 suppositories in 24 hours); CHILD not recommended (see above)
Available from Aurum (who also supply a 150-mg strength)

Caprin® (Sinclair)
Tablets PoM[1], e/c, f/c, pink, aspirin 300 mg, net price 30-tab pack = £1.66, 100-tab pack = £4.89; 75 mg, see section 2.9. Label: 5, 25, 32

Nu-Seals® **Aspirin** (Alliance)
Tablets PoM[1], e/c, aspirin 300 mg, net price 100-tab pack = £5.80; 75 mg, see section 2.9. Label: 5, 25, 32

■ With codeine phosphate 8 mg
[1]**Co-codaprin** (Non-proprietary) PoM [▬]
Dispersible tablets, co-codaprin 8/400 (codeine phosphate 8 mg, aspirin 400 mg). Net price 20 = 78p. Label: 13, 21, 32
Dose: 1–2 tablets in water every 4–6 hours; max. 8 tablets daily
Available from Alpharma
When co-codaprin tablets or dispersible tablets are prescribed and no strength is stated, tablets or dispersible tablets, respectively, containing codeine phosphate 8 mg and aspirin 400 mg should be dispensed

■ Other compound preparations
Aspav® (Alpharma) PoM [▬]
Dispersible tablets, aspirin 500 mg, papaveretum 7.71 mg (providing the equivalent of 5 mg of anhydrous morphine). Net price 30-tab pack = £4.60. Label: 2, 13, 21, 32
Dose: 1–2 tablets in water every 4–6 hours if necessary; max. 8 tablets daily

■ Preparations on sale to the public
For a list of **preparations** containing aspirin and paracetamol **on sale to the public**, see p. 210.

---

1. May be sold to the public provided packs contain no more than 32 capsules or tablets; pharmacists can sell multiple packs up to a total quantity of 100 capsules or tablets in justifiable circumstances; for details see *Medicines, Ethics and Practice*, No. 27, London, Pharmaceutical Press, 2003 (and subsequent editions as available)

PARACETAMOL

(Acetaminophen)

Indications: mild to moderate pain, pyrexia

Cautions: hepatic and renal impairment, alcohol dependence; **interactions:** Appendix 1 (paracetamol)

Side-effects: side-effects rare, but rashes, blood disorders; **important:** liver damage (and less frequently renal damage) following **overdosage**, see Emergency Treatment of Poisoning, p. 22

Dose: *by mouth*, 0.5–1 g every 4–6 hours to a max. of 4 g daily; CHILD 2 months 60 mg for post-immunisation pyrexia; otherwise under 3 months (on doctor's advice only), 10 mg/kg (5 mg/kg if jaundiced); 3 months–1 year 60–120 mg, 1–5 years 120–250 mg, 6–12 years 250–500 mg; these doses may be repeated every 4–6 hours when necessary (max. of 4 doses in 24 hours)

For full Joint Committee on Vaccination and Immunisation recommendation on post-immunisation pyrexia, see section 14.1

Rectal route, see below

Paracetamol (Non-proprietary)

Tablets PoM [1], paracetamol 500 mg. Net price 20 = 15p. Label: 29, 30

Available from Alpharma, APS, IVAX, Sterling Health (*Panadol*® NHS)

Soluble Tablets (= Dispersible tablets) PoM [2], paracetamol 500 mg. Net price 60-tab pack = £2.82. Label: 13, 29, 30

Available from Sterling Health (*Panadol Soluble*® NHS)

Paediatric Soluble Tablets (= Paediatric dispersible tablets), paracetamol 120 mg. Net price 24-tab pack = 82p. Label: 13, 30

Available from R&C (*Disprol*® *Soluble Paracetamol* NHS)

Oral Suspension 120 mg/5 mL (= Paediatric Mixture), paracetamol 120 mg/5 mL. Net price 100 mL = 35p. Label: 30

NOTE. BP directs that when Paediatric Paracetamol Oral Suspension or Paediatric Paracetamol Mixture is prescribed Paracetamol Oral Suspension 120 mg/5 mL should be dispensed; sugar-free versions can be ordered by specifying 'sugar-free'on the prescription

Available from IVAX, R&C (*Disprol*® *Paediatric*, sugar-free), Rosemont (*Paldesic*®), SSL (*Medinol*® *Paediatric*, sugar-free), Sterling Health (*Panadol*® sugar-free), Warner Lambert (*Calpol*® *Paediatric*, *Calpol*® *Paediatric* sugar-free)

Oral Suspension 250 mg/5 mL (= Mixture), paracetamol 250 mg/5 mL. Net price 100 mL = 73p. Label: 30

Available from Hillcross, Rosemont (*Paldesic*®), SSL (*Medinol*® *Over 6* NHS), Warner Wellcome (*Calpol*®6 *Plus* NHS)

Suppositories, paracetamol 60 mg, net price 10 = £9.96; 125 mg, 10 = £11.50; 250 mg, 10 = £23.00; 500 mg, 10 = £9.90. Label: 30

Dose: by rectum, ADULT and CHILD over 12 years 0.5–1 g up to 4 times daily, CHILD 1–5 years 125–250 mg, 6–12 years 250–500 mg

Available from AstraZeneca (Alvedon®, 60 mg, 125 mg, 250 mg), Aurum (120 mg, 240 mg, 500 mg)

1. May be sold to the public provided packs contain no more than 32 capsules or tablets; pharmacists can sell multiple packs up to a total quantity of 100 capsules or tablets in justifiable circumstances; for details see *Medicines, Ethics and Practice*, No. 27, London, Pharmaceutical Press, 2003 (and subsequent editions as available)

2. May be sold to the public under certain circumstances; for exemptions see *Medicines, Ethics and Practice*, No. 27, London, Pharmaceutical Press, 2003 (and subsequent editions as available)

■ Co-codamol 8/500

When co-codamol tablets, dispersible (or effervescent) tablets, or capsules are prescribed and **no strength is stated**, tablets, dispersible (or effervescent) tablets, or capsules, respectively, containing codeine phosphate **8 mg** and paracetamol **500 mg** should be dispensed.

Co-codamol 8/500[2] (Non-proprietary) PoM [image]

Tablets, co-codamol 8/500 (codeine phosphate 8 mg, paracetamol 500 mg) Net price 20 = 23p. Label: 29, 30

Dose: 1–2 tablets every 4–6 hours; max. 8 tablets daily; CHILD 6–12 years ½–1 tablet

Available from Alpharma, APS, Arrow, CP, Generics, IVAX, Sterling Health (*Panadeine*® NHS), Sterwin

Effervescent or *dispersible tablets*, co-codamol 8/500 (codeine phosphate 8 mg, paracetamol 500 mg). Net price 20 = £1.04. Label: 13, 29, 30

Dose: 1–2 tablets in water every 4–6 hours, max. 8 tablets daily; CHILD 6–12 years ½–1 tablet, max 4 daily

Available from Generics, Roche Consumer Health (*Paracodol*® NHS), Sandoz, Sterwin

NOTE. The Drug Tariff allows tablets of co-codamol labelled 'dispersible' to be dispensed against an order for 'effervescent' and *vice versa*

Capsules, co-codamol 8/500 (codeine phosphate 8 mg, paracetamol 500 mg). Net price 30 = £2.49. Label: 29, 30

Dose: 1–2 capsules every 4 hours; max. 8 tablets daily

Available from Roche Consumer Health (*Paracodol*® NHS)

■ Co-codamol 15/500

When co-codamol tablets, dispersible (or effervescent) tablets, or capsules are prescribed and **no strength is stated**, tablets, dispersible (or effervescent) tablets, or capsules, respectively, containing codeine phosphate **8 mg** and paracetamol **500 mg** should be dispensed (see preparations above).

See warnings and notes on p. 208 (**important: special care in elderly—reduce dose**)

Codipar (Goldshield) PoM [image]

Caplets (= tablets), co-codamol 15/500 (codeine phosphate 15 mg, paracetamol 500 mg). Net price 100-tab pack = £7.15. Label: 2, 29, 30

Dose: 1–2 tablets every 4 hours; max. 8 daily; CHILD not recommended

■ Co-codamol 30/500

When co-codamol tablets, dispersible (or effervescent) tablets, or capsules are prescribed and **no strength is stated**, tablets, dispersible (or effervescent) tablets, or capsules, respectively, containing codeine phosphate **8 mg** and on paracetamol **500 mg** should be dispensed (see preparations above).

See warnings and notes on p. 208 (**important: special care in elderly—reduce dose**)

Co-codamol 30/500 (Non-proprietary) PoM [image]

Tablets, co-codamol 30/500 (codeine phosphate 30 mg, paracetamol 500 mg) net price 100-tab pack = £7.38. Label: 2, 29, 30

Dose: 1–2 tablets every 4 hours; max. 8 tablets daily; CHILD not recommended

Available from Arrow, CP, Sterwin

Capsules, co-codamol 30/500 (codeine phosphate 30 mg, paracetamol 500 mg), net price 100-cap pack = £8.21. Label: 2, 29, 30

Dose: 1–2 capsules every 4 hours; max. 8 tablets daily; CHILD not recommended

Available from Goldshield (*Zapain*®), Schwarz (*Medocodene*®)

Kapake® (Galen) PoM ▱

Tablets, scored, co-codamol 30/500 (codeine phosphate 30 mg, paracetamol 500 mg). Net price 30-tab pack = £2.26 (hosp. only), 100-tab pack = £7.53. Label: 2, 29, 30
Dose: 1–2 tablets every 4 hours; max. 8 tablets daily; CHILD not recommended

Capsules, co-codamol 30/500 (codeine phosphate 30 mg, paracetamol 500 mg), net price 100-cap pack = £7.53. Label: 2, 29, 30
Dose: 1–2 capsules every 4 hours; max. 8 capsules daily; CHILD not recommended

Sachets (*Kapake Insts®*), co-codamol 30/500 (codeine phosphate 30 mg, paracetamol 500 mg), net price 30-sachet pack (hosp. only) = £2.56, 100-sachet pack = £8.53. Label: 2, 13, 29, 30
Dose: 1–2 sachets every 4 hours; max. 8 sachets daily; CHILD not recommended
NOTE. Higher strength also available, see under Co-codamol 60/1000

Solpadol® (Sanofi-Synthelabo) PoM ▱

Caplets(= tablets), co-codamol 30/500 (codeine phosphate 30 mg, paracetamol 500 mg). Net price 100-tab pack = £7.54. Label: 2, 29, 30
Dose: 2 tablets every 4 hours; max. 8 daily; CHILD not recommended

Capsules, grey/purple, co-codamol 30/500 (codeine phosphate 30 mg, paracetamol 500 mg). Net price 100-cap pack = £7.54. Label: 2, 29, 30
Dose: 1–2 capsules every 4 hours; max. 8 capsules daily; CHILD not recommended

Effervescent tablets, co-codamol 30/500 (codeine phosphate 30 mg, paracetamol 500 mg). Contains Na^+ 16.9 mmol/tablet; avoid in *renal impairment*. Net price 100-tab pack= £9.05. Label: 2, 13, 29, 30
Dose: 2 tablets in water every 4 hours; max. 8 daily; CHILD not recommended

Tylex® (Schwarz) PoM ▱

Capsules, co-codamol 30/500 (codeine phosphate 30 mg, paracetamol 500 mg). Net price 100-cap pack = £8.21. Label: 2, 29, 30
Dose: 1–2 capsules every 4 hours; max. 8 capsules daily; CHILD not recommended

Effervescent tablets, co-codamol 30/500 (codeine phosphate 30 mg, paracetamol 500 mg). Contains Na^+ 13.6 mmol/tablet; avoid in *renal impairment*. Net price 90-tab pack = £8.15. Label: 2, 13, 29, 30
Excipients: include aspartame 25 mg/tablet (see section 9.4.1)
Dose: 1–2 tablets in water every 4 hours; max. 8 tablets daily; CHILD not recommended

■ Co-codamol 60/1000
See warnings and notes on p. 208 (**important:** special care in elderly—reduce dose)

Kapake® (Galen) PoM ▱

Sachets (*Kapake Insts®*), co-codamol 60/1000 (codeine phosphate 60 mg, paracetamol 1 g), net price 50-sachet pack = £8.53. Label: 2, 13, 30
Dose: 1 sachet every 4 hours; max. 4 sachets daily; CHILD not recommended
NOTE. Lower strength also available, see under Co-codamol 30/500

■ With methionine (co-methiamol)
A mixture of methionine and paracetamol; methionine has no analgesic activity but may prevent paracetamol-induced liver toxicity if overdose taken

Paradote® (Penn)

Tablets, f/c, co-methiamol 100/500 (DL-methionine 100 mg, paracetamol 500 mg). Net price 24-tab pack = £1.05, 96-tab pack = £2.77. Label: 29, 30
Dose: 2 tablets every 4 hours; max. 8 tablets daily; CHILD 12 years and under, not recommended

■ With dihydrocodeine tartrate 10 mg
See notes on p. 208

Co-dydramol (Non-proprietary) PoM ▱

Tablets, scored, co-dydramol 10/500 (dihydrocodeine tartrate 10 mg, paracetamol 500 mg). Net price 20 = 27p. Label: 21, 29, 30
Dose: 1–2 tablets every 4–6 hours; max. 8 tablets daily; CHILD not recommended
Available from Alpharma, APS, Arrow, CP, Generics, IVAX, Sterwin
When co-dydramol tablets are prescribed and no strength is stated tablets containing dihydrocodeine tartrate 10 mg and paracetamol 500 mg should be dispensed.
NOTE. Tablets containing paracetamol 500 mg and dihydrocodeine 7.46 mg (*Paramol®* NHS) are on sale to the public. The name *Paramol®* was formerly applied to a brand of co-dydramol tablets

■ With dihydrocodeine tartrate 20 or 30 mg
See warnings and notes on p. 208 (**important:** special care in elderly—reduce dose)

Remedeine® (Napp) PoM ▱

Tablets, paracetamol 500 mg, dihydrocodeine tartrate 20 mg. Net price 112-tab pack =£12.42. Label: 2, 21, 29, 30
Dose: 1–2 tablets every 4–6 hours; max. 8 tablets daily; CHILD not recommended

Forte tablets, paracetamol 500 mg, dihydrocodeine tartrate 30 mg. Net price 56-tab pack = £7.67. Label: 2, 21, 29, 30
Dose: 1–2 tablets every 4–6 hours; max. 8 tablets daily; CHILD not recommended

■ Other compound preparations
See warnings and notes on p. 208 (**important:** special care in elderly—reduce dose)

Co-proxamol (Non-proprietary) PoM ▱

Tablets, co-proxamol 32.5/325 (dextropropoxyphene hydrochloride 32.5 mg, paracetamol 325 mg). Net price 20 = 24p. Label: 2, 10, patient information leaflet (if available), 29, 30
Dose: 2 tablets 3–4 times daily; max. 8 tablets daily; CHILD not recommended
Available from Alpharma (*Cosalgesic®* NHS), APS, IVAX, Meda (*Distalgesic®* NHS), Sovereign, Sterwin
When co-proxamol tablets are prescribed and no strength is stated tablets containing dextropropoxyphene hydrochloride 32.5 mg and paracetamol 325 mg should be dispensed.

■ Preparations on Sale to the Public
The following is a list of preparations on sale to the public that contain **aspirin** or **paracetamol, alone** or with **other ingredients**. Other significant ingredients (such as codeine and caffeine) are listed. See p. 164 for CSM advice on phenylpropanolamine. For details of preparations containing ibuprofen on sale to the public, see section 10.1.1.

Important: in overdose contact **Poisons Information Services** (p. 20) for full details of the ingredients

Alka-Seltzer® (aspirin), Alka-Seltzer XS® (aspirin, caffeine, paracetamol), Anadin® (aspirin, caffeine), Anadin Cold Control® (paracetamol, caffeine, phenylephrine), Anadin Extra®, Anadin Extra Soluble® (both aspirin, caffeine, paracetamol), Anadin Paracetamol® (paracetamol), Angettes 75® (aspirin), Askit® (aspirin, aloxiprin = polymeric product of aspirin, caffeine), Aspro Clear® (aspirin),

Beechams-All-In-One® (paracetamol, guaifenesin, phenylephrine), Beechams Cold & Flu®, Beechams Flu-Plus Hot Berry Fruits®, Beechams Flu-Plus Powder®, Beechams Hot Lemon®, Hot Lemon and Honey®, Hot Blackcurrant® (all paracetamol, phenylephrine), Beechams Flu-Plus Caplets® (paracetamol, caffeine, phenylephrine), Beechams Lemon Tablets® (aspirin), Beechams Powders® (aspirin, caffeine, phenylephrine), Beechams Powders Capsules® (paracetamol, caffeine, phenylephrine), Benylin 4 Flu® (paracetamol, diphenhydramine, pseudoephedrine), Benylin Day and Night® (day tablets, paracetamol, phenylpropanolamine, night tablets, paracetamol, diphenhydramine), Boots Cold & Flu Relief Tablets® (paracetamol, caffeine, phenylephrine), Boots Pain Relief Paracetamol Suspension 3 Months Plus® (paracetamol), Boots Cold Relief Hot Blackcurrant®, Hot Lemon® (paracetamol), Boots Migraine Relief® (paracetamol, codeine), Boots Seltzer® (aspirin), Boots Tension Headache Relief® (paracetamol, caffeine, codeine, doxylamine)

Calpol Fast Melts®, Calpol Infant®, Calpol 6 Plus® (all paracetamol), Caprin® (aspirin), Codis 500® (aspirin, codeine), Mrs. Cullen's® (aspirin, caffeine)

Day Nurse® (paracetamol, dextromethorphan, phenylpropanolamine), De Witt's Analgesic Pills® (paracetamol, caffeine), Disprin®, Disprin Direct® (all aspirin), Disprin Extra® (aspirin, paracetamol), Disprol® (paracetamol), Doans Backache Pills® (paracetamol, sodium salicylate), Dolvan® (paracetamol, diphenhydramine, ephedrine, caffeine), Dozol® (paracetamol, diphenhydramine)

Feminax® (paracetamol, caffeine, codeine, hyoscine), Fennings Children's Cooling Powders® (paracetamol)

Galpamol® (paracetamol)

Hedex® (paracetamol), Hedex Extra® (paracetamol, caffeine)

Infadrops® (paracetamol)

Lemsip Cold + Flu Breathe Easy® (paracetamol, phenylephrine), Lemsip Cold + Flu Combined Relief Capsules® (paracetamol, caffeine, phenylephrine), Lemsip Cold + Flu Max Strength® (paracetamol, phenylephrine), Lemsip Lemon® or Blackcurrant®, Lemsip Max Strength® (all paracetamol, phenylephrine)

Mandanol® (paracetamol), Maximum Strength Aspro Clear® (aspirin), Medinol® (paracetamol), Medised® (paracetamol, promethazine), Midrid® (paracetamol, isometheptene mucate), Migraleve® (pink tablets, paracetamol, codeine, buclizine, yellow tablets, paracetamol, codeine)

Night Nurse® (paracetamol, dextromethorphan, promethazine), Nirolex Day Cold Comfort® (paracetamol, pholcodine, pseudoephedrine), Nirolex Night Cold Comfort® (paracetamol, pseudoephedrine, diphenhydramine, pholcodeine), Nurse Sykes' Powders® (aspirin, caffeine, paracetamol)

Panadol® (paracetamol), Panadol Extra® (paracetamol, caffeine), Panadol Night® (paracetamol, diphenhydramine), Panadol Soluble® (paracetamol), Panadol Ultra® (paracetamol, codeine), Paracets® (paracetamol), Paracets Plus® (paracetamol, caffeine, phenylephrine), Paracodol® (paracetamol, codeine), Paradote® (co-methiamol (paracetamol, DL-methionine)), Paramol® (paracetamol, dihydrocodeine), Phensic® (aspirin, caffeine), Propain® (paracetamol, caffeine, codeine, diphenhydramine)

Resolve® (paracetamol)

Sinutab® (paracetamol, phenylpropanolamine), Solpadeine® (paracetamol, caffeine, codeine), Solpadeine Max® (paracetamol, codeine), Solpadeine

Soluble® (paracetamol, caffeine, codeine), Sudafed-Co® (paracetamol, pseudoephedrine), Syndol® (paracetamol, caffeine, codeine, doxylamine)

Tixymol® (paracetamol), Tixyplus® (diphenhydramine, paracetamol),

Ultramol Soluble® (paracetamol, codeine, caffeine), Uniflu with Gregovite C® (paracetamol, caffeine, codeine, diphenhydramine, phenylephrine)

Veganin® (caffeine, codeine, paracetamol), Vicks Medinite® (paracetamol, dextromethorphan, doxylamine, ephedrine)

NEFOPAM HYDROCHLORIDE

Indications: moderate pain

Cautions: hepatic or renal disease, elderly, urinary retention; pregnancy and breast-feeding; **interactions:** Appendix 1 (nefopam)

Contra-indications: convulsive disorders; not indicated for myocardial infarction

Side-effects: nausea, nervousness, urinary retention, dry mouth, lightheadedness; less frequently vomiting, blurred vision, drowsiness, sweating, insomnia, tachycardia, headache; confusion and hallucinations also reported; may colour urine (pink)

Dose: *by mouth*, initially 60 mg (elderly, 30 mg) 3 times daily, adjusted according to response; usual range 30–90 mg 3 times daily; CHILD not recommended

By intramuscular injection, 20 mg every 6 hours; CHILD not recommended

NOTE. Nefopam hydrochloride 20 mg by injection ≡ 60 mg by mouth

Acupan® (3M) PoM
Tablets, f/c, nefopam hydrochloride 30 mg. Net price 90-tab pack = £12.02. Label: 2, 14
Injection, nefopam hydrochloride 20 mg/mL. Net price 1-mL amp = 69p

4.7.2   Opioid analgesics

Opioid analgesics are usually used to relieve moderate to severe pain particularly of visceral origin. Repeated administration may cause dependence and tolerance, but this is no deterrent in the control of pain in terminal illness, for guidelines see Prescribing in Palliative Care, p. 13. Regular use of a potent opioid may be appropriate for certain cases of chronic non-malignant pain; treatment should be supervised by a specialist and the patient should be assessed at regular intervals.

SIDE-EFFECTS. Opioid analgesics share many side-effects though qualitative and quantitative differences exist. The most common include nausea, vomiting, constipation, and drowsiness. Larger doses produce respiratory depression and hypotension. **Overdosage**, see Emergency Treatment of Poisoning, p. 24.

INTERACTIONS. See Appendix 1 (opioid analgesics) (**important:** special hazard with *pethidine and possibly other opioids* and MAOIs).

DRIVING. Drowsiness may affect performance of skilled tasks (e.g. driving); effects of alcohol enhanced.

CHOICE. **Morphine** remains the most valuable opioid analgesic for severe pain although it frequently causes nausea and vomiting. It is the standard against which other opioid analgesics are compared. In addition to relief of pain, morphine also confers a state of euphoria and mental detachment.

Morphine is the opioid of choice for the oral treatment of *severe pain in palliative care*. It is given regularly every 4 hours (or every 12 or 24 hours as modified-release preparations). For guidelines on dosage adjustment in palliative care, see p. 13.

Buprenorphine has both opioid agonist and antagonist properties and may precipitate withdrawal symptoms, including pain, in patients dependent on other opioids. It has abuse potential and may itself cause dependence. It has a much longer duration of action than morphine and sublingually is an effective analgesic for 6 to 8 hours. Vomiting may be a problem. Unlike most opioid analgesics its effects are only partially reversed by naloxone.

Codeine is effective for the relief of mild to moderate pain but is too constipating for long-term use.

Diphenoxylate (in combination with atropine, as co-phenotrope) is used in acute diarrhoea (see section 1.4.2).

Dipipanone used alone is less sedating than morphine but the only preparation available contains an anti-emetic and is therefore not suitable for regular regimens in palliative care (see p. 15).

Dextropropoxyphene in combination with paracetamol (co-proxamol) (p. 210)has little more analgesic effect than paracetamol alone. An important disadvantage of co-proxamol is that overdosage (which may be combined with alcohol) is complicated by respiratory depression and acute heart failure due to the dextropropoxyphene and by hepatotoxicity due to the paracetamol. Rapid treatment is essential (see Emergency Treatment of Poisoning, p. 24).

Diamorphine (heroin) is a powerful opioid analgesic. It may cause less nausea and hypotension than morphine. In *palliative care* the greater solubility of diamorphine allows effective doses to be injected in smaller volumes and this is important in the emaciated patient.

Dihydrocodeine has an analgesic efficacy similar to that of codeine. The dose of dihydrocodeine by mouth is usually 30 mg every 4 hours; doubling the dose to 60 mg may provide some additional pain relief but this may be at the cost of more nausea and vomiting. A 40-mg tablet is now also available.

Alfentanil, **fentanyl** and **remifentanil** are used by injection for intra-operative analgesia (section 15.1.4.3); fentanyl is available in a transdermal drug delivery system as a self-adhesive patch which is changed every 72 hours.

Meptazinol is claimed to have a low incidence of respiratory depression. It has a reported length of action of 2 to 7 hours with onset within 15 minutes.

Methadone is less sedating than morphine and acts for longer periods. In prolonged use, methadone should not be administered more often than twice daily to avoid the risk of accumulation and opioid overdosage. Methadone may be used instead of morphine in the occasional patient who experiences excitation (or exacerbation of pain) with morphine.

Nalbuphine has a similar efficacy to that of morphine for pain relief, but may have fewer side-effects and less abuse potential. Nausea and vomiting occur less than with other opioids but respiratory depression is similar to that with morphine.

Oxycodone has an efficacy and side-effect profile similar to that of morphine. It is used primarily for control of *pain in palliative care*. It is used as the pectinate in suppositories (special order from BCM Specials).

Pentazocine has both agonist and antagonist properties and precipitates withdrawal symptoms, including pain in patients dependent on other opioids. By injection it is more potent than dihydrocodeine or codeine, but hallucinations and thought disturbances may occur. It is not recommended and, in particular, should be avoided after myocardial infarction as it may increase pulmonary and aortic blood pressure as well as cardiac work.

Pethidine produces prompt but short-lasting analgesia; it is less constipating than morphine, but even in high doses is a less potent analgesic. It is not suitable for severe continuing pain. It is used for analgesia in labour; however, other opioids, such as morphine or diamorphine, are often preferred for obstetric pain.

Tramadol produces analgesia by two mechanisms: an opioid effect and an enhancement of serotonergic and adrenergic pathways. It has fewer of the typical opioid side-effects (notably, less respiratory depression, less constipation and less addiction potential); psychiatric reactions have been reported.

DOSE. The dose of opioids in the BNF may need to be **adjusted individually** according to the degree of analgesia and side-effects; patients' response to opioids varies widely.

POSTOPERATIVE ANALGESIA. The use of intra-operative opioids affects the prescribing of postoperative analgesics and in many cases delays the need for a postoperative analgesic. A postoperative opioid analgesic should be given with care since it may potentiate any residual respiratory depression (for the treatment of opioid-induced respiratory depression, see section 15.1.7). Non-opioid analgesics are also used for postoperative pain (section 15.1.4.2). **Morphine** and **papaveretum** are used most widely. **Tramadol** is not as effective in severe pain as other opioid analgesics. **Buprenorphine** may antagonise the analgesic effect of previously administered opioids and is generally not recommended. **Pethidine** is metabolised to norpethidine which may accumulate, particularly in renal impairment; norpethidine stimulates the central nervous system and may cause convulsions. **Meptazinol** and **nalbuphine** are rarely used.

Opioids are also given epidurally [unlicensed route] in the postoperative period but are associated with side-effects such as pruritus, urinary retention, nausea and vomiting; respiratory depression can be delayed, particularly with morphine.

For details of patient-controlled analgesia (PCA) to relieve postoperative pain, consult hospital protocols. Formulations specifically designed for PCA are available (*Pharma-Ject® Morphine Sulphate*).

ADDICTS. Although caution is necessary, addicts (and ex-addicts) may be treated with analgesics in the same way as other people when there is a real clinical need. Doctors do not require a special licence to prescribe opioid analgesics for addicts for relief of pain due to organic disease or injury.

MORPHINE SALTS

Indications: see notes above and under Dose; acute diarrhoea (section 1.4.2); cough in terminal care (section 3.9.1)

Cautions: hypotension, hypothyroidism, asthma (avoid during attack) and decreased respiratory reserve, prostatic hypertrophy; pregnancy and breast-feeding; may precipitate coma in hepatic impairment (reduce dose or avoid but many such patients tolerate morphine well); reduce dose or avoid in renal impairment (see also Appendix 3), elderly and debilitated (reduce dose); convulsive disorders, dependence (severe withdrawal symptoms if withdrawn abruptly); use of cough suppressants containing opioid analgesics not generally recommended in children and should be avoided altogether in those under at least 1 year; **interactions:** Appendix 1 (opioid analgesics)
PALLIATIVE CARE. In the control of pain in terminal illness these cautions should not necessarily be a deterrent to the use of opioid analgesics

Contra-indications: avoid in acute respiratory depression, acute alcoholism and where risk of paralytic ileus; also avoid in raised intracranial pressure or head injury (in addition to interfering with respiration, affect pupillary responses vital for neurological assessment); avoid injection in phaeochromocytoma (risk of pressor response to histamine release)

Side-effects: nausea and vomiting (particularly in initial stages), constipation, and drowsiness; larger doses produce respiratory depression and hypotension; other side-effects include difficulty with micturition, ureteric or biliary spasm, dry mouth, sweating, headache, facial flushing, vertigo, bradycardia, tachycardia, palpitations, postural hypotension, hypothermia, hallucinations, dysphoria, mood changes, dependence, miosis, decreased libido or potency, rashes, urticaria and pruritus; **overdosage:** see Emergency Treatment of Poisoning, p. 24; for reversal of opioid-induced respiratory depression, see section 15.1.7.

Dose: acute pain, *by subcutaneous injection* (not suitable for oedematous patients) *or by intramuscular injection*, 10 mg every 4 hours if necessary (15 mg for heavier well-muscled patients); CHILD up to 1 month 150 micrograms/kg, 1–12 months 200 micrograms/kg, 1–5 years 2.5–5 mg, 6–12 years 5–10 mg
By slow intravenous injection, quarter to half corresponding intramuscular dose

Premedication, *by subcutaneous or intramuscular injection*, up to 10 mg 60–90 minutes before operation; CHILD, *by intramuscular injection*, 150 micrograms/kg

Postoperative pain, *by subcutaneous or intramuscular injection*, 10 mg every 2–4 hours if necessary (15 mg for heavier well-muscled patients); CHILD up to 1 month 150 micrograms/kg, 1–12 months 200 micrograms/kg, 1–5 years 2.5–5 mg, 6–12 years 5–10 mg
NOTE. In the postoperative period, the patient should be closely monitored for pain relief as well as for side-effects especially respiratory depression

Patient controlled analgesia (PCA), consult hospital protocols

Myocardial infarction, *by slow intravenous injection* (2 mg/minute), 10 mg followed by a further 5–10 mg if necessary; elderly or frail patients, reduce dose by half

Acute pulmonary oedema, *by slow intravenous injection* (2 mg/minute) 5–10 mg

Chronic pain, *by mouth or by subcutaneous injection* (not suitable for oedematous patients) *or by intramuscular injection*, 5–20 mg regularly every 4 hours; dose may be increased according to needs; oral dose should be approx. double corresponding intramuscular dose and approximately triple corresponding intramuscular *diamorphine* dose (see also Prescribing in Palliative Care, p. 13); *by rectum*, as suppositories, 15–30 mg regularly every 4 hours
NOTE. The doses stated above refer equally to morphine hydrochloride, sulphate, and tartrate; see below for doses of **modified-release** preparations.

■ Oral solutions
NOTE. For advice on transfer from oral solutions of morphine to modified-release preparations of morphine, see Prescribing in Palliative Care, p. 13

Morphine Oral Solutions
PoM or CD
Oral solutions of morphine can be prescribed by writing the formula:
Morphine hydrochloride 5 mg
Chloroform water to 5 mL
NOTE. The proportion of morphine hydrochloride may be altered when specified by the prescriber; if above 13 mg per 5 mL the solution becomes **CD**. For sample prescription see Controlled Drugs and Drug Dependence, p. 7. It is usual to adjust the strength so that the dose volume is 5 or 10 mL.

Oramorph® (Boehringer Ingelheim)
Oramorph® *oral solution* PoM, morphine sulphate 10 mg/5 mL. Net price 100-mL pack = £2.08; 300-mL pack = £5.79; 500-mL pack = £8.73. Label: 2
Oramorph® *Unit Dose Vials 10 mg* PoM (oral vials), sugar-free, morphine sulphate 10 mg/5-mL vial, net price 20 vials = £2.65. Label: 2
Oramorph® *Unit Dose Vials 30 mg* CD (oral vials), sugar-free, morphine sulphate 30 mg/5-mL vial, net price 20 vials = £7.44. Label: 2
Oramorph® *concentrated oral solution* CD, sugar-free, morphine sulphate 100 mg/5 mL. Net price 30-mL pack = £5.82; 120-mL pack = £21.74 (both with calibrated dropper). Label: 2
Oramorph® *Unit Dose Vials 100 mg* CD (oral vials), sugar-free, morphine sulphate 100 mg/5-mL vial, net price 20 vials = £24.80. Label: 2

■ Tablets
Sevredol® (Napp) CD
Tablets, f/c, scored, morphine sulphate 10 mg (blue), net price 56-tab pack = £6.03; 20 mg (pink), 56-tab pack = £12.05; 50 mg (pale green), 56-tab pack = £30.13. Label: 2
Dose: severe pain uncontrolled by weaker opioid, 10–50 mg every 4 hours (dose adjusted according to response); CHILD 3–5 years, 5 mg every 4 hours; 6–12 years, 5–10 mg

■ Modified-release oral preparations
Morcap® **SR** (Sanofi-Synthelabo) CD
Capsules, m/r, clear enclosing ivory and brown pellets, morphine sulphate 20 mg, net price 30-cap pack = £5.45, 60-cap pack = £10.80; 50 mg, 30-cap pack = £13.22, 60-cap pack = £26.40; 100 mg, 30-cap pack = £26.43, 60-cap pack = £50.10. Label: 2, counselling, see below
Dose: adjusted according to daily morphine requirements, for further advice on determining dose, see

Prescribing in Palliative Care, p. 13; dosage requirements may need to be reviewed if the brand is altered
COUNSELLING. Swallow whole or open capsule and sprinkle contents on soft food
NOTE. Prescription must also specify 'capsules' (i.e. 'Morcap SR capsules')

Morphgesic® SR (Amdipharm) [CD]
Tablets, m/r, f/c, morphine sulphate 10 mg (buff), net price 60-tab pack = £4.09; 30 mg (violet), 60-tab pack = £9.81; 60 mg (orange), 60-tab pack = £19.15; 100 mg (grey), 60-tab pack = £30.30. Label: 2, 25
Dose: adjusted according to daily morphine requirements, for further advice on determining dose, see Prescribing in Palliative Care, p. 13; dosage requirements may need to be reviewed if the brand is altered
NOTE. Prescriptions must also specify 'tablets' (i.e. Morphgesic SR tablets)

MST Continus® (Napp) [CD]
Tablets, m/r, f/c, morphine sulphate 5 mg (white), net price 60-tab pack = £3.65; 10 mg (brown), 60-tab pack = £6.09; 15 mg (green), 60-tab pack =£10.68; 30 mg (purple), 60-tab pack = £14.63; 60 mg (orange), 60-tab pack = £28.54; 100 mg (grey), 60-tab pack = £45.18; 200 mg (green), 60-tab pack = £90.38. Label: 2, 25
Suspension (= sachet of granules to mix with water), m/r, pink, morphine sulphate 20 mg/sachet, net price 30-sachet pack = £27.31; 30 mg/sachet, 30-sachet pack = £28.38; 60 mg/sachet, 30-sachet pack = £56.77; 100 mg/sachet, 30-sachet pack = £94.61; 200 mg/sachet pack, 30-sachet pack = £189.22. Label: 2, 13
Dose: adjusted according to daily morphine requirements, for further advice on determining dose, see Prescribing in Palliative Care, p. 13; dosage requirements may need to be reviewed if the brand is altered
NOTE. Prescriptions must also specify 'tablets' or 'suspension' (i.e. 'MST Continus tablets' or 'MST Continus suspension')

MXL® (Napp) [CD]
Capsules, m/r, morphine sulphate 30 mg (light blue), net price 28-cap pack = £11.73; 60 mg (brown), 28-cap pack = £16.07; 90 mg (pink), 28-cap pack = £23.70; 120 mg (green), 28-cap pack = £31.34; 150 mg (blue), 28-cap pack = £39.17; 200 mg (red-brown), 28-cap pack = £49.62. Label: 2, counselling, see below
Dose: adjusted according to daily morphine requirements, for further advice on determining dose, see Prescribing in Palliative Care, p. 13; dosage requirements may need to be reviewed if the brand is altered
COUNSELLING. Swallow whole or open capsule and sprinkle contents on soft food
NOTE. Prescriptions must also specify 'capsules' (i.e. 'MXL capsules')

Zomorph® (Link) [CD]
Capsules, m/r, morphine sulphate 10 mg (yellow/clear enclosing pale yellow pellets), net price 60-cap pack =£4.31; 30 mg (pink/clear enclosing pale yellow pellets), 60-cap pack = £10.33; 60 mg (orange/clear enclosing pale yellow pellets), 60-cap pack = £20.15; 100 mg (white/clear enclosing pale yellow pellets), 60-cap pack = £31.90; 200 mg (clear enclosing pale yellow pellets), 60-cap pack = £63.79. Label: 2, counselling, see below
Dose: adjusted according to daily morphine requirements, for further advice on determining doses, see

Prescribing in Palliative Care, p. 13; dosage requirements may need to be reviewed if the brand is altered
COUNSELLING. Swallow whole or open capsule and sprinkle contents on soft food
NOTE. Prescriptions must also specify 'capsules' (i.e. 'Zomorph capsules')

■ Suppositories
Morphine (Non-proprietary) [CD]
Suppositories, morphine hydrochloride or sulphate 10 mg, net price 12 = £6.90; 15 mg, 12 = £7.13; 20 mg, 12 = £8.50; 30 mg, 12 = £9.96. Label: 2
Available from Aurum, Martindale
NOTE. Both the strength and the morphine salt contained in them must be specified by the prescriber

■ Injections
Morphine Sulphate (Non-proprietary) [CD]
Injection, morphine sulphate 10, 15, 20, and 30 mg/mL, net price 1- and 2-mL amp (all) = 72p–£1.59; 10 mg/mL, 1-mL prefilled syringe = £5.00
Intravenous infusion, morphine sulphate 1 mg/mL, net price 50-mL vial =£5.00; 2 mg/mL, 50-mL vial = £5.10
Available from Aurum, Celltech

Minijet® Morphine Sulphate (Celltech) [CD]
Injection, morphine sulphate 1 mg/mL, net price 10-mL disposable syringe = £5.00

Morphine and Atropine Injection (Non-proprietary) [CD]
Injection, morphine sulphate 10 mg, atropine sulphate 600 micrograms/mL. Net price 1-mL amp = £4.65
Dose: premedication, by subcutaneous injection, 0.5–1 mL

■ Injection with anti-emetic
CAUTION. In myocardial infarction cyclizine may aggravate severe heart failure and counteract the haemodynamic benefits of opioids, see section 4.6. **Not recommended** in palliative care, see Nausea and Vomiting, p. 15
Cyclimorph® (CeNeS) [CD]
Cyclimorph-10® Injection, morphine tartrate 10 mg, cyclizine tartrate 50 mg/mL. Net price 1-mL amp = £1.22
Dose: moderate to severe pain (short-term use only) by subcutaneous, intramuscular, or intravenous injection, 1 mL, repeated not more often than every 4 hours, with not more than 3 doses in any 24-hour period
Cyclimorph-15® Injection, morphine tartrate 15 mg, cyclizine tartrate 50 mg/mL. Net price 1-mL amp = £1.27
Dose: moderate to severe pain (short-term use only) by subcutaneous, intramuscular, or intravenous injection, 1 mL, repeated not more often than every 4 hours, with not more than 3 doses in any 24-hour period

BUPRENORPHINE

Indications: moderate to severe pain; peri-operative analgesia; opioid dependence (section 4.10); moderate to severe cancer pain (patches)
Cautions: see under Morphine Salts and notes above; effects only partially reversed by naloxone: **interactions:** Appendix 1 (opioid analgesics)
FEVER OR EXTERNAL HEAT. Monitor patients using patches for increased side-effects if fever present (increased absorption possible); avoid exposing application site to external heat (may also increase absorption)
Contra-indications: see under Morphine Salts and notes above

Side-effects: see under Morphine Salts and notes above; can give rise to mild withdrawal symptoms in patients dependent on opioids; hiccups, dyspnoea; with patches, local reactions such as erythema and pruritus; delayed local allergic reactions with severe inflammation—discontinue treatment

Dose: moderate to severe pain, *by sublingual administration*, initially 200–400 micrograms every 8 hours, increasing if necessary to 200–400 micrograms every 6–8 hours; CHILD over 6 months, 16–25 kg, 100 micrograms; 25–37.5 kg, 100–200 micrograms; 37.5–50 kg, 200–300 micrograms

By intramuscular or slow intravenous injection, 300–600 micrograms every 6–8 hours; CHILD over 6 months 3–6 micrograms/kg every 6–8 hours (max. 9 micrograms/kg)

Premedication, *by sublingual administration*, 400 micrograms

By intramuscular injection, 300 micrograms

Intra-operative analgesia, *by slow intravenous injection*, 300–450 micrograms

Temgesic® (Schering-Plough) CD
Tablets (sublingual), buprenorphine (as hydrochloride), 200 micrograms, net price 50-tab pack = £5.73; 400 micrograms, 50-tab pack = £11.46. Label: 2, 26
Injection, buprenorphine (as hydrochloride) 300 micrograms/mL, net price 1-mL amp = 53p

Transtec® (Napp) ▼ CD
Patches, self-adhesive, skin-coloured, buprenorphine, '35' patch (releasing 35 micrograms/hour for 72 hours), net price 5 = £28.97; '52.5' patch (releasing 52.5 micrograms/hour for 72 hours), 5 = £43.46; '70' patch (releasing 70 micrograms/hour for 72 hours), 5 = £57.94. Label: 2
Dose: ADULT over 18 years, apply to dry, non-irritated, non-hairy skin on upper torso, removing after 72 hours and siting replacement patch on a different area (avoid same area for at least 6 days). Patients who have not previously received strong opioid analgesic, initially, one '35 micrograms/hour' patch replaced after 72 hours; patients who have received strong opioid analgesic, initial dose based on previous 24-hour opioid requirement, consult product literature
DOSE ADJUSTMENT. When starting, analgesic effect should **not** be evaluated until the system has been worn for **24 hours** (to allow for gradual increase in plasma-buprenorphine concentration)—if necessary, dose should be adjusted at 72-hour intervals using a patch of the next strength *or* using 2 patches of the same strength (applied at *same time* to avoid confusion). Max. 2 patches can be used at any one time. For breakthrough pain, consider 200–400 micrograms buprenorphine sublingually. **Important:** it may take approx. 30 hours for the plasma-buprenorphine concentration to decrease by 50% after patch is removed
LONG DURATION OF ACTION. In view of the long duration of action, patients who have severe side-effects should be monitored for up to 30 hours after removing patch

CODEINE PHOSPHATE

Indications: mild to moderate pain; diarrhoea (section 1.4.2); cough suppression (section 3.9.1)
Cautions: see under Morphine Salts and notes above; use of cough suppressants containing codeine or similar opioid analgesics not generally recommended in children and should be avoided

altogether in those under 1 year; **interactions:** Appendix 1 (opioid analgesics)
Contra-indications: see under Morphine Salts and notes above
Side-effects: see under Morphine Salts and notes above
Dose: *by mouth*, 30–60 mg every 4 hours when necessary, to a max. of 240 mg daily; CHILD 1–12 years, 3 mg/kg daily in divided doses
By intramuscular injection, 30–60 mg every 4 hours when necessary

Codeine Phosphate (Non-proprietary)
Tablets PoM, codeine phosphate 15 mg, net price 20 = 71p; 30 mg, 20 = 95p; 60 mg, 20 = £1.87. Label: 2
NOTE. As for schedule 2 controlled drugs, travellers needing to take codeine phosphate preparations abroad may require a doctor's letter explaining why they are necessary
Syrup PoM, codeine phosphate 25 mg/5 mL. Net price 100 mL = 90p. Label: 2
Injection CD, codeine phosphate 60 mg/mL. Net price 1-mL amp = £2.26

Codeine Linctuses   Section 3.9.1
NOTE. Codeine is an ingredient of some compound analgesic preparations, section 4.7.1 and section 10.1.1 (*Codafen Continus®*)

DIAMORPHINE HYDROCHLORIDE
(Heroin Hydrochloride)
Indications: see notes above; acute pulmonary oedema
Cautions: see under Morphine Salts and notes above; **interactions:** Appendix 1 (opioid analgesics)
Contra-indications: see under Morphine Salts and notes above
Side-effects: see under Morphine Salts and notes above
Dose: acute pain, *by subcutaneous or intramuscular injection*, 5 mg repeated every 4 hours if necessary (up to 10 mg for heavier well-muscled patients)
By slow intravenous injection, quarter to half corresponding intramuscular dose
Myocardial infarction, *by slow intravenous injection* (1 mg/minute), 5 mg followed by a further 2.5–5 mg if necessary; elderly or frail patients, reduce dose by half
Acute pulmonary oedema, *by slow intravenous injection* (1 mg/minute) 2.5–5 mg
Chronic pain, *by mouth or by subcutaneous or intramuscular injection*, 5–10 mg regularly every 4 hours; dose may be increased according to needs; intramuscular dose should be approx. half corresponding oral dose, and approx. one third corresponding oral *morphine* dose—see also Prescribing in Palliative Care, p. 13; *by subcutaneous infusion* (using syringe driver), see Prescribing in Palliative Care, p. 16

Diamorphine (Non-proprietary) CD
Tablets, diamorphine hydrochloride 10 mg. Net price 100-tab pack = £12.30. Label: 2
Available from Aurum
Injection, powder for reconstitution, diamorphine hydrochloride. Net price 5-mg amp = £1.18, 10-mg amp = £1.36, 30-mg amp = £1.62, 100-mg amp = £4.50, 500-mg amp = £20.68
Available from CP, Chiron Vaccines Evans, Hillcross

DIHYDROCODEINE TARTRATE

Indications: moderate to severe pain

Cautions: see under Morphine Salts and notes above; **interactions:** Appendix 1 (opioid analgesics)

Contra-indications: see under Morphine Salts and notes above

Side-effects: see under Morphine Salts and notes above

Dose: *by mouth*, 30 mg every 4–6 hours when necessary (see also notes above); CHILD over 4 years 0.5–1 mg/kg every 4–6 hours

By deep subcutaneous or intramuscular injection, up to 50 mg repeated every 4–6 hours if necessary; CHILD over 4 years 0.5–1 mg/kg every 4–6 hours

Dihydrocodeine (Non-proprietary)
Tablets PoM, dihydrocodeine tartrate 30 mg. Net price 20 = 71p. Label: 2, 21
Available from most generic manufacturers
Oral solution PoM, dihydrocodeine tartrate 10 mg/5 mL. Net price 150 mL =£3.20. Label: 2, 21
Available from Martindale
Injection CD, dihydrocodeine tartrate 50 mg/mL. Net price 1-mL amp = £2.29
Available from Aurum

DF 118 Forte® (Martindale) PoM
Tablets, dihydrocodeine tartrate 40 mg. Net price 100-tab pack = £11.51. Label: 2, 21
Dose: severe pain, 40–80 mg 3 times daily; max. 240 mg daily; CHILD not recommended

■ Modified release

DHC Continus® (Napp) PoM
Tablets, m/r, dihydrocodeine tartrate 60 mg, net price 56-tab pack = £6.69; 90 mg, 56-tab pack = £10.53; 120 mg, 56-tab pack =£14.07. Label: 2, 25
Dose: chronic severe pain, 60–120 mg every 12 hours; CHILD not recommended
NOTE. Dihydrocodeine is an ingredient of some compound analgesic preparations, see section 4.7.1

DIPIPANONE HYDROCHLORIDE

Indications: moderate to severe pain

Cautions: see under Morphine Salts and notes above; **interactions:** Appendix 1 (opioid analgesics)

Contra-indications: see under Morphine Salts and notes above

Side-effects: see under Morphine Salts and notes above

Dose: see preparation below

Diconal® (CeNeS) CD
Tablets, pink, scored, dipipanone hydrochloride 10 mg, cyclizine hydrochloride 30 mg. Net price 50-tab pack = £7.25. Label: 2
Dose: acute pain, 1 tablet gradually increased to 3 tablets every 6 hours; CHILD not recommended
CAUTION. Not recommended in palliative care, see Nausea and vomiting p. 15

FENTANYL

Indications: breakthrough pain in patients already receiving opioid therapy for chronic pain (lozenges); chronic intractable pain (patches), other indications (section 15.1.4.3)

Cautions: see under Morphine Salts and notes above; **interactions:** Appendix 1 (opioid analgesics)

FEVER OR EXTERNAL HEAT. Monitor patients using patches for increased side-effects if fever present (increased absorption possible); avoid exposing application site to external heat (may also increase absorption)

Contra-indications: see under Morphine Salts and notes above

Side-effects: see under Morphine Salts and notes above; with patches, local reactions such as rash, erythema and itching reported

Dose: see under preparation, below
CONVERSION. (from oral morphine to transdermal fentanyl), see Prescribing in Palliative Care, p. 14

Actiq® (Cephalon) CD
Lozenge, (with oromucosal applicator), fentanyl (as citrate) 200 micrograms, net price 3 = £19.44, 30 = £194.40; 400 micrograms, 3 = £19.44, 30 = £194.40; 600 micrograms, 3 = £19.44, 30 = £194.40; 800 micrograms, 3 = £19.44, 30 = £194.40; 1.2 mg, 3 = £19.44, 30 = £194.40; 1.6 mg, 3 = £19.44, 30 = £194.40. Label: 2
Dose: initially 200 micrograms (over 15 minutes) repeated if necessary 15 minutes after first dose (no more than 2 dose units for each pain episode); adjust dose according to response; max. 4 dose units daily
NOTE. If more than 4 episodes of breakthrough pain each day, adjust dose of background analgesic

Durogesic® (Janssen-Cilag) CD
Patches, self-adhesive, transparent, fentanyl, '25' patch (releasing approx. 25 micrograms/hour for 72 hours), net price 5 = £28.97; '50' patch (releasing approx. 50 micrograms/hour for 72 hours), 5 = £54.11; '75' patch (releasing approx. 75 micrograms/hour for 72 hours), 5 = £75.43; '100' patch (releasing approx. 100 micrograms/hour for 72 hours), 5 = £92.97. Label: 2
Dose: apply to dry, non-irritated, non-irradiated, non-hairy skin on torso or upper arm, removing after 72 hours and siting replacement patch on a different area (avoid using the same area for several days). Patients who have not previously received a strong opioid analgesic, initial dose, one '25 micrograms/hour' patch replaced after 72 hours; patients who have received a strong opioid analgesic, initial dose based on previous 24-hour opioid requirement (oral morphine sulphate 90 mg over 24 hours ≈ one '25 micrograms/hour' patch, consult product literature for details); CHILD not recommended
DOSE ADJUSTMENT. When starting, evaluation of the analgesic effect should **not** be made before the system has been worn for **24 hours** (to allow for the gradual increase in plasma-fentanyl concentration)—previous analgesic therapy should be phased out gradually from time of first patch application; if necessary dose should be adjusted at 72-hour intervals in steps of '25 micrograms/hour'. More than one patch may be used at a time for doses greater than '100 micrograms/hour'(but applied at *same time* to avoid confusion)—consider additional or alternative analgesic therapy if dose required exceeds 300 micrograms/hour (**important:** it may take 17 hours or longer for the plasma-fentanyl concentration to decrease by 50%, therefore replacement opioid therapy should be initiated at a low dose, increasing gradually).
LONG DURATION OF ACTION. In view of the long duration of action, patients who have had severe side-effects should be monitored for up to 24 hours after patch removal
NOTE. Prescriptions for fentanyl patches can be written to show the strength in terms of the release rate and it is acceptable to write *'Fentanyl 25 patches'* to prescribe patches that release fentanyl 25 micrograms per hour. The dosage should be expressed in terms of the interval between applying a patch and replacing it with a new one, e.g. *'one patch to be applied every 72 hours'*. The total quantity of patches should be written in words and figures.

HYDROMORPHONE HYDROCHLORIDE

Indications: severe pain in cancer
Cautions: see Morphine Salts and notes above; **interactions:** Appendix 1 (opioid analgesics)
Contra-indications: see Morphine Salts and notes above
Side-effects: see Morphine Salts and notes above
Dose: see under preparations below

Palladone® (Napp) CD
Capsules, hydromorphone hydrochloride 1.3 mg (orange/clear), net price 56-cap pack = £8.82; 2.6 mg (red/clear), 56-cap pack = £17.64. Label: 2, counselling, see below
Dose: 1.3 mg every 4 hours, increased if necessary according to severity of pain; CHILD under 12 years not recommended
COUNSELLING. Swallow whole or open capsule and sprinkle contents on soft food

■ Modified release
Palladone® **SR** (Napp) CD
Capsules, m/r, hydromorphone hydrochloride 2 mg (yellow/clear), net price 56-cap pack = £19.98; 4 mg (pale blue/clear), 56-cap pack = £27.38; 8 mg (pink/clear), 56-cap pack = £53.41; 16 mg (brown/clear), 56-cap pack = £101.46; 24 mg (dark blue/clear), 56-cap pack = £152.21. Label: 2, counselling, see below
Dose: 4 mg every 12 hours, increased if necessary according to severity of pain; CHILD under 12 years not recommended
COUNSELLING. Swallow whole or open capsule and sprinkle contents on soft food

MEPTAZINOL

Indications: moderate to severe pain, including postoperative and obstetric pain and renal colic; peri-operative analgesia, see section 15.1.4.3
Cautions: see under Morphine Salts and notes above; effects only partially reversed by naloxone; **interactions:** Appendix 1 (opioid analgesics)
Contra-indications: see under Morphine Salts and notes above
Side-effects: see under Morphine Salts and notes above
Dose: *by mouth*, 200 mg every 3–6 hours as required; CHILD not recommended
By intramuscular injection, 75–100 mg every 2–4 hours if necessary; obstetric analgesia, 100–150 mg according to patient's weight (2 mg/kg); CHILD not recommended
By slow intravenous injection, 50–100 mg every 2–4 hours if necessary; CHILD not recommended

Meptid® (Shire) PoM
Tablets, orange, f/c, meptazinol 200 mg, net price 112-tab pack = £22.11. Label: 2
Injection, meptazinol 100 mg (as hydrochloride)/mL, net price 1-mL amp = £1.92

METHADONE HYDROCHLORIDE

Indications: severe pain, see notes above; cough in terminal disease (section 3.9.1); adjunct in treatment of opioid dependence (section 4.10)

Cautions: see under Morphine Salts and notes above; **interactions:** Appendix 1 (opioid analgesics)
Contra-indications: see under Morphine Salts and notes above
Side-effects: see under Morphine Salts and notes above
Dose: *by mouth or by subcutaneous or intramuscular injection*, 5–10 mg every 6–8 hours, adjusted according to response; on prolonged use not to be given more frequently than every 12 hours; CHILD not recommended

Methadone (Non-proprietary) CD
Tablets, scored, methadone hydrochloride 5 mg. Net price 50 = £2.97. Label: 2
Available from Martindale (*Physeptone*®)
Injection, methadone hydrochloride, 10 mg/mL, net price 1-mL amp = 86p, 2-mL amp = £1.45, 3.5-mL amp = £1.78, 5-mL amp = £1.92
Available from Auden McKenzie (*Synastone*®) CP, Martindale (*Physeptone*®), Rosemont

NALBUPHINE HYDROCHLORIDE

Indications: moderate to severe pain; premedication; peri-operative analgesia; myocardial infarction
Cautions: see under Morphine Salts and notes above; **interactions:** Appendix 1 (opioid analgesics)
Contra-indications: see under Morphine Salts and notes above
Side-effects: see under Morphine Salts and notes above
Dose: moderate to severe pain, *by subcutaneous, intramuscular, or intravenous injection*, 10–20 mg for 70 kg patient, adjusted as required; CHILD up to 300 micrograms/kg repeated once or twice as necessary
Premedication, *by subcutaneous, intramuscular, or intravenous injection*, 100–200 micrograms/kg
Induction, *by intravenous injection*, 0.3–1 mg/kg over 10–15 minutes
Intra-operative analgesia, *by intravenous injection*, 250–500 micrograms /kg at 30-minute intervals
Myocardial infarction, *by slow intravenous injection*, 10–20 mg repeated after 30 minutes if necessary

Nubain® (Bristol-Myers Squibb) PoM
Injection, nalbuphine hydrochloride 10 mg/mL. Net price 1-mL amp = 70p; 2-mL amp = £1.08

OXYCODONE HYDROCHLORIDE

Indications: moderate to severe pain in patients with cancer; postoperative pain
Cautions: see under Morphine Salts and notes above; avoid in porphyria (section 9.8.2); **interactions:** Appendix 1 (opioid analgesics)
Contra-indications: see under Morphine Salts and notes above; moderate to severe hepatic impairment; severe renal impairment
Side-effects: see under Morphine Salts and notes above
Dose: *by mouth*, initially, 5 mg every 4–6 hours, increased if necessary according to severity of pain, usual max. 400 mg daily, but some patients

may require higher doses; CHILD under 18 years not recommended

By slow intravenous injection, 1–10 mg every 4 hours when necessary

By subcutaneous injection, initially 5 mg every 4 hours when necessary

By subcutaneous infusion, initially 7.5 mg/24 hours adjusted according to response

Patient controlled analgesia (PCA), consult hospital protocols

NOTE. 2 mg oral oxycodone is approximately equivalent to 1 mg parenteral oxycodone

OxyNorm® (Napp) ⟨CD⟩
Capsules, oxycodone hydrochloride 5 mg (orange/beige), net price 56-cap pack = £10.56; 10 mg (white/beige), 56-cap pack = £21.12; 20 mg (pink/beige), 56-cap pack = £42.24. Label: 2
Liquid (= oral solution), oxycodone hydrochloride 5 mg/5 mL, net price 250 mL = £9.43. Label: 2
Concentrate (= concentrated oral solution), sugar-free, oxycodone hydrochloride 10 mg/mL, net price 120 mL = £45.25. Label: 2
Injection ▼, oxycodone hydrochloride 10 mg/mL, net price 1-mL amp = £1.40, 2-mL amp = £2.80

■ Modified release
OxyContin® (Napp) ⟨CD⟩
Tablets, f/c, m/r, oxycodone hydrochloride 5 mg (blue), net price 28-tab pack = £11.58; 10 mg (white), 56-tab pack = £23.14; 20 mg (pink), 56-tab pack = £46.29; 40 mg (yellow), 56-tab pack = £92.59; 80 mg (green), 56-tab pack = £185.18. Label: 2, 25
Dose: initially, 10 mg every 12 hours, increased if necessary according to severity of pain, usual max. 200 mg every 12 hours, but some patients may require higher doses; CHILD under 18 years not recommended

PAPAVERETUM

IMPORTANT. Do **not** confuse with papaverine (section 7.4.5)
A mixture of 253 parts of morphine hydrochloride, 23 parts of papaverine hydrochloride and 20 parts of codeine hydrochloride
The CSM has advised that to avoid confusion the figures of 7.7 mg/ml or 15.4 mg/ml should be used for prescribing purposes

Indications: premedication; enhancement of anaesthesia (but see section 15.1.4.3); postoperative analgesia; severe chronic pain

Cautions: see Morphine Salts and notes above

Contra-indications: see Morphine Salts and notes above

Side-effects: see Morphine Salts and notes above

Dose: *by subcutaneous, intramuscular, or intravenous injection*, 7.7–15.4 mg repeated every 4 hours if necessary (ELDERLY initially 7.7 mg); CHILD up to 1 month 115 micrograms/kg, 1–12 months 154 micrograms/kg, 1–5 years 1.93–3.85 mg, 6–12 years, 3.85–7.7 mg
INTRAVENOUS DOSE. In general the intravenous dose should be 25–50% of the corresponding subcutaneous or intramuscular dose

Papaveretum (Non-proprietary) ⟨CD⟩
Injection, papaveretum 15.4 mg/mL (providing the equivalent of 10 mg of anhydrous morphine/mL), net price 1-mL amp = £1.36
Available from Martindale
NOTE. The name *Omnopon*® was formerly used for papaveretum preparations.

■ With hyoscine
Papaveretum and Hyoscine Injection ⟨CD⟩
Injection, papaveretum 15.4 mg (providing the equivalent of 10 mg of anhydrous morphine), hyoscine hydrobromide 400 micrograms/mL. Net price 1-mL amp = £2.23
Dose: premedication, by subcutaneous or intramuscular injection, 0.5–1 mL
Available from Martindale

■ With aspirin
Section 4.7.1

PENTAZOCINE ⟨CD⟩

Indications: moderate to severe pain, but see notes above

Cautions: see under Morphine Salts and notes above; avoid in porphyria (section 9.8.2); **interactions:** Appendix 1 (opioid analgesics)

Contra-indications: see under Morphine Salts and notes above; patients dependent on opioids; arterial or pulmonary hypertension, heart failure

Side-effects: see under Morphine Salts and notes above; occasional hallucinations

Dose: *by mouth*, pentazocine hydrochloride 50 mg every 3–4 hours preferably after food (range 25–100 mg); max. 600 mg daily; CHILD 6–12 years 25 mg

By subcutaneous, intramuscular, or intravenous injection, moderate pain, pentazocine 30 mg, severe pain 45–60 mg every 3–4 hours when necessary; CHILD over 1 year, *by subcutaneous or intramuscular injection*, up to 1 mg/kg, *by intravenous injection* up to 500 micrograms/kg

By rectum in suppositories, pentazocine 50 mg up to 4 times daily; CHILD not recommended

Pentazocine (Non-proprietary) ⟨CD⟩
Capsules, pentazocine hydrochloride 50 mg. Net price 20 = £3.62. Label: 2, 21
Available from Alpharma, Generics
Tablets, pentazocine hydrochloride 25 mg. Net price 20 = £1.43. Label: 2, 21
Available from Alpharma, Generics
Injection, pentazocine 30 mg (as lactate)/mL. Net price 1-mL amp = £1.67, 2-mL amp = £3.21
Suppositories, pentazocine 50 mg (as lactate). Net price 20 = £19.93. Label: 2
NOTE. The brand name *Fortral*® ⟨NHS⟩ (Sanofi-Synthelabo) is used for all the above preparations of pentazocine

PETHIDINE HYDROCHLORIDE

Indications: moderate to severe pain, obstetric analgesia; peri-operative analgesia

Cautions: see under Morphine Salts and notes above; not suitable for severe continuing pain; **interactions:** Appendix 1 (opioid analgesics)

Contra-indications: see under Morphine Salts and notes above; severe renal impairment

Side-effects: see under Morphine Salts and notes above; convulsions reported in **overdosage**

Dose: acute pain, *by mouth*, 50–150 mg every 4 hours; CHILD 0.5–2 mg/kg

By subcutaneous or intramuscular injection, 25–100 mg, repeated after 4 hours; CHILD, *by intramuscular injection*, 0.5–2 mg/kg

By slow intravenous injection, 25–50 mg, repeated after 4 hours

Obstetric analgesia, *by subcutaneous or intramus-*

cular injection, 50–100 mg, repeated 1–3 hours later if necessary; max. 400 mg in 24 hours

Premedication, *by intramuscular injection*, 25–100 mg 1 hour before operation; CHILD 0.5–2 mg/kg

Postoperative pain, *by subcutaneous or intramuscular injection*, 25–100 mg, every 2–3 hours if necessary; CHILD, *by intramuscular injection*, 0.5–2 mg/kg

NOTE. In the postoperative period, the patient should be closely monitored for pain relief as well as for side-effects especially respiratory depression

Pethidine (Non-proprietary) CD
Tablets, pethidine hydrochloride 50 mg, net price 20 = £1.97. Label: 2
Available from Martindale
Injection, pethidine hydrochloride 50 mg/mL, net price 1-mL amp = 53p, 2-mL amp = 56p; 10 mg/mL, 5-mL amp = £2.06, 10-mL amp = £2.18
Various strengths available from Auden McKenzie, Martindale

Pamergan P100® (Martindale) CD ▰▬
Injection, pethidine hydrochloride 50 mg, promethazine hydrochloride 25 mg/mL. Net price 2-mL amp = 70p
Dose: by intramuscular injection, premedication, 2 mL 60–90 minutes before operation; CHILD 8–12 years 0.75 mL, 13–16 years 1 mL
Obstetric analgesia, 1–2 mL every 4 hours if necessary
Severe pain, 1–2 mL every 4–6 hours if necessary
NOTE. Although usually given intramuscularly, may be given intravenously after dilution to at least 10 mL with water for injections

TRAMADOL HYDROCHLORIDE

Indications: moderate to severe pain

Cautions: see under Morphine Salts and notes above; history of epilepsy (convulsions reported, usually after rapid intravenous injection); manufacturer advises avoid in pregnancy and breast-feeding; not suitable as substitute in opioid-dependent patients; **interactions:** Appendix 1 (opioid analgesics)
GENERAL ANAESTHESIA. Not recommended for analgesia during potentially very light planes of general anaesthesia (possibly increased operative recall reported)

Contra-indications: see under Morphine Salts and notes above

Side-effects: see under Morphine Salts and notes above; also hypotension and occasionally hypertension; anaphylaxis, hallucinations, and confusion reported

Dose: *by mouth*, 50–100 mg not more often than every 4 hours; total of more than 400 mg daily by mouth not usually required; CHILD not recommended

By intramuscular injection or by intravenous injection (over 2–3 minutes) *or by intravenous infusion*, 50–100 mg every 4–6 hours
Postoperative pain, 100 mg initially then 50 mg every 10–20 minutes if necessary during first hour to total max. 250 mg (including initial dose) in first hour, *then* 50–100 mg every 4–6 hours; max. 600 mg daily; CHILD not recommended

Tramadol Hydrochloride (Non-proprietary) PoM
Capsules, tramadol hydrochloride 50 mg. Net price 30-cap pack = £2.21, 100-cap pack = £10.35. Label: 2
Available from Alpharma, APS, Arrow, Galen (*Tramake*®), Generics, Genus, IVAX, PLIVA, Sovereign, Sterwin, Tillomed
Injection, tramadol hydrochloride 50 mg/ml. Net price 2-mL amp = £1.10
Available from Aurum, Sterwin (for intravenous use only)

Tramake Insts® (Galen) PoM
Sachets, effervescent powder, sugar-free, lemon-flavoured, tramadol hydrochloride 50 mg (contains Na$^+$ 9.7 mmol/sachet), net price 60-sachet pack = £8.95; 100 mg (contains Na$^+$ 14.6 mmol/sachet), 60-sachet pack = £17.90. Label: 2, 13
Excipients: include aspartame (section 9.4.1)

Zamadol® (Viatris) PoM
Capsules, tramadol hydrochloride 50 mg, net price 100-cap pack = £8.60. Label: 2
Orodispersible tablets (*Zamadol Melt*®), tramadol hydrochloride 50 mg, net price 100-tab pack = £12.77. Label: 2, counselling, administration
Excipients: include aspartame
COUNSELLING. *Zamadol Melt*® should be sucked and then swallowed. May also be dispersed in water
Injection, tramadol hydrochloride 50 mg/mL, net price 2-mL amp = £1.18

Zydol® (Searle) PoM
Capsules, green/yellow, tramadol hydrochloride 50 mg. Net price 100-cap pack = £16.91. Label: 2
Soluble tablets, tramadol hydrochloride 50 mg, net price 20-tab pack = £3.05, 100-tab pack = £15.23. Label: 2, 13
Injection, tramadol hydrochloride 50 mg/mL. Net price 2-mL amp = £1.24

■ Modified release

Dromadol® **SR** (IVAX) PoM
Tablets, m/r, tramadol hydrochloride 75 mg (grey), net price 60-tab pack = £12.33; 100 mg (white), 60-tab pack = £16.00; 150 mg (beige), 60-tab pack = £24.00; 200 mg (orange), 60-tab pack = £32.00. Label: 2, 25
Dose: initially 75 mg twice daily increased if necessary; usual max. 400 mg daily in 2 divided doses; CHILD under 12 years not recommended

Dromadol® **XL** (IVAX) PoM
Tablets, m/r, tramadol hydrochloride 150 mg, 30-tab pack = £11.83; 200 mg, 30-tab pack = £15.93; 300 mg, 30-tab pack = £24.12; 400 mg, 30-tab pack = £32.38. Label: 2, 25
Dose: 150 mg daily increased if necessary; more than 400 mg once daily not usually required; CHILD under 12 years not recommended

Zamadol® **SR** (Viatris) PoM
Capsules, m/r, tramadol hydrochloride 50 mg (green), net price 60-cap pack = £8.21; 100 mg, net price 60-cap pack = £16.43; 150 mg (dark green), 60-cap pack = £24.64; 200 mg (yellow), 60-cap pack = £32.85. Label: 2
Dose: 50–100 mg twice daily increased if necessary to 150–200 mg twice daily; total of more than 400 mg daily not usually required; CHILD under 12 years not recommended
COUNSELLING. Swallow whole or open capsule and swallow contents immediately without chewing

Zydol SR® (Searle) PoM
Tablets, m/r, f/c, tramadol hydrochloride 100 mg, net price 60-tab pack = £18.26; 150 mg (beige), 60-

tab pack = £27.39; 200 mg (orange), 60-tab pack = £36.52. Label: 2, 25

Dose: 100 mg twice daily increased if necessary to 150–200 mg twice daily; total of more than 400 mg daily not usually required; CHILD not recommended

Zydol XL® (Searle) PoM

Tablets, m/r, f/c, tramadol hydrochloride 150 mg, net price 30-tab pack = £15.22; 200 mg, 30-tab pack = £20.29; 300 mg, 30-tab pack = £30.44; 400 mg, 30-tab pack = £40.59. Label: 2, 25

Dose: 150 mg daily increased if necessary; more than 400 mg once daily not usually required; CHILD not recommended

4.7.3   Neuropathic pain

Neuropathic pain, which occurs as a result of damage to neural tissue, includes *postherpetic neuralgia, phantom limb pain, complex regional pain syndrome* (reflex sympathetic dystrophy, causalgia) *compression neuropathies, peripheral neuropathies* (e.g. due to diabetes, haematological malignancies, rheumatoid arthritis, alcoholism, drug misuse), *trauma, central pain* (e.g. pain following stroke, spinal cord injury and syringomyelia) and *idiopathic neuropathy.* The pain occurs in an area of sensory deficit and may be described as burning, shooting or scalding and is often accompanied by pain that is evoked by a non-noxious stimulus (allodynia).

Trigeminal neuralgia is also caused by dysfunction of neural tissue, but its management is distinct from other forms of neuropathic pain.

Neuropathic pain is generally managed with a tricyclic antidepressant and certain antiepileptic drugs. Neuropathic pain may respond only partially to opioid analgesics. Of the opioids, dextropropoxyphene, methadone, tramadol, and oxycodone are probably the most effective for neuropathic pain and they may be considered when other measures fail. Nerve blocks, transcutaneous electrical nerve stimulation (TENS) and, in selected cases, central electrical stimulation may help. Many patients with chronic neuropathic pain require multidisciplinary management, including physiotherapy and psychological support.

Amitriptyline is prescribed most frequently [unlicensed indication], initially at 10–25 mg each night. The dose may be increased gradually to about 75 mg daily if required (higher doses under specialist supervision); **nortriptyline**, a metabolite of amitriptyline, also given at an initial dose of 10–25 mg at night may produce fewer side-effects. **Gabapentin** (section 4.8.1) is licensed for the treatment of neuropathic pain.

Capsaicin (section 10.3.2) is licensed for neuropathic pain (but the intense burning sensation during initial treatment may limit use). Drugs, that are now generally reserved for use under specialist supervision include **sodium valproate** and occasionally **phenytoin**. **Ketamine** (section 15.1.1), an NMDA antagonist, or **lidocaine (lignocaine)** by intravenous infusion may also be useful in some forms of neuropathic pain [both unlicensed indication; specialist use only].

A **corticosteroid** may help to relieve pressure in compression neuropathy and thereby reduce pain. The management of trigeminal neuralgia and postherpetic neuralgia are outlined below; for the management of neuropathic pain in *palliative care*

see p. 14; for the management of diabetic neuropathy, see section 6.1.5.

Trigeminal neuralgia

Surgery may be the treatment of choice in many patients; a neurological assessment will identify those who stand to benefit. **Carbamazepine** (section 4.8.1) taken during the acute stages of trigeminal neuralgia, reduces the frequency and severity of attacks. Plasma-carbamazepine concentration should be monitored when high doses are given. Small doses should be used initially to reduce the incidence of side-effects e.g. dizziness. **Oxcarbazepine** [unlicensed indication] is an alternative to carbamazepine. **Gabapentin** and **lamotrigine** [unlicensed indication] are also used in trigeminal neuralgia. Some cases respond to **phenytoin** (section 4.8.1); the drug may be given by intravenous infusion (possibly as fosphenytoin) in a crisis (specialist use only).

Postherpetic neuralgia

Postherpetic neuralgia follows acute herpes zoster infection (shingles), particularly in the elderly. If **amitriptyline** fails to manage the pain adequately, **gabapentin** may improve control. A topical analgesic preparation containing **capsaicin** 0.075% (section 10.3.2) is licensed for use in postherpetic neuralgia. Application of topical local anaesthetic preparations may be helpful in some patients.

4.7.4   Antimigraine drugs

4.7.4.1   Treatment of the acute migraine attack
4.7.4.2   Prophylaxis of migraine
4.7.4.3   Cluster headache

4.7.4.1   Treatment of the acute migraine attack

Treatment of a migraine attack should be guided by response to previous treatment and the severity of the attacks. A **simple analgesic** such as aspirin, paracetamol (preferably in a soluble or dispersible form) or an NSAID is often effective; concomitant **antiemetic** treatment may be required. If treatment with an analgesic is inadequate, an attack may be treated with a specific antimigraine compound such as a **5HT₁ agonist** ('triptan'). **Ergot alkaloids** are rarely required now; oral and rectal preparations are associated with many side-effects (including 'ergot headache') and they should be avoided in cerebrovascular or cardiovascular disease.

Analgesics

Most migraine headaches respond to analgesics such as **aspirin** or **paracetamol** (section 4.7.1) but because peristalsis is often reduced during migraine attacks the medication may not be sufficiently well absorbed to be effective; dispersible or effervescent preparations are therefore preferred.

The NSAID **tolfenamic acid** is licensed specifically for the treatment of an acute attack of migraine;

diclofenac potassium, **flurbiprofen, ibuprofen,** and **naproxen sodium** (section 10.1.1) are also licensed for use in migraine. Frequent and prolonged use of analgesics by migraine sufferers may lead to analgesic-induced headache.

ANALGESICS

- Aspirin
Section 4.7.1

- Paracetamol
Section 4.7.1

- Non-steroidal anti-inflammatory drugs (NSAIDs)
Section 10.1.1

- With anti-emetics

Domperamol® (Servier) PoM
Tablets, f/c, paracetamol 500 mg, domperidone (as maleate) 10 mg, net price 16-tab pack = £7.00. Label: 17, 30
Dose: 2 tablets at onset of attack then up to every 4 hours; max. 8 tablets daily; CHILD not recommended

Migraleve® (Pfizer Consumer) ▰▰
Tablets, all f/c, *pink tablets*, buclizine hydrochloride 6.25 mg, paracetamol 500 mg, codeine phosphate 8 mg; *yellow tablets*, paracetamol 500 mg, codeine phosphate 8 mg. Net price 48-tab *Migraleve* PoM (32 pink + 16 yellow) = £5.10; 48 pink (*Migraleve Pink*) = £5.56; 48 yellow (*Migraleve Yellow*) = £4.70. Label: 2, (*Migraleve Pink*), 17, 30
Dose: 2 pink tablets at onset of attack, or if it is imminent, then 2 yellow tablets every 4 hours if necessary; max. in 24 hours 2 pink and 6 yellow; CHILD under 10 years, only under close medical supervision; 10–14 years, half adult dose

MigraMax® (Elan) PoM
Oral powder, aspirin (as lysine acetylsalicylate) 900 mg, metoclopramide hydrochloride 10 mg/sachet, net price 6-sachet pack = £7.00, 20-sachet pack = £23.33. Label: 13, 21, 32
Dose: ADULT over 20 years 1 sachet in water at onset of attack, repeated after 2 hours if necessary (max. 3 sachets in 24 hours); YOUNG ADULT (under 20 years) and CHILD not recommended
IMPORTANT. Metoclopramide can cause **severe extrapyramidal effects**, particularly in children and young adults (for further details, see p. 204)
Excipients: include aspartame (section 9.4.1)

Paramax® (Sanofi-Synthelabo) PoM
Tablets, scored, paracetamol 500 mg, metoclopramide hydrochloride 5 mg. Net price 42-tab pack = £6.69. Label: 17, 30
Sachets, effervescent powder, sugar-free, the contents of 1 sachet = 1 tablet; to be dissolved in ¼ tumblerful of liquid before administration. Net price 42-sachet pack = £8.69. Label: 13, 17, 30
Dose: (tablets or sachets): 2 at onset of attack then every 4 hours when necessary to max. of 6 in 24 hours; YOUNG ADULT 12–19 years, 1 at onset of attack then 1 every 4 hours when necessary to max. of 3 in 24 hours (max. dose of metoclopramide 500 micrograms/kg daily)
IMPORTANT. Metoclopramide can cause **severe extrapyramidal effects**, particularly in children and young adults (for further details, see p. 204)

TOLFENAMIC ACID

Indications: treatment of acute migraine attacks
Cautions: see NSAIDs, section 10.1.1
Contra-indications: see NSAIDs, section 10.1.1

Side-effects: see NSAIDs, section 10.1.1; also dysuria (most commonly in men), tremor, euphoria, and fatigue reported
Dose: 200 mg at onset repeated once after 1–2 hours if necessary

Clotam® (Provalis) PoM
Rapid Tablets, tolfenamic acid 200 mg. Net price 10-tab pack = £15.00

5HT₁ agonists

A 5HT₁ agonist is of considerable value in the treatment of an acute migraine attack. The 5HT₁ agonists ('triptans') act on the 5HT (serotonin) 1B/1D receptors and they are therefore sometimes referred to as $5HT_{1B/1D}$-receptor agonists. A 5HT₁ agonist may be used during the established headache phase of an attack and is the preferred treatment in those who fail to respond to conventional analgesics.

The 5HT₁ agonists available for treating migraine are **almotriptan, eletriptan, frovatriptan, naratriptan, rizatriptan, sumatriptan,** and **zolmitriptan.** Sumatriptan is also of value in cluster headache (section 4.7.4.3).

CAUTIONS. 5HT₁ agonists should be used with caution in conditions which predispose to coronary artery disease (pre-existing cardiac disease, see Contra-indications below); hepatic impairment (see Appendix 2); pregnancy (see Appendix 4) and breast-feeding (see Appendix 5). 5HT₁ agonists are recommended as monotherapy and should not be taken concurrently with other therapies for acute migraine. Little information is available on the use of these drugs in the elderly (over 65 years).

CONTRA-INDICATIONS. 5HT₁ agonists should not be used for prophylaxis and they are contra-indicated in ischaemic heart disease, previous myocardial infarction, coronary vasospasm (including Prinzmetal's angina), and uncontrolled or severe hypertension.

SIDE-EFFECTS. Side-effects of the 5HT₁ agonists include sensations of tingling, heat, heaviness, pressure, or tightness of any part of the body (including throat and chest—discontinue if intense, may be due to coronary vasoconstriction or to anaphylaxis; see also CSM advice under Sumatriptan); flushing, dizziness, feeling of weakness; fatigue; nausea and vomiting also reported.

ALMOTRIPTAN

Indications: treatment of acute migraine attacks
Cautions: see under 5HT₁ agonists above; hepatic impairment (avoid if severe); severe renal impairment (Appendix 3); sensitivity to sulphonamides; not to be taken until 24 hours after stopping an ergotamine-type preparation (ergotamine-type preparations not to be taken until 6 hours after almotriptan); other **interactions:** Appendix 1 (5HT₁ agonists)
Contra-indications: see under 5HT₁ agonists above; previous cerebrovascular accident or transient ischaemic attack; peripheral vascular disease
Side-effects: see under 5HT₁ agonists above; transient increase in blood pressure, drowsiness; also paraesthesia, diarrhoea, dyspepsia, dry mouth, myalgia, headache, tinnitus

Dose: 12.5 mg as soon as possible after onset repeated after 2 hours if migraine recurs (patient not responding should not take second dose for same attack); max. 25 mg in 24 hours; CHILD and ADOLESCENT under 18 years not recommended

Almogran® (Lundbeck) ▼ PoM
Tablets, f/c, almotriptan (as hydrogen malate) 12.5 mg, net price 3-tab pack = £9.75; 6-tab pack = £19.50; 9-tab pack = £29.25. Label: 3

ELETRIPTAN

Indications: treatment of acute migraine attacks

Cautions: see under 5HT₁ agonists above; hepatic impairment (avoid if severe); renal impairment (avoid if severe—Appendix 3); not to be taken until 24 hours after stopping an ergotamine-type preparation (ergotamine-type preparation not to be taken until 24 hours after eletriptan)

Contra-indications: see under 5HT₁ agonists above; previous cerebrovascular accident or transient ischaemic attack; peripheral vascular disease

Side-effects: see under 5HT₁ agonists above; also dry mouth, dyspepsia, abdominal pain, tachycardia, asthenia, drowsiness, ataxia, speech impairment, myasthenia, myalgia, pharyngitis, sweating; less commonly diarrhoea, anorexia, glossitis, thirst, oedema, increased urinary frequency, transient increase in blood pressure, insomnia, depression, confusion, tremor, agitation, euphoria, malaise, arthralgia, dyspnoea, rhinitis, rash, pruritus, visual disturbances, taste disturbance, tinnitus; rarely bradycardia

Dose: 40 mg as soon as possible after onset repeated after 2 hours if migraine recurs (patient not responding should not take second dose for same attack); increase to 80 mg for subsequent attacks if 40-mg dose inadequate; max. 80 mg in 24 hours; CHILD and ADOLESCENT under 18 years not recommended

Relpax® (Pfizer) ▼ PoM
Tablets, f/c, orange, eletriptan (as hydrobromide) 20 mg, net price 6-tab pack = £22.50; 40 mg, 6-tab pack = £22.50. Label: 3

FROVATRIPTAN

Indications: treatment of acute migraine attacks

Cautions: see under 5HT₁ agonists above; not to be taken until 24 hours after stopping an ergotamine-type preparation (ergotamine-type preparation not to be taken until 24 hours after frovatriptan); **interactions:** Appendix 1 (5HT₁ agonists)

Contra-indications: see under 5HT₁ agonists above; severe hepatic impairment; previous cerebrovascular attack or transient ischaemic attack; peripheral vascular disease

Side-effects: see under 5HT₁ agonists above; dry mouth, gastro-intestinal disturbances, palpitations, paraesthesia, drowsiness, sweating; taste disturbances, tachycardia (rarely bradycardia), hypertension, rhinitis, pharyngitis, sinusitis, laryngitis, tremor, muscle spasm, anxiety, insomnia, confusion, nervousness, agitation, impaired concentration, mood disturbances, thirst, micturition disorders, pruritus, tinnitus; rarely bilirubinaemia, stomatitis, hyperventilation, amnesia, abnormal dreams, syncope, hypocalcaemia, hypoglycaemia, urticaria

Dose: 2.5 mg as soon as possible after onset repeated after 2 hours if migraine recurs (patient not responding should not take second dose for same attack); max. 5 mg in 24 hours; CHILD and ADOLESCENT under 18 years not recommended; ELDERLY over 65 years not recommended

Migard® (Menarini) ▼ PoM
Tablets, f/c, frovatriptan (as succinate) 2.5 mg, net price 6-tab pack = £17.70. Label: 3

NARATRIPTAN

Indications: treatment of acute migraine attacks

Cautions: see under 5HT₁ agonists above; renal impairment; sensitivity to sulphonamides; **interactions:** Appendix 1 (5HT₁ agonists)
DRIVING. Drowsiness may affect performance of skilled tasks (e.g. driving)

Contra-indications: see under 5HT₁ agonists above; previous cerebrovascular accident or transient ischaemic attack; peripheral vascular disease

Side-effects: see under 5HT₁ agonists above, bradycardia or tachycardia; visual disturbances; ischaemic colitis reported

Dose: 2.5 mg as soon as possible after onset; if migraine recurs after initial response, dose may be repeated after 4 hours (patient not responding should not take second dose for same attack); max. 5 mg in 24 hours; CHILD and ADOLESCENT under 18 years not recommended

Naramig® (GSK) PoM
Tablets, f/c, green, naratriptan (as hydrochloride) 2.5 mg, net price 6-tab pack = £26.40, 12-tab pack = £52.80. Label: 3

RIZATRIPTAN

Indications: treatment of acute migraine attacks

Cautions: see under 5HT₁ agonists above; renal impairment (Appendix 3); not to be taken until 24 hours after stopping an ergotamine-type preparation (ergotamine-type preparations not to be taken until 6 hours after rizatriptan); other **interactions:** Appendix 1 (5HT₁ agonists)
DRIVING. Drowsiness may affect performance of skilled tasks (e.g. driving)

Contra-indications: see under 5HT₁ agonists above; previous cerebrovascular accident or transient ischaemic attack; peripheral vascular disease

Side-effects: see under 5HT₁ agonists above; drowsiness, palpitations, tachycardia, dry mouth, diarrhoea, dyspepsia, thirst, pharyngeal discomfort, dyspnoea, headache, paraesthesia, decreased alertness, insomnia, tremor, ataxia, nervousness, vertigo, confusion, myalgia and muscle weakness, sweating, urticaria, pruritus, blurred vision; rarely syncope, hypertension; hypersensitivity reactions (including rash, angioedema, and toxic epidermal necrolysis) and taste disturbance reported

Dose: 10 mg as soon as possible after onset repeated after 2 hours if migraine recurs (patient not responding should not take second dose for same attack); max. 20 mg in 24 hours; CHILD and ADOLESCENT under 18 years not recommended
NOTE. Halve dose in patients taking propranolol; not to be taken within 2 hours of taking propranolol

Maxalt® (MSD) PoM
Tablets, pink, rizatriptan (as benzoate) 5 mg, net price 6-tab pack = £26.74; 10 mg, 3-tab pack = £13.37, 6-tab pack = £26.74. Label: 3

Wafers (*Maxalt® Melt*), rizatriptan (as benzoate) 10 mg, net price 3-wafer pack = £13.37, 6-wafer pack = £26.74. Label: 3, counselling, administration

COUNSELLING. *Maxalt® Melt* wafers should be placed on the tongue and allowed to dissolve

Excipients: include aspartame equivalent to phenylalanine 2.1 mg (section 9.4.1)

SUMATRIPTAN

Indications: treatment of acute migraine attacks; cluster headache (subcutaneous injection only)

Cautions: see under $5HT_1$ agonists above; renal impairment; sensitivity to sulphonamides; should not be taken until 24 hours after stopping an ergotamine-containing preparation (ergotamine-containing preparations should not be taken until 6 hours after sumatriptan); other **interactions:** Appendix 1 ($5HT_1$ agonists)

DRIVING. Drowsiness may affect performance of skilled tasks (e.g. driving)

Contra-indications: see under $5HT_1$ agonists above; previous cerebrovascular accident or transient ischaemic attack; peripheral vascular disease; moderate and severe hypertension

Side-effects: see under $5HT_1$ agonists above; drowsiness, transient increase in blood pressure, hypotension, bradycardia or tachycardia, visual disturbances, ischaemic colitis, Raynaud's syndrome, altered liver function tests, seizures reported; erythema at injection site; nasal irritation and taste disturbance with nasal spray

CSM advice. Following reports of chest pain and tightness (coronary vasoconstriction) CSM has emphasised that sumatriptan should **not** be used in ischaemic heart disease or Prinzmetal's angina, and that use with ergotamine should be **avoided** (see also Cautions).

Dose: *by mouth*, 50 mg (some patients may require 100 mg) as soon as possible after onset (patient not responding should not take second dose for same attack); dose may be repeated after not less than 2 hours if migraine recurs; max. 300 mg in 24 hours; CHILD and ADOLESCENT under 18 years not recommended

By subcutaneous injection using auto-injector, 6 mg as soon as possible after onset (patients not responding should not take second dose for same attack); dose may be repeated once after not less than 1 hour if migraine recurs; max. 12 mg in 24 hours; CHILD and ADOLESCENT under 18 years not recommended

IMPORTANT. **Not** for intravenous injection which may cause coronary vasospasm and angina

Intranasally, 10–20 mg (ADOLESCENT 12–17 years 10 mg) into one nostril as soon as possible after onset (patient not responding should not take a second dose for same attack); dose may be repeated once after not less than 2 hours if migraine recurs; max. 40 mg (ADOLESCENT 12–17 years 20 mg) in 24 hours; CHILD under 12 years not recommended

Imigran® (GSK) PoM

Tablets, f/c, sumatriptan (as succinate) 50 mg, net price 6-tab pack = £29.70, 12-tab pack = £56.43; 100 mg, 6-tab pack = £48.00, 12-tab pack = £96.00. Label: 3, 10, patient information leaflet

Injection, sumatriptan (as succinate) 12 mg/mL (= 6 mg/0.5-mL syringe), net price, treatment pack (2 × 0.5-mL prefilled syringes and auto-injector) = £47.52; refill pack 2 × 0.5-mL prefilled cartridges

= £45.21; 6 × 0.5-mL prefilled cartridges = £135.62. Label: 3, 10, patient information leaflet

Nasal spray, sumatriptan 10 mg/0.1-mL actuation, net price 2 unit-dose spray device = £12.00; 20 mg/ 0.1-mL actuation, 2 unit-dose spray device = £12.00, 6 unit-dose spray device = £39.60. Label: 3, 10, patient information leaflet

ZOLMITRIPTAN

Indications: treatment of acute migraine attacks

Cautions: see under $5HT_1$ agonists above; should not be taken within 12 hours of any other $5HT_1$ agonist; should not be taken for at least 24 hours after stopping an ergotamine-containing preparation, and ergotamine-containing preparations should not be taken for at least six hours after stopping zolmitriptan; **interactions:** Appendix 1 ($5HT_1$ agonists)

Contra-indications: see under $5HT_1$ agonists above; Wolff-Parkinson-White syndrome or arrhythmias associated with accessory cardiac conduction pathways; previous cerebrovascular accident or transient ischaemic attack

Side-effects: see under $5HT_1$ agonists above; drowsiness, transient increase in blood pressure, dry mouth, myalgia, muscle weakness, dysaesthesia; rarely, gastro-intestinal ischaemia, angina, myocardial infarction, tachycardia, palpitations, headache; taste disturbance and nasal discomfort with nasal spray

Dose: *by mouth*, 2.5 mg as soon as possible after onset repeated after not less than 2 hours if migraine persists or recurs (increase to 5 mg for subsequent attacks in patients not achieving satisfactory relief with 2.5-mg dose); max. 10 mg in 24 hours; CHILD not recommended

Intranasally, 5 mg (1 spray) into one nostril as soon as possible after onset repeated after not less than 2 hours if migraine persists or recurs; max. 10 mg in 24 hours; CHILD not recommended

Zomig® (AstraZeneca) PoM

Tablets, f/c, yellow, zolmitriptan 2.5 mg, net price 6-tab pack = £24.00, 12-tab pack = £48.00

Orodispersible tablets (*Zomig Rapimelt®*), zolmitriptan 2.5 mg, net-price 6-tab pack = £24.00. Counselling, administration

COUNSELLING. *Zomig Rapimelt®* should be placed on the tongue, allowed to disperse and swallowed

Excipients: include aspartame equivalent to phenylalanine 2.81 mg/ tablet (section 9.4.1)

Nasal spray▼, zolmitriptan 5 mg/0.1-mL unit-dose spray device, net price 6 unit-dose sprays = £40.50

Ergot alkaloids

The value of **ergotamine** for migraine is limited by difficulties in absorption and by its side-effects, particularly nausea, vomiting, abdominal pain, and *muscular cramps*; it is best avoided. The recommended doses of ergotamine preparations should **not** be exceeded and treatment should **not** be repeated at intervals of less than 4 days.

To avoid habituation the frequency of administration of ergotamine should be limited to **no more than** twice a month. It should **never** be prescribed prophylactically but in the management of cluster headache a low dose (e.g. ergotamine 1 mg at night for 6 nights in 7) is occasionally given for 1 to 2 weeks [unlicensed indication].

ERGOTAMINE TARTRATE ◤

Indications: treatment of acute migraine attacks and migraine variants unresponsive to analgesics

Cautions: risk of peripheral vasospasm (see advice below); elderly; dependence (see Ergot alkaloids above), should not be used for migraine prophylaxis; **interactions:** Appendix 1 (ergot alkaloids) and under Sumatriptan (Cautions), below

PERIPHERAL VASOSPASM. Warn patient to stop treatment immediately if numbness or tingling of extremities develops and to contact doctor.

Contra-indications: peripheral vascular disease, coronary heart disease, obliterative vascular disease and Raynaud's syndrome, temporal arteritis, hepatic and renal impairment, sepsis, severe or inadequately controlled hypertension, hyperthyroidism, pregnancy and breast-feeding, porphyria (section 9.8.2)

Side-effects: nausea, vomiting, vertigo, abdominal pain, diarrhoea, muscle cramps, and occasionally headache provoked (usually because of prolonged excessive dosage or abrupt withdrawal); precordial pain, myocardial and intestinal ischaemia, rarely myocardial infarction; repeated high dosage may cause ergotism with gangrene and confusion; pleural, peritoneal and heart-valve fibrosis may occur with excessive use; rectal or anal stricture or ulceration and rectovaginal fistula reported with prolonged use of suppositories

Dose: see under preparations below

Cafergot® (Alliance) PoM ◤
Tablets, ergotamine tartrate 1 mg, caffeine 100 mg. Net price 30-tab pack = £5.90. Label: 18, counselling, dosage
Dose: 1–2 tablets at onset; max. 4 tablets in 24 hours; not to be repeated at intervals of less than 4 days; max. 8 tablets in one week (but see also notes above); CHILD not recommended

Suppositories, ergotamine tartrate 2 mg, caffeine 100 mg. Net price 30 = £13.50. Label: 18, counselling, dosage
Dose: 1 suppository at onset; max. 2 in 24 hours; not to be repeated at intervals of less than 4 days; max. 4 suppositories in one week (but see also notes above); CHILD not recommended

Migril® (CP) PoM ◤
Tablets, scored, ergotamine tartrate 2 mg, cyclizine hydrochloride 50 mg, caffeine hydrate 100 mg. Net price 20 = £11.67. Label: 2, 18, counselling, dosage
Dose: 1 tablet at onset, followed after 30 minutes by ½–1 tablet, repeated every 30 minutes if necessary; max. 4 tablets per attack and 6 tablets in one week (but see also notes above); CHILD not recommended

Anti-emetics

Anti-emetics (section 4.6), such as **metoclopramide** or **domperidone**, or phenothiazine and antihistamine anti-emetics, relieve the nausea associated with migraine attacks. Anti-emetics may be given by intramuscular injection or rectally if vomiting is a problem. Metoclopramide and domperidone have the added advantage of promoting gastric emptying and normal peristalsis; a single dose should be given at the onset of symptoms. Oral analgesic preparations containing metoclopramide or domperidone are a convenient alternative (**important:** for warnings

relating to extrapyramidal effects of metoclopramide particularly in children and young adults, see p. 204).

Other drugs for migraine

Isometheptene mucate (in combination with paracetamol) is licensed for the treatment of acute attacks of migraine; other effective treatments are however available now.

ISOMETHEPTENE MUCATE ◤

Indications: treatment of acute migraine attacks

Cautions: cardiovascular disease, hepatic and renal impairment, diabetes mellitus, hyperthyroidism; **interactions:** Appendix 1 (sympathomimetics)

Contra-indications: glaucoma, severe cardiac, hepatic and renal impairment, severe hypertension, pregnancy and breast-feeding; porphyria (section 9.8.2)

Side-effects: dizziness, circulatory disturbances, rashes, blood disorders also reported

¹**Midrid®** (Shire) PoM ◤
Capsules, red, isometheptene mucate 65 mg, paracetamol 325 mg. Net price 100-cap pack = £13.11. Label: 30, counselling, dosage
Dose: migraine, 2 capsules at onset of attack, followed by 1 capsule every hour if necessary; max. 5 capsules in 12 hours; CHILD not recommended

1. A pack containing 15 capsules may be sold to the public

4.7.4.2 Prophylaxis of migraine

Where migraine attacks are frequent, possible provoking factors such as stress, irregular life-style (e.g. lack of sleep), or chemical triggers (e.g. alcohol and nitrates) should be sought; combined oral contraceptives may also provoke migraine, see section 7.3.1 for advice. Benzodiazepines should be avoided because of the risk of dependence.

Prophylactic therapy is considered for patients who have two or more attacks a month that are disabling. Pizotifen, a beta-blocker, a tricyclic antidepressant (even when the patient is not obviously depressed), or sodium valproate may be used for migraine prophylaxis.

Pizotifen is an antihistamine and serotonin antagonist structurally related to the tricyclic antidepressants. It affords good prophylaxis but may cause weight gain. To avoid undue drowsiness treatment may be started at 500 micrograms at night and gradually increased to 3 mg; it is rarely necessary to exceed this dose.

The **beta-blockers** propranolol, metoprolol, nadolol, and timolol (section 2.4) are all effective. Propranolol is the most commonly used in an initial dose of 40 mg 2 to 3 times daily by mouth. Beta-blockers may also be given as a single daily dose of a long-acting preparation. The value of beta-blockers is limited by their contra-indications (section 2.4) and also by their interactions (see Appendix 1, beta-blockers).

Tricyclic antidepressants (section 4.3.1) [unlicensed] may usefully be prescribed in a dose, for example, of amitriptyline 10 mg at night, increasing to a maintenance dose of 50 to 75 mg at night.

Sodium valproate (section 4.8.1) [unlicensed] may be effective in a dose of 300 mg twice daily.

Cyproheptadine (section 3.4.1), an antihistamine with serotonin-antagonist and calcium channel-blocking properties, may also be tried in refractory cases.

Clonidine (*Dixarit*®) is **not** recommended and may aggravate depression or produce insomnia. **Methysergide**, a semi-synthetic ergot alkaloid, has dangerous side-effects (retroperitoneal fibrosis and fibrosis of the heart valves and pleura); **important:** it should only be administered under hospital supervision.

PIZOTIFEN

Indications: prevention of vascular headache including classical migraine, common migraine, and cluster headache

Cautions: urinary retention; angle-closure glaucoma, renal impairment; pregnancy and breast-feeding; **interactions:** Appendix 1 (pizotifen)
DRIVING. Drowsiness may affect performance of skilled tasks (e.g. driving); effects of alcohol enhanced

Side-effects: antimuscarinic effects, drowsiness, increased appetite and weight gain; occasionally nausea, dizziness; rarely depression; CNS stimulation may occur in children

Dose: 1.5 mg at night *or* 500 micrograms 3 times daily (but see also notes above), adjusted according to response; max. single dose 3 mg, max. daily dose 4.5 mg; CHILD up to 1.5 mg daily in divided doses; max. single dose at night 1 mg

Pizotifen (Non-proprietary) PoM
Tablets, pizotifen (as hydrogen malate), 500 micrograms, net price 28-tab pack = £1.20; 1.5 mg, 28-tab pack = £4.14. Label: 2
Available from Alpharma, APS, IVAX

Sanomigran® (Novartis) PoM
Tablets, both ivory-yellow, s/c, pizotifen (as hydrogen malate), 500 micrograms, net price 60-tab pack = £2.57; 1.5 mg, 28-tab pack = £4.28. Label: 2
Elixir, pizotifen (as hydrogen malate) 250 micrograms/5 mL, net price 300 mL = £4.51. Label: 2

CLONIDINE HYDROCHLORIDE ▰

Indications: prevention of recurrent migraine (but see notes above), vascular headache, menopausal flushing; hypertension (section 2.5.2)

Cautions: depressive illness, concurrent antihypertensive therapy; porphyria (section 9.8.2); **interactions:** Appendix 1 (alpha$_2$-adrenoceptor stimulant)

Side-effects: dry mouth, sedation, dizziness, nausea, nocturnal restlessness; occasionally rashes

Dose: 50 micrograms twice daily, increased after 2 weeks to 75 micrograms twice daily if necessary; CHILD not recommended

Clonidine (Non-proprietary) PoM ▰
Tablets, clonidine hydrochloride 25 micrograms. Net price 112-tab pack = £7.11
Available from Sandoz

Dixarit® (Boehringer Ingelheim) PoM ▰
Tablets, blue, s/c, clonidine hydrochloride 25 micrograms. Net price 112-tab pack = £7.11

Catapres® PoM ▰
(hypertension), section 2.5.2

METHYSERGIDE ▰

Indications: prevention of severe recurrent migraine, cluster headache and other vascular headaches in patients who are refractory to other treatment and whose lives are seriously disrupted (**important:** hospital supervision only, see notes above); diarrhoea associated with carcinoid syndrome

Cautions: history of peptic ulceration; avoid abrupt withdrawal of treatment; after 6 months withdraw (gradually over 2 to 3 weeks) for reassessment for at least 1 month (see also notes above); **interactions:** Appendix 1 (ergot alkaloids)

Contra-indications: renal, hepatic, pulmonary, and cardiovascular disease, severe hypertension, collagen disease, cellulitis, urinary-tract disorders, cachectic or septic conditions, pregnancy, breast-feeding

Side-effects: nausea, vomiting, heartburn, abdominal discomfort, drowsiness, and dizziness occur frequently in initial treatment; mental and behavioural disturbances, insomnia, oedema, weight gain, rashes, loss of scalp hair, cramps, arterial spasm (including coronary artery spasm with angina and possible myocardial infarction), paraesthesias of extremities, postural hypotension, and tachycardia also occur; retroperitoneal and other abnormal fibrotic reactions may occur on prolonged administration, requiring immediate withdrawal of treatment

Dose: initially 1 mg at bedtime, increased gradually over about 2 weeks to 1–2 mg 3 times daily with food (see notes above); CHILD not recommended

Diarrhoea associated with carcinoid syndrome, usual range, 12–20 mg daily (hospital supervision); CHILD not recommended

Deseril® (Alliance) PoM ▰
Tablets, s/c, methysergide (as maleate) 1 mg, net price 60-tab pack = £13.80. Label: 2, 21

4.7.4.3 Cluster headache

Cluster headache rarely responds to standard analgesics. **Sumatriptan** given by subcutaneous injection is the drug of choice for the *treatment* of cluster headache. Alternatively, 100% **oxygen** at a rate of 7–12 litres/minute is useful in aborting an attack.

Prophylaxis of cluster headache is considered if the attacks are frequent, or last over 3 weeks, or if the attacks cannot be treated effectively. **Verapamil** and **lithium** [both unlicensed use] are used for prophylaxis. **Ergotamine**, used on an intermittent basis is an alternative for patients with short bouts, but it should **not** be used for prolonged periods. **Methysergide** is effective but must be used with extreme caution (see section 4.7.4.2) and only if other drugs cannot be used or if they are not effective.

4.8   Antiepileptics

4.8.1   Control of epilepsy
4.8.2   Drugs used in status epilepticus
4.8.3   Febrile convulsions

4.8.1   Control of epilepsy

The object of treatment is to prevent the occurrence of seizures by maintaining an effective dose of one or more antiepileptic drugs. Careful adjustment of doses is necessary, starting with low doses and increasing gradually until seizures are controlled or there are overdose effects.

The frequency of administration is often determined by the plasma half-life, and should be kept as low as possible to encourage better patient compliance. Most antiepileptics, when used in average dosage, may be given twice daily. Phenobarbital and sometimes phenytoin, which have long half-lives, may often be given as a daily dose at bedtime. However, with large doses, some antiepileptics may need to be administered 3 times daily to avoid adverse effects associated with high peak plasma concentrations. Young children metabolise antiepileptics more rapidly than adults and therefore require more frequent doses and a higher amount per kilogram body-weight.

COMBINATION THERAPY. Therapy with two or more antiepileptic drugs concurrently may be necessary; it should preferably only be used when monotherapy with several alternative drugs has proved ineffective. Combination therapy enhances toxicity and drug interactions may occur between antiepileptics (see below).

INTERACTIONS. Interactions between antiepileptics are complex and may enhance toxicity without a corresponding increase in antiepileptic effect. Interactions are usually caused by *hepatic enzyme induction* or *hepatic enzyme inhibition*; *displacement from protein binding sites* is not usually a problem. These interactions are highly variable and unpredictable. Plasma monitoring is therefore often advisable with combination therapy.

Significant interactions that occur **between antiepileptics** themselves are as follows:

> NOTE. Check under each drug for possible interactions when two or more antiepileptic drugs are used

Carbamazepine
often lowers plasma concentration of *clobazam, clonazepam, lamotrigine, an active metabolite of oxcarbazepine*, and of *phenytoin* (but may also raise phenytoin concentration), *tiagabine, topiramate, and valproate*
sometimes lowers plasma concentration of *ethosuximide, and primidone* (but tendency for corresponding increase in phenobarbital level)
Ethosuximide
sometimes raises plasma concentration of *phenytoin*
Gabapentin
no interactions with gabapentin reported

Lamotrigine
sometimes raises plasma concentration of *an active metabolite of carbamazepine* (but evidence is conflicting)
Levetiracetam
no interactions with levetiracetam reported
Oxcarbazepine
sometimes lowers plasma concentration of *carbamazepine* (but may raise concentration of *an active metabolite of carbamazepine*)
sometimes raises plasma concentration of *phenytoin*
often raises plasma concentration of *phenobarbital*
Phenobarbital *or* Primidone
often lowers plasma concentration of *carbamazepine, clonazepam, lamotrigine, an active metabolite of oxcarbazepine*, and of *phenytoin* (but may also raise phenytoin concentration), *tiagabine, and valproate*
sometimes lowers plasma concentration of *ethosuximide*
Phenytoin
often lowers plasma concentration of *clonazepam, carbamazepine, lamotrigine, an active metabolite of oxcarbazepine*, and of *tiagabine, topiramate, and valproate*
often raises plasma concentration of *phenobarbital*
sometimes lowers plasma concentration of *ethosuximide, and primidone* (by increasing conversion to phenobarbital)
Topiramate
sometimes raises plasma concentration of *phenytoin*
Valproate
sometimes lowers plasma concentration of *an active metabolite of oxcarbazepine*
often raises plasma concentration of *an active metabolite of carbamazepine*, and of *lamotrigine, primidone, phenobarbital, and phenytoin* (but may also lower)
sometimes lowers plasma concentration of *ethosuximide, and primidone* (and tendency for significant increase in phenobarbital level)
Vigabatrin
often lowers plasma concentration of *phenytoin*
sometimes lowers plasma concentration of *phenobarbital, and primidone*

For other important interactions see **Appendix 1**, and for FPA guidelines on enzyme-inducing antiepileptics and **oral contraceptives**, see section 7.3.1.

WITHDRAWAL. Abrupt withdrawal of antiepileptics, particularly the barbiturates and benzodiazepines, should be avoided, as this may precipitate severe rebound seizures. Reduction in dosage should be carried out in stages and, in the case of the barbiturates, the withdrawal process may take months. The changeover from one antiepileptic drug regimen to another should be made cautiously, withdrawing the first drug only when the new regimen has been largely established.

The decision to withdraw all antiepileptics from a seizure-free patient, and its timing, is often difficult and may depend on individual patient factors. Even in patients who have been seizure-free for several years, there is a significant risk of seizure recurrence on drug withdrawal.

In patients receiving several antiepileptic drugs, only one drug should be withdrawn at a time.

DRIVING. Patients suffering from epilepsy may drive a motor vehicle (but not a heavy goods or public service vehicle) provided that they have had a seizure-free period of one year or, if subject to attacks only while asleep, have established a 3-year period of asleep attacks without awake attacks. Patients affected by drowsiness should not drive or operate machinery.

Guidance issued by the Drivers Medical Unit of the Driver and Vehicle Licensing Agency (DVLA) recommends that patients should be advised not to drive during withdrawal of antiepileptic drugs, or for 6 months afterwards (see also Drugs and Driving under General Guidance, p. 2).

PREGNANCY AND BREAST-FEEDING. During pregnancy, total plasma concentrations of antiepileptics (particularly of phenytoin) may fall, particularly in the later stages but free plasma concentrations may remain the same (or even rise). There is an increased risk of teratogenicity associated with the use of antiepileptic drugs (reduced if treatment is limited to a single drug). In view of the increased risk of neural tube and other defects associated, in particular, with **carbamazepine, oxcarbazepine, phenytoin** and **valproate** women taking antiepileptic drugs who *may become pregnant* should be **informed of the possible consequences**. Those who *wish to become pregnant* should be referred to an appropriate specialist for advice. Women who become pregnant should be **counselled** and offered **antenatal screening** (alpha-fetoprotein measurement and a second trimester ultrasound scan).

To counteract the risk of neural tube defects adequate folate supplements are advised for women before and during pregnancy; to prevent recurrence of neural tube defects, women should receive folic acid 5 mg daily (section 9.1.2)—this dose may also be appropriate for women receiving antiepileptic drugs.

In view of the risk of neonatal bleeding associated with carbamazepine, phenobarbital and phenytoin, prophylactic vitamin K_1 (section 9.6.6) is recommended for the mother before delivery (as well as for the neonate).

Breast-feeding is acceptable with all antiepileptic drugs, taken in normal doses, with the possible exception of the barbiturates, and also some of the more recently introduced ones, see Appendix 5.

Partial seizures with or without secondary generalisation

Carbamazepine, lamotrigine, sodium valproate and **phenytoin** can be used in monotherapy for secondarily generalised tonic-clonic seizures and for partial (focal) seizures; alternatively **oxcarbazepine** monotherapy can be used. **Phenobarbital** (phenobarbitone) and **primidone** are also effective but they are more sedating and are not used as first-line drugs.

Where a single drug has failed to control the seizures, combination therapy can be tried with the above drugs or with additional drugs, such as gabapentin, tiagabine, topiramate, or vigabatrin; alternatives include acetazolamide, clobazam, and clonazepam.

Generalised seizures

TONIC-CLONIC SEIZURES (GRAND MAL). The drugs of choice for tonic-clonic seizures are **carbamazepine, lamotrigine, phenytoin**, and **sodium valproate**. For those patients who have tonic-clonic seizures as part of the syndrome of primary generalised epilepsy, **sodium valproate** is the drug of choice. **Phenobarbital** and **primidone** are also effective but may be more sedating.

ABSENCE SEIZURES (PETIT MAL). **Ethosuximide** and **sodium valproate** are the drugs of choice in simple absence seizures. Sodium valproate is also highly effective in treating the tonic-clonic seizures which may co-exist with absence seizures in primary generalised epilepsy. **Lamotrigine** may also be effective [unlicensed indication].

MYOCLONIC SEIZURES. Myoclonic seizures (myoclonic jerks) occur in a variety of syndromes, and response to treatment varies considerably. **Sodium valproate** is the drug of choice and **clonazepam, ethosuximide**, or **lamotrigine** may be used. For reference to the adjunctive use of piracetam, see section 4.9.3.

ATYPICAL ABSENCE, ATONIC, AND TONIC SEIZURES. These seizure types are usually seen in childhood, in specific epileptic syndromes, or associated with cerebral damage or mental retardation. They may respond poorly to the traditional drugs. **Phenytoin, sodium valproate, lamotrigine, clonazepam, ethosuximide**, and **phenobarbital** may be tried. Second-line antiepileptic drugs that are occasionally helpful, include **acetazolamide** and **corticosteroids**.

Carbamazepine and oxcarbazepine

Carbamazepine is a drug of choice for simple and complex partial seizures and for tonic-clonic seizures secondary to a focal discharge. It has a wider therapeutic index than phenytoin and the relationship between dose and plasma-carbamazepine concentration is linear, but monitoring of plasma-carbamazepine concentrations may be helpful in determining optimum dosage. It has generally fewer side-effects than phenytoin or the barbiturates, but reversible blurring of vision, dizziness, and unsteadiness are dose-related, and may be dose-limiting. These side-effects may be reduced by altering the timing of medication; use of modified-release tablets also significantly lessens the incidence of dose-related side-effects. It is essential to initiate carbamazepine therapy at a low dose and build this up slowly with increments of 100–200 mg every two weeks.

Oxcarbazepine is licensed for the treatment of partial seizures with or without secondarily generalised tonic-clonic seizures. Oxcarbazepine induces hepatic enzymes to a lesser extent than carbamazepine.

CARBAMAZEPINE

Indications: partial and secondary generalised tonic-clonic seizures, some primary generalised seizures; trigeminal neuralgia; prophylaxis of bipolar disorder unresponsive to lithium

Cautions: hepatic or renal impairment; cardiac disease (see also Contra-indications), skin reactions (see also Blood, hepatic or skin disorders below and under Side-effects), history of haematological reactions to other drugs; manufacturer recommends blood counts and hepatic and renal function tests (but evidence of practical value unsatisfactory); glaucoma; pregnancy (**important:** see p. 227 and Appendix 4 (neural tube screening)), breast-feeding (see p. 227); avoid abrupt withdrawal; **interactions:** see p. 226 and Appendix 1 (carbamazepine)

BLOOD, HEPATIC OR SKIN DISORDERS. Patients or their carers should be told how to recognise signs of blood, liver, or skin disorders, and advised to seek immediate medical attention if symptoms such as fever, sore throat, rash, mouth ulcers, bruising, or bleeding develop. Leucopenia which is severe, progressive or associated with clinical symptoms requires withdrawal (if necessary under cover of suitable alternative).

Contra-indications: AV conduction abnormalities (unless paced); history of bone marrow depression, porphyria (section 9.8.2)

Side-effects: nausea and vomiting, dizziness, drowsiness, headache, ataxia, confusion and agitation (elderly), visual disturbances (especially double vision and often associated with peak plasma concentrations); constipation or diarrhoea, anorexia; mild transient generalised erythematous rash may occur in a large number of patients (withdraw if worsens or is accompanied by other symptoms); leucopenia and other blood disorders (including thrombocytopenia, agranulocytosis and aplastic anaemia); other side-effects include cholestatic jaundice, hepatitis and acute renal failure, Stevens-Johnson syndrome, toxic epidermal necrolysis, alopecia, thromboembolism, arthralgia, fever, proteinuria, lymph node enlargement, cardiac conduction disturbances (sometimes arrhythmias), dyskinesias, paraesthesia, depression, impotence (and impaired fertility), gynaecomastia, galactorrhoea, aggression, activation of psychosis; photosensitivity, pulmonary hypersensitivity (with dyspnoea and pneumonitis), hyponatraemia, oedema, and disturbances of bone metabolism (with osteomalacia) also reported; suppositories may cause occasional rectal irritation

Dose: *by mouth*, epilepsy, initially, 100–200 mg 1–2 times daily, increased slowly (see notes above) to usual dose of 0.8–1.2 g daily in divided doses; in some cases 1.6–2 g daily may be needed; ELDERLY reduce initial dose; CHILD daily in divided doses, up to 1 year 100–200 mg, 1–5 years 200–400 mg, 5–10 years 400–600 mg, 10–15 years 0.6–1 g
Trigeminal neuralgia, initially 100 mg 1–2 times daily (but some patients may require higher initial dose), increased gradually according to response; usual dose 200 mg 3–4 times daily, up to 1.6 g daily in some patients
Prophylaxis of bipolar disorder unresponsive to lithium (see also section 4.2.3), initially 400 mg daily in divided doses increased until symptoms controlled; usual range 400–600 mg daily; max. 1.6 g daily
By rectum, as suppositories, see below
NOTE. Plasma concentration for optimum response 4–12 mg/litre (20–50 micromol/litre)

Carbamazepine (Non-proprietary) PoM
Tablets, carbamazepine 100 mg, net price 20 = 58p; 200 mg, 20 = £1.07; 400 mg, 20 = £2.11. Label: 3, 8, counselling, blood, hepatic or skin disorder symptoms (see above), driving (see notes above)
Available from Alpharma, APS, Generics (*Carbagen*®), Hillcross, IVAX (*Epimaz*®)
NOTE. Different preparations may vary in bioavailability; to avoid reduced effect or excessive side-effects, it may be prudent to avoid changing the formulation (see also notes above on how side-effects may be reduced)

Tegretol® (Cephalon) PoM
Tablets, all scored, carbamazepine 100 mg, net price 84-tab pack = £2.43; 200 mg, 84-tab pack = £4.50; 400 mg, 56-tab pack = £5.90. Label: 3, 8, counselling, blood, hepatic or skin disorder symptoms (see above), driving (see notes above)
Chewtabs, orange, carbamazepine 100 mg, net price 56-tab pack = £3.54; 200 mg, 56-tab pack = £6.59. Label: 3, 8, 21, 24, counselling, blood, hepatic or skin disorder symptoms (see above), driving (see notes above)
Liquid, sugar-free, carbamazepine 100 mg/5 mL. Net price 300-mL pack =£6.86. Label: 3, 8, counselling, blood, hepatic or skin disorder symptoms (see above), driving (see notes above)
Suppositories, carbamazepine 125 mg, net price 5 = £9.00; 250 mg, 5 = £12.00. Label: 3, 8, counselling, blood, hepatic or skin disorder symptoms (see above), driving (see notes above)
Dose: epilepsy, for short-term use (max. 7 days) when oral therapy temporarily not possible; suppositories of 125 mg may be considered to be approximately equivalent in therapeutic effect to tablets of 100 mg but final adjustment should always depend on clinical response (plasma concentration monitoring recommended); max. by rectum 1 g daily in 4 divided doses

■ Modified release
Tegretol® **Retard** (Cephalon) PoM
Tablets, m/r, both scored, carbamazepine 200 mg (beige-orange), net price 56-tab pack = £5.26; 400 mg (brown-orange), 56-tab pack = £10.34. Label: 3, 8, 25, counselling, blood, hepatic or skin disorder symptoms (see above), driving (see notes above)
Dose: epilepsy (ADULT and CHILD over 5 years), as above; trigeminal neuralgia, as above; total daily dose given in 2 divided doses

Teril® **Retard** (Taro) PoM
Tablets, m/r, scored, carbamazepine 200 mg, net price 56-tab pack = £4.85; 400 mg, 56-tab pack = £9.50. Label: 3, 8, 25, counselling, blood, hepatic or skin disorder symptoms (see above), driving (see notes above)
Dose: epilepsy (ADULT and CHILD over 5 years), as above; trigeminal neuralgia, as above; total daily dose given in 1–2 divided doses; bipolar disorder, as above

Timonil® **retard** (CP) PoM
Tablets, m/r, scored, carbamazepine 200 mg, net price 30-tab pack = £2.55; 400 mg, 30-tab pack = £5.05. Label: 3, 8, 25, counselling, blood, hepatic or skin disorder symptoms (see above), driving (see notes above)
Dose: epilepsy (ADULT and CHILD over 1 year), as above; bipolar disorder, as above; trigeminal neuralgia, as above; total daily dose given in 1–2 divided doses

OXCARBAZEPINE

Indications: monotherapy and adjunctive treatment of partial seizures with or without secondarily generalised tonic-clonic seizures

Cautions: hypersensitivity to carbamazepine; avoid abrupt withdrawal; hepatic impairment (Appendix 2), renal impairment (Appendix 3), pregnancy (see p. 227 and Appendix 4), breast-feeding (Appendix 5); elderly, hyponatraemia (monitor plasma-sodium concentration in patients at risk), heart failure (monitor body-weight), cardiac conduction disorders; **interactions:** Appendix 1 (oxcarbazepine)

BLOOD, HEPATIC OR SKIN DISORDERS. Patients or their carers should be told how to recognise signs of blood, liver, or skin disorders, and advised to seek immediate medical attention if symptoms such as lethargy, confusion, muscular twitching, fever, sore throat, rash, blistering, mouth ulcers, bruising, or bleeding develop

Side-effects: nausea, vomiting, constipation, diarrhoea, abdominal pain, dizziness, headache, drowsiness, agitation, amnesia, asthenia, ataxia, confusion, impaired concentration, depression, tremor, hyponatraemia, acne, alopecia, rash, vertigo, nystagmus, visual disorders including diplopia; less commonly urticaria, leucopenia; rarely arrhythmias, Stevens-Johnson syndrome, systemic lupus erythematosus, hepatitis, thrombocytopenia, angioedema, hypersensitivity reactions

Dose: initially 300 mg twice daily increased according to response in steps of up to 600 mg daily at weekly intervals; usual dose range 0.6–2.4 g daily in divided doses; CHILD over 6 years, 8–10 mg/kg daily in 2 divided doses increased according to response in steps of up to 10 mg/kg daily at weekly intervals (in adjunctive therapy, maintenance dose approx. 30 mg/kg daily); max. 46 mg/kg daily in divided doses

NOTE. In adjunctive therapy, patients may require dose reduction of concomitant antiepileptics when using high doses of oxcarbazepine

Trileptal® (Novartis) ▼ PoM
Tablets, f/c, scored, all yellow, oxcarbazepine 150 mg, net price 50-tab pack = £10.00; 300 mg, 50-tab pack = £20.00; 600 mg, 50-tab pack = £40.00. Label: 3, 8, counselling, blood, hepatic or skin disorders (see above), driving (see notes above)
Oral suspension, sugar-free, oxcarbazepine 300 mg/ 5 mL, net price 250 mL (with oral syringe) = £40.00. Label: 3, 8, counselling, blood, hepatic or skin disorders (see above), driving (see notes above)

Ethosuximide

Ethosuximide is sometimes used in simple absence seizures; it may also be used in myoclonic seizures and in atypical absence, atonic, and tonic seizures.

ETHOSUXIMIDE

Indications: absence seizures

Cautions: see notes above; hepatic and renal impairment; manufacturer recommends blood counts and hepatic and renal function tests (but evidence of practical value unsatisfactory); pregnancy (see p. 227 and Appendix 4) and breast-feeding (Appendix 5); avoid sudden with-

drawal; porphyria (see section 9.8.2); **interactions:** Appendix 1 (ethosuximide)

BLOOD DISORDERS. Patients or their carers should be told how to recognise signs of blood disorders, and advised to seek immediate medical attention if symptoms such as fever, sore throat, mouth ulcers, bruising or bleeding develop

Side-effects: gastro-intestinal disturbances, weight loss, drowsiness, dizziness, ataxia, dyskinesia, hiccup, photophobia, headache, depression, and mild euphoria. Psychotic states, rashes, hepatic and renal changes (see Cautions), and haematological disorders such as agranulocytosis and aplastic anaemia occur rarely (blood counts required if signs or symptoms of infection); systemic lupus erythematosus and erythema multiforme (Stevens-Johnson syndrome) reported; other side-effects reported include gum hypertrophy, swelling of tongue, irritability, hyperactivity, sleep disturbances, night terrors, inability to concentrate, aggressiveness, increased libido, myopia, vaginal bleeding

Dose: ADULT and CHILD over 6 years initially, 500 mg daily, increased by 250 mg at intervals of 4–7 days to usual dose of 1–1.5 g daily; occasionally up to 2 g daily may be needed; CHILD up to 6 years initially 250 mg daily, increased gradually to usual dose of 20 mg/kg daily

NOTE. Plasma concentration for optimum response 40–100 mg/litre (300–700 micromol/litre)

Emeside® (LAB) PoM
Capsules, orange, ethosuximide 250 mg. Net price 112-cap pack = £11.15. Label: 8, counselling, blood disorders (see above), driving (see notes above)
Syrup, blackcurrant, ethosuximide 250 mg/5 mL. Net price 200-mL pack = £6.00. Label: 8, counselling, blood disorders (see above), driving (see notes above)

Zarontin® (Parke-Davis) PoM
Capsules, yellow, ethosuximide 250 mg. Net price 56-cap pack = £5.41. Label: 8, counselling, blood disorders (see above), driving (see notes above)
Syrup, yellow, ethosuximide 250 mg/5 mL. Net price 200-mL pack = £4.48. Label: 8, counselling, blood disorders (see above), driving (see notes above)

Gabapentin

Gabapentin can be given as adjunctive therapy in partial epilepsy with or without secondary generalisation. It is also licensed for the treatment of neuropathic pain (section 4.7.3).

GABAPENTIN

Indications: adjunctive treatment of partial seizures with or without secondary generalisation not satisfactorily controlled with other antiepileptics; neuropathic pain (section 4.7.3)

Cautions: avoid sudden withdrawal (taper off over at least 1 week); history of psychotic illness, elderly (may need to reduce dose), renal impairment (Appendix 3), diabetes mellitus, false positive readings with some urinary protein tests; pregnancy (see p. 227 and Appendix 4) and breast-feeding (see p. 227 and Appendix 5); **interactions:** Appendix 1 (gabapentin)

Side-effects: drowsiness, dizziness, ataxia, fatigue; also nystagmus, tremor, diplopia, amblyopia; pharyngitis, dysarthria, weight gain, dyspepsia, amnesia, nervousness, coughing, asthenia, paraesthesia, arthralgia, purpura, leucopenia; rhinitis, myalgia, headache, rarely impotence, urinary incontinence, pancreatitis, altered liver function tests, and Stevens-Johnson syndrome; nausea and vomiting reported

Dose: epilepsy, 300 mg on day 1, then 300 mg twice daily on day 2, then 300 mg 3 times daily (approx. every 8 hours) on day 3, then increased according to response in steps of 300 mg daily (in 3 divided doses) to max. 2.4 g daily, usual range 0.9–1.2 g daily; CHILD 6–12 years (specialist use only) 10 mg/kg on day 1, then 20 mg/kg on day 2, then 25–35 mg/kg daily (in 3 divided doses approx. every 8 hours), maintenance 900 mg daily (body-weight 26–36 kg) or 1.2 g daily (body-weight 37–50 kg)

Neuropathic pain, 300 mg on day 1, then 300 mg twice daily on day 2, then 300 mg 3 times daily on day 3, then increased according to response in steps of 300 mg daily (in 3 divided doses) to max. 1.8 g daily

Neurontin® (Parke-Davis) PoM
Capsules, gabapentin 100 mg (white), net price 100-cap pack = £22.86; 300 mg (yellow), 100-cap pack = £53.00; 400 mg (orange), 100-cap pack = £61.33; titration pack of 40 × 300-mg (yellow) capsules with 10 × 600-mg tablets = £31.80. Label: 3, 5, 8, counselling, driving (see notes above)
Tablets, gabapentin 600 mg, net price 100-tab pack = £106.00; 800 mg, 100-tab pack = £122.66. Label: 3, 5, 8, counselling, driving (see notes above)

Lamotrigine

Lamotrigine is an antiepileptic for partial seizures and primary and secondarily generalised tonic-clonic seizures. It is also used for myoclonic seizures and may be tried for atypical absence, atonic, and tonic seizures in the Lennox-Gastaut syndrome. Lamotrigine may cause serious skin rash especially in children; dose recommendations should be adhered to closely.

Lamotrigine is used either as sole treatment or as an adjunct to treatment with other antiepileptic drugs. Valproate increases plasma-lamotrigine concentration whereas the enzyme inducing antiepileptics reduce it; care is therefore required in choosing the appropriate initial dose and subsequent titration. Where the potential for interaction is not known, treatment should be initiated with lower doses such as those used with valproate.

LAMOTRIGINE

Indications: monotherapy and adjunctive treatment of partial seizures and primary and secondarily generalised tonic-clonic seizures; seizures associated with Lennox-Gastaut syndrome

Cautions: closely monitor (including hepatic, renal and clotting parameters) and consider withdrawal if rash, fever, influenza-like symptoms, drowsiness, or worsening of seizure control develops (although causal relationship not established, lamotrigine given with other antiepileptics has been

associated with rapidly progressive illness with status epilepticus, multi-organ dysfunction, disseminated intravascular coagulation and death); avoid abrupt withdrawal (taper off over 2 weeks or longer) unless serious skin reaction occurs; hepatic impairment (Appendix 2); renal impairment (Appendix 3); elderly; pregnancy and breast-feeding; monitor body-weight in children and review dose if necessary; **interactions:** see p. 226 and Appendix 1 (lamotrigine)

BLOOD DISORDERS. The CSM has advised prescribers to be alert for symptoms and signs suggestive of bone-marrow failure such as anaemia, bruising, or infection. Aplastic anaemia, bone-marrow depression and pancytopenia have been associated rarely with lamotrigine.

Side-effects: commonly rashes (see also below)—fever, malaise, influenza-like symptoms, drowsiness and rarely hepatic dysfunction, lymphadenopathy, leucopenia, and thrombocytopenia reported in conjunction with rash; angioedema, and photosensitivity also reported; diplopia, blurred vision, conjunctivitis, dizziness, drowsiness, insomnia, headache, ataxia, tiredness, gastro-intestinal disturbances (including vomiting), irritability, aggression, tremor, agitation, confusion; headache, nausea, dizziness, diplopia and ataxia in patients also taking carbamazepine usually resolve when dose of either drug reduced

SKIN REACTIONS. Serious skin reactions including Stevens-Johnson syndrome and toxic epidermal necrolysis (rarely with fatalities) have developed especially in children; most rashes occur in the first 8 weeks. The CSM has advised that factors associated with increased risk of serious skin reactions include concomitant use of valproate, initial lamotrigine dosing higher than recommended, and more rapid dose escalation than recommended.

COUNSELLING. Warn patients to see their doctor immediately if rash or influenza-like symptoms associated with hypersensitivity develop

Dose: IMPORTANT. Do not confuse the different combinations; see also notes above

Monotherapy, initially 25 mg daily for 14 days, increased to 50 mg daily for further 14 days, then increased by max. of 50–100 mg every 7–14 days; usual maintenance as monotherapy, 100–200 mg daily in 1–2 divided doses (up to 500 mg daily has been required)

Adjunctive therapy *with valproate*, initially 25 mg every other day for 14 days then 25 mg daily for further 14 days, thereafter increased by max. of 25–50 mg every 7–14 days; usual maintenance, 100–200 mg daily in 1–2 divided doses

Adjunctive therapy (with enzyme inducing drugs) *without valproate*, initially 50 mg daily for 14 days then 50 mg twice daily for further 14 days, thereafter increased by max. of 100 mg every 7–14 days; usual maintenance 200–400 mg daily in 2 divided doses (up to 700 mg daily has been required)

CHILD under 12 years, *monotherapy*, not recommended

CHILD 2–12 years, adjunctive therapy *with valproate*, initially 150 micrograms/kg daily for 14 days (those weighing 17–33 kg may receive 5 mg on alternate days for first 14 days) then 300 micrograms/kg daily for further 14 days, thereafter increased by 300 micrograms/kg every 7–14 days; usual maintenance 1–5 mg/kg daily in 1–2 divided doses

CHILD 2–12 years adjunctive therapy (with enzyme

inducing drugs) *without valproate*, initially 600 micrograms/kg daily in 2 divided doses for 14 days then 1.2 mg/kg daily in 2 divided doses for further 14 days, thereafter increased by 1.2 mg/kg every 7–14 days; usual maintenance 5–15 mg/kg daily in 2 divided doses

Lamictal® (GSK) PoM
Tablets, all yellow, lamotrigine 25 mg, net price 21-tab pack ('*Valproate Add-on therapy' Starter Pack*) = £8.23, 42-tab pack ('*Monotherapy' Starter Pack*) = £16.45, 56-tab pack = £21.95; 50 mg, 42-tab pack ('*Non-valproate Add-on therapy' Starter Pack*) = £27.98, 56-tab pack = £37.31; 100 mg, 56-tab pack = £64.37; 200 mg, 56-tab pack = £109.42. Label: 8, counselling, driving (see notes above)
Dispersible tablets, chewable, lamotrigine 5 mg (scored), net price 28-tab pack = £8.75; 25 mg, 56-tab pack = £21.95; 100 mg, 56-tab pack = £64.37. Label: 8, 13, counselling, driving (see notes above)

Levetiracetam

Levetiracetam is licensed for the adjunctive treatment of partial seizures.

LEVETIRACETAM
Indications: adjunctive treatment of partial seizures with or without secondary generalisation
Cautions: hepatic impairment (Appendix 2); renal impairment (Appendix 3); pregnancy (see p. 227 and Appendix 4); breast-feeding (Appendix 5); avoid sudden withdrawal
Side-effects: drowsiness, asthenia, dizziness; less commonly, anorexia, diarrhoea, dyspepsia, nausea, amnesia, ataxia, depression, emotional lability, aggression, insomnia, nervousness, tremor, vertigo, headache, diplopia, rash; also respiratory-tract infection
Dose: initially 1 g daily in 2 divided doses, adjusted in increments of 1 g every 2 to 4 weeks; max. 3 g daily in 2 divided doses; CHILD under 16 years not recommended

Keppra® (UCB Pharma) ▼ PoM
Tablets, f/c, levetiracetam 250 mg (blue), net price 60-tab pack = £29.70; 500 mg (yellow), 60-tab pack = £49.50; 1 g (white), 60-tab pack = £94.50. Label: 8

Phenobarbital and other barbiturates

Phenobarbital (phenobarbitone) is effective for tonic-clonic and partial seizures but may be sedative in adults and cause behavioural disturbances and hyperkinesia in children. It may be tried for atypical absence, atonic, and tonic seizures. Rebound seizures may be a problem on withdrawal. Monitoring plasma concentrations is less useful than with other drugs because tolerance occurs.

Primidone is largely converted to phenobarbital and this is probably responsible for its antiepileptic action. A small starting dose of primidone (125 mg) is essential, and the drug should be introduced over several weeks.

PHENOBARBITAL
(Phenobarbitone)
Indications: all forms of epilepsy except absence seizures; status epilepticus (section 4.8.2)
Cautions: elderly, debilitated, children, impaired renal or hepatic function, respiratory depression (avoid if severe), pregnancy and breast-feeding (see notes above); avoid sudden withdrawal; see also notes above; avoid in porphyria (see section 9.8.2); **interactions:** see p. 226 and Appendix 1 (barbiturates)
Side-effects: drowsiness, lethargy, mental depression, ataxia and allergic skin reactions; paradoxical excitement, restlessness and confusion in the elderly and hyperkinesia in children; megaloblastic anaemia (may be treated with folic acid); **overdosage:** see Emergency Treatment of Poisoning, p. 25
Dose: *by mouth*, 60–180 mg at night; CHILD 5–8 mg/kg daily
Control of acute seizures, *by intramuscular injection*, 200 mg, repeated after 6 hours if necessary; CHILD 15 mg/kg as a single dose
Status epilepticus, *by intravenous injection* (dilute injection 1 in 10 with water for injections), 10 mg/kg at a rate of not more than 100 mg/minute; max. 1 g
NOTE. For therapeutic purposes phenobarbital and phenobarbital sodium may be considered equivalent in effect. Plasma concentration for optimum response 15–40 mg/litre (60–180 micromol/litre)

[1]**Phenobarbital** (Non-proprietary) CD
Tablets, phenobarbital 15 mg, net price 20 = 45p; 30 mg, 20 = 48p; 60 mg, 20 = 52p. Label: 2, 8, counselling, driving (see notes above)
Elixir, phenobarbital 15 mg/5 mL in a suitable flavoured vehicle, containing alcohol 38%, net price 100 mL = 77p. Label: 2, 8, counselling, driving (see notes above)
NOTE. Some hospitals supply **alcohol-free** formulations of varying phenobarbital strengths
Injection, phenobarbital sodium 200 mg/mL in propylene glycol 90% and water for injections 10%, net price 1-mL amp = £1.74
NOTE. Must be diluted before intravenous administration (see under Dose)
Available from Concord (¹*Gardenal Sodium*® CD), Martindale; other strengths also available from Martindale.

1. See p. 7 for prescribing requirements for phenobarbital

PRIMIDONE
Indications: all forms of epilepsy except absence seizures; essential tremor (also section 4.9.3)
Cautions: see under Phenobarbital; **interactions:** see p. 226 and Appendix 1 (primidone)
Side-effects: see under Phenobarbital; drowsiness, ataxia, nausea, visual disturbances, and rashes, particularly at first, usually reversible on continued administration
Dose: epilepsy, ADULT and CHILD over 9 years, initially, 125 mg daily at bedtime, increased by 125 mg every 3 days to 500 mg daily in 2 divided doses then increased by 250 mg every 3 days to max. 1.5 g daily in divided doses; CHILD under 2 years, 250–500 mg daily in 2 divided doses; 2–5 years, 500–750 mg daily in 2 divided doses; 6–9 years 0.75–1 g daily in 2 divided doses
Essential tremor, initially 50 mg daily increased

gradually over 2–3 weeks according to response; max. 750 mg daily

NOTE. Monitor plasma concentrations of derived phenobarbital. Optimum range as for phenobarbital

Mysoline® (AstraZeneca) PoM

Tablets, scored, primidone 250 mg. Net price 100-tab pack = £1.77. Label: 2, 8, counselling, driving (see notes above)

Phenytoin

Phenytoin is effective in tonic-clonic and partial seizures. It has a narrow therapeutic index and the relationship between dose and plasma concentration is non-linear; small dosage increases in some patients may produce large rises in plasma concentrations with acute toxic side-effects. Monitoring of plasma concentration greatly assists dosage adjustment. A few missed doses or a small change in drug absorption may result in a marked change in plasma concentration.

Phenytoin may cause coarse facies, acne, hirsutism, and gingival hyperplasia and so may be particularly undesirable in adolescent patients.

When only parenteral administration is possible, **fosphenytoin** (section 4.8.2), a pro-drug of phenytoin, may be convenient to give. Whereas phenytoin can be given intravenously only, fosphenytoin may also be given by intramuscular injection.

PHENYTOIN

Indications: all forms of epilepsy except absence seizures; trigeminal neuralgia if carbamazepine inappropriate (see also section 4.7.3)

Cautions: hepatic impairment (reduce dose), pregnancy (**important:** see notes above and Appendix 4), breast-feeding (see notes above); avoid sudden withdrawal; manufacturer recommends blood counts (but evidence of practical value unsatisfactory); avoid in porphyria (section 9.8.2); see also notes above; **interactions:** see p. 226 and Appendix 1 (phenytoin)

BLOOD OR SKIN DISORDERS. Patients or their carers should be told how to recognise signs of blood or skin disorders, and advised to seek immediate medical attention if symptoms such as fever, sore throat, rash, mouth ulcers, bruising, or bleeding develop. Leucopenia which is severe, progressive or associated with clinical symptoms requires withdrawal (if necessary under cover of suitable alternative)

Side-effects: nausea, vomiting, mental confusion, dizziness, headache, tremor, transient nervousness, insomnia occur commonly; rarely dyskinesias, peripheral neuropathy; ataxia, slurred speech, nystagmus and blurred vision are signs of overdosage; rashes (discontinue; if mild re-introduce cautiously but discontinue immediately if recurrence), gingival hypertrophy and tenderness, coarse facies, acne and hirsutism, fever and hepatitis; lupus erythematosus, Stevens-Johnson syndrome, toxic epidermal necrolysis, polyarteritis nodosa; lymphadenopathy; rarely haematological effects, including megaloblastic anaemia (may be treated with folic acid), leucopenia, thrombocytopenia, agranulocytosis, and aplastic anaemia; plasma-calcium concentration may be lowered (rickets and osteomalacia)

Dose: *by mouth*, initially 3–4 mg/kg daily *or* 150–300 mg daily (as a single dose *or* in 2 divided doses) increased gradually as necessary (with plasma-phenytoin concentration monitoring); usual dose 200–500 mg daily (exceptionally, higher doses may be used); CHILD initially 5 mg/kg daily in 2 divided doses, usual dose range 4–8 mg/kg daily (max. 300 mg)

By intravenous injection—section 4.8.2

NOTE. Plasma concentration for optimum response 10–20 mg/litre (40–80 micromol/litre)

COUNSELLING. Take preferably with or after food

Phenytoin (Non-proprietary) PoM

Capsules, phenytoin sodium 50 mg, net price 20 = 48p; 100 mg, 20 = 67p. Label: 8, counselling, administration, blood or skin disorder symptoms (see above), driving (see notes above)

Tablets, coated, phenytoin sodium 50 mg, net price 20 = 89p; 100 mg, 20 = £1.21. Label: 8, counselling, administration, blood or skin disorder symptoms (see above), driving (see notes above)

Available from APS—50-mg tablets may be difficult to obtain

NOTE. On the basis of single dose tests there are no clinically relevant differences in bioavailability between available phenytoin sodium tablets and capsules but there may be a pharmacokinetic basis for maintaining the same brand of phenytoin in some patients

Epanutin® (Parke-Davis) PoM

Capsules, phenytoin sodium 25 mg (white/purple), net price 20 = 47p; 50 mg (white/pink), 20 = 48p; 100 mg (white/orange), 20 = 67p; 300 mg (white/green), 20 = £2.02. Label: 8, counselling, administration, blood or skin disorder symptoms (see above), driving (see notes above)

Infatabs® (= chewable tablets), yellow, scored, phenytoin 50 mg. Net price 20 = £1.32. Label: 8, 24, counselling, blood or skin disorder symptoms (see above), driving (see notes above)

NOTE. Contain phenytoin 50 mg (as against phenytoin sodium) therefore care is needed on changing to capsules or tablets containing phenytoin sodium

Suspension, red, phenytoin 30 mg/5 mL. Net price 100 mL = 71p. Label: 8, counselling, administration, blood or skin disorder symptoms (see above), driving (see notes above)

NOTE. Suspension of phenytoin 90 mg in 15 mL may be considered to be approximately equivalent in therapeutic effect to capsules or tablets containing phenytoin sodium 100 mg, but nevertheless care is needed in making changes

Tiagabine

Tiagabine is used as adjunctive treatment for partial seizures, with or without secondary generalisation.

TIAGABINE

Indications: adjunctive treatment for partial seizures with or without secondary generalisation not satisfactorily controlled with other antiepileptics

Cautions: hepatic impairment (Appendix 2); avoid abrupt withdrawal; **interactions:** Appendix 1 (tiagabine)

DRIVING. May impair performance of skilled tasks (e.g. driving)

Side-effects: diarrhoea, dizziness, tiredness, nervousness, tremor, concentration difficulties, emotional lability, speech impairment; rarely, confusion, depression, drowsiness, psychosis; leucopenia reported

Dose: adjunctive therapy, with *enzyme-inducing* drugs, 5 mg twice daily for 1 week, then increased at weekly intervals in steps of 5–10 mg daily; usual maintenance dose 30–45 mg daily (doses above 30 mg given in 3 divided doses); in patients receiving *non-enzyme-inducing* drugs, initial maintenance dose should be 15–30 mg daily; CHILD under 12 years not recommended

Gabitril® (Cephalon) PoM
Tablets, f/c, scored, tiagabine (as hydrochloride) 5 mg, net price 100-tab pack = £45.37; 10 mg, 100-tab pack = £90.74; 15 mg, 100-tab pack = £136.11. Label: 21

Topiramate

Topiramate can be given alone or as adjunctive treatment in generalised tonic-clonic seizures or partial seizures with or without secondary generalisation. It can also be used as adjunctive treatment for seizures associated with Lennox-Gastaut syndrome.

TOPIRAMATE

Indications: monotherapy and adjunctive treatment of generalised tonic-clonic seizures or partial seizures with or without secondary generalisation; adjunctive treatment of seizures in Lennox-Gastaut syndrome

Cautions: avoid abrupt withdrawal; ensure adequate hydration (especially if predisposition to nephrolithiasis or in strenuous activity or warm environment); pregnancy (see notes above); hepatic impairment (Appendix 2); renal impairment (Appendix 3); **interactions:** see p. 226 and Appendix 1 (topiramate)

CSM ADVICE. Topiramate has been associated with acute myopia with secondary angle-closure glaucoma, typically occurring within 1 month of starting treatment. Choroidal effusions resulting in anterior displacement of the lens and iris have also been reported. The CSM advises that if raised intra-ocular pressure occurs:

- seek specialist ophthalmological advice;
- use appropriate measures to reduce intra-ocular pressure;
- stop topiramate as rapidly as feasible

Contra-indications: breast-feeding
Side-effects: nausea, abdominal pain, weight loss, anorexia; paraesthesia; hypoasthesia, headache, fatigue, dizziness, somnolence, insomnia, impaired memory and concentration, anxiety, depression, nervousness, mood instability; rarely reduced sweating mainly in children, metabolic acidosis

ADJUNCTIVE THERAPY. Commonly agitation, ataxia, asthenia, confusion, cognitive impairment, speech disorders, visual disturbances; also increased salivation, hyperkinesia and personality disorder in children; less commonly taste disturbances; abnormal gait, incoordination, psychotic reactions including hallucinations; leucopenia

Dose: monotherapy, initially 25 mg daily at night for 1 week *then* increased in steps of 25–50 mg daily at intervals of 1–2 weeks taken in 2 divided doses; usual dose 100 mg daily in 2 divided doses; max. 400 mg daily; CHILD 6–16 years, initially 0.5–1 mg/kg daily at night for 1 week *then* increased in steps of 0.5–1 mg/kg daily at intervals of 1–2 weeks taken in 2 divided doses; usual dose 3–

6 mg/kg daily in 2 divided doses; max. 16 mg/kg daily

Adjunctive therapy, initially 25 mg daily for 1 week *then* increased in steps of 25–50 mg daily at intervals of 1–2 weeks; usual dose 200–400 mg daily in 2 divided doses; max. 800 mg daily; CHILD 2–16 years, initially 25 mg daily at night for one week *then* increased in steps of 1–3 mg/kg daily at intervals of 1–2 weeks taken in 2 divided doses; recommended dose range 5–9 mg/kg daily in 2 divided doses; max. 30 mg/kg daily

NOTE. If patient cannot tolerate titration regimen recommended above then smaller steps or longer interval between steps may be used

Topamax® (Janssen-Cilag) PoM
Tablets, f/c, topiramate 25 mg, net price 60-tab pack = £22.02; 50 mg (light yellow), 60-tab pack = £36.17; 100 mg (yellow), 60-tab pack = £64.80; 200 mg (salmon), 60-tab pack = £125.83. Label: 3, 8, counselling, driving (see notes above)
Sprinkle capsules, topiramate 15 mg, net price 60-cap pack = £16.88; 25 mg, 60-cap pack = £25.32; 50 mg, 60-cap pack = £41.60. Label: 3, 8, counselling, administration, driving (see notes above)

COUNSELLING. Swallow whole or open capsule and sprinkle contents on soft food

Valproate

Sodium valproate is effective in controlling tonic-clonic seizures, particularly in primary generalised epilepsy. It is a drug of choice in primary generalised epilepsy, generalised absences and myoclonic seizures, and may be tried in atypical absence, atonic, and tonic seizures. Controlled trials in partial epilepsy suggest that it has similar efficacy to that of carbamazepine and phenytoin. Plasma-valproate concentrations are not a useful index of efficacy, therefore routine monitoring is unhelpful. The drug has widespread metabolic effects, and may have dose-related side-effects.

Valproic acid (as semisodium valproate) (section 4.2.3) is licensed for acute mania associated with bipolar disorder.

SODIUM VALPROATE

Indications: all forms of epilepsy
Cautions: monitor liver function before therapy and during first 6 months especially in patients most at risk (see also below); ensure no undue potential for bleeding before starting and before surgery; renal impairment (Appendix 3); pregnancy (**important** see notes above and Appendix 4 (neural tube screening)); breast-feeding; systemic lupus erythematosus; false-positive urine tests for ketones; avoid sudden withdrawal; see also notes above; **interactions:** see p. 226 and Appendix 1 (valproate)

LIVER TOXICITY. Liver dysfunction (including fatal hepatic failure) has occurred in association with valproate (especially in children under 3 years of age and those with metabolic or degenerative disorders, organic brain disease or severe seizure disorders associated with mental retardation) usually in the first 6 months of therapy and usually involving multiple antiepileptic therapy (monotherapy preferred). Raised liver enzymes are not uncommon during valproate treatment and are usually transient but patients should be reassessed clinically and liver function (including prothrombin time) monitored until return to normal—an abnormally prolonged prothrombin time (particularly in association with other relevant abnormalities) requires discontinuation of treatment. Any concomitant use of salicylates should be stopped.

BLOOD OR HEPATIC DISORDERS. Patients or their carers should be told how to recognise signs of blood or liver disorders, and advised to seek immediate medical attention if symptoms develop (advice is given on patient information leaflet).

PANCREATITIS. Patients or their carers should be told how to recognise signs of pancreatitis, and advised to seek immediate medical attention if symptoms such as abdominal pain, nausea and vomiting develop; discontinue sodium valproate if pancreatitis is diagnosed

Contra-indications: active liver disease, family history of severe hepatic dysfunction, porphyria (section 9.8.2)

Side-effects: gastric irritation, nausea, ataxia and tremor; hyperammonaemia, increased appetite and weight gain; transient hair loss (regrowth may be curly), oedema, thrombocytopenia, and inhibition of platelet aggregation; impaired hepatic function leading rarely to fatal hepatic failure (see also under Cautions—withdraw treatment immediately if vomiting, anorexia, jaundice, drowsiness, or loss of seizure control occurs); rashes; sedation reported (rarely lethargy and confusion associated with too high an initial dose) and also increased alertness (occasionally aggression, hyperactivity and behavioural disturbances); rarely pancreatitis (measure plasma amylase in acute abdominal pain; see also Pancreatitis under Cautions above), extrapyramidal symptoms, dementia, leucopenia, pancytopenia, red cell hypoplasia, fibrinogen reduction; irregular periods, amenorrhoea, gynaecomastia, hearing loss, Fanconi's syndrome, toxic epidermal necrolysis, Stevens-Johnson syndrome, vasculitis, hirsutism and acne also reported

Dose: *by mouth*, initially, 600 mg daily given in 2 divided doses, preferably after food, increasing by 200 mg/day at 3-day intervals to a max. of 2.5 g daily in divided doses, usual maintenance 1–2 g daily (20–30 mg/kg daily); CHILD up to 20 kg, initially 20 mg/kg daily in divided doses, may be increased provided plasma concentrations monitored (above 40 mg/kg daily also monitor clinical chemistry and haematological parameters); over 20 kg, initially 400 mg daily in divided doses increased until control (usually in range of 20–30 mg/kg daily); max. 35 mg/kg daily

By intravenous injection (over 3–5 minutes) or *by intravenous infusion*, continuation of valproate treatment when oral therapy not possible, same as current dose by oral route

Initiation of valproate therapy (when oral valproate not possible), *by intravenous injection* (over 3–5 minutes), 400–800 mg (up to 10 mg/kg) followed by *intravenous infusion* up to max. 2.5 g daily; CHILD, usually 20–30 mg/kg daily, may be increased provided plasma concentrations monitored (above 40 mg/kg daily also monitor clinical chemistry and haematological parameters)

Sodium Valproate (Non-proprietary) PoM
Tablets, e/c, sodium valproate 200 mg, net price 20 = £2.81; 500 mg, 20 = £2.96. Label: 5, 8, 25, counselling, blood or hepatic disorder symptoms (see above), driving (see notes above)
Available from Alpharma, APS, CP (*Orlept®*), Hillcross, IVAX, Sterwin

Oral solution, sodium valproate 200 mg/5 mL. Net price 100 mL = £1.81. Label: 8, counselling, blood or hepatic disorder symptoms (see above), driving (see notes above)
Available from CP, (*Orlept®*, sugar-free), Hillcross, IVAX (sugar-free), Sterwin

Epilim® (Sanofi-Synthelabo) PoM
Tablets (crushable), scored, sodium valproate 100 mg. Net price 20 = 78p. Label: 8, counselling, blood or hepatic disorder symptoms (see above), driving (see notes above)
NOTE. Sodium valproate crushable tablets also available from Hillcross

Tablets, both e/c, lilac, sodium valproate 200 mg, net price 20 = £1.28; 500 mg, 20 = £3.21. Label: 5, 8, 25, counselling, blood or hepatic disorder symptoms (see above), driving (see notes above)

Liquid, red, sugar-free, sodium valproate 200 mg/5 mL. Net price 300-mL pack = £6.48. Label: 8, counselling, blood or hepatic disorder symptoms (see above), driving (see notes above)

Syrup, red, sodium valproate 200 mg/5 mL. Net price 300-mL pack = £6.48. Label: 8, counselling, blood or hepatic disorder symptoms (see above), driving (see notes above)

Epilim Chrono® (Sanofi-Synthelabo) PoM
Tablets, m/r, all lilac, sodium valproate 200 mg (as sodium valproate and valproic acid), net price 100-tab pack = £8.09; 300 mg, 100-tab pack = £12.13; 500 mg, 100-tab pack = £20.21. Label: 8, 25, counselling, blood or hepatic disorder symptoms (see above), driving (see notes above)
Dose: ADULT and CHILD over 20 kg, as above, total daily dose given in 1–2 divided doses

Epilim® Intravenous (Sanofi-Synthelabo) PoM
Injection, powder for reconstitution, sodium valproate. Net price 400-mg vial (with 4-mL amp water for injections) = £9.65

■ Valproic acid

Convulex® (Pharmacia) PoM
Capsules, e/c, valproic acid 150 mg, net price 100-cap pack = £3.68; 300 mg, 100-cap pack = £7.35; 500 mg, 100-cap pack = £12.25. Label: 8, 25, counselling, blood or hepatic disorder symptoms (see above), driving (see notes above)
Dose: ADULT and CHILD initially 15 mg/kg daily in 2–4 divided doses, gradually increasing in steps of 5–10 mg/kg up to 30 mg/kg daily
EQUIVALENCE TO SODIUM VALPROATE. Manufacturer advises that *Convulex®* has a 1:1 dose relationship with products containing sodium valproate, but nevertheless care is needed in making changes.

Vigabatrin

For partial epilepsy with or without secondary generalisation, **vigabatrin** is given in combination with other antiepileptic treatment; its use is restricted to patients in whom all other combinations are inadequate or are not tolerated. It can be used as sole therapy in the management of infantile spasms in West's syndrome.

About one-third of patients treated with vigabatrin have suffered visual field defects; counselling and **careful monitoring** for this side-effect are required (see also Visual Field Defects under Cautions below). Vigabatrin has prominent behavioural side-effects in some patients.

VIGABATRIN

Indications: initiated and supervised by appropriate specialist, adjunctive treatment of partial seizures with or without secondary generalisation not satisfactorily controlled with other antiepileptics; monotherapy for management of infantile spasms (West's syndrome)

Cautions: renal impairment; elderly; closely monitor neurological function; avoid sudden withdrawal (taper off over 2–4 weeks); history of psychosis, depression or behavioural problems; pregnancy (see p. 227 and Appendix 4) and breastfeeding; absence seizures (may be exacerbated); **interactions:** see p. 226 and Appendix 1 (vigabatrin)

VISUAL FIELD DEFECTS. Vigabatrin is associated with visual field defects. The CSM has advised that onset of symptoms varies from 1 month to several years after starting. In most cases, visual field defects have persisted despite discontinuation. Product literature advises visual field testing before treatment and at 6-month intervals; a procedure for testing visual fields in those with a developmental age of less than 9 years is available from the manufacturers. Patients should be warned to report any new visual symptoms that develop and those with symptoms should be referred for an urgent ophthalmological opinion. Gradual withdrawal of vigabatrin should be considered.

Contra-indications: visual field defects

Side-effects: drowsiness (rarely marked sedation, stupor, and confusion with non-specific slow wave EEG), fatigue, visual field defects (see also under Cautions), dizziness, nervousness, irritability, behavioural effects such as excitation and agitation especially in children; depression, abnormal thinking, headache, nystagmus, ataxia, tremor, paraesthesia, impaired concentration; less commonly confusion, aggression, psychosis, mania, memory disturbance, visual disturbance (e.g. diplopia); also weight gain, oedema, gastro-intestinal disturbances, alopecia, rash; less commonly, urticaria, occasional increase in seizure frequency (especially if myoclonic), decrease in liver enzymes, slight decrease in haemoglobin; photophobia and retinal disorders (e.g. peripheral retinal atrophy); optic neuritis, optic atrophy also reported

Dose: with current antiepileptic therapy, initially 1 g daily in single or 2 divided doses then increased according to response in steps of 500 mg at weekly intervals; usual range 2–3 g daily (max. 3 g daily); CHILD initially 40 mg/kg daily in single or 2 divided doses then adjusted according to body-weight 10–15 kg, 0.5–1 g daily; body-weight 15–30 kg, 1–1.5 g daily; body-weight 30–50 kg, 1.5–3 g daily; body-weight over 50 kg, 2–3 g daily

Infantile spasms (West's syndrome), *monotherapy*, 50 mg/kg daily, adjusted according to response over 7 days; up to 150 mg/kg daily used with good tolerability

Sabril® (Aventis Pharma) [PoM]
Tablets, f/c, scored, vigabatrin 500 mg, net price 100-tab pack = £42.83. Label: 3, 8, counselling, driving (see notes above)
Powder, sugar-free, vigabatrin 500 mg/sachet. Net price 50-sachet pack = £23.24. Label: 3, 8, 13, counselling, driving (see notes above)
NOTE. The contents of a sachet should be dissolved in water or a soft drink immediately before taking

Benzodiazepines

Clonazepam is occasionally used in tonic-clonic or partial seizures, but its sedative side-effects may be prominent. **Clobazam** may be used as adjunctive therapy in the treatment of epilepsy (section 4.1.2), but the effectiveness of these and other **benzodiazepines** may wane considerably after weeks or months of continuous therapy.

CLOBAZAM

Indications: adjunct in epilepsy; anxiety (short-term use)
Cautions: see under Diazepam (section 4.1.2)
Contra-indications: see under Diazepam (section 4.1.2)
Side-effects: see under Diazepam (section 4.1.2)
Dose: epilepsy, 20–30 mg daily; max. 60 mg daily; CHILD over 3 years, not more than half adult dose
Anxiety, 20–30 mg daily in divided doses or as a single dose at bedtime, increased in severe anxiety (in hospital patients) to a max. of 60 mg daily in divided doses; ELDERLY (or debilitated) 10–20 mg daily

¹**Clobazam** (Non-proprietary) [PoM] [NHS]
Tablets, clobazam 10 mg. Net price 30-tab pack = £10.98. Label: 2 or 19, 8, counselling, driving (see notes above)
NOTE. The brand name *Frisium*® [NHS] (Hoechst Marion Roussel) is used for clobazam tablets

1. [NHS] except for epilepsy and endorsed 'SLS'

CLONAZEPAM

Indications: all forms of epilepsy; myoclonus; status epilepticus (section 4.8.2)
Cautions: see notes above; respiratory disease; hepatic and renal impairment; elderly and debilitated; pregnancy and breast-feeding (see notes above); avoid sudden withdrawal; porphyria (section 9.8.2); **interactions:** see p. 226 and Appendix 1 (anxiolytics and hypnotics)
DRIVING. Drowsiness may affect performance of skilled tasks (e.g. driving); effects of alcohol enhanced
Contra-indications: respiratory depression; acute pulmonary insufficiency
Side-effects: drowsiness, fatigue, dizziness, muscle hypotonia, coordination disturbances; hypersalivation in infants, paradoxical aggression, irritability and mental changes; rarely, blood disorders, abnormal liver-function tests; **overdosage:** see Emergency Treatment of Poisoning, p. 25
Dose: 1 mg (elderly, 500 micrograms), initially at night for 4 nights, increased over 2–4 weeks to a usual maintenance dose of 4–8 mg daily in divided doses; CHILD up to 1 year 250 micrograms increased as above to 0.5–1 mg, 1–5 years 250 micrograms increased to 1–3 mg, 5–12 years 500 micrograms increased to 3–6 mg

Rivotril® (Roche) [PoM]
Tablets, both scored, clonazepam 500 micrograms (beige), net price 20 = 84p; 2 mg (white), 20 = £1.12. Label: 2, 8, counselling, driving (see notes above)
Injection, section 4.8.2

Other drugs

Acetazolamide (section 11.6), a carbonic anhydrase inhibitor, is a second-line drug for both tonic-clonic and partial seizures. It is occasionally helpful in atypical absence, atonic, and tonic seizures.

Piracetam (section 4.9.3) is used as adjunctive treatment for cortical myoclonus.

4.8.2 Drugs used in status epilepticus

Initial management of status epilepticus includes positioning the patient to avoid injury, supporting respiration including the provision of oxygen, maintaining blood pressure, and the correction of any hypoglycaemia. The use of parenteral **thiamine** should be considered if alcohol abuse is suspected; **pyridoxine** should be administered if the status epilepticus is caused by pyridoxine deficiency.

Major status epilepticus should be treated initially with intravenous **lorazepam**. Intravenous **diazepam** may also be used, but lorazepam has a longer duration of antiepileptic action. Diazepam is associated with a high risk of venous thrombophlebitis which is reduced by using an emulsion (*Diazemuls®*). Alternatively, in prolonged or recurrent seizures, a single dose of **midazolam** (section 15.1.4.1) can be given [unlicensed use] by the buccal route (in a dose of 10 mg) or intranasally (200 micrograms/kg).

Where facilities for resuscitation are not immediately available, small doses of lorazepam or diazepam can be given intravenously, or diazepam can be administered as a rectal solution. Absorption from intramuscular injection or from suppositories is too slow for treatment of status epilepticus.

Clonazepam can also be used as an alternative.

If seizures recur or fail to respond after 30 minutes, phenytoin sodium, fosphenytoin, or phenobarbital sodium should be used.

Phenytoin sodium may be given by slow intravenous injection, with ECG monitoring, followed by the maintenance dosage. Intramuscular use of phenytoin is not recommended (absorption is slow and erratic).

Alternatively, **fosphenytoin**, a pro-drug of phenytoin, can be given more rapidly and when given intravenously causes fewer injection site reactions compared to phenytoin. Intravenous administration requires ECG monitoring. Although it can also be given intramuscularly, absorption is too slow by this route for treatment of status epilepticus. Doses of fosphenytoin should be expressed in terms of phenytoin sodium.

Alternatively, **phenobarbital sodium** can be given by intravenous injection (section 4.8.1).

Paraldehyde also remains a valuable drug. Given rectally it causes little respiratory depression and is therefore useful where facilities for resuscitation are poor.

If the above measures fail to control seizures, anaesthesia with thiopental [unlicensed indication] (section 15.1.1) or in adults, a non-barbiturate anaesthetic such as propofol [unlicensed indication] (section 15.1.1), should be instituted with full intensive care support.

DIAZEPAM

Indications: status epilepticus; convulsions due to poisoning (see Emergency Treatment of Poisoning); other indications (section 4.1.2, section 10.2.2, and section 15.1.4.1)

Cautions: see section 4.1.2; when given intravenously facilities for reversing respiratory depression with mechanical ventilation must be at hand (but see also notes above)
SPECIAL CAUTIONS FOR INTRAVENOUS INFUSION. Intravenous infusion of diazepam is potentially hazardous (especially if prolonged), calling for close and constant observation and best carried out in specialist centres with intensive care facilities. Prolonged infusion may lead to accumulation and delay recovery

Contra-indications: see section 4.1.2

Side-effects: see section 4.1.2; hypotension and apnoea

Dose: *by intravenous injection*, 10–20 mg at a rate of 0.5 mL (2.5 mg) per 30 seconds, repeated if necessary after 30–60 minutes; may be followed by *intravenous infusion* to max. 3 mg/kg over 24 hours; CHILD 200–300 micrograms/kg or 1 mg per year of age

By rectum as rectal solution, ADULT and CHILD over 10 kg 500 micrograms/kg, up to max. 30 mg (ELDERLY 250 micrograms/kg, up to max. 15 mg); repeated after 12 hours if necessary

Diazepam (Non-proprietary) ▼PoM
Injection (solution), diazepam 5 mg/mL. See Appendix 6. Net price 2-mL amp = 32p
Available from CP
Injection (emulsion), diazepam 5 mg/mL (0.5%).
See Appendix 6. Net price 2-mL amp = 73p
Available from Alpharma (*Diazemuls®*)
Rectal tubes (= rectal solution), diazepam 2 mg/mL, net price 1.25-mL (2.5-mg) tube = 90p, 2.5-mL (5-mg) tube = £1.27; 4 mg/mL, 2.5-mL (10-mg) tube = £1.62, 5-mL (20-mg) tube = £2.92
Available from Alpharma (*Stesolid®* 5 mg, 10 mg), CP (*Diazepam Rectubes®* 2.5 mg, 5 mg, 10 mg), Sandoz

■ Oral preparations
Section 4.1.2

CLONAZEPAM

Indications: status epilepticus; other forms of epilepsy, and myoclonus (section 4.8.1)

Cautions: see section 4.8.1; facilities for reversing respiratory depression with mechanical ventilation must be at hand (but see also notes above)
INTRAVENOUS INFUSION. Intravenous infusion of clonazepam is potentially hazardous (especially if prolonged), calling for close and constant observation and best carried out in specialist centres with intensive care facilities. Prolonged infusion may lead to accumulation and delay recovery

Contra-indications: see section 4.8.1; avoid injections containing benzyl alcohol in neonates (see under preparations below)

Side-effects: see section 4.8.1; hypotension and apnoea

Dose: *by intravenous injection* into a large vein (over 30 seconds) *or by intravenous infusion*, 1 mg, repeated if necessary; CHILD all ages, 500 micrograms

Rivotril® (Roche) ▼PoM
Injection, clonazepam 1 mg/mL in solvent, for dilution with 1 mL water for injections immediately before injection or as described in Appendix

6. Net price 1-mL amp (with 1 mL water for injections) = 68p

Excipients: include benzyl alcohol (avoid in neonates, see Excipients, p. 2), ethanol, propylene glycol

■ Oral preparations
Section 4.8.1

FOSPHENYTOIN SODIUM

NOTE. Fosphenytoin is a pro-drug of phenytoin

Indications: status epilepticus; seizures associated with neurosurgery or head injury; when phenytoin by mouth not possible

Cautions: see Phenytoin Sodium; liver impairment (Appendix 2); renal impairment (Appendix 3); resuscitation facilities must be available; **interactions:** see p. 226 and Appendix 1 (phenytoin)

Contra-indications: see Phenytoin Sodium

Side-effects: see Phenytoin Sodium

CSM ADVICE. Intravenous infusion of fosphenytoin has been associated with severe cardiovascular reactions including asystole, ventricular fibrillation, and cardiac arrest. Hypotension, bradycardia, and heart block have also been reported. The CSM advises:

- monitor heart rate, blood pressure, and respiratory function for duration of infusion
- observe patient for at least 30 minutes after infusion
- if hypotension occurs, reduce infusion rate or discontinue
- reduce dose or infusion rate in elderly, and in renal or hepatic impairment.

Dose: expressed as **phenytoin sodium equivalent** (PE); fosphenytoin sodium 1.5 mg ≡ phenytoin sodium 1 mg

Status epilepticus, *by intravenous infusion* (at a rate of 100–150 mg(PE)/minute), initially 15 mg(PE)/kg then *by intramuscular injection* or *by intravenous infusion* (at a rate of 50–100 mg(PE)/minute), 4–5 mg(PE)/kg daily in 1–2 divided doses, dose adjusted according to response and trough plasma-phenytoin concentration

CHILD 5 years and over, *by intravenous infusion* (at a rate of 2–3 mg(PE)/kg/minute), initially 15 mg(PE)/kg then *by intravenous infusion* (at a rate of 1–2 mg(PE)/kg/minute), 4–5 mg(PE)/kg daily in 1–4 divided doses, dose adjusted according to response and trough plasma-phenytoin concentration

Prophylaxis or treatment of seizures associated with neurosurgery or head injury, *by intramuscular injection* or *by intravenous infusion* (at a rate of 50–100 mg(PE)/minute), initially 10–15 mg(PE)/kg then *by intramuscular injection* or *by intravenous infusion* (at a rate of 50–100 mg(PE)/minute), 4–5 mg(PE)/kg daily (in 1–2 divided doses, dose adjusted according to response and trough plasma-phenytoin concentration

CHILD 5 years and over, *by intravenous infusion* (at a rate of 1–2 mg(PE)/kg/minute), initially 10–15 mg(PE)/kg then 4–5 mg(PE)/kg daily in 1–4 divided doses, dose adjusted according to response and trough plasma-phenytoin concentration

Temporary substitution for oral phenytoin, *by intramuscular injection* or *by intravenous infusion* (at a rate of 50–100 mg(PE)/minute), same dose and dosing frequency as oral phenytoin therapy; CHILD 5 years and over, *by intravenous infusion* (at a rate

of 1–2 mg(PE)/kg/minute), same dose and dosing frequency as oral phenytoin therapy

ELDERLY consider 10–25% reduction in dose or infusion rate

> NOTE. Prescriptions for fosphenytoin sodium should state the dose in terms of phenytoin sodium equivalent (PE)

Pro-Epanutin® (Parke-Davis) PoM

Injection concentrate, fosphenytoin sodium 75 mg/mL (equivalent to phenytoin sodium 50 mg/mL), net price 10-mL vial = £40.00

Electrolytes: phosphate 3.7 micromol/mg fosphenytoin sodium (phosphate 5.6 micromol/mg phenytoin sodium)

LORAZEPAM

Indications: status epilepticus; other indications (section 4.1.2)

Cautions: see section 4.1.2; facilities for reversing respiratory depression with mechanical ventilation must be at hand

Contra-indications: see section 4.1.2

Side-effects: see section 4.1.2; hypotension and apnoea

Dose: *by intravenous injection* (into large vein), 4 mg; CHILD 2 mg

■ Preparations
Section 4.1.2

PARALDEHYDE

Indications: status epilepticus

Cautions: bronchopulmonary disease, hepatic impairment; pregnancy (Appendix 4) and breast-feeding (Appendix 5); **interactions:** Appendix 1 (paraldehyde)

Contra-indications: gastric disorders; rectal administration in colitis

Side-effects: rashes; rectal irritation after enema

Dose: *by rectum*, usually 10–20 mL; CHILD up to 3 months 0.5 mL, 3–6 months 1 mL, 6–12 months 1.5 mL, 1–2 years 2 mL, 3–5 years 3–4 mL, 6–12 years 5–6 mL

ADMINISTRATION. Administer as an enema containing 1 part paraldehyde diluted with 9 parts physiological saline (some centres mix paraldehyde with an equal volume of arachis (peanut) oil instead)

NOTE. Do not use paraldehyde if it has a brownish colour or an odour of acetic acid. Avoid contact with rubber and plastics.

Paraldehyde (Non-proprietary) PoM

Injection, sterile paraldehyde, net price 5-mL amp = £9.49

Available from Mayne

PHENYTOIN SODIUM

Indications: status epilepticus; seizures in neurosurgery; arrhythmias, but now obsolete (section 2.3.2)

Cautions: hypotension and heart failure; resuscitation facilities must be available; injection solutions alkaline (irritant to tissues); see also section 4.8.1; **interactions:** see p. 226 and Appendix 1 (phenytoin)

Contra-indications: sinus bradycardia, sino-atrial block, and second- and third-degree heart block; Stokes-Adams syndrome; porphyria (section 9.8.2)

Side-effects: intravenous injection may cause cardiovascular and CNS depression (particularly if injection too rapid) with arrhythmias, hypotension, and cardiovascular collapse; alterations in respiratory function (including respiratory arrest)

Dose: *by slow intravenous injection or infusion* (with blood pressure and ECG monitoring), status epilepticus, 15 mg/kg at a rate not exceeding 50 mg per minute, as a loading dose (see also notes above); maintenance doses of about 100 mg should be given thereafter at intervals of every 6–8 hours, monitored by measurement of plasma concentrations; rate and dose reduced according to weight; CHILD 15 mg/kg as a loading dose (neonate 15–20 mg/kg at rate of 1–3 mg/kg/minute)

Ventricular arrhythmia (but use now obsolete), *by intravenous injection* via caval catheter, 3.5–5 mg/kg at a rate not exceeding 50 mg/minute, with blood pressure and ECG monitoring; repeat once if necessary

NOTE. Phenytoin is licensed for administration by intravenous infusion (at the same rate of administration as the injection—not exceeding 50 mg/minute, for further details of the infusion, see Appendix 6). To avoid local venous irritation each injection or infusion should be preceded and followed by an injection of sterile physiological saline through the same needle or catheter

By intramuscular injection, not recommended (see notes above)

Phenytoin (Non-proprietary) PoM
Injection, phenytoin sodium 50 mg/mL with propylene glycol 40% and alcohol 10% in water for injections, net price 5-mL amp = £3.63
Available from Antigen, Mayne

Epanutin® Ready-Mixed Parenteral (Parke-Davis) PoM
Injection, phenytoin sodium 50 mg/mL with propylene glycol 40% and alcohol 10% in water for injections. Net price 5-mL amp = £4.88

■ Oral preparations
Section 4.8.1

4.8.3   Febrile convulsions

Brief febrile convulsions need only simple treatment such as tepid sponging or bathing, or antipyretic medication, e.g. **paracetamol** (section 4.7.1). *Prolonged febrile convulsions* (those lasting 15 minutes or longer), *recurrent convulsions*, or those occurring in a child at known risk must be treated more actively, as there is the possibility of resulting brain damage. **Diazepam** is the drug of choice given either by slow intravenous injection in a dose of 250 micrograms/kg (section 4.8.2) or preferably rectally in solution (section 4.8.2) in a dose of 500 micrograms/kg (max. 10 mg), repeated if necessary. The rectal route is preferred as satisfactory absorption is achieved within minutes and administration is much easier. Suppositories are not suitable because absorption is too slow.

Intermittent prophylaxis (i.e. the anticonvulsant administered at the onset of fever) is possible in only a small proportion of children. Again **diazepam** is the treatment of choice, orally or rectally.

The exact role of continuous prophylaxis in children at risk from prolonged or complex febrile convulsions is controversial. It is probably indicated in only a small proportion of children, including those whose first seizure occurred at under 14 months or who have pre-existing neurological abnormalities or who have had previous prolonged or focal convulsions. Thus long-term anticonvulsant prophylaxis is rarely indicated.

4.9   Drugs used in parkinsonism and related disorders

4.9.1   Dopaminergic drugs used in parkinsonism

4.9.2   Antimuscarinic drugs used in parkinsonism

4.9.3   Drugs used in essential tremor, chorea, tics, and related disorders

In idiopathic Parkinson's disease, the progressive degeneration of pigmented neurones in the substantia nigra leads to a deficiency of the neurotransmitter dopamine. The resulting neurochemical imbalance in the basal ganglia causes the characteristic signs and symptoms of the illness. Drug therapy does not prevent disease progression, but it improves most patients' quality of life.

When initiating treatment, patients should be advised about its limitations and possible side-effects. About 5–10% of patients with Parkinson's disease respond poorly to treatment.

Symptoms resembling Parkinson's disease can occur in diseases such as progressive supranuclear palsy and multiple system atrophy, but they do not normally respond to the drugs used in the treatment of idiopathic Parkinson's disease.

ELDERLY. Antiparkinsonian drugs can cause confusion in the elderly. It is particularly important to initiate treatment with low doses and to increase the dose gradually.

4.9.1   Dopaminergic drugs used in parkinsonism

Treatment for Parkinson's disease should be initiated under the supervision of a physician specialising in Parkinson's disease. Treatment is usually not started until symptoms cause significant disruption of daily activities.

The dopamine receptor agonists, **bromocriptine**, **cabergoline**, **lisuride** (lysuride), **pergolide**, **pramipexole**, and **ropinirole**, have a direct action on dopamine receptors. The treatment of new patients is often started with dopamine receptor agonists. They are also used with levodopa in more advanced disease.

When used alone, dopamine receptor agonists cause fewer motor complications in long-term treatment compared with levodopa but their improvement on overall motor performance is slightly less. The dopamine receptor agonists are associated with more neuropsychiatric side-effects than levodopa. The ergot-derived dopamine receptor agonists, bromocriptine, cabergoline, lisuride, and pergolide have been associated with fibrotic reactions (see notes below).

Doses of dopamine receptor agonists should be increased slowly according to response and tolerability. They should also be withdrawn gradually.

Apomorphine is a dopamine receptor agonist that is used in advanced disease (see below).

Fibrotic reactions. The CSM has advised that ergot-derived dopamine receptor agonists, bromocriptine, cabergoline, lisuride, and pergolide have been associated with pulmonary, retroperitoneal, and pericardial fibrotic reactions. Before starting treatment with these ergot derivatives it may be appropriate to measure the erythrocyte sedimentation rate and serum creatinine and to obtain a chest X-ray. Patients should be monitored for dyspnoea, persistent cough, chest pain, cardiac failure, and abdominal pain or tenderness. If long-term treatment is expected, then lung-function tests may also be helpful.

Levodopa, the amino-acid precursor of dopamine, acts by replenishing depleted striatal dopamine. It is given with an extracerebral **dopa-decarboxylase inhibitor** that reduces the peripheral conversion of levodopa to dopamine, thereby limiting side-effects such as nausea, vomiting and cardiovascular effects. Additionally, effective brain-dopamine concentrations can be achieved with lower doses of levodopa. The extracerebral dopa-decarboxylase inhibitors used with levodopa are benserazide (in **co-beneldopa**) and carbidopa (in **co-careldopa**).

Levodopa, in combination with a dopa-decarboxylase inhibitor, is useful in the elderly or frail, in patients with other significant illnesses, and in those with more severe symptoms. It is effective and well tolerated in the majority of patients.

Levodopa therapy should be initiated at a low dose and increased in small steps; the final dose should be as low as possible. Intervals between doses should be chosen to suit the needs of the individual patient.

NOTE. When co-careldopa is used, the total daily dose of carbidopa should be at least 70 mg. A lower dose may not achieve full inhibition of extracerebral dopa-decarboxylase, with a resultant increase in side-effects.

Nausea and vomiting with co-beneldopa or co-careldopa are rarely dose-limiting but domperidone (section 4.6) may be useful in controlling these effects.

Levodopa treatment is associated with the development of potentially troublesome motor complications including response fluctuations and dyskinesias. Response fluctuations are characterised by large variations in motor performance, with normal function during the 'on' period, and weakness and restricted mobility during the 'off' period. 'End-of-dose' deterioration also occurs, where the duration of benefit after each dose becomes progressively shorter. Modified-release preparations may help with 'end-of-dose' deterioration or nocturnal immobility and rigidity. Motor complications are particularly problematic in young patients treated with levodopa.

Selegiline is a monoamine-oxidase-B inhibitor used in conjunction with levodopa to reduce 'end-of-dose' deterioration in advanced Parkinson's disease. Early treatment with selegiline alone may delay the need for levodopa therapy for some months but other more effective drugs are preferred. When combined with levodopa, selegiline should be avoided or used with great caution in postural hypotension.

Entacapone prevents the peripheral breakdown of levodopa, allowing more levodopa to reach the brain. It is licensed for use as an adjunct to co-beneldopa or co-careldopa for patients with Parkinson's disease who experience 'end-of-dose' deterioration and cannot be stabilised on these combinations.

Amantadine has modest antiparkinsonian effects. It improves mild bradykinetic disabilities as well as tremor and rigidity. It may also be useful for dyskinesias in more advanced disease. Tolerance to its effects may develop and confusion and hallucinations may occasionally occur. Withdrawal of amantadine should be gradual irrespective of the patient's response to treatment.

Apomorphine is a potent dopamine agonist that is sometimes helpful in advanced disease for patients experiencing unpredictable 'off' periods with levodopa treatment. For the treatment of Parkinson's disease it is only available for parenteral administration. Apomorphine is highly emetogenic; patients must receive domperidone for at least 2 days before starting treatment. Specialist supervision is advisable throughout apomorphine treatment.

Sudden onset of sleep. Excessive daytime sleepiness and sudden onset of sleep can occur with co-careldopa, co-beneldopa, and the dopamine receptor agonists.

Patients starting treatment with these drugs should be warned of the possibility of these effects and of the need to exercise caution when driving or operating machinery.

Patients who have suffered excessive sedation or sudden onset of sleep, should refrain from driving or operating machines, until those effects have stopped recurring.

LEVODOPA

Indications: parkinsonism (but not drug-induced extrapyramidal symptoms), see notes above

Cautions: pulmonary disease, peptic ulceration, cardiovascular disease, diabetes mellitus, osteomalacia, open-angle glaucoma, history of skin melanoma (risk of activation), psychiatric illness (avoid if severe); warn patients about excessive drowsiness (see notes above); in prolonged therapy, psychiatric, hepatic, haematological, renal, and cardiovascular surveillance is advisable; warn patients to resume normal activities gradually; avoid abrupt withdrawal; **interactions:** Appendix 1 (levodopa)

Contra-indications: closed-angle glaucoma; pregnancy (Appendix 4) and breast-feeding (Appendix 5)

Side-effects: anorexia, nausea and vomiting, insomnia, agitation, postural hypotension (rarely labile hypertension), dizziness, tachycardia, arrhythmias, reddish discoloration of urine and other body fluids, rarely hypersensitivity; abnormal involuntary movements and psychiatric symptoms which include hypomania and psychosis may be dose-limiting; depression, drowsiness, headache, flushing, sweating, gastro-intestinal bleeding, peripheral neuropathy, taste disturbance, pruritus, rash, and liver enzyme changes also reported; syndrome resembling neuroleptic malignant syndrome reported on withdrawal

Dose: initially 125–500 mg daily in divided doses after meals, increased according to response (but rarely used alone, see notes above)

Levodopa (Non-proprietary) PoM ▨
Tablets, levodopa 500 mg. Net price 20 = £8.19.
Label: 14, 21, counselling, driving, see notes above
Available from Cambridge

CO-BENELDOPA

A mixture of benserazide hydrochloride and levodopa in mass proportions corresponding to 1 part of benserazide and 4 parts of levodopa

Indications: see under Levodopa and notes above
Cautions: see under Levodopa and notes above
Contra-indications: see under Levodopa
Side-effects: see under Levodopa and notes above
Dose: expressed as levodopa, initially 50 mg 3–4 times daily (100 mg 3 times daily in advanced disease), increased by 100 mg once or twice weekly according to response; usual maintenance dose 400–800 mg daily in divided doses after meals; ELDERLY initially 50 mg once or twice daily, increased by 50 mg every 3–4 days according to response

NOTE. When transferring patients from other levodopa preparations, it is recommended that the previous preparation should be discontinued 12 hours beforehand (although interval can be shorter); 3 capsules co-beneldopa 25/100 (*Madopar 125*®) should be substituted for 2 g levodopa; if transferring from another levodopa/dopa-decarboxylase inhibitor preparation, initial dose, expressed as levodopa, should be 50 mg 3–4 times daily

Madopar® (Roche) PoM
Capsules 62.5, blue/grey, co-beneldopa 12.5/50 (benserazide 12.5 mg (as hydrochloride), levodopa 50 mg). Net price 100-cap pack = £6.67. Label: 14, 21, counselling, driving, see notes above
Capsules 125, blue/pink, co-beneldopa 25/100 (benserazide 25 mg (as hydrochloride), levodopa 100 mg). Net price 100-cap pack=£9.29. Label: 14, 21, counselling, driving, see notes above
Capsules 250, blue/caramel, co-beneldopa 50/200 (benserazide 50 mg (as hydrochloride), levodopa 200 mg). Net price 100-cap pack = £15.84.
Label: 14, 21, counselling, driving, see notes above
Dispersible tablets 62.5, scored, co-beneldopa 12.5/50 (benserazide 12.5 mg (as hydrochloride), levodopa 50 mg). Net price 100-tab pack = £7.92.
Label: 14, 21, counselling, administration, see below, driving see notes above
Dispersible tablets 125, scored, co-beneldopa 25/100 (benserazide 25 mg (as hydrochloride) levodopa 100 mg). Net price 100-tab pack = £14.04.
Label: 14, 21, counselling, administration, see below, driving see notes above
NOTE. The tablets may be dispersed in water or orange squash (not orange juice) or swallowed whole

Madopar® **CR** (Roche) PoM
Capsules 125, m/r, dark green/light blue, co-benel-dopa 25/100 (benserazide 25 mg (as hydro-chloride), levodopa 100 mg). Net price 100-cap pack = £17.16. Label: 5, 14, 25, counselling, driving, see notes above
Dose: Patients not receiving levodopa therapy, initially 1 capsule 3 times daily (max. initial dose 6 capsules daily)
Fluctuations in response related to plasma-levodopa concentration or to timing of dose, initially 1 capsule substituted for every 100 mg of levodopa and given at same dosage frequency, subsequently increased every 2–3 days according to response; average increase of 50%

needed over previous levodopa dose and titration may take up to 4 weeks
Supplementary dose of conventional *Madopar*® may be needed with first morning dose; if response still poor to total daily dose of *Madopar*® CR plus *Madopar*® corresponding to 1.2 g levodopa, consider alternative therapy

CO-CARELDOPA

A mixture of carbidopa and levodopa; the proportions are expressed in the form *x/y* where *x* and *y* are the strengths in milligrams of carbidopa and levodopa respectively
Indications: see under Levodopa and notes above
Cautions: see under Levodopa and notes above
Contra-indications: see under Levodopa
Side-effects: see under Levodopa and notes above
Dose: expressed as levodopa, initially 100 mg (with carbidopa 25 mg, as *Sinemet-Plus*®) 3 times daily, increased by 50–100 mg (with carbidopa 12.5–25 mg, as *Sinemet-62.5*® or *Sinemet-Plus*®) daily or on alternate days according to response, up to 800 mg (with carbidopa 200 mg) daily in divided doses
NOTE. Carbidopa 70–100 mg daily is necessary to achieve full inhibition of peripheral dopa-decarboxylase
Alternatively, initially 50–100 mg (with carbidopa 10–12.5 mg, as *Sinemet-62.5*® or *Sinemet-110*®) 3–4 times daily, increased by 50–100 mg daily or on alternate days according to response, up to 800 mg (with carbidopa 80–100 mg) daily in divided doses
Alternatively, initially 125 mg (with carbidopa 12.5 mg, as ½ tablet of *Sinemet-275*®) 1–2 times daily, increased by 125 mg (with carbidopa 12.5 mg) daily or on alternate days according to response
NOTE. When transferring patients from levodopa, 1 tablet co-careldopa 25/250 (*Sinemet-275*®) 3–4 times daily should be substituted for patients receiving more than 1.5 g levodopa daily; 1 tablet co-careldopa 25/100 (*Sinemet-Plus*®) 3–4 times daily should be substituted for patients receiving less than 1.5 g levodopa daily; levodopa should be discontinued 12 hours beforehand

Sinemet® (Bristol-Myers Squibb) PoM
Sinemet-62.5® *tablets*, yellow, scored, co-careldopa 12.5/50 (carbidopa 12.5 mg (as monohydrate), levodopa 50 mg), net price 90-tab pack = £7.03.
Label: 14, 21, counselling, driving, see notes above
NOTE. 2 tablets *Sinemet-62.5*® ≡ 1 tablet *Sinemet Plus*®; *Sinemet-62.5*® previously known as *Sinemet LS*®
Sinemet-110® *tablets*, blue, scored, co-careldopa 10/100 (carbidopa 10 mg (as monohydrate), levodopa 100 mg), net price 90-tab pack = £7.35. Label: 14, 21, counselling, driving, see notes above
Sinemet-Plus® *tablets*, yellow, scored, co-careldopa 25/100 (carbidopa 25 mg (as monohydrate), levodopa 100 mg), net price 90-tab pack = £10.81.
Label: 14, 21, counselling, driving, see notes above
NOTE. The daily dose of carbidopa required to achieve full inhibition of extracerebral dopa-decarboxylase is 75 mg; co-careldopa 25/100 provides an adequate dose of carbidopa when low doses of levodopa are needed
Sinemet-275® *tablets*, blue, scored, co-careldopa 25/250 (carbidopa 25 mg (as monohydrate), levodopa 250 mg), net price 90-tab pack=£15.36. Label: 14, 21, counselling, driving, see notes above

■ Modified release

Half Sinemet® **CR** (Bristol-Myers Squibb) PoM
Tablets, m/r, pink, co-careldopa 25/100 (carbidopa 25 mg (as monohydrate), levodopa 100 mg), net

price 60-tab pack = £18.99. Label: 14, 25, counselling, driving, see notes above
Dose: for fine adjustment of *Sinemet® CR* dose (see below)

Sinemet® CR (Bristol-Myers Squibb) PoM
Tablets, m/r, peach, co-careldopa 50/200 (carbidopa 50 mg (as monohydrate), levodopa 200 mg), net price 60-tab pack = £22.35. Label: 14, 25, counselling, driving, see notes above
Dose: initial treatment or fluctuations in response to conventional levodopa therapy, 1 *Sinemet® CR* tablet twice daily; both dose and interval then adjusted according to response at intervals of not less than 3 days; if transferring from existing levodopa therapy withdraw 8 hours beforehand; 1 tablet *Sinemet® CR* twice daily can be substituted for a daily dose of levodopa 300–400 mg in conventional *Sinemet®* tablets

■ With entacapone
NOTE. For Parkinson's disease and end-of-dose motor fluctuations not adequately controlled with levodopa and dopa-decarboxylase inhibitor treatment

Stalevo® (Orion) ▼ PoM
Stalevo 50 mg/12.5 mg/200 mg tablets, f/c, brown, levodopa 50 mg, carbidopa 12.5 mg, entacapone 200 mg, net price 30-tab pack = £24.00, 100-tab pack = £80.00. Label: 14 (urine reddish-brown), 25, counselling, driving, see notes above
Stalevo 100 mg/25 mg/200 mg tablets, f/c, brown, levodopa 100 mg, carbidopa 25 mg, entacapone 200 mg, net price 30-tab pack = £24.00, 100-tab pack = £80.00. Label: 14 (urine reddish-brown), 25, counselling, driving, see notes above
Stalevo 150 mg/37.5 mg/200 mg tablets, f/c, brown, levodopa 150 mg, carbidopa 37.5 mg, entacapone 200 mg, net price 30-tab pack = £24.00, 100-tab pack = £80.00. Label: 14 (urine reddish-brown), 25, counselling, driving, see notes above
Dose: only 1 tablet of *Stalevo®* to be taken for each dose
Patients receiving standard-release co-careldopa or co-beneldopa alone, initiate *Stalevo®* at a dose that provides similar (or slightly lower) amount of levodopa
Patients with dyskinesia or receiving more than 800 mg levodopa daily, introduce entacapone before transferring to *Stalevo®* (levodopa dose may need to be reduced by 10–30% initially)
Patients receiving entacapone and standard-release co-careldopa or co-beneldopa, initiate *Stalevo®* at a dose that provides similar (or slightly higher) amount of levodopa

AMANTADINE HYDROCHLORIDE

Indications: Parkinson's disease (but not drug-induced extrapyramidal symptoms); antiviral (section 5.3)
Cautions: hepatic, or renal impairment (Appendix 3), congestive heart disease (may exacerbate oedema), confused or hallucinatory states, elderly; avoid abrupt discontinuation in Parkinson's disease; **interactions:** Appendix 1 (amantadine)
DRIVING. May affect performance of skilled tasks (e.g. driving)
Contra-indications: epilepsy, history of gastric ulceration, severe renal impairment; pregnancy (toxicity in *animals*), breast-feeding
Side-effects: anorexia, nausea, nervousness, inability to concentrate, insomnia, dizziness, convulsions, hallucinations or feelings of detachment, blurred vision, gastro-intestinal disturbances, livedo reticularis and peripheral oedema; rarely leucopenia, rashes

Dose: 100 mg daily increased after one week to 100 mg twice daily, usually in conjunction with other treatment; some patients may require higher doses, max. 400 mg daily
ELDERLY 65 years and over, 100 mg daily adjusted according to response

Symmetrel® (Alliance) PoM
Capsules, red-brown, amantadine hydrochloride 100 mg. Net price 56-cap pack = £15.35. Counselling, driving
NOTE. Also available as *Lysovir®* for the prophylaxis and treatment of influenza A
Syrup, amantadine hydrochloride 50 mg/5 mL. Net price 150-mL pack = £5.05. Counselling, driving

APOMORPHINE HYDROCHLORIDE

Indications: refractory motor fluctuations in Parkinson's disease ('off' episodes) inadequately controlled by levodopa or other dopaminergics (for capable and motivated patients under specialist supervision); erectile dysfunction (section 7.4.5)
Cautions: tendency to nausea and vomiting; pulmonary, cardiovascular or endocrine disease, renal impairment; elderly and debilitated, history of postural hypotension (special care on initiation); hepatic, haemopoietic, renal, and cardiovascular monitoring; *on administration with levodopa* test initially and every 6 months for haemolytic anaemia (development calls for specialist haematological care with dose reduction and possible discontinuation); **interactions:** Appendix 1 (apomorphine)
Contra-indications: respiratory or CNS depression, hepatic impairment, hypersensitivity to opioids; neuropsychiatric problems or dementia; not suitable if 'on' response to levodopa marred by severe dyskinesia, hypotonia or psychiatric effects; pregnancy and breast-feeding; not for intravenous administration
Side-effects: nausea and vomiting (see below under Dose), dyskinesias during 'on' periods (may require discontinuation); postural instability and falls (impaired speech and balance may not improve), increasing cognitive impairment, and personality change during 'on' phase; confusion and hallucinations (if continued, specialist observation required with possible gradual dose reduction), sedation, postural hypotension; also euphoria, light-headedness, restlessness, tremors; haemolytic anaemia with levodopa (see Cautions) and rarely eosinophilia; local reactions common (include nodule formation and possible ulceration)—rotate injection sites, dilute with sodium chloride 0.9%, consider ultrasound, ensure no infection
Dose: *by subcutaneous injection,* usual range (after initiation as below) 3–30 mg daily in divided doses; subcutaneous infusion may be preferable in those requiring division of injections into more than 10 doses daily; max. single dose 10 mg; ADOLESCENT (under 18 years) and CHILD not recommended
By continuous subcutaneous infusion (those requiring division into more than 10 injections daily) initially 1 mg/hour daily increased according to

response (not more often than every 4 hours) in max. steps of 500 micrograms/hour to max. 4 mg/hour (15–60 micrograms/kg/hour); change infusion site every 12 hours and give during waking hours only (24-hour infusions not advised unless severe night-time symptoms)—intermittent bolus boosts also usually needed (in those with severe dyskinesias only when absolutely necessary)

Total daily dose by either route (or combined routes) max. 100 mg

REQUIREMENTS FOR INITIATION. *Hospital admission* and at least 2 days of pretreatment with domperidone for nausea and vomiting, *after at least 3 days* withhold existing antiparkinsonian medication overnight to provoke 'off' episode, *determine* threshold dose, *re-establish* other antiparkinsonian drugs, *determine* effective apomorphine regimen, *teach* to administer by subcutaneous injection into lower abdomen or outer thigh at first sign of 'off' episode, *discharge* from hospital, *monitor* frequently and *adjust* dosage regimen as appropriate (domperidone may normally be withdrawn over several weeks or longer)—for full details of initiation requirements, consult product literature

APO-go® (Britannia) PoM
Injection, apomorphine hydrochloride 10 mg/mL, net price 2-mL amp = £7.59, 5-mL amp = £15.23
Injection (APO-go® Pen), apomorphine hydrochloride 10 mg/mL, net price 3-mL pen injector = £24.78

BROMOCRIPTINE

Indications: parkinsonism (but not drug-induced extrapyramidal symptoms); endocrine disorders, section 6.7.1

Cautions: section 6.7.1; fibrotic reactions—see CSM advice in notes above
HYPOTENSIVE REACTIONS. Hypotensive reactions in some patients may be disturbing during the first few days of treatment and particular care should be exercised when driving or operating machinery; tolerance may be reduced by alcohol

Contra-indications: section 6.7.1

Side-effects: section 6.7.1

Dose: first week 1–1.25 mg at night, second week 2–2.5 mg at night, third week 2.5 mg twice daily, fourth week 2.5 mg 3 times daily then increasing by 2.5 mg every 3–14 days according to response to a usual range of 10–40 mg daily; taken with food

■ Preparations
Section 6.7.1

CABERGOLINE

Indications: adjunct to levodopa (with dopa-decarboxylase inhibitor) in Parkinson's disease; endocrine disorders (section 6.7.1)

Cautions: section 6.7.1; fibrotic reactions—see CSM advice in notes above
HYPOTENSIVE REACTIONS. Hypotensive reactions in some patients may be disturbing during the first few days of treatment; tolerance may be reduced by alcohol

Contra-indications: section 6.7.1

Side-effects: section 6.7.1

Dose: initially 1 mg daily, increased by increments of 0.5–1 mg at 7 or 14 day intervals; usual range 2–6 mg daily
NOTE. Concurrent dose of levodopa may be decreased gradually while dose of cabergoline is increased

Cabaser® (Pharmacia) PoM
Tablets, all scored, cabergoline 1 mg, net price 20-tab pack = £75.45; 2 mg, 20-tab pack = £75.45;

4 mg, 16-tab pack = £75.84. Label: 21, counselling, hypotensive reactions, driving, see notes above
NOTE. Dispense in original container (contains desiccant)

ENTACAPONE

Indications: adjunct to levodopa with dopa-decarboxylase inhibitor in Parkinson's disease and 'end-of-dose' motor fluctuations

Cautions: concurrent levodopa dose may need to be reduced by about 10–30%; **interactions:** Appendix 1 (entacapone)

Contra-indications: pregnancy and breast-feeding; hepatic impairment; phaeochromocytoma; history of neuroleptic malignant syndrome or non-traumatic rhabdomyolysis

Side-effects: nausea, vomiting, abdominal pain, constipation, diarrhoea, urine may be coloured reddish-brown, dry mouth, dyskinesias; dizziness; rarely hepatitis

Dose: 200 mg with each dose of levodopa with dopa-decarboxylase inhibitor; max. 2 g daily

Comtess® (Orion) PoM
Tablets, f/c, brown/orange, entacapone 200 mg, net price 30-tab pack = £18.64, 100-tab pack = £62.14. Label: 14, (urine reddish-brown), counselling, driving, see notes above

LISURIDE MALEATE

(Lysuride maleate)

Indications: Parkinson's disease, used alone or as an adjunct to levodopa

Cautions: history of pituitary tumour; history of psychotic disturbance; pregnancy; porphyria (section 9.8.2); fibrotic reactions—see CSM advice in notes above; **interactions:** Appendix 1 (lisuride)
HYPOTENSIVE REACTIONS. Hypotensive reactions in some patients may be disturbing during the first few days of treatment and particular care should be exercised when driving or operating machinery

Contra-indications: severe disturbances of peripheral circulation; coronary insufficiency

Side-effects: see notes above; nausea and vomiting; dizziness; headache, lethargy, malaise, drowsiness, psychotic reactions (including hallucinations); occasionally severe hypotension, rashes; rarely abdominal pain and constipation; Raynaud's phenomenon reported

Dose: initially 200 micrograms at bedtime with food increased as necessary at weekly intervals to 200 micrograms twice daily (midday and bedtime) then to 200 micrograms 3 times daily (morning, midday, and bedtime); further increases made by adding 200 micrograms each week first to the bedtime dose, then to the midday dose and finally to the morning dose; max. 5 mg daily in 3 divided doses after food

Lisuride Maleate (Non-proprietary) PoM
Tablets, scored, lisuride maleate 200 micrograms. Net price 100-tab pack = £41.92. Label: 21, counselling, hypotensive reactions
Available from Cambridge
NOTE. The brand name *Revanil®* was formerly used for lisuride maleate tablets

PERGOLIDE

Indications: Parkinson's disease, used alone or as adjunct to levodopa

Cautions: arrhythmias or underlying cardiac disease, history of confusion or hallucinations, dyskinesia (may exacerbate), pregnancy (Appendix 4), breast-feeding (Appendix 5); increase dose gradually and avoid abrupt withdrawal; porphyria (section 9.8.2); fibrotic reactions—see CSM advice in notes above; **interactions:** Appendix 1 (pergolide)

HYPOTENSIVE REACTIONS. Hypotensive reactions in some patients may be disturbing during the first few days of treatment and particular care should be exercised when driving or operating machinery

Side-effects: see notes above; hallucinations, confusion, dizziness, dyskinesia, drowsiness, abdominal pain, nausea, vomiting, dyspepsia, diplopia, rhinitis, dyspnoea, pleuritis, pleural effusion, pleural fibrosis, pericarditis, pericardial effusion and retroperitoneal fibrosis, insomnia, constipation or diarrhoea, hypotension, syncope, tachycardia and atrial premature contractions, rash, fever reported; neuroleptic malignant syndrome also reported

Dose: monotherapy, 50 micrograms at night on day 1, then 50 micrograms twice daily on days 2–4, then increased by 100–250 micrograms daily every 3–4 days (given in 3 divided doses) up to a daily dose of 1.5 mg at day 28; after day 30, further increases of up to 250 micrograms twice a week; usual maintenance dose approx. 2–2.5 mg daily (above 5 mg daily not evaluated)

Adjunctive therapy with levodopa, 50 micrograms daily for 2 days, increased gradually by 100–150 micrograms every 3 days over next 12 days, usually given in 3 divided doses; further increases of 250 micrograms every 3 days; usual maintenance dose 3 mg daily (above 5 mg daily not evaluated); during pergolide titration levodopa dose may be reduced cautiously

Celance® (Lilly) PoM
Tablets, all scored, pergolide (as mesilate) 50 micrograms (ivory), net price 100-tab pack = £32.44; 250 micrograms (green), 100-tab pack = £48.92; 1 mg (pink), 100-tab pack = £176.58; 30-day starter pack of 109 × 50-microgram tablets with 57 × 250-microgram tablets = £26.99. Counselling, hypotensive reactions, driving, see notes above

PRAMIPEXOLE

Indications: Parkinson's disease, used alone or as adjunct to levodopa

Cautions: renal impairment (Appendix 3); psychotic disorders; ophthalmological testing recommended (risk of visual disorders); severe cardiovascular disease; pregnancy (Appendix 4); avoid abrupt withdrawal (risk of neuroleptic malignant syndrome); **interactions:** Appendix 1 (pramipexole)

HYPOTENSIVE REACTIONS. Hypotensive reactions may be disturbing in some patients during the first few days of treatment

Contra-indications: breast-feeding (Appendix 5)

Side-effects: nausea, constipation, confusion, drowsiness (including sudden onset of sleep) and insomnia, dizziness, hallucinations (mostly visual), dyskinesia during initial dose titration (more frequent in women—reduce levodopa dose), peripheral oedema

Dose: initially, 264 micrograms daily in 3 divided doses, doubling the dose every 5–7 days to

1.08 mg daily in 3 divided doses; further increased if necessary by 540 micrograms daily at weekly intervals; max. 3.3 mg daily in 3 divided doses

NOTE. During pramipexole dose titration and maintenance, levodopa dose may be reduced

IMPORTANT. Doses and strengths are stated in terms of pramipexole (base); equivalent strengths in terms of pramipexole dihydrochloride monohydrate (salt) are as follows: 88 micrograms base ≡ 125 micrograms salt; 180 micrograms base ≡ 250 micrograms salt; 700 micrograms base ≡ 1 mg salt

Mirapexin® (Pharmacia) ▼ PoM
Tablets, pramipexole (as hydrochloride) 88 micrograms, net price 30-tab pack = £10.00; 180 micrograms (scored), 30-tab pack = £20.00, 100-tab pack = £66.67; 700 micrograms (scored), 30-tab pack = £63.67, 100-tab pack = £212.24. Counselling, hypotensive reactions, driving, see notes above

ROPINIROLE

Indications: Parkinson's disease, either used alone or as an adjunct to levodopa; see also notes above

Cautions: hepatic impairment (Appendix 2); renal impairment (Appendix 3); severe cardiovascular disease, major psychotic disorders, avoid abrupt withdrawal; **interactions:** Appendix 1 (ropinirole)

Contra-indications: pregnancy and breast-feeding

Side-effects: nausea, drowsiness (including sudden onset of sleep), leg oedema, abdominal pain, vomiting and syncope; dyskinesia, hallucinations and confusion reported in adjunctive therapy; occasionally severe hypotension and bradycardia

Dose: initially 750 micrograms daily in 3 divided doses, increased by increments of 750 micrograms at weekly intervals to 3 mg daily; further increased by increments of up to 3 mg at weekly intervals according to response; usual range 3–9 mg daily (but higher doses may be required if used with levodopa); max. 24 mg daily

NOTE. When administered as adjunct to levodopa, concurrent dose of levodopa may be reduced by approx. 20%

Requip® (GSK) PoM
Tablets, f/c, ropinirole (as hydrochloride) 1 mg (green), net price 84-tab pack = £46.20; 2 mg (pink), 84-tab pack = £92.40; 5 mg (blue), 84-tab pack = £184.80; 28-day starter pack of 42 × 250-microgram (white) tablets, 42 × 500-microgram (yellow) tablets, and 21 × 1-mg (green) tablets = £43.12; 28-day follow-on pack of 42 × 500-microgram (yellow) tablets, 42 × 1-mg (green) tablets, and 63 × 2-mg (pink) tablets = £80.00. Label: 21, counselling, driving, see notes above

SELEGILINE HYDROCHLORIDE

Indications: Parkinson's disease, used alone or as adjunct to levodopa

Cautions: gastric and duodenal ulceration (avoid in active ulceration), uncontrolled hypertension, arrhythmias, angina, psychosis, pregnancy and breast-feeding, side-effects of levodopa may be increased, concurrent levodopa dosage may need to be reduced by 10–50%; **interactions:** Appendix 1 (selegiline)

Contra-indications: pregnancy, breast-feeding

Side-effects: nausea, dry mouth; postural hypotension; dyskinesia, vertigo, sleeping disorders, confusion, hallucinations; rarely arrhythmias, agitation, headache, micturition difficulties, skin reactions

Dose: 10 mg in the morning, or 5 mg at breakfast and midday; ELDERLY see below
ELDERLY. To avoid initial confusion and agitation, it may be appropriate to start treatment with a dose of 2.5 mg daily, particularly in the elderly

Selegiline Hydrochloride (Non-proprietary) PoM
Tablets, selegiline hydrochloride 5 mg, net price 56-tab pack = £10.75; 10 mg, 30-tab pack = £11.53
Available from Alpharma, APS, Generics, Hillcross, IVAX, Sandoz, Sanofi-Synthelabo, Sterwin

Eldepryl (Orion) PoM
Tablets, both scored, selegiline hydrochloride 5 mg, net price 60-tab pack = £10.35; 10 mg, 30-tab pack = £10.10
Oral liquid, selegiline hydrochloride 10 mg/5 mL, net price 200 mL = £18.72

- Oral lyophilisate
Zelapar (Athena) PoM
Oral lyophilisates (= freeze-dried tablets), yellow, selegiline hydrochloride 1.25 mg, net price 30-tab pack = £59.95. Counselling, administration
Dose: initially 1.25 mg daily before breakfast
COUNSELLING. Tablets should be placed on the tongue and allowed to dissolve. Advise patient not to drink, rinse, or wash mouth out for 5 minutes after taking the tablet
Excipients: include aspartame (section 9.4.1)
NOTE. Patients receiving 10 mg conventional selegiline hydrochloride tablets can be switched to *Zelapar* 1.25 mg

4.9.2 Antimuscarinic drugs used in parkinsonism

Antimuscarinic drugs exert their antiparkinsonian action by reducing the effects of the central cholinergic excess that occurs as a result of dopamine deficiency. Antimuscarinic drugs are useful in drug-induced parkinsonism, but they are generally not used in idiopathic Parkinson's disease because they are less effective than dopaminergic drugs and they are associated with cognitive impairment.

The antimuscarinic drugs, **benzatropine**, **orphenadrine**, **procyclidine**, and **trihexyphenidyl** (benzhexol), reduce the symptoms of parkinsonism induced by antipsychotic drugs, but there is no justification for giving them routinely in the absence of parkinsonian side-effects. Tardive dyskinesia is not improved by antimuscarinic drugs and may be made worse.

In idiopathic Parkinson's disease, antimuscarinic drugs reduce tremor and rigidity but they have little effect on bradykinesia. They may be useful in reducing sialorrhoea.

No important differences exist between the antimuscarinic drugs, but some patients tolerate one better than another.

Benzatropine may be given parenterally and it is effective emergency treatment for acute drug-induced dystonic reactions which may be severe.

BENZATROPINE MESILATE

(Benztropine mesylate)
Indications: see Trihexyphenidyl Hydrochloride
Cautions: see Trihexyphenidyl Hydrochloride
Contra-indications: see Trihexyphenidyl Hydrochloride; avoid in children under 3 years

Side-effects: see Trihexyphenidyl Hydrochloride, but causes sedation rather than stimulation

Dose: *by mouth*, 0.5–1 mg daily usually at bedtime, gradually increased; max. 6 mg daily; usual maintenance dose 1–4 mg daily in single or divided doses; ELDERLY preferably lower end of range
By intramuscular or intravenous injection, 1–2 mg, repeated if symptoms reappear; ELDERLY preferably lower end of range

Cogentin (MSD) PoM
Injection, benzatropine mesilate 1 mg/mL. Net price 2-mL amp = 92p

ORPHENADRINE HYDROCHLORIDE

Indications: see Trihexyphenidyl Hydrochloride
Cautions: see Trihexyphenidyl Hydrochloride
Contra-indications: see Trihexyphenidyl Hydrochloride; porphyria (section 9.8.2)
Side-effects: see Trihexyphenidyl Hydrochloride; may cause insomnia

Dose: 150 mg daily in divided doses, increased gradually; max. 400 mg daily; ELDERLY preferably lower end of range

Orphenadrine Hydrochloride (Non-proprietary) PoM
Oral solution, orphenadrine hydrochloride 50 mg/5 mL. Net price 200 mL = £9.47. Counselling, driving
Available from Rosemont (sugar-free)

Biorphen (Alliance) PoM
Elixir, sugar-free, orphenadrine hydrochloride 25 mg/5 mL. Net price 200 mL = £7.25. Counselling, driving

Disipal (Yamanouchi) PoM
Tablets, yellow, s/c, orphenadrine hydrochloride 50 mg. Net price 20 = 69p. Counselling, driving
Excipients: include tartrazine

PROCYCLIDINE HYDROCHLORIDE

Indications: see Trihexyphenidyl Hydrochloride
Cautions: see Trihexyphenidyl Hydrochloride
Contra-indications: see Trihexyphenidyl Hydrochloride
Side-effects: see Trihexyphenidyl Hydrochloride

Dose: *by mouth*, 2.5 mg 3 times daily, increased gradually if necessary; usual max. 30 mg daily (60 mg daily in exceptional circumstances); ELDERLY preferably lower end of range
Acute dystonia, *by intramuscular or intravenous injection*, 5–10 mg (occasionally more than 10 mg), usually effective in 5–10 minutes but may need 30 minutes for relief

Procyclidine (Non-proprietary) PoM
Tablets, procyclidine hydrochloride 5 mg. Net price 20 = £1.08. Counselling, driving
Available from Alpharma, APS, Opus (*Mucinil*)

Arpicolin (Rosemont) PoM
Syrup, sugar-free, procyclidine hydrochloride 2.5 mg/5 mL, net price 150 mL = £4.49; 5 mg/5 mL, 150 mL pack = £8.02. Counselling, driving

Kemadrin (GSK) PoM
Tablets, scored, procyclidine hydrochloride 5 mg. Net price 20 = £1.02. Counselling, driving

Kemadrin (Auden Mckenzie) PoM
Injection, procyclidine hydrochloride 5 mg/mL, net price 2-mL amp = £1.49

TRIHEXYPHENIDYL HYDROCHLORIDE

(Benzhexol hydrochloride)

Indications: parkinsonism; drug-induced extra-pyramidal symptoms (but not tardive dyskinesia, see notes above)

Cautions: cardiovascular disease, hepatic or renal impairment; elderly; avoid abrupt discontinuation of treatment; liable to abuse (may produce euphoric effect); pregnancy and breast-feeding; **interactions:** Appendix 1 (antimuscarinics)
DRIVING. May affect performance of skilled tasks (e.g. driving)

Contra-indications: untreated urinary retention, angle-closure glaucoma, gastro-intestinal obstruction, prostatic hypertrophy

Side-effects: dry mouth, gastro-intestinal disturbances, dizziness, blurred vision; less commonly urinary retention, tachycardia, hypersensitivity, nervousness, and with high doses in susceptible patients, confusion, excitement, agitation, hallucinations, insomnia and psychiatric disturbances which may necessitate discontinuation of treatment; impaired memory also reported

Dose: 1 mg daily, increased gradually; usual maintenance dose 5–15 mg daily in 3–4 divided doses (max. 20 mg daily); ELDERLY preferably lower end of range
CHILD not recommended

Trihexyphenidyl (Non-proprietary) PoM
Tablets, trihexyphenidyl hydrochloride 2 mg, net price 20 = 58p; 5 mg, 20 = 78p. Counselling, before or after food (see notes above), driving
Available from Genus

Broflex® (Alliance) PoM
Syrup, pink, trihexyphenidyl hydrochloride 5 mg/5 mL. Net price 200 mL = £6.36. Counselling, before or after food (see notes above), driving

---

4.9.3 Drugs used in essential tremor, chorea, tics, and related disorders

Tetrabenazine is mainly used to control movement disorders in Huntington's chorea and related disorders. It may act by depleting nerve endings of dopamine. It has useful action in only a proportion of patients and its use may be limited by the development of depression.

Haloperidol may be useful in improving motor tics and symptoms of Gilles de la Tourette syndrome and related choreas. **Pimozide** (see section 4.2.1 for CSM warning), **clonidine** (section 4.7.4.2) and **sulpiride** (section 4.2.1) are also used in Gilles de la Tourette syndrome. **Trihexyphenidyl (benzhexol)** (section 4.9.2) at high dosage may also improve some movement disorders; it is sometimes necessary to build the dose up over many weeks, to 20 to 30 mg daily or higher. **Chlorpromazine** and **haloperidol** are used to relieve intractable hiccup (section 4.2.1).

Propranolol or another beta-adrenoceptor blocking drug (section 2.4) may be useful in treating essential tremor or tremors associated with anxiety or thyrotoxicosis. Propranolol is given in a dosage of 40 mg 2 or 3 times daily, increased if necessary; 80 to 160 mg daily is usually required for maintenance.

Primidone (section 4.8.1) in some cases provides relief from benign essential tremor; the dose is increased slowly to reduce side-effects.

Piracetam is used as an adjunctive treatment for myoclonus of cortical origin.

Riluzole is used to extend life or the time to mechanical ventilation in patients with motor neurone disease who have amyotrophic lateral sclerosis.

> **NICE guidance (riluzole).** NICE has recommended (January 2001) riluzole to treat individuals with the amyotrophic lateral sclerosis (ALS) form of motor neurone disease (MND). Treatment should be initiated by a specialist in MND but it can then be supervised under a shared-care arrangement involving the general practitioner.

HALOPERIDOL

Indications: motor tics, adjunctive treatment in choreas and Gilles de la Tourette syndrome; other indications, section 4.2.1

Cautions: section 4.2.1

Contra-indications: section 4.2.1

Side-effects: section 4.2.1

Dose: *by mouth*, 0.5–1.5 mg 3 times daily adjusted according to the response; 10 mg daily or more may occasionally be necessary in Gilles de la Tourette syndrome; CHILD, Gilles de la Tourette syndrome up to 10 mg daily

■ Preparations
Section 4.2.1

PIRACETAM

Indications: adjunctive treatment of cortical myoclonus

Cautions: avoid abrupt withdrawal; elderly; renal impairment (avoid if severe)

Contra-indications: hepatic and severe renal impairment; pregnancy and breast-feeding

Side-effects: diarrhoea, weight gain; somnolence, insomnia, nervousness, depression; hyperkinesia; rash

Dose: initially 7.2 g daily in 2–3 divided doses, increased according to response by 4.8 g daily every 3–4 days to max. 20 g daily (subsequently, attempts should be made to reduce dose of concurrent therapy); CHILD under 16 years not recommended
ORAL SOLUTION. Follow the oral solution with a glass of water (or soft drink) to reduce bitter taste.

Nootropil® (UCB Pharma) PoM
Tablets, f/c, scored, piracetam 800 mg, net price 90-tab pack = £15.80; 1.2 g, 56-tab pack = £14.74. Label: 3
Oral solution, piracetam 333.3 mg/mL, net price 300-mL pack = £21.93. Label: 3

RILUZOLE

Indications: to extend life or the time to mechanical ventilation for patients with amyotrophic lateral sclerosis, initiated by specialists experienced in the management of motor neurone disease

Cautions: history of abnormal hepatic function (consult product literature for details); **interactions:** Appendix 1 (riluzole)
BLOOD DISORDERS. Patients or their carers should be told how to recognise signs of neutropenia and advised to seek

immediate medical attention if symptoms such as fever occur; white blood cell counts should be determined in febrile illness; neutropenia requires discontinuation of riluzole

DRIVING. Dizziness or vertigo may affect performance of skilled tasks (e.g. driving)

Contra-indications: hepatic and renal impairment; pregnancy and breast-feeding

Side-effects: nausea, vomiting, asthenia, tachycardia, somnolence, headache, dizziness, vertigo, abdominal pain, circumoral paraesthesia, alterations in liver function tests

Dose: 50 mg twice daily; CHILD not recommended

Rilutek® (Aventis Pharma) PoM
Tablets, f/c, riluzole 50 mg. Net price 56-tab pack = £220.35. Counselling, blood disorders, driving

TETRABENAZINE

Indications: see under Dose

Cautions: pregnancy; avoid in breast-feeding; **interactions:** Appendix 1 (tetrabenazine)

DRIVING. May affect performance of skilled tasks (e.g. driving)

Side-effects: drowsiness, gastro-intestinal disturbances, depression, extrapyramidal dysfunction, hypotension; rarely parkinsonism; neuroleptic malignant syndrome reported

Dose: movement disorders due to Huntington's chorea, hemiballismus, senile chorea, and related neurological conditions, initially 12.5 mg twice daily (elderly 12.5 mg daily) gradually increased to 12.5–25 mg 3 times daily; max. 200 mg daily

Moderate to severe tardive dyskinesia, initially 12.5 mg daily, gradually increased according to response

Xenazine® **25** (Cambridge) PoM
Tablets, pale yellow-buff, scored, tetrabenazine 25 mg. Net price 112-tab pack = £100.00. Label: 2

Torsion dystonias and other involuntary movements

BOTULINUM A TOXIN-HAEMAGGLUTININ COMPLEX

Indications: dynamic equinus foot deformity caused by spasticity in ambulant paediatric cerebral palsy patients over 2 years; hand and wrist disability associated with stroke; blepharospasm; hemifacial spasm; spasmodic torticollis; severe hyperhidrosis of axillae (all specialist use only)

Cautions: potential for anaphylaxis; history of dysphagia; pregnancy (Appendix 4)

SPECIFIC CAUTIONS FOR BLEPHAROSPASM OR HEMIFACIAL SPASM. Avoid deep or misplaced injections—relevant anatomy (and any alterations due to previous surgery) must be understood before injecting; caution if risk of angle closure glaucoma; reduced blinking can lead to corneal exposure, persistent epithelial defect and corneal ulceration (especially in those with VIIth nerve disorders)—careful testing of corneal sensation in previously operated eyes, avoidance of injection in lower lid area to avoid ectropion and vigorous treatment of epithelial defect needed

SPECIFIC CAUTIONS FOR TORTICOLLIS. Patients with defective neuromuscular transmission (risk of excessive muscle weakness)

COUNSELLING. All patients should be alerted to possible side-effects

Contra-indications: generalised disorders of muscle activity (e.g. myasthenia gravis); breast-feeding

Side-effects: increased electrophysiologic jitter in some distant muscles; misplaced injections may paralyse nearby muscle groups and excessive doses may paralyse distant muscles; influenza-like syndrome, rarely hypersensitivity reactions including rash, pruritus and anaphylaxis; antibody formation (substantial deterioration in response); arrhythmia and myocardial infarction; injection site reactions

SPECIFIC SIDE-EFFECTS IN BLEPHAROSPASM OR HEMIFACIAL SPASM. Ptosis; less frequently keratitis, lagophthalmos, dry eye, irritation, photophobia, lacrimation; ectropion, entropion, diplopia, dizziness, skin rash, facial weakness (including drooping), tiredness, visual disturbance, blurring of vision; rarely eyelid bruising and swelling (minimised by applying gentle pressure at injection site immediately after injection); angle closure glaucoma, corneal ulceration.

SPECIFIC SIDE-EFFECTS IN PAEDIATRIC CEREBRAL PALSY. Myalgia, urinary incontinence, somnolence, malaise, paraesthesia

SPECIFIC SIDE-EFFECTS IN TORTICOLLIS. Dysphagia and pooling of saliva (occurs most frequently after injection into sternomastoid muscle); nausea, dry mouth, rhinitis, drowsiness, headache, dizziness, hypertonia, malaise, stiffness; less frequently dyspnoea, fever, voice alteration, diplopia, and ptosis; rarely respiratory difficulties (associated with high doses); CSM has warned of persistent dysphagia and sequelae (including death)—**important**

Dose: consult product literature (**important:** specific to **each individual preparation** and **not interchangeable**)

Botox® (Allergan) PoM
Injection, powder for reconstitution, botulinum A toxin-haemagglutinin complex, net price 100-unit vial = £128.93

Dysport® (Ipsen) PoM
Injection, powder for reconstitution, botulinum A toxin-haemagglutinin complex, net price 500-unit vial = £164.74

BOTULINUM B TOXIN

Indications: spasmodic torticollis (cervical dystonia)—specialist use only

Cautions: inadvertent injection into a blood vessel; tolerance may occur; **interactions:** Appendix 1 (botulinum toxin)

Contra-indications: neuromuscular or neuromuscular junctional disorders; pregnancy and breast-feeding

Side-effects: increased electrophysiologic jitter in some distant muscles; dry mouth, dysphagia; also dyspepsia, worsening torticollis, neck pain, myasthenia, voice changes, taste disturbances

Dose: *by intramuscular injection*, initially 5000–10 000 units divided between 2–4 most affected muscles; adjust dose and frequency according to response; **important: not** interchangeable with other botulinum toxin preparations

NeuroBloc® (Elan) ▼ PoM
Injection, botulinum B toxin 5000 units/mL, net price 0.5-mL vial = £111.20; 1-mL vial = £148.27; 2-mL vial = £197.69

NOTE. May be diluted with sodium chloride 0.9%

4.10   Drugs used in substance dependence

This section includes drugs used in alcohol dependence, cigarette smoking, and opioid dependence.

The health departments of the UK have produced a report, *Drug Misuse and Dependence* which contains guidelines on clinical management.

Drug Misuse and Dependence, London, The Stationery Office, 1999 can be obtained from:

The Publications Centre
PO Box 276, London SW8 5DT
Telephone orders (087) 0600 5522
Fax (087) 0600 5533

or from The Stationery Office bookshops and through all good booksellers.

It is **important** to be aware that *people who misuse drugs* may be at risk not only from the intrinsic toxicity of the drug itself but also from the practice of injecting preparations intended for administration by mouth. Excipients used in the production of oral dose forms are usually insoluble and may lead to *abscess formation at the site of injection*, or even to *necrosis and gangrene*; moreover, deposits in the heart or lungs may lead to *severe cardiac or pulmonary toxicity*. Additional hazards include *infection* following the use of a dirty needle or an unsterilised diluent.

Alcohol dependence

Disulfiram is used as an adjunct to the treatment of alcohol dependence. It gives rise to extremely unpleasant systemic reactions after the ingestion of even a small amount of alcohol because it leads to accumulation of acetaldehyde in the body. Reactions include flushing of the face, throbbing headache, palpitations, tachycardia, nausea, vomiting, and, with large doses of alcohol, arrhythmias, hypotension, and collapse. Small amounts of alcohol included in many oral medicines may be sufficient to precipitate a reaction (even toiletries and mouthwashes that contain alcohol should be avoided). It may be advisable for patients to carry a card warning of the danger of administration of alcohol.

Long-acting **benzodiazepines** (section 4.1) are used to attenuate withdrawal symptoms but they also have a dependence potential. To minimise the risk of dependence, administration should be for a limited period only (e.g. **chlordiazepoxide** 10–50 mg 4 times daily, gradually reducing over 7–14 days). Benzodiazepines should not be prescribed if the patient is likely to continue drinking alcohol.

Clomethiazole (chlormethiazole) (section 4.1.1) should be used for the management of withdrawal in an **in-patient setting only**. It is associated with a risk of dependence and should not be prescribed if the patient is likely to continue drinking alcohol.

Acamprosate, in combination with counselling, may be helpful in maintaining abstinence in alcohol-dependent patients. It should be initiated as soon as possible *after* abstinence has been achieved and should be maintained if the patient relapses. Continued alcohol abuse, however, negates the therapeutic benefit of acamprosate.

ACAMPROSATE CALCIUM

Indications: maintenance of abstinence in alcohol dependence

Cautions: continued alcohol abuse (risk of treatment failure)

Contra-indications: renal and severe hepatic impairment; pregnancy and breast-feeding

Side-effects: diarrhoea, nausea, vomiting, abdominal pain, pruritus, occasionally maculopapular rash, rarely bullous skin reactions; fluctuation in libido

Dose: ADULT 18–65 years, 60 kg and over, 666 mg 3 times daily; less than 60 kg, 666 mg at breakfast, 333 mg at midday and 333 mg at night

TREATMENT COURSE. Treatment should be initiated as soon as possible after alcohol withdrawal period and maintained if patient relapses; recommended treatment period 1 year

Campral EC® (Merck) [PoM]
Tablet, e/c, acamprosate calcium 333 mg. Net price 168-tab pack = £28.92. Label: 21, 25
Electrolytes: Ca²⁺ 0.8 mmol/tablet

DISULFIRAM

Indications: adjunct in the treatment of chronic alcohol dependence (under specialist supervision)

Cautions: ensure that alcohol not consumed for at least 24 hours before initiating treatment; see also notes above; alcohol challenge **not** recommended on routine basis (if considered essential—specialist units only with resuscitation facilities); hepatic or renal impairment, respiratory disease, diabetes mellitus, epilepsy; **interactions:** Appendix 1 (disulfiram)

ALCOHOL REACTION. Patients should be warned of unpredictable and occasionally severe nature of disulfiram-alcohol interactions. Reactions can occur within 10 minutes and last several hours (may require intensive supportive therapy—oxygen should be available). Patients should not ingest alcohol at all and should be warned of possible presence of alcohol in liquid medicines, remedies, tonics, foods and even in toiletries (alcohol should also be avoided for at least 1 week after stopping)

Contra-indications: cardiac failure, coronary artery disease, history of cerebrovascular accident, hypertension, psychosis, severe personality disorder, suicide risk, pregnancy, breast-feeding

Side-effects: initially drowsiness and fatigue; nausea, vomiting, halitosis, reduced libido; rarely psychotic reactions (depression, paranoia, schizophrenia, mania), allergic dermatitis, peripheral neuritis, hepatic cell damage

Dose: 800 mg as a single dose on first day, reducing over 5 days to 100–200 mg daily; should not be continued for longer than 6 months without review; CHILD not recommended

Antabuse® (Alpharma) [PoM]
Tablets, scored, disulfiram 200 mg. Net price 50-tab pack = £18.38. Label: 2, counselling, alcohol reaction

Cigarette smoking

Smoking cessation interventions are a cost-effective way of reducing ill health and prolonging life. Smokers should be advised to stop and offered help if interested in doing so, with follow-up where appropriate.

Where possible, smokers should have access to a smoking cessation clinic for behavioural support. **Nicotine replacement therapy** and **bupropion** are effective aids to smoking cessation for those smoking more than 10 cigarettes a day. Bupropion has been used as an antidepressant but its mode of action in smoking cessation is not clear and may involve an effect on noradrenaline and dopamine neurotransmission. Nicotine replacement therapy is regarded as the pharmacological treatment of choice in the management of smoking cessation.

NICE guidance (nicotine replacement therapy and bupropion for smoking cessation)
NICE has recommended (March 2002) that nicotine replacement therapy or bupropion should be prescribed only for a smoker who commits to a target stop date. The smoker should be offered advice and encouragement to aid smoking cessation.
Therapy to aid smoking cessation is chosen according to the smoker's likely compliance, availability of counselling and support, previous experience of smoking-cessation aids, contra-indications and adverse effects of the products, and the smoker's preferences.
Initial supply of the prescribed smoking-cessation therapy should be sufficient to last only 2 weeks after the target stop date; normally this will be 2 weeks of nicotine replacement therapy or 3–4 weeks of bupropion. A second prescription should be issued only if the smoker demonstrates a continuing attempt to stop smoking.
If an attempt to stop smoking is unsuccessful, the NHS should not normally fund a further attempt within 6 months.
There is currently insufficient evidence to recommend the combined use of nicotine replacement therapy and bupropion.

CSM advice (bupropion). The CSM has issued a reminder that bupropion is contra-indicated in patients with a history of seizures or of eating disorders, a CNS tumour, or who are experiencing acute symptoms of alcohol or benzodiazepine withdrawal. Bupropion should not be prescribed to patients with other risk factors for seizures unless the potential benefit of smoking cessation clearly outweighs the risk. Factors that increase the risk of seizures include concomitant administration of drugs that can lower the seizure threshold (e.g. antidepressants, antimalarials [such as mefloquine and chloroquine], antipsychotics, quinolones, sedating antihistamines, systemic corticosteroids, theophylline, tramadol], alcohol abuse, history of head trauma, diabetes, and use of stimulants and anorectics.

BUPROPION
(Amfebutamone)

Indications: adjunct to smoking cessation in combination with motivational support

Cautions: elderly; hepatic impairment (Appendix 2, avoid in severe hepatic cirrhosis), renal impairment (Appendix 3); predisposition to seizures (see CSM advice above); measure blood pressure before and during treatment (monitor weekly if used with nicotine products); **interactions**: Appendix 1 (bupropion)

DRIVING. May impair performance of skilled tasks (e.g. driving)

Contra-indications: history of seizures, of eating disorders (see CSM advice above) and of bipolar

disorder; pregnancy (Appendix 4); breast-feeding (Appendix 5)

Side-effects: dry mouth, gastro-intestinal disturbances, insomnia (reduced by avoiding dose at bedtime), tremor, impaired concentration, headache, dizziness, depression, agitation, anxiety, rash, pruritus, sweating, hypersensitivity reactions (may resemble serum sickness), fever, taste disturbances; less commonly chest pain, asthenia, tachycardia, hypertension, flushing, anorexia, tinnitus, visual disturbances; rarely palpitations, postural hypotension, vasodilation, hallucinations, depersonalisation, seizures, abnormal dreams, memory impairment, paraesthesia, incoordination, urinary retention, urinary frequency, Stevens-Johnson syndrome, jaundice, hepatitis, blood-glucose disturbances, exacerbation of psoriasis

Dose: start 1–2 weeks before target stop date, initially 150 mg daily for 6 days then 150 mg twice daily (max. single dose 150 mg, max. daily dose 300 mg; minimum 8 hours between doses); max. period of treatment 7–9 weeks; discontinue if abstinence not achieved at 7 weeks; consider max. 150 mg daily in patients with risk factors for seizures (see CSM advice above); ELDERLY max. 150 mg daily; CHILD and ADOLESCENT under 18 years not recommended

Zyban® (GSK) ▼ [PoM]
Tablets, m/r, f/c, bupropion (as hydrochloride) 150 mg, net price 60-tab pack = £42.85. Label: 25

NICOTINE

Indications: adjunct to smoking cessation

Cautions: cardiovascular disease (avoid if severe); peripheral vascular disease; hyperthyroidism; diabetes mellitus; phaeochromocytoma, renal and hepatic impairment; history of gastritis and peptic ulcers; should not smoke or use nicotine replacement products in combination; pregnancy (Appendix 4); breast-feeding (Appendix 5); *patches*, exercise may increase absorption and side-effects, skin disorders (patches should not be placed on broken skin)

Contra-indications: severe cardiovascular disease (including severe arrhythmias or immediate postmyocardial infarction period); recent cerebrovascular accident (including transient ischaemic attacks)

Side-effects: nausea, dizziness, headache and cold and influenza-like symptoms, palpitations, dyspepsia and other gastro-intestinal disturbances, hiccups, insomnia, vivid dreams, myalgia; other side-effects reported include chest pain, blood pressure changes, anxiety and irritability, somnolence and impaired concentration, abnormal hunger, dysmenorrhoea, rash; *with patches*, skin reactions (discontinue if severe)—vasculitis also reported; *with spray*, nasal irritation, nose bleeds, watering eyes, ear sensations; *with gum, lozenges, sublingual tablets* or *inhalator*, aphthous ulceration (sometimes with swelling of tongue); *with spray, inhalator, lozenges, sublingual tablets* or *gum*, throat irritation; *with inhalator*, cough, rhinitis, pharyngitis, stomatitis, sinusitis, dry mouth; *with lozenges* or *sublingual tablets*, unpleasant taste

Dose: see under preparations, below
NOTE. Proprietary brands of nicotine products on sale to the public include *Boots Nicotine Gum* 2 mg, 4 mg, *Boots*

Nicotine Inhalator 10 mg, and *Boots NRT Patch* 7 mg/24 hours, 14 mg/24 hours, 21 mg/24 hours

Nicorette® (Pharmacia)
Nicorette Microtab (sublingual), nicotine (as a cyclodextrin complex) 2 mg, net price starter pack of 2 × 15-tablet discs with dispenser = £3.57; refill pack of 7 × 15-tablet discs = £9.84. Label: 26
Dose: individuals smoking 20 cigarettes or less daily, *sublingually*, 2 mg each hour; for patients who fail to stop smoking or have significant withdrawal symptoms, consider increasing to 4 mg each hour
Individuals smoking more than 20 cigarettes daily, 4 mg each hour
Max. 80 mg daily; treatment should be continued for at least 3 months followed by a gradual reduction in dosage; max. period of treatment should not exceed 6 months
CHILD under 18 years not recommended
Nicorette chewing gum, sugar-free, nicotine (as resin) 2 mg, net price pack of 15 = £1.71, pack of 30 = £3.25, pack of 105 = £8.89; 4 mg, net price pack of 15 = £2.11, pack of 30 = £3.99, pack of 105 = £10.83
NOTE. Also available in citrus and mint flavour
Dose: individuals smoking 20 cigarettes or fewer daily, initially one 2-mg piece chewed slowly for approx. 30 minutes, when urge to smoke occurs; individuals smoking more than 20 cigarettes daily or needing more than 15 pieces of 2-mg gum daily may need the 4-mg strength; max. 15 pieces of 4-mg strength daily; withdraw gradually after 3 months; CHILD under 18 years not recommended
Nicorette patches, self-adhesive, all beige, nicotine, *'5 mg' patch* (releasing approx. 5 mg/16 hours), net price 7 = £9.07; *'10 mg' patch* (releasing approx. 10 mg/16 hours), 7 = £9.07; *'15 mg' patch* (releasing approx. 15 mg/16 hours), 2 = £2.85, 7 = £9.07
Dose: apply on waking to dry, non-hairy skin on hip, chest or upper arm, removing after approx. 16 hours, usually when retiring to bed; site next patch on different area (avoid using same area on consecutive days); initially '15-mg' patch for 16 hours daily for 8 weeks then if abstinence achieved '10-mg' patch for 16 hours daily for 2 weeks then '5-mg' patch for 16 hours daily for 2 weeks; review treatment if abstinence not achieved in 3 months—further courses may be given if considered beneficial; CHILD under 18 years not recommended
Nicorette nasal spray, nicotine 500 micrograms/ metered spray. Net price 200-spray unit = £10.99
Dose: apply 1 spray into each nostril as required to max. twice an hour for 16 hours daily (max. 64 sprays daily) for 8 weeks, then reduce gradually over next 4 weeks (reduce by half at end of first 2 weeks, stop altogether at end of next 2 weeks); max. treatment length 3 months; CHILD under 18 years not recommended
Nicorette inhalator (nicotine-impregnated plug for use in inhalator mouthpiece), nicotine 10 mg/ cartridge. Net price 6-cartridge (starter) pack = £3.39, 42-cartridge (refill) pack = £11.37
Dose: inhale when urge to smoke occurs; initially use between 6 and 12 cartridges daily for up to 8 weeks, then reduce number of cartridges used by half over next 2 weeks and then stop altogether at end of further 2 weeks; review treatment if abstinence not achieved in 3 months; CHILD under 18 years not recommended

Nicotinell® (Novartis Consumer Health)
Chewing gum, sugar-free, nicotine 2 mg, net price pack of 12 = £1.59, pack of 24 = £3.01, pack of 96 = £8.26; 4 mg, pack of 12 = £1.70, pack of 24 = £3.30, pack of 96 = £10.26
NOTE. Also available in fruit and mint flavours

Dose: initially one 2-mg piece chewed slowly for approx. 30 minutes, when urge to smoke occurs; max. 15 pieces daily; withdraw gradually after 3 months; CHILD under 18 years not recommended
Nicotinell mint lozenge, sugar-free, nicotine (as bitartrate) 1 mg, net price pack of 12 = £1.71, pack of 36 = £4.27, pack of 96 = £9.12. Label: 24
Excipients: include aspartame (section 9.4.1)
Dose: initially 1 lozenge every 1–2 hours, when urge to smoke occurs; max. 25 lozenges daily; withdraw gradually after 3 months; max. period of treatment should not usually exceed 6 months; CHILD under 18 years not recommended
TTS Patches, self-adhesive, all yellowish-ochre, nicotine, *'10' patch* (releasing approx. 7 mg/24 hours), net price 7 = £9.12; *'20' patch* (releasing approx. 14 mg/24 hours), net price 2 = £2.57, 7 = £9.40; *'30' patch* (releasing approx. 21 mg/24 hours), net price 2 = £2.85, 7 = £9.97, 21 = £24.51
Dose: apply to dry, non-hairy skin on trunk or upper arm, removing after 24 hours and siting replacement patch on a different area (avoid using the same area for several days); individuals smoking 20 cigarettes daily or fewer, initially '20' patch daily; individuals smoking more than 20 cigarettes daily, initially '30' patch daily; withdraw gradually, reducing dose every 3–4 weeks; review treatment if abstinence not achieved in 3 months; CHILD under 18 years not recommended

NiQuitin CQ® (GSK Consumer Healthcare)
Chewing gum, sugar-free, mint-flavour, nicotine 2 mg, net price pack of 12 = £1.71, pack of 24 = £3.25, pack of 96 = £9.97; 4 mg, net price pack of 12 = £1.71, pack of 24 = £3.25, pack of 96 = £9.97
Dose: initially 1 piece chewed slowly for approx. 30 minutes, when urge to smoke occurs; max. 15 pieces daily; withdraw gradually after 3 months; CHILD under 18 years not recommended
Lozenges, sugar-free, nicotine (as polocrilex) 2 mg, net price pack of 36 = £5.12, pack of 72 = £9.97; 4 mg, pack of 36 = £5.12, pack of 72 = £9.97.
Contains 0.65 mmol Na$^+$/lozenge
Excipients: include aspartame (section 9.4.1)
Dose: initially 1 lozenge every 1–2 hours (when urge to smoke occurs) (max. 15 lozenges daily) for 6 weeks, then 1 lozenge every 2–4 hours for 3 weeks, then 1 lozenge every 4–8 hours for 3 weeks; withdraw gradually after 3 months; max. period of treatment should not exceed 6 months; CHILD under 18 years not recommended
Patches, self-adhesive, pink/beige, nicotine *'7 mg' patch* (releasing approx. 7 mg/24 hours), net price 7 = £9.97; *'14 mg' patch* (releasing approx. 14 mg/ 24 hours), 7 = £9.97; *'21 mg' patch* (releasing approx. 21 mg/24 hours), 7 = £9.97, 14 = £18.79
NOTE. Also available as a clear patch
Dose: apply on waking to dry, non-hairy skin site, removing after 24 hours and siting replacement patch on different area (avoid using same area for 7 days); individuals smoking 10 or more cigarettes daily, initially '21-mg' patch daily for 6 weeks then '14-mg' patch daily for 2 weeks then '7-mg' patch daily for 2 weeks; review treatment if abstinence not achieved in 10 weeks
Individuals smoking less than 10 cigarettes daily, initially '14-mg' patch daily for 6 weeks then '7-mg' patch daily for 2 weeks
CHILD not recommended
NOTE. Patients using the '21-mg' patch who experience excessive side-effects, which do not resolve within a few days, should change to '14-mg' patch for the remainder of the initial 6 weeks before switching to the '7-mg' patch for the final 2 weeks

Opioid dependence

The management of opioid dependence requires medical, social, and psychological treatment; access to a multidisciplinary team is valuable. Treatment with opioid substitutes or with naltrexone is best initiated under the supervision of an appropriately qualified physician.

Methadone, an opioid *agonist*, can be substituted for opioids such as diamorphine, preventing the onset of withdrawal symptoms; it is itself addictive and should only be prescribed for those who are physically dependent on opioids. It is administered in a single daily dose usually as methadone oral solution 1 mg/mL. The dose is adjusted according to the degree of dependence with the aim of gradual reduction.

Buprenorphine is an opioid partial agonist. Because of its abuse and dependence potential it should be prescribed only for those who are already physically dependent on opioids. It can be used as substitution therapy for patients with moderate opioid dependence. In patients dependent on high doses of opioids, buprenorphine may precipitate withdrawal due to its partial antagonist properties; in these patients, the daily opioid dose should be reduced gradually before initiating therapy with buprenorphine.

Naltrexone, an opioid *antagonist*, blocks the action of opioids and precipitates withdrawal symptoms in opioid-dependent subjects. Because the euphoric action of opioid agonists is blocked by naltrexone it is given to former addicts as an aid to prevent relapse.

Lofexidine is used for the alleviation of symptoms in individuals whose opioid use is well controlled and are undergoing opioid withdrawal. Like clonidine it is an alpha-adrenergic agonist and appears to act centrally to produce a reduction in sympathetic tone, but reduction in blood pressure is less marked.

BUPRENORPHINE

Indications: adjunct in the treatment of opioid dependence; premedication, peri-operative analgesia, analgesia in other situations (section 4.7.2)

Cautions: see section 4.7.2 and notes above; effects only partially reversed by naloxone

Contra-indications: see section 4.7.2; breast-feeding (Appendix 5)

Side-effects: see section 4.7.2

Dose: *by sublingual administration*, initially, 0.8–4 mg as a single daily dose, adjusted according to response; max. 32 mg daily; withdraw gradually; CHILD under 16 years not recommended
NOTE. In those who have not undergone opioid withdrawal, buprenorphine should be administered at least 4 hours after last use of opioid or when signs of craving appear
For those receiving methadone, dose of methadone should be reduced to max. 30 mg daily before starting buprenorphine

Subutex® (Schering-Plough) [CD]
Tablets (sublingual), buprenorphine (as hydrochloride) 400 micrograms, net price 7-tab pack = £1.60; 2 mg, 7-tab pack = £6.72; 8 mg, 7-tab pack = £20.16. Label: 2, 26

LOFEXIDINE HYDROCHLORIDE

Indications: management of symptoms of opioid withdrawal

Cautions: severe coronary insufficiency, recent myocardial infarction, cerebrovascular disease, marked bradycardia (monitor pulse rate frequently); renal impairment; history of depression (on longer treatment); pregnancy and breast-feeding; withdraw gradually over 2–4 days (or longer) to minimise risk of rebound hypertension and associated symptoms; **interactions:** Appendix 1 (lofexidine)

Side-effects: drowsiness, dry mucous membranes (particularly dry mouth, throat and nose), hypotension, bradycardia, rebound hypertension on withdrawal (see Cautions); sedation and coma in overdosage

Dose: initially, 200 micrograms twice daily, increased as necessary in steps of 200–400 micrograms daily to max. 2.4 mg daily; recommended duration of treatment 7–10 days if no opioid use (but longer may be required); withdraw gradually over 2–4 days or longer; CHILD not recommended

BritLofex® (Britannia) [PoM]
Tablets, peach, f/c, lofexidine hydrochloride 200 micrograms. Net price 60-tab pack = £74.44. Label: 2

METHADONE HYDROCHLORIDE

Indications: adjunct in treatment of opioid dependence, see notes above; analgesia (section 4.7.2); cough in terminal disease (section 3.9.1)

Cautions: section 4.7.2

Contra-indications: section 4.7.2

Side-effects: section 4.7.2; **overdosage:** see Emergency Treatment of Poisoning, p. 24
IMPORTANT. Methadone, even in low doses is a **special hazard** for children; non-dependent adults are also at risk of toxicity; dependent adults are at risk if tolerance is incorrectly assessed during induction
INCOMPATIBILITY. Syrup preserved with hydroxybenzoate (parabens) esters may be incompatible with methadone hydrochloride.

Dose: initially 10–20 mg daily, increased by 10–20 mg daily until no signs of withdrawal or intoxication; usual dose 40–60 mg daily; CHILD not recommended (see also important note above)

Methadone (Non-proprietary) [CD]
Oral solution 1 mg/mL, methadone hydrochloride 1 mg/mL, net price 30 mL = 44p, 50 mL = 73p, 100 mL = £1.45, 500 mL = £7.59. Label: 2
Available from Generics (*Methex*®), Hillcross, Martindale (*Physeptone*, also as sugar-free), Rosemont (*Metharose*®, sugar-free), Thornton & Ross—taste and colour of different formulations may vary slightly, also available as sugar-free
IMPORTANT. This preparation is 2½ times the strength of Methadone Linctus; many preparations of this strength are licensed for opioid drug addiction only but some are also licensed for analgesia in severe pain
Injection, methadone hydrochloride 25 mg/mL, net price 2-mL amp = £2.04; 50 mg/mL, 1-mL amp = £2.04
Available from Auden Mckenzie (*Synastone*®)

Methadose® (Rosemont) CD

Oral concentrate, methadone hydrochloride 10 mg/ mL (blue), net price 150 mL = £12.78; 20 mg/mL (brown), 150 mL = £25.56. Label: 2

NOTE. The final strength of the methadone mixture to be dispensed to the patient must be specified on the prescription

IMPORTANT. Care is required in prescribing and dispensing the **correct strength** since any confusion could lead to an overdose; this preparation should be dispensed only **after dilution** as appropriate with *Methadose® Diluent* (life of diluted solution 3 months) and is for drug dependent persons (see also p. 7)

NALTREXONE HYDROCHLORIDE

Indications: adjunct to prevent relapse in detoxified formerly opioid-dependent patients (who have remained opioid-free for at least 7–10 days)

Cautions: hepatic and renal impairment; liver function tests needed before and during treatment; test for opioid dependence with naloxone; avoid concomitant use of opioids but increased dose of opioid analgesic may be required for pain (monitor for opioid intoxication); pregnancy, breast-feeding

WARNING FOR PATIENTS. Patients need to be warned that an attempt to overcome the block could result in acute opioid intoxication

Contra-indications: patients currently dependent on opioids; acute hepatitis or liver failure

Side-effects: nausea, vomiting, abdominal pain; anxiety, nervousness, sleeping difficulty, headache, reduced energy; joint and muscle pain; less frequently, loss of appetite, diarrhoea, constipation, increased thirst; chest pain; increased sweating and lacrimation; increased energy, 'feeling down', irritability, dizziness, chills; delayed ejaculation, decreased potency; rash; occasionally, liver function abnormalities; reversible idiopathic thrombocytopenia reported

Dose: (initiate in specialist clinics only) 25 mg initially then 50 mg daily; the total weekly dose may be divided and given on 3 days of the week for improved compliance (e.g. 100 mg on Monday and Wednesday, and 150 mg on Friday); CHILD not recommended

Nalorex® (Bristol-Myers Squibb) PoM

Tablets, yellow, f/c, scored, naltrexone hydrochloride 50 mg. Net price 28-tab pack = £42.51

4.11 Drugs for dementia

Acetylcholinesterase inhibiting drugs are used in the treatment of Alzheimer's disease, specifically for mild to moderate disease. The evidence to support the use of these drugs relates to their cognitive enhancement.

Treatment with drugs for dementia should be initiated and supervised only by a specialist experienced in the management of dementia.

Benefit is assessed by repeating the cognitive assessment at around 3 months. Such assessment cannot demonstrate how the disease may have progressed in the absence of treatment but it can give a good guide to response. Up to half the patients given these drugs will show a slower rate of cognitive decline. The drug should be discontinued in those thought not to be responding. Many specialists repeat the cognitive assessment 4 to 6 weeks after discontinuation to assess deterioration; if significant dete-

rioration occurs during this short period, consideration should be given to restarting therapy.

Donepezil is a reversible inhibitor of acetylcholinesterase that can be given once daily. **Galantamine** is a reversible inhibitor of acetylcholinesterase and it also has nicotinic receptor agonist properties. It is given twice daily. **Rivastigmine** is a reversible noncompetitive inhibitor of acetylcholinesterases, which is given twice daily.

Acetylcholinesterase inhibitors can cause unwanted dose-related cholinergic effects and should be started at a low dose and the dose increased according to response and tolerability.

Memantine is a NMDA-receptor antagonist that affects glutamate transmission; it is licensed for treating moderate to severe Alzheimer's disease.

> **NICE guidance (Alzheimer's disease).** NICE has recommended (January 2001) that, for the adjunctive treatment of mild and moderate Alzheimer's disease in those whose mini mental-state examination (MMSE) score is above 12 points, donepezil, galantamine, and rivastigmine should be available under the following conditions:
>
> • Alzheimer's disease must be diagnosed in a specialist clinic; the clinic should also assess cognitive, global and behavioural functioning, activities of daily living, and the likelihood of compliance with treatment;
>
> • treatment should be initiated by specialists but may be continued by general practitioners under a shared-care protocol;
>
> • the carers' views of the condition should be sought before and during drug treatment;
>
> • the patient should be assessed 2–4 months after maintenance dose is established; drug treatment should continue only if MMSE score has improved or has not deteriorated *and* if behavioural or functional assessment shows improvement;
>
> • the patient should be assessed every 6 months and drug treatment should normally continue only if MMSE score remains above 12 points and if treatment is considered to have a worthwhile effect on the global, functional and behavioural condition.

DONEPEZIL HYDROCHLORIDE

Indications: mild to moderate dementia in Alzheimer's disease

Cautions: sick sinus syndrome or other supraventricular conduction abnormalities; susceptibility to peptic ulcers; asthma, chronic obstructive pulmonary disease; may exacerbate extrapyramidal symptoms; hepatic impairment; **interactions:** Appendix 1 (parasympathomimetics)

Contra-indications: pregnancy and breast-feeding

Side-effects: nausea, vomiting, anorexia, diarrhoea, fatigue, insomnia, headache, dizziness, syncope, psychiatric disturbances, muscle cramps, urinary incontinence, rash, pruritus; less frequently, bradycardia, convulsions, gastric and duodenal ulcers, gastro-intestinal haemorrhage; rarely, sino-atrial block, AV block, hepatitis reported; potential for bladder outflow obstruction

Dose: 5 mg once daily at bedtime, increased if necessary after one month to 10 mg daily; max. 10 mg daily

Aricept® (Pfizer, Eisai) PoM
Tablets, f/c, donepezil hydrochloride 5 mg, net price 28-tab pack = £68.32; 10 mg (yellow), 28-tab pack = £95.76.

GALANTAMINE

Indications: mild to moderate dementia in Alzheimer's disease

Cautions: hepatic impairment (Appendix 2—avoid if severe); sick sinus syndrome or other supraventricular conduction abnormalities; susceptibility to peptic ulcers; asthma, chronic obstructive pulmonary disease; pregnancy (Appendix 4); avoid in urinary retention and gastro-intestinal obstruction; **interactions:** Appendix 1 (parasympathomimetics)

Contra-indications: severe renal impairment; breast-feeding (Appendix 5); metabolic disorders of galactose metabolism

Side-effects: nausea, vomiting (transient), diarrhoea, abdominal pain, dyspepsia, anorexia, fatigue, dizziness, headache, drowsiness, weight loss; less commonly confusion, insomnia, rhinitis, urinary tract infection; tremor; syncope and severe bradycardia reported; potential for bladder outflow obstruction, convulsions

Dose: initially 4 mg twice daily for 4 weeks increased to 8 mg twice daily for 4 weeks; maintenance 8–12 mg twice daily

Reminyl® (Shire) PoM
Tablets, all f/c, galantamine (as hydrobromide) 4 mg (white), net price 56-tab pack = £54.60; 8 mg (pink), 56-tab pack = £68.32; 12 mg (orange-brown), 56-tab pack = £84.00 Label: 21
Oral solution, galantamine (as hydrobromide) 4 mg/mL, net price 100 mL with pipette = £120.00. Label: 21

MEMANTINE HYDROCHLORIDE

Indications: moderate to severe dementia in Alzheimer's disease

Cautions: renal impairment (avoid if severe—Appendix 3); epilepsy; pregnancy (Appendix 4); **interactions:** Appendix 1 (memantine)

Contra-indications: breast-feeding

Side-effects: dizziness, confusion, headache, hallucinations, tiredness; less commonly, vomiting, anxiety, hypertonia, cystitis, increased libido

Dose: initially, 5 mg in the morning, increased in steps of 5 mg at intervals of 1 week up to max. 10 mg twice daily

Ebixa® (Lundbeck) ▼ PoM
Tablets, f/c, scored, memantine hydrochloride 10 mg, net price 28-tab pack = £37.10, 56-tab pack = £74.20, 112-tab pack = £148.40
Oral drops, memantine hydrochloride 10 mg/g, net price 50 g = £66.25, 100 g = £132.50
NOTE. 5 mg ≡ 10 drops of memantine hydrochloride oral drops

RIVASTIGMINE

Indications: mild to moderate dementia in Alzheimer's disease

Cautions: renal impairment, mild to moderate hepatic impairment (Appendix 2); sick sinus syndrome, conduction abnormalities; gastric or duodenal ulcers (and those at risk of developing ulcers); history of asthma or chronic obstructive pulmonary disease; history of seizures, bladder outflow obstruction, pregnancy (Appendix 4); may exacerbate extrapyramidal symptoms (including worsening of Parkinson's disease); monitor body-weight; **interactions:** Appendix 1 (parasympathomimetics)
NOTE. If treatment interrupted for more than several days, re-introduce with initial dose and increase gradually (see Dose)

Contra-indications: breast-feeding

Side-effects: nausea, vomiting, diarrhoea, dyspepsia, anorexia, abdominal pain; dizziness, headache, drowsiness, tremor, asthenia, malaise, agitation, confusion; sweating; less commonly, syncope, depression, insomnia; rarely gastric or duodenal ulceration, gastro-intestinal haemorrhage, pancreatitis, angina pectoris, arrhythmias, bradycardia, hypertension, convulsions, hallucinations, urinary infection, rash
NOTE. Gastro-intestinal side-effects may occur more commonly in women

Dose: initially 1.5 mg twice daily, increased in steps of 1.5 mg twice daily at intervals of at least 2 weeks according to response and tolerance; usual range 3–6 mg twice daily; max. 6 mg twice daily

Exelon® (Novartis) PoM
Capsules, rivastigmine (as hydrogen tartrate) 1.5 mg (yellow), net price 28-cap pack = £34.02, 56-cap pack = £68.04; 3 mg (orange), 28-cap pack = £34.02, 56-cap pack = £68.04; 4.5 mg (red), 28-cap pack = £34.02, 56-cap pack = £68.04; 6 mg (red/orange), 28-cap pack = £34.02, 56-cap pack = £68.04. Label: 21, 25
Oral solution, rivastigmine (as hydrogen tartrate) 2 mg/mL, net price 120 mL (with oral syringe) = £116.64. Label: 21

5: Infections

Notifiable diseases

Doctors must notify the Proper Officer of the local authority (usually the consultant in communicable disease control) when attending a patient suspected of suffering from any of the diseases listed below; a form is available from the Proper Officer.

Anthrax	Ophthalmia neonatorum
Cholera	Paratyphoid fever
Diphtheria	Plague
Dysentery (amoebic or bacillary)	Poliomyelitis, acute
Encephalitis, acute	Rabies
Food poisoning	Relapsing fever
Haemorrhagic fever (viral)	Rubella
Hepatitis, viral	Scarlet fever
Leprosy	Smallpox
Leptospirosis	Tetanus
Malaria	Tuberculosis
Measles	Typhoid fever
Meningitis	Typhus
Meningococcal septicaemia (without meningitis)	Whooping cough
Mumps	Yellow fever

NOTE. It is good practice for doctors to also inform the consultant in communicable disease control of instances of other infections (e.g. psittacosis) where there could be a public health risk.

5.1   Antibacterial drugs

CHOICE OF A SUITABLE DRUG. Before selecting an antibacterial the clinician must first consider two factors—the patient and the known or likely causative organism. Factors related to the patient which must be considered include history of allergy, renal and hepatic function, resistance to infection (i.e. whether immunocompromised), ability to tolerate drugs by mouth, severity of illness, ethnic origin, age and, if female, whether pregnant, breast-feeding or taking an oral contraceptive.

The known or likely organism and its antibacterial sensitivity, in association with the above factors, will suggest one or more antibacterials, the final choice depending on the microbiological, pharmacological, and toxicological properties.

An example of a rational approach to the selection of an antibacterial is treatment of a urinary-tract infection in a patient complaining of nausea in early pregnancy. The organism is reported as being resistant to ampicillin but sensitive to nitrofurantoin (can cause nausea), gentamicin (can be given only by injection and best avoided in pregnancy), tetracycline (causes dental discoloration) and trimethoprim (folate antagonist therefore theoretical teratogenic risk), and cefalexin. The safest antibiotics in pregnancy are the penicillins and cephalosporins; therefore, cefalexin would be indicated for this patient.

The principles involved in selection of an antibacterial must allow for a number of variables including changing renal and hepatic function, increasing bacterial resistance, and new information on side-effects. Duration of therapy, dosage, and route of administration depend on site, type and severity of infection and response.

ANTIBACTERIAL POLICIES. Local policies often limit the antibacterials that may be used to achieve reasonable economy consistent with adequate cover, and to reduce the development of resistant organisms. A policy may indicate a range of drugs for general use, and permit other drugs only on the advice of the microbiologist or physician responsible for the control of infectious diseases.

BEFORE STARTING THERAPY. The following precepts should be considered before starting:

- Viral infections should not be treated with antibacterials;
- Samples should be taken for culture and sensitivity testing; 'blind' antibacterial prescribing for unexplained pyrexia usually leads to further difficulty in establishing the diagnosis;
- Knowledge of **prevalent organisms** and their current sensitivity is of great help in choosing an antibacterial before bacteriological confirmation is available;
- The **dose** of an antibacterial varies according to a number of factors including age, weight, renal function, and severity of infection. The prescribing of the so-called 'standard' dose in serious infections may result in failure of treatment or even death of the patient; therefore it is important to prescribe a dose appropriate to the condition. An inadequate dose may also increase the likelihood of antibacterial resistance. On the other hand, for an antibacterial with a narrow margin between the toxic and therapeutic dose (e.g. an aminoglycoside) it is also important to avoid an excessive dose and the concentration of the drug in the plasma may need to be monitored;
- The **route** of administration of an antibacterial often depends on the severity of the infection. Life-threatening infections require intravenous therapy. Whenever possible painful intramuscular injections should be avoided in children;
- **Duration** of therapy depends on the nature of the infection and the response to treatment. Courses should not be unduly prolonged because they encourage resistance, they may lead to side-effects and they are costly. However, in certain infections such as tuberculosis or chronic osteomyelitis it is necessary to treat for prolonged periods. Conversely a single dose of an antibacterial may cure uncomplicated urinary-tract infections.

SUPERINFECTION. In general, broad-spectrum antibacterial drugs such as the cephalosporins are more likely to be associated with adverse reactions related to the selection of resistant organisms e.g. *fungal infections* or *antibiotic-associated colitis* (pseudomembranous colitis); other problems associated with superinfection include vaginitis and pruritus ani.

THERAPY. Suggested treatment is shown in table 1. When the pathogen has been isolated treatment may be changed to a more appropriate antibacterial if necessary. If no bacterium is cultured the antibacterial can be continued or stopped on clinical grounds. Infections for which prophylaxis is useful are listed in table 2.

Table 1. Summary of antibacterial therapy

> If treating a patient suspected of suffering from a notifiable disease, the consultant in communicable disease control should be informed (see p. 253)

Gastro-intestinal system

Gastro-enteritis
Antibacterial not usually indicated
Frequently self-limiting and may not be bacterial

Campylobacter enteritis
Ciprofloxacin *or* erythromycin

Invasive salmonellosis
Ciprofloxacin *or* trimethoprim
Includes severe infections which may be invasive

Shigellosis
Ciprofloxacin *or* trimethoprim
Antibacterial not indicated for mild cases. Ciprofloxacin should be used for trimethoprim-resistant strains

Typhoid fever
Ciprofloxacin *or* cefotaxime *or* chloramphenicol
Infections from Indian subcontinent, Middle-East, and South-East Asia may be multiple-antibacterial-resistant and sensitivity should be tested; azithromycin [unlicensed indication] may be an option in mild or moderate disease caused by multiple antibacterial-resistant organisms

Antibiotic-associated colitis (pseudomembranous colitis)
Oral metronidazole *or* oral vancomycin
Give metronidazole by intravenous infusion if oral treatment inappropriate

Biliary-tract infection
A cephalosporin *or* gentamicin

Peritonitis
A cephalosporin (*or* gentamicin) + metronidazole (*or* clindamycin)

Peritoneal dialysis-associated peritonitis
Either vancomycin[1] + ceftazidime added to dialysis fluid *or* vancomycin added to dialysis fluid + ciprofloxacin by mouth
Treat for 14 days or longer

Cardiovascular system

Endocarditis caused by streptococci (e.g. viridans streptococci)
Benzylpenicillin (*or* vancomycin[1] if penicillin-allergic) + low-dose gentamicin (i.e. 80 mg twice daily)
Treat for up to 4 weeks; stop after 2 weeks if organism fully sensitive to penicillin; treat penicillin-allergic patients with vancomycin for 4 weeks + low-dose gentamicin for first 2 weeks

Endocarditis caused by enterococci (e.g. *Enterococcus faecalis*)
Amoxicillin[2] (*or* vancomycin[1] if penicillin-allergic) + low-dose gentamicin (i.e. 80 mg twice daily)
Treat for 4 weeks; if gentamicin-resistant, substitute streptomycin for gentamicin and treat for at least 6 weeks

Endocarditis caused by staphylococci (including *Staph. aureus, Staph. epidermidis*)
Flucloxacillin (*or* benzylpenicillin if penicillin-sensitive *or* vancomycin if penicillin-allergic or if methicillin-resistant staphylococci) + gentamicin (*or* fusidic acid)
Treat for 4 weeks; stop gentamicin (or fusidic acid) after 1 week

---

1. Where vancomycin is suggested teicoplanin may be used.

2. Where amoxicillin is suggested ampicillin may be used.

Respiratory system

Haemophilus influenzae epiglottitis
Cefotaxime or chloramphenicol
Give intravenously

Exacerbations of chronic bronchitis
Amoxicillin[1] or tetracycline (or erythromycin[2])
Some pneumococci and Haemophilus influenzae strains tetracycline-resistant; 15% H. influenzae strains amoxicillin-resistant

Uncomplicated community-acquired pneumonia
Amoxicillin[1] (or benzylpenicillin if previously healthy chest or erythromycin[2] if penicillin-allergic)
Add flucloxacillin if staphylococci suspected, e.g. in influenza or measles; treat for 7 days (14–21 days for infections caused by staphylococci); pneumococci with decreased penicillin sensitivity being isolated but not yet common in UK; add erythromycin[2] if atypical pathogens suspected

Severe community-acquired pneumonia of unknown aetiology
Cefuroxime (or cefotaxime) + erythromycin[2]
Add flucloxacillin if staphylococci suspected; treat for 10 days (14–21 days if staphylococci, legionella, or Gram-negative enteric bacilli suspected)

Pneumonia possibly caused by atypical pathogens
Erythromycin[2]
Severe Legionella infections may require addition of rifampicin; tetracycline is an alternative for chlamydial and mycoplasma infections; treat for at least 14 days (14–21 days for legionella)

Hospital-acquired pneumonia
A broad-spectrum cephalosporin (e.g. cefotaxime or ceftazidime) or an antipseudomonal penicillin or another antipseudomonal beta-lactam
An aminoglycoside may be added in severe illness

Central nervous system

Meningitis: Initial 'blind' therapy
- Transfer patient urgently to hospital.
- If bacterial meningitis and especially if meningococcal disease suspected, general practitioners should give benzylpenicillin (see p. 259 for dose) before urgent transfer to hospital; cefotaxime (section 5.1.2) may be an alternative in penicillin allergy; chloramphenicol (section 5.1.7) may be used if history of anaphylaxis to penicillin or to cephalosporins

Meningitis caused by meningococci
Benzylpenicillin or cefotaxime
Treat for at least 5 days; substitute chloramphenicol if history of anaphylaxis to penicillin or to cephalosporins; give rifampicin for 2 days before hospital discharge to patients treated with benzylpenicillin or chloramphenicol

Meningitis caused by pneumococci
Cefotaxime
Treat for 10–14 days; substitute benzylpenicillin if organism penicillin-sensitive; if organism highly penicillin- and cephalosporin-resistant, add vancomycin and if necessary rifampicin; consider early adjunctive treatment with dexamethasone (but may reduce penetration of vancomycin into cerebrospinal fluid)

Meningitis caused by Haemophilus influenzae
Cefotaxime
Treat for at least 10 days; substitute chloramphenicol if history of anaphylaxis to penicillin or to cephalosporins or if organism resistant to cefotaxime; consider early adjunctive treatment with dexamethasone; for H. influenzae type b give rifampicin for 4 days before hospital discharge

Meningitis caused by Listeria
Amoxicillin[1] + gentamicin
Treat for 10–14 days

---

1. Where amoxicillin is suggested ampicillin may be used.

2. Where erythromycin is suggested another macrolide (e.g. azithromycin or clarithromycin) may be used.

Urinary tract

Acute pyelonephritis
A broad-spectrum cephalosporin or a quinolone
Treat for 14 days; longer treatment may be necessary in complicated pyelonephritis

Acute prostatitis
A quinolone or trimethoprim
Treat for 28 days; in severe infection, start treatment with a high dose broad-spectrum cephalosporin (e.g. cefuroxime or cefotaxime) + gentamicin

'Lower' urinary-tract infection
Trimethoprim or amoxicillin[1] or nitrofurantoin or oral cephalosporin
Treat for 7 days but a short course (e.g. 3 days) of trimethoprim or amoxicillin is usually adequate for uncomplicated urinary-tract infections in women

Genital system

Syphilis
Procaine benzylpenicillin [unlicensed] or doxycycline or erythromycin
Treat early syphilis for 14 days (10 days with procaine benzylpenicillin); treat late latent syphilis with procaine benzylpenicillin for 17 days (or with doxycycline for 28 days); treat asymptomatic contacts of patients with infectious syphilis with doxycycline for 14 days or with a single dose of azithromycin; contact tracing recommended

Uncomplicated gonorrhoea
Cefixime [unlicensed indication] or ciprofloxacin
Single-dose treatment in uncomplicated infection; choice depends on locality where infection acquired; use ciprofloxacin only if organism sensitive; contact-tracing recommended; remember chlamydia; pharyngeal infection requires treatment with ciprofloxacin or ofloxacin if sensitive

Uncomplicated genital chlamydial infection, non-gonococcal urethritis and non-specific genital infection
Doxycycline or azithromycin
Treat with doxycycline for 7 days or with azithromycin as a single dose; alternatively treat with erythromycin for 14 days; contact tracing recommended

Pelvic inflammatory disease
Ofloxacin + metronidazole
Treat for at least 14 days; in severely ill patients substitute initial treatment with doxycycline + cefoxitin, then switch to oral treatment with doxycycline + metronidazole to complete 14 days' treatment; contact tracing recommended; remember gonorrhoea

Blood

Septicaemia: Initial 'blind' therapy
Community-acquired septicaemia, aminoglycoside + a broad-spectrum penicillin or a broad-spectrum cephalosporin alone (e.g. cefotaxime)
Hospital-acquired septicaemia, aminoglycoside + a broad-spectrum antipseudomonal beta-lactam antibiotic (e.g. ceftazidime, Tazocin®, Timentin®), or meropenem alone, or imipenem (with cilastatin as Primaxin®) alone
Choice depends on local resistance patterns and clinical presentation; use aminoglycoside + broad-spectrum antipseudomonal beta-lactam antibiotic if pseudomonas suspected; add metronidazole if anaerobic infection suspected; add flucloxacillin or vancomycin[3] if Gram-positive infection suspected

Septicaemia related to vascular catheter
Vancomycin[3]
Add an aminoglycoside + a broad-spectrum antipseudomonal beta-lactam if Gram-negative sepsis suspected, especially in the immunocompromised; consider removing vascular catheter, particularly if infection caused by Staphylococcus aureus, pseudomonas, or candida

---

3. Where vancomycin is suggested teicoplanin may be used.

Meningococcal septicaemia

Benzylpenicillin *or* cefotaxime

If meningococcal disease suspected, general practitioners advised to give a single dose of benzylpenicillin before urgent transportation to hospital (see under Benzylpenicillin, section 5.1.1.1); give rifampicin for 2 days before hospital discharge

Musculoskeletal system

Osteomyelitis

Flucloxacillin *or* clindamycin if penicillin-allergic (*or* vancomycin[1] if resistant *Staphylococcus epidermidis* or methicillin-resistant *Staph. aureus*)

Treat acute infection for 4–6 weeks and chronic infection for at least 12 weeks; combine vancomycin[1] with either fusidic acid or rifampicin if prostheses present or if life-threatening condition

Septic arthritis

Flucloxacillin + fusidic acid (*or* rifampicin) *or* clindamycin alone if penicillin-allergic (*or* vancomycin[1] if resistant *Staphylococcus epidermidis* or methicillin-resistant *Staph. aureus*)

Treat for 6–12 weeks; combine vancomycin[1] with either fusidic acid or rifampicin if prostheses present or if life-threatening condition

Eye

Purulent conjunctivitis

Chloramphenicol *or* gentamicin eye-drops

Ear, nose, and oropharynx

Dental infections

Phenoxymethylpenicillin (*or* amoxicillin[2]) *or* erythromycin *or* metronidazole

Tetracycline for chronic destructive forms of periodontal disease

Sinusitis

Amoxicillin[2] *or* doxycycline *or* erythromycin[3]

Antibacterial should usually be used only for persistent symptoms and purulent discharge lasting at least 7 days or if severe symptoms; treat for 3–7 days

Otitis externa

Flucloxacillin

Use ciprofloxacin (or an aminoglycoside) if pseudomonas suspected, see section 12.1.1

Otitis media

Amoxicillin[2] (*or* erythromycin[3] if penicillin-allergic)

Many infections caused by viruses; most uncomplicated cases resolve without antibacterial treatment; in children without systemic features, antibacterial treatment may be started after 72 hours if no improvement, or earlier if deterioration; treat for 5 days (longer if severely ill); initial parenteral therapy in severe infections; consider co-amoxiclav or ceftriaxone if no improvement after 24–48 hours

Throat infections

Phenoxymethylpenicillin (*or* erythromycin[3] if penicillin-allergic) *or* oral cephalosporin

Most throat infections are caused by viruses and many do not require antibiotic therapy; prescribe antibacterial for beta-haemolytic streptococcal pharyngitis (treat for 10 days), if history of valvular heart disease, if marked systemic upset, if peritonsillar cellulitis or if at increased risk from acute infection (e.g. in immunosuppression, diabetes); **avoid** amoxicillin if possibility of glandular fever, see section 5.1.1.3; initial parenteral therapy (in severe infection) with benzylpenicillin, then oral therapy with phenoxymethylpenicillin *or* amoxicillin[2]

Skin

Impetigo

Topical fusidic acid (*or* mupirocin if methicillin-resistant *Staphylococcus aureus*); oral flucloxacillin *or* erythromycin if widespread

Topical treatment for 7 days usually adequate; max. duration of topical treatment 10 days; seek local micro-

biology advice before using topical treatment in hospital; add phenoxymethylpenicillin to flucloxacillin if streptococcal infection suspected

Erysipelas

Phenoxymethylpenicillin

Add flucloxacillin if staphylococcus suspected

Cellulitis

Phenoxymethylpenicillin + flucloxacillin (*or* erythromycin alone if penicillin-allergic)

Severe cellulitis may require parenteral benzylpenicillin + flucloxacillin

Animal bites

Co-amoxiclav alone

Cleanse wound thoroughly; for tetanus-prone wound, give human tetanus immunoglobulin (with adsorbed tetanus vaccine if necessary, according to immunisation history and risk of infection), see under Tetanus Vaccines, section 14.4

Acne—see section 13.6

Table 2. Summary of antibacterial prophylaxis

Prevention of recurrence of rheumatic fever

Phenoxymethylpenicillin 250 mg twice daily *or* sulfadiazine 1 g daily (500 mg daily for patients under 30 kg)

Prevention of secondary case of meningococcal meningitis[4]

Rifampicin 600 mg every 12 hours for 2 days; CHILD 10 mg/kg (under 1 year, 5 mg/kg) every 12 hours for 2 days

or ciprofloxacin [not licensed for this indication] 500 mg as a single dose; CHILD 5–12 years 250 mg *or* i/m ceftriaxone [not licensed for this indication] 250 mg as a single dose; CHILD under 12 years 125 mg

Prevention of secondary case of *Haemophilus influenzae* type b disease[4]

Rifampicin 600 mg once daily for 4 days (regimen of choice for adults); CHILD 1–3 months 10 mg/kg once daily for 4 days, over 3 months 20 mg/kg once daily for 4 days (max. 600 mg daily)

Prevention of secondary case of diphtheria in non-immune patient

Erythromycin 500 mg every 6 hours for 7 days; CHILD up to 2 years 125 mg every 6 hours, 2–8 years 250 mg every 6 hours

Treat for further 10 days if nasopharyngeal swabs positive after first 7 days' treatment

Prevention of pertussis

ADULT and CHILD erythromycin 50 mg/kg (max. 2 g) daily in 4 divided doses for 14 days

NOTE. Pertussis vaccine inappropriate for outbreak since 3 injections required for protection

Prevention of pneumococcal infection in asplenia or in patients with sickle cell disease

Phenoxymethylpenicillin 500 mg every 12 hours; CHILD under 5 years 125 mg every 12 hours, 6–12 years 250 mg every 12 hours—if cover also

---

1. Where vancomycin is suggested teicoplanin may be used.

2. Where amoxicillin is suggested ampicillin may be used.

3. Where erythromycin is suggested another macrolide (e.g. azithromycin or clarithromycin) may be used.

4. For details of those who should receive chemoprophylaxis contact a consultant in communicable disease control (or a consultant in infectious diseases or the local public health laboratory). Unless there has been mouth-to-mouth contact (or direct exposure to infectious droplets from a patient with meningococcal disease), healthcare workers do not generally require chemoprophylaxis.

needed for *H. influenzae* in CHILD give amoxicillin instead (under 5 years 125 mg every 12 hours, over 5 years 250 mg every 12 hours)

NOTE. Antibiotic prophylaxis is not fully reliable

Prevention of endocarditis[1] in patients with heart-valve lesion, septal defect, patent ductus, prosthetic valve, or history of endocarditis

Dental procedures[2] *under local or no anaesthesia*, patients who have not received more than a single dose of a penicillin[3] in the previous month, including those with a prosthetic valve (but not those who have had endocarditis), oral amoxicillin 3 g 1 hour before procedure; CHILD under 5 years quarter adult dose; 5–10 years half adult dose

patients who are penicillin-allergic or have received more than a single dose of a penicillin[3] in the previous month, oral clindamycin[4] 600 mg 1 hour before procedure; CHILD under 5 years clindamycin[4] 150 mg *or* azithromycin[5] 200 mg; 5–10 years clindamycin[4] 300 mg *or* azithromycin[5] 300 mg

patients who have had endocarditis, amoxicillin + gentamicin, as under general anaesthesia

Dental procedures[2] *under general anaesthesia,*
no special risk (including patients who have not received more than a single dose of a penicillin in the previous month),
either i/v amoxicillin 1 g at induction, then oral amoxicillin 500 mg 6 hours later; CHILD under 5 years quarter adult dose; 5–10 years half adult dose *or* oral amoxicillin 3 g 4 hours before induction then oral amoxicillin 3 g as soon as possible after procedure; CHILD under 5 years quarter adult dose; 5–10 years half adult dose

special risk (patients with a prosthetic valve or who have had endocarditis), i/v amoxicillin 1 g + i/v gentamicin 120 mg at induction, then oral amoxicillin 500 mg 6 hours later; CHILD under 5 years amoxicillin quarter adult dose, gentamicin 2 mg/kg; 5–10 years amoxicillin half adult dose, gentamicin 2 mg/kg

patients who are penicillin-allergic or who have received more than a single dose of a penicillin in the previous month,
either i/v vancomycin 1 g over at least 100 minutes then i/v gentamicin 120 mg at induction or 15 minutes before procedure; CHILD under 10 years vancomycin 20 mg/kg, gentamicin 2 mg/kg *or* i/v teicoplanin 400 mg + gentamicin 120 mg at induction or 15 minutes before procedure; CHILD under 14 years teicoplanin 6 mg/kg, gentamicin 2 mg/kg *or* i/v clindamycin[4] 300 mg over at least 10 minutes at induction or 15 minutes before procedure then oral or i/v clindamycin 150 mg 6 hours later; CHILD under 5 years quarter adult dose; 5–10 years half adult dose

Upper respiratory-tract procedures, as for dental procedures; post-operative dose may be given parenterally if swallowing is painful

Genito-urinary procedures, as for *special risk* patients undergoing dental procedures under general anaesthesia except that clindamycin is not given, see above; if urine infected, prophylaxis should also cover infective organism

Obstetric, gynaecological and gastro-intestinal procedures (prophylaxis required for patients with prosthetic valves or those who have had endocarditis only), as for genito-urinary procedures

---

Joint prostheses and dental treatment. Advice of a Working Party of the British Society for Antimicrobial Chemotherapy is that patients with prosthetic joint implants (including total hip replacements) do not require antibiotic prophylaxis for dental treatment. The Working Party considers that it is unacceptable to expose patients to the adverse effects of antibiotics when there is no evidence that such prophylaxis is of any benefit, but that those who develop any intercurrent infection require prompt treatment with antibiotics to which the infecting organisms are sensitive.
The Working Party has commented that joint infections have rarely been shown to follow dental procedures and are even more rarely caused by oral streptococci.

Dermatological procedures. Advice of a Working Party of the British Society for Antimicrobial Chemotherapy is that patients who undergo dermatological procedures[6] do not require antibacterial prophylaxis against endocarditis.

Immunosuppression and indwelling intraperitoneal catheters. Advice of a Working Party of the British Society for Antimicrobial Chemotherapy is that patients who are immunosuppressed (including transplant patients) and patients with indwelling intraperitoneal catheters do not require antibiotic prophylaxis for dental treatment provided there is no other indication for prophylaxis.
The Working Party has commented that there is little evidence that dental treatment is followed by infection in immunosuppressed and immunodeficient patients nor is there evidence that dental treatment is followed by infection in patients with indwelling intraperitoneal catheters.

---

1. Advice on the prevention of endocarditis reflects the recommendations of a Working Party of the British Society for Antimicrobial Chemotherapy, *Lancet*, 1982, **2**, 1323–26; *idem*, 1986, **1**, 1267; *idem*, 1990, **335**, 88–9; *idem*, 1992, **339**, 1292–93; *idem*, 1997, **350**, 1100; also *J Antimicrob Chemother*, 1993; **31**, 437–8

2. Dental procedures that require antibiotic prophylaxis are, *extractions, scaling,* and *surgery involving gingival tissues.* Antibiotic prophylaxis for dental procedures may be supplemented with *chlorhexidine gluconate gel 1%* or *chlorhexidine gluconate mouthwash 0.2%,* used 5 minutes before procedure

3. For multistage procedures a max. of 2 single doses of a penicillin may be given in a month; alternative drugs should be used for further treatment and the penicillin should not be used again for 3–4 months

4. If **clindamycin** is used, periodontal or other multistage procedures should not be repeated at intervals of less than 2 weeks; clindamycin is not licensed for use in endocarditis prophylaxis

5. Azithromycin is not licensed for use in endocarditis prophylaxis

6. The British Association of Dermatologists Therapy Guidelines and Audit Subcommittee advise that such dermatological procedures include skin biopsies and excision of moles or of malignant lesions

Prevention of gas-gangrene in high lower-limb amputations or following major trauma

Benzylpenicillin 300–600 mg every 6 hours for 5 days *or* if penicillin-allergic metronidazole 500 mg every 8 hours

Prevention of tuberculosis in susceptible close contacts or those who have become tuberculin positive[1]

Isoniazid 300 mg daily for 6 months; CHILD 5–10 mg/kg daily (max. 300 mg daily) *or* isoniazid 300 mg daily + rifampicin 600 mg daily (450 mg if less than 50 kg) for 3 months; CHILD isoniazid 5–10 mg/kg daily (max. 300 mg daily) + rifampicin 10 mg/kg daily (max. 600 mg daily)

Prevention of infection in gastro-intestinal procedures

Operations on stomach or oesophagus for carcinoma, or cholecystectomy in patients with possibly infected bile
Single dose[2] of i/v gentamicin *or* i/v cefuroxime
Resections in colon and rectum for carcinoma, and resections in inflammatory bowel disease, and appendicectomy
Single dose[2] of i/v gentamicin + i/v metronidazole[3] *or* i/v cefuroxime + i/v metronidazole[3] *or* i/v co-amoxiclav alone
Endoscopic retrograde cholangiopancreatography
Single dose of i/v gentamicin *or* oral *or* i/v ciprofloxacin
Prophylaxis particularly recommended if bile stasis, pancreatic pseudocyst, previous cholangitis or neutropenia

Prevention of infection in orthopaedic surgery

Joint replacement including hip and knee
Single dose[2] of i/v cefuroxime *or* i/v flucloxacillin
Substitute i/v vancomycin if history of allergy to penicillins or to cephalosporins

Prevention of infection in urological procedures

Transrectal prostate biopsy
Single dose[2] of i/v cefuroxime + i/v metronidazole[3] *or* i/v gentamicin + i/v metronidazole[3]
Transurethral resection of prostate
Single dose[2] of oral ciprofloxacin *or* i/v gentamicin *or* i/v cefuroxime

Prevention of infection in obstetric and gynaecological surgery

Caesarean section in women at high risk of infection
Single dose[2] of i/v amoxicillin or i/v cefuroxime
Administer immediately after umbilical cord is clamped; substitute i/v clindamycin if history of allergy to penicillins or cephalosporins
Hysterectomy
Single dose[2] of i/v cefuroxime + i/v metronidazole[3] *or* i/v gentamicin + i/v metronidazole[3] *or* i/v co-amoxiclav alone

---

5.1.1 Penicillins

5.1.1.1	Benzylpenicillin and phenoxymethylpenicillin
5.1.1.2	Penicillinase-resistant penicillins
5.1.1.3	Broad-spectrum penicillins
5.1.1.4	Antipseudomonal penicillins
5.1.1.5	Mecillinams

The penicillins are bactericidal and act by interfering with bacterial cell wall synthesis. They diffuse well into body tissues and fluids, but penetration into the cerebrospinal fluid is poor except when the meninges are inflamed. They are excreted in the urine in therapeutic concentrations.

The most important side-effect of the penicillins is hypersensitivity which causes rashes and anaphylaxis and can be fatal. Allergic reactions to penicillins occur in 1–10% of exposed individuals; anaphylactic reactions occur in fewer than 0.05% of treated patients. Individuals with a history of anaphylaxis, urticaria, or rash immediately after penicillin administration are at risk of immediate hypersensitivity to a penicillin; these individuals should not receive a penicillin, a cephalosporin or another beta-lactam antibiotic. Patients who are allergic to one penicillin will be allergic to all because the hypersensitivity is related to the basic penicillin structure. Individuals with a history of a minor rash (i.e. non-confluent rash restricted to a small area of the body) or a rash that occurs more than 72 hours after penicillin administration are probably not allergic to penicillin and in these individuals a penicillin should not be withheld unnecessarily for serious infections; the possibility of an allergic reaction should, however, be borne in mind.

A rare but serious toxic effect of the penicillins is encephalopathy due to cerebral irritation. This may result from excessively high doses or in patients with severe renal failure. The penicillins should **not** be given by intrathecal injection because they can cause encephalopathy which may be fatal.

Another problem relating to high doses of penicillin, or normal doses given to patients with renal failure, is the accumulation of electrolyte since most

---

1. The Joint Tuberculosis Committee recommends chemoprophylaxis for patients with documented recent tuberculin conversion, for some tuberculin-positive children identified in BCG schools programme, for children under 2 years in close contact with smear-positive tuberculosis (including those previously vaccinated with BCG but now showing strongly positive Heaf test), for children under 16 years showing a positive Heaf test at new immigrant or contact screening; chemoprophylaxis should be considered in immigrant adults 16–34 years without a BCG scar but with strongly positive Heaf test. See also section 5.1.9, for advice on immunocompromised patients and on prevention of tuberculosis.

2. Additional intra-operative or postoperative doses of antibacterial may be given for prolonged procedures or if there is major blood loss

3. Metronidazole may alternatively be given by suppository but to allow adequate absorption, it should be given 2 hours before surgery

injectable penicillins contain either sodium or potassium.

Diarrhoea frequently occurs during oral penicillin therapy. It is most common with broad-spectrum penicillins, which can also cause antibiotic-associated colitis.

5.1.1.1 Benzylpenicillin and phenoxymethylpenicillin

Benzylpenicillin (Penicillin G) remains an important and useful antibiotic but is inactivated by bacterial beta-lactamases. It is effective for many streptococcal (including pneumococcal), gonococcal, and meningococcal infections and also for anthrax (section 5.1.12), diphtheria, gas-gangrene, leptospirosis, and treatment of Lyme disease (section 5.1.1.3) in children. Pneumococci, meningococci, and gonococci which have decreased sensitivity to penicillin have been isolated; benzylpenicillin is no longer the drug of first choice for pneumococcal meningitis. Although benzylpenicillin is effective in the treatment of tetanus, metronidazole (section 5.1.11) is preferred. Benzylpenicillin is inactivated by gastric acid and absorption from the gut is low; therefore it is best given by injection.

Procaine benzylpenicillin (procaine penicillin) (available on a named-patient basis from IDIS) is used for the treatment of early syphilis and late latent syphilis; it is given in a dose of 600 mg daily by intramuscular injection.

Phenoxymethylpenicillin (Penicillin V) has a similar antibacterial spectrum to benzylpenicillin, but is less active. It is gastric acid-stable, so is suitable for oral administration. It should not be used for serious infections because absorption can be unpredictable and plasma concentrations variable. It is indicated principally for respiratory-tract infections in children, for streptococcal tonsillitis, and for continuing treatment after one or more injections of benzylpenicillin when clinical response has begun. It should not be used for meningococcal or gonococcal infections. Phenoxymethylpenicillin is used for prophylaxis against streptococcal infections following rheumatic fever and against pneumococcal infections following splenectomy or in sickle cell disease.

BENZYLPENICILLIN
(Penicillin G)

Indications: throat infections, otitis media, streptococcal endocarditis, meningococcal disease, pneumonia (Table 1, section 5.1); anthrax; prophylaxis in limb amputation (Table 2, section 5.1)

Cautions: history of allergy; renal impairment (Appendix 3); false-positive urinary glucose (if tested for reducing substances); **interactions:** Appendix 1 (penicillins)

Contra-indications: penicillin hypersensitivity

Side-effects: hypersensitivity reactions including urticaria, fever, joint pains, rashes, angioedema, anaphylaxis, serum sickness-like reactions, haemolytic anaemia and interstitial nephritis; neutropenia, thrombocytopenia, coagulation disorders and central nervous system toxicity including convulsions reported (especially with high doses or in severe renal impairment); diarrhoea and antibiotic-associated colitis

Dose: *by intramuscular or by slow intravenous injection or by infusion*, 2.4–4.8 g daily in 4 divided doses, increased if necessary in more serious infections (see also below); PREMATURE INFANT and NEONATE, 50 mg/kg daily in 2 divided doses; INFANT 1–4 weeks, 75 mg/kg daily in 3 divided doses; CHILD 1 month–12 years, 100 mg/ kg daily in 4 divided doses (higher doses may be required, see also below)

Bacterial endocarditis, *by slow intravenous injection or by infusion*, 7.2 g daily in 6 divided doses

Anthrax (in combination with other antibacterials, see also section 5.1.12), *by slow intravenous injection or by infusion*, 2.4 g every 4 hours; CHILD 150 mg/kg daily in 4 divided doses

Meningococcal disease, *by slow intravenous injection or by infusion*, 2.4 g every 4 hours; PREMATURE INFANT and NEONATE, 100 mg/kg daily in 2 divided doses; INFANT 1–4 weeks, 150 mg/kg daily in 3 divided doses; CHILD 1 month–12 years, 180–300 mg/kg daily in 4–6 divided doses

Important. If bacterial meningitis and especially if meningococcal disease is suspected general practitioners are advised to give a single injection of benzylpenicillin by intravenous injection (or by intramuscular injection) before transferring the patient urgently to hospital. Suitable doses are: ADULT 1.2 g; INFANT 300 mg; CHILD 1–9 years 600 mg, 10 years and over as for adult. In **penicillin allergy**, cefotaxime (section 5.1.2) may be an alternative; chloramphenicol may be used if there is a history of anaphylaxis to penicillins

By intrathecal injection, **not** recommended

NOTE. Benzylpenicillin doses in BNF may differ from those in product literature

Crystapen® (Britannia) PoM
Injection, powder for reconstitution, benzylpenicillin sodium (unbuffered), net price 600-mg vial = 42p, 2-vial 'GP pack' = £1.90; 1.2-g vial = 84p
Electrolytes: Na⁺ 1.68 mmol/600-mg vial; 3.36 mmol/1.2-g vial

---

PHENOXYMETHYLPENICILLIN
(Penicillin V)

Indications: tonsillitis, otitis media, erysipelas; rheumatic fever and pneumococcal infection prophylaxis (Table 2, section 5.1)

Cautions: see under Benzylpenicillin; **interactions:** Appendix 1 (penicillins)

Contra-indications: see under Benzylpenicillin

Side-effects: see under Benzylpenicillin

Dose: 500 mg every 6 hours increased up to 1 g every 6 hours in severe infections; CHILD, every 6 hours, up to 1 year 62.5 mg, 1–5 years 125 mg, 6–12 years 250 mg

NOTE. Phenoxymethylpenicillin doses in the BNF may differ from those in product literature

Phenoxymethylpenicillin (Non-proprietary) PoM
Tablets, phenoxymethylpenicillin (as potassium salt) 250 mg, net price 28-tab pack = £1.78.
Label: 9, 23
Available from Alpharma, APS (*Apsin®*), Arrow, Berk, Generics, Kent, Sovereign
Oral solution, phenoxymethylpenicillin (as potassium salt) for reconstitution with water, net price 125 mg/5 mL, 100 mL = £1.66; 250 mg/5 mL, 100 mL = £2.29. Label: 9, 23
Available from Alpharma, APS (*Apsin®*), Arrow, Generics, Kent, Sandoz, Sovereign

5.1.1.2 Penicillinase-resistant penicillins

Most staphylococci are now resistant to benzylpenicillin because they produce penicillinases. **Flucloxacillin**, however, is not inactivated by these enzymes and is thus effective in infections caused by penicillin-resistant staphylococci, which is the sole indication for its use. Flucloxacillin is acid-stable and can, therefore, be given by mouth as well as by injection.

Flucloxacillin is well absorbed from the gut. For CSM warning on cholestatic jaundice see under Flucloxacillin.

MRSA. *Staphylococcus aureus* strains resistant to methicillin [now discontinued] (methicillin-resistant *Staph. aureus*, MRSA) and to flucloxacillin have emerged in many hospitals; some of these organisms may be sensitive to vancomycin or teicoplanin (section 5.1.7). Strains may be susceptible to rifampicin, sodium fusidate, tetracyclines, aminoglycosides, and macrolides. Rifampicin or sodium fusidate should not be used alone because resistance may develop rapidly. Trimethoprim alone may be used for urinary-tract infections caused by some MRSA strains. Linezolid (section 5.1.7) and the combination of the streptogramin antibiotics quinupristin and dalfopristin (section 5.1.7) are active against MRSA but these antibacterial drugs should be reserved for organisms resistant to other antibacterials or for patients who cannot tolerate other antibacterial drugs. Treatment is guided by the sensitivity of the infecting strain. For eradication of nasal carriage of MRSA see section 12.2.3.

FLUCLOXACILLIN

Indications: infections due to beta-lactamase-producing staphylococci including otitis externa; adjunct in pneumonia, impetigo, cellulitis, osteomyelitis and in staphylococcal endocarditis (Table 1, section 5.1)

Cautions: see under Benzylpenicillin (section 5.1.1.1); porphyria (section 9.8.2)

CHOLESTATIC JAUNDICE. CSM has advised that cholestatic jaundice may occur up to several weeks after treatment with flucloxacillin has been stopped. Administration for more than 2 weeks and increasing age are risk factors

Contra-indications: see under Benzylpenicillin (section 5.1.1.1)

Side-effects: see under Benzylpenicillin (section 5.1.1.1); also hepatitis and cholestatic jaundice reported (see also CSM advice above)

Dose: *by mouth*, 250–500 mg every 6 hours, at least 30 minutes before food; CHILD under 2 years quarter adult dose; 2–10 years half adult dose

By intramuscular injection, 250–500 mg every 6 hours; CHILD under 2 years quarter adult dose; 2–10 years half adult dose

By slow intravenous injection or by intravenous infusion, 0.25–2 g every 6 hours; CHILD under 2 years quarter adult dose; 2–10 years half adult dose

Endocarditis (see Table 1, section 5.1), 12 g daily in 6 divided doses for 4 weeks

Osteomyelitis (see Table 1, section 5.1), up to 8 g daily in 3–4 divided doses

NOTE. Flucloxacillin doses in BNF may differ from those in product literature

Flucloxacillin (Non-proprietary) ▣ᴏᴍ

Capsules, flucloxacillin (as sodium salt) 250 mg, net price 20 = £2.09; 500 mg, 20 = £3.38. Label: 9, 23

Available from Alpharma, APS, Arrow, Ashbourne (*Fluclomix®*), Berk (*Ladropen®*), Galen (*Galfloxin®*), IVAX, Kent

Oral solution (= elixir or syrup), flucloxacillin (as sodium salt) for reconstitution with water, 125 mg/5 mL, net price 100 mL = £3.23; 250 mg/5 mL, 100 mL = £6.97. Label: 9, 23

Available from Alpharma, APS, Arrow, Berk (*Ladropen®*), IVAX, Kent, Sandoz

Injection, powder for reconstitution, flucloxacillin (as sodium salt). Net price 250-mg vial = £1.02; 500-mg vial = £2.04; 1-g vial = £4.08

Available from Berk (*Ladropen®*), CP

Floxapen® (GSK) ▣ᴏᴍ

Capsules, both black/caramel, flucloxacillin (as sodium salt) 250 mg, net price 28-cap pack = £6.79; 500 mg, 28-cap pack = £13.61. Label: 9, 23

Syrup, flucloxacillin (as magnesium salt) for reconstitution with water, 125 mg/5 mL, net price 100 mL = £3.49; 250 mg/5 mL, 100 mL = £6.97. Label: 9, 23

Excipients: include sucrose

Injection, powder for reconstitution, flucloxacillin (as sodium salt). Net price 250-mg vial = 98p; 500-mg vial = £1.95; 1-g vial = £3.90

Electrolytes: Na^+ 0.57 mmol/250-mg vial, 1.13 mmol/500-mg vial, 2.26 mmol/1-g vial

5.1.1.3 Broad-spectrum penicillins

Ampicillin is active against certain Gram-positive and Gram-negative organisms but is inactivated by penicillinases including those produced by *Staphylococcus aureus* and by common Gram-negative bacilli such as *Escherichia coli*. Almost all staphylococci, 50% of *E. coli* strains and 15% of *Haemophilus influenzae* strains are now resistant. The likelihood of resistance should therefore be considered before using ampicillin for the 'blind' treatment of infections; in particular, it should not be used for hospital patients without checking sensitivity.

Ampicillin is well excreted in the bile and urine. It is principally indicated for the treatment of exacerbations of chronic bronchitis and middle ear infections, both of which are usually due to *Streptococcus pneumoniae* and *H. influenzae*, and for urinary-tract infections (section 5.1.13).

Ampicillin can be given by mouth but less than half the dose is absorbed, and absorption is further decreased by the presence of food in the gut.

Maculopapular rashes commonly occur with ampicillin (and amoxicillin) but are not usually related to true penicillin allergy. They almost always occur in patients with glandular fever; broad-spectrum penicillins should not therefore be used for 'blind' treatment of a sore throat. Rashes are also common in patients with acute or chronic lymphocytic leukaemia or in cytomegalovirus infection.

Amoxicillin (amoxycillin) is a derivative of ampicillin and has a similar antibacterial spectrum. It is better absorbed than ampicillin when given by mouth, producing higher plasma and tissue concentrations; unlike ampicillin, absorption is not affected by the presence of food in the stomach. Amoxicillin is used for endocarditis prophylaxis (section 5.1, table 2); it may also be used for the treatment of Lyme disease [not licensed], see below.

Co-amoxiclav consists of amoxicillin with the beta-lactamase inhibitor clavulanic acid. Clavulanic acid itself has no significant antibacterial activity but, by inactivating beta-lactamases, it makes the combination active against beta-lactamase-producing bacteria that are resistant to amoxicillin. These include resistant strains of *Staph. aureus*, *E. coli*, and *H. influenzae*, as well as many *Bacteroides* and *Klebsiella* spp. Co-amoxiclav should be reserved for infections likely, or known, to be caused by amoxicillin-resistant beta-lactamase-producing strains; for CSM warning on cholestatic jaundice see under Co-amoxiclav.

A combination of ampicillin with flucloxacillin (as co-fluampicil) is available to treat infections involving either streptococci or staphylococci (e.g. cellulitis).

LYME DISEASE. Lyme disease should generally be treated by those experienced in its management. **Doxycycline** is the antibacterial of choice for *early Lyme disease*. **Amoxicillin** [unlicensed indication], **cefuroxime axetil**, or **azithromycin** [unlicensed indication] are alternatives if doxycycline is contraindicated. Intravenous administration of **cefotaxime**, **ceftriaxone**, or **benzylpenicillin** is recommended for Lyme disease associated with moderate to severe *cardiac* or neurological abnormalities, *late Lyme disease*, and *Lyme arthritis*. The duration of treatment is generally 2–4 weeks; Lyme arthritis requires longer treatment with oral antibacterial drugs.

AMOXICILLIN

(Amoxycillin)

Indications: see under Ampicillin; also endocarditis prophylaxis (Table 2, section 5.1); and treatment (Table 1, section 5.1); anthrax (section 5.1.12); adjunct in listerial meningitis (Table 1, section 5.1); *Helicobacter pylori* eradication (section 1.3)

Cautions: see under Ampicillin

Contra-indications: see under Ampicillin

Side-effects: see under Ampicillin

Dose: *by mouth*, 250 mg every 8 hours, doubled in severe infections; CHILD up to 10 years, 125 mg every 8 hours, doubled in severe infections
Pneumonia, 0.5–1 g every 8 hours
Anthrax (treatment and post-exposure prophylaxis—see also section 5.1.12), 500 mg every 8 hours; CHILD body-weight under 20 kg, 80 mg/kg daily in 3 divided doses, body-weight over 20 kg, adult dose

Short-course oral therapy
Dental abscess, 3 g repeated after 8 hours
Urinary-tract infections, 3 g repeated after 10–12 hours

By intramuscular injection, 500 mg every 8 hours; CHILD, 50–100 mg/kg daily in divided doses

By intravenous injection or infusion, 500 mg every 8 hours increased to 1 g every 6 hours in severe infections; CHILD, 50–100 mg/kg daily in divided doses

Listerial meningitis (in combination with another antibiotic, see Table 1, section 5.1), *by intravenous infusion*, 2 g every 4 hours for 10–14 days
Enterococcal endocarditis (in combination with

another antibiotic if necessary, see Table 1, section 5.1), *by intravenous infusion*, 2 g every 4 hours
NOTE. Amoxicillin doses in BNF may differ from those in product literature

Amoxicillin (Non-proprietary) PoM
Capsules, amoxicillin (as trihydrate) 250 mg, net price 21 = £1.85; 500 mg, 21 = £1.08 Label: 9
Available from Alpharma, APS, Arrow, Ashbourne (*Amix*®), Bristol, DDSA, Eastern (*Amoram*®), Galen (*Galenamox*®), Hillcross, IVAX, Kent, Ranbaxy (*Rimoxallin*®)

Oral suspension, amoxicillin (as trihydrate) for reconstitution with water, 125 mg/5 mL, net price 100 mL = £1.15; 250 mg/5 mL, 100 mL = £1.80. Label: 9
NOTE. Sugar-free versions are available and can be ordered by specifying 'sugar-free' on the prescription
Available from Alpharma, APS, Arrow, Ashbourne (*Amix*®), Berk (*Almodan*®), Bristol, Eastern (*Amoram*®), Galen (*Galenamox*®), Hillcross, IVAX, Kent, Ranbaxy (*Rimoxallin*®)

Sachets, sugar-free, amoxicillin (as trihydrate) 3 g/sachet, net price 2-sachet pack = £4.69, 14-sachet pack = £31.94. Label: 9, 13
Available from Hillcross, IVAX, Kent

Injection, powder for reconstitution, amoxicillin (as sodium salt), net price 250-mg vial = 36p; 500-mg vial = 66p; 1-g vial = £1.31
Available from CP

Amoxil® (GSK) PoM
Capsules, both maroon/gold, amoxicillin (as trihydrate), 250 mg, net price 21-cap pack = £3.86; 500 mg, 21-cap pack = £7.73. Label: 9

Syrup SF, both sugar-free, peach- strawberry- and lemon-flavoured, amoxicillin (as trihydrate) for reconstitution with water, 125 mg/5 mL, net price 100 mL = £2.31; 250 mg/5 mL, 100 mL = £4.62. Label: 9

Paediatric suspension, amoxicillin 125 mg (as trihydrate)/1.25 mL when reconstituted with water, net price 20 mL (peach- strawberry- and lemon-flavoured) = £3.63. Label: 9, counselling , use of pipette
Excipients: include sucrose 600 mg/1.25 mL

Sachets SF, powder, sugar-free, amoxicillin (as trihydrate) 3 g/sachet, 2-sachet pack (peach-strawberry- and lemon-flavoured) = £4.97. Label: 9, 13

Injection, powder for reconstitution, amoxicillin (as sodium salt), net price 250-mg vial = 34p; 500-mg vial = 63p; 1-g vial = £1.25
Electrolytes: Na⁺ 3.3 mmol/g

AMPICILLIN

Indications: urinary-tract infections, otitis media, sinusitis, bronchitis, uncomplicated community-acquired pneumonia (Table 1, section 5.1), *Haemophilus influenzae* infections, invasive salmonellosis; listerial meningitis (Table 1, section 5.1)

Cautions: history of allergy; renal impairment (Appendix 3); erythematous rashes common in glandular fever, cytomegalovirus infection, and acute or chronic lymphocytic leukaemia (see notes above); **interactions:** Appendix 1 (penicillins)

Contra-indications: penicillin hypersensitivity

Side-effects: nausea, vomiting, diarrhoea; rashes (discontinue treatment); rarely, antibiotic-associated colitis; see also under Benzylpenicillin (section 5.1.1.1)

Dose: *by mouth*, 0.25–1 g every 6 hours, at least 30 minutes before food; CHILD under 10 years, half adult dose

Urinary-tract infections, 500 mg every 8 hours; CHILD under 10 years, half adult dose

By intramuscular injection or intravenous injection or infusion, 500 mg every 4–6 hours; CHILD under 10 years, half adult dose

Listerial meningitis (in combination with another antibiotic), *by intravenous infusion*, 2 g every 4 hours for 10–14 days; INFANT under 1 month, 50 mg/kg every 6 hours; 1–3 months, 50–100 mg/kg every 6 hours; CHILD 3 months–12 years, 100 mg/kg every 6 hours (max. 12 g daily)

NOTE. Ampicillin doses in BNF may differ from those in product literature

Ampicillin (Non-proprietary) PoM
Capsules, ampicillin 250 mg, net price 20 = 62p; 500 mg, 20 = £1.20. Label: 9, 23
Available from Alpharma, Arrow, IVAX, Kent, Ranbaxy (*Rimacillin®*)
Oral suspension, ampicillin 125 mg/5 mL when reconstituted with water, net price 100 mL = £1.75; 250 mg/5 mL, 100 mL = £3.25. Label: 9, 23
Available from Alpharma, IVAX, Kent, Ranbaxy (*Rimacillin®*)

Penbritin® (GSK) PoM
Capsules, both black/red, ampicillin (as trihydrate) 250 mg, net price 28-cap pack = £2.26. Label: 9, 23
Injection, powder for reconstitution, ampicillin (as sodium salt). Net price 500-mg vial = 74p
Electrolytes: Na⁺ 1.47 mmol/500-mg vial

■ With flucloxacillin
See Co-fluampicil

CO-AMOXICLAV

A mixture of amoxicillin (as the trihydrate or as the sodium salt) and clavulanic acid (as potassium clavulanate); the proportions are expressed in the form *x/y* where *x* and *y* are the strengths in milligrams of amoxicillin and clavulanic acid respectively

Indications: infections due to beta-lactamase-producing strains (where amoxicillin alone not appropriate) including respiratory-tract infections, genito-urinary and abdominal infections, cellulitis, animal bites, severe dental infection with spreading cellulitis

Cautions: see under Ampicillin and notes above; also caution in hepatic impairment (monitor hepatic function), pregnancy
CHOLESTATIC JAUNDICE. CSM has advised that cholestatic jaundice can occur either during or shortly after the use of co-amoxiclav. An epidemiological study has shown that the risk of acute liver toxicity was about 6 times greater with co-amoxiclav than with amoxicillin. Cholestatic jaundice is more common in patients above the age of 65 years and in men; these reactions have only rarely been reported in children. Jaundice is usually self-limiting and very rarely fatal. The duration of treatment should be appropriate to the indication and should not usually exceed 14 days

Contra-indications: penicillin hypersensitivity, history of co-amoxiclav-associated or penicillin-associated jaundice or hepatic dysfunction

Side-effects: see under Ampicillin; hepatitis, cholestatic jaundice (see above); erythema multiforme (including Stevens-Johnson syndrome), toxic epidermal necrolysis, exfoliative dermatitis, vasculitis reported; rarely prolongation of bleeding time, dizziness, headache, convulsions (particularly with

high doses or in renal impairment); superficial staining of teeth with suspension, phlebitis at injection site

Dose: *by mouth*, expressed as amoxicillin, 250 mg every 8 hours, dose doubled in severe infections; CHILD see under preparations below (under 6 years *Augmentin®* '125/31 SF' suspension; 6–12 years *Augmentin®* '250/62 SF' suspension *or* for short-term treatment with twice daily dosage in CHILD 2 months–12 years *Augmentin-Duo®* 400/57 suspension)

Severe dental infections (but not generally first-line, see notes above), expressed as amoxicillin, 250 mg every 8 hours for 5 days

By intravenous injection over 3–4 minutes *or by intravenous infusion*, expressed as amoxicillin, 1 g every 8 hours increased to 1 g every 6 hours in more serious infections; INFANTS up to 3 months 25 mg/kg every 8 hours (every 12 hours in the perinatal period and in premature infants); CHILD 3 months–12 years, 25 mg/kg every 8 hours increased to 25 mg/kg every 6 hours in more serious infections

Surgical prophylaxis, expressed as amoxicillin, 1 g at induction; for high risk procedures (e.g. colorectal surgery) up to 2–3 further doses of 1 g may be given every 8 hours

Co-amoxiclav (Non-proprietary) PoM
Tablets, co-amoxiclav 250/125 (amoxicillin 250 mg as trihydrate, clavulanic acid 125 mg as potassium salt), net price 21-tab pack = £9.74. Label: 9
Available from Alpharma, APS, Ashbourne (*Amiclav®*), Generics, IVAX, Sterwin
Tablets, co-amoxiclav 500/125 (amoxicillin 500 mg as trihydrate, clavulanic acid 125 mg as potassium salt), net price 21-tab pack = £15.72. Label: 9
Available from APS, IVAX, Sterwin
Oral suspension, co-amoxiclav 125/31 (amoxicillin 125 mg as trihydrate, clavulanic acid 31.25 mg as potassium salt)/5 mL when reconstituted with water, net price 100 mL = £4.57. Label: 9
Excipients: include aspartame 12.5 mg/5 mL (section 9.4.1)
Available from APS, Generics, IVAX
Oral suspension, co-amoxiclav 250/62 (amoxicillin 250 mg as trihydrate, clavulanic acid 62.5 mg as potassium salt)/5 mL when reconstituted with water, net price 100 mL = £6.42. Label: 9
Available from APS, Generics, IVAX (*excipients:* include aspartame 12.5mg/5mL (section 9.4.1)), Sterwin

Augmentin® (GSK) PoM
Tablets 375 mg, f/c, co-amoxiclav 250/125 (amoxicillin 250 mg as trihydrate, clavulanic acid 125 mg as potassium salt), net price 21-tab pack = £9.79. Label: 9
Tablets 625 mg, f/c, co-amoxiclav 500/125 (amoxicillin 500 mg as trihydrate, clavulanic acid 125 mg as potassium salt). Net price 21-tab pack = £15.73. Label: 9
Dispersible tablets, sugar-free, co-amoxiclav 250/125 (amoxicillin 250 mg as trihydrate, clavulanic acid 125 mg as potassium salt). Net price 21-tab pack = £10.99. Label: 9, 13
Suspension '125/31 SF', sugar-free, co-amoxiclav 125/31 (amoxicillin 125 mg as trihydrate, clavulanic acid 31 mg as potassium salt)/5 mL when reconstituted with water. Net price 100 mL = £4.57. Label: 9
Excipients: include aspartame 12.5 mg/5 mL (section 9.4.1)
Dose: CHILD 1–6 years (10–18 kg) 5 mL every 8 hours *or* INFANT and CHILD up to 6 years 0.8 mL/kg daily in 3

divided doses; in severe infections dose increased to
1.6 mL/kg daily in 3 divided doses
Suspension '250/62 SF', sugar-free, co-amoxiclav
250/62 (amoxicillin 250 mg as trihydrate, clavulanic acid 62 mg as potassium salt)/5 mL when
reconstituted with water. Net price 100 mL = £6.42.
Label: 9
Excipients: include aspartame 12.5 mg/5 mL (section 9.4.1)
Dose: CHILD 6–12 years (18–40 kg) 5 mL every 8 hours
or 0.4 mL/kg daily in 3 divided doses; in severe infections
dose increased to 0.8 mL/kg daily in 3 divided doses
Injection 600 mg, powder for reconstitution, co-
amoxiclav 500/100 (amoxicillin 500 mg as sodium
salt, clavulanic acid 100 mg as potassium salt). Net
price per vial = £1.49
Electrolytes: Na$^+$ 1.6 mmol, K$^+$ 0.5 mmol/600-mg vial
Injection 1.2 g, powder for reconstitution, co-
amoxiclav 1000/200 (amoxicillin 1 g as sodium
salt, clavulanic acid 200 mg as potassium salt). Net
price per vial = £2.97
Electrolytes: Na$^+$ 3.1 mmol, K$^+$ 1 mmol/1.2-g vial

Augmentin-Duo® (GSK) PoM
Suspension '400/57', sugar-free, strawberry-flavoured, co-amoxiclav 400/57 (amoxicillin 400 mg
as trihydrate, clavulanic acid 57 mg as potassium
salt)/5 mL when reconstituted with water. Net price
35 mL = £4.71, 70 mL = £6.61. Label: 9
Excipients: include aspartame 12.5 mg/5 mL (section 9.4.1)
Dose: CHILD 2 months–2 years 0.15 mL/kg twice daily,
2–6 years (13–21 kg) 2.5 mL twice daily, 7–12 years (22–
40 kg) 5 mL twice daily, doubled in severe infections

CO-FLUAMPICIL

A mixture of equal parts by mass of flucloxacillin and
ampicillin
Indications: mixed infections involving beta-lactamase-producing staphylococci
Cautions: see under Ampicillin and Flucloxacillin
Contra-indications: see under Ampicillin and
Flucloxacillin
Side-effects: see under Ampicillin and Flucloxacillin
Dose: *by mouth*, co-fluampicil, 250/250 every 6
hours, dose doubled in severe infections; CHILD
under 10 years half adult dose, dose doubled in
severe infections
*By intramuscular or slow intravenous injection or by
intravenous infusion*, co-fluampicil 250/250 every
6 hours, dose doubled in severe infections; CHILD
under 2 years quarter adult dose, 2–10 years half
adult dose, dose doubled in severe infections

Co-fluampicil (Non-proprietary) PoM
Capsules, co-fluampicil 250/250 (flucloxacillin
250 mg as sodium salt, ampicillin 250 mg as
trihydrate), net price 28-cap pack = £8.85. Label: 9,
22
Available from Alpharma, CP, Generics (*Flu-Amp*®),
IVAX, Kent

Magnapen® (CP) PoM
Capsules, black/turquoise, co-fluampicil 250/250
(flucloxacillin 250 mg as sodium salt, ampicillin
250 mg as trihydrate), net price 20-cap pack =
£6.15. Label: 9, 22
Syrup, co-fluampicil 125/125 (flucloxacillin
125 mg as magnesium salt, ampicillin 125 mg as
trihydrate)/5 mL when reconstituted with water,
net price 100 mL = £4.99. Label: 9, 22
Excipients: include sucrose 3.14 g/5 mL
Injection 500 mg, powder for reconstitution, co-
fluampicil 250/250 (flucloxacillin 250 mg as sod-

ium salt, ampicillin 250 mg as sodium salt), net
price per vial = £1.33
Electrolytes: Na$^+$ 1.3 mmol/vial

5.1.1.4 Antipseudomonal penicillins

The carboxypenicillin, **ticarcillin**, is principally
indicated for serious infections caused by *Pseudomonas aeruginosa* although it also has activity
against certain other Gram-negative bacilli including
Proteus spp. and *Bacteroides fragilis*.

Ticarcillin is now available only in combination
with clavulanic acid (section 5.1.1.3); the combination (*Timentin*®) is active against beta-lactamase-
producing bacteria resistant to ticarcillin.

Tazocin® contains the ureidopenicillin **piperacillin**
with the beta-lactamase inhibitor tazobactam. Piperacillin is more active than ticarcillin against *Ps.
aeruginosa*. The spectrum of activity of *Tazocin*® is
comparable to that of the carbapenems, imipenem
and meropenem (section 5.1.2).

For pseudomonas septicaemias (especially in neutropenia or endocarditis) these antipseudomonal
penicillins should be given with an aminoglycoside
(e.g. gentamicin or netilmicin, section 5.1.4) since
they have a synergistic effect. Penicillins and aminoglycosides must not, however, be mixed in the same
syringe or infusion.

Owing to the sodium content of many of these
antibiotics, high doses may lead to hypernatraemia.

PIPERACILLIN

Indications: see preparations
Cautions: see under Benzylpenicillin (section
5.1.1.1); renal impairment (Appendix 3)
Contra-indications: see under Benzylpenicillin
(section 5.1.1.1)
Side-effects: see under Benzylpenicillin (section
5.1.1.1); also nausea and vomiting; rarely stomatitis, dyspepsia, abdominal pain, constipation, dry
mouth, hepatitis, jaundice, oedema, hypotension,
fatigue, myalgia, Stevens-Johnson syndrome,
toxic epidermal necrolysis, eosinophilia, pancytopenia, hypoglycaemia, hypokalaemia, injection-
site reactions
Dose: see preparations

■ With tazobactam

Tazocin® (Lederle) PoM
Injection 2.25 g, powder for reconstitution, piperacillin 2 g (as sodium salt), tazobactam 250 mg (as
sodium salt). Net price per vial = £7.96
Electrolytes: Na$^+$ 4.69 mmol/2.25-g vial
Injection 4.5 g, powder for reconstitution, piperacillin 4 g (as sodium salt), tazobactam 500 mg (as
sodium salt). Net price per vial = £15.79; infusion
pack (4.5-g infusion bottle, 50-mL bottle water for
injections and transfer needle) = £14.48
Electrolytes: Na$^+$ 9.37 mmol/4.5-g vial
Dose: lower respiratory-tract, urinary-tract, intra-abdominal and skin infections, and septicaemia, ADULT and
CHILD over 12 years, *by intravenous injection* over 3–5
minutes *or by intravenous infusion*, 2.25–4.5 g every 6–8
hours, usually 4.5 g every 8 hours
Complicated appendicitis, *by intravenous injection* over
3–5 minutes or *by intravenous infusion*, CHILD 2–12 years,
112.5 mg/kg every 8 hours (max. 4.5 g every 8 hours) for
5–14 days; CHILD 2–12 years, not recommended
Infections in neutropenic patients (in combination with an
aminoglycoside), *by intravenous injection* over 3–5

minutes *or by intravenous infusion*, ADULT and CHILD over 50 kg, 4.5 g every 6 hours; CHILD less than 50 kg, 90 mg/kg every 6 hours

TICARCILLIN

Indications: infections due to *Pseudomonas* and *Proteus* spp, see notes above

Cautions: see under Benzylpenicillin (section 5.1.1.1)

Contra-indications: see under Benzylpenicillin (section 5.1.1.1)

Side-effects: see under Benzylpenicillin (section 5.1.1.1); also nausea, vomiting, coagulation disorders, haemorrhagic cystitis (more frequent in children), injection-site reactions, Stevens-Johnson syndrome, toxic epidermal necrolysis, hypokalaemia, eosinophilia

Dose: see under preparation

■ With clavulanic acid

NOTE. For a CSM warning on cholestatic jaundice possibly associated with clavulanic acid, see under Co-amoxiclav p. 262.

Timentin® (GSK) [PoM]

Injection 3.2 g, powder for reconstitution, ticarcillin 3 g (as sodium salt), clavulanic acid 200 mg (as potassium salt). Net price per vial = £6.08

Electrolytes: Na⁺ 16 mmol, K⁺ 1 mmol/3.2-g vial

Dose: by intravenous infusion, 3.2 g every 6–8 hours increased to every 4 hours in more severe infections; CHILD 80 mg/kg every 6–8 hours (every 12 hours in neonates)

5.1.1.5 Mecillinams

Pivmecillinam has significant activity against many Gram-negative bacteria including *Escherichia coli*, klebsiella, enterobacter, and salmonellae. It is not active against *Pseudomonas aeruginosa* or enterococci. Pivmecillinam is hydrolysed to mecillinam, which is the active drug.

PIVMECILLINAM HYDROCHLORIDE

Indications: see under Dose below

Cautions: see under Benzylpenicillin (section 5.1.1.1); also liver and renal function tests required in long-term use; pregnancy; **interactions:** Appendix 1 (penicillins)

Contra-indications: see under Benzylpenicillin (section 5.1.1.1); also carnitine deficiency, oesophageal strictures, gastro-intestinal obstruction, infants under 3 months

Side-effects: see under Benzylpenicillin (section 5.1.1.1); nausea, vomiting, dyspepsia; also reduced serum and total body carnitine (especially with long-term or repeated use)

Dose: acute uncomplicated cystitis, ADULT and CHILD over 40 kg, initially 400 mg then 200 mg every 8 hours for 3 days

Chronic or recurrent bacteriuria, ADULT and CHILD over 40 kg, 400 mg every 6–8 hours

Urinary-tract infections, CHILD under 40 kg, 20–40 mg/kg daily in 3–4 divided doses

Salmonellosis, not recommended therefore no dose stated

COUNSELLING. Tablets should be swallowed whole with plenty of fluid during meals while sitting or standing

Selexid® (Leo) [PoM]

Tablets, f/c, pivmecillinam hydrochloride 200 mg, net price 10-tab pack = £4.50. Label 9, 21, 27, counselling, posture (see Dose above)

5.1.2 Cephalosporins, cephamycins, and other beta-lactams

Antibiotics in this section include the **cephalosporins**, such as cefotaxime, ceftazidime, cefuroxime, cefalexin and cefradine, the **cephamycin**, cefoxitin, the **monobactam**, aztreonam, and the **carbapenems**, imipenem (a thienamycin derivative) and meropenem.

Cephalosporins and cephamycins

The cephalosporins are broad-spectrum antibiotics which are used for the treatment of septicaemia, pneumonia, meningitis, biliary-tract infections, peritonitis, and urinary-tract infections. All have a similar antibacterial spectrum although individual agents have differing activity against certain organisms. The pharmacology of the cephalosporins is similar to that of the penicillins, excretion being principally renal. Cephalosporins penetrate the cerebrospinal fluid poorly unless the meninges are inflamed; cefotaxime is a suitable cephalosporin for infections of the CNS (e.g meningitis).

The principal side-effect of the cephalosporins is hypersensitivity and about 10% of penicillin-sensitive patients will also be allergic to the cephalosporins. Haemorrhage due to interference with blood clotting factors has been associated with several cephalosporins.

Cefradine (cephradine) has generally been replaced by the newer cephalosporins.

Cefuroxime is a 'second generation' cephalosporin that is less susceptible than the earlier cephalosporins to inactivation by beta-lactamases. It is, therefore, active against certain bacteria which are resistant to the other drugs and has greater activity against *Haemophilus influenzae* and *Neisseria gonorrhoeae*.

Cefotaxime, ceftazidime and **ceftriaxone** are 'third generation' cephalosporins with greater activity than the 'second generation' cephalosporins against certain Gram-negative bacteria. However, they are less active than cefuroxime against Gram-positive bacteria, most notably *Staphylococcus aureus*. Their broad antibacterial spectrum may encourage superinfection with resistant bacteria or fungi.

Ceftazidime has good activity against pseudomonas. It is also active against other Gram-negative bacteria.

Ceftriaxone has a longer half-life and therefore only needs once daily administration. Indications include serious infections such as septicaemia, pneumonia, and meningitis. The calcium salt of ceftriaxone forms a precipitate in the gall bladder which may rarely cause symptoms but these usually resolve when the antibiotic is stopped.

Cefpirome is indicated for urinary-tract, lower respiratory-tract and skin infections, bacteraemia, and infections associated with neutropenia.

Cefoxitin, a cephamycin antibiotic, is active against bowel flora including *Bacteroides fragilis*

and because of this it has been recommended for abdominal sepsis such as peritonitis.

ORALLY ACTIVE CEPHALOSPORINS. The orally active 'first generation' cephalosporins, **cefalexin** (cephalexin), **cefradine**, and **cefadroxil** and the 'second generation' cephalosporins, **cefaclor** and **cefprozil**, have a similar antimicrobial spectrum. They are useful for urinary-tract infections which do not respond to other drugs or which occur in pregnancy, respiratory-tract infections, otitis media, sinusitis, and skin and soft-tissue infections. Cefaclor has good activity against *H. influenzae*, but it is associated with protracted skin reactions especially in children. Cefadroxil has a long duration of action and can be given twice daily; it has poor activity against *H. influenzae*. **Cefuroxime axetil**, an ester of the 'second generation' cephalosporin cefuroxime, has the same antibacterial spectrum as the parent compound; it is poorly absorbed.

Cefixime has a longer duration of action than the other cephalosporins that are active by mouth. It is presently only licensed for acute infections.

Cefpodoxime proxetil is more active than the other oral cephalosporins against respiratory bacterial pathogens and it is licensed for upper and lower respiratory-tract infections.

For treatment of Lyme disease, see section 5.1.1.3.

CEFACLOR

Indications: infections due to sensitive Gram-positive and Gram-negative bacteria, but see notes above

Cautions: penicillin sensitivity; renal impairment (Appendix 3); pregnancy and breast-feeding (but appropriate to use); false positive urinary glucose (if tested for reducing substances) and false positive Coombs' test; **interactions:** Appendix 1 (cephalosporins)

Contra-indications: cephalosporin hypersensitivity; porphyria (section 9.8.2)

Side-effects: diarrhoea and rarely antibiotic-associated colitis (CSM has warned both more likely with higher doses), nausea and vomiting, abdominal discomfort, headache; allergic reactions including rashes, pruritus, urticaria, serum sickness-like reactions with rashes, fever and arthralgia, and anaphylaxis; erythema multiforme, toxic epidermal necrolysis reported; disturbances in liver enzymes, transient hepatitis and cholestatic jaundice; other side-effects reported include eosinophilia and blood disorders (including thrombocytopenia, leucopenia, agranulocytosis, aplastic anaemia and haemolytic anaemia); reversible interstitial nephritis, hyperactivity, nervousness, sleep disturbances, hallucinations, confusion, hypertonia, and dizziness

Dose: 250 mg every 8 hours, doubled for severe infections; max. 4 g daily; CHILD over 1 month, 20 mg/kg daily in 3 divided doses, doubled for severe infections, max. 1 g daily; *or* 1 month–1 year, 62.5 mg every 8 hours; 1–5 years, 125 mg; over 5 years, 250 mg; doses doubled for severe infections

Cefaclor (Non-proprietary) [PoM]
Capsules, cefaclor (as monohydrate) 250 mg, net price 21-cap pack = £6.54; 500 mg 50-cap pack = £24.46. Label: 9
Available from Alpharma, APS, Galen (*Keftid*®), Hillcross

Suspension, cefaclor (as monohydrate) for reconstitution with water, 125 mg/5 mL, net price 100 mL = £4.90; 250 mg/5 mL, 100 mL = £9.80. Label: 9
NOTE. Sugar-free versions are available and can be ordered by specifying 'sugar-free' on the prescription
Available from Alpharma, APS, Galen (*Keftid*®), Generics, Genus, Hillcross

Distaclor® (Dista) [PoM]
Capsules, cefaclor (as monohydrate) 500 mg (violet/grey), net price 20 = £21.66. Label: 9
Suspension, both pink, cefaclor (as monohydrate) for reconstitution with water, 125 mg/5 mL, net price 100 mL = £5.16; 250 mg/5 mL, 100 mL = £10.32. Label: 9

Distaclor MR® (Dista) [PoM]
Tablets, m/r, both blue, cefaclor (as monohydrate) 375 mg. Net price 14-tab pack = £6.93. Label: 9, 21, 25
Dose: 375 mg every 12 hours with food, dose doubled for pneumonia
Lower urinary-tract infections, 375 mg every 12 hours with food
NOTE. Modified-release tablets containing cefaclor (as monohydrate) 375 mg available from Ranbaxy

CEFADROXIL

Indications: see under Cefaclor; see also notes above

Cautions: see under Cefaclor

Contra-indications: see under Cefaclor

Side-effects: see under Cefaclor

Dose: patients over 40 kg, 0.5–1 g twice daily; skin, soft tissue, and simple urinary-tract infections, 1 g daily; CHILD under 1 year, 25 mg/kg daily in divided doses; 1–6 years, 250 mg twice daily; over 6 years, 500 mg twice daily

Baxan® (Bristol-Myers Squibb) [PoM]
Capsules, cefadroxil (as monohydrate) 500 mg, net price 20-cap pack = £5.64. Label: 9
Suspension, cefadroxil (as monohydrate) for reconstitution with water, 125 mg/5 mL, net price 60 mL = £1.75; 250 mg/5 mL, 60 mL = £3.48; 500 mg/5 mL, 60 mL = £5.21. Label: 9

CEFALEXIN

(Cephalexin)

Indications: see under Cefaclor

Cautions: see under Cefaclor

Contra-indications: see under Cefaclor

Side-effects: see under Cefaclor

Dose: 250 mg every 6 hours *or* 500 mg every 8–12 hours increased to 1–1.5 g every 6–8 hours for severe infections; CHILD 25 mg/kg daily in divided doses, doubled for severe infections, max. 100 mg/kg daily; *or* under 1 year 125 mg every 12 hours, 1–5 years 125 mg every 8 hours, 6–12 years 250 mg every 8 hours
Prophylaxis of recurrent urinary-tract infection, ADULT 125 mg at night

Cefalexin (Non-proprietary) [PoM]
Capsules, cefalexin 250 mg, net price 28-cap pack = £2.47; 500 mg, 21-cap pack = £3.46. Label: 9
Available from Alpharma, APS, Arrow, Generics, Hillcross, IVAX, Kent, Ranbaxy

Tablets, cefalexin 250 mg, net price 28-tab pack = £2.59; 500 mg, 21-tab pack = £3.72. Label: 9
Available from Alpharma, APS, Arrow, Hillcross, IVAX, Kent

Oral suspension, cefalexin for reconstitution with water, 125 mg/5 mL, net price 100 mL = £1.28; 250 mg/5 mL, 100 mL = £2.19. Label: 9
Available from Alpharma, APS, Arrow, Hillcross, IVAX, Kent

Ceporex® (Galen) PoM
Capsules, both caramel/grey, cefalexin 250 mg, net price 28-cap pack = £4.47; 500 mg, 28-cap pack = £8.72. Label: 9
Tablets, all pink, f/c, cefalexin 250 mg, net price 28-tab pack = £4.47; 500 mg, 28-tab pack = £8.72. Label: 9
Syrup, all orange, cefalexin for reconstitution with water, 125 mg/5 mL, net price 100 mL = £1.59; 250 mg/5 mL, 100 mL = £3.19; 500 mg/5 mL, 100 mL = £6.19. Label: 9

Keflex® (Lilly) PoM
Capsules, cefalexin 250 mg (green/white), net price 28-cap pack = £1.89; 500 mg (pale green/dark green), 21-cap pack = £2.66. Label: 9
Tablets, both peach, cefalexin 250 mg, net price 28-tab pack = £2.25; 500 mg (scored), 21-tab pack = £2.66. Label: 9
Suspension, cefalexin for reconstitution with water, 125 mg/5 mL, net price 100 mL = 88p; 250 mg/5 mL, 100 mL = £1.51. Label: 9

CEFIXIME

Indications: see under Cefaclor (acute infections only); gonorrhoea [unlicensed indication] (Table 1, section 5.1)
Cautions: see under Cefaclor
Contra-indications: see under Cefaclor
Side-effects: see under Cefaclor
Dose: ADULT and CHILD over 10 years, 200–400 mg daily in 1–2 divided doses; CHILD over 6 months 8 mg/kg daily in 1–2 divided doses *or* 6 months–1 year 75 mg daily; 1–4 years 100 mg daily; 5–10 years 200 mg daily
Gonorrhoea [unlicensed indication], 400 mg as a single dose

Suprax® (Rhône-Poulenc Rorer) PoM
Tablets, f/c, scored, cefixime 200 mg. Net price 7-tab pack = £12.03. Label: 9
Paediatric oral suspension, cefixime 100 mg/5 mL when reconstituted with water. Net price 37.5 mL (with double-ended spoon for measuring 3.75 mL or 5 mL since dilution not recommended) = £7.90; 75 mL = £14.18. Label: 9

CEFOTAXIME

Indications: see under Cefaclor; gonorrhoea; surgical prophylaxis; Haemophilus epiglottitis and meningitis (section 5.1, table 1); see also notes above
Cautions: see under Cefaclor
Contra-indications: see under Cefaclor
Side-effects: see under Cefaclor; rarely arrhythmias following rapid injection reported
Dose: *by intramuscular or intravenous injection or by intravenous infusion*, 1 g every 12 hours increased in severe infections (e.g. meningitis) to 8 g daily in 4 divided doses; higher doses (up to 12 g daily in 3–4 divided doses) may be required; NEONATE 50 mg/kg daily in 2–4 divided doses increased to 150–200 mg/kg daily in severe infections; CHILD 100–150 mg/kg daily in 2–4 divided

doses increased up to 200 mg/kg daily in very severe infections
Gonorrhoea, 500 mg as a single dose
Important. If bacterial meningitis and especially if meningococcal disease is suspected the patient should be transferred urgently to hospital. If benzylpenicillin cannot be given (e.g. because of an allergy), a single dose of cefotaxime may be given (if available) before urgent transfer to hospital. Suitable doses of cefotaxime by intravenous injection (or by intramuscular injection) are ADULT and CHILD over 12 years 1 g; CHILD under 12 years 50 mg/kg; chloramphenicol (section 5.1.7) may be used if there is a history of anaphylaxis to penicillins or cephalosporins

Cefotaxime (Non-proprietary) PoM
Injection, powder for reconstitution, cefotaxime (as sodium salt), net price 500-mg vial = £2.30; 1-g vial = £4.63; 2-g vial = £9.22
Available from Genus

Claforan® (Aventis Pharma) PoM
Injection, powder for reconstitution, cefotaxime (as sodium salt), net price 500-mg vial = £2.30; 1-g vial (with or without infusion connector) = £4.63; 2-g vial (with or without infusion connector) = £9.22
Electrolytes: Na+ 2.09 mmol/g

CEFOXITIN

Indications: see under Cefaclor; surgical prophylaxis; more active against Gram-negative bacteria
Cautions: see under Cefaclor
Contra-indications: see under Cefaclor
Side-effects: see under Cefaclor
Dose: *by deep intramuscular or by slow intravenous injection or by infusion*, 1–2 g every 6–8 hours, increased up to 12 g daily in divided doses for infections requiring higher doses; CHILD up to 1 week 20–40 mg/kg every 12 hours, 1–4 weeks 20–40 mg/kg every 8 hours, over 1 month 20–40 mg/kg every 6–8 hours, increased up to 200 mg/kg daily in divided doses (max. 12 g daily) in severe infections; intravenous route recommended for children
Uncomplicated urinary-tract infection, *by deep intramuscular injection*, 1 g every 12 hours for 10 days
Surgical prophylaxis, *by deep intramuscular injection or by intravenous injection or infusion*, 2 g at induction; further doses may be given every 6 hours for up to 24 hours for high-risk procedures; CHILD 30–40 mg/kg at induction; further doses may be given every 6 hours (every 8–12 hours in NEONATES) for up to 24 hours for high-risk procedures; intravenous route recommended for children

Mefoxin® (MSD) PoM
Injection, powder for reconstitution, cefoxitin (as sodium salt). Net price 1-g vial = £4.92; 2-g vial = £9.84
Electrolytes: Na+ 2.3 mmol/g

CEFPIROME

Indications: see under Cefaclor and notes above
Cautions: see under Cefaclor; interference with creatinine assays using picrate method
Contra-indications: see under Cefaclor
Side-effects: see under Cefaclor; taste disturbance shortly after injection reported
Dose: *by intravenous injection or infusion*, complicated upper and lower urinary-tract, skin and soft-

tissue infections, 1 g every 12 hours increased to 2 g every 12 hours in very severe infections
Lower respiratory-tract infections, 1–2 g every 12 hours
Severe infections including bacteraemia and septicaemia and infections in neutropenic patients, 2 g every 12 hours
CHILD under 12 years not recommended

Cefrom® (Hoechst Marion Roussel) [PoM]
Injection, powder for reconstitution, cefpirome (as sulphate), net price 1-g vial = £10.75; 2-g vial = £21.50

CEFPODOXIME

Indications: see under Dose
Cautions: see under Cefaclor
Contra-indications: see under Cefaclor
Side-effects: see under Cefaclor
Dose: upper respiratory-tract infections (but in pharyngitis and tonsillitis reserved for infections which are recurrent, chronic, or resistant to other antibacterials), 100 mg twice daily (200 mg twice daily in sinusitis)
Lower respiratory-tract infections (including bronchitis and pneumonia), 100–200 mg twice daily
Skin and soft tissue infections, 200 mg twice daily
Uncomplicated urinary-tract infections, 100 mg twice daily (200 mg twice daily in uncomplicated upper urinary-tract infections)
Uncomplicated gonorrhoea, 200 mg as a single dose
CHILD 15 days–6 months 4 mg/kg every 12 hours, 6 months–2 years 40 mg every 12 hours, 3–8 years 80 mg every 12 hours, over 9 years 100 mg every 12 hours

Orelox® (Hoechst Marion Roussel) [PoM]
Tablets, f/c, cefpodoxime 100 mg (as proxetil), net price 10-tab pack = £9.26. Label: 5, 9, 21
Oral suspension, cefpodoxime (as proxetil) for reconstitution with water, 40 mg/5 mL, net price 100 mL = £10.89. Label: 5, 9, 21
Excipients: include aspartame (section 9.4.1)

CEFPROZIL

Indications: see under Dose
Cautions: see under Cefaclor
Contra-indications: see under Cefaclor
Side-effects: see under Cefaclor
Dose: upper respiratory-tract infections and skin and soft tissue infections, 500 mg once daily usually for 10 days; CHILD 6 months–12 years, 20 mg/kg (max. 500 mg) once daily
Acute exacerbation of chronic bronchitis, 500 mg every 12 hours usually for 10 days
Otitis media, CHILD 6 months–12 years, 20 mg/kg (max. 500 mg) every 12 hours

Cefzil® (Bristol-Myers Squibb) ▼ [PoM]
Tablets, cefprozil, 250 mg (orange), net price 20-tab pack = £14.95; 500 mg, 10-tab pack = £14.95. Label: 9
Suspension, cefprozil, 250 mg/5 mL when reconstituted with water, net price 100 mL = £15.22. Label: 9
Excipients: include aspartame equivalent to phenylalanine 28 mg/5 mL (section 9.4.1)

CEFRADINE
(Cephradine)

Indications: see under Cefaclor; surgical prophylaxis
Cautions: see under Cefaclor
Contra-indications: see under Cefaclor
Side-effects: see under Cefaclor
Dose: *by mouth*, 250–500 mg every 6 hours *or* 0.5–1 g every 12 hours; up to 1 g every 6 hours in severe infections; CHILD, 25–50 mg/kg daily in 2–4 divided doses
By deep intramuscular injection or by intravenous injection over 3–5 minutes *or by intravenous infusion*, 0.5–1 g every 6 hours, increased to 8 g daily in severe infections; CHILD 50–100 mg/kg daily in 4 divided doses
Surgical prophylaxis, *by deep intramuscular injection or by intravenous injection* over 3–5 minutes, 1–2 g at induction

Cefradine (Non-proprietary) [PoM]
Capsules, cefradine 250 mg, net price 20-cap pack = £3.48; 500 mg, 20-cap pack = £6.90. Label: 9
Available from APS, Galen (*Nicef®*), Generics, IVAX

Velosef® (Squibb) [PoM]
Capsules, cefradine 250 mg (orange/blue), net price 20-cap pack = £3.55; 500 mg (blue), 20-cap pack = £7.00. Label: 9
Syrup, cefradine 250 mg/5 mL when reconstituted with water. Net price 100 mL = £4.22. Label: 9
Injection, powder for reconstitution, cefradine. Net price 500-mg vial = 99p; 1-g vial = £1.95

CEFTAZIDIME

Indications: see under Cefaclor; see also notes above
Cautions: see under Cefaclor
Contra-indications: see under Cefaclor
Side-effects: see under Cefaclor
Dose: *by deep intramuscular injection or intravenous injection or infusion*, 1 g every 8 hours *or* 2 g every 12 hours; 2 g every 8–12 hours *or* 3 g every 12 hours in severe infections; single doses over 1 g intravenous route only; ELDERLY usual max. 3 g daily; CHILD, up to 2 months 25–60 mg/kg daily in 2 divided doses, over 2 months 30–100 mg/kg daily in 2–3 divided doses; up to 150 mg/kg daily (max. 6 g daily) in 3 divided doses if immunocompromised or meningitis; intravenous route recommended for children
Urinary-tract and less serious infections, 0.5–1 g every 12 hours
Pseudomonal lung infection in cystic fibrosis, ADULT 100–150 mg/kg daily in 3 divided doses; CHILD up to 150 mg/kg daily (max. 6 g daily) in 3 divided doses; intravenous route recommended for children
Surgical prophylaxis, prostatic surgery, 1 g at induction of anaesthesia repeated if necessary when catheter removed

Fortum® (GSK) [PoM]
Injection, powder for reconstitution, ceftazidime (as pentahydrate), with sodium carbonate, net price 250-mg vial = £2.37, 500-mg vial = £4.73, 1-g vial = £9.45, 2-g vial (for injection and for infusion, both) = £18.91, 3-g vial (for injection or infusion) = £27.70; *Monovial*, 2 g vial (with transfer needle) = £18.91
Electrolytes: Na$^+$ 2.3 mmol/g

Kefadim® (Lilly) [PoM]
Injection, powder for reconstitution, ceftazidime (as pentahydrate), with sodium carbonate, net price 1-g vial = £9.90, 2-g vial = £19.80
Electrolytes: Na⁺ 2.3 mmol/g

CEFTRIAXONE

Indications: see under Cefaclor and notes above; surgical prophylaxis; prophylaxis of meningococcal meningitis [unlicensed indication] (Table 2, section 5.1)

Cautions: see under Cefaclor; severe renal impairment (Appendix 3); hepatic impairment if accompanied by renal impairment (Appendix 2); premature neonates; may displace bilirubin from serum albumin, administer over 60 minutes in neonates (see also Contra-indications); treatment longer than 14 days, renal failure, dehydration, or concomitant total parenteral nutrition—risk of ceftriaxone precipitation in gall bladder

Contra-indications: see under Cefaclor; neonates with jaundice, hypoalbuminaemia, acidosis or impaired bilirubin binding

Side-effects: see under Cefaclor; calcium ceftriaxone precipitates in urine (particularly in very young, dehydrated or those who are immobilised) or in gall bladder—consider discontinuation if symptomatic; rarely prolongation of prothrombin time, pancreatitis

Dose: *by deep intramuscular injection, or by intravenous injection over at least 2–4 minutes, or by intravenous infusion,* 1 g daily; 2–4 g daily in severe infections; intramuscular doses over 1 g divided between more than one site
NEONATE *by intravenous infusion* over 60 minutes, 20–50 mg/kg daily (max. 50 mg/kg daily) INFANT and CHILD under 50 kg, *by deep intramuscular injection, or by intravenous injection over 2–4 minutes, or by intravenous infusion,* 20–50 mg/kg daily; up to 80 mg/kg daily in severe infections; doses of 50 mg/kg and over by intravenous infusion only; 50 kg and over, adult dose
Uncomplicated gonorrhoea, *by deep intramuscular injection,* 250 mg as a single dose
Surgical prophylaxis, *by deep intramuscular injection or by intravenous injection over at least 2–4 minutes,* 1 g at induction; colorectal surgery, *by deep intramuscular injection or by intravenous injection over at least 2–4 minutes or by intravenous infusion,* 2 g at induction; intramuscular doses over 1 g divided between more than one site

Ceftriaxone (Non-proprietary) [PoM]
Injection, powder for reconstitution, ceftriaxone (as sodium salt), net price 1-g vial = £10.94; 2-g vial = £21.89
Available from Genus, PLIVA

Rocephin® (Roche) [PoM]
Injection, powder for reconstitution, ceftriaxone (as sodium salt), net price 250-mg vial = £2.74; 1-g vial = £10.94; 2-g vial = £21.89
Electrolytes: Na⁺ 3.6 mmol/g

CEFUROXIME

Indications: see under Cefaclor; surgical prophylaxis; more active against *Haemophilus influenzae* and *Neisseria gonorrhoeae*; Lyme disease

Cautions: see under Cefaclor

Contra-indications: see under Cefaclor

Side-effects: see under Cefaclor

Dose: *by mouth* (as cefuroxime axetil), 250 mg twice daily in most infections including mild to moderate lower respiratory-tract infections (e.g. bronchitis); doubled for more severe lower respiratory-tract infections or if pneumonia suspected
Urinary-tract infection, 125 mg twice daily, doubled in pyelonephritis
Gonorrhoea, 1 g as a single dose
CHILD over 3 months, 125 mg twice daily, if necessary doubled in child over 2 years with otitis media
Lyme disease, ADULT and CHILD over 12 years, 500 mg twice daily for 20 days
By intramuscular injection or intravenous injection or infusion, 750 mg every 6–8 hours; 1.5 g every 6–8 hours in severe infections; single doses over 750 mg intravenous route only
CHILD usual dose 60 mg/kg daily (range 30–100 mg/kg daily) in 3–4 divided doses (2–3 divided doses in neonates)
Gonorrhoea, 1.5 g as a single dose *by intramuscular injection* (divided between 2 sites)
Surgical prophylaxis, 1.5 g *by intravenous injection* at induction; up to 3 further doses of 750 mg may be given *by intramuscular or intravenous* injection every 8 hours for high-risk procedures
Meningitis, 3 g intravenously every 8 hours; CHILD, 200–240 mg/kg daily (in 3–4 divided doses) reduced to 100 mg/kg daily after 3 days or on clinical improvement; NEONATE, 100 mg/kg daily reduced to 50 mg/kg daily

Cefuroxime (Non-proprietary) [PoM]
Injection, powder for reconstitution, cefuroxime (as sodium salt), net price 750-mg vial = £2.64; 1.5-g vial = £5.29
Available from Lilly

Zinacef® (GSK) [PoM]
Injection, powder for reconstitution, cefuroxime (as sodium salt). Net price 250-mg vial = 93p; 750-mg vial = £2.52; 1.5-g vial = £5.05
Electrolytes: Na⁺ 1.8 mmol/750-mg vial

Zinnat® (GSK) [PoM]
Tablets, both f/c, cefuroxime (as axetil) 125 mg, net price 14-tab pack = £5.20; 250 mg, 14-tab pack = £10.40. Label: 9, 21, 25
Suspension, cefuroxime (as axetil) 125 mg/5 mL when reconstituted with water, net price 70 mL = £5.94. Label: 9, 21
Sachets, cefuroxime (as axetil) 125 mg/sachet, net price 14-sachet pack = £5.94. Label: 9, 13, 21

Other beta-lactam antibiotics

Aztreonam is a monocyclic beta-lactam ('monobactam') antibiotic with an antibacterial spectrum limited to Gram-negative aerobic bacteria including *Pseudomonas aeruginosa, Neisseria meningitidis,* and *Haemophilus influenzae*; it should not be used alone for 'blind' treatment since it is not active against Gram-positive organisms. Aztreonam is also effective against *Neisseria gonorrhoeae* (but not against concurrent chlamydial infection). Side-effects are similar to those of the other beta-lactams although aztreonam may be less likely to cause hypersensitivity in penicillin-sensitive patients.

Imipenem, a carbapenem, has a broad spectrum of activity which includes many aerobic and anaerobic

Gram-positive and Gram-negative bacteria. Imipenem is partially inactivated in the kidney by enzymatic activity and is therefore administered in combination with **cilastatin**, a specific enzyme inhibitor, which blocks its renal metabolism. Side-effects are similar to those of other beta-lactam antibiotics; neurotoxicity has been observed at very high dosage or in renal failure.

Meropenem is similar to imipenem but is stable to the renal enzyme which inactivates imipenem and therefore can be given without cilastatin. Meropenem has less seizure-inducing potential and can be used to treat central nervous system infection.

Ertapenem has a broad spectrum of activity, which covers Gram-positive and Gram-negative organisms and anaerobes. It is licensed for treating abdominal and gynaecological infections and for community-acquired pneumonia, but it is not active against atypical respiratory pathogens and it has limited activity against penicillin-resistant pneumococci. Unlike imipenem and meropenem, ertapenem is not active against *Pseudomonas* or against *Acinetobacter* spp.

AZTREONAM

Indications: Gram-negative infections including *Pseudomonas aeruginosa*, *Haemophilus influenzae*, and *Neisseria meningitidis*

Cautions: hypersensitivity to beta-lactam antibiotics; hepatic impairment; reduce dose in renal impairment; breast-feeding (Appendix 5); **interactions:** Appendix 1 (aztreonam)

Contra-indications: aztreonam hypersensitivity; pregnancy

Side-effects: nausea, vomiting, diarrhoea, abdominal cramps; mouth ulcers, altered taste; jaundice and hepatitis; blood disorders (including thrombocytopenia and neutropenia); urticaria and rashes

Dose: *by deep intramuscular injection or by intravenous injection* over 3–5 minutes *or by intravenous infusion,* 1 g every 8 hours *or* 2 g every 12 hours; 2 g every 6–8 hours for severe infections (including systemic *Pseudomonas aeruginosa* and lung infections in cystic fibrosis); single doses over 1 g intravenous route only

CHILD over 1 week, *by intravenous injection or infusion,* 30 mg/kg every 6–8 hours increased in severe infections for child of 2 years or older to 50 mg/kg every 6–8 hours; max. 8 g daily

Urinary-tract infections, 0.5–1 g every 8–12 hours

Gonorrhoea, cystitis, *by intramuscular injection,* 1 g as a single dose

Azactam® (Squibb) PoM
Injection, powder for reconstitution, aztreonam. Net price 500-mg vial = £4.48; 1-g vial = £8.95; 2-g vial = £17.90

ERTAPENEM

Indications: abdominal infections; acute gynaecological infections; community-acquired pneumonia

Cautions: renal impairment (Appendix 3); pregnancy (Appendix 4); **interactions:** Appendix 1 (ertapenem)

Contra-indications: hypersensitivity to beta-lactam antibiotics; breast-feeding (Appendix 5)

Side-effects: diarrhoea, nausea, vomiting, headache, injection-site reactions, rash, pruritus, raised platelet count; less frequently dry mouth, taste disturbances, dyspepsia, abdominal pain, anorexia, constipation, antibiotic-associated colitis, hypotension, chest pain, oedema, pharyngeal discomfort, dyspnoea, dizziness, sleep disturbances, confusion, asthenia, seizures, vaginitis, raised glucose; rarely dysphagia, cholecystitis, liver disorder (including jaundice), arrhythmia, increase in blood pressure, syncope, nasal congestion, cough, wheezing, hypersensitivity reactions, anxiety, depression, agitation, tremor, pelvic peritonitis, renal impairment, muscle cramp, scleral disorder, blood disorders (including neutropenia, thrombocytopenia, haemorrhage), hypoglycaemia, electrolyte disturbances

Dose: *by intravenous infusion,* ADULT over 18 years, 1 g once daily

Invanz® (MSD) ▼ PoM
Intravenous infusion, powder for reconstitution, ertapenem (as sodium salt), net price 1-g vial = £31.65
Electrolytes: Na$^+$ 6 mmol/1-g vial

IMIPENEM WITH CILASTATIN

Indications: aerobic and anaerobic Gram-positive and Gram-negative infections; surgical prophylaxis; hospital-acquired septicaemia (Table 1, section 5.1); not indicated for CNS infections

Cautions: renal impairment (Appendix 3); CNS disorders (e.g. epilepsy); pregnancy (Appendix 4); **interactions:** Appendix 1 (imipenem with cilastatin)

Contra-indications: hypersensitivity to beta-lactam antibiotics; breast-feeding (Appendix 5)

Side-effects: nausea, vomiting, diarrhoea (antibiotic-associated colitis reported), taste disturbances, tooth or tongue discoloration, hearing loss; blood disorders, positive Coombs' test; allergic reactions (with rash, pruritus, urticaria, Stevens-Johnson syndrome, fever, anaphylactic reactions, rarely toxic epidermal necrolysis, exfoliative dermatitis); myoclonic activity, convulsions, confusion and mental disturbances reported; slight increases in liver enzymes and bilirubin reported, rarely hepatitis; increases in serum creatinine and blood urea; red coloration of urine in children reported; local reactions: erythema, pain and induration, and thrombophlebitis

Dose: *by deep intramuscular injection,* mild to moderate infections, in terms of imipenem, 500–750 mg every 12 hours

By intravenous infusion, in terms of imipenem, 1–2 g daily (in 3–4 divided doses); less sensitive organisms, up to 50 mg/kg daily (max. 4 g daily) in 3–4 divided doses; CHILD 3 months and older, 60 mg/kg (up to max. of 2 g) daily in 4 divided doses; over 40 kg, adult dose

Surgical prophylaxis, *by intravenous infusion,* 1 g at induction repeated after 3 hours, supplemented in high risk (e.g. colorectal) surgery by doses of 500 mg 8 and 16 hours after induction

Primaxin® (MSD) PoM
Intramuscular injection, powder for reconstitution, imipenem (as monohydrate) 500 mg with cilastatin (as sodium salt) 500 mg, net price per vial = £12.00
Electrolytes: Na$^+$ 1.47 mmol/vial

Intravenous infusion, powder for reconstitution, imipenem (as monohydrate) 500 mg with cilastatin (as sodium salt) 500 mg, net price per vial =

£12.00; *Monovial* (vial with transfer needle) =
£12.00
Electrolytes: Na⁺ 1.72 mmol/vial

MEROPENEM

Indications: aerobic and anaerobic Gram-positive and Gram-negative infections

Cautions: hepatic impairment (monitor liver function); renal impairment (Appendix 3); pregnancy and breast-feeding; **interactions:** Appendix 1 (meropenem)

Contra-indications: hypersensitivity to beta-lactam antbiotics

Side-effects: nausea, vomiting, diarrhoea (antibiotic-associated colitis reported), abdominal pain; disturbances in liver function tests; thrombocytopenia (reduction in partial thromboplastin time reported), positive Coombs' test, eosinophilia, leucopenia, neutropenia; headache, paraesthesia; hypersensitivity reactions including rash, pruritus, urticaria, angioedema, and anaphylaxis; also reported, convulsions, Stevens-Johnson syndrome and toxic epidermal necrolysis; local reactions including pain and thrombophlebitis at injection site

Dose: *by intravenous injection* over 5 minutes *or by intravenous infusion*, 500 mg every 8 hours, dose doubled in hospital-acquired pneumonia, peritonitis, septicaemia and infections in neutropenic patients; CHILD 3 months–12 years [not licensed for infection in neutropenia] 10–20 mg/kg every 8 hours, over 50 kg body weight adult dose

Meningitis, 2 g every 8 hours; CHILD 3 months–12 years 40 mg/kg every 8 hours, over 50 kg body weight adult dose

Exacerbations of chronic lower respiratory-tract infection in cystic fibrosis, up to 2 g every 8 hours; CHILD 4–18 years 25–40 mg/kg every 8 hours

Meronem® (AstraZeneca) PoM
Injection, powder for reconstitution, meropenem (as trihydrate), net price 500-mg vial = £14.33; 1-g vial = £28.65
Electrolytes: Na⁺ 3.9 mmol/g

5.1.3 Tetracyclines

The tetracyclines are broad-spectrum antibiotics whose value has decreased owing to increasing bacterial resistance. They remain, however, the treatment of choice for infections caused by chlamydia (trachoma, psittacosis, salpingitis, urethritis, and lymphogranuloma venereum), rickettsia (including Q-fever), brucella (doxycycline with either streptomycin or rifampicin), and the spirochaete, *Borrelia burgdorferi* (Lyme disease—see section 5.1.1.3). They are also used in respiratory and genital mycoplasma infections, in acne, in destructive (refractory) periodontal disease, in exacerbations of chronic bronchitis (because of their activity against *Haemophilus influenzae*), and for leptospirosis in penicillin hypersensitivity (as an alternative to erythromycin).

Microbiologically, there is little to choose between the various tetracyclines, the only exception being **minocycline** which has a broader spectrum; it is active against *Neisseria meningitidis* and has been used for meningococcal prophylaxis but is no longer

recommended because of side-effects including dizziness and vertigo (see section 5.1, table 2 for current recommendations). *Deteclo®* (a combination of tetracycline, chlortetracycline and demeclocycline) does not have any advantages over preparations containing a single tetracycline

CAUTIONS. Tetracyclines should be used with caution in patients with hepatic impairment (Appendix 2) or those receiving potentially hepatotoxic drugs. Tetracyclines may increase muscle weakness in patients with myasthenia gravis, and exacerbate systemic lupus erythematosus. Antacids, and aluminium, calcium, iron, magnesium and zinc salts decrease the absorption of tetracyclines; milk also reduces the absorption of demeclocycline, oxytetracycline, and tetracycline. Other **interactions:** Appendix 1 (tetracyclines).

CONTRA-INDICATIONS. Deposition of tetracyclines in growing bone and teeth (by binding to calcium) causes staining and occasionally dental hypoplasia, and they should **not** be given to children under 12 years, or to pregnant or breast-feeding women (Appendixes 4 and 5). However, doxycycline may be used in children for treatment and post-exposure prophylaxis of anthrax when an alternative antibacterial cannot be given [unlicensed indication]. With the exception of **doxycycline** and **minocycline**, the tetracyclines may exacerbate renal failure and should **not** be given to patients with kidney disease (Appendix 3).

SIDE-EFFECTS. Side-effects of the tetracyclines include nausea, vomiting, diarrhoea (antibiotic-associated coltis reported occasionally), dysphagia, and oesophageal irritation. Other rare side-effects include hepatotoxicity, blood dyscrasias, photosensitivity (particularly with demeclocycline), and hypersensitivity reactions (including rash, exfoliative dermatitis, urticaria, angioedema, anaphylaxis, pericarditis). Headache and visual disturbances may indicate benign intracranial hypertension (discontinue treatment); bulging fontanelles have been reported in infants.

TETRACYCLINE

Indications: see notes above; acne vulgaris, rosacea (section 13.6)

Cautions: see notes above

Contra-indications: see notes above

Side-effects: see notes above; also reported, pancreatitis, acute renal failure, skin discoloration

Dose: *by mouth*, 250 mg every 6 hours, increased in severe infections to 500 mg every 6–8 hours

Acne, see section 13.6.2

Non-gonococcal urethritis, 500 mg every 6 hours for 7–14 days (21 days if failure or relapse after first course)

COUNSELLING. Tablets should be swallowed whole with plenty of fluid while sitting or standing

Tetracycline (Non-proprietary) PoM
Tablets, coated, tetracycline hydrochloride 250 mg, net price 28–tab pack = £1.06. Label: 7, 9, 23, counselling, posture
Available from Alpharma, Hillcross, IVAX

■ Compound preparations
Deteclo® (Goldshield) PoM ▣

Tablets, blue, f/c, tetracycline hydrochloride
115.4 mg, chlortetracycline hydrochloride
115.4 mg, demeclocycline hydrochloride 69.2 mg,
net price 14-tab pack = £1.83. Label: 7, 9, 11, 23,
counselling, posture
Dose: 1 tablet every 12 hours; 3–4 tablets daily in more
severe infections

DEMECLOCYCLINE HYDROCHLORIDE

Indications: see notes above; also inappropriate
secretion of antidiuretic hormone, section 6.5.2
Cautions: see notes above, but photosensitivity
more common (avoid exposure to sunlight or sun
lamps)
Contra-indications: see notes above
Side-effects: see notes above; also reported, pancreatitis, reversible nephrogenic diabetes insipidus,
acute renal failure
Dose: 150 mg every 6 hours *or* 300 mg every 12
hours

Ledermycin® (Goldshield) PoM
Capsules, red, demeclocycline hydrochloride
150 mg, net price 28-cap pack = £5.78. Label: 7, 9,
11, 23

DOXYCYCLINE

Indications: see notes above; chronic prostatitis;
sinusitis, syphilis, pelvic inflammatory disease
(Table 1, section 5.1); treatment and prophylaxis
of anthrax [unlicensed indication]; malaria treatment and prophylaxis (section 5.4.1); rosacea
[unlicensed indication], acne vulgaris (section
13.6)
Cautions: see notes above, but may be used in renal
impairment; alcohol dependence; photosensitivity
reported (avoid exposure to sunlight or sun lamps);
avoid in porphyria (section 9.8.2)
Contra-indications: see notes above
Side-effects: see notes above; also anorexia
Dose: 200 mg on first day, then 100 mg daily; severe
infections (including refractory urinary-tract infections), 200 mg daily
Early syphilis, 100 mg twice daily for 14 days; late
latent syphilis 200 mg twice daily for 28 days
Uncomplicated genital chlamydia, non-gonococcal
urethritis, 100 mg twice daily for 7 days (14 days in
pelvic inflammatory disease, see also Table 1,
section 5.1)
Anthrax (treatment or post-exposure prophylaxis;
see also section 5.1.12), 100 mg twice daily; CHILD
(only if alternative antibacterial cannot be given)
[unlicensed dose] 5 mg/kg daily in 2 divided doses
(max. 200 mg daily)
COUNSELLING. Capsules should be swallowed whole with
plenty of fluid during meals while sitting or standing
NOTE. Doxycycline doses in BNF may differ from those in
product literature

Doxycycline (Non-proprietary) PoM
Capsules, doxycycline (as hyclate) 50 mg, net price
28-cap pack = £6.77; 100 mg, 8-cap pack = £2.49.
Label: 6, 9, 11, 27, counselling, posture
Available from Alpharma, APS, Hillcross, IVAX, Kent,
PLIVA, Sandoz (*Doxylar*®)

Vibramycin® (Pfizer) PoM
Capsules, doxycycline (as hyclate) 50 mg (green/
ivory), net price 28-cap pack = £7.74, 56-cap pack
(*Acne Pack*) = £17.80; 100 mg (green), 8-cap pack
= £4.18. Label: 6, 9, 11, 27, counselling, posture

Vibramycin-D® (Pfizer) PoM
Dispersible tablets, off-white, doxycycline 100 mg.
Net price 8-tab pack = £4.91. Label: 6, 9, 11, 13

LYMECYCLINE

Indications: see notes above
Cautions: see notes above
Contra-indications: see notes above
Side-effects: see notes above; also reported, pan-
creatitis
Dose: 408 mg every 12 hours, increased to 1.224–
1.632 g daily in severe infections
Acne, 408 mg daily for at least 8 weeks

Tetralysal 300® (Galderma) PoM
Capsules, red/yellow, lymecycline 408 mg (= tetra-
cycline 300 mg). Net price 28-cap pack = £7.16.
Label: 6, 9

MINOCYCLINE

Indications: see notes above; meningococcal carrier
state; acne vulgaris (section 13.6.2)
Cautions: see notes above, but may be used in renal
impairment; if treatment continued for longer than
6 months, monitor every 3 months for hepatotoxicity, pigmentation and for systemic lupus erythematosus—discontinue if these develop or if pre-
existing systemic lupus erythematosus worsens
Contra-indications: see notes above
Side-effects: see notes above; also anorexia, pancreatitis, dizziness, tinnitus and vertigo (more
common in women), acute renal failure; pigmentation (sometimes irreversible), discoloration of
conjunctiva, tears and sweat, systemic lupus
erythematosus
Dose: 100 mg twice daily
Acne, see section 13.6.2
Prophylaxis of asymptomatic meningococcal carrier state (but no longer recommended, see notes
above), 100 mg twice daily for 5 days usually
followed by rifampicin
COUNSELLING. Tablets or capsules should be swallowed
whole with plenty of fluid while sitting or standing

Minocycline (Non-proprietary) PoM
Capsules, minocycline (as hydrochloride) 50 mg,
net price 56-cap pack = £17.20; 100 mg, 28-cap
pack = £14.74. Label: 6, 9, counselling, posture
Available from Crookes (*Aknemin*®)
Tablets, minocycline (as hydrochloride) 50 mg, net
price 28-tab pack = £7.57, 84-tab pack = £32.39;
100 mg, 28-tab pack = £11.41. Label: 6, 9,
counselling, posture
Available from Alpharma, Ashbourne (*Blemix*®), CP,
Generics, Hillcross, IVAX, Lederle (*Minocin*®), PLIVA,
Tillomed

Minocin MR® (Lederle) PoM
Capsules, m/r, orange/brown (enclosing yellow and
white pellets), minocycline (as hydrochloride)
100 mg. Net price 56-cap pack = £42.27. Label: 6,
25
Dose: acne, 1 capsule daily

OXYTETRACYCLINE

Indications: see notes above; acne vulgaris, rosacea
(section 13.6)

Cautions: see notes above; porphyria (section 9.8.2)
Contra-indications: see notes above
Side-effects: see notes above
Dose: 250–500 mg every 6 hours
Acne, see section 13.6.2

Oxytetracycline (Non-proprietary) [PoM]
Tablets, coated, oxytetracycline dihydrate 250 mg, net price 28-tab pack = 81p. Label: 7, 9, 23
Available from Alpharma, APS, Ashbourne (*Oxytetramix*®), DDSA (*Oxymycin*®), IVAX

5.1.4   Aminoglycosides

These include amikacin, gentamicin, neomycin, netilmicin, streptomycin, and tobramycin. All are bactericidal and active against some Gram-positive and many Gram-negative organisms. Amikacin, gentamicin, and tobramycin are also active against *Pseudomonas aeruginosa*; streptomycin is active against *Mycobacterium tuberculosis* and is now almost entirely reserved for tuberculosis (section 5.1.9).

The aminoglycosides are not absorbed from the gut (although there is a risk of absorption in inflammatory bowel disease and liver failure) and must therefore be given by injection for systemic infections.

Excretion is principally via the kidney and accumulation occurs in renal impairment.

Most side-effects of this group of antibiotics are dose-related therefore care must be taken with dosage and whenever possible treatment should not exceed 7 days. The important side-effects are ototoxicity, and nephrotoxicity; they occur most commonly in the elderly and in patients with renal failure.

If there is impairment of renal function (or high predose serum concentrations) the interval between doses must be increased; if the renal impairment is severe the dose itself should be reduced as well.

Aminoglycosides may impair neuromuscular transmission and should not be given to patients with myasthenia gravis; large doses given during surgery have been responsible for a transient myasthenic syndrome in patients with normal neuromuscular function.

Aminoglycosides should preferably not be given with potentially ototoxic diuretics (e.g. furosemide (frusemide)); if concurrent use is unavoidable administration of the aminoglycoside and of the diuretic should be separated by as long a period as practicable.

SERUM CONCENTRATIONS. Serum concentration monitoring avoids both excessive and subtherapeutic concentrations thus preventing toxicity and ensuring efficacy. In patients with normal renal function, aminoglycoside concentrations should be measured after 3 or 4 doses; patients with renal impairment may require earlier and more frequent measurement of aminoglycoside concentration.

Blood samples should be taken approximately 1 hour after intramuscular or intravenous administration ('peak' concentration) and also just before the next dose ('trough' concentration).

Serum aminoglycoside concentrations should be measured in all patients and **must** be determined in infants, in the elderly, in obesity, and in cystic fibrosis, *or* if high doses are being given, *or* if there is renal impairment.

ONCE DAILY DOSAGE. Although aminoglycosides are generally given in 2–3 divided doses during the 24 hours, *once daily administration* is more convenient (while ensuring adequate serum concentration) but **expert advice** about dosage and serum concentrations should be obtained.

ENDOCARDITIS. **Gentamicin** is used in combination with other antibiotics for the treatment of bacterial endocarditis (Table 1, section 5.1). Serumgentamicin concentration should be determined twice each week (more often in renal impairment).

For *streptococcal* and *enterococcal endocarditis* see under Gentamicin. **Streptomycin** may be used as an alternative in gentamicin-resistant enterococcal endocarditis.

In *staphylococcal endocarditis*, gentamicin is given in conventional doses to achieve a one-hour ('peak') serum-gentamicin concentration of 5–10 mg/litre and a pre-dose ('trough') concentration of less than 2 mg/litre.

Gentamicin is the aminoglycoside of choice in the UK and is used widely for the treatment of serious infections. It has a broad spectrum but is inactive against anaerobes and has poor activity against haemolytic streptococci and pneumococci. When used for the 'blind' therapy of undiagnosed serious infections it is usually given in conjunction with a penicillin or metronidazole (or both). Gentamicin is used together with another antibiotic for the treatment of endocarditis (see above and Table 1, section 5.1).

In adults the dose of gentamicin for most infections is up to 5 mg/kg daily given in divided doses every 8 hours (if renal function is normal); whenever possible treatment should not exceed 7 days. Higher doses are occasionally indicated for serious infections, especially in the neonate or the immunocompromised patient. Loading and maintenance doses may be calculated on the basis of the patient's weight and renal function (e.g. using a nomogram); adjustments are then made according to serum-gentamicin concentrations.

Amikacin is a derivative of kanamycin and has one important advantage over gentamicin in that it is more stable than gentamicin to enzyme inactivation. Amikacin is used in the treatment of serious infections caused by gentamicin-resistant Gram-negative bacilli.

Netilmicin has similar activity to gentamicin, but may cause less ototoxicity in those needing treatment for longer than 10 days. Netilmicin is active against a number of gentamicin-resistant Gram-negative bacilli but is less active against *Ps. aeruginosa* than gentamicin or tobramycin.

Tobramycin has similar activity to gentamicin. It is slightly more active against *Ps. aeruginosa* but shows less activity against certain other Gram-negative bacteria. Tobramycin may be administered by nebuliser on a cyclical basis (28 days of tobramycin followed by a 28-day tobramycin-free interval) for the treatment of chronic pulmonary *Ps. aeruginosa* infection in cystic fibrosis; however, resistance may develop and some patients do not respond to treatment.

Neomycin is too toxic for parenteral administration and can only be used for infections of the skin or mucous membranes or to reduce the bacterial population of the colon prior to bowel surgery or in hepatic failure. Oral administration may lead to malabsorption. Small amounts of neomycin may be absorbed from the gut in patients with hepatic failure and, as these patients may also be uraemic, cumulation may occur with resultant ototoxicity.

GENTAMICIN

Indications: septicaemia and neonatal sepsis; meningitis and other CNS infections; biliary-tract infection, acute pyelonephritis or prostatitis, endocarditis (see notes above); pneumonia in hospital patients, adjunct in listerial meningitis (Table 1, section 5.1); eye (section 11.3.1); ear (section 12.1.1)

Cautions: pregnancy (Appendix 4), renal impairment, infants and elderly (adjust dose and monitor renal, auditory and vestibular function together with serum gentamicin concentrations); avoid prolonged use; conditions characterised by muscular weakness; significant obesity (monitor serum-gentamicin concentration closely and possibly reduce dose); see also notes above; **interactions:** Appendix 1 (aminoglycosides)

Contra-indications: myasthenia gravis

Side-effects: vestibular and auditory damage, nephrotoxicity; rarely, hypomagnesaemia on prolonged therapy, antibiotic-associated colitis; also reported, nausea, vomiting, rash; see also notes above

Dose: *by intramuscular or by slow intravenous injection* over at least 3 minutes *or by intravenous infusion*, 3–5 mg/kg daily (in divided doses every 8 hours), see also notes above

CHILD up to 2 weeks, 3 mg/kg every 12 hours; 2 weeks–12 years, 2 mg/kg every 8 hours

Streptococcal or enterococcal endocarditis in combination with other drugs, 80 mg twice daily

Endocarditis prophylaxis, Table 2, section 5.1

By intrathecal injection, seek specialist advice, 1 mg daily (increased if necessary to 5 mg daily)

NOTE. One-hour ('peak') serum concentration should be 5–10 mg/litre (3–5 mg/litre for streptococcal or enterococcal endocarditis); pre-dose ('trough') concentration should be less than 2 mg/litre (less than 1 mg/litre for streptococcal or enterococcal endocarditis)

Gentamicin (Non-proprietary) PoM
Injection, gentamicin (as sulphate), net price 40 mg/mL, 1-mL amp = £1.40, 2-mL amp = £1.54, 2-mL vial = £1.54
Available from Mayne

Cidomycin® (Hoechst Marion Roussel) PoM
Injection, gentamicin 40 mg (as sulphate)/mL. Net price 2-mL amp or vial = £1.48
Paediatric injection, gentamicin 10 mg (as sulphate)/mL. Net price 2-mL vial = 62p
Intrathecal injection, gentamicin 5 mg (as sulphate)/mL. Net price 1-mL amp = 74p

Genticin® (Roche) PoM
Injection, gentamicin 40 mg (as sulphate)/mL. Net price 2-mL amp = £1.51

Isotonic Gentamicin Injection (Baxter) PoM
Intravenous infusion, gentamicin 800 micrograms (as sulphate)/mL in sodium chloride intravenous infusion 0.9%. Net price 100-mL (80-mg) *Viaflex®* bag = £1.61
Electrolytes: Na^+ 15.4 mmol/100-mL bag

AMIKACIN

Indications: serious Gram-negative infections resistant to gentamicin

Cautions: see under Gentamicin

Contra-indications: see under Gentamicin

Side-effects: see under Gentamicin

Dose: *by intramuscular or by slow intravenous injection or by infusion,* 15 mg/kg daily in 2 divided doses, increased to 22.5 mg/kg daily in 3 divided doses in severe infections; max. 1.5 g daily for up to 10 days (max. cumulative dose 15 g); CHILD 15 mg/kg daily in 2 divided doses; NEONATE loading dose of 10 mg/kg then 15 mg/kg daily in 2 divided doses

NOTE. One-hour ('peak') serum concentration should not exceed 30 mg/litre; pre-dose ('trough') concentration should be less than 10 mg/litre

Amikacin (Non-proprietary) PoM
Injection, amikacin (as sulphate) 250 mg/mL. Net price 2-mL vial = £10.14
Electrolytes: Na^+ 0.56 mmol/500-mg vial
Available from Mayne

Amikin® (Bristol-Myers Squibb) PoM
Injection, amikacin (as sulphate) 250 mg/mL. Net price 2-mL vial = £10.14
Electrolytes: Na^+ < 0.5 mmol/vial
Paediatric injection, amikacin (as sulphate) 50 mg/mL. Net price 2-mL vial = £2.36
Electrolytes: Na^+ < 0.5 mmol/vial

NEOMYCIN SULPHATE

Indications: bowel sterilisation before surgery, see also notes above

Cautions: see under Gentamicin but too toxic for systemic use, see notes above

Contra-indications: see under Gentamicin; intestinal obstruction

Side-effects: see under Gentamicin but poorly absorbed on oral administration; increased salivation, stomatitis

Dose: *by mouth,* pre-operative bowel sterilisation, 1 g every hour for 4 hours, then 1 g every 4 hours for 2–3 days
Hepatic coma, up to 4 g daily in divided doses usually for max. 14 days

Neomycin (Non-proprietary) PoM
Tablets, neomycin sulphate 500 mg. Net price 20 = £3.44
Available from APS, Sovereign (*Nivemycin®*)

NETILMICIN

Indications: serious Gram-negative infections resistant to gentamicin

Cautions: see under Gentamicin

Contra-indications: see under Gentamicin

Side-effects: see under Gentamicin

Dose: *by intramuscular injection or by intravenous injection over 3–5 minutes or by intravenous infusion,* 4–6 mg/kg daily, as a single daily dose or in divided doses every 8 or 12 hours; in severe infections, up to 7.5 mg/kg daily in divided doses every 8 hours (reduced as soon as clinically indicated, usually within 48 hours) NEONATE up to 1 week, 3 mg/kg every 12 hours; INFANT over 1 week, 2.5–3 mg/kg every 8 hours; CHILD 2–2.5 mg/kg every 8 hours

Urinary-tract infection, 150 mg as a single daily dose for 5 days

Gonorrhoea, 300 mg as a single dose

NOTE. For divided daily dose regimens, one-hour ('peak') serum concentration should not exceed 12 mg/litre; pre-dose ('trough') concentration should be less than 2 mg/litre

Netillin® (Schering-Plough) [PoM]
Injection, netilmicin (as sulphate) 10 mg/mL, net price 1.5-mL (15-mg) amp = £1.42; 50 mg/mL, 1-mL (50-mg) amp = £2.11; 100 mg/mL, 1-mL (100-mg) amp = £2.75; 1.5-mL (150-mg) amp = £3.92, 2-mL (200-mg) amp = £5.09

TOBRAMYCIN

Indications: see under Gentamicin and notes above
Cautions: see under Gentamicin
SPECIFIC CAUTIONS FOR INHALED TREATMENT. Other inhaled drugs should be administered before tobramycin; monitor for bronchospasm with initial dose, measure peak flow before and after nebulisation—if bronchospasm occurs, repeat test using bronchodilator; monitor renal function before treatment and then annually; severe haemoptysis
Contra-indications: see under Gentamicin
Side-effects: see under Gentamicin; *on inhalation*, mouth ulcers, voice alteration, cough, bronchospasm (see Cautions)
Dose: *by intramuscular injection or by slow intravenous injection or by intravenous infusion*, 3 mg/kg daily in divided doses every 8 hours, see also notes above; in severe infections up to 5 mg/kg daily in divided doses every 6–8 hours (reduced to 3 mg/kg as soon as clinically indicated); NEONATE 2 mg/kg every 12 hours; CHILD over 1 week 2–2.5 mg/kg every 8 hours
Urinary-tract infection, *by intramuscular injection*, 2–3 mg/kg daily as a single dose
NOTE. One-hour ('peak') serum concentration should not exceed 10 mg/litre; pre-dose ('trough') concentration should be less than 2 mg/litre
Chronic pulmonary *Pseudomonas aeruginosa* infection in cystic fibrosis patients, *by inhalation of nebulised solution*, ADULT and CHILD over 6 years, 300 mg every 12 hours for 28 days, courses repeated after 28-day interval

Tobramycin (Non-proprietary) [PoM]
Injection, tobramycin (as sulphate) 40 mg/mL, net price 1-mL (40-mg) vial = £2.46, 2-mL (80-mg) vial = £3.77, 6-mL (240-mg) vial = £12.47
Available from Alpharma, Mayne

Nebcin® (King) [PoM]
Injection, tobramycin (as sulphate) 10 mg/mL, net price 2-mL (20-mg) vial = £2.27; 40 mg/mL, 2-mL (80-mg) vial = £5.52

Tobi® (Chiron) [PoM]
Nebuliser solution, tobramycin 60 mg/mL, net price 56 × 5-mL (300-mg) unit = £1540.00

5.1.5   Macrolides

Erythromycin has an antibacterial spectrum that is similar but not identical to that of penicillin; it is thus an alternative in penicillin-allergic patients.

Indications for erythromycin include respiratory infections, whooping cough, legionnaires' disease, and campylobacter enteritis. It is active against many penicillin-resistant staphylococci but some are now also resistant to erythromycin; it has poor activity against *Haemophilus influenzae*. Erythromycin is also active against chlamydia and mycoplasmas.

Erythromycin causes nausea, vomiting, and diarrhoea in some patients; in mild to moderate infections this can be avoided by giving a lower dose (250 mg 4 times daily) but if a more serious infection, such as Legionella pneumonia, is suspected higher doses are needed.

Azithromycin is a macrolide with slightly less activity than erythromycin against Gram-positive bacteria but enhanced activity against some Gram-negative organisms including *H. influenzae*. Plasma concentrations are very low but tissue concentrations are much higher. It has a long tissue half-life and once daily dosage is recommended. For treatment of Lyme disease, see section 5.1.1.3. Azithromycin is also used in the treatment of trachoma [unlicensed indication] (section 11.3.1).

Clarithromycin is an erythromycin derivative with slightly greater activity than the parent compound. Tissue concentrations are higher than with erythromycin. It is given twice daily.

Azithromycin and clarithromycin cause fewer gastro-intestinal side-effects than erythromycin.

Spiramycin is also a macrolide (section 5.4.7).

The ketolide **telithromycin** is a derivative of erythromycin. The antibacterial spectrum of telithromycin is similar to that of macrolides and it is also active against penicillin- and erythromycin-resistant *Streptococcus pneumoniae*.

ERYTHROMYCIN

Indications: alternative to penicillin in hypersensitive patients; campylobacter enteritis, pneumonia, legionnaires' disease, syphilis, non-gonococcal urethritis, chronic prostatitis, diphtheria and whooping cough prophylaxis; acne vulgaris and rosacea (section 13.6)
Cautions: hepatic and renal impairment; prolongation of QT interval (ventricular tachycardia reported); porphyria (section 9.8.2); pregnancy (not known to be harmful) and breast-feeding (only small amounts in milk); **interactions:** Appendix 1 (macrolides)
ARRHYTHMIAS. Avoid concomitant administration with pimozide or terfenadine [other interactions, Appendix 1]
Side-effects: nausea, vomiting, abdominal discomfort, diarrhoea (antibiotic-associated colitis reported); urticaria, rashes and other allergic reactions; reversible hearing loss reported after large doses; cholestatic jaundice, cardiac effects (including chest pain and arrhythmias), myasthenia-like syndrome, Stevens-Johnson syndrome, and toxic epidermal necrolysis also reported
Dose: *by mouth*, ADULT and CHILD over 8 years, 250–500 mg every 6 hours or 0.5–1 g every 12 hours (see notes above); up to 4 g daily in severe infections; CHILD up to 2 years 125 mg every 6 hours, 2–8 years 250 mg every 6 hours, doses doubled for severe infections
Early syphilis, 500 mg 4 times daily for 14 days
Uncomplicated genital chlamydia, non-gonococcal urethritis, 500 mg twice daily for 14 days
By intravenous infusion, ADULT and CHILD severe infections, 50 mg/kg daily by continuous infusion or in divided doses every 6 hours; mild infections (oral treatment not possible), 25 mg/kg daily; NEONATE 30–45 mg/kg daily in 3 divided doses

Erythromycin (Non-proprietary) PoM
Capsules, enclosing e/c microgranules, erythromycin 250 mg, net price 28-cap pack = £5.95.
Label: 5, 9, 25
Available from PLIVA, Tillomed (*Tiloryth*®)
Tablets, e/c, erythromycin 250 mg, net price 20 = £2.20. Label: 5, 9, 25
Available from, Alpharma, APS, Ashbourne (*Rommix*®), Generics, IVAX, Kent

Erythromycin Ethyl Succinate (Non-proprietary) PoM
Oral suspension, erythromycin (as ethyl succinate) for reconstitution with water 125 mg/5 mL, net price 100 mL = £1.15; 250 mg/5 mL, 100 mL = £1.80; 500 mg/5 mL, 100 mL = £2.89. Label: 9
NOTE. Sugar-free versions are available and can be ordered by specifying 'sugar-free' on the prescription
Available from Alpharma, APS, Generics, Hillcross, IVAX, Kent, Pinewood (*Primacine*®)

Erythromycin Lactobionate (Non-proprietary) PoM
Intravenous infusion, powder for reconstitution, erythromycin (as lactobionate), net price 1-g vial = £9.39
Available from Abbott, Mayne

Erymax® (Elan) PoM
Capsules, opaque orange/clear orange, enclosing orange and white e/c pellets, erythromycin 250 mg, net price 28-cap pack = £5.95, 112-cap pack = £23.80. Label: 5, 9, 25
Dose: 1 capsule every 6 hours *or* 2 capsules every 12 hours; acne, 1 capsule twice daily for 1 month then 1 capsule daily

Erythrocin® (Abbott) PoM
Tablets, both f/c, erythromycin (as stearate), 250 mg, net price 20 = £2.99; 500 mg, 20 = £6.01. Label: 9

Erythroped® (Abbott) PoM
Suspension SF, sugar-free, banana-flavoured, erythromycin (as ethyl succinate) for reconstitution with water, 125 mg/5 mL (*Suspension PI SF*), net price 140 mL = £3.18; 250 mg/5 mL, 140 mL = £6.20; 500 mg/5 mL (*Suspension SF Forte*), 140 mL = £10.99. Label: 9

Erythroped A® (Abbott) PoM
Tablets, yellow, f/c, erythromycin 500 mg (as ethyl succinate). Net price 28-tab pack = £10.19. Label: 9

AZITHROMYCIN

Indications: respiratory-tract infections; otitis media; skin and soft-tissue infections; uncomplicated genital chlamydial infections and non-gonococcal urethritis (Table 1, section 5.1); mild or moderate typhoid due to multiple-antibacterial-resistant organisms
Cautions: see under Erythromycin; pregnancy and breast-feeding; **interactions:** Appendix 1 (macrolides)
Contra-indications: hepatic impairment
Side-effects: see under Erythromycin; anorexia, dyspepsia, constipation; dizziness, headache, drowsiness; photosensitivity; hepatitis, interstitial nephritis, acute renal failure, asthenia, paraesthesia, convulsions and mild neutropenia reported; rarely tinnitus, hepatic necrosis, hepatic failure, and taste disturbances
Dose: 500 mg once daily for 3 days; CHILD over 6 months 10 mg/kg once daily for 3 days; *or* body-

weight 15–25 kg, 200 mg once daily for 3 days; body-weight 26–35 kg, 300 mg once daily for 3 days; body-weight 36–45 kg, 400 mg once daily for 3 days
Uncomplicated genital chlamydial infections and non-gonococcal urethritis, 1 g as a single dose
Typhoid [unlicensed indication], 500 mg once daily for 7 days

Zithromax® (Pfizer) PoM
Capsules, azithromycin (as dihydrate) 250 mg, net price 4-cap pack = £8.95, 6-cap pack = £13.43. Label: 5, 9, 23
Oral suspension, cherry/banana-flavoured, azithromycin (as dihydrate) 200 mg/5 mL when reconstituted with water. Net price 15-mL pack = £5.08, 22.5-mL pack = £7.62, 30-mL pack = £13.80. Label: 5, 9

CLARITHROMYCIN

Indications: respiratory-tract infections, mild to moderate skin and soft tissue infections, otitis media; *Helicobacter pylori* eradication (section 1.3)
Cautions: see under Erythromycin; renal impairment (Appendix 3); pregnancy and breast-feeding; **interactions:** Appendix 1 (macrolides)
ARRHYTHMIAS. Avoid concomitant administration with pimozide or terfenadine [other interactions, Appendix 1]
Side-effects: see under Erythromycin; also reported, dyspepsia, headache, smell and taste disturbances, tooth and tongue discoloration, stomatitis, glossitis, pancreatitis, arthralgia, myalgia, dizziness, vertigo, tinnitus, anxiety, insomnia, nightmares, confusion, psychosis, convulsions, paraesthesia, hypoglycaemia, hepatitis, renal failure, leucopenia, and thrombocytopenia; on intravenous infusion, local tenderness, phlebitis
Dose: *by mouth*, 250 mg every 12 hours for 7 days, increased in severe infections to 500 mg every 12 hours for up to 14 days; CHILD body-weight under 8 kg, 7.5 mg/kg twice daily; 8–11 kg (1–2 years), 62.5 mg twice daily; 12–19 kg (3–6 years), 125 mg twice daily; 20–29 kg (7–9 years), 187.5 mg twice daily; 30–40 kg (10–12 years), 250 mg twice daily
By intravenous infusion into larger proximal vein, 500 mg twice daily; CHILD not recommended

Klaricid® (Abbott) PoM
Tablets, both yellow, f/c, clarithromycin 250 mg, net price 14-tab pack = £11.76; 500 mg, 14-tab pack = £23.55, 20-tab pack = £33.64. Label: 9
Paediatric suspension, clarithromycin for reconstitution with water 125 mg/5 mL, net price 70 mL = £6.00, 100 mL = £10.32; 250 mg/5 mL, 70 mL = £12.00. Label: 9
Granules, clarithromycin 250 mg/sachet, net price 14-sachet pack = £12.56. Label: 9, 13
Intravenous infusion, powder for reconstitution, clarithromycin. Net price 500-mg vial = £12.32
Electrolytes: Na$^+$ < 0.5 mmol/500-mg vial

Klaricid XL® (Abbott) PoM
Tablets, m/r, yellow, clarithromycin 500 mg, net price 7-tab pack = £10.65, 14-tab pack = £21.30. Label: 9, 21, 25
Dose: 500 mg once daily (doubled in severe infections) for 7–14 days

TELITHROMYCIN

Indications: community-acquired pneumonia; exacerbation of chronic bronchitis; sinusitis; beta-haemolytic streptococcal pharyngitis or tonsillitis when beta-lactam antibiotics are inappropriate

Cautions: hepatic impairment; renal impairment (Appendix 3); pregnancy (Appendix 4); coronary heart disease, ventricular arrhythmias, bradycardia, hypokalaemia, hypomagnesaemia—risk of QT interval prolongation; concomitant administration of drugs that prolong QT-interval; myasthenia gravis (risk of exacerbation—use only if no other alternative); **interactions:** Appendix 1 (telithromycin)

Contra-indications: breast-feeding (Appendix 5); prolongation of QT interval; congenital or family history of QT interval prolongation (if not excluded by ECG)

ARRHYTHMIAS. Avoid concomitant administration with pimozide or terfenadine [other interactions, Appendix 1]

Side-effects: diarrhoea; nausea, vomiting, flatulence, abdominal pain, taste disturbances, dizziness, headache; less frequently constipation, stomatitis, anorexia, flushing, palpitations, drowsiness, insomnia, nervousness, rash, urticaria, pruritus, blurred vision, eosinophilia; rarely cholestatic jaundice, paraesthesia, arrhythmias, hypotension; also reported, antibiotic-associated colitis, hepatitis, face oedema, altered sense of smell, muscle cramp, erythema multiforme

Dose: 800 mg once daily for 5 days for sinusitis or exacerbation of chronic bronchitis *or* for 7–10 days in community-acquired pneumonia; CHILD under 18 years safety and efficacy not established

Beta-haemolytic streptococcal pharyngitis or tonsillitis, ADULT and CHILD over 12 years, 800 mg once daily for 5 days

Ketek® (Aventis Pharma) ▼ PoM
Tablets, orange, f/c, telithromycin 400 mg, net price 10-tab pack = £19.21. Label: 9

5.1.6   Clindamycin

Clindamycin has only a limited use because of serious side-effects. Its most serious toxic effect is antibiotic-associated colitis (section 1.5) which may be fatal and is most common in middle-aged and elderly women, especially following operation. Although it can occur with most antibacterials it is more frequently seen with clindamycin. Patients should therefore discontinue treatment immediately if diarrhoea develops.

Clindamycin is active against Gram-positive cocci, including penicillin-resistant staphylococci and also against many anaerobes, especially *Bacteroides fragilis*. It is well concentrated in bone and excreted in bile and urine.

Clindamycin is recommended for staphylococcal joint and bone infections such as osteomyelitis, and intra-abdominal sepsis. Clindamycin is also used for endocarditis prophylaxis (section 5.1, table 2).

CLINDAMYCIN

Indications: staphylococcal bone and joint infections, peritonitis; endocarditis prophylaxis [unlicensed indication], table 2, section 5.1

Cautions: discontinue immediately if diarrhoea or colitis develops; hepatic or renal impairment; monitor liver and renal function on prolonged therapy and in neonates and infants; pregnancy; breast-feeding (Appendix 5); avoid rapid intravenous administration; **interactions:** Appendix 1 (clindamycin)

Contra-indications: diarrhoeal states; avoid injections containing benzyl alcholol in neonates (see under preparations below)

Side-effects: diarrhoea (discontinue treatment), abdominal discomfort, nausea, vomiting, antibiotic-associated colitis; jaundice and altered liver function tests; neutropenia, eosinophilia, agranulocytosis and thrombocytopenia reported; rash, pruritus, urticaria, anaphylactoid reactions, erythema multiforme, exfoliative and vesiculobullous dermatitis reported; pain, induration, and abscess after intramuscular injection; thrombophlebitis after intravenous injection

Dose: *by mouth*, 150–300 mg every 6 hours; up to 450 mg every 6 hours in severe infections; CHILD, 3–6 mg/kg every 6 hours

COUNSELLING. Patients should discontinue immediately and contact doctor if diarrhoea develops; capsules should be swallowed with a glass of water.

By deep intramuscular injection or by intravenous infusion, 0.6–2.7 g daily (in 2–4 divided doses); life-threatening infection, up to 4.8 g daily; single doses above 600 mg by intravenous infusion only; single doses by intravenous infusion not to exceed 1.2 g

CHILD over 1 month, 15–40 mg/kg daily in 3–4 divided doses; severe infections, at least 300 mg daily regardless of weight

Clindamycin (Non-proprietary) PoM
Capsules, clindamycin (as hydrochloride) 150 mg, net price 24-cap pack = £13.72. Label: 9, 27, counselling, see above (diarrhoea)
Available from Sandoz

Dalacin C® (Pharmacia) PoM
Capsules, clindamycin (as hydrochloride) 75 mg (lavender), net price 24-cap pack = £7.45; 150 mg, (lavender/maroon), 24-cap pack = £13.72. Label: 9, 27, counselling, see above (diarrhoea)
Injection, clindamycin (as phosphate) 150 mg/mL, net price 2-mL amp = £6.20; 4-mL amp = £9.83
Excipients: include benzyl alcohol (avoid in neonates, see Excipients, p. 2)

5.1.7   Some other antibacterials

Antibacterials discussed in this section include chloramphenicol, fusidic acid, glycopeptide antibiotics (vancomycin and teicoplanin), the streptogramins (quinupristin and dalfopristin) and the polymyxin, colistin.

Chloramphenicol

Chloramphenicol is a potent broad-spectrum antibiotic; however, it is associated with serious haematological side-effects when given systemically and should therefore be reserved for the treatment of life-threatening infections, particularly those caused by *Haemophilus influenzae*, and also for typhoid fever.

Chloramphenicol eye drops (section 11.3.1) and chloramphenicol ear drops (section 12.1.1) are also available.

CHLORAMPHENICOL

Indications: see notes above

Cautions: avoid repeated courses and prolonged treatment; reduce doses in hepatic impairment (Appendix 2); renal impairment (Appendix 3); blood counts required before and periodically during treatment; monitor plasma-chloramphenicol concentration in neonates (see below); **interactions:** Appendix 1 (chloramphenicol)

Contra-indications: pregnancy (see also Appendix 4), breast-feeding, porphyria (section 9.8.2)

Side-effects: blood disorders including reversible and irreversible aplastic anaemia (with reports of resulting leukaemia), peripheral neuritis, optic neuritis, headache, depression, urticaria, erythema multiforme, nausea, vomiting, diarrhoea, stomatitis, glossitis, dry mouth; nocturnal haemoglobinuria reported; grey syndrome (abdominal distension, pallid cyanosis, circulatory collapse) may follow excessive doses in neonates with immature hepatic metabolism

Dose: *by mouth or by intravenous injection or infusion*, 50 mg/kg daily in 4 divided doses (exceptionally, can be doubled for severe infections such as septicaemia and meningitis, providing high doses reduced as soon as clinically indicated); CHILD, haemophilus epiglottitis and pyogenic meningitis, 50–100 mg/kg daily in divided doses (high dosages decreased as soon as clinically indicated); INFANTS under 2 weeks 25 mg/kg daily (in 4 divided doses), 2 weeks–1 year 50 mg/kg daily (in 4 divided doses)

NOTE. Plasma concentration monitoring required in neonates and preferred in those under 4 years of age, in the elderly, and in hepatic impairment; recommended peak plasma concentration (approx. 1 hour after intravenous injection or infusion) 15–25 mg/litre; pre-dose ('trough') concentration should not exceed 15 mg/litre

Chloramphenicol (Non-proprietary) PoM
Capsules, chloramphenicol 250 mg. Net price 60 = £20.73
Available from Sussex

Kemicetine® (Pharmacia) PoM
Injection, powder for reconstitution, chloramphenicol (as sodium succinate). Net price 1-g vial = £1.39
Electrolytes: Na$^+$ 3.14 mmol/g

Fusidic acid

Fusidic acid and its salts are narrow-spectrum antibiotics. The only indication for their use is in infections caused by penicillin-resistant staphylococci, especially osteomyelitis, as they are well concentrated in bone; they are also used for staphylococcal endocarditis (section 5.1, table 1). A second antistaphylococcal antibiotic is usually required to prevent emergence of resistance.

SODIUM FUSIDATE

Indications: penicillin-resistant staphylococcal infection including osteomyelitis; staphylococcal endocarditis in combination with other antibacterials (Table 1, section 5.1)

Cautions: hepatic impairment (Appendix 2)— monitor liver function with high doses, on prolonged therapy or in hepatic impairment; elimination may be reduced in hepatic impairment or biliary disease or biliary obstruction; pregnancy (Appendix 4); breast-feeding (Appendix 5)

Side-effects: nausea, vomiting, reversible jaundice, especially after high dosage or rapid infusion (withdraw therapy if persistent); rarely rashes, acute renal failure (usually with jaundice), blood disorders

Dose: see under Preparations, below

Fucidin® (Leo) PoM
Tablets, f/c, sodium fusidate 250 mg, net price 10-tab pack = £6.47. Label: 9
Dose: as sodium fusidate, 500 mg every 8 hours, doubled for severe infections
Skin infection, as sodium fusidate, 250 mg every 12 hours for 5–10 days
Suspension, off-white, banana- and orange-flavoured, fusidic acid 250 mg/5 mL, net price 50 mL = £7.24. Label: 9, 21
Dose: as fusidic acid, ADULT 750 mg every 8 hours; CHILD up to 1 year 50 mg/kg daily (in 3 divided doses), 1–5 years 250 mg every 8 hours, 5–12 years 500 mg every 8 hours
NOTE. Fusidic acid is incompletely absorbed and doses recommended for suspension are proportionately higher than those for sodium fusidate tablets
Intravenous infusion, powder for reconstitution, sodium fusidate 500 mg (= fusidic acid 480 mg), with buffer, net price per vial (with diluent) = £7.78
Electrolytes: Na$^+$ 3.1 mmol/vial when reconstituted with buffer
Dose: as sodium fusidate, by intravenous infusion, ADULT over 50 kg, 500 mg 3 times daily; ADULT under 50 kg and CHILD, 6–7 mg/kg 3 times daily

Vancomycin and teicoplanin

The glycopeptide antibiotics vancomycin and teicoplanin have bactericidal activity against aerobic and anaerobic Gram-positive bacteria.

Vancomycin is used *by the intravenous route* in the prophylaxis and treatment of endocarditis and other serious infections caused by Gram-positive cocci including multi-resistant staphylococci; however, there are increasing reports of vancomycin-resistant enterococci. It has a relatively long duration of action and can therefore be given every 12 hours. Vancomycin (added to dialysis fluid) is also used in the treatment of peritonitis associated with peritoneal dialysis [unlicensed route] (Table 1 section 5.1).

Vancomycin given *by mouth* is effective in the treatment of antibiotic-associated colitis (pseudomembranous colitis, see also section 1.5); a dose of 125 mg every 6 hours for 7 to 10 days is considered adequate (higher dose may be considered if the infection fails to respond or if it is severe). Vancomycin should **not** be given by mouth for systemic infections since it is not significantly absorbed.

Teicoplanin is very similar to vancomycin but has a significantly longer duration of action allowing once-daily administration. Unlike vancomycin, teicoplanin can be given by intramuscular as well as by intravenous injection; it is not given by mouth.

VANCOMYCIN

Indications: see notes above

Cautions: avoid rapid infusion (risk of anaphylactoid reactions, see Side-effects); rotate infusion sites; renal impairment (Appendix 3); elderly; avoid if history of deafness; all patients require plasma-vancomycin measurement (after 3 or 4 doses if renal function normal, earlier if renal impairment), blood counts, urinalysis, and renal function tests; monitor auditory function in elderly or if renal impairment; pregnancy and breast-feeding (Appendixes 4 and 5); systemic absorption may follow oral administration especially in inflammatory bowel disorders or following multiple doses; **interactions:** Appendix 1 (vancomycin)

Side-effects: after parenteral administration: nephrotoxicity including renal failure and interstitial nephritis; ototoxicity (discontinue if tinnitus occurs); blood disorders including neutropenia (usually after 1 week or cumulative dose of 25 g), rarely agranulocytosis and thrombocytopenia; nausea; chills; fever; eosinophilia, anaphylaxis, rashes (including exfoliative dermatitis, Stevens-Johnson syndrome, toxic epidermal necrolysis, and vasculitis); phlebitis (irritant to tissue); on rapid infusion, severe hypotension (including shock and cardiac arrest), wheezing, dyspnoea, urticaria, pruritus, flushing of the upper body ('red man' syndrome), pain and muscle spasm of back and chest

Dose: *by mouth*, antibiotic-associated colitis, 125 mg every 6 hours for 7–10 days, see notes above; CHILD 5 mg/kg every 6 hours, over 5 years, half adult dose

NOTE. Oral paediatric dose is lower than that on product literature but is adequate

By intravenous infusion, 500 mg every 6 hours *or* 1 g every 12 hours; ELDERLY over 65 years, 500 mg every 12 hours *or* 1 g once daily; NEONATE up to 1 week, 15 mg/kg initially then 10 mg/kg every 12 hours; INFANT 1–4 weeks, 15 mg/kg initially then 10 mg/kg every 8 hours; CHILD over 1 month, 10 mg/kg every 6 hours

Endocarditis prophylaxis, section 5.1, table 2

NOTE. Plasma concentration monitoring required; pre-dose ('trough') concentration should be 5–10 mg/litre; vancomycin doses in BNF may differ from those in product literature

Vancomycin (Non-proprietary) PoM

Capsules, vancomycin (as hydrochloride) 125 mg, net price 28-cap pack = £66.23; 250 mg, 28-cap pack = £132.47. Label: 9

Available from Alpharma

Injection, powder for reconstitution, vancomycin (as hydrochloride), for use as an infusion, net price 500-mg vial = £6.67; 1-g vial = £15.12

NOTE. Can be used to prepare solution for oral administration

Available from Alpharma, Mayne

Vancocin® (Lilly) PoM

Matrigel capsules, vancomycin (as hydrochloride) 125 mg (blue/peach), net price 20-cap pack = £63.08; 250 mg (blue/grey), 20-cap pack = £126.16. Label: 9

Injection, powder for reconstitution, vancomycin (as hydrochloride), for use as an infusion, net price 500-mg vial = £8.66; 1-g vial = £17.32

NOTE. Can be used to prepare solution for oral administration

TEICOPLANIN

Indications: potentially serious Gram-positive infections including endocarditis, dialysis-associated peritonitis, and serious infections due to *Staphylococcus aureus*; prophylaxis in endocarditis [unlicensed indication] and in orthopaedic surgery at risk of infection with Gram-positive organisms

Cautions: vancomycin sensitivity; blood counts and liver and kidney function tests required; renal impairment (Appendix 3)—monitor renal and auditory function on prolonged administration or if other nephrotoxic or neurotoxic drugs given; pregnancy (Appendix 4) and breast-feeding; **interactions:** Appendix 1 (teicoplanin)

Side-effects: nausea, vomiting, diarrhoea; rash, pruritus, fever, bronchospasm, rigors, urticaria, angioedema, anaphylaxis; dizziness, headache; blood disorders including eosinophilia, leucopenia, neutropenia, and thrombocytopenia; disturbances in liver enzymes, transient increase of serum creatinine, renal failure; tinnitus, mild hearing loss, and vestibular disorders also reported; rarely exfoliative dermatitis, Stevens-Johnson syndrome, toxic epidermal necrolysis; local reactions include erythema, pain, thrombophlebitis, injection site abscess and rarely flushing with infusion

Dose: *by intramuscular injection or by intravenous injection or infusion*, initially 400 mg (for severe infections, *by intravenous injection or infusion*, initially 400 mg every 12 hours for 3 doses), then 200 mg daily (400 mg daily for severe infections); higher doses may be required in patients of over 85 kg and in severe burns or endocarditis (consult product literature)

CHILD over 2 months *by intravenous injection or infusion*, initially 10 mg/kg every 12 hours for 3 doses, subsequently 6 mg/kg daily (severe infections or in neutropenia, 10 mg/kg daily); subsequent doses can be given *by intramuscular injection* (but intravenous administration preferred in children); NEONATE *by intravenous infusion*, initially a single dose of 16 mg/kg, subsequently 8 mg/kg daily

Orthopaedic surgery prophylaxis, *by intravenous injection*, 400 mg at induction of anaesthesia

Endocarditis prophylaxis [unlicensed indication], section 5.1, table 2

Targocid® (Aventis Pharma) PoM

Injection, powder for reconstitution, teicoplanin, net price 200-mg vial (with diluent) = £18.90; 400-mg vial (with diluent) = £38.30

Electrolytes: Na⁺ < 0.5 mmol/200- and 400-mg vial

Linezolid

Linezolid, an oxazolidinone antibacterial, is active against Gram-positive bacteria including methicillin-resistant *Staphylococcus aureus* (MRSA), and vancomycin-resistant enterococci. Resistance to linezolid can develop with prolonged treatment or if the dose is less than that recommended. Linezolid should be reserved for infections resistant to other antibacterials or when other antibacterials are not tolerated. Linezolid is not sufficiently active against common Gram-negative organisms.

LINEZOLID

Indications: pneumonia, complicated skin and soft-tissue infections caused by Gram-positive bacteria (initiated under expert supervision)

Cautions: hepatic impairment (Appendix 2); renal impairment (Appendix 3); pregnancy (Appendix 4); monitor full blood count (including platelet count) weekly (see also CSM Advice below); unless close observation and blood-pressure monitoring possible, avoid in uncontrolled hypertension, phaeochromocytoma, carcinoid tumour, thyrotoxicosis, bipolar depression, schizophrenia, or acute confusional states; **interactions:** Appendix 1 (MAOIs)

CSM advice. Haematopoietic disorders (including thrombocytopenia, anaemia, leucopenia, and pancytopenia) have been reported in patients receiving linezolid. It is recommended that full blood counts are monitored weekly. Close monitoring is recommended in patients who:

- receive treatment for more than 10–14 days;
- have pre-existing myelosuppression;
- are receiving drugs that may have adverse effects on haemoglobin, blood counts, or platelet function;
- have severe renal impairment.

If significant myelosuppression occurs, treatment should be stopped unless it is considered essential, in which case intensive monitoring of blood counts and appropriate management should be implemented.

MONOAMINE OXIDASE INHIBITION. Linezolid is a reversible, non-selective monoamine oxidase inhibitor (MAOI). Patients should avoid consuming large amounts of tyramine-rich foods (such as mature cheese, yeast extracts, undistilled alcoholic beverages, and fermented soya bean products). In addition, linezolid should not be given with another MAOI or within 2 weeks of stopping another MAOI. Unless close observation and blood-pressure monitoring is possible, avoid in those receiving SSRIs, $5HT_1$ agonists ('triptans'), tricyclic antidepressants, sympathomimetics, dopaminergics, buspirone, pethidine and possibly other opioid analgesics. For other interactions see Appendix 1 (MAOIs)

Contra-indications: breast-feeding (Appendix 5); see also Monoamine oxidase inhibition above

Side-effects: diarrhoea (antibiotic-associated colitis reported), nausea, vomiting, taste disturbances, headache; less frequently thirst, dry mouth, glossitis, stomatitis, tongue discoloration, abdominal pain, dyspepsia, gastritis, constipation, pancreatitis, hypertension, fever, fatigue, dizziness, insomnia, neuropathy, tinnitus, polyuria, rash, pruritus, diaphoresis, blurred vision, anaemia, leucopenia, thrombocytopenia, pancytopenia, eosinophilia, electrolyte disturbances; injection-site reactions

Dose: *by mouth*, ADULT over 18 years, 600 mg every 12 hours for 10–14 days

By intravenous infusion over 30–120 minutes, ADULT over 18 years, 600 mg every 12 hours

Zyvox (Pharmacia) ▼ PoM
Tablets, f/c, linezolid 600 mg, net price 10-tab pack = £445.00. Label: 9, 10, patient information leaflet
Suspension, yellow, orange-flavoured, linezolid 100 mg/5 mL when reconstituted with water, net price 150 mL = £222.50. Label: 9, 10 patient information leaflet
Excipients: include aspartame 20 mg/5 mL (section 9.4.1); $Na^+ < 0.5$ mmol/5 mL

Intravenous infusion, linezolid 2 mg/mL, net price 300-mL *Excel®* bag = £44.50
Excipients: include Na^+ 5 mmol/300-mL bag, glucose 13.71 g/300-mL bag

---

Quinupristin and dalfopristin

A combination of the streptogramin antibiotics, **quinupristin** and **dalfopristin** (as *Synercid®*) has recently been licensed for infections due to Gram-positive bacteria. The combination should be reserved for treating infections which have failed to respond to other antibacterials (e.g. methicillin-resistant *Staphylococcus aureus*, MRSA) or for patients who cannot be treated with other antibacterials. Quinupristin and dalfopristin are not active against *Enterococcus faecalis* and they need to be given in combination with other antibacterials for mixed infections which also involve Gram-negative organisms.

QUINUPRISTIN WITH DALFOPRISTIN

A mixture of quinupristin and dalfopristin (both as mesilate salts) in the proportions 3 parts to 7 parts

Indications: serious Gram-positive infections where no alternative antibacterial is suitable including hospital-acquired pneumonia, skin and soft-tissue infections, infections due to vancomycin-resistant *Enterococcus faecium*

Cautions: hepatic impairment (avoid if severe; Appendix 2); pregnancy (Appendix 4); predisposition to cardiac arrhythmias (including congenital QT syndrome, concomitant use of drugs that prolong QT interval, cardiac hypertrophy, dilated cardiomyopathy, hypokalaemia, hypomagnesaemia, bradycardia); **interactions**: Appendix 1 (quinupristin with dalfopristin)

Contra-indications: plasma-bilirubin concentration greater than 3 times upper limit of reference range; breast-feeding (Appendix 5)

Side-effects: nausea, vomiting, diarrhoea, headache, arthralgia, myalgia, asthenia, rash, pruritus, anaemia, leucopenia, eosinophilia, raised urea and creatinine; injection-site reactions on peripheral venous administration; less frequently oral candidiasis, stomatitis, constipation, abdominal pain, antibiotic-associated colitis, anorexia, peripheral oedema, hypotension, chest pain, arrhythmias, dyspnoea, hypersensitivity reactions (including anaphylaxis and urticaria), insomnia, anxiety, confusion, dizziness, paraesthesia, hypertonia, hepatitis, jaundice, pancreatitis, gout; also reported, thrombocytopenia, pancytopenia, electrolyte disturbances

Dose: expressed as a combination of quinupristin and dalfopristin (in a ratio of 3:7)

ADULT over 18 years, by *intravenous infusion* into central vein, 7.5 mg/kg every 8 hours for 7 days in skin and soft-tissue infections; for 10 days in hospital-acquired pneumonia; duration of treatment in *E. faecium* infection depends on site of infection

NOTE. In emergency, first dose may be administered *via* peripheral line until central venous catheter in place

Synercid® (Aventis Pharma) PoM
Intravenous infusion, powder for reconstitution, quinupristin (as mesilate) 150 mg, dalfopristin (as mesilate) 350 mg, net price 500-mg vial = £37.00
Electrolytes: Na⁺ approx. 16 mmol/500-mg vial

Polymyxins

The polymyxin antibiotic, **colistin**, is active against Gram-negative organisms, including *Pseudomonas aeruginosa*. It is **not** absorbed by mouth and thus needs to be given by injection to obtain a systemic effect; however, it is toxic and has few, if any, indications for systemic use.

Colistin is used by mouth in bowel sterilisation regimens in neutropenic patients (usually with nystatin); it is **not** recommended for gastro-intestinal infections. It is also given by inhalation of a nebulised solution as an adjunct to standard antibacterial therapy in patients with cystic fibrosis.

Both colistin and polymyxin B are included in some preparations for topical application.

COLISTIN

Indications: see notes above

Cautions: renal impairment (Appendix 3); porphyria (section 9.8.2); risk of bronchospasm on inhalation—may be prevented or treated with a selective beta₂ agonist; **interactions:** Appendix 1 (polymyxins)

Contra-indications: myasthenia gravis; pregnancy; breast-feeding

Side-effects: neurotoxicity reported especially with excessive doses (including apnoea, perioral and peripheral paraesthesia, vertigo; rarely vasomotor instability, slurred speech, confusion, psychosis, visual disturbances); nephrotoxicity; hypersensitivity reactions including rash; injection-site reactions; inhalation may cause sore throat, sore mouth, cough, bronchospasm

Dose: *by mouth,* bowel sterilisation, 1.5–3 million-units every 8 hours

By intravenous injection into a totally implantable venous access device, *or by intravenous infusion* (but see notes above), ADULT and CHILD body-weight under 60 kg, 50 000–75 000 units/kg daily in 3 divided doses; body-weight over 60 kg, 1–2 million units every 8 hours

NOTE. Plasma concentration monitoring required in neonates, renal impairment, and in cystic fibrosis; recommended 'peak' plasma-colistin concentration (approx. 30 minutes after intravenous injection or infusion) 10–15 mg/litre (125–200 units/mL)

By inhalation of nebulised solution, ADULT and CHILD over 2 years, 1–2 million units every 12 hours; CHILD under 2 years, 0.5–1 million units every 12 hours

Colomycin® (Forest) PoM
Tablets, scored, colistin sulphate 1.5 million units. Net price 50 = £62.18
Syrup, colistin sulphate 250 000 units/5 mL when reconstituted with water. Net price 80 mL = £3.71
Injection, powder for reconstitution, colistimethate sodium (colistin sulphomethate sodium). Net price 500 000-unit vial = £1.22; 1 million-unit vial = £1.79; 2 million-unit vial = £3.30
Electrolytes: (before reconstitution) Na⁺ < 0.5 mmol/500 000-unit, 1 million-unit, and 2 million-unit vial

Promixin (Profile) PoM
Powder for nebuliser solution, colistimethate sodium (colistin sulphomethate sodium), net price 1 million-unit vial = £2.30
Injection, powder for reconstitution, colistimethate sodium (colistin sulphomethate sodium), net price 1 million unit-vial = £2.30
Electrolytes: (before reconstitution) Na⁺ < 0.5 mmol/1 million-unit vial

5.1.8 Sulphonamides and trimethoprim

The importance of the sulphonamides has decreased as a result of increasing bacterial resistance and their replacement by antibacterials which are generally more active and less toxic.

Sulfamethoxazole (sulphamethoxazole) and trimethoprim are used in combination (as **co-trimoxazole**) because of their synergistic activity. However, co-trimoxazole is associated with rare but serious side-effects (e.g. Stevens-Johnson syndrome and blood dyscrasias, notably bone marrow depression and agranulocytosis) especially in the elderly (see CSM recommendations below).

> **CSM recommendations.** Co-trimoxazole should be limited to the role of drug of choice in *Pneumocystis carinii* pneumonia; it is also indicated for *toxoplasmosis* and *nocardiasis*. It should now only be considered for use in *acute exacerbations of chronic bronchitis* and *infections of the urinary tract* when there is good bacteriological evidence of sensitivity to co-trimoxazole and good reason to prefer this combination to a single antibacterial; similarly it should only be used in *acute otitis media in children* when there is good reason to prefer it.

Trimethoprim can be used alone for urinary- and respiratory-tract infections and for prostatitis, shigellosis, and invasive salmonella infections. Trimethoprim has side-effects similar to co-trimoxazole but they are less severe and occur less frequently.

For *topical preparations* of sulphonamides used in the treatment of burns see section 13.10.1.1.

CO-TRIMOXAZOLE

A mixture of trimethoprim and sulfamethoxazole in the proportions of 1 part to 5 parts

Indications: see CSM recommendations above

Cautions: hepatic impairment (avoid if severe); renal impairment (avoid if severe; Appendix 3); maintain adequate fluid intake; avoid in blood disorders (unless under specialist supervision); monitor blood counts on prolonged treatment; discontinue immediately if blood disorders or rash develop; predisposition to folate deficiency; elderly (see CSM recommendations above); asthma; G6PD deficiency (section 9.1.5); pregnancy (Appendix 4) and breast-feeding (Appendix 5); avoid in infants under 6 weeks (except for treatment or prophylaxis of pneumocystis pneumonia); **interactions:** Appendix 1 (trimethoprim, sulfamethoxazole)

Contra-indications: porphyria (section 9.8.2)

Side-effects: nausea, vomiting; rash (including Stevens-Johnson syndrome, toxic epidermal necrolysis, photosensitivity)—discontinue immediately; blood disorders (including neutropenia, thrombocytopenia, rarely agranulocytosis and purpura)—discontinue immediately; rarely, allergic reactions, systemic lupus erythematosus, myocarditis, serum sickness, diarrhoea, glossitis, stomatitis, anorexia, arthralgia, myalgia; also reported, liver damage including jaundice and hepatic necrosis, pancreatitis, antibiotic-associated colitis, eosinophilia, cough and shortness of breath, pulmonary infiltrates, aseptic meningitis, headache, depression, convulsions, peripheral neuropathy, ataxia, tinnitus, vertigo, dizziness, hallucinations, megaloblastic anaemia, electrolyte disturbances, crystalluria, renal disorders including interstitial nephritis

Dose: *by mouth*, 960 mg every 12 hours; CHILD, every 12 hours, 6 weeks–5 months, 120 mg; 6 months–5 years, 240 mg; 6–12 years, 480 mg

By intravenous infusion, 960 mg every 12 hours increased to 1.44 g every 12 hours in severe infections; CHILD 36 mg/kg daily in 2 divided doses increased to 54 mg/kg daily in severe infections

Treatment of *Pneumocystis carinii* infections (undertaken where facilities for appropriate monitoring available—consult microbiologist and product literature), *by mouth or by intravenous infusion*, ADULT and CHILD over 4 weeks 120 mg/kg daily in 2–4 divided doses for 14 days

Prophylaxis of *Pneumocystis carinii* infections, *by mouth*, 960 mg once daily (may be reduced to 480 mg once daily to improve tolerance) *or* 960 mg on alternate days (3 times a week) *or* 960 mg twice daily on alternate days (3 times a week); CHILD 6 weeks–5 months 120 mg twice daily on 3 consecutive days *or* 7 days per week; 6 months–5 years 240 mg; 6–12 years 480 mg
NOTE. 480 mg of co-trimoxazole consists of sulfamethoxazole 400 mg and trimethoprim 80 mg

Co-trimoxazole (Non-proprietary) PoM
Tablets, co-trimoxazole 480 mg, net price 28-tab pack = £4.08; 960 mg, 20 = £5.05. Label: 9
Available from Alpharma, DDSA (*Fectrim®*, *Fectrim® Forte*), Hillcross, IVAX
Paediatric oral suspension, co-trimoxazole 240 mg/5 mL, net price 100 mL = £1.12. Label: 9
Available from IVAX
Oral suspension, co-trimoxazole 480 mg/5 mL. Net price 100 mL = £3.50. Label: 9
Available from Kent
Strong sterile solution, co-trimoxazole 96 mg/mL. For dilution and use as an intravenous infusion. Net price 5-mL amp = £1.58, 10-mL amp = £3.06
Available from Mayne

Septrin® (GSK) PoM
Tablets, co-trimoxazole 480 mg. Net price 20 = £3.34. Label: 9
Forte tablets, scored, co-trimoxazole 960 mg. Net price 20 = £5.05. Label: 9
Adult suspension, vanilla-flavoured, co-trimoxazole 480 mg/5 mL. Net price 100 mL = £4.74. Label: 9
Paediatric suspension, sugar-free, banana- and vanilla-flavoured, co-trimoxazole 240 mg/5 mL. Net price 100 mL = £2.63. Label: 9
Intravenous infusion, co-trimoxazole 96 mg/mL. To be diluted before use. Net price 5-mL amp = £1.59

SULFADIAZINE
(Sulphadiazine)

Indications: prevention of rheumatic fever recurrence, toxoplasmosis [unlicensed]—see section 5.4.7

Cautions: see under Co-trimoxazole; renal impairment (avoid if severe; Appendix 3); **interactions:** Appendix 1 (sulphonamides)

Contra-indications: see under Co-trimoxazole

Side-effects: see under Co-trimoxazole

Dose: prevention of rheumatic fever, *by mouth*, 1 g daily (500 mg daily for patients less than 30 kg)

Sulfadiazine (Non-proprietary) PoM
Tablets, sulfadiazine 500 mg, net price 56-tab pack = £17.60. Label: 9, 27
Available from CP
Injection, sulfadiazine (as sodium salt) 250 mg/mL, net price 4-mL amp = £4.97
Available from Concord

TRIMETHOPRIM

Indications: urinary-tract infections, acute and chronic bronchitis

Cautions: renal impairment (Appendix 3); pregnancy (Appendix 4); breast-feeding (Appendix 5); predisposition to folate deficiency; elderly; manufacturer recommends blood counts on long-term therapy (but evidence of practical value unsatisfactory); neonates (specialist supervision required); porphyria (section 9.8.2); **interactions:** Appendix 1 (trimethoprim)
BLOOD DISORDERS. On long-term treatment, patients and their carers should be told how to recognise signs of blood disorders and advised to seek immediate medical attention if symptoms such as fever, sore throat, rash, mouth ulcers, purpura, bruising or bleeding develop

Contra-indications: blood dyscrasias

Side-effects: gastro-intestinal disturbances including nausea and vomiting, pruritus, rashes, hyperkalaemia, depression of haematopoiesis; rarely erythema multiforme, toxic epidermal necrolysis, photosensitivity and other allergic reactions including angioedema and anaphylaxis; aseptic meningitis reported

Dose: acute infections, 200 mg every 12 hours; CHILD, every 12 hours, 6 weeks–5 months 25 mg, 6 months–5 years 50 mg, 6–12 years 100 mg
Chronic infections and prophylaxis, 100 mg at night; CHILD 1–2 mg/kg at night

Trimethoprim (Non-proprietary) PoM
Tablets, trimethoprim 100 mg, net price 20 = 49p; 200 mg, 20 = 97p. Label: 9
Available from Alpharma, APS, Berk (*Trimopan®*), IVAX, Kent

Monotrim® (Solvay) PoM
Suspension, sugar-free, trimethoprim 50 mg/5 mL. Net price 100 mL = £1.77. Label: 9

Trimopan® (APS) PoM
Suspension, sugar-free, trimethoprim 50 mg/5 mL. Net price 100 mL = £1.77. Label: 9

5.1.9   Antituberculous drugs

Tuberculosis is treated in two phases—an *initial phase* using at least three drugs and a *continuation phase* using two drugs in fully sensitive cases. Treatment requires specialised knowledge, particularly where the disease involves resistant organisms or non-respiratory organs.

The regimens given below are based on the Joint Tuberculosis Committee of the British Thoracic Society guidelines for the treatment of tuberculosis in the UK; variations occur in other countries. Either the unsupervised regimen or the supervised regimen described below should be used; the two regimens should **not** be used concurrently.

INITIAL PHASE. The concurrent use of at least three drugs during the initial phase is designed to reduce the bacterial population as rapidly as possible and to prevent the emergence of drug-resistant bacteria. The drugs are best given as combination preparations unless one of the components cannot be given because of resistance or intolerance. The treatment of choice for the initial phase is the daily use of isoniazid, rifampicin, pyrazinamide and ethambutol; ethambutol can be omitted from the regimen if the risk of resistance to isoniazid is low (e.g. those who have not been treated previously for tuberculosis, those who are not immunosuppressed, and those who have not been in contact with organisms likely to be drug resistant). Streptomycin is rarely used in the UK although it may be used in the initial phase of treatment if resistance to isoniazid has been established before therapy is commenced. The initial phase drugs should be continued for 2 months. Where a positive culture for *M. tuberculosis* has been obtained, but susceptibility results are not available after 2 months, treatment with pyrazinamide (and ethambutol if appropriate) should be continued until full susceptibility is confirmed, even if this is for longer than 2 months.

CONTINUATION PHASE. After the initial phase, treatment is continued for a further 4 months with isoniazid and rifampicin (preferably given as a combination preparation). Longer treatment is necessary for meningitis and for resistant organisms which may also require modification of the regimen.

UNSUPERVISED TREATMENT. The following regimen should be used for patients who are likely to take antituberculous drugs reliably **without supervision**. Patients who are unlikely to comply with daily administration of antituberculous drugs should be treated with the regimen described under Supervised Treatment.

Recommended dosage for standard unsupervised 6-month treatment
Rifater® [rifampicin, isoniazid, and pyrazinamide] (for 2-month initial phase only)
ADULT under 40 kg 3 tablets daily, 40–49 kg 4 tablets daily, 50–64 kg 5 tablets daily, over 65 kg 6 tablets daily
¹**Ethambutol** (for 2-month initial phase only)
ADULT AND CHILD 15 mg/kg daily
Rifinah® or **Rimactazid**® [rifampicin and isoniazid] (for 4-month continuation phase following initial treatment with *Rifater*®)
ADULT under 50 kg 3 tablets daily of *Rifinah*®-150 or *Rimactazid*®-150, 50 kg and over, 2 tablets daily of *Rifinah*®-300 or *Rimactazid*®-300
or (if combination preparations not appropriate):
Isoniazid (for 2-month initial and 4-month continuation phases)
ADULT 300 mg daily; CHILD 5–10 mg/kg (max. 300 mg) daily

---

1. Ethambutol may be omitted from the regimen if the risk of isoniazid resistance is low

Rifampicin (for 2-month initial and 4-month continuation phases)
ADULT under 50 kg 450 mg daily, 50 kg and over 600 mg daily; CHILD 10 mg/kg (max. 600 mg) daily
Pyrazinamide (for 2-month initial phase only)
ADULT under 50 kg 1.5 g daily, 50 kg and over 2 g daily; CHILD 35 mg/kg daily
¹**Ethambutol** (for 2-month initial phase only)
ADULT AND CHILD 15 mg/kg daily

PREGNANCY AND BREAST-FEEDING. The standard regimen (above) may be used during pregnancy and breast-feeding. Streptomycin should not be given in pregnancy.

CHILDREN. Children are given isoniazid, rifampicin, and pyrazinamide for the first 2 months followed by isoniazid and rifampicin during the next 4 months. Ethambutol should be included in the first 2 months in children with a high risk of resistant infection (see Initial Phase, above). However, care is needed in young children because of the difficulty in testing eyesight and in obtaining reports of visual symptoms (see below).

SUPERVISED TREATMENT. Drug administration needs to be **fully supervised** (directly observed therapy, DOT) in patients who cannot comply reliably with the treatment regimen. These patients are given isoniazid, rifampicin, pyrazinamide and ethambutol (or streptomycin) 3 times a week under supervision for the first 2 months followed by isoniazid and rifampicin 3 times a week for a further 4 months.

Recommended dosage for intermittent supervised 6-month treatment
Isoniazid (for 2-month initial and 4-month continuation phases)
ADULT AND CHILD 15 mg/kg (max. 900 mg) 3 times a week
Rifampicin (for 2-month initial and 4-month continuation phases)
ADULT 600–900 mg 3 times a week; CHILD 15 mg/kg (max. 900 mg) 3 times a week
Pyrazinamide (for 2-month initial phase only)
ADULT under 50 kg 2 g 3 times a week, 50 kg and over 2.5 g 3 times a week; CHILD 50 mg/kg 3 times a week
¹**Ethambutol** (for 2-month initial phase only)
ADULT AND CHILD 30 mg/kg 3 times a week

IMMUNOCOMPROMISED PATIENTS. Multi-resistant *Mycobacterium tuberculosis* may be present in immunocompromised patients. The organism should always be cultured to confirm its type and drug sensitivity. Confirmed *M. tuberculosis* infection sensitive to first-line drugs should be treated with a standard 6-month regimen; after completing treatment, patients should be closely monitored. The regimen may need to be modified if infection is caused by resistant organisms, and specialist advice is needed.

Specialist advice should be sought about tuberculosis treatment or chemoprophylaxis in a HIV-positive individual; care is required in choosing the regimen and in avoiding potentially hazardous interactions.

Infection may also be caused by other mycobacteria e.g. *M. avium* complex in which case specialist advice on management is needed.

PREVENTION OF TUBERCULOSIS. Some individuals may develop tuberculosis owing to reactivation of previously latent disease. Chemoprophylaxis may be required in those who have evidence of latent tuberculosis and are receiving treatment with immunosuppressants (including cytotoxics and possibly long-term treatment with systemic corticosteroids). In these cases, isoniazid chemoprophylaxis may be given for 6 months; longer chemoprophylaxis is not recommended.

For prevention of tuberculosis in susceptible close contacts or those who have become tuberculin-positive, see Table 2, section 5.1. For advice on immunisation against tuberculosis, see section 14.4

MONITORING. Since isoniazid, rifampicin and pyrazinamide are associated with liver toxicity (see Appendix 2), *hepatic function* should be checked before treatment with these drugs. Those with pre-existing liver disease or alcohol dependence should have frequent checks particularly in the first 2 months. If there is no evidence of liver disease (and pre-treatment liver function is normal), further checks are only necessary if the patient develops fever, malaise, vomiting, jaundice or unexplained deterioration during treatment. In view of the need to comply fully with antituberculous treatment on the one hand and to guard against serious liver damage on the other, patients and their carers should be informed carefully how to recognise signs of liver disorders and advised to discontinue treatment and seek **immediate** medical attention should symptoms of liver disease occur.

Renal function should be checked before treatment with antituberculous drugs and appropriate dosage adjustments made. Streptomycin or ethambutol should preferably be avoided in patients with renal impairment, but if used, the dose should be reduced and the plasma-drug concentration monitored.

Visual acuity should be tested before ethambutol is used (see below).

> Major causes of treatment failure are incorrect prescribing by the physician and inadequate compliance by the patient. Monthly tablet counts and urine examination (rifampicin imparts an orange-red coloration) may be useful indicators of compliance with treatment. Avoid both excessive and inadequate dosage. Treatment should be supervised by a specialist physician.

Isoniazid is cheap and highly effective. Like rifampicin it should always be included in any antituberculous regimen unless there is a specific contra-indication. Its only common side-effect is peripheral neuropathy which is more likely to occur where there are pre-existing risk factors such as diabetes, alcohol dependence, chronic renal failure, malnutrition and HIV infection. In these circumstances pyridoxine 10 mg daily (or 20 mg daily if suitable product not available) (section 9.6.2) should be given prophylactically from the start of treatment. Other side-effects such as hepatitis (important: see Monitoring above) and psychosis are rare.

Rifampicin, a rifamycin, is a key component of any antituberculous regimen. Like isoniazid it should always be included unless there is a specific contra-indication.

During the first two months ('initial phase') of rifampicin administration transient disturbance of liver function with elevated serum transaminases is common but generally does not require interruption of treatment. Occasionally more serious liver toxicity requires a change of treatment particularly in those with pre-existing liver disease (important: see Monitoring above).

On intermittent treatment six toxicity syndromes have been recognised—influenza-like, abdominal, and respiratory symptoms, shock, renal failure, and thrombocytopenic purpura—and can occur in 20 to 30% of patients.

Rifampicin induces hepatic enzymes which accelerate the metabolism of several drugs including oestrogens, corticosteroids, phenytoin, sulphonylureas, and anticoagulants; **interactions:** Appendix 1 (rifamycins). **Important:** the effectiveness of oral contraceptives is reduced and alternative family planning advice should be offered (section 7.3.1).

Rifabutin, a newly introduced rifamycin, is indicated for *prophylaxis* against *M. avium* complex infections in patients with a low CD4 count; it is also licensed for the *treatment* of non-tuberculous mycobacterial disease and pulmonary tuberculosis. As with rifampicin it induces hepatic enzymes and the effectiveness of oral contraceptives is reduced requiring alternative family planning methods.

Pyrazinamide is a bactericidal drug only active against intracellular dividing forms of *Mycobacterium tuberculosis*; it exerts its main effect only in the first two or three months. It is particularly useful in tuberculous meningitis because of good meningeal penetration. It is not active against *M. bovis*. Serious liver toxicity may occasionally occur (important: see Monitoring above).

Ethambutol is included in a treatment regimen if isoniazid resistance is suspected; it can be omitted if the risk of resistance is low.

Side-effects of ethambutol are largely confined to visual disturbances in the form of loss of acuity, colour blindness, and restriction of visual fields. These toxic effects are more common where excessive dosage is used or if the patient's renal function is impaired. The earliest features of ocular toxicity are subjective and patients should be advised to discontinue therapy immediately if they develop deterioration in vision and promptly seek further advice. Early discontinuation of the drug is almost always followed by recovery of eyesight. Patients who cannot understand warnings about visual side-effects should, if possible, be given an alternative drug. In particular, ethambutol should be used with caution in children until they are at least 5 years old and capable of reporting symptomatic visual changes accurately.

Visual acuity should be tested by Snellen chart before treatment with ethambutol.

Streptomycin is now rarely used in the UK except for resistant organisms. It is given intramuscularly in a dose of 15 mg/kg (max. 1 g) daily; the dose is reduced in those under 50 kg, those over 40 years or those with renal impairment. Plasma-drug concentration should be measured in patients with impaired renal function in whom streptomycin must be used with great care. Side-effects increase after a cumulative dose of 100 g, which should only be exceeded in exceptional circumstances.

Drug-resistant tuberculosis should be treated by a specialist physician with experience in such cases, and where appropriate facilities for infection-control exist. Second-line drugs available for infections caused by resistant organisms, or when first-line drugs cause unacceptable side-effects, include amikacin, capreomycin, cycloserine, newer macrolides (e.g. azithromycin and clarithromycin), quinolones (e.g. ciprofloxacin and ofloxacin) and protionamide (prothionamide) (no longer on UK market).

CAPREOMYCIN

Indications: in combination with other drugs, tuberculosis resistant to first-line drugs

Cautions: renal, hepatic, or auditory impairment; monitor renal, hepatic, auditory, and vestibular function and electrolytes; pregnancy (teratogenic in *animals*) and breast-feeding; **interactions:** Appendix 1 (capreomycin)

Side-effects: hypersensitivity reactions including urticaria and rashes; leucocytosis or leucopenia, rarely thrombocytopenia; changes in liver function tests; nephrotoxicity, electrolyte disturbances; hearing loss with tinnitus and vertigo; neuromuscular block after large doses, pain and induration at injection site

Dose: by deep intramuscular injection, 1 g daily (not more than 20 mg/kg) for 2–4 months, then 1 g 2–3 times each week

Capastat® (King) PoM
Injection, powder for reconstitution, capreomycin sulphate 1 million units (= capreomycin approx. 1 g). Net price per vial = £16.47

CYCLOSERINE

Indications: in combination with other drugs, tuberculosis resistant to first-line drugs

Cautions: reduce dose in renal impairment (avoid if severe); monitor haematological, renal, and hepatic function; pregnancy and breast-feeding; **interactions:** Appendix 1 (cycloserine)

Contra-indications: severe renal impairment, epilepsy, depression, severe anxiety, psychotic states, alcohol dependence, porphyria (section 9.8.2)

Side-effects: mainly neurological, including headache, dizziness, vertigo, drowsiness, tremor, convulsions, confusion, psychosis, depression (discontinue or reduce dose if symptoms of CNS toxicity); rashes, allergic dermatitis (discontinue or reduce dose); megaloblastic anaemia; changes in liver function tests; heart failure at high doses reported

Dose: initially 250 mg every 12 hours for 2 weeks increased according to blood concentration and response to max. 500 mg every 12 hours; CHILD initially 10 mg/kg daily adjusted according to blood concentration and response
NOTE. Blood concentration monitoring required especially in renal impairment or if dose exceeds 500 mg daily or if signs of toxicity; blood concentration should not exceed 30 mg/litre

Cycloserine (King) PoM
Capsules, red/grey cycloserine 250 mg, net price 100-cap pack = £220.69. Label: 2, 8

ETHAMBUTOL HYDROCHLORIDE

Indications: tuberculosis, in combination with other drugs

Cautions: reduce dose in renal impairment and if creatinine clearance less than 30 mL/minute, also monitor plasma-ethambutol concentration; elderly; pregnancy; test visual acuity before treatment and warn patients to report visual changes—see notes above; young children (see notes above)—routine ophthalmological monitoring recommended

Contra-indications: optic neuritis, poor vision

Side-effects: optic neuritis, red/green colour blindness, peripheral neuritis, rarely rash, pruritus, urticaria, thrombocytopenia

Dose: see notes above
NOTE. 'Peak' concentration (2–2.5 hours after dose) should be 2–6 mg/litre (7–22 micromol/litre); 'trough' (pre-dose) concentration should be less than 1 mg/litre (4 micromol/litre); for advice on laboratory assay of ethambutol contact the Poisons Unit at New Cross Hospital (Tel (020) 7771 5360)

Ethambutol (Non-proprietary) PoM
Tablets, ethambutol hydrochloride 100 mg (yellow), net price 56-tab pack = £11.50; 400 mg (grey), 56-tab pack = £42.73. Label: 8
Available from Genus

ISONIAZID

Indications: tuberculosis, in combination with other drugs; prophylaxis—Table 2, section 5.1

Cautions: hepatic impairment (monitor hepatic function, see below); renal impairment; slow acetylator status (increased risk of side-effects); epilepsy; history of psychosis; alcohol dependence, malnutrition, diabetes mellitus, HIV infection (risk of peripheral neuritis); pregnancy and breast-feeding; porphyria (section 9.8.2); **interactions:** Appendix 1 (isoniazid)
HEPATIC DISORDERS. Patients or their carers should be told how to recognise signs of liver disorder, and advised to discontinue treatment and seek immediate medical attention if symptoms such as persistent nausea, vomiting, malaise or jaundice develop

Contra-indications: drug-induced liver disease

Side-effects: nausea, vomiting, constipation, dry mouth; peripheral neuritis with high doses (pyridoxine prophylaxis, see notes above); optic neuritis, convulsions, psychotic episodes, vertigo; hypersensitivity reactions including fever, erythema multiforme, purpura; blood disorders including agranulocytosis, haemolytic anaemia, aplastic anaemia; hepatitis (especially over age of 35 years); systemic lupus erythematosus-like syndrome, pellagra, hyperreflexia, difficulty with micturition, hyperglycaemia, and gynaecomastia reported

Dose: by mouth or by intramuscular or intravenous injection, see notes above

Isoniazid (Non-proprietary) PoM
Tablets, isoniazid 50 mg, net price 56-tab pack = £5.78; 100 mg, 28-tab pack = £5.77. Label: 8, 22
Available from Celltech
Elixir (BPC), isoniazid 50 mg, citric acid monohydrate 12.5 mg, sodium citrate 60 mg, concentrated anise water 0.05 mL, compound tartrazine solution 0.05 mL, glycerol 1 mL, double-strength chloroform water 2 mL, water to 5 mL. Label: 8, 22
'Special order' [unlicensed] product; contact Martindale, Rosemont, or regional hospital manufacturing unit
Injection, isoniazid 25 mg/mL, net price 2-mL amp = £7.11
Available from Cambridge

■ Combined preparations

Rifater® (Aventis Pharma) [PoM]
Tablets, pink, s/c, rifampicin 120 mg, isoniazid 50 mg, pyrazinamide 300 mg. Net price 20 = £4.72. Label: 8, 14, 22, counselling, see lenses above
Dose: initial treatment of pulmonary tuberculosis, patients up to 40 kg 3 tablets daily preferably before breakfast, 40–49 kg 4 tablets daily, 50–64 kg 5 tablets daily, 65 kg or more, 6 tablets daily; not suitable for use in children

Rifinah 150® (Aventis Pharma) [PoM]
Tablets, pink, s/c, rifampicin 150 mg, isoniazid 100 mg, net price 84-tab pack = £17.80. Label: 8, 14, 22, counselling, see lenses above
Dose: ADULT under 50 kg, 3 tablets daily, preferably before breakfast

Rifinah 300® (Aventis Pharma) [PoM]
Tablets, orange, s/c, rifampicin 300 mg, isoniazid 150 mg, net price 56-tab pack = £23.52. Label: 8, 14, 22, counselling, see lenses above
Dose: ADULT 50 kg and over, 2 tablets daily, preferably before breakfast

Rimactazid 150® (Swedish Orphan) [PoM]
Tablets, pink, s/c, rifampicin 150 mg, isoniazid 100 mg, net price 84-tab pack = £16.42. Label: 8, 14, 22, counselling, see lenses above
Dose: ADULT under 50 kg, 3 tablets daily, preferably before breakfast

Rimactazid 300® (Swedish Orphan) [PoM]
Tablets, orange, s/c, rifampicin 300 mg, isoniazid 150 mg, net price 56-tab pack = £21.71. Label: 8, 14, 22, counselling, see lenses above
Dose: ADULT 50 kg and over, 2 tablets daily, preferably before breakfast

STREPTOMYCIN

Indications: tuberculosis, in combination with other drugs; adjunct to doxycycline in brucellosis
Cautions: see under Aminoglycosides, section 5.1.4; **interactions:** Appendix 1 (aminoglycosides)
Contra-indications: see under Aminoglycosides, section 5.1.4
Side-effects: see under Aminoglycosides, section 5.1.4; also hypersensitivity reactions, paraesthesia of mouth
Dose: *by deep intramuscular injection*, tuberculosis, see notes above; brucellosis, expert advice essential
NOTE. One-hour ('peak') concentration should be 15–40 mg/litre; pre-dose ('trough') concentration should be less than 5 mg/litre (less than 1 mg/litre in renal impairment or in those over 50 years)

Streptomycin Sulphate (Celltech) [PoM]
Injection, powder for reconstitution, streptomycin (as sulphate), net price 1-g vial = £8.25

5.1.10 Antileprotic drugs

Advice from a member of the Panel of Leprosy Opinion is essential for the treatment of leprosy (Hansen's disease). Details of the Panel can be obtained from the Department of Health telephone (020) 7972 4480.
The World Health Organization has made recommendations to overcome the problem of dapsone resistance and to prevent the emergence of resistance to other antileprotic drugs. Drugs recommended are

dapsone, rifampicin (section 5.1.9), and **clofazimine**. Other drugs with significant activity against *Mycobacterium leprae* include ofloxacin, minocycline and clarithromycin, but none of these are as active as rifampicin; at present they should be reserved as second-line drugs for leprosy.
A three-drug regimen is recommended for *multibacillary leprosy* (lepromatous, borderline-lepromatous, and borderline leprosy) and a two-drug regimen for *paucibacillary leprosy* (borderline-tuberculoid, tuberculoid, and indeterminate). The following regimens are widely used throughout the world (with minor local variations):

Multibacillary leprosy (3-drug regimen)

Rifampicin	600 mg once-monthly, supervised (450 mg for adults weighing less than 35 kg)
Dapsone	100 mg daily, self-administered (50 mg daily or 1–2 mg/kg daily for adults weighing less than 35 kg)
Clofazimine	300 mg once-monthly, supervised, *and* 50 mg daily (or 100 mg on alternate days), self-administered

Multibacillary leprosy should be treated for at least 2 years. Treatment should be continued unchanged during both type I (reversal) or type II (erythema nodosum leprosum) reactions. During reversal reactions neuritic pain or weakness can herald the rapid onset of permanent nerve damage. Treatment with prednisolone (initially 40–60 mg daily) should be instituted at once. Mild type II reactions may respond to aspirin or chloroquine. Severe type II reactions may require corticosteroids; thalidomide [unlicensed] is also useful in men and post-menopausal women who have become corticosteroid dependent, but it should be used under **specialist supervision** and it should **never** be used in women of childbearing potential (significant teratogenic risk—for CSM guidance on prescribing, see *Current Problems in Pharmacovigilance* 1994; **20**, 8). Increased doses of clofazimine 100 mg 3 times daily for the first month with subsequent reductions, are also useful but may take 4–6 weeks to attain full effect.

Paucibacillary leprosy (2-drug regimen)

Rifampicin	600 mg once-monthly, supervised (450 mg for those weighing less than 35 kg)
Dapsone	100 mg daily, self-administered (50 mg daily or 1–2 mg/kg daily for adults weighing less than 35 kg)

Paucibacillary leprosy should be treated for 6 months. If treatment is interrupted the regimen should be recommenced where it was left off to complete the full course.
Neither the multibacillary nor the paucibacillary antileprosy regimen is sufficient to treat tuberculosis.

DAPSONE

Indications: leprosy, dermatitis herpetiformis; *Pneumocystis carinii* pneumonia (section 5.4.8)
Cautions: cardiac or pulmonary disease; anaemia (treat severe anaemia before starting); susceptibility to haemolysis including G6PD deficiency (section 9.1.5)—susceptible breast-feeding infants also at risk (Appendix 5); pregnancy (Appendix 4); avoid in porphyria (section 9.8.2); **interactions:** Appendix 1 (dapsone)
BLOOD DISORDERS. On long-term treatment, patients and their carers should be told how to recognise signs of blood

disorders and advised to seek immediate medical attention if symptoms such as fever, sore throat, rash, mouth ulcers, purpura, bruising or bleeding develop

Side-effects: (dose-related and uncommon at doses used for leprosy), haemolysis, methaemoglobinaemia, neuropathy, allergic dermatitis (rarely including toxic epidermal necrolysis and Stevens-Johnson syndrome), anorexia, nausea, vomiting, tachycardia, headache, insomnia, psychosis, hepatitis, agranulocytosis; dapsone syndrome (rash with fever and eosinophilia)—discontinue immediately (may progress to exfoliative dermatitis, hepatitis, hypoalbuminaemia, psychosis and death)

Dose: leprosy, 1–2 mg/kg daily, see notes above

Dermatitis herpetiformis, see specialist literature

Dapsone (Non-proprietary) PoM
Tablets, dapsone 50 mg, net price 28-tab pack = £2.07; 100 mg, 28-tab pack = £2.96. Label: 8
Available from Alpharma

CLOFAZIMINE

Indications: leprosy

Cautions: hepatic and renal impairment; pregnancy and breast-feeding; may discolour soft contact lenses; avoid if persistent abdominal pain and diarrhoea

Side-effects: nausea, vomiting (hospitalise if persistent), abdominal pain; headache, tiredness; brownish-black discoloration of lesions and skin including areas exposed to light; reversible hair discoloration; dry skin; red discoloration of faeces, urine and other body fluids; also rash, pruritus, photosensitivity, acne-like eruptions, anorexia, eosinophilic enteropathy, bowel obstruction, dry eyes, dimmed vision, macular and subepithelial corneal pigmentation; elevation of blood sugar, weight loss, splenic infarction, lymphadenopathy

Dose: leprosy, see notes above

Lepromatous lepra reactions, dosage increased to 300 mg daily for max. of 3 months

Lamprene® (Alliance) PoM
Capsules, brown, clofazimine 100 mg, net price 100-cap pack = £23.50. Label: 8, 14, 21

5.1.11 Metronidazole and tinidazole

Metronidazole is an antimicrobial drug with high activity against anaerobic bacteria and protozoa; indications include trichomonal vaginitis (section 5.4.3), bacterial vaginosis (notably *Gardnerella vaginalis* infections), and *Entamoeba histolytica* and *Giardia lamblia* infections (section 5.4.2). It is also used for surgical and gynaecological sepsis in which its activity against colonic anaerobes, especially *Bacteroides fragilis*, is important. Metronidazole is also effective in the treatment of antibiotic-associated colitis (pseudomembranous colitis, see also section 1.5). Metronidazole by the rectal route is an effective alternative to the intravenous route when oral administration is not possible. Intravenous metronidazole is used for the treatment of established cases of tetanus; diazepam (section 10.2.2) and tetanus immunoglobulin (section 14.5) are also used.

Topical metronidazole (section 13.10.1.2) reduces the odour produced by anaerobic bacteria in fungating tumours; it is also used in the management of rosacea (section 13.6).

Tinidazole is similar to metronidazole but has a longer duration of action.

METRONIDAZOLE

Indications: anaerobic infections (including dental), see under Dose below; protozoal infections (section 5.4.2); *Helicobacter pylori* eradication (section 1.3); skin (section 13.10.1.2)

Cautions: disulfiram-like reaction with alcohol, hepatic impairment and hepatic encephalopathy (Appendix 2); pregnancy and breast-feeding (Appendixes 4 and 5); clinical and laboratory monitoring advised if treatment exceeds 10 days; **interactions:** Appendix 1 (metronidazole)

Side-effects: nausea, vomiting, unpleasant taste, furred tongue, and gastro-intestinal disturbances; rashes; rarely drowsiness, headache, dizziness, ataxia, darkening of urine, erythema multiforme, pruritus, urticaria, angioedema, and anaphylaxis; also reported abnormal liver function tests, hepatitis, jaundice, thrombocytopenia, aplastic anaemia, myalgia, arthralgia; on prolonged or intensive therapy peripheral neuropathy, transient epileptiform seizures, and leucopenia

Dose: anaerobic infections (usually treated for 7 days and for 10 days in antibiotic-associated colitis), *by mouth, either* 800 mg initially then 400 mg every 8 hours *or* 500 mg every 8 hours, CHILD 7.5 mg/kg every 8 hours; *by rectum*, 1 g every 8 hours for 3 days, then 1 g every 12 hours, CHILD every 8 hours for 3 days, then every 12 hours, age up to 1 year 125 mg, 1–5 years 250 mg, 5–10 years 500 mg, over 10 years, adult dose; *by intravenous infusion* over 20 minutes, 500 mg every 8 hours; CHILD 7.5 mg/kg every 8 hours

Leg ulcers and pressure sores, *by mouth*, 400 mg every 8 hours for 7 days

Bacterial vaginosis, *by mouth*, 400–500 mg twice daily for 5–7 days *or* 2 g as a single dose

Pelvic inflammatory disease (see also Table 1, section 5.1), *by mouth*, 400 mg twice daily for 14 days

Acute ulcerative gingivitis, *by mouth*, 200–250 mg every 8 hours for 3 days; CHILD 1–3 years 50 mg every 8 hours for 3 days; 3–7 years 100 mg every 12 hours; 7–10 years 100 mg every 8 hours

Acute dental infections, *by mouth*, 200 mg every 8 hours for 3 days

Surgical prophylaxis, *by mouth*, 400–500 mg 2 hours before surgery; up to 3 further doses of 400–500 mg may be given every 8 hours for high-risk procedures; CHILD 7.5 mg/kg 2 hours before surgery; up to 3 further doses of 7.5 mg/kg may be given every 8 hours for high-risk procedures
By rectum, 1 g 2 hours before surgery; up to 3 further doses of 1 g may be given every 8 hours for high-risk procedures; CHILD 5–10 years 500 mg 2 hours before surgery; up to 3 further doses of 500 mg may be given every 8 hours for high-risk procedures
By intravenous infusion (if rectal administration inappropriate), 500 mg at induction; up to 3 further doses of 500 mg may be given every 8 hours for high-risk procedures; CHILD 7.5 mg/kg at induc-

tion; up to 3 further doses of 7.5 mg/kg may be given every 8 hours for high-risk procedures
NOTE. Metronidazole doses in BNF may differ from those in product literature

Metronidazole (Non-proprietary) PoM
Tablets, metronidazole 200 mg, net price 20 =40p; 400 mg, 20 =83p. Label: 4, 9, 21, 25, 27
Available from Alpharma, APS, Arrow, DDSA (*Vaginyl®*), Hillcross, IVAX, Kent, Rosemont
Tablets, metronidazole 500 mg, net price 21-tab pack = £3.50. Label: 4, 9, 21, 25, 27
Available from Alpharma
Suspension, metronidazole (as benzoate) 200 mg/5 mL. Net price 100 mL = £7.70. Label: 4, 9, 23
Available from Hillcross, Rosemont (*Norzol®*)
Intravenous infusion, metronidazole 5 mg/mL. Net price 20-mL amp = £1.53, 100-mL container = £3.57
Available from Braun, Galen, Phoenix

Flagyl® (Hawgreen) PoM
Tablets, both f/c, ivory, metronidazole 200 mg, net price 21-tab pack = £3.89; 400 mg, 14-tab pack = £5.50. Label: 4, 9, 21, 25, 27
Suppositories, metronidazole 500 mg, net price 10 = £13.17; 1 g, 10 = £20.00. Label: 4, 9

Flagyl® (Aventis Pharma) PoM
Intravenous infusion, metronidazole 5 mg/mL, net price 100-mL *Viaflex®* bag = £3.41
Electrolytes: Na+ 13.6 mmol/100-mL bag

Flagyl S® (Hawgreen) PoM
Suspension, orange- and lemon-flavoured, metronidazole (as benzoate) 200 mg/5 mL. Net price 100 mL = £9.69. Label: 4, 9, 23

Metrolyl® (Sandoz) PoM
Intravenous infusion, metronidazole 5 mg/mL, net price 100-mL Steriflex® bag = £12.22
Electrolytes: Na+ 14.53 mmol/100-mL bag
Suppositories, metronidazole 500 mg, net price 10 = £13.27; 1 g, 10 = £19.76. Label: 4, 9

TINIDAZOLE

Indications: anaerobic infections, see under Dose below; protozoal infections (section 5.4.2); *Helicobacter pylori* eradication (section 1.3)
Cautions: see under Metronidazole; pregnancy (manufacturer advises avoidance in first trimester); avoid in porphyria (section 9.8.2); **interactions:** Appendix 1 (tinidazole)
Side-effects: see under Metronidazole
Dose: anaerobic infections *by mouth*, 2 g initially, followed by 1 g daily *or* 500 mg twice daily, usually for 5–6 days
Bacterial vaginosis and acute ulcerative gingivitis, a single 2-g dose
Abdominal surgery prophylaxis, a single 2-g dose approximately 12 hours before surgery

Fasigyn® (Pfizer) PoM
Tablets, f/c, tinidazole 500 mg. Net price 20-tab pack = £11.50. Label: 4, 9, 21, 25

5.1.12 Quinolones

Nalidixic acid and **norfloxacin** are effective in uncomplicated urinary-tract infections.
Ciprofloxacin is active against both Gram-positive and Gram-negative bacteria. It is particularly active against Gram-negative bacteria, including salmonella, shigella, campylobacter, neisseria, and pseudo-

monas. Ciprofloxacin has only moderate activity against Gram-positive bacteria such as *Streptococcus pneumoniae* and *Enterococcus faecalis*; it is not the drug of first choice for pneumococcal pneumonia. It is active against chlamydia and some mycobacteria. Most anaerobic organisms are not susceptible. Uses for ciprofloxacin include infections of the respiratory tract (but not for pneumococcal pneumonia) and of the urinary tract, and of the gastro-intestinal system (including typhoid fever), and gonorrhoea and septicaemia caused by sensitive organisms.

Ofloxacin is used for urinary-tract infections, lower respiratory-tract infections, gonorrhoea, and non-gonococcal urethritis and cervicitis.

Levofloxacin is active against Gram-positive and Gram-negative organisms. It has greater activity against pneumococci than ciprofloxacin.

Although ciprofloxacin, levofloxacin and ofloxacin are licensed for skin and soft-tissue infections, many staphylococci are resistant to the quinolones and their use should be avoided in MRSA infections.

Moxifloxacin is licensed for respiratory-tract infections; it is active against Gram-positive and Gram-negative organisms. It has greater activity against Gram-positive organisms including pneumococci than ciprofloxacin. Moxifloxacin is not active against *Pseudomonas aeruginosa* or methicillin-resistant *Staphylococcus aureus* (MRSA).
SCOTTISH MEDICINES CONSORTIUM ADVICE. The Scottish Medicines Consortium has advised (October 2003) that moxifloxacin should be used in NHS Scotland for treating acute exacerbations of chronic bronchitis **only** if conventional treatment has failed or is contra-indicated, and for **second-line treatment** of community-acquired pneumonia.

ANTHRAX. *Inhalation* or *gastro-intestinal anthrax* should be treated initially with either **ciprofloxacin** or **doxycycline** [unlicensed indication] (section 5.1.3) combined with one or two other antibacterials (such as amoxicillin, benzylpenicillin, chloramphenicol, clarithromycin, clindamycin, imipenem with cilastatin, rifampicin [unlicensed indication], and vancomycin). When the condition improves and the sensitivity of the *Bacillus anthracis* strain is known, treatment may be switched to a single antibacterial. Treatment should continue for 60 days because germination may be delayed.
Cutaneous anthrax should be treated with either ciprofloxacin [unlicensed indication] or doxycycline [unlicensed indication] (section 5.1.3) for 7 days. Treatment may be switched to amoxicillin (section 5.1.1.3) if the infecting strain is susceptible. Treatment may need to be extended to 60 days if exposure is due to aerosol. A combination of antibacterials for 14 days is recommended for cutaneous anthrax with systemic features, extensive oedema, or lesions of the head or neck.
Ciprofloxacin or doxycycline may be given for *post-exposure prophylaxis*. If exposure is confirmed, antibacterial prophylaxis should continue for 60 days. Antibacterial prophylaxis may be switched to amoxicillin after 10–14 days if the strain of *B. anthracis* is susceptible. Vaccination against anthrax (section 14.4) may allow the duration of antibacterial prophylaxis to be shortened.

CAUTIONS. Quinolones should be used with caution in patients with a history of epilepsy or conditions that predispose to seizures, in G6PD deficiency (section 9.1.5), myasthenia gravis (risk of exacerbation), in pregnancy (Appendix 4), during breast-feeding (Appendix 5), and in children or adolescents (arthropathy has developed in weight-bearing joints in young *animals*—see below). Exposure to excessive sunlight should be avoided (discontinue if photosensitivity occurs). The CSM has warned that quinolones may induce **convulsions** in patients with or without a history of convulsions; taking NSAIDs at the same time may also induce them. Other **interactions:** Appendix 1 (quinolones). USE IN CHILDREN. Quinolones cause arthropathy in the weight-bearing joints of immature *animals* and are therefore generally not recommended in children and growing adolescents. However, the significance of this effect in humans is uncertain and in some specific circumstances short-term use of a quinolone in children may be justified. Nalidixic acid is used for urinary-tract infections in children over 3 months of age. Ciprofloxacin is licensed for pseudomonal infections in cystic fibrosis (for children above 5 years of age), and for treatment and prophylaxis of inhalational anthrax.

CSM advice (tendon damage). Tendon damage (including rupture) has been reported rarely in patients receiving quinolones. Tendon rupture may occur within 48 hours of starting treatment. The CSM has reminded that:

- quinolones are contra-indicated in patients with a history of tendon disorders related to quinolone use;
- elderly patients are more prone to tendinitis;
- the risk of tendon rupture is increased by the concomitant use of corticosteroids;
- if tendinitis is suspected, the quinolone should be discontinued immediately.

SIDE-EFFECTS. Side-effects of the quinolones include nausea, vomiting, dyspepsia, abdominal pain, diarrhoea (rarely antibiotic-associated colitis), headache, dizziness, sleep disorders, rash (rarely Stevens-Johnson syndrome and toxic epidermal necrolysis), and pruritus. Less frequent side-effects include anorexia, increase in blood urea and creatinine; drowsiness, restlessness, asthenia, depression, confusion, hallucinations, convulsions, paraesthesia; photosensitivity, hypersensitivity reactions including fever, urticaria, angioedema, arthralgia, myalgia, and anaphylaxis; blood disorders (including eosinophilia, leucopenia, thrombocytopenia); disturbances in vision, taste, hearing and smell. Also isolated reports of tendon inflammation and damage (especially in the elderly and in those taking corticosteroids, see also CSM advice above). Other side-effects that have been reported include haemolytic anaemia, renal failure, interstitial nephritis, and hepatic dysfunction (including hepatitis and cholestatic jaundice). The drug should be **discontinued** if psychiatric, neurological or hypersensitivity reactions (including severe rash) occur.

CIPROFLOXACIN

Indications: see notes above and under Dose; eye infections (section 11.3.1)

Cautions: see notes above; renal impairment (Appendix 3); avoid excessive alkalinity of urine and ensure adequate fluid intake (risk of crystalluria); **interactions:** Appendix 1 (quinolones).
DRIVING. May impair performance of skilled tasks (e.g. driving); effects enhanced by alcohol

Side-effects: see notes above; also reported flatulence, dysphagia, tremor, hyperglycaemia, vasculitis, erythema nodosum, petechiae, haemorrhagic bullae, tinnitus, tenosynovitis, tachycardia, oedema, syncope, hot flushes and sweating; pain and phlebitis at injection site

Dose: *by mouth*, respiratory-tract infections, 250–750 mg twice daily
Urinary-tract infections, 250–500 mg twice daily (100 mg twice daily for 3 days in acute uncomplicated cystitis in women)
Chronic prostatitis, 500 mg twice daily for 28 days
Gonorrhoea, 500 mg as a single dose
Pseudomonal lower respiratory-tract infection in cystic fibrosis, 750 mg twice daily; CHILD 5–17 years (see Cautions above), up to 20 mg/kg twice daily (max. 1.5 g daily)
Most other infections, 500–750 mg twice daily
Surgical prophylaxis, 750 mg 60–90 minutes before procedure
Prophylaxis of meningococcal meningitis [not licensed], Table 2, section 5.1
By intravenous infusion (over 30–60 minutes; 400 mg over 60 minutes), 200–400 mg twice daily
Pseudomonal lower respiratory-tract infection in cystic fibrosis, 400 mg twice daily; CHILD 5–17 years (see Cautions above), up to 10 mg/kg 3 times daily (max. 1.2 g daily)
Urinary-tract infections, 100 mg twice daily
Gonorrhoea, 100 mg as a single dose
CHILD not recommended (see Cautions above) but where benefit outweighs risk, *by mouth*, 10–30 mg/kg daily in 2 divided doses *or by intravenous infusion*, 8–16 mg/kg daily in 2 divided doses
Anthrax (treatment and post-exposure prophylaxis, see notes above), *by mouth*, 500 mg twice daily; CHILD 30 mg/kg daily in 2 divided doses (max. 1g daily)
By intravenous infusion, 400 mg twice daily; CHILD 20 mg/kg daily in 2 divided doses (max. 800 mg daily)

Ciprofloxacin (Non-proprietary) [PoM]
Tablets, ciprofloxacin (as hydrochloride) 100 mg, net price 6-tab pack = £2.64; 250 mg, 10-tab pack = £6.31, 20-tab pack = £12.30; 500 mg, 10-tab pack = £12.02, 20–tab pack = £24.07; 750 mg, 10-tab pack = £17.59. Label: 7, 9, 25, counselling, driving
Available from Alpharma, APS, Arrow, Chemidex, Generics, PLIVA, Sandoz, Sterwin, Tillomed

Ciproxin® (Bayer) [PoM]
Tablets, all f/c, ciprofloxacin (as hydrochloride) 100 mg, net price 6-tab pack = £2.80; 250 mg (scored), 10-tab pack = £7.50, 20-tab pack = £15.00; 500 mg (scored), 10-tab pack = £14.20, 20-tab pack = £28.40; 750 mg, 10-tab pack = £20.00. Label: 7, 9, 25, counselling, driving
Suspension, strawberry-flavoured, ciprofloxacin for reconstitution with diluent provided, 250 mg/ 5 mL, net price 100 mL = £15.00. Label: 7, 9, 25, counselling, driving
Intravenous infusion, ciprofloxacin (as lactate) 2 mg/mL, in sodium chloride 0.9%, net price 50-mL bottle = £8.65
Electrolytes: Na⁺ 15.4 mmol/100-mL bottle
Intravenous infusion (Flexibag), ciprofloxacin (as lactate) 2 mg/mL, in glucose 5%, net price 100-mL infusion bag = £16.89, 200-mL infusion bag = £25.70

LEVOFLOXACIN

Indications: see under Dose

Cautions: see notes above; renal impairment (Appendix 3); **interactions:** Appendix 1 (quinolones)

DRIVING. May impair performance of skilled tasks (e.g. driving)

Side-effects: see notes above; rarely tremor, anxiety, tachycardia, hypotension, hypoglycaemia, pneumonitis, rhabdomyolysis; local reactions and transient hypotension reported with infusion

Dose: *by mouth*, acute sinusitis, 500 mg daily for 10–14 days

Exacerbation of chronic bronchitis, 250–500 mg daily for 7–10 days

Community-acquired pneumonia, 500 mg once or twice daily for 7–14 days

Urinary-tract infections, 250 mg daily for 7–10 days (for 3 days in uncomplicated infection)

Skin and soft tissue infections, 250 mg daily *or* 500 mg once or twice daily for 7–14 days

By intravenous infusion (over at least 60 minutes for 500 mg), community-acquired pneumonia, 500 mg once or twice daily

Complicated urinary-tract infections, 250 mg daily, increased in severe infections

Skin and soft tissue infections, 500 mg twice daily

Tavanic® (Hoechst Marion Roussel) PoM

Tablets, yellow-red, f/c, scored, levofloxacin 250 mg, net price 5-tab pack = £7.77, 10-tab pack = £15.54; 500 mg, 5-tab pack = £13.90, 10-tab pack = £27.80. Label: 6, 9, 25, counselling, driving

Intravenous infusion, levofloxacin 5 mg/mL, net price 100-mL bottle = £28.39

Electrolytes: Na^+ 15.4 mmol/100-mL bottle

MOXIFLOXACIN

Indications: see notes above for Scottish Medicines Consortium advice; community-acquired pneumonia; exacerbation of chronic bronchitis; sinusitis

Cautions: see notes above; renal impairment (Appendix 3); conditions pre-disposing to arrhythmias, including myocardial ischaemia; **interactions:** Appendix 1 (quinolones)

DRIVING. May impair performance of skilled tasks (e.g. driving)

Contra-indications: see notes above; severe hepatic impairment; history of QT-interval prolongation, bradycardia, history of symptomatic arrhythmias, heart failure with reduced left ventricular ejection fraction, electrolyte disturbances, concomitant use with other drugs known to prolong QT-interval

Side-effects: see notes above; also reported dry mouth, stomatitis, glossitis, flatulence, constipation, arrhythmias, palpitations, syncope, peripheral oedema, angina, blood pressure changes, vasodilatation, dyspnoea, anxiety, agitation, tremor, abnormal dreams, incoordination, dry skin, sweating, hyperglycaemia, hyperlipidaemia, and altered prothrombin concentration

Dose: 400 mg once daily for 10 days in community-acquired pneumonia, for 5–10 days in exacerbation of chronic bronchitis, for 7 days in sinusitis

Avelox® (Bayer) ▼ PoM

Tablets, f/c, moxifloxacin (as hydrochloride) 400 mg, net price 5-tab pack = £10.95. Label: 6, 9, counselling, driving

NALIDIXIC ACID

Indications: urinary-tract infections

Cautions: see notes above; avoid in porphyria (section 9.8.2); liver disease; renal impairment (Appendix 3); false positive urinary glucose (if tested for reducing substances); monitor blood counts, renal and liver function if treatment exceeds 2 weeks; **interactions:** Appendix 1 (quinolones)

Side-effects: see notes above; also reported toxic psychosis, weakness, increased intracranial pressure, cranial nerve palsy, metabolic acidosis

Dose: 1 g every 6 hours for 7 days, reduced in chronic infections to 500 mg every 6 hours; CHILD over 3 months max. 50 mg/kg daily in divided doses; reduced in prolonged therapy to 30 mg/kg daily

Mictral® (Sanofi-Synthelabo) PoM

Granules, effervescent, nalidixic acid 660 mg, sodium citrate (as sodium citrate and citric acid) 4.1 g/sachet (Na^+ 41 mmol/sachet). Net price 9-sachet pack = £5.48. Label: 9, 11, 13

Dose: 1 sachet in water 3 times daily for 3 days

Negram® (Sanofi-Synthelabo) PoM

Tablets, beige, nalidixic acid 500 mg. Net price 56-tab pack = £12.83. Label: 9, 11, 23

Suspension, pink, sugar-free, nalidixic acid 300 mg/ 5 mL (raspberry-flavoured), net price 120 mL = £10.28. Label: 9, 11, 23

Uriben® (Rosemont) PoM

Suspension, pink, nalidixic acid 300 mg/5 mL, net price 150 mL = £12.15. Label: 9, 11

NORFLOXACIN

Indications: see under Dose

Cautions: see notes above; renal impairment (Appendix 3); **interactions:** Appendix 1 (quinolones)

DRIVING. May impair performance of skilled tasks (e.g. driving)

Side-effects: see notes above; also reported euphoria, anxiety, tinnitus, polyneuropathy, exfoliative dermatitis, pancreatitis, vasculitis

Dose: urinary-tract infections, 400 mg twice daily for 7–10 days (for 3 days in uncomplicated lower urinary-tract infections)

Chronic relapsing urinary-tract infections, 400 mg twice daily for up to 12 weeks; may be reduced to 400 mg once daily if adequate suppression within first 4 weeks

Chronic prostatitis, 400 mg twice daily for 28 days

Norfloxacin (Non-proprietary) PoM

Tablets, norfloxacin 400 mg, net price 6-tab pack = £2.13, 14-tab pack = £4.95. Label: 7, 9, 23, counselling, driving

Available from Genus, Ratiopharm

Utinor® (MSD) PoM

Tablets, scored, norfloxacin 400 mg. Net price 6-tab pack = £2.19, 14-tab pack = £5.11. Label: 7, 9, 23, counselling, driving

OFLOXACIN

Indications: see under Dose

Cautions: see notes above; hepatic and renal impairment (Appendixes 2 and 3); history of psychiatric illness; **interactions:** Appendix 1 (quinolones)

DRIVING. May affect performance of skilled tasks (e.g. driving); effects enhanced by alcohol

Side-effects: see notes above; also reported, tachycardia, transient hypotension, vasculitic reactions, anxiety, unsteady gait and tremor, hypaesthesia, neuropathy, extrapyramidal symptoms, psychotic reactions (discontinue treatment—see notes above); very rarely changes in blood sugar; isolated cases of pneumonitis; on intravenous infusion, hypotension and local reactions (including thrombophlebitis)

Dose: *by mouth*, urinary-tract infections, 200–400 mg daily preferably in the morning, increased if necessary in upper urinary-tract infections to 400 mg twice daily

Chronic prostatitis, 200 mg twice daily for 28 days

Lower respiratory-tract infections, 400 mg daily preferably in the morning, increased if necessary to 400 mg twice daily

Skin and soft-tissue infections, 400 mg twice daily

Uncomplicated gonorrhoea, 400 mg as a single dose

Uncomplicated genital chlamydial infection, nongonococcal urethritis, 400 mg daily in single or divided doses for 7 days

Pelvic inflammatory disease (see also section 5.1, table 1), 400 mg twice daily for 14 days

By intravenous infusion (over at least 30 minutes for each 200 mg), complicated urinary-tract infection, 200 mg daily

Lower respiratory-tract infection, 200 mg twice daily

Septicaemia, 200 mg twice daily

Skin and soft-tissue infections, 400 mg twice daily

Severe or complicated infections, dose may be increased to 400 mg twice daily

Ofloxacin (Non-proprietary) PoM
Tablets, ofloxacin 200 mg, net price 10-tab pack = £10.72; 400 mg, 5-tab pack = £10.74, 10-tab pack = £21.80. Label: 6, 9, 11, counselling, driving
Available from APS, Dexcel, Generics

Tarivid® (Aventis Pharma) PoM
Tablets, f/c, scored, ofloxacin 200 mg, net price 10-tab pack = £9.80, 20-tab pack = £19.58; 400 mg (yellow), 5-tab pack = £9.78, 10-tab pack = £19.50. Label: 6, 9, 11, counselling, driving
Intravenous infusion, ofloxacin (as hydrochloride) 2 mg/mL, net price 50-mL bottle = £16.95; 100-mL bottle = £21.02 (both hosp. only)

5.1.13 Urinary-tract infections

Urinary-tract infection is more common in women than in men; when it occurs in men there is frequently an underlying abnormality of the renal tract. Recurrent episodes of infection are an indication for radiological investigation especially in children in whom untreated pyelonephritis may lead to permanent kidney damage.

Escherichia coli is the most common cause of urinary-tract infection; *Staphylococcus saprophyticus* is also common in sexually active young women. Less common causes include Proteus and Klebsiella spp. *Pseudomonas aeruginosa* infections are almost invariably associated with functional or anatomical abnormalities of the renal tract. *Staphylococcus epidermidis* and *Enterococcus faecalis* infection may complicate catheterisation or instrumentation.

> Whenever possible a specimen of urine should be collected for culture and sensitivity testing before starting antibacterial therapy. The antibacterial chosen should reflect local antibacterial sensitivity, which needs to be reviewed regularly.

Uncomplicated lower urinary-tract infections often respond to amoxicillin, nalidixic acid, nitrofurantoin, or trimethoprim given for 7 days (3 days of trimethoprim or amoxicillin may be adequate for infections in women); those caused by fully sensitive bacteria respond to two 3-g doses of amoxicillin (section 5.1.1.3). Widespread bacterial resistance, especially to ampicillin or amoxicillin has increased the importance of urine culture before therapy. Alternatives for resistant organisms include co-amoxiclav (amoxicillin with clavulanic acid), an oral cephalosporin, pivmecillinam, or a quinolone.

Long-term low dose therapy may be required in selected patients to prevent *recurrence of infection*; indications include frequent relapses and significant kidney damage. Trimethoprim, nitrofurantoin and cefalexin have been recommended for long-term therapy.

Methenamine (hexamine) should **not** generally be used because it requires an acidic urine for its antimicrobial activity and it is ineffective for upper urinary-tract infections; it may, however, have a role in chronic bacteriuria particularly in infection caused by highly resistant Gram-negative bacteria or by yeasts.

Acute pyelonephritis can lead to septicaemia and is best treated initially by injection of a broad-spectrum antibacterial such as cefuroxime or a quinolone especially if the patient is severely ill; gentamicin can also be used.

Prostatitis can be difficult to cure and requires treatment for several weeks with an antibacterial which penetrates prostatic tissue such as trimethoprim, or some quinolones.

Where infection is localised and associated with an indwelling *catheter* a bladder instillation is often effective (section 7.4.4).

Patients with *heart-valve lesions* undergoing instrumentation of the urinary tract should be given a parenteral antibiotic to prevent bacteraemia and endocarditis (section 5.1, table 2).

Urinary-tract infection in *pregnancy* may be asymptomatic and requires prompt treatment to prevent progression to acute pyelonephritis. Penicillins and cephalosporins are suitable for treating urinary-tract infection during pregnancy. Nitrofurantoin may also be used but it should be avoided at term. Sulphonamides, quinolones, and tetracyclines should be avoided during pregnancy; trimethoprim should also preferably be avoided particularly in the first trimester..

In *renal failure* antibacterials normally excreted by the kidney accumulate with resultant toxicity unless the dose is reduced. This applies especially to the aminoglycosides which should be used with great caution; tetracyclines, hexamine, and nitrofurantoin should be avoided altogether.

CHILDREN. Urinary-tract infections in children require prompt antibacterial treatment to minimise the risk of renal scarring. For the first infection, treatment may be initiated with trimethoprim or co-amoxiclav and the choice of antibacterial is reviewed when sensitivity results are available; full doses of the antibacterial drug should be given for 5–7 days. Antibacterial prophylaxis with low doses of trimethoprim or nitrofurantoin should then be given until investigations for the infection are complete; long-term prophylaxis may be necessary in some cases (e.g. vesicoureteric reflux or renal scarring).

Seriously ill children should be transferred to hospital and treated initially with intravenous antibacterial drugs such as ampicillin with gentamicin or cefotaxime alone until the infection responds; full doses of oral antibacterials are then given for a further period. Antibacterial prophylaxis should then be given as above.

NITROFURANTOIN

Indications: urinary-tract infections

Cautions: anaemia; diabetes mellitus; electrolyte imbalance; vitamin B and folate deficiency; pulmonary disease; hepatic impairment; monitor lung and liver function on long-term therapy, especially in the elderly (discontinue if deterioration in lung function); susceptibility to peripheral neuropathy; false positive urinary glucose (if tested for reducing substances); urine may be coloured yellow or brown; **interactions:** Appendix 1 (nitrofurantoin)

Contra-indications: impaired renal function, infants less than 3 months old, G6PD deficiency (including pregnancy at term, and breast-feeding of affected infants, see section 9.1.5 and Appendixes 4 and 5), porphyria (section 9.8.2)

Side-effects: anorexia, nausea, vomiting, and diarrhoea; acute and chronic pulmonary reactions (pulmonary fibrosis reported; possible association with lupus erythematosus-like syndrome); peripheral neuropathy; also reported, hypersensitivity reactions (including angioedema, anaphylaxis, sialadenitis, urticaria, rash and pruritus); rarely, cholestatic jaundice, hepatitis, exfoliative dermatitis, erythema multiforme, pancreatitis, arthralgia, blood disorders (including agranulocytosis, thrombocytopenia, and aplastic anaemia), benign intracranial hypertension, and transient alopecia

Dose: acute uncomplicated infection, 50 mg every 6 hours with food for 7 days; CHILD over 3 months, 3 mg/kg daily in 4 divided doses
Severe chronic recurrent infection, 100 mg every 6 hours with food for 7 days (dose reduced or discontinued if severe nausea)
Prophylaxis (but see Cautions), 50–100 mg at night; CHILD over 3 months, 1 mg/kg at night

Nitrofurantoin (Non-proprietary) ▣PoM▣
Tablets, nitrofurantoin 50 mg, net price 20 = £1.58; 100 mg, 20 = £2.97. Label: 9, 14, 21
Available from Alpharma, APS
Oral suspension, nitrofurantoin 25 mg/5 mL, net price 300 mL = £65.00. Label: 9, 14, 21
Available from Goldshield

Furadantin® (Goldshield) ▣PoM▣
Tablets, all yellow, scored, nitrofurantoin 50 mg, net price 20 = £1.96; 100 mg, 20 = £3.62. Label: 9, 14, 21

Macrobid® (Goldshield) ▣PoM▣
Capsules, m/r, blue/yellow, nitrofurantoin 100 mg (as nitrofurantoin macrocrystals and nitrofurantoin monohydrate). Net price 14-cap pack = £4.89. Label: 9, 14, 21, 25
Dose: uncomplicated urinary-tract infection, 1 capsule twice daily with food
Genito-urinary surgical prophylaxis, 1 capsule twice daily on day of procedure and for 3 days after

Macrodantin® (Goldshield) ▣PoM▣
Capsules, nitrofurantoin 50 mg (yellow/white), net price 30-cap pack = £3.05; 100 mg (yellow), 20 = £3.84. Label: 9, 14, 21

METHENAMINE HIPPURATE ▣▬◢▣

(Hexamine hippurate)

Indications: prophylaxis and long-term treatment of chronic or recurrent lower urinary-tract infections

Cautions: pregnancy; avoid concurrent administration with sulphonamides (risk of crystalluria) or urinary alkalinising agents; **interactions:** Appendix 1 (methenamine)

Contra-indications: hepatic impairment, severe renal impairment, severe dehydration, gout, metabolic acidosis

Side-effects: gastro-intestinal disturbances, bladder irritation, rash

Dose: 1 g every 12 hours (may be increased in patients with catheters to 1 g every 8 hours); CHILD 6–12 years 500 mg every 12 hours

Hiprex® (3M) ▣▬◢▣
Tablets, scored, methenamine hippurate 1 g. Net price 60-tab pack = £7.07. Label: 9

5.2   Antifungal drugs

Treatment of fungal infections

The systemic treatment of common fungal infections is outlined below; specialist treatment is required in most forms of systemic or disseminated fungal infections. For local treatment of fungal infections, see section 7.2.2 (genital), section 7.4.4 (bladder), section 11.3.2 (eye), section 12.1.1 (ear), section 12.3.2 (oropharynx), and section 13.10.2 (skin).

ASPERGILLOSIS. Aspergillosis most commonly affects the respiratory tract but in severely immuno-compromised patients, invasive forms can affect the sinuses, heart, brain, and skin. **Amphotericin** by intravenous infusion is the drug of choice but response can be variable; liposomal amphotericin, **itraconazole**, or **voriconazole** are alternatives in patients in whom initial treatment has failed. **Caspofungin** is licensed for invasive aspergillosis unresponsive to amphotericin or to itraconazole, or in patients who cannot tolerate amphotericin or itraconazole.

CANDIDIASIS. Many superficial candidal infections are treated locally including infections of the vagina (section 7.2.2) and of the skin (section 13.10.2).

Oropharyngeal candidiasis generally responds to topical therapy (section 12.3.2); an imidazole or triazole antifungal is given by mouth for unresponsive infections. Fluconazole is effective and is reliably absorbed.

For *deep and disseminated candidiasis*, **amphotericin** by intravenous infusion is used alone or with **flucytosine** by intravenous infusion; an alternative is **fluconazole** given alone, particularly in AIDS patients (in whom flucytosine is best avoided because of its bone marrow toxicity). **Voriconazole** is licensed for infections caused by fluconazole-resistant *Candida* spp. (including *C. krusei*). **Caspofungin** is licensed for the treatment of invasive candidiasis.

CRYPTOCOCCOSIS. Cryptococcosis is uncommon but infection in the immunocompromised, especially in AIDS patients, can be life-threatening; cryptococcal meningitis is the most common form of fungal meningitis. The treatment of choice is **amphotericin** by intravenous infusion with or without **flucytosine** by intravenous infusion. **Fluconazole** given alone is an alternative particularly in AIDS patients with no disturbance of consciousness. Following successful treatment, fluconazole can be used for prophylaxis against relapse until immunity recovers.

HISTOPLASMOSIS. Histoplasmosis is rare in temperate climates; it can be life-threatening, particularly in HIV-infected persons. **Itraconazole** or **ketoconazole** can be used for the treatment of immunocompetent patients with indolent non-meningeal infection including chronic pulmonary histoplasmosis. **Amphotericin** by intravenous infusion is preferred in patients with fulminant or severe infections. Intravenous itraconazole is also licensed for histoplasmosis.

SKIN AND NAIL INFECTIONS. Mild localised fungal infections of the skin (including tinea corporis, tinea cruris, and tinea pedis) respond to topical therapy (section 13.10.2). Systemic therapy (itraconazole, fluconazole, or terbinafine) is appropriate if topical therapy fails, if many areas are affected, or if the site of infection is difficult to treat such as in infections of the nails (onychomycosis) and of the scalp (tinea capitis).

Griseofulvin is used for tinea capitis in adults and children; it was used extensively in tinea of various other sites but it has largely been replaced by newer antifungals. Oral imidazole or triazole antifungals (particularly **itraconazole**) and **terbinafine** are used more commonly because they have a broader spectrum of activity and require a shorter duration of treatment; the role of terbinafine in the management of microsporum species (cat or dog ringworm) is uncertain.

Pityriasis versicolor may be treated with **itraconazole** by mouth if topical therapy is ineffective; **fluconazole** by mouth is an alternative. Oral **terbinafine** is **not** effective for pityriasis versicolor.

Terbinafine and **itraconazole** have largely replaced griseofulvin for the systemic treatment of onychomycosis, particularly of the toenail; terbinafine is considered to be the drug of choice. Itraconazole can be administered as intermittent 'pulse' therapy.

IMMUNOCOMPROMISED PATIENTS. Immunocompromised patients are at particular risk of fungal infections and may receive antifungal drugs prophylactically; oral imidazole or triazole antifungals are the drugs of choice for prophylaxis. **Fluconazole** is more reliably absorbed than itraconazole and ketoconazole; fluconazole is considered to be less toxic than ketoconazole on long-term use.

Amphotericin by intravenous infusion is used for the empirical *treatment* of serious fungal infections. Fluconazole is used for treatment of *Candida albicans* infection.

Drugs used in fungal infections

POLYENE ANTIFUNGALS. The polyene antifungals include amphotericin and nystatin; neither drug is absorbed when given by mouth. They are used for oral, oropharyngeal, and perioral infections by local application in the mouth (section 12.3.2).

Amphotericin by intravenous infusion is used for the treatment of systemic fungal infections and is active against most fungi and yeasts. It is highly protein bound and penetrates poorly into body fluids and tissues. When given parenterally amphotericin is toxic and side-effects are common. Lipid formulations of amphotericin (*Abelcet*®, *AmBisome*®, and *Amphocil*®) are significantly less toxic and are recommended when the conventional formulation of amphotericin is contra-indicated because of toxicity, especially nephrotoxicity; lipid formulations are more expensive.

Nystatin is used principally for *Candida albicans* infections of the skin and mucous membranes, including oesophageal and intestinal candidiasis.

IMIDAZOLE ANTIFUNGALS. Clotrimazole, econazole, fenticonazole, sulconazole, and tioconazole are used for the local treatment of vaginal candidiasis (section 7.2.2) and for dermatophyte infections (section 13.10.2).

Ketoconazole is better absorbed by mouth than other imidazoles. It has been associated with fatal hepatotoxicity; the CSM has advised that prescribers should weigh the potential benefits of ketoconazole treatment against the risk of liver damage and should carefully monitor patients both clinically and biochemically. It should not be used for superficial fungal infections.

Miconazole can be used locally for oral infections; it is also effective in intestinal infections. Systemic absorption may follow use of miconazole oral gel and may result in significant drug interactions.

TRIAZOLE ANTIFUNGALS. **Fluconazole** is very well absorbed after oral administration. It also achieves good penetration into the cerebrospinal fluid to treat fungal meningitis.

Itraconazole is active against a wide range of dermatophytes. Itraconazole capsules require an acid environment in the stomach for optimal absorption.

Itraconazole has been associated with liver damage and should not be given to patients with a history of liver disease; fluconazole is less frequently associated with hepatotoxicity.

Voriconazole is a broad-spectrum antifungal drug which is licensed for use in life-threatening infections.

OTHER ANTIFUNGALS. **Caspofungin** is active against *Aspergillus* spp. It is given by intravenous infusion for invasive infection. The Scottish Medicines Consortium (March 2003) does not recommend the use of caspofungin in NHS Scotland because of a lack of robust data on efficacy and safety in the treatment of invasive aspergillosis. **Flucytosine** is often used with amphotericin in a synergistic combination. Bone marrow depression can occur which limits its use, particularly in AIDS patients; weekly blood counts are necessary during prolonged therapy. Resistance to flucytosine can develop during therapy and sensitivity testing is essential before and during treatment.

Griseofulvin is effective for widespread or intractable dermatophyte infections but has been superseded by newer antifungals, particularly for nail infections. It is usually well tolerated and is licensed for use in children. Duration of therapy is dependent on the site of the infection and may be required for a number of months.

Terbinafine is the drug of choice for fungal nail infections and is also used for ringworm infections where oral treatment is considered appropriate.

AMPHOTERICIN

(Amphotericin B)

Indications: See under Dose

Cautions: when given parenterally, toxicity common (close supervision necessary and test dose required); renal impairment (Appendix 3); hepatic and renal-function tests, blood counts, and plasma electrolyte monitoring required; corticosteroids (avoid except to control reactions); pregnancy and breast-feeding; avoid rapid infusion (risk of arrhythmias); **interactions:** Appendix 1 (amphotericin)

ANAPHYLAXIS. The CSM has advised that anaphylaxis occurs rarely with any intravenous amphotericin product and a test dose is advisable before the first infusion; the patient should be carefully observed for about 30 minutes after the test dose. Prophylactic antipyretics or hydrocortisone should only be used in patients who have previously experienced acute adverse reactions (in whom continued treatment with amphotericin is essential)

Side-effects: when given parenterally, anorexia, nausea and vomiting, diarrhoea, epigastric pain; febrile reactions, headache, muscle and joint pain; anaemia; disturbances in renal function (including hypokalaemia and hypomagnesaemia) and renal toxicity; also cardiovascular toxicity (including arrhythmias), blood disorders, neurological disorders (including hearing loss, diplopia, convulsions, peripheral neuropathy), abnormal liver function (discontinue treatment), rash, anaphylactoid reactions (see Anaphylaxis, above); pain and thrombophlebitis at injection site

Dose: *by mouth,* intestinal candidiasis, 100–200 mg every 6 hours; INFANT and CHILD, 100 mg 4 times daily

Prophylaxis NEONATE 100 mg once daily

Oral and perioral infections, see section 12.3.2

By intravenous infusion, see under preparations, below

Fungilin® (Squibb) PoM

Tablets, yellow, scored, amphotericin 100 mg, Net price 56-tab pack = £8.32. Label: 9

Suspension, yellow, sugar-free, amphotericin 100 mg/mL, net price 12 mL = £2.31. Label: 9, counselling, use of pipette

Fungizone® (Squibb) PoM

Intravenous infusion, powder for reconstitution, amphotericin (as sodium deoxycholate complex). Net price 50-mg vial = £3.70

Electrolytes: Na$^+$ < 0.5 mmol/vial

Dose: by intravenous infusion, systemic fungal infections, initial test dose of 1 mg over 20–30 minutes then 250 micrograms/kg daily, gradually increased if tolerated to 1 mg/kg daily; max. (severe infection) 1.5 mg/kg daily or on alternate days

NOTE. Prolonged treatment usually necessary; if interrupted for longer than 7 days recommence at 250 micrograms/kg daily and increase gradually

■ Lipid formulations

Abelcet® (Elan) PoM

Intravenous infusion, amphotericin 5 mg/mL as lipid complex with L-α-dimyristoylphosphatidylcholine and L-α-dimyristoylphosphatidylglycerol. Net price 10-mL vial = £50.00, 20-mL vial = £82.13 (hosp. only)

Dose: severe invasive candidiasis; severe systemic fungal infections in patients not responding to conventional amphotericin or to other antifungal drugs or where toxicity or renal impairment precludes conventional amphotericin, including invasive aspergillosis, cryptococcal meningitis and disseminated cryptococcosis in HIV patients, by intravenous infusion, ADULT and CHILD, initial test dose 1 mg over 15 minutes then 5 mg/kg daily for at least 14 days

AmBisome® (Gilead) PoM

Intravenous infusion, powder for reconstitution, amphotericin 50 mg encapsulated in liposomes. Net price 50-mg vial = £138.47

Electrolytes: Na$^+$ < 0.5 mmol/vial

Dose: severe systemic or deep mycoses where toxicity (particularly nephrotoxicity) precludes use of conventional amphotericin, by intravenous infusion, ADULT and CHILD initial test dose 1 mg over 10 minutes then 1 mg/kg daily as a single dose increased gradually if necessary to 3 mg/kg daily as a single dose

Infections in febrile neutropenic patients unresponsive to broad-spectrum antibacterials, ADULT and CHILD, initial test dose 1 mg over 10 minutes then 3 mg/kg daily as a single dose until afebrile for 3 consecutive days; max. period of treatment 42 days

Visceral leishmaniasis, see section 5.4.5 and product literature

Amphocil® (Cambridge) PoM

Intravenous infusion, powder for reconstitution, amphotericin as a complex with sodium cholesteryl sulphate. Net price 50-mg vial = £104.10, 100-mg vial = £190.05

Electrolytes: Na$^+$ < 0.5 mmol/vial

Dose: severe systemic or deep mycoses where toxicity or renal failure preclude use of conventional amphotericin, by intravenous infusion, ADULT and CHILD initial test dose 2 mg over 10 minutes then 1 mg/kg daily as a single dose increased gradually if necessary to 3–4 mg/kg daily as a single dose

CASPOFUNGIN

Indications: invasive aspergillosis either unresponsive to amphotericin or itraconazole or in patients intolerant of amphotericin or itraconazole; invasive candidiasis

Cautions: hepatic impairment (Appendix 2); pregnancy (Appendix 4); **interactions:** Appendix 1 (caspofungin)

Contra-indications: breast-feeding (Appendix 5)

Side-effects: nausea, vomiting, abdominal pain, diarrhoea, flushing, fever, headache, injection-site

reactions, rash, pruritus, anaemia, decrease in serum potassium; also reported, pulmonary oedema, adult respiratory distress syndrome, hypersensitivity reactions (including anaphylaxis)
Dose: *by intravenous infusion*, ADULT over 18 years, 70 mg on first day then 50 mg once daily (70 mg once daily if body-weight over 80 kg)

Cancidas® (MSD) ▼ PoM
Intravenous infusion, powder for reconstitution, caspofungin (as acetate), net price 50-mg vial = £327.67; 70-mg vial = £416.78

FLUCONAZOLE

Indications: see under Dose
Cautions: renal impairment (Appendix 3); pregnancy (Appendix 4) and breast-feeding (Appendix 5); monitor liver function—discontinue if signs or symptoms of hepatic disease (risk of hepatic necrosis); **interactions:** Appendix 1 (antifungals, triazole)
Side-effects: nausea, abdominal discomfort, diarrhoea, flatulence, headache, rash (discontinue treatment or monitor closely if infection invasive or systemic); less frequently dyspepsia, vomiting, taste disturbance, hepatic disorders, angioedema, anaphylaxis, dizziness, seizures, alopecia, pruritus, toxic epidermal necrolysis, Stevens-Johnson syndrome (severe cutaneous reactions more likely in AIDS patients), hyperlipidaemia, leucopenia, thrombocytopenia, and hypokalaemia reported
Dose: vaginal candidiasis and candidal balanitis, *by mouth*, a single dose of 150 mg
Mucosal candidiasis (except genital), *by mouth*, 50 mg daily (100 mg daily in unusually difficult infections) given for 7–14 days in oropharyngeal candidiasis (max. 14 days except in severely immunocompromised patients); for 14 days in atrophic oral candidiasis associated with dentures; for 14–30 days in other mucosal infections (e.g. oesophagitis, candiduria, non-invasive bronchopulmonary infections); CHILD *by mouth or by intravenous infusion*, 3–6 mg/kg on first day then 3 mg/kg daily (every 72 hours in NEONATE up to 2 weeks old, every 48 hours in neonate 2–4 weeks old)
Tinea pedis, corporis, cruris, pityriasis versicolor, and dermal candidiasis, *by mouth*, 50 mg daily for 2–4 weeks (for 6 weeks in tinea pedis); max. duration of treatment 6 weeks
Invasive candidal infections (including candidaemia and disseminated candidiasis) and cryptococcal infections (including meningitis), *by mouth or intravenous infusion*, 400 mg initially then 200 mg daily, increased if necessary to 400 mg daily; treatment continued according to response (at least 6–8 weeks for cryptococcal meningitis); CHILD 6–12 mg/kg daily (every 72 hours in NEONATE up to 2 weeks old, every 48 hours in NEONATE 2–4 weeks old); max. 400 mg daily
Prevention of relapse of cryptococcal meningitis in AIDS patients after completion of primary therapy, *by mouth or by intravenous infusion*, 100–200 mg daily
Prevention of fungal infections in immunocompromised patients following cytotoxic chemotherapy or radiotherapy, *by mouth or by intravenous infusion*, 50–400 mg daily adjusted according to risk; 400 mg daily if high risk of systemic infec-

tions e.g. following bone-marrow transplantation; commence treatment before anticipated onset of neutropenia and continue for 7 days after neutrophil count in desirable range; CHILD according to extent and duration of neutropenia, 3–12 mg/kg daily (every 72 hours in NEONATE up to 2 weeks old, every 48 hours in NEONATE 2–4 weeks old); max. 400 mg daily

Fluconazole (Non-proprietary) PoM
[1]*Capsules*, fluconazole 50 mg, net price 7-cap pack = £13.99; 150 mg, single-capsule pack = £6.48; 200 mg, 7-cap pack = £59.52. Label: 9, (50 and 200 mg)
Available from Alpharma, APS, Generics, IVAX, PLIVA, Sandoz, Sterwin
Intravenous infusion, fluconazole 2 mg/mL, net price 25-mL bottle = £7.31; 100-mL bottle = £29.27
Available from PLIVA

Diflucan® (Pfizer) PoM
[1]*Capsules*, fluconazole 50 mg (blue/white), net price 7-cap pack = £16.61; 150 mg (blue), single-capsule pack = £7.12; 200 mg (purple/white), 7-cap pack = £66.42. Label: 9, (50 and 200 mg)
Oral suspension, orange-flavoured, fluconazole for reconstitution with water, 50 mg/5 mL, net price 35 mL = £16.61; 200 mg/5 mL, 35 mL = £66.42. Label: 9
Intravenous infusion, fluconazole 2 mg/mL in sodium chloride intravenous infusion 0.9%, net price 25-mL bottle = £7.32; 100-mL bottle = £29.28
Electrolytes: Na$^+$ 15 mmol/100-mL bottle

FLUCYTOSINE

Indications: systemic yeast and fungal infections; adjunct to amphotericin (or fluconazole) in cryptococcal meningitis, adjunct to amphotericin in severe systemic candidiasis and in other severe or long-standing infections
Cautions: renal impairment (Appendix 3); elderly; blood disorders; liver- and kidney-function tests and blood counts required (weekly in renal impairment or blood disorders); pregnancy, breast-feeding; **interactions:** Appendix 1 (flucytosine)
Side-effects: nausea, vomiting, diarrhoea, rashes; less frequently confusion, hallucinations, convulsions, headache, sedation, vertigo, alterations in liver function tests (hepatitis and hepatic necrosis reported); blood disorders including thrombocytopenia, leucopenia, and aplastic anaemia reported
Dose: *by intravenous infusion* over 20–40 minutes, ADULT and CHILD, 200 mg/kg daily in 4 divided doses usually for not more than 7 days; extremely sensitive organisms, 100–150 mg/kg daily may be sufficient; treat for at least 4 months in cryptococcal meningitis
NOTE. For plasma concentration monitoring blood should be taken shortly before starting the next infusion; plasma concentration for optimum response 25–50 mg/litre (200–400 micromol/litre)—should not be allowed to exceed 80 mg/litre (620 micromol/litre)

---

1. Capsules can be sold to the public for vaginal candidiasis and associated candidal balanitis in those aged 16–60 years, in a container or packaging containing not more than 150 mg and labelled to show a max. dose of 150 mg; proprietary brands on sale to the public include *Canesten*® *Oral*, *Diflucan*® *One*

Ancotil® (ICN) [PoM]
Intravenous infusion, flucytosine 10 mg/mL. Net price 250-mL infusion bottle = £35.69 (hosp. only)
Electrolytes: Na⁺ 34.5 mmol/250-mL bottle
NOTE. Flucytosine tablets may be available on a named-patient basis from Bell and Croyden; the brand name *Alcobon®* was used formerly for flucytosine infusion

GRISEOFULVIN

Indications: dermatophyte infections of the skin, scalp, hair and nails where topical therapy has failed or is inappropriate

Cautions: interactions: Appendix 1 (griseofulvin)
DRIVING. May impair performance of skilled tasks (e.g. driving); effects of alcohol enhanced

Contra-indications: severe liver disease; systemic lupus erythematosus (risk of exacerbation); porphyria (section 9.8.2); pregnancy (**avoid** pregnancy **during** and for **1 month after** treatment; men should not father children within 6 months of treatment); breast-feeding (Appendix 5)

Side-effects: headache, nausea, vomiting, rashes, photosensitivity; dizziness, fatigue, and leucopenia reported; systemic lupus erythematosus, erythema multiforme, toxic epidermal necrolysis, peripheral neuropathy, confusion and impaired co-ordination also reported

Dose: 500 mg daily in divided doses or as a single dose, in severe infection dose may be doubled, reducing when response occurs; CHILD, 10 mg/kg daily in divided doses or as a single dose

Grisovin® (GSK) [PoM]
Tablets, both f/c, griseofulvin 125 mg, net price 20 = 51p; 500 mg, 20 = £1.93. Label: 9, 21, counselling, driving

ITRACONAZOLE

Indications: see under Dose

Cautions: liver disease (Appendix 2); liver function tests required if history of liver disease or if treatment exceeds 1 month or if anorexia, nausea, vomiting, fatigue, abdominal pain or dark urine develop (discontinue if test abnormal); renal impairment (Appendix 3); absorption reduced in AIDS and neutropenia (monitor plasma-itraconazole concentration and increase dose if necessary); history of congestive heart failure (see also CSM advice, below); pregnancy (Appendix 4) and breast-feeding (Appendix 5); **interactions:** Appendix 1 (antifungals, triazole)

CSM advice (heart failure). Following rare reports of heart failure, the CSM has advised caution when prescribing itraconazole to patients at high risk of heart failure. Those at risk include:

- patients receiving high doses and longer treatment courses;

- older patients and those with cardiac disease;

- patients receiving treatment with negative inotropic drugs, e.g. calcium channel blockers.

Side-effects: nausea, abdominal pain, dyspepsia, constipation (vomiting and diarrhoea with oral liquid or intravenous infusion), headache, dizziness, raised liver enzymes, menstrual disorders; allergic reactions (including pruritus, rash, urticaria and angioedema), hepatitis and cholestatic jaundice (especially if treatment exceeds 1 month),

heart failure, peripheral neuropathy (discontinue treatment), and Stevens-Johnson syndrome reported; on prolonged use hypokalaemia, oedema and hair loss reported

Dose: *by mouth*, oropharyngeal candidiasis, 100 mg daily (200 mg daily in AIDS or neutropenia) for 15 days; see also under *Sporanox®* oral liquid below

Vulvovaginal candidiasis, 200 mg twice daily for 1 day

Pityriasis versicolor, 200 mg daily for 7 days

Tinea corporis and tinea cruris, *either* 100 mg daily for 15 days *or* 200 mg daily for 7 days

Tinea pedis and tinea manuum, *either* 100 mg daily for 30 days *or* 200 mg twice daily for 7 days

Onychomycosis, *either* 200 mg daily for 3 months *or* course ('pulse') of 200 mg twice daily for 7 days, subsequent courses repeated after 21-day interval; fingernails 2 courses, toenails 3 courses

Histoplasmosis, 200 mg 1–2 times daily

Systemic aspergillosis, candidiasis and cryptococcosis including cryptococcal meningitis where other antifungal drugs inappropriate or ineffective, 200 mg once daily (candidiasis 100–200 mg once daily) increased in invasive or disseminated disease and in cryptococcal meningitis to 200 mg twice daily

Maintenance in AIDS patients to prevent relapse of underlying fungal infection and prophylaxis in neutropenia when standard therapy inappropriate, 200 mg once daily, increased to 200 mg twice daily if low plasma-itraconazole concentration (see Cautions)

Prophylaxis in patients with haematological malignancy or undergoing bone-marrow transplant, see under *Sporanox®* oral liquid below

CHILD and ELDERLY safety and efficacy not established

By intravenous infusion, systemic aspergillosis, candidiasis and cryptococcosis including cryptococcal meningitis where other antifungal drugs inappropriate or ineffective, histoplasmosis, 200 mg every 12 hours for 2 days, then 200 mg once daily for max. 12 days; CHILD and ELDERLY safety and efficacy not established

Sporanox® (Janssen-Cilag) [PoM]
Capsules, blue/pink, enclosing coated beads, itraconazole 100 mg, net price 4-cap pack = £4.19; 15-cap pack = £15.72; 28-cap pack (*Sporanox®-Pulse*)= £29.35; 60-cap pack = £62.89. Label: 5, 9, 21, 25
Oral liquid, sugar-free, itraconazole 10 mg/mL, net price 150 mL (with 10-mL measuring cup) = £52.28. Label: 9, 23, counselling, administration
Dose: oral or oesophageal candidiasis in HIV-positive or other immunocompromised patients, 20 mL (2 measuring cups) daily in 1–2 divided doses for 1 week (continue for another week if no response)
Fluconazole-resistant oral or oesophageal candidiasis, 10–20 mL (1–2 measuring cups) twice daily for 2 weeks (continue for another 2 weeks if no response; the higher dose should not be used for longer than 2 weeks if no signs of improvement)
Prophylaxis of deep fungal infections (when standard therapy is inappropriate) in patients with haematological malignancy or undergoing bone-marrow transplantation who are expected to become neutropenic, 5 mg/kg daily in 2 divided doses; start 1 week before transplantation or immediately before chemotherapy and continue until

neutrophil count recovers; CHILD and ELDERLY safety and efficacy not established

COUNSELLING. Do not take with food; swish around mouth and swallow, do not rinse afterwards

Concentrate for intravenous infusion▼, itraconazole 10 mg/mL. For dilution before use. Net price 25-mL amp (with infusion bag and filter) = £71.43
Excipients: include propylene glycol

KETOCONAZOLE

Indications: systemic mycoses, serious chronic resistant mucocutaneous candidiasis, serious resistant gastro-intestinal mycoses, chronic resistant vaginal candidiasis, resistant dermatophyte infections of skin or finger nails (not toe nails); prophylaxis of mycoses in immunosuppressed patients

Cautions: monitor liver function clinically and biochemically—for treatment lasting longer than 14 days perform liver function tests before starting, 14 days after starting, then at monthly intervals (for details consult product literature)—for CSM advice see p. 293; avoid in porphyria (section 9.8.2); **interactions:** Appendix 1 (antifungals, imidazole)

Contra-indications: hepatic impairment; pregnancy (Appendix 4) and breast-feeding

Side-effects: nausea, vomiting, abdominal pain; headache; rashes, urticaria, pruritus; rarely angioedema, thrombocytopenia, paraesthesia, photophobia, dizziness, alopecia, gynaecomastia and oligospermia; fatal liver damage—see also under Cautions, risk of developing hepatitis greater if given for longer than 14 days

Dose: 200 mg once daily with food, usually for 14 days; if response inadequate after 14 days continue until at least 1 week after symptoms have cleared and cultures negative; max. 400 mg (ELDERLY 200 mg) daily

CHILD 3 mg/kg daily

Chronic resistant vaginal candidiasis, 400 mg once daily with food for 5 days

Prophylaxis and maintenance treatment in immunosuppressed patients, 200 mg daily

Nizoral® (Janssen-Cilag) P̶o̶M̶
Tablets, scored, ketoconazole 200 mg. Net price 30-tab pack = £15.69. Label: 5, 9, 21

MICONAZOLE

Indications: see under Dose

Cautions: pregnancy and breast-feeding; avoid in porphyria (section 9.8.2); **interactions:** Appendix 1 (antifungals, imidazole)

Contra-indications: hepatic impairment

Side-effects: nausea and vomiting, diarrhoea (usually on long-term treatment); rarely allergic reactions; isolated reports of hepatitis

Dose: prevention and treatment of oral and intestinal fungal infections, 5–10 mL in the mouth after food 4 times daily; retain near lesions before swallowing; CHILD under 2 years, 2.5 mL twice daily, 2–6 years, 5 mL twice daily, over 6 years, 5 mL 4 times daily

Localised lesions, smear on affected area with clean finger (dental prostheses should be removed at night and brushed with gel); treatment continued for 48 hours after lesions have resolved

¹**Daktarin**® (Janssen-Cilag) P̶o̶M̶
Oral gel, sugar-free, orange-flavoured, miconazole 24 mg/mL (20 mg/g). Net price 15-g tube = £2.37, 80-g tube = £5.00. Label: 9, counselling advised, hold in mouth, after food

1. 15-g tube can be sold to public

NYSTATIN

Indications: candidiasis; vaginal infection (section 7.2.2); oral infection (section 12.3.2); skin infection (section 13.10.2)

Side-effects: nausea, vomiting, diarrhoea at high doses; oral irritation and sensitisation; rash (including urticaria) and rarely Stevens-Johnson syndrome reported

Dose: *by mouth,* intestinal candidiasis 500 000 units every 6 hours, doubled in severe infections; CHILD 100 000 units 4 times daily

Prophylaxis, 1 million units once daily; NEONATE 100 000 units once daily

NOTE. Unlicensed for treatment of candidiasis in NEONATE under 1 month

Nystatin (Non-proprietary) P̶o̶M̶
Oral suspension, nystatin 100 000 units/mL. Net price 30 mL = £2.05. Label: 9, counselling, use of pipette

Available from Hillcross, Rosemont (sugar-free, *Nystamont*®)

Nystan® (Squibb) P̶o̶M̶
Tablets, brown, s/c, nystatin 500 000 units, net price 56-tab pack = £4.70. Label: 9
Suspension, yellow, nystatin 100 000 units/mL, net price 30 mL with pipette = £2.05. Label: 9, counselling, use of pipette

TERBINAFINE

Indications: dermatophyte infections of the nails, ringworm infections (including tinea pedis, cruris, and corporis) where oral therapy appropriate (due to site, severity or extent)

Cautions: hepatic and renal impairment (Appendixes 2 and 3); pregnancy, breast-feeding (Appendix 5); psoriasis (risk of exacerbation); autoimmune disease (risk of lupus-erythematosus-like effect) **interactions:** Appendix 1 (terbinafine)

Side-effects: abdominal discomfort, anorexia, nausea, diarrhoea; headache; rash and urticaria occasionally with arthralgia or myalgia; less frequently taste disturbance; rarely liver toxicity (including jaundice, cholestasis and hepatitis) — discontinue treatment, angioedema, dizziness, malaise, paraesthesia, hypoaesthesia, photosensitivity, serious skin reactions (including Stevens-Johnson syndrome and toxic epidermal necrolysis) —discontinue treatment if progressive skin rash; also reported, psychiatric disturbances, blood disorders (including leucopenia and thrombocytopenia)

Dose: 250 mg daily usually for 2–6 weeks in tinea pedis, 2–4 weeks in tinea cruris, 4 weeks in tinea corporis, 6 weeks–3 months in nail infections (occasionally longer in toenail infections); CHILD [unlicensed] usually for 2 weeks, tinea capitis, over 1 year, body-weight 10–20 kg, 62.5 mg once daily; body-weight 20–40 kg, 125 mg once daily; body-weight over 40 kg, 250 mg once daily

Lamisil® (Novartis) PoM
Tablets, off-white, scored, terbinafine 250 mg (as hydrochloride), net price 14-tab pack = £23.16, 28-tab pack = £44.66. Label: 9

VORICONAZOLE
Indications: invasive aspergillosis; serious infections caused by *Scedosporium* spp., *Fusarium* spp., or invasive fluconazole-resistant *Candida* spp. (including *C. krusei*)
Cautions: monitor liver function before treatment and during treatment; haematological malignancy (increased risk of hepatic reactions); hepatic impairment (Appendix 2); monitor renal function; renal impairment (Appendix 3); pregnancy (ensure effective contraception during treatment—Appendix 4); electrolyte disturbances, cardiomyopathy, bradycardia, symptomatic arrhythmias, history of QT interval prolongation, concomitant use with other drugs that prolong QT interval; avoid exposure to sunlight; **interactions:** Appendix 1 (antifungals, triazole)
Contra-indications: breast-feeding (Appendix 5)
Side-effects: nausea, vomiting, abdominal pain, diarrhoea, peripheral oedema, headache, fever, visual disturbances including altered perception, blurred vision, changes in coloured vision and photophobia (usually transient and reversible), rash; also commonly jaundice, cheilitis, hypotension, chest pain, respiratory distress syndrome, pulmonary oedema, influenza-like symptoms, dizziness, asthenia, anxiety, depression, confusion, agitation, hallucinations, paraesthesia, tremor, acute renal failure, haematuria, pruritus, exfoliative dermatitis, injection-site reactions and infusion-related reactions including flushing, photosensitivity, alopecia, blood disorders (including anaemia, thrombocytopenia, leucopenia, pancytopenia), hypokalaemia, hypoglycaemia; less commonly taste disturbances, gingivitis, glossitis, dyspepsia, duodenitis, constipation, cholecystitis, pancreatitis, hepatitis, arrhythmias (including QT interval prolongation), syncope, adrenocortical insufficiency, hypersensitivity reactions (including anaphylactoid reactions, urticaria, angioedema, dyspnoea), hypoaesthesia, ataxia, nystagmus, diplopia, cerebral oedema, arthritis, psoriasis, Stevens-Johnson syndrome, blepharitis, optic neuritis, papilloedema, scleritis, raised serum cholesterol; rarely pseudomembranous colitis, extrapyramidal effects, hypertonia, hypothyroidism, hyperthyroidism, discoid lupus erythematosus, toxic epidermal necrolysis, retinal haemorrhage, optic atrophy
Dose: *by mouth*, ADULT and ADOLESCENT over 12 years, body-weight over 40 kg, 400 mg every 12 hours for 2 doses then 200 mg every 12 hours, increased if necessary to 300 mg every 12 hours; body-weight under 40 kg, 200 mg every 12 hours for 2 doses then 100 mg every 12 hours, increased if necessary to 150 mg every 12 hours; CHILD 2–11 years, 6 mg/kg every 12 hours for 2 doses, then 4 mg/kg every 12 hours
By intravenous infusion, ADULT and CHILD over 2 years, 6 mg/kg every 12 hours for 2 doses, then 4 mg/kg every 12 hours (reduced in ADULT and ADOLESCENT over 12 years to 3 mg/kg every 12 hours if not tolerated) for max. 6 months

Vfend® (Pfizer) ▼ PoM
Tablets, f/c, voriconazole 50 mg, net price 28-tablet pack = £227.84; 200 mg, 28-tab pack = £911.36.
Label: 11, counselling, administration
COUNSELLING. Tablets to be taken at least 1 hour before or one hour after food
Intravenous infusion, powder for reconstitution, voriconazole, net price 200-mg vial = £77.14
Excipients: include sulphobutylether beta cyclodextrin sodium (risk of accumulation in renal impairment)
Electrolytes: Na⁺ 9.62 mmol/vial

5.3 Antiviral drugs

The majority of virus infections resolve spontaneously in immunocompetent subjects. A number of specific treatments for viral infections are available, particularly for the immunocompromised. This section includes notes on herpes simplex and varicella-zoster, human immunodeficiency virus, cytomegalovirus, respiratory syncytial virus, viral hepatitis and influenza.

Herpes simplex and varicella–zoster

Aciclovir is active against herpes viruses but does not eradicate them. It is effective only if started at the onset of the episode. Uses of aciclovir include the systemic treatment of varicella–zoster (chickenpox—shingles) and the systemic and topical treatment of herpes simplex infections of the skin and mucous membranes (including initial and recurrent genital herpes); it is also used topically in the eye. It can be life-saving in herpes simplex and varicella–zoster infections in the immunocompromised, and is also used for prevention of recurrence and for herpes simplex prophylaxis in the immunocompromised. Aciclovir may also be given by mouth to immunocompetent adults and older adolescents with chickenpox; it is not generally indicated for immunocompetent children in whom the disease is milder. See also section 11.3.3 (eye) and section 13.10.3 (skin, including herpes labialis).

Famciclovir, a prodrug of penciclovir, is similar to aciclovir and it is recommended for herpes zoster and initial and recurrent genital herpes. Penciclovir itself is used as a cream for herpes simplex labialis (section 13.10.3). **Valaciclovir** is an ester of aciclovir which is licensed for herpes zoster and for herpes simplex infections of the skin and mucous membranes (including initial and recurrent genital herpes). Valaciclovir is also licensed for preventing cytomegalovirus disease following renal transplantation.

Idoxuridine (section 13.10.3) is also only effective if started at the onset of infection; it is too toxic for systemic use. It has been used topically in the treatment of herpes simplex lesions of the skin and external genitalia with variable results; it has also been used topically in the treatment of zoster, but evidence of its value is dubious.

Inosine pranobex has been used by mouth for herpes simplex infections; its effectiveness has not been established.

ACICLOVIR
(Acyclovir)
Indications: herpes simplex and varicella–zoster (see also under Dose)

Cautions: maintain adequate hydration (especially with infusion or high doses); renal impairment (Appendix 3); pregnancy and breast-feeding; **interactions:** Appendix 1 (aciclovir)

Side-effects: nausea, vomiting, abdominal pain, diarrhoea, headache, fatigue, rash, urticaria, pruritus, photosensitivity; rarely hepatitis, jaundice, dyspnoea, angioedema, anaphylaxis, neurological reactions (including dizziness, confusion, hallucinations and drowsiness), acute renal failure, decreases in haematological indices; on *intravenous infusion*, severe local inflammation (sometimes leading to ulceration), fever, and rarely agitation, tremors, psychosis and convulsions

Dose: *by mouth*, herpes simplex, treatment, 200 mg (400 mg in the immunocompromised or if absorption impaired) 5 times daily, usually for 5 days; CHILD under 2 years, half adult dose, over 2 years, adult dose

Herpes simplex, prevention of recurrence, 200 mg 4 times daily *or* 400 mg twice daily possibly reduced to 200 mg 2 or 3 times daily and interrupted every 6–12 months

Herpes simplex, prophylaxis in the immunocompromised, 200–400 mg 4 times daily; CHILD under 2 years, half adult dose, over 2 years, adult dose

Varicella and herpes zoster, treatment, 800 mg 5 times daily for 7 days; CHILD, varicella, 20 mg/kg (max. 800 mg) 4 times daily for 5 days *or* under 2 years 200 mg 4 times daily, 2–5 years 400 mg 4 times daily, over 6 years 800 mg 4 times daily

By intravenous infusion, treatment of herpes simplex in the immunocompromised, severe initial genital herpes, and varicella–zoster, 5 mg/kg every 8 hours usually for 5 days, doubled to 10 mg/kg every 8 hours in varicella–zoster in the immunocompromised and in simplex encephalitis (usually given for 10 days in encephalitis); prophylaxis of herpes simplex in the immunocompromised, 5 mg/kg every 8 hours

NEONATE and INFANT up to 3 months, herpes simplex, 10 mg/kg every 8 hours usually for 10 days; CHILD 3 months–12 years, herpes simplex or varicella–zoster, 250 mg/m² every 8 hours usually for 5 days, doubled to 500 mg/m² every 8 hours for varicella–zoster in the immunocompromised and in simplex encephalitis (usually given for 10 days in encephalitis)

By topical application, see sections 13.10.3 (skin) and 11.3.3 (eye)

Aciclovir (Non-proprietary) PoM
Tablets, aciclovir 200 mg, net price 25-tab pack = £4.46; 400 mg, 56-tab pack = £7.41; 800 mg, 35-tab pack = £45.10. Label: 9
Available from Alpharma, CP, Opus (*Virovir*®), Sovereign, Sterwin, Zurich
Dispersible tablets, aciclovir 200 mg, net price 25-tab pack = £6.25; 400 mg, 56-tab pack = £22.56; 800 mg, 35-tab pack = £22.52. Label: 9
Available from Hillcross, IVAX, Pharmacia, Ranbaxy, Sanofi-Synthelabo, Sterwin
Intravenous infusion, powder for reconstitution, aciclovir (as sodium salt). Net price 250-mg vial = £10.09; 500-mg vial = £14.11
Electrolytes: Na⁺ 1.1 mmol/250-mg vial
Available from Genus, Sovereign, Zurich
Intravenous infusion, aciclovir (as sodium salt), 25 mg/mL, net price 10-mL (250-mg) vial =

£10.37; 20-mL (500-mg) vial = £19.21; 40-mL (1-g) vial = £40.44
Electrolytes: Na⁺ 1.16 mmol/250-mg vial
Available from Mayne

Zovirax® (GSK) PoM
Tablets, all dispersible, f/c, aciclovir 200 mg (blue), net price 25-tab pack = £20.22; 400 mg (pink), 56-tab pack = £74.17; 800 mg (scored, *Shingles Treatment Pack*), 35-tab pack = £75.11. Label: 9
Suspension, both off-white, sugar-free, aciclovir 200 mg/5 mL (banana-flavoured), net price 125 mL = £31.78; 400 mg/5 mL (*Double Strength Suspension*, orange-flavoured) 100 mL = £35.51. Label: 9
Intravenous infusion, powder for reconstitution, aciclovir (as sodium salt). Net price 250-mg vial = £10.91; 500-mg vial = £20.22
Electrolytes: Na⁺ 1.1 mmol/250-mg vial

FAMCICLOVIR

NOTE. Famciclovir is a pro-drug of penciclovir

Indications: treatment of herpes zoster, acute genital herpes simplex and suppression of recurrent genital herpes

Cautions: renal impairment (Appendix 3); pregnancy and breast-feeding; **interactions:** Appendix 1 (famciclovir)

Side-effects: nausea, vomiting; headache; rarely dizziness, confusion, hallucinations, rash; abdominal pain and fever have been reported in immunocompromised patients

Dose: herpes zoster, 250 mg 3 times daily for 7 days *or* 750 mg once daily for 7 days (in immunocompromised, 500 mg 3 times daily for 10 days)
Genital herpes, first episode, 250 mg 3 times daily for 5 days; recurrent infection, 125 mg twice daily for 5 days (in immunocompromised, all episodes, 500 mg twice daily for 7 days)
Genital herpes, suppression, 250 mg twice daily (in HIV patients, 500 mg twice daily) interrupted every 6–12 months
CHILD not recommended

Famvir® (Novartis) PoM
Tablets, all f/c, famciclovir 125 mg, net price 10-tab pack = £28.12; 250 mg, 15-tab pack = £84.35, 21-tab pack = £118.08; 56-tab pack = £314.90; 500 mg, 14-tab pack = £157.47, 30-tab pack = £337.34, 56-tab pack = £629.89; 750 mg, 7-tab pack = £112.72. Label: 9

INOSINE PRANOBEX

Indications: see under Dose

Cautions: avoid in renal impairment; history of gout or hyperuricaemia

Contra-indications: pregnancy

Side-effects: reversible increase in serum and urinary uric acid

Dose: mucocutaneous herpes simplex, 1 g 4 times daily for 7–14 days
Adjunctive treatment of genital warts, 1 g 3 times daily for 14–28 days
Subacute sclerosing panencephalitis, 50–100 mg/kg daily in 6 divided doses

Imunovir® (Ardern) PoM
Tablets, inosine pranobex 500 mg. Net price 100 = £39.50. Label: 9

VALACICLOVIR

NOTE. Valaciclovir is a pro-drug of aciclovir

Indications: treatment of herpes zoster; treatment of initial and suppression of recurrent herpes simplex infections of skin and mucous membranes including initial and recurrent genital herpes; prevention of cytomegalovirus disease following renal transplantation

Cautions: see under Aciclovir; hepatic impairment (Appendix 2)

Side-effects: see under Aciclovir but neurological reactions more frequent with high doses

Dose: herpes zoster, 1 g 3 times daily for 7 days

Herpes simplex, first episode, 500 mg twice daily for 5 days (up to 10 days if severe); recurrent infection, 500 mg twice daily for 5 days

Herpes simplex, suppression, 500 mg daily in 1–2 divided doses (in immunocompromised, 500 mg twice daily)

Prevention of cytomegalovirus disease following renal transplantation (preferably starting within 72 hours of transplantation), 2 g 4 times daily usually for 90 days

CHILD not recommended

Valtrex® (GSK) PoM

Tablets, f/c, valaciclovir (as hydrochloride) 500 mg, net price 10-tab pack = £23.50, 42-tab pack = £98.50. Label: 9

Human immunodeficiency virus

There is no cure for infection caused by the human immunodeficiency virus (HIV) but a number of drugs slow or halt disease progression. Drugs for HIV infection (antiretrovirals) increase life expectancy considerably but they are toxic. Treatment should be undertaken only by those experienced in their use. Advice on the management of HIV changes rapidly .

PRINCIPLES OF TREATMENT. Treatment is aimed at reducing the plasma viral load as much as possible and for as long as possible; it should be started before the immune system is irreversibly damaged. The need for early drug treatment should, however, be balanced against the development of toxicity. Commitment to treatment and strict adherence over many years are required; the regimen chosen should take into account convenience and patient tolerance. The development of drug resistance is reduced by using a combination of drugs; such combinations should have synergistic or additive activity while ensuring that their toxicity is not additive. Testing for resistance to antiviral drugs particularly in therapeutic failure should be considered.

INITIATION OF TREATMENT. The optimum time for initiation of antiviral treatment will depend primarily on the CD4 cell count; the plasma viral load and clinical symptoms may also help. Initiating treatment with a combination of drugs ('highly active antiretroviral therapy' which includes 2 nucleoside reverse transcriptase inhibitors with *either* a non-nucleoside reverse transcriptase inhibitor *or* 1 or 2 protease inhibitors) is recommended.

SWITCHING THERAPY. Deterioration of the condition (including clinical and virological changes) may require either switching therapy or adding another antiviral drug. The choice of an alternative regimen depends on factors such as the response to previous treatment, tolerance and the possibility of cross-resistance.

PREGNANCY AND BREAST-FEEDING. Treatment of HIV infection in pregnancy aims to reduce the risk of toxicity to the fetus (although the teratogenic potential of most antiretroviral drugs is unknown), to minimise the viral load and disease progression in the mother, and to prevent transmission of infection to the neonate. **All treatment options require careful assessment by a specialist.** Zidovudine monotherapy reduces transmission of infection to the neonate. However, combination antiretroviral therapy maximises the chance of preventing transmission and represents optimal therapy for the mother.

Breast-feeding by HIV-positive mothers may cause HIV infection in the infant and should be avoided.

POST-EXPOSURE PROPHYLAXIS. Post-exposure prophylaxis with antiretroviral drugs [unlicensed indication] may be appropriate following occupational exposure to HIV-contaminated material. Immediate expert advice should be sought in such cases; national guidelines on post-exposure prophylaxis for healthcare workers have been developed (by the Chief Medical Officer's Expert Advisory Group on AIDS) and local ones may also be available. Treatment is chosen on the basis of efficacy and antiretrovirals with a high potential for toxicity are not appropriate for prophylaxis.

DRUGS USED FOR HIV INFECTION. **Zidovudine**, a nucleoside reverse transcriptase inhibitor (or 'nucleoside analogue'), was the first anti-HIV drug to be introduced. Higher doses of zidovudine alone were used to prevent the AIDS dementia complex but combination therapy including zidovudine at standard doses is now preferred. Other nucleoside reverse transcriptase inhibitors include **abacavir**, **didanosine**, **emtricitabine**, **lamivudine**, **stavudine**, **tenofovir**, and **zalcitabine**.

The protease inhibitors include **amprenavir**, **indinavir**, **lopinavir**, **nelfinavir**, **ritonavir**, and **saquinavir**. Ritonavir in low doses (typically 100 mg twice daily) boosts the activity of amprenavir, indinavir, lopinavir, and saquinavir increasing the persistence of plasma concentrations of these drugs; at such a low dose, ritonavir has no intrinsic antiviral activity. A combination of lopinavir with low-dose ritonavir is available. The protease inhibitors are metabolised by cytochrome P450 enzyme systems and therefore have a significant potential for drug interactions. Protease inhibitors are associated with lipodystrophy and metabolic effects (see below).

The non-nucleoside reverse transcriptase inhibitors **efavirenz** and **nevirapine** may interact with a number of drugs metabolised in the liver. Nevirapine is associated with a high incidence of rash (including Stevens-Johnson syndrome) and occasionally fatal hepatitis. Rash is also associated with efavirenz but it is usually milder. Efavirenz treatment has also been associated with an increased plasma cholesterol concentration.

Enfuvirtide, which inhibits HIV from fusing to the host cell, is licensed for managing infection that has failed to respond to a regimen of other antiretroviral drugs; enfuvirtide should be combined with other potentially active antiretroviral drugs.

LIPODYSTROPHY AND METABOLIC EFFECTS. The MHRA (formerly MCA) has advised that combination antiretroviral therapy, including regimens containing a protease inhibitor, is associated with redistribution of body fat in some patients (e.g. decreased fat under the skin, increased abdominal fat, 'buffalo humps' and breast enlargement). Protease inhibitors are also associated with metabolic abnormalities such as hyperlipidaemia, insulin resistance, and hyperglycaemia. Clinical examination should include an evaluation of fat distribution; measurement of serum lipids and blood glucose should be considered.

Nucleoside reverse transcriptase inhibitors

ABACAVIR
Indications: HIV infection in combination with other antiretroviral drugs
Cautions: hepatic impairment (see below and Appendix 2); renal impairment (Appendix 3); **interactions:** Appendix 1 (abacavir)
HYPERSENSITIVITY REACTIONS. Life-threatening hypersensitivity reactions reported—characterised by fever or rash and possibly nausea, vomiting, diarrhoea, abdominal pain, lethargy, malaise, headache, myalgia and renal failure; less frequently mouth ulceration, oedema, hypotension, dyspnoea, sore throat, cough, paraesthesia, arthralgia, conjunctivitis, lymphadenopathy, lymphocytopenia and anaphylaxis (CSM has identified hypersensitivity reactions presenting as sore throat, influenza-like illness, cough and breathlessness); rarely myolysis; laboratory abnormalities may include raised liver function tests (see below) and creatine phosphokinase; symptoms usually appear in the first 6 weeks, but may occur at any time; monitor for symptoms every 2 weeks for 2 months; discontinue immediately if any symptom of hypersensitivity develops and do not rechallenge (risk of more severe hypersensitivity reaction); discontinue if hypersensitivity cannot be ruled out, even when other diagnoses possible—if rechallenge necessary it must be carried out in hospital setting; if abacavir is stopped for any reason other than hypersensitivity, exclude hypersensitivity reaction as the cause and rechallenge only if medical assistance is readily available; care needed with concomitant use of drugs which cause skin toxicity
COUNSELLING. Patients should be told the importance of regular dosing (intermittent therapy may increase the risk of sensitisation), how to recognise signs of hypersensitivity, and advised to seek immediate medical attention if symptoms develop or before re-starting treatment; patients should be advised to keep Alert card with them at all times
HEPATIC DISEASE. Potentially life-threatening lactic acidosis and severe hepatomegaly with steatosis reported therefore caution in liver disease, liver enzyme abnormalities, or risk factors for liver disease (particularly in obese women); suspend or discontinue if deterioration in liver function tests, hepatic steatosis, progressive hepatomegaly or unexplained lactic acidosis
Contra-indications: pregnancy (Appendix 4); breast-feeding
Side-effects: hypersensitivity reactions (see above), nausea, vomiting, diarrhoea, anorexia, lethargy, fatigue, fever, headache, pancreatitis, lactic acidosis (see above), hepatitis (see above); rash and gastro-intestinal disturbances more common in children
Dose: 300 mg every 12 hours; CHILD 3 months–12 years, 8 mg/kg every 12 hours (max. 600 mg daily)

Ziagen® (GSK) [PoM]
Tablets, yellow, f/c, abacavir (as sulphate) 300 mg, net price 60-tab pack = £238.50. Counselling, hypersensitivity reactions
Oral solution, sugar-free, banana and strawberry flavoured, abacavir (as sulphate) 20 mg/ml, net price 240-mL = £63.60. Counselling, hypersensitivity reactions

■ With lamivudine and zidovudine
Trizivir® (GSK) [PoM]
Tablets, blue-green, f/c, abacavir (as sulphate) 300 mg, lamivudine 150 mg, zidovudine 300 mg, net price 60-tab pack = £581.08. Counselling, hypersensitivity reactions
Dose: ADULT over 18 years, 1 tablet twice daily
NOTE. For patients stabilised (for 6–8 weeks) on the individual components in the same proportions. For cautions, contra-indications and side-effects of individual drugs see Abacavir, Lamivudine and Zidovudine

DIDANOSINE
(ddI, DDI)
Indications: HIV infection in combination with other antiretroviral drugs
Cautions: history of pancreatitis (preferably avoid, otherwise extreme caution, see also below); peripheral neuropathy or hyperuricaemia (see under Side-effects); history of liver disease (see below); hepatic and renal impairment (see Appendixes 2 and 3); pregnancy; dilated retinal examinations recommended (especially in children) every 6 months, or if visual changes occur; **interactions:** Appendix 1 (didanosine)
PANCREATITIS. If symptoms of pancreatitis develop or if serum amylase or lipase is raised (even if asymptomatic) suspend treatment until diagnosis of pancreatitis excluded; on return to normal values re-initiate treatment only if essential (using low dose increased gradually if appropriate). Whenever possible avoid concomitant treatment with other drugs known to cause pancreatic toxicity (e.g. intravenous pentamidine isetionate); monitor closely if concomitant therapy unavoidable. Since significant elevations of triglycerides cause pancreatitis monitor closely if elevated
HEPATIC DISEASE. Potentially life-threatening lactic acidosis and severe hepatomegaly with steatosis reported therefore caution in liver disease (especially in hepatitis C treated with interferon alfa and ribavirin), excessive alcohol intake liver enzyme abnormalities, or risk factors for liver disease (particularly in obese women); suspend or discontinue if deterioration in liver function tests, hepatic steatosis, progressive hepatomegaly or lactic acidosis
Contra-indications: breast-feeding
Side-effects: diarrhoea, nausea, vomiting, abdominal pain, peripheral neuropathy especially in advanced HIV infection—suspend (reduced dose may be tolerated when symptoms resolve), headache, fatigue, rash, hyperuricaemia (suspend if raised significantly); less frequently, pancreatitis (see also under Cautions), abnormal liver function tests (see also under Cautions); rarely, flatulence, dry mouth, parotid gland enlargement, anorexia, sialadenitis, hepatitis, liver failure, anaphylactic reactions, fever, arthralgia, mylagia, rhabdomyolysis, dry eyes, retinal and optic nerve changes (especially in children), alopecia, diabetes mellitus, hypoglycaemia, anaemia, leucopenia, and thrombocytopenia
Dose: ADULT under 60 kg 250 mg daily in 1–2 divided doses, 60 kg and over 400 mg daily in 1–2

divided doses; CHILD over 3 months (under 6 years *Videx*® tablets only), 240 mg/m² daily (180 mg/m² daily in combination with zidovudine) in 1–2 divided doses

Videx® (Bristol-Myers Squibb) PoM
Tablets, both with calcium and magnesium antacids, didanosine 25 mg, net price 60-tab pack = £28.60; 200 mg, 60-tab pack = £176.00. Label: 23, counselling, administration, see below
Excipients: include aspartame equivalent to phenylalanine 36.5 mg per tablet (section 9.4.1)
NOTE. Antacids in formulation may affect absorption of other drugs—see **interactions:** Appendix 1 (antacids)
COUNSELLING. To ensure sufficient antacid, each dose to be taken as 2 tablets (CHILD under 1 year 1 tablet) chewed thoroughly, crushed or dispersed in water; clear apple juice may be added to flavour
Videx® *EC capsules*, enclosing e/c granules, didanosine 125 mg, net price 30-cap pack = £55.00; 200 mg, 30-cap pack = £88.00; 250 mg, 30-cap pack = £110.00; 400 mg, 30-cap pack = £176.00. Label: 25, counselling, administration, see below
COUNSELLING. Capsules to be taken at least 2 hours before or 2 hours after food; if tenofovir also used, both may be given with food

EMTRICITABINE

Indications: HIV infection in combination with other antiretroviral drugs

Cautions: chronic hepatitis B or C; (increased risk of hepatic side-effects; see also Hepatic Disease below); renal impairment (Appendix 3); pregnancy (Appendix 4); **interactions:** Appendix 1 (emtricitabine)
HEPATIC DISEASE. Potentially life-threatening lactic acidosis and severe hepatomegaly with steatosis reported, therefore, caution in liver disease (especially in hepatitis C treated with interferon alfa and ribavirin), liver enzyme abnormalities, or risk factors for liver disease (particularly in obese women); suspend or discontinue if deterioration in liver function, hepatic steatosis, progressive hepatomegaly or lactic acidosis. On discontinuation, monitor closely patients with hepatitis B—risk of exacerbation of hepatitis

Contra-indications: breast-feeding

Side-effects: see cautions above; diarrhoea, nausea, headache, raised creatine kinase; less frequently vomiting, dyspepsia, abdominal pain, dizziness, asthenia, insomnia, abnormal dreams, rash, pruritus, urticaria, hyperpigmentation, raised serum amylase and lipase, raised liver enzymes (see Hepatic Disease above), hypertriglyceridaemia, hyperglycaemia, neutropenia, anaemia

Dose: ADULT and CHILD body-weight over 33 kg, 200 mg once daily

Emtriva® (Gilead) ▼ PoM
Capsules, white/blue, emtricitabine 200 mg, net price 30-cap pack = £163.50

LAMIVUDINE
(3TC)
Indications: see preparations below
Cautions: renal impairment (Appendix 3), hepatic disease (see below); pregnancy (Appendix 4); **interactions:** Appendix 1 (lamivudine)
HEPATIC DISEASE. Potentially life-threatening lactic acidosis and severe hepatomegaly with steatosis reported therefore caution (particularly in obese women) in liver disease, liver enzyme abnormalities, or risk factors for liver disease; suspend or discontinue if deterioration in liver function tests, hepatic steatosis, progressive hepatomegaly or unexplained lactic acidosis. Recurrent hepatitis

in patients with chronic hepatitis B may occur on discontinuation of lamivudine. When treating chronic hepatitis B with lamivudine, monitor liver function tests at least every 3 months and serological markers of hepatitis B every 6 months, more frequently in patients with advanced liver disease or following transplantation (monitoring to continue after discontinuation)—consult product literature

Contra-indications: breast-feeding
Side-effects: nausea, vomiting, diarrhoea, abdominal pain; cough; headache, fatigue, insomnia; malaise, fever, rash, alopecia, muscle disorders; nasal symptoms; peripheral neuropathy reported; rarely pancreatitis (discontinue); neutropenia, anaemia, thrombocytopenia, and red cell aplasia; lactic acidosis; raised liver enzymes and serum amylase reported

Dose: see preparations below

Epivir® (GSK) PoM
Tablets, f/c, lamivudine 150 mg, net price 60-tab pack = £163.59; 300 mg, 30-tab pack = £179.80
Oral solution, banana- and strawberry-flavoured, lamivudine 50 mg/5 mL, net price 240-mL pack = £44.53
Excipients: include sucrose 1 g/5 mL
Dose: HIV infection in combination with other antiretroviral drugs, 150 mg every 12 hours *or* 300 mg once daily; CHILD 3 months–12 years, 4 mg/kg every 12 hours; max. 300 mg daily

Zeffix® (GSK) PoM
Tablets, brown, f/c, lamivudine 100 mg, net price 28-tab pack = £83.97
Oral solution, banana and strawberry flavoured, lamivudine 25 mg/5 mL, net price 240-mL pack = £24.50
Excipients: include sucrose 1 g/5 mL
Dose: chronic hepatitis B infection (with evidence of viral replication and histology of active liver inflammation or fibrosis), 100 mg daily; CHILD [unlicensed indication] 2–11 years, 3 mg/kg once daily (max. 100 mg daily); 12–17 years, adult dose; patients receiving lamivudine for concomitant HIV infection should continue to receive lamivudine in a dose appropriate for HIV infection

■ With zidovudine
See under Zidovudine

■ With abacavir and zidovudine
See under Abacavir

STAVUDINE
(d4T)
Indications: HIV infection in combination with other antiretroviral drugs
Cautions: history of peripheral neuropathy (see below); history of pancreatitis or concomitant use with other drugs associated with pancreatitis; hepatic disease (see below); renal impairment (Appendix 3); pregnancy (Appendix 4); **interactions:** Appendix 1 (stavudine)
PERIPHERAL NEUROPATHY. Suspend if peripheral neuropathy develops—characterised by persistent numbness, tingling or pain in feet or hands; if symptoms resolve satisfactorily on withdrawal and if stavudine needs to be continued, resume treatment at half previous dose
HEPATIC DISEASE. Potentially life-threatening lactic acidosis and severe hepatomegaly with steatosis reported therefore caution in liver disease (especially in hepatitis treated with interferon alfa and ribavirin), liver enzyme abnormalities, or risk factors for liver disease (particularly in obese women); suspend or discontinue if deterioration in liver function tests, hepatic steatosis, progressive hepatomegaly or lactic acidosis

Contra-indications: breast-feeding

Side-effects: diarrhoea, nausea, abdominal pain, dyspepsia; peripheral neuropathy, dizziness, headache, drowsiness, insomnia, abnormal dreams, depression, fatigue; lipodystrophy; rash, pruritus; less commonly pancreatitis, hepatitis, jaundice, anorexia, lactic acidosis (see Hepatic Disease under Cautions), anxiety, mood disorders, gynaecomastia, arthralgia, myalgia; very rarely thrombocytopenia

Dose: ADULT under 60 kg, 30 mg every 12 hours preferably at least 1 hour before food; 60 kg and over, 40 mg every 12 hours; CHILD over 3 months, under 30 kg, 1 mg/kg every 12 hours; 30 kg and over, adult dose

Zerit® (Bristol-Myers Squibb) [PoM]
Capsules, stavudine 15 mg (yellow/red), net price 56-cap pack = £153.87; 20 mg (brown), 56-cap pack = £159.19; 30 mg (light orange/dark orange), 56-cap pack = £166.94; 40 mg (dark orange), 56-cap pack = £171.98 (all hosp. only)
Oral solution, cherry-flavoured, stavudine for reconstitution with water, 1 mg/mL, net price 200 mL = £24.50

TENOFOVIR DISOPROXIL

Indications: HIV infection in combination with other antiretroviral drugs

Cautions: renal impairment (Appendix 3)—test renal function and serum phosphate before treatment, then every 4 weeks (weekly if given with nephrotoxic drug e.g. cidofovir or in patients with renal impairment), interrupt treatment if renal function deteriorates or serum phosphate decreases; pregnancy (Appendix 4); **interactions:** Appendix 1 (tenofovir)
HEPATIC DISEASE. Potentially life-threatening lactic acidosis and severe hepatomegaly with steatosis reported, therefore, caution in liver disease (especially in hepatitis C treated with interferon alfa and ribavirin), liver enzyme abnormalities, or risk factors for liver disease (particularly in obese women); suspend or discontinue if deterioration in liver function tests, hepatic steatosis, progressive hepatomegaly or lactic acidosis

Contra-indications: breast-feeding

Side-effects: diarrhoea, nausea, vomiting, flatulence, dizziness, hypophosphataemia; also reported, pancreatitis, lactic acidosis (see Cautions above), dyspnoea, asthenia, rash, renal failure

Dose: ADULT over 18 years, 245 mg once daily

Viread® (Gilead) ▼ [PoM]
Tablets, f/c, blue, tenofovir disoproxil (as fumarate) 245 mg, net price 30-tab pack = £255.00. Label: 21, counselling, administration
COUNSELLING. Patients with swallowing difficulties may disperse tablet in half a glass of water or orange juice

---

ZALCITABINE

(ddC, DDC)

Indications: HIV infection in combination with other antiretroviral drugs

Cautions: patients at risk of developing peripheral neuropathy (see below); pancreatitis (see also below)—monitor serum amylase in those with history of elevated serum amylase, pancreatitis, alcohol abuse, or receiving parenteral nutrition; cardiomyopathy, history of congestive cardiac failure; hepatotoxicity (see below); pregnancy (women of childbearing age should use effective contraception during treatment); renal impairment

(Appendix 3); **interactions:** Appendix 1 (zalcitabine)
PERIPHERAL NEUROPATHY. Discontinue immediately if peripheral neuropathy develops—characterised by numbness and burning dysaesthesia possibly followed by sharp shooting pains or severe continuous burning and potentially irreversible pain; extreme caution and close monitoring required in those at risk of peripheral neuropathy (especially those with low CD4 cell count for whom risk is greater and those receiving another drug known to cause peripheral neuropathy)
PANCREATITIS. Discontinue permanently if clinical pancreatitis develops; suspend if raised serum amylase associated with dysglycaemia, rising triglyceride, decreasing serum calcium or other signs of impending pancreatitis until pancreatitis excluded; suspend if treatment required with another drug known to cause pancreatic toxicity (e.g. intravenous pentamidine isetionate); caution and close monitoring if history of pancreatitis (or of elevated serum amylase) or if at risk of pancreatitis
HEPATIC DISEASE. Potentially life-threatening lactic acidosis and severe hepatomegaly with steatosis reported therefore caution in liver disease, liver enzyme abnormalities, or history of alcohol abuse or hepatitis; suspend or discontinue if deterioration in liver function tests, hepatic steatosis, progressive hepatomegaly or unexplained lactic acidosis

Contra-indications: peripheral neuropathy (see also above); breast-feeding

Side-effects: peripheral neuropathy (discontinue immediately, see also above); oral ulcers, nausea, vomiting, dysphagia, anorexia, diarrhoea, abdominal pain, constipation; pharyngitis; headache, dizziness; myalgia, arthralgia; rash, pruritus, sweating, weight loss, fatigue, fever, rigors, chest pain, anaemia, leucopenia, neutropenia, thrombocytopenia, disorders of liver function; less frequently pancreatitis (see also above), oesophageal ulcers (suspend treatment if no response to treatment for specific organisms), rectal ulcers, jaundice and hepatocellular damage (see also under Cautions); other less frequent side-effects include taste, hearing and visual disturbances, tachycardia, cardiomyopathy, congestive heart failure, dyspnoea, seizures, tremor, movement disorders, mood changes, sleep disturbances, alopecia, hyperuricaemia and renal disorders

Dose: 750 micrograms every 8 hours; CHILD under 13 years safety and efficacy not established

Hivid® (Roche) [PoM]
Tablets, both f/c, zalcitabine 375 micrograms (beige), net price 100-tab pack = £99.51; 750 micrograms (grey), 100-tab pack = £151.57

ZIDOVUDINE

(Azidothymidine, AZT)

NOTE. The abbreviation AZT which has sometimes been used for zidovudine has also been used for another drug

Indications: HIV infection in combination with other antiretroviral drugs; for prevention of maternal-fetal HIV transmission (see notes above under Pregnancy and Breast-feeding)

Cautions: haematological toxicity (blood tests at least every 2 weeks for first 3 months then at least once a month, early disease with good bone marrow reserves may require less frequent tests e.g. every 1–3 months); vitamin B_{12} deficiency (increased risk of neutropenia); reduce dose or interrupt treatment according to product literature if anaemia or myelosuppression; renal impairment (Appendix 3); hepatic impairment (see below and Appendix 2); risk of lactic acidosis, (see below);

elderly; pregnancy; **interactions:** Appendix 1 (zidovudine)

HEPATIC DISEASE. Potentially life threatening lactic acidosis and severe hepatomegaly with steatosis reported therefore caution in liver disease (especially in chronic hepatitis C treated with interferon alfa and ribavirin), liver enzyme abnormalities, or risk factors for liver disease (particularly in obese women), suspend or discontinue if deterioration in liver function tests, hepatic steatosis, progressive hepatomegaly or lactic acidosis

Contra-indications: abnormally low neutrophil counts or haemoglobin values (consult product literature); neonates with hyperbilirubinaemia requiring treatment other than phototherapy, or with raised transaminase (consult product literature); breast-feeding

Side-effects: anaemia (may require transfusion), neutropenia, and leucopenia (all more frequent with high dose and advanced disease); also include, nausea and vomiting, abdominal pain, dyspepsia, diarrhoea, flatulence, taste disturbance, pancreatitis, liver disorders including fatty change and raised bilirubin and liver enzymes (see also under Cautions); chest pain, dyspnoea, cough; influenza-like symptoms, headache, fever, paraesthesia, neuropathy, convulsions, dizziness, somnolence, insomnia, anxiety, depression, loss of mental acuity, malaise, anorexia, asthenia, myopathy, myalgia; pancytopenia, thrombocytopenia; gynaecomastia; urinary frequency; rash, pruritus, pigmentation of nail, skin and oral mucosa

Dose: *by mouth*, 500–600 mg daily in 2–3 divided doses; CHILD over 3 months 360–480 mg/m^2 daily in 3–4 divided doses; max. 200 mg every 6 hours

Prevention of maternal-fetal HIV transmission, seek specialist advice (combination therapy preferred)

Patients temporarily unable to take zidovudine by mouth, *by intravenous infusion* over 1 hour, 1–2 mg/kg every 4 hours (approximating to 1.5–3 mg/kg every 4 hours by mouth) usually for not more than 2 weeks; CHILD 80–160 mg/m^2 every 6 hours (120 mg/m^2 every 6 hours approximates to 180 mg/m^2 every 6 hours by mouth)

Retrovir® (GSK) PoM
Capsules, zidovudine 100 mg (white/blue band), net price 100-cap pack = £119.33; 250 mg (blue/white/dark blue band), 40-cap pack = £119.33
Oral solution, sugar-free, strawberry-flavoured, zidovudine 50 mg/5 mL, net price 200-mL pack with 10-mL oral syringe = £23.87
Injection, zidovudine 10 mg/mL. For dilution and use as an intravenous infusion. Net price 20-mL vial = £11.98

▪ With lamivudine
For cautions, contra-indications, and side-effects of lamivudine, see Lamivudine
Combivir® (GSK) PoM
Tablets, f/c, zidovudine 300 mg, lamivudine 150 mg, net price 60-tab pack = £342.58
Dose: 1 tablet twice daily

▪ With abacavir and lamivudine
See under Abacavir

Protease inhibitors

SIDE-EFFECTS. Side-effects of the protease inhibitors include gastro-intestinal disturbances (including diarrhoea, nausea, vomiting, abdominal pain, flatulence), hepatic dysfunction, pancreatitis; blood dis-

orders including anaemia, neutropenia, and thrombocytopenia; sleep disturbances, fatigue, headache, dizziness, paraesthesia, myalgia, myositis, rhabdomyolysis; taste disturbances; rash, pruritus, Stevens-Johnson syndrome, hypersensitivity reactions including anaphylaxis; see also notes above for lipodystrophy and metabolic effects.

AMPRENAVIR

Indications: HIV infection in combination with other antiretroviral drugs in patients previously treated with other protease inhibitors

Cautions: diabetes, haemophilia; hepatic impairment (Appendix 2); severe renal impairment (Appendix 3); pregnancy (Appendix 4); **interactions:** Appendix 1 (amprenavir)

RASH. Rash may occur, usually in the second week of therapy; discontinue permanently if severe rash with systemic or allergic symptoms or, mucosal involvement; if rash mild or moderate, may continue without interruption—rash usually resolves within 2 weeks and may respond to antihistamines

Contra-indications: breast-feeding

Side-effects: see notes above; also reported, rash including rarely Stevens-Johnson syndrome (see also above); tremors, oral or perioral paraesthesia, mood disorders including depression

Dose: see preparations below

Agenerase® (GSK) PoM
Capsules, both ivory, amprenavir 50 mg, net price 480-cap pack = £150.00; 150 mg, 240-cap pack = £225.00. Label: 5
Excipients: include vitamin E 36 units/50 mg amprenavir (avoid vitamin E supplements)
Dose: ADULT over 12 years, body-weight over 50 kg, 1.2 g every 12 hours; ADULT over 12 years, body-weight under 50 kg and CHILD over 4 years, 20 mg/kg every 12 hours (max. 2.4 g daily), CHILD under 4 years safety and efficacy not established
With low-dose ritonavir, ADULT over 12 years, body-weight over 50 kg, amprenavir 600 mg every 12 hours with ritonavir 100–200 mg every 12 hours
Oral solution, grape-bubblegum- and peppermint-flavoured, amprenavir 15 mg/mL, net price 240-mL pack = £36.00. Label: 4, 5
Excipients: include vitamin E 46 units/mL (avoid vitamin E supplements), propylene glycol 550 mg/mL (see Excipients, p. 2)
Dose: ADULT and CHILD over 4 years, 17 mg/kg every 8 hours (max. 2.8 g daily); CHILD under 4 years not recommended
NOTE. The bioavailability of *Agenerase*® oral solution is lower than that of capsules; the two formulations are **not** interchangeable on a milligram-for-milligram basis

INDINAVIR

Indications: HIV infection in combination with nucleoside reverse transcriptase inhibitors

Cautions: hepatic impairment (Appendix 2); ensure adequate hydration (risk of nephrolithiasis especially in children); patients at risk of nephrolithiasis (monitor for nephrolithiasis); diabetes; haemophilia; pregnancy (Appendix 4); metabolism of many drugs inhibited if administered concomitantly, **interactions:** Appendix 1 (indinavir)

Contra-indications: breast-feeding

Side-effects: see notes above; also reported, dry mouth, hypoaesthesia, dry skin, hyperpigmentation, alopecia, paronychia, interstitial nephritis (with medullary calcification and cortical atrophy in asymptomatic severe leucocyturia), nephrolithiasis (may require interruption or discontinuation; more frequent in children), dysuria, haematuria, crystalluria, proteinuria, pyuria (in children); haemolytic anaemia

Dose: 800 mg every 8 hours; CHILD and ADOLESCENT 4–17 years, 500 mg/m^2 every 8 hours (max. 800 mg every 8 hours); CHILD under 4 years, safety and efficacy not established

Crixivan® (MSD) ▣PoM▣

Capsules, indinavir (as sulphate), 200 mg, net price 360-cap pack = £226.28; 400 mg, 90-cap pack = £113.15, 180-cap pack = £226.28. Label: 27, counselling, administration

COUNSELLING. Administer 1 hour before or 2 hours after a meal; may be administered with a low-fat, light meal; in combination with didanosine tablets, allow 1 hour between each drug (antacids in didanosine tablets reduce absorption of indinavir)

NOTE. Bottles include desiccant canisters

LOPINAVIR WITH RITONAVIR

Indications: HIV infection in combination with other antiretroviral drugs

Cautions: hepatic impairment—avoid if severe (Appendix 2, *Kaletra*®); renal impairment (Appendix 3, *Kaletra*®); haemophilia; pregnancy (Appendix 4, *Kaletra*®); diabetes; pancreatitis (see below); **interactions:** Appendix 1 (lopinavir, ritonavir)

PANCREATITIS. Signs and symptoms suggestive of pancreatitis (including raised serum amylase and lipase) should be evaluated—discontinue if pancreatitis diagnosed

Contra-indications: breast-feeding (Appendix 5, *Kaletra*®)

Side-effects: see notes and Cautions above; also reported, dry mouth, influenza-like syndrome, appetite changes, hypertension, palpitations, thrombophlebitis, vasculitis, chest pain, dyspnoea, agitation, anxiety, ataxia, hypertonia, confusion, depression, dyskinesia, peripheral neuritis; Cushing's syndrome, hypothyroidism, sexual dysfunction, dehydration, oedema, lactic acidosis, arthralgia, abnormal vision, otitis media, tinnitus, acne, alopecia, dry skin, skin discoloration, nail disorders, sweating; raised bilirubin and lowered sodium also reported in children

Dose: see preparations below

Kaletra® (Abbott) ▼ ▣PoM▣

Capsules, orange, lopinavir 133.3 mg, ritonavir 33.3 mg, net price 180-cap pack = £332.31. Label: 21

Dose: ADULT and ADOLESCENT with body surface area of 1.3 m^2 or greater, 3 capsules twice daily with food; CHILD with body surface area less than 1.3 m^2, see under Oral Solution

Oral solution, lopinavir 400 mg, ritonavir 100 mg/ 5 mL, net price 5×60-mL packs = £332.31. Label: 21

Excipients: include propylene glycol 153 mg/mL (see Excipients, p. 2), alcohol 42%

Dose: ADULT and ADOLESCENT with body surface area of 1.3 m^2 or greater, 5 mL twice daily with food; CHILD over 2 years 2.9 mL/m^2 twice daily with food, max. 5 mL twice daily; CHILD under 2 years, safety and efficacy not established

NOTE. 5 mL oral solution ≡ 3 capsules; where appropriate, capsules may be used instead of oral solution

NELFINAVIR

Indications: HIV infection in combination with other antiretroviral drugs

Cautions: hepatic and renal impairment; diabetes; haemophilia; pregnancy; **interactions:** Appendix 1 (nelfinavir)

Contra-indications: breast-feeding

Side-effects: see notes above; also reported, fever

Dose: 1.25 g twice daily *or* 750 mg 3 times daily; CHILD 3–13 years, initially 50–55 mg/kg twice daily (max. 1.25 g twice daily) *or* 25–30 mg/kg 3 times daily (max. 750 mg 3 times daily)

Viracept® (Roche) ▣PoM▣

Tablets, f/c, nelfinavir (as mesilate) 250 mg, net price 300-tab pack = £321.37. Label: 21

Oral powder, nelfinavir (as mesilate) 50 mg/g. Net price 144 g (with 1-g and 5-g scoop) = £30.88. Label: 21, counselling, administration

Excipients: include aspartame (section 9.4.1)

COUNSELLING. Powder may be mixed with water, milk, formula feeds or pudding; it should **not** be mixed with acidic foods or juices owing to its taste

RITONAVIR

Indications: progressive or advanced HIV infection in combination with nucleoside reverse transcriptase inhibitors; low doses used to increase effect of some protease inhibitors

Cautions: hepatic impairment; diabetes; haemophilia; pregnancy; pancreatitis (see below); **interactions:** Appendix 1 (ritonavir)

PANCREATITIS. Signs and symptoms suggestive of pancreatitis (including raised serum amylase and lipase) should be evaluated—discontinue if pancreatitis diagnosed

Contra-indications: severe hepatic impairment; breast-feeding

Side-effects: see notes and Cautions above; also reported, diarrhoea (may impair absorption—close monitoring required), throat irritation, vasodilatation, syncope, hypotension; circumoral and peripheral paraesthesia, hyperaesthesia, seizures, raised uric acid, dry mouth and ulceration, cough, anxiety, fever, pain, decreased thyroxine, sweating, electrolyte disturbances, increased prothrombin time

Dose: 600 mg every 12 hours; CHILD over 2 years initially 250 mg/m^2 every 12 hours, increased by 50 mg/m^2 at intervals of 2–3 days to 350 mg/m^2 every 12 hours (max. 600 mg every 12 hours)

Low-dose booster to increase effect of other protease inhibitors, 100 mg every 12 hours

Norvir® (Abbott) ▣PoM▣

Capsules, ritonavir 100 mg, net price 336-cap pack = £377.39. Label 21

Excipients: include alcohol 12%

Oral solution, sugar-free, ritonavir 400 mg/5 mL, net price 5 × 90-mL packs (with measuring cup) = £403.20. Label: 21, counselling, administration

COUNSELLING. Oral solution contains 43% alcohol; bitter taste can be masked by mixing with chocolate milk; do not mix with water, measuring cup must be dry

■ With lopinavir
See under Lopinavir with ritonavir

SAQUINAVIR

Indications: HIV infection in combination with other antiretroviral drugs

Cautions: hepatic impairment (Appendix 2); renal impairment (Appendix 3); diabetes; haemophilia; pregnancy (Appendix 4); **interactions:** Appendix 1 (saquinavir)

Contra-indications: severe hepatic impairment (Appendix 2), breast-feeding

Side-effects: see notes above; also buccal and mucosal ulceration, chest pain, peripheral neuropathy, mood changes, fever, changes in libido, verruca, nephrolithiasis

Dose: see preparations below

NOTE. To avoid confusion between the different formulations of saquinavir, prescribers should specify the brand to be dispensed; absorption from *Fortovase®* is much greater than from *Invirase®*. Treatment should generally be initiated with *Fortovase®*

Fortovase® (Roche) PoM

Capsules (gel-filled), beige, saquinavir 200 mg, net price 180-cap pack = £104.34. Label: 21

Dose: ADULT over 16 years, 1.2 g every 8 hours (within 2 hours after a meal)

With low-dose ritonavir, ADULT over 16 years, 1 g every 12 hours (within 2 hours after a meal)

Invirase® (Roche) PoM

Capsules, brown/green, saquinavir (as mesilate) 200 mg, net price 270-cap pack = £289.23. Label: 21

Dose: With low-dose ritonavir, ADULT over 16 years, 1 g every 12 hours (within 2 hours after a meal)

Non-nucleoside reverse transcriptase inhibitors

EFAVIRENZ

Indications: HIV infection in combination with other antiretroviral drugs

Cautions: hepatic impairment (avoid if severe; Appendix 2); severe renal impairment; pregnancy (Appendix 4); elderly; history of mental illness or seizures; **interactions:** Appendix 1 (efavirenz)

RASH. Rash, usually in the first 2 weeks, is the most common side-effect; discontinue if severe rash with blistering, desquamation, mucosal involvement or fever; if rash mild or moderate, may continue without interruption—rash usually resolves within 1 month

Contra-indications: breast-feeding

Side-effects: rash including Stevens-Johnson syndrome (see also above); dizziness, headache, insomnia, somnolence, abnormal dreams, fatigue, impaired concentration (administration at bedtime especially in first 2–4 weeks reduces CNS effects); nausea; less frequently vomiting, diarrhoea, hepatitis, depression, anxiety, psychosis, amnesia, ataxia, stupor, vertigo; also reported abdominal pain, raised serum cholesterol, elevated liver enzymes (especially if seropositive for hepatitis B or C), hepatic failure, pancreatitis, convulsions, gynaecomastia, pruritus, blurred vision

Dose: *see preparations below*

Sustiva (Bristol-Myers Squibb) ▼ PoM

Capsules, efavirenz 50 mg (yellow/white), net price 30-cap pack = £18.72; 100 mg (white), 30-cap pack = £37.39; 200 mg (yellow), 90-cap pack = £224.09

Dose: ADULT and CHILD over 3 years, body-weight 13–14 kg, 200 mg once daily; body-weight 15–19 kg, 250 mg once daily; body-weight 20–24 kg, 300 mg once daily; body-weight 25–32.4 kg, 350 mg once daily; body-weight 32.5–39 kg, 400 mg once daily; body-weight 40 kg and over, 600 mg once daily

Tablets, f/c, yellow, efavirenz 600 mg, net price 30-tab pack = £224.09

Dose: ADULT and ADOLESCENT over 12 years, body-weight over 40 kg, 600 mg once daily

Oral solution, sugar-free, strawberry and mint flavour, efavirenz 30 mg/mL, net price 180-mL pack = £56.02

Dose: ADULT and CHILD over 5 years, body-weight 13–14 kg, 270 mg once daily; body-weight 15–19 kg, 300 mg once daily; body-weight 20–24 kg, 360 mg once daily; body-weight 25–32.4 kg, 450 mg once daily; body-weight 32.5–39 kg, 510 mg once daily; body-weight 40 kg and over, 720 mg once daily; CHILD 3–4 years, body-weight 13–14 kg, 360 mg once daily; body-weight 15–19 kg, 390 mg once daily; body-weight 20–24 kg, 450 mg once daily; body-weight 25–32.4 kg, 510 mg once daily

NOTE. The bioavailability of *Sustiva®* oral solution is lower than that of the capsules and tablets; the oral solution is **not** interchangeable with either capsules or tablets on a milligram-for-milligram basis

NEVIRAPINE

Indications: progressive or advanced HIV infection, in combination with at least two other antiretroviral drugs

Cautions: hepatic impairment (see below and Appendix 2); history of chronic hepatitis (greater risk of hepatic side-effects), pregnancy (Appendix 4); **interactions:** Appendix 1 (nevirapine)

HEPATIC DISEASE. Potentially life-threatening hepatotoxicity including fatal fulminant hepatitis reported usually occurring in first 8 weeks; monitor liver function before treatment then every 2 weeks for 2 months then after 1 month and then every 3–6 months; discontinue permanently if abnormalities in liver function tests accompanied by hypersensitivity reaction (rash, fever, arthralgia, myalgia, lymphadenopathy, hepatitis, renal impairment, eosinophilia, granulocytopenia); suspend if severe abnormalities in liver function tests but no hypersensitivity reaction—discontinue permanently if significant liver function abnormalities recur; monitor patient closely if mild to moderate abnormalities in liver function tests with no hypersensitivity reaction

NOTE. If treatment interrupted for more than 7 days reintroduce with 200 mg daily (CHILD 4 mg/kg daily) and increase dose cautiously

RASH. Rash, usually occurring in first 8 weeks, is most common side-effect; incidence reduced if introduced at low dose and dose increased gradually; discontinue permanently if severe rash or if rash accompanied by blistering, oral lesions, conjunctivitis, swelling, general malaise or hypersensitivity reactions; if rash mild or moderate may continue without interruption but dose should not be increased until rash resolves

COUNSELLING. Patients should be told how to recognise hypersensitivity reactions and advised to seek immediate medical attention if symptoms develop

Contra-indications: breast-feeding; severe hepatic impairment; post-exposure prophylaxis

Side-effects: rash including Stevens-Johnson syndrome and rarely, toxic epidermal necrolysis (see also Cautions above); hepatitis or jaundice reported (see also Cautions above); nausea, vomiting, abdominal pain, diarrhoea, headache, drowsiness, fatigue, fever; hypersensitivity reactions (may involve hepatic reactions and rash, see Cautions above); also reported, anaphylaxis, angioedema, urticaria, neuropsychiatric reactions, anaemia

Dose: 200 mg once daily for first 14 days then (if no rash present) 200 mg twice daily; CHILD 2 months–8 years, 4 mg/kg once daily for first 14 days then (if no rash present) 7 mg/kg twice daily (max. 400 mg daily); 8–16 years (but under 50 kg), 4 mg/kg once daily for first 14 days then (if no rash present) 4 mg/kg twice daily (max. 400 mg daily); over 50 kg, adult dose

Viramune® (Boehringer Ingelheim) ▼ PoM
Tablets, nevirapine 200 mg, net price 60-tab pack = £168.00. Counselling, hypersensitivity reactions
Suspension, nevirapine 50 mg/5 mL, net price 240-mL pack = £50.40. Counselling, hypersensitivity reactions

Other antiretrovirals

ENFUVIRTIDE

Indications: HIV infection in combination with other antiretroviral drugs for resistant infection or for patients intolerant to other antiretroviral regimens

Cautions: chronic hepatitis B or C (possibly greater risk of hepatic side-effects); hepatic impairment (Appendix 2); renal impairment (Appendix 3); pregnancy (Appendix 4)
HYPERSENSITIVITY REACTIONS. Hypersensitivity reactions reported—characterised by rash, fever, nausea, vomiting, chills, rigors, low blood pressure, respiratory distress, glomerulonephritis, and raised liver function tests; discontinue immediately if any signs or symptoms of systemic hypersensitivity develop and do not rechallenge
COUNSELLING. Patients should be told how to recognise signs of hypersensitivity, and advised to discontinue treatment and seek immediate medical attention if symptoms of systemic hypersensitivity reaction develop

Contra-indications: breast-feeding (Appendix 5)
Side-effects: injection-site reactions; headache, insomnia, eosinophilia; less frequently abdominal pain, constipation, taste disturbance, oral candidiasis, pancreatitis, cough, sore throat, sinusitis, asthenia, anxiety, depression, dizziness, peripheral neuropathy, anorexia, weight loss, herpes simplex infection, influenza-like illness, pneumonia, myalgia, arthralgia, conjunctivitis, pruritus, dry skin, skin papilloma, sweating, folliculitis, lymphadenopathy; rarely hypersensitivity reactions (see Cautions)
Dose: *by subcutaneous injection*, ADULT and ADOLESCENT over 16 years, 90 mg twice daily; CHILD 6–15 years, 2 mg/kg twice daily (max. 90 mg twice daily)

Fuzeon® (Roche) ▼ PoM
Injection, powder for reconstitution, enfuvirtide 108 mg (= enfuvirtide 90 mg/mL when reconstituted with 1.1 mL water for injections), net price 108-mg vial = £19.93 (with solvent, syringe, and alcohol swabs). Counselling, hypersensitivity reactions

Cytomegalovirus (CMV)

Recommendations for the optimum maintenance therapy of cytomegalovirus (CMV) infections and the duration of treatment are subject to rapid change.
Ganciclovir is related to aciclovir but it is more active against cytomegalovirus; it is also much more toxic than aciclovir and should therefore be prescribed only when the potential benefit outweighs the risks. Ganciclovir is administered by intravenous infusion for the *initial treatment* of CMV retinitis. Ganciclovir causes profound myelosuppression when given with zidovudine; the two should not normally be given together particularly during initial ganciclovir therapy. The likelihood of ganciclovir resistance increases in patients with a high viral load

or in those who receive the drug over a long duration; cross-resistance to cidofovir is common.
Valaciclovir (see p. 300) is licensed for prevention of cytomegalovirus disease following renal transplantation.
Valganciclovir is an ester of ganciclovir which is licensed for the *initial treatment* and *maintenance treatment* of CMV retinitis in AIDS patients. Valganciclovir is also licensed for preventing CMV disease following solid organ transplantation from a cytomegalovirus-positive donor.
Foscarnet is also active against cytomegalovirus; it is toxic and can cause renal impairment.
Cidofovir is a DNA polymerase chain inhibitor which is given for CMV retinitis in AIDS patients when ganciclovir and foscarnet are contra-indicated; it is given in combination with probenecid. It is nephrotoxic.
For local treatment of CMV retinitis, see section 11.3.3.

CIDOFOVIR

Indications: cytomegalovirus retinitis in AIDS patients for whom other drugs are inappropriate
Cautions: monitor renal function (serum creatinine and urinary protein) and neutrophil count within 24 hours before each dose; co-treatment with probenecid and prior hydration with intravenous fluids necessary to minimise potential nephrotoxicity (see below); diabetes mellitus (increased risk of ocular hypotony); **interactions:** Appendix 1 (cidofovir)
NEPHROTOXICITY. Do not initiate treatment in renal impairment (assess creatinine clearance and proteinuria—consult product literature); discontinue treatment and give intravenous fluids if renal function deteriorates—consult product literature
OCULAR DISORDERS. Regular ophthalmological examinations recommended; iritis and uveitis have been reported which may respond to a topical corticosteroid with or without a cycloplegic drug—discontinue cidofovir if no response to topical corticosteroid or if condition worsens, or if iritis or uveitis recurs after successful treatment

Contra-indications: renal impairment (creatinine clearance 55 mL/minute or less); concomitant administration of potentially nephrotoxic drugs (discontinue potentially nephrotoxic drugs at least 7 days before starting cidofovir); pregnancy (avoid pregnancy during and for 1 month after treatment, men should not father a child during or within 3 months of treatment), breast-feeding
Side-effects: nephrotoxicity (see Cautions above); neutropenia, fever, asthenia, alopecia, nausea, vomiting, hypotony, decreased intra-ocular pressure, iritis, uveitis (see Cautions above)
Dose: *by intravenous infusion* over 1 hour, initial (induction) treatment, 5 mg/kg once weekly for 2 weeks (give probenecid and intravenous fluids with each dose, see below); CHILD not recommended
Maintenance treatment, beginning 2 weeks after completion of induction, *by intravenous infusion* over 1 hour, 5 mg/kg once every 2 weeks (give probenecid and intravenous fluids with each dose, see below)
PROBENECID CO-TREATMENT. *By mouth* (preferably after food), probenecid 2 g 3 hours before cidofovir infusion followed by probenecid 1 g at 2 hours and 1 g at 8 hours after the end of cidofovir infusion (total probenecid 4 g);

for cautions, contra-indications and side-effects of probenecid see section 10.1.4

PRIOR HYDRATION. Sodium chloride 0.9%, *by intravenous infusion*, 1 litre over 1 hour immediately before cidofovir infusion (if tolerated an additional 1 litre may be given over 1–3 hours, starting at the same time as the cidofovir infusion or immediately afterwards)

Vistide® (Pharmacia) PoM
Intravenous infusion, cidofovir 75 mg/mL, net price 5-mL vial = £653.22
CAUTION IN HANDLING. Cidofovir is toxic and personnel should be adequately protected during handling and administration; if solution comes into contact with skin or mucosa, wash off immediately with water

GANCICLOVIR

Indications: life-threatening or sight-threatening cytomegalovirus infections in immunocompromised patients only; prevention of cytomegalovirus disease during immunosuppressive therapy following organ transplantation; local treatment of CMV retinitis (section 11.3.3)

Cautions: close monitoring of blood counts (dose adjustment or interruption may be required—consult product literature); history of cytopenia; low platelet count; potential carcinogen and teratogen; renal impairment (consult product literature); ensure adequate hydration during intravenous administration; vesicant—infuse into vein with adequate flow preferably using a plastic cannula; limited experience in children (possible risk of long-term carcinogenic or reproductive toxicity—not for neonatal or congenital cytomegalovirus disease); **interactions:** Appendix 1 (ganciclovir)

Contra-indications: pregnancy (ensure effective contraception during treatment and barrier contraception for men during and for at least 90 days after treatment); breast-feeding; hypersensitivity to ganciclovir or aciclovir; abnormally low neutrophil or platelet counts (see product literature)

Side-effects: nausea, diarrhoea, asthenia, leucopenia, anaemia; less frequently, vomiting, abdominal pain, flatulence, anorexia, headache, paraesthesia, rash, alopecia, injection-site reactions, neutropenia, thrombocytopenia; rarely, mouth ulcers, dry mouth, dysphagia, dyspepsia, gastrointestinal haemorrhage, faecal incontinence, constipation, pancreatitis, hepatitis, chest pain, arrhythmias, hypertension, hypotension, vasodilatation, oedema, thrombophlebitis, dyspnoea, fever, migraine, dizziness, sleep disturbances, abnormal dreams, anxiety, confusion, ataxia, depression, euphoria, mania, psychosis, abnormal gait, seizures, tremor, neuropathy, coma, breast pain, urinary frequency, haematuria, renal impairment, myalgia, myasthenia, urticaria, pruritus, acne, photosensitivity, sweating, disturbances in taste, hearing, and vision, eye pain, changes in blood glucose, hypokalaemia, eosinophilia, pancytopenia

Dose: *by intravenous infusion*, initially (induction) 5 mg/kg every 12 hours for 14–21 days for treatment or for 7–14 days for prevention; maintenance (for patients at risk of relapse of retinitis) 6 mg/kg daily on 5 days per week *or* 5 mg/kg daily until adequate recovery of immunity; if retinitis progresses initial induction treatment may be repeated

Cymevene® (Roche) PoM
Intravenous infusion, powder for reconstitution, ganciclovir (as sodium salt). Net price 500-mg vial = £33.98
Electrolytes: Na⁺ 2 mmol/500-mg vial
CAUTION IN HANDLING. Ganciclovir is toxic and personnel should be adequately protected during handling and administration; if solution comes into contact with skin or mucosa, wash off immediately with soap and water

FOSCARNET SODIUM

Indications: cytomegalovirus retinitis in AIDS patients; mucocutaneous herpes simplex virus infections unresponsive to aciclovir in immunocompromised patients

Cautions: renal impairment (reduce dose or avoid if severe); monitor electrolytes, particularly calcium and magnesium; monitor serum creatinine every second day during induction and every week during maintenance; ensure adequate hydration; avoid rapid infusion; **interactions:** Appendix 1 (foscarnet)

Contra-indications: pregnancy, breast-feeding

Side-effects: nausea, vomiting, diarrhoea (occasionally constipation and dyspepsia), abdominal pain, anorexia; changes in blood pressure and ECG; headache, fatigue, mood disturbances (including psychosis), asthenia, paraesthesia, convulsions, tremor, dizziness, and other neurological disorders; rash; impairment of renal function including acute renal failure; hypocalcaemia (sometimes symptomatic) and other electrolyte disturbances; abnormal liver function tests; decreased haemoglobin concentration, leucopenia, granulocytopenia, thrombocytopenia; thrombophlebitis if given undiluted by peripheral vein; genital irritation and ulceration (due to high concentrations excreted in urine); isolated reports of pancreatitis

Dose: CMV retinitis induction, *by intravenous infusion*, 60 mg/kg every 8 hours for 2–3 weeks then maintenance, 60 mg/kg daily, increased to 90–120 mg/kg if tolerated; if retinitis progresses on maintenance dose, repeat induction regimen
Mucocutaneous herpes simplex infection, *by intravenous infusion*, 40 mg/kg every 8 hours for 2–3 weeks or until lesions heal

Foscavir® (AstraZeneca) PoM
Intravenous infusion, foscarnet sodium hexahydrate 24 mg/mL, net price 250-mL bottle = £34.49

VALGANCICLOVIR

NOTE. Valganciclovir is a pro-drug of ganciclovir

Indications: induction and maintenance treatment of cytomegalovirus retinitis in AIDS patients; prevention of cytomegalovirus disease following solid organ transplantation from a cytomegalovirus-positive donor.

Cautions: see under Ganciclovir

Side-effects: see under Ganciclovir

Dose: CMV retinitis, induction, 900 mg twice daily for 21 days then 900 mg once daily; induction regimen may be repeated if retinitis progresses
Prevention of cytomegalovirus disease following solid organ transplantation (starting within 10 days of transplantation), 900 mg once daily for 100 days
CHILD and ADOLESCENT not recommended
NOTE. Oral valganciclovir 900 mg twice daily is equivalent to intravenous ganciclovir 5 mg/kg twice daily

Valcyte® (Roche) ▼ [PoM]
Tablets, pink, f/c, valganciclovir (as hydrochloride) 450 mg , net price 60-tab pack = £1195.89.
Label: 21
CAUTION IN HANDLING. Valganciclovir is a potential teratogen and carcinogen and caution is advised for handling of broken tablets; if broken tablets come into contact with skin or mucosa, wash off immediately with water

Viral hepatitis

The management of uncomplicated acute viral hepatitis is largely symptomatic. Early treatment of acute hepatitis C with interferon alfa [unlicensed indication] may reduce the risk of chronic infection. Hepatitis B and hepatitis C viruses are major causes of chronic hepatitis. For details on immunisation against hepatitis A and B infections, see section 14.4 (active immunisation) and section 14.5 (passive immunisation).

CHRONIC HEPATITIS B. **Interferon alfa** (section 8.2.4) is used in the treatment of chronic hepatitis B but its use is limited by a response rate of less than 50%, and relapse is frequent. If no improvement occurs after 3–4 months of treatment, interferon alfa should be discontinued. Interferon alfa is contra-indicated in patients receiving immunosuppressant treatment (or who have received it recently). The manufacturers of interferon alfa contra-indicate its use in decompensated liver disease but low doses can be used with great caution in these patients.
Lamivudine (see p. 302) is used for the initial treatment of chronic hepatitis B. It can also be used in patients with decompensated liver disease. Treatment should be continued if there is no loss of efficacy and until adequate seroconversion is achieved (consult product literature); it is continued long-term in decompensated liver disease. Hepatitis B viruses with reduced susceptibility to lamivudine have emerged following extended therapy. In patients infected with HIV and hepatitis B, lamivudine should be given only as part of combination antiretroviral therapy and in a dose appropriate for treating HIV; the use of lamivudine alone is likely to result in lamivudine-resistant HIV.
Adefovir dipivoxil is licensed for the treatment of chronic hepatitis B. It is effectve in lamivudine-resistant chronic hepatitis B. Treatment should be continued, if there is no loss in efficacy, until adequate seroconversion has occurred (consult product literature); it is continued long-term in patients with decompensated liver disease or cirrhosis.

CHRONIC HEPATITIS C. A combination of **ribavirin** (see p. 311) and **peginterferon alfa** (section 8.2.4) is used for the treatment of chronic hepatitis C. Consider discontinuing treatment after 12 weeks if the circulating viral RNA has not decreased to less than 1% of the count at the start of treatment. In those responding to treatment, the combination should be continued for a total of 6 months. For some viral genotypes it may be necessary to extend treatment by a further 6 months (consult product literature). Combination therapy can also be used in patients who have not responded to monotherapy with interferon alfa or peginterferon alfa. The combination of ribavirin and interferon alfa is less effective

than the combination of peginterferon alfa and ribavirin. Ribavirin monotherapy is ineffective.
Peginterferon alfa alone may be used in the treatment of chronic hepatitis C if ribavirin is not tolerated or is contra-indicated, but monotherapy is less effective and relapse is more common. Interferon alfa alone has also been used but it is less effective than peginterferon alfa.

> **NICE guidance (ribavirin and interferon alfa for hepatitis C).** NICE has recommended (October 2000) that the combination of interferon alfa [peginterferon alfa now also available—see above] and ribavirin should be used for the treatment of moderate to severe hepatitis C (as determined by liver histology or, if biopsy too risky, determined on clinical grounds) in patients aged over 18 years who have:
>
> - not previously been treated with combination therapy;
> - previously responded to interferon alfa monotherapy, but have since relapsed.
>
> Combination therapy with interferon alfa and ribavirin should be continued for 6 months. Extension of treatment by a further 6 months is recommended only in patients infected with hepatitis C virus of genotype 1 and who have responded to treatment during the first 6 months (as judged by clearance of circulating viral RNA).
> Interferon alfa monotherapy should be considered when ribavirin is contra-indicated or not tolerated. Treatment with interferon alfa alone or in combination with ribavirin is not recommended in patients who continue to abuse intravenous drugs and are at risk of reinfection or who are heavy users of alcohol (risk of exacerbating liver damage).

ADEFOVIR DIPIVOXIL

Indications: chronic hepatitis B infection with *either* compensated liver disease with evidence of viral replication, and histologically documented active liver inflammation and fibrosis *or* decompensated liver disease

Cautions: monitor liver function and viral, and serological markers for hepatitis B every 6 months; discontinue if deterioration in liver function, hepatic steatosis, progressive hepatomegaly or unexplained lactic acidosis; recurrent hepatitis may occur on discontinuation; monitor renal function every 3 months, more frequently in renal impairment (Appendix 3) or in patients receiving nephrotoxic drugs; pregnancy (Appendix 4); elderly; HIV infection (particularly if uncontrolled—theoretical risk of HIV resistance)

Contra-indications: breast-feeding

Side-effects: nausea, dyspepsia, abdominal pain, flatulence, diarrhoea, asthenia, headache, renal failure

Dose: ADULT over 18 years, 10 mg once daily

Hepsera (Gilead) ▼ [PoM]
Tablets, adefovir dipivoxil 10 mg, net price 30-tab pack = £315.00

Influenza

For advice on immunisation against influenza, see section 14.4.
Oseltamivir and **zanamivir** reduce replication of influenza A and B viruses by inhibiting viral

neuraminidase. They are most effective for the treatment of influenza if started within a few hours of the onset of symptoms; they are licensed for use within 48 hours of the first symptoms. In otherwise healthy individuals they reduce the duration of symptoms by about 1–1.5 days. The effect of oseltamivir or zanamivir on hospitalisation or on mortality is not clear in those at risk of serious complications from influenza. Oseltamivir is also licensed for prophylaxis when used within 48 hours of exposure to influenza and when influenza is circulating in the community; it is also licensed for use in exceptional circumstances (e.g. when vaccination does not cover the infecting strain) to prevent influenza in an epidemic.

NICE guidance (oseltamivir, zanamivir, and amantadine for prophylaxis and treatment of influenza). NICE has recommended (February and September 2003) that the drugs described here are not a substitute for vaccination, which remains the most effective way of preventing illness from influenza. When influenza A or influenza B is circulating in the community:

- amantadine is **not** recommended for post-exposure prophylaxis, seasonal prophylaxis, or treatment of influenza;

- oseltamivir and zanamivir are **not** recommended for seasonal prophylaxis against influenza;

- oseltamivir or zanamivir are **not** recommended for the post-exposure prophylaxis, or treatment of otherwise healthy individuals with influenza;

- oseltamivir is recommended for post-exposure prophylaxis in at-risk adults and adolescents over 13 years who are not effectively protected by influenza vaccine and who can commence oseltamivir within 48 hours of close contact with someone suffering from influenza-like illness; prophylaxis is also recommended for residents in care establishments (regardless of prior influenza vaccination) who can commence oseltamivir within 48 hours if influenza-like illness is present in the establishment;

- oseltamivir and zanamivir are recommended (in accordance with UK licensing) to treat at-risk adults who can start treatment within 48 hours of the onset of symptoms; oseltamivir is recommended for at-risk children who can start treatment within 48 hours of the onset of symptoms;

At-risk patients are defined as those aged over 65 years or those who have one or more of the following conditions:

- chronic respiratory disease (including chronic obstructive pulmonary disease and asthma) [but see cautions under Zanamivir below];

- significant cardiovascular disease (excluding hypertension);

- chronic renal disease;

- immunosuppression;

- diabetes mellitus.

Community-based virological surveillance schemes including those run by the Health Protection Agency and the Royal College of General Practitioners should be used to indicate when influenza is circulating in the community.

Amantadine is licensed for prophylaxis and treatment of influenza A but it is no longer recommended (see NICE guidance). Amantadine has also been used by mouth for herpes zoster, but its effectiveness has not been established.

AMANTADINE HYDROCHLORIDE

Indications: see under Dose; parkinsonism (section 4.9.1)
Cautions: see section 4.9.1
Contra-indications: see section 4.9.1
Side-effects: see section 4.9.1
Dose: herpes zoster (but see notes above), 100 mg twice daily for 14 days, if necessary extended for a further 14 days for post-herpetic pain

Influenza A (see also notes above), ADULT and CHILD over 10 years, treatment, 100 mg daily for 4–5 days; prophylaxis, 100 mg daily usually for 6 weeks or with influenza vaccination for 2–3 weeks after vaccination

ELDERLY 100 mg daily

Lysovir® (Alliance) PoM
Capsules, red-brown, amantadine hydrochloride 100 mg, net price 5-cap pack = £2.40, 14-cap pack = £4.80. Counselling, driving

Symmetrel® (Alliance) PoM
Section 4.9.1

OSELTAMIVIR

Indications: see notes above
Cautions: renal impairment (Appendix 3); pregnancy (Appendix 4); breast-feeding (Appendix 5)
Side-effects: nausea, vomiting, abdominal pain, dyspepsia, diarrhoea; headache, fatigue, insomnia, dizziness; conjunctivitis, epistaxis; ear disorder; rash; rarely hepatitis
Dose: prevention of influenza, 75 mg once daily for at least 7 days for post-exposure prophylaxis; for up to 6 weeks during an epidemic; CHILD under 12 years safety and efficacy not established

Treatment of influenza, 75 mg every 12 hours for 5 days; CHILD over 1 year, body-weight 15 kg or under, 30 mg every 12 hours, body-weight 16–23 kg, 45 mg every 12 hours, body-weight 24–40 kg, 60 mg every 12 hours, body-weight over 40 kg, adult dose

Tamiflu® (Roche) ▼ PoM
Capsules, grey/yellow, oseltamivir (as phosphate) 75 mg, net price 10-cap pack = £18.18. Label: 9
Suspension, sugar-free, tutti-frutti-flavoured, oseltamivir (as phosphate) for reconstitution with water, 60 mg/5 mL, net price 75 mL = £18.18. Label: 9

ZANAMIVIR

Indications: see notes above
Cautions: asthma and chronic pulmonary disease (risk of bronchospasm—short-acting bronchodilator should be available; avoid in severe asthma unless close monitoring possible and appropriate facilities available to treat bronchospasm); uncontrolled chronic illness; other inhaled drugs should be administered before zanamivir; pregnancy (Appendix 4)
Contra-indications: breast-feeding

Side-effects: gastro-intestinal disturbances; reported rarely, bronchospasm, respiratory impairment, angioedema, and rash
Dose: *by inhalation of powder*, 10 mg twice daily for 5 days, CHILD under 12 years not recommended

Relenza® (GSK) PoM
Dry powder for inhalation disks containing 4 blisters of zanamivir 5mg/blister, net price 5 disks with *Diskhaler®* device = £26.40

Respiratory syncytial virus

Ribavirin (tribavirin) inhibits a wide range of DNA and RNA viruses. It is licensed for administration by inhalation for the treatment of severe bronchiolitis caused by the respiratory syncytial virus (RSV) in infants, especially when they have other serious diseases. However, there is no clear evidence that ribavirin produces clinically relevant benefit in RSV bronchiolitis. Ribavirin is given by mouth with peginterferon alfa or interferon alfa for the treatment of chronic hepatitis C infection (see Viral Hepatitis, p. 309). It is also effective in Lassa fever [unlicensed indication].

Palivizumab is a monoclonal antibody indicated for the prevention of respiratory syncytial virus infection in infants at high risk of infection. It is licensed for monthly use during the RSV season; the first dose should be administered before the start of the RSV season.

PALIVIZUMAB

Indications: prevention of serious lower respiratory-tract infection caused by respiratory syncytial virus (RSV) requiring hospitalisation in children born at 35 weeks gestation or less and who are less than 6 months old at onset of RSV season, or in children less than 2 years old who have received treatment for bronchopulmonary dysplasia within the last 6 months, or in children under 2 years with haemodynamically significant congenital heart disease
Cautions: moderate to severe acute infection or febrile illness; thrombocytopenia; serum-palivizumab concentration may be reduced after cardiac surgery
Contra-indications: hypersensitivity to humanised monoclonal antibodies
Side-effects: fever, injection site reactions, nervousness; less frequently diarrhoea, vomiting, constipation, haemorrhage, rhinitis, cough, wheeze, pain, drowsiness, asthenia, hyperkinesia, rash, leucopenia; rarely apnoea, hypersensitivity reactions (including anaphylaxis)
Dose: *by intramuscular injection* (preferably in anterolateral thigh), 15 mg/kg once a month during season of RSV risk (children undergoing cardiac bypass surgery, 15 mg/kg as soon as stable after surgery, then at monthly intervals during season of risk); injection volume over 1 mL should be divided between more than one site

Synagis® (Abbott) ▼ PoM
Injection, powder for reconstitution, palivizumab, net price 50-mg vial = £424.00; 100-mg vial = £706.00

RIBAVIRIN
(Tribavirin)

Indications: severe respiratory syncytial virus bronchiolitis in infants and children; in combination with peginterferon alfa or interferon alfa for chronic hepatitis C not previously treated in patients without liver decompensation and who have fibrosis or high inflammatory activity or for relapse following previous response to interferon alfa

Cautions:
SPECIFIC CAUTIONS FOR INHALED TREATMENT. Maintain standard supportive respiratory and fluid management therapy; monitor electrolytes closely; monitor equipment for precipitation; pregnant women (and those planning pregnancy) should avoid exposure to aerosol
SPECIFIC CAUTIONS FOR ORAL TREATMENT. Exclude pregnancy before treatment; effective contraception essential during treatment and for 6 months after treatment in women and in men; routine monthly pregnancy tests recommended; condoms must be used if partner of male patient is pregnant (ribavirin excreted in semen); renal impairment (Appendix 3); cardiac disease (assessment including ECG recommended before and during treatment—discontinue if deterioration); gout; determine full blood count, platelets, electrolytes, serum creatinine, liver function tests and uric acid before starting treatment and then on weeks 2 and 4 of treatment, then as indicated clinically—adjust dose if adverse reactions or laboratory abnormalities develop (consult product literature)

Interactions: Appendix 1 (Ribavirin)

Contra-indications: pregnancy (**important teratogenic risk**: see Cautions and Appendix 4); breast-feeding
SPECIFIC CONTRA-INDICATIONS FOR ORAL TREATMENT. Severe cardiac disease, including unstable or uncontrolled cardiac disease in previous 6 months; haemoglobinopathies; severe debilitating medical conditions; severe hepatic dysfunction or decompensated cirrhosis (Appendix 2); autoimmune disease (including autoimmune hepatitis); history of severe psychiatric condition

Side-effects:
SPECIFIC SIDE-EFFECTS FOR INHALED TREATMENT. Worsening respiration, bacterial pneumonia, and pneumothorax reported; rarely non-specific anaemia and haemolysis
SPECIFIC SIDE-EFFECTS FOR ORAL TREATMENT. Haemolytic anaemia (may be reversed by epoetin); also reported (in combination with peginterferon alfa or interferon alfa) nausea, vomiting, dry mouth, stomatitis, glossitis, dyspepsia, abdominal pain, gastritis, peptic ulcer, flatulence, diarrhoea, constipation, pancreatitis, anorexia, weight loss; chest pain, tachycardia, palpitations, syncope, peripheral oedema, flushing; dyspnoea, cough, rhinitis, pharyngitis, interstitial pneumonitis; sleep disturbances, asthenia, impaired concentration and memory, irritability, aggression, anxiety, depression, dizziness, tremor, hypertonia, myalgia, arthralgia, paraesthesia, peripheral neuropathy, influenza-like symptoms, headache; thyroid disorders, menstrual disturbances, reduced libido, impotence; rash, pruritus, urticaria, photosensitivity, alopecia, dry skin; taste disturbance, eye changes including blurred vision, tinnitus; neutropenia, thrombocytopenia, aplastic anaemia, lymphadenopathy, hyperuricaemia

Dose: see preparations below

Copegus® (Roche) ▼ PoM
Tablets, f/c, pink, ribavirin 200 mg, net price 42-tab pack = £124.32, 112-tab pack = £331.52, 168-tab pack = £497.28. Label: 21
Dose: chronic hepatitis C (in combination with interferon alfa or peginterferon alfa), ADULT over 18 years, body-weight under 75 kg, 400 mg in the morning and 600 mg in

the evening; body-weight 75 kg and over, 600 mg twice daily

NOTE. Chronic hepatitis C genotype 2 or 3 requires a lower dose of *Copegus*® (in combination with peginterferon alfa), usual dose 400 mg twice daily

Rebetol® (Schering-Plough) ▼ PoM
Capsules, ribavirin 200 mg, net price 84-cap pack = £296.40, 140-cap pack = £494.00, 168-cap pack = £592.80. Label: 21
Dose: chronic hepatitis C (in combination with interferon alfa or peginterferon alfa), ADULT over 18 years, body-weight under 65 kg, 400 mg twice daily; body-weight 65–85 kg, 400 mg in the morning and 600 mg in the evening; body-weight over 85 kg, 600 mg twice daily

Virazole® (ICN) PoM
Inhalation, ribavirin 6 g for reconstitution with 300 mL water for injections. Net price 3 × 6-g vials = £349.00
Dose: bronchiolitis, *by aerosol inhalation or nebulisation* (via small particle aerosol generator) of solution containing 20 mg/mL for 12–18 hours for at least 3 days; max. 7 days

5.4   Antiprotozoal drugs

5.4.1   Antimalarials
5.4.2   Amoebicides
5.4.3   Trichomonacides
5.4.4   Antigiardial drugs
5.4.5   Leishmaniacides
5.4.6   Trypanocides
5.4.7   Drugs for toxoplasmosis
5.4.8   Drugs for pneumocystis pneumonia

Advice on specific problems available from:

HPA (Health Protection Agency) Malaria Reference Laboratory (for healthcare professionals **only**)	(020) 7636 3924 (prophylaxis only)
National Travel Health Network and Centre (for healthcare professionals **only**)	(020) 7380 9234
Scottish Centre for Infection and Environmental Health (registered users of Travax only) www.travax.scot.nhs.uk (for registered users of the NHS Travax website only)	(0141) 300 1130 (weekdays 2–4 p.m. only)
Birmingham	(0121) 424 0357
Liverpool	(0151) 708 9393
London	(020) 7387 9300 (treatment)
Oxford	(01865) 225 214
Recorded advice for Travellers (£1.00/minute standard rate)	09065 508 908
Hospital for Tropical Diseases Travel Healthline (50p/minute)	09061 337 733
NHS advice for travellers www.fitfortravel.scot.nhs.uk	09061 337 733

WHO advice on international travel and health
www.who.int/ith

5.4.1   Antimalarials

Recommendations on the prophylaxis and treatment of malaria reflect guidelines agreed by UK malaria specialists.
   The centres listed above should be consulted for advice on special problems.

Treatment of malaria

If the infective species is **not known**, or if the infection is **mixed**, initial treatment should be as for *falciparum malaria* with quinine, mefloquine, *Malarone*® (proguanil with atovaquone), or *Riamet*® (artemether with lumefantrine). Falciparum malaria can progress rapidly in unprotected individuals and antimalarial treatment should be considered in those with features of severe malaria and possible exposure, even if the initial blood tests for the organism are negative.

Falciparum malaria (treatment)

Falciparum malaria (malignant malaria) is caused by *Plasmodium falciparum*. In most parts of the world *P. falciparum* is now resistant to chloroquine which should not therefore be given for treatment.[1]
   Quinine, **mefloquine**, *Malarone*® (proguanil with atovaquone), or *Riamet*® (artemether with lumefantrine) can be given *by mouth* if the patient can swallow and retain tablets and there are no serious manifestations (e.g. impaired consciousness); quinine should be given *by intravenous infusion* (see below) if the patient is seriously ill or unable to take tablets. Specialist advice should be sought in difficult cases since other drugs such as **artesunate** (given intravenously) and intramuscular **artemether** may be available for 'named-patient use'.

Oral. The adult dosage regimen for **quinine** *by mouth* is:
600 mg (of quinine salt[2]) every 8 hours for 7 days *and* (if quinine resistance known or suspected) *followed by*
either **Fansidar**® 3 tablets as a single dose
or (if *Fansidar*®-resistant) **doxycycline** 200 mg daily for at least 7 days.

Alternatively **mefloquine**, *Malarone*®, or *Riamet*® may be given instead of quinine but resistance to mefloquine has been reported in several countries. It is not necessary to give *Fansidar*® or doxycycline after mefloquine, *Malarone*®, or *Riamet*® treatment.

---

1. For chloroquine-sensitive strains of falciparum malaria chloroquine is effective *by mouth* in the dosage schedule outlined under benign malarias but it should **not** be used unless there is an **unambiguous exposure history** in one of the few remaining areas of chloroquine sensitivity.

If the patient with a *chloroquine-sensitive infection* is seriously ill, chloroquine is given *by continuous intravenous infusion*. The dosage (for adults and children) is chloroquine 10 mg/kg (of base) infused over 8 hours, followed by three 8-hour infusions of 5 mg/kg (of base) each. *Oral therapy* is started as soon as possible to complete the course; the total cumulative dose for the course should be 25 mg/kg of base.

2. Valid for quinine hydrochloride, dihydrochloride, and sulphate; not valid for quinine bisulphate which contains a correspondingly smaller amount of quinine.

The adult dosage regimen for **mefloquine** *by mouth* is:

20–25 mg/kg (of mefloquine base) as a single dose (up to maximum 1.5 g) *or preferably* as 2–3 divided doses 6–8 hours apart.

The adult dose of ***Malarone*** *by mouth* is:
4 ('standard') tablets once daily for 3 days.

The dose of ***Riamet*** *by mouth* for adult with body-weight of over 35 kg is:
4 tablets initially, followed by 5 further doses of 4 tablets each given at 8, 24, 36, 48, and 60 hours (total 24 tablets over 60 hours).

Parenteral. If the patient is seriously ill, **quinine** should be given *by intravenous infusion*. The adult dosage regimen for quinine *by infusion* is:
loading dose[1] of 20 mg/kg[2] (up to maximum 1.4 g) of quinine salt[3] infused over 4 hours *then after 8–12 hours* maintenance dose of 10 mg/kg[4] (up to maximum 700 mg) of quinine salt[3] infused over 4 hours every 8–12 hours (until patient can swallow tablets to complete the 7-day course) *followed by either Fansidar* or doxycycline as above. Alternatively, after at least 2–3 days' treatment with a parenteral quinine salt, treatment may be completed with mefloquine by mouth started at least 12 hours after parenteral quinine salt has been administered.

CHILDREN.

Oral. **Quinine** is well tolerated by children although the salts are bitter. The dosage regimen for quinine *by mouth* for children is:
10 mg/kg (of quinine salt[3]) every 8 hours for 7 days *then* (if quinine resistance known or suspected) *either*
Fansidar as a single dose: up to 4 years ½ tablet, 5–6 years 1 tablet, 7–9 years 1½ tablets, 10–14 years 2 tablets
or clindamycin 10–40 mg/kg every 8 hours for 5 days [unlicensed indication]

Alternatively **mefloquine**, ***Malarone***, or ***Riamet*** may be given instead of quinine; it is not necessary to give *Fansidar* after mefloquine, *Malarone*, or *Riamet* treatment. The dose regimen for mefloquine *by mouth* for children is calculated on a mg/kg basis as for adults (see above). The dose regimen for *Malarone* *by mouth* for children over 40 kg is the same as for adults (see above); the dose regimen for *Malarone* for smaller children is reduced as follows:

weight under 11 kg, no suitable dose form
weight 11–20 kg, 1 ('standard') tablet daily for 3 days; weight 21–30 kg, 2 ('standard') tablets daily

for 3 days; weight 31–40 kg, 3 ('standard') tablets daily for 3 days.

The dose regimen of *Riamet* *by mouth* for children over 12 years and body-weight over 35 kg is the same as for adults (see above).

Parenteral. The dose regimen for quinine *by intravenous infusion* for children is calculated on a mg/kg basis as for adults (see above).

PREGNANCY. Falciparum malaria is particularly dangerous in pregnancy, especially in the last trimester. The adult treatment doses of oral and intravenous quinine given above (including the loading dose) can safely be given to pregnant women. Alternatively, clindamycin, 900 mg every 8 hours for 5 days [unlicensed indication] can be given in combination with quinine. Doxycycline should be avoided in pregnancy (causes dental discoloration); *Fansidar*, mefloquine, and *Malarone* are also best avoided until more information is available.

Benign malarias (treatment)

Benign malaria is usually caused by *Plasmodium vivax* and less commonly by *P. ovale* and *P. malariae*. **Chloroquine**[5] is the drug of choice for the treatment of benign malarias (but chloroquine-resistant *P. vivax* infection has been reported from New Guinea and some adjacent islands).
The adult dosage regimen for **chloroquine** *by mouth* is:

initial dose of 600 mg (of base) *then*
a single dose of 300 mg after 6 to 8 hours *then*
a single dose of 300 mg daily for 2 days
(approximate total cumulative dose of 25 mg/kg of base)

Chloroquine alone is adequate for *P. malariae* infections but in the case of *P. vivax* and *P. ovale*, a *radical cure* (to destroy parasites in the liver and thus prevent relapses) is required. This is achieved with **primaquine**[6] in an adult dosage of 15 mg daily for 14 to 21 days given after the chloroquine; a 21-day (or even longer) course may be needed for Chesson-type strains of *P. vivax* from south-east Asia and western Pacific.

CHILDREN. The dosage regimen of chloroquine for benign malaria in children is:
initial dose of 10 mg/kg (of base) *then*
a single dose of 5 mg/kg after 6–8 hours *then*
a single dose of 5 mg/kg daily for 2 days
For a *radical cure* children are then given primaquine[6] in a dose of 250 micrograms/kg daily.

PREGNANCY. The adult treatment doses of chloroquine can be given for benign malaria. In the case of

---

1. In intensive care units the loading dose can alternatively be given as quinine salt[3] 7 mg/kg infused over 30 minutes followed immediately by 10 mg/kg over 4 hours then (after 8 hours) maintenance dose as described.

2. **Important:** the loading dose of 20 mg/kg should **not** be used if the patient has received quinine (or quinidine) or mefloquine during the previous 24 hours

3. Valid for quinine hydrochloride, dihydrochloride, and sulphate; not valid for quinine bisulphate which contains a correspondingly smaller amount of quinine.

4. Maintenance dose should be reduced to 5–7 mg/kg of salt in patients with renal impairment or if parenteral treatment is required for more than 48 hours.

5. Mefloquine is also active in benign malarias (but is not required since chloroquine is usually effective); as with chloroquine a radical cure is required for *P. vivax* and *P. ovale* infections.

6. Before starting primaquine blood should be tested for glucose-6-phosphate dehydrogenase (G6PD) activity since the drug can cause haemolysis in G6PD-deficient patients. In G6PD deficiency primaquine, in a dose for adults of 30 mg once a week (children 500–750 micrograms/kg once a week) for 8 weeks, has been found useful and without undue harmful effects.

P. vivax or *P. ovale*, however, the radical cure with primaquine should be **postponed** until the pregnancy is over; instead chloroquine should be continued at a dose of 600 mg each week during the pregnancy.

Prophylaxis against malaria

The recommendations on prophylaxis reflect guidelines agreed by UK malaria specialists; the advice is aimed at residents of the UK who travel to endemic areas. The choice of drug for a particular individual should take into account:

risk of exposure to malaria;
extent of drug resistance;
efficacy of the recommended drugs;
side-effects of the drugs;
patient-related factors (e.g. age, pregnancy, renal or hepatic impairment).

PROTECTION AGAINST BITES. **Prophylaxis is not absolute**, and breakthrough infection can occur with any of the drugs recommended. Personal protection against being bitten is very important. Mosquito nets impregnated with permethrin provide the most effective barrier protection against insects; coils, mats and vaporised insecticides are also useful. Diethyltoluamide (DEET) in lotions, sprays or roll-on formulations is safe and effective when applied to the skin but the protective effect only lasts for a few hours. Long sleeves and trousers worn after dusk also provide protection.

LENGTH OF PROPHYLAXIS. In order to determine tolerance and to establish habit, prophylaxis should generally be started one week (preferably 2–3 weeks in the case of mefloquine) before travel into an endemic area (or if not possible at earliest opportunity up to 1 or 2 days before travel); *Malarone*® prophylaxis should be started 1–2 days before travel. Prophylaxis should be continued for **4 weeks after leaving** (except for *Malarone*® prophylaxis which should be stopped 1 week after leaving).

In those requiring long-term prophylaxis, chloroquine and proguanil may be used for periods of over 5 years. Mefloquine is licensed for up to 1 year (although it has been used for up to 3 years without undue problems). Doxycycline can be used for up to 2 years while *Malarone*® is licensed for up to 28 days but can probably be used for up to 3 months. Specialist advice should be sought for long-term prophylaxis.

RETURN FROM MALARIAL REGION. It is important to be aware that **any illness** that occurs within 1 year and **especially within 3 months of return might be malaria** even if all recommended precautions against malaria were taken. Travellers should be **warned** of this and told that if they develop any illness **particularly within 3 months** of their return they should go **immediately** to a doctor and specifically mention their exposure to malaria.

CHILDREN. Prophylactic doses are based on guidelines agreed by UK malaria experts and may differ from advice in product literature. Weight is a better guide than age. If in doubt telephone centres listed on p. 312.

EPILEPSY. Both chloroquine and mefloquine are unsuitable for malaria prophylaxis in individuals with a history of epilepsy. In areas *without chloro-*

quine resistance proguanil 200 mg daily alone is recommended; in areas *with chloroquine resistance*, doxycycline or *Malarone*® may be considered; the metabolism of doxycycline may be influenced by antiepileptics (see **interactions:** Appendix 1 (tetracyclines)).

ASPLENIA. Asplenic individuals (or those with severe splenic dysfunction) are at particular risk of severe malaria. If travel to malarious areas is unavoidable, rigorous precautions are required against contracting the disease.

RENAL IMPAIRMENT. Avoidance (or dosage reduction) of proguanil is recommended since it is excreted by the kidneys. *Malarone*® should not be used for prophylaxis in patients with creatinine clearance less than 30 mL/minute. Chloroquine is only partially excreted by the kidneys and reduction of the dose for prophylaxis is not required except in severe impairment. Mefloquine is considered to be appropriate to use in renal impairment and does not require dosage reduction. Doxycycline is also considered to be appropriate.

PREGNANCY. Travel to malarious areas should be avoided during pregnancy; if travel is unavoidable, effective prophylaxis must be used. Chloroquine and proguanil may be given in usual doses in areas where *P. falciparum* strains are sensitive; in the case of proguanil, folic acid 5 mg daily should be given. The manufacturer advises that prophylaxis with mefloquine should be avoided as a matter of principle but studies of mefloquine in pregnancy (including use in the first trimester) indicate that it can be considered for travel to chloroquine-resistant areas. Doxycycline is contra-indicated during pregnancy. *Malarone*® should be avoided during pregnancy unless there is no suitable alternative. The centres listed on p. 312 should be consulted for advice on prophylaxis in resistant areas.

BREAST-FEEDING. Prophylaxis is required in **breast-fed infants**; although antimalarials are present in milk, the amounts are too variable to give reliable protection.

Specific recommendations

Where a journey requires two regimens, the regimen for the higher risk area should be used for the whole journey. Those travelling to remote or little-visited areas may require expert advice.

Risk may vary in different parts of a country—check under all risk levels

WARNING. Settled immigrants (or long-term visitors) to the UK may be unaware that they will have **lost some of their immunity** and also that the areas where they previously lived **may now be malarious**

North Africa, the Middle East, and Central Asia

VERY LOW RISK. Risk *very low* in Algeria, Egypt (tourist areas malaria-free), Georgia (south-east,

July–October), Kyrgystan (southern and western areas), Libya, rural Morocco, most tourist areas of Turkey, Uzbekistan (extreme south-east only):

> chemoprophylaxis not recommended but avoid mosquito bites and consider malaria if fever presents

LOW RISK. Risk *low* in Armenia (June–October), Azerbaijan (southern border areas, June–September), Egypt (El Fayoum only, June–October), rural north Iraq and Basrah Province (May–November), north border of Syria (May–October), Turkey (plain around Adana, Side, south-east Anatolia, March–November), Turkmenistan (south-east only, June–October):

preferably

> chloroquine *or* (if chloroquine not appropriate) proguanil hydrochloride

RISK. Risk *present* and *chloroquine resistance present* in Afghanistan (below 2000 m, May–November), Iran, Oman (remote rural areas only), Saudi Arabia (except northern, eastern and central provinces, Asir plateau, and western border cities where very little risk, no risk in Mecca), Tajikistan (June–October), Yemen (no risk in Sana'a):

> chloroquine + proguanil hydrochloride

Sub-Saharan Africa

No chemoprophylaxis recommended for Cape Verde and non-rural areas of Mauritius (but avoid mosquito bites and consider malaria if fever presents); *chloroquine prophylaxis* appropriate for rural areas of **Mauritius**

SEASONAL RISK. Risk *present* (in parts of country) and *some chloroquine resistance* in northern half of Botswana (November–June), Mauritania (all year in south; July–November in north), Namibia (all year along Kavango and Kunene rivers; November–June in northern third), areas below 1200 m in Zimbabwe (November–June; all year in Zambezi valley where prophylaxis as for *Very High Risk*, below; risk negligible in Harare and Bulawayo):

> chloroquine + proguanil hydrochloride *or* (if chloroquine + proguanil not appropriate) mefloquine *or* doxycycline *or* Malarone®

NOTE. In Zimbabwe and neighbouring countries, pyrimethamine with dapsone (also known as *Deltaprim®*) prophylaxis is used by local residents (sometimes with chloroquine).

VERY HIGH RISK. Risk *very high* (or *locally very high*) and *chloroquine resistance very widespread* in Angola, Benin, Burkina Faso, Burundi, Cameroon, Central African Republic, Chad, Comoros, Congo, Democratic Republic of the Congo (formely Zaïre), Djibouti, Equatorial Guinea, Eritrea, Ethiopia (below

2200 m; no risk in Addis Ababa), Gabon, Gambia, Ghana, Guinea, Guinea-Bissau, Ivory Coast, Kenya, Liberia, Madagascar, Malawi, Mali, Mozambique, Niger, Nigeria, Principe, Rwanda, São Tomé, Senegal, Sierra Leone, Somalia, South Africa (Kruger Park, north-east, low-altitude areas of Northern Province and Mpumalanga, and north-east Kwa-Zulu-Natal as far south as Tugela river), Sudan, Swaziland, Tanzania, Togo, Uganda, Zambia, Zimbabwe (Zambezi valley, see also above):

> mefloquine *or* doxycycline *or* Malarone®

South Asia

VARIABLE RISK. Risk *variable* and *chloroquine resistance usually moderate* in Bangladesh (except in Chittagong Hill Tracts, see below; no risk in Dhaka city), southern districts of Bhutan, India (no risk in parts of mountain states of north), Nepal (below 1500 m, especially Terai districts; no risk in Kathmandu), Pakistan (below 2000 m), Sri Lanka (no risk in and just south of Colombo):

> chloroquine + proguanil hydrochloride

HIGH RISK. Risk *high* and *chloroquine resistance high* in Bangladesh (only in Chittagong Hill Tracts):

> mefloquine *or* doxycycline *or* Malarone®

South-East Asia

VERY LOW RISK. Risk *very low* in Bali, main tourist areas of China (but *substantial risk* in Yunnan and Hainan, see below; *chloroquine prophylaxis* appropriate for other remote areas), Hong Kong, Korea (both Democratic People's Republic and Republic), Malaysia (but *substantial risk* in Sabah, and *variable risk* in deep forests, see below), Sarawak (but *variable risk* in deep forests, see below), Thailand (Bangkok, main tourist centres—**important**: regional risk exists, see under *Great risk*, below):

> chemoprophylaxis not recommended but avoid mosquito bites and consider malaria if fever presents

VARIABLE RISK. Risk *variable* and *some chloroquine resistance* in Indonesia (very low risk in Bali, and cities but *substantial risk* in Irian Jaya and Lombok, see below), rural Philippines below 600 m (no risk in cities, Cebu, Bohol, and Catanduanes), deep forests of peninsular Malaysia and Sarawak (but *substantial risk* in Sabah, see below):

> chloroquine + proguanil hydrochloride

SUBSTANTIAL RISK. Risk *substantial* and *drug resistance common* in Cambodia (no risk in Phnom Penh; for western provinces, see below), China (Yunnan and Hainan; *chloroquine prophylaxis* appropriate for other remote areas), East Timor, Irian Jaya, Laos (no risk in Vientiane), Lombok, Malaysia (Sabah; see also *Very low risk* and *Variable risk* above), Myanmar (formerly Burma; see also *Great risk* below), Vietnam (no risk in cities, Red River delta area, coastal plain north of Nha Trang):

mefloquine *or* doxycycline *or* Malarone®

GREAT RISK AND DRUG RESISTANCE PRESENT. Risk *great and mefloquine resistance present* in western provinces of Cambodia, borders of Thailand with Cambodia and Myanmar, and Ko Chang, Myanmar (eastern Shan State):

doxycycline *or* Malarone®

Oceania

RISK. Risk *high* and *chloroquine resistance high* in Papua New Guinea (below 1800 m), Solomon Islands, Vanuatu:

doxycycline *or* mefloquine *or* Malarone®

Central and South America and the Caribbean

VARIABLE TO LOW RISK. Risk *variable to low* in Argentina (rural areas along northern borders only), rural Belize (except Belize district), rural Costa Rica (below 500 m), Dominican Republic, El Salvador (Santa Ana province in west), Guatemala (below 1500 m), Haiti, Honduras, some rural areas of Mexico (not regularly visited by tourists), Nicaragua, Panama (west of Panama Canal but *variable to high risk* east of Panama Canal, see below), rural Paraguay:

chloroquine *or* (if chloroquine not appropriate) proguanil hydrochloride

VARIABLE TO HIGH RISK. Risk *variable to high* and *chloroquine resistance present* in rural areas of Bolivia (below 2500 m), Ecuador (below 1500 m; no malaria in Galapagos Islands and Guayaquil; see below for Esmeraldas Province), Panama (east of Panama Canal), rural areas of Peru (below 1500 m; see below for Amazon basin area), rural areas of Venezuela (except on coast, Caracas free of malaria):

chloroquine + proguanil hydrochloride *or* (if chloroquine + proguanil not appropriate) mefloquine *or* doxycycline *or* Malarone®

HIGH RISK. Risk *high* and *marked chloroquine resistance* in Bolivia (Amazon basin area), Brazil (throughout 'Legal Amazon' area which includes the Amazon basin area, Mato Grosso and Maranhao only; elsewhere *very low risk*—no chemoprophylaxis), Colombia (most areas below 800 m), Ecuador

(Esmeraldas Province), French Guiana, all interior regions of Guyana, Peru (Amazon basin area), Surinam (except Paramaribo and coast), Venezuela (Amazon basin area):

mefloquine *or* doxycycline *or* Malarone®

Standby treatment

Adults travelling for prolonged periods to areas of chloroquine-resistance who are unlikely to have easy access to medical care should carry a standby treatment course. Self-medication should be **avoided** if medical help is accessible; prophylaxis should be continued during and after the attack.

In order to avoid excessive self-medication, the traveller should be provided with **written instructions** that urgent medical attention should be sought if fever (38°C or more) develops 7 days (or more) after arriving in a malarious area and that self-treatment is indicated if medical help is not immediately available or the condition is worsening.

In view of the continuing emergence of resistant strains and of the different regimens required for different areas expert advice should be sought on the best treatment course for an individual traveller. A drug used for chemoprophylaxis should not be considered for standby treatment.

Artemether with lumefantrine

Artemether with lumefantrine is licensed for the *treatment of acute uncomplicated falciparum malaria*.

ARTEMETHER WITH LUMEFANTRINE

Indications: treatment of acute uncomplicated falciparum malaria

Cautions: electrolyte disturbances, concomitant use with other drugs known to cause QT-interval prolongation; hepatic impairment (Appendix 2); renal impairment (Appendix 3); pregnancy (Appendix 4); monitor patients unable to take food (greater risk of recrudescence); concomitant use with drugs that are metabolised by cytochrome P450 2D6; **interactions:** Appendix 1 (artemether with lumefantrine)

DRIVING. Dizziness may affect performance of skilled tasks (e.g. driving)

Contra-indications: history of arrhythmias, of clinically relevant bradycardia, and of congestive heart failure accompanied by reduced left ventricular ejection fraction; family history of sudden death or of congenital QT interval prolongation; breast-feeding (Appendix 5)

Side-effects: abdominal pain, anorexia, diarrhoea, vomiting, nausea, palpitations, cough, headache, dizziness, sleep disturbances, asthenia, arthralgia, myalgia, pruritus and rash

Dose: see notes above

Riamet® (Novartis) ▼ PoM
Tablets, yellow, artemether 20 mg, lumefantrine 120 mg, net price 24-tab pack = £22.50. Label: 21, counselling, driving

Chloroquine

Chloroquine is used for the *prophylaxis of malaria* in areas of the world where the *risk of chloroquine-resistant falciparum malaria is still low*. It is also used with proguanil when chloroquine-resistant falciparum malaria is present but this regimen may not give optimal protection (see specific recommendations by country, p. 314).

Chloroquine is **no longer recommended** for the *treatment of falciparum malaria* owing to widespread resistance, nor is it recommended if the infective species is *not known* or if the infection is *mixed*; in these cases treatment should be with quinine, mefloquine, *Malarone®*, or *Riamet®* (for details, see p. 312). It is still recommended for the *treatment of benign malarias* (for details, see p. 313).

CHLOROQUINE

Indications: chemoprophylaxis and treatment of malaria, see notes above; rheumatoid arthritis and lupus erythematosus (section 10.1.3)

Cautions: renal impairment (see notes above), pregnancy (but for malaria benefit outweighs risk, see Appendix 4, Antimalarials), may exacerbate psoriasis, neurological disorders (avoid for prophylaxis if history of epilepsy, see notes above), may aggravate myasthenia gravis, severe gastrointestinal disorders, G6PD deficiency (see section 9.1.5); ophthalmic examination and long-term therapy, see under Chloroquine, section 10.1.3; avoid concurrent therapy with hepatotoxic drugs—other **interactions:** Appendix 1 (chloroquine and hydroxychloroquine)

Side-effects: gastro-intestinal disturbances, headache; also convulsions, visual disturbances, depigmentation or loss of hair, skin reactions (rashes, pruritus); rarely, bone-marrow suppression, hypersensitivity reactions such as urticaria and angioedema; other side-effects (not usually associated with malaria prophylaxis or treatment), see under Chloroquine, section 10.1.3; very toxic in **overdosage**—immediate advice from poisons centres essential (see also p. 24)

Dose: expressed as chloroquine base

Prophylaxis of malaria, preferably started 1 week before entering endemic area and continued for 4 weeks after leaving (see notes above), 300 mg once weekly; INFANT up to 12 weeks body-weight under 6 kg, 37.5 mg once weekly; 12 weeks–11 months body-weight 6–10 kg, 75 mg once weekly; CHILD 1–3 years body-weight 10–16 kg, 112.5 mg once weekly; 4–7 years body-weight 16–25 kg, 150 mg once weekly; 8–12 years body-weight 25–45 kg, 225 mg once weekly; over 13 years body-weight over 45 kg, adult dose

Treatment of malaria, see notes above
COUNSELLING. Warn travellers about **importance** of avoiding mosquito bites, **importance** of taking prophylaxis regularly, and **importance** of immediate visit to doctor if ill within 1 year and **especially** within 3 months of return. For details, see notes above
NOTE. Chloroquine doses in BNF may differ from those in product literature

Chloroquine sulphate (Non-proprietary) [PoM]
Injection, chloroquine sulphate 54.5 mg/mL (≡ chloroquine base 40 mg/mL), net price 5-mL amp = 79p
Available from Beacon

[1]**Avloclor®** (AstraZeneca) [PoM]
Tablets, scored, chloroquine phosphate 250 mg (≡ chloroquine base 155 mg). Net price 20-tab pack = £1.22. Label: 5, counselling, prophylaxis, see above

[1]**Nivaquine®** (Beacon)
Tablets, f/c, yellow, chloroquine sulphate 200 mg (≡ chloroquine base 150 mg), net price 28-tab pack = £2.00. Label: 5, counselling, prophylaxis, see above
Syrup, golden, chloroquine sulphate 68 mg/5 mL (≡ chloroquine base 50 mg/5 mL), net price 100 mL = £4.77. Label: 5, counselling, prophylaxis, see above

■ With proguanil
For cautions and side-effects of proguanil see Proguanil; for dose see notes above
Paludrine/Avloclor® (AstraZeneca)
Tablets, travel pack of 14 tablets of chloroquine phosphate 250 mg (≡ chloroquine base 155 mg) and 98 tablets of proguanil hydrochloride 100 mg, net price 112-tab pack = £8.79. Label: 5, 21, counselling, prophylaxis, see above
Available as a generic from Boots

Mefloquine

Mefloquine is used for the *prophylaxis of malaria* in areas of the world where there is a *high risk of chloroquine-resistant falciparum malaria* (for details, see specific recommendations by country, p. 314).

Mefloquine is used for the *treatment of falciparum malaria* or if the infective species is *not known* or if the infection is *mixed* (for details, see p. 312.). It is also effective for the *treatment of benign malarias*, but is not required as chloroquine is usually effective. Mefloquine should not be used for treatment if it has been used for prophylaxis.

The CSM has advised that travellers should be informed about adverse reactions of mefloquine and, if they occur, medical advice should be sought on alternative antimalarials before the next dose is due; the patient information leaflet, which describes adverse reactions should always be provided when dispensing mefloquine

MEFLOQUINE

Indications: chemoprophylaxis of malaria, treatment of uncomplicated falciparum malaria and chloroquine-resistant vivax malaria, see notes above

Cautions: pregnancy (see notes under Treatment of malaria and under Prophylaxis against malaria)—manufacturer advises **avoid** pregnancy during and for 3 months after; breast-feeding (Appendix 5); avoid for chemoprophylaxis in severe hepatic

1. Can be sold to the public provided it is licensed and labelled for the prophylaxis of malaria. Drugs for malaria prophylaxis not prescribable on the NHS; health authorities may investigate circumstances under which antimalarials are prescribed

impairment; cardiac conduction disorders; epilepsy (avoid for prophylaxis); not recommended in infants under 3 months (5 kg); other **interactions:** Appendix 1 (mefloquine)

DRIVING. Dizziness or a disturbed sense of balance may affect performance of skilled tasks (e.g. driving); effects may persist for up to 3 weeks

Contra-indications: history of neuropsychiatric disorders, including depression, or convulsions; hypersensitivity to quinine

Side-effects: nausea, vomiting, diarrhoea, abdominal pain; dizziness, loss of balance, headache, sleep disorders (insomnia, drowsiness, abnormal dreams); also neuropsychiatric reactions (including sensory and motor neuropathies, tremor, ataxia, anxiety, depression, suicidal ideation, panic attacks, agitation, hallucinations, psychosis, convulsions), tinnitus and vestibular disorders, visual disturbances, circulatory disorders (hypotension and hypertension), chest pain, tachycardia, bradycardia, cardiac conduction disorders, dyspnoea, muscle weakness, myalgia, arthralgia, rash, urticaria, pruritus, alopecia, asthenia, malaise, fatigue, fever, loss of appetite, leucopenia or leucocytosis, thrombocytopenia; rarely Stevens-Johnson syndrome, AV block, encephalopathy and anaphylaxis

Dose: prophylaxis of malaria, preferably started 2–3 weeks before entering endemic area and continued for 4 weeks after leaving (see notes above), ADULT and CHILD body-weight over 45 kg, 250 mg once weekly; body-weight 6–16 kg, 62.5 mg once weekly; body-weight 16–25 kg, 125 mg once weekly; body-weight 25–45 kg, 187.5 mg once weekly

LONG-TERM CHEMOPROPHYLAXIS. Mefloquine prophylaxis can be taken for up to 1 year

Treatment of malaria, see notes above

COUNSELLING. See CSM advice in notes above. Also warn travellers about **importance** of avoiding mosquito bites, **importance** of taking prophylaxis regularly, and **importance** of immediate visit to doctor if ill within 1 year and **especially** within 3 months of return. For details, see notes above

¹**Lariam**® (Roche) PoM
Tablets, scored, mefloquine (as hydrochloride) 250 mg. Net price 8-tab pack = £14.53. Label: 21, 25, 27, counselling, driving, prophylaxis, see above

Primaquine

Primaquine is used to eliminate the liver stages of *P. vivax* or *P. ovale following chloroquine treatment* (for details, see p. 313).

PRIMAQUINE

Indications: adjunct in the treatment of *Plasmodium vivax* and *P. ovale* malaria (eradication of liver stages)

Cautions: G6PD deficiency (see notes above); systemic diseases associated with granulocytopenia (e.g. rheumatoid arthritis, lupus erythematosus); pregnancy and breast-feeding; **interactions:** Appendix 1 (primaquine)

1. Drugs for malaria prophylaxis not prescribable on the NHS; health authorities may investigate circumstances under which antimalarials prescribed

Side-effects: nausea, vomiting, anorexia, abdominal pain; less commonly methaemoglobinaemia, haemolytic anaemia especially in G6PD deficiency, leucopenia

Dose: see notes above

Primaquine (Non-proprietary)
Tablets, primaquine (as phosphate) 7.5 mg or 15 mg Available on a named-patient basis from Durbin, IDIS

Proguanil

Proguanil is used (usually *with chloroquine*, but occasionally *alone*) for the *prophylaxis of malaria*, (for details, see specific recommendations by country, p. 314).

Proguanil used alone is not suitable for the *treatment of malaria*; *Malarone*® (a combination of atovaquone with proguanil) is, however, licensed for the treatment of acute uncomplicated falciparum malaria. *Malarone*® is also used for the *prophylaxis of falciparum malaria* in areas of *widespread mefloquine or chloroquine resistance*. *Malarone*® is also used as an alternative to mefloquine or doxycycline. *Malarone*® is particularly suitable for short trips to highly chloroquine-resistant areas because it needs to be taken only for 7 days after leaving an endemic area.

PROGUANIL HYDROCHLORIDE

Indications: chemoprophylaxis of malaria
Cautions: renal impairment (see notes under Prophylaxis against malaria and Appendix 3); pregnancy (folate supplements needed); **interactions:** Appendix 1 (proguanil)
Side-effects: mild gastric intolerance and diarrhoea; occasionally mouth ulcers and stomatitis; skin reactions and hair loss reported; rarely hypersensitivity reactions such as urticaria and angioedema
Dose: prophylaxis of malaria, preferably started 1 week before entering endemic area and continued for 4 weeks after leaving (see notes above), 200 mg once daily; INFANT up to 12 weeks body-weight under 6 kg, 25 mg once daily; 12 weeks–11 months body-weight 6–10 kg, 50 mg once daily; CHILD 1–3 years body-weight 10–16 kg, 75 mg once daily; 4–7 years body-weight 16–25 kg, 100 mg once daily; 8–12 years, body-weight 25–45 kg, 150 mg once daily; over 13 years body-weight over 45 kg, adult dose

COUNSELLING. Warn travellers about **importance** of avoiding mosquito bites, **importance** of taking prophylaxis regularly, and **importance** of immediate visit to doctor if ill within 1 year and **especially** within 3 months of return. For details, see notes above

NOTE. Proguanil doses in BNF may differ from those in product literature

¹**Paludrine**® (AstraZeneca)
Tablets, scored, proguanil hydrochloride 100 mg. Net price 98-tab pack = £7.43. Label: 21, counselling, prophylaxis, see above

■ With chloroquine
See under Chloroquine

PROGUANIL HYDROCHLORIDE WITH ATOVAQUONE

Indications: treatment of acute uncomplicated falciparum malaria and prophylaxis of falciparum malaria, particularly where resistance to other antimalarial drugs suspected

Cautions: renal impairment (Appendix 3), diarrhoea or vomiting (reduced absorption of atovaquone), pregnancy (Appendix 4) and breast-feeding (Appendix 5); efficacy not evaluated in cerebral or complicated malaria (including hyperparasitaemia, pulmonary oedema or renal failure); **interactions:** see Appendix 1 (proguanil, atovaquone)

Side-effects: nausea, vomiting, mouth ulcers and stomatitis, diarrhoea, abdominal pain, anorexia, fever; headache, dizziness, abnormal dreams, insomnia, cough, visual disturbances, pruritus, rash, urticaria, angioedema; blood disorders, hyponatraemia, and hair loss reported

Dose: see under preparation

COUNSELLING. Warn travellers about **importance** of avoiding mosquito bites, **importance** of taking prophylaxis regularly, and **importance** of immediate visit to doctor if ill within 1 year and **especially** within 3 months of return. For details, see notes above

¹**Malarone**® (GSK) ▼ PoM

Tablets ('standard'), pink, f/c, proguanil hydrochloride 100 mg, atovaquone 250 mg. Net price 12-tab pack = £22.92. Label: 21, counselling, prophylaxis, see below

Dose: prophylaxis of malaria, started 1–2 days before entering endemic area and continued for 1 week after leaving, ADULT and CHILD over 40 kg, 1 tablet daily
Treatment of falciparum malaria, ADULT and CHILD bodyweight over 40 kg, 4 tablets once daily for 3 days; CHILD body-weight 11–20 kg 1 tablet daily for 3 days; body-weight 21–30 kg 2 tablets once daily for 3 days; body-weight 31–40 kg 3 tablets once daily for 3 days

¹**Malarone**® **Paediatric** (GSK) ▼ PoM

Paediatric tablets, pink, f/c proguanil hydrochloride 25 mg, atovaquone 62.5 mg, net price 12-tab pack = £7.64. Label: 21, counselling, prophylaxis, see above

Dose: prophylaxis of malaria, started 1–2 days before entering endemic area and continued for 1 week after leaving, CHILD body-weight 11–20 kg, 1 tablet once daily; body-weight 21–30 kg, 2 tablets once daily; body-weight 31–40 kg, 3 tablets once daily; body-weight over 40 kg use Malarone® ('standard') tablets, see p. 314
Treatment of falciparum malaria, see above

Pyrimethamine

Pyrimethamine should not be used alone, but is used with sulfadoxine (in Fansidar®).

Fansidar® is not recommended for the prophylaxis of malaria, but it is used in the treatment of falciparum malaria and can be used with (or following) quinine.

PYRIMETHAMINE

Indications: malaria (but used only in combined preparations incorporating sulfadoxine); toxoplasmosis—section 5.4.7

Cautions: hepatic or renal impairment, pregnancy (Appendix 4); breast-feeding (Appendix 5); blood counts required with prolonged treatment; history of seizures—avoid large loading doses; **interactions:** Appendix 1 (pyrimethamine)

1. Drugs for malaria prophylaxis not prescribable on the NHS; health authorities may investigate circumstances under which antimalarials prescribed

Side-effects: depression of haematopoiesis with high doses, rashes, insomnia

Dose: malaria, no dose stated because not recommended alone
Toxoplasmosis, section 5.4.7

Daraprim® (GSK) PoM ▱

Tablets, scored, pyrimethamine 25 mg. Net price 30-tab pack = £2.33

PYRIMETHAMINE WITH SULFADOXINE

Indications: adjunct to quinine in treatment of Plasmodium falciparum malaria (see notes above); **not** recommended for prophylaxis

Cautions: see under Pyrimethamine and under Co-trimoxazole (section 5.1.8); pregnancy and breast-feeding (Appendixes 4 and 5); not recommended for prophylaxis (severe side-effects on long-term use); **interactions:** Appendix 1 (pyrimethamine, sulphonamides)

Contra-indications: see under Pyrimethamine and under Co-trimoxazole (section 5.1.8); sulphonamide allergy

Side-effects: see under Pyrimethamine and under Co-trimoxazole (section 5.1.8); pulmonary infiltrates (e.g. eosinophilic or allergic alveolitis) reported—discontinue if cough or shortness of breath

Dose: treatment, see notes above
Prophylaxis, not recommended by UK malaria experts

Fansidar® (Roche) PoM

Tablets, scored, pyrimethamine 25 mg, sulfadoxine 500 mg, net price 3-tab pack = 80p

Quinine

Quinine is not suitable for the prophylaxis of malaria.

Quinine is used for the treatment of falciparum malaria or if the infective species is not known or if the infection is mixed (for details see p. 312).

QUININE

Indications: falciparum malaria; nocturnal leg cramps, see section 10.2.2

Cautions: atrial fibrillation, conduction defects, heart block, pregnancy (but appropriate for treatment of malaria); monitor blood glucose concentration during parenteral treatment; G6PD deficiency (see section 9.1.5); **interactions:** Appendix 1 (quinine)

Contra-indications: haemoglobinuria, myasthenia gravis, optic neuritis

Side-effects: cinchonism, including tinnitus, headache, hot and flushed skin, nausea, abdominal pain, rashes, visual disturbances (including temporary blindness), confusion; hypersensitivity reactions including angioedema, blood disorders (including thrombocytopenia and intravascular coagulation), and acute renal failure; hypoglycaemia (especially after parenteral administration); cardiovascular effects (see Cautions); very toxic in **overdosage**—immediate advice from poisons centres essential (see also p. 24)

Dose: see notes above
NOTE. Quinine (anhydrous base) 100 mg ≡ quinine bisulphate 169 mg ≡ quinine dihydrochloride 122 mg ≡ quinine hydrochloride 122 mg ≡ quinine sulphate 121 mg. Quinine bisulphate 300-mg tablets are available but provide less quinine than 300 mg of the dihydrochloride, hydrochloride, or sulphate

Quinine Sulphate (Non-proprietary) [PoM]
Tablets, coated, quinine sulphate 200 mg, net price 28-tab pack = £1.46; 300 mg, 28-tab pack = £1.34
Available from Alpharma, APS, Bristol, CP, Generics, Hillcross, Kent

Quinine Dihydrochloride (Non-proprietary) [PoM]
Injection, quinine dihydrochloride 300 mg/mL. For dilution and use as an infusion. 1- and 2-mL amps
Available from Martindale (special order) or from specialist centres (see p. 312)
NOTE. Intravenous injection of quinine is so hazardous that it has been superseded by infusion

Tetracyclines

Doxycycline (section 5.1.3) is used for the *prophylaxis of malaria* in areas of *widespread mefloquine or chloroquine resistance*. Doxycycline is also used as an alternative to mefloquine or *Malarone®* (for details, see specific recommendations by country, p. 314).

Doxycycline is also used as an *adjunct to quinine in the treatment of falciparum malaria* (for details see p. 312).

DOXYCYCLINE

Indications: prophylaxis of malaria; adjunct to quinine in treatment of *Plasmodium falciparum* malaria; see also section 5.1.3
Cautions: section 5.1.3
Contra-indications: section 5.1.3
Side-effects: section 5.1.3
Dose: prophylaxis of malaria, preferably started 1 week before entering endemic area and continued for 4 weeks after leaving (see notes above), 100 mg once daily; CHILD over 12 years body-weight 25–45 kg, 75 mg once daily
Treatment of falciparum malaria, see notes above

■ Preparations
Section 5.1.3

5.4.2   Amoebicides

Metronidazole is the drug of choice for *acute invasive amoebic dysentery* since it is very effective against vegetative forms of *Entamoeba histolytica* in ulcers; it is given in an adult dose of 800 mg three times daily for 5 days. **Tinidazole** is also effective. Metronidazole and tinidazole are also active against amoebae which may have migrated to the liver. Treatment with metronidazole (or tinidazole) is followed by a 10-day course of diloxanide furoate.

Diloxanide furoate is the drug of choice for asymptomatic patients with *E. histolytica* cysts in the faeces; metronidazole and tinidazole are relatively ineffective. Diloxanide furoate is relatively free from toxic effects and the usual course is of 10 days, given alone for chronic infections or following metronidazole or tinidazole treatment.

For *amoebic abscesses* of the liver **metronidazole** is effective in doses of 400 mg 3 times daily for 5–10 days; tinidazole is an alternative. The course may be repeated after 2 weeks if necessary. Aspiration of the abscess is indicated where it is suspected that it may rupture or where there is no improvement after 72 hours of metronidazole; the aspiration may need to be repeated. Aspiration aids penetration of metronidazole and, for abscesses with more than 100 mL of pus, if carried out in conjunction with drug therapy, may reduce the period of disability.

Diloxanide furoate is not effective against hepatic amoebiasis, but a 10-day course should be given at the completion of metronidazole or tinidazole treatment to destroy any amoebae in the gut.

DILOXANIDE FUROATE

Indications: see notes above; chronic amoebiasis and as adjunct to metronidazole or tinidazole in acute amoebiasis
Contra-indications: pregnancy (Appendix 4), breast-feeding (Appendix 5)
Side-effects: flatulence, vomiting, urticaria, pruritus
Dose: 500 mg every 8 hours for 10 days; CHILD over 25 kg, 20 mg/kg daily in 3 divided doses for 10 days
See also notes above

Diloxanide (Non-proprietary) [PoM]
Tablets, diloxanide furoate 500 mg, net price 30-tab pack = £32.95. Label: 9
Available from Sovereign

METRONIDAZOLE

Indications: see under Dose below; anaerobic infections, section 5.1.11
Cautions: section 5.1.11
Side-effects: section 5.1.11
Dose: *by mouth*, invasive intestinal amoebiasis, 800 mg every 8 hours for 5 days; CHILD 1–3 years 200 mg every 8 hours; 3–7 years 200 mg every 6 hours; 7–10 years 400 mg every 8 hours
Extra-intestinal amoebiasis (including liver abscess) and symptomless amoebic cyst passers, 400–800 mg every 8 hours for 5–10 days; CHILD 1–3 years 100–200 mg every 8 hours; 3–7 years 100–200 mg every 6 hours; 7–10 years 200–400 mg every 8 hours
Urogenital trichomoniasis, 200 mg every 8 hours for 7 days *or* 400–500 mg every 12 hours for 5–7 days, *or* 2 g as a single dose; CHILD 1–3 years 50 mg every 8 hours for 7 days; 3–7 years 100 mg every 12 hours; 7–10 years 100 mg every 8 hours
Giardiasis, 2 g daily for 3 days *or* 400 mg 3 times daily for 5 days *or* 500 mg twice daily for 7–10 days; CHILD 1–3 years 500 mg daily for 3 days; 3–7 years 600–800 mg daily; 7–10 years 1 g daily

■ Preparations
Section 5.1.11

TINIDAZOLE

Indications: see under Dose below; anaerobic infections, section 5.1.11
Cautions: section 5.1.11
Side-effects: section 5.1.11
Dose: intestinal amoebiasis, 2 g daily for 2–3 days; CHILD 50–60 mg/kg daily for 3 days
Amoebic involvement of liver, 1.5–2 g daily for 3–6 days; CHILD 50–60 mg/kg daily for 5 days
Urogenital trichomoniasis and giardiasis, single

2 g dose; CHILD single dose of 50–75 mg/kg (repeated once if necessary)

■ Preparations
Section 5.1.11

5.4.3 Trichomonacides

Metronidazole (section 5.4.2) is the treatment of choice for *Trichomonas vaginalis* infection. Contact tracing is recommended and sexual contacts should be treated simultaneously.

If metronidazole is ineffective, **tinidazole** may be tried; it is usually given as a single 2-g dose, with food. A further 2-g dose may be given if there is no clinical improvement.

5.4.4 Antigiardial drugs

Metronidazole (section 5.4.2) is the treatment of choice for *Giardia lamblia* infections, given by mouth in a dosage of 2 g daily for 3 days or 400 mg every 8 hours for 5 days.

Alternative treatments are **tinidazole** (section 5.4.2) 2 g as a single dose or **mepacrine hydrochloride** 100 mg every 8 hours for 5–7 days [unlicensed indication].

MEPACRINE HYDROCHLORIDE

Indications: giardiasis; discoid lupus erythematosus—(Antimalarials, section 10.1.3)
Cautions: hepatic impairment, elderly, history of psychosis; avoid in psoriasis; **interactions:** Appendix 1 (mepacrine)
Side-effects: gastro-intestinal disturbances; dizziness, headache; with large doses nausea, vomiting and occasionally transient acute toxic psychosis and CNS stimulation; on prolonged treatment yellow discoloration of skin and urine, chronic dermatoses (including severe exfoliative dermatitis), hepatitis, aplastic anaemia; also reported blue/black discoloration of palate and nails and corneal deposits with visual disturbances
Dose: giardiasis, 100 mg every 8 hours for 5–7 days; CHILD 2 mg/kg every 8 hours

Mepacrine Hydrochloride
Tablets, mepacrine hydrochloride 100 mg. Label: 4, 9, 14, 21
Available from BCM Specials [unlicensed—special order]

5.4.5 Leishmaniacides

Cutaneous leishmaniasis frequently heals spontaneously but if skin lesions are extensive or unsightly, treatment is indicated, as it is in visceral leishmaniasis (kala-azar).

Sodium stibogluconate, an organic pentavalent antimony compound, is the treatment of choice for visceral leishmaniasis. The dose is 20 mg/kg daily (max. 850 mg) for at least 20 days by intramuscular or intravenous injection; the dosage varies with different geographical regions and expert advice should be obtained. Skin lesions are treated for 10 days.

Amphotericin is used with or after an antimony compound for visceral leishmaniasis unresponsive to the antimonial alone; side-effects may be reduced by

using liposomal amphotericin (*AmBisome*®—section 5.2) at a dose of 1–3 mg/kg daily for 10–21 days to a cumulative dose of 21–30 mg/kg. Other lipid formulations of amphotericin (*Abelcet*® and *Amphocil*®) are also likely to be effective but less information is available.

Pentamidine isetionate (pentamidine isethionate) (section 5.4.8) has been used in antimony-resistant visceral leishmaniasis, but although the initial response is often good, the relapse rate is high; it is associated with serious side-effects. Other treatments include paromomycin (available on named-patient basis from IDIS).

SODIUM STIBOGLUCONATE

Indications: leishmaniasis
Cautions: hepatic impairment; pregnancy; intravenous injections must be given slowly over 5 minutes (to reduce risk of local thrombosis) and stopped if coughing or substernal pain; mucocutaneous disease (see below); heart disease (withdraw if conduction disturbances occur); treat intercurrent infection (e.g. pneumonia)
MUCOCUTANEOUS DISEASE. Successful treatment of mucocutaneous leishmaniasis may induce severe inflammation around the lesions (may be life-threatening if pharyngeal or tracheal involvement)—may require corticosteroid
Contra-indications: significant renal impairment; breast-feeding
Side-effects: anorexia, nausea, vomiting, abdominal pain; ECG changes; headache, lethargy, myalgia; raised liver enzymes; coughing and substernal pain (see Cautions); rarely anaphylaxis; also reported, fever, sweating, flushing, vertigo, bleeding from nose or gum, jaundice, rash; pain and thrombosis on intravenous administration, intramuscular injection is painful
Dose: see notes above

Pentostam® (GSK) PoM
Injection, sodium stibogluconate equivalent to pentavalent antimony 100 mg/mL. Net price 100-mL bottle = £71.43

5.4.6 Trypanocides

The prophylaxis and treatment of trypanosomiasis is difficult and differs according to the strain of organism. Expert advice should therefore be obtained.

5.4.7 Drugs for toxoplasmosis

Most infections caused by *Toxoplasma gondii* are self-limiting, and treatment is not necessary. Exceptions are patients with eye involvement (toxoplasma choroidoretinitis), and those who are immunosuppressed. Toxoplasmic encephalitis is a common complication of AIDS. The treatment of choice is a combination of pyrimethamine and sulfadiazine (sulphadiazine), given for several weeks (expert advice **essential**). Pyrimethamine is a folate antagonist, and adverse reactions to this combination are relatively common (folinic acid supplements and weekly blood counts needed). Alternative regimens use combinations of pyrimethamine with clindamycin or clarithromycin or azithromycin. Long-term secondary prophylaxis is required after treatment of toxoplasmosis in AIDS.

If toxoplasmosis is acquired in pregnancy, transplacental infection may lead to severe disease in the fetus. Spiramycin (available on named-patient basis from IDIS) may reduce the risk of transmission of maternal infection to the fetus.

5.4.8 Drugs for pneumocystis pneumonia

Pneumonia caused by *Pneumocystis carinii* occurs in immunosuppressed patients; it is a common cause of pneumonia in AIDS. Pneumocystis pneumonia should generally be treated by those experienced in its management. Blood gas measurement is used to assess disease severity.

Treatment

MILD TO MODERATE DISEASE. **Co-trimoxazole** (section 5.1.8) in high dosage is the drug of choice for the treatment of mild to moderate pneumocystis pneumonia.

Atovaquone is licensed for the treatment of mild to moderate pneumocystis infection in patients who cannot tolerate co-trimoxazole. A combination of **dapsone** 100 mg daily (section 5.1.10) with **trimethoprim** 5 mg/kg every 6–8 hours (section 5.1.8) is given by mouth for the treatment of mild to moderate disease [unlicensed indication].

A combination of **clindamycin** 600 mg by mouth every 6 hours (section 5.1.6) and **primaquine** 15 mg daily by mouth (section 5.4.1) is used in the treatment of mild to moderate disease [unlicensed indication]; this combination is associated with considerable toxicity.

Inhaled **pentamidine isetionate** is sometimes used for mild disease. It is better tolerated than parenteral pentamidine but systemic absorption may still occur.

SEVERE DISEASE. **Co-trimoxazole** (section 5.1.8) in high dosage, given by mouth or by intravenous infusion, is the drug of choice for the treatment of severe pneumocystis pneumonia. **Pentamidine isetionate** given by intravenous infusion is an alternative for patients who cannot tolerate co-trimoxazole, or who have not responded to it. Pentamidine isetionate is a potentially toxic drug that can cause severe hypotension during or immediately after infusion.

Corticosteroid treatment can be lifesaving in those with severe pneumocystis pneumonia (see Adjunctive Therapy below).

ADJUNCTIVE THERAPY. In moderate to severe infections associated with HIV infection, prednisolone 50–80 mg daily is given by mouth for 5 days (alternatively, hydrocortisone may be given parenterally); the dose is then reduced to complete 21 days of treatment. Corticosteroid treatment should ideally be started at the same time as the anti-pneumocystis therapy and certainly no later than 24–72 hours afterwards. The corticosteroid should be withdrawn before anti-pneumocystis treatment is complete.

Prophylaxis

Prophylaxis against pneumocystis pneumonia should be given to all patients with a history of the infection. Prophylaxis against pneumocystis pneumonia should also be considered for severely immunocompromised patients. Prophylaxis should continue until immunity recovers sufficiently. It should not be discontinued if the patient has oral candidiasis, continues to lose weight, or is receiving cytotoxic therapy or long-term immunosuppressant therapy.

Co-trimoxazole by mouth is the drug of choice for prophylaxis against pneumocystis pneumonia. It is given in a dose of 960 mg daily or 960 mg on alternate days (3 times a week); the dose may be reduced to co-trimoxazole 480 mg daily to improve tolerance.

Intermittent inhalation of **pentamidine isetionate** is used for prophylaxis against penumocystis pneumonia in patients unable to tolerate co-trimoxazole. It is effective but patients may be prone to extrapulmonary infection. Alternatively, **dapsone** 100 mg daily (section 5.1.10) can be used. **Atovaquone** 750 mg twice daily has also been used for prophylaxis [unlicensed indication].

ATOVAQUONE

Indications: treatment of mild to moderate *Pneumocystis carinii* pneumonia in patients intolerant of co-trimoxazole

Cautions: initial diarrhoea and difficulty in taking with food may reduce absorption (and require alternative therapy); other causes of pulmonary disease should be sought and treated; elderly; hepatic and renal impairment; pregnancy; avoid breast-feeding; **interactions:** Appendix 1 (atovaquone)

Side-effects: diarrhoea, nausea, vomiting; headache, insomnia; rash, fever; elevated liver enzymes and amylase; anaemia, neutropenia; hyponatraemia

Dose: 750 mg twice daily with food (particularly high fat) for 21 days; CHILD not recommended

Wellvone® (GSK) [PoM]
Suspension, sugar-free, fruit-flavoured, atovaquone 750 mg/5 mL, net price 210 mL = £435.82.
Label: 21

▪ With proguanil hydrochloride
See section 5.4.1

PENTAMIDINE ISETIONATE

Indications: see under Dose (should only be given by specialists)

Cautions: risk of severe hypotension following administration (establish baseline blood pressure and administer with patient lying down; monitor blood pressure closely during administration, and at regular intervals, until treatment concluded); hepatic and renal impairment; hypertension or hypotension; hyperglycaemia or hypoglycaemia; leucopenia, thrombocytopenia, or anaemia; pregnancy and breast-feeding; carry out laboratory monitoring according to product literature; care required to protect personnel during handling and administration; **interactions:** Appendix 1 (pentamidine isetionate)

Side-effects: severe reactions, sometimes fatal, due to hypotension, hypoglycaemia, pancreatitis, and arrhythmias; also leucopenia, thrombocytopenia, acute renal failure, hypocalcaemia; also reported: azotaemia, abnormal liver-function tests, anaemia, hyperkalaemia, nausea and vomiting, dizziness, syncope, flushing, hyperglycaemia, rash, and taste disturbances; Stevens-Johnson syndrome reported; on inhalation, bronchoconstriction (may be prevented by prior use of bronchodilators), cough, shortness of breath, and wheezing; discomfort, pain, induration, abscess formation, and muscle necrosis at injection site

Dose: *Pneumocystis carinii* pneumonia, *by intravenous infusion*, 4 mg/kg daily for at least 14 days (reduced according to product literature in renal impairment)

By inhalation of nebulised solution (using suitable equipment—consult product literature) 600 mg pentamidine isetionate daily for 3 weeks; secondary prevention, 300 mg every 4 weeks *or* 150 mg every 2 weeks

Visceral leishmaniasis (kala-azar, section 5.4.5), *by deep intramuscular injection*, 3–4 mg/kg on alternate days to max. total of 10 injections; course may be repeated if necessary

Cutaneous leishmaniasis, *by deep intramuscular injection*, 3–4 mg/kg once or twice weekly until condition resolves (but see also section 5.4.5)

Trypanosomiasis, *by deep intramuscular injection or intravenous infusion*, 4 mg/kg daily or on alternate days to total of 7–10 injections

NOTE. Direct bolus intravenous injection should be avoided whenever possible and **never** given rapidly; intramuscular injections should be deep and preferably given into the buttock

Pentacarinat® (JHC) PoM
Injection, powder for reconstitution, pentamidine isetionate, net price 300-mg vial = £32.74
Nebuliser solution, pentamidine isetionate, net price 300-mg bottle = £34.57
CAUTION IN HANDLING. Pentamidine isetionate is toxic and personnel should be adequately protected during handling and administration—consult product literature

5.5 Anthelmintics

Advice on prophylaxis and treatment of helminth infections is available from:

Birmingham	(0121) 424 0357
Scottish Centre for Infection and Environmental Health (registered users of Travax only)	(0141) 300 1130 (weekdays 2–4 p.m. only)
Liverpool	(0151) 708 9393
London	(020) 7387 9300 (treatment)

5.5.1 Drugs for threadworms
(pinworms, *Enterobius vermicularis*)

Anthelmintics are effective in threadworm infections, but their use needs to be combined with hygienic measures to break the cycle of auto-infection. All members of the family require treatment.

Adult threadworms do not live for longer than 6 weeks and for development of fresh worms, ova must be swallowed and exposed to the action of digestive juices in the upper intestinal tract. Direct multiplication of worms does not take place in the large bowel. Adult female worms lay ova on the perianal skin which causes pruritus; scratching the area then leads to ova being transmitted on fingers to the mouth, often via food eaten with unwashed hands. Washing hands and scrubbing nails before each meal and after each visit to the toilet is essential. A bath taken immediately after rising will remove ova laid during the night.

Mebendazole is the drug of choice for treating threadworm infection in patients of all ages over 2 years. It is given as a single dose; as reinfection is very common, a second dose may be given after 2–3 weeks.

Piperazine is available in combination with sennosides as a single-dose preparation.

MEBENDAZOLE

Indications: threadworm, roundworm, whipworm, and hookworm infections

Cautions: pregnancy (toxicity in *rats*), breast-feeding; **interactions:** Appendix 1 (mebendazole)
NOTE. The package insert in the *Vermox®* pack includes the statement that it is not suitable for women known to be pregnant or children under 2 years

Side-effects: rarely abdominal pain, diarrhoea; hypersensitivity reactions (including exanthema, rash, urticaria, and angioedema) reported

Dose: threadworms, ADULT and CHILD over 2 years, 100 mg as a single dose; if reinfection occurs second dose may be needed after 2–3 weeks; CHILD under 2 years, not yet recommended

Whipworms, ADULT and CHILD over 2 years, 100 mg twice daily for 3 days; CHILD under 2 years, not yet recommended

Roundworms—section 5.5.2
Hookworms—section 5.5.4

[1]**Mebendazole** (Non-proprietary) PoM
Tablets, chewable, mebendazole 100 mg

1. Can be sold to the public if supplied for oral use in the treatment of enterobiasis in adults and children over 2 years provided its container or package is labelled to show a max. single dose of 100 mg and it is supplied in a container or package containing not more than 800 mg; proprietary brands on sale to the public include *Boots Threadworm Tablets 2 Years Plus®*, *Ovex®* and *Pripsen® Mebendazole*

Vermox® (Janssen-Cilag) PoM
Tablets, orange, scored, chewable, mebendazole 100 mg. Net price 6-tab pack = £1.53
Suspension, mebendazole 100 mg/5 mL. Net price 30 mL = £1.77

PIPERAZINE

Indications: threadworm and roundworm infections

Cautions: liver impairment (Appendix 2); renal impairment (Appendix 3); epilepsy; pregnancy (Appendix 4); packs on sale to the general public carry a warning to avoid in epilepsy, liver or kidney disease, and to seek medical advice in pregnancy

Side-effects: nausea, vomiting, colic, diarrhoea, allergic reactions including urticaria, broncho-spasm, and rare reports of arthralgia, fever, Ste-vens-Johnson syndrome and angioedema; rarely dizziness, muscular incoordination ('worm wob-ble'); drowsiness, nystagmus, vertigo, blurred vision, confusion and clonic contractions in patients with neurological or renal abnormalities

Dose: see under Preparation, below

■ **With sennosides**
For cautions, contra-indications, side-effects of senna see section 1.6.2

Pripsen® (Thornton & Ross)
Oral powder, piperazine phosphate 4 g, total sennosides (calculated as sennoside B) 15.3 mg/sachet. Net price two-dose sachet pack = £1.31. Label: 13
Dose: threadworms, stirred into milk or water, ADULT and CHILD over 6 years, content of 1 sachet as a single dose (bedtime in adults or morning in children), repeated after 14 days; INFANT 3 months–1 year, 1 level 2.5-mL spoonful in the morning, repeated after 14 days; CHILD 1–6 years, 1 level 5-mL spoonful in the morning, repeated after 14 days
Roundworms, first dose as for threadworms; repeat at monthly intervals for up to 3 months if reinfection risk

Levamisole (available on named-patient basis from IDIS) is very effective against *Ascaris lumbricoides* and is generally considered to be the drug of choice. It is very well tolerated; mild nausea or vomiting has been reported in about 1% of treated patients; it is given as a single dose of 120–150 mg in adults.

Mebendazole (section 5.5.1) is also active against ascaris; the usual dose is 100 mg twice daily for 3 days. **Piperazine** may be given in a single adult dose, see Piperazine, above.

Taenicides

Niclosamide (available on named-patient basis from IDIS) is the most widely used drug for tapeworm infections and side-effects are limited to occasional gastro-intestinal upset, lightheadedness, and pru-ritus; it is not effective against larval worms. Fears of developing cysticercosis in *Taenia solium* infec-tions have proved unfounded. All the same, it is wise to anticipate this possibility by using an anti-emetic on wakening.

Praziquantel (available on named-patient basis from Merck (*Cysticide®*)) is as effective as niclos-amide and is given as a single dose of 10–20 mg/kg after a light breakfast (a single dose of 25 mg/kg for *Hymenolepis nana*).

Hydatid disease

Cysts caused by *Echinococcus granulosus* grow slowly and asymptomatic patients do not always require treatment. Surgical treatment remains the method of choice in many situations. **Albendazole** (available on named-patient basis from IDIS (*Zen-tel®*)) is used in conjunction with surgery to reduce the risk of recurrence or as primary treatment in inoperable cases. Alveolar echinococcosis due to *E. multilocularis* is usually fatal if untreated. Surgical removal with albendazole cover is the treatment of choice, but where effective surgery is impossible, repeated cycles of albendazole (for a year or more) may help. Careful monitoring of liver function is particularly important during drug treatment.

Hookworms live in the upper small intestine and draw blood from the point of their attachment to their host. An iron-deficiency anaemia may thereby be produced and, if present, effective treatment of the infection requires not only expulsion of the worms but treatment of the anaemia.

Mebendazole (section 5.5.1) has a useful broad-spectrum activity, and is effective against hook-worms; the usual dose is 100 mg twice daily for 3 days.

Adult *Schistosoma haematobium* worms live in the genito-urinary veins and adult *S. mansoni* in those of the colon and mesentery. *S. japonicum* is more widely distributed in veins of the alimentary tract and portal system.

Praziquantel (available on named-patient basis from Merck (*Cysticide®*)) is effective against all human schistosomes. The dose is 40 mg/kg in 2 divided doses 4–6 hours apart on one day (60 mg/kg in 3 divided doses on one day for *S. japonicum* infections). No serious toxic effects have been reported. Of all the available schistosomicides, it has the most attractive combination of effectiveness, broad-spectrum activity, and low toxicity.

Hycanthone, lucanthone, niridazole, oxamniquine, and sodium stibocaptate have now been superseded.

Diethylcarbamazine (not on UK market) is effec-tive against microfilariae and adults of *Loa loa*, *Wuchereria bancrofti*, and *Brugia malayi*. To mini-mise reactions treatment is commenced with a dose of diethylcarbamazine citrate 1 mg/kg on the first day and increased gradually over 3 days to 6 mg/kg daily in divided doses; this dosage is maintained for 21 days and usually gives a radical cure for these infections. Close medical supervision is necessary particularly in the early phase of treatment.

In heavy infections there may be a febrile reaction, and in heavy *Loa loa* infection there is a small risk of encephalopathy. In such cases treatment must be given under careful in-patient supervision and stopped at the first sign of cerebral involvement (and specialist advice sought).

Ivermectin (*Mectizan*®, MSD, available on named-patient basis) is very effective in *onchocerciasis* and it is now the drug of choice. A single dose of 150 micrograms/kg by mouth produces a prolonged reduction in microfilarial levels. Retreatment at intervals of 6 to 12 months depending on symptoms must be given until the adult worms die out. Reactions are usually slight and most commonly take the form of temporary aggravation of itching and rash. Diethylcarbamazine or suramin should no longer be used for onchocerciasis because of their toxicity.

5.5.7 Drugs for cutaneous larva migrans
(creeping eruption)

Dog and cat hookworm larvae may enter human skin where they produce slowly extending itching tracks usually on the foot. Single tracks can be treated with topical tiabendazole (no commercial preparation available). Multiple infections respond to **ivermectin** (*Mectizan*®, MSD, available on named-patient basis), **albendazole** (available on named-patient basis from IDIS (*Zentel*®)) or **tiabendazole** (thiabendazole) (available on a named-patient basis from IDIS (*Mintezol*®, *Triasox*®)) by mouth.

5.5.8 Drugs for strongyloidiasis

Adult *Strongyloides stercoralis* live in the gut and produce larvae which penetrate the gut wall and invade the tissues, setting up a cycle of auto-infection. **Tiabendazole** (thiabendazole) (available on a named-patient basis from IDIS (*Mintezol*®, *Triasox*®)) is the drug of choice for adults (but side-effects are much more marked in the elderly); it is given at a dosage of 25 mg/kg (max. 1.5 g) every 12 hours for 3 days. **Albendazole** is an alternative (available on named-patient basis from IDIS (*Zentel*®)) with fewer side-effects; it is given in a dose of 400 mg twice daily for 3 days, repeated after 3 weeks if necessary. **Ivermectin** (*Mectizan*®, MSD, available on named-patient basis) in a dose of 200 micrograms/kg daily for 2 days may be the most effective drug for chronic *Strongyloides* infection.

6: Endocrine system

6.1 Drugs used in diabetes

Diabetes mellitus occurs because of a lack of insulin or resistance to its action. Diabetes is clinically defined by measurement of fasting or random blood-glucose concentration (and occasionally by glucose tolerance test). There are two principal classes of diabetes (and many subtypes not listed here):

TYPE 1 DIABETES. Type 1 diabetes, also referred to as insulin-dependent diabetes mellitus (IDDM), is due to a deficiency of insulin following autoimmune destruction of pancreatic beta cells. Patients with type 1 diabetes require administration of insulin.

TYPE 2 DIABETES. Type 2 diabetes, also referred to as non-insulin-dependent diabetes (NIDDM), is due to reduced secretion of insulin or to peripheral resistance to the action of insulin. Although patients may be controlled on diet alone, many require oral antidiabetic drugs or insulin to maintain satisfactory control. In overweight individuals, type 2 diabetes may be prevented by losing weight and increasing physical activity; use of drugs such as orlistat (section 4.5.1) may be considered in obese patients.

Treatment should be aimed at alleviating symptoms and minimising the risk of long-term complications by appropriate control of diabetes. Other risk factors for cardiovascular disease (smoking, hypertension, obesity and hyperlipidaemia) should be addressed.

Diabetes is a strong risk factor for cardiovascular disease. The use of an ACE inhibitor (section 2.5.5.1), of low-dose aspirin (section 2.9) and of a lipid-regulating drug (section 2.12) can be beneficial in patients with diabetes and a high cardiovascular risk. For reference to the use of an ACE inhibitor in the management of diabetic nephropathy, see section 6.1.5.

PREVENTION OF DIABETIC COMPLICATIONS. Optimal glycaemic control in both type 1 diabetes and type 2 diabetes reduces, in the long term, the risk of microvascular complications including retinopathy, development of proteinuria and to some extent neuropathy. However, a temporary deterioration in established diabetic retinopathy may occur when normalising blood-glucose concentration.

A measure of the total glycated (or glycosylated) haemoglobin (HbA_1) or a specific fraction (HbA_{1c}) provides a good indication of long-term glycaemic control. The ideal HbA_{1c} concentration is between 6.5 and 7.5% but this cannot always be achieved, and for those on insulin there are significantly increased risks of severe hypoglycaemia. Tight control of blood pressure in hypertensive patients with type 2 diabetes reduces mortality significantly and protects visual acuity (by reducing considerably the risks of maculopathy and retinal photocoagulation) (see also section 2.5).

6.1.1 Insulins

6.1.1.1	Short-acting insulins
6.1.1.2	Intermediate- and long-acting insulins
6.1.1.3	Hypodermic equipment

Insulin plays a key role in the regulation of carbohydrate, fat, and protein metabolism. It is a polypeptide hormone of complex structure. There are differences in the amino-acid sequence of animal insulins, human insulins and the human insulin analogues. Insulin may be extracted from pork pancreas and purified by crystallisation; it may also be extracted from beef pancreas, but beef insulins are now rarely used. Human sequence insulin may be produced semisynthetically by enzymatic modification of porcine insulin (emp) or biosynthetically by recombinant DNA technology using bacteria (crb, prb) or yeast (pyr).

All insulin preparations are to a greater or lesser extent immunogenic in man but immunological resistance to insulin action is uncommon. Preparations of human sequence insulin should theoretically be less immunogenic, but no real advantage has been shown in trials.

Insulin is inactivated by gastro-intestinal enzymes, and must therefore be given by injection; the subcutaneous route is ideal in most circumstances. It is usually injected into the upper arms, thighs, buttocks, or abdomen; there may be increased absorption from a limb site if the limb is used in strenuous exercise following the injection. Generally subcutaneous insulin injections cause few problems; fat hypertrophy does however occur but can be minimised by rotating the injection sites. Local allergic reactions are now rare.

Insulin is needed by all patients with ketoacidosis, and it is likely to be needed by most patients with:

- rapid onset of symptoms;
- substantial loss of weight;
- weakness;
- ketonuria.

If the condition worsens, vomiting can occur and patients may rapidly develop ketoacidosis. Insulin is required by almost all children with diabetes. It is also needed for type 2 diabetes when other methods have failed to achieve good control, and temporarily in the presence of intercurrent illness or perioperatively. Pregnant women with type 2 diabetes should be treated with insulin when diet alone fails. The majority of those who are obese can be managed by dietary changes or, if diet alone fails to achieve adequate control, by also administering oral hypoglycaemic drugs (section 6.1.2).

MANAGEMENT OF DIABETES WITH INSULIN. The aim of treatment is to achieve the best possible control of blood-glucose concentration without making the patient obsessional and to avoid disabling hypoglycaemia; close co-operation is needed between the patient and the medical team since good control reduces the risk of complications. Mixtures of insulin preparations may be required and appropriate combinations have to be determined for the individual patient. For patients with acute-onset diabetes, treatment should be started with soluble insulin given 3 times daily with medium-acting insulin at bedtime. For those less severely ill, treatment is usually started with a mixture of premixed short- and medium-acting insulins (most commonly in a proportion of 30% soluble insulin and 70% isophane insulin) given twice daily; 8 units twice daily is a suitable initial dose for most ambulant patients. The proportion of the short-acting soluble component can be increased in those with excessive postprandial hyperglycaemia.

The dose of insulin is adjusted on an individual basis, by gradually increasing the dose but avoiding troublesome hypoglycaemic reactions.

There are 3 main types of insulin preparations:

- those of **short** duration which have a relatively rapid onset of action, namely soluble insulin, insulin lispro and insulin aspart;
- those with an **intermediate** action, e.g. isophane insulin and insulin zinc suspension; and
- those whose action is slower in onset and lasts for **long** periods, e.g. crystalline insulin zinc suspension

The duration of action of a particular type of insulin varies considerably from one patient to another, and needs to be assessed individually.

EXAMPLES OF RECOMMENDED INSULIN REGIMENS.

- Short-acting insulin mixed with intermediate-acting insulin: twice daily (before meals)
- Short-acting insulin mixed with intermediate-acting insulin: before breakfast
  Short-acting insulin: before evening meal
  Intermediate-acting insulin: at bedtime
- Short-acting insulin: three times daily (before breakfast, midday and evening meal)
  Intermediate-acting insulin: at bedtime
- Intermediate-acting insulin with or without short-acting insulin: once daily either before breakfast or at bedtime suffices for some patients with type 2 diabetes who need insulin, sometimes in combination with oral hypoglycaemic drugs

Insulin requirements may be increased by infection, stress, accidental or surgical trauma, puberty, and during the second and third trimesters of pregnancy. Requirements may be decreased in patients with renal or hepatic impairment and in those with some endocrine disorders (e.g. Addison's disease, hypopituitarism) or coeliac disease. In pregnancy insulin requirements should be assessed frequently by an experienced diabetes physician.

INSULIN ADMINISTRATION. Insulin is generally given by *subcutaneous injection*. Injection devices ('pens') (section 6.1.1.3) which hold the insulin in a cartridge and meter the required dose are convenient to use. The conventional syringe and needle is still the preferred method of insulin administration by many and is also required for insulins not available in cartridge form.

For intensive insulin regimens multiple subcutaneous injections (3 to 4 times daily) are usually recommended.

Short-acting insulins (soluble insulin, insulin aspart and insulin lispro) can also be given by *continuous subcutaneous infusion* using a portable infusion pump. This device delivers a continuous basal insulin infusion and patient-activated bolus doses at meal times. This technique is appropriate only for patients who suffer recurrent hypoglycaemia or marked morning rise in blood-glucose concentration despite optimised multiple-injection regimens. NICE (February 2003) has also recommended continuous subcutaneous infusion as an option in those who suffer repeated or unpredictable hypoglycaemia despite optimal multiple-injection regimens (including the use of insulin glargine where appropriate). Patients on subcutaneous insulin infusion must be highly motivated, able to monitor their blood-glucose concentration, and have expert training, advice and supervision from an experienced healthcare team.

Soluble insulin by the *intravenous route* is reserved for urgent treatment, and for fine control in serious illness and in the perioperative period (see under Diabetes and Surgery, below).

UNITS. The word 'unit' should **not** be abbreviated.

MONITORING. Many patients now monitor their own blood-glucose concentrations (section 6.1.6). Since blood-glucose concentrations vary substantially throughout the day, 'normoglycaemia' cannot always be achieved throughout a 24-hour period without causing damaging hypoglycaemia. It is therefore best to recommend that patients should maintain a blood-glucose concentration of between 4 and 10 mmol/litre for most of the time, while accepting that on occasions, for brief periods, it will be above these values; strenuous efforts should be made to prevent the blood-glucose concentration from falling below 4 mmol/litre. Patients should be advised to look for 'peaks' and 'troughs' of blood glucose, and to adjust their insulin dosage only once or twice weekly. Overall it is ideal to aim for an HbA_{1c} (glycosylated haemoglobin) concentration of 6.5–7.5% or less (normal range 4–6%) although this is not always possible without causing disabling hypoglycaemia. Fructosamine can also be used for assessment of control; this is simpler and cheaper but the measurement of HbA_{1c} is generally a more reliable method.

The intake of energy and of simple and complex carbohydrates should be adequate to allow normal growth and development but obesity must be avoided. The carbohydrate intake needs to be regulated and should be distributed throughout the day. Fine control of plasma glucose can be achieved by moving portions of carbohydrate from one meal to another without altering the total intake.

HYPOGLYCAEMIA. Hypoglycaemia is a potential problem for all patients receiving insulin and careful instruction to the patient must be directed towards avoiding it.

Loss of warning of hypoglycaemia is common among insulin-treated patients and can be a serious hazard, especially for drivers and those in dangerous occupations. Very tight control of diabetes lowers the blood-glucose concentration needed to trigger hypoglycaemic symptoms; increase in the frequency of hypoglycaemic episodes reduces the warning symptoms experienced by the patient. Beta-blockers can also blunt hypoglycaemic awareness (and also delay recovery).

To restore the warning signs, episodes of hypoglycaemia must be reduced to a minimum; this involves appropriate adjustment of insulin type, dose and frequency together with suitable timing and quantity of meals and snacks.

Some patients have reported loss of hypoglycaemia warning after transfer to human insulin. Clinical studies do not confirm that human insulin decreases hypoglycaemia awareness. If a patient believes that human insulin is responsible for the loss of warning it is reasonable to revert to animal insulin and essential to educate the patient about avoiding hypoglycaemia. Great care should be taken to specify whether a human or an animal preparation is required.

Few patients are now treated with beef insulins; when undertaking conversion from beef to human insulin, the total dose should be reduced by about 10% with careful monitoring for the first few days. When changing between pork and human sequence insulins, a dose change is not usually needed, but careful monitoring is still advised.

DRIVING. Drivers treated with insulin or oral antidiabetic drugs are required to notify the Driver and Vehicle Licensing Agency of their condition, as are drivers of Group 2 vehicles (heavy goods vehicles or public service vehicles) whose diabetes is controlled by diet alone; the Agency's Drivers Medical Unit provides guidance on eligibility to drive. Driving is not permitted when hypoglycaemic awareness is impaired.

Drivers need to be particularly careful to avoid hypoglycaemia (see also above) and should be warned of the problems. They should normally check their blood-glucose concentration before driving and, on long journeys, at 2-hour intervals. Drivers treated with insulin should ensure that a supply of sugar is always available in the vehicle and they should avoid driving if they are late for a meal. If hypoglycaemia occurs, or warning signs develop, the driver should:

- stop the vehicle in a safe place;
- switch off the ignition;
- eat or drink a suitable source of sugar;
- wait until recovery is complete before continuing journey; recovery may take 15 minutes or longer and should preferably be confirmed by checking blood-glucose concentration.

DIABETES AND SURGERY. The following regimen is suitable when surgery in a patient with type 1 diabetes requires intravenous infusion of insulin for 12 hours or longer.

- Give an injection of the patient's usual insulin on the night before the operation.
- Early on the day of the operation, start an intravenous infusion of glucose 5% or 10% containing potassium chloride 10 mmol/litre (provided that the patient is not hyperkalaemic) and infuse at a constant rate appropriate to the patient's fluid requirements (usually 125 mL per hour); make up a solution of soluble insulin 1 unit/mL in sodium chloride 0.9% and infuse intravenously using a syringe pump piggy-backed to the intravenous infusion.

- The rate of the insulin infusion should normally be:

Blood glucose < 4 mmol/litre, give 0.5 units/ hour

Blood glucose 4–15 mmol/litre, give 2 units/ hour

Blood glucose 15–20 mmol/litre, give 4 units/ hour

Blood glucose > 20 mmol/litre, review.

In resistant cases (such as patients who are in shock or severely ill or those receiving corticosteroids or sympathomimetics) 2–4 times these rates or even more may be needed.

If a syringe pump is not available soluble insulin 16 units/litre should be added to the intravenous infusion of glucose 5% or 10% containing potassium chloride 10 mmol per litre (provided the patient is not hyperkalaemic) and the infusion run at the rate appropriate to the patient's fluid requirements (usually 125 mL per hour) with the insulin dose adjusted as follows:

Blood glucose < 4 mmol/litre, give 8 units/litre

Blood glucose 4–15 mmol/litre, give 16 units/litre

Blood glucose 15–20 mmol/litre, give 32 units/litre

Blood glucose > 20 mmol/litre, review.

The rate of intravenous infusion depends on the volume depletion, cardiac function, age, and other factors. Blood-glucose concentration should be measured pre-operatively and then hourly until stable, thereafter every 2 hours. The duration of action of intravenous insulin is only a few minutes and the infusion must not be stopped unless the patient becomes overtly hypoglycaemic (blood glucose < 3 mmol/litre) in which case it should be stopped for up to 30 minutes. The amount of potassium chloride required in the infusion needs to be assessed by regular measurement of plasma electrolytes. Sodium chloride 0.9% infusion should replace glucose 5% or 10% if the blood glucose is persistently above 15 mmol/litre.

Once the patient starts to eat and drink, give subcutaneous insulin before breakfast and stop intravenous insulin 30 minutes later; the dose may need to be 10–20% more than usual if the patient is still in bed or unwell. If the patient was not previously receiving insulin, an appropriate initial dose is 30–40 units daily in four divided doses using soluble insulin before meals and intermediate-acting insulin at bedtime and the dose adjusted from day to day. Patients with hyperglycaemia often relapse after conversion back to subcutaneous insulin calling for one of the following approaches:

- additional doses of soluble insulin at any of the four injection times (before meals or bedtime) or
- temporary addition of intravenous insulin infusion (while continuing the subcutaneous regimen) until blood-glucose concentration is satisfactory or
- complete reversion to the intravenous regimen (especially if the patient is unwell).

6.1.1.1 Short-acting insulins

Soluble insulin is a short-acting form of insulin. For maintenance regimens it is usual to inject it 15 to 30 minutes before meals.

Soluble insulin is the most appropriate form of insulin for use in diabetic emergencies and at the time of surgery. It can be given intravenously and intramuscularly, as well as subcutaneously.

When injected subcutaneously, soluble insulin has a rapid onset of action (30 to 60 minutes), a peak action between 2 and 4 hours, and a duration of action of up to 8 hours. Human sequence preparations tend to act more rapidly and they have a shorter duration of action.

When injected intravenously, soluble insulin has a very short half-life of only about 5 minutes and its effect disappears within 30 minutes.

The human insulin analogues, **insulin lispro** and **insulin aspart**, have a faster onset and shorter duration of action than soluble insulin; as a result, compared to soluble insulin, fasting and preprandial blood-glucose concentration is a little higher, postprandial blood-glucose concentration is a little lower, and hypoglycaemia occurs slightly less frequently. Subcutaneous injection of insulin lispro or of insulin aspart may be convenient for those who wish to inject shortly before or, when necessary, shortly after a meal. They may also help those prone to pre-lunch hypoglycaemia and those who eat late in the evening and are prone to nocturnal hypoglycaemia. Insulin aspart and insulin lispro may also be administered by subcutaneous infusion.

SOLUBLE INSULIN
(Insulin Injection; Neutral Insulin)

A sterile solution of insulin (i.e. bovine or porcine) or of human insulin; pH 6.6–8.0

Indications: diabetes mellitus; diabetic ketoacidosis (section 6.1.3)

Cautions: see notes above; reduce dose in renal impairment; **interactions:** Appendix 1 (antidiabetics)

Side-effects: see notes above; transient oedema; local reactions and fat hypertrophy at injection site; overdose causes hypoglycaemia

Dose: *by subcutaneous, intramuscular, or intravenous injection or intravenous infusion*, according to requirements

COUNSELLING. Show container to patient and confirm that patient is expecting the version dispensed

■ Highly purified animal

Hypurin® Bovine Neutral (CP) PoM

Injection, soluble insulin (bovine, highly purified) 100 units/mL. Net price 10-mL vial = £18.48; cartridges (for *Autopen®* devices) 5 × 1.5 mL = £13.86, 5 × 3 mL = £27.72

Hypurin® Porcine Neutral (CP) PoM

Injection, soluble insulin (porcine, highly purified) 100 units/mL. Net price 10-mL vial = £16.80; cartridges (for *Autopen®* devices) 5 × 1.5 mL = £12.60, 5 × 3 mL = £25.20

Pork Actrapid® (Novo Nordisk) PoM

Injection, soluble insulin (porcine, highly purified) 100 units/mL. Net price 10-mL vial = £6.58

NOTE. Not recommended for use in subcutaneous insulin infusion pumps—may precipitate in catheter or needle

■ Human sequence

Actrapid® (Novo Nordisk) PoM

Injection, soluble insulin (human, pyr) 100 units/ mL. Net price 10-mL vial = £10.50; *Actrapid Penfill®* cartridge (for *Innovo®* and *NovoPen®*

devices) 5 × 3 mL = £22.27; 5 × 3-mL *Actrapid Novolet* ® prefilled disposable injection devices (range 2–78 units, allowing 2-unit dosage adjustment) = £26.50
NOTE. Not recommended for use in subcutaneous insulin infusion pumps—may precipitate in catheter or needle

Velosulin® (Novo Nordisk) [PoM]
Injection, soluble insulin (human, pyr) 100 units/mL. Net price 10-mL vial = £10.50

Humulin S® (Lilly) [PoM]
Injection, soluble insulin (human, prb) 100 units/mL. Net price 10-mL vial = £13.75; 5 × 3-mL cartridge (for *Autopen*® *3 mL* or *HumaPen*®) = £23.43; 5 × 3-mL *Humaject S*® prefilled disposable injection devices (range 2–96 units, allowing 2-unit dosage adjustment) = £24.95

Insuman® **Rapid** (Aventis Pharma) ▼ [PoM]
Injection, soluble insulin (human, crb) 100 units/mL, net price 5-mL vial = £5.31; 5 × 3-mL cartridge (for *OptiPen*® *Pro* [NHS]) = £21.30; 5 × 3-mL *Insuman*® *Rapid OptiSet*® prefilled disposable injection devices (range 2–40 units, allowing 2-unit dosage adjustment) = £25.37
NOTE. Not recommended for use in subcutaneous insulin infusion pumps

■ Mixed preparations
See Biphasic Isophane Insulin (section 6.1.1.2)

INSULIN ASPART
(Recombinant human insulin analogue)
Indications: diabetes mellitus
Cautions: see under Soluble Insulin; children (use only if benefit likely compared to soluble insulin)
Side-effects: see under Soluble Insulin
Dose: *by subcutaneous injection*, immediately before meals or when necessary shortly after meals, according to requirements
By subcutaneous infusion, intravenous injection or intravenous infusion, according to requirements
COUNSELLING. Show container to patient and confirm that patient is expecting the version dispensed

NovoRapid® (Novo Nordisk) ▼ [PoM]
Injection, insulin aspart (recombinant human insulin analogue) 100 units/mL, net price 10-mL vial = £15.71; *Penfill*® cartridge (for *Innovo*® and *Novo-Pen*® devices) 5 × 3-mL = £26.78; 5 × 3-mL *FlexPen*® prefilled disposable injection devices (range 1–60 units, allowing 1-unit dosage adjustment) = £29.59; 5 × 3-mL *NovoLet*® prefilled disposable injection devices (range 2–78 units, allowing 2-unit dosage adjustment) = £28.31

INSULIN LISPRO
(Recombinant human insulin analogue)
Indications: diabetes mellitus
Cautions: see under Soluble Insulin; children (use only if benefit likely compared to soluble insulin)
Side-effects: see under Soluble Insulin
Dose: *by subcutaneous injection* shortly before meals or when necessary shortly after meals, according to requirements
By subcutaneous infusion, or intravenous injection, or intravenous infusion, according to requirements
COUNSELLING. Show container to patient and confirm that patient is expecting the version dispensed

Humalog® (Lilly) [PoM]
Injection, insulin lispro (recombinant human insulin analogue) 100 units/mL. Net price 10-mL vial = £17.82; 5 × 3-mL cartridge (for *Autopen*® *3 mL* or *HumaPen*®) = £29.46; 5 × 3-mL *Humalog*®-*Pen* prefilled disposable injection devices (range 1–60 units, allowing 1-unit dosage adjustment) = £29.46

6.1.1.2   Intermediate- and long-acting insulins

When given by subcutaneous injection, intermediate- and long-acting insulins have an onset of action of approximately 1–2 hours, a maximal effect at 4–12 hours, and a duration of 16–35 hours. Some are given twice daily in conjunction with short-acting (soluble) insulin, and others are given once daily, particularly in elderly patients. They can be mixed with soluble insulin in the syringe, essentially retaining the properties of the two components, although there may be some blunting of the initial effect of the soluble insulin component (especially on mixing with protamine zinc insulin, see below).

Isophane insulin is a suspension of insulin with protamine which is of particular value for initiation of twice-daily insulin regimens. Patients usually mix isophane with soluble insulin but ready-mixed preparations may be appropriate (**biphasic isophane insulin**, **biphasic insulin aspart**, or **biphasic insulin lispro**).

Insulin zinc suspension (crystalline) has a more prolonged duration of action; it may be used independently or in **insulin zinc suspension** (30% amorphous, 70% crystalline).

Protamine zinc insulin is usually given once daily with short-acting (soluble) insulin. It has the drawback of binding with the soluble insulin when mixed in the same syringe, and is now rarely used.

Insulin glargine, a human insulin analogue with a prolonged duration of action, has recently been introduced; it is given once daily.

> **NICE guidance (insulin glargine).** NICE has recommended (December 2002) that insulin glargine should be available as an option for patients with type 1 diabetes.
>
> Insulin glargine is **not** recommended for routine use in patients with type 2 diabetes who require insulin, but it may be considered in type 2 diabetes for those:
>
> - who require assistance with injecting their insulin; *or*
> - whose lifestyle is significantly restricted by recurrent symptomatic hypoglycaemia; *or*
> - who would otherwise need twice-daily basal insulin injections in combination with oral anti-diabetic drugs

INSULIN GLARGINE
(Recombinant human insulin analogue—long acting)
Indications: diabetes mellitus
Cautions: see under Soluble Insulin (section 6.1.1.1)
Side-effects: see under Soluble Insulin (section 6.1.1.1)
Dose: *by subcutaneous injection*, ADULT and CHILD over 6 years, according to requirements
COUNSELLING. Show container to patient and confirm that patient is expecting the version dispensed

Lantus® (Aventis Pharma) ▼ PoM

Injection, insulin glargine (recombinant human insulin analogue) 100 units/mL, net price 10-mL vial = £22.29; 5 × 3-mL cartridge (for *OptiPen® Pro* NHS) = £37.89; 5 × 3-mL *Lantus® OptiSet®* prefilled disposable injection devices (range 2–40 units, allowing 2-unit dosage adjustment) = £39.00

INSULIN ZINC SUSPENSION

(Insulin Zinc Suspension (Mixed); I. Z. S.—long acting)
A sterile neutral suspension of bovine and/or porcine insulin or of human insulin in the form of a complex obtained by the addition of a suitable zinc salt; consists of rhombohedral crystals (10–40 microns) and of particles of no uniform shape (not exceeding 2 microns)

Indications: diabetes mellitus

Cautions: see under Soluble Insulin (section 6.1.1.1)

Side-effects: see under Soluble Insulin (section 6.1.1.1)

Dose: *by subcutaneous injection*, according to requirements
COUNSELLING. Show container to patient and confirm that patient is expecting the version dispensed

■ Highly purified animal

Hypurin® Bovine Lente (CP) PoM

Injection, insulin zinc suspension (bovine, highly purified) 100 units/mL. Net price 10-mL vial = £18.48

■ Human sequence

Monotard® (Novo Nordisk) PoM

Injection, insulin zinc suspension (human, pyr) 100 units/mL. Net price 10-mL vial = £10.50

Humulin Lente® (Lilly) PoM

Injection, insulin zinc suspension (human, prb) 100 units/mL. Net price 10-mL vial = £13.75

INSULIN ZINC SUSPENSION (CRYSTALLINE)

(Cryst. I. Z. S.—long acting)
A sterile neutral suspension of bovine insulin or of human insulin in the form of a complex obtained by the addition of a suitable zinc salt; consists of rhombohedral crystals (10–40 microns)

Indications: diabetes mellitus

Cautions: see under Soluble Insulin (section 6.1.1.1)

Side-effects: see under Soluble Insulin (section 6.1.1.1)

Dose: *by subcutaneous injection*, according to requirements
COUNSELLING. Show container to patient and confirm that patient is expecting the version dispensed

■ Human sequence

Ultratard® (Novo Nordisk) PoM

Injection, insulin zinc suspension, crystalline (human, pyr) 100 units/mL. Net price 10-mL vial = £10.50

Humulin Zn® (Lilly) PoM

Injection, insulin zinc suspension, crystalline (human, prb) 100 units/mL. Net price 10-mL vial = £13.75

ISOPHANE INSULIN

(Isophane Insulin Injection; Isophane Protamine Insulin Injection; Isophane Insulin (NPH)—intermediate acting)
A sterile suspension of bovine or porcine insulin or of human insulin in the form of a complex obtained by the addition of protamine sulphate or another suitable protamine

Indications: diabetes mellitus

Cautions: see under Soluble Insulin (section 6.1.1.1)

Side-effects: see under Soluble Insulin (section 6.1.1.1); protamine may cause allergic reactions

Dose: *by subcutaneous injection*, according to requirements
COUNSELLING. Show container to patient and confirm that patient is expecting the version dispensed

■ Highly purified animal

Hypurin® Bovine Isophane (CP) PoM

Injection, isophane insulin (bovine, highly purified) 100 units/mL. Net price 10-mL vial = £18.48; cartridges (for *Autopen®* devices) 5 × 1.5 mL = £13.86, 5 × 3 mL = £27.72

Hypurin® Porcine Isophane (CP) PoM

Injection, isophane insulin (porcine, highly purified) 100 units/mL. Net price 10-mL vial = £16.80; cartridges (for *Autopen®* devices) 5 × 1.5 mL = £12.60, 5 × 3 mL = £25.20

Pork Insulatard® (Novo Nordisk) PoM

Injection, isophane insulin (porcine, highly purified) 100 units/mL. Net price 10-mL vial = £6.58

■ Human sequence

Insulatard® (Novo Nordisk) PoM

Injection, isophane insulin (human, pyr) 100 units/mL. Net price 10-mL vial = £10.50; *Insulatard Penfill®* cartridge (for *Innovo®*, or *Novopen®* devices) 5 × 3 mL = £22.27; 5 × 3-mL *Insulatard FlexPen®* prefilled disposable injection devices (range 1–60 units, allowing 1-unit dosage adjustment) = £29.59; 5 × 3-mL *Insulatard Novolet®* prefilled disposable injection devices (range 2–78 units, allowing 2-unit dosage adjustment) = £26.50; 5 × 3-mL *Insulatard InnoLet®* prefilled disposable injection devices (range 1–50 units, allowing 1-unit dosage adjustment) = £26.84

Humulin I® (Lilly) PoM

Injection, isophane insulin (human, prb) 100 units/mL. Net price 10-mL vial = £13.75; 5 × 3-mL cartridge (for *Autopen® 3 mL* or *HumaPen®*) = £24.95; 5 × 3-mL *Humulin I-Pen®* prefilled disposable injection devices (range 1–60 units, allowing 1-unit dosage adjustment) = £24.95

Insuman® Basal (Aventis Pharma) ▼ PoM

Injection, isophane insulin (human, crb) 100 units/mL, net price 5-mL vial = £5.31; 5 × 3-mL cartridge (for *OptiPen® Pro* NHS) = £21.30; 5 × 3-mL *Insuman® Basal OptiSet®* prefilled disposable injection devices (range 2–40 units, allowing 2-unit dosage adjustment) = £25.37

■ Mixed preparations
See Biphasic Isophane Insulin (p. 332)

PROTAMINE ZINC INSULIN

(Protamine Zinc Insulin Injection—long acting)
A sterile suspension of insulin in the form of a complex obtained by the addition of a suitable protamine and zinc chloride; this preparation was included in BP 1980 but is not included in BP 1988

Indications: diabetes mellitus

Cautions: see under Soluble Insulin (section 6.1.1.1); see also notes above

Side-effects: see under Soluble Insulin (section 6.1.1.1); protamine may cause allergic reactions
Dose: *by subcutaneous injection,* according to requirements
COUNSELLING. Show container to patient and confirm that patient is expecting the version dispensed

Hypurin® Bovine Protamine Zinc (CP) PoM
Injection, protamine zinc insulin (bovine, highly purified) 100 units/mL. Net price 10-mL vial = £18.48

Biphasic insulins

BIPHASIC INSULIN ASPART
(Intermediate-acting insulin)
Indications: diabetes mellitus
Cautions: see under Soluble Insulin and Insulin Aspart (section 6.1.1.1)
Side-effects: see under Soluble Insulin (section 6.1.1.1); protamine may cause allergic reactions
Dose: *by subcutaneous injection,* up to 10 minutes before or soon after a meal, according to requirements
COUNSELLING. Show container to patient and confirm that patient is expecting the version dispensed; the proportions of the two components should be checked **carefully** (the order in which the proportions are stated may not be the same in other countries)

NovoMix® 30 (Novo Nordisk) ▼ PoM
Injection, biphasic insulin aspart (recombinant human insulin analogue), 30% insulin aspart, 70% insulin aspart protamine, 100 units/mL, net price 5 × 3-mL *Penfill®* cartridges (for *Innovo®* and *NovoPen®* devices) = £26.78; 5 × 3-mL *FlexPen®* prefilled disposable injection devices (range 1–60 units, allowing 1-unit dosage adjustment) = £29.59

BIPHASIC INSULIN LISPRO
(Intermediate-acting insulin)
Indications: diabetes mellitus
Cautions: see under Soluble Insulin and Insulin Lispro (section 6.1.1.1)
Side-effects: see under Soluble Insulin (section 6.1.1.1); protamine may cause allergic reactions
Dose: *by subcutaneous injection,* up to 15 minutes before or soon after a meal, according to requirements
COUNSELLING. Show container to patient and confirm that patient is expecting the version dispensed; the proportions of the two components should be checked **carefully** (the order in which the proportions are stated may not be the same in other countries)

Humalog® Mix25 (Lilly) PoM
Injection, biphasic insulin lispro (recombinant human insulin analogue), 25% insulin lispro, 75% insulin lispro protamine, 100 units/mL, net price 5 × 3-mL cartridge (for *Autopen® 3 mL* or *Huma-Pen®*) = £29.46; 5 × 3-mL prefilled disposable injection devices (range 1–60 units, allowing 1-unit dosage adjustment) = £30.98

Humalog® Mix50 (Lilly) PoM
Injection, biphasic insulin lispro (recombinant human insulin analogue), 50% insulin lispro, 50% insulin lispro protamine, 100 units/mL, net price 5 × 3-mL prefilled disposable injection devices

(range 1–60 units, allowing 1-unit dosage adjustment) = £30.98

BIPHASIC ISOPHANE INSULIN
(Biphasic Isophane Insulin Injection—intermediate acting)
A sterile buffered suspension of either porcine or human insulin complexed with protamine sulphate (or another suitable protamine) in a solution of insulin of the same species
Indications: diabetes mellitus
Cautions: see under Soluble Insulin (section 6.1.1.1)
Side-effects: see under Soluble Insulin (section 6.1.1.1); protamine may cause allergic reactions
Dose: *by subcutaneous injection,* according to requirements
COUNSELLING. Show container to patient and confirm that patient is expecting the version dispensed; the proportions of the two components should be checked **carefully** (the order in which the proportions are stated may not be the same in other countries)

■ Highly purified animal

Hypurin® Porcine 30/70 Mix (CP) PoM
Injection, biphasic isophane insulin (porcine, highly purified), 30% soluble, 70% isophane, 100 units/mL. Net price 10-mL vial = £16.80; cartridges (for *Autopen®* devices) 5 × 1.5 ml = £12.60, 5 × 3 mL = £25.20

Pork Mixtard 30® (Novo Nordisk) PoM
Injection, biphasic isophane insulin (porcine, highly purified), 30% soluble, 70% isophane, 100 units/mL. Net price 10-mL vial = £6.58

■ Human sequence

Mixtard® 10 (Novo Nordisk) PoM
Injection, biphasic isophane insulin (human, pyr), 10% soluble, 90% isophane, 100 units/mL. Net price *Mixtard 10 Penfill®* cartridge (for *Innovo®* or *Novopen®* devices) 5 × 3 mL = £22.27; 5 × 3-mL *Mixtard 10 Novolet®* prefilled disposable injection devices (range 2–78 units, allowing 2-unit dosage adjustment) = £26.50

Mixtard® 20 (Novo Nordisk) PoM
Injection, biphasic isophane insulin (human, pyr), 20% soluble, 80% isophane, 100 units/mL. Net price *Mixtard 20 Penfill®* cartridge (for *Innovo®* or *Novopen®* devices) 5 × 3 mL = £22.27; 5 × 3-mL *Mixtard 20 Novolet®* prefilled disposable injection devices (range 2–78 units, allowing 2-unit dosage adjustment) = £26.50

Mixtard® 30 (Novo Nordisk) PoM
Injection, biphasic isophane insulin (human, pyr), 30% soluble, 70% isophane, 100 units/mL. Net price 10-mL vial = £10.50; *Mixtard 30 Penfill®* cartridge (for *Innovo®* or *Novopen®* devices) 5 × 3 mL = £22.27; 5 × 3-mL *Mixtard 30 Novolet®* prefilled disposable injection devices (range 2–78 units, allowing 2-unit dosage adjustment) = £26.50; 5 × 3-mL *Mixtard 30 InnoLet®* prefilled disposable injection devices (range 1–50 units allowing 1-unit dosage adjustment) = £26.84

Mixtard® 40 (Novo Nordisk) PoM
Injection, biphasic isophane insulin (human, pyr), 40% soluble, 60% isophane, 100 units/mL. Net price *Mixtard 40 Penfill®* cartridge (for *Innovo®* or *Novopen®* devices) 5 × 3 mL = £22.27; 5 × 3-mL *Mixtard 40 Novolet®* prefilled disposable injection

devices (range 2–78 units, allowing 2-unit dosage adjustment) = £26.50

Mixtard® 50 (Novo Nordisk) PoM
Injection, biphasic isophane insulin (human, pyr), 50% soluble, 50% isophane, 100 units/mL. Net price 10-mL vial = £10.50; *Mixtard 50 Penfill®* cartridge (for *Innovo®* or *Novopen®* devices) 5 × 3 mL = £22.27; 5 × 3-mL *Mixtard 50 Novolet®* prefilled disposable injection devices (range 2–78 units, allowing 2-unit dosage adjustment) = £26.50

Humulin M2® (Lilly) PoM
Injection, biphasic isophane insulin (human, prb), 20% soluble, 80% isophane, 100 units/mL. Net price 5 × 3-mL cartridge (for *Autopen® 3 mL* or *HumaPen®*) = £23.43

Humulin M3® (Lilly) PoM
Injection, biphasic isophane insulin (human, prb), 30% soluble, 70% isophane, 100 units/mL. Net price 10-mL vial = £13.75; 5 × 3-mL cartridge (for *Autopen® 3 mL* or *HumaPen®*) = £23.43; 5 × 3-mL *Humaject M3®* prefilled disposable injection devices (range 2–96 units, allowing 2-unit dosage adjustment) = £24.95

Humulin M5® (Lilly) PoM
Injection, biphasic isophane insulin (human, prb), 50% soluble, 50% isophane, 100 units/mL. Net price 10-mL vial = £13.75

Insuman® Comb 15 (Aventis Pharma) ▼ PoM
Injection, biphasic isophane insulin (human, crb), 15% soluble, 85% isophane, 100 units/mL, net price 5-mL vial = £5.31; 5 × 3-mL cartridge (for *OptiPen® Pro* NHS) = £21.30; 5 × 3-mL *Insuman® Comb 15 OptiSet®* prefilled disposable injection devices (range 2–40 units, allowing 2-unit dosage adjustment) = £25.37

Insuman® Comb 25 (Aventis Pharma) ▼ PoM
Injection, biphasic isophane insulin (human, crb), 25% soluble, 75% isophane, 100 units/mL, net price 5-mL vial = £5.31; 5 × 3-mL cartridge (for *OptiPen® Pro* NHS) = £21.30; 5 × 3-mL *Insuman® Comb 25 OptiSet®* prefilled disposable injection devices (range 2–40 units, allowing 2-unit dosage adjustment) = £25.37

Insuman® Comb 50 (Aventis Pharma) ▼ PoM
Injection, biphasic isophane insulin (human, crb), 50% soluble, 50% isophane, 100 units/mL, net price 5-mL vial = £5.31; 5 × 3-mL cartridge (for *OptiPen®Pro* NHS) = £21.30; 5 × 3-mL *Insuman® Comb 50 OptiSet®* prefilled disposable injection devices (range 2–40 units, allowing 2-unit dosage adjustment) = £25.37

6.1.1.3   Hypodermic equipment

Patients should be advised on the safe disposal of lancets, single-use syringes, and needles. Suitable arrangements for the safe disposal of contaminated waste must be made before these products are prescribed for patients who are carriers of infectious diseases.

■ Injection devices
Autopen® (Owen Mumford)
Injection device; Autopen® 1.5 mL (for use with CP and Lilly 1.5-mL insulin cartridges), allows adjustment of dosage in multiples of 1 unit, max. 16 units (single-unit version) or 2 units, max. 32 units (2-unit version), net price (both) =

£14.42; *Autopen® 3 mL*, *Autopen® Special Edition*, *Autopen® Junior* (for use with Lilly 3-mL insulin cartridges), and *Autopen® 24* (for use with Aventis 3-mL insulin cartridges), all allow adjustment of dosage in multiples of 1 unit, max. 21 units (single-unit version) or 2 units, max. 42 units (2-unit version), net price = £14.42

HumaPen® Ergo (Lilly)
Injection device, for use with *Humulin®* and *Humalog®* 3-mL cartridges; allows adjustment of dosage in multiples of 1 unit, max. 60 units, net price = £22.39 (available in burgundy and teal)

Innovo® (Novo Nordisk)
Injection device, for use with 3-mL *Penfill®* insulin cartridges; allows adjustment of dosage in multiples of 1 unit, max. 70 units, net price = £25.91 (available in green or orange)

mhi-500® (Medical House)
Needle-free insulin delivery device for use with any 10-mL vial of insulin, allows adjustment of dosage in multiples of 0.5 units, max. 50 units, net price *starter pack (mhi-500®* device, 5 nozzles, 2 insulin vial adaptors) = £120.00, *3-month consumables pack* (13 nozzles, 5 insulin vial adaptors) = £22.15, *vial adaptor pack* (6 insulin vial adaptors) = £7.38, *nozzle pack* (6 nozzles) = £7.38

NovoPen® (Novo Nordisk)
Injection device; for use with *Penfill®* insulin cartridges; *NovoPen® Junior* (for 3-mL cartridges), allows adjustment of dosage in multiples of 0.5 units, max. 35 units, net price = £22.80; *NovoPen® 3 Demi* (for 3-mL cartridges), allows adjustment of dosage in multiples of 0.5 units, max. 35 units, net price = £23.20; *NovoPen® 3 Classic* or *Fun* (for 3-mL cartridges), allows adjustment of dosage in multiples of 1 unit, max. 70 units, net price = £23.20

OptiPen® Pro (Aventis Pharma) NHS
Injection device, for use with *Insuman®* insulin cartridges; allows adjustment of dosage in multiples of 1 unit, max. 60 units (available free of charge from Aventis and clinics)

■ Lancets—sterile, single use
Type A (Drug Tariff)
Cylindrical mount fluted longitudinally; compatible with *B-D Lancer®* NHS (Becton Dickinson), *Glucolet®* NHS (Bayer Diagnostics), *Monoject®* NHS (Tyco), *Penlet®* II (Lifescan) and *Soft Touch®* NHS (Roche Diagnostics) finger-pricking devices
Available from Bayer (*Microlet®*, net price 100-lancet pack = £3.42; 200-lancet pack = £6.52), Becton Dickinson (*Microfine®+*, net price 200-lancet pack = £6.13), Entaco (*Milward® Steri-Let*, 0.66 mm/23-gauge, net price 100-lancet pack = £3.00, 200-lancet pack = £5.70; 0.36 mm/28-gauge, net price 100-lancet pack = £3.00, 200-lancet pack = £5.70) Hypoguard (*Hypoguard Supreme®*, net price 100-lancet pack = £2.75), LifeScan (*Finepoint®*, net price 100-lancet pack = £3.42; *One Touch UltraSoft®*, net price 100-lancet pack = £3.36), MediSense (*MediSense® Thin*, net price 200-lancet pack = £6.51), Menarini (*GlucoMen® Fine*, net price 100-lancet pack = £3.30; 200-lancet pack = £6.39), Owen Mumford (*Unilet General Purpose®*, net price 100-lancet pack = £3.40; 200-lancet pack = £6.47; *Unilet General Purpose® Superlite*, net price 100-lancet pack = £3.34; 200-lancet pack = £6.33; *Unilet® ComforTouch*, net price 100-lancet pack = £3.34; 200-lancet pack = £6.33), Therasense (*Freestyle®*, net price 100-lancet pack = £3.30), Tyco (*Monolet®*, net price 100-lancet pack = £3.28; 200-lancet pack = £6.24; *Monolet Extra®*, net price 100-lancet pack = £3.28), Vitrex Medical (*Vitrex Soft®*, 0.65 mm/23-gauge, net price 100-lancet pack = £3.00, 200-lancet pack = £5.70; 0.36 mm/28-gauge, net price 100-lancet pack = £3.19, 200-lancet pack = £6.13), Zygo Medica (*Cleanlet® Fine*, net price 100-lancet pack = £3.19, 200-lancet pack = £6.13)

Type B (Drug Tariff)
Cylindrical mount with concentric ribs; compatible with
Autolet® [NHS] (Owen Mumford) and *Glucolet®* [NHS] (Bayer
Diagnostics) finger-pricking devices
Available from Owen Mumford (*Unilet® Superlite*, net
price 100-lancet pack = £3.34; 200-lancet pack = £6.33;
Unilet® ComferTouch, net price 100-lancet pack = £3.34;
200-lancet pack = £6.33))

Type C (Drug Tariff)
Device specific; compatible with *Softclix®* [NHS] (Roche
Diagnostics) finger-pricking device
Available from Roche Diagnostics (*Softclix®*, net price
200-lancet pack = £6.68)

■ Needles
Hypodermic Needle, Sterile single use (Drug Tariff)
For use with reusable glass syringe, sizes 0.5 mm (25G), 0.45
mm (26G), 0.4 mm (27G). Net price 100-needle pack = £2.44
Available from Becton Dickinson (*Microlance®*), Tyco
(*Monoject®*)

Needles for Prefilled and Reusable Pen Injectors
(Drug Tariff)
Screw on, needle length 6.1 mm or less, net price 100-needle
pack = £11.67; 6.2–9.9 mm, 100-needle pack = £8.27; 10 mm
or more, 100-needle pack = £8.27
Available from Becton Dickinson (*BD Microfine®+*),
Exelint, Novo Nordisk (*NovoFine®*), Owen Mumford
(*Unifine® Pentips*)
Snap on, needle length 6.1 mm or less, net price 100-needle
pack = £11.42; 6.2–9.9 mm, 100-needle pack = £8.10; 10 mm
or more, 100-needle pack = £8.10
Available from Disetronic (*Penfine®*)

■ Syringes
Hypodermic Syringe (Drug Tariff)
Calibrated glass with Luer taper conical fitting, for use with
U100 insulin. Net price 0.5 mL and 1 mL = £14.66
Available from Rand Rocket (*Abcare®*)

Pre-Set U100 Insulin Syringe (Drug Tariff)
Calibrated glass with Luer taper conical fitting, supplied with
dosage chart and strong box, for blind patients. Net price 1 mL
= £21.99
Available from Rand Rocket

U100 Insulin Syringe with Needle (Drug Tariff)
Disposable with fixed or separate needle for single use or single
patient-use, colour coded orange. Needle length 8 mm,
diameters 0.33 mm (29G), 0.3 mm (30G), net price 10 (with
needle), 0.3 mL = £1.23, 0.5 mL = £1.19; needle length
12 mm, diameters 0.45 mm (26G), 0.4 mm (27G), 0.36 mm
(28G), 0.33 mm (29G), net price 10 (with needle), 0.3 mL =
£1.32; 0.5 mL = £1.28; 1 mL = £1.29
Available from Becton Dickinson (*B-D Micro-Fine®+
Plastipak®*), Braun (*Omnikan®*), Codan (*Insupak®*),
Exelint, Owen Mumford (*Unifine®*), Rand Rocket (*Clin-
ipak®*), Tyco (*Monoject® Ultra*)

■ Accessories
Needle Clipping (Chopping) Device (Drug Tariff)
Consisting of a clipper to remove needle from its hub and
container from which cut-off needles cannot be retrieved;
designed to hold 1200 needles, not suitable for use with
lancets. Net price = £1.20
Available from Becton Dickinson (*B-D Safe-clip®*)

Sharpsbin (Drug Tariff)
Net price 1-litre sharpsbin = 85p

6.1.2 Oral antidiabetic drugs

6.1.2.1	Sulphonylureas
6.1.2.2	Biguanides
6.1.2.3	Other antidiabetics

Oral antidiabetic drugs are used for the treatment of
type 2 (non-insulin-dependent) diabetes mellitus.

They should be prescribed only if the patient fails
to respond adequately to at least 3 months' restriction
of energy and carbohydrate intake and an increase in
physical activity. They should be used to augment
the effect of diet and exercise, and not to replace
them.

For patients not adequately controlled by diet and
oral hypoglycaemic drugs, insulin may be added to
the treatment regimen or substituted for oral therapy.
When insulin is added to oral therapy, it is generally
given at bedtime as isophane insulin, and when
insulin replaces an oral regimen it is generally given
as twice-daily injections of a biphasic insulin (or
isophane insulin mixed with soluble insulin). Weight
gain and hypoglycaemia may be complications of
insulin therapy but weight gain may be reduced if the
insulin is given in combination with oral therapy.

6.1.2.1 Sulphonylureas

The sulphonylureas act mainly by augmenting insulin secretion and consequently are effective only
when some residual pancreatic beta-cell activity is
present; during long-term administration they also
have an extrapancreatic action. All may cause
hypoglycaemia but this is uncommon and usually
indicates excessive dosage. Sulphonylurea-induced
hypoglycaemia may persist for many hours and must
always be treated in hospital.

Sulphonylureas are considered for patients who are
not overweight, or in whom metformin is contra-
indicated or not tolerated. Several sulphonylureas are
available and choice is determined by side-effects
and the duration of action as well as the patient's age
and renal function. The long-acting sulphonylureas
chlorpropamide and **glibenclamide** are associated
with a greater risk of hypoglycaemia; for this reason
they should be avoided in the elderly and shorter-
acting alternatives, such as **gliclazide** or **tolbutamide**, should be used instead. Chlorpropamide also
has more side-effects than the other sulphonylureas
(see below) and therefore it is no longer recommended.

When the combination of strict diet and sulphonylurea treatment fails other options include:

- combining with metformin (section 6.1.2.2)
  (reports of increased hazard with this combination remain unconfirmed);
- combining with acarbose (section 6.1.2.3),
  which may have a small beneficial effect, but
  flatulence can be a problem;
- combining with pioglitazone or rosiglitazone,
  but see section 6.1.2.3;
- combining with bedtime isophane insulin (section 6.1.1) but weight gain and hypoglycaemia
  can occur.

Insulin therapy should be instituted temporarily
during intercurrent illness (such as myocardial
infarction, coma, infection, and trauma). Sulphonylureas should be omitted on the morning of surgery;
insulin is often required because of the ensuing
hyperglycaemia in these circumstances.

CAUTIONS. Sulphonylureas can encourage weight
gain and should be prescribed only if poor control
and symptoms persist despite adequate attempts at
dieting; metformin (section 6.1.2.2) is considered the
drug of choice in obese patients. Caution is needed in

the elderly and in those with mild to moderate hepatic (Appendix 2) and renal impairment (Appendix 3) because of the hazard of hypoglycaemia. The short-acting tolbutamide may be used in renal impairment, as may gliquidone and gliclazide which are principally metabolised in the liver, but careful monitoring of blood-glucose concentration is essential; care is required to choose the smallest possible dose that produces adequate control of blood glucose.

CONTRA-INDICATIONS. Sulphonylureas should be avoided where possible in severe hepatic (Appendix 2) and renal (Appendix 3) impairment and in porphyria (section 9.8.2). They should not be used while breast-feeding and insulin therapy should be substituted during pregnancy (see also Appendix 4). Sulphonylureas are contra-indicated in the presence of ketoacidosis.

SIDE-EFFECTS. Side-effects of sulphonylureas are generally mild and infrequent and include gastro-intestinal disturbances such as nausea, vomiting, diarrhoea and constipation.

Chlorpropamide has appreciably more side-effects, mainly because of its very prolonged duration of action and the consequent hazard of hypoglycaemia and it should no longer be used. It may also cause facial flushing after drinking alcohol; this effect does not normally occur with other sulphonylureas. Chlorpropamide may also enhance antidiuretic hormone secretion and very rarely cause hyponatraemia (hyponatraemia is also reported with glimepiride and glipizide).

Sulphonylureas can occasionally cause a disturbance in liver function, which may rarely lead to cholestatic jaundice, hepatitis and hepatic failure. Hypersensitivity reactions can occur, usually in the first 6–8 weeks of therapy, they consist mainly of allergic skin reactions which progress rarely to erythema multiforme and exfoliative dermatitis, fever and jaundice; photosensitivity has rarely been reported with chlorpropamide and glipizide. Blood disorders are also rare but may include leucopenia, thrombocytopenia, agranulocytosis, pancytopenia, haemolytic anaemia, and aplastic anaemia.

CHLORPROPAMIDE

Indications: type 2 diabetes mellitus (for use in diabetes insipidus, see section 6.5.2)
Cautions: see notes above; **interactions:** Appendix 1 (antidiabetics)
Contra-indications: see notes above
Side-effects: see notes above
Dose: initially 250 mg daily with breakfast (ELDERLY 100–125 mg but avoid—see notes above), adjusted according to response; max. 500 mg daily

Chlorpropamide (Non-proprietary) PoM
Tablets, chlorpropamide 100 mg, net price 20 = £1.70; 250 mg, 20 = £2.00. Label: 4
Available from Sussex

GLIBENCLAMIDE

Indications: type 2 diabetes mellitus
Cautions: see notes above; **interactions:** Appendix 1 (antidiabetics)
Contra-indications: see notes above
Side-effects: see notes above

Dose: initially 5 mg daily with or immediately after breakfast (ELDERLY 2.5 mg, but avoid—see notes above), adjusted according to response; max. 15 mg daily

Glibenclamide (Non-proprietary) PoM
Tablets, glibenclamide 2.5 mg, net price 28-tab pack = 96p; 5 mg, 28-tab pack = £1.22
Available from Alpharma, APS, Arrow, Ashbourne (*Diabetamide*®), CP, Generics, Hillcross, IVAX, Kent

Daonil® (Hoechst Marion Roussel) PoM
Tablets, scored, glibenclamide 5 mg. Net price 28-tab pack = £2.63

Semi-Daonil® (Hoechst Marion Roussel) PoM
Tablets, scored, glibenclamide 2.5 mg. Net price 28-tab pack = £1.58

Euglucon® (Aventis Pharma) PoM
Tablets, glibenclamide 2.5 mg, net price 28-tab pack = £1.58; 5 mg (scored), 28-tab pack = £2.63

GLICLAZIDE

Indications: type 2 diabetes mellitus
Cautions: see notes above; **interactions:** Appendix 1 (antidiabetics)
Contra-indications: see notes above
Side-effects: see notes above
Dose: initially, 40–80 mg daily, adjusted according to response; up to 160 mg as a single dose, with breakfast; higher doses divided; max. 320 mg daily

Gliclazide (Non-proprietary) PoM
Tablets, scored, gliclazide 80 mg, net price 28-tab pack = £2.59, 60-tab pack = £6.05
Available from Alpharma, APS, Arrow, Generics (*DIAGLYK*®), Genus, Hillcross, IVAX, PLIVA

Diamicron® (Servier) PoM
Tablets, scored, gliclazide 80 mg, net price 60-tab pack = £7.00

■ Modified release

Diamicron® **MR** (Servier) PoM
Tablets, m/r, gliclazide 30 mg, net price 28-tab pack = £4.00, 56-tab pack = £8.00, 84-tab pack = £12.00, 112-tab pack = £16.00
Dose: initially 30 mg daily with breakfast, adjusted according to response every 4 weeks (after 2 weeks if no decrease in blood glucose); max. 120 mg daily
NOTE. *Diamicron*® *MR* 30 mg may be considered to be approximately equivalent in therapeutic effect to standard formulation *Diamicron*® 80 mg

GLIMEPIRIDE

Indications: type 2 diabetes mellitus
Cautions: see notes above; manufacturer recommends regular hepatic and haematological monitoring but limited evidence of clinical value; **interactions**: Appendix 1 (antidiabetics)
Contra-indications: see notes above
Side-effects: see notes above
Dose: initially 1 mg daily, adjusted according to response in 1-mg steps at 1–2 week intervals; usual max. 4 mg daily (exceptionally, up to 6 mg daily may be used); taken shortly before or with first main meal

Amaryl® (Hoechst Marion Roussel) PoM
Tablets, all scored, glimepiride 1 mg (pink), net price 30-tab pack = £4.41; 2 mg (green), 30-tab pack = £7.25; 3 mg (yellow), 30-tab pack = £10.94; 4 mg (blue), 30-tab pack = £14.49

GLIPIZIDE

Indications: type 2 diabetes mellitus

Cautions: see notes above; **interactions:** Appendix 1 (antidiabetics)

Contra-indications: see notes above

Side-effects: see notes above; also dizziness, drowsiness

Dose: initially 2.5–5 mg daily shortly before breakfast or lunch, adjusted according to response; max. 20 mg daily; up to 15 mg may be given as a single dose; higher doses divided

Glipizide (Non-proprietary) [PoM]
Tablets, glipizide 5 mg, 56-tab pack = £4.58
Available from Alpharma, Generics, Hillcross, IVAX

Glibenese® (Pfizer) [PoM]
Tablets, scored, glipizide 5 mg. Net price 56-tab pack = £4.36

Minodiab® (Pharmacia) [PoM]
Tablets, glipizide 2.5 mg, net price 28-tab pack = £1.48; 5 mg (scored), 28-tab pack = £1.26

GLIQUIDONE

Indications: type 2 diabetes mellitus

Cautions: see notes above; **interactions:** Appendix 1 (antidiabetics)

Contra-indications: see notes above

Side-effects: see notes above

Dose: initially 15 mg daily before breakfast, adjusted to 45–60 mg daily in 2 or 3 divided doses; max. single dose 60 mg, max. daily dose 180 mg

Glurenorm® (Sanofi-Synthelabo) [PoM]
Tablets, scored, gliquidone 30 mg. Net price 100-tab pack = £17.54

TOLBUTAMIDE

Indications: type 2 diabetes mellitus

Cautions: see notes above; **interactions:** Appendix 1 (antidiabetics)

Contra-indications: see notes above

Side-effects: see notes above; also headache, tinnitus

Dose: 0.5–1.5 g (max. 2 g) daily in divided doses (see notes above); with or immediately after breakfast

Tolbutamide (Non-proprietary) [PoM]
Tablets, tolbutamide 500 mg. Net price 28 = £1.10
Available from Alpharma, APS, Hillcross

6.1.2.2 Biguanides

Metformin, the only available biguanide, has a different mode of action from the sulphonylureas, and is not interchangeable with them. It exerts its effect mainly by decreasing gluconeogenesis and by increasing peripheral utilisation of glucose; since it acts only in the presence of endogenous insulin it is effective only if there are some residual functioning pancreatic islet cells.

Metformin is the drug of first choice in overweight patients in whom strict dieting has failed to control diabetes, if appropriate it may also be considered as an option in patients who are not overweight. It is also used when diabetes is inadequately controlled with sulphonylurea treatment. When the combination of strict diet and metformin treatment fails, other options include:

- combining with acarbose (section 6.1.2.3), which may have a small beneficial effect, but flatulence can be a problem;

- combining with insulin (section 6.1.1) but weight gain and hypoglycaemia can be problems (weight gain minimised if insulin given at night);

- combining with a sulphonylurea (section 6.1.2.1) (reports of increased hazard with this combination remain unconfirmed);

- combining with pioglitazone or rosiglitazone (section 6.1.2.3);

- combining with repaglinide or nateglinide (section 6.1.2.3).

Insulin treatment is almost always required in medical and surgical emergencies; insulin should also be substituted before elective surgery (omit metformin the evening before surgery and give insulin if required).

Hypoglycaemia does not usually occur with metformin; other advantages are the lower incidence of weight gain and lower plasma-insulin concentration. It does not exert a hypoglycaemic action in non-diabetic subjects unless given in overdose.

Gastro-intestinal side-effects are initially common with metformin, and may persist in some patients, particularly when very high doses such as 3 g daily are given.

Metformin may provoke lactic acidosis which is most likely to occur in patients with renal impairment; it should not be used in patients with even mild renal impairment.

METFORMIN HYDROCHLORIDE

Indications: diabetes mellitus (see notes above)

Cautions: see notes above; measure serum creatinine before treatment and once or twice annually during treatment; **interactions:** Appendix 1 (antidiabetics)

Contra-indications: renal impairment (Appendix 3), ketoacidosis, withdraw if tissue hypoxia likely (e.g. sepsis, respiratory failure, recent myocardial infarction, hepatic impairment), use of iodine-containing X-ray contrast media (do not restart metformin until renal function returns to normal) and use of general anaesthesia (suspend metformin 2 days beforehand and restart when renal function returns to normal), pregnancy and breast-feeding

Side-effects: anorexia, nausea, vomiting, diarrhoea (usually transient), abdominal pain, metallic taste; rarely lactic acidosis (withdraw treatment), decreased vitamin-B_{12} absorption, erythema

Dose: initially 500 mg with breakfast for at least 1 week then 500 mg with breakfast and evening meal for at least 1 week then 500 mg with breakfast, lunch and evening meal; max. 3 g daily in divided doses but most physicians limit this to 2 g daily (see notes above)
NOTE. Metformin doses in the BNF may differ from those in the product literature

Metformin (Non-proprietary) [PoM]
Tablets, coated, metformin hydrochloride 500 mg, net price 28 = 77p, 84 = £2.31; 850 mg, 56-tab pack = £2.37 Label: 21
Available from Alpharma, APS, Arrow, Auden McKenzie, CP, Generics, Hillcross, IVAX, Kent, Sovereign, Sterwin, Taro

Glucophage® (Merck) [PoM]
Tablets, f/c, metformin hydrochloride 500 mg, net price 84-tab pack = £2.40; 850 mg, 56-tab pack = £2.67. Label: 21

■ With rosiglitazone
See section 6.1.2.3

6.1.2.3 Other antidiabetics

Acarbose, an inhibitor of intestinal alpha glucosidases, delays the digestion and absorption of starch and sucrose. It has a small but significant effect in lowering blood glucose and is used either on its own or as an adjunct to metformin or to sulphonylureas when they prove inadequate. Postprandial hyperglycaemia in type 1 (insulin-dependent) diabetes can be reduced by acarbose, but it has been little used for this purpose. Flatulence deters some from using acarbose although this side-effect tends to decrease with time.

Nateglinide and **repaglinide** stimulate insulin release. Both drugs have a rapid onset of action and short duration of activity, and should be administered shortly before each main meal. Repaglinide may be given as monotherapy for patients who are not overweight or for those in whom metformin is contra-indicated or not tolerated, or it may be given in combination with metformin. Nateglinide is licensed only for use with metformin.

The thiazolidinediones, **pioglitazone** and **rosiglitazone**, reduce peripheral insulin resistance, leading to a reduction of blood-glucose concentration. Either drug may be used alone or in combination with metformin or with a sulphonylurea (if metformin inappropriate); the combination of a thiazolidinedione plus metformin is preferred to a thiazolidinedione plus sulphonylurea, particularly for obese patients. Inadequate response to a combination of metformin and sulphonylurea may indicate failing insulin release; the introduction of pioglitazone or rosiglitazone has a limited role in these circumstances and insulin treatment should not be delayed. Blood-glucose control may deteriorate temporarily when a thiazolidinedione is substituted for an oral antidiabetic drug that is being used in combination with another. Long-term benefits of the thiazolidinediones have not yet been demonstrated.

> **NICE guidance (pioglitazone and rosiglitazone for type 2 diabetes mellitus).** NICE has advised (August 2003) that the use of a thiazolidinedione (pioglitazone or rosiglitazone) as second-line therapy added to either metformin or a sulphonylurea is **not** recommended [see also notes above], except for:
> - patients who are unable to tolerate metformin and sulphonylurea combination therapy, *or*
> - patients in whom either metformin or a sulphonylurea is contra-indicated.
>
> In such cases, the thiazolidinedione should replace whichever drug in the combination is poorly tolerated or contra-indicated.

ACARBOSE

Indications: diabetes mellitus inadequately controlled by diet or by diet with oral hypoglycaemic agents

Cautions: monitor liver function; may enhance hypoglycaemic effects of insulin and sulphonylureas (hypoglycaemic episodes may be treated with oral glucose but not with sucrose); **interactions:** Appendix 1 (antidiabetics)

Contra-indications: pregnancy and breast-feeding; inflammatory bowel disease (e.g. ulcerative colitis, Crohn's disease), partial intestinal obstruc-

tion (or predisposition); hepatic impairment, severe renal impairment; hernia, history of abdominal surgery

Side-effects: flatulence, soft stools, diarrhoea (may need to reduce dose or withdraw), abdominal distention and pain; rarely nausea, abnormal liver function tests and skin reactions; ileus, oedema, jaundice and hepatitis reported

NOTE. Antacids not recommended for treating side-effects (unlikely to be beneficial)

Dose: 50 mg daily initially (to minimise side-effects) increased to 50 mg 3 times daily, then increased if necessary after 6–8 weeks to 100 mg 3 times daily; max. 200 mg 3 times daily; CHILD under 12 years not recommended

COUNSELLING. Tablets should be chewed with first mouthful of food or swallowed whole with a little liquid immediately before food. To counteract possible hypoglycaemia, patients receiving insulin or a sulphonylurea as well as acarbose need to carry glucose (not sucrose—acarbose interferes with sucrose absorption)

Glucobay® (Bayer) PoM

Tablets, acarbose 50 mg, net price 90-tab pack = £9.68; 100 mg (scored), 90-tab pack = £12.51. Counselling, administration

NATEGLINIDE

Indications: type 2 diabetes mellitus in combination with metformin when metformin alone inadequate

Cautions: substitute insulin during intercurrent illness (such as myocardial infarction, coma, infection, and trauma) and during surgery; debilitated and malnourished patients; moderate hepatic impairment (avoid if severe—Appendix 2); **interactions:** Appendix 1 (antidiabetics)

Contra-indications: ketoacidosis; pregnancy (Appendix 4) and breast-feeding (Appendix 5)

Side-effects: hypoglycaemia; hypersensitivity reactions including pruritus, rashes and urticaria

Dose: initially 60 mg 3 times daily within 30 minutes before main meals, adjusted according to response up to max. 180 mg 3 times daily; CHILD and ADOLESCENT under 18 years not recommended

Starlix® (Novartis) PoM

Tablets, f/c, nateglinide 60 mg (pink), net price 84-tab pack = £19.75; 120 mg (yellow), 84-tab pack = £22.50; 180 mg (red), 84-tab pack = £22.50

PIOGLITAZONE

Indications: type 2 diabetes mellitus (alone or combined with metformin or a sulphonylurea—see notes above)

Cautions: monitor liver function (see below); cardiovascular disease (risk of heart failure); **interactions:** Appendix 1 (antidiabetics)

LIVER TOXICITY. Rare reports of liver dysfunction; monitor liver function before treatment, then every 2 months for 12 months and periodically thereafter; advise patients to seek immediate medical attention if symptoms such as nausea, vomiting, abdominal pain, fatigue and dark urine develop; discontinue if jaundice occurs

Contra-indications: hepatic impairment, history of heart failure, combination with insulin (risk of heart failure), pregnancy (Appendix 4), breast-feeding (Appendix 5)

Side-effects: gastro-intestinal disturbances, weight gain, oedema, anaemia, headache, visual disturbances, dizziness, arthralgia, hypoaesthesia, hae-

maturia, impotence; less commonly hypoglycaemia, fatigue, insomnia, vertigo, sweating, altered
blood lipids, proteinuria; see also Liver Toxicity
above

Dose: initially 15–30 mg once daily increased to
45 mg once daily according to response

Actos® (Takeda) ▼ PoM
Tablets, pioglitazone (as hydrochloride) 15 mg, net
price 28-tab pack = £26.60; 30 mg, 28-tab pack =
£36.96; 45 mg, 28-tab pack = £36.96

REPAGLINIDE

Indications: type 2 diabetes mellitus (as monotherapy or in combination with metformin when
metformin alone inadequate)

Cautions: substitute insulin during intercurrent
illness (such as myocardial infarction, coma,
infection, and trauma) and during surgery; debilitated and malnourished patients; renal impairment;
interactions: Appendix 1 (antidiabetics)

Contra-indications: ketoacidosis; severe hepatic
impairment; pregnancy (Appendix 4) and breast-
feeding

Side-effects: abdominal pain, diarrhoea, constipation, nausea, vomiting; hypoglycaemia, hypersensitivity reactions including pruritus, rashes
and urticaria

Dose: initially 500 micrograms within 30 minutes
before main meals (1 mg if transferring from
another oral hypoglycaemic), adjusted according
to response at intervals of 1–2 weeks; up to 4 mg
may be given as a single dose, max. 16 mg daily
CHILD and ADOLESCENT under 18 years and ELDERLY
over 75 years, not recommended

NovoNorm® (Novo Nordisk) ▼ PoM
Tablets, repaglinide 500 micrograms, net price 30-
tab pack = £4.03, 90-tab pack = £12.09; 1 mg
(yellow), 30-tab pack = £4.08, 90-tab pack =
£12.24; 2 mg (peach), 90-tab pack = £12.24

ROSIGLITAZONE

Indications: type 2 diabetes mellitus (alone or
combined with metformin or a sulphonylurea—
see also notes above)

Cautions: monitor liver function (see below);
cardiovascular disease (risk of heart failure), renal
impairment (Appendix 3); **interactions:** Appendix
1 (antidiabetics)
LIVER TOXICITY. Rare reports of liver dysfunction
reported; monitor liver function before treatment, then
every 2 months for 12 months and periodically thereafter;
advise patients to seek immediate medical attention if
symptoms such as nausea, vomiting, abdominal pain,
fatigue and dark urine develop; discontinue if jaundice
occurs

Contra-indications: hepatic impairment, history
of heart failure, combination with insulin (risk of
heart failure), pregnancy (Appendix 4), breast-
feeding (Appendix 5)

Side-effects: gastro-intestinal disturbances, headache, anaemia, altered blood lipids, weight gain,
oedema, hypoglycaemia; less commonly fatigue,
paraesthesia, alopecia, dyspnoea; rarely pulmonary oedema; very rarely angioedema, urticaria;
see also Liver Toxicity above

Dose: initially 4 mg daily; if used alone or in
combination with metformin may increase to

8 mg daily (in 1 or 2 divided doses) after 8 weeks
according to response

Avandia® (GSK) ▼ PoM
Tablets, f/c, rosiglitazone (as maleate) 4 mg
(orange), net price 28-tab pack = £26.60, 56-tab
pack = £53.20; 8 mg (red/brown), 28-tab pack =
£54.60

■ With metformin
For cautions, contra-indications and side-effects of
metformin see section 6.1.2.2

Avandamet (GSK) ▼ PoM
Avandamet® *1 mg/500 mg tablets*, f/c, yellow,
rosiglitazone (as maleate) 1 mg, metformin hydrochloride 500 mg, net price 112-tab pack = £29.80.
Label: 21
Avandamet® *2 mg/500 mg tablets*, f/c, pink, rosiglitazone (as maleate) 2 mg, metformin hydrochloride
500 mg, net price 112-tab pack = £56.40. Label: 21
Dose: type 2 diabetes mellitus not controlled by metformin
alone, initially 2 *Avandamet*® 1 mg/500 mg tablets twice
daily, increased after 8 weeks according to response up to 2
Avandamet® 2 mg/500 mg tablets twice daily; max. 8 mg
rosiglitazone and 2 g metformin hydrochloride daily
NOTE. Titration with the individual components (rosiglitazone and metformin) may be desirable before initiation
of *Avandamet*®

6.1.3   Diabetic ketoacidosis

Soluble insulin, used intravenously, is the most
appropriate form of insulin for the management of
diabetic ketoacidotic and hyperosmolar non-ketotic
coma. It is preferable to use the type of soluble
insulin that the patient has been using previously. It is
necessary to achieve and to maintain an adequate
plasma-insulin concentration until the metabolic
disturbance is brought under control.

Insulin is best given by intravenous infusion, using
an infusion pump, and diluted to 1 unit/mL (care in
mixing, see Appendix 6). Adequate plasma-insulin
concentration can usually be maintained with infusion rates of 6 units/hour for adults and 0.1 units/kg/
hour for children. Blood glucose is expected to
decrease by about 5 mmol/litre/hour; if the response
is inadequate the infusion rate can be doubled or
quadrupled. When the blood-glucose concentration
has fallen to 10 mmol/litre the infusion rate can be
reduced to 3 units/hour for adults (about 0.02 units/
kg/hour for children) and continued until the patient
is ready to take food by mouth. The insulin infusion
should not be stopped before subcutaneous insulin
has been started.

No matter how large, a bolus intravenous injection
of insulin can provide an adequate plasma concentration for a short time only; therefore if facilities for
intravenous infusion are not available the insulin is
given by *intramuscular injection*. An initial loading
dose of 20 units intramuscularly is followed by
6 units intramuscularly every hour until the blood-
glucose concentration falls to 10 mmol/litre; intramuscular injections are then given every 2 hours.
Although absorption of insulin is usually rapid after
intramuscular injection, it may be impaired in the
presence of hypotension and poor tissue perfusion;
moreover insulin may accumulate during treatment
and late hypoglycaemia should be watched for and
treated appropriately.

Intravenous replacement of fluid and electrolytes
(section 9.2.2) with **sodium chloride** intravenous

infusion is an essential part of the management of ketoacidosis; **potassium chloride** is included in the infusion as appropriate to prevent the hypokalaemia induced by the insulin. **Sodium bicarbonate** infusion (1.26% or 2.74%) is used only in cases of extreme acidosis and shock since the acid-base disturbance is normally corrected by the insulin. **Glucose** solution (5%) is infused once the blood glucose has decreased below 10 mmol/litre but insulin infusion must continue.

6.1.4 Treatment of hypoglycaemia

Initially glucose 10–20 g is given by mouth either in liquid form or as granulated sugar or sugar lumps. Approximately 10 g of glucose is available from 2 teaspoons sugar, 3 sugar lumps, *Hypostop®* Gel (glucose 9.2 g/23-g oral ampoule, available from Bio Diagnostics), milk 200 mL, and non-diet versions of *Lucozade®* Sparkling Glucose Drink 50–55 mL, *Coca-Cola®* 90 mL, *Ribena®* Original 15 mL (to be diluted). If necessary this may be repeated in 10–15 minutes.

Hypoglycaemia which causes unconsciousness is an emergency. **Glucagon** can be given for acute insulin-induced hypoglycaemia; it is not appropriate for chronic hypoglycaemia. It is a polypeptide hormone produced by the alpha cells of the islets of Langerhans. It increases plasma-glucose concentration by mobilising glycogen stored in the liver. It can be injected by any route (intramuscular, subcutaneous, or intravenous) in a dose of 1 mg (1 unit) in circumstances when an intravenous injection of glucose would be difficult or impossible to administer. It may be issued to close relatives of insulin-treated patients for emergency use in hypoglycaemic attacks. It is often advisable to prescribe on an 'if necessary' basis to hospitalised insulin-treated patients, so that it may be given rapidly by the nurses during an hypoglycaemic emergency. If not effective in 10 minutes intravenous glucose should be given.

Alternatively, 50 mL of **glucose intravenous infusion 20%** (section 9.2.2) may be given intravenously into a large vein through a large-gauge needle; care is required since this concentration is irritant especially if extravasation occurs. Alternatively, 25 mL of glucose intravenous infusion 50% may be given, but this higher concentration is more irritant and viscous making administration difficult. Glucose intravenous infusion 10% may also be used but larger volumes are needed. Close monitoring is necessary in the case of an overdose with a long-acting insulin because further administration of glucose may be required. Patients whose hypoglycaemia is caused by an oral antidiabetic drug should be transferred to hospital because the hypoglycaemic effects of these drugs may persist for many hours.

GLUCAGON

Indications: see notes above and under Dose

Cautions: see notes above, insulinoma, glucagonoma; ineffective in chronic hypoglycaemia, starvation, and adrenal insufficiency

Contra-indications: phaeochromocytoma

Side-effects: nausea, vomiting, diarrhoea, hypokalaemia, rarely hypersensitivity reactions

Dose: *by subcutaneous, intramuscular, or intravenous injection*, ADULT and CHILD over 8 years (or body-weight over 25 kg), 1 mg; CHILD under 8 years (or body-weight under 25 kg), 500 micrograms; if no response within 10 minutes intravenous glucose must be given

Diagnostic aid, consult product literature

Beta-blocker poisoning, see p. 24

NOTE. 1 unit of glucagon = 1 mg of glucagon

GlucaGen® HypoKit (Novo Nordisk) PoM
Injection, powder for reconstitution, glucagon (rys) as hydrochloride with lactose, net price 1-mg vial with prefilled syringe containing water for injection = £19.95

Chronic hypoglycaemia

Diazoxide, administered by mouth, is useful in the management of patients with chronic hypoglycaemia from excess endogenous insulin secretion, either from an islet cell tumour or islet cell hyperplasia. It has no place in the management of acute hypoglycaemia.

DIAZOXIDE

Indications: chronic intractable hypoglycaemia (for use in hypertensive crisis see section 2.5.1)

Cautions: ischaemic heart disease, pregnancy, labour, impaired renal function; haematological examinations and blood pressure monitoring required during prolonged treatment; growth, bone, and developmental checks in children; interactions: Appendix 1 (diazoxide)

Side-effects: anorexia, nausea, vomiting, hyperuricaemia, hypotension, oedema, tachycardia, arrhythmias, extrapyramidal effects; hypertrichosis on prolonged treatment

Dose: *by mouth*, ADULT and CHILD, initially 5 mg/kg daily in 2–3 divided doses

Eudemine® (Celltech) PoM
Tablets, diazoxide 50 mg. Net price 20 = £7.68

6.1.5 Treatment of diabetic nephropathy and neuropathy

Diabetic nephropathy

Regular review of diabetic patients should include an annual test for urinary protein (using *Albustix®*) and serum creatinine measurement. If the urinary protein test is negative, the urine should be tested for microalbuminuria (the earliest sign of nephropathy). If reagent strip tests (*Micral-Test II®* NHS or *Microbumintest®* NHS) are used and prove positive, the result should be confirmed by laboratory analysis of a urine sample. Provided there are no contra-indications, all diabetic patients with nephropathy causing proteinuria or with established microalbuminuria (at least 3 positive tests) should be treated with an ACE inhibitor (section 2.5.5.1) or an angiotensin-II receptor antagonist (section 2.5.5.2) even if the blood pressure is normal; in any case, to minimise the risk of renal deterioration, blood pressure should be carefully controlled (section 2.5).

ACE inhibitors may potentiate the hypoglycaemic effect of insulin and oral antidiabetic drugs; this effect is more likely during the first weeks of combined treatment and in patients with renal impairment.

For the treatment of hypertension in diabetes, see section 2.5.

Diabetic neuropathy

Optimal diabetic control is beneficial for the management of *painful neuropathy* in patients with type 1 diabetes (see also section 4.7.3). **Paracetamol** or a **non-steroidal anti-inflammatory drug** such as ibuprofen (section 10.1.1) may relieve *mild to moderate pain*.

The **tricyclic antidepressants** amitriptyline and nortriptyline (section 4.3.1) are the drugs of choice for painful diabetic neuropathy [unlicensed use]; amitriptyline is given in a dose of 25–75 mg daily (higher doses under specialist supervision). Other classes of antidepressants do not appear to be effective. **Gabapentin** (section 4.8.1) is licensed for the treatment of neuropathic pain and is an effective alternative to a tricyclic antidepressant.

Carbamazepine and **phenytoin** [both unlicensed] (section 4.8.1) may be useful for shooting or stabbing pain, but adverse effects are common; carbamazepine 200–800 mg daily in divided doses has been used.

Capsaicin cream 0.075% (section 10.3.2) is licensed for painful diabetic neuropathy and may have some effect, but it produces an intense burning sensation during the initial treatment period.

Neuropathic pain may respond partially to some **opioid analgesics**, such as dextropropoxyphene, methadone, oxycodone and tramadol, and they may have a role when other treatments have failed.

In *autonomic neuropathy* diabetic diarrhoea can often be managed by 2 or 3 doses of **tetracycline** 250 mg [unlicensed use] (section 5.1.3). Otherwise **codeine phosphate** (section 1.4.2) is the best drug, but other antidiarrhoeal preparations can be tried. An **antiemetic** which promotes gastric transit, such as metoclopramide or domperidone (section 4.6), is helpful for gastroparesis. In rare cases when an antiemetic does not help, erythromycin (especially when given intravenously) may be beneficial but this needs confirmation.

For the management of erectile dysfunction, see section 7.4.5.

In *neuropathic postural hypotension* increased salt intake and the use of the **mineralocorticoid** fludrocortisone 100–400 micrograms daily [unlicensed use] (section 6.3.1) help by increasing plasma volume, but uncomfortable oedema is a common side-effect. Fludrocortisone can also be combined with **flurbiprofen** (section 10.1.1) and **ephedrine hydrochloride** (section 3.1.1.2) [both unlicensed]. **Midodrine** [unlicensed], an alpha agonist, may also be useful in postural hypotension.

Gustatory sweating can be treated with an **antimuscarinic** such as propantheline bromide (section 1.2); side-effects are common. For the management of hyperhidrosis, see section 13.12.

In some patients with *neuropathic oedema*, **ephedrine hydrochloride** [unlicensed use] 30–60 mg 3 times daily offers effective relief.

6.1.6 Diagnostic and monitoring agents for diabetes mellitus

Blood glucose monitoring

Blood glucose monitoring gives a direct measure of the glucose concentration at the time of the test and can detect hypoglycaemia as well as hyperglycaemia. Patients should be properly trained in the use of blood glucose monitoring systems and to take appropriate action on the results obtained. Inadequate understanding of the normal fluctuations in blood glucose may lead to confusion and inappropriate action. It is ideal for patients to observe the 'peaks' and 'troughs' of blood glucose over 24 hours and make adjustments of their insulin no more than once or twice weekly. Daily alterations to the insulin dose are highly undesirable (except during illness).

Blood glucose monitoring is best carried out by means of a meter. Visual colour comparison is sometimes used but is much less satisfactory. Meters give a more precise reading and are useful for patients with poor eyesight or who are colour blind. NOTE. In the UK blood-glucose concentration is expressed in mmol/litre and Diabetes UK advises that these units should be used for self-monitoring of blood glucose. In other European countries units of mg/100 mL (or mg/dL) are commonly used.

It is advisable to check that the meter is pre-set in the correct units.

■ Test strips

Active® (Roche Diagnostics)
Reagent strips, for blood glucose monitoring, range 0.6– 33.3 mmol/litre, for use with *Glucotrend*® and *Accu-Chek*® *Active* [NHS] meters only. Net price 50-strip pack = £15.55

Advantage II® (Roche Diagnostics)
Reagent strips, for blood glucose monitoring, range 0.6– 33.3 mmol/litre, for use with *Accu-Chek*® *Advantage* [NHS] meter only. Net price 50-strip pack = £15.55

Ascensia® **Autodisc** (Bayer Diagnostics)
Sensor discs, for blood glucose monitoring, range 0.6– 33.3 mmol/litre, for use with *Ascensia Breeze*® [NHS] and *Ascensia Esprit*® 2 [NHS] meters only. Net price 5 × 10-disc pack = £15.40

Ascensia® **Glucodisc** (Bayer Diagnostics)
Sensor discs, for blood glucose monitoring, range 0.6– 33.3 mmol/L, for use with *Ascensia Esprit*® 2 [NHS] meter only. Net price 5 × 10-disc pack = £15.26

BM-Accutest® (Roche Diagnostics)
Reagent strips, for blood glucose monitoring, range 1.1– 33.3 mmol/litre, for use with *Accutrend*® [NHS] meters only. Net price 50-strip pack = £15.07

BM-Test 1–44® (Roche Diagnostics)
Reagent strips, for blood glucose monitoring, visual range 1– 44 mmol/litre, meter range 0.5–27.7 mmol/litre, suitable for use with *Reflolux*® *S* [NHS]. Net price 50-strip pack = £15.87

Compact® (Roche Diagnostics)
Reagent strips, for blood glucose monitoring, range 0.6– 33.3 mmol/litre, for use with *Accu-Chek*® *Compact* [NHS] meter only. Net price 3 × 17-strip pack = £15.67

FreeStyle® (TheraSense)
Reagent strips, for blood glucose monitoring, range 1.1– 27.8 mmol/litre, for use with *FreeStyle*® [NHS] meter only. Net price 50-strip pack = £15.40

GlucoMen® (Menarini Diagnostics)
Sensor strips, for blood glucose monitoring, range 1.1–33.3 mmol/litre, for use with *GlucoMen*® *Glycó* [NHS] meter only. Net price 50-strip pack = £14.43

Glucostix® (Bayer Diagnostics)
Reagent strips, for blood glucose monitoring, visual range 1–44 mmol/litre, meter range 2–22 mmol/litre, suitable for use with *Glucometer*® *GX* [NHS]. Net price 50-strip pack = £15.84

Glucotide® (Bayer Diagnostics)
Reagent strips, for blood glucose monitoring, range 0.6–33.3 mmol/litre, for use with *Glucometer*® *4* [NHS] meter only. Net price 50-strip pack = £15.06

Hypoguard® **Supreme** (Hypoguard)
Reagent strips, for blood glucose monitoring, range 2.2–27.7 mmol/litre, for use with *Hypoguard*® *Supreme* meters. Net price 50-strip pack = £13.64

Hypoguard® **Supreme Spectrum** (Hypoguard)
Reagent strips, for blood glucose monitoring, visual range 2.2–27.8 mmol/litre. Net price 50-strip pack = £10.34

MediSense G2® (MediSense)
Sensor strips, for blood glucose monitoring, range 1.1–33.3 mmol/litre. for use with *MediSense Card*® [NHS] or *MediSense Pen*® [NHS] meters only. Net price 50-strip pack = £14.40

MediSense® **Optium Plus** (MediSense)
Sensor strips, for blood glucose monitoring, range 1.1–27.7 mmol/litre, for use with *MediSense*® *Optium* [NHS] meter only. Net price 50-strip pack = £15.30

MediSense® **Soft-Sense** (MediSense)
Sensor strips, for blood glucose monitoring, range 1.7–25 mmol/litre, for use with *MediSense*® *Soft-Sense* [NHS] meter only. Net price 50-strip pack = £15.28

One Touch® (LifeScan)
Reagent strips, for blood glucose monitoring, range 0–33.3 mmol/litre, for use with *One Touch*® *II*, *Profile* and *Basic* [NHS] meters only. Net price 50-strip pack = £15.14

One Touch® **Ultra** (LifeScan)
Reagent strips, for blood glucose monitoring, range 1.1–33.3 mmol/litre, for use with *One Touch*® *Ultra* [NHS] meter only. Net price 50-strip pack = £15.30

PocketScan® (LifeScan)
Reagent strips, for blood glucose monitoring, range 1.1–33.3 mmol/litre, for use with *PocketScan*® [NHS] meter only. Net price 50-strip pack = £14.94

Prestige® **Smart System** (DiagnoSys)
Reagent strips, for blood glucose monitoring, range 1.4–33.3 mmol/litre, for use with *Prestige*® *Smart System* [NHS] meter only. Net price 50-strip pack = £15.01

■ Meters

Accu-Chek® **Active** (Roche Diagnostics) [NHS]
Meter, for blood glucose monitoring (for use with *Active*® test strips). *Accu-Chek*® *Active* system = £15.00

Accu-Chek® **Advantage** (Roche Diagnostics) [NHS]
Meter, for blood glucose monitoring (for use with *Advantage II*® test strips). *Accu-Chek*® *Advantage* system = £4.20

Accu-Chek® **Compact** (Roche Diagnostics) [NHS]
Meter, for blood glucose monitoring (for use with *Compact*® test strips). *Accu-Chek*® *Compact* system = £6.00

Ascensia Breeze® (Bayer Diagnostics) [NHS]
Meter, for blood glucose monitoring (for use with *Ascensia*® *Autodisc* test sensor discs)

Ascensia Esprit® **2** (Bayer Diagnostics) [NHS]
Meter, for blood glucose monitoring (for use with *Ascensia*® *Glucodisc* test sensor discs) = £17.49

FreeStyle® (TheraSense)
Meter for blood glucose monitoring (for use with *FreeStyle*® test strips) = £25.00

GlucoMen® **Glycó** (Menarini Diagnostics) [NHS]
Meter, for blood glucose monitoring (for use with *GlucoMen*® sensor strips)

GlucoMen® **PC** (Menarini Diagnostics) [NHS]
Meter, for blood glucose monitoring (for use with *GlucoMen*® sensor strips)

Glucotrend® (Roche Diagnostics) [NHS]
Meters, for blood glucose monitoring (for use with *Gluco-trend*® test strips). *Glucotrend*® *2 Soft Test System* pack [NHS] = £25.00; *Glucotrend*® *Premium* pack [NHS] = £36.74

Hypoguard® **Supreme** (Hypoguard) [NHS]
Meters, for blood glucose monitoring (for use with *Hypoguard*® *Supreme* test strips). *Hypoguard*® *Supreme Plus* meter = £35.00; *Hypoguard*® *Supreme Extra* meter = £45.00

MediSense® (MediSense) [NHS]
Meters (Sensor), for blood glucose monitoring. *MediSense Card* = £15.31, *MediSense*® card starter pack = £17.50, *MediSense*® *Pen* = £30.63, *MediSense*® pen starter pack = £39.38, *MediSense*® *Precision QID* starter pack = £12.00 (all for use with *MediSense G2*® test strips); *MediSense*® *Optium* starter pack (for use with *MediSense*® *Optium* test strips) = £17.50; *MediSense*® *Soft-Sense* meter (for use with *MediSense*® *Soft-Sense* test strips)

One Touch® (LifeScan) [NHS]
Meters, for blood glucose monitoring (for use with *One Touch*® test strips). *One Touch*® *Basic* system pack = £9.38, *One Touch*® *Profile* system pack = £18.38

One Touch® **Ultra** (LifeScan) [NHS]
Meter, for blood glucose monitoring (for use with *One Touch*® *Ultra* test strips) = £10.00

PocketScan® (LifeScan) [NHS]
Meter, for blood glucose monitoring (for use with *PocketScan*® test strips). *Complete PocketScan*® *System* = £17.50

Prestige® **Smart System** (DiagnoSys) [NHS]
Meter, for blood glucose monitoring (for use with *Prestige*® *Smart System* test strips) = £5.63

Urinalysis

Urine testing for glucose is useful in patients who find blood glucose monitoring difficult. Tests for glucose range from reagent strips specific to glucose to reagent tablets which detect all reducing sugars. Few patients still use *Clinitest*®; *Clinistix*® is suitable for screening purposes only. Tests for ketones by patients are rarely required unless they become unwell.

Microalbuminuria can be detected with *Micral-Test II*® [NHS] or *Microbumintest*® [NHS] but this should be followed by confirmation in the laboratory, since false positive results are common.

■ Glucose

Clinistix® (Bayer Diagnostics)
Reagent strips, for detection of glucose in urine. Net price 50-strip pack = £3.13

Clinitest® (Bayer Diagnostics)
Reagent tablets, for detection of glucose and other reducing substances in urine. Pocket set [NHS] (test tube, dropper and 36 tablets), net price = £4.02, 36-tab pack = £2.00, 6-test tube pack [NHS] = £3.70, 6-dropper pack [NHS] = £3.80

Diabur-Test 5000® (Roche Diagnostics)
Reagent strips, for detection of glucose in urine. Net price 50-strip pack = £2.59

Diastix® (Bayer Diagnostics)
Reagent strips, for detection of glucose in urine. Net price 50-strip pack = £2.66

Medi-Test® **Glucose** (BHR)
Reagent strips, for detection of glucose in urine. Net price 50-strip pack = £2.17

■ Ketones

Acetest® (Bayer Diagnostics)
Reagent tablets, for detection of ketones in urine. Net price 100-tab pack = £3.53

Ketostix® (Bayer Diagnostics)
Reagent strips, for detection of ketones in urine. Net price 50-strip pack = £2.82

Ketur Test® (Roche Diagnostics)
Reagent strips, for detection of ketones in urine. Net price 50-strip pack = £2.49

■ Protein

Albustix® (Bayer Diagnostics)
Reagent strips, for detection of protein in urine. Net price 50-strip pack = £3.87

Medi-Test® Protein 2 (BHR)
Reagent strips, for detection of protein in urine. Net price 50-strip pack = £3.03

■ Other reagent strips available for urinalysis include:

Combur-3 Test® NHS (glucose and protein—Roche Diagnostics), *Clinitek Microalbumin®* NHS (albumin and creatinine—Bayer Diagnostics), *Ketodiastix®* NHS (glucose and ketones—Bayer Diagnostics), *Medi-Test Combi 2®* NHS (glucose and protein—BHR), *Micral-Test II®* NHS (albumin—Roche Diagnostics), *Microalbustix®* NHS (albumin and creatinine—Bayer Diagnostics), *Microbumintest®* NHS (albumin—Bayer Diagnostics), *Uristix®* NHS (glucose and protein—Bayer Diagnostics)

Glucose tolerance test

The **glucose** tolerance test is now rarely needed for the diagnosis of diabetes when symptoms of hyperglycaemia are present, though it is still required to establish the presence of gestational diabetes. This generally involves giving anhydrous glucose 75 g (equivalent to Glucose BP 82.5 g) by mouth to the fasting patient, and measuring blood-glucose concentrations at intervals.

The appropriate amount of glucose should be given with 200–300 mL fluid. Anhydrous glucose 75 g may alternatively be given as 113 mL *Polycal®* (Nutricia Clinical) with extra fluid to administer a total volume of 200–300 mL.

6.2   Thyroid and antithyroid drugs

6.2.1   Thyroid hormones
6.2.2   Antithyroid drugs

6.2.1   Thyroid hormones

Thyroid hormones are used in hypothyroidism (myxoedema), and also in diffuse non-toxic goitre, Hashimoto's thyroiditis (lymphadenoid goitre), and thyroid carcinoma. Neonatal hypothyroidism requires prompt treatment for normal development.

Levothyroxine sodium (thyroxine sodium) is the treatment of choice for *maintenance* therapy. The initial dose should not exceed 100 micrograms daily, preferably before breakfast, or 25 to 50 micrograms in elderly patients or those with cardiac disease, increased by 25 to 50 micrograms at intervals of at least 4 weeks. The usual maintenance dose to relieve

hypothyroidism is 100 to 200 micrograms daily which can be administered as a single dose.

In infants and children doses of thyroxine, for congenital hypothyroidism and juvenile myxoedema, should be titrated according to clinical response, growth assessment, and measurements of plasma thyroxine and thyroid-stimulating hormone.

Liothyronine sodium has a similar action to levothyroxine but is more rapidly metabolised and has a more rapid effect; 20 micrograms is equivalent to 100 micrograms of levothyroxine. Its effects develop after a few hours and disappear within 24 to 48 hours of discontinuing treatment. It may be used in *severe hypothyroid states* when a rapid response is desired.

Liothyronine by intravenous injection is the treatment of choice in *hypothyroid coma*. Adjunctive therapy includes intravenous fluids, hydrocortisone, and treatment of infection; assisted ventilation is often required.

LEVOTHYROXINE SODIUM
(Thyroxine sodium)

Indications: hypothyroidism

Cautions: panhypopituitarism or predisposition to adrenal insufficiency from other causes (initiate corticosteroid therapy before starting levothyroxine), elderly, cardiovascular disorders (myocardial insufficiency or ECG evidence of myocardial infarction, see Initial Dosage below), long-standing hypothyroidism, diabetes insipidus, diabetes mellitus (dosage increase may be needed for antidiabetic drugs including insulin); pregnancy (Appendix 4) and breast-feeding (Appendix 5); **interactions:** Appendix 1 (thyroid hormones)
INITIAL DOSAGE. A pre-therapy ECG is valuable as changes induced by hypothyroidism may be confused with evidence of ischaemia. If too rapid an increase of metabolism is produced (causing diarrhoea, nervousness, rapid pulse, insomnia, tremors and sometimes anginal pain where there is latent myocardial ischaemia), reduce dose or withhold for 1–2 days and start again at a lower dose

Contra-indications: thyrotoxicosis

Side-effects: usually at excessive dosage (see Initial Dosage above) include anginal pain, arrhythmias, palpitation, skeletal muscle cramps, tachycardia, diarrhoea, vomiting, tremors, restlessness, excitability, insomnia, headache, flushing, sweating, fever, heat intolerance, excessive loss of weight and muscular weakness

Dose: ADULT, initially 50–100 micrograms (50 micrograms for those over 50 years) daily, preferably before breakfast, adjusted in steps of 50 micrograms every 3–4 weeks until normal metabolism maintained (usually 100–200 micrograms daily); where there is cardiac disease, initially 25 micrograms daily *or* 50 micrograms on alternate days, adjusted in steps of 25 micrograms every 4 weeks

Congenital hypothyroidism and juvenile myxoedema, CHILD up to 1 month initially 5–10 micrograms/kg daily, over 1 month initially 5 micrograms/kg daily adjusted in steps of 25 micrograms every 2–4 weeks until mild toxic symptoms appear then reduce dose slightly

Levothyroxine (Non-proprietary) PoM

Tablets, levothyroxine sodium 25 micrograms, net price 28-tab pack = 85p; 50 micrograms, 28-tab pack = 57p; 100 micrograms, 28-tab pack = 86p Available from Alpharma, APS, CP, Goldshield (*Eltroxin®*), Hillcross, IVAX

LIOTHYRONINE SODIUM

(L-Tri-iodothyronine sodium)

Indications: see notes above

Cautions: see under Levothyroxine Sodium; **interactions:** Appendix 1 (thyroid hormones)

Contra-indications: see under Levothyroxine Sodium

Side-effects: see under Levothyroxine Sodium

Dose: *by mouth,* initially 10–20 micrograms daily gradually increased to 60 micrograms daily in 2–3 divided doses; elderly patients should receive smaller initial doses; CHILD, adult dose reduced in proportion to body-weight

By slow intravenous injection, hypothyroid coma, 5–20 micrograms repeated every 12 hours or as often as every 4 hours if necessary; alternatively 50 micrograms initially then 25 micrograms every 8 hours reducing to 25 micrograms twice daily

Tertroxin® (Goldshield) PoM

Tablets, scored, liothyronine sodium 20 micrograms, net price 100-tab pack = £15.92

Triiodothyronine (Goldshield) PoM

Injection, powder for reconstitution, liothyronine sodium (with dextran). Net price 20-microgram amp = £37.92

6.2.2 Antithyroid drugs

Antithyroid drugs are used for hyperthyroidism either to prepare patients for thyroidectomy or for long-term management. In the UK carbimazole is the most commonly used drug. Propylthiouracil may be used in patients who suffer sensitivity reactions to carbimazole as sensitivity is not necessarily displayed to both drugs. Both drugs act primarily by interfering with the synthesis of thyroid hormones.

> **CSM warning (neutropenia and agranulocytosis)**
> Doctors are reminded of the importance of recognising bone marrow suppression induced by carbimazole and the need to stop treatment promptly.
>
> 1. Patient should be asked to report symptoms and signs suggestive of infection, especially sore throat.
> 2. A white blood cell count should be performed if there is any clinical evidence of infection.
> 3. Carbimazole should be stopped promptly if there is clinical or laboratory evidence of neutropenia.

Carbimazole is given in a dose of 15 to 40 mg daily; occasionally a larger dose may be required. This dose is continued until the patient becomes euthyroid, usually after 4 to 8 weeks and the dose is then gradually reduced to a maintenance dose of 5 to 15 mg. Therapy is usually given for 12 to 18 months. Children may be given carbimazole in an initial dose of 250 micrograms/kg three times daily, adjusted according to response; treatment in children should be undertaken by a specialist. Rashes and pruritus are common but they can be treated with antihistamines

without discontinuing therapy; alternatively propylthiouracil may be substituted. All patients should be advised to report any sore throat immediately because of the rare complication of agranulocytosis (see CSM warning, above).

Propylthiouracil is given in a dose of 200 to 400 mg daily in adults and this dose is maintained until the patient becomes euthyroid; the dose may then be gradually reduced to a maintenance dose of 50 to 150 mg daily.

Antithyroid drugs only need to be given once daily because of their prolonged effect on the thyroid. Over-treatment can result in the rapid development of hypothyroidism and should be avoided particularly during pregnancy because it can cause fetal goitre.

A combination of carbimazole, 40 to 60 mg daily with levothyroxine, 50 to 150 micrograms daily, may be used in a *blocking-replacement regimen*; therapy is usually given for 18 months. The blocking-replacement regimen is **not** suitable during pregnancy.

Iodine has been used as an adjunct to antithyroid drugs for 10 to 14 days before partial thyroidectomy; however, there is little evidence of a beneficial effect. Iodine should not be used for long-term treatment because its antithyroid action tends to diminish.

Radioactive sodium iodide (^{131}I) solution is used increasingly for the treatment of thyrotoxicosis at all ages, particularly where medical therapy or compliance is a problem, in patients with cardiac disease, and in patients who relapse after thyroidectomy.

Propranolol is useful for rapid relief of thyrotoxic symptoms and may be used in conjunction with antithyroid drugs or as an adjunct to radioactive iodine. Beta-blockers are also useful in neonatal thyrotoxicosis and in supraventricular arrhythmias due to hyperthyroidism. Propranolol has been used in conjunction with iodine to prepare mildly thyrotoxic patients for surgery but it is preferable to make the patient euthyroid with carbimazole. Laboratory tests of thyroid function are not altered by beta-blockers. Most experience in treating thyrotoxicosis has been gained with propranolol but **nadolol** is also used. For doses and preparations of beta-blockers see section 2.4.

Thyrotoxic crisis ('thyroid storm') requires emergency treatment with intravenous administration of fluids, propranolol (5 mg) and hydrocortisone (100 mg every 6 hours, as sodium succinate), as well as oral iodine solution and carbimazole or propylthiouracil which may need to be administered by nasogastric tube.

PREGNANCY AND BREAST-FEEDING. Radioactive iodine therapy is contra-indicated during pregnancy. Propylthiouracil and carbimazole can be given but the blocking-replacement regimen (see above) is **not** suitable. Both propylthiouracil and carbimazole cross the placenta and in high doses may cause fetal goitre and hypothyroidism—the lowest dose that will control the hyperthyroid state should be used (requirements in Graves' disease tend to fall during pregnancy). Rarely, carbimazole has been associated with aplasia cutis of the neonate.

Carbimazole and propylthiouracil appear in breast milk but this does not preclude breast-feeding as long as neonatal development is closely monitored and the lowest effective dose is used.

CARBIMAZOLE

Indications: hyperthyroidism

Cautions: liver disorders, pregnancy, breast-feeding (see notes above)

Side-effects: nausea, mild gastro-intestinal disturbances, headache, rashes and pruritus, arthralgia; rarely myopathy, alopecia, bone marrow suppression (including pancytopenia and agranulocytosis, see **CSM warning** above), jaundice

Dose: see notes above

COUNSELLING. Warn patient to tell doctor **immediately** if sore throat, mouth ulcers, bruising, fever, malaise, or non-specific illness develops

Neo-Mercazole® (Roche) PoM

Tablets, both pink, carbimazole 5 mg, net price 100-tab pack = £3.30; 20 mg, 100-tab pack = £12.25. Counselling, blood disorder symptoms

IODINE AND IODIDE

Indications: thyrotoxicosis (pre-operative)

Cautions: pregnancy, children; not for long-term treatment

Contra-indications: breast-feeding

Side-effects: hypersensitivity reactions including coryza-like symptoms, headache, lacrimation, conjunctivitis, pain in salivary glands, laryngitis, bronchitis, rashes; on prolonged treatment depression, insomnia, impotence; goitre in infants of mothers taking iodides

Aqueous Iodine Oral Solution

(Lugol's Solution), iodine 5%, potassium iodide 10% in purified water, freshly boiled and cooled, total iodine 130 mg/mL. Net price 100 mL = £1.90. Label: 27

Dose: 0.1–0.3 mL 3 times daily well diluted with milk or water

PROPYLTHIOURACIL

Indications: hyperthyroidism

Cautions: see under Carbimazole; hepatic impairment (Appendix 2), renal impairment (Appendix 3)

Side-effects: see under Carbimazole; leucopenia; rarely cutaneous vasculitis, thrombocytopenia, aplastic anaemia, hypoprothrombinaemia, hepatitis, encephalopathy, hepatic necrosis, nephritis, lupus erythematosus-like syndromes

Dose: see notes above

Propylthiouracil (Non-proprietary) PoM

Tablets, propylthiouracil 50 mg. Net price 56-tab pack = £24.95

Available from Celltech, CP, Hillcross, IVAX

6.3　Corticosteroids

6.3.1　　Replacement therapy
6.3.2　　Glucocorticoid therapy

6.3.1　Replacement therapy

The adrenal cortex normally secretes hydrocortisone (cortisol) which has glucocorticoid activity and weak mineralocorticoid activity. It also secretes the mineralocorticoid aldosterone.

In deficiency states, physiological replacement is best achieved with a combination of **hydrocortisone** (section 6.3.2) and the mineralocorticoid **fludrocortisone**; hydrocortisone alone does not usually provide sufficient mineralocorticoid activity for complete replacement.

In *Addison's disease* or following adrenalectomy, **hydrocortisone** 20 to 30 mg daily by mouth is usually required. This is given in 2 doses, the larger in the morning and the smaller in the evening, mimicking the normal diurnal rhythm of cortisol secretion. The optimum daily dose is determined on the basis of clinical response. Glucocorticoid therapy is supplemented by fludrocortisone 50 to 300 micrograms daily.

In *acute adrenocortical insufficiency*, **hydrocortisone** is given intravenously (preferably as sodium succinate) in doses of 100 mg every 6 to 8 hours in sodium chloride intravenous infusion 0.9%.

In *hypopituitarism* glucocorticoids should be given as in adrenocortical insufficiency, but since the production of aldosterone is also regulated by the renin-angiotensin system a mineralocorticoid is not usually required. Additional replacement therapy with levothyroxine (section 6.2.1) and sex hormones (section 6.4) should be given as indicated by the pattern of hormone deficiency.

FLUDROCORTISONE ACETATE

Indications: mineralocorticoid replacement in adrenocortical insufficiency

Cautions: section 6.3.2; **interactions:** Appendix 1 (corticosteroids)

Contra-indications: section 6.3.2

Side-effects: section 6.3.2

Dose: 50–300 micrograms daily; CHILD 5 micrograms/kg daily

Florinef® (Squibb) PoM

Tablets, pink, scored, fludrocortisone acetate 100 micrograms. Net price 56-tab pack = £2.69. Label: 10, steroid card

6.3.2　Glucocorticoid therapy

In comparing the relative potencies of corticosteroids in terms of their anti-inflammatory (glucocorticoid) effects it should be borne in mind that high glucocorticoid activity in itself is of no advantage unless it is accompanied by relatively low mineralocorticoid activity (see Disadvantages of Corticosteroids below). The mineralocorticoid activity of **fludrocortisone** (section 6.3.1) is so high that its anti-inflammatory activity is of no clinical relevance. The table below shows equivalent anti-inflammatory doses.

Equivalent anti-inflammatory doses of corticosteroids

This table takes no account of mineralocorticoid effects, nor does it take account of variations in duration of action

Prednisolone 5 mg

≡	Betamethasone 750 micrograms
≡	Cortisone acetate 25 mg
≡	Deflazacort 6 mg
≡	Dexamethasone 750 micrograms
≡	Hydrocortisone 20 mg
≡	Methylprednisolone 4 mg
≡	Triamcinolone 4 mg

The relatively high mineralocorticoid activity of **cortisone** and **hydrocortisone**, and the resulting fluid retention, make them unsuitable for disease suppression on a long-term basis. However, they can be used for adrenal replacement therapy (section 6.3.1); hydrocortisone is preferred because cortisone requires conversion in the liver to hydrocortisone. Hydrocortisone is used on a short-term basis by intravenous injection for the emergency management of some conditions. The relatively moderate anti-inflammatory potency of hydrocortisone also makes it a useful topical corticosteroid for the management of inflammatory skin conditions because side-effects (both topical and systemic) are less marked (section 13.4); cortisone is not active topically.

Prednisolone has predominantly glucocorticoid activity and is the corticosteroid most commonly used by mouth for long-term disease suppression.

Betamethasone and **dexamethasone** have very high glucocorticoid activity in conjunction with insignificant mineralocorticoid activity. This makes them particularly suitable for high-dose therapy in conditions where fluid retention would be a disadvantage (e.g. cerebral oedema).

Betamethasone and dexamethasone also have a long duration of action and this, coupled with their lack of mineralocorticoid action makes them particularly suitable for conditions which require suppression of corticotropin (corticotrophin) secretion (e.g. congenital adrenal hyperplasia). Some esters of betamethasone and of **beclometasone** (beclomethasone) exert a considerably more marked topical effect (e.g. on the skin or the lungs) than when given by mouth; use is made of this to obtain topical effects whilst minimising systemic side-effects (e.g. for skin applications and asthma inhalations).

Deflazacort has a high glucocorticoid activity; it is derived from prednisolone.

Disadvantages of corticosteroids

Overdosage or prolonged use may exaggerate some of the normal physiological actions of corticosteroids leading to mineralocorticoid and glucocorticoid side-effects.

Mineralocorticoid side-effects include hypertension, sodium and water retention and potassium loss. They are most marked with fludrocortisone, but are significant with cortisone, hydrocortisone, corticotropin, and tetracosactide (tetracosactrin). Mineralocorticoid actions are negligible with the high potency glucocorticoids, betamethasone and dexamethasone, and occur only slightly with methylprednisolone, prednisolone, and triamcinolone.

Glucocorticoid side-effects include diabetes and osteoporosis (section 6.6), which is a danger, particularly in the elderly, as it may result in osteoporotic fractures for example of the hip or vertebrae; in addition high doses are associated with avascular necrosis of the femoral head. Mental disturbances may occur; a serious paranoid state or depression with risk of suicide may be induced, particularly in patients with a history of mental disorder. Euphoria is frequently observed. Muscle wasting (proximal myopathy) may also occur. Corticosteroid therapy is also weakly linked with peptic ulceration (the potential advantage of soluble or enteric-coated preparations to reduce the risk is speculative only).

High doses of corticosteroids may cause Cushing's syndrome, with moon face, striae, and acne; it is usually reversible on withdrawal of treatment, but this must always be gradually tapered to avoid symptoms of acute adrenal insufficiency (**important:** see also Adrenal Suppression below).

In children, administration of corticosteroids may result in suppression of growth. For the effect of corticosteroids given in pregnancy, see Pregnancy and Breast-feeding, below.

Adrenal Suppression

During prolonged therapy with corticosteroids, adrenal atrophy develops and may persist for years after stopping. Abrupt withdrawal after a prolonged period may lead to acute adrenal insufficiency, hypotension or death (see Withdrawal of Corticosteroids, below). Withdrawal may also be associated with fever, myalgia, arthralgia, rhinitis, conjunctivitis, painful itchy skin nodules and weight loss.

To compensate for a diminished adrenocortical response caused by prolonged corticosteroid treatment, any significant intercurrent illness, trauma, or surgical procedure requires a temporary increase in corticosteroid dose, or if already stopped, a temporary re-introduction of corticosteroid treatment. Anaesthetists **must** therefore know whether a patient is taking or has been taking a corticosteroid, to avoid a precipitous fall in blood pressure during anaesthesia or in the immediate postoperative period. A suitable regimen for corticosteroid replacement, in patients who have taken more than 10 mg prednisolone daily (or equivalent) within 3 months of surgery, is:

- *Minor surgery under general anaesthesia*—usual oral corticosteroid dose on the morning of surgery or hydrocortisone 25–50 mg (usually the sodium succinate) intravenously at induction; the usual oral corticosteroid dose is recommenced after surgery

- *Moderate or major surgery*—usual oral corticosteroid dose on the morning of surgery and hydrocortisone 25–50 mg intravenously at induction, followed by hydrocortisone 25–50 mg 3 times a day by intravenous injection for 24 hours after moderate surgery or for 48–72 hours after major surgery; the usual pre-operative oral corticosteroid dose is recommenced on stopping hydrocortisone injections

Patients on long-term corticosteroid treatment should carry a Steroid Treatment Card (see p. 346) which gives guidance on minimising risk and provides details of prescriber, drug, dosage and duration of treatment.

Infections

Prolonged courses of corticosteroids increase susceptibility to infections and severity of infections; clinical presentation of infections may also be atypical. Serious infections e.g. *septicaemia* and *tuberculosis* may reach an advanced stage before being recognised, and *amoebiasis* or *strongyloidiasis* may be activated or exacerbated (exclude before initiating a corticosteroid in those at risk or with suggestive symptoms). Fungal or viral *ocular infections* may also be exacerbated (see also section 11.4.1).

CHICKENPOX. Unless they have had chickenpox, patients receiving oral or parenteral corticosteroids for purposes other than replacement should be regarded as being *at risk of severe chickenpox* (see Steroid Treatment Card). Manifestations of fulminant illness include pneumonia, hepatitis and disseminated intravascular coagulation; rash is not necessarily a prominent feature.

Passive immunisation with varicella–zoster immunoglobulin (section 14.5) is needed for exposed non-immune patients receiving systemic corticosteroids or for those who have used them within the previous 3 months; varicella–zoster immunoglobulin should preferably be given within 3 days of exposure and no later than 10 days. Confirmed chickenpox warrants specialist care and urgent treatment (section 5.3). Corticosteroids should not be stopped and dosage may need to be increased.

Topical, inhaled or rectal corticosteroids are less likely to be associated with an increased risk of severe chickenpox.

MEASLES. Patients taking corticosteroids should be advised to take particular care to avoid exposure to measles and to seek immediate medical advice if exposure occurs. Prophylaxis with intramuscular normal immunoglobulin (section 14.5) may be needed.

Following concern about severe chickenpox associated with systemic corticosteroids, the CSM has issued a notice that **every** patient prescribed a *systemic* corticosteroid should receive the patient information leaflet supplied by the manufacturer.

Steroid treatment cards (see below) should also be issued where appropriate. Doctors and pharmacists can obtain supplies of the card from:

England and Wales
Department of Health
PO Box 777
London, SEI 6XH
Tel: (08701) 555 455

Scotland
Banner Business Supplies
20 South Gyle Crescent
Edinburgh, EHI2 9EB
Tel: (01506) 448 440
Fax: (01256) 448 400

For other references to the adverse effects of corticosteroids see section 11.4 (eye) and section 13.4 (skin).

Use of corticosteroids

Dosage of corticosteroids varies widely in different diseases and in different patients. If the use of a corticosteroid can save or prolong life, as in exfoliative dermatitis, pemphigus, acute leukaemia or acute transplant rejection, high doses may need to be given, because the complications of therapy are likely to be less serious than the effects of the disease itself.

When long-term corticosteroid therapy is used in some chronic diseases, the adverse effects of treatment may become greater than the disabilities caused by the disease. To minimise side-effects the maintenance dose should be kept as low as possible.

When potentially less harmful measures are ineffective corticosteroids are used topically for the treatment of inflammatory conditions of the skin (section 13.4). Corticosteroids should be avoided or used only under specialist supervision in psoriasis (section 13.5).

Corticosteroids are used both topically (by rectum) and systemically (by mouth or intravenously) in the management of ulcerative colitis and Crohn's disease (section 1.5 and section 1.7.2).

Use can be made of the mineralocorticoid activity of fludrocortisone to treat postural hypotension in autonomic neuropathy (section 6.1.5).

Although very high doses of corticosteroids have been given by intravenous injection in septic shock, a study of high-dose methylprednisolone sodium succinate did not demonstrate efficacy and, moreover, suggested a higher mortality in some subsets of patients given the high-dose corticosteroid therapy. However, there is evidence that administration of

STEROID TREATMENT CARD

I am a patient on STEROID treatment which must not be stopped suddenly

- If you have been taking this medicine for more than three weeks, the dose should be reduced gradually when you stop taking steroids unless your doctor says otherwise.

- Read the patient information leaflet given with the medicine.

- Always carry this card with you and show it to anyone who treats you (for example a doctor, nurse, pharmacist or dentist). For one year after you stop the treatment, you must mention that you have taken steroids.

- If you become ill, or if you come into contact with anyone who has an infectious disease, consult your doctor promptly. If you have never had chickenpox, you should avoid close contact with people who have chickenpox or shingles. If you do come into contact with chickenpox, see your doctor urgently.

- Make sure that the information on the card is kept up to date.

lower doses of hydrocortisone (50 mg intravenously every 6 hours) and fludrocortisone (50 micrograms daily by mouth) is of benefit in patients who have adrenocortical insufficiency as a consequence of septic shock.

Dexamethasone and betamethasone have little if any mineralocorticoid action and their long duration of action makes them particularly suitable for suppressing corticotropin secretion in congenital adrenal hyperplasia where the dose should be tailored to clinical response and by measurement of adrenal androgens and 17-hydroxyprogesterone. In common with all glucocorticoids their suppressive action on the hypothalamic-pituitary-adrenal axis is greatest and most prolonged when they are given at night. In most normal subjects a single dose of 1 mg of dexamethasone at night, depending on weight, is sufficient to inhibit corticotropin secretion for 24 hours. This is the basis of the 'overnight dexamethasone suppression test' for diagnosing Cushing's syndrome.

Betamethasone and dexamethasone are also appropriate for conditions where water retention would be a disadvantage, as for example in treating traumatic cerebral oedema with doses of 12 to 20 mg daily.

In acute hypersensitivity reactions such as angioedema of the upper respiratory tract and anaphylactic shock, corticosteroids are indicated as an adjunct to emergency treatment with adrenaline (epinephrine) (section 3.4.3). In such cases hydrocortisone (as sodium succinate) by intravenous injection in a dose of 100 to 300 mg may be required.

Corticosteroids are preferably used by inhalation in the management of asthma (section 3.2) but systemic therapy in association with bronchodilators is required for the emergency treatment of severe acute asthma (section 3.1.1).

Corticosteroids may also be useful in conditions such as chronic active hepatitis, and sarcoidosis; they may also lead to remissions of acquired haemolytic anaemia (section 9.1.3), and some cases of the nephrotic syndrome (particularly in children) and thrombocytopenic purpura (section 9.1.4).

Corticosteroids can improve the prognosis of serious conditions such as systemic lupus erythematosus, temporal arteritis, and polyarteritis nodosa; the effects of the disease process may be suppressed and symptoms relieved, but the underlying condition is not cured, although it may ultimately remit. It is usual to begin therapy in these conditions at fairly high dose, such as 40 to 60 mg prednisolone daily, and then to reduce the dose to the lowest commensurate with disease control.

For other references to the use of corticosteroids see Prescribing in Palliative Care, section 8.2.2 (immunosuppresion), section 10.1.2 (rheumatic diseases), section 11.4 (eye), section 12.1.1 (otitis externa), section 12.2.1 (allergic rhinitis), and section 12.3.1 (aphthous ulcers).

Pregnancy and breast-feeding
Following a review of the data on the safety of systemic corticosteroids used in pregnancy and breast-feeding the CSM has concluded:

- corticosteroids vary in their ability to cross the placenta; betamethasone and dexamethasone cross the placenta readily while 88% of prednisolone is inactivated as it crosses the placenta;

- there is no convincing evidence that systemic corticosteroids increase the incidence of congenital abnormalities such as cleft palate or lip;
- when administration is prolonged or repeated during pregnancy, systemic corticosteroids increase the risk of intra-uterine growth retardation; there is no evidence of intra-uterine growth retardation following short-term treatment (e.g. prophylactic treatment for neonatal respiratory distress syndrome);
- any adrenal suppression in the neonate following prenatal exposure usually resolves spontaneously after birth and is rarely clinically important;
- prednisolone appears in small amounts in breast milk but doses of up to 40 mg daily are unlikely to cause systemic effects in the infant; infants should be monitored for adrenal suppression if the mothers are taking a higher dose.

See also Appendix 4.

Administration
Whenever possible *local treatment* with creams, intra-articular injections, inhalations, eye-drops, or enemas should be used in preference to *systemic treatment*. The suppressive action of a corticosteroid on cortisol secretion is least when it is given as a single dose in the morning. In an attempt to reduce pituitary-adrenal suppression further, the total dose for two days can sometimes be taken as a single dose on alternate days; alternate-day administration has not been very successful in the management of asthma (section 3.2). Pituitary-adrenal suppression can also be reduced by means of intermittent therapy with short courses. In some conditions it may be possible to reduce the dose of corticosteroid by adding a small dose of an immunosuppressive drug (section 8.2.1).

Withdrawal of corticosteroids
The CSM has recommended that *gradual* withdrawal of systemic corticosteroids should be considered in those whose disease is unlikely to relapse and have

- recently received repeated courses (particularly if taken for longer than 3 weeks)
- taken a short course within 1 year of stopping long-term therapy
- other possible causes of adrenal suppression
- received more than 40 mg daily prednisolone (or equivalent)
- been given repeat doses in the evening
- received more than 3 weeks' treatment

Systemic corticosteroids may be stopped abruptly in those whose disease is unlikely to relapse *and* who have received treatment for 3 weeks or less *and* who are not included in the patient groups described above.

During corticosteroid withdrawal the dose may be reduced rapidly down to physiological doses (equivalent to prednisolone 7.5 mg daily) and then reduced more slowly. Assessment of the disease may be needed during withdrawal to ensure that relapse does not occur.

PREDNISOLONE
Indications: suppression of inflammatory and allergic disorders; see also notes above; inflammatory bowel disease, section 1.5; asthma, section 3.2; immunosuppression, section 8.2.2; rheumatic disease, section 10.1.2

Cautions: adrenal suppression and infection (see notes above), children and adolescents (growth retardation possibly irreversible), elderly (close supervision required particularly on long-term treatment); frequent monitoring required if history of tuberculosis (or X-ray changes), hypertension, recent myocardial infarction (rupture reported), congestive heart failure, liver failure, renal impairment, diabetes mellitus including family history, osteoporosis (post-menopausal women at special risk), glaucoma (including family history), corneal perforation, severe affective disorders (particularly if history of steroid-induced psychosis), epilepsy, peptic ulcer, hypothyroidism, history of steroid myopathy; pregnancy and breast-feeding (see notes above); **interactions:** Appendix 1 (corticosteroids)

Contra-indications: systemic infection (unless specific antimicrobial therapy given); avoid live virus vaccines in those receiving immunosuppressive doses (serum antibody response diminished)

Side-effects: minimised by using lowest effective dose for minimum period possible; *gastro-intestinal effects* include dyspepsia, peptic ulceration (with perforation), abdominal distension, acute pancreatitis, oesophageal ulceration and candidiasis; *musculoskeletal effects* include proximal myopathy, osteoporosis, vertebral and long bone fractures, avascular osteonecrosis, tendon rupture; *endocrine effects* include adrenal suppression, menstrual irregularities and amenorrhoea, Cushing's syndrome (with high doses, usually reversible on withdrawal), hirsutism, weight gain, negative nitrogen and calcium balance, increased appetite; increased susceptibility to and severity of infection; *neuropsychiatric effects* include euphoria, psychological dependence, depression, insomnia, increased intracranial pressure with papilloedema in children (usually after withdrawal), psychosis and aggravation of schizophrenia, aggravation of epilepsy; *ophthalmic effects* include glaucoma, papilloedema, posterior subcapsular cataracts, corneal or scleral thinning and exacerbation of ophthalmic viral or fungal disease; *other side-effects* include impaired healing, skin atrophy, bruising, striae, telangiectasia, acne, myocardial rupture following recent myocardial infarction, fluid and electrolyte disturbance, leucocytosis, hypersensitivity reactions (including anaphylaxis), thromboembolism, nausea, malaise, hiccups

Dose: *by mouth,* initially, up to 10–20 mg daily (severe disease, up to 60 mg daily), preferably taken in the morning after breakfast; can often be reduced within a few days but may need to be continued for several weeks or months

Maintenance, usual range, 2.5–15 mg daily, but higher doses may be needed; cushingoid side-effects increasingly likely with doses above 7.5 mg daily

By intramuscular injection, prednisolone acetate (section 10.1.2.2), 25–100 mg once or twice weekly

Prednisolone (Non-proprietary) PoM
Tablets, prednisolone 1 mg, net price 28-tab pack = 53p; 5 mg, 28-tab pack = 68p; 25 mg, 56-tab pack = £9.30. Label: 10, steroid card, 21
Available from Alpharma, APS, Arrow, Beacon, CP, Hillcross, IVAX

Tablets, both e/c, prednisolone 2.5 mg (brown), net price 30-tab pack = 31p; 5 mg (red), 30-tab pack = 51p. Label: 5, 10, steroid card, 25
Available from Alpharma, APS Berk, IVAX (2.5 mg), Pfizer (*Deltacortril Enteric*®)

Soluble tablets, prednisolone 5 mg (as sodium phosphate), net price 30-tab pack = £2.20.
Label: 10, steroid card, 13, 21
Available from Sovereign

Injection, see section 10.1.2.2

BETAMETHASONE

Indications: suppression of inflammatory and allergic disorders; congenital adrenal hyperplasia; cerebral oedema; see also notes above; ear (section 12.1.1); eye (section 11.4.1); nose (section 12.2.1)

Cautions: see notes above and under Prednisolone

Contra-indications: see notes above and under Prednisolone

Side-effects: see notes above and under Prednisolone

Dose: *by mouth,* usual range 0.5–5 mg daily; see also Administration (above)

By intramuscular injection or slow intravenous injection or infusion, 4–20 mg, repeated up to 4 times in 24 hours; CHILD, *by slow intravenous injection,* up to 1 year 1 mg, 1–5 years 2 mg, 6–12 years 4 mg

Betnelan® (Celltech) PoM
Tablets, scored, betamethasone 500 micrograms. Net price 100-tab pack = £3.63. Label: 10, steroid card, 21

Betnesol® (Celltech) PoM
Soluble tablets, pink, scored, betamethasone 500 micrograms (as sodium phosphate). Net price 100-tab pack = £4.10. Label: 10, steroid card, 13, 21
Injection, betamethasone 4 mg (as sodium phosphate)/mL. Net price 1-mL amp = 97p. Label: 10, steroid card

CORTISONE ACETATE

Indications: see under Dose but now superseded, see also notes above

Cautions: see notes above and under Prednisolone

Contra-indications: see notes above and under Prednisolone

Side-effects: see notes above and under Prednisolone

Dose: for replacement therapy, 25–37.5 mg daily in divided doses

Cortisone acetate (Non-proprietary) PoM
Tablets, cortisone acetate 25 mg, net price 56-tab pack = £10.30. Label: 10, steroid card, 21
Available from Beacon

DEFLAZACORT

Indications: suppression of inflammatory and allergic disorders

Cautions: see notes above and under Prednisolone

Contra-indications: see notes above and under Prednisolone

Side-effects: see notes above and under Prednisolone

Dose: usual maintenance 3–18 mg daily (acute disorders, initially up to 120 mg daily); see also Administration (above)
CHILD 0.25–1.5 mg/kg daily (or on alternate days); see also Administration (above)

Calcort® (Shire) PoM

Tablets, deflazacort 1 mg, net price 100-tab pack = £8.00; 6 mg, 60-tab pack = £16.46; 30 mg, 30-tab pack = £22.80. Label: 5, 10, steroid card

DEXAMETHASONE

Indications: suppression of inflammatory and allergic disorders; diagnosis of Cushing's disease, congenital adrenal hyperplasia; cerebral oedema; nausea and vomiting with chemotherapy (section 8.1); rheumatic disease (section 10.1.2); eye (section 11.4.1); see also notes above

Cautions: see notes above and under Prednisolone

Contra-indications: see notes above and under Prednisolone

Side-effects: see notes above and under Prednisolone; perineal irritation may follow intravenous administration of the phosphate ester

Dose: *by mouth*, usual range 0.5–10 mg daily; CHILD 10–100 micrograms/kg daily; see also Administration (above)

By intramuscular injection or slow intravenous injection or infusion (as dexamethasone phosphate), initially 0.5–24 mg; CHILD 200–400 micrograms/kg daily

Cerebral oedema (as dexamethasone phosphate), *by intravenous injection*, 10 mg initially, then 4 mg *by intramuscular injection* every 6 hours as required for 2–4 days then gradually reduced and stopped over 5–7 days

NOTE. Dexamethasone 1 mg ≡ dexamethasone phosphate 1.2 mg ≡ dexamethasone sodium phosphate 1.3 mg

Dexamethasone (Non-proprietary) PoM

Tablets, dexamethasone 500 micrograms, net price 20 = 64p; 2 mg, 20 = £2.20. Label: 10, steroid card, 21
Available from Organon

Oral solution, sugar-free, dexamethasone (as dexamethasone sodium phosphate) 2 mg/5 mL, net price 150-mL = £45.00
Available from Rosemont (*Dexsol®*)

Injection, dexamethasone phosphate (as dexamethasone sodium phosphate) 4 mg/mL, net price 1-mL amp = £1.00, 2-mL vial = £1.98; 24 mg/mL, 5-mL vial = £16.66. Label: 10, steroid card
Available from Mayne

Injection, dexamethasone sodium phosphate 5 mg/mL, net price 1-mL amp = £1.00, 2-mL vial = £1.98. Label: 10, steroid card
Available from Organon

Decadron® (MSD) PoM

Tablets, scored, dexamethasone 500 micrograms, net price 30-tab pack = 96p. Label: 10, steroid card, 21

HYDROCORTISONE

Indications: adrenocortical insufficiency (section 6.3.1); shock; see also notes above; hypersensitivity reactions e.g. anaphylactic shock and angioedema (section 3.4.3); inflammatory bowel disease (section 1.5); haemorrhoids (section 1.7.2); rheumatic disease (section 10.1.2); eye (section 11.4.1); skin (section 13.4)

Cautions: see notes above and under Prednisolone

Contra-indications: see notes above and under Prednisolone

Side-effects: see notes above and under Prednisolone; phosphate ester associated with paraesthesia and pain (particularly in the perineal region)

Dose: *by mouth*, replacement therapy, 20–30 mg daily in divided doses—see section 6.3.1; CHILD 10–30 mg

By intramuscular injection or slow intravenous injection or infusion, 100–500 mg, 3–4 times in 24 hours or as required; CHILD *by slow intravenous injection* up to 1 year 25 mg, 1–5 years 50 mg, 6–12 years 100 mg

Efcortesol® (Sovereign) PoM ◼

Injection, hydrocortisone 100 mg (as sodium phosphate)/mL, net price 1-mL amp = 75p, 5-mL amp = £3.40. Label: 10, steroid card

NOTE. Paraesthesia and pain (particularly in the perineal region) may follow intravenous injection of the phosphate ester

Hydrocortone® (MSD) PoM

Tablets, hydrocortisone 10 mg, net price 30-tab pack = 70p; 20 mg, 30-tab pack = £1.07. Label: 10, steroid card, 21

Solu-Cortef® (Pharmacia) PoM

Injection, powder for reconstitution, hydrocortisone (as sodium succinate). Net price 100-mg vial = 92p, 100-mg vial with 2-mL amp water for injections = £1.16. Label: 10, steroid card

METHYLPREDNISOLONE

Indications: suppression of inflammatory and allergic disorders; cerebral oedema; see also notes above; rheumatic disease (section 10.1.2); skin (section 13.4)

Cautions: see notes above and under Prednisolone; rapid intravenous administration of large doses associated with cardiovascular collapse

Contra-indications: see notes above and under Prednisolone

Side-effects: see notes above and under Prednisolone

Dose: *by mouth*, usual range 2–40 mg daily; see also Administration (above)

By intramuscular injection or slow intravenous injection or infusion, initially 10–500 mg; graft rejection, up to 1 g daily *by intravenous infusion* for up to 3 days

Medrone® (Pharmacia) PoM

Tablets, scored, methylprednisolone 2 mg (pink), net price 30-tab pack = £3.23; 4 mg, 30-tab pack = £6.19; 16 mg, 30-tab pack = £17.17; 100 mg (blue), 20-tab pack = £48.32. Label: 10, steroid card, 21

Solu-Medrone® (Pharmacia) PoM

Injection, powder for reconstitution, methylprednisolone (as sodium succinate) (all with solvent). Net price 40-mg vial = £1.58; 125-mg vial = £4.75; 500-mg vial = £9.60; 1-g vial = £17.30; 2-g vial = £32.86. Label: 10, steroid card

■ Intramuscular depot

Depo-Medrone® (Pharmacia) PoM

Injection (aqueous suspension), methylprednisolone acetate 40 mg/mL. Net price 1-mL vial = £2.87; 2-mL vial = £5.15; 3-mL vial = £7.47. Label: 10, steroid card

Dose: by deep intramuscular injection into gluteal muscle, 40–120 mg, a second injection may be given after 2–3 weeks if required

TRIAMCINOLONE

Indications: suppression of inflammatory and allergic disorders; see also notes above; rheumatic disease, section 10.1.2; mouth, section 12.3.1; skin, section 13.4

Cautions: see notes above and under Prednisolone; high dosage may cause proximal myopathy, avoid in chronic therapy

Contra-indications: see notes above and under Prednisolone

Side-effects: see notes above and under Prednisolone

Dose: *by deep intramuscular injection*, into gluteal muscle, 40 mg of acetonide for depot effect, repeated at intervals according to the patient's response; max. single dose 100 mg

Kenalog® Intra-articular/Intramuscular (Squibb) PoM

Injection (aqueous suspension), triamcinolone acetonide 40 mg/mL, net price 1-mL vial = £1.70; 1-mL prefilled syringe = £2.11; 2-mL prefilled syringe = £3.66. Label: 10, steroid card

NOTE. Intramuscular needle with prefilled syringe should be replaced for intra-articular injection

6.4   Sex hormones

6.4.1	Female sex hormones
6.4.2	Male sex hormones and antagonists
6.4.3	Anabolic steroids

6.4.1   Female sex hormones

6.4.1.1	Oestrogens and HRT
6.4.1.2	Progestogens

6.4.1.1   Oestrogens and HRT

Oestrogens are necessary for the development of female secondary sexual characteristics; they also stimulate myometrial hypertrophy with endometrial hyperplasia.

In terms of oestrogenic activity *natural oestrogens* (estradiol (oestradiol), estrone (oestrone), and estriol (oestriol)) have a more appropriate profile for hormone replacement therapy (HRT) than *synthetic oestrogens* (ethinylestradiol (ethinyloestradiol) and mestranol). Tibolone has oestrogenic, progestogenic and weak androgenic activity.

Oestrogen therapy is given cyclically or continuously for a number of gynaecological conditions. If long-term therapy is required a progestogen should normally be added to reduce the risk of cystic hyperplasia of the endometrium (or of endometriotic foci in women who have had a hysterectomy) and possible transformation to cancer.

Oestrogens are no longer used to *suppress lactation* because of their association with thromboembolism.

Hormone replacement therapy

Hormone replacement therapy (HRT) with small doses of an oestrogen (together with a progestogen in women with an intact uterus) is appropriate for alleviating menopausal symptoms such as *vaginal atrophy* or *vasomotor instability*. Small doses of oestrogen given systemically in the perimenopausal and postmenopausal period also diminish postme-

nopausal *osteoporosis* (section 6.6.1) but other drugs (section 6.6) are preferred. Menopausal atrophic vaginitis may respond to a short course of topical vaginal oestrogen preparation (section 7.2.1) given for a few weeks and repeated if necessary.

Systemic therapy with an oestrogen alleviates the symptoms of oestrogen deficiency such as *vasomotor symptoms*. However, HRT increases the risk of *venous thromboembolism,* of *stroke* and, after some years of use, HRT increases the risk of *endometrial cancer* (reduced by a progestogen) and of *breast cancer* (see below). The CSM advises that the minium effective dose should be used for the shortest duration. Treatment should be reviewed at least annually and for osteoporosis alternative treatments considered (section 6.6). HRT does not reduce the incidence of coronary heart disease and it should **not** be prescribed for this purpose.

Clonidine (section 4.7.4.2) may be used to reduce vasomotor symptoms in women who cannot take an oestrogen, but clonidine may cause unacceptable side-effects.

HRT may be used in women with *early natural or surgical menopause (before age 45 years)*, since they are at high risk of osteoporosis. For early menopause, HRT can be given until the approximate age of natural menopause (i.e. until age 50 years). Alternatives to HRT should be considered if osteoporosis is the main concern (section 6.6).

In women with an intact uterus, the addition of a progestogen reduces the risk of endometrial cancer but this should be weighed against the increased risk of breast cancer.

In healthy women without symptoms, the risk of using HRT outweighs the potential benefit of preventing osteoporosis.

RISK OF BREAST CANCER. The CSM has estimated that using *all* types of HRT, including tibolone, increases the risk of breast cancer within 1–2 years of initiating treatment. The increased risk is related to the duration of HRT use (but not to the age at which HRT is started) and this excess risk disappears within about 5 years of stopping.

About 32 in every 1000 women aged 50–65 years not using HRT have breast cancer diagnosed over 15 or 20 years. In those using *oestrogen-only HRT* for 5 years, breast cancer is diagnosed in about 1.5 extra cases in 1000 and about 5 extra cases in 1000 after 10 years use. In those using oestrogen and progestogen *combined HRT* for 5 years, breast cancer is diagnosed in 6 extra cases in 1000 and 19 extra cases in 1000 after 10 years use. Tibolone increases the risk of breast cancer but to a lesser extent than with *combined HRT.*

RISK OF VENOUS THROMBOEMBOLISM. Women on combned or oestrogen-only HRT are at an increased risk of deep vein thrombosis and of pulmonary embolism especially in the first year.

The CSM has estimated that about 3 in every 1000 *women aged 50–60 years* not using HRT develop venous thromboembolism over 5 years; this figure rises by about 4 extra cases in 1000 in those using oestrogen HRT for 5 years. About 8 in every 1000 *women aged 60–70 years* not using HRT develop venous thromboembolism over 5 years; this figure rises by about 9 extra cases in 1000 in those using oestrogen HRT for 5 years. It is not known if tibolone increases the risk of venous thromboembolism.

In *women who have predisposing factors* (such as a personal or family history of deep vein thrombosis or pulmonary embolism, severe varicose veins, obesity, trauma, or prolonged bed-rest) it may be prudent to review the need for HRT as in some cases the risks of HRT may exceed the benefits. See below for advice on surgery.

Travel may increase the risk of deep vein thrombosis, see under Travel in section 7.3.1.

OTHER RISKS. Combined oestrogen-progestogen or oestrogen-only HRT slightly increases the risk of *stroke*. The CSM has estimated that about 3 in every 1000 *women aged 50–60 years* not using HRT have a stroke over 5 years; this figure rises by about 1 extra case in 1000 in those using HRT for 5 years. About 11 in every *1000 women aged 60–70 years* not using HRT have a stroke over 5 years; this figure rises by about 4 extra cases in 1000 in those using HRT for 5 years.

HRT does not prevent *coronary heart disease* and should not be prescribed for this purpose. HRT possibly increases the risk of coronary heart disease in the first year.

The CSM has estimated that about 5 in every 1000 women aged 50–64 years not using HRT have *endometrial cancer* diagnosed over 15 or 20 years; in those using *oestrogen-only HRT* for 5 years endometrial cancer is diagnosed in about 4 extra cases in 1000 and about 10 extra cases in 1000 after 10 years use. In those using oestrogen and progestogen *combined HRT* for 10 years endometrial cancer is diagnosed in about 2 extra cases in 1000. The risk of endometrial cancer may be different for sequential and continuous combined HRT. The risk of endometrial cancer with tibolone is not known.

The CSM has estimated that about 9 in every 1000 women aged 50–69 years not using HRT have *ovarian cancer* diagnosed over 15 or 20 years; this figure rises by about 1 extra case in 1000 in those using *oestrogen-only HRT* for 5 years and by about 3 extra cases in 1000 in those using *oestrogen-only HRT* for 10 years; the risks in women using combined HRT are unclear.

CHOICE. The choice of HRT for an individual depends on an overall balance of indication, risk, and convenience. A woman with an intact uterus normally requires oestrogen with cyclical progestogen for the last 12 to 14 days of the cycle *or* a preparation which involves continuous administration of an oestrogen and a progestogen (*or* one which provides both oestrogenic and progestogenic activity in a single preparation). Continuous combined preparations or tibolone are **not suitable** for use in the *perimenopause* or within 12 months of the last menstrual period; women who use such preparations may bleed irregularly in the early stages of treatment—if bleeding continues endometrial abnormality should be ruled out and consideration given to changing to cyclical HRT.

An oestrogen alone is suitable for continuous use in women without a uterus. However, in endometriosis, endometrial foci may remain despite hysterectomy and the addition of a progestogen should be considered in these circumstances.

An oestrogen may be given by mouth or it may be given by subcutaneous or transdermal administration, which avoids first-pass metabolism. In the case of subcutaneous implants, recurrence of vasomotor symptoms at supraphysiological plasma concentrations may occur; moreover, there is evidence of prolonged endometrial stimulation after discontinuation (calling for continued cyclical progestogen). For the use of topical HRT preparations see section 7.2.1.

CONTRACEPTION. HRT does **not** provide contraception and a woman is considered potentially fertile for *2 years after her last menstrual period* if she is *under 50 years*, and for *1 year* if she is *over 50 years*. A woman who is under 50 years and free of all risk factors for venous and arterial disease can use a low-oestrogen combined oral contraceptive pill (section 7.3.1) to provide both *relief of menopausal symptoms* and *contraception*; it is recommended that the oral contraceptive be stopped at 50 years of age since there are more suitable alternatives. If any potentially fertile woman needs HRT, *non-hormonal contraceptive measures* (such as condoms, or by this age, contraceptive foam, section 7.3.3) are necessary.

Measurement of follicle-stimulating hormone can help to determine fertility, but high measurements alone (particularly in women aged under 50 years) do not necessarily preclude the possibility of becoming pregnant.

SURGERY. Major surgery under general anaesthesia, including orthopaedic and vascular leg surgery, is a predisposing factor for venous thromboembolism and it may be prudent to stop HRT 4–6 weeks before surgery (see Risk of Venous Thromboembolism, above); it should be restarted only after full mobilisation. If HRT is continued or if discontinuation is not possible (e.g. in non-elective surgery), prophylaxis with heparin and graduated compression hosiery is advised. Oestrogenic activity may persist after removing an estradiol implant (see above).

REASONS TO STOP HRT. For circumstances in which HRT should be stopped, see p. 389.

OESTROGENS FOR HRT

NOTE. Relates only to small amounts of oestrogens given for hormone replacement therapy

Indications: see notes above and under preparations

Cautions: prolonged exposure to unopposed oestrogens may increase risk of developing endometrial cancer (see notes above); migraine (or migraine-like headaches); diabetes (increased risk of heart disease); history of breast nodules or fibrocystic disease—closely monitor breast status (risk of breast cancer, see notes above); risk factors for oestrogen-dependent tumours (e.g. breast cancer in first-degree relative); uterine fibroids may increase in size, symptoms of endometriosis may be exacerbated; factors predisposing to thromboembolism (see notes above); presence of antiphospholipid antibodies (increased risk of thrombotic events); increased risk of gall-bladder disease reported; hypophyseal tumours; porphyria (see section 9.8.2); **interactions:** Appendix 1 (oestrogens)

OTHER CONDITIONS. The product literature advises caution in other conditions including hypertension, renal disease, asthma, epilepsy, sickle-cell disease, melanoma, otosclerosis, multiple sclerosis, and systemic lupus erythematosus (but care required if antiphospholipid antibodies present, see above). Evidence for caution in these conditions is unsatisfactory and many women with these conditions may stand to benefit from HRT.

Contra-indications: pregnancy; oestrogen-dependent cancer, history of breast cancer, active thrombophlebitis, active or recent arterial thromboembolic disease (e.g. angina or myocardial infarction), venous thromboembolism, or history of recurrent venous thromboembolism (unless already on anticoagulant treatment), liver disease (where liver function tests have failed to return to normal), Dubin-Johnson and Rotor syndromes (or monitor closely), untreated endometrial hyperplasia, undiagnosed vaginal bleeding, breast-feeding

Side-effects: see notes above for risks of long-term use; nausea and vomiting, abdominal cramps and bloating, weight changes, breast enlargement and tenderness, premenstrual-like syndrome, sodium and fluid retention, cholestatic jaundice, glucose intolerance, altered blood lipids–may lead to pancreatitis, rashes and chloasma, changes in libido, depression, mood changes, headache, migraine, dizziness, leg cramps (rule out venous thrombosis), vaginal candidiasis, contact lenses may irritate; transdermal delivery systems may cause contact sensitisation (possible severe hypersensitivity reaction on continued exposure), and headache has been reported on vigorous exercise; nasal spray may cause local irritation, rhinorrhoea and epistaxis

WITHDRAWAL BLEEDING. Cyclical HRT (where a progestogen is taken for 12–14 days of each 28-day oestrogen treatment cycle) usually results in *regular withdrawal bleeding* towards the end of the progestogen. The aim of continuous combined HRT (where a combination of oestrogen and progestogen is taken, usually in a single tablet, throughout each 28-day treatment cycle) is to avoid bleeding, but *irregular bleeding* may occur during the early treatment stages (if it continues endometrial abnormality should be excluded and consideration given to cyclical HRT instead)

Dose: see under preparations

COUNSELLING ON PATCHES. Patch should be removed after 3–4 days (or once a week in case of 7-day patch) and replaced with fresh patch on slightly different site; recommended sites: clean, dry, unbroken areas of skin on trunk below waistline; not to be applied on or near breasts or under waistband. If patch falls off in bath allow skin to cool before applying new patch

■ Conjugated oestrogens with progestogen

Premique® (Wyeth) PoM
Premique® tablets, s/c, blue, conjugated oestrogen (equine) 625 micrograms and medroxyprogesterone acetate 5 mg. Net price 3 × 28-tab pack = £27.14
Dose: menopausal symptoms and osteoporosis prophylaxis, in women with intact uterus, 1 tablet daily continuously (starting on day 1 of menstruation if cycles have not ceased)
Premique® Cycle Calendar pack, all s/c, 14 white tablets, conjugated oestrogens (equine) 625 micrograms; 14 green tablets, conjugated oestrogens (equine) 625 micrograms and medroxyprogesterone acetate 10 mg, net price 3 × 28-tab pack = £24.87
Dose: menopausal symptoms and osteoporosis prophylaxis, 1 white tablet daily for 14 days, starting on day 1 of menstruation (or at any time if cycles have ceased or are infrequent) then 1 green tablet daily for 14 days; subsequent courses are repeated without interval

Prempak-C® (Wyeth) PoM
Prempak C® 0.625 Calendar pack, s/c, 28 maroon tablets, conjugated oestrogens (equine) 625 micrograms; 12 light brown tablets, norgestrel 150 micrograms (≡ levonorgestrel 75 micrograms). Net price 3 × 40-tab pack = £17.67
Dose: menopausal symptoms and osteoporosis prophylaxis, in women with intact uterus, 1 maroon tablet daily continuously, starting on day 1 of menstruation (or at any time if cycles have ceased or are infrequent), and 1 brown tablet daily on days 17–28 of each 28-day treatment cycle; subsequent courses are repeated without interval
Prempak C® 1.25 Calendar pack, s/c, 28 yellow tablets, conjugated oestrogens (equine) 1.25 mg; 12 light brown tablets, norgestrel 150 micrograms (≡ levonorgestrel 75 micrograms). Net price 3 × 40-tab pack = £17.67
Dose: see under 0.625 Calendar pack, but taking 1 yellow tablet daily continuously (instead of 1 maroon tablet) if symptoms not fully controlled with lower strength

■ Estradiol with progestogen

Climagest® (Novartis) PoM
Climagest® 1-mg tablets, 16 grey-blue, estradiol valerate 1 mg; 12 white, estradiol valerate 1 mg and norethisterone 1 mg. Net price 28-tab pack = £4.78; 3 × 28-tab pack = £13.92
Dose: menopausal symptoms, 1 grey-blue tablet daily for 16 days, starting on day 1 of menstruation (or at any time if cycles have ceased or are infrequent) then 1 white tablet for 12 days; subsequent courses are repeated without interval
Climagest® 2-mg tablets, 16 blue, estradiol valerate 2 mg; 12 yellow, estradiol valerate 2 mg and norethisterone 1 mg. Net price 28-tab pack = £4.78; 3 × 28-tab pack = £13.92
Dose: see *Climagest® 1-mg*, but starting with 1 blue tablet daily (instead of 1 grey-blue tablet) if symptoms not controlled with lower strength

Climesse® (Novartis) PoM
Tablets, pink, estradiol valerate 2 mg, norethisterone 700 micrograms. Net price 1 × 28-tab pack = £8.62; 3 × 28-tab pack = £25.86
Dose: menopausal symptoms and osteoporosis prophylaxis, in women with intact uterus, 1 tablet daily continuously
NOTE. Unsuitable for use in perimenopausal women or within 12 months of last menstrual period—see Choice above

Cyclo-Progynova® (Viatris) PoM
Cyclo-Progynova® 1-mg tablets, all s/c, 11 beige, estradiol valerate 1 mg; 10 brown, estradiol valerate 1 mg and levonorgestrel 250 micrograms. Net price per pack = £3.34
Dose: menopausal symptoms, in women with intact uterus, 1 beige tablet daily for 11 days, starting on day 5 of menstruation (or at any time if cycles have ceased or are infrequent), then 1 brown tablet daily for 10 days, followed by a 7-day interval
Cyclo-Progynova® 2-mg tablets, all s/c, 11 white, estradiol valerate 2 mg; 10 brown, estradiol valerate 2 mg and norgestrel 500 micrograms (≡ levonorgestrel 250 micrograms). Net price per pack = £3.34
Dose: menopausal symptoms and osteoporosis prophylaxis as *Cyclo-Progynova® 1-mg*, but starting with 1 white tablet daily for 11 days, then 1 brown tablet daily for 10 days, followed by a 7-day interval

Elleste-Duet® (Pharmacia) PoM
Elleste-Duet® 1-mg tablets, 16 white, estradiol 1 mg; 12 green, estradiol 1 mg and norethisterone acetate 1 mg. Net price 3 × 28-tab pack = £9.72
Dose: menopausal symptoms, 1 white tablet daily for 16 days starting on day 1 of menstruation (or at any time if cycles have ceased or are infrequent), then 1 green tablet daily for 12 days; subsequent courses are repeated without interval

Elleste-Duet® 2-mg tablets, 16 orange, estradiol 2 mg; 12 grey, estradiol 2 mg, norethisterone acetate 1 mg. Net price 3 × 28-tab pack = £9.72

Dose: menopausal symptoms and osteoporosis prophylaxis, 1 orange tablet daily for 16 days, starting on day 1 of menstruation (or at any time if cycles have ceased or are infrequent) then 1 grey tablet daily for 12 days; subsequent courses are repeated without interval

Elleste-Duet Conti® tablets, f/c, grey, estradiol 2 mg, norethisterone acetate 1 mg. Net price 3 × 28-tab pack = £17.97

Dose: menopausal symptoms and osteoporosis prophylaxis, in women with intact uterus, 1 tablet daily on a continuous basis (if changing from cyclical HRT begin treatment at the end of scheduled bleed)

NOTE. Unsuitable for use in perimenopausal women or within 12 months of last menstrual period—see Choice above

Estracombi® (Novartis) PoM

Combination pack, self-adhesive patches of *Estraderm TTS®* 50 (releasing estradiol approx. 50 micrograms/24 hours) and of *Estragest TTS®* (releasing estradiol approx. 50 micrograms/24 hours and norethisterone acetate 250 micrograms/24 hours); net price 1-month pack (4 of each) = £11.14, 3-month pack (12 of each) = £33.42. Counselling, administration

Dose: menopausal symptoms and osteoporosis prophylaxis, in women with intact uterus, starting within 5 days of onset of menstruation (or any time if cycles have ceased or are infrequent), 1 *Estraderm TTS® 50* patch to be applied twice weekly for 2 weeks followed by 1 *Estragest TTS®* patch twice weekly for 2 weeks; subsequent courses are repeated without interval

Evorel® (Janssen-Cilag) PoM

Evorel® Conti patches, self-adhesive, (releasing estradiol approx. 50 micrograms/24 hours and norethisterone acetate approx. 170 micrograms/24 hours), net price 8-patch pack = £12.90, 24-patch pack = £38.70. Counselling, administration

Dose: menopausal symptoms and osteoporosis prophylaxis, in women with intact uterus, 1 patch to be applied twice weekly continuously

Evorel® Pak calendar pack, 8 self-adhesive patches (releasing estradiol approx. 50 micrograms/24 hours) and 12 tablets, norethisterone 1 mg, net price per pack = £8.45. Counselling, administration

Dose: menopausal symptoms and osteoporosis prophylaxis, in women with intact uterus, apply 1 patch twice weekly continuously (increased if necessary for menopausal symptoms to 2 patches twice weekly after first month) and take 1 tablet daily on days 15–26 of each 28-day treatment cycle

Evorel® Sequi combination pack, 4 self-adhesive patches of *Evorel® 50* (releasing estradiol approx. 50 micrograms/24 hours) and 4 self-adhesive patches of *Evorel® Conti* (releasing estradiol approx. 50 micrograms/24 hours and norethisterone acetate approx. 170 micrograms/24 hours), net price 8-patch pack = £11.00. Counselling, administration

Dose: menopausal symptoms and osteoporosis prophylaxis, in women with intact uterus, 1 *Evorel® 50* patch to be applied twice weekly for 2 weeks followed by 1 *Evorel® Conti* patch twice weekly for 2 weeks; subsequent courses are repeated without interval

Femapak® (Solvay) PoM

Femapak® 40 combination pack of 8 self-adhesive patches of *Fematrix® 40* (releasing estradiol approx. 40 micrograms/24 hours) and 14 tablets of *Duphaston®* (dydrogesterone 10 mg). Net price per pack = £8.45. Counselling, administration

Dose: see under *Femapak® 80*

Femapak® 80 combination pack of 8 self-adhesive patches of *Fematrix® 80* (releasing estradiol approx. 80 micrograms/24 hours) and 14 tablets of *Duphaston®* (dydrogesterone 10 mg). Net price per pack = £8.95. Counselling, administration

Dose: menopausal symptoms (and osteoporosis prophylaxis in case of *Femapak® 80* **only**), in women with intact uterus, starting within 5 days of onset of menstruation (or any time if cycles have ceased or are infrequent), apply 1 patch twice weekly continuously and take 1 tablet daily on days 15–28 of each 28-day treatment cycle; therapy should be initiated with *Femapak® 40* in those with menopausal symptoms, prolonged oestrogen deficiency or anticipated intolerance to higher strengths, subsequently adjusted to lowest effective dose

Femoston® (Solvay) PoM

Femoston® 1/10 tablets, both f/c, 14 white, estradiol 1 mg; 14 grey, estradiol 1 mg, dydrogesterone 10 mg. Net price 3 × 28-tab pack = £14.97

Dose: menopausal symptoms and osteoporosis prophylaxis, in women with intact uterus, 1 white tablet daily for 14 days, starting within 5 days of onset of menstruation (or any time if cycles have ceased or are infrequent) then 1 grey tablet for 14 days; subsequent courses repeated without interval

Femoston® 2/10 tablets, both f/c, 14 red, estradiol 2 mg; 14 yellow, estradiol 2 mg, dydrogesterone 10 mg. Net price 3 × 28-tab pack = £14.97

Dose: menopausal symptoms and osteoporosis prophylaxis, in women with intact uterus, 1 red tablet daily for 14 days, starting within 5 days of onset of menstruation (or any time if cycles have ceased or are infrequent) then 1 yellow tablet daily for 14 days; subsequent courses repeated without interval; where therapy required for menopausal symptoms alone, *Femston® 1/10* given initially and *Femston® 2/10* substituted if symptoms not controlled

Femoston® 2/20 tablets, both f/c, 14 red, estradiol 2 mg; 14 blue, estradiol 2 mg, dydrogesterone 20 mg. Net price 3 × 28-tab pack = £22.44

Dose: see *Femoston® 2/10*, but taking 1 blue tablet (instead of 1 yellow tablet) if withdrawal bleed is early or endometrial biopsy shows inadequate progestational response

Femoston®-conti tablets, f/c, salmon, estradiol 1 mg, dydrogesterone 5 mg, net price 3 × 28-tab pack = £22.62

Dose: menopausal symptoms and osteoporosis prophylaxis, in women with intact uterus, 1 tablet daily continuously (if changing from cyclical HRT begin treatment the day after finishing oestrogen plus progestogen phase)

NOTE. Unsuitable for use in perimenopausal women or within 12 months of last menstrual period—see Choice above

FemSeven® Conti (Merck) PoM

Patches, self-adhesive (releasing estradiol approx. 50 micrograms/24 hours and levonorgestrel approx. 7 micrograms/24 hours); net price 4-patch pack = £12.90, 12-patch pack = £ 36.77. Counselling, administration

Dose: menopausal symptoms in women with intact uterus, 1 patch to be applied once a week continuously

NOTE. Unsuitable for use in perimenopausal women or within 12 months of last menstrual period—see Choice above

FemSeven® Sequi (Merck) PoM

Combination pack, self-adhesive patches of *FemSeven® Sequi Phase 1* (releasing estradiol approx.

50 micrograms/24 hours) and of *FemSeven®Sequi Phase 2* (releasing estradiol approx. 50 micrograms/24 hours and levonorgestrel approx. 10 micrograms/24 hours); net price 1-month pack (2 of each) = £9.98, 3-month pack (6 of each) = £28.44. Counselling, administration
Dose: menopausal symptoms in women with intact uterus, 1 *Phase 1* patch applied once a week for 2 weeks followed by 1 *Phase 2* patch once a week for 2 weeks; subsequent courses are repeated without interval

FemTab® Continuous (Merck) PoM
Tablets, f/c, pink, estradiol 2 mg, norethisterone acetate 1 mg, net price 3 × 28-tab pack = £18.02
Dose: menopausal symptoms and osteoporosis prophylaxis, in women with intact uterus, 1 tablet daily continuously; start at end of scheduled bleed if changing from cyclical HRT
NOTE. Unsuitable for use in perimenopausal women or within 12 months of last menstrual period—see Choice above

FemTab® Sequi (Merck) PoM
Tablets, both s/c, 16 white, estradiol valerate 2 mg; 12 pink, estradiol valerate 2 mg, levonorgestrel 75 micrograms, net price 3 × 28-tab pack = £15.15
Dose: menopausal symptoms and osteoporosis prophylaxis, in women with intact uterus, 1 white tablet daily for 16 days, starting on day 5 of menstruation (or any time if cycles have ceased or are infrequent) then 1 pink tablet daily for 12 days; subsequent courses are repeated without interval

Indivina® (Orion) ▼ PoM
Indivina® 1 mg/2.5 mg tablets, estradiol valerate 1 mg, medroxyprogesterone acetate 2.5 mg, net price 3 × 28-tab pack = £22.62
Indivina® 1 mg/5 mg tablets, estradiol valerate 1 mg, medroxyprogesterone acetate 5 mg, net price 3 × 28-tab pack = £22.62
Indivina® 2 mg/5 mg tablets, estradiol valerate 2 mg, medroxyprogesterone acetate 5 mg, net price 3 × 28-tab pack = £22.62
Dose: menopausal symptoms and osteoporosis prophylaxis, in women with intact uterus, 1 tablet daily continuously; initiate therapy with *Indivina® 1 mg/2.5 mg* tablets and adjust according to response; start at end of scheduled bleed if changing from cyclical HRT
NOTE. Less suitable for use in perimenopausal women or within 3 years of last menstrual period—see Choice above

Kliofem® (Novo Nordisk) PoM
Tablets, f/c yellow, estradiol 2 mg, norethisterone acetate 1 mg. Net price 3 × 28-tab pack = £15.45
Dose: menopausal symptoms and osteoporosis prophylaxis, in women with intact uterus, 1 tablet daily continuously; start at end of scheduled bleed if changing from cyclical HRT
NOTE. Unsuitable for use in perimenopausal women or within 12 months of last menstrual period—see Choice above

Kliovance® (Novo Nordisk) PoM
Tablets, f/c, estradiol 1mg, norethisterone acetate 500 micrograms, net price 3 × 28-tab pack = £15.45
Dose: menopausal symptoms and osteoporosis prophylaxis, in women with intact uterus, 1 tablet daily continuously; start at end of scheduled bleed if changing from cyclical HRT
NOTE. Unsuitable for use in perimenopausal women or within 12 months of last menstrual period—see Choice above

Novofem (Novo Nordisk) PoM
Tablets, f/c, 16 red, estradiol 1 mg; 12 white, estradiol 1 mg, norethisterone acetate 1 mg, net price 3 × 28-tab pack = £13.50
Dose: menopausal symptoms and osteoporosis prophylaxis in women with intact uterus, 1 red tablet daily for 16 days then 1 white tablet daily for 12 days; subsequent courses are repeated without interval; start treatment with red tablet at any time or if changing from cyclical HRT, start treatment the day after finishing oestrogen plus progestogen phase

Nuvelle® (Schering Health) PoM
Nuvelle® tablets, all s/c, 16 white, estradiol valerate 2 mg; 12 pink, estradiol valerate 2 mg and levonorgestrel 75 micrograms. Net price 3 × 28-tab pack = £15.15
Dose: menopausal symptoms and osteoporosis prophylaxis, in women with intact uterus, 1 white tablet daily for 16 days, starting on day 5 of menstruation (or any time if cycles have ceased or are infrequent) then 1 pink tablet daily for 12 days; subsequent courses are repeated without interval
Nuvelle® Continuous tablets, f/c, pink, estradiol 2 mg, norethisterone acetate 1 mg, net price 3 × 28-tab pack = £18.02
Dose: menopausal symptoms and osteoporosis prophylaxis, in women with intact uterus, 1 tablet daily continuously; start at end of scheduled bleed if changing from cyclical HRT
NOTE. Unsuitable for use in perimenopausal women or within 12 months of last menstrual period—see Choice above

Tridestra® (Orion) PoM
Tablets, 70 white, estradiol valerate 2 mg; 14 blue, estradiol valerate 2 mg and medroxyprogesterone acetate 20 mg; 7 yellow, inactive. Net price 91-tab pack = £23.78
Dose: menopausal symptoms and osteoporosis prophylaxis, in women with intact uterus, 1 white tablet daily for 70 days, then 1 blue tablet daily for 14 days, then 1 yellow tablet daily for 7 days; subsequent courses are repeated without interval

Trisequens® (Novo Nordisk) PoM
Trisequens® tablets, 12 blue, estradiol 2 mg; 10 white, estradiol 2 mg, norethisterone acetate 1 mg; 6 red, estradiol 1 mg, net price 3 × 28-tab pack = £14.40
Dose: menopausal symptoms and osteoporosis prophylaxis, in women with intact uterus, 1 blue tablet daily, starting on day 5 of menstruation (or at any time if cycles have ceased or are infrequent), then 1 tablet daily in sequence (without interruption)
Trisequens Forte® tablets, 12 yellow, estradiol 4 mg; 10 white, estradiol 4 mg, norethisterone acetate 1 mg; 6 red, estradiol 1 mg, net price 3 × 28-tab pack = £14.40
Dose: menopausal symptoms, see under *Trisequens®*, starting with 1 yellow tablet daily (instead of 1 blue tablet) if symptoms not fully controlled with lower strength

■ Conjugated oestrogens only
Premarin® (Wyeth) PoM
Tablets, all s/c, conjugated oestrogens (equine) 625 micrograms (maroon), net price 3 × 28-tab pack = £9.72; 1.25 mg (yellow), 3 × 28-tab pack = £13.19
Dose: menopausal symptoms and osteoporosis prophylaxis, (with progestogen for 12–14 days per cycle in women with intact uterus), 0.625–1.25 mg daily

■ Estradiol only

Estradiol Implants (Organon) PoM
Implant, estradiol 25 mg, net price each = £9.59;
50 mg, each = £19.16; 100 mg, each = £33.40
Dose: by implantation, oestrogen replacement, and osteoporosis prophylaxis (with cyclical progestogen for 10–13
days of each cycle in women with intact uterus, see notes
above), 25–100 mg as required (usually every 4–8
months) according to oestrogen levels—check before
each implant
NOTE. On removing implant for the last time from those
with intact uterus, cyclical progesterone should be
continued until withdrawal bleed stops

Aerodiol® (Servier) ▼ PoM
Nasal spray, estradiol 150 micrograms/metered
spray, net price 4.2-mL unit (60 metered sprays) =
£7.25
Dose: menopausal symptoms, initially 1 spray into each
nostril daily at the same time each day *either* continuously
or for 21–28 days followed by a 2–7 day treatment-free
interval; daily dose adjusted according to response to 1–4
sprays daily in divided doses; with cyclical progestogen
for at least 12 days of each cycle in women with intact
uterus; not to be used immediately after nasal corticosteroid or nasal vasoconstrictor
NOTE. If patient has a severely blocked nose, *Aerodiol*®
may be temporarily administered into the mouth between
the cheek and the gum above the upper teeth; in this
situation the normal dose should be doubled

Climaval® (Novartis) PoM
Tablets, estradiol valerate 1 mg (grey-blue), net
price 1 × 28-tab pack = £2.55, 3 × 28-tab pack =
£7.66; 2 mg (blue), 1 × 28-tab pack = £2.55, 3 ×
28-tab pack = £7.66
Dose: menopausal symptoms (if patient has had a
hysterectomy), 1–2 mg daily

Elleste-Solo® (Pharmacia) PoM
Elleste-Solo® 1-mg tablets, estradiol 1 mg. Net price
3 × 28-tab pack = £5.34
Dose: menopausal symptoms, with cyclical progestogen
for 12–14 days of each cycle in women with intact uterus,
1 mg daily starting on day 1 of menstruation (or at any
time if cycles have ceased or are infrequent)
Elleste-Solo® 2-mg tablets, orange, estradiol 2 mg.
Net price 3 × 28-tab pack = £5.34
Dose: menopausal symptoms not controlled with lower
strength and osteoporosis prophylaxis, with cyclical
progestogen for 12–14 days of each cycle in women with
intact uterus, 2 mg daily starting on day 1 of menstruation
(or at any time if cycles have ceased or are infrequent)

Elleste Solo® MX (Pharmacia) PoM
Patches, self-adhesive, estradiol, *MX 40 patch*
(releasing approx. 40 micrograms/24 hours), net
price 8-patch pack = £5.19; *MX 80 patch* (releasing
approx. 80 micrograms/24 hours), 8-patch pack =
£5.99. Counselling, administration.
Dose: menopausal symptoms (and osteoporosis prophylaxis in case of *Elleste Solo MX 80*® **only**), 1 patch to be
applied twice weekly continuously starting within 5 days
of onset of menstruation (or at any time if cycles have
ceased or are infrequent); with cyclical progestogen for
12–14 days of each cycle in women with intact uterus;
therapy should be initiated with *MX 40* in those with
menopausal symptoms, prolonged oestrogen deficiency
or anticipated intolerance to higher strength, dosage may
be increased if required, subsequently adjusted to lowest
effective dose

Estraderm MX® (Novartis) PoM
Patches, self-adhesive, estradiol, *MX 25 patch*
(releasing approx. 25 micrograms/24 hours), net
price 8-patch pack = £5.20, 24-patch pack =

£15.59; *MX 50 patch* (releasing approx. 50 micr-
ograms/24 hours), 8-patch pack = £5.22, 24-patch
pack = £15.65, 20-patch pack (hosp. only) =
£13.04; *MX 75 patch* (releasing approx. 75 micr-
ograms/24 hours), 8-patch pack = £6.08, 24-patch
pack = £18.25; *MX 100 patch* (releasing approx.
100 micrograms/24 hours), 8-patch pack = £6.31,
24-patch pack = £18.94. Counselling, administration
Dose: menopausal symptoms (and osteoporosis prophylaxis in case of *Estraderm MX® 50* and *75* **only**), 1 patch
to be applied twice weekly continuously, with cyclical
progestogen for 12 days of each cycle in women with
intact uterus; therapy should be initiated with *MX 50* for
first month, subsequently adjusted to lowest effective
dose

Estraderm TTS® (Novartis) PoM
Patches, self-adhesive, estradiol, *TTS 25 patch*
(releasing approx. 25 micrograms/24 hours), net
price, 8-patch pack = £6.21, 24-patch pack =
£18.63; *TTS 50 patch* (releasing approx. 50 micr-
ograms/24 hours), 8-patch pack = £6.23, 24-patch
pack = £18.69; *TTS 100 patch* (releasing approx.
100 micrograms/24 hours), 8-patch pack = £7.52,
24-patch pack = £22.63, 20-patch pack (hosp.
only) = £16.76. Counselling, administration
Dose: menopausal symptoms (and osteoporosis prophylaxis in case of *Estraderm TTS® 50* **only**), 1 patch to be
applied twice weekly continuously, with cyclical progestogen for 12 days of each cycle in women with intact
uterus; therapy should be initiated with *TTS 50* for first
month, subsequently adjusted to lowest effective dose

Evorel® (Janssen-Cilag) PoM
Patches, self-adhesive, estradiol, *'25' patch*
(releasing approx. 25 micrograms/24 hours), net
price 8-patch pack = £3.07; *'50' patch* (releasing
approx. 50 micrograms/24 hours), 8-patch pack =
£3.48, 24-patch pack = £10.45; *'75' patch*
(releasing approx. 75 micrograms/24 hours), 8-
patch pack = £3.70; *'100' patch* (releasing approx.
100 micrograms/24 hours), 8-patch pack = £3.84.
Counselling, administration
Dose: menopausal symptoms and osteoporosis prophylaxis (except *Evorel®* 25), 1 patch to be applied twice
weekly continuously, with cyclical progestogen for at
least 12 days of each cycle in women with intact uterus;
therapy should be initiated with *'50' patch* for first month,
subsequently adjusted to lowest effective dose

Fematrix® (Solvay) PoM
Fematrix® 40 patch, self-adhesive, estradiol, *'40'*
patch (releasing approx. 40 micrograms/24 hours).
Net price 8-patch pack = £5.50. Counselling,
administration
Dose: menopausal symptoms, 1 patch to be applied twice
weekly continuously starting within 5 days of onset of
menstruation (or at any time if cycles have ceased or are
infrequent), with cyclical progestogen for 12–14 days of
each cycle in women with intact uterus; *'80' patch* may be
used if required (subsequently adjusted to lowest effective
dose)
Fematrix® 80 patch, self-adhesive, estradiol (releasing approx. 80 micrograms/24 hours). Net price 8-
patch pack = £6.00. Counselling, administration
Dose: menopausal symptoms and osteoporosis prophylaxis, as for *Fematrix® 40*; therapy should be initiated
with *Fematrix® 40* in those with menopausal symptoms,
prolonged oestrogen deficiency or anticipated intolerance
to higher strength

FemSeven® (Merck) PoM

Patches, self-adhesive, estradiol, *'50' patch* (releasing approx. 50 micrograms/24 hours), net price 4-patch pack = £4.57, 12-patch pack = £13.65; *'75' patch* (releasing approx. 75 micrograms/24 hours), net price 4-patch pack = £5.29; *'100' patch* (releasing approx. 100 micrograms/24 hours), net price 4-patch pack = £5.52. Counselling, administration

Dose: menopausal symptoms and osteoporosis prophylaxis, 1 patch to be applied once a week continuously, with cyclical progestogen for at least 10 days of each cycle in women with intact uterus; therapy should be initiated with *FemSeven*® *50* patches for the first few months, subsequently adjusted according to response

FemTab® (Merck) PoM

Tablets, s/c, estradiol valerate 1 mg, net price 3 × 28-tab pack = £7.72; 2 mg, 3 × 28-tab pack = £7.72

Dose: menopausal symptoms, 1–2 mg daily continuously; osteoporosis prophylaxis, 2 mg daily continuously; with cyclical progestogen for 12 days of each cycle in women with intact uterus

Menorest® (Novartis) PoM

Patches, self-adhesive, estradiol, *'50' patch* (releasing approx. 50 micrograms/24 hours), 8-patch pack = £7.69; *'75' patch* (releasing approx. 75 micrograms/24 hours), 8-patch pack = £8.95. Counselling administration

Dose: menopausal symptoms and osteoporosis prophylaxis, 1 patch to be applied twice weekly continuously, with cyclical progestogen for at least 12 days of each cycle in women with intact uterus; therapy should be initiated with *'50' patch* for first month, subsequently adjusted to lowest effective dose

Menoring® **50** (Galen) PoM

Vaginal ring, releasing estradiol approx. 50 micrograms/24 hours, net price 1-ring pack = £29.50. Label: 10, patient information leaflet

Dose: for postmenopausal vasomotor and urogenital symptoms in women without a uterus, to be inserted into upper third of vagina and worn continuously; replace after 3 months

Oestrogel® (Hoechst Marion Roussel) PoM

Gel, estradiol 0.06%, net price 64-dose pump pack = £7.95. Counselling, administration

Dose: menopausal symptoms and osteoporosis prophylaxis, 2 measures (estradiol 1.5 mg) to be applied over an area twice that of the template provided once daily continuously, starting within 5 days of menstruation (or anytime if cycles have ceased or are infrequent), with cyclical progestogen for 12 days of each cycle in women with intact uterus; for menopausal symptoms may be increased if necessary after 1 month to max. 4 measures daily

COUNSELLING. Apply gel to clean, dry, intact skin such as arms, shoulders or inner thighs and allow to dry for 5 minutes before covering with clothing. Not to be applied on or near breasts or on vulval region. Avoid skin contact with another person (particularly male) and avoid other skin products or washing the area for at least 1 hour after application

Progynova® (Schering Health) PoM

Tablets, both s/c, estradiol valerate 1 mg (beige), net price 3 × 28-tab pack = £7.72; 2 mg (blue), 3 × 28-tab pack = £7.72

Dose: menopausal symptoms, 1–2 mg daily continuously; osteoporosis prophylaxis, 2 mg daily continuously; with cyclical progestogen for 12 days of each cycle in women with intact uterus

Progynova® **TS** (Schering Health) PoM

Patches, self-adhesive, *Progynova*® *TS 50* (releasing estradiol approx. 50 micrograms/24 hours), net price 12-patch pack = £17.88; *Progynova*® *TS 100* (releasing estradiol approx. 100 micrograms/24 hours), 12-patch pack = £19.68. Counselling, administration

Dose: menopausal symptoms, 1 patch to be applied once a week on a continuous or cyclical basis (1 patch per week for three weeks followed by a 7-day patch-free interval); therapy should be initiated with *Progynova*® *TS 50* and adjusted to lowest effective dose; osteoporosis prophylaxis, 1 *Progynova*® *TS 50* patch to be applied once a week on a continuous basis (with cyclical progestogen for 10–14 days of each cycle in women with intact uterus)

NOTE. Women receiving *Progynova*® *TS 100* patches for menopausal symptoms may continue with this strength for osteoporosis prophylaxis

Sandrena® (Organon) PoM

Gel, estradiol (0.1%), 500 microgram/500 mg sachet, net price 28-sachet pack = £5.68, 1 mg/1 g sachet, 28-sachet pack = £6.54. Counselling, administration

Dose: menopausal symptoms, estradiol 1 mg (1 g gel) to be applied once daily over area 1–2 times size of hand; with cyclical progestogen for 12–14 days of each cycle in women with intact uterus; dose may be adjusted after 2–3 cycles to a usual dose of estradiol 0.5–1.5 mg (0.5–1.5 g gel) daily

COUNSELLING. Apply gel to intact areas of skin such as lower trunk or thighs, using right and left sides on alternate days. Wash hands after application. Not to be applied on the breasts or face and avoid contact with eyes. Allow area of application to dry for 5 minutes and do not wash area for at least 1 hour

Zumenon® (Solvay) PoM

Tablets, f/c, estradiol 1 mg, net price 84-tab pack = £7.65; 2 mg (red), 84-tab pack = £7.65

Dose: menopausal symptoms, initially 1 mg daily starting on day 5 of menstruation (or any time if cycles have ceased or are infrequent) adjusted to 1–4 mg daily according to response; osteoporosis prophylaxis, 2 mg daily; with cyclical progestogen for 10–14 days of each cycle in women with intact uterus

■ Estradiol, estriol and estrone

Hormonin® (Shire) PoM

Tablets, pink, estradiol 600 micrograms, estriol 270 micrograms, estrone 1.4 mg. Net price 84-tab pack = £6.61

Dose: menopausal symptoms and osteoporosis prophylaxis, 1–2 tablets daily, with cyclical progestogen for 12–14 days of each cycle in women with intact uterus

NOTE. *Hormonin*® tablets can be given continuously or cyclically (21 days out of 28)

■ Estriol only

Ovestin® (Organon) PoM

Tablets, scored, estriol 1 mg. Net price 30-tab pack = £4.20. Label: 25

Dose: genito-urinary symptoms associated with oestrogen-deficiency states, 0.5–3 mg daily, as single dose, for up to 1 month, then 0.5–1 mg daily until restoration of epithelial integrity (short-term use)

■ Estropipate only

Harmogen® (Pharmacia) PoM

Tablets, peach, scored, estropipate 1.5 mg. Net price 28-tab pack = £3.77

Dose: menopausal symptoms and osteoporosis prophylaxis, 1.5 mg daily continuously (with cyclical progestogen for 10–13 days of each cycle in women with intact uterus); up to 3 mg daily (in single or divided doses) for vasomotor symptoms and menopausal vaginitis

Raloxifene

Raloxifene is licensed for the treatment and prevention of *postmenopausal osteoporosis*; unlike hormone replacement therapy, raloxifene does not reduce menopausal vasomotor symptoms.

Raloxifene may reduce the incidence of oestrogen-receptor-positive breast cancer but its role in established breast cancer is not yet clear. The manufacturer advises avoiding its use during treatment for breast cancer.

RALOXIFENE HYDROCHLORIDE

Indications: treatment and prevention of postmenopausal osteoporosis

Cautions: risk factors for venous thromboembolism (discontinue if prolonged immobilisation); breast cancer (see notes above); history of oestrogen-induced hypertriglyceridaemia (monitor serum triglycerides); **interactions:** Appendix 1 (raloxifene)

Contra-indications: history of venous thromboembolism, undiagnosed uterine bleeding, endometrial cancer, hepatic impairment, cholestasis, severe renal impairment; pregnancy and breast-feeding

Side-effects: venous thromboembolism, thrombophlebitis, hot flushes, leg cramps, peripheral oedema, influenza-like symptoms; rarely rashes, gastro-intestinal disturbances, hypertension, headache (including migraine), breast discomfort

Dose: 60 mg once daily

Evista® (Lilly) ▼ PoM
Tablets, f/c, raloxifene hydrochloride 60 mg, net price 28-tab pack = £21.74; 84-tab pack = £65.21

Tibolone

Tibolone combines oestrogenic and progestogenic activity with weak androgenic activity. It is used for the treatment of vasomotor symptoms of the menopause and for osteoporosis prophylaxis if other drugs (section 6.6) cannot be used.

Tibolone increases the risk of breast cancer though the risk is less than that with combined oestrogen and progestogen HRT (see section 6.4.1.1).

Tibolone is given continuously, without cyclical progestogen.

TIBOLONE

Indications: short-term treatment of symptoms of oestrogen deficiency (including women being treated with gonadotrophin releasing hormone analogues); osteoporosis prophylaxis in women at risk of fractures (second-line)

Cautions: renal impairment, history of liver disease, epilepsy, migraine, diabetes mellitus, hypercholesterolaemia; withdraw if signs of thromboembolic disease, abnormal liver function tests or cholestatic jaundice; see also Note below; **interactions:** Appendix 1 (tibolone)

Contra-indications: hormone-dependent tumours, history of cardiovascular or cerebrovascular disease (e.g. thrombophlebitis, thromboembolism),

uninvestigated vaginal bleeding, severe liver disease, pregnancy, breast-feeding

Side-effects: see notes above; weight changes, oedema, dizziness, seborrhoeic dermatitis, vaginal bleeding, headache, abdominal pain, gastro-intestinal disturbances, increased facial hair; depression, arthralgia, myalgia, migraine, breast cancer (see notes above and section 6.4.1.1), visual disturbances, liver-function changes, rash and pruritus also reported

Dose: 2.5 mg daily

NOTE. Unsuitable for use in the premenopause (unless being treated with gonadotrophin-releasing hormone analogue) and as (or with) an oral contraceptive; also unsuitable for use within 12 months of last menstrual period (may cause irregular bleeding); induce withdrawal bleed with progestogen if transferring from another form of HRT

Livial® (Organon) PoM
Tablets, tibolone 2.5 mg. Net price 28-tab pack = £13.05; 3 × 28-tab pack = £39.14

Ethinylestradiol

Ethinylestradiol (ethinyloestradiol) has been used as hormone replacement for menopausal symptoms in a dose of 10–20 micrograms daily. This has now been largely replaced by more appropriate forms of oestrogen.

Ethinylestradiol is occasionally used, under **specialist supervision**, for the management of *hereditary haemorrhagic telangiectasia* (but evidence of any beneficial effect is uncertain). Side-effects include nausea, fluid retention, and thrombosis. Impotence and gynaecomastia occur in men.

For use in breast cancer, see section 8.3.1.

ETHINYLESTRADIOL

(Ethinyloestradiol)

Indications: see notes above

Cautions: cardiovascular disease (sodium retention with oedema, thromboembolism), hepatic impairment (jaundice); see also under Combined Hormonal Contraceptives (section 7.3.1) and under Oestrogen for HRT (above)

Contra-indications: see under Combined Hormonal Contraceptives (section 7.3.1) and under Oestrogen for HRT (above)

Side-effects: feminising effects in men; see also under Combined Hormonal Contraceptives (section 7.3.1) and under Oestrogen for HRT (above)

Dose: see notes above

Ethinylestradiol (Non-proprietary) PoM
Tablets, ethinylestradiol 10 micrograms, net price 21-tab pack = £12.92; 50 micrograms, 21-tab pack = £15.32; 1 mg, 28-tab pack = £28.85
Available from Celltech

6.4.1.2 Progestogens

There are two main groups of progestogen, *progesterone and its analogues* (dydrogesterone and medroxyprogesterone) and *testosterone analogues* (norethisterone and norgestrel). The newer progestogens (desogestrel, norgestimate, and gestodene) are all derivatives of norgestrel; levonorgestrel is the active isomer of norgestrel and has twice its potency. Progesterone and its analogues are less androgenic than the testosterone derivatives and neither progesterone nor dydrogesterone causes virilisation.

Where *endometriosis* requires drug treatment, it may respond to a progestogen, e.g. norethisterone, administered on a continuous basis. Danazol, gestrinone, and gonadorelin analogues are also available (section 6.7.2).

Although oral progestogens have been used widely for *menorrhagia* they are relatively ineffective compared with tranexamic acid (section 2.11) or, particularly where dysmenorrhoea is also a factor, mefenamic acid (section 10.1.1); the levonorgestrel-releasing intra-uterine system (section 7.3.2.3) may be particularly useful for women also requiring contraception. Oral progestogens have also been used for *severe dysmenorrhoea*, but where contraception is also required in younger women the best choice is a combined oral contraceptive (section 7.3.1).

Progestogens have also been advocated for the alleviation of *premenstrual symptoms*, but no convincing physiological basis for such treatment has been shown.

Progestogens have been used for the prevention of spontaneous abortion in women with a history of *recurrent miscarriage* (habitual abortion) but there is no evidence of benefit and they are **not** recommended for this purpose. In pregnant women with antiphospholipid antibody syndrome who have suffered recurrent miscarriage, administration of low-dose aspirin (section 2.9) and a prophylactic dose of a low molecular weight heparin (section 2.8.1) may decrease the risk of fetal loss (use under specialist supervision only).

HORMONE REPLACEMENT THERAPY. In women with a uterus a progestogen needs to be added to *long-term oestrogen therapy for hormone replacement*, to prevent cystic hyperplasia of the endometrium and possible transformation to cancer; it can be added on a cyclical or a continuous basis (see section 6.4.1.1). Combined packs incorporating suitable progestogen tablets are available, see p. 352.

ORAL CONTRACEPTION. Desogestrel, etynodiol (ethynodiol), gestodene, levonorgestrel, norethisterone, and norgestimate are used in *combined oral contraceptives* and in *progestogen-only contraceptives* (section 7.3.1 and section 7.3.2).

CANCER. Progestogens also have a role in *neoplastic disease* (section 8.3.2).

CAUTIONS. Progestogens should be used with caution in conditions that may worsen with fluid retention e.g. epilepsy, hypertension, migraine, asthma, cardiac or renal dysfunction, and in those susceptible to thromboembolism (particular caution with high dose). Care is also required in liver impairment (avoid if severe), and in those with a history of depression. Progestogens can decrease glucose tolerance and diabetes should be monitored closely. For **interactions** see Appendix 1 (progestogens).

CONTRA-INDICATIONS. Progestogens should be avoided in patients with a history of liver tumours, and in severe liver impairment. They are also contra-indicated in those with genital or breast cancer (unless progestogens are being used in the management of these conditions), severe arterial disease,

undiagnosed vaginal bleeding and porphyria (section 9.8.2). Progestogens should not be used if there is a history during pregnancy of idiopathic jaundice, severe pruritus, or pemphigoid gestationis.

SIDE-EFFECTS. Side-effects of progestogens include menstrual disturbances, premenstrual-like syndrome (including bloating, fluid retention, breast tenderness), weight gain, nausea, headache, dizziness, insomnia, drowsiness, depression; also skin reactions (including urticaria, pruritus, rash, and acne), hirsutism and alopecia. Jaundice and anaphylactoid reactions have also been reported.

DYDROGESTERONE

Indications: see under Dose and notes above
Cautions: see notes above; breast-feeding (Appendix 5)
Contra-indications: see notes above
Side-effects: see notes above
Dose: endometriosis, 10 mg 2–3 times daily from day 5 to 25 of cycle or continuously

Infertility, irregular cycles, 10 mg twice daily from day 11 to 25 for at least 6 cycles (but not recommended)

Recurrent miscarriage, 10 mg twice daily from day 11 to 25 of cycle until conception, then continuously until week 20 of pregnancy and then gradually reduced (but not recommended, see notes above)

Dysfunctional uterine bleeding, 10 mg twice daily (together with an oestrogen) for 5–7 days to arrest bleeding; 10 mg twice daily (together with an oestrogen) from day 11 to 25 of cycle to prevent bleeding

Dysmenorrhoea (but see notes above), 10 mg twice daily from day 5 to 25 of cycle

Amenorrhoea, 10 mg twice daily from day 11 to 25 of cycle with oestrogen therapy from day 1 to 25 of cycle

Premenstrual syndrome, 10 mg twice daily from day 12 to 26 of cycle increased if necessary (but not recommended, see notes above)

Hormone replacement therapy, with continuous oestrogen therapy, see under *Duphaston® HRT* below

Duphaston® (Solvay) [PoM]
Tablets, scored, dydrogesterone 10 mg. Net price 60-tab pack = £4.49

Duphaston® HRT (Solvay) [PoM]
Tablets, scored, dydrogesterone 10 mg. Net price 42-tab pack = £3.14
Dose: 10 mg daily on days 15–28 of each 28-day oestrogen HRT cycle, increased to 10 mg twice daily if withdrawal bleed is early or endometrial biopsy shows inadequate progestational response

MEDROXYPROGESTERONE ACETATE

Indications: see under Dose; contraception (section 7.3.2.2); malignant disease (section 8.3.2)
Cautions: see notes above; breast-feeding (Appendix 5)
Contra-indications: see notes above; pregnancy (Appendix 4)
Side-effects: see notes above; indigestion
Dose: *by mouth,* 2.5–10 mg daily for 5–10 days beginning on day 16 to 21 of cycle, repeated for 2

cycles in dysfunctional uterine bleeding and 3 cycles in secondary amenorrhoea

Mild to moderate endometriosis, 10 mg 3 times daily for 90 consecutive days, beginning on day 1 of cycle

Progestogenic opposition of oestrogen HRT, 10 mg daily for the last 14 days of each 28-day oestrogen HRT cycle

Provera® (Pharmacia) PoM

Tablets, all scored, medroxyprogesterone acetate 2.5 mg (orange), net price 30-tab pack = £1.84; 5 mg (blue), 10-tab pack = £1.23; 10 mg (white), 10-tab pack = £2.47, 90-tab pack = £22.16

■ Combined preparations
Section 6.4.1.1

NORETHISTERONE

Indications: see under Dose; HRT (section 6.4.1.1); contraception (section 7.3.1 and section 7.3.2); malignant disease (section 8.3.2)

Cautions: see notes above; breast-feeding (Appendix 5)

Contra-indications: see notes above; pregnancy (Appendix 4)

Side-effects: see notes above

Dose: endometriosis, 10–15 mg daily for 4–6 months or longer, starting on day 5 of cycle (if spotting occurs increase dose to 20–25 mg daily, reduced once bleeding has stopped)

Dysfunctional uterine bleeding, menorrhagia (but see notes above), 5 mg 3 times daily for 10 days to arrest bleeding; to prevent bleeding 5 mg twice daily from day 19 to 26

Dysmenorrhoea (but see notes above), 5 mg 3 times daily from day 5 to 24 for 3–4 cycles

Premenstrual syndrome, 5 mg 2–3 times daily from day 19 to 26 for several cycles (but not recommended, see notes above)

Postponement of menstruation, 5 mg 3 times daily starting 3 days before anticipated onset (menstruation occurs 2–3 days after stopping)

Progestogenic opposition of menopausal oestrogen HRT, see under *Micronor® HRT* , below

■ Tablets of 5 mg

Norethisterone (Non-proprietary) PoM

Tablets, norethisterone 5 mg, net price 30-tab pack = £2.16; 100-tab pack = £7.17
Available from Alpharma, CP, Sandoz

Primolut N® (Schering Health) PoM

Tablets, norethisterone 5 mg. Net price 30-tab pack = £2.16

Utovlan® (Pharmacia) PoM

Tablets, norethisterone 5 mg, net price 30-tab pack = £1.40, 90-tab pack = £4.21

■ Tablets of 1 mg for HRT

Micronor® **HRT** (Janssen-Cilag) PoM

Tablets, norethisterone 1 mg. Net price 3 × 12-tab pack = £3.75
Dose: 1 tablet daily on days 15–26 of each 28-day oestrogen HRT cycle

■ Combined preparations
Section 6.4.1.1

PROGESTERONE

Indications: see under preparations

Cautions: see notes above; breast-feeding (Appendix 5)

Contra-indications: see notes above; missed or incomplete abortion

Side-effects: see notes above; injection-site reactions; pain, diarrhoea and flatulence can occur with rectal administration

Crinone® (Serono) PoM

Vaginal gel, progesterone 90 mg/application (8%), 15 = £38.51
Dose: by vagina, infertility due to inadequate luteal phase, insert 1 applicatorful daily starting either after documented ovulation or on day 18–21 of cycle. *In vitro* fertilisation, daily application continued for 30 days after laboratory evidence of pregnancy

Cyclogest® (Shire) PoM �037

Pessaries, progesterone 200 mg, net price 15 = £5.22; 400 mg, 15 = £7.55
Dose: by vagina or rectum, premenstrual syndrome and post-natal depression, 200 mg daily to 400 mg twice daily; for premenstrual syndrome start on day 12–14 and continue until onset of menstruation (but not recommended, see notes above); rectally if barrier methods of contraception are used, in patients who have recently given birth or in those who suffer from vaginal infection or recurrent cystitis

Gestone® (Nordic) PoM

Injection, progesterone 50 mg/mL, 1-mL amp = 57p, 2-mL amp = 75p
Dose: by deep intramuscular injection into buttock, dysfunctional uterine bleeding, 5–10 mg daily for 5–10 days until 2 days before expected onset of menstruation
Recurrent miscarriage due to inadequate luteal phase (but not recommended, see notes above) or following *in vitro* fertilisation *or* gamete intra-fallopian transfer, 25–100 mg 2–7 times a week from day 15, or day of embryo or gamete transfer, until 8–16 weeks of pregnancy; max. 200 mg daily

6.4.2 Male sex hormones and antagonists

Androgens cause masculinisation; they may be used as replacement therapy in castrated adults and in those who are hypogonadal due to either pituitary or testicular disease. In the normal male they inhibit pituitary gonadotrophin secretion and depress spermatogenesis. Androgens also have an anabolic action which led to the development of anabolic steroids (section 6.4.3).

Androgens are useless as a treatment of impotence and impaired spermatogenesis unless there is associated hypogonadism; they should not be given until the hypogonadism has been properly investigated. Treatment should be under expert supervision.

When given to patients with hypopituitarism they can lead to normal sexual development and potency but not to fertility. If fertility is desired, the usual treatment is with gonadotrophins or pulsatile gonadotrophin-releasing hormone (section 6.5.1) which will stimulate spermatogenesis as well as androgen production.

Caution should be used when androgens or chorionic gonadotrophin are used in treating boys with delayed puberty since the fusion of epiphyses is hastened and may result in short stature.

Intramuscular depot preparations of **testosterone esters** are preferred for replacement therapy. Testosterone enantate or propionate or alternatively *Sustanon*®, which consists of a mixture of testosterone esters and has a longer duration of action, may be used. Satisfactory replacement therapy can sometimes be obtained with 1 mL of *Sustanon 250*®, given by intramuscular injection once a month, although more frequent dose intervals are often necessary. Implants of testosterone can be used for hypogonadism; the implants are replaced every 4 to 5 months. Menopausal women are also sometimes given implants of testosterone (in a dose of 50–100 mg every 4–8 months) as an adjunct to hormone replacement therapy.

Testosterone undecanoate and **mesterolone** are available for oral administration. Testosterone patches and topical gel are also available.

TESTOSTERONE AND ESTERS

Indications: see under preparations

Cautions: cardiac, renal, or hepatic impairment (Appendix 2), elderly, ischaemic heart disease, hypertension, epilepsy, migraine, diabetes mellitus, skeletal metastases (risk of hypercalcaemia), undertake regular examination of the prostate during treatment; pre-pubertal boys (see notes above and under Side-effects); **interactions:** Appendix 1 (testosterone)

Contra-indications: breast cancer in men, prostate cancer, history of primary liver tumours, hypercalcaemia, pregnancy, breast-feeding, nephrosis

Side-effects: prostate abnormalities and prostate cancer, headache, depression, gastro-intestinal bleeding, nausea, cholestatic jaundice, changes in libido, gynaecomastia, polycythaemia, anxiety, asthenia, paraesthesia, hypertension, electrolyte disturbances including sodium retention with oedema and hypercalcaemia; increased bone growth; androgenic effects such as hirsutism, male-pattern baldness, seborrhoea, acne, excessive frequency and duration of penile erection, precocious sexual development and premature closure of epiphyses in pre-pubertal males, suppression of spermatogenesis in men and virilism in women; rarely liver tumours; *with patches and gel*, local irritation and allergic reactions

■ Oral

Restandol® (Organon) [PoM]
Capsules, red-brown, testosterone undecanoate 40 mg in oily solution. Net price 28-cap pack = £8.30; 56-cap pack = £16.60. Label: 21, 25
Dose: androgen deficiency, 120–160 mg daily for 2–3 weeks; maintenance 40–120 mg daily

■ Intramuscular

Testosterone Enantate (Non-proprietary) [PoM]
Injection (oily), testosterone enantate 250 mg/mL.
Net price 1-mL amp = £8.33
Available from Cambridge
The brand name *Primoteston Depot*® was formerly used for testosterone enantate injection
Dose: by slow intramuscular injection, hypogonadism, initially 250 mg every 2–3 weeks; maintenance 250 mg every 3–6 weeks
Breast cancer, 250 mg every 2–3 weeks

Sustanon 100® (Organon) [PoM]
Injection (oily), testosterone propionate 20 mg, testosterone phenylpropionate 40 mg, and testo-

sterone isocaproate 40 mg/mL. Net price 1-mL amp = £1.17
NOTE. Contains arachis (peanut) oil
Dose: by deep intramuscular injection, androgen deficiency, 1 mL every 2 weeks

Sustanon 250® (Organon) [PoM]
Injection (oily), testosterone propionate 30 mg, testosterone phenylpropionate 60 mg, testosterone isocaproate 60 mg, and testosterone decanoate 100 mg/mL. Net price 1-mL amp = £2.74
NOTE. Contains arachis (peanut) oil
Dose: by deep intramuscular injection, androgen deficiency, 1 mL usually every 3 weeks

Virormone® (Nordic) [PoM]
Injection, testosterone propionate 50 mg/mL. Net price 2-mL amp = 59p
Dose: by intramuscular injection, androgen deficiency, 50 mg 2–3 times weekly
Delayed puberty, 50 mg weekly
Breast cancer in women, 100 mg 2–3 times weekly

■ Implant

Testosterone (Organon) [PoM]
Implant, testosterone 100 mg, net price = £7.40; 200 mg = £13.79
Dose: by implantation, male hypogonadism, 100–600 mg; 600 mg usually maintains plasma-testosterone concentration within the normal range for 4–5 months
Menopausal women, see notes above

■ Transdermal preparations

Andropatch® (GSK) [PoM]
Patches, self-adhesive, releasing testosterone approx. 2.5 mg/24 hours, net price 60-patch pack = £52.80; releasing testosterone approx. 5 mg/24 hours, net price 30-patch pack = £52.80.
Counselling, administration
Dose: androgen deficiency in men (over 15 years) associated with primary or secondary hypogonadism, apply to clean, dry, unbroken skin on back, abdomen, upper arms or thighs, removing after 24 hours and siting replacement patch on a different area (with an interval of 7 days before using the same site); initially apply patches equivalent to testosterone 5 mg/24 hours (2.5 mg/24 hours in non-virilised patients) at night (approx. 10 p.m.), then adjust to 2.5 mg to 7.5 mg every 24 hours according to plasma-testosterone concentration (those with a body-weight over 130 kg may require 7.5 mg every 24 hours)

Testogel® (Schering Health) ▼ [PoM]
Gel, testosterone 50 mg/5 g sachet, net price 30-sachet pack = £33.00. Counselling, administration
Dose: hypogonadism due to androgen deficiency in men (over 18 years), 50 mg testosterone (5 g gel) to be applied once daily; subsequent application adjusted according to response in 25-mg (2.5 g gel) increments to max. 100 mg (10 g gel) daily
COUNSELLING. Apply thin layer of gel on clean, dry, healthy skin such as shoulders, arms or abdomen, immediately after sachet is opened. Not to be applied on genital area as high alcohol content may cause local irritation. Allow to dry for 3–5 minutes before dressing. Wash hands with soap and water after applying gel, avoid shower or bath for at least 6 hours
Avoid skin contact with gel application sites to prevent testosterone transfer to other people, especially pregnant women and children—consult product literature

MESTEROLONE

Indications: see under Dose

Cautions: see under Testosterone and Esters

Contra-indications: see under Testosterone and Esters

Side-effects: see under Testosterone and Esters but spermatogenesis unimpaired
Dose: androgen deficiency and male infertility associated with hypogonadism, 25 mg 3–4 times daily for several months, reduced to 50–75 mg daily in divided doses for maintenance; CHILD not recommended

Pro-Viron® (Schering Health) PoM
Tablets, scored, mesterolone 25 mg. Net price 30-tab pack = £4.75

Anti-androgens

Cyproterone acetate

Cyproterone acetate is an anti-androgen used in the treatment of severe hypersexuality and sexual deviation in the male. It inhibits spermatogenesis and produces reversible infertility (but is not a male contraceptive); abnormal sperm forms are produced. Fully informed consent is recommended and an initial spermatogram. As hepatic tumours have been produced in *animal* studies, careful consideration should be given to the risk/benefit ratio before treatment. Cyproterone acetate is also used as an adjunct in prostatic cancer (section 8.3.4.2) and in the treatment of acne and hirsutism in women (section 13.6.2).

CYPROTERONE ACETATE

Indications: see notes above; prostate cancer (section 8.3.4.2)
Cautions: ineffective for male hypersexuality in chronic alcoholism (relevance to prostate cancer not known); blood counts initially and throughout treatment; monitor hepatic function regularly (liver function tests should be performed before treatment, see also under Side-effects below); monitor adrenocortical function regularly; diabetes mellitus (see also Contra-indications)
DRIVING. Fatigue and lassitude may impair performance of skilled tasks (e.g. driving)
Contra-indications: (do not apply in prostate cancer) hepatic disease, severe diabetes (with vascular changes); sickle-cell anaemia, malignant or wasting disease, severe depression, history of thrombo-embolic disorders; youths under 18 years (may arrest bone maturation and testicular development)
Side-effects: fatigue and lassitude, breathlessness, weight changes, reduced sebum production (may clear acne), changes in hair pattern, gynaecomastia (rarely leading to galactorrhoea and benign breast nodules); rarely hypersensitivity reactions, rash and osteoporosis; inhibition of spermatogenesis (see notes above); hepatotoxicity reported (including jaundice, hepatitis and hepatic failure usually in men given 200–300 mg daily for prostatic cancer, see section 8.3.4.2 for details and warnings)
Dose: male hypersexuality, 50 mg twice daily after food

Cyproterone Acetate (Non-proprietary) PoM
Tablets, cyproterone acetate 50 mg, net price 56-tab pack = £32.23. Label 21
Available from Generics

Androcur® (Schering Health) PoM
Tablets, scored, cyproterone acetate 50 mg. Net price 56-tab pack = £30.46. Label: 21

Dutasteride and finasteride

Dutasteride and **finasteride** are specific inhibitors of the enzyme 5α-reductase, which metabolises testosterone into the more potent androgen, dihydrotestosterone. This inhibition of testosterone metabolism leads to reduction in prostate size, with improvement in urinary flow rate and in obstructive symptoms. Dutasteride and finasteride are alternatives to alpha-blockers (section 7.4.1) particularly in men with a significantly enlarged prostate.

A low strength of finasteride is licensed for treating male-pattern baldness in men (section 13.9).

CAUTIONS. Dutasteride and finasteride decrease serum concentration of prostate cancer markers such as prostate-specific antigen; reference values may need adjustment. Both dutasteride and finasteride are excreted in semen and use of a condom is recommended if sexual partner is pregnant or likely to become pregnant. Women of childbearing potential should avoid handling crushed or broken tablets of finasteride and leaking capsules of dutasteride.

CONTRA-INDICATIONS. Dutasteride and finasteride are contra-indicated in women, children, and adolescents.

SIDE-EFFECTS. The side-effects of dutasteride and finasteride include impotence, decreased libido, ejaculation disorders, and breast tenderness and enlargement.

DUTASTERIDE

Indications: benign prostatic hyperplasia
Cautions: see notes above; **interactions:** Appendix 1 (dutasteride)
Contra-indications: see notes above; also severe hepatic impairment
Side-effects: see notes above
Dose: 500 micrograms daily (may require 6 months' treatment before benefit is obtained)

Avodart® (GSK) ▼ PoM
Capsules, yellow, dutasteride 500 micrograms, net price 30-cap pack = £26.68. Label: 25

FINASTERIDE

Indications: benign prostatic hyperplasia; male-pattern baldness in men (section 13.9)
Cautions: see notes above; also obstructive uropathy
Side-effects: see notes above; also testicular pain, hypersensitivity reactions (including lip and face swelling, pruritus and rash)
Dose: 5 mg daily, review treatment after 6 months (may require several months' treatment before benefit is obtained)

Proscar® (MSD) PoM
Tablets, blue, f/c, finasteride 5 mg. Net price 28-tab pack = £24.90

6.4.3   Anabolic steroids

Anabolic steroids have some androgenic activity but they cause less virilisation than androgens in women.

They are used in the treatment of some *aplastic anaemias* (section 9.1.3). Anabolic steroids have been given for osteoporosis in women but they are no longer advocated for this purpose.

The protein-building properties of anabolic steroids have not proved beneficial in the clinical setting. Their use as body builders or tonics is quite unjustified; some athletes abuse them.

NANDROLONE

Indications: osteoporosis in postmenopausal women (but not recommended, see notes above); aplastic anaemia (section 9.1.3)

Cautions: cardiac and renal impairment, hepatic impairment (see Appendix 2), hypertension, diabetes mellitus, epilepsy, migraine; monitor skeletal maturation in young patients; skeletal metastases (risk of hypercalcaemia); **interactions:** Appendix 1 (anabolic steroids)

Contra-indications: severe hepatic impairment, prostate cancer, male breast cancer, pregnancy and breast-feeding, porphyria (section 9.8.2)

Side-effects: acne, sodium retention with oedema, virilisation with high doses including voice changes (sometimes irreversible), amenorrhoea, inhibition of spermatogenesis, premature epiphyseal closure; abnormal liver-function tests reported with high doses; liver tumours reported occasionally on prolonged treatment with anabolic steroids

Dose: see below

Deca-Durabolin® (Organon) PoM ▭
Injection (oily), nandrolone decanoate 50 mg/mL, net price 1-mL amp = £3.54
Excipients: include arachis (peanut) oil and benzyl alcohol (see Excipients, p. 2)
Dose: by deep intramuscular injection, 50 mg every 3 weeks

6.5 Hypothalamic and pituitary hormones and anti-oestrogens

6.5.1   Hypothalamic and anterior pituitary hormones and anti-oestrogens
6.5.2   Posterior pituitary hormones and antagonists

> Use of preparations in these sections requires detailed prior investigation of the patient and *should be reserved for specialist centres.*

6.5.1 Hypothalamic and anterior pituitary hormones and anti-oestrogens

Anti-oestrogens

The anti-oestrogens **clomifene** (clomiphene) and **tamoxifen** (section 8.3.4.1) are used in the treatment of female infertility due to oligomenorrhoea or secondary amenorrhoea (e.g. associated with poly-cystic ovarian disease). They induce gonadotrophin release by occupying oestrogen receptors in the hypothalamus, thereby interfering with feedback mechanisms; chorionic gonadotrophin is sometimes used as an adjunct. Patients should be warned that there is a risk of multiple pregnancy (*rarely* more than twins).

CLOMIFENE CITRATE
(Clomiphene Citrate)

Indications: anovulatory infertility—see notes above

Cautions: see notes above; polycystic ovary syndrome (cysts may enlarge during treatment), ovarian hyperstimulation syndrome, uterine fibroids, ectopic pregnancy, incidence of multiple births increased (consider ultrasound monitoring), visual symptoms (discontinue and initiate ophthalmological examination); breast-feeding (Appendix 5)

CSM Advice. The CSM has recommended that clomifene should not normally be used for longer than 6 cycles (possibly increased risk of ovarian cancer)

Contra-indications: hepatic disease, ovarian cysts, hormone dependent tumours or abnormal uterine bleeding of undetermined cause, pregnancy (exclude before treatment)

Side-effects: visual disturbances (withdraw), ovarian hyperstimulation (withdraw), hot flushes, abdominal discomfort, occasionally nausea, vomiting, depression, insomnia, breast tenderness, headache, intermenstrual spotting, menorrhagia, endometriosis, convulsions, weight gain, rashes, dizziness, hair loss

Dose: 50 mg daily for 5 days, starting within about 5 days of onset of menstruation (preferably on 2nd day) or at any time (normally preceded by a progestogen-induced withdrawal bleed) if cycles have ceased; second course of 100 mg daily for 5 days may be given in absence of ovulation; most patients who are going to respond will do so to first course; 3 courses should constitute adequate therapeutic trial; long-term cyclical therapy not recommended—see CSM advice, above

Clomifene (Non-proprietary) PoM
Tablets, clomifene citrate 50 mg, net price 30-tab pack = £11.25
Available from CP

Clomid® (Aventis Pharma) PoM
Tablets, yellow, scored, clomifene citrate 50 mg. Net price 30-tab pack = £11.27

Anterior pituitary hormones

Corticotrophins

Tetracosactide (tetracosactrin), an analogue of corticotropin (ACTH), is used to test adrenocortical function; failure of the plasma cortisol concentration to rise after administration of tetracosactide indicates adrenocortical insufficiency.

Both corticotropin and tetracosactide were formerly used as alternatives to corticosteroids in conditions such as Crohn's disease or rheumatoid arthritis; their value was limited by the variable and unpredictable therapeutic response and by the waning of their effect with time.

TETRACOSACTIDE
(Tetracosactrin)

Indications: see notes above

Cautions: as for corticosteroids, section 6.3.2; **important:** risk of anaphylaxis (medical supervision; consult product literature); **interactions:** Appendix 1 (corticosteroids)

Contra-indications: as for corticosteroids, section 6.3.2; avoid injections containing benzyl alcohol in neonates (see under preparations)

Side-effects: as for corticosteroids, section 6.3.2

Dose: see under preparations below

Synacthen® (Alliance) PoM
Injection, tetracosactide 250 micrograms (as acetate)/mL. Net price 1-mL amp = £3.00
Dose: diagnostic (30-minute test), *by intramuscular or intravenous injection,* 250 micrograms as a single dose

Synacthen Depot® (Alliance) PoM
Injection (aqueous suspension), tetracosactide acetate 1 mg/mL, with zinc phosphate complex. Net price 1-mL amp = £4.29
Excipients: include benzyl alcohol (avoid in neonates, see Excipients p. 2)
Dose: diagnostic (5-hour test), *by intramuscular injection,* 1 mg as a single dose
NOTE. Formerly used therapeutically by intramuscular injection, in an initial dose of 1 mg daily (or every 12 hours in acute cases); reduced to 1 mg every 2–3 days, then 1 mg weekly (or 500 micrograms every 2–3 days) but value was limited (see notes above)

Gonadotrophins

Follicle-stimulating hormone (FSH) and luteinising hormone (LH) together (as in **human menopausal gonadotrophin**), follicle-stimulating hormone alone (as in **follitropin**), or chorionic gonadotrophin, are used in the treatment of infertility in women with proven hypopituitarism or who have not responded to clomifene, or in superovulation treatment for assisted conception (such as *in vitro* fertilisation).

The gonadotrophins are also occasionally used in the treatment of hypogonadotrophic hypogonadism and associated oligospermia. There is no justification for their use in primary gonadal failure.

Chorionic gonadotrophin has also been used in delayed puberty in the male to stimulate endogenous testosterone production, but has little advantage over testosterone (section 6.4.2).

CHORIONIC GONADOTROPHIN
(Human Chorionic Gonadotrophin; HCG)
A preparation of a glycoprotein fraction secreted by the placenta and obtained from the urine of pregnant women having the action of the pituitary luteinising hormone

Indications: see notes above

Cautions: cardiac or renal impairment, asthma, epilepsy, migraine; prepubertal boys (risk of premature epiphyseal closure or precocious puberty)

Contra-indications: androgen-dependent tumours

Side-effects: oedema (particularly in males—reduce dose), headache, tiredness, mood changes, gynaecomastia, local reactions; may aggravate ovarian hyperstimulation, multiple pregnancy

Dose: *by subcutaneous or intramuscular injection,* according to patient's response

Choragon® (Ferring) PoM
Injection, powder for reconstitution, chorionic gonadotrophin. Net price 5000-unit amp (with solvent) = £3.50. For intramuscular injection

Pregnyl® (Organon) PoM
Injection, powder for reconstitution, chorionic gonadotrophin. Net price 1500-unit amp = £2.37; 5000-unit amp = £3.52 (both with solvent). For subcutaneous or intramuscular injection

CHORIOGONADOTROPIN ALFA
(Human chorionic gonadotropin)

Indications: see notes above

Cautions: rule out infertility caused by hypothyroidism, adrenocortical deficiency, hyperprolactinaemia, tumours of the pituitary or hypothalamus

Contra-indications: ovarian enlargement or cyst (unless caused by polycystic ovarian disease); ectopic pregnancy in previous 3 months; active thromboembolic disorders; hypothalamus, pituitary, ovarian, uterine or mammary malignancy

Side-effects: nausea, vomiting, abdominal pain; headache, tiredness; injection-site reactions; ovarian hyperstimulation syndrome; rarely diarrhoea, depression, irritability, breast pain; ectopic pregnancy and ovarian torsion reported

Dose: *by subcutaneous injection,* according to patient's response

Ovitrelle® (Serono) ▼ PoM
Injection, choriogonadotropin alfa, net price 6500-unit/0.5 mL (250-micrograms/0.5 mL) prefilled syringe = £39.19

FOLLITROPIN ALFA and BETA
(Recombinant human follicle stimulating hormone)

Indications: see notes above

Cautions: see under Human Menopausal Gonadotrophins

Contra-indications: see under Human Menopausal Gonadotrophins

Side-effects: see under Human Menopausal Gonadotrophins

Dose: *by subcutaneous or intramuscular injection,* according to patient's response

■ Follitropin alfa

Gonal-F® (Serono) PoM
Injection, powder for reconstitution, follitropin alfa. Net price 75-unit amp = £26.25; 450 units/0.75 mL, multidose vial = £157.50; 1050 units/1.75 mL, multidose vial = £367.50 (all with diluent). For subcutaneous injection

■ Follitropin beta

Puregon® (Organon) PoM
Injection, follitropin beta 100 units/mL, net price 0.5-mL (50-unit) vial = £20.15; 200 units/mL, 0.5-mL (100-unit) vial = £40.30; 300 units/mL, 0.5-mL (150-unit) vial = £54.43; 400 units/mL, 0.5-mL (200-unit) vial = £72.57. For subcutaneous or intramuscular injection
Excipients: may include neomycin and streptomycin

HUMAN MENOPAUSAL GONADOTROPHINS

Purified extract of human post-menopausal urine containing follicle-stimulating hormone (FSH) and luteinising hormone (LH); the relative *in vivo* activity is designated as a ratio; the 1:1 ratio is also known as menotrophin

Indications: see notes above

Cautions: rule out infertility caused by adrenal or thyroid disorders, hyperprolactinaemia or tumours of the pituitary or hypothalamus

Contra-indications: ovarian cysts (not caused by polycystic ovarian syndrome); tumours of breast, uterus, ovaries, testes or prostate; vaginal bleeding of unknown cause; pregnancy and breast-feeding

Side-effects: ovarian hyperstimulation, increased risk of multiple pregnancy and miscarriage, hypersensitivity reactions, nausea, vomiting, joint pain, fever, injection site reactions, very rarely thromboembolism; gynaecomastia, acne, and weight gain reported in men

Dose: *by deep intramuscular or subcutaneous injection*, according to patient's response

Menogon® (Ferring) [PoM]
Injection, powder for reconstitution, menotrophin as follicle-stimulating hormone 75 units, luteinising hormone 75 units, net price per amp (with solvent) = £10.64. For intramuscular injection

Menopur® (Ferring) [PoM]
Injection, powder for reconstitution, menotrophin as follicle-stimulating hormone 75 units, luteinising hormone 75 units, net price per amp (with solvent) = £14.00. For intramuscular or subcutaneous injection

Merional® (Denfleet) [PoM]
Injection, powder for reconstitution, menotrophin as follicle-stimulating hormone 75 units, luteinising hormone 75 units, net price per vial (with solvent) = £13.95; menotrophin as follicle-stimulating hormone 150 units, luteinising hormone 150 units, net price per vial (with solvent) = £27.90. For intramuscular injection

---

LUTROPIN ALFA

(Recombinant human luteinising hormone)

Indications: see notes above

Cautions: rule out infertility caused by hypothyroidism, adrenocortical deficiency, hyperprolactinaemia, tumours of the pituitary or hypothalamus

Contra-indications: ovarian enlargement or cyst (unless caused by polycystic ovarian disease); undiagnosed vaginal bleeding; tumours of hypothalamus and pituitary; ovarian, uterine or mammary carcinoma

Side-effects: nausea, vomiting, abdominal and pelvic pain; headache, somnolence; injection-site reactions; ovarian hyperstimulation syndrome, ovarian cyst, breast pain, ectopic pregnancy; thromboembolism, adnexal torsion, and haemoperitoneum

Dose: *by subcutaneous injection*, in conjunction with follicle-stimulating hormone, according to response

Luveris® (Serono) ▼ [PoM]
Injection, powder for reconstitution, lutropin alfa, net price 75-unit vial = £39.19 (with solvent)

Growth hormone

Growth hormone is used to treat deficiency of the hormone. In children it is used in Prader-Willi syndrome, Turner syndrome and in chronic renal insufficiency (see NICE guidance below).

Growth hormone of human origin (HGH; somatotrophin) has been replaced by a growth hormone of human sequence, **somatropin**, produced using recombinant DNA technology.

NICE guidance (somatropin in children with growth failure). NICE has recommended (May 2002) treatment with somatropin for children with:

- proven growth-hormone deficiency;
- Turner syndrome;
- Prader-Willi syndrome;
- chronic renal insufficiency before puberty.

Treatment should be initiated and monitored by a paediatrician with expertise in managing growth-hormone disorders; treatment can be continued under a shared-care protocol by a general practitioner.

Treatment should be discontinued if the response is poor (i.e. an increase in growth velocity of less than 50% from baseline) in the first year of therapy.

In children with chronic renal insufficiency, treatment should be stopped after renal transplantation and not restarted for at least a year

---

NICE guidance (somatropin for adults with growth hormone deficiency). NICE has recommended (August 2003) somatropin in adults **only** if the following 3 criteria are fulfilled:

- Severe growth hormone deficiency, established by an appropriate method,
- Impaired quality of life, measured by means of a specific questionnaire,
- Already receiving treatment for another pituitary hormone deficiency.

Somatropin treatment should be discontinued if the quality of life has not improved sufficiently by 9 months.

Severe growth hormone deficiency developing after linear growth is complete but before the age of 25 years should be treated with growth hormone; treatment should continue until adult peak bone mass has been achieved. Treatment for adult-onset growth hormone deficiency should be stopped only when the patient and the patient's physician consider it appropriate.

Treatment with somatropin should be initiated and managed by a physician with expertise in growth hormone disorders; maintenance treatment can be prescribed in the community under a shared-care protocol.

SOMATROPIN

(Synthetic Human Growth Hormone)

Indications: see under Dose

Cautions: diabetes mellitus (adjustment of antidiabetic therapy may be necessary), papilloedema (see under Side-effects), relative deficiencies of other pituitary hormones (notably hypothyroidism—manufacturers recommend periodic thyroid function tests but limited evidence of clinical value), history of malignant disease, disorders of the epiphysis of the hip (monitor for limping), resolved intracranial hypertension (monitor closely), rotate subcutaneous injection sites to prevent lipoatrophy; breast-feeding; **interactions:** Appendix 1 (somatropin)

Contra-indications: evidence of tumour activity (complete antitumour therapy and ensure intracranial lesions inactive before starting); not to be used after renal transplantation in seriously ill patients or for growth promotion in children with closed epiphyses (or near closure in Prader-Willi syndrome); pregnancy (interrupt treatment if pregnancy occurs)

Side-effects: headache, funduscopy for papilloedema recommended if severe or recurrent headache, visual problems, nausea and vomiting occur—if papilloedema confirmed consider benign intracranial hypertension (rare cases reported); fluid retention (peripheral oedema), arthralgia, myalgia, carpal tunnel syndrome, paraesthesia, antibody formation, hypothyroidism, hyperglycaemia, hypoglycaemia, reactions at injection site; leukaemia in children with growth hormone deficiency also reported

Dose: Gonadal dysgenesis (Turner syndrome), *by subcutaneous injection*, 45–50 micrograms/kg daily *or* 1.4 mg/m^2 daily

Deficiency of growth hormone in children, *by subcutaneous or intramuscular injection*, 23–39 micrograms/kg daily *or* 0.7–1 mg/m^2 daily

Prader-Willi syndrome, *by subcutaneous injection* in children with growth velocity greater than 1 cm/ year, in combination with energy-restricted diet, 35 micrograms/kg daily *or* 1 mg/m^2 daily; max. 2.7 mg daily

Chronic renal insufficiency in children (renal function decreased to less than 50%), *by subcutaneous injection*, 45–50 micrograms/kg daily *or* 1.4 mg/ m^2 daily (higher doses may be needed) adjusted if necessary after 6 months

Adult growth hormone deficiency, *by subcutaneous injection*, initially 150–300 micrograms daily, gradually increased if required to max. 1 mg daily; use minimum effective dose (requirements may decrease with age)

NOTE. Dose formerly expressed in units; somatropin 1 mg ≡ 3 units

Genotropin® (Pharmacia) PoM

Injection, two-compartment cartridge containing powder for reconstitution, somatropin (rbe) and diluent, net price 5.3-mg (16-unit) cartridge = £122.87, 12-mg (36-unit) cartridge = £278.20. For use with *Genotropin*® *Pen* NHS device (available free of charge from clinics). For subcutaneous injection

MiniQuick injection, two-compartment single-dose syringe containing powder for reconstitution, somatropin (rbe) and diluent, net price 0.2-mg (0.6-unit) syringe = £4.64; 0.4-mg (1.2-unit) syringe = £9.27; 0.6-mg (1.8-unit) syringe = £13.91; 0.8-mg (2.4-unit) syringe = £18.55; 1-mg (3-unit) syringe = £23.18; 1.2-mg (3.6-unit) syringe = £27.82; 1.4-mg (4.2-unit) syringe = £32.46; 1.6-mg (4.8-unit) syringe = £37.09; 1.8-mg (5.4-unit) syringe = £41.73; 2-mg (6-unit) syringe = £46.37. For subcutaneous injection

Humatrope® (Lilly) PoM

Injection, powder for reconstitution, somatropin (rbe), net price 1.33-mg (4-unit) vial (with diluent) = £30.50; 6-mg (18-unit) vial = £137.25; 12-mg (36-unit) cartridge = £274.50; 24-mg (72-unit) cartridge = £549.00; all supplied with diluent. For subcutaneous or intramuscular injection; cartridges for intramuscular injection

Norditropin® (Novo Nordisk) PoM

SimpleXx injection, somatropin (epr) 3.3 mg (10 units)/mL, net price 1.5-mL (5-mg, 15-unit) cartridge = £115.90; 6.7 mg (20 units)/mL, 1.5-mL (10-mg, 30-unit) cartridge = £231.80; 10 mg

(30 units)/mL, 1.5-mL (15-mg, 45-unit) cartridge = £347.70. For use with appropriate *NordiPen*® NHS device (available free of charge from clinics). For subcutaneous injection

Saizen® (Serono) PoM

Injection, powder for reconstitution, somatropin (rmc), net price 1.33-mg (4-unit) vial (with diluent) = £30.50; 3.33-mg (10-unit) vial (with diluent) = £76.25. For subcutaneous or intramuscular injection

Click.easy®, powder for reconstitution, somatropin (rmc), net price 8-mg (24-unit) vial (in *Click.easy*® device with diluent) = £183.00. For use with *One.click*® NHS autoinjector device *or* *Cool.Click*® NHS needle-free device (both available free of charge from clinics). For subcutaneous injection

Zomacton® (Ferring) PoM

Injection, powder for reconstitution, somatropin (rbe), net price 4-mg (12-unit) vial (with diluent) = £87.44. For use with *ZomaJet*® *2* NHS needle-free device or with *Auto-Jector*® NHS (both available free of charge from clinics) or with needles and syringes. For subcutaneous injection

Hypothalamic hormones

Gonadorelin when injected intravenously in normal subjects leads to a rapid rise in plasma concentrations of both luteinising hormone (LH) and follicle-stimulating hormone (FSH). It has not proved to be very helpful, however, in distinguishing hypothalamic from pituitary lesions. **Gonadorelin analogues** are indicated in endometriosis and infertility (section 6.7.2) and in breast and prostate cancer (section 8.3.4).

Protirelin is a hypothalamic releasing hormone which stimulates the release of thyrotrophin from the pituitary. It is indicated for the diagnosis of mild hyperthyroidism or hypothyroidism, but its use has been superseded by immunoassays for thyroid-stimulating hormone.

Sermorelin, an analogue of growth hormone releasing hormone (somatorelin, GHRH), is licensed as a diagnostic test for secretion of growth hormone.

GONADORELIN

(Gonadotrophin-releasing hormone; GnRH; LH–RH)

Indications: see preparations below

Cautions: pituitary adenoma

Side-effects: rarely, nausea, headache, abdominal pain, increased menstrual bleeding; rarely, hypersensitivity reaction on repeated administration of large doses; irritation at injection site

Dose: see under preparations

HRF® (Intrapharm) PoM

Injection, powder for reconstitution, gonadorelin. Net price 100-microgram vial (with diluent) = £13.45 (hosp. only)

Dose: for assessment of pituitary function (adults), *by subcutaneous or intravenous injection*, 100 micrograms

PROTIRELIN

(Thyrotrophin-releasing hormone; TRH)

Indications: assessment of thyroid function and thyroid stimulating hormone reserve

Cautions: severe hypopituitarism, myocardial ischaemia, bronchial asthma and obstructive airways disease, pregnancy, breast-feeding (Appendix 5)

Side-effects: after rapid intravenous administration desire to micturate, flushing, dizziness, nausea, strange taste; transient increase in pulse rate and blood pressure; rarely bronchospasm

Dose: *by intravenous injection*, 200 micrograms; CHILD 1 microgram/kg

Protirelin (Non-proprietary) [PoM]
Injection, protirelin 100 micrograms/mL. Net price 2-mL amp = £8.68
Available from Cambridge
The brand name *TRH-Cambridge®* was formerly used for protirelin injection

SERMORELIN

Indications: see notes above

Cautions: epilepsy; discontinue growth hormone therapy 1–2 weeks before test; untreated hypothyroidism, antithyroid drugs; obesity, hyperglycaemia, elevated plasma fatty acids; avoid preparations which affect release of growth hormone (includes those affecting release of somatostatin, insulin or glucocorticoids and cyclo-oxygenase inhibitors such as aspirin and indometacin); **interactions:** Appendix 1 (sermorelin)

Contra-indications: pregnancy and breast-feeding

Side-effects: occasional facial flushing and pain at injection site

Dose: *by intravenous injection*, 1 microgram/kg in the morning after an overnight fast

Geref 50® (Serono) [PoM]
Injection, powder for reconstitution, sermorelin 50 micrograms (as acetate). Net price per amp (with solvent) = £52.53

6.5.2 Posterior pituitary hormones and antagonists

Posterior pituitary hormones

DIABETES INSIPIDUS. **Vasopressin** (antidiuretic hormone, ADH) is used in the treatment of *pituitary* ('cranial') *diabetes insipidus* as is its analogue **desmopressin**. Dosage is tailored to produce a slight diuresis every 24 hours to avoid water intoxication. Treatment may be required for a limited period only in diabetes insipidus following trauma or pituitary surgery.

Desmopressin is more potent and has a longer duration of action than vasopressin; unlike vasopressin it has no vasoconstrictor effect. It is given by mouth or intranasally for maintenance therapy, and by injection in the postoperative period or in unconscious patients. Desmopressin is also used in the differential diagnosis of diabetes insipidus. Following a dose of 2 micrograms intramuscularly or 20 micrograms intranasally, restoration of the ability to concentrate urine after water deprivation confirms a diagnosis of cranial diabetes insipidus. Failure to respond occurs in nephrogenic diabetes insipidus.

In *nephrogenic* and *partial pituitary diabetes insipidus* benefit may be gained from the paradoxical antidiuretic effect of thiazides (section 2.2.1) e.g. chlortalidone 100 mg twice daily reduced to maintenance dose of 50 mg daily.

Chlorpropamide (section 6.1.2.1) is also useful in partial pituitary diabetes insipidus, and probably acts by sensitising the renal tubules to the action of remaining endogenous vasopressin; it is given in doses of up to 350 mg daily in adults and 200 mg daily in children, care being taken to avoid hypoglycaemia. Carbamazepine (section 4.8.1) is also sometimes useful (in a dose of 200 mg once or twice daily) [unlicensed]; its mode of action may be similar to that of chlorpropamide.

OTHER USES. Desmopressin injection is also used to boost factor VIII concentrations in mild to moderate haemophilia. For a comment on use of desmopressin in nocturnal enuresis see section 7.4.2.

Vasopressin infusion is used to control variceal bleeding in portal hypertension, prior to more definitive treatment and with variable results. Terlipressin, a derivative of vasopressin, is used similarly.

Oxytocin, another posterior pituitary hormone, is indicated in obstetrics (section 7.1.1).

VASOPRESSIN

Indications: pituitary diabetes insipidus; bleeding from oesophageal varices

Cautions: heart failure, hypertension, asthma, epilepsy, migraine or other conditions which might be aggravated by water retention; renal impairment (see also Contra-indications); pregnancy (Appendix 4); avoid fluid overload

Contra-indications: vascular disease (especially disease of coronary arteries) unless extreme caution, chronic nephritis (until reasonable blood nitrogen concentrations attained)

Side-effects: fluid retention, pallor, tremor, sweating, vertigo, headache, nausea, vomiting, belching, abdominal cramps, desire to defaecate, hypersensitivity reactions (including anaphylaxis), constriction of coronary arteries (may cause anginal attacks and myocardial ischaemia), peripheral ischaemia and rarely gangrene

Dose: *by subcutaneous or intramuscular injection*, diabetes insipidus, 5–20 units every four hours
By intravenous infusion, initial control of variceal bleeding, 20 units over 15 minutes

■ Synthetic vasopressin

Pitressin® (Goldshield) [PoM]
Injection, argipressin (synthetic vasopressin) 20 units/mL. Net price 1-mL amp = £16.99 (hosp. only)

DESMOPRESSIN

Indications: see under Dose

Cautions: see under Vasopressin; less pressor activity, but still considerable caution in renal impairment, in cardiovascular disease and in hypertension (not indicated for nocturnal enuresis or nocturia in these circumstances); elderly (avoid for nocturnal enuresis and nocturia in those over 65 years); also considerable caution in cystic fibrosis; in nocturia and nocturnal enuresis limit fluid intake to minimum from 1 hour before dose until 8 hours afterwards; in nocturia periodic blood pressure and weight checks needed to monitor for fluid overload; pregnancy (Appendix 4) **interactions:** Appendix 1 (desmopressin)

HYPONATRAEMIC CONVULSIONS. The CSM has advised that patients being treated for primary nocturnal enuresis should be warned to avoid fluid overload (including during swimming) and to stop taking desmopressin during an episode of vomiting or diarrhoea (until fluid balance normal). The risk of hyponatraemic convulsions can also be minimised by keeping to the recommended starting doses and by avoiding concomitant use of drugs which increase secretion of vasopressin (e.g. tricyclic antidepressants)

Contra-indications: cardiac insufficiency and other conditions treated with diuretics; psychogenic polydipsia and polydipsia in alcohol dependence

Side-effects: fluid retention, and hyponatraemia (in more serious cases with convulsions) on administration without restricting fluid intake; stomach pain, headache, nausea, vomiting, allergic reactions, and emotional disturbance in children also reported; epistaxis, nasal congestion, rhinitis with nasal spray

Dose: *by mouth*

Diabetes insipidus, treatment, ADULT and CHILD initially 300 micrograms daily (in 3 divided doses); maintenance, 300–600 micrograms daily in 3 divided doses; range 0.2–1.2 mg daily

Primary nocturnal enuresis (if urine concentrating ability normal), ADULT (under 65 years) and CHILD over 5 years (preferably over 7 years) 200 micrograms at bedtime, only increased to 400 micrograms if lower dose not effective (**important:** see also Cautions); withdraw for at least 1 week for reassessment after 3 months

Postoperative polyuria or polydipsia, adjust dose according to urine osmolality

Intranasally

Diabetes insipidus, diagnosis, ADULT and CHILD 20 micrograms (limit fluid intake to 500 mL from 1 hour before to 8 hours after administration)

Diabetes insipidus, treatment, ADULT 10–40 micrograms daily (in 1–2 divided doses); CHILD 5–20 micrograms daily; infants may require lower doses

Primary nocturnal enuresis (if urine concentrating ability normal), ADULT (under 65 years) and CHILD over 5 years (preferably over 7 years) initially 20 micrograms at bedtime, only increased to 40 micrograms if lower dose not effective (**important:** see also Cautions); withdraw for at least 1 week for reassessment after 3 months

Nocturia associated with multiple sclerosis (when other treatments have failed), ADULT (under 65 years) 10–20 micrograms at bedtime (**important:** see also Cautions), dose not to be repeated within 24 hours

Renal function testing (empty bladder at time of administration and limit fluid intake to 500 mL from 1 hour before until 8 hours after administration), ADULT 40 micrograms; INFANT under 1 year 10 micrograms (restrict fluid intake to 50% at next 2 feeds to avoid fluid overload), CHILD 1–15 years 20 micrograms

By injection

Diabetes insipidus, diagnosis (*subcutaneous or intramuscular*), ADULT and CHILD 2 micrograms (limit fluid intake to 500 mL from 1 hour before to 8 hours after administration)

Diabetes insipidus, treatment (*subcutaneous, intramuscular or intravenous*), ADULT 1–4 micrograms daily; CHILD 400 nanograms

Renal function testing (empty bladder at time of administration and limit fluid intake to 500 mL from 1 hour before until 8 hours after administration) (*subcutaneous or intramuscular*), ADULT and CHILD 2 micrograms; INFANT 400 nanograms (restrict fluid intake to 50% at next 2 feeds)

Mild to moderate haemophilia and von Willebrand disease, post lumbar puncture headache, fibrinolytic response testing, consult product literature

Desmopressin acetate (Non-proprietary) [PoM]
Nasal spray, desmopressin acetate 10 micrograms/ metered spray, net price 6-mL unit (60 metered sprays) = £28.00. Counselling, fluid intake, see above
Available from Alpharma, PLIVA (*Presinex*®)
NOTE. Children requiring dose of less than 10 micrograms should be given *DDAVP*® intranasal solution

DDAVP® (Ferring) [PoM]
Tablets, both scored, desmopressin acetate 100 micrograms, net price 90-tab pack = £46.57; 200 micrograms, 90-tab pack = £93.15. Counselling, fluid intake, see above
Intranasal solution, desmopressin acetate 100 micrograms/mL. Net price 2.5-mL dropper bottle and catheter = £10.45. Counselling, fluid intake, see above
Injection, desmopressin acetate 4 micrograms/mL. Net price 1-mL amp = £1.18

Desmotabs® (Ferring) [PoM]
Tablets, scored, desmopressin acetate 200 micrograms, net price 30-tab pack = £31.07. Counselling, fluid intake, see above

Desmospray® (Ferring) [PoM]
Nasal spray, desmopressin acetate 10 micrograms/ metered spray. Net price 6-mL unit (60 metered sprays) = £28.00. Counselling, fluid intake, see above
NOTE. Children requiring dose of less than 10 micrograms should be given *DDAVP*® intranasal solution

Nocutil® (Norgine) [PoM]
Nasal spray, desmopressin acetate 10 micrograms/ metered spray, net price 5-mL unit (50 metered sprays) = £21.17. Counselling, fluid intake, see above

---

TERLIPRESSIN

Indications: bleeding from oesophageal varices
Cautions: see under Vasopressin
Contra-indications: see under Vasopressin
Side-effects: see under Vasopressin, but effects milder

Dose: *by intravenous injection*, 2 mg followed by 1 or 2 mg every 4 to 6 hours until bleeding is controlled, for up to 72 hours

Glypressin® (Ferring) [PoM]
Injection, terlipressin, powder for reconstitution. Net price 1-mg vial with 5 mL diluent = £20.90 (hosp. only)

Antidiuretic hormone antagonists

Demeclocycline (section 5.1.3) may be used in the treatment of hyponatraemia resulting from inappropriate secretion of antidiuretic hormone. It is thought to act by directly blocking the renal tubular effect of antidiuretic hormone. Initially 0.9 to 1.2 g is given daily in divided doses, reduced to 600–900 mg daily for maintenance.

6.6 Drugs affecting bone metabolism

6.6.1 Calcitonin and teriparatide
6.6.2 Bisphosphonates

See also calcium (section 9.5.1.1), phosphorus (section 9.5.2), vitamin D (section 9.6.4), and oestrogens in postmenopausal osteoporosis (section 6.4.1.1).

Osteoporosis

Osteoporosis occurs most commonly in postmenopausal women and in those taking long-term oral corticosteroids (glucocorticosteroids). Other risk factors for osteoporosis include low body weight, cigarette smoking, excess alcohol intake, lack of physical activity, family history of osteoporosis, and early menopause.

> Those at risk of osteoporosis should maintain an adequate intake of **calcium and vitamin D** and any deficiency should be corrected by increasing dietary intake or taking supplements.

Elderly patients, especially those who are housebound or live in residential or nursing homes, are at increased risk of calcium and vitamin D deficiency and may benefit from supplements (section 9.5.1.1 and section 9.6.4). Reversible secondary causes of osteoporosis such as hyperthyroidism, hyperparathyroidism, osteomalacia or hypogonadism should be excluded, in both men and women, before treatment for osteoporosis is initiated.

POSTMENOPAUSAL OSTEOPOROSIS. **Hormone replacement therapy** (HRT, section 6.4.1.1) is of most benefit *for the prophylaxis* of postmenopausal osteoporosis if started early in menopause and continued for up to 5 years, but bone loss resumes (possibly at an accelerated rate) on stopping HRT. The CSM has advised that HRT should **not** be considered first-line therapy for long-term prevention of osteoporosis in women over 50 years of age. HRT remains an option where other therapies are contra-indicated, cannot be tolerated, or if there is a lack of response; however, the risks and benefits should be carefully assessed. Women of Afro-Caribbean origin appear to be less susceptible to osteoporosis than those who are white or of Asian origin. The **bisphosphonates** (alendronate, etidronate and risedronate, section 6.6.2) are also effective for preventing osteoporosis. **Calcitonin** (section 6.6.1) may be considered for those at high risk of osteoporosis for whom HRT or a bisphosphonate is unsuitable.

Postmenopausal osteoporosis may be *treated* with a **bisphosphonate** (section 6.6.2). The bisphosphonates (such as alendronate, etidronate, and risedronate) decrease the risk of vertebral fracture; alendronate and risedronate have also been shown to reduce non-vertebral fractures. If bisphosphonates

are unsuitable **calcitriol** (section 9.6.4) or **calcitonin** may be considered. Calcitonin may also be useful for pain relief for up to 3 months after a vertebral fracture if other analgesics are ineffective. **Teriparatide** (section 6.6.1) has been introduced for the treatment of postmenopausal oestoporosis.

Raloxifene (section 6.4.1.1) is licensed for the *prophylaxis* and *treatment* of vertebral fractures in postmenopausal women.

CORTICOSTEROID-INDUCED OSTEOPOROSIS. To reduce the risk of osteoporosis doses of oral corticosteroids should be as low as possible and courses of treatment as short as possible. The risk of osteoporosis may be related to cumulative dose of corticosteroids; even intermittent courses can therefore increase the risk. The greatest rate of bone loss occurs during the first 6–12 months of corticosteroid use and so early steps to prevent the development of osteoporosis are important. Long-term use of high-dose inhaled corticosteroids may also contribute to corticosteroid-induced osteoporosis(section 3.2).

Patients taking (or who are likely to take) the equivalent of prednisolone 7.5 mg or more each day for 3 months or longer should be assessed and where necessary given prophylactic treatment; those aged over 65 years are at greater risk. Patients taking oral corticosteroids who have sustained a low-trauma fracture should receive treatment for osteoporosis. The therapeutic options for *prophylaxis* and *treatment* of corticosteroid-induced osteoporosis are the same:

- a bisphosphonate such as alendronate, etidronate or risedronate;
- calcitriol.
- hormone replacement (HRT in women, (section 6.4.1) testosterone in men (section 6.4.2))

6.6.1 Calcitonin and teriparatide

Calcitonin is involved with parathyroid hormone in the regulation of bone turnover and hence in the maintenance of calcium balance and homoeostasis. **Calcitonin (salmon)** (salcatonin, synthetic or recombinant salmon calcitonin) is used to lower the plasma-calcium concentration in some patients with hypercalcaemia (notably when associated with malignant disease). In the treatment of severe Paget's disease of bone it is used mainly for relief of pain but it is also effective in relieving some of the neurological complications, for example deafness. Calcitonin can also be used in the prevention and treatment of postmenopausal osteoporosis (see section 6.6).

Teriparatide, a recombinant, fragment of parathyroid hormone, has been introduced for the treatment of postmenopausal osteoporosis.

CALCITONIN (SALMON)/ SALCATONIN

Indications: see under Dose
Cautions: history of allergy (skin test advised); renal impairment; heart failure; children—use for short periods only and monitor bone growth; pregnancy (Appendix 4), breast-feeding (Appendix 5)

Side-effects: nausea, vomiting, diarrhoea, flushing, dizziness, tingling of hands, unpleasant taste, rash, abdominal pain; allergic reactions including anaphylaxis reported; inflammatory reactions at injection site; nasal spray may cause local irritation and ulceration, rhinitis, sinusitis, epistaxis

Dose: hypercalcaemia, *by subcutaneous or intramuscular injection*, range from 5–10 units/kg daily (in 1–2 divided doses) *to* 400 units every 6–8 hours adjusted according to clinical and biochemical response (no additional benefit with over 8 units/kg every 6 hours); *by slow intravenous infusion* (*Forcaltonin®* and *Miacalcic®* ampoules only), 5–10 units/kg over at least 6 hours

Paget's disease of bone, *by subcutaneous or intramuscular injection*, dose range 50 units 3 times weekly to 100 units daily, in single or divided doses

Bone pain in neoplastic disease, *by subcutaneous or intramuscular injection*, 200 units every 6 hours *or* 400 units every 12 hours for 48 hours; may be repeated at discretion of physician

Postmenopausal osteoporosis, *by subcutaneous or intramuscular injection*, 100 units daily with dietary calcium and vitamin D supplements (see section 9.5.1.1 and section 9.6.4)

Intranasally, 200 units (1 spray) into one nostril daily, with dietary calcium and vitamin D supplements (see section 9.5.1.1 and section 9.6.4)

Forcaltonin® (Strakan) PoM
Injection, calcitonin (salmon) (recombinant) 100 units/mL, net price 1-mL amp = £3.56
For subcutaneous or intramuscular injection and for dilution and use as an intravenous infusion

Miacalcic® (Novartis) PoM
Nasal spray▼, calcitonin (salmon) 200 units/metered spray, net price 2-mL unit (approx. 14 metered sprays) = £20.99
Injection, calcitonin (salmon) 50 units/mL, net price 1-mL amp = £4.27; 100 units/mL, 1-mL amp = £8.55; 200 units/mL, 2-mL vial = £30.75
For subcutaneous or intramuscular injection and for dilution and use as an intravenous infusion

TERIPARATIDE

Indications: treatment of postmenopausal osteoporosis

Cautions: moderate renal impairment, (avoid if severe)

Contra-indications: pre-existing hypercalcaemia, metabolic bone diseases, including Paget's disease and hyperparathyroidism, unexplained raised levels of alkaline phosphatase, previous radiation therapy to the skeleton, pregnancy and breast-feeding

Side-effects: gastro-intestinal disorders (including nausea, reflux and haemorrhoids); postural hypotension; dysponea; depression, dizziness, vertigo; urinary disorders, polyuria; muscle cramps, sciatica; increased sweating; injection-site reactions

Dose: *by subcutaneous injection*, 20 micrograms daily; max. duration of treatment 18 months

Foresteo® (Lilly) ▼ PoM
Injection, teriparatide 250 micrograms/mL, net price 3-mL prefilled pen = £271.88
NOTE. 3-ml prefilled pen intended for 28 doses

6.6.2   Bisphosphonates

Bisphosphonates are adsorbed onto hydroxyapatite crystals in bone, slowing both their rate of growth and dissolution, and therefore reducing the rate of bone turnover. Bisphosphonates have an important role in the prophylaxis and treatment of osteoporosis and corticosteroid-induced osteoporosis; **alendronic acid** or **risedronate sodium** are considered the drugs of choice for these conditions, but **disodium etidronate** may be considered if these drugs are unsuitable or not tolerated (see also section 6.6).

Bisphosphonates are also used in the treatment of *Paget's disease* and hypercalcaemia of malignancy (section 9.5.1.2). Disodium etidronate can impair bone mineralisation when used continuously or in high doses (such as in the treatment of *Paget's disease*).

ALENDRONIC ACID

Indications: see under Dose

Cautions: upper gastro-intestinal disorders (dysphagia, symptomatic oesophageal disease, gastritis, duodenitis, or ulcers—see also under Contra-indications and Side-effects); history (within 1 year) of ulcers, active gastro-intestinal bleeding, or surgery of the upper gastro-intestinal tract; renal impairment (manufacturer advises avoid if creatinine clearance is less than 35 mL/minute); correct disturbances of calcium and mineral metabolism (e.g. vitamin-D deficiency, hypocalcaemia) before starting; exclude other causes of osteoporosis; **interactions:** Appendix 1 (bisphosphonates)

Contra-indications: abnormalities of oesophagus and other factors which delay emptying (e.g. stricture or achalasia), hypocalcaemia, pregnancy and breast-feeding

Side-effects: oesophageal reactions (see below), abdominal pain and distension, diarrhoea or constipation, flatulence, musculoskeletal pain, headache; rarely rash, erythema, photosensitivity, uveitis, transient decrease in serum phosphate; nausea, vomiting, peptic ulceration and hypersensitivity reactions (including urticaria and angioedema) also reported

OESOPHAGEAL REACTIONS. Severe oesophageal reactions (oesophagitis, oesophageal ulcers, oesophageal stricture and oesophageal erosions) have been reported; patients should be advised to stop taking the tablets and to seek medical attention if they develop symptoms of oesophageal irritation such as dysphagia, new or worsening heartburn, pain on swallowing or retrosternal pain

Dose: treatment of postmenopausal osteoporosis and osteoporosis in men, 10 mg daily *or* (in postmenopausal osteoporosis) 70 mg once weekly

Prevention of postmenopausal osteoporosis, 5 mg daily

Prevention and treatment of corticosteroid-induced osteoporosis, 5 mg daily (postmenopausal women not receiving hormone replacement therapy, 10 mg daily)

COUNSELLING. Swallow the tablets whole with a full glass of water on an empty stomach at least 30 minutes before breakfast (and any other oral medication); stand or sit upright for at least 30 minutes and do not lie down until after eating breakfast. Do not take the tablets at bedtime or before rising.

Fosamax® (MSD) [PoM]
Tablets, alendronic acid (as sodium alendronate)
5 mg, net price 28-tab pack = £25.43; 10 mg, 28-tab
pack = £23.12. Counselling, administration

Fosamax® **Once Weekly** (MSD) ▼ [PoM]
Tablets, alendronic acid (as sodium alendronate)
70 mg, net price 4-tab pack = £23.12. Counselling,
administration

DISODIUM ETIDRONATE
Indications: see under Dose
Cautions: renal impairment (Appendix 3); **interactions:** Appendix 1 (bisphosphonates)
Contra-indications: moderate to severe renal impairment; pregnancy and breast-feeding; not indicated for osteoporosis in presence of hypercalcaemia or hypercalciuria or for osteomalacia
Side-effects: nausea, diarrhoea or constipation, abdominal pain; increased bone pain in Paget's disease, also increased risk of fractures with high doses in Paget's disease (discontinue if fractures occur); rarely exacerbation of asthma, skin reactions (including angioedema, rash, urticaria and pruritus), transient hyperphosphataemia, headache, paraesthesia, peripheral neuropathy reported; blood disorders (including leucopenia, agranulocytosis and pancytopenia) also reported
Dose: Paget's disease of bone, *by mouth*, 5 mg/kg as a single daily dose for up to 6 months; doses above 10 mg/kg daily for up to 3 months may be used with caution but doses above 20 mg/kg daily are not recommended; after interval of not less than 3 months may be repeated where evidence of reactivation—including biochemical indices (avoid premature retreatment)
MONITORING. Serum phosphate, serum alkaline phosphatase and (if possible) urinary hydroxyproline should be measured before starting and at intervals of 3 months—consult product literature for further details
Osteoporosis, see under *Didronel PMO*®
COUNSELLING. Avoid food for at least 2 hours before and after oral treatment, particularly calcium-containing products (e.g. milk); also avoid iron and mineral supplements and antacids

Didronel® (Procter & Gamble Pharm.) [PoM]
Tablets, disodium etidronate 200 mg. Net price 60-tab pack = £37.30. Counselling, food and calcium (see above)

■ With calcium carbonate
For cautions and side-effects of calcium carbonate see section 9.5.1.1
Didronel PMO® (Procter & Gamble Pharm.) [PoM]
Tablets, 14 white, disodium etidronate 400 mg; 76 pink, effervescent, calcium carbonate 1.25 g (*Cacit*®). Net price per pack = £40.20. Label: 10, patient information leaflet, counselling, food and calcium (see above)
Dose: treatment of osteoporosis, prevention of bone loss in postmenopausal women (particularly if hormone replacement therapy inappropriate), and prevention and treatment of corticosteroid-induced osteoporosis, given in 90-day cycles, 1 *Didronel*® tablet daily for 14 days, then 1 *Cacit*® tablet daily for 76 days

---

DISODIUM PAMIDRONATE
Disodium pamidronate was formerly called aminohydroxypropylidenediphosphonate disodium (APD)
Indications: see under Dose
Cautions: renal impairment (Appendix 3)—monitor renal function in renal disease or predisposition to renal impairment (e.g. in multiple myeloma or tumour-induced hypercalcaemia); cardiac disease (especially in elderly); previous thyroid surgery (risk of hypocalcaemia); monitor serum electrolytes, calcium and phosphate—possibility of convulsions due to electrolyte changes; avoid concurrent use with other bisphosphonates; **interactions:** Appendix 1 (bisphosphonates)
DRIVING. Patients should be warned against driving or operating machinery immediately after treatment (somnolence or dizziness may occur)
Contra-indications: pregnancy and breast-feeding
Side-effects: hypophosphataemia, transient rise in body temperature, fever and influenza-like symptoms (sometimes accompanied by malaise, rigors, fatigue and flushes); occasionally transient bone pain, arthralgia, myalgia, nausea, vomiting, headache, lymphocytopenia, hypomagnesaemia; rarely muscle cramps, anorexia, abdominal pain, diarrhoea, constipation, dyspepsia, agitation, confusion, dizziness, insomnia, somnolence, lethargy, anaemia, leucopenia, hypotension or hypertension, rash, pruritus, hyperkalaemia or hypokalaemia, hypernatraemia; isolated cases of seizures, hallucinations, thrombocytopenia, haematuria, acute renal failure, deterioration of pre-existing renal disease, conjunctivitis and other ocular symptoms, abnormal liver function tests, reactivation of herpes simplex and zoster also reported; also local reactions at injection site
Dose: *by slow intravenous infusion* (via cannula in a relatively large vein), see also Appendix 6
Hypercalcaemia of malignancy, according to serum calcium concentration 15–60 mg in single infusion or in divided doses over 2–4 days; max. 90 mg per treatment course
Osteolytic lesions and bone pain in bone metastases associated with breast cancer or multiple myeloma, 90 mg every 4 weeks (or every 3 weeks to coincide with chemotherapy in breast cancer)
Paget's disease of bone, 30 mg once a week for 6 weeks (total dose 180 mg) *or* 30 mg in first week then 60 mg every other week (total dose 210 mg); max. total 360 mg (in divided doses of 60 mg) per treatment course; may be repeated every 6 months
CHILD not recommended
CALCIUM AND VITAMIN D SUPPLEMENTS. Oral supplements are advised for those with Paget's disease at risk of calcium or vitamin D deficiency (e.g. through malabsorption or lack of exposure to sunlight) to minimise potential risk of hypocalcaemia

Disodium pamidronate (Non-proprietary) [PoM]
Concentrate for intravenous infusion, disodium pamidronate 3 mg/mL, net price 5-mL vial = £27.50, 10-mL vial = £55.00; 6 mg/mL, 10-mL vial = £110.00; 9 mg/mL, 10-mL vial = £165.00
Available from Mayne

Aredia Dry Powder® (Novartis) [PoM]
Injection, powder for reconstitution, disodium pamidronate, for use as an infusion. Net price 15-mg vial = £29.83; 30-mg vial = £59.66; 90-mg vial = £170.45 (all with diluent)

IBANDRONIC ACID

Indications: hypercalcaemia of malignancy

Cautions: hepatic impairment (Appendix 2); monitor renal function and serum calcium, phosphate and magnesium; cardiac disease (avoid fluid overload); **interactions:** Appendix 1 (bisphosphonates)

Contra-indications: moderate to severe renal impairment (Appendix 3), pregnancy (Appendix 4), breast-feeding (Appendix 5)

Side-effects: hypocalcaemia, hypophosphataemia, influenza-like symptoms including fever, chills, muscle and bone pain reported; rarely hypersensitivity reactions (bronchospasm and angioedema reported)

Dose: *by intravenous infusion*, according to serum calcium concentration, 2–4 mg in single infusion CHILD not recommended

Bondronat® (Roche) ▼ PoM
Concentrate for intravenous infusion, ibandronic acid 1 mg/mL, net price 2–mL amp = £94.86

RISEDRONATE SODIUM

Indications: see under Dose

Cautions: oesophageal abnormalities and other factors which delay transit or emptying (e.g. stricture or achalasia—see also under Side-effects); renal impairment (manufacturer advises avoid if creatinine clearance is less than 30 mL/minute); correct hypocalcaemia before starting, correct other disturbances of bone and mineral metabolism (e.g. vitamin-D deficiency) at onset of treatment; **interactions:** Appendix 1 (bisphosphonates)

Contra-indications: hypocalcaemia (see Cautions above), pregnancy and breast-feeding

Side-effects: gastro-intestinal effects (including dyspepsia, nausea, diarrhoea, constipation, oesophageal stricture, and duodenitis); dizziness, headache; influenza-like symptoms, musculoskeletal pain; rarely glossitis, oedema, weight loss, apnoea, bronchitis, sinusitis, rash, nocturia, ambylopia, corneal lesion, dry eye, tinnitus, iritis

Dose: Paget's disease of bone, 30 mg daily for 2 months; may be repeated if necessary after at least 2 months

Treatment of postmenopausal osteoporosis to reduce risk of vertebral or hip fractures, 5 mg daily *or* 35 mg once weekly

Prevention of osteoporosis (including corticosteroid-induced osteoporosis) in postmenopausal women, 5 mg daily

COUNSELLING. Swallow tablets whole with full glass of water; on rising, take on an empty stomach at least 30 minutes before first food or drink of the day **or**, if taking at any other time of the day, avoid food and drink for at least 2 hours before or after risedronate (particularly avoid calcium-containing products e.g. milk, also avoid iron and mineral supplements and antacids; stand or sit upright for at least 30 minutes; do not take tablets at bedtime or before rising

Actonel® (Procter & Gamble Pharm.) PoM
Tablets, f/c, risedronate sodium 5 mg (yellow), net price 28-tab pack = £21.83; 30 mg (white), 28-tab pack = £152.81. Counselling, administration, food and calcium (see above)

Actonel Once a Week® (Procter & Gamble Pharm.)
▼ PoM
Tablets, f/c, risedronate sodium 35 mg (orange), net price 4-tab pack = £21.83. Counselling, administration, food and calcium (see above)

SODIUM CLODRONATE

Indications: see under Dose

Cautions: monitor renal and hepatic function and white cell count; also monitor serum calcium and phosphate periodically; renal dysfunction reported in patients receiving concomitant NSAIDs; maintain adequate fluid intake during treatment; **interactions:** Appendix 1 (bisphosphonates)

Contra-indications: moderate to severe renal impairment; pregnancy and breast-feeding

Side-effects: nausea, diarrhoea; skin reactions

Dose: osteolytic lesions, hypercalcaemia and bone pain associated with skeletal metastases in patients with breast cancer or multiple myeloma, *by mouth*, 1.6 g daily in single or 2 divided doses increased if necessary to a max. of 3.2 g daily

COUNSELLING. Avoid food for 1 hour before and after treatment, particularly calcium-containing products e.g. milk; also avoid iron and mineral supplements and antacids; maintain adequate fluid intake

Hypercalcaemia of malignancy, *by slow intravenous infusion*, 300 mg daily for max. 7–10 days *or* by single-dose infusion of 1.5 g

Bonefos® (Boehringer Ingelheim) PoM
Capsules, yellow, sodium clodronate 400 mg. Net price 30-cap pack = £43.54, 120-cap pack = £174.16. Counselling, food and calcium
Tablets, f/c, scored, sodium clodronate 800 mg. Net price 10-tab pack = £30.40; 60-tab pack = £182.39. Counselling, food and calcium
Concentrate (= intravenous solution), sodium clodronate 60 mg/mL, for dilution and use as infusion. Net price 5-mL amp = £13.78

Loron® (Roche) PoM
Loron® *capsules*, sodium clodronate 400 mg. Net price 30-cap pack = £43.54. Label: 10, patient information leaflet, counselling, food and calcium
Loron 520® *tablets*, f/c, scored, sodium clodronate 520 mg. Net price 60-tab pack = £174.18. Label: 10, patient information leaflet, counselling, food and calcium
Dose: 2 tablets daily in single or two divided doses; may be increased to max. 4 tablets daily
NOTE. Due to greater bioavailability one *Loron 520*® tablet (520 mg) is equivalent to two *Loron*® capsules (2 × 400 mg)

TILUDRONIC ACID

Indications: Paget's disease of bone

Cautions: renal impairment (monitor renal function regularly, see under Contra-indications); correct disturbances of calcium metabolism (e.g. vitamin D deficiency, hypocalcaemia) before starting; avoid concomitant use of indometacin; **interactions:** Appendix 1 (bisphosphonates)

Contra-indications: severe renal impairment, juvenile Paget's disease, pregnancy and breast-feeding

Side-effects: stomach pain, nausea, diarrhoea; rarely asthenia, dizziness, headache and skin reactions

Dose: 400 mg daily as a single dose for 12 weeks; may be repeated if necessary after 6 months
COUNSELLING. Avoid food for 2 hours before and after treatment, particularly calcium-containing products e.g. milk; also avoid antacids

Skelid® (Sanofi-Synthelabo) PoM
Tablets, tiludronic acid (as tiludronate disodium) 200 mg. Net price 28-tab pack = £99.00. Counselling, food and calcium

ZOLEDRONIC ACID

Indications: see under Dose
Cautions: monitor serum electrolytes, calcium, phosphate and magnesium; assess renal function before each dose; ensure adequate hydration; renal impairment (Appendix 3); severe hepatic impairment (Appendix 2); cardiac disease (avoid fluid overload); **interactions:** Appendix 1 (bisphosphonates)
Contra-indications: pregnancy (Appendix 4), breast-feeding
Side-effects: hypophosphataemia, anaemia, influenza-like symptoms including bone pain; myalgia, arthralgia, fever and rigors; gastro-intestinal effects including nausea, vomiting, and anorexia; headache, conjunctivitis, renal impairment (rarely acute renal failure); rarely diarrhoea, constipation, taste disturbance, dry mouth, stomatitis, chest pain, dyspnoea, cough, dizziness, paraesthesia, tremor, anxiety, sleep disturbance, blurred vision, weight gain, pruritus, rash, sweating, haematuria, proteinuria, hypersensitivity reactions (including angioedema), asthenia, peripheral oedema, hypertension, thrombocytopenia, leucopenia, hypomagnesaemia, also injection-site reactions; very rarely bradycardia, confusion, hyperkalaemia, hypokaleamia, hypernatraemia, pancytopenia
Dose: reduction of bone damage in advanced malignancies involving bone (with calcium and vitamin D supplement), *by intravenous infusion*, 4 mg every 3–4 weeks
Hypercalcaemia of malignancy, *by intravenous infusion*, 4 mg as a single dose
CHILD not recommended

Zometa® (Novartis) ▼ PoM
Injection, powder for reconstitution, zoledronic acid, for use as an infusion, net price 4-mg vial (with water for injections) = £195.00

6.7   Other endocrine drugs

6.7.1   Bromocriptine and other dopaminergic drugs

Bromocriptine is a stimulant of dopamine receptors in the brain; it also inhibits release of prolactin by the pituitary. Bromocriptine is used for the treatment of galactorrhoea and cyclical benign breast disease, and for the treatment of prolactinomas (when it reduces both plasma prolactin concentration and tumour size). Bromocriptine also inhibits the release of growth hormone and is sometimes used in the treatment of acromegaly, but somatostatin analogues (such as octreotide, section 8.3.4.3) are more effective.

Cabergoline has actions and uses similar to those of bromocriptine, but its duration of action is longer. Its side-effects appear to differ from that of bromocriptine and patients intolerant of bromocriptine may be able to tolerate cabergoline (and *vice versa*).

> **Fibrotic reactions.** The CSM has advised that ergot-derived dopamine-receptor agonists, bromocriptine, cabergoline, lisuride, and pergolide have been associated with pulmonary, retroperitoneal, and pericardial fibrotic reactions.
> Before starting treatment with these ergot derivatives it may be appropriate to measure the erythrocyte sedimentation rate and serum creatinine and to obtain a chest X-ray. Patients should be monitored for dyspnoea, persistent cough, chest pain, cardiac failure, and abdominal pain or tenderness. If long-term treatment is expected, then lung-function tests may also be helpful.

Quinagolide has actions and uses similar to those of ergot-derived dopamine agonists, but its side-effects differ slightly.

SUPPRESSION OF LACTATION. Although bromocriptine and cabergoline are licensed to suppress lactation, they are **not** recommended for routine suppression (or for the relief of symptoms of postpartum pain and engorgement) that can be adequately treated with simple analgesics and breast support. If a dopamine-receptor agonist is required, cabergoline is preferred. Quinagolide is not licensed for the suppression of lactation.

> **Sudden onset of sleep.** Excessive daytime sleepiness and sudden onset of sleep can occur with dopaminergic drugs.
> Patients starting treatment with these drugs should be warned of the possibility of these effects and of the need to exercise caution when driving or operating machinery.
> Patients who have suffered excessive sedation or sudden onset of sleep, should refrain from driving or operating machines, until those effects have stopped recurring.

BROMOCRIPTINE

Indications: see notes above and under Dose; parkinsonism (section 4.9.1)

Cautions: specialist evaluation—monitor for pituitary enlargement, particularly during pregnancy, annual gynaecological assessment (postmenopausal, every 6 months), monitor for peptic ulceration in acromegalic patients; contraceptive advice if appropriate (oral contraceptives may increase prolactin concentration); avoid breast-feeding for about 5 days if lactation prevention fails; history of serious mental disorders (especially psychotic disorders) or cardiovascular disease or Raynaud's syndrome; monitor for retroperitoneal fibrosis (see Fibrotic Reactions in notes above); porphyria (section 9.8.2); **interactions:** Appendix 1 (bromocriptine)

HYPOTENSIVE REACTIONS. Hypotensive reactions may be disturbing in some patients during the first few days of treatment and particular care should be exercised when driving or operating machinery; tolerance may be reduced by alcohol

Contra-indications: hypersensitivity to bromocriptine or other ergot alkaloids; toxaemia of pregnancy and hypertension in postpartum women or in puerperium (see also below)

POSTPARTUM OR PUERPERIUM. Should not be used postpartum or in puerperium in women with high blood pressure, coronary artery disease or symptoms (or history) of serious mental disorder; monitor blood pressure carefully (especially during first few days) in postpartum women. Very rarely hypertension, myocardial infarction, seizures or stroke (both sometimes preceded by severe headache) and mental disorders have been reported in postpartum women given bromocriptine for lactation suppression—caution with antihypertensive therapy and avoid other ergot alkaloids. Discontinue immediately if hypertension, unremitting headache or signs of CNS toxicity develop

Side-effects: nausea, vomiting, constipation, headache, dizziness, postural hypotension, drowsiness, vasospasm of fingers and toes particularly in patients with Raynaud's syndrome; also, particularly with *high doses*, confusion, psychomotor excitation, hallucinations, dyskinesia, dry mouth, leg cramps, pleural effusions (may necessitate withdrawal of treatment), retroperitoneal fibrosis reported (monitoring required)–see Fibrotic Reactions in notes above

Dose: prevention or suppression of lactation (but see notes above and under Cautions), 2.5 mg on day 1 (prevention) or daily for 2–3 days (suppression); then 2.5 mg twice daily for 14 days

Hypogonadism, galactorrhoea, infertility, initially 1–1.25 mg at bedtime, increased gradually; usual dose 7.5 mg daily in divided doses, increased if necessary to max. 30 mg daily, usual dose in infertility without hyperprolactinaemia, 2.5 mg twice daily

Cyclical benign breast disease (see also Breast Pain, section 6.7.2) and cyclical menstrual disorders (particularly breast pain), 1–1.25 mg at bedtime, increased gradually; usual dose 2.5 mg twice daily

Acromegaly, initially 1–1.25 mg at bedtime, increase gradually to 5 mg every 6 hours

Prolactinoma, initially 1–1.25 mg at bedtime; increased gradually to 5 mg every 6 hours (occasional patients may require up to 30 mg daily)

CHILD under 15 years, not recommended

Bromocriptine (Non-proprietary) PoM

Tablets, bromocriptine (as mesilate) 2.5 mg, net price 30-tab pack = £5.04. Label: 21, counselling, hypotensive reactions, driving, see notes above
Available from IVAX

Parlodel® (Novartis) PoM

Tablets, both scored, bromocriptine (as mesilate) 1 mg, net price 100-tab pack = £9.90; 2.5 mg, 30-tab pack = £5.78. Label: 21, counselling, hypotensive reactions, driving, see notes above
Capsules, bromocriptine (as mesilate) 5 mg (blue/white), net price 100-cap pack = £37.57; 10 mg (white), 100-cap pack = £69.50. Label: 21, counselling, hypotensive reactions, driving, see notes above

CABERGOLINE

Indications: see notes above and under Dose

Cautions: see under Bromocriptine; peptic ulcer, gastro-intestinal bleeding; severe hepatic impairment; fibrotic lung disease (see Fibrotic Reactions in notes above); monthly pregnancy tests during the amenorrhoeic period; advise non-hormonal contraception if pregnancy not desired (see also Contra-indications); **interactions:** Appendix 1 (cabergoline)

HYPOTENSIVE REACTIONS. Hypotensive reactions may be disturbing in some patients during the first few days of treatment and particular care should be exercised when driving or operating machinery; tolerance may be reduced by alcohol

Contra-indications: see under Bromocriptine; exclude pregnancy before starting and discontinue 1 month before intended conception (ovulatory cycles persist for 6 months)—discontinue if pregnancy occurs during treatment (specialist advice needed); avoid breast-feeding if lactation prevention fails

Side-effects: see under Bromocriptine; also dyspepsia, epigastric and abdominal pain, breast pain, palpitations, angina, epistaxis, peripheral oedema, hemianopia, asthenia, paraesthesia, erythromelagia, hot flushes, depression

Dose: prevention of lactation (but see notes above and under Contra-indications), during first day postpartum, 1 mg as a single dose; suppression of established lactation (but see notes above) 250 micrograms every 12 hours for 2 days

Hyperprolactinaemic disorders, 500 micrograms weekly (as a single dose *or* as 2 divided doses on separate days) increased at monthly intervals in steps of 500 micrograms until optimal therapeutic response (usually 1 mg weekly, range 0.25–2 mg weekly) with monthly monitoring of serum prolactin levels; reduce initial dose and increase more gradually if patient intolerant; over 1 mg weekly give as divided doses; up to 4.5 mg weekly has been used in hyperprolactinaemic patients

Parkinsonism, section 4.9.1

CHILD under 16 years, not recommended

Dostinex® (Pharmacia) PoM

Tablets, scored, cabergoline 500 micrograms. Net price 8-tab pack = £30.04. Label: 21, counselling, hypotensive reactions, driving, see notes above

QUINAGOLIDE

Indications: see notes above and under Dose

Cautions: see under Bromocriptine; advise non-hormonal contraception if pregnancy not desired; discontinue if pregnancy occurs during treatment (specialist advice needed); **interactions:** Appendix 1 (quinagolide)

HYPOTENSIVE REACTIONS. Hypotensive reactions may be disturbing in some patients during the first few days of treatment—monitor blood pressure for a few days after starting treatment and following dosage increases; particular care should be exercised when driving or operating machinery; tolerance may be reduced by alcohol

Contra-indications: see under Bromocriptine; hypersensitivity to quinagolide (but not ergot alkaloids); hepatic or renal impairment; breast-feeding

Side-effects: nausea, vomiting, headache, dizziness, fatigue; less frequently anorexia, abdominal pain, constipation or diarrhoea, oedema, flushing, hypotension, nasal congestion, insomnia; rarely psychosis

Dose: hyperprolactinaemia, 25 micrograms at bedtime for 3 days; increased at intervals of 3 days in steps of 25 micrograms to usual maintenance dose of 75–150 micrograms daily; for doses higher than 300 micrograms daily increase in steps of 75–150 micrograms at intervals of not less than 4 weeks

CHILD not recommended

Norprolac® (Novartis) PoM
Tablets, quinagolide (as hydrochloride) 75 micrograms (white), net price 30-tab pack = £62.36; starter pack of 3 × 25-microgram tabs (pink) with 3 × 50-microgram tabs (blue) = £5.47. Label: 21, counselling, hypotensive reactions

---

6.7.2 Drugs affecting gonadotrophins

Danazol inhibits pituitary gonadotrophins; it combines androgenic activity with antioestrogenic and antiprogestogenic activity. It is licensed for the treatment of *endometriosis* and for the relief of severe pain and tenderness in *benign fibrocystic breast disease* where other measures have proved unsatisfactory. It may also be effective in the long-term management of *hereditary angioedema* [unlicensed indication].

Gestrinone has general actions similar to those of danazol and is indicated for the treatment of endometriosis.

Cetrorelix and **ganirelix** are luteinising hormone releasing hormone antagonists, which inhibit the release of gonadotrophins (luteinising hormone and follicle-stimulating hormone). They are used in the treatment of infertility by assisted reproductive techniques.

CETRORELIX

Indications: adjunct in the treatment of female infertility (under specialist supervision)

Contra-indications: pregnancy, breast-feeding, moderate renal impairment, moderate hepatic impairment

Side-effects: nausea, headache, injection site reactions; rarely hypersensitivity reactions

Dose: *by subcutaneous injection* into the lower abdominal wall,

either 250 micrograms in the morning, starting on day 5 or 6 of ovarian stimulation with gonadotrophins (*or* each evening starting on day 5 of ovarian stimulation); continue throughout administration of gonadotrophin including day of ovulation induction (*or* evening before ovulation induction)

or 3 mg on day 7 of ovarian stimulation with gonadotrophins; if ovulation induction not possible on day 5 after 3-mg dose, additional 250 micrograms once daily until day of ovulation induction

Cetrotide® (Serono) ▼ PoM
Injection, powder for reconstitution, cetrorelix (as acetate), net price 250-micrograms vial = £24.00; 3-mg vial = £168.00 (both with solvent)

DANAZOL

Indications: see notes above and under Dose

Cautions: cardiac, hepatic, or renal impairment (avoid if severe), elderly, polycythaemia, epilepsy, diabetes mellitus, hypertension, migraine, lipoprotein disorder, history of thrombosis or thromboembolic disease; withdraw if virilisation (may be irreversible on continued use); non-hormonal contraceptive methods should be used, if appropriate; **interactions:** Appendix 1 (danazol)

Contra-indications: pregnancy (Appendix 4), ensure that patients with amenorrhoea are not pregnant; breast-feeding; severe hepatic, renal or cardiac impairment; thromboembolic disease; undiagnosed genital bleeding; androgen-dependent tumours; porphyria (section 9.8.2)

Side-effects: nausea, dizziness, skin reactions including rashes, photosensitivity and exfoliative dermatitis, fever, backache, nervousness, mood changes, anxiety, changes in libido, vertigo, fatigue, epigastric and pleuritic pain, headache, weight gain; menstrual disturbances, vaginal dryness and irritation, flushing and reduction in breast size; musculo-skeletal spasm, joint pain and swelling, hair loss; androgenic effects including acne, oily skin, oedema, hirsutism, voice changes and rarely clitoral hypertrophy (see also Cautions); temporary alteration in lipoproteins and other metabolic changes, insulin resistance; thrombotic events; leucopenia, thrombocytopenia, eosinophilia, reversible erythrocytosis or polycythaemia reported; headache and visual disturbances may indicate benign intracranial hypertension; rarely cholestatic jaundice, pancreatitis, peliosis hepatis and benign hepatic adenomata

Dose: in women of child-bearing potential, treatment should start during menstruation, preferably on day 1

Endometriosis, 200–800 mg daily in up to 4 divided doses, adjusted to achieve amenorrhoea, usually for 3–6 months

Severe pain and tenderness in benign fibrocystic breast disease not responding to other treatment, 300 mg daily in divided doses usually for 3–6 months

Hereditary angioedema [unlicensed indication], intially 200 mg 2–3 times daily, then reduced according to response

Danazol (Non-proprietary) PoM
Capsules, danazol 100 mg, net price 60-cap pack = £14.70; 200 mg, net price 56-cap pack = £26.39
Available from Alpharma, Generics, Hillcross, IVAX, Sterwin

Danol® (Sanofi-Synthelabo) PoM
Capsules, danazol 100 mg (grey/white), net price 60-cap pack = £17.04; 200 mg (pink/white), 60-cap pack = £33.75

GANIRELIX

Indications: adjunct in the treatment of female infertility (under specialist supervision)

Contra-indications: pregnancy, breast-feeding, moderate renal impairment, moderate hepatic impairment

Side-effects: nausea, headache, injection site reactions; dizziness and malaise also reported

Dose: *by subcutaneous injection* preferably into the upper leg (rotate injection sites to prevent lipoatrophy), 250 micrograms in the morning (or each afternoon) starting on day 6 of ovarian stimulation with gonadotrophins; continue throughout administration of gonadotrophins including day of ovulation induction (if administering in afternoon, give last dose in afternoon *before* ovulation induction)

Orgalutran® (Organon) ▼ PoM
Injection, ganirelix, 500 micrograms/mL, net price 0.5-mL prefilled syringe = £24.00

GESTRINONE

Indications: endometriosis
Cautions: cardiac and renal impairment; **interactions:** Appendix 1 (gestrinone)
Contra-indications: pregnancy (use non-hormonal method of contraception) and breast-feeding; severe cardiac, renal or hepatic impairment; metabolic or vascular disorders associated with previous sex hormone treatment
Side-effects: spotting; acne, oily skin, fluid retention, weight gain, hirsutism, voice change; liver enzyme disturbances; headache; gastro-intestinal disturbances; change in libido, flushing, decrease in breast size; nervousness, depression, change in appetite; muscle cramp
Dose: 2.5 mg twice weekly starting on first day of cycle with second dose 3 days later, repeated on same two days preferably at same time each week; duration of treatment usually 6 months
MISSED DOSES. One missed dose—2.5 mg as soon as possible and maintain original sequence; two or more missed doses—discontinue, re-start on first day of new cycle (following negative pregnancy test)

Dimetriose® (Florizel) PoM
Capsules, gestrinone 2.5 mg, net price 8-cap pack = £111.73

Gonadorelin analogues

Administration of **gonadorelin analogues** produces an initial phase of stimulation; continued administration is followed by down-regulation of gonadotrophin-releasing hormone receptors, thereby reducing the release of gonadotrophins (follicle stimulating hormone and luteinising hormone) which in turn leads to inhibition of androgen and oestrogen production.

Gonadorelin analogues are used in the treatment of endometriosis, infertility, anaemia due to uterine fibroids (together with iron supplementation), breast cancer (section 8.3.4.1) and prostate cancer (section 8.3.4.2) and before intra-uterine surgery. Use of leuprorelin and triptorelin for 3 to 4 months before surgery reduces the uterine volume, fibroid size and associated bleeding. For women undergoing hysterectomy or myomectomy, a vaginal procedure is made more feasible following the use of a gonadorelin analogue.

CAUTIONS. Non-hormonal, barrier methods of contraception should be used during entire treatment period with gonadorelin analogues; also use with caution in patients with metabolic bone disease because decrease in bone mineral density can occur.

CONTRA-INDICATIONS. Gonadorelin analogues are contra-indicated for use longer than 6 months (do not repeat), where there is undiagnosed vaginal bleeding, in pregnancy (Appendix 4; exclude pregnancy—also give first injection during menstruation or shortly afterwards *or* use barrier contraception for 1 month beforehand) and in breast-feeding.

SIDE-EFFECTS. Side-effects of the gonadorelin analogues related to the inhibition of oestrogen production include menopausal-like symptoms (e.g. hot flushes, increased sweating, vaginal dryness, dyspareunia and loss of libido) and a decrease in trabecular bone density; these effects can be reduced by hormone replacement (e.g. with an oestrogen and a progestogen or with tibolone). Side-effects of gonadorelin analogues also include headache (rarely migraine) and hypersensitivity reactions including urticaria, pruritus, skin rashes, asthma and anaphylaxis; when treating uterine fibroids bleeding associated with fibroid degeneration can occur; spray formulations can cause irritation of the nasal mucosa including nose bleeds; local reactions at injection site can occur; other side-effects also reported with some gonadorelin analogues include palpitations, hypertension, ovarian cysts (may require withdrawal), changes in breast size, musculoskeletal pain or weakness, visual disturbances, paraesthesia, changes in scalp and body hair, oedema of the face and extremities, weight changes, and mood changes including depression.

BUSERELIN

Indications: see under Dose; prostate cancer (section 8.3.4.2)
Cautions: see notes above; polycystic ovarian disease, depression, hypertension, diabetes
Contra-indications: see notes above; hormone-dependent tumours
Side-effects: see notes above; initially withdrawal bleeding and subsequently breakthrough bleeding, leucorrhoea; nausea, vomiting, constipation, diarrhoea; anxiety, memory and concentration disturbances, sleep disturbances, nervousness, dizziness, drowsiness; breast tenderness, lactation; abdominal pain; fatigue; increased thirst, changes in appetite; acne, dry skin, splitting nails, dry eyes; altered blood lipids, leucopenia, thrombocytopenia; hearing disturbances; reduced glucose tolerance
Dose: endometriosis, *intranasally*, 300 micrograms (one 150-microgram spray in each nostril) 3 times daily (starting on days 1 or 2 of menstruation); max. duration of treatment 6 months (do not repeat)
Pituitary desensitisation before induction of ovulation by gonadotrophins for *in vitro* fertilisation (under specialist supervision), *by subcutaneous injection*, 200–500 micrograms daily given as a single injection (occasionally up to 500 micrograms twice daily may be needed) starting in early follicular phase (day 1) *or*, after exclusion of pregnancy, in midluteal phase (day 21) and continued until down-regulation achieved (usually about 1–3 weeks) then maintained during gonadotrophin administration (stopping gonadotrophin and buserelin on administration of chorionic gonadotrophin at appropriate stage of follicular development)
Intranasally, 150 micrograms (one spray in one nostril) 4 times daily during waking hours (occa-

sionally up to 300 micrograms 4 times daily may be needed) starting in early follicular phase (day 1) *or*, after exclusion of pregnancy, in midluteal phase (day 21) and continued until down-regulation achieved (usually about 2–3 weeks) then maintained during gonadotrophin administration (stopping gonadotrophin and buserelin on administration of chorionic gonadotrophin at appropriate stage of follicular development)

COUNSELLING. Avoid use of nasal decongestants before and for at least 30 minutes after treatment

Suprecur® (Aventis Pharma) PoM
Nasal spray, buserelin (as acetate) 150 micrograms/ metered spray. Net price 2 × 100-dose pack (with metered dose pumps) = £75.43. Counselling, nasal decongestants
Injection, buserelin (as acetate) 1 mg/mL. Net price 5.5-mL vial = £11.85

GOSERELIN

Indications: see under Dose; prostate cancer (section 8.3.4.2); early and advanced breast cancer (section 8.3.4.1)
Cautions: see notes above; polycystic ovarian disease
Contra-indications: see notes above
Side-effects: see notes above; withdrawal bleeding
Dose: *by subcutaneous injection* into anterior abdominal wall, endometriosis, 3.6 mg every 28 days; max. duration of treatment 6 months (do not repeat); endometrial thinning before intra-uterine surgery, 3.6 mg (may be repeated after 28 days if uterus is large or to allow flexible surgical timing); before surgery in women who have anaemia due to uterine fibroids, 3.6 mg every 28 days (with supplementary iron); max. duration of treatment 3 months
Pituitary desensitisation before induction of ovulation by gonadotrophins for *in vitro* fertilisation (under specialist supervision), after exclusion of pregnancy, 3.6 mg to achieve pituitary down-regulation (usually 1–3 weeks) then gonadotrophin is administered (stopping gonadotrophin on administration of chorionic gonadotrophin at appropriate stage of follicular development)

■ Preparation
Section 8.3.4.2

LEUPRORELIN ACETATE

Indications: see under Dose; prostate cancer (section 8.3.4.2)
Cautions: see notes above; family history of osteoporosis; chronic use of other drugs which reduce bone density including alcohol and tobacco; diabetes
Contra-indications: see notes above
Side-effects: see notes above; breast tenderness; nausea, vomiting, diarrhoea, anorexia; fever, chills; sleep disturbances, dizziness, fatigue, leucopenia, thrombocytopenia; altered blood lipids, pulmonary embolism; spinal fracture, paralysis, hypotension and worsening of depression also reported
Dose: *by subcutaneous or intramuscular injection*, endometriosis, 3.75 mg as a single dose in first 5 days of menstrual cycle then every month for max. 6 months (course not to be repeated)

Endometrial thinning before intra-uterine surgery, 3.75 mg as a single dose (given between days 3 and 5 of menstrual cycle) 5–6 weeks before surgery
Reduction of size of uterine fibroids and of associated bleeding before surgery, 3.75 mg as a single dose every month usually for 3–4 months (max. 6 months)

■ Preparation
Section 8.3.4.2

NAFARELIN

Indications: see under Dose
Cautions: see notes above
Contra-indications: see notes above
Side-effects: see notes above; acne
Dose: women over 18 years, endometriosis, 200 micrograms twice daily as one spray in one nostril in the morning and one spray in the other nostril in the evening (starting on days 2–4 of menstruation), max. duration of treatment 6 months (do not repeat)
Pituitary desensitisation before induction of ovulation by gonadotrophins for *in vitro* fertilisation (under specialist supervision), 400 micrograms (one spray in each nostril) twice daily starting in early follicular phase (day 2) or, after exclusion of pregnancy, in midluteal phase (day 21) and continued until down-regulation achieved (usually within 4 weeks) then maintained (usually for 8–12 days) during gonadotrophin administration (stopping gonadotrophin and nafarelin on administration of chorionic gonadotrophin at follicular maturity); discontinue if down-regulation not achieved within 12 weeks

COUNSELLING. Avoid use of nasal decongestants before and for at least 30 minutes after treatment; repeat dose if sneezing occurs during or immediately after administration

Synarel® (Pharmacia) PoM
Nasal spray, nafarelin (as acetate) 200 micrograms/ metered spray. Net price 30-dose unit = £32.28; 60-dose unit = £55.66. Label: 10, patient information leaflet, counselling, see above

TRIPTORELIN

Indications: see under Dose; prostate cancer (section 8.3.4.2)
Cautions: see notes above
Contra-indications: see notes above
Side-effects: see notes above; asthenia
Dose: *by intramuscular injection*, endometriosis and reduction in size of uterine fibroids, 3 mg every 4 weeks starting during the first 5 days of menstrual cycle; for uterine fibroids continue treatment for at least 3 months; max. duration of treatment 6 months (do not repeat)

■ Preparations
Section 8.3.4.2

Breast pain (mastalgia)

Once any serious underlying cause for breast pain has been ruled out, most women will respond to reassurance and reduction in dietary fat; withdrawal of an oral contraceptive or of hormone replacement therapy may help to resolve the pain.

Mild, non-cyclical breast pain is treated with simple analgesics (section 4.7.1); moderate to severe pain, cyclical pain or symptoms that persist for longer than 6 months may require specific drug treatment. **Bromocriptine** (section 6.7.1) is used in the management of breast pain but is associated with unpleasant side-effects; it acts within 2 months.

Danazol (section 6.7.2) is licensed for the relief of severe pain and tenderness in benign fibrocystic breast disease which has not responded to other treatment.

Tamoxifen (section 8.3.4.1) may be a useful adjunct in the treatment of mastalgia [unlicensed indication] especially when symptoms can definitely be related to cyclic oestrogen production; it may be given on the days of the cycle when symptoms are predicted.

Treatment for breast pain should be reviewed after 6 months and continued if necessary. Symptoms recur in about 50% of women within 2 years of withdrawal of therapy but may be less severe.

6.7.3 Metyrapone and trilostane

Metyrapone is a competitive inhibitor of 11β-hydroxylation in the adrenal cortex; the resulting inhibition of cortisol (and to a lesser extent aldosterone) production leads to an increase in ACTH production which, in turn, leads to increased synthesis and release of cortisol precursors. It may be used as a test of anterior pituitary function.

Although most types of *Cushing's syndrome* are treated surgically, that which occasionally accompanies carcinoma of the bronchus is not usually amenable to surgery. Metyrapone has been found helpful in controlling the symptoms of the disease; it is also used in other forms of Cushing's syndrome to prepare the patient for surgery. The dosages used are either low, and tailored to cortisol production, or high, in which case corticosteroid replacement therapy is also needed.

Trilostane reversibly inhibits 3β-hydroxysteroid dehydrogenase/delta 5-4 isomerase in the adrenal cortex; the resulting inhibition of the synthesis of mineralocorticoids and glucocorticoids may be useful in *Cushing's syndrome* and *primary hyperaldosteronism*. Trilostane appears to be less effective than metyrapone for Cushing's syndrome (where it is tailored to corticosteroid production). It also has a minor role in post-menopausal breast cancer that has relapsed following initial oestrogen antagonist therapy (corticosteroid replacement therapy is also required). **Ketoconazole** (section 5.2) is also used by specialists for the management of *Cushing's syndrome* [unlicensed indication].

See also aminoglutethimide (section 8.3.4)

METYRAPONE

Indications: see notes above and under Dose (specialist supervision in hospital)

Cautions: gross hypopituitarism (risk of precipitating acute adrenal failure); hypertension on long-term administration; hypothyroidism or hepatic impairment (delayed response); many drugs interfere with diagnostic estimation of steroids; avoid in porphyria (section 9.8.2)

DRIVING. Drowsiness may affect the performance of skilled tasks (e.g. driving)

Contra-indications: adrenocortical insufficiency (see Cautions); pregnancy (Appendix 4), breast-feeding (Appendix 5)

Side-effects: occasional nausea, vomiting, dizziness, headache, hypotension, sedation; rarely abdominal pain, allergic skin reactions, hypoadrenalism, hirsutism

Dose: differential diagnosis of ACTH-dependent Cushing's syndrome, 750 mg every 4 hours for 6 doses; CHILD 15 mg/kg (minimum 250 mg) every 4 hours for 6 doses

Management of Cushing's syndrome, range 0.25–6 g daily, tailored to cortisol production; see notes above

Resistant oedema due to increased aldosterone secretion in cirrhosis, nephrosis, and congestive heart failure (with glucocorticoid replacement therapy) 3 g daily in divided doses

Metopirone® (Alliance) PoM
Capsules, ivory, metyrapone 250 mg. Net price 100-tab pack = £42.50. Label: 21, counselling, driving

TRILOSTANE

Indications: see notes above and under Dose (specialist supervision)

Cautions: breast cancer (concurrent corticosteroid replacement therapy needed, see under Dose), adrenal cortical hyperfunction (tailored to cortisol and electrolytes, concurrent corticosteroid therapy may be needed, see under Dose); hepatic and renal impairment; **interactions:** Appendix 1 (trilostane)

Contra-indications: pregnancy (use non-hormonal method of contraception) and breast-feeding; children

Side-effects: flushing, tingling and swelling of mouth, rhinorrhoea, nausea, vomiting, diarrhoea, and rashes reported; rarely granulocytopenia

Dose: adrenal cortical hyperfunction, 240 mg daily in divided doses for at least 3 days then tailored according to response with regular monitoring of plasma electrolytes and circulating corticosteroids (both mineralocorticoid and glucocorticoid replacement therapy may be needed); usual dose: 120–480 mg daily (may be increased to 960 mg)

Postmenopausal breast cancer (with glucocorticoid replacement therapy) following relapse to initial oestrogen receptor antagonist therapy, initially 240 mg daily increased every 3 days in steps of 240 mg to a maintenance dose of 960 mg daily (720 mg daily if not tolerated)

Modrenal® (Wanskerne) PoM
Capsules, trilostane 60 mg (pink/black), net price 100-cap pack = £49.50; 120 mg (pink/yellow), 100-cap pack = £98.50. Label: 21

7: Obstetrics, gynaecology, and urinary-tract disorders

For hormonal therapy of gynaecological disorders see section 6.4.1, section 6.5.1 and section 6.7.2.

7.1 Drugs used in obstetrics

7.1.1	Prostaglandins and oxytocics
7.1.2	Mifepristone
7.1.3	Myometrial relaxants

Because of the complexity of dosage regimens in obstetrics, in all cases **detailed specialist literature** should be consulted.

7.1.1 Prostaglandins and oxytocics

Prostaglandins and oxytocics are used to induce abortion or induce or augment labour and to minimise blood loss from the placental site. They include oxytocin, ergometrine, and the prostaglandins. All induce uterine contractions with varying degrees of pain according to the strength of contractions induced.

INDUCTION OF ABORTION. **Gemeprost**, administered vaginally as pessaries is the preferred prostaglandin for the medical induction of late therapeutic abortion. Gemeprost ripens and softens the cervix before surgical abortion, particularly in primigravida. The prostaglandin **misoprostol** is given by mouth or by vaginal administration to induce medical abortion [unlicensed indication]; intravaginal use ripens the cervix before surgical abortion [unlicensed indication]. Extra-amniotic **dinoprostone** is rarely used nowadays.

Pre-treatment with **mifepristone** (section 7.1.2) can facilitate the process of medical abortion. It sensitises the uterus to subsequent administration of a prostaglandin and, therefore, abortion occurs in a shorter time and with a lower dose of prostaglandin.

INDUCTION AND AUGMENTATION OF LABOUR. **Dinoprostone** is available as vaginal tablets, pessaries and vaginal gels for the induction of labour. The intravenous solution is rarely used; it is associated with more side-effects.

Oxytocin (*Syntocinon*®) is administered by slow intravenous infusion, using an infusion pump, to induce or augment labour, usually in conjunction with amniotomy. Uterine activity must be monitored carefully and hyperstimulation avoided. Large doses of oxytocin may result in excessive fluid retention.

Misoprostol is given orally or vaginally for the induction of labour [unlicensed indication].

NICE guidance (induction of labour). NICE has recommended (June 2001) that:

- dinoprostone is preferable to oxytocin for induction of labour in women with intact membranes, regardless of parity or cervical favourability;

- dinoprostone or oxytocin are equally effective for the induction of labour in women with ruptured membranes, regardless of parity or cervical favourability;

- oxytocin should not be started for 6 hours following administration of vaginal prostaglandins;

- when used to induce labour, the recommended dose of oxytocin by intravenous infusion[1] is initially 0.001–0.002 units/minute increased at intervals of at least 30 minutes until a maximum of 3–4 contractions occur every 10 minutes (0.012 units/minute is often adequate); the maximum recommended rate is 0.032 units/minute (licensed max. 0.02 units/minute)

1. Oxytocin should be used in standard dilutions of 10 units/500 mL (infusing 3 mL/hour delivers 0.001 unit/minute) or, for higher doses, 30 units/500 mL (infusing 1 mL/hour delivers 0.001 unit/minute).

PREVENTION AND TREATMENT OF HAEMORRHAGE. Bleeding due to incomplete abortion can be controlled with **ergometrine** and **oxytocin** (*Syntometrine*®) given intramuscularly, the dose is adjusted according to the patient's condition and blood loss. This is commonly used before surgical evacuation of the uterus, particularly when surgery is delayed. Oxytocin and ergometrine combined are more effective in early pregnancy than either drug alone.

For the routine management of the third stage of labour ergometrine 500 micrograms with oxytocin 5 units (*Syntometrine*® 1 mL) is given by intramuscular injection on delivery of the anterior shoulder or, at the latest, immediately after the baby is delivered. If ergometrine is inappropriate (e.g. in pre-eclampsia), oxytocin may be given by intramuscular injection [unlicensed indication].

In excessive uterine bleeding, any placental products remaining in the uterus should be removed. In bleeding caused by uterine atony oxytocic drugs are used in turn as follows:

- oxytocin 5–10 units by intravenous injection
- ergometrine 250–500 micrograms by intravenous injection
- oxytocin 5–30 units in 500 mL infusion fluid given by intravenous infusion at a rate that controls uterine atony

Carboprost has an important role in severe postpartum haemorrhage unresponsive to ergometrine and oxytocin.

Mild secondary postpartum haemorrhage has been treated in domiciliary practice with ergometrine by mouth, but it is rarely used now.

CARBOPROST

Indications: postpartum haemorrhage due to uterine atony in patients unresponsive to ergometrine and oxytocin

Cautions: history of glaucoma or raised intra-ocular pressure, asthma, hypertension, hypotension, anaemia, jaundice, diabetes, epilepsy; uterine scars; excessive dosage may cause uterine rupture; **interactions:** Appendix 1 (prostaglandins)

Contra-indications: untreated pelvic infection; cardiac, renal, pulmonary, or hepatic disease

Side-effects: nausea, vomiting and diarrhoea, hyperthermia and flushing, bronchospasm; less frequent effects include raised blood pressure, dyspnoea, and pulmonary oedema; chills, headache, diaphoresis, dizziness; cardiovascular collapse also reported; erythema and pain at injection site reported

Dose: *by deep intramuscular injection*, 250 micrograms repeated if necessary at intervals of 1½ hours (in severe cases the interval may be reduced but should not be less than 15 minutes); total dose should not exceed 2 mg (8 doses)

Hemabate® (Pharmacia) PoM
Injection, carboprost as trometamol salt (tromethamine salt) 250 micrograms/mL, net price 1-mL amp = £18.20 (hosp. only)

DINOPROSTONE

Indications: see notes above and under preparations below

Cautions: history of asthma, glaucoma and raised intra-ocular pressure; cardiac, hepatic or renal impairment; hypertension; history of epilepsy; uterine scarring; monitor uterine activity and fetal status (particular care if history of uterine hypertony); uterine rupture; see also notes above; effect of oxytocin enhanced (care needed in monitoring uterine activity when used in sequence)—see also under *Propess*® and Appendix 1 (prostaglandins)

Contra-indications: active cardiac, pulmonary, renal or hepatic disease; placenta praevia or unexplained vaginal bleeding during pregnancy; ruptured membranes, major cephalopelvic disproportion or fetal malpresentation, history of caesarean section or major uterine surgery, untreated pelvic infection, fetal distress, grand multiparas and multiple pregnancy, history of difficult or traumatic delivery; avoid extra-amniotic route in cervicitis or vaginitis

Side-effects: nausea, vomiting, diarrhoea; other side-effects include uterine hypertonus, severe uterine contractions, pulmonary or amniotic fluid embolism, abruptio placenta, fetal distress, maternal hypertension, bronchospasm, rapid cervical dilation, fever, backache; uterine hypercontractility with or without fetal bradycardia, low Apgar scores; cardiac arrest, uterine rupture, stillbirth or neonatal death also reported; vaginal symptoms (warmth, irritation, pain); after intravenous administration—flushing, shivering, headache, dizziness, temporary pyrexia and raised white blood cell count; also local tissue reaction and erythema after intravenous administration and possibility of infection after extra-amniotic administration

Dose: see under preparations, below
IMPORTANT. Do not confuse dose of *Prostin E2*® vaginal **gel** with that of *Prostin E2*® vaginal **tablets**—not bioequivalent.

Propess® (Ferring) PoM
Pessaries (within retrieval system), releasing dinoprostone approx. 5 mg over 12 hours. Net price 1-pessary pack = £43.44
Dose: by vagina, cervical ripening and induction of labour at term, 1 pessary inserted high into posterior fornix; if cervical ripening insufficient, remove pessary 8–12 hours later and replace with a second pessary (which should also be removed not more than 12 hours later); max. 2 consecutive pessaries
IMPORTANT. Effect of oxytocin enhanced—particular care needed to monitor uterine activity when oxytocin used in sequence (remove pessary beforehand)

Prostin E2® (Pharmacia) PoM
Intravenous solution ▬, for dilution and use as an infusion, dinoprostone 1 mg/mL, net price 0.75-mL amp = £8.52; 10 mg/mL, 0.5-mL amp = £18.40 (both hosp. only; rarely used, consult product literature for dose and indications)
Extra-amniotic solution ▬, dinoprostone 10 mg/mL. Net price 0.5-mL amp (with diluent) = £18.40 (hosp. only; less commonly used nowadays, consult product literature for dose and indications)
Vaginal gel, dinoprostone 400 micrograms/mL, net price 2.5 mL (1 mg) = £15.25; 800 micrograms/mL, 2.5 mL (2 mg) = £16.80
Dose: by vagina, induction of labour, inserted high into posterior fornix (avoid administration into cervical canal), 1 mg (unfavourable primigravida 2 mg), followed after 6 hours by 1–2 mg if required; max. [gel] 3 mg (unfavourable primigravida 4 mg)
Vaginal tablets, dinoprostone 3 mg. Net price 8-vaginal tab pack = £78.05
Dose: by vagina, induction of labour, inserted high into posterior fornix, 3 mg, followed after 6–8 hours by 3 mg if labour is not established; max. 6 mg [vaginal tablets]
NOTE. *Prostin E2 Vaginal Gel* and *Vaginal Tablets* are **not** bioequivalent

---

ERGOMETRINE MALEATE

Indications: see notes above
Cautions: cardiac disease, hypertension, hepatic, and renal impairment, multiple pregnancy; porphyria (section 9.8.2); **interactions:** Appendix 1 (ergot alkaloids)
Contra-indications: induction of labour, first and second stages of labour, vascular disease, severe cardiac disease, severe hepatic and renal impairment, sepsis, severe hypertension, eclampsia
Side-effects: nausea, vomiting, headache, dizziness, tinnitus, abdominal pain, chest pain, palpitation, dyspnoea, bradycardia, transient hypertension, vasoconstriction, stroke, myocardial infarction and pulmonary oedema also reported
Dose: see notes above

Ergometrine (Non-proprietary) PoM
Tablets ▬, ergometrine maleate 500 micrograms, net price 21-tab pack = £25.00
Available from IVAX, Celltech
Injection, ergometrine maleate 500 micrograms/mL. Net price 1-mL amp = 60p
Available from Antigen, Phoenix

■ With oxytocin
Syntometrine® (Alliance) PoM
Injection, ergometrine maleate 500 micrograms, oxytocin 5 units/mL. Net price 1-mL amp = £1.38
Dose: by intramuscular injection, 1 mL; by intravenous injection, no longer recommended

GEMEPROST

Indications: see under Dose
Cautions: obstructive airways disease, cardiovascular insufficiency, raised intra-ocular pressure, cervicitis or vaginitis; **interactions:** Appendix 1 (prostaglandins)
IMPORTANT. For warnings relating to use of gemeprost in a patient undergoing induction of abortion with mifepristone, see under Mifepristone and Note below
Contra-indications: unexplained vaginal bleeding
Side-effects: vaginal bleeding and uterine pain; nausea, vomiting, or diarrhoea; headache, muscle weakness, dizziness, flushing, chills, backache, dyspnoea, chest pain, palpitations and mild pyrexia; uterine rupture reported (most commonly in multiparas or if history of uterine surgery or if given with intravenous oxytocics); also reported severe hypotension, coronary artery spasm and myocardial infarction
Dose: *by vagina* in pessaries, softening and dilation of the cervix to facilitate transcervical operative procedures in first trimester, inserted into posterior fornix, 1 mg 3 hours before surgery
Second trimester abortion, inserted into posterior fornix, 1 mg every 3 hours for max. of 5 administrations; second course may begin 24 hours after start of treatment (if treatment fails pregnancy should be terminated by another method)
Second trimester intra-uterine death, inserted into posterior fornix, 1 mg every 3 hours for max. of 5 administrations only; monitor for coagulopathy
NOTE. If used in combination with mifepristone, carefully monitor blood pressure and pulse for 6 hours

Gemeprost (Non-proprietary) PoM
Pessaries, gemeprost 1 mg. Net price 5-pessary pack = £215.00
Available from Beacon

OXYTOCIN

Indications: see under Dose and notes above
Cautions: particular caution needed when given for *induction or enhancement of labour* in presence of borderline cephalopelvic disproportion (avoid if significant), mild or moderate pregnancy-induced hypertension or cardiac disease, women over 35 years or with history of lower-uterine segment caesarean section (see also under Contra-indications below); if fetal death *in utero* or meconium-stained amniotic fluid avoid tumultuous labour (may cause amniotic fluid embolism); water intoxication and hyponatraemia—avoid large infusion volumes and restrict fluid intake (see also Appendix 6); effects enhanced by concomitant prostaglandins (very careful monitoring), caudal block anaesthesia (may enhance hypertensive effects of sympathomimetic vasopressors), see also **interactions:** Appendix 1 (oxytocin)
Contra-indications: hypertonic uterine contractions, mechanical obstruction to delivery, fetal distress; any condition where spontaneous labour or vaginal delivery inadvisable (e.g. significant cephalopelvic disproportion, malpresentation, placenta praevia, vasa praevia, placental abruption, cord presentation or prolapse, predisposition to uterine rupture as in multiple pregnancy, polyhydramnios, grand multiparity and presence of uterine scar from major surgery—including caesarean section); avoid prolonged administration in

oxytocin-resistant uterine inertia, severe pre-eclamptic toxaemia or severe cardiovascular disease

Side-effects: uterine spasm (may occur at low doses), uterine hyperstimulation (usually with excessive doses—may cause fetal distress, asphyxia and death, or may lead to hypertonicity, tetanic contractions, soft-tissue damage or uterine rupture); water intoxication and hyponatraemia associated with high doses with large infusion volumes of electrolyte-free fluid (see also under Dose below); also nausea, vomiting, arrhythmias; rashes and anaphylactoid reactions (with dyspnoea, hypotension or shock) also reported; placental abruption and amniotic fluid embolism also reported on overdose

Dose: induction of labour for medical reasons or stimulation of labour in hypotonic uterine inertia, *by intravenous infusion*, see NICE guidance above; do not use total of more than 5 units in any one day (may be repeated the following day starting again at 0.001–0.002 units/minute)

IMPORTANT. Careful monitoring of fetal heart rate and uterine motility essential for dose titration (never give intravenous bolus injection during labour); discontinue immediately in uterine hyperactivity or fetal distress

Caesarean section, *by slow intravenous injection* immediately after delivery, 5 units

Prevention of postpartum haemorrhage, after delivery of placenta, *by slow intravenous injection*, 5 units (if infusion used for induction or enhancement of labour, increase rate during third stage and for next few hours)

NOTE. May be given in a dose of 10 units by intramuscular injection [unlicensed route] instead of oxytocin with ergometrine (*Syntometrine*®), see notes above

Treatment of postpartum haemorrhage, *by slow intravenous injection*, 5–10 units, followed in severe cases *by intravenous infusion* of 5–30 units in 500 mL infusion fluid at a rate sufficient to control uterine atony

IMPORTANT. Avoid rapid intravenous injection (may cause short-lasting drop in blood pressure); prolonged administration, see warning below

Incomplete, inevitable or missed abortion, *by slow intravenous injection*, 5 units followed if necessary *by intravenous infusion*, 0.02–0.04 units/minute or faster

IMPORTANT. Prolonged intravenous administration at high doses with large volume of fluid (as possible in inevitable or missed abortion or postpartum haemorrhage) may cause water intoxication with hyponatraemia. To avoid: use electrolyte-containing diluent (i.e. not glucose), increase oxytocin concentration to reduce fluid, restrict fluid intake by mouth; monitor fluid and electrolytes

NOTE. Oxytocin doses in the BNF may differ from those in the product literature

Syntocinon® (Alliance) [PoM]
Injection, oxytocin, net price 5 units/mL, 1-mL amp = £1.23; 10 units/mL, 1-mL amp = £1.40

■ With ergometrine
See Syntometrine®, p. 380

7.1.1.1   Ductus arteriosus

Maintenance of patency

Alprostadil (prostaglandin E₁) is used to maintain patency of the ductus arteriosus in neonates with congenital heart defects, prior to corrective surgery in centres where intensive care is immediately available.

ALPROSTADIL

Indications: congenital heart defects in neonates prior to corrective surgery; erectile dysfunction (section 7.4.5)

Cautions: see notes above; history of haemorrhage, avoid in hyaline membrane disease, monitor arterial pressure; **interactions:** Appendix 1 (alprostadil)

Side-effects: apnoea (particularly in infants under 2 kg), flushing, bradycardia, hypotension, tachycardia, cardiac arrest, oedema, diarrhoea, fever, convulsions, disseminated intravascular coagulation, hypokalaemia; cortical proliferation of long bones, weakening of the wall of the ductus arteriosus and pulmonary artery may follow prolonged use; gastric-outlet obstruction reported

Dose: *by intravenous infusion*, initially 50–100 nanograms/kg/minute, then decreased to lowest effective dose

Prostin VR® (Pharmacia) [PoM]
Intravenous solution, alprostadil 500 micrograms/mL in alcohol. For dilution and use as an infusion. Net price 1-mL amp = £75.19 (hosp. only)

Closure of ductus arteriosus

Indometacin (indomethacin) is used to close a patent ductus arteriosus in premature babies, probably by inhibiting prostaglandin synthesis.

INDOMETACIN
(Indomethacin)

Indications: patent ductus arteriosus in premature babies (under specialist supervision in neonatal intensive care unit); rheumatoid disease (section 10.1.1)

Cautions: may mask symptoms of infection; may reduce urine output by 50% or more (monitor carefully—see also under Anuria or Oliguria, below) and precipitate renal impairment especially if extracellular volume depleted, heart failure, sepsis, or hepatic impairment, or if receiving nephrotoxic drugs; may induce hyponatraemia; monitor renal function and electrolytes; inhibition of platelet aggregation (monitor for bleeding); **interactions:** Appendix 1 (NSAIDs)

ANURIA OR OLIGURIA. If anuria or marked oliguria (urinary output less than 0.6 mL/kg/hour) at time of scheduled second or third dose, delay until renal function returns to normal

Contra-indications: untreated infection, bleeding (especially with active intracranial haemorrhage or gastro-intestinal bleeding); thrombocytopenia, coagulation defects, necrotising enterocolitis, renal impairment

Side-effects: include haemorrhagic, renal, gastro-intestinal, metabolic, and coagulation disorders; pulmonary hypertension, intracranial bleeding, fluid retention, and exacerbation of infection

Dose: *by intravenous injection*, over 20–30 minutes (using a suitable syringe driver), 3 doses at intervals of 12–24 hours (provided urine output remains adequate), age less than 48 hours, 200 micrograms/kg then 100 micrograms/kg then

100 micrograms/kg; age 2–7 days, 200 micrograms/kg then 200 micrograms/kg then 200 micrograms/kg; age over 7 days, 200 micrograms/kg then 250 micrograms/kg then 250 micrograms/kg; solution prepared with 1–2 mL sodium chloride 0.9% or water for injections (not glucose and no preservatives)

If ductus arteriosus reopens a second course of 3 injections may be given 48 hours after first course

Indocid PDA® (MSD) PoM
Injection, powder for reconstitution, indometacin (as sodium trihydrate). Net price 3 × 1-mg vials = £22.50 (hosp. only)

7.1.2   Mifepristone

Mifepristone, an antiprogestogenic steroid, sensitises the myometrium to prostaglandin-induced contractions and it softens and dilates the cervix. For the termination of pregnancy, a single dose of mifepristone is followed by vaginal administration of the prostaglandin gemeprost. Although the licensed dose of mifepristone is 600 mg, there is evidence that lower doses are effective for medical abortion in pregnancy of up to 20 weeks' gestation. The Royal College of Obstetricians and Gynaecologists' guidelines for both early and mid-trimester medical abortions include the following [unlicensed] regimens:

- For gestation up to 7 weeks (and as an option for gestation of 7–9 weeks), mifepristone 200 mg by mouth followed 36 hours later by gemeprost 500 micrograms by vagina
- For mid-trimester medical abortion (gestation up to 20 weeks), mifepristone 200 mg by mouth followed 36 hours later by gemeprost 1 mg every 6 hours by vagina

MIFEPRISTONE

Indications: see under dose

Cautions: asthma (avoid if severe); haemorrhagic disorders and anticoagulant therapy; prosthetic heart valve or history of endocarditis (prophylaxis recommended, see section 5.1 table 2); smokers aged over 35 years (increased risk of cardiovascular events); adrenal suppression (may require corticosteroid); not recommended in hepatic or renal impairment; breast-feeding (Appendix 5); avoid aspirin and NSAIDs for analgesia; **interactions:** Appendix 1 (mifepristone)

IMPORTANT. For warnings relating to use of gemeprost in a patient undergoing induction of abortion with mifepristone, see under Gemeprost

Contra-indications: uncontrolled severe asthma; suspected ectopic pregnancy (use other specific means of termination); chronic adrenal failure, porphyria (section 9.8.2)

Side-effects: vaginal bleeding (sometimes severe) may occur between administration of mifepristone and surgery, and rarely abortion may occur before surgery; malaise, faintness, headache, nausea, vomiting, rashes; uterine pain after gemeprost (may be severe and require parenteral opioids)

Dose: medical termination of intra-uterine pregnancy of up to 63 days gestation, *by mouth*, mifepristone 600 mg as a single dose under medical supervision, followed 36–48 hours later (unless abortion already complete) by gemeprost

1 mg *by vagina* and observed for at least 6 hours (or until bleeding or pain at acceptable level) with follow-up visit 10–14 days later to verify complete expulsion (if treatment fails essential that pregnancy be terminated by another method)

Softening and dilatation of cervix before mechanical cervical dilatation for termination of pregnancy, 36–48 hours before procedure, *by mouth*, mifepristone 600 mg as a single dose under medical supervision

Termination of pregnancy of 13–24 weeks gestation (in combination with gemeprost), *by mouth*, mifepristone 600 mg as a single dose under medical supervision followed 36–48 hours later by gemeprost 1 mg *by vagina* every 3 hours up to max. 5 mg; if abortion does not occur, 24 hours after start of treatment repeat course of gemeprost 1 mg *by vagina* up to max. 5 mg (if treatment fails pregnancy should be terminated by another method); follow-up visit after appropriate interval to assess vaginal bleeding recommended

NOTE. Careful monitoring essential for 6 hours after administration of gemeprost pessary (risk of profound hypotension)

Labour induction in fetal death *in utero*, *by mouth*, mifepristone 600 mg daily as a single dose for 2 days under medical supervision; if labour not started within 72 hours of first dose, another method should be used

Mifegyne® (Exelgyn) PoM
Tablets, yellow, mifepristone 200 mg. Net price 3-tab pack = £41.83 (supplied to NHS hospitals and premises approved under Abortion Act 1967).
Label: 10, patient information leaflet

7.1.3   Myometrial relaxants

Beta₂ agonists (beta₂-sympathomimetics, beta₂-adrenoceptor stimulants) relax uterine muscle and are used in selected cases to inhibit *premature delivery*.

Beta₂ agonists are indicated for the inhibition of *uncomplicated* premature labour *between 24 and 33 weeks* of gestation and they may permit a delay in delivery of at least 48 hours; no statistically significant effect on perinatal mortality has as yet been observed. The greatest benefit is gained by using the delay to administer corticosteroid therapy (with care to avoid fluid overload) or to implement other measures which improve perinatal health (including transfer to a unit with neonatal intensive care facility). Prolonged therapy should be avoided since risks to the mother (see under Ritodrine Hydrochloride, below) increase after 48 hours and there is a lack of evidence of benefit from further treatment; oral therapy following initial parenteral treatment is therefore not recommended.

The oxytocin receptor antagonist, **atosiban**, is also licensed for the inhibition of *uncomplicated* premature labour *between 24 and 33 weeks* of gestation. Atosiban has fewer side-effects than other licensed myometrial relaxants and may be useful when a beta₂ agonist is not appropriate e.g. in cardiac disease.

Indometacin (indomethacin) (section 10.1.1), a cyclo-oxygenase inhibitor, also inhibits labour [unlicensed indication] and it may be useful in situations where a beta₂ agonist is not appropriate; however, there are concerns about neonatal complications such as transient impairment of renal function and premature closure of ductus arteriosus.

ATOSIBAN

Indications: uncomplicated premature labour (see notes above)

Cautions: monitor blood loss after delivery; intrauterine growth retardation; hepatic and renal impairment

Contra-indications: eclampsia and severe preeclampsia, intra-uterine infection, intra-uterine fetal death, antepartum haemorrhage (requiring immediate delivery), placenta praevia, abruptio placenta, intra-uterine growth retardation with abnormal fetal heart rate, premature rupture of membranes after 30 weeks' gestation

Side-effects: nausea, vomiting, tachycardia, hypotension, headache, dizziness, hot flushes, hyperglycaemia, injection site reaction; less commonly pruritus, rash, fever, insomnia

Dose: *by intravenous injection*, initially 6.75 mg over 1 minute, then *by intravenous infusion* 18 mg/hour for 3 hours, then 6 mg/hour for up to 45 hours; max. duration of treatment 48 hours

Tractocile® (Ferring) ▼ PoM
Injection, atosiban (as acetate) 7.5 mg/mL, net price 0.9-mL (6.75-mg) vial = £20.00
Concentrate for intravenous infusion, atosiban (as acetate) 7.5 mg/mL, net price 5-mL vial = £55.00

RITODRINE HYDROCHLORIDE

Indications: uncomplicated premature labour (see notes above)

Cautions: suspected cardiac disease (physician experienced in cardiology to assess), hypertension, hyperthyroidism, hypokalaemia (special risk with potassium-depleting diuretics), diabetes mellitus (closely monitor blood glucose during intravenous treatment); mild to moderate pre-eclampsia, monitor blood pressure and pulse rate (should not exceed 140 beats per minute) and avoid overhydration (Appendix 6); **important:** closely monitor state of hydration (discontinue immediately and institute diuretic therapy if pulmonary oedema occurs); concomitant beta-blocker treatment; drugs likely to enhance sympathomimetic side-effects or induce arrhythmias, see also **interactions**, Appendix 1 (sympathomimetics *and* sympathomimetics, beta₂)

Contra-indications: cardiac disease, eclampsia and severe pre-eclampsia, intra-uterine infection, intra-uterine fetal death, antepartum haemorrhage (requires immediate delivery), placenta praevia, cord compression

Side-effects: nausea, vomiting, flushing, sweating, tremor; hypokalaemia, tachycardia, palpitations, and hypotension (left lateral position throughout infusion to minimise risk), uterine bleeding (may be reversed with a non-selective beta-blocker); pulmonary oedema (see below and under Cautions); chest pain or tightness (with or without ECG changes) and arrhythmias reported; salivary gland enlargement also reported; on prolonged administration (several weeks) leucopenia and agranulocytosis reported; liver function abnormalities (including increased transaminases and hepatitis) reported

Dose: *by intravenous infusion* (**important:** minimum fluid volume, see below), initially 50 micrograms/minute, increased gradually according to response by 50 micrograms/minute every 10 minutes until contractions stop or maternal heart rate reaches 140 beats per minute; continue for 12–48 hours after contractions cease (usual rate 150–350 micrograms/minute); max. rate 350 micrograms/minute; or *by intramuscular injection*, 10 mg every 3–8 hours continued for 12–48 hours after contractions have ceased; then *by mouth* (but see notes above), 10 mg 30 minutes before termination of intravenous infusion, repeated every 2 hours for 24 hours, followed by 10–20 mg every 4–6 hours, max. oral dose 120 mg daily

IMPORTANT. Manufacturer states that although *fatal pulmonary oedema* associated with ritodrine infusion is almost certainly multifactorial in origin evidence suggests that **fluid overload** may be the most important single factor. The volume of infusion should therefore be kept to a minimum; for further guidance see Appendix 6. For specific guidance on infusion rates, consult product literature

Yutopar® (Durbin) PoM
Tablets▭, yellow, scored, ritodrine hydrochloride 10 mg. Net price 90-tab pack = £25.55
Injection, ritodrine hydrochloride 10 mg/mL. Net price 5-mL amp = £2.98

SALBUTAMOL

Indications: uncomplicated premature labour (see notes above); asthma (section 3.1.1)

Cautions: see under Ritodrine Hydrochloride; **interactions:** Appendix 1 (sympathomimetics, beta₂)

Contra-indications: see under Ritodrine Hydrochloride

Side-effects: see under Ritodrine Hydrochloride; headache, rarely muscle cramps; hypersensitivity reactions including bronchospasm, urticaria, and angioedema reported

Dose: *by intravenous infusion*, initially 10 micrograms/minute, rate increased gradually according to response at 10-minute intervals until contractions diminish then increase rate slowly until contractions cease (max. rate 45 micrograms/minute); maintain rate for 1 hour after contractions have stopped, then gradually reduce by 50% every 6 hours; then *by mouth* (but see notes above), 4 mg every 6–8 hours

■ Preparations
Section 3.1.1.1

TERBUTALINE SULPHATE

Indications: uncomplicated premature labour (see notes above); asthma (section 3.1.1)

Cautions: see under Ritodrine Hydrochloride; **interactions:** Appendix 1 (sympathomimetics, beta₂)

Contra-indications: see under Ritodrine Hydrochloride

Side-effects: see under Ritodrine Hydrochloride

Dose: *by intravenous infusion*, 5 micrograms/minute for 20 minutes, increased every 20 minutes in steps of 2.5 micrograms/minute until contractions have ceased (more than 10 micrograms/minute should **seldom** be given—20 micrograms/minute should **not** be exceeded), continue for 1 hour then decrease every 20 minutes in steps of 2.5 micrograms/minute to lowest dose that maintains suppression, continue at this level for 12 hours then *by mouth* (but see notes above), 5 mg every 8 hours for as long as is desirable to prolong pregnancy (or alternatively follow the *intravenous infusion* by *subcutaneous injection* 250 micrograms every 6 hours for a few days then *by mouth* as above)

▪ Preparations
Section 3.1.1.1

7.2 Treatment of vaginal and vulval conditions

7.2.1 Preparations for vaginal atrophy
7.2.2 Anti-infective drugs

Symptoms are primarily referable to the vulva, but infections almost invariably involve the vagina which should also be treated. Applications to the vulva alone are likely to give only symptomatic relief without cure.

Aqueous medicated douches may disturb normal vaginal acidity and bacterial flora.

Topical anaesthetic agents give only symptomatic relief and may cause sensitivity reactions. They are indicated only in cases of pruritus where specific local causes have been excluded.

Systemic drugs are required in the treatment of infections such as gonorrhoea and syphilis (section 5.1).

7.2.1 Preparations for vaginal atrophy

Topical HRT

Application of cream containing an oestrogen may be used on a short-term basis to improve the quality of the vaginal epithelium in *menopausal atrophic vaginitis*. It is **important** to bear in mind that topical oestrogens should be used in the **minimum effective** amount to minimise systemic effects. Modified-release vaginal tablets and an impregnated vaginal ring are now also available.

The risk of endometrial hyperplasia and carcinoma is increased when *systemic* oestrogens are administered alone for prolonged periods. The endometrial safety of long-term or repeated use of *topical* vaginal oestrogens is uncertain; treatment should be reviewed at least annually, with special consideration given to any symptoms of endometrial hyperplasia or carcinoma.

Topical oestrogens are also used before vaginal surgery in postmenopausal women for prolapse when there is epithelial atrophy.

For a general comment on hormone replacement therapy, including the role of topical oestrogens, see section 6.4.1.1.

OESTROGENS, TOPICAL

Indications: see notes above
Cautions: see Oestrogens for HRT (section 6.4.1.1); interrupt treatment periodically to assess need for continued treatment
Contra-indications: see Oestrogens for HRT (section 6.4.1.1); pregnancy and breast-feeding
Side-effects: see Oestrogens for HRT (section 6.4.1.1); local irritation

Ortho-Gynest® (Janssen-Cilag) PoM
Intravaginal cream, estriol 0.01%. Net price 80 g with applicator = £2.72
Excipients: include arachis (peanut) oil
Condoms: damages latex condoms and diaphragms
Dose: insert 1 applicatorful daily, preferably in evening; reduced to 1 applicatorful twice a week; attempts to reduce or discontinue should be made at 3–6 month intervals with re-examination
Pessaries, estriol 500 micrograms. Net price 15 pessaries = £5.29
Excipients: include butylated hydroxytoluene
Condoms: damages latex condoms and diaphragms
Dose: insert 1 pessary daily, preferably in the evening, until improvement occurs; maintenance 1 pessary twice a week; attempts to reduce or discontinue should be made at 3–6 month intervals with re-examination

Ovestin® (Organon) PoM
Intravaginal cream, estriol 0.1%. Net price 15 g with applicator = £4.98
Excipients: include cetyl alcohol, polysorbates, stearyl alcohol
Condoms: effect on latex condoms and diaphragms not yet known
Dose: insert 1 applicator-dose daily for 2–3 weeks, then reduce to twice a week (discontinue every 2–3 months for 4 weeks to assess need for further treatment); vaginal surgery, 1 applicator-dose daily for 2 weeks before surgery, resuming 2 weeks after surgery

Premarin® (Wyeth) PoM
Vaginal cream, conjugated oestrogens (equine) 625 micrograms/g. Net price 42.5 g with calibrated applicator = £2.19
Excipients: include cetyl alcohol, propylene glycol
Condoms: effect on latex condoms and diaphragms not yet known
Dose: insert 1–2 g daily, starting on day 5 of cycle (or at any time if cycles have ceased), for 3 weeks, repeated after a 1-week interval

Vagifem® (Novo Nordisk) PoM
Vaginal tablets, f/c, m/r, estradiol 25 micrograms in disposable applicators. Net price 15-applicator pack = £6.62
Excipients: none as listed in section 13.1.3
Condoms: no evidence of damage to latex condoms and diaphragms
Dose: insert 1 tablet daily for 2 weeks then reduce to 1 tablet twice weekly; discontinue after 3 months to assess need for further treatment

▪ Vaginal ring
Estring® (Pharmacia) PoM
Vaginal ring, releasing estradiol approx. 7.5 micrograms/24 hours. Net price 1-ring pack = £31.42.
Label: 10, patient information leaflet
Dose: for postmenopausal urogenital conditions (not suitable for vasomotor symptoms or osteoporosis prophylaxis), to be inserted into upper third of vagina and worn continuously; replace after 3 months; max. duration of continuous treatment 2 years

Non-hormonal preparations

Non-hormonal vaginal preparations include *Replens MD*® NHS which has an acid pH and provides a high moisture content for up to 3 days, and *Sen-selle*® NHS which is a water-based lubricant.

See section 7.2.2 for the pH-modifying preparation *Aci-jel*®.

7.2.2 Anti-infective drugs

Effective specific treatments are available for the common vaginal infections.

Fungal infections

Candidal vulvitis can be treated locally with cream but is almost invariably associated with vaginal infection which should also be treated. *Vaginal candidiasis* is treated primarily with antifungal pessaries or cream inserted high into the vagina (including during menstruation). Single-dose preparations offer an advantage when compliance is a problem. Local irritation may occur on application of vaginal antifungal products

Imidazole drugs (clotrimazole, econazole, fenticonazole, and miconazole) are effective in short courses of 3 to 14 days according to the preparation used. Vaginal applications may be supplemented with antifungal cream for vulvitis and to treat other superficial sites of infection.

Nystatin is a well established antifungal drug. One or two pessaries are inserted for 14 to 28 nights; a cream is also used in cases of vulvitis and infection of other superficial sites. Nystatin stains clothing yellow.

Oral treatment of vaginal infection with fluconazole or itraconazole (section 5.2) is also effective; oral ketoconazole has been associated with fatal hepatotoxicity (see section 5.2 for CSM warning).

RECURRENT VULVOVAGINAL CANDIDIASIS. Recurrence is particularly likely if there are predisposing factors such as antibacterial therapy, pregnancy, diabetes mellitus and possibly oral contraceptive use. Possible reservoirs of infection may also lead to recontamination and should be treated; these include other skin sites such as the digits, nail beds, and umbilicus as well as the gastro-intestinal tract and the bladder. The partner may also be the source of re-infection and, if symptomatic, should be treated with cream at the same time.

Treatment against candida may need to be extended for 6 months in recurrent vulvovaginal candidiasis. Some recommended regimens [all unlicensed] include:

- fluconazole (section 5.2) by mouth 100 mg (as a single dose) every week for 6 months
- clotrimazole vaginally 500-mg pessary (as a single dose) every week for 6 months
- itraconazole (section 5.2) by mouth 400 mg (as 2 divided doses on one day) every month for 6 months.

PREPARATIONS FOR VAGINAL AND VULVAL CANDIDIASIS

Side-effects: occasional local irritation

Clotrimazole (Non-proprietary)
Cream (topical), clotrimazole 1%, net price 20 g = £1.77, 50 g = £3.80
Condoms: effect on latex condoms and diaphragms not yet known
Dose: apply to anogenital area 2–3 times daily
Available from Akita (*Candiden*®), APS, Ashbourne (*Abtrim*®), PLIVA, Generics
Pessary, clotrimazole 500 mg, net price 1 pessary with applicator = £3.43
Dose: insert 1 at night as a single dose
Available from Akita (*Candiden*®), APS, Ashbourne (*Abtrim*®), Tillomed

Canesten® (Bayer Consumer Care)
Cream (topical), clotrimazole 1%. Net price 20 g = £2.14; 50 g = £3.80
Excipients: include benzyl alcohol, cetostearyl alcohol, polysorbates
Condoms: damages latex condoms and diaphragms
Dose: apply to anogenital area 2–3 times daily
Thrush Cream (topical), clotrimazole 2%, net price 20 g = £3.02
Excipients: include benzyl alcohol, cetostearyl alcohol, polysorbates
Condoms: damages latex condoms and diaphragms
Dose: apply to anogenital area 2–3 times daily
Vaginal cream (10% VC®) PoM, clotrimazole 10%. Net price 5-g applicator pack = £4.50
Excipients: include benzyl alcohol, cetostearyl alcohol, polysorbates
Condoms: damages latex condoms and diaphragms
Dose: insert 5 g at night as a single dose; may be repeated once if necessary
NOTE. Available for sale to the public as *Canesten*®*Once*
Pessaries, clotrimazole 100 mg, net price 6 pessaries with applicator = £3.62; 200 mg, 3 pessaries with applicator = £3.89
Condoms: damages latex condoms and diaphragms
Dose: insert 200 mg for 3 nights *or* 100 mg for 6 nights
Pessary, clotrimazole 500 mg. Net price 1 with applicator = £3.48
Excipients: none as listed in section 13.1.3
Condoms: damages latex condoms and diaphragms
Dose: insert 1 at night as a single dose
Combi, clotrimazole 500-mg pessary and cream (topical) 2%. Net price 1 pessary and 10 g cream = £4.95
Condoms: damages latex condoms and diaphragms

Ecostatin® (Squibb)
Cream (topical), econazole nitrate 1%. Net price 15 g = £1.49; 30 g = £2.75
Excipients: include butylated hydroxyanisole, fragrance
Condoms: damages latex condoms and diaphragms
Dose: apply to anogenital area twice daily
Pessaries PoM, econazole nitrate 150 mg. Net price 3 with applicator = £3.35
Excipients: none as listed in section 13.1.3
Condoms: damages latex condoms and diaphragms
Dose: insert 1 pessary for 3 nights
Pessary (Ecostatin 1®) PoM, econazole nitrate 150 mg, formulated for single-dose therapy. Net price 1 pessary with applicator = £3.35
Excipients: none as listed in section 13.1.3
Condoms: damages latex condoms and diaphragms
Dose: insert 1 pessary at night as a single dose
Twinpack PoM, econazole nitrate 150-mg pessaries and cream 1%. Net price 3 pessaries and 15 g cream = £4.35
Condoms: damages latex condoms and diaphragms

Gyno-Daktarin® (Janssen-Cilag) PoM
Intravaginal cream, miconazole nitrate 2%. Net price 78 g with applicators = £4.95
Excipients: include butylated hydroxyanisole
Condoms: damages latex condoms and diaphragms
Dose: insert 5-g applicatorful once daily for 10–14 days *or* twice daily for 7 days; *topical,* apply to anogenital area twice daily

Pessaries, miconazole nitrate 100 mg. Net price 14 = £3.35
Excipients: none as listed in section 13.1.3
Condoms: damages latex condoms and diaphragms
Dose: insert 1 pessary daily for 14 days or 1 pessary twice daily for 7 days
Combipack, miconazole nitrate 100-mg pessaries and cream (topical) 2%. Net price 14 pessaries and 15 g cream = £4.35
Condoms: damages latex condoms and diaphragms
Ovule (= vaginal capsule) (*Gyno-Daktarin 1*®), miconazole nitrate 1.2 g in a fatty basis. Net price 1 ovule (with finger stall) = £3.35
Excipients: include hydroxybenzoates (parabens)
Condoms: damages latex condoms and diaphragms
Dose: insert 1 ovule at night as a single dose

Gyno-Pevaryl® (Janssen-Cilag)
Cream, econazole nitrate 1%. Net price 15 g = £1.50; 30 g = £3.45
Excipients: none as listed in section 13.1.3
Condoms: damages latex condoms and diaphragms
Dose: insert 5-g applicatorful intravaginally and apply to vulva at night for at least 14 nights
Pessaries, econazole nitrate 150 mg. Net price 3 pessaries = £3.17
Excipients: none as listed in section 13.1.3
Condoms: damages latex condoms and diaphragms
Dose: insert 1 pessary for 3 nights
Pessary (*Gyno-Pevaryl 1*®), econazole nitrate 150 mg, formulated for single-dose therapy. Net price 1 pessary with applicator = £3.37
Excipients: none as listed in section 13.1.3
Condoms: damages latex condoms and diaphragms
Dose: insert 1 pessary at night as a single dose
Combipack, econazole nitrate 150-mg pessaries, econazole nitrate 1% cream. Net price 3 pessaries and 15 g cream = £4.35
Condoms: damages latex condoms and diaphragms
CP pack (*Gyno-Pevaryl 1*®), econazole nitrate 150-mg pessary, econazole nitrate 1% cream. Net price 1 pessary and 15 g cream = £4.35
Condoms: damages latex condoms and diaphragms

Lomexin® (Akita) [PoM]
Pessaries, fenticonazole nitrate 200 mg, net price 3 pessaries = £2.83; 600 mg, 1 pessary = £2.83
Excipients: include hydroxybenzoates (parabens)
Condoms: damages latex condoms and diaphragms
Dose: insert 600 mg for 1 night *or* 200 mg for 3 nights

Nizoral® (Janssen-Cilag) [PoM]
Cream (topical), ketoconazole 2%. Net price 30 g = £3.81
Excipients: include polysorbates, propylene glycol, stearyl alcohol
Dose: apply to anogenital area once or twice daily

Nystan® (Squibb) [PoM]
Cream and *Ointment,* see section 13.10.2
Vaginal cream, nystatin 100 000 units/4-g application. Net price 60 g with applicator = £2.77
Excipients: include benzyl alcohol, propylene glycol
Condoms: damages latex condoms and diaphragms
Dose: insert 1–2 applicatorfuls at night for at least 14 nights
Pessaries, yellow, nystatin 100 000 units. Net price 28-pessary pack = £1.96
Excipients: none as listed in section 13.1.3
Condoms: no evidence of damage to latex condoms and diaphragms
Dose: insert 1–2 pessaries at night for at least 14 nights

Pevaryl® (Janssen-Cilag)
Cream, econazole nitrate 1%. Net price 30 g = £2.65
Excipients: include butylated hydroxyanisole, fragrance
Condoms: effect on latex condoms and diaphragms not yet known
Dose: apply to anogenital area twice daily

Other infections

Vaginal preparations intended to restore normal acidity (*Aci-Jel*®) may prevent recurrence of vaginal infections and permit the re-establishment of the normal vaginal flora.

Trichomonal infections commonly involve the lower urinary tract as well as the genital system and need systemic treatment with metronidazole or tinidazole (section 5.1.11).

Bacterial infections with Gram-negative organisms are particularly common in association with gynaecological operations and trauma. Metronidazole is effective against certain Gram-negative organisms, especially *Bacteroides* spp. and may be used prophylactically in gynaecological surgery.

Topical vaginal products containing povidone–iodine can be used to treat vaginitis due to candidal, trichomonal, non-specific or mixed infections; they are also used for the pre-operative preparation of the vagina. Clindamycin cream and metronidazole gel are also indicated for bacterial vaginosis; *Sultrin*® cream is licensed for the treatment of infections due to *Haemophilus vaginalis* only.

The antiviral drugs aciclovir, famciclovir and valaciclovir may be used in the treatment of genital infection due to *herpes simplex virus,* the HSV type 2 being a major cause of genital ulceration. They have a beneficial effect on virus shedding and healing, generally giving relief from pain and other symptoms. See section 5.3 for systemic preparations, and section 13.10.3 for topical preparations.

PREPARATIONS FOR OTHER VAGINAL INFECTIONS

Aci-Jel® (Janssen-Cilag)
Vaginal jelly, glacial acetic acid 0.94% in a buffered (pH 4) basis. Net price 85 g with applicator = £3.37
Excipients: include hydroxybenzoates (parabens), fragrance
Condoms: effect on latex condoms and diaphragms not yet known
Dose: non-specific infections, insert 1 applicatorful once or twice daily for up to 2 weeks to restore vaginal acidity

Betadine® (SSL)
Cautions: avoid in pregnancy (also if planned) and in breast-feeding; renal impairment (see Appendix 3); avoid regular use in thyroid disorders
Side-effects: rarely sensitivity; may interfere with thyroid function
Vaginal Cleansing Kit, solution, povidone-iodine 10%. Net price 250 mL with measuring bottle and applicator = £2.79
Excipients: include fragrance
Condoms: effect on latex condoms and diaphragms not yet known
Dose: to be diluted and used once daily, preferably in the morning; may be used with Betadine® pessaries or vaginal gel
Pessaries, brown, povidone-iodine 200 mg. Net price 28 pessaries with applicator = £6.06
Condoms: effect on latex condoms and diaphragms not yet known
Vaginal gel, brown, povidone-iodine 10%. Net price 80 g with applicator = £2.79
Excipients: none as listed in section 13.1.3
Condoms: effect on latex condoms and diaphragms not yet known
Dose: vaginal infections or pre-operatively, insert 1 moistened pessary night and morning for up to 14 days *or* use morning pessary with one applicatorful of gel at night *or* morning douche with pessary (or one applicatorful of gel) at night

Dalacin® (Pharmacia) [PoM]
Cream, clindamycin 2% (as phosphate). Net price
40-g pack with 7 applicators = £10.86
Excipients: include benzyl alcohol, cetostearyl alcohol, polysorbates, propylene glycol
Condoms: damages latex condoms and diaphrags
Side-effects: irritation, cervicitis and vaginitis; poorly absorbed into the blood—very low likelihood of systemic effects (section 5.1.6)
Dose: bacterial vaginosis, insert 5-g applicatorful at night for 3–7 nights

Sultrin® (Janssen-Cilag) [PoM] [▭]
Cream, sulfathiazole 3.42%, sulfacetamide 2.86%, sulfabenzamide 3.7%. Net price 80 g with applicator = £3.48
Excipients: include arachis (peanut) oil, cetyl alcohol, hydroxybenzoates (parabens), propylene glycol, wool fat
Condoms: damages latex condoms and diaphrags
Cautions: absorption of sulphonamides may produce systemic effects
Contra-indications: pregnancy and breast-feeding; hypersensitivity to peanuts
Side-effects: sensitivity
Dose: bacterial vaginosis, insert 1 applicatorful of cream twice daily for 10 days, then once daily if necessary (but see also notes above)

Zidoval® (3M) [PoM]
Vaginal gel, metronidazole 0.75%. Net price 40-g pack with 5 applicators = £4.63
Excipients: include disodium edetate, hydroxybenzoates (parabens), propylene glycol
Cautions: not recommended during menstruation; some absorption may occur, see section 5.1.11 for systemic effects
Side-effects: local effects including irritation, candidiasis, abnormal discharge, pelvic discomfort
Dose: bacterial vaginosis, insert 5-g applicatorful at night for 5 nights

7.3 Contraceptives

7.3.1 Combined hormonal contraceptives
7.3.2 Progestogen-only contraceptives
7.3.3 Spermicidal contraceptives
7.3.4 Contraceptive devices

The criteria by which contraceptive methods should be judged are effectiveness, acceptability, and freedom from side-effects.

Hormonal contraception is the most effective method of fertility control, short of sterilisation, but has unwanted major and minor side-effects, especially for certain groups of women.

Intra-uterine devices have a high use-effectiveness but may produce undesirable local side-effects. They are most suitable for older parous women, but less appropriate for younger nulliparous women and for those with an increased risk of pelvic inflammatory disease.

Barrier methods alone (condoms, diaphragms, and caps) are less effective but can be very reliable for well-motivated couples if used in conjunction with a **spermicide**. Occasionally sensitivity reactions occur. The female condom (*Femidom*®) is now also available; it is prelubricated but does not contain a spermicide.

7.3.1 Combined hormonal contraceptives

Oral contraceptives containing an oestrogen and a progestogen ('combined oral contraceptives') are the most effective preparations for general use. Advantages of combined oral contraceptives include:

- reliable and reversible;
- reduced dysmenorrhoea and menorrhagia;
- reduced incidence of premenstrual tension;
- less symptomatic fibroids and functional ovarian cysts;
- less benign breast disease;
- reduced risk of ovarian and endometrial cancer;
- reduced risk of pelvic inflammatory disease, which may be a risk with intra-uterine devices.

Combined oral contraceptives containing a fixed amount of an oestrogen and a progestogen in each active tablet are termed 'monophasic'; those with varying amounts of the two hormones according to the stage of the cycle are termed 'biphasic' and 'triphasic'. A transdermal patch containing an oestrogen with a progestogen has been introduced recently.

CHOICE. The oestrogen content of combined oral contraceptives ranges from 20 to 40 micrograms and generally a preparation with the lowest oestrogen and progestogen content which gives good cycle control and minimal side-effects in the individual woman is chosen.

- *Low strength preparations* (containing ethinylestradiol 20 micrograms) are particularly appropriate for women with risk factors for circulatory disease, provided a combined oral contraceptive is otherwise suitable. It is recommended that the combined oral contraceptive is not continued beyond 50 years of age since more suitable alternatives exist.

- *Standard strength preparations* (containing ethinylestradiol 30 or 35 micrograms or in 30/40 microgram *phased* preparations) are appropriate for standard use—but see Risk of Venous Thromboembolism below. Phased preparations are generally reserved for women who *either* do not have withdrawal bleeding *or* who have breakthrough bleeding with monophasic products.

The progestogens desogestrel, drospirenone, and gestodene (in combination with ethinylestradiol) may be considered for women who have side-effects (such as acne, headache, depression, weight gain, breast symptoms, and breakthrough bleeding) with other progestogens. However, women should be advised that desogestrel and gestodene have also been associated with an increased risk of *venous thromboembolism*. Drospirenone, a derivative of spironolactone, has anti-androgenic and anti-mineralocorticoid activity; it should be used with care if an increased concentration of potassium might be hazardous. The progestogen norelgestromin is combined with ethinylestradiol in a transdermal patch.

RISK OF VENOUS THROMBOEMBOLISM. There is an increased risk of venous thromboembolic disease (particularly during the first year) in users of oral contraceptives but this risk is considerably smaller than that associated with pregnancy (about 60 cases of venous thromboembolic disease per 100 000 pregnancies). In all cases the risk of venous thromboembolism increases with age and in the presence of other risk factors for venous thromboembolism (e.g. obesity). The risk of venous thromboembolism with transdermal patches is not yet known.

The incidence of venous thromboembolism in healthy, non-pregnant women who are not taking an oral contraceptive is about 5 cases per 100 000 women per year. For those using combined oral contraceptives containing second generation progestogens e.g. levonorgestrel, this incidence is about 15 per 100 000 women per year of use. Some studies have reported a greater risk of venous thromboembolism in women using preparations containing the third generation progestogens desogestrel and gestodene; the incidence in these women is about 25 per 100 000 women per year of use.

The absolute risk of venous thromboembolism in women using combined oral contraceptives containing these third generation progestogens remains very small and well below the risk associated with pregnancy. Provided that women are informed of and accept the relative risks of venous thromboembolism, the choice of oral contraceptive is for the woman together with the prescriber jointly to decide in the light of her individual medical history and any contra-indications.

TRAVEL. Women taking oral contraceptives, or using the patch may be at an increased risk of deep-vein thrombosis during travel involving long periods of immobility (over 5 hours). The risk may be reduced by appropriate exercise during the journey and possibly by wearing elastic hosiery.

MISSED PILL. It is important to bear in mind that the critical time for loss of protection is when a pill is omitted at the *beginning* or *end* of a cycle (which lengthens the pill-free interval). The following is now recommended by family planning organisations:

'If you forget a pill, take it as soon as you remember, and the next one at your normal time. If you are 12 or more hours late with any pill (especially the first in the packet) the pill may not work. As soon as you remember, continue normal pill taking. However, you will not be protected for the next seven days and must either not have sex or use another method such as the condom. If these seven days run beyond the end of your packet, start the next packet at once when you have finished the present one, i.e. do not have a gap between packets. This will mean you may not have a period until the end of two packets but this does you no harm. Nor does it matter if you see some bleeding on tablet-taking days. If you are using everyday (ED) pills—miss out the seven inactive pills. If you are not sure which these are, ask your doctor.'

In addition to these precautions, emergency contraception is recommended if:

- 2 or more combined oral contraceptive tablets are missed from the first 7 tablets in a packet;
- 4 or more consecutive tablets are missed mid-packet.

DELAYED APPLICATION OR DETACHED PATCH. If a patch remains partly detached for less than 24 hours, reapply to the same site or replace with a new patch immediately; no additional contraception is needed and the next patch should be applied on the usual 'change day'. If a patch remains detached for more than 24 hours or if the user is not aware when the patch became detached then stop the current

contraceptive cycle and start a new cycle by applying a new patch, giving a new 'Day 1'; an additional non-hormonal contraceptive must be used concurrently for the first 7 days of the new cycle.

If application of a new patch at the start of a new cycle is delayed, protection is lost. A new patch should be applied as soon as remembered giving a new 'Day 1'; additional non-hormonal methods of contraception should be used concurrently for the first 7 days of the new cycle. If intercourse has occurred during this extended patch-free interval, a possibility of fertilisation should be considered. If application of a patch in the middle of the cycle is delayed (i.e. the patch is not changed on day 8 or day 15):

- for up to 48 hours, apply a new patch immediately; next patch change day remains the same and no additional contraception is required.
- for more than 48 hours, protection may have been lost. Stop the current cycle and start a new four-week cycle immediately by applying a new patch giving a new 'Day 1'; additional non-hormonal contraception should be used concurrently for the first 7 days of the new cycle.

If the patch is not removed at the end of the cycle (day 22), remove it as soon as possble and start the next cycle on the usual 'change day', after day 28; no additional contraception is required.

DIARRHOEA AND VOMITING. Vomiting up to 3 hours after taking an oral contraceptive *or* very severe diarrhoea can interfere with its absorption. Additional precautions should therefore be used during and for 7 days after recovery. If the vomiting and diarrhoea occurs during the last 7 tablets, the next pill-free interval should be omitted (in the case of ED tablets the inactive ones should be omitted).

INTERACTIONS. The effectiveness of both *combined* and *progestogen-only* oral contraceptives may be considerably reduced by interaction with drugs that induce hepatic enzyme activity (e.g. **carbamazepine, griseofulvin, modafinil, nelfinavir, nevirapine, oxcarbazepine, phenytoin, phenobarbital, ritonavir, topiramate**, and, above all, **rifabutin** and **rifampicin**); advice on the possibility of interaction with newer antiretroviral drugs should be sought from HIV specialists.

Family Planning Association (FPA) advice relating to a *short-term course of an enzyme-inducing drug* (for rifampicin and rifabutin, see also below) is that additional contraceptive precautions should be taken whilst taking the enzyme-inducing drug and for at least 7 days after stopping it; if these 7 days run beyond the end of a packet the new packet should be started immediately without a break (in the case of ED tablets the inactive ones should be omitted). It should be noted that **rifampicin** and **rifabutin** are such potent enzyme-inducing drugs that even if a course lasts for less than 7 days the additional contraceptive precautions should be continued for at least 4 weeks after stopping.

FPA advice relating to a *long-term course of an enzyme-inducing drug* (for rifampicin and rifabutin, see also below) in a woman unable to use an alternative method of contraception is to take a combination of oral contraceptives to provide a daily intake of ethinylestradiol 50 micrograms or more [unlicensed use]; 'tricycling' (i.e. taking 3 or 4 packets of monophasic tablets without a break followed by a short tablet-free interval of 4 days) is recommended [but women should be warned of uncertainty about the effectiveness of this regimen]. **Rifampicin** and **rifabutin** are such potent enzyme-inducing drugs that an alternative method of contraception (such as an IUD) is **always** recommended. Since the excretory function of the liver does not return to normal for several weeks after stopping an enzyme-inducing drug, FPA advice relating to *withdrawal* is that appropriate contraceptive measures are required for 4 to 8 weeks after stopping.

The effectiveness of contraceptive patches may also be reduced by drugs that induce hepatic enzyme activity. Additional contraceptive precautions are required whilst taking the enzyme–inducing drug and for 4 weeks after stopping. For women taking long term enzyme–inducing drugs another method of contraception should be considered.

Some **broad-spectrum antibacterials** (e.g. ampicillin, doxycycline) may reduce the efficacy of *combined* oral contraceptives by impairing the bacterial flora responsible for recycling of ethinylestradiol from the large bowel. FPA advice is that additional contraceptive precautions should be taken whilst taking a *short course of a broad-spectrum antibiotic* and for 7 days after stopping. If these 7 days run beyond the end of a packet the next packet should be started immediately without a break (in the case of ED tablets the inactive ones should be omitted). If the antibiotic course *exceeds 3 weeks*, the bacterial flora develops antibiotic resistance and additional precautions become unnecessary; additional precautions are also unnecessary if a woman starting a *combined* oral contraceptive has been on a course of antibiotics for 3 weeks or more.

It is possible that some antibacterials affect the efficacy of contraceptive patches. Additional contraceptive precautions are recommended during concomitant use and for 7 days after discontinuation of the antibacterial (except tetracycline). If concomitant administration runs beyond the 3 weeks of patch treatment, a new treatment cycle should be started immediately without a patch-free break.

SURGERY. Oestrogen-containing contraceptives should preferably be discontinued (and adequate alternative contraceptive arrangements made) 4 weeks before major elective surgery and all surgery to the legs or surgery which involves prolonged immobilisation of a lower limb; they should normally be recommenced at the first menses occurring at least 2 weeks after full mobilisation. A depot injection of a progestogen-only contraceptive may be offered and the oestrogen-containing contraceptive restarted later—if preferred before the next injection would be due. When discontinuation of an oestrogen-containing contraceptive is not possible, e.g. after trauma or if a patient admitted for an elective procedure is still on an oestrogen-containing contraceptive, thromboprophylaxis (with heparin and graduated compression hosiery) is advised. These recommendations do not apply to minor surgery with short duration of anaesthesia, e.g. laparoscopic sterilisation or tooth extraction, or to women using oestrogen-free hormonal contraceptives (whether by mouth or by injection).

REASON TO STOP IMMEDIATELY. Combined hormonal contraceptives or hormone replacement therapy (HRT) should be stopped (pending investigation and treatment), if any of the following occur:

- sudden severe chest pain (even if not radiating to left arm);
- sudden breathlessness (or cough with blood-stained sputum);
- unexplained severe pain in calf of one leg;
- severe stomach pain;
- serious neurological effects including unusual severe, prolonged headache especially if first time or getting progressively worse *or* sudden partial or complete loss of vision *or* sudden disturbance of hearing or other perceptual disorders *or* dysphasia *or* bad fainting attack or collapse *or* first unexplained epileptic seizure *or* weakness, motor disturbances, very marked numbness suddenly affecting one side or one part of body;
- hepatitis, jaundice, liver enlargement;
- severe depression;
- blood pressure above systolic 160 mmHg and diastolic 100 mmHg;
- detection of a risk factor see Cautions and Contraindications under Combined Hormonal Contraceptives

COMBINED HORMONAL CONTRACEPTIVES

Indications: contraception; menstrual symptoms (section 6.4.1.2)

Cautions: risk factors for venous thromboembolism (see below and also notes above), arterial disease and migraine, see below; hyperprolactinaemia (seek specialist advice); severe depression, sickle-cell disease, inflammatory bowel disease including Crohn's disease; **interactions:** see above and Appendix 1 (oestrogens, progestogens)

RISK FACTORS FOR VENOUS THROMBOEMBOLISM (SEE ALSO NOTES ABOVE). Use with **caution** if any of following factors present but **avoid** if two or more factors present:

- *family history of venous thromboembolism* in first degree relative aged under 45 years (avoid contraceptive containing desogestrel or gestodene, *or* if known prothrombotic coagulation abnormality e.g. factor V Leiden or antiphospholipid antibodies (including lupus anticoagulant));
- *obesity*—body mass index above 30 kg/m^2 (avoid if body mass index above 39 kg/m^2);
- *long-term immobilisation* e.g. in a wheelchair (avoid if confined to bed or leg in plaster cast);
- *varicose veins* (avoid during sclerosing treatment or where definite history of thrombosis).

RISK FACTORS FOR ARTERIAL DISEASE. Use with **caution** if any one of following factors present but **avoid** if two or more factors present:

- *family history of arterial disease* in first degree relative aged under 45 years (avoid if atherogenic lipid profile);
- *diabetes mellitus* (avoid if diabetes complications present);
- *hypertension*—blood pressure above *systolic 140 mmHg* and *diastolic 90 mmHg* (avoid if blood pressure above *systolic 160 mmHg* and *diastolic 100 mmHg*);
- *smoking* (avoid if smoking 40 or more cigarettes daily);
- *age* over 35 years (avoid if over 50 years);
- *obesity* (avoid if body mass index above 39 kg/m^2);
- *migraine*—see below.

MIGRAINE. Subject should report any increase in headache frequency or onset of focal symptoms (discontinue immediately and refer urgently to neurology expert if focal neurological symptoms not typical of aura persist for more than 1 hour—see also Reason to stop immediately in notes above); **contra-indicated** in

- migraine with typical focal aura,
- severe migraine regularly lasting over 72 hours despite treatment,
- migraine treated with ergot derivatives;

use with **caution** in

- migraine without focal aura,
- migraine controlled with $5HT_1$ agonist (section 4.7.4.1).

Contra-indications: pregnancy; personal history of venous or arterial thrombosis, severe or multiple risk factors for arterial disease or for venous thromboembolism (see above), heart disease associated with pulmonary hypertension or risk of embolus; migraine (see above), transient cerebral ischaemic attacks without headaches; liver disease including disorders of hepatic excretion (e.g. Dubin-Johnson or Rotor syndromes), infective hepatitis (until liver function returns to normal); systemic lupus erythematosus; porphyria (section 9.8.2); liver adenoma; gallstones; after evacuation of hydatidiform mole (until return to normal of urine and plasma gonadotrophin concentration); history of haemolytic uraemic syndrome or history during pregnancy of pruritus, cholestatic jaundice, chorea or deterioration of otosclerosis, pemphigoid gestationis; breast or genital-tract carcinoma; undiagnosed vaginal bleeding; breast-feeding (until weaning or for 6 months after birth)

Side-effects: nausea, vomiting, headache, breast tenderness, changes in body weight, fluid retention, thrombosis (more common when factor V Leiden present or in blood groups A, B, and AB; see also notes above), changes in libido, depression, chorea, skin reactions, chloasma, hypertension, contact lenses may irritate, impairment of liver function, hepatic tumours, reduced menstrual loss, 'spotting' in early cycles, absence of withdrawal bleeding; rarely photosensitivity

BREAST CANCER. There is a small increase in the risk of having breast cancer diagnosed in women taking the combined oral contraceptive pill; this relative risk may be due to an earlier diagnosis. In users of combined oral contraceptive pills the cancers are more likely to be localised to the breast. The most important factor for diagnosing breast cancer appears to be the age at which the contraceptive is stopped rather than the duration of use; any increase in the rate of diagnosis diminishes gradually during the 10 years after stopping and disappears by 10 years. The CSM has advised that a possible small increase in the risk of breast cancer should be weighed against the benefits and evidence of the protective effect against cancers of the ovary and endometrium

Dose: *by mouth*, each tablet should be taken at approximately same time each day; if delayed by longer than 12 hours contraceptive protection may be lost

21-day combined (monophasic) preparations, 1 tablet daily for 21 days; subsequent courses repeated after a 7-day interval (during which withdrawal bleeding occurs); first course usually started on day 1 of cycle—if starting on day 4 of cycle or later additional precautions (barrier methods) necessary during first 7 days

Every day (ED) combined (monophasic) preparations, 1 *active* tablet starting on day 1 of cycle (see also under preparations below)—if starting on day 4 of cycle or later additional precautions (barrier methods) necessary during first 7 days; if starting with *inactive* tablet on day 1 additional precautions required for 14 days; withdrawal bleeding occurs when *inactive* tablets being taken; subsequent courses repeated without interval

Biphasic and triphasic preparations, see under individual preparations below

CHANGING TO COMBINED PREPARATION CONTAINING DIFFERENT PROGESTOGEN. *21-day combined preparations:* continue current pack until last tablet and start first tablet of new brand the next day. If a 7-day break is taken before starting new brand, additional precautions (barrier methods) should be used during first 7 days of taking the new brand. *Every Day (ED) combined preparations:* start the new brand (first tablet of a *21-day preparation* or the first *active* tablet of an *ED preparation*) the day after taking the last *active* tablet of previous brand (omitting the *inactive* tablets). If not possible to avoid taking the *inactive* tablets of an *ED preparation*, additional precautions (barrier methods) necessary during first 14 days of taking the new brand.

CHANGING FROM PROGESTOGEN-ONLY TABLET. Start on day 1 of menstruation or any day if amenorrhoea present and pregnancy has been excluded.

SECONDARY AMENORRHOEA (EXCLUDE PREGNANCY). Start any day, additional precautions (barrier methods) necessary during first 7 days.

AFTER CHILDBIRTH (NOT BREAST-FEEDING). Start 3 weeks after birth (increased risk of thrombosis if started earlier); later than 3 weeks postpartum additional precautions (barrier methods) necessary for first 7 days.

Not recommended if woman breast-feeding—oral progestogen-only contraceptive preferred.

AFTER ABORTION OR MISCARRIAGE. Start same day.

By transdermal application, apply first patch on day 1 of cycle, change patch on days 8 and 15; remove third patch on day 22 and apply new patch after 7-day patch-free interval to start subsequent contraceptive cycle

CHANGING FROM COMBINED ORAL CONTRACEPTIVE. Apply patch on the first day of withdrawal bleeding; if no withdrawal bleeding within 5 days of taking last *active* tablet, rule out pregnancy before applying first patch. Unless patch is applied on first day of withdrawal bleeding, additional precautions (barrier methods) should be used concurrently for first 7 days

CHANGING FROM PROGESTOGEN-ONLY METHOD. From an implant, apply first patch on the day implant removed; from an injection, apply first patch when next injection due; from oral progestogen, first patch may be started on any day after stopping pill. For all methods additional precautions (barrier methods) should be used concurrently for first 7 days

AFTER CHILDBIRTH (NOT BREAST-FEEDING). Start 4 weeks after birth; if started later than 4 weeks after birth additional precautions (barrier methods) should be used for first 7 days

AFTER ABORTION OR MISCARRIAGE. Before 20 weeks' gestation start immediately; no additional contraception required if started immediately. After 20 weeks' gestation start on day 21 after abortion or on the first day of first spontaneous menstruation; additional precautions (barrier methods) should be used for first 7 days after applying the patch

---

Low strength (oral)

■ Ethinylestradiol with Norethisterone

Loestrin 20® (Galen) <u>PoM</u>

Tablets, norethisterone acetate 1 mg, ethinylestradiol 20 micrograms. Net price 3 × 21-tab pack = £2.73

Dose: 1 tablet daily for 21 days; subsequent courses repeated after 7-day tablet-free interval (during which withdrawal bleeding occurs); for starting routines see under Dose above

■ Ethinylestradiol with Desogestrel

See Risk of venous thromboembolism in notes above before prescribing

Mercilon® (Organon) PoM

Tablets, desogestrel 150 micrograms, ethinylestradiol 20 micrograms. Net price 3 × 21-tab pack = £8.57

Dose: 1 tablet daily for 21 days; subsequent courses repeated after 7-day tablet-free interval (during which withdrawal bleeding occurs); for starting routines see under Dose above

■ Ethinylestradiol with Gestodene

See Risk of venous thromboembolism in notes above before prescribing

Femodette® (Schering Health) PoM

Tablets, s/c, gestodene 75 micrograms, ethinylestradiol 20 micrograms, net price 3 × 21-tab pack = £8.25

Dose: 1 tablet daily for 21 days; subsequent courses repeated after 7-day tablet-free interval (during which withdrawal bleeding occurs); for starting routines see under Dose above

Low strength (transdermal)

■ Ethinylestradiol with Norelgestromin

The Scottish Medicines Consortium has advised (September 2003) that *Evra*® patches should be restricted for use in women who are likely to comply poorly with combined oral contraceptives

Evra® (Janssen-Cilag) ▼ PoM

Patches, self-adhesive (releasing ethinylestradiol approx. 20 micrograms/24 hours and norelgestromin approx. 150 micrograms/24 hours); net price 9-patch pack = £23.23. Counselling, administration

Dose: 1 patch to be applied once weekly for three weeks, followed by a 7-day patch-free interval; subsequent courses repeated after 7-day patch-free interval (during which withdrawal bleeding occurs); for starting routines see under Dose above

NOTE. Adhesives or bandages should not be used to hold patch in place. If patch no longer sticky do not reapply but use a new patch.

Standard strength

■ Ethinylestradiol with Levonorgestrel

Eugynon 30® (Schering Health) PoM

Tablets, levonorgestrel 250 micrograms, ethinylestradiol 30 micrograms. Net price 3 × 21-tab pack = £2.48

Dose: 1 tablet daily for 21 days; subsequent courses repeated after 7-day tablet-free interval (during which withdrawal bleeding occurs); for starting routines see under Dose above

Logynon® (Schering Health) PoM

6 light brown tablets, ethinylestradiol 30 micrograms, levonorgestrel 50 micrograms;

5 white tablets, ethinylestradiol 40 micrograms, levonorgestrel 75 micrograms;

10 ochre tablets, ethinylestradiol 30 micrograms, levonorgestrel 125 micrograms.

Net price 3 × 21-tab pack = £3.92

Dose: 1 tablet daily for 21 days, starting with light brown tablet marked 1 on day 1 of cycle; repeat after 7-day tablet-free interval

Logynon ED® (Schering Health) PoM

6 light brown tablets, ethinylestradiol 30 micrograms, levonorgestrel 50 micrograms;

5 white tablets, ethinylestradiol 40 micrograms, levonorgestrel 75 micrograms;

10 ochre tablets, ethinylestradiol 30 micrograms, levonorgestrel 125 micrograms;

7 white, inactive tablets.

Net price 3 × 28-tab pack = £3.92

Dose: 1 tablet daily for 28 days, starting on day 1 of cycle with active tablet (withdrawal bleeding occurs when inactive tablets being taken); subsequent courses repeated without interval; for starting routines see under Dose above

Microgynon 30® (Schering Health) PoM

Tablets, s/c, levonorgestrel 150 micrograms, ethinylestradiol 30 micrograms. Net price 21-tab pack = 94p

Dose: 1 tablet daily for 21 days; subsequent courses repeated after 7-day tablet-free interval (during which withdrawal bleeding occurs); for starting routines see under Dose above

Microgynon 30 ED® (Schering Health) PoM

Tablets, beige, levonorgestrel 150 micrograms, ethinylestradiol 30 micrograms, white inactive tablets. Net price 3 × 28-tab (7 are inactive) pack = £2.56

Dose: 1 tablet daily for 28 days starting on day 1 of cycle with active tablet (withdrawal bleeding occurs when inactive tablets being taken); subsequent courses repeated without interval; for starting routines see also under Dose above

Ovranette® (Wyeth) PoM

Tablets, levonorgestrel 150 micrograms, ethinylestradiol 30 micrograms. Net price 3 × 21-tab pack = £2.46

Dose: 1 tablet daily for 21 days; subsequent courses repeated after 7-day tablet-free interval (during which withdrawal bleeding occurs); for starting routines see under Dose above

Trinordiol® (Wyeth) PoM

6 light brown tablets, ethinylestradiol 30 micrograms, levonorgestrel 50 micrograms;

5 white tablets, ethinylestradiol 40 micrograms, levonorgestrel 75 micrograms;

10 ochre tablets, ethinylestradiol 30 micrograms, levonorgestrel 125 micrograms.

Net price 3 × 21-tab pack = £4.34

Dose: 1 tablet daily for 21 days, starting with light brown tablet marked 1 on day 1 of cycle; repeat after 7-day tablet-free interval

■ Ethinylestradiol with Norethisterone

BiNovum® (Janssen-Cilag) PoM

7 white tablets, ethinylestradiol 35 micrograms, norethisterone 500 micrograms;

14 peach tablets, ethinylestradiol 35 micrograms, norethisterone 1mg.

Net price 3 × 21-tab pack = £2.24

Dose: 1 tablet daily for 21 days, starting with white tablet on day 1 of cycle; repeat after 7-day tablet-free interval

Brevinor® (Pharmacia) PoM

Tablets, blue, norethisterone 500 micrograms, ethinylestradiol 35 micrograms. Net price 3 × 21-tab pack = £1.99

Dose: 1 tablet daily for 21 days; subsequent courses repeated after 7-day tablet-free interval (during which withdrawal bleeding occurs); for starting routines see under Dose above

Loestrin 30® (Parke-Davis) PoM
Tablets, norethisterone acetate 1.5 mg, ethinylestradiol 30 micrograms. Net price 3 × 21-tab pack = £3.93
Dose: 1 tablet daily for 21 days; subsequent courses repeated after 7-day tablet-free interval (during which withdrawal bleeding occurs); for starting routines see under Dose above

Norimin® (Pharmacia) PoM
Tablets, norethisterone 1 mg, ethinylestradiol 35 micrograms. Net price 3 × 21-tab pack = £2.28
Dose: 1 tablet daily for 21 days; subsequent courses repeated after 7-day tablet-free interval (during which withdrawal bleeding occurs); for starting routines see under Dose above

Ovysmen® (Janssen-Cilag) PoM
Tablets, norethisterone 500 micrograms, ethinylestradiol 35 micrograms. Net price 3 × 21-tab pack = £1.70
Dose: 1 tablet daily for 21 days; subsequent courses repeated after 7-day tablet-free interval (during which withdrawal bleeding occurs); for starting routines see under Dose above

Synphase® (Pharmacia) PoM
7 blue tablets, ethinylestradiol 35 micrograms, norethisterone 500 micrograms;
9 white tablets, ethinylestradiol 35 micrograms, norethisterone 1 mg;
5 blue tablets, ethinylestradiol 35 micrograms, norethisterone 500 micrograms.
Net price 21-tab pack = £1.20
Dose: 1 tablet daily for 21 days, starting with blue tablet marked 1 on day 1 of cycle; repeat after 7-day tablet-free interval

TriNovum® (Janssen-Cilag) PoM
7 white tablets, ethinylestradiol 35 micrograms, norethisterone 500 micrograms;
7 light peach tablets, ethinylestradiol 35 micrograms, norethisterone 750 micrograms;
7 peach tablets, ethinylestradiol 35 micrograms, norethisterone 1 mg.
Net price 3 × 21-tab pack = £3.11
Dose: 1 tablet daily for 21 days, starting with white tablet on day 1 of cycle; repeat after 7-day tablet-free interval

■ Ethinylestradiol with Norgestimate
Cilest® (Janssen-Cilag) PoM
Tablets, blue, norgestimate 250 micrograms, ethinylestradiol 35 micrograms. Net price 3 × 21-tab pack = £6.42, 6 × 21-tab pack = £12.84
Dose: 1 tablet daily for 21 days; subsequent courses repeated after 7-day tablet-free interval (during which withdrawal bleeding occurs); for starting routines see under Dose above

■ Ethinylestradiol with Desogestrel
See Risk of venous thromboembolism in notes above before prescribing
Marvelon® (Organon) PoM
Tablets, desogestrel 150 micrograms, ethinylestradiol 30 micrograms. Net price 3 × 21-tab pack = £6.70
Dose: 1 tablet daily for 21 days; subsequent courses repeated after 7-day tablet-free interval (during which withdrawal bleeding occurs); for starting routines see under Dose above

■ Ethinylestradiol with Drospirenone
The Scottish Medicines Consortium has advised (March 2003) that *Yasmin*® is not recommended
Yasmin® (Schering Health) ▼ PoM
Tablets, f/c, yellow, drospirenone 3 mg, ethinylestradiol 30 micrograms. Net price 3 × 21-tab pack = £14.70
Dose: 1 tablet daily for 21 days; subsequent courses repeated after 7-day tablet-free interval (during which withdrawal bleeding occurs); for starting routines see under Dose above

■ Ethinylestradiol with Gestodene
See Risk of venous thromboembolism in notes above before prescribing
Femodene® (Schering Health) PoM
Tablets, s/c, gestodene 75 micrograms, ethinylestradiol 30 micrograms. Net price 3 × 21-tab pack = £6.84
Dose: 1 tablet daily for 21 days; subsequent courses repeated after 7-day tablet-free interval (during which withdrawal bleeding occurs); for starting routines see under Dose above

Femodene® **ED** (Schering Health) PoM
Tablets, s/c, gestodene 75 micrograms, ethinylestradiol 30 micrograms. Net price 3 × 28-tab (7 are inactive) pack = £6.84
Dose: 1 tablet daily for 28 days, starting on day 1 of cycle with active tablet (withdrawal bleeding occurs when inactive tablets being taken); subsequent courses repeated without interval; for starting routines see under Dose above

Minulet® (Wyeth) PoM
Tablets, gestodene 75 micrograms, ethinylestradiol 30 micrograms. Net price 3 × 21-tab pack = £6.84
Dose: 1 tablet daily for 21 days; subsequent courses repeated after 7-day tablet-free interval (during which withdrawal bleeding occurs); for starting routines see under Dose above

Triadene® (Schering Health) PoM
6 beige tablets, ethinylestradiol 30 micrograms, gestodene 50 micrograms;
5 dark brown tablets, ethinylestradiol 40 micrograms, gestodene 70 micrograms;
10 white tablets, ethinylestradiol 30 micrograms, gestodene 100 micrograms.
Net price 3 × 21-tab pack = £9.54
Dose: 1 tablet daily for 21 days, starting with beige tablet marked 'start' on day 1 of cycle; repeat after 7-day tablet-free interval

Tri-Minulet® (Wyeth) PoM
6 beige tablets, ethinylestradiol 30 micrograms, gestodene 50 micrograms;
5 dark brown tablets, ethinylestradiol 40 micrograms, gestodene 70 micrograms;
10 white tablets, ethinylestradiol 30 micrograms, gestodene 100 micrograms.
Net price 3 × 21-tab pack = £9.54
Dose: 1 tablet daily for 21 days, starting with beige tablet marked '1' on day 1 of the cycle; repeat after 7-day tablet-free interval

■ Mestranol with Norethisterone
Norinyl-1® (Pharmacia) PoM
Tablets, norethisterone 1 mg, mestranol 50 micrograms. Net price 3 × 21-tab pack = £2.19
Dose: 1 tablet daily for 21 days; subsequent courses repeated after 7-day tablet-free interval (during which withdrawal bleeding occurs); for starting routines see under Dose above

■ Ethinylestradiol with cyproterone acetate
See co-cyprindiol (section 13.6.2)

Emergency contraception

Hormonal methods

Hormonal emergency contraception involves the use of **levonorgestrel**. It is effective if dose is taken within 72 hours (3 days) of unprotected intercourse; taking the dose as soon as possible increases efficacy. Levonorgestrel may also be used between 72 and 120 hours after unprotected intercourse [unlicensed use] but efficacy decreases with time. Hormonal emergency contraception is less effective than insertion of an intra-uterine device (see below).

If vomiting occurs within 3 hours of taking levonorgestrel, a replacement dose can be given. If an anti-emetic is required domperidone is preferred.

When prescribing hormonal emergency contraception the doctor should explain:

- that the next period may be early or late;
- that a barrier method of contraception needs to be used until the next period;
- the need to return promptly if any lower abdominal pain occurs because this could signify an ectopic pregnancy (and also in 3 to 4 weeks if the subsequent menstrual bleed is abnormally light, heavy or brief, or is absent, or if she is otherwise concerned).

Intrauterine pregnancy despite treatment: see Appendix 4 (levonorgestrel).

INTERACTIONS. The effectiveness of the hormonal method of emergency contraception is reduced by enzyme-inducing drugs; a copper intra-uterine device may be offered or, otherwise, the dose of levonorgestrel should be increased to 2.25 mg (i.e. 3 tablets) taken as a single dose. There is no need to increase the dose for emergency contraception if the patient is taking antibacterials that are not enzyme inducers.

LEVONORGESTREL

Indications: emergency contraception
Cautions: see notes above; past ectopic pregnancy; severe malabsorption syndromes, severe liver disease, pregnancy (see notes above and appendix 4); breast-feeding (Appendix 5); **interactions:** see notes above and Appendix 1 (progestogens)
Contra-indications: porphyria (section 9.8.2)
Side-effects: menstrual irregularities (see also notes above), nausea, low abdominal pain, fatigue, headache, dizziness, breast tenderness, vomiting
Dose: 1.5 mg (2 tablets) as a single dose as soon as possible after coitus (preferably within 12 hours but no later than after 72 hours)

[1]**Levonelle®-2** (Schering Health) [PoM]
Tablets, levonorgestrel 750 micrograms, net price 2-tab pack = £5.50
1. Can be sold to women over 16 years as *Levonelle®*; when supplying emergency contraception to the public, pharmacists should refer to guidance issued by the Royal Pharmaceutical Society of Great Britain

Intra-uterine device

Insertion of an intra-uterine device is more effective than the hormonal methods of emergency contraception. A copper intra-uterine contraceptive device (section 7.3.4) can be inserted up to 120 hours (5 days) after unprotected intercourse; sexually transmitted diseases should be tested for and insertion of the device should usually be covered by antibacterial prophylaxis (e,g, azithromycin 1 g as a single dose). If intercourse has occurred more than 5 days previously, the device can still be inserted up to 5 days after the earliest likely calculated ovulation (i.e. within the minimum period before implantation).

7.3.2   Progestogen-only contraceptives

7.3.2.1   Oral progestogen-only contraceptives
7.3.2.2   Parenteral progestogen-only contraceptives
7.3.2.3   Intra-uterine progestogen-only device

7.3.2.1   Oral progestogen-only contraceptives

Oral progestogen-only preparations may offer a suitable alternative when oestrogens are contra-indicated (including those patients with venous thrombosis or a past history or predisposition to venous thrombosis), but have a higher failure rate than combined preparations. They are suitable for older women, for heavy smokers, and for those with hypertension, valvular heart disease, diabetes mellitus, and migraine. Menstrual irregularities (oligomenorrhoea, menorrhagia) are more common but tend to resolve on long-term treatment.

INTERACTIONS. Effectiveness of oral progestogen-only preparations is not affected by broad-spectrum antibiotics but is reduced by enzyme-inducing drugs—see p. 388 and Appendix 1 (progestogens).

SURGERY. All progestogen-only contraceptives (including those given by injection) are suitable for use as an alternative to combined oral contraceptives before major elective surgery, before all surgery to the legs, or before surgery which involves prolonged immobilisation of a lower limb.

STARTING ROUTINE. One tablet daily, on a continuous basis, starting on day 1 of cycle and taken at the same time each day (if delayed by longer than 3 hours contraceptive protection may be lost). Additional contraceptive precautions are not necessary when initiating treatment.

Changing from a combined oral contraceptive: start on the day following completion of the combined oral contraceptive course without a break (or in the case of ED tablets omitting the inactive ones).

After childbirth: start any time after 3 weeks postpartum (increased risk of breakthrough bleeding if started earlier)—lactation is not affected.

MISSED PILL. The following advice is now recommended by family planning organisations:

'If you forget a pill, take it as soon as you remember and carry on with the next pill at the right time. If the pill was more than three hours overdue you are not protected. Continue normal pill-taking but you must also use another method, such as the condom, for the next 7 days.'

The Faculty of Family Planning and Reproductive Health Care recommends emergency contraception (see p. 393) if one or more progestogen-only contraceptive tablets are missed or taken more than 3 hours late.

DIARRHOEA AND VOMITING. Vomiting up to 3 hours after taking an oral contraceptive *or* very severe diarrhoea can interfere with its absorption. Additional precautions should be used during and for 7 days after recovery.

ORAL PROGESTOGEN-ONLY CONTRACEPTIVES

(Progestogen-only pill, 'POP')

Indications: contraception

Cautions: heart disease, sex-steroid dependent cancer, past ectopic pregnancy, malabsorption syndromes, functional ovarian cysts, active liver disease, recurrent cholestatic jaundice, history of jaundice in pregnancy; **interactions:** p. 388 and Appendix 1 (progestogens)

OTHER CONDITIONS. The product literature advises caution in patients with history of thromboembolism, hypertension, diabetes mellitus and migraine; evidence for caution in these conditions is unsatisfactory

Contra-indications: pregnancy, undiagnosed vaginal bleeding; severe arterial disease; liver adenoma, porphyria (section 9.8.2); after evacuation of hydatidiform mole (until return to normal of urine and plasma gonadotrophin values); history of breast cancer but evidence for contra–indication uncertain

Side-effects: menstrual irregularities (see also notes above); nausea, vomiting, headache, dizziness, breast discomfort, depression, skin disorders, disturbance of appetite, weight changes, changes in libido

BREAST CANCER. There is a small increase in the risk of having breast cancer diagnosed in women using, or who have recently used, a progestogen-only contraceptive pill; this relative risk may be due to an earlier diagnosis. The most important risk factor appears to be the age at which the contraceptive is stopped rather than the duration of use; the risk disappears gradually during the 10 years after stopping and there is no excess risk by 10 years. The CSM has advised that a possible small increase in the risk of breast cancer should be weighed against the benefits

Dose: 1 tablet daily at same time each day, starting on day 1 of cycle then continuously; if administration delayed for 3 hours or more it should be regarded as a 'missed pill', see notes above

Cerazette® (Organon) ▼ PoM
Tablets, f/c, desogestrel 75 micrograms. Net price 3 × 28-tab pack = £8.85

Femulen® (Pharmacia) PoM
Tablets, etynodiol diacetate 500 micrograms. Net price 3 × 28-tab pack = £3.31

Micronor® (Janssen-Cilag) PoM
Tablets, norethisterone 350 micrograms. Net price 3 × 28-tab pack = £1.89

Microval® (Wyeth) PoM
Tablets, levonorgestrel 30 micrograms. Net price 35-tab pack = 90p

Neogest® (Schering Health) PoM
Tablets, brown, s/c, norgestrel 75 micrograms (≡ levonorgestrel 37.5 micrograms). Net price 35-tab pack = 98p

Norgeston® (Schering Health) PoM
Tablets, s/c, levonorgestrel 30 micrograms. Net price 35-tab pack = 98p

Noriday® (Pharmacia) PoM
Tablets, norethisterone 350 micrograms. Net price 3 × 28-tab pack = £2.10

7.3.2.2 Parenteral progestogen-only contraceptives

Medroxyprogesterone acetate (*Depo-Provera®*) is a long-acting progestogen given by intramuscular injection; it is as effective as the combined oral preparations but because of its prolonged action it should never be given without *full counselling backed by the patient information leaflet.* It may be used as a short-term or long-term contraceptive for women who have been counselled about the likelihood of menstrual disturbance and the potential for a delay in return to full fertility. Delayed return of fertility and irregular cycles may occur after discontinuation of treatment but there is no evidence of permanent infertility. Heavy bleeding has been reported in patients given medroxyprogesterone acetate in the immediate puerperium (the first dose is best delayed until 6 weeks after birth). If the woman is not breast-feeding, the first injection may be given within 5 days postpartum (she should be warned that the risk of heavy or prolonged bleeding may be increased). Reduction in bone mineral density has also been reported. **Norethisterone enantate** (*Noristerat®*) is a long-acting progestogen given as an oily injection which provides contraception for 8 weeks; it is used as short-term interim contraception e.g. before vasectomy becomes effective. The **cautions** and **contra-indications** of oral progestogen-only contraceptives apply except that because the injection also reliably inhibits ovulation, it protects against ectopic pregnancy and functional ovarian cysts.

An **etonogestrel-releasing implant** (*Implanon®*), consisting of a single flexible rod, is also available; the rod is inserted subdermally into the lower surface of the upper arm and it provides effective contraception for up to 3 years. In women with a body mass index greater than 35 kg/m^2, blood etonogestrel concentrations are lower and therefore the implant may not provide effective contraception during the third year; earlier replacement should be considered in such patients. Local reactions such as bruising and itching may occur at the insertion site. The **cautions, contra-indications** and **side-effects** of oral preparations apply; the contraceptive effect of *Implanon®* is rapidly reversed on removal of the implant. *The doctor or nurse administering (or removing) the system should be fully trained in the technique and should provide full counselling backed by the patient information leaflet.*

The **levonorgestrel-releasing implant system** (*Norplant®*, Hoechst Marion Roussel) has been discontinued, but some women may have the system in place until 2004. Unlike the injectable progestogen-only contraceptive method, the effects of *Norplant®* are almost immediately reversible on removal of the implants. *The doctor removing the system should be fully trained in the technique.*

INTERACTIONS. Effectiveness of parenteral progestogen-only contraceptives is not affected by broad-spectrum antibiotics. However, effectiveness of norethisterone and etonogestrel (but not medroxyprogesterone acetate) may be reduced by enzyme-inducing drugs; alternative contraceptive method should be considered or an additional contraceptive method used while the enzyme-inducing drug is being taken.

PARENTERAL PROGESTOGEN-ONLY CONTRACEPTIVES

Indications: contraception, see also notes above and under preparations (roles vary according to preparation)

Cautions: see notes above and under preparations; possible risk of breast cancer, see oral progestogen-only contraceptives (section 7.3.2.1); history during pregnancy of pruritus or of deterioration of otosclerosis, disturbances of lipid metabolism; **interactions:** see notes above and Appendix 1 (progestogens)

COUNSELLING. Full counselling backed by *patient information leaflet* required before administration

Contra-indications: see notes above; history of breast cancer

Side-effects: see notes above

Dose: see under preparations

■ Injectable preparations

Depo-Provera® (Pharmacia) PoM

Injection (aqueous suspension), medroxyprogesterone acetate 150 mg/mL, net price 1-mL prefilled syringe = £5.01, 1-mL vial = £5.01. Counselling, see patient information leaflet

*Dose: by deep intramuscular injection,*150 mg within first 5 days of cycle or within first 5 days after parturition (delay until 6 weeks after parturition if breast-feeding); for long-term contraception, repeated every 12 weeks (if interval greater than 12 weeks and 5 days, exclude pregnancy before next injection and advise patient to use additional contraceptive measures (e.g. barrier) for 14 days after the injection)

Noristerat® (Schering Health) PoM

Injection (oily), norethisterone enantate 200 mg/mL. Net price 1-mL amp = £3.59. Counselling, see patient information leaflet

Dose: by deep intramuscular injection given very slowly *into gluteal muscle,* short-term contraception, 200 mg within first 5 days of cycle or immediately after parturition (duration 8 weeks); may be repeated once after 8 weeks (withhold breast-feeding for neonates with severe or persistent jaundice requiring medical treatment)

■ Implants

Implanon® (Organon) PoM

Implant, containing etonogestrel 68 mg in each flexible rod, net price = £90.00. Counselling, see patient information leaflet

Dose: by subdermal implantation, no previous hormonal contraceptive, 1 implant inserted during first 5 days of cycle; parturition or abortion in second trimester, 1 implant inserted between days 21–28 after delivery or abortion (if inserted after 28 days additional precautions necessary for next 7 days); abortion in first trimester, 1 implant inserted immediately; changing from an oral contraceptive, consult product literature; remove within 3 years of insertion

7.3.2.3 Intra-uterine progestogen-only device

The progestogen-only intra-uterine system, *Mirena®*, releases **levonorgestrel** directly into the uterine cavity. It is licensed for use as a contraceptive and for the treatment of primary menorrhagia. This may therefore be a contraceptive method of choice for women who have excessively heavy menses. The effects of the intra-uterine system are mainly local and hormonal including prevention of endometrial proliferation, thickening of cervical mucus, and suppression of ovulation in some women (in some cycles). In addition to the progestogenic activity, the intra-uterine system itself may contribute slightly to the contraceptive effect. Return of fertility after removal is rapid and appears to be complete. Advantages over copper intra-uterine devices are that there may be an improvement in any dysmenorrhoea and a reduction in blood loss; there is also evidence that the frequency of pelvic inflammatory disease may be reduced (particularly in the youngest age groups who are most at risk).

In primary menorrhagia, menstrual bleeding is reduced significantly within 3–6 months of inserting the levonorgestrel intra-uterine system, probably because it prevents endometrial proliferation. Another treatment should be considered if menorrhagia does not improve within this period (section 6.4.1.2).

Generally the **cautions** and **contra-indications** are as for standard intra-uterine devices (section 7.3.4) but the risk of ectopic pregnancy is considerably smaller. Moreover, since the progestogen is released close to the site of the main contraceptive action (on cervical mucus and endometrium) progestogenic side-effects and interactions are less likely to be a problem—in particular, enzyme-inducing drugs are unlikely to significantly reduce the contraceptive effect. Initially changes in the pattern and duration of menstrual bleeding (spotting or prolonged bleeding) are common and the patient should be fully counselled (and provided with a patient information leaflet) before insertion. Improvement in progestogenic side-effects, such as mastalgia and mood changes, and in the bleeding pattern usually occurs a few months after insertion and bleeding may often become very light or absent. Functional ovarian cysts (usually asymptomatic) may occur and usually resolve spontaneously (ultrasound monitoring recommended).

INTRA-UTERINE PROGESTOGEN-ONLY SYSTEM

Indications: contraception, primary menorrhagia

Cautions: see notes above; in case of pregnancy—remove system (teratogenicity cannot be excluded); not suitable for emergency contraception; **interactions:** see notes above and Appendix 1 (progestogens)

Contra-indications: see notes above

Side-effects: see notes above

Mirena® (Schering Health) PoM

Intra-uterine system, T-shaped plastic frame (impregnated with barium sulphate and with threads attached to base) with polydimethylsiloxane reservoir releasing levonorgestrel 20 micrograms/24 hours. Net price = £98.18. Counselling, see patient information leaflet

Dose: Insert into uterine cavity within 7 days of onset of menstruation (anytime if replacement) or immediately after first-trimester termination by curettage; postpartum insertions should be delayed until 6 weeks after delivery; effective for 5 years

7.3.3 Spermicidal contraceptives

Spermicidal contraceptives are useful additional safeguards but do **not** give adequate protection if used alone except where fertility is already significantly diminished (section 6.4.1.1); they are suitable for use with barrier methods. They have two components: a spermicide and a vehicle which itself may have some inhibiting effect on sperm activity.

> **CSM advice.** Products such as petroleum jelly (*Vaseline®*), baby oil and oil-based vaginal and rectal preparations are likely to damage condoms and contraceptive diaphragms made from latex rubber, and may render them less effective as a barrier method of contraception and as a protection from sexually transmitted diseases (including HIV).

Condoms: no evidence of harm to latex condoms and diaphragms with the products listed below

Delfen® (Janssen-Cilag)
Foam, nonoxinol '9' 12.5%, pressurised aerosol unit in a water-miscible basis. Net price 20 g (with applicator) = £4.65
Excipients: include cetyl alcohol, hydroxybenzoates (parabens), propylene glycol, fragrance

Duragel® (SSL)
Gel, nonoxinol '9' 2% in a water-soluble basis. Net price 100-g tube = £3.45
Excipients: include propylene glycol

Gynol II® (Janssen-Cilag)
Jelly, nonoxinol '9' 2% in a water-soluble basis. Net price 81 g = £2.61; applicator = 75p
Excipients: include hydroxybenzoates (parabens), propylene glycol, sorbic acid

Ortho-Creme® (Janssen-Cilag)
Cream, nonoxinol '9' 2% in a water-miscible basis. Net price 70 g = £2.44; applicator = 75p
Excipients: include cetyl alcohol, hydroxybenzoates (parabens), propylene glycol, sorbic acid, fragrance

Orthoforms® (Janssen-Cilag)
Pessaries, nonoxinol '9' 5% in a water-soluble basis. Net price 15 pessaries = £2.40
Excipients: none as listed in section 13.1.3

7.3.4 Contraceptive devices

Intra-uterine devices

The intra-uterine device (IUD) is suitable for older parous women and as a second-line contraceptive in young nulliparous women who should be carefully screened because they have an increased background risk of pelvic inflammatory disease.

Smaller devices have been introduced to minimise side-effects; these consist of a plastic carrier wound with copper wire or fitted with copper bands; some also have a central core of silver to prevent fragmentation of the copper. Fertility declines with age and therefore a copper intra-uterine device which is fitted in a woman over the age of 40, may remain in the uterus until menopause. The intra-uterine device *Gyne-T 380®* (Janssen-Cilag) is no longer available, but some women may have the device in place until 2009.

A frameless, copper-bearing intra-uterine device (*GyneFix®*) has been introduced recently. It consists of a knotted, polypropylene thread with 6 copper sleeves; the device is anchored in the uterus by inserting the knot into the uterine fundus. *The healthcare professional inserting (or removing) the device should be fully trained in the technique and should provide full counselling backed by the patient information leaflet.*

The timing and technique of fitting an intra-uterine device are critical for its subsequent performance and call for proper training and experience. Devices should not be fitted during the heavy days of the period; they are best fitted after the end of menstruation and before the calculated time of implantation. The main excess risk of infection occurs in the first 20 days after insertion and is believed to be related to existing carriage of a sexually transmitted disease, therefore pre-screening (at least for chlamydia) should ideally be performed. The woman should be advised to attend *as an emergency* if she experiences sustained pain during the next 20 days.

An intra-uterine device should not be removed in mid-cycle unless an additional contraceptive was used for the previous 7 days. If removal is essential post-coital contraception should be considered.

If an intra-uterine device fails and the woman wishes to continue to full-term the device should be removed in the first trimester if possible.

INTRA-UTERINE CONTRACEPTIVE DEVICES

Indications: see notes above

Cautions: anaemia, heavy menses (progestogen intra-uterine system might be preferable, section 7.3.2.3), endometriosis, severe primary dysmenorrhoea, history of pelvic inflammatory disease, history of ectopic pregnancy or tubal surgery, diabetes, fertility problems, nulliparity and young age, severely scarred uterus (including after endometrial resection) or severe cervical stenosis, valvular heart disease (antibacterial cover needed—section 5.1 table 2)—avoid if prosthetic valve or history of infective endocarditis; drug- or disease-induced immunosuppression (risk of infection—avoid if marked immunosuppression); joint and other prostheses (increased risk of infection); epilepsy; increased risk of expulsion if inserted before uterine involution; gynaecological examination before insertion, 6–8 weeks after then annually but counsel women to see doctor promptly in case of significant symptoms, especially pain; anticoagulant therapy (avoid if possible); remove if pregnancy occurs; if pregnancy occurs, increased likelihood that it may be ectopic

Contra-indications: pregnancy, severe anaemia, recent sexually transmitted infection (if not fully investigated and treated), unexplained uterine bleeding, distorted or small uterine cavity, genital malignancy, active trophoblastic disease, pelvic inflammatory disease, established or marked immunosuppression; *copper devices:* copper allergy, Wilson's disease, medical diathermy

Side-effects: uterine or cervical perforation, displacement, expulsion; pelvic infection may be exacerbated, heavy menses, dysmenorrhoea, allergy; *on insertion:* pain (alleviated by NSAID such as ibuprofen 30 minutes before insertion) and bleeding, occasionally, epileptic seizure, vasovagal attack

Flexi-T® 300 (FP)
Intra-uterine device, copper wire, surface area approx. 300 mm² wound on vertical stem of T-shaped plastic carrier, impregnated with barium sulphate for radio-opacity, monofilament thread attached to base of vertical stem; preloaded in inserter, net price = £8.65
For uterine length over 5 cm; replacement every 5 years (see also notes above)

GyneFix® (FP)
Intra-uterine device, 6 copper sleeves with surface area of 330 mm² on polypropylene thread, net price = £24.75
Suitable for all uterine sizes; replacement every 5 years

Multiload® Cu250 (Organon)
Intra-uterine device, copper wire, surface area approx. 250 mm² wound on vertical stem of plastic carrier, 3.5 cm length, with 2 down-curving flexible arms, monofilament thread attached to base of vertical stem; preloaded in inserter, net price = £7.13
For uterine length 6–9 cm; replacement every 3 years (but see notes above)

Multiload® Cu250 Short (Organon)
Intra-uterine device, as above, with vertical stem length 2.4 cm, net price = £7.13
For uterine length 5–7 cm; replacement every 3 years (but see notes above)

Multiload® Cu375 (Organon)
Intra-uterine device, as above, with copper surface area approx. 375 mm² and vertical stem length 3.5 cm, net price = £9.24
For uterine length 6–9 cm; replacement every 5 years (see notes above)

Nova-T® 380 (Schering Health)
Intra-uterine device, copper wire with silver core, surface area approx. 380 mm² wound on vertical stem of T-shaped plastic carrier, impregnated with barium sulphate for radio-opacity, threads attached to base of vertical stem, net price = £13.50
For uterine length 6.5–9 cm; replacement every 5 years (see notes above)

T-Safe® CU 380 A (FP)
Intra-uterine device, copper wire, wound on vertical stem of T-shaped plastic carrier with copper collar on the distal portion of each arm, total surface area approx. 380 mm², impregnated with barium sulphate for radio-opacity, threads attached to base of vertical stem, net price = £9.40
For uterine length 6.5–9 cm; replacement every 8 years (see notes above)

Other contraceptive devices

■ Contraceptive caps
Type A contraceptive pessary
Opaque rubber, sizes 1 to 5 (55–75 mm rising in steps of 5 mm), net price = £7.03
Available from Lamberts (*Dumas Vault Cap®*)

Type B contraceptive pessary
Opaque rubber, sizes 22 to 31 mm (rising in steps of 3 mm), net price = £8.20
Available from Lamberts (*Prentif Cavity Rim Cervical Cap®*)

Type C contraceptive pessary
Opaque rubber, sizes 1 to 3 (42, 48 and 54 mm), net price = £7.03
Available from Lamberts (*Vimule Cap®*)

■ Contraceptive diaphragms
Type A Diaphragm with flat metal spring
Transparent rubber with flat metal spring, sizes 55–95 mm (rising in steps of 5 mm), net price = £5.59
Available from Lamberts (*Reflexions®*)

Type B Diaphragm with coiled metal rim
Opaque rubber with coiled metal rim, sizes 60–100 mm (rising in steps of 5 mm), net price = £6.14
Available from Janssen-Cilag (*Ortho®*)

Type C Arcing Spring Diaphragm
Opaque rubber with arcing spring, sizes 60–95 mm (rising in steps of 5 mm), net price = £6.98
Available from Janssen-Cilag (*All-Flex®*)

■ Fertility thermometer
Fertility (Ovulation) Thermometer (Zeal)
Mercury in glass thermometer, range 35 to 39°C (graduated in 0.1°C), net price = £1.76
For monitoring ovulation for the fertility awareness method of contraception

7.4 Drugs for genito-urinary disorders

7.4.1 Drugs for urinary retention
7.4.2 Drugs for urinary frequency, enuresis, and incontinence
7.4.3 Drugs used in urological pain
7.4.4 Bladder instillations and urological surgery
7.4.5 Drugs for erectile dysfunction

For drugs used in the treatment of urinary-tract infections see section 5.1.13.

7.4.1 Drugs for urinary retention

Acute retention is painful and is treated by catheterisation.

Chronic retention is painless and often long-standing. Catheterisation is unnecessary unless there is deterioration of renal function. After the cause has initially been established and treated, drugs may be required to increase detrusor muscle tone.

Benign prostatic hyperplasia is treated either surgically or medically with alpha-blockers (see below) or with the anti-androgen finasteride (section 6.4.2).

Alpha-blockers

The selective alpha-blockers, **alfuzosin**, **doxazosin**, **indoramin**, **prazosin**, **tamsulosin** and **terazosin** relax smooth muscle in benign prostatic hyperplasia producing an increase in urinary flow-rate and an improvement in obstructive symptoms.

CAUTIONS. Since selective alpha-blockers reduce blood pressure, patients receiving antihypertensive treatment may require reduced dosage and specialist supervision. Caution may be required in the elderly and in patients with hepatic impairment (Appendix 2) and severe renal impairment (Appendix 3). For **interactions** see Appendix 1 (alpha-blockers).

CONTRA-INDICATIONS. Alpha-blockers should be avoided in patients with a history of postural hypotension and micturition syncope.

SIDE-EFFECTS. Side-effects of selective alpha-blockers include drowsiness, hypotension (notably postural hypotension), syncope, asthenia, depression, headache, dry mouth, gastro-intestinal disturbances (including nausea, vomiting, diarrhoea, constipation), oedema, blurred vision, rhinitis, erectile disorders (including priapism), tachycardia, and palpitations. Hypersensitivity reactions including rash, pruritus and angioedema have also been reported.

ALFUZOSIN HYDROCHLORIDE

Indications: see notes above
Cautions: see notes above
Contra-indications: see notes above; severe liver impairment
Side-effects: see notes above; flushes, chest pain
Dose: 2.5 mg 3 times daily, max. 10 mg daily; ELDERLY initially 2.5 mg twice daily
FIRST DOSE EFFECT. First dose may cause collapse due to hypotensive effect (therefore should be taken on retiring to bed). Patient should be warned to lie down if symptoms such as dizziness, fatigue or sweating develop, and to remain lying down until they abate completely

Xatral® (Sanofi-Synthelabo) [PoM]
Tablets, f/c, alfuzosin hydrochloride 2.5 mg, net price 60-tab pack = £22.80. Label: 3, counselling, see dose above

■ Modified release
Xatral® **XL** (Sanofi-Synthelabo) [PoM]
Tablets, m/r, yellow/white, alfuzosin hydrochloride 10 mg, net price 10-tab pack = £7.93, 30-tab pack = £23.80. Label: 3, 21, 25, counselling, see above
Dose: 10 mg once daily

DOXAZOSIN

Indications: see notes above and section 2.5.4
Cautions: see notes above and section 2.5.4
Contra-indications: see notes above
Side-effects: see notes above and section 2.5.4
Dose: initially 1 mg daily; dose may be doubled at intervals of 1–2 weeks according to response, up to max. 8 mg daily; usual maintenance 2–4 mg daily

■ Preparations
Section 2.5.4

INDORAMIN

Indications: see notes above and section 2.5.4
Cautions: see notes above and section 2.5.4
Contra-indications: see notes above and section 2.5.4
Side-effects: see notes above and section 2.5.4
Dose: 20 mg twice daily; increased if necessary by 20 mg every 2 weeks to max. 100 mg daily in divided doses; ELDERLY, 20 mg at night may be adequate

Doralese® (GSK) [PoM]
Tablets, yellow, f/c, indoramin 20 mg, net price 60-tab pack = £12.30. Label: 2

PRAZOSIN HYDROCHLORIDE

Indications: see notes above and section 2.5.4
Cautions: see notes above and section 2.5.4
Contra-indications: see notes above and section 2.5.4
Side-effects: see notes above and section 2.5.4; paraesthesia, arthralgia, epistaxis, nervousness, dyspnoea, hallucinations, alopecia
Dose: initially 500 micrograms twice daily for 3–7 days, subsequently adjusted according to response; usual maintenance (and max.) 2 mg twice daily; ELDERLY initiate with lowest possible dose
FIRST DOSE EFFECT. First dose may cause collapse due to hypotensive effect (therefore should be taken on retiring to bed). Patient should be warned to lie down if symptoms such as dizziness, fatigue or sweating develop, and to remain lying down until they abate completely

■ Preparations
Section 2.5.4

TAMSULOSIN HYDROCHLORIDE

Indications: see notes above
Cautions: see notes above
Contra-indications: see notes above; severe liver impairment
Side-effects: see notes above
Dose: 400 micrograms daily as a single dose after food

Flomax® **MR** (Yamanouchi) [PoM]
Capsules, m/r, tamsulosin hydrochloride 400 micrograms. Net price 30-cap pack = £22.00. Label: 25

TERAZOSIN

Indications: see notes above and section 2.5.4
Cautions: see notes above and section 2.5.4
Contra-indications: see notes above
Side-effects: see notes above and section 2.5.4; weight gain, paraesthesia, dyspnoea, thrombocytopenia, nervousness, decreased libido, back pain and pain in extremities
Dose: initially 1 mg at bedtime; if necessary dose may be doubled at intervals of 1–2 weeks according to response, up to max. 10 mg once daily; usual maintenance 5–10 mg daily
FIRST DOSE EFFECT. First dose may cause collapse due to hypotensive effect (therefore should be taken on retiring to bed). Patient should be warned to lie down if symptoms such as dizziness, fatigue or sweating develop, and to remain lying down until they abate completely

Terazosin (Non-proprietary) [PoM]
Tablets, terazosin (as hydrochloride) 2 mg, net price 28-tab pack = £7.75; 5 mg, 28-tab pack = £12.58; 10 mg, 28-tab pack = £25.73
Available from Alpharma, APS, Generics, Ratiopharm

Hytrin BPH® (Abbott) [PoM]
Tablets, terazosin (as hydrochloride) 2 mg (yellow) net price, 28-tab pack = £8.07; 5 mg (tan), 28-tab pack = £13.07; 10 mg (blue), 28-tab pack = £26.59; starter pack of 7 × 1-mg tab with 14 × 2-mg tab and 7 × 5-mg tab = £10.97. Label: 3, counselling, see dose above

Parasympathomimetics

The parasympathomimetic **bethanechol** increases detrusor muscle contraction. However, it has only a limited role in the relief of urinary retention; its use has been superseded by catheterisation.

Distigmine inhibits the breakdown of acetylcholine. It may help patients with an upper motor neurone neurogenic bladder.

CAUTIONS and CONTRA-INDICATIONS. Parasympathomimetics should be used with caution or avoided in hyperthyroidism or in cardiac disorders including bradycardia, arrhythmias and recent myocardial infarction. They are contra-indicated in intestinal or urinary obstruction or where increased motility of the gastro-intestinal or urinary tract could be harmful. Parasympathomimetics should also be avoided in gastro-intestinal ulceration, asthma, hypotension, epilepsy, parkinsonism, pregnancy, and breast-feeding. **Interactions**: Appendix 1 (parasympathomimetics)

SIDE-EFFECTS. Parasympathomimetic side-effects such as nausea, vomiting, intestinal colic, bradycardia, blurred vision, and sweating may occur, particularly in the elderly.

BETHANECHOL CHLORIDE

Indications: urinary retention, but see notes above
Cautions: see notes above
Contra-indications: see notes above
Side-effects: see notes above
Dose: 10–25 mg 3–4 times daily half an hour before food

Myotonine® (Glenwood) PoM
Tablets, both scored, bethanechol chloride 10 mg, net price 20 = £1.01; 25 mg, 20 = £1.30 Label: 22

DISTIGMINE BROMIDE

Indications: postoperative urinary retention (see notes above), neurogenic bladder; myasthenia gravis (section 10.2.1)
Cautions: see notes above; also pregnancy (Appendix 4), breast-feeding
Contra-indications: see notes above; also severe postoperative shock, serious circulatory insufficiency
Side-effects: see notes above, but action slower than bethamechol chloride (therefore side-effects less acute; see also Neostigmine (section 10.2.1); also dyspnoea, muscle twitching, and urinary frequency
Dose: urinary retention, 5 mg daily, half an hour before breakfast
Neurogenic bladder, 5 mg daily or on alternate days, half an hour before breakfast

Ubretid® (Rhône-Poulenc Rorer) PoM
Tablets, scored, distigmine bromide 5 mg. Net price 30-tab pack = £31.26. Label: 22

7.4.2 Drugs for urinary frequency, enuresis, and incontinence

Urinary incontinence

Incontinence in adults which arises from detrusor instability is managed by combining drug therapy with conservative methods for managing urge incontinence such as pelvic floor exercises and bladder training; stress incontinence is generally managed by non-drug methods.

Involuntary detrusor contractions cause urgency and urge incontinence, usually with frequency and nocturia. Antimuscarinic drugs reduce these contractions and increase bladder capacity. **Oxybutynin** also has a direct relaxant effect on urinary smooth muscle. Side-effects limit the use of oxybutynin but they may be reduced by starting at a lower dose; a modified-release preparation of oxybutynin is effective and has fewer side-effects. The efficacy and side-effects of **tolterodine** are comparable to those of modified-release oxybutynin. **Flavoxate** has less marked side-effects but it is also less effective. **Propiverine** and **trospium** are newer antimuscarinic drugs licensed for urinary frequency, urgency, and incontinence. The need for continuing antimuscarinic drug therapy should be reviewed after 6 months.

Propantheline and tricyclic antidepressants were used for urge incontinence but they are little used now because of their side-effects. The use of imipramine is limited by its potential to cause cardiac side-effects.

Purified bovine collagen implant (*Contigen®*, Bard) is indicated for *urinary incontinence* caused by intrinsic sphincter deficiency (poor or non-functioning bladder outlet mechanism). The implant should be inserted only by surgeons or physicians trained in the technique for injection of the implant.

CAUTIONS. Antimuscarinic drugs should be used with caution in the elderly (especially if frail) and in those with autonomic neuropathy. They should also be used with caution in hiatus hernia with reflux oesophagitis, and in hepatic impairment (Appendix 2; avoid propiverine) and renal impairment (Appendix 3). Antimuscarinics may worsen hyperthyroidism, coronary artery disease, congestive heart failure, prostatic hypertrophy, arrhythmias and tachycardia. For **interactions** see Appendix 1 (antimuscarinics).

CONTRA-INDICATIONS. Antimuscarinic drugs should be avoided in patients with myasthenia gravis, glaucoma, significant bladder outflow obstruction or urinary retention, severe ulcerative colitis, toxic megacolon, and in gastro-intestinal obstruction or intestinal atony.

SIDE-EFFECTS. Side-effects of antimuscarinic drugs include dry mouth, constipation, blurred vision, drowsiness, nausea, vomiting, abdominal discomfort, difficulty in micturition (less commonly urinary retention), palpitations, and skin reactions (including dry skin, rash, and photosensitivity); also headache, diarrhoea, angioedema, arrhythmias and tachycardia. Central nervous system stimulation, such as restlessness, disorientation, hallucination and convulsion may occur; children are at higher risk of these effects. Antimuscarinic drugs may reduce sweating leading to heat sensations and fainting in hot environments.

FLAVOXATE HYDROCHLORIDE

Indications: urinary frequency and incontinence, dysuria, urgency; bladder spasms due to catheterisation

Cautions: see notes above; pregnancy (Appendix 4), breast-feeding (Appendix 5)

Contra-indications: see notes above; gastro-intestinal haemorrhage

Side-effects: see notes above; also vertigo, fatigue, eosinophilia

Dose: 200 mg 3 times daily; CHILD under 12 years not recommended

Urispas 200® (Shire) [PoM]
Tablets, f/c, flavoxate hydrochloride 200 mg, net price 90-tab pack = £11.87

OXYBUTYNIN HYDROCHLORIDE

Indications: urinary frequency, urgency and incontinence, neurogenic bladder instability and nocturnal enuresis

Cautions: see notes above; pregnancy (Appendix 4), porphyria (section 9.8.2)

Contra-indications: see notes above; breast-feeding (Appendix 5)

Side-effects: see notes above; also anorexia, facial flushing (more marked in children) and dizziness

Dose: initially 2.5–5 mg 2–3 times daily increased if necessary to max. 5 mg 4 times daily

ELDERLY initially 2.5–3 mg twice daily, increased to 5 mg twice daily according to response and tolerance

CHILD over 5 years, neurogenic bladder instability, 2.5–3 mg twice daily increased to 5 mg twice daily (max. 5 mg 3 times daily); nocturnal enuresis (preferably over 7 years, see notes below), 2.5–3 mg twice daily increased to 5 mg 2–3 times daily (last dose before bedtime)

Oxybutynin Hydrochloride (Non-proprietary) [PoM]
Tablets, oxybutynin hydrochloride 2.5 mg, net price 56-tab pack = £3.43; 3 mg, 56-tab pack = £8.49; 5 mg, 56-tab pack = £9.50, 84-tab pack = £20.52. Label: 3

Cystrin® (Sanofi-Synthelabo) [PoM]
Tablets, oxybutynin hydrochloride 3 mg, net price 56-tab pack = £9.15; 5 mg (scored), 84-tab pack = £22.88. Label: 3

Ditropan® (Sanofi-Synthelabo) [PoM]
Tablets, both blue, scored, oxybutynin hydrochloride 2.5 mg, net price 84-tab pack = £6.86; 5 mg, 84-tab pack = £13.34. Label: 3
Elixir, oxybutynin hydrochloride 2.5 mg/5 mL. Net price 150-mL pack= £4.78. Label: 3

■ Modified release

Lyrinel® **XL** (Janssen-Cilag) [PoM]
Tablets, m/r, oxybutynin hydrochloride 5 mg (yellow), net price 30-tab pack = £12.34; 10 mg (pink), 30-tab pack = £24.68. Label: 3, 25
Dose: ADULT over 18 years, initially 5 mg daily, adjusted according to response in 5-mg steps at weekly intervals; max. 30 mg daily taken as a single dose
NOTE. Patients taking immediate-release oxybutynin may be transferred to the nearest equivalent daily dose of *Lyrinel*® *XL*

PROPANTHELINE BROMIDE

Indications: adult enuresis

Cautions: see notes above; ulcerative colitis, pregnancy (Appendix 4) and breast-feeding (Appendix 5)

Contra-indications: see notes above

Side-effects: see notes above; also facial flushing

Dose: initially 15 mg 3 times daily at least one hour before food and 30 mg at bedtime, subsequently adjusted according to response (max. 120 mg daily)

■ Preparations
Section 1.2

PROPIVERINE HYDROCHLORIDE

Indications: urinary frequency, urgency and incontinence; neurogenic bladder instability

Cautions: see notes above

Contra-indications: see notes above; pregnancy (Appendix 4) and breast-feeding (Appendix 5)

Side-effects: see notes above

Dose: 15 mg 1–3 times daily, increased if necessary to max. 15 mg 4 times daily
CHILD not recommended

Detrunorm® (Schering-Plough) [PoM]
Tablets, pink, s/c, propiverine hydrochloride 15 mg, net price 28-tab pack = £15.28, 56-tab pack = £30.56. Label: 3

TOLTERODINE TARTRATE

Indications: urinary frequency, urgency and incontinence

Cautions: see notes above

Contra-indications: see notes above; pregnancy (Appendix 4) and breast-feeding (Appendix 5)

Side-effects: see notes above; also dyspepsia, fatigue, flatulence, chest pain, dry eyes, peripheral oedema, paraesthesia

Dose: 2 mg twice daily; reduce to 1mg twice daily if necessary to minimise side-effects
CHILD not recommended

Detrusitol® (Pharmacia) [PoM]
Tablets, f/c, tolterodine tartrate 1 mg, net price 56-tab pack = £29.03; 2 mg, 56-tab pack = £30.56

■ Modified release

Detrusitol® **XL** (Pharmacia) [PoM]
Capsules, blue, m/r, tolterodine tartrate 4 mg, net price 28-cap pack = £29.03. Label: 25
Dose: 4 mg once daily (dose form not appropriate for hepatic and renal impairment)

TROSPIUM CHLORIDE

Indications: urinary frequency, urgency and incontinence

Cautions: see notes above; pregnancy and breast-feeding

Contra-indications: see notes above

Side-effects: see notes above; also flatulence, chest pain, dyspnoea, rash and asthenia

Dose: 20 mg twice daily before food
CHILD not recommended

Regurin® (Galen) ▼ PoM
Tablets, brown, f/c, trospium chloride 20 mg, net price 60-tab pack = £25.00. Label 23

Nocturnal enuresis

Nocturnal enuresis is a common occurrence in young children but persists in as many as 5% by 10 years of age. Treatment is not appropriate in children under 5 years and it is usually not needed in those aged under 7 years and in cases where the child and parents are not anxious about the bedwetting; however, children over 10 years usually require prompt treatment. An **enuresis alarm** should be first-line treatment for well-motivated children aged over 7 years because it may achieve a more sustained reduction of enuresis than use of drugs. Use of an alarm may be combined with drug therapy if either method alone is unsuccessful.

Drug therapy is not usually appropriate for children under 7 years of age; it can be used when alternative measures have failed, preferably on a short-term basis, to cover periods away from home for example. The possible side-effects of the various drugs should be borne in mind when they are prescribed.

Desmopressin (section 6.5.2), an analogue of vasopressin, is used for nocturnal enuresis; it is given intranasally or it may be given by mouth as tablets. Particular care is needed to avoid fluid overload and treatment should not be continued for longer than 3 months without stopping for a week for full re-assessment.

Tricyclics (section 4.3.1) such as **amitriptyline**, **imipramine**, and less often **nortriptyline** are also used but behaviour disturbances may occur and relapse is common after withdrawal. Treatment should not normally exceed 3 months unless a full physical examination is given and the child is fully re-assessed; toxicity following overdosage with tricyclics is of particular concern.

7.4.3 Drugs used in urological pain

The acute pain of *ureteric colic* may be relieved with **pethidine** (section 4.7.2). **Diclofenac** by injection or as suppositories (section 10.1.1) is also effective and compares favourably with pethidine; other non-steroidal anti-inflammatory drugs are occasionally given by injection.

Lidocaine (lignocaine) gel is a useful topical application in *urethral pain* or to relieve the discomfort of catheterisation (section 15.2).

Alkalinisation of urine

Alkalinisation of urine may be undertaken with **potassium citrate**. The alkalinising action may relieve the discomfort of *cystitis* caused by lower urinary tract infections. **Sodium bicarbonate** is used as a urinary alkalinising agent in some metabolic and renal disorders (section 9.2.1.3).

POTASSIUM CITRATE

Indications: relief of discomfort in mild urinary-tract infections; alkalinisation of urine

Cautions: renal impairment, cardiac disease; elderly; **interactions:** Appendix 1 (potassium salts)

Side-effects: hyperkalaemia on prolonged high dosage, mild diuresis

Potassium Citrate Mixture BP
(Potassium Citrate Oral Solution)
Oral solution, potassium citrate 30%, citric acid monohydrate 5% in a suitable vehicle with a lemon flavour. Extemporaneous preparations should be recently prepared according to the following formula: potassium citrate 3 g, citric acid monohydrate 500 mg, syrup 2.5 mL, quillaia tincture 0.1 mL, lemon spirit 0.05 mL, double-strength chloroform water 3 mL, water to 10 mL. Contains about 28 mmol K^+/10 mL. Label: 27
Dose: 10 mL 3 times daily well diluted with water
NOTE. Concentrates for preparation of Potassium Citrate Mixture BP are available from Hillcross
Proprietary brands of potassium citrate on sale to the public for the relief of discomfort in mild urinary-tract infections include *Cystopurin*® (Roche Consumer Health) and *Effercitrate*® (Typharm)

SODIUM BICARBONATE

Indications: relief of discomfort in mild urinary-tract infections; alkalinisation of urine

Cautions: hepatic and renal impairment, cardiac disease, pregnancy; patients on sodium-restricted diet; elderly; avoid prolonged use; **interactions:** Appendix 1 (antacids)

Side-effects: belching, alkalosis on prolonged use

Dose: 3 g in water every 2 hours until urinary pH exceeds 7; maintenance of alkaline urine 5–10 g daily

■ Preparations
Section 9.2.1.3

SODIUM CITRATE

Indications: relief of discomfort in mild urinary-tract infections

Cautions: renal impairment, cardiac disease, hypertension, pregnancy, patients on a sodium-restricted diet; elderly

Side-effects: mild diuresis
NOTE. Proprietary brands of sodium citrate on sale to the public for the relief of discomfort in mild urinary-tract infections include *Boots Cystitis Relief Sachets and Tablets*, *Canesten*® *Oasis* (Bayer), *Cymalon*® (Thornton & Ross), and *Cystemme*® (Abbott)

Acidification of urine

Urine acidification is difficult; it is very occasionally used in the management of recurrent urinary-tract infections and to prevent renal stone formation, especially in patients with paraplegia or with a neurogenic bladder. Methenamine (section 5.1.13) requires acid urine for its antimicrobial activity.

Ammonium chloride may be used for urinary acidification but tolerance can develop rapidly. Vomiting and, with large doses, hypokalaemia and acidosis can also occur. Ammonium chloride oral solution needs to be prepared extemporaneously and may not be readily available. **Ascorbic acid** is less suitable for urine acidification because it is not always reliable and high doses, which can lead to renal stones in those with hyperoxaluria, are required.

For pH-modifying solutions for the maintenance of indwelling urinary catheters, see section 7.4.4.

Other preparations for urinary disorders

A terpene mixture (*Rowatinex®*) is claimed to be of benefit in *urolithiasis* for the expulsion of calculi.

Rowatinex® (Rowa) [PoM] ▭
Capsules, yellow, e/c, anethol 4 mg, borneol 10 mg, camphene 15 mg, cineole 3 mg, fenchone 4 mg, pinene 31 mg. Net price 50 = £7.35. Label: 25
Dose: 1–2 capsules 3–4 times daily before food; CHILD not recommended

7.4.4 Bladder instillations and urological surgery

BLADDER INFECTION. Various solutions are available as irrigations or washouts.

Aqueous **chlorhexidine** (section 13.11.2) may be used in the management of common infections of the bladder but it is ineffective against most *Pseudomonas* spp. Solutions containing chlorhexidine 1 in 5000 (0.02%) are used but they may irritate the mucosa and cause burning and haematuria (in which case they should be discontinued); sterile **sodium chloride solution 0.9%** (physiological saline) is usually adequate and is preferred as a mechanical irrigant.

Continuous bladder irrigation with **amphotericin** 50 micrograms/mL (section 5.2) may be of value in mycotic infections.

DISSOLUTION OF BLOOD CLOTS. Clot retention is usually treated by irrigation with sterile **sodium chloride solution 0.9%** but sterile **sodium citrate solution for bladder irrigation 3%** may also be helpful. **Streptokinase-streptodornase** (*Varidase Topical®*, section 13.11.7) is an alternative.

BLADDER CANCER. Bladder instillations of **doxorubicin** (section 8.1.2), **mitomycin** (section 8.1.2), and **thiotepa** (section 8.1.1) are used for recurrent superficial bladder tumours. Such instillations reduce systemic side-effects; adverse effects on the bladder (e.g. micturition disorders and reduction in bladder capacity) may occur.

Instillation of **epirubicin** (section 8.1.2) is used for treatment and prophylaxis of certain forms of superficial bladder cancer; instillation of **doxorubicin** (section 8.1.2) is also used for some papillary tumours.

Instillation of **BCG** (Bacillus Calmette-Guérin), a live attenuated strain derived from *Mycobacterium bovis* (section 8.2.4), has been licensed recently for the treatment of primary or recurrent bladder carcinoma *in-situ* and for the prevention of recurrence following transurethral resection.

INTERSTITIAL CYSTITIS. **Dimethyl sulfoxide** (dimethyl sulphoxide) may be used for symptomatic relief in patients with interstitial cystitis (Hunner's ulcer). 50 mL of a 50% solution (*Rimso-50®*— available on named-patient basis from Britannia) is instilled into the bladder, retained for 15 minutes, and voided by the patient. Treatment is repeated at intervals of 2 weeks. Bladder spasm and hypersensitivity reactions may occur and long-term use requires ophthalmic, renal, and hepatic assessment at intervals of 6 months.

SODIUM CITRATE

Indications: bladder washouts, see notes above

Sterile Sodium Citrate Solution for Bladder Irrigation sodium citrate 3%, dilute hydrochloric acid 0.2%, in purified water, freshly boiled and cooled, and sterilised

Urological surgery

There is a high risk of fluid absorption from the irrigant used in endoscopic surgery within the urinary tract; if this occurs in excess, hypervolaemia, haemolysis, and renal failure may result. **Glycine irrigation solution 1.5%** is the irrigant of choice for transurethral resection of the prostate gland and bladder tumours; **sterile sodium chloride solution 0.9%** (physiological saline) is used for percutaneous renal surgery.

GLYCINE

Indications: bladder irrigation during urological surgery; see notes above
Cautions: see notes above
Side-effects: see notes above

Glycine Irrigation Solution (Non-proprietary)
Irrigation solution, glycine 1.5% in water for injections
Available from Baxter, Fresenius

Maintenance of indwelling urinary catheters

The deposition which occurs in catheterised patients is usually chiefly composed of phosphate and to minimise this the catheter (if latex) should be changed at least as often as every 6 weeks. If the catheter is to be left for longer periods a silicone catheter should be used together with the appropriate use of catheter maintenance solutions. Repeated blockage usually indicates that the catheter needs to be changed.

CATHETER PATENCY SOLUTIONS

Chlorhexidine 0.02%
Available from Braun (*Uro-Tainer Chlorhexidine®*, 100-mL sachet = £2.60), SSL (*Uriflex C®*, 100-mL sachet = £2.40)

Mandelic acid 1%
Available from Braun (*Uro-Tainer Mandelic Acid®*, 100-mL sachet = £2.60)

Sodium chloride 0.9%
Available from Bard (*OptiFlo S®*, 50-and 100-mL sachets = £3.04), Braun (*Uro-Tainer Sodium*

Chloride®, 50- and 100-mL sachets = £2.45, *Uro-Tainer M®*, with integral drug additive port, 50- and 100-mL sachets = £2.90), SSL (*Uriflex S®*, 100-mL sachet = £2.40, *Uriflex SP®* with integral drug additive port, 100-mL sachet = £2.40)

Solution G

Citric acid 3.23%, magnesium oxide 0.38%, sodium bicarbonate 0.7%, disodium edetate 0.01%.
Available from Bard (*OptiFlo G®*, 50- and 100-mL sachets = £3.23), Braun (*Uro-Tainer Suby G®*, 50- and 100-mL sachets = £2.60), SSL (*Uriflex G®*, 100-mL sachet = £2.40)

Solution R

Citric acid 6%, gluconolactone 0.6%, magnesium carbonate 2.8%, disodium edetate 0.01%. Available from Bard (*OptiFlo R®*, 50- and 100-mL sachets = £3.23), Braun (*Uro-Tainer Solution R®*, 50- and 100-mL sachets = £2.60), SSL (*Uriflex R®*, 100-mL sachet = £2.40)

7.4.5 Drugs for erectile dysfunction

Reasons for failure to produce a satisfactory erection include *psychogenic, vascular, neurogenic,* and *endocrine abnormalities;* impotence can also be drug-induced. Intracavernosal injection or urethral application of vasoactive drugs under careful medical supervision is used for both diagnostic and therapeutic purposes.

Erectile disorders may also be treated with drugs given by mouth which increase the blood flow to the penis. Drugs should be used with caution if the penis is deformed (e.g. in angulation, cavernosal fibrosis, and Peyronie's disease).

Drug treatments for erectile dysfunction may only be prescribed on the NHS under certain circumstances (see individual preparations). The Department of Health (England) has recommended that treatment should also be available from specialist services (commissioned by Health Authorities and Primary Care Groups, and operating under local agreement) when the condition is causing severe distress; specialist centres should use form FP10(HP) or form HBP in Scotland or form WP10HP in Wales and endorse them 'SLS' if the treatment is to be dispensed in the community. The following criteria should be considered when assessing distress:

- significant disruption to normal social and occupational activities;
- a marked effect on mood, behaviour, social and environmental awareness;
- a marked effect on interpersonal relationships.

Alprostadil

Alprostadil (prostaglandin E₁) is given by intracavernosal injection or intraurethral application for the management of erectile dysfunction (after exclusion of treatable medical causes); it is also used as a diagnostic test.

ALPROSTADIL

Indications: erectile dysfunction (including aid to diagnosis); neonatal congenital heart defects (section 7.1.1.1)

Cautions: priapism—patients should be instructed to report any erection lasting 4 hours or longer—for recommendations, see below; anatomical deformations of penis (painful erection more likely)—follow up regularly to detect signs of penile fibrosis (consider discontinuation if angulation, cavernosal fibrosis or Peyronie's disease develop); **interactions:** Appendix 1 (alprostadil)

Contra-indications: predisposition to prolonged erection (as in sickle cell anaemia, multiple myeloma or leukaemia); not for use with other agents for erectile dysfunction, in patients with penile implants or when sexual activity medically inadvisable; urethral application also contra-indicated in urethral stricture, severe hypospadia, severe curvature, balanitis, urethritis

Side-effects: penile pain, priapism (see below and under Cautions); reactions at injection site include haematoma, haemosiderin deposits, penile rash, penile oedema, penile fibrosis, haemorrhage, inflammation; other local reactions include urethral burning and bleeding, penile warmth, numbness, penile or urinary-tract infection, irritation, sensitivity, phimosis, pruritus, erythema, venous leak, abnormal ejaculation; systemic effects reported include testicular pain and swelling, scrotal disorders, changes in micturition (including haematuria), nausea, dry mouth, fainting, hypotension (very rarely circulatory collapse) or hypertension, rapid pulse, vasodilatation, chest pain, supraventricular extrasystole, peripheral vascular disorder, dizziness, weakness, localised pain (buttocks, legs, genital, perineal, abdominal), headache, pelvic pain, back pain, influenza-like syndrome, swelling of the leg veins

PRIAPISM. If priapism should occur treatment should not be delayed more than 6 hours and is as follows:
Initial therapy by penile aspiration—using aseptic technique a 19–21 gauge butterfly needle inserted into the corpus cavernosum and 20–50 mL of blood aspirated; if necessary the procedure may be repeated on the opposite side.
If aspiration unsuccessful, *cautious* intracavernosal injection of a sympathomimetic with action on alpha-adrenergic receptors, continuously monitoring blood pressure and pulse (*extreme caution:* coronary heart disease, hypertension, cerebral ischaemia or if taking antidepressant) as follows:

- intracavernosal injections of phenylephrine 100–200 micrograms (0.5–1 mL of a 200 microgram/mL solution) every 5–10 minutes; max. total dose 1 mg [unlicensed indication] [*important:* if suitable strength of phenylephrine injection not available may be specially prepared by diluting 0.1 mL of the phenylephrine 1% (10 mg/mL) injection to 5 mL with sodium chloride 0.9%]; *alternatively*
- intracavernosal injections of adrenaline 10–20 micrograms (0.5–1mL of a 20 microgram/mL solution) every 5–10 minutes; max. total dose 100 micrograms [*important:* if suitable strength of adrenaline not available may be specially prepared by diluting 0.1 mL of the adrenaline 1 in 1000 (1mg/mL) injection to 5 mL with sodium chloride 0.9%]; *alternatively*
- intracavernosal injection of metaraminol (*caution: has been associated with fatal hypertensive crises*); metaraminol 1 mg (0.1 mL of 10 mg/mL metaraminol injection) is diluted to 50 mL with sodium chloride 0.9% and given carefully by slow injection into the corpora in 5-mL injections every 15 minutes [unlicensed indication].

If necessary the sympathomimetic injections can be

followed by further aspiration of blood through the same butterfly needle.

If sympathomimetics unsuccessful, urgent surgical referral for management (possibly including shunt procedure).

Dose: see under preparations below

■ Intracavernosal injection

¹**Caverject**® (Pharmacia) PoM NHS

Injection, powder for reconstitution, alprostadil, net price 5-microgram vial = £7.33; 10-microgram vial = £9.24; 20-microgram vial = £11.94; 40-microgram vial = £21.58 (all with diluent-filled syringe, needles and swabs)

Caverject® Dual Chamber, double-chamber cartridges (containing alprostadil and diluent), net price 10-microgram cartridge (for doses 2.5–10 micrograms) = £7.35; 20-microgram cartridge (for doses 5–20 micrograms) = £9.50 (both with needles)

Dose: by direct intracavernosal injection, erectile dysfunction, first dose 2.5 micrograms, second dose 5 micrograms (if some response to first dose) *or* 7.5 micrograms (if no response to first dose), increasing in steps of 5–10 micrograms to obtain dose suitable for producing erection not lasting more than 1 hour (neurological dysfunction, first dose 1.25 micrograms, second dose 2.5 micrograms, third dose 5 micrograms, increasing in steps of 5 micrograms to obtain suitable dose); if no response to dose then next higher dose can be given within 1 hour, if there is a response the next dose should not be given for at least 24 hours; usual range 5–20 micrograms; max. 60 micrograms (max. frequency of injection not more than once daily and not more than 3 times in any 1 week)

NOTE. The first dose must be given by medically trained personnel; self-administration may only be undertaken after proper training

Aid to diagnosis, 20 micrograms as a single dose (where evidence of neurological dysfunction, initially 5 micrograms and max. 10 micrograms)—consult product literature for details

¹**Viridal**® Duo (Schwarz) PoM NHS

Starter Pack (hosp. only), contents as for *Continuation Pack* below plus *Duoject* applicator, 10-microgram starter pack = £21.65, 20-microgram starter pack = £26.39, 40-microgram starter pack = £32.08; *Continuation Pack*, 2 double-chamber cartridges (containing alprostadil and diluent), 2 needles, swabs, 10-microgram continuation pack = £16.18, 20-microgram continuation pack = £20.91, 40-microgram continuation pack = £26.61; *Duoject*® applicator available free of charge from Schwarz

Dose: by direct intracavernosal injection, erectile dysfunction, initially 2.5 micrograms (1.25 micrograms in

1. NHS except to treat erectile dysfunction in men who:

- have diabetes, multiple sclerosis, Parkinson's disease, poliomyelitis, prostate cancer, severe pelvic injury, single gene neurological disease, spina bifida or spinal cord injury;

- are receiving dialysis for renal failure;

- have had radical pelvic surgery, prostatectomy, or kidney transplant;

- were receiving *Caverject*®, *Erecnos*®, *MUSE*®, *Viagra*® or *Viridal*® for erectile dysfunction, at the expense of the NHS, on 14 September 1998;

- are suffering severe distress as a result of impotence (prescribed by specialist centres only, see notes above).

The prescription must be endorsed 'SLS'.

neurogenic erectile dysfunction) increasing in steps of 2.5–5 micrograms to obtain dose suitable for producing erection not lasting more than 1 hour; usual range 10–20 micrograms; max. 40 micrograms (max. frequency of injection not more than 2–3 times per week with at least 24 hour interval between injections); erection lasting longer than 2 hours—re-titrate dose; patient should report to doctor erection lasting longer than 4 hours

NOTE. The first dose must be given by medically trained personnel; self-administration may only be undertaken after proper training

■ Urethral application

COUNSELLING. If partner pregnant barrier contraception should be used

¹**MUSE**® (Meda) PoM NHS

Urethral application, alprostadil, net price 125-microgram single-use applicator = £9.89, 250-microgram single-use applicator = £10.76, 500-microgram single-use applicator = £10.76, 1-mg single-use applicator = £11.01 (all strengths also available in packs of 6 applicators)

Condoms: no evidence of harm to latex condoms and diaphragms

Dose: by direct urethral application, erectile dysfunction, initially 250 micrograms adjusted according to response (usual range 0.125–1 mg); max. 2 doses in 24 hours and 7 doses in 7 days)

NOTE. The first dose must be given by medically trained personnel; self-administration may only be undertaken after proper training

Aid to diagnosis, 500 micrograms as a single dose

Apomorphine

Apomorphine is licensed for the treatment of erectile dysfunction; it is given as sublingual tablets. Compared to subcutaneous injection, absorption from the sublingual site is limited.

APOMORPHINE HYDROCHLORIDE

Indications: erectile dysfunction; Parkinson's disease (section 4.9.1)

Cautions: hepatic impairment (Appendix 2), renal impairment (Appendix 3); uncontrolled hypertension, hypotension; elderly; anatomical deformation of penis (e.g. angulation, cavernosal fibrosis, Peyronie's disease); not recommended for use in combination with other treatments for erectile dysfunction; **interactions:** Appendix 1 (apomorphine)

DRIVING. May impair performance of skilled tasks (e.g. driving)

Contra-indications: recent myocardial infarction; severe unstable angina, severe heart failure or hypotension; conditions where sexual activity is medically inadvisable

Side-effects: nausea, dyspepsia, headache, dizziness, yawning, drowsiness, rhinitis, pharyngitis, cough, flushing, taste disturbance, sweating; vasovagal syndrome; less frequently syncope, stomatitis, mouth ulcers; rarely hypersensitivity reactions including angioedema

Dose: *by sublingual administration*, initially 2 mg approx. 20 minutes before sexual activity, subsequent doses may be increased to 3 mg if necessary; minimum of 8 hours between doses

¹**Uprima**® (Abbott) ▼ PoM NHS

Sublingual tablets, both red, apomorphine hydrochloride 2 mg, net price 2-tab pack = £10.67; 3 mg, 4-tab pack = £21.34. Counselling, driving

Phosphodiesterase type-5 inhibitors

Sildenafil, **tadalafil** and **vardenafil** are phosphodiesterase type-5 inhibitors licensed for the treatment of erectile dysfunction; they are not recommended for use with other treatments for erectile dysfunction. The patient should be assessed appropriately before prescribing sildenafil, tadalafil or vardenafil. Since these drugs are given by mouth there is a potential for drug interactions.

CAUTIONS. Sildenafil, tadalafil and vardenafil should be used with caution in cardiovascular disease, anatomical deformation of the penis (e.g. angulation, cavernosal fibrosis, Peyronie's disease), and in those with a predisposition to prolonged erection (e.g. in sickle-cell anaemia, multiple myeloma, or leukaemia).

CONTRA-INDICATIONS. Sildenafil, tadalafil and vardenafil are contra-indicated in patients receiving nitrates or in patients in whom vasodilation or sexual activity are inadvisable. In the absence of information, manufacturers contra-indicate these drugs in hypotension, recent stroke, unstable angina, and myocardial infarction.

SIDE-EFFECTS. The side-effects of sildenafil, tadalafil and vardenafil include dyspepsia, vomiting, headache, flushing, dizziness, visual disturbances, raised intra-ocular pressure, and nasal congestion. Hypersensitivity reactions (including rash), priapism, and painful red eyes have been reported.

SILDENAFIL

Indications: erectile dysfunction

Cautions: see notes above; also hepatic impairment (Appendix 2—avoid if severe); renal impairment (Appendix 3); bleeding disorders or active peptic ulceration; **interactions:** Appendix 1 (sildenafil)

Contra-indications: see notes above; also hereditary degenerative retinal disorders

Side-effects: see notes above; also serious cardiovascular events reported

Dose: initially 50 mg (ELDERLY 25 mg) approx. 1 hour before sexual activity, subsequent doses adjusted according to response to 25–100 mg as a single dose as needed; max. 1 dose in 24 hours (max. single dose 100 mg)

NOTE. Onset of effect may be delayed if taken with food

1. [NHS] except to treat erectile dysfunction in men who:

- have diabetes, multiple sclerosis, Parkinson's disease, poliomyelitis, prostate cancer, severe pelvic injury, single gene neurological disease, spina bifida or spinal cord injury;
- are receiving dialysis for renal failure;
- have had radical pelvic surgery, prostatectomy, or kidney transplant;
- were receiving *Caverject®*, *Erecnos®*, *MUSE®*, *Viagra®* or *Viridal®* for erectile dysfunction, at the expense of the NHS, on 14 September 1998;
- are suffering severe distress as a result of impotence (prescribed by specialist centres only, see notes above).

The prescription must be endorsed 'SLS'.

[1]**Viagra**® (Pfizer) [PoM] [NHS]

Tablets, all blue, f/c, sildenafil (as citrate), 25 mg, net price 4-tab pack = £16.59, 8-tab pack = £33.19; 50 mg, 4-tab pack = £19.34, 8-tab pack = £38.67; 100 mg, 4-tab pack = £23.50, 8-tab pack = £46.99

TADALAFIL

Indications: erectile dysfunction

Cautions: see notes above; also hepatic impairment (Appendix 2); renal impairment (Appendix 3); **interactions:** Appendix 1 (tadalafil)

Contra-indications: see notes above; also moderate heart failure, uncontrolled arrhythmias, uncontrolled hypertension

Side-effects: see notes above; also back pain, myalgia

Dose: initially 10 mg approx. 30 minutes–12 hours before sexual activity, subsequent doses adjusted according to response to 20 mg as a single dose; max. 1 dose in 24 hours (but daily use not recommended)

NOTE. Effect may persist for up to 24 hours

[1]**Cialis**® (Lilly) ▼ [PoM] [NHS]

Tablets, f/c, tadalafil 10 mg (light yellow), net price 4-tab pack = £19.34; 20 mg (yellow), 4-tab pack = £19.34; 8-tab pack = £38.67

VARDENAFIL

Indications: erectile dysfunction

Cautions: see notes above; also hepatic impairment (Appendix 2—avoid if severe); renal impairment (Appendix 3); bleeding disorders or active peptic ulceration; **interactions:** Appendix 1 (vardenafil)

Contra-indications: see notes above; also hereditary degenerative retinal disorders

Side-effects: see notes above; also nausea, hypertension, photosensitivity reactions rarely hypertonia, hypotension, syncope

Dose: initially 10 mg (ELDERLY 5 mg) approx. 25–60 minutes before sexual activity, subsequent doses adjusted according to response up to max. 20 mg as a single dose; max. 1 dose in 24 hours

NOTE. Onset of effect may be delayed if taken with high-fat meal

[1]**Levitra**® (Bayer) ▼ [PoM] [NHS]

Tablets, all orange, f/c, vardenafil (as hydrochloride trihydrate) 5 mg, net price 4-tab pack = £16.59, 8-tab pack = £33.19; 10 mg, 4-tab pack = £19.34, 8-tab pack = £38.67; 20 mg, 4-tab pack = £23.50, 8-tab pack = £46.99

Papaverine and phentolamine

Although not licensed the smooth muscle relaxant **papaverine** has also been given by intracavernosal injection for erectile dysfunction. Patients with neurological or psychogenic impotence are more sensitive to the effect of papaverine than those with vascular abnormalities. **Phentolamine** is added if the response is inadequate [unlicensed indication].

Persistence of the erection for longer than 4 hours is an emergency, see advice under Alprostadil, above.

8: Malignant disease and immunosuppression

8.1   Cytotoxic drugs

8.1.1   Alkylating drugs
8.1.2   Cytotoxic antibiotics
8.1.3   Antimetabolites
8.1.4   Vinca alkaloids and etoposide
8.1.5   Other antineoplastic drugs

The chemotherapy of cancer is complex and should be confined to specialists in oncology. Cytotoxic drugs have both anti-cancer activity and the potential for damage to normal tissue. Chemotherapy may be given with a curative intent or it may aim to prolong life or to palliate symptoms. In an increasing number of cases chemotherapy may be combined with radiotherapy or surgery or both as either neoadjuvant treatment (initial chemotherapy aimed at shrinking the primary tumour, thereby rendering local therapy less destructive or more effective) or as adjuvant treatment (which follows definitive treatment of the primary disease, when the risk of sub-clinical metastatic disease is known to be high). All chemotherapy drugs cause side-effects and a balance has to be struck between likely benefit and acceptable toxicity.

CRM guidelines on handling cytotoxic drugs:

1. Trained personnel should reconstitute cytotoxics;
2. Reconstitution should be carried out in designated areas;
3. Protective clothing (including gloves) should be worn;
4. The eyes should be protected and means of first aid should be specified;
5. Pregnant staff should not handle cytotoxics;
6. Adequate care should be taken in the disposal of waste material, including syringes, containers, and absorbent material.

Intrathecal chemotherapy. A Health Service Circular (HSC 2003/010) provides guidance on the introduction of safe practice in NHS Trusts where intrathecal chemotherapy is administered. Support for training programmes is also available.
Copies, and further information may be obtained from:
Department of Health
PO Box 777
London SE1 6XH
Fax: 01623 724524
www.doh.gov.uk/intrathecalchemotherapy/

Combinations of cytotoxic drugs are frequently more toxic than single drugs but have the advantage in certain tumours of enhanced response, reduced development of drug resistance and increased survival. However for some tumours, single-agent chemotherapy remains the treatment of choice.

> Most cytotoxic drugs are teratogenic, and all may cause life-threatening toxicity; administration should, where possible, be confined to those experienced in their use.
>
> Because of the complexity of dosage regimens in the treatment of malignant disease, dose statements have been omitted from some of the drug entries in this chapter. *In all cases detailed specialist literature should be consulted.*
>
> Prescriptions should **not** be repeated except on the instructions of a specialist.

Cytotoxic drugs fall naturally into a number of classes, each with characteristic antitumour action, sites of action, and toxicity. A knowledge of sites of metabolism and excretion is important because impaired drug handling as a result of disease is not uncommon and may result in enhanced toxicity.

Side-effects of cytotoxic drugs

Side-effects commonly encountered with cytotoxic drugs are discussed below whilst side-effects characteristic of a particular drug or class of drugs (e.g. neurotoxicity with vinca alkaloids) are described in the appropriate sections. Manufacturers' product literature should be consulted for full details of side-effects associated with individual drugs.

EXTRAVASATION OF INTRAVENOUS DRUGS. A number of cytotoxic drugs will cause severe local tissue necrosis if leakage into the extravascular compartment occurs. To reduce the risk of extravasation injury it is recommended that cytotoxic drugs are administered by appropriately trained staff. For information on the prevention and management of extravasation injury see section 10.3.

ORAL MUCOSITIS. A sore mouth is a common complication of cancer chemotherapy; it is most often associated with fluorouracil, methotrexate, and the anthracyclines. It is best to prevent the complication. Good mouth care (rinsing the mouth frequently and effective brushing of the teeth with a soft brush 2–3 times daily) is probably effective. For fluorouracil, sucking ice chips during short infusions of the drug is also helpful.

Once a sore mouth has developed, treatment is much less effective. Saline mouthwashes should be used but there is no good evidence to support the use of antiseptic or anti-inflammatory mouthwashes. In general, mucositis is self-limiting but with poor oral hygiene it can be a focus for blood-borne infection.

HYPERURICAEMIA. Hyperuricaemia, which can result in uric acid crystal formation in the urinary tract with associated renal dysfunction is a complication of the treatment of non-Hodgkin's lymphoma and leukaemia. Allopurinol (see section 10.1.4) should be started 24 hours before treating such tumours; patients should be adequately hydrated. The dose of mercaptopurine or azathioprine should be reduced if allopurinol needs to be given concomitantly (see Appendix 1).

Rasburicase (section 10.1.4) is a recombinant urate oxidase, which has been licensed recently for hyperuricaemia in patients with haematological malignancy, for details, see p. 498.

NAUSEA AND VOMITING. Nausea and vomiting cause considerable distress to many patients who receive chemotherapy, and to a lesser extent abdominal radiotherapy, and may lead to refusal of further treatment. Symptoms may be acute (occurring within 24 hours of treatment), delayed (first occurring more than 24 hours after treatment) or anticipatory (occurring prior to subsequent doses). Delayed and anticipatory symptoms are more difficult to control than acute symptoms and require different management.

Patients vary in their susceptibility to drug-induced nausea and vomiting; those affected more often include women, patients under 50 years of age, anxious patients, and those who experience motion sickness. Susceptibility also increases with repeated exposure to the drug.

Drugs may be divided according to their emetogenic potential and some examples are given below, but the symptoms vary according to the dose, to other drugs administered and to individual susceptibility.

Mildly emetogenic treatment—fluorouracil, etoposide, methotrexate (less than $100 \, \text{mg/m}^2$), the vinca alkaloids, and abdominal radiotherapy.

Moderately emetogenic treatment—doxorubicin, intermediate and low doses of cyclophosphamide, mitoxantrone (mitozantrone), and high doses of methotrexate ($0.1–1.2 \, \text{g/m}^2$).

Highly emetogenic treatment—cisplatin, dacarbazine, and high doses of cyclophosphamide.

Prevention of acute symptoms. For patients at *low risk of emesis*, pretreatment with domperidone or, in adults over 20 years, with metoclopramide, continued for up to 24 hours after chemotherapy, is often effective (section 4.6). If metoclopramide or domperidone are not sufficiently effective, additional drugs such as dexamethasone (6–10 mg by mouth) or lorazepam (1–2 mg by mouth) may be used.

For patients at *high risk of emesis* or when other treatment is inadequate, a specific (5HT$_3$) serotonin antagonist (section 4.6), usually given by mouth, is often highly effective, particularly when used with dexamethasone.

Prevention of delayed symptoms. Dexamethasone, given by mouth, is the drug of choice for preventing delayed symptoms; it is used alone or with metoclopramide or prochlorperazine. The 5HT$_3$ antagonists may be less effective for delayed symptoms.

Prevention of anticipatory symptoms. Good symptom control is the best way to prevent anticipatory symptoms. The addition of lorazepam to antiemetic therapy is helpful because of its amnesic, sedative and anxiolytic effects.

BONE-MARROW SUPPRESSION. All cytotoxic drugs except vincristine and bleomycin cause bone-marrow depression. This commonly occurs 7 to 10 days after administration, but is delayed for certain drugs, such as carmustine, lomustine, and melphalan. Peripheral blood counts must be checked before each treatment, and doses should be reduced or therapy delayed if bone-marrow has not recovered.

Fever in a neutropenic patient (neutrophil count less than 1.0×10^9/litre) requires immediate broad-spectrum antibacterial therapy. Patients at low risk (those receiving chemotherapy for solid tumours, lymphoma or chronic leukaemia) can be treated with oral ciprofloxacin with or without co-amoxiclav (initially in hospital). All other patients should receive parenteral broad-spectrum antibacterial therapy. Appropriate bacteriological investigations should be conducted as soon as possible.

In selected patients, the duration and the severity of neutropenia can be reduced by the use of bone marrow growth factors (colony stimulating factors, section 9.1.6) or (in patients with ovarian carcinoma receiving cisplatin and cyclophosphamide) by the use of amifostine (see p. 409).

Symptomatic anaemia is usually treated with red blood cell transfusions. Epoetin administered subcutaneously is also effective but not widely used.

ALOPECIA. Reversible hair loss is a common complication, although it varies in degree between drugs and individual patients. No pharmacological methods of preventing this are available.

REPRODUCTIVE FUNCTION. Most cytotoxic drugs are teratogenic and should not be administered during pregnancy, especially during the first trimester.

Contraceptive advice should be offered where appropriate before cytotoxic therapy begins (and should cover the duration of contraception required after therapy has ended). Regimens that do not contain an alkylating drug may have less effect on fertility, but those with an alkylating drug carry the risk of causing permanent male sterility (there is no effect on potency). Pre-treatment counselling and consideration of sperm storage may be appropriate. Women are less severely affected, though the span of reproductive life may be shortened by the onset of a premature menopause. No increase in fetal abnormalities or abortion-rate has been recorded in patients who remain fertile after cytotoxic chemotherapy.

Drugs for cytotoxic-induced side-effects

Methotrexate-induced mucositis and myelosuppression

Folinic acid (given as calcium folinate) is used to counteract the folate-antagonist action of methotrexate and thus speed recovery from methotrexate-induced mucositis or myelosuppression. It is generally given 24 hours after the methotrexate, in a dose of 15 mg by mouth every 6 hours, for 2–8 doses (depending on the dose of methotrexate). It does not counteract the antibacterial activity of folate antagonists such as trimethoprim.

When folinic acid and fluorouracil are used together in metastatic colorectal cancer the response-rate improves compared to that with fluorouracil alone.

The calcium salt of **levofolinic acid**, a single isomer of folinic acid, is also used for rescue therapy following methotrexate administration and for use with fluorouracil for colorectal cancer. The dose of calcium levofolinate is generally half that of calcium folinate.

The disodium salt of folinic acid is also licensed for rescue therapy following methotrexate therapy and for use with fluorouracil for colorectal cancer.

CALCIUM FOLINATE

(Calcium leucovorin)

Indications: see notes above

Cautions: avoid simultaneous administration of methotrexate; **not** indicated for pernicious anaemia or other megaloblastic anaemias due to vitamin B$_{12}$ deficiency; pregnancy and breast-feeding; **interactions:** Appendix 1 (folates)

IMPORTANT. Intrathecal injection **contra-indicated**

Side-effects: hypersensitivity reactions; rarely pyrexia after parenteral use

Dose: expressed in terms of folinic acid

As an antidote to methotrexate (usually started 24 hours after the beginning of methotrexate infusion), usually up to 120 mg in divided doses over 12–24 hours *by intramuscular or intravenous injection or by intravenous infusion*, followed by 12–15 mg *intramuscularly or* 15 mg *by mouth* every 6 hours for the next 48–72 hours

Suspected methotrexate overdosage, immediate administration of folinic acid at a rate not exceeding 160 mg/minute in a dose equal to (or higher than) the dose of methotrexate

Adjunct to fluorouracil in colorectal cancer, consult product literature

Calcium Folinate (Non-proprietary) PoM
Tablets, scored, folinic acid (as calcium salt) 15 mg, net price 10-tab pack = £41.10, 30-tab pack = £85.74
Available from APS, Goldshield, Hillcross, Mayne, Pharmacia (*Refolinon*®)
NOTE. Not all strengths and pack sizes are available from all manufacturers
Injection, folinic acid (as calcium salt) 3 mg/mL, net price 1-mL amp = £2.28, 10-mL amp = £4.62; 7.5 mg/mL, net price 2-mL amp = £7.80; 10 mg/mL, net price 5-mL vial = £19.41, 10-mL vial = £35.09, 30-mL vial = £94.69, 35-mL vial = £90.98
Available from CP, Lederle (*Lederfolin*®), Mayne
NOTE. Not all strengths and pack sizes are available from all manufacturers
Injection, powder for reconstitution, folinic acid (as calcium salt), net price 15-mg vial = £4.46; 30-mg vial = £8.36
Available from Goldshield

CALCIUM LEVOFOLINATE

(Calcium levoleucovorin)

Indications: see notes above

Cautions: see Calcium Folinate

Side-effects: see Calcium Folinate

Dose: expressed in terms of levofolinic acid

As an antidote to methotrexate (usually started 24 hours after the beginning of methotrexate infusion), usually 7.5 mg, *by intramuscular injection, or by intravenous injection or by intravenous infusion* every 6 hours for 10 doses

Suspected methotrexate overdosage, immediate administration of levofolinic acid at a rate not exceeding 160 mg/minute in a dose which is at least 50% of the dose of methotrexate

Adjunct to fluorouracil in colorectal cancer, consult product literature

Isovorin® (Wyeth) ▼ PoM
Injection, levofolinic acid (as calcium salt) 10 mg/mL, net price 2.5-mL vial = £13.00, 5-mL vial = £26.00, 17.5-mL vial = £91.00

DISODIUM FOLINATE

Indications: see notes above
Cautions: see Calcium Folinate
Side-effects: see Calcium Folinate
Dose: as an antidote to methotrexate, see Calcium Folinate

Adjunct to fluorouracil in colorectal cancer, consult product literature

Sodiofolin® (Medac) [PoM]
Injection, folinic acid (as disodium salt) 50 mg/mL, net price 2-mL vial = £35.09, 8-mL vial = £126.25, 18-mL vial = £284.07

Platinum-induced neutropenic infection and nephrotoxicity

Amifostine is licensed for the reduction of risk of infection associated with cisplatin- and cyclophosphamide-induced neutropenia in advanced ovarian carcinoma, and for the reduction of nephrotoxicity caused by cisplatin. Amifostine is also licensed for protection against xerostomia during radiotherapy for head and neck cancer.

Other drugs for the reduction of risk of infection associated with neutropenia include granulocyte-colony stimulating factor and granulocyte macrophage-colony stimulating factor (section 9.1.6).

AMIFOSTINE

Indications: (specialist use only) see under Dose
Cautions: ensure adequate hydration before treatment; infuse with patient supine and monitor arterial blood pressure (interrupt infusion if blood pressure decreases significantly, consult product literature); during chemotherapy interrupt antihypertensive therapy 24 hours before treatment with amifostine and monitor closely, during radiotherapy monitor closely if concomitant antihypertensive therapy; monitor serum calcium in patients at risk of hypocalcaemia; not recommended in renal and hepatic impairment; pregnancy and breast-feeding; **interactions:** Appendix 1 (amifostine)
Side-effects: hypotension (reversed by infusion of physiological saline and postural management), nausea, vomiting, flushing, chills, dizziness, drowsiness, hiccups, sneezing; rarely convulsions, clinical hypocalcaemia; allergic reactions
Dose: reduction of neutropenia-related risk of infection due to cyclophosphamide and cisplatin treatment in patients with advanced ovarian carcinoma, *by intravenous infusion* over 15 minutes, ADULT 910 mg/m² once daily started within 30 minutes before chemotherapy (reduced to 740 mg/m² for subsequent cycles if full dose could not be given first time due to hypotension lasting more than 5 minutes after interruption, consult product literature)

Reduction of nephrotoxicity associated with cisplatin in patients with advanced solid tumours of non-germ-cell origin, consult product literature

Prevention of xerostomia during radiotherapy for head and neck cancer, *by intravenous infusion* over 3 minutes, ADULT 200 mg/m² once daily starting 15–30 minutes before radiotherapy

CHILD and ELDERLY (over 70 years) not recommended

Ethyol® (Schering-Plough) [PoM]
Intravenous infusion, powder for reconstitution, amifostine, net price 375-mg vial = £108.00; 500-mg vial = £144.00

Urothelial toxicity

Haemorrhagic cystitis is a common manifestation of urothelial toxicity which occurs with the oxazaphosphorines, cyclophosphamide and ifosfamide; it is caused by the metabolite acrolein. **Mesna** reacts specifically with this metabolite in the urinary tract, preventing toxicity. Mesna is used routinely (preferably by mouth) in patients receiving ifosfamide, and in patients receiving cyclophosphamide by the intravenous route at a high dose (e.g. more than 2 g) or in those who experienced urothelial toxicity when given cyclophosphamide previously.

MESNA

Indications: see notes above
Contra-indications: hypersensitivity to thiol-containing compounds
Side-effects: nausea, vomiting, colic, diarrhoea, fatigue, headache, limb and joint pains, depression, irritability, rash, hypotension and tachycardia; rarely hypersensitivity reactions (more common in patients with auto-immune disorders)
Dose: calculated according to oxazaphosphorine (cyclophosphamide or ifosfamide) treatment—for details consult product literature; when given *by mouth*, dose is given 2 hours *before* oxazaphosphorine treatment and repeated 2 and 6 hours *after* treatment; when given *by intravenous injection*, dose is given *with* oxazaphosphorine treatment and repeated 4 and 8 hours *after* treatment

Uromitexan® (Baxter Oncology) [PoM]
Tablets, f/c, mesna 400 mg, net price 10-tab pack = £17.43; 600 mg, 10-tab pack = £22.63
Injection, mesna 100 mg/mL. Net price 4-mL amp = £1.61; 10-mL amp = £3.62
NOTE. For oral administration contents of ampoule are taken in a flavoured drink such as orange juice or cola which may be stored in a refrigerator for up to 24 hours in a sealed container

8.1.1 Alkylating drugs

Extensive experience is available with these drugs, which are among the most widely used in cancer chemotherapy. They act by damaging DNA, thus interfering with cell replication. In addition to the side-effects common to many cytotoxic drugs (section 8.1), there are two problems associated with prolonged usage. Firstly, gametogenesis is often severely affected (section 8.1). Secondly, prolonged use of these drugs, particularly when combined with extensive irradiation, is associated with a marked increase in the incidence of acute non-lymphocytic leukaemia.

Cyclophosphamide is widely used in the treatment of chronic lymphocytic leukaemia, the lymphomas, and solid tumours. It is given by mouth or intravenously and is inactive until metabolised by the liver. A urinary metabolite of cyclophosphamide, acrolein, may cause haemorrhagic cystitis; this is a rare but very serious complication. An increased fluid intake, for 24–48 hours after intravenous injection, will help avoid this complication. When high-dose therapy (e.g. more than 2 g intravenously) is used or when the patient is considered to be at high risk of cystitis (e.g. previous pelvic irradiation) mesna (given initially intravenously then by mouth) will also help prevent this—see under Urothelial toxicity (section 8.1).

Ifosfamide is related to cyclophosphamide and is given intravenously; mesna (section 8.1) is routinely given with it to reduce urothelial toxicity.

Chlorambucil is used to treat chronic lymphocytic leukaemia, non-Hodgkin's lymphoma, Hodgkin's disease, and Waldenstrom's macroglobulinaemia. It is given by mouth. Side-effects, apart from bone-marrow suppression, are uncommon. However, patients occasionally develop severe widespread rashes which can progress to Stevens-Johnson syndrome or to toxic epidermal necrolysis. If a rash occurs further chlorambucil is contra-indicated and cyclophosphamide is substituted.

Melphalan is licensed for the treatment of multiple myeloma, advanced ovarian adenocarcinoma, advanced breast cancer, childhood neuroblastoma, and polycythaemia vera. Melphalan is also licensed for regional arterial perfusion in localised malignant melanoma of the extremities and localised soft-tissue sarcoma of the extremities.

Busulfan (busulphan) is given by mouth to treat chronic myeloid leukaemia. Busulphan given intravenously, followed by cyclophosphamide, is also licensed as conditioning treatment before haemato-poietic stem-cell transplantation in adults. Frequent blood tests are necessary because excessive myelo-suppression may result in irreversible bone-marrow aplasia. Rarely, progressive pulmonary fibrosis is associated with busulfan. Skin hyperpigmentation is a common side-effect of oral therapy.

Lomustine is a lipid-soluble nitrosourea and is given by mouth. It is mainly used to treat Hodgkin's disease and certain solid tumours. Bone marrow toxicity is delayed, and the drug is therefore given at intervals of 4 to 6 weeks. Permanent bone marrow damage may occur with prolonged use. Nausea and vomiting are common and moderately severe.

Carmustine is given intravenously. It has similar activity and toxicity to lomustine and is most commonly given to patients with myeloma, lymphoma, and brain tumours. Cumulative renal damage and delayed pulmonary fibrosis may occur.

Chlormethine (mustine) is used in some regimens for the management of Hodgkin's disease. It is a very toxic drug which causes severe vomiting. The freshly prepared injection must be given into a fast-running intravenous infusion. Local extravasation causes severe tissue necrosis.

Estramustine is a combination of an oestrogen and chlormethine used predominantly in prostate cancer. It is given by mouth and has both an antimitotic effect and (by reducing testosterone concentration) a hormonal effect.

Treosulfan is given by mouth or intravenously and is used to treat ovarian cancer. Skin pigmentation is a common side-effect and allergic alveolitis, pulmonary fibrosis and haemorrhagic cystitis occur rarely.

Thiotepa is usually used as an intracavitary drug for the treatment of malignant effusions or bladder cancer (section 7.4.4). It is also occasionally used to

treat breast cancer, but requires parenteral administration.

Mitobronitol is occasionally used to treat chronic myeloid leukaemia; it is available on a named-patient basis only (as *Myelobromol®*, Durbin).

BUSULFAN
(Busulphan)

Indications: see notes above

Cautions: see section 8.1 and notes above; avoid in porphyria (section 9.8.2); **interactions:** Appendix 1 (busulfan)

Side-effects: see section 8.1 and notes above

Dose: *by mouth*, chronic myeloid leukaemia, induction of remission, 60 micrograms/kg to max. 4 mg daily; maintenance, 0.5–2 mg daily

By intravenous infusion, consult product literature

Busilvex® (Fabre) ▼ PoM
Concentrate for intravenous infusion, busulfan 6 mg/mL, net price 10-mL vial = £201.25

Myleran® (GSK) PoM
Tablets, f/c, busulfan 2 mg, net price 25-tab pack = £5.59

CARMUSTINE

Indications: see notes above

Cautions: see section 8.1 and notes above

Side-effects: see section 8.1 and notes above; irritant to tissues

BiCNU® (Bristol-Myers Squibb) PoM
Injection, powder for reconstitution, carmustine. Net price 100-mg vial (with diluent) = £12.50

CHLORAMBUCIL

Indications: see notes above

Cautions: see section 8.1 and notes above; avoid in porphyria (section 9.8.2)

Side-effects: see section 8.1 and notes above

Dose: Hodgkin's disease, used alone, 200 micrograms/kg daily for 4–8 weeks

Non-Hodgkin's lymphoma, used alone, initially 100–200 micrograms/kg daily for 4–8 weeks then dose reduced or given intermittently

Chronic lymphocytic leukaemia, initially 150 micrograms/kg daily until leucocyte count sufficiently reduced; maintenance (started 4 weeks after end of first course) 100 micrograms/kg daily

Waldenstrom's macroglobulinaemia, 6–12 mg daily until leucopenia occurs, then reduce to 2–8 mg daily

Leukeran® (GSK) PoM
Tablets, f/c, brown, chlorambucil 2 mg, net price 25-tab pack = £8.99

CHLORMETHINE HYDROCHLORIDE
(Mustine hydrochloride)

Indications: Hodgkin's disease—see notes above

Cautions: see section 8.1 and notes above; caution in handling

Side-effects: see section 8.1 and notes above; irritant to tissues

Chlormethine Hydrochloride (Sovereign) PoM
Injection, powder for reconstitution, chlormethine hydrochloride, net price 10-mg vial = £43.99

CYCLOPHOSPHAMIDE

Indications: see notes above
Cautions: see section 8.1 and notes above; hepatic and renal impairment (Appendixes 2 and 3); avoid in porphyria (section 9.8.2); **interactions:** Appendix 1 (cyclophosphamide)
Side-effects: see section 8.1 and notes above

Cyclophosphamide (Non-proprietary) PoM
Tablets, s/c, cyclophosphamide (anhydrous) 50 mg, net price 20 = £2.12. Label: 27
Available from Pharmacia
Injection, powder for reconstitution, cyclophosphamide, net price 500-mg vial = £2.88; 1-g vial = £5.04
Available from Pharmacia

Endoxana® (Baxter Oncology) PoM
Tablets, s/c, cyclophosphamide 50 mg, net price 100-tab pack = £10.03. Label: 27
Injection, powder for reconstitution, cyclophosphamide. Net price 200-mg vial = £1.54; 500-mg vial = £2.68; 1-g vial = £4.68

ESTRAMUSTINE PHOSPHATE

Indications: prostate cancer
Cautions: see section 8.1; renal impairment
Contra-indications: peptic ulceration, severe liver disease (Appendix 2), cardiac disease
Side-effects: see section 8.1; also gynaecomastia, altered liver function, cardiovascular disorders (angina and rare reports of myocardial infarction)
Dose: 0.14–1.4 g daily in divided doses (usual initial dose 560 mg daily)
COUNSELLING. Each dose should be taken not less than 1 hour before or 2 hours after meals and should not be taken with dairy products

Estracyt® (Pharmacia) PoM
Capsules, estramustine phosphate 140 mg (as disodium salt). Net price 100-cap pack = £171.28. Label: 23, counselling, see above

IFOSFAMIDE

Indications: see notes above
Cautions: see section 8.1 and notes above; renal impairment (Appendix 3); **interactions:** Appendix 1 (ifosfamide)
Contra-indications: hepatic impairment
Side-effects: see section 8.1 and notes above

Mitoxana® (Baxter Oncology) PoM
Injection, powder for reconstitution, ifosfamide. Net price 1-g vial = £20.31; 2-g vial = £37.59 (hosp. only)

LOMUSTINE

Indications: see notes above
Cautions: see section 8.1 and notes above
Side-effects: see section 8.1 and notes above
Dose: used alone, 120–130 mg/m² body-surface every 6–8 weeks

Lomustine (Medac) PoM
Capsules, blue/clear, lomustine 40 mg. Net price 20-cap pack = £254.95
NOTE. The brand name *CCNU*® has been used for lomustine capsules

MELPHALAN

Indications: see notes above
Cautions: see section 8.1 and notes above; renal impairment (Appendix 3); **interactions:** Appendix 1 (melphalan)
Side-effects: see section 8.1 and notes above
Dose: *by mouth*, multiple myeloma, dose may vary according to regimen; typical dose 150 micrograms/kg daily for 4 days, repeated every 6 weeks
Ovarian adenocarcinoma, 200 micrograms/kg daily for 5 days, repeated every 4–8 weeks
Advanced breast cancer, 150 micrograms/kg daily for 5 days, repeated every 6 weeks
Polycythaemia vera, initially, 6–10 mg daily reduced after 5–7 days to 2–4 mg daily until satisfactory response then further reduce to 2–6 mg **per week**
By intravenous injection or infusion and regional arterial perfusion, consult product literature

Alkeran® (GSK) PoM
Tablets, melphalan 2 mg, net price 25 = £12.32
Injection, powder for reconstitution, melphalan 50 mg (as hydrochloride). Net price 50-mg vial (with solvent-diluent) = £29.69

THIOTEPA

Indications: see notes above and section 7.4.4
Cautions: see section 8.1; **interactions:** Appendix 1 (thiotepa)
Side-effects: see section 8.1

Thiotepa (Goldshield) PoM
Injection, powder for reconstitution, thiotepa, net price 15-mg vial = £5.20

TREOSULFAN

Indications: see notes above
Cautions: see section 8.1
Side-effects: see section 8.1 and notes above
Dose: *by mouth*, courses of 1–2 g daily in 3–4 divided doses to provide total dose of 21–28 g over initial 8 weeks (with treatment-free intervals during this period—consult product literature)
By intravenous injection or by intraperitoneal administration, consult product literature

Treosulfan (Medac) PoM
Capsules, treosulfan 250 mg. Net price 20 = £50.85. Label: 25
Injection, powder for reconstitution, treosulfan. Net price 1 g = £31.18; 5 g = £120.48 (both in infusion bottle with transfer needle)

8.1.2 Cytotoxic antibiotics

Drugs in this group are widely used. Many cytotoxic antibiotics act as radiomimetics and simultaneous use of radiotherapy should be **avoided** as it may result in markedly enhanced toxicity.

Aclarubicin, daunorubicin, doxorubicin, epirubicin and idarubicin are anthracycline antibiotics. Mitoxantrone (mitozantrone) is an anthracycline derivative.

Doxorubicin is used to treat the acute leukaemias, lymphomas, and a variety of solid tumours. It is given by injection into a fast-running infusion, commonly at 21-day intervals. Extravasation can cause severe tissue necrosis. Doxorubicin is largely excreted by the biliary tract, and an elevated bilirubin concentration is an indication for reducing the dose. Supraventricular tachycardia related to drug administration is an uncommon complication. Higher cumulative doses are associated with cardiomyopathy and it is usual to limit total cumulative doses to 450 mg/m^2 because symptomatic and potentially fatal heart failure is common above this dose. Patients with cardiac disease, the elderly, and those who have received myocardial irradiation should be treated cautiously. Cardiac monitoring may assist in determining safe dosage. Some evidence suggests that weekly low-dose administration may be less cardiotoxic. Doxorubicin is also given by bladder instillation for the treatment of transitional cell carcinoma, papillary bladder tumours and carcinoma *in-situ*.

Liposomal formulations of doxorubicin for intravenous use are also available. They may reduce the incidence of cardiotoxicity and lower the potential for local necrosis, but infusion reactions, sometimes severe, may occur. Hand-foot syndrome (painful, macular reddening skin eruptions) occurs commonly with liposomal doxorubicin and may be dose limiting. It can occur after 2–3 treatment cycles and may be prevented by cooling hands and feet and avoiding socks, gloves, or tight-fitting footwear for 4–7 days after treatment.

NICE guidance (pegylated liposomal doxorubicin). NICE has recommended (July 2002) that pegylated liposomal doxorubicin be considered an option for the second-line (or subsequent) treatment of advanced ovarian cancer where the disease is initially resistant or refractory to first-line platinum-based combination therapy or it has become resistant after successive courses of platinum-based combination therapy.

Pegylated liposomal doxorubicin is not recommended in patients with poor performance status (Eastern Cooperative Oncology Group score 3 or worse) or bowel obstruction, or in patients who have previously not responded to pegylated liposomal doxorubicin.

Epirubicin is structurally related to doxorubicin and clinical trials suggest that it is as effective in the treatment of breast cancer. A maximum cumulative dose of 0.9–1 g/m^2 is recommended to help avoid cardiotoxicity. Like doxorubicin it is given intravenously and by bladder instillation.

Aclarubicin and **idarubicin** are anthracyclines with general properties similar to those of doxorubicin. They are both given intravenously. Idarubicin may also be given by mouth.

Daunorubicin also has general properties similar to those of doxorubicin. It should be given by intravenous infusion and is indicated for acute leukaemias. A liposomal formulation for intravenous use is licensed for AIDS-related Kaposi's sarcoma.

Use with trastuzumab. Concomitant use of anthracyclines with trastuzumab (section 8.1.5) is associated with cardiotoxicity; for details, see p. 422.

Mitoxantrone (mitozantrone) is structurally related to doxorubicin; it is used for metastatic breast cancer. Mitoxantrone is also licensed for use in the treatment of non-Hodgkin's lymphoma and adult non-lymphocytic leukaemia. It is given intravenously and is well tolerated but myelosuppression and dose-related

cardiotoxicity occur; cardiac examinations are recommended after a cumulative dose of 160 mg/m^2.

Bleomycin is given intravenously or intramuscularly to treat metastatic germ cell cancer and, in some regimens, non-Hodgkin's lymphoma. It causes little bone-marrow suppression but dermatological toxicity is common and increased pigmentation particularly affecting the flexures and subcutaneous sclerotic plaques may occur. Mucositis is also relatively common and an association with Raynaud's phenomenon is reported. Hypersensitivity reactions manifest by chills and fevers commonly occur a few hours after drug administration and may be prevented by simultaneous administration of a corticosteroid, for example hydrocortisone intravenously. The principal problem associated with the use of bleomycin is progressive pulmonary fibrosis. This is dose-related, occurring more commonly at cumulative doses greater than 300 000 units (see Bleomycin, below) and in the elderly. Basal lung crepitations or suspicious chest X-ray changes are an indication to stop therapy with this drug. Patients who have received extensive treatment with bleomycin (e.g. cumulative dose more than 100 000 units—see Bleomycin below) may be at risk of developing respiratory failure if a general anaesthetic is given with high inspired oxygen concentrations. Anaesthetists should be warned of this.

Dactinomycin is principally used to treat paediatric cancers; it is given intravenously. Its side-effects are similar to those of doxorubicin, except that cardiac toxicity is not a problem.

Mitomycin is given intravenously to treat upper gastro-intestinal and breast cancers and by bladder instillation for superficial bladder tumours. It causes delayed bone-marrow toxicity and therefore it is usually administered at 6-weekly intervals. Prolonged use may result in permanent bone-marrow damage. It may also cause lung fibrosis and renal damage.

ACLARUBICIN

Indications: acute non-lymphocytic leukaemia in patients who have relapsed or are resistant or refractory to first-line chemotherapy

Cautions: see section 8.1 and notes above; hepatic and renal impairment; irritant to tissues

Side-effects: see section 8.1 and notes above

Aclarubicin (Medac) PoM
Injection, powder for reconstitution, aclarubicin 20 mg (as hydrochloride). Net price 20-mg vial = £98.55
NOTE. The brand names *Aclacin*® and *Aclaplastin*® have been used for aclarubicin preparations

BLEOMYCIN

Indications: squamous cell carcinoma; see also notes above

Cautions: see section 8.1 and notes above; renal impairment (Appendix 3); caution in handling—irritant to tissues

Side-effects: see section 8.1 and notes above

Bleomycin (Non-proprietary) PoM
Injection, powder for reconstitution, bleomycin (as sulphate). Net price 15 000-unit vial = £15.56
NOTE. To conform to the European Pharmacopoeia vials previously labelled as containing '15 units' of bleomycin

are now labelled as containing 15 000 units. The amount of bleomycin in the vial has not changed.

Available from Kyowa Hakko (*Bleo-Kyowa®*), Mayne

DACTINOMYCIN

(Actinomycin D)

Indications: see notes above

Cautions: see section 8.1 and notes above; caution in handling—irritant to tissues

Side-effects: see section 8.1 and notes above

Cosmegen Lyovac® (MSD) PoM
Injection, powder for reconstitution, dactinomycin, net price 500-microgram vial = £1.50

DAUNORUBICIN

Indications: see notes above

Cautions: see section 8.1 and notes above; hepatic impairment (Appendix 2), renal impairment (Appendix 3); caution in handling—irritant to tissues

Side-effects: see section 8.1 and notes above

Daunorubicin (Non-proprietary) PoM
Injection, powder for reconstitution, daunorubicin (as hydrochloride), net price 20-mg vial = £39.26
Available from Beacon
NOTE. The brand name *Cerubidin®* was formerly used.

■ Lipid formulation

DaunoXome® (Gilead) PoM
Concentrate for intravenous infusion, daunorubicin encapsulated in liposomes. For dilution before use. Net price 50-mg vial = £148.03
For advanced AIDS-related Kaposi's sarcoma

DOXORUBICIN HYDROCHLORIDE

Indications: see notes above and section 7.4.4

Cautions: see section 8.1 and notes above; hepatic impairment (Appendix 2); caution in handling—irritant to tissues; **interactions:** Appendix 1 (doxorubicin)

Side-effects: see section 8.1 and notes above

Doxorubicin Rapid Dissolution (Pharmacia) PoM
Injection, powder for reconstitution, doxorubicin hydrochloride, net price 10-mg vial = £18.72; 50-mg vial = £93.60
NOTE. This preparation has replaced *Adriamycin®*
Various strengths also available from Medac

Doxorubicin Solution for Injection (Pharmacia) PoM
Injection, doxorubicin hydrochloride 2 mg/mL, net price 5-mL vial = £20.60, 25-mL vial = £103.00, 100-mL vial = £412.00
Various strengths and sizes also available from Mayne, Medac

■ Lipid formulation

Caelyx® (Schering-Plough) PoM
Concentrate for intravenous infusion, doxorubicin hydrochloride 2 mg/mL encapsulated in liposomes. For dilution before use. Net price 10-mL vial = £411.30, 25-mL vial = £813.49
For AIDS-related Kaposi's sarcoma in patients with low CD4 count and extensive mucocutaneous or visceral disease, for advanced ovarian cancer when platinum-based chemotherapy has failed, and as monotherapy for metastatic breast cancer with increased cardiac risk

Myocet® (Elan) ▼ PoM
Injection, powder for reconstitution, doxorubicin hydrochloride (as doxorubicin–citrate complex)

encapsulated in liposomes, net price 50-mg vial (with vials of liposomes and buffer) = £464.50
For use with cyclophosphamide for metastatic breast cancer

EPIRUBICIN HYDROCHLORIDE

Indications: see notes above and section 7.4.4

Cautions: see section 8.1 and notes above; hepatic impairment (Appendix 2); caution in handling—irritant to tissues

Side-effects: see section 8.1 and notes above

Pharmorubicin® Rapid Dissolution (Pharmacia) PoM
Injection, powder for reconstitution, epirubicin hydrochloride. Net price 10-mg vial = £19.31; 20-mg vial = £38.62; 50-mg vial = £96.54

Pharmorubicin® Solution for Injection (Pharmacia) PoM
Injection, epirubicin hydrochloride 2 mg/mL, net price 5-mL vial = £19.31, 25-mL vial = £96.54

IDARUBICIN HYDROCHLORIDE

Indications: advanced breast cancer after failure of first-line chemotherapy (not including anthracyclines); acute leukaemias—see notes above

Cautions: see section 8.1 and notes above; hepatic impairment (Appendix 2); renal impairment (Appendix 3); caution in handling—irritant to tissues

Side-effects: see section 8.1 and notes above

Dose: *by mouth*, acute non-lymphocytic leukaemia, 30 mg/m² daily for 3 days alone *or* 15–30 mg/m² daily for 3 days in combination therapy

Advanced breast cancer, 45 mg/m² alone, as a single dose *or* divided over 3 consecutive days; repeat every 3–4 weeks

Max. cumulative dose *by mouth* (for all indications) 400 mg/m²

By intravenous administration, consult product literature

Zavedos® (Pharmacia) PoM
Capsules, idarubicin hydrochloride, 5 mg (red), net price 1-cap pack = £34.56; 10 mg (red/white), 1-cap pack = £69.12; 25 mg (white), 1-cap pack = £172.80. Label: 25
Injection, powder for reconstitution, idarubicin hydrochloride, net price 5-mg vial = £87.36; 10-mg vial = £174.72

MITOMYCIN

Indications: see notes above and section 7.4.4

Cautions: see section 8.1 and notes above; caution in handling—irritant to tissues

Side-effects: see section 8.1 and notes above

Mitomycin (Non-proprietary) PoM
Injection, powder for reconstitution, mitomycin. Net price 10-mg vial = £22.67; 20-mg vial = £41.70
Available from Mayne
NOTE. May be difficult to obtain

Mitomycin C Kyowa® (Kyowa Hakko) PoM
Injection, powder for reconstitution, mitomycin. Net price 2-mg vial = £5.88; 10-mg vial = £19.37; 20-mg vial = £36.94; 40-mg vial = £73.88 (hosp. only)

MITOXANTRONE
(Mitozantrone)
Indications: see notes above
Cautions: see section 8.1 and notes above; intrathecal administration not recommended
Side-effects: see section 8.1 and notes above

Mitoxantrone (Non-proprietary) PoM
Concentrate for intravenous infusion, mitoxantrone (as hydrochloride) 2 mg/mL, net price 10-mL vial = £100.00
Available from Mayne

Novantrone® (Lederle) PoM
Concentrate for intravenous infusion, mitoxantrone (as hydrochloride) 2 mg/mL, net price 10-mL vial = £150.43, 12.5-mL vial = £188.05, 15-mL vial = £225.60

Onkotrone® (Baxter Oncology) PoM
Concentrate for intravenous infusion, mitoxantrone (as hydrochloride) 2 mg/mL, net price 10-mL vial = £135.39, 12.5-mL vial = £169.25, 15-mL vial = £203.04

8.1.3   Antimetabolites

Antimetabolites are incorporated into new nuclear material or combine irreversibly with vital cellular enzymes, preventing normal cellular division.

Methotrexate inhibits the enzyme dihydrofolate reductase, essential for the synthesis of purines and pyrimidines. It is given by mouth, intravenously, intramuscularly, or intrathecally.

Methotrexate is used as maintenance therapy for childhood acute lymphoblastic leukaemia. Other uses include choriocarcinoma, non-Hodgkin's lymphoma, and a number of solid tumours. Intrathecal methotrexate is used in the CNS prophylaxis of childhood acute lymphoblastic leukaemia, and as a therapy for established meningeal cancer or lymphoma.

Methotrexate causes myelosuppression, mucositis, and rarely pneumonitis. It is **contra-indicated** in significant renal impairment because it is excreted primarily by the kidney. It is also contra-indicated in patients with severe hepatic impairment. It should also be **avoided** if a significant pleural effusion or ascites is present because it tends to accumulate in these fluids, and its subsequent return to the circulation will be associated with myelosuppression. Systemic toxicity may occur following intrathecal administration and blood counts should be carefully monitored.

Folinic acid (section 8.1) following methotrexate administration helps to prevent methotrexate-induced mucositis or myelosuppression.

Capecitabine, which is metabolised to fluorouracil, is given by mouth. It is used as monotherapy for metastatic colorectal cancer; it has been shown to be of similar efficacy as a combination of fluorouracil and folinic acid. It is also licensed for second-line treatment of locally advanced or metastatic breast cancer either in combination with docetaxel (where previous therapy included an anthracycline) or alone (after failure of a taxane and anthracycline regimen or where further anthracycline treatment is not indicated).

> **NICE guidance (capecitabine and tegafur with uracil for metastatic colorectal cancer).** NICE has recommended (May 2003) capecitabine or tegafur with uracil (in combination with folinic acid) as an option for the first-line treatment of metastatic colorectal cancer.

> **NICE guidance (capecitabine for locally advanced or metastatic breast cancer).** NICE has recommended (May 2003) capecitabine in combination with docetaxel in preference to docetaxel monotherapy for locally advanced or metastatic breast cancer in people for whom anthracycline-containing regimens are unsuitable or have failed.
> Capecitabine monotherapy is recommended as an option for people with locally advanced or metastatic breast cancer who have not previously received capecitabine in combination therapy and for whom anthracycline and taxane-containing regimens have failed or further anthracycline therapy is contra-indicated.

Cytarabine acts by interfering with pyrimidine synthesis. It is given subcutaneously, intravenously, or intrathecally. Its predominant use is in the induction of remission of acute myeloblastic leukaemia. It is a potent myelosuppressant and requires careful haematological monitoring.

Fludarabine is licensed for the initial treatment of advanced B-cell chronic lymphocytic leukaemia (CLL) or after first-line treatment in patients with sufficient bone-marrow reserves; it is given daily by mouth for 5 days every 28 days. Fludarabine is generally well tolerated but it does cause myelosuppression, which may be cumulative. Immunosuppression is also common (see panel on cladribine and fludarabine below) and co-trimoxazole is often used to prevent pneumocystis infection. Immune-mediated haemolytic anaemia, thrombocytopenia, and neutropenia are less common side-effects.

> **NICE guidance (fludarabine).** NICE has recommended (September 2001) oral fludarabine as second-line therapy for B-cell chronic lymphocytic leukaemia (CLL) for patients who have either failed, or are intolerant of, first-line chemotherapy.

Cladribine is an effective but potentially toxic drug given by intravenous infusion for the treatment of hairy cell leukaemia. It is also licensed for chronic lymphocytic leukaemia in patients who have failed to respond to standard regimens containing an alkylating agent; it is given by intravenous infusion. Myelosuppression may be severe and serious neurotoxicity has been reported rarely.

> **Cladribine** and **fludarabine** have a potent and prolonged immunosuppressive effect and only irradiated blood products should be administered to prevent potentially fatal graft-versus-host reaction. Prescribers should consult specialist literature when using highly immunosuppressive drugs.

Gemcitabine is used intravenously; it is given alone for palliative treatment or with cisplatin as a first-line treatment for locally advanced or metastatic non-small cell lung cancer. It is also used in the treatment of locally advanced or metastatic pancreatic cancer. Combined with cisplatin, gemcitabine is also licensed for the treatment of advanced bladder cancer. It is generally well tolerated but may cause mild gastro-intestinal side-effects and rashes; renal impairment, pulmonary toxicity and influenza-like symptoms have also been reported. Haemolytic uraemic syndrome has been reported rarely and gemcitabine should be discontinued if signs of microangiopathic haemolytic anaemia occur.

NICE guidance (gemcitabine). NICE has recommended (May 2001) that gemcitabine is an option for first-line chemotherapy for patients with advanced or metastatic adenocarcinoma of the pancreas and a Karnofsky score of at least 50 [Karnofsky score is a measure of the ability to perform ordinary tasks]. Gemcitabine is not recommended for patients who can have potentially curative surgery. There is insufficient evidence about its use for second-line treatment of pancreatic adenocarcinoma.

NICE guidance (docetaxel, paclitaxel, gemcitabine and vinorelbine for non-small cell lung cancer). NICE has recommended (June 2001) that chemotherapy should be considered for non-small cell lung cancer in patients who are unsuitable for curative treatment or who are unlikely to respond to such treatment.
Gemcitabine, paclitaxel, or vinorelbine should be considered as first-line chemotherapy for advanced non-small cell lung cancer. Combination of each of these drugs with platinum-based chemotherapy, where tolerated, is likely to be most effective.
Docetaxel monotherapy should be considered for locally advanced or metastatic non-small cell lung cancer which relapses after previous chemotherapy.

Fluorouracil is usually given intravenously because absorption following oral administration is unpredictable. It is used to treat a number of solid tumours, including gastro-intestinal tract cancers and breast cancer. It is commonly used with folinic acid in advanced colorectal cancer. It may also be used topically for certain malignant and pre-malignant skin lesions. Toxicity is unusual, but may include myelosuppression, mucositis, and rarely a cerebellar syndrome. On prolonged infusion, a desquamative hand–foot syndrome may occur.

Raltitrexed, a thymidylate synthase inhibitor, is given intravenously for palliation of advanced colorectal cancer when fluorouracil and folinic acid cannot be used. It is probably of similar efficacy to fluorouracil. Raltitrexed is generally well tolerated, but can cause marked myelosuppression and gastro-intestinal side-effects.

NICE guidance (irinotecan, oxaliplatin and raltitrexed for advanced colorectal cancer). See p. 420

Mercaptopurine is used as maintenance therapy for the acute leukaemias and in the management of ulcerative colitis and Crohn's disease (section 1.5). Azathioprine, which is metabolised to mercaptopurine, is generally used as an immunosuppressant (section 8.2.1 and section 10.1.3). The dose of both drugs should be reduced if the patient is receiving allopurinol since it interferes with their metabolism.

Tegafur (in combination with uracil) is given by mouth, together with calcium folinate, in the management of metastatic colorectal cancer. Tegafur is a prodrug of fluorouracil; uracil inhibits the degradation of fluorouracil. Tegafur (with uracil) has been shown to be of similar efficacy as a combination of fluorouracil and folinic acid for metastatic colorectal cancer. For NICE guidance on capecitabine and tegafur with uracil for metastatic colorectal cancer, see above

Tioguanine (thioguanine) is given by mouth to induce remission in acute myeloid leukaemia.

CAPECITABINE

Indications: see notes above
Cautions: see section 8.1; **interactions:** Appendix 1 (fluorouracil)
Contra-indications: hepatic impairment, renal impairment (Appendix 3)
Side-effects: see section 8.1 and notes above; hand–foot (desquamative) syndrome
Dose: ADULT over 18 years, 1.25 g/m^2 twice daily for 14 days; subsequent courses repeated after a 7-day interval

Xeloda® (Roche) ▼ PoM
Tablets, f/c, peach, capecitabine 150 mg, net price 60-tab pack = £44.47; 500 mg, 120-tab pack = £295.06. Label: 21

CLADRIBINE

Indications: see notes above
Cautions: see section 8.1 and notes above; use irradiated blood only
Side-effects: see section 8.1 and notes above

Leustat® (Janssen-Cilag) PoM
Injection, cladribine 1 mg/mL. For dilution and use as an infusion, net price 10-mL vial = £182.29

CYTARABINE

Indications: acute leukaemias
Cautions: see section 8.1 and notes above; hepatic impairment (Appendix 2); **interactions:** Appendix 1 (cytarabine)
Side-effects: see section 8.1 and notes above

Cytarabine (Non-proprietary) PoM
Injection (for intravenous, subcutaneous or intrathecal use), cytarabine 20 mg/mL, net price 5-mL vial (Mayne) = £4.00
Injection (for intravenous or subcutaneous use), cytarabine 20 mg/mL, net price 5-mL vial (Pharmacia) = £3.90, 25-mL vial (Pharmacia) = £19.50
Injection (for intravenous or subcutaneous use), cytarabine 100 mg/mL, net price 1-mL vial (Mayne) = £4.00; 5-mL vial (Mayne) = £20.00; 10-mL vial (Mayne) = £40.00, (Pharmacia) = £39.00; 20-mL vial (Mayne) = £79.00, (Pharmacia) = £77.50; 20-mL _Onco-vial®_ (Mayne) = £79.00

FLUDARABINE PHOSPHATE

Indications: see notes above
Cautions: see section 8.1 and notes above; use irradiated blood only; renal impairment (Appendix 3) **interactions:** Appendix 1 (fludarabine)
Side-effects: see section 8.1 and notes above
Dose: _by mouth_, ADULT 40 mg/m^2 for 5 days every 28 days usually for 6 cycles
By intravenous injection or infusion, consult product literature

Fludara® (Schering Health) PoM
Tablets▼, f/c, pink, fludarabine phosphate 10 mg,
net price 15-tab pack = £279.00, 20-tab pack =
£372.00
Injection, powder for reconstitution, fludarabine
phosphate. Net price 50-mg vial = £143.00

FLUOROURACIL

Indications: see notes above
Cautions: see section 8.1 and notes above; caution
in handling—irritant to tissues; **interactions:**
Appendix 1 (fluorouracil)
Side-effects: see section 8.1 and notes above; also
local irritation with topical preparation
Dose: *by mouth*, maintenance 15 mg/kg weekly;
max. in one day 1 g
*By intravenous injection or infusion or by intra-
arterial infusion*, consult product literature

Fluorouracil (Non-proprietary) PoM
Capsules, fluorouracil 250 mg.
Available from Cambridge on a named-patient basis
Injection, fluorouracil (as sodium salt) 25 mg/mL,
net price 10-mL vial = £3.20, 20-mL vial = £6.40,
100-mL vial = £32.00; 50 mg/mL, 10-mL vial =
£6.40, 20-mL vial = £12.80, 50-mL vial = £32.00,
100-mL vial = £64.00
Available from Mayne, Medac

■ Topical preparations
Efudix® (ICN) PoM
Cream, fluorouracil 5%. Net price 20 g = £18.27
Excipients: include hydroxybenzoates (parabens)
Dose: malignant and pre-malignant skin lesions, apply
thinly to the affected area once or twice daily; cover with
occlusive dressing in malignant conditions; max. area of
skin treated at one time, 500 cm², usual duration of initial
therapy, 3–4 weeks

GEMCITABINE

Indications: see notes above
Cautions: see section 8.1 and notes above
Side-effects: see section 8.1 and notes above

Gemzar® (Lilly) PoM
Injection, powder for reconstitution, gemcitabine
(as hydrochloride), net price 200-mg vial = £32.55;
1-g vial = £162.76 (both hosp. only)

MERCAPTOPURINE

Indications: acute leukaemias; inflammatory bowel
disease [unlicensed indication] (section 1.5)
Cautions: see section 8.1 and notes above; monitor
liver function—hepatic impairment (Appendix 2);
renal impairment (Appendix 3); **interactions:**
Appendix 1 (mercaptopurine)
Side-effects: see section 8.1 and notes above; also
hepatotoxicity; rarely pancreatitis
Dose: initially 2.5 mg/kg daily

Puri-Nethol® (GSK) PoM
Tablets, fawn, scored, mercaptopurine 50 mg. Net
price 25 = £20.19

METHOTREXATE

Indications: see notes above and under Dose;
rheumatoid arthritis (section 10.1.3); psoriasis
(section 13.5.3)
Cautions: see section 8.1, notes above and section
10.1.3; **interactions:** Appendix 1 (methotrexate)

Side-effects: see section 8.1, notes above and
section 10.1.3
Dose: *by mouth*, leukaemia in children (maintenance), 15 mg/m² weekly in combination with
other drugs

Important. Note that the above dose is a **weekly**
dose. The CSM has received reports of prescription
and dispensing errors including fatalities. Attention
should be paid to the **strength** of methotrexate
tablets prescribed and the **frequency** of dosing

---

*By intravenous injection or infusion, by intra-arte-
rial infusion, or by intramuscular injection, or
intrathecal administration*, consult product literature

Methotrexate (Non-proprietary) PoM
Injection, methotrexate 2.5 mg (as sodium salt)/mL.
Net price 2-mL vial (Mayne) = £1.68
Injection, methotrexate 25 mg (as sodium salt)/mL.
Net price 2-mL vial (Mayne) = £4.58, (Goldshield)
= £2.62; 8-mL vial (Goldshield) = £10.02; 20-mL
vial (Mayne) = £39.09, (Goldshield) = £25.07; 40-
mL vial (Goldshield) = £44.57; 200-mL vial
(Goldshield) = £200.57
Injection, methotrexate 100 mg/mL (not for
intrathecal use). Net price 10-mL vial (Mayne) =
£78.33; 50-mL vial (Mayne) = £380.07

■ Oral preparations
Section 10.1.3

RALTITREXED

Indications: see notes above
Cautions: see section 8.1 and notes above; hepatic
and renal impairment (Appendixes 2 and 3)
Side-effects: see section 8.1 and notes above

Tomudex® (AstraZeneca) PoM
Injection, powder for reconstitution, raltitrexed. Net
price 2-mg vial = £121.86

TEGAFUR WITH URACIL

Indications: see notes above
Cautions: see section 8.1; cardiac disease; renal
impairment; hepatic impairment (avoid if severe—
Appendix 2); **interactions:** Appendix 1 (fluorouracil)
Side-effects: see section 8.1 and notes above
Dose: ADULT, tegafur 300 mg/m² (with uracil
672 mg/m²) daily in 3 divided doses for 28 days;
subsequent courses repeated after 7-day interval;
for dose adjustment due to toxicity, consult product
literature

Uftoral® (Bristol-Myers Squibb) ▼ PoM
Capsules, tegafur 100 mg, uracil 224 mg, net price
21-cap pack = £66.57, 28-cap pack = £88.76, 35-
cap pack = £110.95, 42-cap pack = £133.14.
Label: 23

TIOGUANINE

(Thioguanine)
Indications: acute leukaemias; chronic myeloid
leukaemia
Cautions: see section 8.1 and notes above; renal
impairment (Appendix 3)
Side-effects: see section 8.1 and notes above

Dose: induction, 100–200 mg/m^2 in 1–2 divided doses for 5–20 days; maintenance, usually 60–200 mg/m^2 daily

Lanvis® (GSK) PoM
Tablets, yellow, scored, tioguanine 40 mg. Net price 25-tab pack = £48.83

8.1.4 Vinca alkaloids and etoposide

The vinca alkaloids, **vinblastine**, **vincristine**, and **vindesine**, are used to treat the acute leukaemias, lymphomas, and some solid tumours (e.g. breast and lung cancer). **Vinorelbine**, a semi-synthetic vinca alkaloid, is used for advanced breast cancer (see also NICE guidance below) and for advanced non-small cell lung cancer (see also NICE guidance, p. 415).

Neurotoxicity, usually as peripheral or autonomic neuropathy, occurs with all vinca alkaloids and is a limiting side-effect of vincristine; it occurs less often with vindesine, vinblastine, and vinorelbine. Patients with neurotoxicity commonly have peripheral paraesthesia, loss of deep tendon reflexes, abdominal pain, and constipation. If symptoms of neurotoxicity are severe, doses should be reduced. Motor weakness can also occur, and increasing motor weakness calls for discontinuation of these drugs. Recovery from neurotoxic effects is usually slow but complete.

Myelosuppression is the dose-limiting side-effect of vinblastine, vindesine, and vinorelbine; vincristine causes negligible myelosuppression. The vinca alkaloids may cause reversible alopecia. They cause severe local irritation and care must be taken to avoid extravasation.

> Vinblastine, vincristine, vindesine, and vinorelbine are for **intravenous administration only**. Inadvertent intrathecal administration can cause severe neurotoxicity, which is usually fatal.

> **NICE guidance (vinorelbine for advanced breast cancer).** NICE has recommended (December 2002) that vinorelbine be considered as an option for the second-line (or subsequent) treatment of advanced breast cancer where anthracycline-based regimens have failed or are unsuitable.
> Vinorelbine monotherapy is not recommended as first-line treatment for advanced breast cancer.
> Insufficient information is available to recommend the routine use of vinorelbine in combination with other therapies for advanced breast cancer.

Etoposide may be given orally or by slow intravenous infusion, the oral dose being double the intravenous dose. A preparation containing etoposide phosphate can be given by intravenous injection or infusion. Etoposide is usually given daily for 3–5 days and courses should not be repeated more frequently than at intervals of 21 days. It has particularly useful activity in small cell carcinoma of the bronchus, the lymphomas, and testicular cancer. Toxic effects include alopecia, myelosuppression, nausea, and vomiting.

ETOPOSIDE

Indications: see notes above
Cautions: see section 8.1 and notes above

Contra-indications: see section 8.1 and notes above; severe hepatic impairment
Side-effects: see section 8.1 and notes above; irritant to tissues
Dose: *by mouth*, 120–240 mg/m^2 daily for 5 days
By intravenous infusion, consult product literature

Etoposide (Non-proprietary) PoM
Concentrate for intravenous infusion, etoposide 20 mg/mL, net price 5-mL vial (Mayne; Medac, *Eposin*®) = £14.50, 10-mL vial (APS; Mayne) = £29.00, 25-mL vial (Medac, *Eposin*®) = £67.50

Etopophos® (Bristol-Myers Squibb) PoM
Injection, powder for reconstitution, etoposide (as phosphate), net price 100-mg vial = £29.87 (hosp. only)

Vepesid® (Bristol-Myers Squibb) PoM
Capsules, both pink, etoposide 50 mg, net price 20 = £113.95; 100 mg, 10-cap pack = £99.57 (hosp. only). Label: 23
Concentrate for intravenous infusion, etoposide 20 mg/mL, net price 5-mL vial = £14.58 (hosp. only)

VINBLASTINE SULPHATE

Indications: see notes above
Cautions: see section 8.1 and notes above; hepatic impairment (Appendix 2); caution in handling; **interactions:** Appendix 1 (vinblastine)
Contra-indications: see section 8.1 and notes above
IMPORTANT. Intrathecal injection **contra-indicated**
Side-effects: see section 8.1 and notes above; irritant to tissues

Vinblastine (Non-proprietary) PoM
Injection, vinblastine sulphate 1 mg/mL. Net price 10-mL vial = £13.09
Available from Mayne

Velbe® (Clonmel) PoM
Injection, powder for reconstitution, vinblastine sulphate. Net price 10-mg amp = £14.15

VINCRISTINE SULPHATE

Indications: see notes above
Cautions: see section 8.1 and notes above; hepatic impairment (Appendix 2); caution in handling; **interactions:** Appendix 1 (vincristine)
Contra-indications: see section 8.1 and notes above
IMPORTANT. Intrathecal injection **contra-indicated**
Side-effects: see section 8.1 and notes above; irritant to tissues

Vincristine (Non-proprietary) PoM
Injection, vincristine sulphate 1 mg/mL. Net price 1-mL vial = £10.92; 2-mL vial = £21.17; 5-mL vial = £44.16
Available from Mayne

Oncovin® (Clonmel) PoM
Injection, vincristine sulphate 1 mg/mL, net price 1-mL vial = £14.18; 2-mL vial = £28.05

VINDESINE SULPHATE

Indications: see notes above
Cautions: see section 8.1 and notes above; hepatic impairment (Appendix 2); caution in handling
Contra-indications: see section 8.1 and notes above
IMPORTANT. Intrathecal injection **contra-indicated**

Side-effects: see section 8.1 and notes above; irritant to tissues

Eldisine® (Clonmel) PoM
Injection, powder for reconstitution, vindesine sulphate, net price 5-mg vial = £78.30 (hosp. only)

VINORELBINE

Indications: see notes above
Cautions: see section 8.1 and notes above; hepatic impairment (Appendix 2); caution in handling
Contra-indications: see section 8.1 and notes above
IMPORTANT. Intrathecal injection **contra-indicated**
Side-effects: see section 8.1 and notes above; irritant to tissues

Navelbine® (Fabre) PoM
Injection concentrate, vinorelbine (as tartrate) 10 mg/mL. Net price 1-mL vial = £31.25; 5-mL vial = £147.06

8.1.5 Other antineoplastic drugs

Amsacrine

Amsacrine has an action and toxic effects similar to those of doxorubicin (section 8.1.2) and is given *intravenously*. It is occasionally used in acute myeloid leukaemia. Side-effects include myelosuppression and mucositis; electrolytes should be monitored as fatal arrhythmias have occurred in association with hypokalaemia.

AMSACRINE

Indications: see notes above
Cautions: see section 8.1 and notes above; reduce dose in renal or hepatic impairment; also caution in handling—irritant to skin and tissues
Side-effects: see section 8.1 and notes above

Amsidine® (Goldshield) PoM
Concentrate for intravenous infusion, amsacrine 5 mg (as lactate)/mL, when reconstituted by mixing two solutions. Net price 1.5-mL (75-mg) amp with 13.5-mL diluent vial = £49.17 (hosp. only)
NOTE. Use glass apparatus for reconstitution

Bexarotene

Bexarotene is an agonist at the retinoid X receptor, which is involved in the regulation of cell differentiation and proliferation. It is generally well tolerated when given by mouth and it is associated with little myelosuppression or immunosuppression. Bexarotene can cause regression of cutaneous T-cell lymphoma. The main adverse effects are hyperlipidaemia, hypothyroidism, leucopenia, headache, rash, and pruritus.

BEXAROTENE

Indications: skin manifestations of cutaneous T-cell lymphoma refractory to previous systemic treatment

Cautions: see section 8.1 and notes above; hyperlipidaemia (avoid if uncontrolled), hypothyroidism (avoid if uncontrolled); hypersensitivity to retinoids
Contra-indications: see section 8.1 and notes above; history of pancreatitis, hypervitaminosis A, hepatic impairment
Side-effects: see section 8.1 and notes above
Dose: initially 300 mg/m² daily as a single dose with a meal; adjust dose according to response

Targretin® (Elan) ▼ PoM
Capsules, bexarotene 75 mg in a liquid suspension, net price 100-cap pack = £937.50

Crisantaspase

Crisantaspase is the enzyme asparaginase produced by *Erwinia chrysanthemi*. It is given *intramuscularly* or *subcutaneously* almost exclusively in acute lymphoblastic leukaemia. Facilities for the management of anaphylaxis should be available. Side-effects also include nausea, vomiting, CNS depression, and liver function and blood lipid changes; careful monitoring is therefore necessary and the urine is tested for glucose because of a risk of hyperglycaemia.

CRISANTASPASE

Indications: see notes above
Cautions: see notes above
Side-effects: see notes above

Erwinase® (Ipsen) PoM
Injection, powder for reconstitution, crisantaspase. Net price 10 000-unit vial = £39.94

Dacarbazine and temozolomide

Dacarbazine is used to treat metastatic melanoma and, in combination therapy, soft tissue sarcomas. It is also a component of a commonly used combination for Hodgkin's disease (ABVD—doxorubicin [previously *Adriamycin®*], bleomycin, vinblastine, and dacarbazine). It is given *intravenously*. The predominant side-effects are myelosuppression and severe nausea and vomiting.

Temozolomide is structurally related to dacarbazine and is licensed for second-line treatment of malignant glioma.

> **NICE guidance (temozolomide).** NICE has recommended (April 2001) that temozolomide may be considered for the treatment of recurrent malignant glioma, which has not responded to first-line chemotherapy.

DACARBAZINE

Indications: see notes above
Cautions: see section 8.1; hepatic and renal impairment (Appendixes 2 and 3); caution in handling
Side-effects: see section 8.1 and notes above; rarely liver necrosis due to hepatic vein thrombosis; irritant to skin and tissues

Dacarbazine (Non-proprietary) PoM
Injection, powder for reconstitution, dacarbazine (as citrate), net price 100-mg vial = £5.11 (Medac); 200-mg vial = £7.24 (Medac) or £7.50 (Mayne);

500-mg vial = £16.50 (Medac); 600-mg vial =
£22.50 (Mayne); 1-g vial = £31.80 (Medac)
Available from Mayne, Medac

DTIC-Dome® (Bayer) [PoM]
Injection, powder for reconstitution, dacarbazine.
Net price 200-mg vial = £7.40

TEMOZOLOMIDE
Indications: see notes above
Cautions: see section 8.1; severe hepatic impairment and renal impairment; **interactions:** Appendix 1 (temozolomide)
Side-effects: see section 8.1
Dose: 200 mg/m^2 once daily for 5 days of a 28-day
cycle; for patients previously treated with chemotherapy—consult product literature; CHILD
under 3 years not recommended

Temodal® (Schering-Plough) ▼ [PoM]
Capsules, temozolomide 5 mg, net price 5-cap pack
= £17.30; 20 mg, 5-cap pack = £69.20; 100 mg, 5-
cap pack = £346.00; 250 mg, 5-cap pack = £865.00.
Label: 23, 25

Hydroxycarbamide

Hydroxycarbamide (hydroxyurea) is an orally
active drug used mainly in the treatment of chronic
myeloid leukaemia. It is occasionally used for
polycythaemia (the usual treatment is venesection).
Myelosuppression, nausea, and skin reactions are the
most common toxic effects.

HYDROXYCARBAMIDE
(Hydroxyurea)
Indications: see notes above
Cautions: see section 8.1 and notes above
Side-effects: see section 8.1 and notes above
Dose: 20–30 mg/kg daily *or* 80 mg/kg every third
day

Hydroxycarbamide (Non-proprietary) [PoM]
Capsules, hydroxycarbamide 500 mg, net price 20 =
£2.39
Available from Medac

Hydrea® (Squibb) [PoM]
Capsules, pink/green, hydroxycarbamide 500 mg.
Net price 20 = £2.39

Imatinib

Imatinib is a protein–tyrosine kinase inhibitor,
which is licensed for the treatment of newly
diagnosed chronic myeloid leukaemia where bone
marrow transplantation is not considered first-line
treatment and for chronic myeloid leukaemia in
chronic phase after failure of interferon alfa, or in
accelerated phase, or in blast crisis. It is also licensed
for Kit-positive unresectable or metastatic malignant
gastro-intestinal stromal tumours (GIST). The most
frequent side-effects of imatinib are nausea, vomiting, diarrhoea, oedema, abdominal pain, fatigue,
myalgia, headache, and rash; gynaecomastia because
of reduced testosterone has been reported.

**NICE guidance (imatinib for chronic myeloid
leukaemia).** NICE has recommended (October
2003) imatinib as first-line treatment for Philadel-
phia-chromosome-positive chronic myeloid leukaemia in the chronic phase and as an option for
patients presenting in the accelerated phase or with
blast crisis, provided that imatinib has not been used
previously.
Where imatinib has failed to stop disease progression
from chronic phase to accelerated phase or blast
crisis, continued use is recommended only as part of
further clinical study.

IMATINIB
Indications: see notes above
Cautions: consult product literature; pregnancy
(Appendix 4 and section 8.1); **interactions:**
Appendix 1 (imatinib)
Contra-indications: breast-feeding
Side-effects: see section 8.1 and notes above
Dose: consult product literature

Glivec® (Novartis) ▼ [PoM]
Capsules, orange, imatinib (as mesilate) 100 mg, net
price 120-cap pack = £1557.36

Pentostatin

Pentostatin is highly active in hairy cell leukaemia.
It is given *intravenously* on alternate weeks and is
capable of inducing prolonged complete remission.
It is potentially toxic, causing myelosuppression,
immunosuppression and a number of other side-
effects which may be severe. Its use is probably best
confined to specialist centres.

PENTOSTATIN
Indications: see notes above
Cautions: see section 8.1 and notes above; **inter-
actions:** Appendix 1 (pentostatin)
Side-effects: see section 8.1 and notes above

Nipent® (Lederle) [PoM]
Injection, powder for reconstitution, pentostatin.
Net price 10-mg vial = £928.80

Platinum compounds

Carboplatin is widely used in the treatment of
advanced ovarian cancer and lung cancer (particularly the small cell type). It is given *intravenously*.
The dose of carboplatin is determined according to
renal function rather than body surface area. Carboplatin can be given on an outpatient basis and is
better tolerated than cisplatin; nausea and vomiting
are reduced in severity and nephrotoxicity, neurotoxicity, and ototoxicity are much less of a problem
than with cisplatin. It is, however, more myelosuppressive than cisplatin.

Cisplatin is of value in patients with metastatic
germ cell cancers (seminoma and teratoma). It is also
used in the treatment of bladder, lung, upper gastro-
intestinal and ovarian cancer (although carboplatin is
preferred for ovarian cancer). It is given *intravenously*. Cisplatin requires intensive intravenous
hydration and treatment may be complicated by
severe nausea and vomiting. Cisplatin is toxic,
causing nephrotoxicity (monitoring of renal function
is essential), ototoxicity, peripheral neuropathy,

hypomagnesaemia and myelosuppression. It is, however, increasingly given in a day-care setting.

Oxaliplatin is licensed for the treatment of metastatic colorectal cancer in combination with fluorouracil and folinic acid; it is given by intravenous infusion. Neurotoxic side-effects (including sensory peripheral neuropathy) are dose limiting. Other side-effects include gastro-intestinal disturbances, ototoxicity, and myelosuppression. Manufacturers advise renal function monitoring in moderate impairment.

> **NICE guidance (irinotecan, oxaliplatin, and raltitrexed for advanced colorectal cancer).**
> NICE has recommended (March 2002) that oxaliplatin, in combination with fluorouracil and folinic acid, should be considered first-line treatment for advanced colorectal cancer **only** in patients with metastases which are confined to the liver and which could be resected following treatment.
> Irinotecan monotherapy is recommended in patients who have failed to respond to an established fluorouracil-containing treatment.
> A combination of fluorouracil and folinic acid with either irinotecan or oxaliplatin is **not** recommended for *routine* first-line treatment of advanced colorectal cancer.
> Raltitrexed is **not** recommended for the treatment of advanced colorectal cancer. Its use should be confined to clinical studies.

CARBOPLATIN

Indications: see notes above
Cautions: see section 8.1 and notes above; renal impairment (Appendix 3); **interactions:** Appendix 1 (platinum compounds)
Side-effects: see section 8.1 and notes above

Carboplatin (Non-proprietary) PoM
Injection, carboplatin 10 mg/mL, net price 5-mL vial = £22.86 (Mayne), 15-mL vial = £56.29 (APS) or £65.83 (Mayne), 15-mL *Onco-vial®* = £72.41 (Mayne), 45-mL vial = £168.85 (APS) or £197.48 (Mayne), 45-mL *Onco-vial®* = £217.23 (Mayne), 60-mL vial = £260.00 (Mayne)
Available from APS, Mayne

Paraplatin® (Bristol-Myers Squibb) PoM
Injection, carboplatin 10 mg/mL, net price 5-mL vial = £22.86, 15-mL vial = £65.83, 45-mL vial = £197.48, 60-mL vial = £263.31

CISPLATIN

Indications: see notes above
Cautions: see section 8.1 and notes above; renal impairment (Appendix 3); **interactions:** Appendix 1 (platinum compounds)
Side-effects: see section 8.1 and notes above

Cisplatin (Non-proprietary) PoM
Injection, cisplatin 1 mg/mL. Net price 10-mL vial = £5.85; 50-mL vial = £25.37 (APS) or £28.11 (Bristol-Myers Squibb, Mayne); 100-mL vial = £50.22 (APS) or £55.64 (Bristol-Myers Squibb, Mayne)
Available from APS, Mayne
Injection, powder for reconstitution, cisplatin, net price 50-mg vial = £17.00
Available from Pharmacia

OXALIPLATIN

Indications: metastatic colorectal cancer in combination with fluorouracil and folinic acid
Cautions: see section 8.1 and notes above; renal impairment (Appendix 3); **interactions:** Appendix 1 (platinum compounds)
Contra-indications: see section 8.1; peripheral neuropathy with functional impairment
Side-effects: see section 8.1 and notes above

Eloxatin® (Sanofi-Synthelabo) PoM
Injection, powder for reconstitution, oxaliplatin, net price 50-mg vial = £165.00, 100-mg vial = £330.00

Porfimer sodium and temoporfin

Porfimer sodium and **temoporfin** are used in the photodynamic treatment of various tumours. The drugs accumulate in malignant tissue and are activated by laser light to produce a cytotoxic effect.

Porfimer sodium is licensed for photodynamic therapy of non-small cell lung cancer and obstructing oesophageal cancer. Temoporfin is licensed for photodynamic therapy of advanced head and neck cancer.

PORFIMER SODIUM

Indications: non-small cell lung cancer; oesophageal cancer; see notes above
Cautions: see section 8.1; avoid exposure of skin and eyes to direct sunlight or bright indoor light for at least 30 days
Contra-indications: see section 8.1; severe hepatic impairment; tracheo-oesophageal or broncho-oesophageal fistula; porphyria (section 9.8.2)
Side-effects: see section 8.1; photosensitivity (see Cautions above—sunscreens offer no protection), constipation
Dose: *by intravenous injection* over 3 to 5 minutes, 2 mg/kg
NOTE. For further information on administration and light activation, consult product literature

Photofrin (Sinclair) ▼ PoM
Injection, powder for reconstitution, porfimer sodium, net price 15-mg vial = £154.00; 75-mg vial = £770.00

TEMOPORFIN

Indications: advanced head and neck squamous cell carcinoma refractory to, or unsuitable for, other treatments
Cautions: see section 8.1; avoid exposure of skin and eyes to direct sunlight or bright indoor light for at least 15 days after administration; **interactions:** Appendix 1 (temoporfin)
Contra-indications: see section 8.1; porphyria (section 9.8.2) or other diseases exacerbated by light; elective surgery or ophthalmic slit-lamp examination for 30 days after administration; existing photosensitising treatment; pregnancy (Appendix 4); breast-feeding (Appendix 5)
Side-effects: see section 8.1; photosensitivity (see Cautions above—sunscreens offer no protection), constipation, local haemorrhage, facial pain and oedema, scarring, dysphagia

Dose: *by intravenous injection* over at least 6 minutes, ADULT 150 microgram/kg

NOTE. For use undiluted; for further information on administration and light activation, consult product literature

Foscan® (Biolitec) ▼ PoM
Injection, temoporfin 4 mg/mL, net price 5-mL vial = £4400.00

Procarbazine

Procarbazine is most often used in Hodgkin's disease, for example in MOPP (chlormethine (mustine), vincristine [*Oncovin®*], procarbazine, and prednisolone) chemotherapy. It is given *by mouth*. Toxic effects include nausea, myelosuppression, and a hypersensitivity rash preventing further use of this drug. It is a mild monoamine-oxidase inhibitor but dietary restriction is not considered necessary. Alcohol ingestion may cause a disulfiram-like reaction.

PROCARBAZINE

Indications: see notes above
Cautions: see section 8.1 and notes above; hepatic impairment—avoid if severe; renal impairment—avoid if severe; **interactions:** Appendix 1 (procarbazine)
Side-effects: see section 8.1 and notes above
Dose: used alone, initially 50 mg daily, increased by 50 mg daily to 250–300 mg daily in divided doses; maintenance (on remission) 50–150 mg daily to cumulative total of at least 6 g

Procarbazine (Cambridge) PoM
Capsules, ivory, procarbazine (as hydrochloride) 50 mg, net price 50-cap pack = £37.44. Label: 4

Razoxane

Razoxane has limited activity in the leukaemias, and is little used.

RAZOXANE

Indications: see notes above
Cautions: see section 8.1
Side-effects: see section 8.1
Dose: acute leukaemias, 150–500 mg/m^2 daily for 3–5 days

Razoxane (Cambridge) PoM
Tablets, scored, razoxane 125 mg. Net price 30-tab pack = £74.56

Taxanes

Paclitaxel is a member of the taxane group of drugs. It is given by *intravenous infusion*. Paclitaxel given with carboplatin or cisplatin is used for the treatment of ovarian cancer (see NICE guidance below); the combination is also considered appropriate for women whose ovarian cancer is initially considered inoperable. Paclitaxel is also used in the secondary treatment of metastatic breast cancer (see NICE guidance below). There is limited evidence to support its use in non-small cell lung cancer. Routine premedication with a corticosteroid, an antihistamine and a histamine H$_2$-receptor antagonist is recom-

mended to prevent severe hypersensitivity reactions; hypersensitivity reactions may occur rarely despite premedication, although more commonly only bradycardia or asymptomatic hypotension occur.

Other side-effects of paclitaxel include myelosuppression, peripheral neuropathy, and cardiac conduction defects with arrhythmias (which are nearly always asymptomatic). It also causes alopecia and muscle pain; nausea and vomiting is mild to moderate.

Docetaxel is used in the treatment of advanced or metastatic breast cancer (see NICE guidance below) and non-small cell lung cancer. Docetaxel is also licensed for initial chemotherapy with doxorubicin for advanced breast cancer. Its side-effects are similar to those of paclitaxel but persistent fluid retention (commonly as leg oedema that worsens during treatment) can be resistant to treatment; hypersensitivity reactions also occur. Dexamethasone by mouth for 3 days, starting on the day before each course of docetaxel, is recommended for reducing fluid retention and hypersensitivity reactions.

NICE guidance (paclitaxel for ovarian cancer). NICE has recommended (January 2003) that *either* paclitaxel in combination with a platinum compound (cisplatin or carboplatin) *or* a platinum compound alone be used for the first-line treatment of ovarian cancer (usually following surgery).

On relapse, additional courses of the first-line treatment should be considered if the previous response was adequate. When the tumour fails to respond, a different regimen should be considered as second-line treatment.

Paclitaxel should be considered an option for second-line treatment only in women who have not already received the drug.

NICE guidance (breast cancer). NICE has recommended (September 2001) that both docetaxel and paclitaxel should be available for the treatment of advanced breast cancer where initial cytotoxic chemotherapy (including an anthracycline) has failed or is inappropriate. The use of taxanes for adjuvant treatment of early breast cancer or for the first-line treatment of advanced breast cancer should be limited to clinical trials [but see notes above].

NICE guidance (docetaxel, paclitaxel, gemcitabine and vinorelbine for non-small cell lung cancer). See p. 415.

DOCETAXEL

Indications: with doxorubicin for initial chemotherapy of advanced or metastatic breast cancer; advanced or metastatic breast cancer where adjuvant cytotoxic chemotherapy (with anthracycline or alkylating drug) has failed; advanced or metastatic non-small cell lung cancer where first-line chemotherapy has failed
Cautions: see section 8.1 and notes above; hepatic impairment (Appendix 2); **interactions:** Appendix 1 (docetaxel)
Side-effects: see section 8.1 and notes above

Taxotere® (Aventis Pharma) PoM
Concentrate for intravenous infusion, docetaxel 40 mg/mL. Net price 0.5-mL vial = £175.00, 2-mL vial = £575.00 (both with diluent) (hosp. only)

PACLITAXEL

Indications: primary ovarian cancer (advanced or residual disease following laparotomy) in combination with cisplatin; metastatic ovarian cancer where standard platinum-containing therapy has failed; advanced or metastatic breast cancer (in combination with trastuzumab) when an anthracycline not appropriate; metastatic breast cancer where standard anthracycline-containing therapy has failed or is inappropriate; non-small cell lung cancer (in combination with cisplatin) when surgery or radiotherapy not appropriate

Cautions: see section 8.1 and notes above; **interactions:** Appendix 1 (paclitaxel)

Contra-indications: see section 8.1 and notes above; severe hepatic impairment

Side-effects: see section 8.1 and notes above

Taxol® (Bristol-Myers Squibb) PoM
Concentrate for intravenous infusion, paclitaxel 6 mg/mL, net price 5-mL vial = £124.79, 16.7-mL vial = £374.00, 50-mL vial = £1122.00 (hosp. only)
Excipients: include polyoxyl castor oil (risk of anaphylaxis, see Excipients, p. 2)

Topoisomerase I inhibitors

Irinotecan and topotecan inhibit topoisomerase I, an enzyme involved in DNA replication.

Irinotecan is licensed for metastatic colorectal cancer in combination with fluorouracil and folinic acid or as monotherapy when treatment containing fluorouracil has failed; it is given by intravenous infusion.

> **NICE guidance (irinotecan, oxaliplatin and raltitrexed for advanced colorectal cancer).** See p. 420

Topotecan is given by intravenous infusion in metastatic ovarian cancer when first-line or subsequent therapy has failed.

In addition to dose-limiting myelosuppression, side-effects of irinotecan and topotecan include gastro-intestinal effects (delayed diarrhoea requiring prompt treatment may follow irinotecan treatment), asthenia, alopecia, and anorexia.

> **NICE guidance (topotecan).** NICE has recommended (August 2001) that topotecan be considered as one option for the second-line (or subsequent) treatment of advanced ovarian cancer where the disease is initially refractory to first-line platinum-based combination therapy or it has become resistant after successive courses of platinum-based combination therapy.
> Topotecan is not recommended in patients with poor performance status (Eastern Cooperative Oncology Group score 3 or worse), bowel obstruction, or after previous exposure to topotecan or another drug in the same class.

IRINOTECAN HYDROCHLORIDE

Indications: metastatic colorectal cancer in combination with fluorouracil and folinic acid or where treatment containing fluorouracil has failed

Cautions: see section 8.1 and notes above; raised plasma-bilirubin concentration (see under Contra-indications and Appendix 2)

Contra-indications: see section 8.1 and notes above, also chronic inflammatory bowel disease, bowel obstruction; plasma bilirubin concentration more than 1.5 times the upper limit of reference range; avoid conception for at least 3 months after cessation of treatment

Side-effects: see section 8.1 and notes above; also acute cholinergic syndrome (with early diarrhoea) and delayed diarrhoea (consult product literature)

Campto® (Aventis Pharma) PoM
Concentrate for intravenous infusion, irinotecan hydrochloride 20 mg/mL, net price 2-mL vial = £53.00; 5-mL vial = £130.00

TOPOTECAN

Indications: metastatic ovarian cancer where first-line or subsequent therapy has failed

Cautions: see section 8.1 and notes above

Contra-indications: see section 8.1 and notes above

Side-effects: see section 8.1 and notes above

Hycamtin® (Merck) ▼ PoM
Intravenous infusion, powder for reconstitution, topotecan (as hydrochloride), net price 1-mg vial = £105.00; 4-mg vial = £312.50

Trastuzumab

Trastuzumab is licensed, in combination with paclitaxel, for metastatic breast cancer in patients with tumours overexpressing the human epidermal growth factor receptor 2 (HER2) who have not received chemotherapy for metastatic breast cancer and in whom anthracycline treatment is inappropriate.

Trastuzumab is also licensed as monotherapy for metastatic breast cancer in patients with tumours that overexpress HER2 who have received at least 2 chemotherapy regimens including, where appropriate, an anthracycline and a taxane; women with oestrogen-receptor-positive breast cancer should also have received hormonal therapy.

Trastuzumab is given by intravenous infusion. Resuscitation facilities should be available and treatment should be initiated by a specialist.

> **NICE guidance (trastuzumab for advanced breast cancer).** NICE has recommended (March 2002) that trastuzumab, used in accordance with the licensed indications for *Herceptin®*, is an option in the management of metastatic breast cancer.

USE WITH ANTHRACYCLINES. Concomitant use of trastuzumab with anthracyclines (section 8.1.2) is associated with cardiotoxicity. The EMEA has advised that the use of anthracyclines even after stopping trastuzumab may carry a higher risk of cardiotoxicity and if possible should be avoided for up to 22 weeks. If anthracyclines need to be used, cardiac function should be monitored.

TRASTUZUMAB

Indications: see notes above and product literature

Cautions: symptomatic heart failure, history of hypertension, coronary artery disease; pregnancy (Appendix 4)

CARDIOTOXICITY. Monitor cardiac function of all patients before and during treatment—for details of monitoring and managing cardiotoxicity, consult product literature

Contra-indications: severe dyspnoea at rest; breast-feeding (Appendix 5)

Side-effects: infusion-related side-effects including chills, fever, hypersensitivity reactions such as anaphylaxis, urticaria and angioedema, pulmonary events (possibly delayed onset); cardiotoxicity (see also above); gastro-intestinal symptoms, asthenia, headache, chest pains, arthralgia, myalgia, hypotension

Herceptin® (Roche) ▼ PoM

Injection, powder for reconstitution, trastuzumab, net price 150-mg vial = £407.40. For intravenous infusion

Tretinoin

Tretinoin is licensed for the induction of remission in acute promyelocytic leukaemia. It is used in previously untreated patients as well as in those who have relapsed after standard chemotherapy or who are refractory to it.

TRETINOIN

NOTE. Tretinoin is the acid form of vitamin A

Indications: see notes above; acne (section 13.6.1); photodamage (section 13.8.1)

Cautions: exclude pregnancy before starting treatment and avoid pregnancy during and for at least 1 month after treatment; monitor haematological and coagulation profile, liver function, serum calcium and plasma lipids before and during treatment; increased risk of thrombo-embolism during first month of treatment; hepatic and renal impairment (Appendixes 2 and 3); **interactions:** Appendix 1 (retinoids)

Contra-indications: pregnancy (**important teratogenic risk:** see Cautions and Appendix 4) and breast-feeding

Side-effects: retinoic acid syndrome (fever, dyspnoea, acute respiratory distress, pulmonary infiltrates, pleural effusion, hyperleukocytosis, hypotension, oedema, weight gain, hepatic, renal and multi-organ failure) requires immediate treatment—consult product literature; gastro-intestinal disturbances, pancreatitis; arrhythmias, flushing, oedema; headache, benign intracranial hypertension (mainly in children—consider dose reduction if intractable headache in children), shivering, dizziness, confusion, anxiety, depression, insomnia, paraesthesia, visual and hearing disturbances; raised liver enzymes, serum creatinine and lipids; bone and chest pain, alopecia, erythema, rash, pruritus, sweating, dry skin and mucous membranes, cheilitis; thromboembolism, hypercalcaemia, and genital ulceration reported

Dose: ADULT and CHILD 45 mg/m² daily in 2 divided doses, max. duration of treatment 90 days (consult product literature for details of concomitant chemotherapy)

Vesanoid® (Roche) PoM

Capsules, yellow/brown, tretinoin 10 mg. Net price 100-cap pack = £183.36. Label: 21

8.2 Drugs affecting the immune response

8.2.1 Antiproliferative immunosuppressants
8.2.2 Corticosteroids and other immunosuppressants
8.2.3 Rituximab and alemtuzumab
8.2.4 Other immunomodulating drugs

Immunosuppressant therapy

Immunosuppressants are used to suppress rejection in organ transplant recipients and to treat a variety of chronic inflammatory and autoimmune diseases. Solid organ transplant patients are usually maintained on a corticosteroid combined with a calcineurin inhibitor (ciclosporin or tacrolimus), *or* with an antiproliferative drug (azathioprine or mycophenolate mofetil), *or* with both. Specialist management is required and other immunomodulators may be used to initiate treatment or to treat rejection.

IMPAIRED IMMUNE RESPONSIVENESS. Modification of tissue reactions caused by corticosteroids and other immunosuppressants may result in the rapid *spread of infection*. Corticosteroids may suppress clinical signs of infection and allow diseases such as septicaemia or tuberculosis to reach an advanced stage before being recognised—**important:** for advice on measles and chickenpox (varicella) exposure, see Immunoglobulins (section 14.5). For general comments and warnings relating to corticosteroids and immunosuppressants see section 6.3.2 (under Prednisolone).

PREGNANCY. Transplant patients immunosuppressed with azathioprine should not discontinue it on becoming pregnant; there is no evidence that azathioprine is teratogenic. However, there have been reports of premature birth and low birth-weight following exposure to azathioprine, particularly in combination with corticosteroids. Spontaneous abortion has been reported following maternal or paternal exposure.

There is less experience of ciclosporin in pregnancy but it does not appear to be any more harmful than azathioprine. The use of these drugs during pregnancy needs to be supervised in specialist units.

Manufacturers contra-indicate the use of tacrolimus and mycophenolate in pregnancy (Appendix 4).

8.2.1 Antiproliferative immunosuppressants

Azathioprine is widely used for transplant recipients and it is also used to treat a number of autoimmune conditions, usually when corticosteroid therapy alone provides inadequate control. It is metabolised to mercaptopurine, and doses should be reduced when allopurinol is given concurrently.

Blood tests and monitoring for signs of myelosuppression are essential in long-term treatment with azathioprine. The enzyme thiopurine methyltransferase (TPMT) metabolises azathioprine; the risk of myelosuppression is increased in those with a low activity of the enzyme, particularly in the very few individuals who are homozygous for low TPMT activity.

Mycophenolate mofetil is metabolised to mycophenolic acid which has a more selective mode of action than azathioprine. It is licensed for the prophylaxis of acute rejection in renal or cardiac transplantation when used in combination with ciclosporin and corticosteroids. There is evidence that compared with similar regimens incorporating azathioprine, mycophenolate mofetil reduces the risk of acute rejection episodes; the risk of opportunistic infections (particularly due to tissue-invasive cytomegalovirus) and the occurrence of blood disorders such as leucopenia may be higher.

Cyclophosphamide (section 8.1.1) is less commonly prescribed as an immunosuppressant.

AZATHIOPRINE

Indications: see notes above; also rheumatoid arthritis (section 10.1.3)

Cautions: monitor for toxicity throughout treatment; monitor full blood count weekly (more frequently with higher doses or if hepatic or renal impairment) for first 4 weeks (manufacturer advises weekly monitoring for 8 weeks but evidence of practical value unsatisfactory), thereafter reduce frequency of monitoring to at least every 3 months; hepatic impairment (Appendix 2); renal impairment (Appendix 3); reduce dose in elderly; pregnancy (see section 8.2)—treatment should not generally be initiated during pregnancy; **interactions:** Appendix 1 (azathioprine)
BONE MARROW SUPPRESSION. Patients should be warned to report immediately any signs or symptoms of bone marrow suppression e.g. inexplicable bruising or bleeding, infection

Contra-indications: hypersensitivity to azathioprine or mercaptopurine

Side-effects: hypersensitivity reactions (including malaise, dizziness, vomiting, diarrhoea, fever, rigors, myalgia, arthralgia, rash, hypotension and interstitial nephritis—calling for immediate withdrawal); dose-related bone marrow suppression (see also Cautions); liver impairment, cholestatic jaundice, hair loss and increased susceptibility to infections and colitis in patients also receiving corticosteroids; nausea; rarely pancreatitis, pneumonitis, hepatic veno-occlusive disease

Dose: by mouth, or (if oral administration not possible—intravenous solution very irritant, see below) by intravenous injection over at least 1 minute (followed by 50 mL sodium chloride intravenous infusion), or by intravenous infusion, autoimmune conditions, 1–3 mg/kg daily, adjusted according to response (consider withdrawal if no improvement in 3 months)

Suppression of transplant rejection, initially up to 5 mg/kg then 1–4 mg/kg daily according to response
NOTE. Intravenous injection is alkaline and very irritant, intravenous route should therefore be used **only** if oral route not feasible, see also Appendix 6

Azathioprine (Non-proprietary) PoM
Tablets, azathioprine 25 mg, net price 28-tab pack = £9.28; 50 mg, 56-tab pack = £9.97. Label: 21
Available from Alpharma, Ashbourne (*Immunoprin®*), Hillcross, IVAX, Kent, Opus (*Oprisine®*), Penn (*Azamune®*)

Imuran® (GSK) PoM
Tablets, both f/c, azathioprine 25 mg (orange), net price 100-tab pack = £39.35; 50 mg (yellow), 100-tab pack = £65.61. Label: 21
Injection, powder for reconstitution, azathioprine (as sodium salt). Net price 50-mg vial = £16.54

MYCOPHENOLATE MOFETIL

Indications: prophylaxis of acute renal, cardiac, or hepatic transplant rejection (in combination with ciclosporin and corticosteroids) under specialist supervision

Cautions: full blood counts every week for 4 weeks then twice a month for 2 months then every month in the first year (possibly interrupt treatment if neutropenia develops); elderly (increased risk of infection, gastro-intestinal haemorrhage and pulmonary oedema); children (higher incidence of side-effects may call for temporary reduction of dose or interruption); active serious gastro-intestinal disease (risk of haemorrhage, ulceration and perforation); delayed graft function; increased susceptibility to skin cancer (avoid exposure to strong sunlight); **interactions:** Appendix 1 (mycophenolate mofetil)
BONE MARROW SUPPRESSION. Patients should be warned to report immediately any signs or symptoms of bone marrow suppression e.g. infection and inexplicable bruising or bleeding

Contra-indications: pregnancy (exclude before starting and avoid for 6 weeks after discontinuation) (Appendix 4); breast-feeding (Appendix 5)

Side-effects: diarrhoea, vomiting, constipation, nausea, dyspepsia, pancreatitis, abdominal pain; hypertension, oedema, chest pain; dyspnoea, cough, rhinitis; dizziness, insomnia, headache, tremor; infection (including cytomegalovirus viraemia, herpes simplex, candidiasis, aspergillosis, sepsis, urinary-tract infection and pneumonia); leucopenia (see also Cautions), anaemia, thrombocytopenia, leucocytosis, polycythaemia; electrolyte disturbances, hyperglycaemia, hypercholesterolaemia; asthenia; renal damage, haematuria; acne; lymphoproliferative disease; less frequently, gastro-intestinal perforation, colitis, abnormal liver-function tests, hepatitis, gingivitis, mouth ulceration, haemorrhage, influenza-like syndrome, hypotension, arrhythmias, tachycardia, hypoglycaemia, weight gain; allergic reactions, benign neoplasm of skin and skin carcinoma reported

Dose: renal transplantation, by mouth, 1 g twice daily starting within 72 hours of transplantation or by intravenous infusion, 1 g twice daily starting within 24 hours of transplantation for up to max. 14 days (then transfer to oral therapy); CHILD and ADOLESCENT 2–18 years (and body-surface area over 1.25 m²) 600 mg/m² twice daily (max. 2 g daily)
NOTE. Tablets and capsules not appropriate for dose titration in young children

Cardiac transplantation, by mouth, 1.5 g twice daily starting within 5 days of transplantation

Hepatic transplantation, *by intravenous infusion*, 1 g twice daily starting within 24 hours of transplantation for 4 days (up to max. 14 days), then *by mouth*, 1.5 g twice daily as soon as is tolerated

CellCept® (Roche) ▼ PoM

Capsules, blue/brown, mycophenolate mofetil 250 mg, net price 100-cap pack = £113.41
Tablets, lavender, mycophenolate mofetil 500 mg, net price 50-tab pack = £113.41
Oral suspension, mycophenolate mofetil 1 g/5 mL when reconstituted with water, net price 175 mL = £158.77
Intravenous infusion, powder for reconstitution, mycophenolate mofetil (as hydrochloride), net price 500-mg vial = £9.69

8.2.2 Corticosteroids and other immunosuppressants

Prednisolone (section 6.3.2) is widely used in oncology. It has a marked antitumour effect in acute lymphoblastic leukaemia, Hodgkin's disease, and the non-Hodgkin lymphomas. It has a role in the palliation of symptomatic end-stage malignant disease when it may enhance appetite and produce a sense of well-being (see also Prescribing in Palliative Care, p. 14).

The corticosteroids are also powerful immunosuppressants. They are used to prevent organ transplant rejection, and in high dose to treat rejection episodes.

Ciclosporin (cyclosporin), a calcineurin inhibitor, is a potent immunosuppressant which is virtually non-myelotoxic but markedly nephrotoxic. It has an important role in organ and tissue transplantation, for prevention of graft rejection following bone marrow, kidney, liver, pancreas, heart, lung, and heart-lung transplantation, and for prophylaxis and treatment of graft-versus-host disease.

Tacrolimus is also a calcineurin inhibitor. Although not chemically related to ciclosporin it has a similar mode of action and side-effects, but the incidence of neurotoxicity and nephrotoxicity appears to be greater; cardiomyopathy has also been reported. Disturbance of glucose metabolism also appears to be significant; hypertrichosis appears to be less of a problem than with ciclosporin.

Sirolimus is a potent non-calcineurin inhibiting immunosuppressant introduced recently for renal transplantation. It can cause hyperlipidaemia.

Basiliximab and **daclizumab** are monoclonal antibodies that prevent T-lymphocyte proliferation; they are used for prophylaxis of acute rejection in allogenic renal transplantation. They are given with ciclosporin and corticosteroid immunosuppression regimens; their use should be confined to specialist centres.

BASILIXIMAB

Indications: see notes above

Contra-indications: pregnancy (Appendix 4) and breast-feeding

Side-effects: severe hypersensitivity reactions reported rarely; for side-effects of regimen see under Ciclosporin (below) and Prednisolone (section 6.3.2)

Dose: *by intravenous injection or by intravenous infusion*, 20 mg within 2 hours before transplant surgery and 20 mg 4 days after surgery; CHILD and ADOLESCENT under 35 kg, 10 mg within 2 hours before transplant surgery and 10 mg 4 days after surgery; withhold second dose if severe hypersensitivity or graft loss occurs

Simulect® (Novartis) PoM

Injection, powder for reconstitution, basiliximab, net price 10-mg vial = £758.69, 20-mg vial = £842.38 (both with water for injections) . For intravenous infusion

CICLOSPORIN

(Cyclosporin)

Indications: see notes above, and under Dose; atopic dermatitis and psoriasis (section 13.5.3); rheumatoid arthritis (section 10.1.3)

Cautions: monitor kidney function—dose dependent increase in serum creatinine and urea during first few weeks may necessitate dose reduction in transplant patients (exclude rejection if kidney transplant) or discontinuation in non-transplant patients; monitor liver function (dosage adjustment based on bilirubin and liver enzymes may be needed); monitor blood pressure—discontinue if hypertension develops that cannot be controlled by antihypertensives; hyperuricaemia; monitor serum potassium especially in renal dysfunction (risk of hyperkalaemia); monitor serum magnesium; measure blood lipids before treatment and thereafter as appropriate; pregnancy (see p. 423) and breast-feeding (Appendix 5); porphyria (section 9.8.2); use with tacrolimus specifically contra-indicated and apart from specialist use in transplant patients preferably avoid other immunosuppressants with the exception of corticosteroids (increased risk of infection and lymphoma); **interactions:** Appendix 1 (ciclosporin)

ADDITIONAL CAUTIONS IN NEPHROTIC SYNDROME. **Contra-indicated** in uncontrolled hypertension, uncontrolled infections, and malignancy; reduce dose by 25–50% if serum creatinine more than 30% above baseline on more than one measurement; in renal impairment initially 2.5 mg/kg daily; in long-term management, perform renal biopsies at yearly intervals

ADDITIONAL CAUTIONS. Atopic Dermatitis and Psoriasis, section 13.5.3; Rheumatoid Arthritis, section 10.1.3

Side-effects: dose-dependent increase in serum creatinine and urea during first few weeks (see also under Cautions); less commonly renal structural changes on long-term administration; also hypertrichosis, headache, tremor, hypertension (especially in heart transplant patients), hepatic dysfunction, fatigue, gingival hypertrophy, gastrointestinal disturbances, burning sensation in hands and feet (usually during first week); *occasionally* rash (possibly allergic), mild anaemia, hyperkalaemia, hyperuricaemia, gout, hypomagnesaemia, hypercholesterolaemia, hyperglycaemia, weight increase, oedema, pancreatitis, neuropathy, confusion, paraesthesia, convulsions, benign intracranial hypertension (discontinue), dysmenorrhoea or amenorrhoea; myalgia, muscle weakness, cramps, myopathy, gynaecomastia (in patients receiving concomitant spironolactone), colitis and cortical blindness also reported; thrombocytopenia (sometimes with haemolytic uraemic syndrome) also reported; incidence of malignancies and lymphoproliferative disorders similar to that with other immunosuppressive therapy

Dose: organ transplantation, used alone, ADULT and CHILD over 3 months 10–15 mg/kg *by mouth* 4–12 hours before transplantation followed by 10–15 mg/kg daily for 1–2 weeks postoperatively then reduced gradually to 2–6 mg/kg daily for maintenance (dose should be adjusted according to blood-ciclosporin concentration and renal function); dose lower if given concomitantly with other immunosuppressant therapy (e.g. corticosteroids); if necessary one-third corresponding oral dose can be given *by intravenous infusion* over 2–6 hours

Bone-marrow transplantation, prevention and treatment of graft-versus-host disease, ADULT and CHILD over 3 months 3–5 mg/kg daily *by intravenous infusion* over 2–6 hours from day before transplantation to 2 weeks postoperatively (or 12.5–15 mg/kg daily *by mouth*) then 12.5 mg/kg daily *by mouth* for 3–6 months then tailed off (may take up to a year after transplantation)

Nephrotic syndrome, *by mouth*, 5 mg/kg daily in 2 divided doses; CHILD 6 mg/kg daily in 2 divided doses; maintenance treatment reduce to lowest effective dose according to proteinuria and serum creatinine measurements; discontinue after 3 months if no improvement in glomerulonephritis or glomerulosclerosis (after 6 months in membranous glomerulonephritis)

CONVERSION. Any conversion between brands should be undertaken very carefully and the manufacturer contacted for further information. Currently only *Neoral®* remains available for oral use; *Sandimmun®* capsules and oral solution and *SangCya®* oral solution are available on named-patient basis only for patients who cannot be transferred to another brand of oral ciclosporin

> Because of differences in bioavailability, the brand of ciclosporin to be dispensed should be specified by the prescriber

Neoral® (Novartis) PoM
Capsules, ciclosporin 10 mg (yellow/white), net price 30-cap pack = £8.22; 25 mg (blue/grey), 30-cap pack = £20.54; 50 mg (yellow/white), 30-cap pack = £40.22; 100 mg (blue/grey), 30-cap pack = £76.33. Counselling, administration
Oral solution, yellow, sugar-free, ciclosporin 100 mg/mL, net price 50 mL = £114.38. Counselling, administration
COUNSELLING. Total daily dose should be taken in 2 divided doses. Avoid grapefruit or grapefruit juice for 1 hour before dose
Mix solution with orange juice (or squash) or apple juice (to improve taste) or with water immediately before taking (and rinse with more to ensure total dose). Do not mix with grapefruit juice. Keep medicine measure away from other liquids (including water)

Sandimmun® (Novartis) PoM
Concentrate for intravenous infusion (oily), ciclosporin 50 mg/mL. To be diluted before use. Net price 1-mL amp = £1.94; 5-mL amp = £9.17
Excipients: include polyoxyl castor oil (risk of anaphylaxis, see Excipients, p. 2)
NOTE. Observe for at least 30 minutes after starting infusion and at frequent intervals thereafter

DACLIZUMAB

Indications: see notes above
Contra-indications: pregnancy and breast-feeding
Side-effects: severe hypersensitivity reactions reported rarely; for side-effects of regimen see under Ciclosporin (above) and Prednisolone (section 6.3.2)

Dose: *by intravenous infusion,* ADULT and CHILD, 1 mg/kg within the 24-hour period before transplantation, then 1 mg/kg every 14 days for a total of 5 doses

Zenapax® (Roche) ▼ PoM
Concentrate for intravenous infusion, daclizumab 5 mg/mL, net price 5-mL = £240.52

SIROLIMUS

Indications: prophylaxis of organ rejection in kidney allograft recipients (initially in combination with ciclosporin and corticosteroid, then with corticosteroid only); see also under Dose

Cautions: monitor kidney function when given with ciclosporin; Afro-Caribbean patients may require higher doses; hepatic impairment (Appendix 2); food may affect absorption (administer at the same time with respect to food); **interactions:** Appendix 1 (sirolimus)

Contra-indications: pregnancy (Appendix 4); breast-feeding (Appendix 5)

Side-effects: lymphocele, oedema, abdominal pain, diarrhoea, tachycardia, anaemia, fever, thrombocytopenia, neutropenia, leucopenia, thrombotic thrombocytopenic purpura, hyperlipidaemias (including hypercholesterolaemia, hypertriglyceridaemia), increase in serum creatinine in patients also receiving ciclosporin, hypokalaemia, arthralgia, acne; less commonly, venous thromboembolism, epistaxis, interstitial lung disease, impaired healing, increased susceptibility to infection, stomatitis, haemolytic uraemia, bone necrosis, rash, pyelonephritis; rarely, pancreatitis, susceptibility to lymphoma and other malignancies particularly of the skin, pancytopenia, hepatic necrosis, hypersensitivity reactions including anaphylaxis

Dose: initially 6 mg, after surgery, then 2 mg once daily (dose adjusted according to blood-sirolimus concentration) in combination with ciclosporin and corticosteroid for 2–3 months (sirolimus given 4 hours after ciclosporin); ciclosporin should then be withdrawn over 4–8 weeks (if not possible, sirolimus should be discontinued and an alternate immunosuppressive regimen used)
NOTE. Pre-dose ('trough') blood-sirolimus concentration (using chromatographic assay) when used with ciclosporin should be 4–12 micrograms/litre; after withdrawal of ciclosporin pre-dose blood-sirolimus concentration should be 12–20 micrograms/litre; close monitoring of blood-sirolimus concentration required in hepatic impairment, during treatment with potent inducers or inhibitors of metabolism and after discontinuing them
When changing between oral solution and tablets, measurement of serum 'trough' blood-sirolimus concentration after 1–2 weeks is recommended

Rapamune® (Wyeth) ▼ PoM
Tablets, coated, sirolimus 1 mg, net price 30-tab pack = £90.00, 100-tab pack = £300.00; 2 mg, 30-tab pack = £180.00, 100-tab pack = £600.00
Oral solution, sirolimus 1 mg/mL, net price 60 mL = £169.00. Counselling, administration
COUNSELLING. Mix solution with at least 60 mL water or orange juice in a glass or plastic container immediately before taking; refill container with at least 120 mL and drink immediately (to ensure total dose). Do not mix with any other liquids

TACROLIMUS

Indications: primary immunosuppression in liver and kidney allograft recipients and allograft rejection resistant to conventional immunosuppressive regimens, see also notes above; moderate to severe atopic eczema (section 13.5.3)

Cautions: see under Ciclosporin; also monitor ECG (**important:** also echocardiography, see CSM warning below), visual status, blood glucose, haematological and neurological parameters; **interactions:** Appendix 1 (tacrolimus)

DRIVING. May affect performance of skilled tasks (e.g. driving)

Contra-indications: hypersensitivity to macrolides; pregnancy (exclude before starting—if contraception needed non-hormonal methods should be used), breast-feeding; avoid concurrent administration with ciclosporin (care if patient has previously received ciclosporin)

Side-effects: include gastro-intestinal disturbances including dyspepsia, and inflammatory and ulcerative disorders; hepatic dysfunction, jaundice, bile-duct and gall-bladder abnormalities; hypertension (less frequently hypotension), tachycardia, angina, arrhythmias, thromboembolic and ischaemic events, rarely myocardial hypertrophy, cardiomyopathy (**important:** see CSM warning below); dyspnoea, pleural effusion, tremor, headache, insomnia, paraesthesia, confusion, depression, dizziness, anxiety, convulsions, incoordination, encephalopathy, psychosis; visual and hearing abnormalities; haematological effects including anaemia, leucocytosis, leucopenia, thrombocytopaenia, coagulation disorders; altered acid-base balance and glucose metabolism, electrolyte disturbances including hyperkalaemia (less frequently hypokalaemia); altered renal function including increased serum creatinine; hypophosphataemia, hypercalcaemia, hyperuricaemia; muscle cramps, arthralgia; pruritus, alopecia, rash, sweating, acne, photosensitivity; susceptibility to lymphoma and other malignancies particularly of the skin; less commonly ascites, pancreatitis, atelectasis, kidney damage and renal failure, myasthenia, hirsutism, rarely Stevens-Johnson syndrome

CSM WARNING. Cardiomyopathy has been reported in children given tacrolimus after transplantation. Patients should be monitored carefully by echocardiography for hypertrophic changes; dose reduction or discontinuation should be considered if these occur

Dose: liver transplantation, starting 6 hours after transplantation, *by mouth*, 100–200 micrograms/kg daily in 2 divided doses *or by intravenous infusion* over 24 hours, 10–50 micrograms/kg; CHILD *by mouth*, 300 micrograms/kg daily in 2 divided doses *or by intravenous infusion* over 24 hours, 50 micrograms/kg

Renal transplantation, starting within 24 hours of transplantation, *by mouth*, 150–300 micrograms/kg daily in 2 divided doses *or by intravenous infusion* over 24 hours, 50–100 micrograms/kg; CHILD *by mouth*, 300 micrograms/kg daily in 2 divided doses *or by intravenous infusion* over 24 hours, 100 micrograms/kg

Maintenance treatment, dose adjusted according to response

Prograf® (Fujisawa) [PoM]
Capsules, tacrolimus 500 micrograms (yellow), net price 50-cap pack = £71.56; 1 mg (white), 50-cap pack = £92.93, 100-cap pack = £185.86; 5 mg (greyish-red), 50-cap pack =£343.34. Label: 23, counselling, driving

Concentrate for intravenous infusion, tacrolimus 5 mg/mL. To be diluted before use. Net price 1-mL amp = £67.67

Excipients: include polyoxyl castor oil (risk of anaphylaxis, see Excipients, p. 2)

8.2.3 Rituximab and alemtuzumab

Rituximab, a monoclonal antibody which causes lysis of B lymphocytes, is licensed for the treatment of chemotherapy-resistant advanced follicular lymphoma (see NICE guidance below) and for diffuse large B-cell non-Hodgkin's lymphoma in combination with other chemotherapy (see NICE guidance below). Full resuscitation facilities should be at hand and as with other cytotoxics, treatment should be undertaken under the close supervision of a specialist.

Rituximab should be used with caution in patients receiving cardiotoxic chemotherapy or with a history of cardiovascular disease because exacerbation of angina, arrhythmia, and heart failure have been reported. Transient hypotension occurs frequently during infusion and antihypertensives may need to be withheld for 12 hours before infusion.

Infusion-related side-effects (including cytokine release syndrome) are reported commonly with rituximab and occur predominantly during the first infusion; they include fever and chills, nausea and vomiting, allergic reactions (such as rash, pruritus, angioedema, bronchospasm and dyspnoea), flushing and tumour pain. Patients should be given an analgesic and an antihistamine before each dose of rituximab to reduce these effects. Premedication with a corticosteroid should also be considered. The infusion may have to be stopped temporarily and the infusion-related effects treated—consult product literature for appropriate management. Evidence of pulmonary infiltration and features of tumour lysis syndrome should be sought if infusion-related effects occur.

Fatalities following **severe** cytokine release syndrome (characterised by severe dyspnoea) and associated with features of tumour lysis syndrome have occurred 1–2 hours after infusion of rituximab. Patients with a high tumour burden as well as those with pulmonary insufficiency or infiltration are at increased risk and should be monitored **very closely** (and a slower rate of infusion considered).

NICE guidance (rituximab for follicular non-Hodgkin's lymphoma). NICE has recommended (March 2002) that for stage III or IV follicular lymphoma, rituximab is used only if the disease is resistant to other chemotherapy or if the patient cannot tolerate such treatment. In these circumstances rituximab should be used as part of a prospective study.

NICE guidance (rituximab for aggressive non-Hodgkin's lymphoma). NICE has recommended (September 2003) rituximab, in combination with cyclophosphamide, doxorubicin, vincristine and prednisolone, for first-line treatment of CD20-positive diffuse large-B-cell lymphoma at clinical stage II, III or IV.
The use of rituximab for localised (stage I) disease should be limited to clinical trials.

Alemtuzumab, another monoclonal antibody that causes lysis of B lymphocytes, is licensed for use in patients with chronic lymphocytic leukaemia which has failed to respond to treatment with an alkylating drug, or which has remitted for only a short period (less than 6 months) following fludarabine treatment. In common with rituximab, it causes infusion-related side-effects including cytokine release syndrome (see above).

ALEMTUZUMAB

Indications: see notes above
Cautions: see notes above—for full details (including monitoring) consult product literature
Contra-indications: pregnancy (Appendix 4) and breast-feeding (Appendix 5); for full details consult product literature
Side-effects: see notes above—for full details (including monitoring and management of side-effects) consult product literature
Dose: consult product literature

MabCampath® (Schering Health) ▼ PoM
Concentrate for intravenous infusion, alemtuzumab 10 mg/mL, net price 3-mL amp = £283.33

RITUXIMAB

Indications: see notes above
Cautions: see notes above—but for full details (including monitoring) consult product literature; pregnancy (Appendix 4)
Contra-indications: breast-feeding
Side-effects: see notes above—but for full details (including monitoring and management of side-effects) consult product literature

MabThera® (Roche) ▼ PoM
Concentrate for intravenous infusion, rituximab 10 mg/mL, net price 10-mL vial = £174.63, 50-mL vial = £873.15

8.2.4 Other immunomodulating drugs

Interferon alfa

Interferon alfa has shown some antitumour effect in certain lymphomas and solid tumours. Interferon alfa preparations are also used in the treatment of chronic hepatitis B, and chronic hepatitis C ideally in combination with ribavirin (section 5.3). Side-effects are dose-related, but commonly include anorexia, nausea, influenza-like symptoms, and lethargy. Ocular side-effects and depression (including suicidal behaviour) have also been reported. Myelosuppression may occur, particularly affecting granulocyte counts. Cardiovascular problems (hypotension, hypertension, and arrhythmias), nephrotoxicity and hepatotoxicity have been reported. Hypertriglyceridaemia, sometimes severe, has been observed; monitoring of lipid concentration is recommended. Other side-effects include hypersensitivity reactions, thyroid abnormalities, hyperglycaemia, alopecia, psoriasiform rash, confusion, coma and seizures (usually with high doses in the elderly).

Polyethylene glycol-conjugated ('pegylated') derivatives of interferon alfa (**peginterferon alfa-2a** and **peginterferon alfa-2b**) are available; pegylation increases the persistence of the interferon in the blood. The peginterferons are licensed for the treatment of chronic hepatitis C, ideally in combination with ribavirin (see section 5.3).

INTERFERON ALFA

Indications: see under preparations
Cautions: consult product literature; **interactions:** Appendix 1 (interferons)
Contra-indications: consult product literature; avoid injections containing benzyl alcohol in neonates (see under preparations below)
Side-effects: see notes above and consult product literature
Dose: consult product literature

IntronA® (Schering-Plough) PoM
Injection, interferon alfa-2b (rbe) 10 million units/mL, net price 2.5-mL vial = £135.00. For subcutaneous or intravenous injection
Injection, powder for reconstitution, interferon alfa-2b (rbe), net price 10-million unit vial (with injection equipment and water for injections) = £53.96. For subcutaneous or intravenous injection
Injection pen, interferon alfa-2b (rbe), net price 15 million units/mL, 1.5-mL cartridge = £97.20; 25 million units/mL, 1.5-mL cartridge = £162.00; 50 million units/mL, 1.5-mL cartridge = £324.00. For subcutaneous injection
NOTE. Each 1.5-mL multidose cartridge delivers 6 doses of 0.2 mL i.e. a total of 1.2 mL
For chronic myelogenous leukaemia (as monotherapy or in combination with cytarabine), hairy cell leukaemia, follicular lymphoma, lymph or liver metastases of carcinoid tumour, chronic hepatitis B, chronic hepatitis C, adjunct to surgery in malignant melanoma and maintenance of remission in multiple myeloma

Roferon-A® (Roche) PoM
Injection, interferon alfa-2a (rbe). Net price 6 million units/mL, 0.5-mL (3 million-unit) prefilled syringe = £16.20; 9 million units/mL, 0.5-mL (4.5 million-unit) prefilled syringe = £24.30; 12 million units/mL, 0.5-mL (6 million-unit) prefilled syringe = £32.39; 18 million units/mL, 0.5-mL (9 million-unit) prefilled syringe = £48.59; 36 million units/mL, 0.5-mL (18 million-unit) prefilled syringe = £97.19; 30 million units/mL, 0.6-mL (18 million-unit) cartridge = £97.19, for use with *Roferon* pen device. For subcutaneous injection (cartridges, vials, and prefilled syringes) and intramuscular injection (cartridges and vials)
Excipients: include benzyl alcohol (avoid in neonates, see Excipients, p. 2)
For AIDS-related Kaposi's sarcoma, hairy cell leukaemia, chronic myelogenous leukaemia, recurrent or metastatic renal cell carcinoma, progressive cutaneous T-cell lymphoma, chronic hepatitis B and chronic hepatitis C, follicular non-Hodgkin's lymphoma, adjunct to surgery in malignant melanoma

Viraferon® (Schering-Plough) PoM
Injection, interferon alfa-2b (rbe) 6 million units/mL, net price 3-mL vial = £97.20. For subcutaneous injection
Injection pen, interferon alfa-2b (rbe), net price 15 million units/mL, 1.5-mL cartridge = £97.20. For subcutaneous injection
NOTE. 1.5-mL multidose cartridge delivers 6 doses of 0.2 mL each
For chronic hepatitis B and chronic hepatitis C

PEGINTERFERON ALFA

Indications: combined with ribavirin for chronic hepatitis C; as monotherapy if ribavirin not tolerated or contra-indicated (see section 5.3)
Cautions: consult product literature; **interactions:** Appendix 1 (interferons)
Contra-indications: consult product literature
Side-effects: see notes above and consult product literature
Dose: consult product literature

Pegasys® (Roche) ▼ PoM
Injection, peginterferon alfa-2a, net price 135-microgram prefilled syringe = £123.00, 180-microgram prefilled syringe = £142.00. For subcutaneous injection

PegIntron® (Schering-Plough) ▼ PoM
Injection, powder for reconstitution, peginterferon alfa-2b (rbe), net price 50-microgram vial = £67.50, 80-microgram vial = £108.00, 100-microgram vial = £135.00, 120-microgram vial = £162.00, 150-microgram vial = £202.50 (all with injection equipment and water for injections). For subcutaneous injection

ViraferonPeg® (Schering-Plough) ▼ PoM
Injection, powder for reconstitution, peginterferon alfa-2b (rbe), net price 50-microgram vial = £67.50, 80-microgram vial = £108.00, 100-microgram vial = £135.00, 120-microgram vial = £162.00, 150-microgram vial = £202.50 (all with injection equipment and water for injections). For subcutaneous injection
Injection, prefilled pen, powder for reconstitution, peginterferon alfa-2b (rbe), net price 50-microgram pen = £74.25, 80-microgram pen = £118.80, 100-microgram pen = £148.50, 120-microgram pen = £178.20, 150-microgram pen = £222.75 (all with needles and swabs). For subcutaneous injection

Interferon beta

Interferon beta is licensed for use in patients with *relapsing, remitting multiple sclerosis* (characterised by at least two attacks of neurological dysfunction over the previous 2 or 3 years, followed by complete or incomplete recovery) who are able to walk unaided. Not all patients respond and a deterioration in the bouts has been observed in some. Interferon beta-1b is also licensed for use in patients with *secondary progressive multiple sclerosis* but its role in this condition has not been confirmed.

Interferon beta should not be used in those with a history of severe depressive illness (or of suicidal ideation), in those with inadequately controlled epilepsy, or in decompensated hepatic impairment; caution is advised in those with a history of these conditions or with cardiac disorders or myelosuppression. Side-effects reported most frequently include irritation at injection site (including inflammation, hypersensitivity, necrosis) and influenza-like symptoms (fever, chills, myalgia, or malaise) but these decrease over time; nausea and vomiting occur occasionally. Other side-effects include hypersensitivity reactions (including anaphylaxis and urticaria), blood disorders, menstrual disorders, mood and personality changes, suicide attempts, confusion and convulsions; alopecia, hepatitis, and thyroid

dysfunction have been reported rarely with interferon beta-1b.

NICE guidance (interferon beta and glatiramer for multiple sclerosis). NICE does not recommend (January 2002) either interferon beta or glatiramer acetate for the treatment of multiple sclerosis in the NHS in England and Wales. Patients who are currently receiving interferon beta or glatiramer acetate for multiple sclerosis, whether as routine therapy or as part of a clinical trial, should have the option to continue treatment until they and their consultant consider it appropriate to stop, having regard to the established criteria for withdrawal from treatment.

Provision of disease-modifying therapies for multiple sclerosis. The Department of Health, the National Assembly for Wales, the Scottish Executive, the Northern Ireland Department of Health, Social Services & Public Safety, and the manufacturers have reached agreement on a risk-sharing scheme for the NHS supply of interferon beta and glatiramer acetate for multiple sclerosis. Health Service Circular (HSC 2002/004) explains how patients can participate in the scheme (www.doh.gov.uk/publications/coinh.html).

INTERFERON BETA

Indications: see notes above
Cautions: see notes above and consult product literature
Contra-indications: consult product literature; pregnancy (Appendix 4—advise contraceptive measures if appropriate), breast-feeding (Appendix 5)
Side-effects: see notes above and consult product literature
Dose: consult product literature

■ Interferon beta-1a

Avonex® (Biogen) PoM
Injection, interferon beta-1a 60 micrograms (12 million units)/mL, net price 0.5-mL (30-microgram, 6 million-unit) prefilled syringe = £163.50. For intramuscular injection

Rebif® (Serono) PoM
Injection, interferon beta-1a, net price 22-microgram (6 million-unit) prefilled syringe = £58.26; 44-microgram (12 million-unit) prefilled syringe = £77.36. For subcutaneous injection

■ Interferon beta-1b

Betaferon® (Schering Health) PoM
Injection, powder for reconstitution, interferon beta-1b. Net price 300-microgram (9.6 million-unit) vial with diluent = £39.78. For subcutaneous injection
NOTE. An autoinjector device (*Betaject*® *Light*) is available from Schering Health

Aldesleukin

Aldesleukin (recombinant interleukin-2) is licensed for metastatic renal cell carcinoma; it is usually given by subcutaneous injection. It is now rarely given by intravenous infusion because of an association with a capillary leak syndrome, which can cause pulmonary oedema and hypotension. Aldesleukin produces tumour shrinkage in a small proportion of patients, but it has not been shown to increase survival. Bone-

marrow, hepatic, renal, thyroid, and CNS toxicity is common. It is for use in **specialist units** only.
Interactions: Appendix 1 (aldesleukin)

Proleukin® (Chiron) PoM
Injection, powder for reconstitution, aldesleukin. Net price 18-million unit vial = £140.00. For subcutaneous injection
Injection, powder for reconstitution, aldesleukin. Net price 18-million unit vial = £140.00. For intravenous infusion but see notes above
For metastatic renal cell carcinoma, **excluding** patients in whom all three of the following prognostic factors are present: performance status of Eastern Co-operative Oncology Group of 1 or greater, more than one organ with metastatic disease sites, and a period of less than 24 months between initial diagnosis of primary tumour and date of evaluation of treatment.

BCG bladder instillation

BCG (**Bacillus Calmette-Guérin**) is a live attenuated strain derived from *Mycobacterium bovis*. It is licensed as a bladder instillation for the treatment of primary or recurrent bladder carcinoma and for the prevention of recurrence following transurethral resection.

BACILLUS CALMETTE-GUÉRIN

Indications: see notes above; BCG immunisation (section 14.4)
Cautions: screen for active tuberculosis (contra-indicated if tuberculosis confirmed); traumatic catheterisation (delay administration until mucosal damage healed)
Contra-indications: impaired immune response, HIV infection, urinary-tract infection, tuberculosis, fever of unknown origin; pregnancy and breast-feeding
Side-effects: cystitis, dysuria, urinary frequency, haematuria, malaise, fever, influenza-like syndrome; also systemic BCG infection (with fatalities)—consult product literature; rarely hypersensitivity reactions (such as arthralgia and rash), orchitis, transient urethral obstruction, bladder contracture, renal abscess; ocular symptoms reported
Dose: consult product literature

ImmuCyst® (Cambridge) ▼ PoM
Bladder instillation, freeze-dried powder containing attenuated *Mycobacterium bovis* prepared from the Connaught strain of bacillus of Calmette and Guérin, net price 81-mg vial = £89.00

OncoTICE® (Organon) ▼ PoM
Bladder instillation, freeze-dried powder containing attenuated *Mycobacterium bovis* prepared from the TICE strain of bacillus of Calmette and Guérin, net price 12.5-mg vial = £80.00

Glatiramer acetate

Glatiramer is an immunomodulating drug comprising synthetic polypeptides. It is licensed for reducing the frequency of relapses in ambulatory patients with relapsing-remitting multiple sclerosis who have had at least one clinical relapse in the past two years. Initiation of treatment with glatiramer should be supervised by a specialist.

NICE guidance (interferon beta and glatiramer for multiple sclerosis). See p. 429

Provision of disease-modifying therapies for multiple sclerosis. See p. 429

GLATIRAMER ACETATE

Indications: see notes above
Cautions: cardiac disorders; renal impairment; pregnancy (Appendix 4) and breast-feeding (Appendix 5)
Side-effects: flushing, chest pain, palpitations, tachycardia, and dyspnoea may occur within minutes of injection; injection site reactions; nausea, peripheral and face oedema, syncope, asthenia, headache, tremor, sweating, lymphadenopathy, hypertonia, arthralgia, rash; convulsions, hypersensitivity reactions including anaphylaxis, bronchospasm and urticaria reported rarely
Dose: *by subcutaneous injection*, ADULT over 18 years, 20 mg daily

Copaxone® (Teva) ▼ PoM
Injection, powder for reconstitution, glatiramer acetate, net price 20-mg vial with diluent = £18.22

8.3 Sex hormones and hormone antagonists in malignant disease

8.3.1	Oestrogens
8.3.2	Progestogens
8.3.3	Androgens
8.3.4	Hormone antagonists

Hormonal manipulation has an important role in the treatment of breast, prostate, and endometrial cancer, and a more marginal role in the treatment of hypernephroma. These treatments are not curative, but may provide excellent palliation of symptoms in selected patients, sometimes for a period of years. Tumour response, and treatment toxicity should be carefully monitored and treatment changed if progression occurs or side-effects exceed benefit.

8.3.1 Oestrogens

Diethylstilbestrol (stilboestrol) is rarely used to treat prostate cancer because of its side-effects. It is occasionally used in postmenopausal women with breast cancer. Toxicity is common and dose-related side-effects include nausea, fluid retention, and venous and arterial thrombosis. Impotence and gynaecomastia always occur in men, and withdrawal bleeding may be a problem in women. Hypercalcaemia and bone pain may also occur in breast cancer.
Ethinylestradiol (ethinyloestradiol) is the most potent oestrogen available; unlike other oestrogens it is only slowly metabolised in the liver. It is used in breast cancer [unlicensed indication].

DIETHYLSTILBESTROL

(Stilboestrol)

Indications: see notes above

Cautions: cardiovascular disease; hepatic impairment

Side-effects: sodium retention with oedema, thromboembolism, jaundice, feminising effects in men; see also notes above

Dose: breast cancer, 10–20 mg daily
Prostate cancer, 1–3 mg daily

Diethylstilbestrol (Non-proprietary) PoM
Tablets, diethylstilbestrol 1 mg, net price 28 = £26.40; 5 mg, 28 = £36.64
Available from APS (*Apstil®*)

ETHINYLESTRADIOL

(Ethinyloestradiol)

Indications: see notes above; other indications (section 6.4.1.1)

Cautions: see under Diethylstilbestrol and notes above; **interactions:** Appendix 1 (oestrogens)

Side-effects: see under Diethylstilbestrol and notes above

Dose: breast cancer [unlicensed indication], 1–3 mg daily

■ Preparations
Section 6.4.1.1

8.3.2   Progestogens

Progestogens have a role in the treatment of endometrial cancer; their use in breast cancer and renal cell cancer has declined. Progestogens are now rarely used to treat prostate cancer. **Medroxyprogesterone** or **megestrol** are usually chosen and can be given orally; high-dose or parenteral treatment cannot be recommended. Side-effects are mild but may include nausea, fluid retention, and weight gain.

GESTONORONE CAPROATE

(Gestronol Hexanoate)

Indications: see notes above; benign prostatic hypertrophy

Cautions: see section 6.4.1.2 and notes above; **interactions:** Appendix 1 (gestonorone)

Contra-indications: see section 6.4.1.2 and notes above

Side-effects: see section 6.4.1.2 and notes above

Dose: endometrial cancer, *by intramuscular injection*, 200–400 mg every 5–7 days
Benign prostatic hypertrophy, *by intramuscular injection*, 200 mg every week, increased to 300–400 mg every week if necessary

Gestonorone Caproate (Non-proprietary) PoM
Injection (oily), gestonorone caproate 100 mg/mL. Net price 2-mL amp = £12.50
Available from Cambridge

MEDROXYPROGESTERONE ACETATE

Indications: see notes above; contraception (section 7.3.2.2); other indications (section 6.4.1.2)

Cautions: see section 6.4.1.2 and notes above; **interactions:** Appendix 1 (progestogens)

Contra-indications: see section 6.4.1.2 and notes above

Side-effects: see section 6.4.1.2 and notes above; glucocorticoid effects at high dose may lead to a cushingoid syndrome

Dose: see preparations below

Farlutal® and *Provera®* tablets may **not** be bioequivalent

Farlutal® (Pharmacia) PoM
Tablets, both scored, medroxyprogesterone acetate 100 mg, net price 100-tab pack = £48.70; 250 mg, 50 = £60.88
Tablets, scored, medroxyprogesterone acetate 500 mg. Net price 56 = £136.36. Label: 27
Injection, medroxyprogesterone acetate 200 mg/mL. Net price 2.5-mL vial = £13.26
Dose: by mouth, breast cancer, 1–1.5 g daily, up to 2 g daily has been used; other hormone-dependent cancers, 100–500 mg daily
By deep intramuscular injection into the gluteal muscle, breast carcinoma, initially 0.5–1 g daily for 4 weeks; maintenance, 500 mg twice a week
Endometrial carcinoma, initially 500 mg twice weekly for 3 months; maintenance, 500 mg once weekly
Renal adenocarcinoma, initially 500 mg on alternate days for 30 days; maintenance, 500 mg twice weekly until day 60, then 250 mg once weekly
Prostatic adenocarcinoma, initially 500 mg twice weekly; maintenance, 500 mg once weekly

Provera® (Pharmacia) PoM
Tablets, medroxyprogesterone acetate 100 mg (scored), net price 60-tab pack = £29.98, 100-tab pack = £49.94; 200 mg (scored), 30-tab pack = £29.65, 100-tab pack = £98.82; 400 mg, 30-tab pack = £58.67
Dose: endometrial and renal cell cancer, 200–400 mg daily; breast cancer, 400–800 mg daily
Tablets, medroxyprogesterone acetate 2.5 mg, 5 mg and 10 mg, see section 6.4.1.2

MEGESTROL ACETATE

Indications: see notes above

Cautions: see under Medroxyprogesterone acetate (section 6.4.1.2) and notes above; **interactions:** Appendix 1 (progestogens)

Contra-indications: see under Medroxyprogesterone acetate (section 6.4.1.2) and notes above

Side-effects: see under Medroxyprogesterone acetate (section 6.4.1.2) and notes above

Dose: breast cancer, 160 mg daily in single or divided doses; endometrial cancer, 40–320 mg daily in divided doses

Megace® (Bristol-Myers Squibb) PoM
Tablets, both scored, megestrol acetate 40 mg, net price 20 = £5.08; 160 mg (off-white), 30-tab pack = £29.30

NORETHISTERONE

Indications: see notes above; other indications (section 6.4.1.2)

Cautions: see section 6.4.1.2 and notes above; **interactions:** Appendix 1 (progestogens)

Contra-indications: see section 6.4.1.2 and notes above

Side-effects: see section 6.4.1.2 and notes above

Dose: breast cancer, 40 mg daily, increased to 60 mg daily if required

■ Preparations
Section 6.4.1.2

8.3.3   Androgens

Testosterone esters (section 6.4.2) have largely been superseded by other drugs for breast cancer.

8.3.4   Hormone antagonists

8.3.4.1   Breast cancer

The management of patients with breast cancer involves surgery, radiotherapy, drug therapy, or a combination of these.

EARLY BREAST CANCER. All women should be considered for adjuvant therapy following surgical removal of the tumour. Adjuvant therapy is used to eradicate the micrometastases that cause relapses. Choice of adjuvant treatment is determined by the risk of recurrence, oestrogen-receptor status of the primary tumour, and menopausal status.

Tamoxifen is an oestrogen-receptor antagonist and is the adjuvant hormonal treatment of choice in all women with oestrogen-receptor-positive breast cancer; it is supplemented in selected cases by cytotoxic chemotherapy. Premenopausal women may also benefit from treatment with a gonadorelin analogue or ovarian ablation.

Treatment with tamoxifen delays the growth of metastases and increases survival; if tolerated it should be continued for 5 years. Tamoxifen also reduces risk of developing cancer in the other breast.

Anastrozole is licensed for the adjuvant treatment of oestrogen-receptor-positive early breast cancer in postmenopausal women who are unable to take tamoxifen therapy because of high risk of thromboembolism or endometrial abnormalities.

Cytotoxic chemotherapy is preferred for both premenopausal and postmenopausal women with oestrogen-receptor-negative breast cancer.

ADVANCED BREAST CANCER. Tamoxifen is used in postmenopausal women with oestrogen-receptor-positive tumours, long disease-free interval following treatment for early breast cancer, and disease limited to bone or soft tissues. However, aromatase inhibitors, such as anastrozole or letrozole, may be more effective and are regarded as preferred treatment in postmenopausal women. Ovarian ablation or a gonadorelin analogue (section 8.3.4.2) should be considered in premenopausal women.

Progestogens such as medroxyprogesterone acetate continue to have a role in postmenopausal women with advanced breast cancer. They are as effective as tamoxifen, but they are not as well tolerated; they are less effective than the aromatase inhibitors.

Cytotoxic chemotherapy is preferred for advanced oestrogen-receptor-negative tumours and for aggressive disease, particularly where metastases involve visceral sites (e.g. the liver) or where the disease-free interval following treatment for early breast cancer is short.

CHEMOPREVENTION. Recent evidence suggests that tamoxifen prophylaxis can reduce breast cancer in women at high risk of the disease. However, the adverse effects of tamoxifen preclude its routine use in most women.

CYTOTOXIC DRUGS USED IN BREAST CANCER. The most common cytotoxic chemotherapy regimen for both adjuvant use and metastatic disease has been cyclophosphamide (section 8.1.1), methotrexate and fluorouracil (both section 8.1.3). However, anthracycline-containing regimens are now increasingly used and should be regarded as standard therapy unless contra-indicated (e.g. in cardiac disease).

Metastatic disease. The choice of chemotherapy regimen will be influenced by whether the patient has previously received adjuvant treatment and the presence of any co-morbidity.

For women who have not previously received chemotherapy, *either* cyclophosphamide, methotrexate and fluorouracil *or* an anthracycline-containing regimen is the standard initial therapy for metastatic breast disease.

Patients with anthracycline-refractory or resistant disease should be considered for treatment with a taxane (section 8.1.5) either alone or in combination with trastuzumab if they have tumours that overexpress HER2 (human epidermal growth factor-2). Other cytotoxic drugs with activity against breast cancer include capecitabine (section 8.1.3), mitoxantrone, mitomycin (both section 8.1.2), and vinorelbine (section 8.1.4). In cancers that overexpress HER2, trastuzumab (section 8.1.5) is an option for chemotherapy-resistant disease.

OESTROGEN-RECEPTOR ANTAGONISTS. **Tamoxifen** is an oestrogen-receptor antagonist that is licensed for breast and anovulatory infertility (section 6.5.1).

Toremifene is licensed for hormone-dependent metastatic breast cancer in postmenopausal women, but it is not often used.

AROMATASE INHIBITORS. Aromatase inhibitors act predominantly by blocking the conversion of androgens to oestrogens in the peripheral tissues. They do not inhibit ovarian oestrogen synthesis and should not be used in premenopausal women.

Anastrozole and **letrozole** are non-steroidal aromatase inhibitors; **exemestane** is a steroidal aromatase inhibitor. Anastrozole and letrozole are at least as effective as tamoxifen for first-line treatment of metastatic breast cancer in postmenopausal women. However, it is not yet known whether the benefits of aromatase inhibitors persist over the long term.

Aminoglutethimide has largely been replaced by the newer, more selective aromatase inhibitors, which are better tolerated. Aminoglutethimide causes adrenal hypofunction and corticosteroid replacement therapy is needed.

GONADORELIN ANALOGUES. **Goserelin** (section 8.3.4.2), a gonadorelin analogue is licensed for the management of advanced breast cancer in premenopausal women.

OTHER DRUGS USED IN BREAST CANCER. **Trilostane** (section 6.7.3) is licensed for postmenopausal breast cancer. It is quite well tolerated but diarrhoea and abdominal discomfort may be a problem. Trilostane causes adrenal hypofunction and corticosteroid replacement therapy is needed.

The use of **bisphosphonates** (section 6.6.2) in patients with metastatic breast cancer may prevent skeletal complications of bone metastases.

TAMOXIFEN

Indications: see under Dose and notes above; mastalgia [unlicensed indication] (section 6.7.2)

Cautions: occasional cystic ovarian swellings in premenopausal women, occasional hypercalcaemia if bony metastases; increased risk of thromboembolic events when used with cytotoxics (see also below); breast-feeding (Appendix 5); endometrial changes (**important:** see below); porphyria (section 9.8.2); **interactions:** Appendix 1 (tamoxifen)

ENDOMETRIAL CHANGES. Increased endometrial changes, including hyperplasia, polyps, cancer, and uterine sarcoma reported; prompt investigation required if abnormal vaginal bleeding including menstrual irregularities, vaginal discharge, and pelvic pain or pressure in those receiving (or who have received) tamoxifen.

Contra-indications: pregnancy (exclude before commencing and advise non-hormonal contraception if appropriate—Appendix 4)

Side-effects: hot flushes, vaginal bleeding and vaginal discharge (**important:** see also Endometrial Changes under Cautions), suppression of menstruation in some premenopausal women, pruritus vulvae, gastro-intestinal disturbances, headache, light-headedness, tumour flare, decreased platelet counts; occasionally oedema, alopecia, rashes, uterine fibroids; also visual disturbances (including corneal changes, cataracts, retinopathy); leucopenia (sometimes with anaemia and thrombocytopenia, rarely neutropenia; hypertriglyceridaemia reported (sometimes with pancreatitis); thromboembolic events reported (see below); liver enzyme changes (rarely fatty liver, cholestasis, hepatitis); rarely interstitial pneumonitis, hypersensitivity reactions including angioedema, Stevens-Johnson syndrome, bullous pemphigoid; see also notes above

RISK OF THROMBOEMBOLISM. Tamoxifen can increase the risk of thromboembolism particularly during and immediately after major surgery or periods of immobility. Patients should be made aware of the symptoms of thromboembolism and advised to report sudden breathlessness and any pain in the calf of one leg

Dose: breast cancer, 20 mg daily

CSM ADVICE. The CSM has advised that tamoxifen in a dose of 20 mg daily substantially increases survival in early breast cancer, and that no further benefit has been demonstrated with higher doses. Patients should be told of the small risk of endometrial cancer (see under Cautions above) and encouraged to report relevant symptoms early. They can, however, be reassured that the benefits of treatment far outweigh the risks

Anovulatory infertility, 20 mg daily on days 2, 3, 4 and 5 of cycle; if necessary the daily dose may be increased to 40 mg then 80 mg for subsequent courses; if cycles irregular, start initial course on any day, with subsequent course starting 45 days later *or* on day 2 of cycle if menstruation occurs

Tamoxifen (Non-proprietary) PoM
Tablets, tamoxifen (as citrate) 10 mg, net price 30-tab pack = £1.97; 20 mg, 30-tab pack = £2.24; 40 mg, 30-tab pack = £8.42
Available from Alpharma, APS, CP, Hillcross, IVAX, Kent
Oral solution, tamoxifen (as citrate) 10 mg/5 mL, net price 150 mL = £31.50
Available from Rosemont (*Soltamox*®)

Nolvadex® (AstraZeneca) PoM
Tablets, tamoxifen (as citrate) 10 mg, net price 30-tab pack = £5.78; 20 mg (*Nolvadex-D*®), 30-tab pack = £8.71

AMINOGLUTETHIMIDE

Indications: see notes above and under Dose

Cautions: see notes above; adrenal hypofunction (see below); monitor blood pressure, plasma electrolytes, blood counts, and thyroid function; **interactions:** Appendix 1 (aminoglutethimide)

ADRENAL HYPOFUNCTION. May cause adrenal hypofunction especially under conditions of stress (such as surgery, trauma, or acute illness), therefore corticosteroid replacement therapy is necessary (section 6.3.1). If a synthetic glucocorticoid such as dexamethasone is used instead of hydrocortisone a relatively high dose may be needed (metabolism of synthetic corticosteroids accelerated)

Contra-indications: pregnancy (advise non-hormonal contraceptive methods if appropriate) and breast-feeding; porphyria (section 9.8.2)

Side-effects: see notes above; drowsiness, lethargy, rash (sometimes with fever—usually in first 2 weeks and resolves despite continued administration); occasionally dizziness, nausea; other side-effects reported include ataxia, headache, depression, insomnia, pruritus, urticaria, diarrhoea, vomiting, constipation, anorexia, sweating, hypotension, adrenal insufficiency, hyponatraemia, hypoglycaemia, agranulocytosis, leucopenia, thrombocytopenia, hyperkalaemia, exfoliative dermatitis, Stevens-Johnson syndrome, hypothyroidism, inappropriate ADH-secretion, masculinisation and hirsutism in females, renal impairment, pancytopenia, allergy, anaphylactic reactions, allergic alveolitis (withdraw immediately if suspected), cholestatic hepatitis, confusion

Dose: advanced breast or prostate cancer, 250 mg daily, increased once a week to max. 250 mg 4 times daily (in breast cancer 250 mg twice daily has proved sufficient in some patients; in prostate cancer up to 750 mg daily is usually satisfactory); given with a glucocorticoid (and sometimes with a mineralocorticoid as well)

Cushing's syndrome due to malignant disease, 250 mg daily, increased gradually to 1 g daily in divided doses (occasionally 1.5–2 g daily); glucocorticoid given only if necessary

Orimeten® (Novartis) PoM
Tablets, scored, aminoglutethimide 250 mg. Net price 56-tab pack = £24.27. Label: 2

ANASTROZOLE

Indications: adjuvant treatment of oestrogen-receptor-positive early breast cancer in postmenopausal women who are unable to take tamoxifen because of high risk of thromboembolism or endometrial abnormalities; advanced breast cancer in postmenopausal women

Cautions: laboratory test for menopause if doubt; susceptibility to osteoporosis (assess bone mineral density before treatment and at regular intervals)

Contra-indications: pregnancy and breast-feeding; moderate or severe hepatic disease, moderate or severe renal impairment; not for premenopausal women

Side-effects: hot flushes, vaginal dryness, vaginal bleeding, hair thinning, anorexia, nausea, vomiting, diarrhoea, headache, arthralgia, bone fractures, rash (including Stevens-Johnson syndrome); asthenia and drowsiness—may initially affect ability to drive or operate machinery; slight increases in total cholesterol levels reported; very rarely allergic reactions including angioedema and anaphylaxis

Dose: 1 mg daily; for early disease, recommended duration 5 years

Arimidex® (AstraZeneca) PoM
Tablets, f/c, anastrozole 1 mg. Net price 28-tab pack = £83.16

EXEMESTANE

Indications: advanced breast cancer in postmenopausal women in whom anti-oestrogen therapy has failed

Cautions: hepatic and renal impairment

Contra-indications: pregnancy and breast-feeding; not indicated for premenopausal women

Side-effects: hot flushes, nausea, dizziness, fatigue, sweating; less frequently vomiting, dyspepsia, constipation, abdominal pain, anorexia, peripheral oedema, headache, depression, insomnia, alopecia, rash; rarely thrombocytopenia, leucopenia

Dose: 25 mg daily

Aromasin® (Pharmacia) ▼ PoM
Tablets, s/c, exemestane 25 mg, net price 15-tab pack = £44.40, 30-tab pack = £88.80, 90-tab pack = £266.40. Label: 21

LETROZOLE

Indications: advanced breast cancer in postmenopausal women; pre-operative treatment in postmenopausal women with localised hormone-receptor-positive breast cancer to allow subsequent breast conserving surgery

Cautions: severe renal impairment

Contra-indications: severe hepatic impairment; not indicated for premenopausal women; pregnancy and breast-feeding

Side-effects: hot flushes, nausea, vomiting, fatigue, dizziness, headache, dyspepsia, constipation, diarrhoea, anorexia, appetite increase, alopecia, increased sweating, rash, peripheral oedema, musculoskeletal pain; less frequently hypertension, palpitations, tachycardia, dyspnoea, drowsiness, insomnia, depression, anxiety, memory impairment, dysaesthesia, taste disturbance, pruritus, dry skin, urticaria, thrombophlebitis, abdominal pain, urinary frequency, urinary-tract infection, vaginal bleeding, vaginal discharge, breast pain, pyrexia, mucosal dryness, stomatitis, cataract, eye irritation, tumour pain, leucopenia, hypercholesterolaemia, general oedema; rarely pulmonary embolism, arterial thrombosis, cerebrovascular infarction

Dose: 2.5 mg daily; discontinue if tumour progression occurs

Femara® (Novartis) PoM
Tablets, f/c, letrozole 2.5 mg. Net price 14-tab pack = £41.58, 28-tab pack = £83.16

TOREMIFENE

Indications: hormone-dependent metastatic breast cancer in postmenopausal women

Cautions: hypercalcaemia may occur (especially if bone metastases and usually at beginning of treatment); **interactions:** Appendix 1 (toremifene) ENDOMETRIAL CHANGES. There is a risk of increased endometrial changes including hyperplasia, polyps and cancer. Abnormal vaginal bleeding including menstrual irregularities, vaginal discharge and symptoms such as pelvic pain or pressure should be promptly investigated

Contra-indications: endometrial hyperplasia, severe hepatic impairment, history of severe thromboembolic disease; pregnancy and breast-feeding

Side-effects: hot flushes, vaginal bleeding or discharge (**important:** see also Cautions), dizziness, oedema, sweating, nausea, vomiting, chest or back pain, fatigue, headache, skin discoloration, weight increase, insomnia, constipation, dyspnoea, paresis, tremor, vertigo, pruritus, anorexia, corneal opacity (reversible), asthenia; thromboembolic events reported; rarely dermatitis, alopecia, emotional lability, depression, jaundice, stiffness

Dose: 60 mg daily

Fareston® (Orion) PoM
Tablets, toremifene (as citrate) 60 mg. Net price 30-tab pack = £30.37

8.3.4.2 Prostate cancer and gonadorelin analogues

Metastatic cancer of the prostate usually responds to hormonal treatment aimed at androgen depletion. Standard treatments include bilateral subcapsular orchidectomy or use of a gonadorelin analogue (**buserelin**, **goserelin**, **leuprorelin**, or **triptorelin**). Response in most patients lasts for 12 to 18 months. No entirely satisfactory therapy exists for disease progression despite this treatment (hormone-refractory prostate cancer), but occasional patients respond to other hormone manipulation e.g. with an anti-androgen. Bone disease can often be palliated with irradiation or, if widespread, with strontium, aminoglutethimide (section 8.3.4.1), or prednisolone (section 6.3.2).

Gonadorelin analogues

Gonadorelin analogues are as effective as orchidectomy or **diethylstilbestrol** (section 8.3.1) but are expensive and require parenteral administration, at least initially. They cause initial stimulation then depression of luteinising hormone release by the pituitary. During the initial stage (1–2 weeks) increased production of testosterone may be associated with progression of prostate cancer. In susceptible patients this tumour 'flare' may cause spinal cord compression, ureteric obstruction or increased bone pain. When such problems are anticipated, alternative treatments (e.g. orchidectomy) or concomitant use of an anti-androgen such as cyproterone acetate or flutamide (see below) are recommended; anti-androgen treatment should be started 3 days before the gonadorelin analogue and continued for 3 weeks. Gonadorelin analogues are also used in women for breast cancer (section 8.3.4.1) and other indications (section 6.7.2).

CAUTIONS. Men at risk of tumour 'flare' (see above) should be monitored closely during the first month of therapy. Caution is required in women with metabolic bone disease because decreases in bone mineral density may occur. The injection site should be rotated.

SIDE-EFFECTS. The gonadorelin analogues cause side-effects similar to the menopause in women and orchidectomy in men and include hot flushes and sweating, sexual dysfunction, vaginal dryness or bleeding, and gynaecomastia or changes in breast size. Signs and symptoms of prostate or breast cancer may worsen initially (managed in prostate cancer with anti-androgens, see above). Other side-effects include hypersensitivity reactions (rashes, pruritus, asthma, and rarely anaphylaxis); injection site reactions (see Cautions), headache (rarely migraine), visual disturbances, dizziness, arthralgia and possibly myalgia, hair loss, peripheral oedema, gastrointestinal disturbances, weight changes, sleep disorders, and mood changes.

Anti-androgens

Cyproterone acetate, **flutamide** and **bicalutamide** are anti-androgens that inhibit the tumour 'flare' which may occur after commencing gonadorelin analogue administration. Cyproterone acetate and flutamide are also licensed for use alone in patients with metastatic prostate cancer refractory to gonadorelin analogue therapy. Bicalutamide is used for prostate cancer either alone or as an adjunct to other therapy, according to the clinical circumstances.

BICALUTAMIDE

Indications: advanced prostate cancer in combination with a gonadorelin analogue or surgical castration; locally advanced prostate cancer either alone or as adjuvant treatment

Cautions: hepatic impairment (Appendix 2), also consider periodic liver function tests; **interactions:** Appendix 1 (bicalutamide)

Side-effects: nausea, vomiting, diarrhoea, asthenia, gynaecomastia, breast tenderness, hot flushes, pruritus, dry skin, alopecia, hirsutism, decreased libido, impotence, weight gain; rarely abdominal pain, cardiovascular disorders (including angina, heart failure and arrhythmias), depression, dyspepsia, haematuria, cholestasis, jaundice, thrombocytopenia

Dose: advanced prostate cancer, with orchidectomy or gonadorelin therapy, 50 mg daily (in gonadorelin therapy, started 3 days beforehand, see also notes above)
Locally advanced prostate cancer, 150 mg once daily
NOTE. The CSM has advised (October 2003) that bicalutamide should no longer be used for the treatment of localised prostate cancer

Casodex® (AstraZeneca) [PoM]
Tablets, f/c, bicalutamide 50 mg, net price 28-tab pack = £128.00; 150 mg, 28-tab pack = £240.00

BUSERELIN

Indications: advanced prostate cancer; other indications (section 6.7.2)

Cautions: depression, see also notes above

Side-effects: see notes above; worsening hypertension, palpitations, glucose intolerance, altered blood lipids, thrombocytopenia, leucopenia, nervousness, fatigue, memory and concentration disturbances, anxiety, increased thirst, hearing disorders, musculoskeletal pain; nasal irritation, nose bleeds and altered sense of taste and smell (spray formulation only)

Dose: *by subcutaneous injection*, 500 micrograms every 8 hours for 7 days, then *intranasally*, 1 spray into each nostril 6 times daily (see also notes above)
COUNSELLING. Avoid use of nasal decongestants before and for at least 30 minutes after treatment.

Suprefact® (Aventis Pharma) [PoM]
Injection, buserelin (as acetate) 1 mg/mL. Net price 2 × 5.5-mL vial = £23.69
Nasal spray, buserelin (as acetate) 100 micrograms/metered spray. Net price treatment pack of 4 × 10-g bottle with spray pump = £87.68. Counselling, see above

CYPROTERONE ACETATE

Indications: prostate cancer, see under Dose and also notes above; other indications, see section 6.4.2

Cautions: in prostate cancer, blood counts initially and throughout treatment, hepatic impairment (Appendix 2); monitor hepatic function (liver function tests should be performed before treatment, see also under Side-effects below); monitor adrenocortical function regularly; risk of recurrence of thromboembolic disease; diabetes mellitus, sickle-cell anaemia, severe depression (in other indications some of these are contra-indicated, see section 6.4.2)
DRIVING. Fatigue and lassitude may impair performance of skilled tasks (e.g. driving).

Contra-indications: none in prostate cancer; for contra-indications relating to other indications see section 6.4.2

Side-effects: see section 6.4.2
HEPATOTOXICITY. Direct hepatic toxicity including jaundice, hepatitis and hepatic failure have been reported (usually after several months) in patients treated with cyproterone acetate 200–300 mg daily. Liver function tests should be performed before treatment and whenever symptoms suggestive of hepatotoxicity occur—if confirmed cyproterone should normally be withdrawn unless the hepatotoxicity can be explained by another cause such as metastatic disease (in which case cyproterone should be continued only if the perceived benefit exceeds the risk)

Dose: flare with initial gonadorelin therapy, 300 mg daily in 2–3 divided doses, reduced to 200 mg daily in 2–3 divided doses if necesssary
Long-term palliative therapy where gonadorelin analogues or orchidectomy contra-indicated, not tolerated, or where oral therapy preferred, 200–300 mg daily in 2–3 divided doses
Hot flushes with gonadorelin therapy or after orchidectomy, initially 50 mg daily, adjusted according to response to 50–150 mg daily in 1–3 divided doses

Cyproterone Acetate (Non-proprietary) [PoM]
Tablets, cyproterone acetate 50 mg, net price 56-tab pack = £31.54; 100 mg, 84-tab pack = £91.39. Label: 21
Available from Generics

Cyprostat® (Schering Health) [PoM]
Tablets, scored, cyproterone acetate 50 mg, net price 168-tab pack = £91.39; 100 mg, 84-tab pack = £91.39. Label: 21

FLUTAMIDE

Indications: advanced prostate cancer, see also notes above

Cautions: cardiac disease (oedema reported); hepatic impairment (Appendix 2), also liver function tests, monthly for first 4 months, periodically thereafter and at the first sign or symptom of liver disorder (e.g. pruritus, dark urine, persistent anorexia, jaundice, abdominal pain, unexplained influenza-like symptoms); avoid excessive alcohol consumption; **interactions:** Appendix 1 (flutamide)

Side-effects: gynaecomastia (sometimes with galactorrhoea); nausea, vomiting, diarrhoea, increased appetite, insomnia, tiredness; other side-effects reported include decreased libido, reduced sperm count, gastric and chest pain, headache, dizziness, oedema, blurred vision, thirst, rash, pruritus, haemolytic anaemia, systemic lupus erythematosus-like syndrome, and lymphoedema; hepatic injury (with transaminase abnormalities, cholestatic jaundice, hepatic necrosis, hepatic encephalopathy and occasional fatality) reported

Dose: 250 mg 3 times daily (see also notes above)

Flutamide (Non-proprietary) [PoM]
Tablets, flutamide 250 mg. Net price 84-tab pack = £66.63
Available from Alpharma, Chiron (*Chimax®*), Generics, Hillcross, Tillomed

Drogenil® (Schering-Plough) [PoM]
Tablets, yellow, scored, flutamide 250 mg, net price 84-tab pack = £70.00

GOSERELIN

Indications: prostate cancer; advanced breast cancer; oestrogen-receptor positive early breast cancer (section 8.3.4.1); other indications (section 6.7.2)

Cautions: see notes above; breast-feeding (Appendix 5)

Contra-indications: pregnancy (Appendix 4); undiagnosed vaginal bleeding

Side-effects: see notes above; also transient changes in blood pressure, paraesthesia, rarely hypercalcaemia (in patients with metastatic breast cancer)

Dose: see under preparations below

Zoladex® (AstraZeneca) [PoM]
Implant, goserelin 3.6 mg (as acetate) in syringe applicator. Net price each = £122.27
Dose: breast cancer and prostate cancer *by subcutaneous injection* into anterior abdominal wall, 3.6 mg every 28 days (see also notes above)

Zoladex® LA (AstraZeneca) [PoM]
Implant, goserelin 10.8 mg (as acetate) in syringe applicator. Net price each = £366.81
Dose: prostate cancer, *by subcutaneous injection* into anterior abdominal wall, 10.8 mg every 12 weeks (see also notes above)

LEUPRORELIN ACETATE

Indications: advanced prostate cancer; other indications (section 6.7.2)

Cautions: see notes above and section 6.7.2

Side-effects: see notes above and section 6.7.2; also fatigue, muscle weakness, paraesthesia, hypertension, palpitations, alteration of glucose tolerance and of blood lipids; thrombocytopenia and leucopenia reported

Dose: see under preparations below

Prostap® SR (Wyeth) [PoM]
Injection (microsphere powder for reconstitution), leuprorelin acetate, net price 3.75-mg vial with 1-mL vehicle-filled syringe = £125.40
Dose: advanced prostate cancer , *by subcutaneous or by intramuscular injection*, 3.75 mg every 4 weeks (see also notes above)

Prostap® 3 (Wyeth) [PoM]
Injection (microsphere powder for reconstitution), leuprorelin acetate, net price 11.25-mg vial with 2-mL vehicle-filled syringe = £376.20
Dose: advanced prostate cancer, *by subcutaneous injection*, 11.25 mg every three months (see also notes above)

TRIPTORELIN

Indications: advanced prostate cancer; endometriosis (section 6.7.2)

Cautions: see notes above

Side-effects: see notes above; transient hypertension, dry mouth, excessive salivation, paraesthesia, increased dysuria

Dose: *by intramuscular injection*, 3 mg every 4 weeks (see also notes above)

De-capeptyl® sr (Ipsen) [PoM]
Injection (copolymer microsphere powder for aqueous suspension), triptorelin. Net price 4.2-mg vial (with diluent) = £105.05
NOTE. Each 4.2-mg vial includes an overage to allow administration of a 3-mg dose

8.3.4.3 Somatostatin analogues

Octreotide and **lanreotide** are analogues of the hypothalamic release-inhibiting hormone somatostatin. They are indicated for the relief of symptoms associated with neuroendocrine (particularly carcinoid) tumours and acromegaly. Additionally, lanreotide is licensed for the treatment of thyroid tumours and octreotide is also licensed for the prevention of complications following pancreatic surgery; octreotide may also be valuable in reducing vomiting in palliative care (see p. 15) and in stopping variceal bleeding [unlicensed indication]—see also vasopressin and terlipressin (section 6.5.2).

CAUTIONS. Growth hormone-secreting pituitary tumours can expand causing serious complications; during treatment with somatostatin analogues patients should be monitored for signs of tumour expansion (e.g. visual field defects). Ultrasound examination of the gallbladder is recommended before treatment and at intervals of 6–12 months during treatment (avoid abrupt withdrawal of short-acting octreotide—see Side-effects below). In insulinoma an increase in the depth and duration of hypoglycaemia may occur (observe patients when initiating treatment and changing doses); in diabetes mellitus, insulin or oral antidiabetic requirements may be reduced.

SIDE-EFFECTS. Gastro-intestinal disturbances including anorexia, nausea, vomiting, abdominal pain and bloating, flatulence, diarrhoea, and steatorrhoea may occur. Postprandial glucose tolerance may be impaired and rarely persistent hyperglycaemia occurs with chronic administration; hypoglycaemia has also been reported. Gallstones have been reported after long-term treatment (abrupt withdrawal of subcutaneous octreotide is associated with biliary colic and pancreatitis). Pain and irritation may occur at the injection site and sites should be rotated. Rarely, pancreatitis has been reported shortly after administration.

OCTREOTIDE

Indications: see under Dose

Cautions: see notes above; hepatic impairment; pregnancy and breast-feeding (Appendixes 4 and 5); monitor thyroid function on long-term therapy; **interactions:** Appendix 1 (octreotide)

Side-effects: see notes above; rarely altered liver function tests, hepatitis and transient alopecia

Dose: symptoms associated with carcinoid tumours with features of carcinoid syndrome, VIPomas, glucagonomas, *by subcutaneous injection*, initially 50 micrograms once or twice daily, gradually increased according to response to 200 micrograms 3 times daily (higher doses required exceptionally); maintenance doses variable; in carcinoid tumours discontinue after 1 week if no effect; if rapid response required, initial dose *by intravenous injection* (with ECG monitoring and after dilution to a concentration of 10–50% with sodium chloride 0.9% injection)

Acromegaly, short-term treatment before pituitary surgery *or* long-term treatment in those inadequately controlled by other treatment *or* until radiotherapy becomes fully effective *by subcutaneous injection*, 100–200 micrograms 3 times daily; discontinue if no improvement within 3 months

Prevention of complications following pancreatic surgery, consult product literature

Sandostatin® (Novartis) PoM
Injection, octreotide (as acetate) 50 micrograms/ mL, net price 1-mL amp = £3.47; 100 micrograms/ mL, 1-mL amp = £6.53; 200 micrograms/mL 5-mL vial = £65.10; 500 micrograms/mL, 1-mL amp = £31.65

■ Depot preparation

Sandostatin LAR® (Novartis) PoM
Injection (microsphere powder for aqueous suspension), octreotide (as acetate) 10-mg vial = £637.50; 20-mg vial = £850.00; 30-mg vial = £1062.50 (all supplied with 2.5-mL diluent-filled syringe)
Dose: acromegaly and neuroendocrine tumours in patients adequately controlled on subcutaneous octreotide, *by deep intramuscular injection* (into the gluteal muscle), initially 20 mg every 4 weeks for 3 months, then adjusted according to symptoms and laboratory tests; max. 30 mg every 4 weeks
For acromegaly, start depot octreotide 1 day after the last dose of subcutaneous octreotide; for neuroendocrine tumours, continue subcutaneous octreotide for 2 weeks after first dose of depot octreotide

LANREOTIDE

Indications: see notes above

Cautions: see notes above; pregnancy and breast-feeding (Appendixes 4 and 5); **interactions:** Appendix 1 (lanreotide)

Side-effects: see notes above; also reported asthenia, fatigue, raised bilirubin; less commonly skin nodule, hot flushes, leg pain, malaise, headache, tenesmus, decreased libido, drowsiness, pruritus, increased sweating; rarely hypothyroidism (monitor as necessary)

Dose: see under preparations

Somatuline® **LA** (Ipsen) PoM
Injection (copolymer microparticles for aqueous suspension), lanreotide (as acetate) 30-mg vial (with vehicle) = £334.25
Dose: by intramuscular injection, acromegaly and neuroendocrine (particularly carcinoid) tumours, initially 30 mg every 14 days, frequency increased to every 7–10 days according to response
Thyroid tumours, 30 mg every 14 days, frequency increased to every 10 days according to response

Somatuline Autogel® (Ipsen)
Injection, prefilled syringe, lanreotide (as acetate) 60 mg = £542.00; 90 mg = £722.00; 120 mg = £932.00
Dose: by deep subcutaneous injection into the gluteal region, acromegaly (if somatostatin analogue not given previously), initially 60 mg every 28 days, adjusted according to response; for patients treated previously with somatostatin analogue, consult product literature for initial dose
Neuroendocrine (particularly carcinoid) tumours, initially 60–120 mg every 28 days, adjusted according to response

9: Nutrition and blood

9.1 Anaemias and some other blood disorders

Before initiating treatment for anaemia it is essential to determine which type is present. Iron salts may be harmful and result in iron overload if given alone to patients with anaemias other than those due to iron deficiency.

9.1.1 Iron-deficiency anaemias

Treatment with an iron preparation is justified only in the presence of a demonstrable iron-deficiency state. Before starting treatment, it is important to exclude any serious underlying cause of the anaemia (e.g. gastric erosion, gastro-intestinal cancer).

Prophylaxis with an iron preparation is justifiable in individuals who have additional risk factors for iron deficiency (e.g. poor diet). Prophylaxis may also be appropriate in malabsorption, menorrhagia, pregnancy, after subtotal or total gastrectomy, and in the management of low birth-weight infants such as premature babies, twins, and in infants delivered by caesarean section.

9.1.1.1 Oral iron

Iron salts should be given by mouth unless there are good reasons for using another route.

Ferrous salts show only marginal differences between one another in efficiency of absorption of iron, but ferric salts are much less well absorbed. Haemoglobin regeneration rate is little affected by the type of salt used provided sufficient iron is given, and in most patients the speed of response is not critical. Choice of preparation is thus usually decided by incidence of side-effects and cost.

The oral dose of elemental iron for deficiency should be 100 to 200 mg daily. It is customary to give this as dried **ferrous sulphate**, 200 mg ($\equiv$ 65 mg elemental iron) three times daily; a dose of ferrous sulphate 200 mg once or twice daily may be effective for prophylaxis or for mild iron deficiency. Ferrous sulphate 200–300 mg 3 times daily may be required to produce an optimum response to epoetin in iron-deficient patients with chronic renal failure.

Iron content of different iron salts

Iron salt	Amount	Content of ferrous iron
Ferrous fumarate	200 mg	65 mg
Ferrous gluconate	300 mg	35 mg
Ferrous succinate	100 mg	35 mg
Ferrous sulphate	300 mg	60 mg
Ferrous sulphate, dried	200 mg	65 mg

THERAPEUTIC RESPONSE. The haemoglobin concentration should rise by about 100–200 mg/100 mL (1–2 g/litre) per day or 2 g/100 mL (20 g/litre) over 3–4 weeks. When the haemoglobin is in the normal range, treatment should be continued for a further 3 months to replenish the iron stores. Epithelial tissue changes such as atrophic glossitis and koilonychia are usually improved, but the response is often slow.

COMPOUND PREPARATIONS. Some oral preparations contain ascorbic acid to aid absorption of the iron but the therapeutic advantage of such preparations is minimal and cost may be increased..

There is no justification for the inclusion of other ingredients, such as the B group of vitamins (except folic acid for pregnant women, see Iron and Folic Acid, p. 440 and on p. 442).

MODIFIED-RELEASE PREPARATIONS. Modified-release preparations are designed to release iron gradually so that a smaller amount of iron is present in the gastro-intestinal tract at any one time. These preparations are licensed for once-daily dosage.

However, modified-release preparations are likely to carry the iron past the first part of the duodenum into an area of the gut where iron absorption may be poor. The low incidence of side-effects may reflect the small amounts of iron available for absorption under these conditions and so the preparations have no therapeutic advantage and should not be used.

SIDE-EFFECTS. Gastro-intestinal irritation may occur with iron salts. Nausea and epigastric pain are dose-related but the relationship between dose and altered bowel habit (constipation or diarrhoea) is less clear. Oral iron, particularly modified-release preparations, may exacerbate diarrhoea in patients with inflammatory bowel disease; care is also needed in patients with intestinal strictures and diverticula.

Iron preparations taken orally may be constipating, particularly in older patients, occasionally leading to faecal impaction.

If side-effects occur, the dose may be reduced; alternatively, another iron salt may be used but an improvement in tolerance may simply be a result of a lower content of elemental iron. The incidence of side-effects due to ferrous sulphate is no greater than with other iron salts when compared on the basis of equivalent amounts of elemental iron.

Iron preparations are an important cause of accidental overdose in children. For the treatment of **iron overdose**, see Emergency Treatment of Poisoning, p. 25.

FERROUS SULPHATE

Indications: iron-deficiency anaemia

Cautions: pregnancy (see section 9.1.1); **interactions:** Appendix 1 (iron)

Side-effects: see notes above

Dose: see under preparations below and notes above
COUNSELLING. Although iron preparations are best absorbed on an empty stomach they may be taken after food to reduce gastro-intestinal side-effects; they may discolour stools

Ferrous Sulphate (Non-proprietary)

Tablets, coated, dried ferrous sulphate 200 mg (65 mg iron), net price 20 = 63p

Dose: prophylactic, 1 tablet daily; therapeutic, 1 tablet 2–3 times daily

■ Modified-release preparations

Feospan® (Intrapharm) NHS ▭

Spansule® (= capsules m/r), clear/red, enclosing green and brown pellets, dried ferrous sulphate 150 mg (47 mg iron). Net price 30-cap pack = 90p. Label: 25

Dose: 1–2 capsules daily; CHILD over 1 year 1 capsule daily; can be opened and sprinkled on food

Ferrograd® (Abbott) ▭

Filmtabs® (= tablets f/c), m/r, red, dried ferrous sulphate 325 mg (105 mg iron). Net price 30-tab pack = 54p. Label: 25

Dose: 1 tablet daily before food

Slow-Fe® (Novartis Consumer Health) ▭

Tablets, m/r, dried ferrous sulphate 160 mg (50 mg iron). Net price 28-tab pack = 24p. Label: 25

Dose: prophylactic, 1 tablet daily; therapeutic, 2 tablets daily; CHILD over 6 years, 1 tablet daily

FERROUS FUMARATE

Indications: iron-deficiency anaemia

Cautions: pregnancy (see section 9.1.1); **interactions:** Appendix 1 (iron)

Side-effects: see notes above

Dose: see under preparations below and notes above

Fersaday® (Goldshield)

Tablets, brown, f/c, ferrous fumarate 322 mg (100 mg iron). Net price 28-tab pack = 50p

Dose: prophylactic, 1 tablet daily; therapeutic, 1 tablet twice daily

Fersamal® (Goldshield)

Tablets, brown, ferrous fumarate 210 mg (68 mg iron). Net price 20 = 24p

Dose: 1–2 tablets 3 times daily

Syrup, brown, ferrous fumarate approx. 140 mg (45 mg iron)/5 mL. Net price 200 mL = £2.35

Dose: 10–20 mL twice daily; PREMATURE INFANT 0.6–2.4 mL/kg daily; CHILD up to 6 years 2.5–5 mL twice daily

Galfer® (Thornton & Ross)

Capsules, red/green, ferrous fumarate 305 mg (100 mg iron). Net price 20 = 36p

Dose: 1 capsule 1–2 times daily before food

Syrup, brown, sugar-free ferrous fumarate 140 mg (45 mg iron)/5 mL. Net price 300 mL = £4.86

Dose: 10 mL 1–2 times daily before food; CHILD (full-term infant and young child) 2.5–5 mL 1–2 times daily

FERROUS GLUCONATE

Indications: iron-deficiency anaemia

Cautions: pregnancy (see section 9.1.1); **interactions:** Appendix 1 (iron)

Side-effects: see notes above

Dose: see under preparation below and notes above

Ferrous Gluconate (Non-proprietary)

Tablets, red, coated, ferrous gluconate 300 mg (35 mg iron). Net price 20 = 73p

Dose: prophylactic, 2 tablets daily before food; therapeutic, 4–6 tablets daily in divided doses before food; CHILD 6–12 years, prophylactic and therapeutic, 1–3 tablets daily

FERROUS GLYCINE SULPHATE

Indications: iron-deficiency anaemia
Cautions: pregnancy (see section 9.1.1); **interactions:** Appendix 1 (iron)
Side-effects: see notes above
Dose: see under preparation below and notes above

Plesmet® (Link)
Syrup, ferrous glycine sulphate equivalent to 25 mg iron/5 mL. Net price 100 mL = 62p
Dose: 5–10 mL 3 times daily; CHILD 2.5–5 mL 1–3 times daily, according to age

POLYSACCHARIDE-IRON COMPLEX

Indications: iron-deficiency anaemia
Cautions: pregnancy (see section 9.1.1); **interactions:** Appendix 1 (iron)
Side-effects: see notes above
Dose: see under preparation below and notes above

Niferex® (Tillomed)
Elixir, brown, sugar-free, polysaccharide-iron complex equivalent to 100 mg of iron/5 mL. Net price 240-mL pack = £6.06; [NHS]¹ 30-mL dropper bottle for paediatric use = £2.16. Counselling, use of dropper
Dose: prophylactic, 2.5 mL daily; therapeutic, 5 mL 1–2 times daily (once daily if required during second and third trimester of pregnancy); PREMATURE INFANT and INFANT, (from dropper bottle) 1 drop (approx. 500 micrograms iron) per 450 g body-weight 3 times daily; CHILD 2–6 years 2.5 mL daily, 6–12 years 5 mL daily

1. except 30 mL paediatric dropper bottle for prophylaxis and treatment of iron deficiency in infants born prematurely and endorsed 'SLS'

SODIUM FEREDETATE

(Sodium ironedetate)
Indications: iron-deficiency anaemia
Cautions: pregnancy (see section 9.1.1); **interactions:** Appendix 1 (iron)
Side-effects: see notes above
Dose: see under preparation below and notes above

Sytron® (Link)
Elixir, sugar-free, sodium feredetate 190 mg equivalent to 27.5 mg of iron/5 mL. Net price 100 mL = 94p
Dose: 5 mL increasing gradually to 10 mL 3 times daily; INFANT and PREMATURE INFANT 2.5 mL twice daily (smaller doses should be used initially); CHILD 1–5 years 2.5 mL 3 times daily, 6–12 years 5 mL 3 times daily

Iron and folic acid

These preparations are used during pregnancy in women who are at high risk of developing iron and folic acid deficiency; they should be distinguished from those used for the prevention of neural tube defects in women planning a pregnancy (see p. 442).

It is important to note that the small doses of folic acid contained in these preparations are inadequate for the treatment of megaloblastic anaemias.

Fefol® (Intrapharm) [NHS] ▇
Spansule® (= capsules m/r), clear/green, enclosing brown, yellow, and white pellets, dried ferrous sulphate 150 mg (47 mg iron), folic acid 500 micrograms. Net price 30-cap pack = £1.69. Label: 25
Dose: 1 capsule daily

Ferrograd Folic® (Abbott) ▇
Filmtabs® (= tablets f/c), red/yellow, dried ferrous sulphate 325 mg (105 mg iron) for sustained release, folic acid 350 micrograms. Net price 30-tab pack = 60p. Label: 25
Dose: 1 tablet daily before food

Galfer FA® (Thornton & Ross)
Capsules, red/yellow, ferrous fumarate 305 mg (100 mg iron), folic acid 350 micrograms. Net price 20 = 40p
Dose: 1 capsule daily before food

Lexpec with Iron-M® (Rosemont) [PoM]
Syrup, brown, sugar-free, ferric ammonium citrate equivalent to 80 mg iron, folic acid 500 micrograms/5 mL. Net price 125 mL = £3.63
Dose: 5–10 mL daily before food
NOTE. *Lexpec with Iron-M*® contains five times less folic acid than *Lexpec with Iron*®

Pregaday® (Celltech)
Tablets, brown, f/c, ferrous fumarate equivalent to 100 mg (50 mg iron), folic acid 350 micrograms. Net price 28-tab pack = 96p
Dose: 1 tablet daily

Slow-Fe Folic® (Novartis Consumer Health) [PoM] ▇
Tablets, m/r, ivory, f/c, dried ferrous sulphate 160 mg (50 mg iron), folic acid 400 micrograms. Net price 28-tab pack = 27p. Label: 25
Dose: 1–2 tablets daily

■ Higher folic acid content
Appropriate in context of prevention of *recurrence of neural tube defects*, see recommendations on p. 442. *Cautions:* theoretical possibility of masking anaemia due to vitamin-B_{12} deficiency (which could allow vitamin-B_{12} neuropathy to develop).

Ferfolic SV® (Durbin) [PoM] [NHS]
Tablets, pink, ferrous gluconate 250 mg (30 mg iron), folic acid 4 mg, ascorbic acid 10 mg. Net price 100-tab pack = £2.50
Dose: anaemia, 1–3 tablets daily after food
Prophylaxis of neural tube defects in women known to be at risk, 1 tablet daily started before conception and continued for at least first trimester; see also recommendations on p. 442

Lexpec with Iron® (Rosemont) [PoM]
Syrup, brown, sugar-free, ferric ammonium citrate equivalent to 80 mg iron, folic acid 2.5 mg/5 mL. Net price 150 mL = £4.35
Dose: 5–10 mL daily before food
NOTE. *Lexpec with Iron*® contains five times as much folic acid as *Lexpec with Iron-M*®

Compound iron preparations

There is no justification for prescribing compound iron preparations, except for preparations of iron and folic acid for prophylactic use in pregnancy (see above).

Ferrograd C® (Abbott) [NHS] ▇
Filmtabs® (= tablets f/c), red, dried ferrous sulphate 325 mg (105 mg iron) for sustained release, ascorbic acid 500 mg (as sodium salt). Net price 30-tab pack = £1.71. Label: 25
Dose: 1 tablet daily before food

Givitol® (Galen) NHS ▭

Capsules, red/maroon, ferrous fumarate 305 mg (100 mg iron) with vitamins B group and C. Net price 20 = 88p

Dose: 1 capsule daily before food

9.1.1.2   Parenteral iron

Iron may be administered parenterally as iron dextran, or iron sucrose. Parenteral iron is generally reserved for use when oral therapy is unsuccessful because the patient cannot tolerate oral iron, or does not take it reliably, or if there is continuing blood loss, or in malabsorption.

Also, many patients with chronic renal failure who are receiving haemodialysis (and some who are receiving peritoneal dialysis) require iron by the intravenous route on a regular basis (see also Erythropoietin, section 9.1.3).

With the exception of patients with severe renal failure receiving haemodialysis, parenteral iron does not produce a faster haemoglobin response than oral iron provided that the oral iron preparation is taken reliably and is absorbed adequately.

Iron dextran, a complex of ferric hydroxide with dextrans, and **iron sucrose**, a complex of ferric hydroxide with sucrose, are given either by *slow intravenous injection* or by *intravenous infusion*. Anaphylactoid reactions can occur and patients should be given a small test dose initially.

IRON DEXTRAN

A complex of ferric hydroxide with sucrose containing 5% (50 mg/mL) of iron

Indications: iron-deficiency anaemia, see notes above

Cautions: facilities for cardiopulmonary resuscitation must be at hand; increased risk of allergic reaction in immune or inflammatory conditions; hepatic impairment (Appendix 2); renal impairment; oral iron not to be given until 5 days after last injection; pregnancy (Appendix 4)

Contra-indications: history of allergic disorders including asthma and eczema; infection; active rheumatoid arthritis

Side-effects: nausea, dyspepsia, diarrhoea, chest pains, hypotension, dyspnoea, arthralgia, myalgia, pruritus, urticaria, rash, fever, shivering, flushing, headache; rarely anaphylactoid reactions; injection site reactions including phlebitis reported

Dose: *by slow intravenous injection* or *by intravenous infusion*, calculated according to body-weight and iron deficit, consult product literature CHILD under 14 years, not recommended

CosmoFer® (Vitaline) ▼ PoM
Injection, iron (as iron dextran) 50 mg/mL, net price 2-mL amp = £7.97

IRON SUCROSE

A complex of ferric hydroxide with sucrose containing 2% (20 mg/mL) of iron

Indications: iron-deficiency anaemia, see notes above

Cautions: oral iron therapy should not be given until 5 days after last injection; facilities for cardiopulmonary resuscitation must be at hand; pregnancy (Appendix 4)

Contra-indications: history of allergic disorders including asthma, eczema and anaphylaxis; liver disease; infection

Side-effects: nausea, vomiting, taste disturbances, headache, hypotension; less frequently paraesthesia, abdominal disorders, myalgia, fever, flushing, urticaria, peripheral oedema; rarely anaphylactoid reactions; injection site reactions including phlebitis reported

Dose: *by slow intravenous injection* or *by intravenous infusion*, calculated according to body-weight and iron deficit, consult product literature CHILD not recommended

Venofer® (Syner-Med) PoM
Injection, iron (as iron sucrose) 20 mg/mL, net price 5-mL amp = £8.98

9.1.2   Drugs used in megaloblastic anaemias

Most megaloblastic anaemias result from a lack of either vitamin B_{12} or folate, and it is essential to establish in every case which deficiency is present and the underlying cause. In emergencies, where delay might be dangerous, it is sometimes necessary to administer both substances after the bone marrow test while plasma assay results are awaited. Normally, however, appropriate treatment should be instituted only when the results of tests are available.

One cause of megaloblastic anaemia in the UK is *pernicious anaemia* in which lack of gastric intrinsic factor resulting from an auto-immune gastritis causes malabsorption of vitamin B_{12}.

Vitamin B_{12} is also needed in the treatment of megaloblastosis caused by *prolonged nitrous oxide anaesthesia*, which inactivates the vitamin, and in the rare syndrome of *congenital transcobalamin II deficiency*.

Vitamin B_{12} should be given prophylactically after *total gastrectomy* or *total ileal resection* (or after *partial gastrectomy* if a vitamin B_{12} absorption test shows vitamin B_{12} malabsorption).

Apart from dietary deficiency, all other causes of vitamin-B_{12} deficiency are attributable to malabsorption. There is little place for the use of low-dose vitamin B_{12} orally and none for vitamin B_{12} intrinsic factor complexes given by mouth. Vitamin B_{12} in larger oral doses of 1–2 mg daily [unlicensed] may be effective.

Hydroxocobalamin has completely replaced cyanocobalamin as the form of vitamin B_{12} of choice for therapy; it is retained in the body longer than cyanocobalamin and thus for maintenance therapy can be given at intervals of up to 3 months. Treatment is generally initiated with frequent administration of intramuscular injections to replenish the depleted body stores. Thereafter, maintenance treatment, which is usually for life, can be instituted. There is no evidence that doses larger than those recommended provide any additional benefit in vitamin-B_{12} neuropathy.

Folic acid has few indications for long-term therapy since most causes of folate deficiency are self-limiting or will yield to a short course of treatment. It should not be used in undiagnosed megaloblastic anaemia unless vitamin B_{12} is administered concurrently otherwise neuropathy may be precipitated (see above).

In *folate-deficient megaloblastic anaemia* (e.g. because of poor nutrition, pregnancy, or antiepileptics), standard treatment to bring about a haematological remission and replenish body stores, is oral administration of folic acid 5 mg daily for 4 months; up to 15 mg daily may be necessary in malabsorption states. In pregnancy folic acid 5 mg is continued to term.

For *prophylaxis in chronic haemolytic states or in renal dialysis*, it is sufficient to give folic acid 5 mg daily or even weekly, depending on the diet and the rate of haemolysis.

For *prophylaxis in pregnancy* the dose of folic acid is 200–500 micrograms daily (see Iron and Folic Acid, section 9.1.1.1). See also Prevention of Neural Tube Defects below.

Folinic acid is also effective in the treatment of folate-deficient megaloblastic anaemia but it is generally used in association with cytotoxic drugs (see section 8.1); it is given as calcium folinate.

PREVENTION OF NEURAL TUBE DEFECTS. Recommendations of an expert advisory group of the Department of Health include the advice that:

To prevent *recurrence of neural tube defect* (in a child of a man or woman with spina bifida or if there is a history of neural tube defect in a previous child) women who wish to become pregnant (or who are at risk of becoming pregnant) should be advised to take folic acid supplements at a dose of 5 mg daily (reduced to 4 mg daily if a suitable preparation becomes available); supplementation should continue until week 12 of pregnancy. Women receiving antiepileptic therapy need individual counselling by their doctor before starting folic acid.

To prevent *first occurrence of neural tube defect* women who are planning a pregnancy should be advised to take folic acid as a medicinal or food supplement at a dose of 400 micrograms daily before conception and during the first 12 weeks of pregnancy. Women who have not been taking supplements and who suspect they are pregnant should start at once and continue until week 12 of pregnancy.

There is **no** justification for prescribing multiple-ingredient vitamin preparations containing vitamin B_{12} or folic acid.

HYDROXOCOBALAMIN

Indications: see under dose below

Cautions: should not be given before diagnosis fully established but see also notes above

Side-effects: itching, exanthema; fever, chills, hot flushes; nausea, dizziness; initial hypokalaemia; rarely acneform and bullous eruptions; anaphylaxis

Dose: *by intramuscular injection*, pernicious anaemia and other macrocytic anaemias without neurological involvement, initially 1 mg 3 times a week for 2 weeks then 1 mg every 3 months

Pernicious anaemia and other macrocytic anaemias with neurological involvement, initially 1 mg on alternate days until no further improvement, then 1 mg every 2 months

Prophylaxis of macrocytic anaemias associated with vitamin-B_{12} deficiency, 1 mg every 2–3 months

Tobacco amblyopia and Leber's optic atrophy, initially 1 mg daily for 2 weeks, then 1 mg twice weekly until no further improvement, thereafter 1 mg every 1–3 months

CHILD, doses as for adult

Hydroxocobalamin (Non-proprietary) PoM

Injection, hydroxocobalamin 1 mg/mL. Net price 1-mL amp = £2.46

NOTE. The BP directs that when vitamin B_{12} injection is prescribed or demanded hydroxocobalamin injection shall be dispensed or supplied

Available from Celltech (*Neo-Cytamen*® NHS), Goldshield, Link (*Cobalin-H*® NHS)

CYANOCOBALAMIN

Indications: see notes above

Dose: *by mouth*, vitamin-B_{12} deficiency of dietary origin, 50–150 micrograms or more daily taken between meals; CHILD 50–105 micrograms daily in 1–3 divided doses

By intramuscular injection, initially 1 mg repeated 10 times at intervals of 2–3 days, maintenance 1 mg every month, but see notes above

Cyanocobalamin (Non-proprietary)

[1] *Tablets* NHS, cyanocobalamin 50 micrograms. Net price 50-tab pack = £3.04

Available from Goldshield (*Cytacon*® NHS)

Liquid NHS, cyanocobalamin 35 micrograms/5 mL. Net price 200 mL = £2.77

Available from Goldshield (*Cytacon*® NHS)

Injection PoM, cyanocobalamin 1 mg/mL. Net price 1-mL amp = £1.67

NOTE. The BP directs that when vitamin B_{12} injection is prescribed or demanded hydroxocobalamin injection shall be dispensed or supplied

Available from Celltech (*Cytamen*® NHS)

1. NHS except to treat or prevent vitamin-B_{12} deficiency in a patient who is a vegan or who has a proven vitamin-B_{12} deficiency of dietary origin and endorsed 'SLS'

FOLIC ACID

Indications: see notes above

Cautions: should never be given alone for pernicious anaemia and other vitamin-B_{12} deficiency states (may precipitate subacute combined degeneration of the spinal cord); **interactions:** Appendix 1 (folates)

Dose: *by mouth*, initially, 5 mg daily for 4 months (see notes above); maintenance, 5 mg every 1–7 days depending on underlying disease; CHILD up to 1 year, 500 micrograms/kg daily; over 1 year, as adult dose

Prevention of neural tube defects, see notes above

[1] **Folic Acid** (Non-proprietary) PoM

Tablets, folic acid 400 micrograms, net price = 90-tab pack = £2.24; 5 mg, 20 = 31p

NOTE. 400-microgram tablets available from Lane (*Preconceive*®), 5-mg tablets available from various suppliers

Syrup, folic acid 2.5 mg/5 mL, net price 150 mL = £9.74; 400 micrograms/5 mL, 150 mL = £1.49

NOTE. 2.5 mg/5 mL syrup available from Hillcross and Rosemont (*Lexpec*®, sugar-free); 400 micrograms/5 mL oral solution available from Rosemont (*Folicare*®)

Injection, folic acid 15 mg, net price 1–mL amp = £1.24

Available from BCM Specials [unlicensed—special order]

1. Can be sold to the public provided daily doses do not exceed 500 micrograms

Drugs used in hypoplastic, haemolytic, and renal anaemias

Anabolic steroids (section 6.4.3), pyridoxine, antilymphocyte immunoglobulin, and various corticosteroids are used in hypoplastic and haemolytic anaemias.

Antilymphocyte globulin given intravenously through a central line over 12–18 hours each day for 5 days produces a response in about 50% of cases of acquired *aplastic anaemia*; the response rate may be increased when ciclosporin is given as well. Severe reactions are common in the first 2 days and profound immunosuppression can occur; antilymphocyte globulin should be given under specialist supervision with appropriate resuscitation facilities. Alternatively, oxymetholone tablets (available on a named-patient basis only) may be used in aplastic anaemia at a dose of 1–5 mg/kg daily for 3 to 6 months.

It is unlikely that dietary deprivation of **pyridoxine** (section 9.6.2) produces clinically relevant haematological effects. However, certain forms of *sideroblastic anaemia* respond to pharmacological doses, possibly reflecting its role as a co-enzyme during haemoglobin synthesis. Pyridoxine is indicated in both *idiopathic acquired* and *hereditary sideroblastic anaemias*. Although complete cures have not been reported, some increase in haemoglobin may occur; the dose required is usually high, up to 400 mg daily. *Reversible sideroblastic anaemias* respond to treatment of the underlying cause but in pregnancy, haemolytic anaemias, and alcohol dependence, or during isoniazid treatment, pyridoxine is also indicated.

Hydroxycarbamide (hydroxyurea, section 8.1.5) can reduce the rate of crises in *sickle cell disease* and reduce the need for blood transfusions [unlicensed indication].

Corticosteroids (see section 6.3) have an important place in the management of a wide variety of haematological disorders. They include conditions with an immune basis such as *autoimmune haemolytic anaemia*, *immune thrombocytopenias* and *neutropenias*, and *major transfusion reactions*. They are also used in chemotherapy schedules for many types of *lymphoma*, *lymphoid leukaemias*, and *paraproteinaemias*, including *multiple myeloma*.

Erythropoietin

Epoetin (recombinant human erythropoietin) is used for the anaemia associated with erythropoietin deficiency in chronic renal failure, to increase the yield of autologous blood in normal individuals and to shorten the period of anaemia in patients receiving cytotoxic chemotherapy. The clinical efficacy of epoetin alfa and epoetin beta is similar. Epoetin beta is also used for the prevention of anaemia in premature infants of low-birth-weight.

Darbepoetin, is a hyperglycosylated derivative of epoetin which has a longer half-life and may be administered less frequently than epoetin.

Other factors which contribute to the anaemia of chronic renal failure such as iron or folate deficiency should be corrected before treatment and monitored during therapy. Supplemental iron may improve the response in resistant patients. Aluminium toxicity, concurrent infection or other inflammatory disease may impair the response to erythropoietin.

> **CSM advice.** There have been very rare reports of pure red cell aplasia in patients treated with epoetin alfa. The CSM has advised that in patients developing epoetin alfa failure with a diagnosis of pure red cell aplasia, treatment with epoetin alfa must be discontinued and testing for erythropoietin antibodies considered. Patients who develop pure red cell aplasia should **not** be switched to another erythropoietin.

DARBEPOETIN ALFA

Indications: see under Dose below

Cautions: see Epoetin; sickle cell anaemia; hepatic disease (Appendix 2); pregnancy (Appendix 4); **interactions:** Appendix 1 (epoetin)

Contra-indications: see Epoetin; breast-feeding (Appendix 5)

Side-effects: see Epoetin; also, peripheral oedema; injection site pain

Dose: anaemia associated with chronic renal failure, *by intravenous* or *subcutaneous injection*, ADULT and CHILD over 11 years, initially 450 nanograms/kg once weekly adjusted according to response by approx. 25% of initial dose at intervals of at least 4 weeks; reduce dose by 25–50% if haemoglobin rise exceeds 2.5 g/100 mL per month; suspend if haemoglobin exceeds 14 g/100 mL until it falls below 13 g/100 mL and then restart with dose at 25% below previous dose

NOTE. When changing route give same dose then adjust according to weekly or fortnightly haemoglobin measurements

Anaemia in adults with non-myeloid malignancies receiving chemotherapy, *by subcutaneous injection*, initially 2.25 micrograms/kg once weekly, if appropriate rise in haemoglobin not achieved after 4 weeks, double initial dose; if response remains inadequate after further 4 weeks discontinue treatment; suspend if haemoglobin exceeds 14 g/100 mL until concentration falls below 13 g/100 mL and reinstate at 50% of previous dose

Aranesp® (Amgen) ▼ PoM

Injection, prefilled syringe, darbepoetin alfa, net price 10 micrograms = £16.76; 15 micrograms = £25.14; 20 micrograms = £33.52; 30 micrograms = £50.28; 40 micrograms = £67.04; 50 micrograms = £83.80; 60 micrograms = £100.56; 80 micrograms = £134.08; 100 micrograms = £167.60; 150 micrograms = £251.40; 300 micrograms = £502.80.

EPOETIN ALFA and BETA

(Recombinant human erythropoietins)

NOTE. Although epoetin alfa and beta are clinically indistinguishable the prescriber must specify which is required

Indications: see under preparations, below

Cautions: inadequately treated or poorly controlled blood pressure (monitor closely blood pressure, haemoglobin, and electrolytes), interrupt treatment if blood pressure uncontrolled; sudden stabbing migraine-like pain is warning of hypertensive crisis; exclude other causes of anaemia (e.g. folic acid or vitamin B_{12} deficiency) and give iron supplements if necessary (see also notes above); ischaemic vascular disease; thrombocytosis (monitor platelet count for first 8 weeks); epilepsy; malignant disease; chronic liver failure; increase in heparin dose may be needed; risk of thrombosis may be increased when used for anaemia before orthopaedic surgery—avoid in cardiovascular disease including recent myocardial infarction or cerebrovascular accident; pregnancy (Appendix 4) and breast-feeding (Appendix 5); **interactions:** Appendix 1 (epoetin)

Contra-indications: uncontrolled hypertension; avoid injections containing benzyl alcohol in neonates (see under preparations, below)

Side-effects: dose-dependent increase in blood pressure or aggravation of hypertension; in isolated patients with normal or low blood pressure, hypertensive crisis with encephalopathy-like symptoms and generalised tonic-clonic seizures requiring immediate medical attention; dose-dependent increase in platelet count (but thrombocytosis rare) regressing during treatment; influenza-like symptoms (may be reduced if intravenous injection given over 5 minutes); shunt thrombosis especially if tendency to hypotension or arteriovenous shunt complications; isolated reports of hyperkalaemia, skin reactions; very rarely sudden loss of response because of pure red cell aplasia, particularly following subcutaneous administration in patients with chronic renal failure (discontinue erythropoietin therapy)—see also CSM advice above

Dose: aimed at increasing haemoglobin concentration at rate not exceeding 2 g/100 mL/month to stable level of 10–12 g/100 mL (9.5–11 g/100 mL in children); see under preparations, below

■ Epoetin alfa

Eprex® (Janssen-Cilag) PoM
Injection, epoetin alfa 40 000 units/mL, net price 1-mL (40 000-unit) vial = £335.20
Injection, prefilled syringe, epoetin alfa, net price 1000 units = £8.38; 2000 units = £16.76; 3000 units = £25.14; 4000 units = £33.52; 5000 units = £41.90; 6000 units = £50.28; 8000 units = £67.04; 10 000 units = £83.80. An auto-injector device is available for use with 10 000-units prefilled syringes
Dose: anaemia associated with chronic renal failure in patients on haemodialysis, *by intravenous injection* over 1–5 minutes, initially 50 units/kg 3 times weekly adjusted according to response in steps of 25 units/kg 3 times weekly at intervals of at least 4 weeks; maintenance dose (when haemoglobin concentration of 10–12 g/100 mL achieved), usually a total of 75–300 units/kg weekly (as a single dose or in divided doses); CHILD initially as for adults; maintenance dose (when haemoglobin concentration of 9.5–11 g/100 mL achieved), body-weight under 10 kg usually 75–150 units/kg 3 times weekly, body-weight 10–30 kg usually 60–150 units/kg 3 times weekly, body-weight over 30 kg usually 30–100 units/kg 3 times weekly
IMPORTANT. Subcutaneous injection **contra-indicated** in patients with chronic renal failure
Anaemia associated with chronic renal failure in adults on peritoneal dialysis, *by intravenous injection* over 1–5 minutes, initially 50 units/kg twice weekly; maintenance dose (when haemoglobin concentration of 10–12 g/100 mL achieved), 25–50 units/kg twice weekly
IMPORTANT. Subcutaneous injection **contra-indicated** in patients with chronic renal failure
Severe symptomatic anaemia of renal origin in adults with renal insufficiency not yet on dialysis, *by intravenous injection* over 1–5 minutes, initially 50 units/kg 3 times weekly increased according to response in steps of 25 units/kg 3 times weekly at intervals of at least 4 weeks; maintenance dose (when haemoglobin concentration of 10–12 g/100 mL achieved), 17–33 units/kg 3 times weekly; max. 200 units/kg 3 times weekly;
IMPORTANT. Subcutaneous injection **contra-indicated** in patients with chronic renal failure
Anaemia in adults receiving cancer chemotherapy, *by subcutaneous injection* (max. 1 mL per injection site), initially 150 units/kg 3 times weekly, increased if appropriate rise in haemoglobin (or reticulocyte count) not achieved after 4 weeks to 300 units/kg 3 times weekly; discontinue if inadequate response after 4 weeks at higher dose; reduce dose by 25–50% if haemoglobin rise exceeds 2 g/100 mL per month; suspend if haemoglobin exceeds 14 g/100 mL until it falls below 12 g/100 mL and reinstate with dose at 25% below previous dose; continue epoetin for 1 month after end of chemotherapy
To increase yield of autologous blood (to avoid homologous blood) in predonation programme in moderate anaemia *either* when large volume of blood required *or* when sufficient blood cannot be saved for elective major surgery, *by intravenous injection* over 1–5 minutes, 600 units/kg twice weekly for 3 weeks before surgery; consult product literature for details and advice on ensuring high iron stores
Moderate anaemia (haemoglobin concentration 10–13 g/100 mL) before elective orthopaedic surgery in adults with expected moderate blood loss to reduce exposure to allogeneic transfusion or if autologous transfusion unavailable, *by subcutaneous injection* (max. 1 mL per injection site), 600 units/kg every week for 3 weeks before surgery and on day of surgery *or* 300 units/kg daily for 15 days starting 10 days before surgery; consult product literature for details

■ Epoetin beta

NeoRecormon® (Roche) PoM
Injection, prefilled syringe, epoetin beta, net price 500 units = £4.19; 1000 units = £8.38; 2000 units = £16.76; 3000 units = £25.14; 4000 units = £33.52; 5000 units = £41.90; 6000 units = £50.28; 10 000 units = £83.80
Excipients: include phenylalanine up to 300 micrograms/syringe (section 9.4.1)
Multidose injection, powder for reconstitution, epoetin beta, net price 50 000-unit vial = £419.01; 100 000-unit vial = £838.01 (both with solvent)
Excipients: include phenylalanine up to 5 mg/vial (section 9.4.1), benzyl alcohol (avoid in neonates, see Excipients p. 2)
NOTE. Avoid contact of reconstituted injection with glass; use only plastic materials
Reco-Pen, (for subcutaneous use), double-chamber cartridges (containing epoetin beta and solvent), net price 10 000-unit cartridge = £83.80; 20 000-unit cartridge = £167.60; 60 000-unit cartridge = £502.81; for use with *Reco-Pen* injection device and needles (both available free from Roche)
Excipients: include phenylalanine up to 500 micrograms/cartridge (section 9.4.1), benzyl alcohol (avoid in neonates, see Excipients, p. 2)
Dose: anaemia associated with chronic renal failure in dialysis patients, symptomatic anaemia of renal origin in patients not yet on dialysis, ADULT and CHILD
By subcutaneous injection, initially 20 units/kg weekly (in 1–7 divided doses) for 4 weeks, increased according to response at intervals of 4 weeks in steps of 60 units/kg; maintenance dose (when haemoglobin concentration of

10–12 g/100 mL achieved), initially reduce dose by half then adjust according to response at intervals of 1–2 weeks; max. 720 units/kg weekly

By intravenous injection over 2 minutes, initially 40 units/kg 3 times weekly for 4 weeks, increased according to response to 80 units/kg 3 times weekly with further increases if needed at intervals of 4 weeks in steps of 20 units/kg 3 times weekly; maintenance dose (when haemoglobin concentration of 10–12 g/100 mL achieved), initially reduce dose by half then adjust according to response at intervals of 1–2 weeks; max. 720 units/kg weekly

Prevention of anaemias of prematurity in infants with birth-weight of 0.75–1.5 kg and gestational age of less than 34 weeks, *by subcutaneous injection* (of single-dose, unpreserved injection), 250 units/kg 3 times weekly preferably starting within 3 days of birth and continued for 6 weeks

Anaemia in adults with solid tumours receiving platinum-containing chemotherapy, *by subcutaneous injection*, initially 450 units/kg weekly (in 3–7 divided doses), increased if appropriate rise in haemoglobin not achieved after 4 weeks to 900 units/kg weekly (in 3–7 divided doses); reduce dose by half if haemoglobin rise exceeds 2 g/100 mL per month; suspend if haemoglobin exceeds 14 g/100 mL until concentration falls below 12 g/100 mL and reinstate at 50% of the previous weekly dose; continue for up to 3 weeks after end of chemotherapy

NOTE. If haemoglobin concentration falls by more than 1 g/100 mL in the first cycle of chemotherapy despite treatment with epoetin beta, further treatment may not be effective

Dose: To increase yield of autologous blood (to avoid homologous blood) in predonation programme in moderate anaemia when blood conserving procedures are insufficient or unavailable, consult product literature

Anaemia in adults with multiple myeloma, low-grade non-Hodgkin's lymphoma or chronic lymphocytic leukaemia receiving chemotherapy, *by subcutaneous injection*, initially 450 units/kg weekly (as a single dose or in 3–7 divided doses), increased if rise in haemoglobin of at least 1 g/100 mL not achieved after 4 weeks to 900 units/kg weekly (in 2–7 divided doses); reduce dose by half if haemoglobin rise exceeds 2 g/100 mL per month; suspend if haemoglobin exceeds 14 g/100 mL until concentration falls below 13 g/100 mL and reinstate at 50% of previous dose; max. 900 units/kg weekly; continue for up to 4 weeks after end of chemotherapy

NOTE. Discontinue treatment if haemoglobin concentration does not increase by at least 1 g/100 mL after 8 weeks of therapy

Iron overload

Severe tissue iron overload may occur in aplastic and other refractory anaemias, mainly as the result of repeated blood transfusions. It is a particular problem in refractory anaemias with hyperplastic bone marrow, especially *thalassaemia major*, where excessive iron absorption from the gut and inappropriate iron therapy may add to the tissue siderosis.

Iron overload associated with haemochromatosis may be treated with repeated venesection. Venesection may also be used for patients who have received multiple transfusions and whose bone marrow has recovered. Where venesection is contra-indicated, the long-term administration of the iron chelating compound **desferrioxamine mesilate** is useful. Subcutaneous infusions of desferrioxamine are given over 8–12 hours, 3–7 times a week. The dose should reflect the degree of iron overload. For children starting therapy (and who have low iron overload) the dose should not exceed 30 mg/kg. For established

overload the dose is usually between 20 and 50 mg/kg daily. Desferrioxamine (up to 2 g per unit of blood) may also be given at the time of blood transfusion, provided that the desferrioxamine is **not** added to the blood and is **not** given through the same line as the blood (but the two may be given through the same cannula).

Iron excretion induced by desferrioxamine is enhanced by administration of ascorbic acid (vitamin C, section 9.6.3) in a dose of 200 mg daily (100 mg in infants); it should be given separately from food since it also enhances iron absorption. Ascorbic acid should not be given to patients with cardiac dysfunction; in patients with normal cardiac function ascorbic acid should be introduced 1 month after starting desferrioxamine.

Infusion of desferrioxamine may be used to treat *aluminium overload* in dialysis patients; theoretically 100 mg of desferrioxamine binds with 4.1 mg of aluminium.

Deferiprone, an oral iron chelator, is licensed for the treatment of iron overload in patients with thalassaemia major in whom desferrioxamine is contra-indicated or is not tolerated. Blood dyscrasias, particularly agranulocytosis, have been reported with deferiprone.

DEFERIPRONE

Indications: see notes above

Cautions: neutropenia (monitor neutrophil count weekly and discontinue treatment if neutropenia develops); hepatic and renal impairment; limited experience in children 6–10 years

BLOOD DISORDERS. Patients or their carers should be told how to recognise signs of neutropenia and advised to seek immediate medical attention if symptoms such as fever or sore throat develop

Contra-indications: pregnancy (Appendix 4) and breast-feeding

Side-effects: gastro-intestinal disturbances; red-brown urine discoloration; arthropathy; neutropenia, agranulocytosis

Dose: ADULT and CHILD over 6 years 25 mg/kg (to the nearest 250 mg) 3 times daily (max. 100 mg/kg daily); CHILD under 6 years not recommended

Ferriprox® (Swedish Orphan) ▼ PoM
Tablets, f/c, scored, deferiprone 500 mg, net price 100-tab pack = £152.39. Label: 14, counselling, blood disorders

DESFERRIOXAMINE MESILATE
(Deferoxamine Mesilate)

Indications: see notes above; iron poisoning, see Emergency Treatment of Poisoning

Cautions: renal impairment; eye and ear examinations before treatment and at 3-month intervals during treatment; aluminium-related encephalopathy (may exacerbate neurological dysfunction); pregnancy (Appendix 4), breast-feeding; **interactions:** Appendix 1 (desferrioxamine)

Side-effects: hypotension (especially when given too rapidly by intravenous injection), disturbances of hearing and vision (including lens opacity and retinopathy); injection site reactions, gastro-intestinal disturbances, asthma, fever, headache, arthralgia and myalgia; very rarely anaphylaxis, acute respiratory distress syndrome, neurological disturbances (including dizziness, neuropathy and paraesthesia), Yersinia and mucormycosis infections, rash, renal impairment, and blood dyscrasias

Dose: see notes above; iron poisoning, see Emergency Treatment of Poisoning

NOTE. For full details and warnings relating to administration, consult product literature

Desferal® (Novartis) [PoM]
Injection, powder for reconstitution, desferrioxamine mesilate, net price 500-mg vial = £4.44, 2-g vial = £17.77

9.1.4 Drugs used in autoimmune thrombocytopenic purpura

It is usual to treat autoimmune (idiopathic) thrombocytopenic purpura with a **corticosteroid**, e.g. prednisolone 1 mg/kg daily, gradually reducing the dose over several weeks. Splenectomy is considered if a satisfactory platelet count is not achieved or if there is a relapse on reducing the dose of corticosteroid or withdrawing it.

Immunoglobulin preparations (section 14.5), are also used in autoimmune thrombocytopenic purpura or where a temporary rapid rise in platelets is needed, as in pregnancy or pre-operatively; they are also used for children often in preference to a corticosteroid. Anti-D immunoglobulin is licensed for the management of autoimmune thrombocytopenic purpura.

In autoimmune thrombocytopenic purpura refractory to corticosteroid treatment or in chronic cases where splenectomy is inappropriate, **danazol** (section 6.7.2) may be used [unlicensed indication], particularly in older patients. Danazol may also allow the dose of corticosteroid to be reduced.

Other therapy that has been tried in refractory autoimmune thrombocytopenic purpura includes azathioprine (section 8.2.1), cyclophosphamide (section 8.1.1), vincristine (section 8.1.4), and ciclosporin (section 8.2.2). For patients with chronic severe thrombocytopenia refractory to other therapy, tranexamic acid (section 2.11) may be given to reduce the severity of haemorrhage.

9.1.5 G6PD deficiency

Glucose 6-phosphate dehydrogenase (G6PD) deficiency is highly prevalent in individuals originating from most parts of Africa, from most parts of Asia, from Oceania, and from Southern Europe; it can also occur, rarely, in any other individuals.

Individuals with G6PD deficiency are susceptible to developing acute haemolytic anaemia on taking a number of common drugs. They are also susceptible to developing acute haemolytic anaemia upon ingestion of fava beans (broad beans, *Vicia faba*); this is termed *favism* and can be more severe in children or when the fresh fava beans are eaten raw.

When prescribing drugs for patients with G6PD deficiency, the following three points should be kept in mind:

- G6PD deficiency is genetically heterogeneous; susceptibility to the haemolytic risk from drugs varies; thus, a drug found to be safe in some

G6PD-deficient individuals may not be equally safe in others;

- manufacturers do not routinely test drugs for their effects in G6PD-deficient individuals;
- the risk and severity of haemolysis is almost always dose-related.

The lists below should be read with these points in mind. Ideally, information about G6PD deficiency should be available before prescribing a drug listed below. However, in the absence of this information, the possibility of haemolysis should be considered, especially if the patient belongs to a group in which G6PD deficiency is common.

A very few G6PD-deficient individuals with chronic non-spherocytic haemolytic anaemia have haemolysis even in the absence of an exogenous trigger. These patients must be regarded as being at high risk of severe exacerbation of haemolysis following administration of any of the drugs listed below.

Drugs with definite risk of haemolysis in most G6PD-deficient individuals. Dapsone and other sulphones (higher doses for dermatitis herpetiformis more likely to cause problems)
Methylthioninium chloride (methylene blue)
Niridazole [not on UK market]
Nitrofurantoin
Pamaquin [not on UK market]
Primaquine (30 mg weekly for 8 weeks has been found to be without undue harmful effects in African and Asian people, see section 5.4.1)
Quinolones (including ciprofloxacin, moxifloxacin, nalidixic acid, norfloxacin, and ofloxacin)
Sulphonamides (including co-trimoxazole; some sulphonamides, e.g. sulfadiazine, have been tested and found not to be haemolytic in many G6PD-deficient individuals)

Drugs with possible risk of haemolysis in some G6PD-deficient individuals. Aspirin (acceptable up to a dose of at least 1 g daily in most G6PD-deficient individuals)
Chloroquine (acceptable in acute malaria)
Menadione, water-soluble derivatives (e.g. menadiol sodium phosphate)
Probenecid [not on UK market]
Quinidine (acceptable in acute malaria)
Quinine (acceptable in acute malaria)

NOTE. Mothballs may contain naphthalene which also causes haemolysis in individuals with G6PD-deficiency.

9.1.6 Drugs used in neutropenia

Recombinant human granulocyte-colony stimulating factor (rhG-CSF) stimulates the production of neutrophils and may reduce the duration of chemotherapy-induced neutropenia and thereby reduce the incidence of associated sepsis; there is as yet no evidence that it improves overall survival. **Filgrastim** (unglycosylated rhG-CSF) and **lenograstim** (glycosylated rhG-CSF) have similar effects; both have been used in a variety of clinical settings but they do not have any clear-cut routine indications. In congenital neutropenia filgrastim usually elevates the neutrophil count with appropriate clinical response. Prolonged use may be associated with an increased risk of myeloid malignancy. **Pegfilgrastim**, a polyethylene glycol-conjugated ('pegylated') derivative of filgrastim has been introduced recently. Pegylation increases the duration of filgrastim activity.

Molgramostim (recombinant human granulocyte macrophage-colony stimulating factor) stimulates the production of all granulocytes and monocytes. It has more side-effects than granulocyte-colony stimulating factor and is ineffective in congenital neutropenia.

Treatment with recombinant human growth factors should only be prescribed by those experienced in their use.

For the use of **amifostine** in cytotoxic-induced neutropenic infection, see section 8.1.

CAUTIONS. Granulocyte-colony stimulating factors should be used with caution during pregnancy (Appendix 4) and breast-feeding (Appendix 5). Blood counts (including differential white cell count and platelet count) should be monitored.

SIDE-EFFECTS. Side-effects of granulocyte-colony stimulating factors include gastro-intestinal disturbances (including nausea, vomiting, and diarrhoea), anorexia, headache, asthenia, fever, musculoskeletal pain, bone pain, rash, alopecia, injection-site reactions, and leucocytosis. Less frequent side-effects include chest pain, hypersensitivity reactions (including anaphylaxis and bronchospasm) and arthralgia. There have been reports of pulmonary infiltrates leading to acute respiratory distress syndrome.

FILGRASTIM

(Recombinant human granulocyte-colony stimulating factor, G-CSF)

Indications: (specialist use only) reduction in duration of neutropenia and incidence of febrile neutropenia in cytotoxic chemotherapy for malignancy (except chronic myeloid leukaemia and myelodysplastic syndromes); reduction in duration of neutropenia (and associated sequelae) in myeloablative therapy followed by bone-marrow transplantation; mobilisation of peripheral blood progenitor cells for harvesting and subsequent autologous or allogeneic infusion; severe congenital neutropenia, cyclic neutropenia, or idiopathic neutropenia and history of severe or recurrent infections (distinguish carefully from other haematological disorders, consult product literature); persistent neutropenia in advanced HIV infection

Cautions: see notes above; also reduced myeloid precursors; regular morphological and cytogenetic bone-marrow examinations recommended in severe congenital neutropenia (possible risk of myelodysplastic syndromes or leukaemia); secondary acute myeloid leukaemia, sickle cell disease; monitor spleen size (risk of rupture); osteoporotic bone disease (monitor bone density if given for more than 6 months); **interactions:** Appendix 1 (filgrastim)

Contra-indications: severe congenital neutropenia (Kostman's syndrome) with abnormal cytogenetics

Side-effects: see notes above; also splenic enlargement, hepatomegaly, transient hypotension, epistaxis, urinary abnormalities (including dysuria, proteinuria, and haematuria), osteoporosis, exacerbation of rheumatoid arthritis, cutaneous vasculitis, thrombocytopenia, anaemia, transient decrease in blood glucose, raised uric acid

Dose: cytotoxic-induced neutropenia, preferably *by subcutaneous injection or by intravenous infusion* (over 30 minutes), ADULT and CHILD, 500 000 units/kg daily started not less than 24 hours after cytotoxic chemotherapy, continued until neutrophil count in normal range, usually for up to 14 days (up to 38 days in acute myeloid leukaemia)

Myeloablative therapy followed by bone-marrow transplantation, *by intravenous infusion* over 30 minutes or over 24 hours *or by subcutaneous infusion* over 24 hours, 1 million units/kg daily, started not less than 24 hours following cytotoxic chemotherapy (and within 24 hours of bone-marrow infusion), then adjusted according to absolute neutrophil count (consult product literature)

Mobilisation of peripheral blood progenitor cells for autologous infusion, used alone, *by subcutaneous injection or by subcutaneous infusion* over 24 hours, 1 million units/kg daily for 5-7 days; used following adjunctive myelosuppressive chemotherapy (to improve yield), *by subcutaneous injection*, 500 000 units/kg daily, started the day after completion of chemotherapy and continued until neutrophil count in normal range; for timing of leukapheresis consult product literature

Mobilisation of peripheral blood progenitor cells in normal donors for allogeneic infusion, *by subcutaneous injection*, ADULT under 60 years and ADOLESCENT over 16 years, 1 million units/kg daily for 4–5 days; for timing of leukapheresis consult product literature

Severe chronic neutropenia, *by subcutaneous injection*, ADULT and CHILD, in severe congenital neutropenia, initially 1.2 million units/kg daily in single or divided doses (initially 500 000 units/kg daily in idiopathic or cyclic neutropenia), adjusted according to response (consult product literature)

Persistent neutropenia in HIV infection, *by subcutaneous injection*, initially 100 000 units/kg daily, increased as necessary until absolute neutrophil count in normal range (usual max. 400 000 units/kg daily), then adjusted to maintain absolute neutrophil count in normal range (consult product literature)

Neupogen® (Amgen) PoM
Injection, filgrastim 30 million units (300 micrograms)/mL; net price 1-mL vial = £73.56, 1.6-mL (48 million-unit) vial = £117.32
Injection (Singleject®), filgrastim 60 million units (600 micrograms)/mL, net price 0.5-mL prefilled syringe = £73.56; 96 million units (960 micrograms)/mL, 0.5-mL prefilled syringe = £117.32

LENOGRASTIM

(Recombinant human granulocyte-colony stimulating factor, rHuG-CSF)

Indications: (specialist use only) reduction in the duration of neutropenia and associated complications following bone-marrow transplantation for non-myeloid malignancy or following treatment with cytotoxic chemotherapy associated with a significant incidence of febrile neutropenia; mobilisation of peripheral blood progenitor cells for harvesting and subsequent infusion

Cautions: see notes above; also pre-malignant myeloid conditions; reduced myeloid precursors; sickle cell disease; monitor spleen size (risk of rupture)

Side-effects: see notes above; also splenic rupture, cutaneous vasculitis, Sweet's syndrome, toxic epidermal necrolysis

Dose: following bone-marrow transplantation, *by intravenous infusion,* ADULT and CHILD over 2 years 19.2 million units/m^2 daily started the day after transplantation, continued until neutrophil count stable in acceptable range (max. 28 days)

Cytotoxic-induced neutropenia, *by subcutaneous injection,* ADULT 19.2 million units/m^2 daily started the day after completion of chemotherapy, continued until neutrophil count stable in acceptable range (max. 28 days)

Mobilisation of peripheral blood progenitor cells, used alone, *by subcutaneous injection,* ADULT 1.28 million units/kg daily for 4–6 days (5–6 days in healthy donors); used following adjunctive myelosuppressive chemotherapy (to improve yield), *by subcutaneous injection,* 19.2 million-units/m^2 daily, started the day after completion of chemotherapy and continued until neutrophil count in acceptable range; for timing of leukapheresis consult product literature

Granocyte® (Chugai) PoM
Injection, powder for reconstitution, lenograstim, net price 13.4 million-unit (105-microgram) vial = £40.11; 33.6 million-unit (263-microgram) vial = £73.56 (both with 1-mL amp or 1-mL prefilled syringe water for injections)

MOLGRAMOSTIM
(Recombinant human granulocyte macrophage-colony stimulating factor, GM-CSF)

Indications: (specialist use only) reduction of severity of neutropenia (and risk of infection) in cytotoxic chemotherapy; acceleration of myeloid recovery following bone-marrow transplantation; neutropenia in patients treated with ganciclovir in AIDS-related cytomegalovirus retinitis

Cautions: see notes above; also myeloid malignancies; monitor serum albumin concentration; monitor closely patients with pulmonary disease; history of or predisposition to autoimmune disease

Contra-indications: concomitant use with widefield radiotherapy

Side-effects: see notes above; also stomatitis, flushing, peripheral oedema, cardiac failure, capillary leak syndrome, hypotension, arrhythmias, pericardial effusion, pericarditis, cerebrovascular disorders, intracranial hypertension, pleural effusion, pulmonary oedema, syncope, dyspnoea, dizziness, paraesthesia, confusion, convulsions, pruritus, increased sweating

Dose: (first dose under medical supervision)
Cytotoxic chemotherapy, *by subcutaneous injection,* 60 000–110 000 units/kg daily, starting 24 hours after last dose of chemotherapy, continued for 7–10 days

Bone-marrow transplantation, *by intravenous infusion,* 110 000 units/kg daily, starting day after transplantation, continued until absolute neutro-

phil count in desirable range (see product literature); max. duration of treatment 30 days

Adjunct in ganciclovir treatment, *by subcutaneous injection,* 60 000 units/kg daily for 5 days then adjusted to maintain desirable absolute neutrophil count and white blood cell count

Leucomax® (Schering-Plough) PoM
Injection, powder for reconstitution, molgramostim, net price 1.67 million unit (150 microgram) vial = £42.13; 3.33 million unit (300 microgram) vial = £84.26; 4.44 million unit (400 microgram) vial = £112.34
NOTE. May be difficult to obtain

PEGFILGRASTIM
(Pegylated recombinant methionyl human granulocyte-colony stimulating factor)

Indications: (specialist use only) reduction in duration of neutropenia and incidence of febrile neutropenia in cytotoxic chemotherapy for malignancy (except chronic myeloid leukaemia and myelodysplastic syndromes)

Cautions: see notes above; also acute leukaemia and myelosuppressive chemotherapy; sickle-cell disease; monitor spleen size (risk of rupture); **interactions:** Appendix 1 (filgrastim)

Side-effects: see notes above; also raised uric acid

Dose: (expressed as filgrastim) *by subcutaneous injection,* ADULT over 18 years, 6 mg (0.6 mL) for each chemotherapy cycle, starting 24 hours after chemotherapy

Neulasta® (Amgen) ▼ PoM
Injection, pegfilgrastim (expressed as filgrastim) 10 mg/mL, net price 0.6-mL (6-mg) prefilled syringe = £768.00

9.2   Fluids and electrolytes

9.2.1   Oral preparations for fluid and electrolyte imbalance

9.2.2   Parenteral preparations for fluid and electrolyte imbalance

The following tables give a selection of useful electrolyte values:

Electrolyte concentrations —intravenous fluids

Intravenous infusion	Millimoles per litre				
	Na$^+$	K$^+$	HCO$_3^-$	Cl$^-$	Ca^{2+}
Normal plasma values	142	4.5	26	103	2.5
Sodium Chloride 0.9%	150	—	—	150	—
Compound Sodium Lactate (Hartmann's)	131	5	29	111	2
Sodium Chloride 0.18% and Glucose 4%	30	—	—	30	—
Potassium Chloride 0.3% and Glucose 5%	—	40	—	40	—
Potassium Chloride 0.3% and Sodium Chloride 0.9%	150	40	—	190	—
To correct metabolic acidosis					
Sodium Bicarbonate 1.26%	150	—	150	—	—
Sodium Bicarbonate 8.4% for cardiac arrest	1000	—	1000	—	—
Sodium Lactate (m/6)	167	—	167	—	—

Electrolyte content —gastro-intestinal secretions

Type of fluid	Millimoles per litre				
	H^+	Na^+	K^+	HCO_3^-	Cl^-
Gastric	40–60	20–80	5–20	—	100–150
Biliary	—	120–140	5–15	30–50	80–120
Pancreatic	—	120–140	5–15	70–110	40–80
Small bowel	—	120–140	5–15	20–40	90–130

Faeces, vomit, or aspiration should be saved and analysed where possible if abnormal losses are suspected; where this is impracticable the approximations above may be helpful in planning replacement therapy

9.2.1 Oral preparations for fluid and electrolyte imbalance

9.2.1.1 Oral potassium
9.2.1.2 Oral sodium and water
9.2.1.3 Oral bicarbonate

Sodium and potassium salts, which may be given by mouth to prevent deficiencies or to treat established deficiencies of mild or moderate degree, are discussed in this section. Oral preparations for removing excess potassium and preparations for oral rehydration therapy are also included here. Oral bicarbonate, for metabolic acidosis, is also described in this section.

For reference to calcium, magnesium, and phosphate, see section 9.5.

9.2.1.1 Oral potassium

Compensation for potassium loss is especially necessary:

- in those taking digoxin or anti-arrhythmic drugs, where potassium depletion may induce arrhythmias;
- in patients in whom secondary hyperaldosteronism occurs, e.g. renal artery stenosis, cirrhosis of the liver, the nephrotic syndrome, and severe heart failure;
- in patients with excessive losses of potassium in the faeces, e.g. chronic diarrhoea associated with intestinal malabsorption or laxative abuse.

Measures to compensate for potassium loss may also be required in the elderly since they frequently take inadequate amounts of potassium in the diet (but see below for **warning** on **renal insufficiency**). Measures may also be required during long-term administration of drugs known to induce potassium loss (e.g. corticosteroids). Potassium supplements are **seldom required** with the small doses of diuretics given to treat hypertension; **potassium-sparing diuretics** (rather than potassium supplements) are recommended for prevention of hypokalaemia due to diuretics such as furosemide (frusemide) or the thiazides when these are given to eliminate oedema.

DOSAGE. If potassium salts are used for the *prevention of hypokalaemia*, then doses of potassium chloride 2 to 4 g (approx. 25 to 50 mmol) daily by mouth are suitable in patients taking a normal diet. *Smaller doses* must be used if there is *renal*

insufficiency (common in the elderly) otherwise there is **danger of hyperkalaemia**. Potassium salts cause nausea and vomiting therefore poor compliance is a major limitation to their effectiveness; where appropriate, potassium-sparing diuretics are preferable (see also above). When there is *established potassium depletion* larger doses may be necessary, the quantity depending on the severity of any continuing potassium loss (monitoring of plasma-potassium concentration and specialist advice would be required). Potassium depletion is frequently associated with chloride depletion and with metabolic alkalosis, and these disorders require correction.

ADMINISTRATION. Potassium salts are preferably given as a liquid (or effervescent) preparation, rather than modified-release tablets; they should be given as the chloride (the use of effervescent potassium tablets BPC 1968 should be restricted to *hyperchloraemic states*, section 9.2.1.3).

Salt substitutes. A number of salt substitutes which contain significant amounts of potassium chloride are readily available as health food products (e.g. *LoSalt®* and *Ruthmol®*). These should not be used by patients with renal failure as potassium intoxication may result.

POTASSIUM CHLORIDE

Indications: potassium depletion (see notes above)
Cautions: elderly, mild to moderate renal impairment (close monitoring required), intestinal stricture, history of peptic ulcer, hiatus hernia (for sustained-release preparations); **important:** special hazard if given with drugs liable to raise plasma potassium concentration such as potassium-sparing diuretics, ACE inhibitors, or ciclosporin, for other **interactions:** Appendix 1 (potassium salts)
Contra-indications: severe renal impairment, plasma potassium concentrations above 5 mmol/litre
Side-effects: nausea and vomiting (severe symptoms may indicate obstruction), oesophageal or small bowel ulceration
Dose: see notes above

NOTE. Do not confuse Effervescent Potassium Tablets BPC 1968 (section 9.2.1.3) with effervescent potassium chloride tablets. Effervescent Potassium Tablets BPC 1968 do not contain chloride ions and their use should be restricted to hyperchloraemic states (section 9.2.1.3). Effervescent Potassium Chloride Tablets BP are usually available in two strengths, one containing 6.7 mmol each of K^+ and Cl^- (corresponding to *Kloref®*), the other containing 12 mmol K^+ and 8 mmol Cl^- (corresponding to *Sando-K®*). Generic prescriptions must specify the strength required.

Kay-Cee-L® (Geistlich)
Syrup, red, sugar-free, potassium chloride 7.5% (1 mmol/mL each of K^+ and Cl^-). Net price 500 mL = £3.56. Label: 21

Kloref® (Alpharma)
Tablets, effervescent, betaine hydrochloride, potassium benzoate, bicarbonate, and chloride, equivalent to potassium chloride 500 mg (6.7 mmol each of K^+ and Cl^-). Net price 50 = £1.90. Label: 13, 21
NOTE. May be difficult to obtain

Sando-K® (HK Pharma)
Tablets, effervescent, potassium bicarbonate and chloride equivalent to potassium 470 mg (12 mmol of K^+) and chloride 285 mg (8 mmol of Cl^-). Net price 20 = £1.53. Label: 13, 21

■ Modified-release preparations

Avoid unless effervescent tablets or liquid preparations inappropriate

Slow-K® (Alliance)

Tablets, m/r, orange, s/c, potassium chloride 600 mg (8 mmol each of K⁺ and Cl⁻). Net price 20 = 55p. Label: 25, 27, counselling, swallow whole with fluid during meals while sitting or standing

Potassium removal

Ion-exchange resins may be used to remove excess potassium in *mild hyperkalaemia* or in *moderate hyperkalaemia* when there are no ECG changes; intravenous therapy is required in emergencies (section 9.2.2).

POLYSTYRENE SULPHONATE RESINS

Indications: hyperkalaemia associated with anuria or severe oliguria, and in dialysis patients

Cautions: children (impaction of resin with excessive dosage or inadequate dilution); monitor for electrolyte disturbances (stop if plasma-potassium concentration below 5 mmol/litre); pregnancy and breast-feeding; sodium-containing resin in congestive heart failure, hypertension, renal impairment, and oedema

Contra-indications: obstructive bowel disease; oral administration or reduced gut motility in neonates; avoid calcium-containing resin in hyperparathyroidism, multiple myeloma, sarcoidosis, or metastatic carcinoma

Side-effects: rectal ulceration following rectal administration; colonic necrosis reported following enemas containing sorbitol; sodium retention, hypercalcaemia, gastric irritation, anorexia, nausea and vomiting, constipation (discontinue treatment—avoid magnesium-containing laxatives), diarrhoea; calcium-containing resin may cause hypercalcaemia (in dialysed patients and occasionally in those with renal impairment), hypomagnesaemia

Dose: *by mouth*, 15 g 3–4 times daily in water (not fruit squash which has a high potassium content) or as a paste; CHILD 0.5–1 g/kg daily in divided doses

By rectum, as an enema, 30 g in methylcellulose solution, retained for 9 hours followed by irrigation to remove resin from colon; NEONATE and CHILD, 0.5–1 g/kg daily

Calcium Resonium® (Sanofi-Synthelabo)

Powder, buff, calcium polystyrene sulphonate. Net price 300 g = £47.55. Label: 13

Resonium A® (Sanofi-Synthelabo)

Powder, buff, sodium polystyrene sulphonate. Net price 454 g = £58.53. Label: 13

9.2.1.2 Oral sodium and water

Sodium chloride is indicated in states of sodium depletion and usually needs to be given intravenously (section 9.2.2). In chronic conditions associated with mild or moderate degrees of sodium depletion, e.g. in salt-losing bowel or renal disease, oral supplements of sodium chloride or sodium bicarbonate (section 9.2.1.3), according to the acid-base status of the patient, may be sufficient.

SODIUM CHLORIDE

Indications: sodium depletion; see also section 9.2.2

Slow Sodium® (HK Pharma)

Tablets, m/r, sodium chloride 600 mg (approx. 10 mmol each of Na⁺ and Cl⁻). Net price 100-tab pack = £6.05. Label: 25

Dose: prophylaxis of sodium chloride deficiency 4–8 tablets daily with water (in severe depletion up to max. 20 tablets daily)

Chronic renal salt wasting, up to 20 tablets daily with appropriate fluid intake

CHILD, according to requirements

Oral rehydration therapy (ORT)

As a worldwide problem *diarrhoea* is by far the most important indication for fluid and electrolyte replacement. Intestinal absorption of sodium and water is enhanced by glucose (and other carbohydrates). Replacement of fluid and electrolytes lost through diarrhoea can therefore be achieved by giving solutions containing sodium, potassium, and glucose or another carbohydrate such as rice starch.

Oral rehydration solutions should:

- enhance the absorption of water and electrolytes;
- replace the electrolyte deficit adequately and safely;
- contain an alkalinising agent to counter acidosis;
- be slightly hypo-osmolar (about 250 mmol/litre) to prevent the possible induction of osmotic diarrhoea;
- be simple to use in hospital and at home;
- be palatable and acceptable, especially to children;
- be readily available.

It is the policy of the World Health Organization (WHO) to promote a single oral rehydration solution but to use it flexibly (e.g. by giving extra water between drinks of oral rehydration solution to moderately dehydrated infants).

Oral rehydration solutions used in the UK are lower in sodium (50–60 mmol/litre) than the WHO formulation since, in general, patients suffer less severe sodium loss.

Rehydration should be rapid over 3 to 4 hours (except in hypernatraemic dehydration in which case rehydration should occur more slowly over 12 hours). The patient should be reassessed after initial rehydration and if still dehydrated rapid fluid replacement should continue.

Once rehydration is complete further dehydration is prevented by encouraging the patient to drink normal volumes of an appropriate fluid and by replacing continuing losses with an oral rehydration solution; in infants, breast-feeding or formula feeds should be offered between oral rehydration drinks.

For intravenous rehydration see section 9.2.2.

ORAL REHYDRATION SALTS (ORS)

Indications: fluid and electrolyte loss in diarrhoea, see notes above

Dose: according to fluid loss, usually 200–400 mL solution after every loose motion; INFANT 1–1½ times usual feed volume; CHILD 200 mL after every loose motion

■ UK formulations

NOTE. After reconstitution any unused solution should be discarded no later than 1 hour after preparation unless stored in a refrigerator when it may be kept for up to 24 hours. Proprietary brands of oral rehydration salts on sale to the public include *Boots Oral Rehydration Treatment*.

Dioralyte® (Rhône-Poulenc Rorer)
Effervescent tablets, sodium chloride 117 mg, sodium bicarbonate 336 mg, potassium chloride 186 mg, citric acid anhydrous 384 mg, anhydrous glucose 1.62 g. Net price 10-tab pack (blackcurrant- or citrus-flavoured) = £1.42
Dose: reconstitute 2 tablets with 200 mL of water (only for adults and for children over 1 year)
NOTE. Ten tablets when reconstituted with 1 litre of water provide Na$^+$ 60 mmol, K$^+$ 25 mmol, Cl$^-$ 45 mmol, citrate 20 mmol, and glucose 90 mmol
Oral powder, sodium chloride 470 mg, potassium chloride 300 mg, disodium hydrogen citrate 530 mg, glucose 3.56 g/sachet, net price 6-sachet pack = £1.96, 20-sachet pack (blackcurrant- or citrus-flavoured or natural) = £5.68
Dose: reconstitute one sachet with 200 mL of water (freshly boiled and cooled for infants)
NOTE. Five sachets reconstituted with 1 litre of water provide Na$^+$ 60 mmol, K$^+$ 20 mmol, Cl$^-$ 60 mmol, citrate 10 mmol, and glucose 90 mmol

Dioralyte® Relief (Rhône-Poulenc Rorer)
Oral powder, sodium chloride 350 mg, potassium chloride 300 mg, sodium citrate 580 mg, cooked rice powder 6 g/sachet, net price 6-sachet pack (apricot-, blackcurrant- or raspberry-flavoured) = £2.20, 20-sachet pack (apricot-flavoured) = £6.81
Dose: reconstitute one sachet with 200 mL of water (freshly boiled and cooled for infants)
NOTE. 5 sachets when reconstitued with 1 litre of water provide Na$^+$ 60 mmol, K$^+$ 20 mmol, Cl$^-$ 50 mmol and citrate 20 mmol; contains aspartame (section 9.4.1)

Electrolade® (Eastern)
Oral powder, sodium chloride 236 mg, potassium chloride 300 mg, sodium bicarbonate 500 mg, anhydrous glucose 4 g/sachet (banana-, blackcurrant-, melon-, or orange-flavoured). Net price 6-sachet (plain or multiflavoured) pack = £1.33, 20-sachet (single- or multiflavoured) pack = £4.99
Dose: reconstitute one sachet with 200 mL of water (freshly boiled and cooled for infants)
NOTE. Five sachets when reconstituted with 1 litre of water provide Na$^+$ 50 mmol, K$^+$ 20 mmol, Cl$^-$ 40 mmol, HCO$_3^-$ 30 mmol, and glucose 111 mmol

Rapolyte® (Provalis)
Oral powder, sodium chloride 350 mg, potassium chloride 300 mg, sodium citrate 600 mg, anhydrous glucose 4 g, net price 20-sachet pack (blackcurrant-, natural-, raspberry-, or tutti-frutti-flavoured) = £4.60
Dose: reconstitute one sachet with 200 mL of water (freshly boiled and cooled for infants)
NOTE. Five sachets when reconstituted with 1 litre of water provide Na$^+$ 60 mmol, K$^+$ 20 mmol, Cl$^-$ 50 mmol, citrate 10 mmol, and glucose 110 mmol

Rehidrat® (Pharmacia)
Oral powder, sodium chloride 440 mg, potassium chloride 380 mg, sodium bicarbonate 420 mg, citric acid 440 mg, glucose 4.09 g, sucrose 8.07 g, fructose 70 mg/sachet. Net price 24-sachet pack

(orange, blackcurrant or lemon and lime flavour) = £7.73; 16-sachet pack (mixed flavours) = £5.15
NOTE. Lemon and lime version stains vomit green; blackcurrant version contains greater amounts of glucose (4.13 g) and sucrose (8.17 g), and less fructose (10 mg)
Dose: reconstitute one sachet with 250 mL of water (freshly boiled and cooled for infants)
NOTE. Four sachets when reconstituted with 1 litre of water provide Na$^+$ 50 mmol, K$^+$ 50 mmol, HCO$_3^-$ 20 mmol, citrate 9 mmol, glucose approx. 91 mmol, sucrose approx. 94 mmol, and fructose approx. 1–2 mmol

■ WHO formulation

Oral Rehydration Salts (Non-proprietary)
Oral powder, sodium chloride 2.6 g, potassium chloride 1.5 g, sodium citrate 2.9 g, anhydrous glucose 13.5 g. To be dissolved in sufficient water to produce 1 litre (providing Na$^+$ 75 mmol, K$^+$ 20 mmol, Cl$^-$ 65 mmol, citrate 10 mmol, glucose 75 mmol/litre)
NOTE. Recommended by the WHO and the United Nations Children's Fund but not commonly used in the UK.

9.2.1.3   Oral bicarbonate

Sodium bicarbonate is given by mouth for *chronic acidotic states* such as uraemic acidosis or renal tubular acidosis. The dose for correction of metabolic acidosis is not predictable and the response must be assessed; sodium bicarbonate 4.8 g daily (57 mmol each of Na$^+$ and HCO$_3^-$) or more may be required. For severe metabolic acidosis, sodium bicarbonate can be given intravenously (section 9.2.2).

Sodium bicarbonate may also be used to increase the pH of the urine (see section 7.4.3); for use in dyspepsia see section 1.1.1.

Sodium supplements may increase blood pressure or cause fluid retention and pulmonary oedema in those at risk; hypokalaemia may be exacerbated.

Where *hyperchloraemic acidosis* is associated with potassium deficiency, as in some renal tubular and gastro-intestinal disorders it may be appropriate to give oral **potassium bicarbonate**, although acute or severe deficiency should be managed by intravenous therapy.

SODIUM BICARBONATE

Indications: see notes above
Cautions: see notes above; avoid in respiratory acidosis; **interactions:** Appendix 1 (antacids)
Dose: see notes above

Sodium Bicarbonate (Non-proprietary)
Capsules, sodium bicarbonate 500 mg (approx. 6 mmol each of Na$^+$ and HCO$_3^-$). Net price 20 = £6.08
Available from IVAX
Tablets, sodium bicarbonate 600 mg, net price 20 tabs = 50p
IMPORTANT. Oral solutions of sodium bicarbonate are required occasionally; these need to be obtained on special order and the strength of sodium bicarbonate should be stated on the prescription

POTASSIUM BICARBONATE

Indications: see notes above
Cautions: cardiac disease, renal impairment; **interactions:** Appendix 1 (potassium salts)

Contra-indications: hypochloraemia; plasma potassium concentration above 5 mmol/litre
Side-effects: nausea and vomiting
Dose: see notes above

Potassium Tablets, Effervescent (Non-proprietary)
Effervescent tablets, potassium bicarbonate 500 mg, potassium acid tartrate 300 mg, each tablet providing 6.5 mmol of K^+. To be dissolved in water before administration. Net price 56 = £4.20.
Label: 13, 21
Available from Alpharma, Hillcross
NOTE. These tablets do not contain chloride; for effervescent tablets containing potassium and chloride, see under Potassium Chloride, section 9.2.1.1

9.2.2 Parenteral preparations for fluid and electrolyte imbalance

9.2.2.1 Electrolytes and water
9.2.2.2 Plasma and plasma substitutes

9.2.2.1 Electrolytes and water

Solutions of electrolytes are given intravenously, to meet normal fluid and electrolyte requirements or to replenish substantial deficits or continuing losses, when the patient is nauseated or vomiting and is unable to take adequate amounts by mouth. When intravenous administration is not possible large volumes of fluid can also be given subcutaneously by hypodermoclysis.

In an individual patient the nature and severity of the electrolyte imbalance must be assessed from the history and clinical and biochemical examination. Sodium, potassium, chloride, magnesium, phosphate, and water depletion can occur singly and in combination with or without disturbances of acid-base balance; for reference to the use of magnesium and phosphates, see section 9.5.

Isotonic solutions may be infused safely into a peripheral vein. Solutions more concentrated than plasma, for example 20% glucose are best given through an indwelling catheter positioned in a large vein.

Intravenous sodium

Sodium chloride in isotonic solution provides the most important extracellular ions in near physiological concentration and is indicated in *sodium depletion* which may arise from such conditions as gastro-enteritis, diabetic ketoacidosis, ileus, and ascites. In a severe deficit of from 4 to 8 litres, 2 to 3 litres of isotonic sodium chloride may be given over 2 to 3 hours; thereafter infusion can usually be at a slower rate. Excessive administration should be avoided; the jugular venous pressure should be assessed, the bases of the lungs should be examined for crepitations, and in elderly or seriously ill patients it is often helpful to monitor the right atrial (central) venous pressure.

Chronic hyponatraemia should ideally be corrected by fluid restriction. However, if sodium chloride is required, the deficit should be corrected slowly to avoid the risk of osmotic demyelination syndrome; the rise in plasma-sodium concentration should be limited to no more than 10 mmol/litre in 24 hours.

Compound sodium lactate (Hartmann's solution) can be used instead of isotonic sodium chloride solution during surgery or in the initial management of the injured or wounded.

Sodium chloride and glucose solutions are indicated when there is combined *water and sodium depletion*. A 1:1 mixture of isotonic sodium chloride and 5% glucose allows some of the water (free of sodium) to enter body cells which suffer most from dehydration while the sodium salt with a volume of water determined by the normal plasma Na^+ remains extracellular. Maintenance fluid should accurately reflect daily requirements and close monitoring is required to avoid fluid and electrolyte imbalance. Illness or injury increase the secretion of anti-diuretic hormone and therefore the ability to excrete excess water may be impaired. Injudicious use of solutions such as sodium chloride 0.18% and glucose 4% may also cause dilutional hyponatraemia especially in children and the elderly; if necessary, guidance should be sought from a clinician experienced in the management of fluid and electrolytes.

Combined sodium, potassium, chloride, and water depletion may occur, for example, with severe diarrhoea or persistent vomiting; replacement is carried out with sodium chloride intravenous infusion 0.9% and glucose intravenous infusion 5% with potassium as appropriate.

SODIUM CHLORIDE

Indications: electrolyte imbalance, also section 9.2.1.2
Cautions: restrict intake in impaired renal function, cardiac failure, hypertension, peripheral and pulmonary oedema, toxaemia of pregnancy
Side-effects: administration of large doses may give rise to sodium accumulation and oedema
Dose: see notes above

Sodium Chloride Intravenous Infusion (Non-proprietary) PoM
Intravenous infusion, usual strength sodium chloride 0.9% (9 g, 150 mmol each of Na^+ and Cl^-/litre), this strength being supplied when normal saline for injection is requested. Net price 2-mL amp = 25p; 5-mL amp = 33p; 10-mL amp = 36p; 20-mL amp = £1.03; 50-mL amp = £2.01
In hospitals, 500- and 1000-mL packs, and sometimes other sizes, are available
NOTE. The term 'normal saline' should **not** be used to describe sodium chloride intravenous infusion 0.9%; the term 'physiological saline' is acceptable but it is preferable to give the composition (i.e. sodium chloride intravenous infusion 0.9%).

■ With other ingredients
Sodium Chloride and Glucose Intravenous Infusion (Non-proprietary) PoM
Intravenous infusion, sodium chloride 0.18% (Na^+ and Cl^- each 30 mmol/litre), glucose 4%
In hospitals, usually 500-mL packs and sometimes other sizes are available

Intravenous infusion, sodium chloride 0.9% (Na$^+$ and Cl$^-$ each 150 mmol/litre), glucose 5%
In hospitals, usually 500-mL packs and sometimes other sizes are available

Intravenous infusion, sodium chloride 0.45% (Na$^+$ and Cl$^-$ each 75 mmol/litre), glucose 2.5%
In hospitals, usually 500-mL packs and sometimes other sizes are available

Ringer's Solution for Injection [PoM]

Calcium chloride (dihydrate) 322 micrograms, potassium chloride 300 micrograms, sodium chloride 8.6 mg/mL, providing the following ions (in mmol/litre), Ca^{2+} 2.2, K$^+$ 4, Na$^+$ 147, Cl$^-$ 156
In hospitals, 500- and 1000-mL packs, and sometimes other sizes, are available

Sodium Lactate Intravenous Infusion, Compound (Non-proprietary) [PoM]

(Hartmann's Solution for Injection; Ringer-Lactate Solution for Injection)
Intravenous infusion, sodium chloride 0.6%, sodium lactate 0.25%, potassium chloride 0.04%, calcium chloride 0.027% (containing Na$^+$ 131 mmol, K$^+$ 5 mmol, Ca^{2+} 2 mmol, HCO$_3^-$ (as lactate) 29 mmol, Cl$^-$ 111 mmol/litre)
In hospitals, 500- and 1000-mL packs, and sometimes other sizes are available

Intravenous glucose

Glucose solutions (5%) are mainly used to replace water deficits and should be given alone when there is no significant loss of electrolytes. Average water requirements in a healthy adult are 1.5 to 2.5 litres daily and this is needed to balance unavoidable losses of water through the skin and lungs and to provide sufficient for urinary excretion. Water depletion (dehydration) tends to occur when these losses are not matched by a comparable intake, as for example may occur in coma or dysphagia or in the aged or apathetic who may not drink water in sufficient amount on their own initiative.

Excessive loss of water without loss of electrolytes is uncommon, occurring in fevers, hyperthyroidism, and in uncommon water-losing renal states such as diabetes insipidus or hypercalcaemia. The volume of glucose solution needed to replace deficits with the severity of the disorder, but usually lies within the range of 2 to 6 litres.

Glucose solutions are also given in regimens with calcium, bicarbonate, and insulin for the emergency management of *hyperkalaemia*. They are also given, after correction of hyperglycaemia, during treatment of diabetic ketoacidosis, when they must be accompanied by continuing insulin infusion.

GLUCOSE

(Dextrose Monohydrate)
NOTE. Glucose BP is the monohydrate but Glucose Intravenous Infusion BP is a sterile solution of anhydrous glucose or glucose monohydrate, potency being expressed in terms of anhydrous glucose
Indications: fluid replacement (see notes above), provision of energy (section 9.3)
Side-effects: glucose injections especially if hypertonic may have a low pH and may cause venous irritation and thrombophlebitis
Dose: water replacement, see notes above; energy source, 1–3 litres daily of 20–50% solution

Glucose Intravenous Infusion (Non-proprietary) [PoM]

Intravenous infusion, glucose or anhydrous glucose (potency expressed in terms of anhydrous glucose), usual strength 5% (50 mg/mL). 25% solution, net price 25-mL amp = £2.21; 50% solution, 25-mL amp = £3.80, 50-mL amp = £1.63
In hospitals, 500- and 1000-mL packs, and sometimes other sizes and strengths, are available; also available from Celltech (*Min-I-Jet® Glucose*, 50% in 50-mL disposable syringe)

Intravenous potassium

Potassium chloride and sodium chloride intravenous infusion is the initial treatment for the correction of *severe hypokalaemia* and when sufficient potassium cannot be taken by mouth. Ready-mixed infusion solutions should be used when possible; alternatively, potassium chloride concentrate, as ampoules containing 1.5 g (K$^+$ 20 mmol) in 10 mL, is **thoroughly mixed** with 500 mL of sodium chloride 0.9% intravenous infusion and given slowly over 2 to 3 hours, with specialist advice and ECG monitoring in difficult cases. Higher concentrations of potassium chloride may be given in very severe depletion, but require specialist advice.

Repeated measurements of plasma-potassium concentration are necessary to determine whether further infusions are required and to avoid the development of hyperkalaemia, which is especially likely in renal impairment.

Initial potassium replacement therapy should **not** involve glucose infusions, because glucose may cause a further decrease in the plasma-potassium concentration.

POTASSIUM CHLORIDE

Indications: electrolyte imbalance; see also oral potassium supplements, section 9.2.1.1
Cautions: for intravenous infusion the concentration of solution should not usually exceed 3.2 g (43 mmol)/litre; specialist advice and ECG monitoring (see notes above); **interactions:** Appendix 1 (potassium salts)
Side-effects: rapid infusion toxic to heart
Dose: *by slow intravenous infusion*, depending on the deficit or the daily maintenance requirements, see also notes above

Potassium Chloride and Glucose Intravenous Infusion (Non-proprietary) [PoM]

Intravenous infusion, usual strength potassium chloride 0.3% (3 g, 40 mmol each of K$^+$ and Cl$^-$/litre) with 5% of anhydrous glucose
In hospitals, 500- and 1000-mL packs, and sometimes other sizes, are available

Potassium Chloride and Sodium Chloride Intravenous Infusion (Non-proprietary) [PoM]

Intravenous infusion, usual strength potassium chloride 0.3% (3 g/litre) and sodium chloride 0.9% (9 g/litre), containing K$^+$ 40 mmol, Na$^+$ 150 mmol, and Cl$^-$ 190 mmol/litre
In hospitals, 500- and 1000-mL packs, and sometimes other sizes, are available

Potassium Chloride, Sodium Chloride, and Glucose Intravenous Infusion (Non-proprietary) [PoM]

Intravenous infusion, sodium chloride 0.18% (1.8 g, Na$^+$ 30 mmol/litre) with 4% of anhydrous glucose and usually sufficient potassium chloride to provide K$^+$ 10–40 mmol/litre (to be specified by the prescriber)

In hospitals, 500- and 1000-mL packs, and sometimes other sizes, are available

Potassium Chloride Concentrate, Sterile (Non-proprietary) PoM

Sterile concentrate, potassium chloride 15% (150 mg, approximately 2 mmol each of K$^+$ and Cl$^-$/mL). Net price 10-mL amp = 42p

IMPORTANT. Must be diluted with **not less** than 50 times its volume of sodium chloride intravenous infusion 0.9% or other suitable diluent and **mixed well**

Solutions containing 10 and 20% of potassium chloride are also available in both 5- and 10-mL ampoules

---

Bicarbonate and lactate

Sodium bicarbonate is used to control severe *metabolic acidosis* (as in renal failure). Since this condition is usually attended by sodium depletion, it is reasonable to correct this first by the administration of isotonic sodium chloride intravenous infusion, provided the kidneys are not primarily affected and the degree of acidosis is not so severe as to impair renal function. In these circumstances, isotonic sodium chloride alone is usually effective as it restores the ability of the kidneys to generate bicarbonate. In renal acidosis or in severe metabolic acidosis of any origin (for example blood pH < 7.1) sodium bicarbonate (1.26%) may be infused in isotonic sodium chloride when the acidosis remains unresponsive to correction of anoxia or fluid depletion; a total volume of up to 6 litres (4 litres of sodium chloride and 2 litres of sodium bicarbonate) may be necessary in the adult. In severe shock due for example to cardiac arrest (see section 2.7), metabolic acidosis may develop without sodium depletion; in these circumstances sodium bicarbonate is best given in a small volume of hypertonic solution, such as 50 mL of 8.4% solution intravenously; plasma pH should be monitored.

Sodium bicarbonate infusion is also used in the emergency management of *hyperkalaemia* (see also under Glucose).

Sodium lactate intravenous infusion is obsolete in metabolic acidosis, and carries the risk of producing lactic acidosis, particularly in seriously ill patients with poor tissue perfusion or impaired hepatic function.

SODIUM BICARBONATE

Indications: metabolic acidosis
Dose: *by slow intravenous injection,* a strong solution (up to 8.4%), or *by continuous intravenous infusion,* a weaker solution (usually 1.26%), an amount appropriate to the body base deficit (see notes above)

Sodium Bicarbonate Intravenous Infusion PoM
Usual strength sodium bicarbonate 1.26% (12.6 g, 150 mmol each of Na$^+$ and HCO$_3^-$/litre); various other strengths available

In hospitals, 500- and 1000-mL packs, and sometimes other sizes, are available

Min-I-Jet® Sodium Bicarbonate (Celltech) PoM
Intravenous injection, sodium bicarbonate in disposable syringe, net price 4.2%, 10 mL = £5.29; 8.4%, 10 mL = £5.71, 50 mL = £7.75

SODIUM LACTATE ▱

Indications: see notes above

Sodium Lactate (Non-proprietary) PoM ▱
Intravenous infusion, sodium lactate M/6, contains the following ions (in mmol/litre), Na$^+$ 167, HCO$_3^-$ (as lactate) 167

Water

Water for Injections. PoM Net price 1-mL amp = 18p; 2-mL amp = 17p; 5-mL amp = 28p; 10-mL amp = 31p; 20-mL amp = 55p; 50-mL amp = £1.91; 100-mL amp = 23p

---

9.2.2.2 Plasma and plasma substitutes

Albumin solutions, prepared from whole blood, contain soluble proteins and electrolytes but no clotting factors, blood group antibodies, or plasma cholinesterases; they may be given without regard to the recipient's blood group.

Albumin solutions are used for the treatment of severe hypoproteinaemia, particularly when associated with a low plasma volume. Concentrated albumin solutions may also be used to obtain a diuresis in hypoalbuminaemic patients (e.g. in hepatic cirrhosis). The use of albumin solutions in acute plasma or blood loss may be wasteful; plasma substitutes are more appropriate. Albumin solutions have been linked with increased mortality in patients with hypovolaemia or hypoalbuminaemia such as those with acute blood loss or burns; it is uncertain whether albumin is responsible for the extra deaths.

> Plasma and plasma substitutes are often used in very ill patients whose condition is unstable. Therefore, close monitoring is required and fluid and electrolyte therapy should be adjusted according to the patient's condition at all times.

CSM advice. Following the publication of a meta-analysis in July 1998 concerning the safety of human albumin solution, the CSM has asked that product literature for albumin products should reflect the following:

- indications should focus on the use of albumin to replace lost fluids rather than the underlying cause of hypovolaemia; hypoalbuminaemia itself is not an appropriate indication;
- warnings should be added about the risks of hypervolaemia and cardiovascular overload, and the importance of monitoring patients receiving albumin to avoid these complications;
- special care is needed when administering albumin in conditions where capillary integrity is affected.

ALBUMIN SOLUTION

(Human Albumin Solution)

A solution containing protein derived from plasma, serum, or normal placentas; at least 95% of the protein is albumin. The solution may be isotonic (containing 4–5% protein) or concentrated (containing 15–25% protein).

Indications: see under preparations, below and also CSM advice above

Cautions: history of cardiac or circulatory disease (administer slowly to avoid rapid rise in blood pressure and cardiac failure, and monitor cardiovascular and respiratory function); correct dehydration when administering concentrated solution

Contra-indications: cardiac failure; severe anaemia

Side-effects: hypersensitivity reactions (including anaphylaxis) with nausea, vomiting, increased salivation, fever, tachycardia, hypotension and chills reported

■ Isotonic solutions

Indications: acute or sub-acute loss of plasma volume e.g. in burns, pancreatitis, trauma, and complications of surgery; plasma exchange

Available as: *Human Albumin Solution 4.5%* (50-, 100-, 250- and 400-mL bottles—Baxter Bioscience); *Human Albumin Solution 5%* (100-, 250- and 500-mL bottles—Grifols); *ALBA®* 4.5% (100- and 400-mL bottles—SNBTS); *Albutein®* 5% (250- and 500-mL bottles—Grifols); *Octalbin®* 5% (100- and 200-mL bottles—Octapharm); *Zenalb®* 4.5% (50-, 100-, 250-, and 500-mL bottles—BPL)

■ Concentrated solutions (20–25%)

Indications: severe hypoalbuminaemia associated with low plasma volume and generalised oedema where salt and water restriction with plasma volume expansion are required; adjunct in the treatment of hyperbilirubinaemia by exchange transfusion in the newborn

Available as: *Human Albumin Solution 20%* (50- and 100-mL vials—Baxter Bioscience); *Human Albumin Solution 20%* (50- and 100-mL bottles—Grifols); *ALBA®* 20% (100-mL vials—SNBTS); *Albutein®* 20% (50- and 100-mL bottles—Grifols); *Albutein®* 25% (20-, 50-, and 100-mL vials—Grifols); *Octalbin®* 20% (50- and 100-mL bottles—Octapharm); *Zenalb®* 20% (50- and 100-mL bottles—BPL)

Plasma substitutes

Dextrans, gelatin, and the etherified starches, **hexastarch, hydroxyethyl starch** and **pentastarch** are macromolecular substances which are metabolised slowly; they may be used at the outset to expand and maintain blood volume in shock arising from conditions such as burns or septicaemia. Plasma substitutes may be used as an immediate short-term measure to treat haemorrhage until blood is available. They are rarely needed when shock is due to sodium and water depletion because, in these circumstances, the shock responds to water and electrolyte repletion. See also section 2.7.1 for the management of shock.

Plasma substitutes should **not** be used to maintain plasma volume in conditions such as burns or peritonitis where there is loss of plasma protein, water and electrolytes over periods of several days or weeks. In these situations, plasma or plasma protein fractions containing large amounts of albumin should be given.

Large volumes of *some* plasma substitutes can increase the risk of bleeding through depletion of coagulation factors; however, the risk is reduced if 1–2 litres of a substitute such as hexastarch are used.

Dextran 70 by intravenous infusion is used predominantly for volume expansion. Dextran 40 intravenous infusion is used in an attempt to improve peripheral blood flow in ischaemic disease of the limbs. Dextrans 40 and 70 have also been used in the prophylaxis of thromboembolism but are now rarely used for this purpose.

Dextrans may interfere with blood group crossmatching or biochemical measurements and these should be carried out before infusion is begun.

> Plasma and plasma substitutes are often used in very ill patients whose condition is unstable. Therefore, close monitoring is required and fluid and electrolyte therapy should be adjusted according to the patient's condition at all times.

CAUTIONS. Plasma substitutes should be used with caution in patients with cardiac disease or renal impairment; urine output should be monitored. Care should be taken to avoid haematocrit concentration from falling below 25–30% and the patient should be monitored for hypersensitivity reactions.

SIDE-EFFECTS. Hypersensitivity reactions may occur including, rarely, severe anaphylactoid reactions. Transient increase in bleeding time may occur.

DEXTRAN 40

Dextrans of weight average molecular weight about '40 000'

Indications: conditions associated with peripheral local slowing of the blood flow; prophylaxis of post-surgical thromboembolic disease (but see notes above)

Cautions: see notes above; can interfere with some laboratory tests (see also above); correct dehydration beforehand, give adequate fluids during therapy and, where possible, monitor central venous pressure; pregnancy (Appendix 4)

Side-effects: see notes above

Dose: *by intravenous infusion,* initially 500–1000 mL; further doses are given according to the patient's condition (see notes above)

Dextran 40® (Baxter) PoM

Intravenous infusion, dextran 40 intravenous infusion in glucose intravenous infusion 5% or in sodium chloride intravenous infusion 0.9%. Net price 500-mL bag (both) = £4.56

DEXTRAN 70

Dextrans of weight average molecular weight about '70 000'

Indications: short-term blood volume expansion; prophylaxis of post-surgical thromboembolic disease (but see notes above)

Cautions: see notes above; can interfere with some laboratory tests (see also above); where possible, monitor central venous pressure; pregnancy (Appendix 4)

Side-effects: see notes above

Dose: *by intravenous infusion,* after moderate to severe haemorrhage or in the shock phase of burn injury (initial 48 hours), 500–1000 mL rapidly initially followed by 500 mL later if necessary (see also notes above); total dosage should not exceed 20 mL/kg during initial 24 hours; CHILD total dosage should not exceed 20 mL/kg

Dextran 70® (Baxter) **PoM**

Intravenous infusion, dextran 70 intravenous infusion in glucose intravenous infusion 5% or in sodium chloride intravenous infusion 0.9%. Net price 500-mL bag (both) = £4.56

■ Hypertonic solution

RescueFlow® (Vitaline) **PoM**

Intravenous infusion, dextran 70 intravenous infusion 6% in sodium chloride intravenous infusion 7.5%. Net price 250-mL bag = £28.50

Indications: initial treatment of hypovolaemia with hypotension induced by traumatic injury
Cautions: see notes above; severe hyperglycaemia and hyperosmolality
Dose: by intravenous infusion over 2–5 minutes, 250 mL, followed immediately by administration of isotonic fluids

---

GELATIN

NOTE. The gelatin is partially degraded

Indications: low blood volume

Cautions: see notes above

Side-effects: see notes above

Dose: *by intravenous infusion*, initially 500–1000 mL of a 3.5–4% solution (see notes above)

Gelofusine® (Braun) **PoM**

Intravenous infusion, succinylated gelatin (modified fluid gelatin, average molecular weight 30 000) 40 g (4%), Na^+ 154 mmol, Cl^- 120 mmol/litre, net price 500-mL *Ecobag*® = £4.63, 1-litre *Ecobag*® = £9.45

Volplex® (Cambridge) **PoM**

Intravenous infusion, succinylated gelatin (modified fluid gelatin, average molecular weight 30 000) 40 g (4%), Na^+ 154 mmol, Cl^- 125 mmol/litre, net price 500-mL bag = £5.05

ETHERIFIED STARCH

A starch composed of more than 90% of amylopectin that has been etherified with hydroxyethyl groups; hetastarch has a higher degree of etherification than pentastarch

Indications: low blood volume

Cautions: see notes above; children

Side-effects: see notes above

Dose: see under preparations below

■ Hexastarch

eloHAES® (Fresenius Kabi) **PoM**

Intravenous infusion, hexastarch (weight average molecular weight 200 000) 6% in sodium chloride intravenous infusion 0.9%. Net price 500-mL *Steriflex*® bag = £12.50

Dose: by intravenous infusion, 500–1000 mL; usual daily max. 1500 mL (see notes above)

■ Pentastarch

HAES-steril® (Fresenius Kabi) **PoM**

Intravenous infusion, pentastarch (weight average molecular weight 200 000), net price (both in sodium chloride intravenous infusion 0.9%) 6%, 500 mL = £10.50; 10%, 500 mL = £16.50

Dose: by intravenous infusion, pentastarch 6%, up to 2500 mL daily; pentastarch 10%, up to 1500 mL daily (see notes above)

Hemohes® (Braun) **PoM**

Intravenous infusion, pentastarch (weight average molecular weight 200 000), net price (both in

sodium chloride intravenous infusion 0.9%) 6%, 500 mL = £12.50; 10%, 500 mL = £16.50

Dose: by intravenous infusion, pentastarch 6%, up to 2500 mL daily; pentastarch 10%, up to 1500 mL daily (see notes above)

■ Tetrastarch

Voluven® (Fresenius Kabi) **PoM**

Intravenous infusion, hydroxyethyl starch (weight average molecular weight 130 000) 6% in sodium chloride intravenous infusion 0.9%, net price 500-mL bag = £12.50

Dose: by intravenous infusion, up to 50 mL/kg daily (see notes above)

9.3   Intravenous nutrition

When adequate feeding through the alimentary tract is not possible, nutrients may be given by intravenous infusion. This may be in addition to ordinary oral or tube feeding—**supplemental parenteral nutrition**, or may be the sole source of nutrition—**total parenteral nutrition** (TPN). Indications for this method include preparation of undernourished patients for surgery, chemotherapy, or radiation therapy; severe or prolonged disorders of the gastro-intestinal tract; major surgery, trauma, or burns; prolonged coma or refusal to eat; and some patients with renal or hepatic failure. The composition of proprietary preparations available is given in the table below.

Total parenteral nutrition requires the use of a solution containing amino acids, glucose, fat, electrolytes, trace elements, and vitamins. This is now commonly provided by the pharmacy in the form of a 3-litre bag. A single dose of vitamin B_{12}, as hydroxocobalamin, is given by intramuscular injection; regular vitamin B_{12} injections are not usually required unless total parenteral nutrition continues for many months. Folic acid is given in a dose of 15 mg once or twice each week, usually in the nutrition solution. Other vitamins are usually given daily; they are generally introduced in the parenteral nutrition solution. Alternatively, if the patient is able to take small amounts by mouth, vitamins may be given orally.

The nutrition solution is infused through a central venous catheter inserted under full surgical precautions. Alternatively infusion through a peripheral vein is used for supplementary as well as total parenteral nutrition for periods of up to a month, depending on the availability of peripheral veins; factors prolonging cannula life and preventing thrombophlebitis include the use of soft polyurethane paediatric cannulas and use of feeds of low osmolality and neutral pH. Only nutritional fluids should be given by the dedicated intravenous line.

Before starting, the patient should be well oxygenated with a near normal circulating blood volume and attention should be given to renal function and acid-base status. Appropriate biochemical tests should have been carried out beforehand and serious deficits corrected. Nutritional and electrolyte status must be monitored throughout treatment.

Complications of long-term TPN include gall bladder sludging, gall stones, cholestasis and abnormal liver function tests. For details of the prevention

Proprietary Infusion Fluids for Parenteral Feeding

Preparation	Nitrogen g/litre	[1]Energy kJ/litre	Electrolytes mmol/litre					Other components/litre
			K$^+$	Mg^{2+}	Na$^+$	Acet$^-$	Cl$^-$	
Aminoplasmal 5% E (Braun) Net price 500 mL = £9.02	8		25	2.6	43	59	29	dihydrogen phosphate 9 mmol, malic acid 1.01 g
Aminoplasmal 10% (Braun) Net price 500 mL = £17.06	16						57	
Clinimix N9G20E (Baxter) Net price (dual compartment bag of amino acids with electrolytes 1000 mL and glucose 20% with calcium 1000 mL) = £29.00	4.55	1680	30	2.5	35	50	40	Ca^{2+} 2.25 mmol, phosphate 15 mmol, anhydrous glucose 100 g
Clinimix N14G30E (Baxter) Net price (dual compartment bag of amino acids with electrolytes 1000 mL and glucose 30% with calcium 1000 mL) = £33.00	7	2520	30	2.5	35	70	40	Ca^{2+} 2.25 mmol, phosphate 15 mmol, anhydrous glucose 150 g
ClinOleic 20% (Baxter) Net price 100 mL = £6.28; 250 mL = £10.08; 500 mL = £13.88		8360						purified olive and soya oil 200 g, glycerol 22.5 g, egg phosphatides 12 g
Compleven (Fresenius Kabi) Net price (2500-mL triple compartment bag of amino acids 1000 mL, glucose 1000 mL, lipid emulsion 500 mL) = £67.00	4.8	3275	20	2	32		32.4	Ca^{2+} 2 mmol, Zn^{2+} 0.04 mmol, glycerophosphate 8 mmol, anhydrous glucose 96 g, soya oil 40 g, egg lecithin 2.4 g, glycerol 2.4 g
Glamin (Fresenius Kabi) Net price 250 mL = £14.16; 500 mL = £26.38	22.4				62			
Hyperamine 30 (Braun) Net price 500 mL = £23.67	30				5			
Intrafusin 11 (Fresenius Kabi) Net price 1000 mL = £14.24	11.4		40	5	80		76	Ca^{2+} 3 mmol, phosphate 20 mmol, citrate 6 mmol
Intrafusin 22 (Fresenius Kabi) Net price 500 mL = £14.24	22.8							
Intralipid 10% (Fresenius Kabi) Net price 100 mL = £3.90; 500 mL = £8.58		4600						soya oil 100 g, glycerol 22 g, purified egg phospholipids 12 g, phosphate 15 mmol
Intralipid 20% (Fresenius Kabi) Net price 100 mL = £5.85; 250 mL = £9.65; 500 mL = £12.87		8400						soya oil 200 g, glycerol 22 g, purified egg phospholipids 12 g, phosphate 15 mmol
Intralipid 30% (Fresenius Kabi) Net price 333 mL = £14.40		12600						soya oil 300 g, glycerol 16.7 g, purified egg phospholipids 12 g, phosphate 15 mmol
Ivelip 10% (Baxter) Net price 500 mL = £9.08		4600						soya oil 100 g, glycerol 25 g
Ivelip 20% (Baxter) Net price 100 mL = £6.28; 500 mL = £13.88		8400						soya oil 200 g, glycerol 25 g
Kabiven (Fresenius Kabi) Net price (triple compartment bag of amino acids and electrolytes 300 mL, 450 mL, 600 mL, or 750 mL; glucose 526 mL, 790 mL, 1053 mL, or 1316 mL; lipid emulsion 200 mL, 300 mL, 400 mL, or 500 mL) 1026 mL = £35.00, 1540 mL = £50.00, 2053 mL = £67.00, 2566 mL = £70.00	5.3	3275	23	4	31	38	45	Ca^{2+} 2 mmol, phosphate 9.7 mmol, anhydrous glucose 97 g, soya oil 39 g
Kabiven Peripheral (Fresenius Kabi) Net price (triple compartment bag of amino acids and electrolytes 300 mL, 400 mL, or 500 mL; glucose 885 mL, 1180 mL, or 1475 mL; lipid emulsion 255 mL, 340 mL, or 425 mL) 1440 mL = £35.00, 1920 mL = £50.00, 2400 mL = £64.00	3.75	2625	17	2.8	22	27	33	Ca^{2+} 1.4 mmol, phosphate 7.5 mmol, anhydrous glucose 67.5 g, soya oil 35.4 g
Lipofundin MCT/LCT 10% (Braun) Net price 100 mL = £7.70; 500 mL = £12.90		4430						soya oil 50 g, medium chain triglycerides 50 g
Lipofundin MCT/LCT 20% (Braun) Net price 100 mL = £12.51; 250 mL = £11.30; 500 mL = £19.18		8000						soya oil 100 g, medium chain triglycerides 100 g

1. Excludes protein- or amino acid-derived energy
Note. 1000 kcal = 4200 kJ; 1000 kJ = 238.8 kcal. All entries are PoM

Proprietary Infusion Fluids for Parenteral Feeding

Preparation	Nitrogen g/litre	[1]Energy kJ/litre	K+	Mg2+	Na+	Acet-	Cl-	Other components/litre
Lipofundin N 10% (Braun) Net price 100 mL = £7.10; 250 mL = £9.50; 500 mL = £11.76		4470						soya oil 100 g, glycerol 25 g, egg lethicin 8 g
Lipofundin N 20% (Braun) Net price 100 mL = £8.10; 250 mL = £9.99; 500 mL = £18.38		8520						soya oil 200 g, glycerol 25 g, egg lethicin 12 g
Nutracel 400 (Baxter) Net price 500 mL = £2.43		3400			18	0.16	66	Ca2+ 15 mmol, Mn2+ 0.01 mmol, Zn2+ 0.08 mmol, anhydrous glucose 200 g
Nutracel 800 (Baxter) Net price 1000 mL = £4.19		3400			9	0.08	33	Ca2+ 7.5 mmol, Mn2+ 0.005 mmol, Zn2+ 0.04 mmol, anhydrous glucose 200 g
NuTRIflex Lipid basal (Braun) Net price (triple compartment bag of amino acids 500 mL, 750 mL or 1000 mL; glucose 500 mL, 750 mL or 1000 mL; lipid emulsion 20% 250 mL, 375 mL or 500 mL) 1250 mL = £41.50, 1875 mL = £56.20, 2500 mL = £64.00	3.68	3268	28	3.2	40	36	32	Ca2+ 3.2 mmol, anhydrous glucose 100 g, phosphate 12 mmol, soya oil 20 g, medium chain trigylcerides 20 g
NuTRIflex Lipid peri (Braun) Net price (triple compartment bag of amino acids 500 mL or 1000 mL; glucose 500 mL or 1000 mL; lipid emulsion 20% 250 mL or 500 mL) 1250 mL = £43.38, 2500 mL = £65.05	4.56	2664	24	2.4	40	32	38.4	Ca2+ 2.4 mmol, Zn2+ 0.024 mmol, phosphate 6 mmol, anhydrous glucose 64 g, soya oil 20 g, medium chain triglycerides 20 g
NuTRIflex Lipid plus (Braun) Net price (triple compartment bag of amino acids 500 mL, 750 mL or 1000 mL; glucose 500 mL, 750 mL or 1000 mL; lipid emulsion 20% 250 mL, 375 mL or 500 mL) 1250 mL = £47.17, 1875 mL = £60.23, 2500 mL = £69.27	5.44	3600	28	3.2	40	36	36	Ca2+ 3.2 mmol, Zn2+ 0.024 mmol, phosphate 12 mmol, anhydrous glucose 120 g, soya oil 20 g, medium chain triglycerides 20 g
NuTRIflex Lipid plus without Electrolytes (Braun) Net price (triple compartment bag of amino acids 500 mL, 750 mL or 1000 mL; glucose 500 mL, 750 mL or 1000 mL; lipid emulsion 20% 250 mL, 375 mL or 500 mL) 1250 mL = £47.17, 1875 mL = £60.23, 2500 mL = £69.27	5.44	3600						anhydrous glucose 120 g, soya oil 20 g, medium chain triglycerides 20 g
NuTRIflex Lipid special (Braun) Net price (triple compartment bag of amino acids 500 mL, 750 mL or 1000 mL; glucose 500 mL, 750 mL or 1000 mL; lipid emulsion 20% 250 mL, 375 mL or 500 mL) 1250 mL = £57.69, 1875 mL = £75.58, 2500 mL = £89.21	8	4004	37.6	4.24	53.6	48	48	Ca2+ 4.24 mmol, Zn2+ 0.032 mmol, phosphate 16 mmol, anhydrous glucose 144 g, soya oil 20 g, medium chain triglycerides 20 g
NuTRIflex Lipid special without Electrolytes (Braun) Net price (triple compartment bag of amino acids 500 mL, 750 mL or 1000 mL; glucose 500 mL, 750 mL or 1000 mL; lipid emulsion 20% 250 mL, 375 mL or 500 mL) 1250 mL = £57.69, 1875 mL = £75.58, 2500 mL = £89.21	8	4004						anhydrous glucose 144 g, soya oil 20 g, medium chain triglycerides 20 g
Nutriflex Basal (Braun) Net price (dual compartment bag of 800 mL and 1200 mL) = £28.35	4.6	2095	30	5.7	49.9	35	50	Ca2+ 3.6 mmol, phosphate 12.8 mmol, anhydrous glucose 125 g
Nutriflex Peri (Braun) Net price (dual compartment bag of 800 mL and 1200 mL) = £33.00	5.7	1340	15	4	27	19.5	31.6	Ca2+ 2.5 mmol, phosphate 5.7 mmol, anhydrous glucose 80 g
Nutriflex Plus (Braun) Net price (dual compartment bag of 800 mL and 1200 mL) = £39.18	6.8	2510	25	5.7	37.2	22.9	35.5	Ca2+ 3.6 mmol, phosphate 20 mmol, anhydrous glucose 150 g
Nutriflex Special (Braun) Net price (dual compartment bag of 750 mL and 750 mL) = £43.30	10	4020	25.7	5	40.5	22	49.5	Ca2+ 4.1 mmol, phosphate 15 mmol, anhydrous glucose 240 g

1. Excludes protein- or amino acid-derived energy
Note. 1000 kcal = 4200 kJ; 1000 kJ = 238.8 kcal. All entries are PoM

Proprietary Infusion Fluids for Parenteral Feeding

Preparation	Nitrogen g/litre	[1]Energy kJ/litre	Electrolytes mmol/litre					Other components/litre
			K^+	Mg^{2+}	Na^+	Acet⁻	Cl⁻	
OliClinomel N4-550E (Baxter) Net price (triple compartment bag of amino acids with electrolytes 1000 mL; glucose 20% 1000 mL; lipid emulsion 10% 500 mL) 2500 mL = £69.30	3.6	2184	16	2.2	21	30	33	Ca^{2+} 2 mmol, phosphate 8.5 mmol, refined olive and soya oil 20 g, anhydrous glucose 80 g
OliClinomel N4-720E (Baxter) Net price (triple compartment bag of amino acids with electrolytes 1000 mL; glucose 20% 1000 mL; lipid emulsion 20% 500 mL) 2500 mL = £69.30	3.64	3024	24	2	28	40	40	Ca^{2+} 1.8 mmol, phosphate 8 mmol, refined olive and soya oil 40 g, anhydrous glucose 80 g
OliClinomel N6-900E (Baxter) Net price (triple compartment bag of amino acids with electrolytes 800 mL or 1000 mL; glucose 30% 800 mL or 1000 mL; lipid emulsion 20% 400 mL or 500 mL) 2000 mL = £70.40, 2500 mL = £75.90	5.6	3696	24	2.2	32	53	46	Ca^{2+} 2 mmol, phosphate 10 mmol, refined olive and soya oil 40 g, anhydrous glucose 120 g
OliClinomel N7-1000 (Baxter) Net price (triple compartment bag of amino acids with electrolytes 400 mL or 600 mL; glucose 40% 400 mL or 600 mL; lipid emulsion 20% 200 mL or 300 mL) 1000 mL = £28.75, 1500 mL = £43.70	6.6	4368				37	16	Phosphate 3 mmol, refined olive and soya oil 40 g, anhydrous glucose 160 g
Plasma-Lyte 148 (water) (Baxter) Net price 1000 mL = £1.59			5	1.5	140	27	98	gluconate 23 mmol
Plasma-Lyte 148 (dextrose 5%) (Baxter) Net price 1000 mL = £1.59		840	5	1.5	140	27	98	gluconate 23 mmol, anhydrous glucose 50 g
Plasma-Lyte M (dextrose 5%) (Baxter) Net price 1000 mL = £1.33		840	16	1.5	40	12	40	Ca^{2+} 2.5 mmol, lactate 12 mmol, anhydrous glucose 50 g
[2]Primene 10% (Baxter) Net price 100 mL = £5.78, 250 mL = £7.92	15						19	
StructoKabiven Electrolyte Free (Fresenius Kabi) Net price (triple compartment bag of amino acids 750 mL or 1000 mL; glucose 42% 446 mL or 595 mL; lipid emulsion 281 mL or 375 mL) 1477 mL = £69.00, 1970 mL = £74.00	8	3685			74.5			Phosphate 2.8 mmol, anhydrous glucose 127 g, glycerol 4.23 g, egg phospholipids 4.56 g, purified structured triglyceride 38.5 g (contains coconut oil, palm kernel oil and soya oil triglycerides)
Structolipid 20% (Fresenius Kabi) Net price 500 mL = £16.09		8200						Purified structured triglyceride 200 g (contains coconut oil, palm kernel oil, and soya oil triglycerides)
Synthamin 9 (Baxter) Net price 500 mL = £6.66; 1000 mL = £12.34	9.1		60	5	70	100	70	acid phosphate 30 mmol
Synthamin 9 EF (electrolyte-free) (Baxter) Net price 500 mL = £6.66; 1000 mL = £12.34	9.1					44	22	
Synthamin 14 (Baxter) Net price 500 mL = £9.64; 1000 mL = £17.13; 3000 mL = £48.98	14		60	5	70	140	70	acid phosphate 30 mmol
Synthamin 14 EF (electrolyte–free) (Baxter) Net price 500 mL = £9.87; 1000 mL = £17.51	14					68	34	
Synthamin 17 (Baxter) Net price 500 mL = £12.66; 1000 mL = £23.00	16.5		60	5	70	150	70	acid phosphate 30 mmol
Synthamin 17 EF (electrolyte–free) (Baxter) Net price 500 mL = £12.66	16.5					82	40	
Vamin 9 (Fresenius Kabi) Net price 500 mL = £5.85; 1000 mL = £10.04	9.4		20	1.5	50		50	Ca^{2+} 2.5 mmol
Vamin 9 Glucose (Fresenius Kabi) Net price 100 mL = £3.02; 500 mL = £6.14; 1000 mL = £11.02	9.4	1700	20	1.5	50		50	Ca^{2+} 2.5 mmol, anhydrous glucose 100 g

1. Excludes protein- or amino acid-derived energy
2. For use in neonates and children only
Note. 1000 kcal = 4200 kJ; 1000 kJ = 238.8 kcal. All entries are PoM

Proprietary Infusion Fluids for Parenteral Feeding

Preparation	Nitrogen g/litre	[1]Energy kJ/litre	Electrolytes mmol/litre					Other components/litre
			K^+	Mg^{2+}	Na^+	Acet⁻	Cl⁻	
Vamin 14 (Fresenius Kabi) Net price 500 mL = £8.63; 1000 mL = £14.67	13.5		50	8	100	135	100	Ca^{2+} 5 mmol, SO_4^{2-} 8 mmol
Vamin 14 (Electrolyte-Free) (Fresenius Kabi) Net price 500 mL = £8.29; 1000 mL = £14.67	13.5				90			
Vamin 18 (Electrolyte-Free) (Fresenius Kabi) Net price 500 mL = £10.97; 1000 mL = £19.74	18				110			
Vaminolact (Fresenius Kabi) Net price 100 mL = £3.36; 500 mL = £7.75	9.3							
Vitrimix KV (Fresenius Kabi) Net price (combined pack of Intralipid 20% 250 mL and Vamin 9 glucose 750 mL) = £19.40	7	3340	15	1.1	38		38	Ca^{2+} 1.9 mmol, anhydrous glucose 75 g, soya oil 50 g, purified egg phospholipids 3 g, glycerol 5.5 g, phosphate 3.75 mmol

and management of TPN complications, specialist literature should be consulted.

Protein is given as mixtures of essential and non-essential synthetic L-amino acids. Ideally, all essential amino acids should be included with a wide variety of non-essential ones to provide sufficient nitrogen together with electrolytes (see also section 9.2.2). Solutions vary in their composition of amino acids; they often contain an energy source (usually glucose) and electrolytes.

Energy is provided in a ratio of 0.6 to 1.1 megajoules (150–250 kcals) per gram of protein nitrogen. Energy requirements must be met if amino acids are to be utilised for tissue maintenance. A mixture of carbohydrate and fat energy sources (usually 30–50% as fat) gives better utilisation of amino acids than glucose alone.

Glucose is the preferred source of carbohydrate, but if more than 180 g is given per day frequent monitoring of blood glucose is required, and insulin may be necessary. Glucose in various strengths from 10 to 50% must be infused through a central venous catheter to avoid thrombosis.

In total parenteral nutrition regimens, it is necessary to provide adequate phosphate in order to allow phosphorylation of the glucose; between 20 and 30 mmol of phosphate is required daily.

Fructose and sorbitol have been used in an attempt to avoid the problem of hyperosmolar hyperglycaemic non-ketotic acidosis but other metabolic problems may occur, as with xylitol and ethanol which are now rarely used.

Fat emulsions have the advantages of a high energy to fluid volume ratio, neutral pH, and iso-osmolarity with plasma, and provide essential fatty acids. Several days of adaptation may be required to attain maximal utilisation. Reactions include occasional febrile episodes (usually only with 20% emulsions) and rare anaphylactic responses. Interference with biochemical measurements such as those for blood gases and calcium may occur if samples are taken before fat has been cleared. Daily checks are necessary to ensure complete clearance from the plasma in conditions where fat metabolism may be disturbed. **Additives may only be mixed with fat emulsions where compatibility is known.**

> **Administration.** Because of the complex requirements relating to parenteral nutrition full details relating to administration have been omitted. In all cases *product literature and other specialist literature should be consulted.*

Supplementary preparations

> Compatibility with the infusion solution must be ascertained before adding supplementary preparations.

Addiphos® (Fresenius Kabi) [PoM]
Solution, sterile, phosphate 40 mmol, K^+ 30 mmol, Na^+ 30 mmol/20 mL. For addition to *Vamin®* solutions and glucose intravenous infusions. Net price 20-mL vial = £1.15

Additrace® (Fresenius Kabi) [PoM]
Solution, trace elements for addition to *Vamin®* solutions and glucose intravenous infusions, traces of Fe^{3+}, Zn^{2+}, Mn^{2+}, Cu^{2+}, Cr^{3+}, Se^{4+}, Mo^{6+}, F⁻, I⁻. For adults and children over 40 kg. Net price 10-mL amp = £1.75

Cernevit® (Baxter) [PoM]
Solution, dl-alpha tocopherol 11.2 units, ascorbic acid 125 mg, biotin 69 micrograms, colecalciferol 220 units, cyanocobalamin 6 micrograms, folic acid 414 micrograms, glycine 250 mg, nicotinamide 46 mg, pantothenic acid (as dexpanthenol) 17.25 mg, pyridoxine hydrochloride 5.5 mg, retinol (as palmitate) 3500 units, riboflavin (as dihydrated sodium phosphate) 4.14 mg, thiamine (as cocarboxylase tetrahydrate) 3.51 mg. Dissolve in 5 mL water for injections. Net price per vial = £2.77

1. Excludes protein- or amino acid-derived energy
Note. 1000 kcal = 4200 kJ; = 238.8 kcal. All entries are PoM

Decan® (Baxter) [PoM]
Solution, trace elements for addition to infusion solutions, Fe^{2+}, Zn^{2+}, Cu^{2+}, Mn^{2+}, F^-, Co^{2+} I^-, Se^{4+}, Mo^{6+}, Cr^{3+}. For adults and children over 40 kg. Net price 40-mL vial = £2.00

Dipeptiven® (Fresenius Kabi) [PoM]
Solution, N(2)-L-alanyl-L-glutamine 200 mg/mL (providing L-alanine 82 mg, L-glutamine 134.6 mg). For addition to infusion solutions containing amino acids. Net price 50 mL = £15.90, 100 mL = £29.60
Dose: amino acid supplement for hypercatabolic or hypermetabolic states, 300–400 mg/kg daily; max. 400 mg/kg daily, dose not to exceed 20% of total amino acid intake

Peditrace® (Fresenius Kabi) [PoM]
Solution, trace elements for addition to *Vaminolact*®, *Vamin*® *14 Electrolyte-Free* solutions and glucose intravenous infusions, traces of Zn^{2+}, Cu^{2+}, Mn^{2+}, Se^{4+}, F^-, I^-. For use in infants (when kidney function established, usually second day of life) and children. Net price 10-mL vial = £3.10
Cautions: reduced biliary excretion especially in cholestatic liver disease or in markedly reduced urinary excretion (careful biochemical monitoring required); total parenteral nutrition exceeding 1 month (measure serum manganese concentration and check liver function before commencing treatment and regularly during treatment)—discontinue if manganese concentration raised or if cholestasis develops

Solivito N® (Fresenius Kabi) [PoM]
Solution, powder for reconstitution, biotin 60 micrograms, cyanocobalamin 5 micrograms, folic acid 400 micrograms, glycine 300 mg, nicotinamide 40 mg, pyridoxine hydrochloride 4.9 mg, riboflavin sodium phosphate 4.9 mg, sodium ascorbate 113 mg, sodium pantothenate 16.5 mg, thiamine mononitrate 3.1 mg. Dissolve in water for injections or glucose intravenous infusion for adding to glucose intravenous infusion or *Intralipid*®; dissolve in *Vitlipid N*® or *Intralipid*® for adding to *Intralipid*® only. Net price per vial = £1.75

Vitlipid N® (Fresenius Kabi) [PoM]
Emulsion, adult, vitamin A 330 units, ergocalciferol 20 units, *dl*-alpha tocopherol 1 unit, phytomenadione 15 micrograms/mL. For addition to *Intralipid*®. For adults and children over 11 years. Net price 10-mL amp = £1.71
Emulsion, infant, vitamin A 230 units, ergocalciferol 40 units, *dl*-alpha tocopherol 0.7 unit, phytomenadione 20 micrograms/mL. For addition to *Intralipid*®. Net price 10-mL amp = £1.71

9.4　Oral nutrition

9.4.1　Foods for special diets
9.4.2　Enteral nutrition

9.4.1　Foods for special diets

These are preparations that have been modified to eliminate a particular constituent from a food or are nutrient mixtures formulated as substitutes for the food. They are for patients who either cannot tolerate or cannot metabolise certain common constituents of food.

PHENYLKETONURIA. Phenylketonuria (phenylalaninaemia), which results from the inability to metabolise phenylalanine, is managed by restricting its dietary intake to a small amount sufficient for tissue building and repair. Aspartame (as a sweetener in some foods and medicines) contributes to the phenylalanine intake and may affect control of phenylketonuria. Where the presence of aspartame is specified in the product literature this is indicated in the BNF against the preparation.

COELIAC DISEASE. Coeliac disease, which results from an intolerance to gluten, is managed by completely eliminating gluten from the diet.

ACBS. In certain clinical conditions some foods may have the characteristics of drugs and the Advisory Committee on Borderline Substances advises as to the circumstances in which such foods may be regarded as drugs and so can be prescribed in the NHS. Prescriptions for these foods issued in accordance with the advice of this committee and endorsed 'ACBS' will normally not be investigated. See Appendix 7 for details of these foods and a listing by clinical condition (consult Drug Tariff for late amendments).

■ Preparations
For preparations on the ACBS list see Appendix 7
Forceval Protein Powder® (Unigreg)
Powder, strawberry, vanilla and natural flavours, protein (calcium caseinate, providing all essential amino acids) 55%, carbohydrate 30%, with vitamins, minerals, trace elements, fat and low electrolytes (lactose- and gluten-free), net price 14 × 30-g sachets = £17.11; chocolate flavour (as above but protein content is 45%), 14 × 36-g sachets = £17.11.
For hypoproteinaemia, malabsorption states and as an adjunct to nutritional support. Not to be prescribed for any CHILD under 2 years or for those with renal or hepatic failure; unsuitable as a sole source of nutrition

9.4.2　Enteral nutrition

The body's reserves of protein rapidly become exhausted in severely ill patients, especially during chronic illness or in those with severe burns, extensive trauma, pancreatitis, or intestinal fistula. Much can be achieved by frequent meals and by persuading the patient to take supplementary snacks of ordinary food between the meals.

However, extra calories, protein, other nutrients, and vitamins are often best given by supplementing ordinary meals with sip or tube feeds of one of the nutritionally complete foods.

When patients cannot feed normally at all, for example patients with severe facial injury, oesophageal obstruction, or coma, a diet composed solely of nutritionally complete foods must be given. This is planned by a dietitian who will take into account the protein and total energy requirement of the patient and decide on the form and relative contribution of carbohydrate and fat to the energy requirements.

There are a number of nutritionally complete foods available and their use reduces an otherwise heavy workload in hospital or in the home. Most contain protein derived from milk or soya. Some contain protein hydrolysates or free amino acids and are only appropriate for patients who have diminished ability to break down protein, as may be the case in inflammatory bowel disease or pancreatic insufficiency.

Even when nutritionally complete feeds are being given it may be important to monitor water and electrolyte balance. Extra minerals (e.g. magnesium and zinc) may be needed in patients where gastro-intestinal secretions are being lost. Additional vitamins may also be needed. Regular haematological and biochemical tests may be needed particularly in the unstable patient.

Some feeds are supplemented with vitamin K; for drug interactions of vitamin K see Appendix 1 (vitamins).

CHILDREN. Infants and young children have special requirements and in most situations liquid feeds prepared for adults are totally unsuitable and should not be given. Expert advice should be sought.

■ Preparations
See Appendix 7

9.5   Minerals

9.5.1   Calcium and magnesium
9.5.2   Phosphorus
9.5.3   Fluoride
9.5.4   Zinc

See section 9.1.1 for iron salts.

9.5.1   Calcium and magnesium

9.5.1.1   Calcium supplements
9.5.1.2   Hypercalcaemia and hypercalciuria
9.5.1.3   Magnesium

9.5.1.1   Calcium supplements

Calcium supplements are usually only required where dietary calcium intake is deficient. This dietary requirement varies with age and is relatively greater in childhood, pregnancy, and lactation, due to an increased demand, and in old age, due to impaired absorption. In osteoporosis, a calcium intake which is double the recommended amount reduces the rate of bone loss. If the actual dietary intake is less than the recommended amount, a supplement of as much as 40 mmol is appropriate.

In hypocalcaemic tetany an initial intravenous injection of 10 mL (2.25 mmol) of calcium gluconate injection 10% should be followed by the continuous infusion of about 40 mL (9 mmol) daily, but plasma calcium should be monitored. This regimen can also be used immediately to temporarily reduce the toxic effects of hyperkalaemia.

CALCIUM SALTS

Indications: see notes above; calcium deficiency
Cautions: renal impairment; sarcoidosis; avoid calcium chloride in respiratory acidosis or respiratory failure; **interactions:** Appendix 1 (antacids, calcium salts)
Contra-indications: conditions associated with

hypercalcaemia and hypercalciuria (e.g. some forms of malignant disease)
Side-effects: gastro-intestinal disturbances; brady-cardia, arrhythmias; *with injection*, peripheral vasodilatation, fall in blood pressure, injection-site reactions
Dose: *by mouth*, daily in divided doses, see notes above

By slow intravenous injection, acute hypocalcaemia, calcium gluconate 1–2 g (Ca^{2+} 2.25–4.5 mmol)
CHILD obtain paediatric advice

■ Oral preparations
Calcium Gluconate (Non-proprietary)
Tablets, calcium gluconate 600 mg (calcium 53.4 mg or Ca^{2+} 1.35 mmol), net price 20 = £1.43. Label: 24
Effervescent tablets, calcium gluconate 1 g (calcium 89 mg or Ca^{2+} 2.25 mmol), net price 28-tab pack = £4.62. Label: 13
NOTE. Each tablet usually contains 4.46 mmol Na^+

Calcium Lactate (Non-proprietary)
Tablets, calcium lactate 300 mg (calcium 39 mg or Ca^{2+} 1 mmol), net price 20 = 62p

Adcal® (Strakan)
Chewable tablets, calcium carbonate 1.5 g (calcium 600 mg or Ca^{2+} 15 mmol), net price 100-tab pack = £7.50. Label: 24

Cacit® (Procter & Gamble Pharm.)
Tablets, effervescent, pink, calcium carbonate 1.25 g, providing calcium citrate when dispersed in water (calcium 500 mg or Ca^{2+} 12.6 mmol), net price 76-tab pack = £16.72. Label: 13

Calcichew® (Shire)
Tablets (chewable), calcium carbonate 1.25 g (calcium 500 mg or Ca^{2+} 12.6 mmol), net price 100-tab pack = £9.33
Forte tablets (chewable), scored, calcium carbonate 2.5 g (calcium 1 g or Ca^{2+} 25 mmol), net price 60-tab pack = £13.16. Label: 24
Excipients: include aspartame

Calcium-500 (Martindale)
Tablets, pink, f/c, calcium carbonate 1.25 g (calcium 500 mg or Ca^{2+} 12.5 mmol). Net price 100-tab pack = £10.17. Label: 25

Calcium-Sandoz® (Alliance)
Syrup, calcium glubionate 1.09 g, calcium lacto-bionate 727 mg (calcium 108.3 mg or Ca^{2+} 2.7 mmol)/5 mL. Net price 300 mL = £3.48

Ossopan® (Sanofi-Synthelabo)
Tablets, buff, f/c, hydroxyapatite 830 mg (calcium 178 mg or Ca^{2+} 4.4 mmol). Net price 50 = £9.64
Granules, brown, hydroxyapatite 3.32 g (calcium 712 mg or Ca^{2+} 17.8 mmol)/sachet, net price 28-sachet pack = £17.23

Sandocal® (Novartis Consumer Health)
Sandocal-400 tablets, effervescent, calcium lactate gluconate 930 mg, calcium carbonate 700 mg, anhydrous citric acid 1.189 g, providing calcium 400 mg (Ca^{2+} 10 mmol). Net price 5 × 20-tab pack = £6.85. Label: 13
Sandocal-1000 tablets, effervescent, calcium lactate gluconate 2.327 g, calcium carbonate 1.75 g, anhydrous citric acid 2.973 g providing 1 g calcium (Ca^{2+} 25 mmol). Net price 3 × 10-tab pack = £6.18. Label: 13

Titralac®   section 9.5.2.2

■ Parenteral preparations

Calcium Gluconate (Non-proprietary) PoM
Injection, calcium gluconate 10% (calcium 8.9 mg or Ca^{2+} 220 micromol)/mL. Net price 10-mL amp = 60p
Available from Phoenix

Calcium Chloride (Non-proprietary) PoM
Injection, calcium chloride 100 mg/mL (calcium 27.3 mg or Ca^{2+} 680 micromol/mL). Net price 10-mL disposable syringe = £4.42
Available from Aurum, Celltech (*Minijet® Calcium Chloride 10%*)

■ With vitamin D
Section 9.6.4

9.5.1.2 Hypercalcaemia and hypercalciuria

SEVERE HYPERCALCAEMIA. Severe hypercalcaemia calls for urgent treatment before detailed investigation of the cause. Dehydration should be corrected first with intravenous infusion of **sodium chloride 0.9%**. Drugs (such as thiazides and vitamin D compounds) which promote hypercalcaemia, should be discontinued and dietary calcium should be restricted.

If *severe hypercalcaemia persists* drugs which inhibit mobilisation of calcium from the skeleton may be required. The **bisphosphonates** are useful and disodium pamidronate (section 6.6.2) is probably the most effective.

Corticosteroids (section 6.3) are widely given, but may only be useful where hypercalcaemia is due to sarcoidosis or vitamin D intoxication; they often take several days to achieve the desired effect.

Calcitonin (section 6.6.1) is relatively non-toxic but is expensive and its effect can wear off after a few days despite continued use; it is rarely effective where bisphosphonates have failed to reduce serum calcium adequately.

Intravenous chelating drugs such as **trisodium edetate** are rarely used; they usually cause pain in the limb receiving the infusion and may cause renal damage; trisodium edetate should no longer be used for the management of hypercalcaemia.

After treatment of severe hypercalcaemia the underlying cause must be established. *Further treatment* is governed by the same principles as for initial therapy. Salt and water depletion and drugs promoting hypercalcaemia should be avoided; oral administration of a bisphosphonate may be useful. Parathyroidectomy may be indicated for hyperparathyroidism.

HYPERCALCIURIA. Hypercalciuria should be investigated for an underlying cause, which should be treated. Where a cause is not identified (idiopathic hypercalciuria), the condition is managed by increasing fluid intake and giving bendroflumethiazide in a dose of 2.5 mg daily (a higher dose is not usually necessary). Reducing dietary calcium intake may be beneficial but severe restriction of calcium intake has not proved beneficial and may even be harmful.

TRISODIUM EDETATE ▰

Indications: hypercalcaemia (but see notes above); lime burns in the eye (see under Preparations)

Cautions: repeated plasma-calcium determinations important; caution in tuberculosis; avoid rapid infusion, see under Dose

Contra-indications: impaired renal function

Side-effects: nausea, diarrhoea, cramp; in overdosage renal damage

Dose: hypercalcaemia, *by intravenous infusion* over 2–3 hours, up to 70 mg/kg daily; CHILD up to 60 mg/kg daily
IMPORTANT. Ensure rate of infusion and concentration correct (see Appendix 6); too rapid a rate or too high a concentration is extremely hazardous and repeated measurements of plasma calcium concentrations are important for control and maintenance of near normal ionised calcium concentrations. Decrease infusion rate on signs of increased muscle reactivity; discontinue if tetany occurs and restart cautiously only after plasma ionised and total calcium concentrations indicate need for further treatment (and tetany has stopped)

Limclair® (Durbin) PoM
Concentrate for infusion, trisodium edetate 200 mg/mL. Net price 5-mL amp = £7.93
NOTE. For topical use in the eye, dilute 1 mL to 50 mL with sterile purified water

9.5.1.3 Magnesium

Magnesium is an essential constituent of many enzyme systems, particularly those involved in energy generation; the largest stores are in the skeleton.

Magnesium salts are not well absorbed from the gastro-intestinal tract, which explains the use of magnesium sulphate (section 1.6.4) as an osmotic laxative.

Magnesium is excreted mainly by the kidneys and is therefore retained in renal failure although significant *hypermagnesaemia* (causing muscle weakness and arrhythmias) is rare.

HYPOMAGNESAEMIA. Since magnesium is secreted in large amounts in the gastro-intestinal fluid, excessive losses in diarrhoea, stoma or fistula are the most common causes of *hypomagnesaemia*; deficiency may also occur in alcoholism or diuretic therapy and it has been reported after prolonged treatment with aminoglycosides. Hypomagnesaemia often causes secondary hypocalcaemia (with which it may be confused) and also hypokalaemia and hyponatraemia.

Symptomatic *hypomagnesaemia* is associated with a deficit of 0.5–1 mmol/kg; up to 160 mmol Mg^{2+} over up to 5 days may be required to replace the deficit (allowing for urinary losses). Magnesium is given initially by intravenous infusion or by intramuscular injection of **magnesium sulphate**; the intramuscular injection is painful. Plasma magnesium concentration should be measured to determine the rate and duration of infusion and the dose should be reduced in renal impairment. To prevent *recurrence of the deficit*, magnesium may be given by mouth in a dose of 24 mmol Mg^{2+} daily in divided doses; a suitable preparation is magnesium glycerophosphate tablets [not licensed, available from IDIS]. For maintenance (e.g. in intravenous nutrition), parenteral doses of magnesium are of the order of 10–20 mmol Mg^{2+} daily (often about 12 mmol Mg^{2+} daily).

ARRHYTHMIAS. Magnesium sulphate has also been recommended for the emergency treatment of *serious arrhythmias*, especially in the presence of hypokalaemia (when hypomagnesaemia may also be present) and when salvos of rapid ventricular tachycardia show the characteristic twisting wave front known as *torsades de pointes*. The usual dose of magnesium sulphate is intravenous injection of 8 mmol Mg^{2+} over 10–15 minutes (repeated once if necessary).

MYOCARDIAL INFARCTION. Evidence suggesting a sustained reduction in mortality in patients with *suspected myocardial infarction* given an initial intravenous injection of magnesium sulphate 8 mmol Mg^{2+} over 20 minutes followed by an intravenous infusion of 65–72 mmol Mg^{2+} over the following 24 hours, has not been borne out by a larger study. Some workers, however, continue to hold the view that magnesium is beneficial if given immediately (and for as long as there is a likelihood of reperfusion taking place).

ECLAMPSIA AND PRE-ECLAMPSIA. Magnesium sulphate is the drug of choice for the prevention of recurrent seizures in *eclampsia*. Regimens may vary between hospitals. Calcium gluconate injection is used for the management of magnesium toxicity.

Magnesium sulphate is also of benefit in women with *pre-eclampsia* in whom there is concern about developing eclampsia. The patient should be monitored carefully (see under Magnesium Sulphate).

MAGNESIUM SULPHATE

Indications: see notes above; constipation (section 1.6.4); severe acute asthma (section 3.1); paste for boils (section 13.10.5)

Cautions: see notes above; hepatic impairment (Appendix 2); renal impairment (Appendix 3); in severe hypomagnesaemia administer initially via controlled infusion device (preferably syringe pump); monitor blood pressure, respiratory rate, urinary output and for signs of overdosage (loss of patellar reflexes, weakness, nausea, sensation of warmth, flushing, drowsiness, double vision, and slurred speech); **interactions:** Appendix 1 (magnesium, parenteral)

Side-effects: generally associated with hypermagnesaemia, nausea, vomiting, thirst, flushing of skin, hypotension, arrhythmias, coma, respiratory depression, drowsiness, confusion, loss of tendon reflexes, muscle weakness; colic and diarrhoea following oral administration

Dose: hypomagnesaemia, see notes above
Prevention of seizure recurrence in eclampsia, initially *by intravenous injection* over 5–15 minutes, 4 g, followed *by intravenous infusion*, 1 g/hour for at least 24 hours after last seizure; if seizure recurs, additional dose *by intravenous injection*, 2 g (4 g if body-weight over 70 kg)
Prevention of seizures in pre-eclampsia [unlicensed indication], initially *by intravenous infusion* over 5–15 minutes, 4 g followed *by intravenous infusion*, 1 g/hour for 24 hours; if seizure occurs, additional dose *by intravenous injection*, 2 g
INTRAVENOUS ADMINISTRATION. For intravenous injection concentration of magnesium sulphate should not exceed 20% (dilute 1 part of magnesium sulphate injection 50% with at least 1.5 parts of water for injections)
NOTE. Magnesium sulphate 1 g equivalent to Mg^{2+} approx. 4 mmol

Magnesium Sulphate (Non-proprietary) PoM
Injection, magnesium sulphate 50% (Mg^{2+} approx. 2 mmol /mL), net price 2-mL (1-g) amp = £2.85, 5-mL (2.5-g) amp = £2.39, 10-mL (5-g) amp = £3.20; prefilled 10-mL (5-g) syringe = £4.72
Available from Auden Mckenzie, Aurum, Celltech

9.5.2 Phosphorus

9.5.2.1 Phosphate supplements
9.5.2.2 Phosphate-binding agents

9.5.2.1 Phosphate supplements

Oral phosphate supplements may be required in addition to vitamin D in a small minority of patients with hypophosphataemic vitamin D-resistant rickets. Diarrhoea is a common side-effect and should prompt a reduction in dosage.

Phosphate infusion is occasionally needed in alcohol dependence or in phosphate deficiency arising from use of parenteral nutrition deficient in phosphate supplements; phosphate depletion also occurs in severe diabetic ketoacidosis. For *established hypophosphataemia*, monobasic potassium phosphate may be infused at a maximum rate of 9 mmol every 12 hours. Excessive doses of phosphates may cause hypocalcaemia and metastatic calcification; it is **essential** to monitor closely plasma concentrations of calcium, phosphate, potassium, and other electrolytes.

For phosphate requirements in *total parenteral nutrition* regimens, see section 9.3.

Phosphate-Sandoz® (HK Pharma)
Tablets, effervescent, anhydrous sodium acid phosphate 1.936 g, sodium bicarbonate 350 mg, potassium bicarbonate 315 mg, equivalent to phosphorus 500 mg (phosphate 16.1 mmol), sodium 468.8 mg (Na^+ 20.4 mmol), potassium 123 mg (K^+ 3.1 mmol). Net price 20 = £3.29. Label: 13
Dose: hypercalcaemia, up to 6 tablets daily adjusted according to response; CHILD under 5 years up to 3 tablets daily
Vitamin D-resistant hypophosphataemic osteomalacia, 4–6 tablets daily; CHILD under 5 years 2–3 tablets daily

9.5.2.2 Phosphate-binding agents

Aluminium-containing and calcium-containing preparations are used as phosphate-binding agents in the management of hyperphosphataemia complicating renal failure. Calcium-containing phosphate-binding agents are contra-indicated in hypercalcaemia or hypercalciuria. Phosphate-binding agents which contain aluminium may increase plasma aluminium in dialysis patients.

Sevelamer is licensed for the treatment of hyperphosphataemia in patients on haemodialysis.

ALUMINIUM HYDROXIDE

Indications: hyperphosphataemia; dyspepsia (section 1.1)

Cautions: hyperaluminaemia; porphyria (section 9.8.2); see also notes above; **interactions:** Appendix 1 (antacids)

Side-effects: see section 1.1.1

Aluminium Hydroxide (Non-proprietary)
Mixture (gel), about 4% w/w Al_2O_3 in water. Net price 200 mL = 41p
Dose: hyperphosphataemia, 20–100 mL according to requirements of patient
NOTE. The brand name *Aludrox* NHS (Pfizer Consumer) is used for aluminium hydroxide mixture, net price 200 mL = £1.42

Alu-Cap® (3M)
Capsules, green/red, dried aluminium hydroxide 475 mg (low Na+). Net price 120-cap pack = £4.03
Dose: phosphate-binding agent in renal failure, 4–20 capsules daily in divided doses with meals

CALCIUM SALTS

Indications: hyperphosphataemia
Cautions: see notes above; **interactions:** Appendix 1 (antacids, calcium salts)
Side-effects: hypercalcaemia

Adcal®, section 9.5.1.1

Calcichew®, section 9.5.1.1

Calcium-500 section 9.5.1.1

Phosex® (Vitaline)
Tablets, yellow, calcium acetate 1 g (calcium 250 mg or Ca^{2+} 6.2 mmol), net price 180-tab pack = £19.79. Label: 25
Dose: phosphate-binding agent (with meals) in renal failure, according to the requirements of the patient

Titralac® (3M)
Tablets, calcium carbonate 420 mg (calcium 168 mg or Ca^{2+} 4.2 mmol), glycine 180 mg. Net price 180-tab pack = £2.81
COUNSELLING. May be chewed, crushed or swallowed whole
Dose: calcium supplement, or phosphate-binding agent (with meals) in renal failure, according to the requirements of the patient

SEVELAMER

Indications: hyperphosphataemia in patients on haemodialysis
Cautions: pregnancy and breast-feeding; gastrointestinal disorders
Contra-indications: bowel obstruction
Dose: initially 2.4–4.836 g (as 6–12 403-mg capsules or 3–6 800-mg tablets) daily in 3 divided doses with meals, then adjusted according to plasma-phosphate concentration

Renagel® (Genzyme) ▼ PoM
Capsules, sevelamer 403 mg, net price 200-cap pack = £73.00. Label: 21
Tablets, f/c, sevelamer 800 mg, net price 180-tab pack = £132.00. Label: 21

9.5.3 Fluoride

Availability of adequate fluoride confers significant resistance to dental caries. It is now considered that the topical action of fluoride on enamel and plaque is more important than the systemic effect.

Where the fluoride content of the drinking water is less than 700 micrograms per litre (0.7 parts per million), daily administration of fluoride tablets or drops is a suitable means of supplementation. Systemic fluoride supplements should not be prescribed without reference to the fluoride content of the local water supply. Infants need not receive fluoride supplements until the age of 6 months.

Dentifrices which incorporate sodium fluoride or monofluorophosphate are also a convenient source of fluoride.

Individuals who are either particularly caries prone or medically compromised may be given additional protection by use of fluoride rinses or by application of fluoride gels. Rinses may be used daily or weekly; daily use of a less concentrated rinse is more effective than weekly use of a more concentrated one. High-strength gels must be applied on a regular basis under professional supervision; extreme caution is necessary to prevent the child from swallowing any excess. Less concentrated gels are available for home use. Varnishes are also available and are particularly valuable for young or handicapped children since they adhere to the teeth and set in the presence of moisture.

FLUORIDES

NOTE. Sodium fluoride 2.2 mg provides approx. 1 mg fluoride ion
Indications: prophylaxis of dental caries—see notes above
Contra-indications: not for areas where drinking water is fluoridated
Side-effects: occasional white flecks on teeth with recommended doses; rarely yellowish-brown discoloration if recommended doses are exceeded
Dose: expressed as fluoride ion (F⁻):
Water content less than F⁻ 300 micrograms/litre (0.3 parts per million), CHILD up to 6 months none; 6 months–3 years F⁻ 250 micrograms daily, 3–6 years F⁻ 500 micrograms daily, over 6 years F⁻ 1 mg daily
Water content between F⁻ 300 and 700 micrograms/litre (0.3–0.7 parts per million), CHILD up to 3 years none, 3–6 years F⁻ 250 micrograms daily, over 6 years F⁻ 500 micrograms daily
Water content above F⁻ 700 micrograms/litre (0.7 parts per million), supplements not advised
NOTE. These doses reflect the recommendations of the British Dental Association, the British Society of Paediatric Dentistry and the British Association for the Study of Community Dentistry (*Br Dent J* 1997; **182**: 6–7)

■ Tablets
COUNSELLING. Tablets should be sucked or dissolved in the mouth and taken preferably in the evening
There are arrangements for health authorities to supply fluoride tablets in the course of pre-school dental schemes, and they may also be supplied in school dental schemes.

En-De-Kay® (Manx)
Fluotabs 3–6 years, orange-flavoured, scored, sodium fluoride 1.1 mg (F⁻ 500 micrograms). Net price 200-tab pack = £1.80
Fluotabs 6+ years, orange-flavoured, scored, sodium fluoride 2.2 mg (F⁻ 1 mg). Net price 200-tab pack = £1.80

Fluor-a-day® (Dental Health)
Tablets, buff, sodium fluoride 1.1 mg (F⁻ 500 micrograms), net price 200-tab pack = £1.91; 2.2 mg (F⁻ 1 mg), 200-tab pack = £1.91

FluoriGard® (Colgate-Palmolive)
Tablets 0.5, purple, grape-flavoured, scored, sodium fluoride 1.1 mg (F⁻ 500 micrograms). Net price 200-tab pack = £1.91
Tablets 1.0, orange, orange-flavoured, scored, sodium fluoride 2.2 mg (F⁻ 1 mg). Net price 200-tab pack = £1.91

■ Oral drops

Note. Fluoride supplements not considered necessary below 6 months of age (see notes above)

En-De-Kay® (Manx)

Fluodrops® (= paediatric drops), sugar-free, sodium fluoride 550 micrograms (F^- 250 micrograms)/0.15 mL. Net price 60 mL = £1.82

NOTE. Corresponds to Sodium Fluoride Oral Drops DPF 0.37% equivalent to sodium fluoride 80 micrograms (F^- 36 micrograms)/drop

■ Mouthwashes

Rinse mouth for 1 minute and spit out

COUNSELLING. Avoid eating, drinking, or rinsing mouth for 15 minutes after use

Duraphat® (Colgate-Palmolive)

Weekly dental rinse (= mouthwash), blue, sodium fluoride 0.2%. Net price 150 mL = £2.42. Counselling, see above

Dose: CHILD 6 years and over, for *weekly* use, rinse with 10 mL

En-De-Kay® (Manx)

Daily fluoride mouthrinse (= mouthwash), blue, sodium fluoride 0.05%. Net price 250 mL = £1.77

Dose: CHILD 6 years and over, for *daily* use, rinse with 10 mL

Fluorinse PoM (= mouthwash), red, sodium fluoride 2%. Net price 100 mL = £3.97. Counselling, see above

Dose: CHILD 8 years and over, for *daily* use, dilute 5 drops to 10 mL of water; for *weekly* use, dilute 20 drops to 10 mL

FluoriGard® (Colgate-Palmolive)

Daily dental rinse (= mouthwash), blue, sodium fluoride 0.05%. Net price 500 mL = £3.11. Counselling, see above

Dose: CHILD 6 years and over, for *daily* use, rinse with 10 mL

■ Gels

FluoriGard® (Colgate-Palmolive)

Gel-Kam (= gel), stannous fluoride 0.4% in glycerol basis. Net price 100 mL = £3.05. Counselling, see below

Dose: ADULT and CHILD 3 years and over, for *daily* use, using a toothbrush, apply onto all tooth surfaces

COUNSELLING. Swish between teeth for 1 minute before spitting out. Avoid eating, drinking, or rinsing mouth for at least 30 minutes after use

■ Toothpastes

Duraphat® (Colgate-Palmolive) PoM

Toothpaste, sodium fluoride 0.619%. Net price 75 mL = £2.86. Counselling, see below

Dose: ADULT and ADOLESCENT over 16 years, apply 1 cm twice daily using a toothbrush

COUNSELLING. Brush teeth for 1 minute before spitting out. Avoid drinking or rinsing mouth for 30 minutes after use

<hr>

9.5.4 Zinc

Zinc supplements should be given only when there is good evidence of deficiency (hypoproteinaemia spuriously lowers plasma-zinc concentration) or in zinc-losing conditions. Zinc deficiency can occur as a result of inadequate diet or malabsorption; excessive loss of zinc can occur in trauma, burns and protein-losing conditions. A zinc supplement is given until clinical improvement occurs but it may

need to be continued in severe malabsorption, metabolic disease or in zinc-losing states.

Total parenteral nutrition regimens usually include trace amounts of zinc. If necessary, further zinc can be added to some intravenous feeding regimens. A suggested dose for intravenous nutrition is elemental zinc 6.5 mg (Zn^{2+} 100 micromol) daily.

ZINC SALTS

Indications: zinc deficiency or supplementation in zinc-losing conditions

Cautions: acute renal failure (may accumulate); **interactions:** Appendix 1 (zinc)

Side-effects: abdominal pain, dyspepsia, nausea, vomiting, diarrhoea, gastric irritation, gastritis; irritability, headache, lethargy

Dose: see preparation below and notes above

Zinc Sulphate (Non-proprietary) PoM

Injection, zinc sulphate 14.6 mg/mL (zinc 50 micromol/mL), net price 10 mL vial = £2.50

Available from Aurum

Solvazinc® (Provalis)

Effervescent tablets, yellow-white, zinc sulphate monohydrate 125 mg (45 mg zinc). Net price 30 = £4.32. Label: 13, 21

Dose: ADULT and CHILD over 30 kg, 1 tablet in water 1–3 times daily after food; CHILD under 10 kg, ½ tablet daily; 10–30 kg, ½ tablet 1–3 times daily

<hr>

9.6 Vitamins

9.6.1	Vitamin A
9.6.2	Vitamin B group
9.6.3	Vitamin C
9.6.4	Vitamin D
9.6.5	Vitamin E
9.6.6	Vitamin K
9.6.7	Multivitamin preparations

Vitamins are used for the prevention and treatment of specific deficiency states or where the diet is known to be inadequate; they may be prescribed in the NHS to prevent or treat deficiency but not as dietary supplements.

Their use as general 'pick-me-ups' is of unproven value and, in the case of preparations containing vitamin A or D, may actually be harmful if patients take more than the prescribed dose. The 'fad' for mega-vitamin therapy with water-soluble vitamins, such as ascorbic acid and pyridoxine, is unscientific and can be harmful.

Dietary reference values for vitamins are available in the Department of Health publication:

Dietary Reference Values for Food Energy and Nutrients for the United Kingdom: Report of the Panel on Dietary Reference Values of the Committee on Medical Aspects of Food Policy. *Report on Health and Social Subjects 41.* London: HMSO, 1991

<hr>

9.6.1 Vitamin A

Deficiency of vitamin A (retinol) is associated with ocular defects (particularly xerophthalmia) and an increased susceptibility to infections, but deficiency is rare in the UK (even in disorders of fat absorption).

Massive overdose can cause rough skin, dry hair, an enlarged liver, and a raised erythrocyte sedimentation rate and raised serum calcium and serum alkaline phosphatase concentrations.

In view of evidence suggesting that high levels of vitamin A may cause birth defects, women who are (or may become) pregnant are advised not to take vitamin A supplements (including tablets and fish-liver oil drops), except on the advice of a doctor or an antenatal clinic; nor should they eat liver or products such as liver paté or liver sausage.

VITAMIN A

(Retinol)

Indications: see notes above
Cautions: see notes above; **interactions:** Appendix 1 (vitamins)
Side-effects: see notes above
Dose: see notes above and under preparations

■ Vitamins A and D

Halibut-liver Oil (Non-proprietary)
Capsules, vitamin A 4000 units [also contains vitamin D]. Net price 20 = 18p
Available from Thornton & Ross

Vitamins A and D (Non-proprietary)
Capsules, vitamin A 4000 units, vitamin D 400 units. Net price 20 = 64p
Available from CP

Halycitrol® (LAB) NHS
Emulsion, vitamin A 4600 units, vitamin D 380 units/5 mL. Net price 114 mL = £1.61
Dose: 5 mL daily but see notes above

■ Vitamins A, C and D

Mothers' and Children's Vitamin Drops (Cupal)
Oral drops, vitamin A 5000 units, vitamin D 2000 units, ascorbic acid 150 mg/mL
Available free of charge to pregnant women and children aged under 5 years in families receiving Income Support or an income-based Jobseeker's Allowance under the Welfare Food Scheme. If prescribed, prescription needs to be endorsed 'ACBS'. Otherwise available direct to the public from maternity and child health clinics
Dose: pregnant and nursing mothers and CHILD 1 month–5 years, 5 drops daily (5 drops contain vitamin A approx. 700 units, ascorbic acid approx. 20 mg, vitamin D approx. 300 units)
NOTE. Recommended by the Department of Health for routine supplementation in all pregnant women (but see notes above) and children from 1 year to 5 years. For breast-fed baby whose mother was in good vitamin status during pregnancy, supplementation may begin at 6 months of age; where there is doubt about the mother's vitamin status during pregnancy, supplementation should begin at 1 month of age; a baby consuming 500 mL infant formula feed or follow-on formula feed daily does not need vitamin supplementation because the formula feeds are fortified with vitamin D

9.6.2 Vitamin B group

Deficiency of the B vitamins, other than deficiency of vitamin B_{12} (section 9.1.2), is rare in the UK and is usually treated by preparations containing thiamine (B_1), riboflavin (B_2), and nicotinamide, which is used in preference to nicotinic acid, as it does not cause vasodilatation. Other members (or substances traditionally classified as members) of the vitamin B complex such as aminobenzoic acid, biotin, choline, inositol, and pantothenic acid or panthenol may be included in vitamin B preparations but there is no evidence of their value.

The severe deficiency states Wernicke's encephalopathy and Korsakoff's psychosis, especially as seen in chronic alcoholism, are best treated initially by the parenteral administration of B vitamins (*Pabrinex*®), followed by oral administration of thiamine in the longer term. Anaphylaxis has been reported with parenteral B vitamins (see CSM advice, below).

As with other vitamins of the B group, pyridoxine (B_6) deficiency is rare, but it may occur during isoniazid therapy (section 5.1.9) and is characterised by peripheral neuritis. High doses of pyridoxine are given in some metabolic disorders, such as hyperoxaluria, and it is also used in sideroblastic anaemia (section 9.1.3). There is evidence to suggest that pyridoxine in a dose not exceeding 100 mg daily may provide some benefit in premenstrual syndrome. It has been tried for a wide variety of other disorders, but there is little sound evidence to support the claims of efficacy, and overdosage induces toxic effects.

Nicotinic acid inhibits the synthesis of cholesterol and triglyceride (see section 2.12). Folic acid and vitamin B_{12} are used in the treatment of megaloblastic anaemia (section 9.1.2). Folinic acid (available as calcium folinate) is used in association with cytotoxic therapy (section 8.1).

RIBOFLAVIN

(Riboflavine, vitamin B_2)

Indications: see notes above

■ Preparations
Injections of vitamins B and C, see under Thiamine

■ Oral vitamin B complex preparations
See below

THIAMINE

(Vitamin B_1)

> **CSM advice.** Since potentially serious allergic adverse reactions may occur during, or shortly after, administration, the CSM has recommended that:
>
> 1. Use be restricted to patients in whom parenteral treatment is essential;
> 2. Intravenous injections should be administered slowly (over 10 minutes);
> 3. Facilities for treating anaphylaxis should be available when administered.

Indications: see notes above
Cautions: anaphylactic shock may occasionally follow injection (see CSM advice above)
Dose: mild chronic deficiency, 10–25 mg daily; severe deficiency, 200–300 mg daily

Thiamine (Non-proprietary)
Tablets, thiamine hydrochloride 50 mg, net price 20 = 80p; 100 mg, 20 = £1.23
Available from Roche Consumer Health (*Benerva*® NHS)

Pabrinex® (Link) PoM
I/M High potency injection, for intramuscular use only, ascorbic acid 500 mg, nicotinamide 160 mg, pyridoxine hydrochloride 50 mg, riboflavin 4 mg,

thiamine hydrochloride 250 mg/7 mL. Net price
7 mL (in 2 amps) = £2.07

I/V High potency injection, for intravenous use only,
ascorbic acid 500 mg, anhydrous glucose 1 g,
nicotinamide 160 mg, pyridoxine hydrochloride
50 mg, riboflavin 4 mg, thiamine hydrochloride
250 mg/10 mL. Net price 10 mL (in 2 amps) =
£2.07

Parenteral vitamins B and C for rapid correction of severe
depletion or malabsorption (e.g. in alcoholism, after acute
infections, postoperatively, or in psychiatric states),
maintenance of vitamins B and C in chronic intermittent
haemodialysis

Dose: see CSM advice above

Coma or delirium from alcohol, from opioids, or from
barbiturates, collapse following narcosis, by intravenous
injection or infusion of *I/V High potency*, 2–3 pairs every
8 hours

Psychosis following narcosis or electroconvulsive therapy, toxicity from acute infections, by intravenous
injection or infusion of *I/V High potency* or by deep
intramuscular injection into the gluteal muscle of *I/M
High potency*, 1 pair twice daily for up to 7 days

Haemodialysis, by intravenous infusion of *I/V High
potency* (in sodium chloride intravenous infusion 0.9%) 1
pair every 2 weeks

■ Oral vitamin B complex preparations
See below

___

PYRIDOXINE HYDROCHLORIDE

(Vitamin B_6)

Indications: see under Dose

Cautions: interactions: Appendix 1 (vitamins)

Dose: deficiency states, 20–50 mg up to 3 times
daily

Isoniazid neuropathy, prophylaxis 10 mg daily [or
20 mg daily if suitable product not available];
therapeutic, 50 mg three times daily

Idiopathic sideroblastic anaemia, 100–400 mg daily
in divided doses

Premenstrual syndrome, 50–100 mg daily (see notes
above)

> **Important.** Concerns about possible toxicity result-
> ing from prolonged use of pyridoxine (vitamin B_6) at
> high dosage have not yet been resolved. The Royal
> Pharmaceutical Society of Great Britain has advised
> that pharmacists should consider how to advise
> customers requesting preparations containing higher
> doses and that they should decide their own policy on
> the display of products containing more than 10 mg
> per daily dose of pyridoxine.

Pyridoxine (Non-proprietary)
Tablets, pyridoxine hydrochloride 10 mg, net price
20 = 34p; 20 mg, 20 = 34p; 50 mg, 20 = 38p
Available from BR, CP, Hillcross

■ Injections of vitamins B and C
See under Thiamine

___

NICOTINAMIDE

Indications: see notes above; acne vulgaris, see
section 13.6.1

Nicotinamide (Non-proprietary)
Tablets, nicotinamide 50 mg. Net price 20 = £1.37

■ Injections of vitamins B and C
See under Thiamine

___

Oral vitamin B complex preparations

NOTE. Other multivitamin preparations are in section 9.6.7.

Vitamin B Tablets, Compound ▭
Tablets, nicotinamide 15 mg, riboflavin 1 mg,
thiamine hydrochloride 1 mg. Net price 20 = 7p
Dose: prophylactic, 1–2 tablets daily

Vitamin B Tablets, Compound, Strong ▭
Tablets, brown, f/c or s/c, nicotinamide 20 mg,
pyridoxine hydrochloride 2 mg, riboflavin 2 mg,
thiamine hydrochloride 5 mg. Net price 28-tab
pack = 42p
Dose: treatment of vitamin-B deficiency, 1–2 tablets 3
times daily

Vigranon B® (Wallace Mfg) **NHS** ▭
Syrup, thiamine hydrochloride 5 mg, riboflavin
2 mg, nicotinamide 20 mg, pyridoxine hydrochloride 2 mg, panthenol 3 mg/5 mL. Net price
150 mL = £2.02

___

Other compounds

Potassium aminobenzoate has been used in the
treatment of various disorders associated with excessive fibrosis such as scleroderma but its therapeutic
value is **doubtful**.

Potaba® (Glenwood) ▭
Capsules, potassium aminobenzoate 500 mg. Net
price 20 = £1.42. Label: 21
Tablets, potassium aminobenzoate 500 mg. Net
price 20 = £1.31. Label: 21
Envules® (= powder in sachets), potassium amino-
benzoate 3 g. Net price 40 sachets = £15.37.
Label: 13, 21
Dose: Peyronie's disease, scleroderma, 12 g daily in
divided doses after food

___

9.6.3   Vitamin C
(Ascorbic acid)

Vitamin C therapy is essential in scurvy, but less
florid manifestations of vitamin C deficiency are
commonly found, especially in the elderly. It is rarely
necessary to prescribe more than 100 mg daily
except early in the treatment of scurvy.

Claims that vitamin C ameliorates colds or promotes wound healing have not been proved.

___

ASCORBIC ACID

Indications: prevention and treatment of scurvy

Dose: prophylactic, 25–75 mg daily; therapeutic,
not less than 250 mg daily in divided doses

Ascorbic Acid (Non-proprietary)
Tablets, ascorbic acid 50 mg, net price 20 = 85p;
100 mg, 20 = 18p; 200 mg, 20 = 22p; 500 mg
(label: 24), 20 = 40p
Available from Alpharma, Roche Consumer Health
(*Redoxon*® **NHS**)
Injection, ascorbic acid 100 mg/mL. Net price 5-mL
amp = £2.51
Available from Celltech

■ For children's welfare vitamin drops containing
vitamin C with A and D
See vitamin A

9.6.4   Vitamin D

NOTE. The term Vitamin D is used for a range of compounds which possess the property of preventing or curing rickets. They include ergocalciferol (calciferol, vitamin D_2), colecalciferol (vitamin D_3), dihydrotachysterol, alfacalcidol (1α-hydroxycholecalciferol), and calcitriol (1,25-dihydroxycholecalciferol).

Simple vitamin D deficiency can be prevented by taking an oral supplement of only 10 micrograms (400 units) of ergocalciferol (calciferol, vitamin D_2) daily. Vitamin D deficiency is not uncommon in Asians consuming unleavened bread and in the elderly living alone and can be prevented by taking an oral supplement of 20 micrograms (800 units) of ergocalciferol daily. Since there is no plain tablet of this strength available **calcium and ergocalciferol tablets** can be given (although the calcium is unnecessary).

Vitamin D deficiency caused by *intestinal malabsorption* or *chronic liver disease* usually requires vitamin D in pharmacological doses, such as **calciferol tablets** up to 1 mg (40 000 units) daily; the hypocalcaemia of *hypoparathyroidism* often requires doses of up to 2.5 mg (100 000 units) daily in order to achieve normocalcaemia. The newer vitamin D derivatives, **alfacalcidol** and **calcitriol**, have a shorter duration of action, and therefore have the advantage that problems associated with hypercalcaemia due to excessive dosage are shorter lasting and easier to treat.

Vitamin D requires hydroxylation by the kidney to its active form therefore the hydroxylated derivatives **alfacalcidol** or **calcitriol** should be prescribed if patients with *severe renal impairment* require vitamin D therapy. Calcitriol is also licensed for the management of postmenopausal osteoporosis.

Important. All patients receiving pharmacological doses of vitamin D should have the plasma-calcium concentration checked at intervals (initially weekly) and whenever nausea or vomiting are present. Breast milk from women taking pharmacological doses of vitamin D may cause hypercalcaemia if given to an infant.

ERGOCALCIFEROL

(Calciferol, Vitamin D_2)

Indications: see notes above

Cautions: take care to ensure correct dose in infants; monitor plasma calcium in patients receiving high doses and in renal impairment; **interactions:** Appendix 1 (vitamins)

Contra-indications: hypercalcaemia; metastatic calcification

Side-effects: symptoms of overdosage include anorexia, lassitude, nausea and vomiting, diarrhoea, weight loss, polyuria, sweating, headache, thirst, vertigo, and raised concentrations of calcium and phosphate in plasma and urine

Dose: see notes above

■ Daily supplements

NOTE. There is no plain vitamin D tablet available for treating simple deficiency (see notes above). Alternatives include vitamins capsules (see 9.6.7), preparations of

vitamins A and D (see 9.6.1), and calcium and ergocalciferol tablets (see below).

Calcium and Ergocalciferol (Non-proprietary)
(Calcium and Vitamin D)
Tablets, calcium lactate 300 mg, calcium phosphate 150 mg (calcium 97 mg or Ca^{2+} 2.4 mmol), ergocalciferol 10 micrograms (400 units). Net price 28-tab pack = 70p. Counselling, crush before administration or may be chewed

Adcal-D₃® (Strakan)
Tablets (chewable), calcium carbonate 1.5 g (calcium 600 mg or Ca^{2+} 15.1 mmol), colecalciferol 10 micrograms (400 units), net price 100-tab pack = £7.50. Label: 24

Cacit® **D3** (Procter & Gamble Pharm.)
Granules, effervescent, calcium carbonate 1.25 g (calcium 500 mg or Ca^{2+} 12.6 mmol), colecalciferol 11 micrograms (440 units)/sachet. Net price 30-sachet pack = £5.03. Label: 13

Calceos® (Provalis)
Tablets (chewable), calcium carbonate 1.25 g (calcium 500 mg or Ca^{2+} 12.6 mmol), colecalciferol 10 micrograms (400 units). Net price 60-tab pack = £5.10. Label: 24

Calcichew® **D3** (Shire)
Tablets (chewable), calcium carbonate 1.25 g (calcium 500 mg or Ca^{2+} 12.6 mmol), colecalciferol 5 micrograms (200 units). Net price 100-tab pack = £15.02. Label: 24
Excipients: include aspartame

Calcichew® **D3 Forte** (Shire)
Tablets (chewable), calcium carbonate 1.25 g (calcium 500 mg or Ca^{2+} 12.6 mmol), colecalciferol 10 micrograms (400 units). Net price 100-tab pack = £9.50. Label: 24
Excipients: include aspartame

Calfovit D3® (Trinity) PoM
Powder, calcium phosphate 3.1 g (calcium 1.2 g or Ca^{2+} 30 mmol), colecalciferol 20 micrograms (800 units), net price 30-sachet pack = £4.32. Label: 13, 21

■ Pharmacological strengths (see notes above)

Calciferol (Non-proprietary)
Tablets, colecalciferol or ergocalciferol 250 micrograms (10 000 units), net price 20 = £4.31; 1.25 mg (50 000 units) may also be available
Available from Celltech (as ergocalciferol)
NOTE. The BP directs that when calciferol tablets qualified by a descriptor relating to strength (such as 'high strength') are prescribed or demanded, the intention of the prescriber or purchaser with respect to the strength expressed in micrograms or milligrams per tablet should be ascertained. To avoid **errors** arising from the use of such titles prescribers are required to **abandon** them and **specify strength required**

Injection PoM, colecalciferol or ergocalciferol, 7.5 mg (300 000 units)/mL in oil. Net price 1-mL amp = £5.92, 2-mL amp = £7.07
Available from Celltech (as ergocalciferol)

ALFACALCIDOL

(1α-Hydroxycholecalciferol)

Indications: see notes above

Cautions: see under Ergocalciferol

Contra-indications: see under Ergocalciferol

Side-effects: see under Ergocalciferol

Dose: *by mouth or by intravenous injection* over 30 seconds, ADULT and CHILD over 20 kg, initially

1 microgram daily (elderly 500 nanograms), adjusted to avoid hypercalcaemia; maintenance, usually 0.25–1 microgram daily; NEONATE and PREMATURE INFANT initially 50–100 nanograms/ kg daily, CHILD under 20 kg initially 50 nanograms/kg daily

Alfacalcidol (Non-proprietary) PoM
Capsules, alfacalcidol 250 nanograms, net price 30-cap pack = £3.29; 500 nanograms 30-cap pack = £6.68; 1 microgram 30-cap pack = £10.01
Available from APS (excipients include arachis (peanut) oil)

One-Alpha® (Leo) PoM
Capsules, alfacalcidol 250 nanograms (white), net price 30-cap pack = £3.37; 500 nanograms (red), 30-cap pack = £6.74; 1 microgram (brown), 30-cap pack = £10.06
Excipients: include sesame oil
Oral drops, sugar-free, alfacalcidol 2 micrograms/ mL (1 drop contains approx. 100 nanograms), net price 10 mL = £24.18
Excipients: include alcohol
NOTE. The concentration of alfacalcidol in *One-Alpha*® *drops* is **10 times greater** than that of the former presentation *One-Alpha*® *solution*.
Injection, alfacalcidol 2 micrograms/mL, net price 0.5-mL amp = £2.32, 1-mL amp = £4.42
NOTE. Contains propylene glycol and should be used with caution in small premature infants

CALCITRIOL

(1,25-Dihydroxycholecalciferol)
Indications: see notes above
Cautions: see under Ergocalciferol; monitor plasma calcium, phosphate, and creatinine during dosage titration
Contra-indications: see under Ergocalciferol
Side-effects: see under Ergocalciferol
Dose: *by mouth*, renal osteodystrophy, initially 250 nanograms daily, or on alternate days (in patients with normal or only slightly reduced plasma-calcium concentration), increased if necessary in steps of 250 nanograms at intervals of 2–4 weeks; usual dose 0.5–1 microgram daily; CHILD not established
Established postmenopausal osteoporosis, 250 nanograms twice daily (monitor plasma-calcium concentration and creatinine, consult product literature)
by intravenous injection (or injection through catheter after haemodialysis), hypocalcaemia in dialysis patients with chronic renal failure, initially 500 nanograms (approx. 10 nanograms/kg) 3 times a week, increased if necessary in steps of 250–500 nanograms at intervals of 2–4 weeks; usual dose 0.5–3 micrograms 3 times a week; CHILD not established
Moderate to severe secondary hyperparathyroidism in dialysis patients, initially 0.5–4 micrograms 3 times a week, increased if necessary in steps of 250–500 nanograms at intervals of 2–4 weeks; max. 8 micrograms 3 times a week

Calcitriol (Non-proprietary) PoM
Capsules, calcitriol 250 nanograms, net price 30-cap pack = £6.18; 500 nanograms, 30-cap pack = £11.05
Available from APS

Rocaltrol® (Roche) PoM
Capsules, calcitriol 250 nanograms (red/white), net price 20 = £4.12; 500 nanograms (red), 20 = £7.36

Calcijex® (Abbott) PoM
Injection, calcitriol 1 microgram/mL, net price 1-mL amp = £5.14; 2 micrograms/mL, 1-mL amp = £10.28

COLECALCIFEROL

(Cholecalciferol, vitamin D₃)
Indications: see under Ergocalciferol—alternative to ergocalciferol in calciferol tablets and injection
Cautions: see under Ergocalciferol
Contra-indications: see under Ergocalciferol
Side-effects: see under Ergocalciferol

DIHYDROTACHYSTEROL

Indications: see under Ergocalciferol
Cautions: see under Ergocalciferol
Contra-indications: see under Ergocalciferol
Side-effects: see under Ergocalciferol

AT 10® (Intrapharm)
Oral solution, dihydrotachysterol 250 micrograms/ mL. Net price 15-mL dropper bottle = £22.87
Excipients: include arachis (peanut) oil
Dose: acute, chronic, and latent forms of hypocalcaemic tetany due to hypoparathyroidism, consult product literature

9.6.5 Vitamin E

(Tocopherols)

The daily requirement of vitamin E has not been well defined but is probably about 3 to 15 mg daily. There is little evidence that oral supplements of vitamin E are essential in adults, even where there is fat malabsorption secondary to cholestasis. In young children with congenital cholestasis, abnormally low vitamin E concentrations may be found in association with neuromuscular abnormalities, which usually respond only to the parenteral administration of vitamin E.

Vitamin E has been tried for various other conditions but there is little scientific evidence of its value.

ALPHA TOCOPHERYL ACETATE

Indications: see notes above
Cautions: predisposition to thrombosis; increased risk of necrotising enterocolitis in premature infants weighing less than 1.5 kg
Side-effects: diarrhoea and abdominal pain with doses more than 1 g daily

Vitamin E Suspension (Cambridge)
Suspension, alpha tocopheryl acetate 500 mg/5 mL. Net price 100 mL = £16.56
Dose: malabsorption in cystic fibrosis, 100–200 mg daily; CHILD under 1 year 50 mg daily; 1 year and over, 100 mg daily
Malabsorption in abetalipoproteinaemia, ADULT and CHILD 50–100 mg/kg daily
Malabsorption in chronic cholestasis, INFANT 150–200 mg/kg daily
NOTE. Tablets containing tocopheryl acetate 100 mg are available on a named-patient basis from Bell and Croyden (*Ephynal*®)

9.6.6 Vitamin K

Vitamin K is necessary for the production of blood clotting factors and proteins necessary for the normal calcification of bone.

Because vitamin K is fat soluble, patients with fat malabsorption, especially in biliary obstruction or hepatic disease, may become deficient. For oral administration to prevent vitamin-K deficiency in malabsorption syndromes, a water-soluble preparation, **menadiol sodium phosphate** must be used; the usual dose is about 10 mg daily.

Oral coumarin anticoagulants act by interfering with vitamin K metabolism in the hepatic cells and their effects can be antagonised by giving vitamin K; for British Society for Haematology Guidelines, see section 2.8.2.

VITAMIN K DEFICIENCY BLEEDING. Infants are relatively deficient in vitamin K and those who do not receive supplements of vitamin K are at risk of serious bleeds including intracranial bleeding. The Chief Medical Officer and the Chief Nursing Officer have recommended that all newborn babies should receive vitamin K to prevent vitamin K deficiency bleeding (haemorrhagic disease of the newborn). An appropriate regimen should be selected after discussion with parents in the antenatal period.

Vitamin K (as **phytomenadione**) 1 mg may be given by a single intramuscular injection at birth; this prevents vitamin K deficiency bleeding in virtually all babies. Fears about the safety of parenteral vitamin K appear to be unfounded.

Alternatively, vitamin K may be given by mouth, and arrangements must be in place to ensure the appropriate regimen is followed. Two doses of a colloidal (mixed micelle) preparation of phytomenadione 2 mg should be given in the first week. For breast-fed babies, a third dose of phytomenadione 2 mg is given at 1 month of age; the third dose is omitted in formula-fed babies because formula feeds contain vitamin K.

MENADIOL SODIUM PHOSPHATE

Indications: see notes above

Cautions: G6PD deficiency (section 9.1.5) and vitamin E deficiency (risk of haemolysis); **interactions:** Appendix 1 (vitamins)

Contra-indications: neonates and infants, late pregnancy

Dose: see notes above

Menadiol Phosphate (Non-proprietary)

Tablets, menadiol sodium phosphate equivalent to 10 mg of menadiol phosphate. Net price 100-tab pack = £35.56
Available from Cambridge

PHYTOMENADIONE

(Vitamin K$_1$)

Indications: see notes above

Cautions: intravenous injections should be given very slowly (see also below); pregnancy (Appendix 4); **interactions:** Appendix 1 (vitamins)

Dose: see notes above and section 2.8.2

Konakion® (Roche) PoM

Tablets, s/c, phytomenadione 10 mg, net price 10-tab pack = £1.77. To be chewed or allowed to dissolve slowly in the mouth (Label: 24)

Injection (Konakion® Neonatal), phytomenadione 2 mg/mL, net price 0.5-mL amp = 23p
Excipients: include polyoxyl castor oil (risk of anaphylaxis, see Excipients, p. 2)
NOTE. *Konakion® Neonatal* is for use in healthy neonates of over 36 weeks gestation; for intramuscular injection only

■ Colloidal formulation

Konakion® MM (Roche) PoM

Injection, phytomenadione 10 mg/mL in a mixed micelles vehicle. Net price 1-mL amp = 43p
Excipients: include glycocholic acid 54.6 mg/amp, lecithin
CAUTIONS. reduce dose in elderly; liver impairment (glycocholic acid may displace bilirubin); reports of anaphylactoid reactions
NOTE. *Konakion® MM* may be administered by slow intravenous injection or by intravenous infusion in glucose 5% (see Appendix 6); **not** for intramuscular injection

Konakion® MM Paediatric (Roche) PoM

Injection, phytomenadione 10 mg/mL in a mixed micelles vehicle. Net price 0.2-mL amp = £1.55
Excipients: include glycocholic acid 10.9 mg/amp, lecithin
CAUTIONS. parenteral administration in premature infants of less than 2.5 kg (increased risk of kernicterus)
NOTE. *Konakion® MM Paediatric* may be administered *by mouth* or *by intramuscular injection* or *by intravenous injection*

9.6.7 Multivitamin preparations

Vitamins

Capsules, ascorbic acid 15 mg, nicotinamide 7.5 mg, riboflavin 500 micrograms, thiamine hydrochloride 1 mg, vitamin A 2500 units, vitamin D 300 units. Net price 20 = 21p

Abidec® (W-L)

Drops, vitamins A, B group, C, and D. Net price 25 mL (with dropper) = £1.84
Excipients: include arachis (peanut) oil

Dalivit® (Eastern)

Oral drops, vitamins A, B group, C, and D, net price 25 mL = £1.60, 50 mL = £2.86

Vitamin and mineral supplements and adjuncts to synthetic diets

Forceval® (Unigreg)

Capsules, brown/red, vitamins (ascorbic acid 60 mg, biotin 100 micrograms, cyanocobalamin 3 micrograms, folic acid 400 micrograms, nicotinamide 18 mg, pantothenic acid 4 mg, pyridoxine 2 mg, riboflavin 1.6 mg, thiamine 1.2 mg, vitamin A 2500 units, vitamin D$_2$ 400 units, vitamin E 10 mg, minerals and trace elements (calcium 100 mg, chromium 200 micrograms, copper 2 mg, iodine 140 micrograms, iron 12 mg, magnesium 30 mg, manganese 3 mg, molybdenum 250 micrograms, phosphorus 77 mg, potassium 4 mg, selenium 50 micrograms, zinc 15 mg). Net price 30-cap pack = £5.15, 45-cap pack = £7.35; 90-cap pack = £14.04
Dose: vitamin and mineral deficiency and as adjunct in synthetic diets, 1 capsule daily

Junior capsules, brown, vitamins (ascorbic acid 25 mg, biotin 50 micrograms, cyanocobalamin 2 micrograms, folic acid 100 micrograms, nicotinamide 7.5 mg, pantothenic acid 2 mg, pyridoxine 1 mg, riboflavin 1 mg, thiamine 1.5 mg, vitamin A 1250 units, vitamin D$_2$ 200 units, vitamin E 5 mg, vitamin K$_1$ 25 micrograms), minerals and trace elements (chromium 50 micrograms, copper 1 mg, iodine 75 micrograms, iron 5 mg, magnesium 1 mg, manganese 1.25 mg, molybdenum 50 micrograms, selenium 25 micrograms, zinc 5 mg). Net price 30-cap pack = £3.87, 60-cap pack = £7.35
Dose: vitamin and mineral deficiency and as adjunct in synthetic diets, CHILD over 5 years, 2 capsules daily

Ketovite® (Paines & Byrne)
Tablets PoM, yellow, ascorbic acid 16.6 mg, riboflavin 1 mg, thiamine hydrochloride 1 mg, pyridoxine hydrochloride 330 micrograms, nicotinamide 3.3 mg, calcium pantothenate 1.16 mg, alpha tocopheryl acetate 5 mg, inositol 50 mg, biotin 170 micrograms, folic acid 250 micrograms, acetomenaphthone 500 micrograms. Net price 100-tab pack = £4.17
Dose: prevention of vitamin deficiency in disorders of carbohydrate or amino-acid metabolism and adjunct in restricted, specialised, or synthetic diets, 1 tablet 3 times daily; use with *Ketovite® Liquid* for complete vitamin supplementation
Liquid, pink, sugar-free, vitamin A 2500 units, ergocalciferol 400 units, choline chloride 150 mg, cyanocobalamin 12.5 micrograms/5 mL. Net price 150-mL pack = £2.70
Dose: prevention of vitamin deficiency in disorders of carbohydrate or amino-acid metabolism and adjunct in restricted, specialised, or synthetic diets, 5 mL daily; use with *Ketovite® Tablets* for complete vitamin supplementation

Vivioptal® (Pharma-Global)
Capsules, brown, vitamins (biotin 50 micrograms, calcium ascorbate 60 mg, colecalciferol 400 units, cyanocobalamin 3 micrograms, dexpanthenol 10 mg, folic acid 400 micrograms, inositol 30 mg, nicotinamide 25 mg, pyridoxine 6.08 mg, riboflavin 3 mg, rutoside 20 mg, thiamine nitrate 5 mg, vitamin A 5000 units, vitamin E 10 mg), minerals and trace elements (calcium hydrogen phosphate 35 mg, cobalt sulphate 100 micrograms, copper sulphate 500 micrograms, iron 3.25 mg, magnesium glycerophosphate 40 mg, manganese sulphate 500 micrograms, potassium sulphate 8 mg, sodium molybdate 80 micrograms, zinc oxide 500 micrograms); also contains adenosine, choline hydrogen tartrate, ethyl linoleate, lecithin, lysine hydrochloride, and orotic acid, net price 30-cap pack = £5.62
Dose: vitamin and mineral deficiency and as an adjunct in synthetic diets, 1 capsule daily
Excipients: include arachis (peanut) oil

9.7 Bitters and tonics

Mixtures containing simple and aromatic bitters, such as alkaline gentian mixture, are traditional remedies for loss of appetite. All depend on suggestion.

Gentian Mixture, Acid, BP
Mixture, concentrated compound gentian infusion 10%, dilute hydrochloric acid 5% in a suitable vehicle. Extemporaneous preparations should be recently prepared according to the following formula: concentrated compound gentian infusion 1 mL, dilute hydrochloric acid 0.5 mL, double-strength chloroform water 5 mL, water to 10 mL
Dose: 10 mL 3 times daily in water before meals

Gentian Mixture, Alkaline, BP
(Alkaline Gentian Oral Solution)
Mixture, concentrated compound gentian infusion 10%, sodium bicarbonate 5% in a suitable vehicle. Extemporaneous preparations should be recently prepared according to the following formula: concentrated compound gentian infusion 1 mL, sodium bicarbonate 500 mg, double-strength chloroform water 5 mL, water to 10 mL
Dose: 10 mL 3 times daily in water before meals

Effico® (Forest) NHS ▭
Tonic, orange-red, thiamine hydrochloride 180 micrograms, nicotinamide 2.1 mg, caffeine 20.2 mg, compound gentian infusion 0.31 mL/5 mL. Net price 300-mL pack = £2.42, 500-mL pack = £3.07

Labiton® (LAB) NHS ▭
Tonic, brown, thiamine hydrochloride 375 micrograms, caffeine 3.5 mg, kola nut dried extract 3.025 mg, alcohol 1.4 mL/5 mL. Net price 200 mL = £2.38

Metatone® (W-L) NHS ▭
Tonic, thiamine hydrochloride 500 micrograms, calcium glycerophosphate 45.6 mg, manganese glycerophosphate 5.7 mg, potassium glycerophosphate 45.6 mg, sodium glycerophosphate 22.8 mg/5 mL. Net price 300 mL = £2.79

9.8 Metabolic disorders

9.8.1   Drugs used in metabolic disorders
9.8.2   Acute porphyrias

This section covers drugs used in metabolic disorders and not readily classified elsewhere.

9.8.1 Drugs used in metabolic disorders

Wilson's disease

Penicillamine (see also section 10.1.3) is used in Wilson's disease (hepatolenticular degeneration) to aid the elimination of copper ions. See below for other indications.

Trientine is used for the treatment of Wilson's disease only, in patients intolerant of penicillamine; it is **not** an alternative to penicillamine for rheumatoid arthritis or cystinuria. Penicillamine-induced systemic lupus erythematosus may not resolve on transfer to trientine.

PENICILLAMINE

Indications: see under Dose below
Cautions: see section 10.1.3
Contra-indications: see section 10.1.3
Side-effects: see section 10.1.3
Dose: Wilson's disease, 1.5–2 g daily in divided doses before food; max. 2 g daily for 1 year;

maintenance 0.75–1 g daily; ELDERLY 20 mg/kg daily in divided doses, adjusted according to response; CHILD up to 20 mg/kg daily in divided doses, minimum 500 mg daily

Autoimmune hepatitis (used rarely; after disease controlled with corticosteroids), initially 500 mg daily in divided doses increased slowly over 3 months; usual maintenance dose 1.25 g daily; ELDERLY not recommended

Cystinuria, therapeutic, 1–3 g daily in divided doses before food, adjusted to maintain urinary cystine below 200 mg/litre; prophylactic (maintain urinary cystine below 300 mg/litre) 0.5–1 g at bedtime; maintain adequate fluid intake (at least 3 litres daily); CHILD and ELDERLY minimum dose to maintain urinary cystine below 200 mg/litre

Severe active rheumatoid arthritis, section 10.1.3

Copper and lead poisoning, see Emergency Treatment of Poisoning

■ Preparations
Section 10.1.3

TRIENTINE DIHYDROCHLORIDE

Indications: Wilson's disease in patients intolerant of penicillamine

Cautions: see notes above; pregnancy; **interactions:** Appendix 1 (trientine)

Side-effects: nausea, rash; rarely anaemia

Dose: 1.2–2.4 g daily in 2–4 divided doses before food; CHILD initially 0.6–1.5 g daily in 2–4 divided doses before food, adjusted according to response

Trientine Dihydrochloride PoM
Capsules, trientine dihydrochloride 300 mg. Label: 6, 22
Available from Univar
NOTE. The CSM has requested that in addition to the usual CSM reporting request special records should also be kept by the pharmacist

Carnitine deficiency

Carnitine is available for the management of primary carnitine deficiency due to inborn errors of metabolism or of secondary deficiency in haemodialysis patients.

CARNITINE

Indications: primary and secondary carnitine deficiency

Cautions: renal impairment; monitoring of free and acyl carnitine in blood and urine recommended; pregnancy (but appropriate to use) and breast-feeding

Side-effects: nausea, vomiting, abdominal pain, diarrhoea, body odour; side-effects may be dose-related—monitor tolerance during first week and after any dose increase

Dose: primary deficiency, *by mouth*, up to 200 mg/kg daily in 2–4 divided doses; higher doses of up to 400 mg/kg daily occasionally required; *by intravenous injection*, up to 100 mg/kg daily in 3–4 divided doses

Secondary deficiency, *by intravenous injection*, 20 mg/kg after each dialysis session (dosage adjusted according to carnitine concentration); maintenance, *by mouth*, 1 g daily

Carnitor® (Shire) PoM
Oral liquid, L-carnitine 1 g/10-mL single-dose bottle. Net price 10 × 10-mL single-dose bottle = £35.00

Paediatric solution, L-carnitine 30%. Net price 20 mL = £21.00

Injection, L-carnitine 200 mg/mL. Net price 5-mL amp = £11.90

Gaucher's disease

Imiglucerase, an enzyme produced by recombinant DNA technology, is administered as enzyme replacement therapy in Gaucher's disease, a familial disorder affecting principally the liver, spleen, bone marrow, and lymph nodes.

IMIGLUCERASE

Indications: (specialist use only) type I Gaucher's disease

Cautions: pregnancy and breast-feeding; monitor for imiglucerase antibodies; when stabilised monitor all parameters and response to treatment at intervals of 6–12 months

Side-effects: pruritus, pain, swelling or sterile abscess at injection site; hypersensitivity reactions; also reported nausea, vomiting, diarrhoea, abdominal pain, fatigue, headache, dizziness, fever, rash

Dose: *by intravenous infusion*, initially 60 units/kg once every 2 weeks (2.5 units/kg 3 times a week or 15 units/kg once every 2 weeks may improve haematological parameters and organomegaly, but not bone parameters); maintenance, adjust dose according to response

Cerezyme® (Genzyme) PoM
Intravenous infusion, powder for reconstitution, imiglucerase, net price 200-unit vial = £595.00; 400-unit vial = £1190.00

Nephropathic cystinosis

Mercaptamine (cysteamine) is available for the treatment of nephropathic cystinosis.

MERCAPTAMINE
(Cysteamine)

Indications: (specialist use only) nephropathic cystinosis

Cautions: leucocyte-cystine concentration and haematological monitoring required—consult product literature; dose of phosphate supplement may need to be adjusted

Contra-indications: pregnancy and breast-feeding; hypersensitivity to mercaptamine or penicillamine

Side-effects: breath and body odour, nausea, vomiting, diarrhoea, anorexia, lethargy, fever, rash; also reported dehydration, hypertension, abdominal discomfort, gastroenteritis, drowsiness, encephalopathy, headache, nervousness, depression; anaemia, leucopenia, increases in liver enzymes; rarely gastro-intestinal ulceration and bleeding, seizures, hallucinations, urticaria, interstitial nephritis

Dose: initial doses should be one-sixth to one-quarter of the expected maintenance dose, increased gradually over 4–6 weeks

Maintenance, ADULT and CHILD over 50 kg body-weight, 2 g daily in 4 divided doses

CHILD up to 12 years, 1.3 g/m^2 (approx. 50 mg/kg) daily in 4 divided doses

Cystagon® (Orphan Europe) ▼ PoM
Capsules, mercaptamine (as bitartrate) 50 mg, net price 100-cap pack = £44.00; 150 mg, 100-cap pack = £125.00
NOTE. CHILD under 6 years at risk of aspiration, capsules can be opened and contents sprinkled on food (at a temperature suitable for eating); avoid adding to acidic drinks (e.g. orange juice)

Urea cycle disorders

Sodium phenylbutyrate has recently become available for the management of urea cycle disorders. It is indicated as adjunctive therapy in all patients with neonatal-onset disease and in those with late-onset disease who have a history of hyperammonaemic encephalopathy.
  Carglumic acid is licensed for the treatment of hyperammonaemia due to *N*-acetylglutamate synthase deficiency.

CARGLUMIC ACID

Indications: hyperammonaemia due to *N*-acetyl-glutamate synthase deficiency (initiated under specialist supervision)
Cautions: pregnancy (Appendix 4) and breast-feeding (Appendix 5)
Side-effects: occasionally, raised transaminases, sweating
Dose: ADULT and CHILD initially 100 mg/kg daily in 2–4 divided doses immediately before food (max. 250 mg/kg daily), adjusted according to plasma–ammonia concentration; maintenance 10–100 mg/kg daily in 2–4 divided doses

Carbaglu® (Orphan Europe) ▼ PoM
Dispersible tablets, carglumic acid 200 mg, net price 60-tab pack = £2685.00. Label: 13

SODIUM PHENYLBUTYRATE

Indications: adjunct in long-term treatment of urea cycle disorders (under specialist supervision)
Cautions: congestive heart failure, hepatic and renal impairment
Contra-indications: pregnancy (Appendix 4) and breast-feeding
Side-effects: amenorrhoea and irregular menstrual cycles, decreased appetite, body odour, taste disturbances; less commonly nausea, vomiting, abdominal pain, peptic ulcer, pancreatitis, rectal bleeding, arrhythmia, oedema, syncope, depression, headache, rash, weight gain, renal tubular acidosis, aplastic anaemia, ecchymoses
Dose: ADULT and CHILD over 20 kg, 9.9–13 g/m^2 daily in divided doses with meals (max. 20 g daily); CHILD less than 20 kg, 450–600 mg/kg daily in divided doses with meals

Ammonaps® (Orphan Europe) ▼ PoM
Tablets, sodium phenylbutyrate 500 mg. Contains Na$^+$ 2.7 mmol/tablet. Net price 250-tab pack = £493.00
Granules, sodium phenylbutyrate 940 mg/g. Contains Na$^+$ 5.4 mmol/g. Net price 266-g pack = £860.00
NOTE. Granules should be mixed with food before taking

9.8.2   Acute porphyrias

The acute porphyrias (acute intermittent porphyria, variegate porphyria, hereditary coproporphyria and 5-aminolaevulinic acid dehydratase deficiency porphyria) are hereditary disorders of haem biosynthesis; they have a prevalence of about 1 in 10 000 of the population.
  Great care must be taken when prescribing for patients with acute porphyria since many drugs can induce acute porphyric crises. Since acute porphyrias are hereditary, relatives of affected individuals should be screened and advised about the potential danger of certain drugs.
  Treatment of serious or life-threatening conditions should not be withheld from patients with acute porphyria. Where there is no safe alternative, urinary porphobilinogen excretion should be measured regularly; if it increases or symptoms occur, the drug can be withdrawn and the acute attack treated.
  Haem arginate is administered by short intravenous infusion as haem replacement in moderate, severe or unremitting acute porphyria crises.

Supplies of haem arginate may be obtained outside office hours from the on-call pharmacist at:
St. James University Hospital, Leeds   (0113) 243 3144
                                                           or (0113) 283 7010

St Thomas' Hospital, London   (020) 7928 9292

HAEM ARGINATE

(Human hemin)
Indications: acute porphyrias (acute intermittent porphyria, porphyria variegata, hereditary copro-porphyria)
Cautions: pregnancy and breast feeding
Side-effects: rarely hypersensitivity reactions and fever; pain and thrombophlebitis at injection site
Dose: *by intravenous infusion*, ADULT and CHILD 3 mg/kg once daily (max. 250 mg daily) for 4 days; if response inadequate, repeat 4-day course with close biochemical monitoring

Normosang® (Orphan Europe) ▼ PoM
Concentrate for intravenous infusion, haem arginate 25 mg/mL, net price 10-mL amp = £281.25

Drugs unsafe for use in acute porphyrias

The following list contains drugs on the UK market that have been classified as 'unsafe' in porphyria because they have been shown to be porphyrinogenic in animals or *in vitro*, or have been associated with acute attacks in patients.
  Further information may be obtained from:

Welsh Medicines Information Centre
University Hospital of Wales
Cardiff CF14 4XW
Telephone (029) 2074 2979

NOTE. Quite modest changes in chemical structure can lead to changes in porphyrinogenicity but where possible general statements have been made about groups of drugs; these should be checked first

Drug groups (check first)

Amphetamines	Diuretics[6]
Anabolic Steroids	Ergot Derivatives[7]
Antidepressants[1]	Gold Salts
Antihistamines[2]	Hormone Replacement Therapy[5]
Barbiturates[3]	Menopausal Steroids[5]
Benzodiazepines[4]	Progestogens[5]
Cephalosporins	Sulphonamides[8]
Contraceptives, steroid[5]	Sulphonylureas[9]

Individual Drugs (check groups above first)

Alcohol	Lidocaine (lignocaine)[13]
Aluminium-containing antacids[10]	Mebeverine
Aminoglutethimide	Mefenamic Acid
Amiodarone	Meprobamate
Azapropazone	Methotrexate
Baclofen	Methyldopa
Bromocriptine	Metoclopramide[14]
Busulfan	Metyrapone
Captopril	Miconazole
Carbamazepine	Mifepristone
Carisoprodol	Minoxidil[14]
Chloral Hydrate[11]	Nalidixic Acid
Chlorambucil	Nifedipine
Chloramphenicol	Nitrofurantoin
Chloroform[12]	Orphenadrine
Ciclosporin	Oxybutynin
Clonidine	Oxycodone
Cocaine	Oxymetazoline
Colistin	Oxytetracycline
Cyclophosphamide	Pentazocine[15]
Cycloserine	Pentoxifylline (oxpentifylline)
Danazol	Phenoxybenzamine
Dapsone	Phenylbutazone
Dexfenfluramine	Phenytoin
Diclofenac	Piroxicam
Doxycycline	Porfimer
Econazole	Prilocaine
Enflurane	Probenecid
Erythromycin	Pyrazinamide
Etamsylate	Ranitidine
Ethionamide	Rifabutin[16]
Ethosuximide	Rifampicin[16]
Etomidate	Simvastatin
Fenfluramine	Sulfinpyrazone
Flucloxacillin	Sulpiride
Flupentixol	Tamoxifen
Griseofulvin	Temoporfin
Halothane	Theophylline[17]
Hydralazine	Thioridazine
Hyoscine	Tinidazole
Isometheptene Mucate	Triclofos[11]
Isoniazid	Trimethoprim
Ketoconazole	Valproate[4]
Ketorolac	Verapamil
	Zuclopenthixol

1. Includes tricyclic (and related) and MAOIs; fluoxetine thought to be safe.

2. Cetirizine, chlorphenamine, cyclizine, diphenhydramine, doxylamine, ketotifen, loratadine, and alimemazine (trimeprazine) thought to be safe.

3. Includes methohexital, primidone, and thiopental.

4. Status epilepticus has been treated successfully with intravenous diazepam; temazepam is thought to be safe; where essential, seizure prophylaxis has been undertaken with clonazepam or valproate. Clobazam, lorazepam, and midazolam probably safe.

5. Progestogens are more porphyrinogenic than oestrogens; oestrogens may be safe at least in replacement doses. Progestogens should be avoided whenever possible by all women susceptible to acute porphyria; however, where non-hormonal contraception is inappropriate, progestogens may be used with extreme caution if the potential benefit outweighs risk. The risk of an acute attack is greatest in women who have had a previous attack or are aged under 30 years. Long-acting progestogen preparations should never be used in those at risk of acute porphyria.

6. Acetazolamide, amiloride, bumetanide, cyclopenthiazide and triamterene have been used.

7. Includes ergometrine (oxytocin probably safe), lisuride and pergolide.

8. Includes co-trimoxazole and sulfasalazine.

9. Glipizide is thought to be safe.

10. Absorption limited but magnesium-containing antacids preferable.

11. Although evidence of hazard is uncertain, manufacturer advises avoid.

12. Small amounts in medicines probably safe.

13. Bupivacaine is thought to be safe; lidocaine (lignocaine) and prilocaine may be used with caution.

14. May be used with caution if safer alternative not available.

15. Buprenorphine, codeine, diamorphine, dihydrocodeine, fentanyl, morphine, and pethidine are thought to be safe.

16. Rifamycins have been used in a few patients without evidence of harm—use with caution if safer alternative not available.

17. Includes aminophylline.

10: Musculoskeletal and joint diseases

For treatment of septic arthritis see section 5.1, table 1.

10.1 Drugs used in rheumatic diseases and gout

10.1.1 Non-steroidal anti-inflammatory drugs

10.1.2 Corticosteroids

10.1.3 Drugs which suppress the rheumatic disease process

10.1.4 Gout and cytotoxic-induced hyperuricaemia

Rheumatoid arthritis and other inflammatory disorders

Most rheumatic diseases require symptomatic treatment to relieve pain. A non-steroidal anti-inflammatory drug (NSAID) is indicated when pain and stiffness are due to inflammatory rheumatic disease. Drugs are also used to influence the disease process itself (section 10.1.3). For rheumatoid arthritis these include penicillamine, gold salts, antimalarials (chloroquine and hydroxychloroquine), drugs that affect the immune response (anakinra, azathioprine, ciclosporin, cyclophosphamide, etanercept, infliximab, leflunomide, and methotrexate), and sulfasalazine—they are known as disease-modifying antirheumatic drugs; corticosteroids may also reduce the rate of joint destruction (section 10.1.2.1). Drugs which may affect the disease process in psoriatic arthritis include sulfasalazine, gold salts, azathioprine, and methotrexate (section 10.1.3) and for gout they include uricosuric drugs and allopurinol (section 10.1.4).

Osteoarthritis and soft-tissue disorders

In osteoarthritis (sometimes called degenerative joint disease or osteoarthrosis) non-drug measures such as weight reduction and exercise should be encouraged. For pain relief in osteoarthritis and soft-tissue disorders, paracetamol (section 4.7.1) is often adequate and should be used first. Alternatively a low-dose NSAID (e.g. ibuprofen up to 1.2 g daily) may be used. If pain relief with either drug is inadequate, both paracetamol (in a full dose of 4 g daily) and a low-dose NSAID may be required; if necessary the dose of the NSAID may need to be increased or a low dose of an opioid analgesic given with paracetamol (as co-codamol 8/500 or co-dydramol 10/500).

Topical treatment including application of an NSAID or capsaicin 0.025% (section 10.3.2) may provide some pain relief in osteoarthritis.

Intra-articular corticosteroid injections (section 10.1.2.2) may produce temporary benefit in osteo-arthritis, especially if associated with soft-tissue inflammation.

Hyaluronic acid and its derivatives are available for osteoarthritis of the knee. Sodium hyaluronate (*Arthrease*, DePuy; *Durolane*, Q-Med; *Ferma-thron*, Biomet Merck; *Hyalgan*, Shire; *Orthovisc*, Surgicraft; *Ostenil*, TRB Chemedica; *Supartz*, S&N Hlth.; *Suplasyn*, PLIVA) or hylan G-F 20 (*Synvisc*, Biomatrix) is injected intra-articularly to supplement natural hyaluronic acid in the synovial fluid. These injections may reduce pain over 1–6 months but they are associated with short-term increase in knee inflammation.

10.1.1 Non-steroidal anti-inflammatory drugs

In *single doses* non-steroidal anti-inflammatory drugs (NSAIDs) have analgesic activity comparable to that of paracetamol (section 4.7.1), but paracetamol is preferred, particularly in the elderly (see also Prescribing for the elderly, p. 18).

In regular *full dosage* NSAIDs have both a lasting analgesic and an anti-inflammatory effect which makes them particularly useful for the treatment of continuous or regular pain associated with inflammation. Therefore, although paracetamol often gives adequate pain control in osteoarthritis, NSAIDs are more appropriate than paracetamol or the opioid analgesics in the *inflammatory arthritides* (e.g. rheumatoid arthritis) and in some cases of *advanced osteoarthritis*. They may also be of benefit in the less well defined conditions of *back pain* and *soft-tissue disorders*.

CHOICE. Differences in anti-inflammatory activity between different NSAIDs are small, but there is considerable variation in individual patient tolerance and response. About 60% of patients will respond to any NSAID; of the others, those who do not respond to one may well respond to another. Pain relief starts soon after taking the first dose and a full analgesic effect should normally be obtained within a week, whereas an anti-inflammatory effect may not be achieved (or may not be clinically assessable) for up to 3 weeks. If appropriate responses are not obtained within these times, another NSAID should be tried.

The main differences between NSAIDs are in the incidence and type of side-effects. Before treatment is started the prescriber should weigh efficacy against possible side-effects.

NSAIDs vary in their selectivity for inhibiting different types of cyclo-oxygenase; selective inhibition of cyclo-oxygenase-2 improves gastro-intestinal tolerance. A number of other factors also determine susceptibility to gastro-intestinal effects and an NSAID should be chosen on the basis of the incidence of gastro-intestinal and other side-effects.

Ibuprofen is a propionic acid derivative with anti-inflammatory, analgesic, and antipyretic properties. It has fewer side-effects than other NSAIDs but its anti-inflammatory properties are weaker. Doses of 1.6 to 2.4 g daily are needed for rheumatoid arthritis and it is unsuitable for conditions where inflammation is prominent such as acute gout.

Other propionic acid derivatives:

Naproxen is one of the first choices because it combines good efficacy with a low incidence of side-effects (but more than ibuprofen, see CSM comment below).

Fenbufen is claimed to be associated with less gastro-intestinal bleeding, but there is a high risk of rashes (see p. 482).

Fenoprofen is as effective as naproxen, and **flur-biprofen** may be slightly more effective. Both are associated with slightly more gastro-intestinal side-effects than ibuprofen.

Ketoprofen has anti-inflammatory properties similar to ibuprofen and has more side-effects (see also CSM comment below). **Dexketoprofen**, an isomer of ketoprofen, has been introduced for the short-term relief of mild to moderate pain.

Tiaprofenic acid is as effective as naproxen; it has more side-effects than ibuprofen (**important:** reports of severe cystitis, see CSM advice on p. 486).

Drugs with properties similar to those of propionic acid derivatives:

Azapropazone is similar in effect to naproxen; it has a tendency to cause rashes and is associated with an increased risk of severe gastro-intestinal toxicity (**important:** see CSM restrictions on p. 480).

Diclofenac and **aceclofenac** have actions similar to that of naproxen; their side-effects are also similar to naproxen.

Diflunisal is an aspirin derivative but its clinical effect more closely resembles that of the propionic acid derivatives than that of its parent compound. Its long duration of action allows twice-daily administration.

Indometacin (indomethacin) has an action equal to or superior to that of naproxen, but with a high incidence of side-effects including headaches, dizziness, and gastro-intestinal disturbances (see also CSM comment below).

Mefenamic acid has minor anti-inflammatory properties. Occasionally, it has been associated with diarrhoea and haemolytic anaemia which require discontinuation of treatment.

Nabumetone is comparable in effect to naproxen.

Piroxicam is as effective as naproxen and has a prolonged duration of action which permits once-daily administration. It has more gastro-intestinal side-effects than ibuprofen, especially in the elderly (see also CSM comment below).

Sulindac is similar in tolerance to naproxen.

Tenoxicam is similar in activity and tolerance to naproxen. Its long half-life allows once-daily administration.

Tolfenamic acid is licensed for the treatment of migraine (section 4.7.4.1)

Ketorolac and the selective inhibitor of cyclo-oxygenase-2, **parecoxib** are licensed for the short-term management of postoperative pain (section 15.1.4.2).

Drugs which are selective inhibitors of cyclo-oxygenase-2:

Celecoxib, etodolac, meloxicam, and **rofecoxib** are licensed for symptomatic relief in osteoarthritis and rheumatoid arthritis. Rofecoxib is also licensed for the relief of acute pain. Selective inhibitors of cyclo-oxygenase-2 are as effective as non-selective NSAIDs such as diclofenac and naproxen. They share the side-effects of non-selective NSAIDs. However, the risk of serious upper gastro-intestinal events is lower compared to non-selective NSAIDs; this advantage may be lost in patients who require concomitant low-dose aspirin. The CSM has issued a reminder that celecoxib and rofecoxib do not provide protection against ischaemic cardiovascular events.

Etoricoxib is licensed for symptomatic relief of osteoarthritis, rheumatoid arthritis, and acute gout. **Valdecoxib** is licensed for symptomatic relief of osteoarthritis, rheumatoid arthritis, and dysmenorrhoea. Etoricoxib and valdecoxib do not provide protection against ischaemic cardiovascular events.

NICE guidance (cyclo-oxygenase-2 selective inhibitors). NICE has recommended (July 2001) that, for patients with rheumatoid arthritis or osteoarthritis, cyclo-oxygenase-2 selective inhibitors (celecoxib, etodolac, meloxicam and rofecoxib) should:

- **not** be used routinely in the management of patients with these conditions;
- be used in preference to standard NSAIDs **only** when clearly indicated (and in accordance with UK licensing), for patients with a history of gastroduodenal ulcer or perforation or gastrointestinal bleeding—in these patients even the use of cyclo-oxygenase-2 selective inhibitors should be considered very carefully; they should also be used in preference to standard NSAIDs for other patients at **high risk** of developing serious gastro-intestinal side-effects (e.g. those aged over 65 years, those who are taking other medicines which increase the risk of gastrointestinal effects, those who are debilitated or those receiving long-term treatment with maximal doses of standard NSAIDs);
- **not** be used routinely in preference to standard NSAIDs for patients with cardiovascular disease; the benefit of cyclo-oxygenase-2 selective inhibitors is reduced in patients taking concomitant low-dose aspirin and this combination is **not justified**.

There is no evidence to justify the simultaneous use of gastro-protective drugs with cyclo-oxygenase-2 selective inhibitors as a means of further reducing potential gastro-intestinal side-effects.

CAUTIONS AND CONTRA-INDICATIONS. NSAIDs should be used with caution in the elderly (risk of serious side-effects and fatalities, see also Prescribing for the Elderly p. 18), in allergic disorders (they are **contra-indicated** in patients with a history of hypersensitivity to aspirin or any other NSAID—which includes those in whom attacks of asthma, angioedema, urticaria or rhinitis have been precipitated by aspirin or any other NSAID), during pregnancy and breast-feeding (see Appendixes 4 and 5), and in coagulation defects. Long-term use of

some NSAIDs is associated with reduced female fertility which is reversible on stopping treatment.

In patients with renal, cardiac, or hepatic impairment caution is required since the use of NSAIDs may result in deterioration of renal function (see also under Side-effects, below and Appendixes 2 and 3); the dose should be kept as **low as possible** and renal function should be **monitored**. Celecoxib, etoricoxib, rofecoxib, and valdecoxib are contra-indicated in severe congestive heart failure and caution should be exercised in patients with a history of cardiac failure, left ventricular dysfunction, or hypertension, and in patients with oedema for any other reason.

The CSM has advised that non-selective NSAIDs are contra-indicated in patients with previous or active peptic ulceration and that selective inhibitors of cyclo-oxygenase-2 are contra-indicated in active peptic ulceration (see also **CSM advice** below). While it is preferable to avoid NSAIDs in patients with active or previous gastro-intestinal ulceration or bleeding, and to withdraw them if gastro-intestinal lesions develop, nevertheless patients with serious rheumatic diseases (e.g. rheumatoid arthritis) are usually dependent on NSAIDs for effective relief of pain and stiffness. For advice on the prophylaxis and treatment of NSAID-associated peptic ulcers, see section 1.3.

For **interactions** of NSAIDs, see Appendix 1 (NSAIDs)

SIDE-EFFECTS. The side-effects of NSAIDs vary in severity and frequency. Gastro-intestinal discomfort, nausea, diarrhoea, and occasionally bleeding and ulceration occur (see also CSM advice below). Systemic as well as local effects of NSAIDs contribute to gastro-intestinal damage; taking oral formulations with milk or food, or using enteric-coated formulations, or changing the route of administration may only partially reduce symptoms such as dyspepsia. Those at risk of duodenal or gastric ulceration (including the elderly) who need to continue NSAID treatment should receive either a selective inhibitor of cyclo-oxygenase-2 alone, or a non-selective NSAID with gastroprotective treatment (section 1.3). Other side-effects include hypersensitivity reactions (particularly rashes, angioedema, and bronchospasm—see CSM advice below), headache, dizziness, nervousness, depression, drowsiness, insomnia, vertigo, hearing disturbances such as tinnitus, photosensitivity, and haematuria. Blood disorders have also occurred. Fluid retention may occur (rarely precipitating congestive heart failure in elderly patients); blood pressure may be raised. Renal failure may be provoked by NSAIDs especially in patients with pre-existing renal impairment (**important**, see also under Cautions above). Rarely, papillary necrosis or interstitial fibrosis associated with NSAIDs may lead to renal failure. Hepatic damage, alveolitis, pulmonary eosinophilia, pancreatitis, eye changes, Stevens-Johnson syndrome and toxic epidermal necrolysis are other rare side-effects. Induction of or exacerbation of colitis has been reported. Aseptic meningitis has been reported rarely with NSAIDs; patients with connective tissue disorders such as systemic lupus erythematosus may be especially susceptible.

Overdosage: see Emergency Treatment of Poisoning, p. 22.

CSM advice (gastro-intestinal side-effects). All NSAIDs are associated with serious gastro-intestinal toxicity; the risk is higher in the elderly. Evidence on the relative safety of 7 **non-selective** NSAIDs indicates differences in the risks of serious upper gastro-intestinal side-effects. **Azapropazone** is associated with the *highest risk* (**important:** see also restrictions on p. 480) and **ibuprofen** with the *lowest*; **piroxicam, ketoprofen, indometacin, naproxen** and **diclofenac** are associated with *intermediate risks* (possibly higher in the case of piroxicam). **Selective inhibitors of cyclo-oxygenase-2** are associated with a *lower risk* of serious upper gastro-intestinal side-effects than non-selective NSAIDs.

Recommendations are that NSAIDs associated with low risk e.g. ibuprofen are *generally preferred*, to start at the *lowest recommended dose, not to use more than one* oral NSAID at a time, and to remember that all NSAIDs (including selective inhibitors of cyclo-oxygenase-2) are *contra-indicated* in patients with active peptic ulceration. The CSM also contra-indicates non-selective NSAIDs in patients with a history of peptic ulceration.

The combination of a NSAID and low-dose aspirin may increase the risk of gastro-intestinal side-effects; this combination should only be used if absolutely necessary and the patient monitored closely

CSM warning (asthma). Any degree of worsening of asthma may be related to the ingestion of NSAIDs, either prescribed or (in the case of ibuprofen and others) purchased over the counter.

IBUPROFEN

Indications: pain and inflammation in rheumatic disease (including juvenile arthritis) and other musculoskeletal disorders; mild to moderate pain including dysmenorrhoea; postoperative analgesia; migraine; fever and pain in children; post-immunisation pyrexia (section 14.1)

Cautions: see notes above; **interactions:** Appendix 1 (NSAIDs)

Contra-indications: see notes above

Side-effects: see notes above; **overdosage:** see Emergency Treatment of Poisoning, p. 22

Dose: initially 1.2–1.8 g daily in 3–4 divided doses preferably after food; increased if necessary to max. 2.4 g daily; maintenance dose of 0.6–1.2 g daily may be adequate

Juvenile rheumatoid arthritis, CHILD over 7 kg bodyweight 30–40 mg/kg daily in 3–4 divided doses

Fever and pain in children, CHILD over 7 kg bodyweight 20–30 mg/kg daily in divided doses *or* 1–2 years 50 mg 3–4 times daily, 3–7 years 100 mg 3–4 times daily, 8–12 years 200 mg 3–4 times daily

Ibuprofen (Non-proprietary) PoM
Tablets, coated, ibuprofen 200 mg, net price 84-tab pack = £1.69; 400 mg, 84-tab pack = £2.46; 600 mg, 84-tab pack = £4.60. Label: 21
Various strengths available from Alpharma, APS, Arrow (400-mg strength only), Ashbourne (*Arthrofen*®), Bristol, CP, DDSA (*Ebufac*®), IVAX, Kent, Ranbaxy (*Rimafen*®), Pharmacia (*Motrin*®, 800-mg strength only), Sovereign, Sterwin

Oral suspension, ibuprofen 100 mg/5 mL, net price 100 mL = £1.82, 150 mL = £2.73. Label: 21
NOTE. Sugar-free versions are available and can be ordered by specifying 'sugar-free' on the prescription Available from Crookes (*Nurofen*® *for Children*), Galpharm (*Galprofen*®), Orbis (*Orbifen*® *for Children*), Pfizer Consumer (*Calprofen*®)
NOTE. Proprietary brands of ibuprofen preparations are on sale to the public; brand names include Advil®, Anadin Ibuprofen®, Anadin Ultra®, Arthrofen®, Boots Children's 6 years Plus Fever & Pain Relief®, Cuprofen®, Galprofen®, Hedex® Ibuprofen, Ibrufhalal®, Ibufem®, Inoven®, Librofem®, Migrafen®, Novaprin®, Nurofen®, Nurofen® for Children Singles, Nurofen® Long Lasting, Nurofen® Meltlets, Nurofen® Migraine Pain, Nurofen® Mobile, Nurofen® Recovery, Obifen®, Pacifene®, PhorPain®, Relcofen®; compound proprietary preparations containing ibuprofen include Nurofen® Plus (ibuprofen, codeine), Solpaflex® (ibuprofen, codeine)

Brufen® (Abbott) PoM
Tablets, all magenta, ibuprofen 200 mg (s/c), net price 20 = 82p; 400 mg (s/c), 20 = £1.63; 600 mg (f/c), 20 = £2.45. Label: 21
Syrup, orange, ibuprofen 100 mg/5 mL. Net price 500 mL = £8.07. Label: 21
Granules, effervescent, ibuprofen 600 mg/sachet. Net price 20-sachet pack = £6.80. Label: 13, 21
NOTE. Contains sodium approx. 9 mmol/sachet

■ Topical preparations
Section 10.3.2

■ Modified release
Brufen Retard® (Abbott) PoM
Tablets, m/r, f/c, ibuprofen 800 mg, net price 56-tab pack = £7.24. Label: 25, 27
Dose: 2 tablets daily as a single dose, preferably in the early evening, increased in severe cases to 3 tablets daily in 2 divided doses; CHILD not recommended

Fenbid® (Goldshield) PoM
Spansule® (= capsule m/r), maroon/pink, enclosing off-white pellets, ibuprofen 300 mg. Net price 120-cap pack = £9.64. Label: 25
Dose: 1–3 capsules every 12 hours; CHILD not recommended

■ With codeine
For an adverse comment on compound analgesic preparations, see p. 208. For details of the **side-effects, cautions,** and **contra-indications** of opioid analgesics, see p. 213 (**important:** the elderly are particularly susceptible to opioid side-effects).

Codafen Continus® (Napp) PoM
Tablets, white/pink, ibuprofen 300 mg (m/r), codeine phosphate 20 mg. Net price 56-tab pack = £6.40; 112-tab pack = £12.78. Label: 2, 21, 25
Dose: 1–2 tablets every 12 hours; max. 3 tablets every 12 hours; CHILD not recommended

ACECLOFENAC

Indications: pain and inflammation in rheumatoid arthritis, osteoarthritis and ankylosing spondylitis

Cautions: see notes above; avoid in porphyria (section 9.8.2); **interactions:** Appendix 1 (NSAIDs)

Contra-indications: see notes above

Side-effects: see notes above

Dose: 100 mg twice daily; CHILD not recommended

Preservex® (UCB Pharma) PoM
Tablets, f/c, aceclofenac 100 mg, net price 60-tab pack = £16.44. Label: 21

ACEMETACIN

(Glycolic acid ester of indometacin)

Indications: pain and inflammation in rheumatic disease and other musculoskeletal disorders; post-operative analgesia

Cautions: see under Indometacin and notes above; **interactions:** Appendix 1 (NSAIDs)

DRIVING. Dizziness may affect performance of skilled tasks (e.g. driving)

Contra-indications: see under Indometacin and notes above

Side-effects: see under Indometacin and notes above

Dose: 120 mg daily in divided doses with food, increased if necessary to 180 mg daily; CHILD not recommended

Emflex® (Merck) PoM
Capsules, yellow/orange, acemetacin 60 mg, net price 90-cap pack = £23.50. Label: 21, counselling, driving

---

AZAPROPAZONE

Indications: see under CSM restrictions, below

CSM RESTRICTIONS. CSM *has restricted* azapropazone to use in rheumatoid arthritis, ankylosing spondylitis and acute gout only when other NSAIDs have been tried and failed, *has* **contra-indicated** it in patients with a history of peptic ulceration, and *has reduced* the maximum daily dose to 600 mg for rheumatoid arthritis and ankylosing spondylitis in patients over 60 years

Cautions: see notes above; **interactions:** Appendix 1 (NSAIDs)

Contra-indications: see notes above; porphyria (section 9.8.2); history of peptic ulceration, inflammatory bowel disease or blood disorder; for specific restrictions and contra-indications relating to renal impairment see under Dose

Side-effects: see notes above; photosensitivity, see CSM advice below

PHOTOSENSITIVITY. CSM has reminded of need to advise patients taking azapropazone to avoid direct exposure to sunlight (or to use sunblock preparations)

Dose: rheumatoid arthritis and ankylosing spondylitis, 1.2 g daily in 2 or 4 divided doses; in renal impairment or in ELDERLY over 60 years, 300 mg twice daily, avoid altogether in severe renal impairment; CHILD not recommended

Acute gout (always ensure increased fluid intake), 1.8 g daily in divided doses until acute symptoms subside (usually by day 4) *then* 1.2 g daily in divided doses until symptoms resolve—consider appropriate alternative therapy if they persist; in ELDERLY over 60 years, 1.8 g daily for first 24 hours then 1.2 g daily in divided doses reducing to max. 600 mg daily in divided doses as soon as possible (preferably by day 4) *then* continuing only until acute symptoms resolve—consider appropriate alternative therapy if they persist, and *avoid altogether for gout* in renal impairment; CHILD not recommended

Rheumox® (Goldshield) PoM
Capsules, orange, azapropazone 300 mg. Net price 100-cap pack = £15.50. Label: 11, (also photosensitivity counselling, see above), 21
Tablets, orange, f/c, scored, azapropazone 600 mg. Net price 100-tab pack = £25.50. Label: 11, (also photosensitivity counselling, see above), 21

CELECOXIB

Indications: pain and inflammation in osteoarthritis or rheumatoid arthritis

Cautions: see notes above; **interactions:** Appendix 1 (NSAIDs)

Contra-indications: see notes above; sulphonamide sensitivity; inflammatory bowel disease

Side-effects: see notes above; flatulence, insomnia, pharyngitis, sinusitis; less frequently stomatitis, constipation, palpitations, fatigue, paraesthesia, muscle cramps; rarely taste alteration, alopecia

Dose: osteoarthritis, 200 mg daily in 1–2 divided doses, increased if necessary to max. 200 mg twice daily; CHILD not recommended

Rheumatoid arthritis, 200–400 mg daily in 2 divided doses; ELDERLY initially 200 mg daily in 2 divided doses; max. 200 mg twice daily; CHILD not recommended

Celebrex® (Pharmacia) PoM
Capsules, celecoxib 100 mg (white/blue), net price 60-cap pack = £21.55; 200 mg (white/gold), 30-cap pack = £21.55

DEXKETOPROFEN

Indications: short-term treatment of mild to moderate pain including dysmenorrhoea

Cautions: see notes above; **interactions:** Appendix 1 (NSAIDs)

Contra-indications: see notes above

Side-effects: see notes above

Dose: 12.5 mg every 4–6 hours *or* 25 mg every 8 hours; max. 75 mg daily; ELDERLY initially max. 50 mg daily; CHILD not recommended

Keral® (Menarini) PoM
Tablets, f/c, scored, dexketoprofen (as trometamol) 25 mg, net price 10-tab pack = £1.95 (hosp. only), 20-tab pack = £3.90, 50-tab pack = £9.75. Label: 22

DICLOFENAC SODIUM

Indications: pain and inflammation in rheumatic disease (including juvenile arthritis) and other musculoskeletal disorders; acute gout; postoperative pain

Cautions: see notes above; **interactions:** Appendix 1 (NSAIDs)

Contra-indications: see notes above; porphyria (section 9.8.2)

INTRAVENOUS USE. Additional contra-indications include concomitant NSAID or anticoagulant use (including low-dose heparin), history of haemorrhagic diathesis, history of confirmed or suspected cerebrovascular bleeding, operations with high risk of haemorrhage, history of asthma, moderate or severe renal impairment, hypovolaemia, dehydration

Side-effects: see notes above; suppositories may cause rectal irritation; injection site reactions

Dose: *by mouth*, 75–150 mg daily in 2–3 divided doses

By deep intramuscular injection into the gluteal muscle, acute exacerbations of pain and postoperative pain, 75 mg once daily (twice daily in severe cases) for max. of 2 days

Ureteric colic, 75 mg then a further 75 mg after 30 minutes if necessary

By intravenous infusion (in hospital setting), 75 mg repeated if necessary after 4–6 hours for max. 2 days

Prevention of postoperative pain, initially after surgery 25–50 mg over 15–60 minutes then 5 mg/hour for max. 2 days

By rectum in suppositories, 75–150 mg daily in divided doses

Max. total daily dose by any route 150 mg

CHILD 1–12 years, juvenile arthritis, *by mouth or by rectum*, 1–3 mg/kg daily in divided doses (25 mg e/c tablets, 12.5 mg and 25 mg suppositories only)

Diclofenac Sodium (Non-proprietary) [PoM]
Tablets, both e/c, diclofenac sodium 25 mg, net price 84-tab pack = £2.56; 50 mg, 84-tab pack = £3.70. Label: 5, 25
Available from Alpharma, APS, Arun (*Diclovol*®), Ashbourne (*Diclozip*®), Berk (*Flamrase*®), Dexcel Pharma (*Dicloflex*®), Discovery (*Fenactol*®), Eastern (*Volraman*®), Goldshield (*Acoflam*®), IVAX, Kent, Ranbaxy (*Defenac*®), Sandoz, Sterwin, Trinity (*Lofensaid*®)
Suppositories, diclofenac sodium 100 mg, net price 10 = £3.07
Available from Goldshield (*Econac*®)
Injection, diclofenac sodium 25 mg/mL. Net price 3-mL amp = 74p
Available from Antigen
NOTE. Licensed for intramuscular use

Voltarol® (Novartis) [PoM]
Tablets, both e/c, diclofenac sodium 25 mg (yellow), net price 84-tab pack = £3.94; 50 mg (brown), 84-tab pack = £6.13. Label: 5, 25
Dispersible tablets, sugar-free, pink, diclofenac, equivalent to diclofenac sodium 50 mg, net price 21-tab pack = £5.63. Label: 13, 21
NOTE. Voltarol Dispersible tablets are more suitable for **short-term** use in acute conditions for which treatment required for no more than 3 months (no information on use beyond 3 months)
Injection, diclofenac sodium 25 mg/mL. Net price 3-mL amp = 83p
Excipients: include benzyl alcohol (see Excipients, p. 2)
Suppositories, diclofenac sodium 12.5 mg, net price 10 = 71p; 25 mg, 10 = £1.26; 50 mg, 10 = £2.07; 100 mg, 10 = £3.70
Emulgel® gel, section 10.3.2

■ Diclofenac potassium

Voltarol® **Rapid** (Novartis) [PoM]
Tablets, s/c, diclofenac potassium 25 mg (red), net price 28-tab pack = £3.67; 50 mg (brown), 28-tab pack = £7.03
Dose: rheumatic disease, musculoskeletal disorders, acute gout, post-operative pain, 75–150 mg daily in 2–3 divided doses; CHILD over 14 years, 75–100 mg daily in 2–3 divided doses
Migraine, 50 mg at onset, repeated after 2 hours if necessary then after 4–6 hours; max. 200 mg in 24 hours; CHILD not recommended

■ Modified release

Diclomax SR® (Parke-Davis) [PoM]
Capsules, m/r, yellow, diclofenac sodium 75 mg. Net price 56-cap pack = £13.01. Label: 21, 25
Dose: 1 capsule 1–2 times daily *or* 2 capsules once daily, preferably with food; CHILD not recommended

Diclomax Retard® (Parke-Davis) [PoM]
Capsules, m/r, diclofenac sodium 100 mg. Net price 28-tab pack = £9.36. Label: 21, 25
Dose: 1 capsule daily preferably with food; CHILD not recommended

Motifene® **75 mg** (Sankyo) [PoM]
Capsules, e/c, m/r, diclofenac sodium 75 mg (enclosing e/c pellets containing diclofenac sodium 25 mg and m/r pellets containing diclofenac sodium 50 mg). Net price 56-cap pack = £14.99. Label: 25
Dose: 1 capsule 1-2 times daily; CHILD not recommended

Voltarol® **75 mg SR** (Novartis) [PoM]
Tablets, m/r, pink, diclofenac sodium 75 mg. Net price 28-tab pack = £8.68; 56-tab pack = £17.35. Label: 21, 25
Dose: 75 mg 1–2 times daily preferably with food; CHILD not recommended
NOTE. Modified-release tablets containing diclofenac sodium 75 mg also available from Alpharma (*Flamatak*® MR), APS, Arun (*Diclovol*® SR, *Flamrase*® SR), Dexcel Pharma (*Dicloflex*® 75 SR), Discovery (*Fenactol*® 75 mg SR), Goldshield (*Acoflam*® 75 SR), Hillcross (*Dexomon*® 75 SR), IVAX, Pharmacia (*Flexotard*® MR 75), Ranbaxy (*Defenac*® SR), Sandoz (*Rhumalgan*® CR), Sovereign (*Rheumatac*® Retard 75), Sterwin (*Slofenac*® SR), Trinity (*Volsaid*® Retard 75)

Voltarol® **Retard** (Novartis) [PoM]
Tablets, m/r, red, diclofenac sodium 100 mg. Net price 28-tab pack = £12.72. Label: 21, 25
Dose: 1 tablet daily preferably with food; CHILD not recommended
NOTE. Modified-release tablets containing diclofenac sodium 100 mg available from Alpharma (*Flamatak*® 100 MR), APS, Arun (*Diclovol*® Retard), Berk (*Flamrase*® SR[1]), Dexcel Pharma (*Dicloflex*® Retard), Discovery (*Fenactol*® Retard 100 mg), Goldshield (*Acoflam*® Retard), Hillcross (*Dexomon*® Retard 100), IVAX, Ranbaxy (*Defenac*® Retard), Sandoz (*Rhumalgan*® CR), Sterwin (*Slofenac*® SR), Trinity (*Volsaid*® Retard 100)

1. Also licensed for dysmenorrhoea and associated menorrhagia

■ With misoprostol

For **cautions**, **contra-indications**, and **side-effects** of misoprostol, see section 1.3.4

Arthrotec® (Pharmacia) [PoM]
Arthrotec® *50 tablets*, diclofenac sodium (in e/c core) 50 mg, misoprostol 200 micrograms. Net price 60-tab pack = £13.31; Label: 21, 25
Dose: prophylaxis against NSAID-induced gastroduodenal ulceration in patients requiring diclofenac for rheumatoid arthritis or osteoarthritis, 1 tablet 2–3 times daily with food; CHILD not recommended
Arthrotec® *75 tablets*, diclofenac sodium (in e/c core) 75 mg, misoprostol 200 micrograms. Net price 60-tab pack = £17.59. Label: 21, 25
Dose: prophylaxis against NSAID-induced gastroduodenal ulceration in patients requiring diclofenac for rheumatoid arthritis or osteoarthritis, 1 tablet twice daily with food; CHILD not recommended

DIFLUNISAL

Indications: pain and inflammation in rheumatic disease and other musculoskeletal disorders; mild to moderate pain including dysmenorrhoea
Cautions: see notes above; **interactions:** Appendix 1 (NSAIDs)
Contra-indications: see notes above
Side-effects: see notes above

Dose: mild to moderate pain, initially 1 g, then 500 mg every 12 hours (increased to max. 500 mg every 8 hours if necessary)
Osteoarthritis, rheumatoid arthritis, 0.5–1 g daily as a single daily dose *or* in 2 divided doses
Dysmenorrhoea, initially 1 g, then 500 mg every 12 hours
CHILD not recommended

Dolobid® (MSD) PoM
Tablets, both f/c, diflunisal 250 mg (peach), net price 60-tab pack = £5.41; 500 mg (orange), 60-tab pack = £10.82. Label: 21, 25, counselling, avoid aluminium hydroxide

ETODOLAC

Indications: pain and inflammation in rheumatoid arthritis and osteoarthritis
Cautions: see notes above; **interactions:** Appendix 1 (NSAIDs)
Contra-indications: see notes above
Side-effects: see notes above
Dose: 600 mg daily in 1–2 divided doses; CHILD not recommended

Etodolac (Non-proprietary) PoM
Capsules, etodolac 300 mg, net price 60-cap pack = £8.75
Available from Viatris (*Eccoxolac®*)

Lodine SR® (Shire) PoM
Tablets, m/r, light-grey, etodolac 600 mg. Net price 30-tab pack = £15.50. Label: 25
Dose: 1 tablet daily; CHILD not recommended

ETORICOXIB

Indications: pain and inflammation in osteoarthritis and in rheumatoid arthritis; acute gout
Cautions: see notes above; history of ischaemic heart disease; **interactions:** Appendix 1 (NSAIDs)
Contra-indications: see notes above; inflammatory bowel disease
Side-effects: see notes above; also dry mouth, taste disturbance, mouth ulcers, flatulence, constipation, appetite and weight changes, chest pain, fatigue, paraesthesia, influenza-like syndrome, myalgia
Dose: osteoarthritis, ADULT and ADOLESCENT over 16 years, 60 mg once daily
Rheumatoid arthritis, ADULT and ADOLESCENT over 16 years, 90 mg once daily
Acute gout, ADULT and ADOLESCENT over 16 years, 120 mg once daily

Arcoxia® (MSD) ▼ PoM
Tablets, f/c, etoricoxib 60 mg (green), net price 28-tab pack = £22.96; 90 mg (white), 28-tab pack = £22.96; 120 mg (pale green), 7-tab pack = £5.74

FENBUFEN

Indications: pain and inflammation in rheumatic disease and other musculoskeletal disorders
Cautions: see notes above; **interactions:** Appendix 1 (NSAIDs)
Contra-indications: see notes above
Side-effects: see notes above, but also high risk of rashes especially in seronegative rheumatoid arthritis, psoriatic arthritis and in women (discontinue immediately); erythema multiforme and Stevens-Johnson syndrome reported; also allergic interstitial lung disorders (may follow rashes)

Dose: 300 mg in the morning and 600 mg at bedtime *or* 450 mg twice daily; CHILD under 14 years not recommended

Fenbufen (Non-proprietary) PoM
Capsules, fenbufen 300 mg, net price 84-cap pack = £20.71. Label: 21
Available from Hillcross, IVAX
Tablets, fenbufen 300 mg, net price 84-tab pack = £15.15; 450 mg, 56-tab pack = £13.17. Label: 21
Available from Alpharma, Generics, Hillcross, IVAX, Sterwin

Lederfen® (Goldshield) PoM
Capsules, dark blue, fenbufen 300 mg. Net price 84-cap pack = £20.71. Label: 21
Tablets, both light blue, f/c, fenbufen 300 mg, net price 84-tab pack = £20.71; 450 mg, 56-tab pack = £18.83. Label: 21

FENOPROFEN

Indications: pain and inflammation in rheumatic disease and other musculoskeletal disorders; mild to moderate pain
Cautions: see notes above; **interactions:** Appendix 1 (NSAIDs)
Contra-indications: see notes above
Side-effects: see notes above; upper respiratory-tract infection, nasopharyngitis, and cystitis also reported
Dose: 300–600 mg 3–4 times daily with food; max. 3 g daily; CHILD not recommended

Fenopron® (Typharm) PoM
Tablets, both orange, fenoprofen (as calcium salt) 300 mg (*Fenopron 300*), net price 100-tab pack = £9.45; 600 mg (*Fenopron 600*, scored), 100-tab pack = £18.29. Label: 21

FLURBIPROFEN

Indications: pain and inflammation in rheumatic disease and other musculoskeletal disorders; mild to moderate pain including dysmenorrhoea; migraine; postoperative analgesia; relief of sore throat (section 12.3.1)
Cautions: see notes above; **interactions:** Appendix 1 (NSAIDs)
Contra-indications: see notes above
Side-effects: see notes above; suppositories may cause rectal irritation
Dose: *by mouth or by rectum* in suppositories, 150–200 mg, daily in divided doses, increased in acute conditions to 300 mg daily
Dysmenorrhoea, initially 100 mg, then 50–100 mg every 4–6 hours; max. 300 mg daily
CHILD not recommended

Froben® (Abbott) PoM
Tablets, both yellow, s/c, flurbiprofen 50 mg, net price 20 = £2.18; 100 mg, 20 = £4.13. Label: 21
NOTE. Flurbiprofen tablets also available from Alpharma, Genus, IVAX, Kent
Suppositories, flurbiprofen 100 mg. Net price 12 = £2.90

■ Modified release
Froben SR® (Abbott) PoM
Capsules, m/r, yellow, enclosing off-white beads, flurbiprofen 200 mg. Net price 30-cap pack = £10.88. Label: 21, 25
Dose: rheumatic disease, 1 capsule daily, preferably in the evening; CHILD not recommended

INDOMETACIN
(Indomethacin)

Indications: pain and moderate to severe inflammation in rheumatic disease and other acute musculoskeletal disorders; acute gout; dysmenorrhoea; closure of ductus arteriosus (section 7.1.1.1)

Cautions: see notes above; also epilepsy, parkinsonism, psychiatric disturbances; during prolonged therapy ophthalmic and blood examinations particularly advisable; avoid rectal administration in proctitis and haemorrhoids; **interactions:** Appendix 1 (NSAIDs)
DRIVING. Dizziness may affect performance of skilled tasks (e.g. driving)

Contra-indications: see notes above

Side-effects: see notes above; frequently gastro-intestinal disturbances (including diarrhoea), headache, dizziness, and light-headedness; also gastro-intestinal ulceration and bleeding; rarely, drowsiness, confusion, insomnia, convulsions, psychiatric disturbances, depression, syncope, blood disorders (particularly thrombocytopenia), hypertension, hyperglycaemia, blurred vision, corneal deposits, peripheral neuropathy, and intestinal strictures; suppositories may cause rectal irritation and occasional bleeding

Dose: *by mouth*, rheumatic disease, 50–200 mg daily in divided doses, with food; CHILD not recommended
Acute gout, 150–200 mg daily in divided doses
Dysmenorrhoea, up to 75 mg daily
By rectum in suppositories, 100 mg at night and in the morning if required; CHILD not recommended
Combined oral and rectal treatment, max. total daily dose 150–200 mg

Indometacin (Non-proprietary) PoM
Capsules, indometacin 25 mg, net price 20 = 51p; 50 mg, 20 = 40p. Label: 21, counselling, driving, see above
Available from Alpharma, Ranbaxy (*Rimacid®*)
Suppositories, indometacin 100 mg. Net price 10 = £1.22. Counselling, driving, see above
Available from Alpharma, IVAX

■ Modified release
Indometacin m/r preparations PoM
Capsules, m/r, indometacin 75 mg. Label: 21, 25, counselling, driving, see above
Dose: 1 capsule 1–2 times daily; CHILD not recommended
Available from Alpharma (*Pardelprin®*), Ashbourne (*Indomax 75 SR®*), Generics (*Slo-Indo®*), Hillcross (*Rheumacin LA®*), Pharmacia (*Indomod®*; also 25-mg strength), Sandoz (*Indolar SR®*),
Tablets, m/r, indometacin 25 mg (*Flexin-25 Continus®*, green), net price 56-tab pack = £7.27; 50 mg (*Flexin-50 Continus®*, red), 28-tab pack = £7.27; 75 mg (*Flexin-75 Continus®*, yellow), 28-tab pack = £10.38. Label: 21, 25, counselling, driving, see above
Dose: initially 75 mg daily, adjusted in steps of 25–50 mg; range 25–200 mg daily in 1–2 divided doses; dysmenorrhoea, up to 75 mg daily; CHILD not recommended
Available from Napp

KETOPROFEN

Indications: pain and mild inflammation in rheumatic disease and other musculoskeletal disorders, and after orthopaedic surgery; acute gout; dysmenorrhoea

Cautions: see notes above; **interactions:** Appendix 1 (NSAIDs)

Contra-indications: see notes above

Side-effects: see notes above; pain may occur at injection site (occasionally tissue damage); suppositories may cause rectal irritation

Dose: *by mouth*, rheumatic disease, 100–200 mg daily in 2–4 divided doses with food; CHILD not recommended
Pain and dysmenorrhoea, 50 mg up to 3 times daily; CHILD not recommended
By rectum in suppositories, rheumatic disease, 100 mg at bedtime; CHILD not recommended
Combined oral and rectal treatment, max. total daily dose 200 mg
By deep intramuscular injection into the gluteal muscle, 50–100 mg every 4 hours (max. 200 mg in 24 hours) for up to 3 days; CHILD not recommended

Ketoprofen (Non-proprietary) PoM
Capsules, ketoprofen 50 mg, net price 28-cap pack = £4.50; 100 mg, 100-cap pack = £13.68. Label: 21
Available from Sandoz

Orudis® (Hawgreen) PoM
Capsules, ketoprofen 50 mg (green/purple), net price 112-cap pack = £17.28; 100 mg (pink), 56-cap pack = £17.33.Label: 21
Suppositories, ketoprofen 100 mg. Net price 10 = £7.44

Oruvail® (Hawgreen) PoM
Injection, ketoprofen 50 mg/mL. Net price 2-mL amp = £1.20
Gel, section 10.3.2

■ Modified release
Oruvail® (Hawgreen) PoM
Capsules, all m/r, enclosing white pellets, ketoprofen 100 mg (pink/purple), net price 56-cap pack = £26.77; 150 mg (pink), 28-cap pack = £15.28; 200 mg (pink/white), 28-cap pack = £26.69. Label: 21, 25
Dose: 100–200 mg once daily with food; CHILD not recommended
NOTE. Modified-release capsules containing ketoprofen 100 mg and 200 mg also available from APS (*Ketovail®*), Ashbourne (*Ketozip XL®* 200 mg), Goldshield (*Ketpron XL®* 100 mg, *Ketpron®* 200 mg), Sandoz (*Larafen CR®* 200 mg), Tillomed (*Tiloket® CR*), Trinity (*Ketocid®* 200 mg)

MEFENAMIC ACID

Indications: mild to moderate pain in rheumatoid arthritis (including juvenile arthritis), osteoarthritis, and related conditions; postoperative analgesia; mild to moderate pain; dysmenorrhoea and menorrhagia

Cautions: see notes above; porphyria (section 9.8.2); **interactions:** Appendix 1 (NSAIDs)

Contra-indications: see notes above; inflammatory bowel disease

Side-effects: see notes above; drowsiness; diarrhoea or rashes (withdraw treatment); thrombocytopenia, haemolytic anaemia (positive Coombs' test), and aplastic anaemia reported; convulsions in overdosage

Dose: 500 mg 3 times daily preferably after food; CHILD over 6 months, 25 mg/kg daily in divided doses for not longer than 7 days, except in juvenile arthritis

Mefenamic Acid (Non-proprietary) PoM

Capsules, mefenamic acid 250 mg. Net price 20 =
50p. Label: 21
Available from Arrow, Chemidex (*Ponstan®*), IVAX,
Sanofi-Synthelabo, Sterwin, Tarus

Tablets, mefenamic acid 500 mg, net price 28-tab
pack = £2.54. Label: 21
Available from Alpharma, APS, Ashbourne (*Dysman 500®*), Chemidex (*Ponstan Forte®*), IVAX, Sanofi-Synthelabo, Sterwin, Tarus

Paediatric oral suspension, mefenamic acid 50 mg/
5 mL. Net price 125 mL = £79.98. Label: 21
Available from Chemidex

MELOXICAM

Indications: pain and inflammation in rheumatic
disease; exacerbation of osteoarthritis (short-term);
ankylosing spondylitis

Cautions: see notes above; avoid rectal administration in proctitis or haemorrhoids; **interactions:**
Appendix 1 (NSAIDs)

Contra-indications: see notes above; renal failure
(unless receiving dialysis)

Side-effects: see notes above

Dose: *by mouth*, osteoarthritis, 7.5 mg daily with
food, increased if necessary to max. 15 mg once
daily
Rheumatoid arthritis, ankylosing spondylitis,
15 mg once daily with food, may be reduced to
7.5 mg daily; ELDERLY 7.5 mg daily

By rectum, in suppositories, osteoarthritis, 7.5 mg
daily, increased if necessary to max. 15 mg once
daily
Rheumatoid arthritis, ankylosing spondylitis,
15 mg once daily, may be reduced to 7.5 mg daily;
ELDERLY 7.5 mg daily
CHILD under 15 years not recommended

Mobic® (Boehringer Ingelheim) PoM

Tablets, both yellow, scored, meloxicam 7.5 mg, net
price 30-tab pack = £10.00; 15 mg, 30-tab pack =
£13.90. Label: 21
Suppositories, meloxicam 7.5 mg, net price 12 =
£4.00; 15 mg, 12 = £6.00

NABUMETONE

Indications: pain and inflammation in osteoarthritis
and rheumatoid arthritis

Cautions: see notes above; **interactions:** Appendix
1 (NSAIDs)

Contra-indications: see notes above

Side-effects: see notes above

Dose: 1 g at night, in severe conditions 0.5–1 g in
morning as well; elderly 0.5–1 g daily; CHILD not
recommended

Nabumetone (Non-proprietary) PoM

Tablets, nabumetone 500 mg, net price 56-tab pack
= £17.28. Label: 21
Available from Alpharma, APS, Generics

Relifex® (Meda) PoM

Tablets, red, f/c, nabumetone 500 mg. Net price 56-
tab pack = £14.83. Label: 21
Dispersible tablets, nabumetone 500 mg, net price
10-tab pack = £2.65, 60-tab pack = £15.89.
Label: 13, 21
Suspension, sugar-free, nabumetone 500 mg/5 mL.
Net price 300-mL pack = £24.08. Label: 21

NAPROXEN

Indications: pain and inflammation in rheumatic
disease (including juvenile arthritis) and other
musculoskeletal disorders; dysmenorrhoea; acute
gout

Cautions: see notes above; **interactions:** Appendix
1 (NSAIDs)

Contra-indications: see notes above

Side-effects: see notes above

Dose: 0.5–1 g daily in 1–2 divided doses; CHILD
(over 5 years), juvenile arthritis, 10 mg/kg daily in
2 divided doses
Acute musculoskeletal disorders and dysmenorrhoea, 500 mg initially, then 250 mg every 6–8
hours as required; max. dose after first day 1.25 g
daily; CHILD under 16 years not recommended
Acute gout, 750 mg initially, then 250 mg every 8
hours until attack has passed; CHILD under 16 years
not recommended

Naproxen (Non-proprietary) PoM

Tablets, naproxen 250 mg, net price 28-tab pack =
£1.57; 500 mg, 28-tab pack = £3.51. Label: 21
Available from Alpharma, APS, Arrow, Ashbourne
(*Arthrosin®*), CP (*Arthroxen®*), Hillcross, IVAX, Sterwin

Tablets, e/c, naproxen 250 mg, net price 56-tab pack
= £4.44; 375 mg, 56-tab pack = £6.96; 500 mg, 56-
tab pack = £8.14. Label: 5, 25
Available from Alpharma, Ardern (*Nycopren®*), APS,
Ashbourne (*Arthrosin® EC*), Berk (*Timpron® EC*), Cox,
Generics, IVAX

Naprosyn® (Roche) PoM

Tablets, all scored, naproxen 250 mg (buff), net
price 56-tab pack = £4.89; 500 mg (buff), 56-tab
pack = £9.77. Label: 21
Tablets, e/c, (*Naprosyn EC®*), naproxen 250 mg, net
price 56-tab pack = £4.89; 375 mg, 56-tab pack =
£7.33; 500 mg, 56-tab pack = £9.77. Label: 5, 25

Synflex® (Roche) PoM

Tablets, blue, naproxen sodium 275 mg. Net price
60-tab pack = £8.11. Label: 21
NOTE. 275 mg naproxen sodium ≡ 250 mg naproxen
Dose: musculoskeletal disorders, postoperative analgesia,
550 mg twice daily when necessary, preferably after food;
max. 1.1 g daily; CHILD under 16 years not recommended
Dysmenorrhoea and acute gout, initially 550 mg then
275 mg every 6–8 hours as required; max. of 1.375 g on
first day and 1.1 g daily thereafter; CHILD under 16 years
not recommended
Migraine, 825 mg at onset, then 275–550 mg at least 30
minutes after initial dose; max 1.375 g in 24 hours; CHILD
under 16 years not recommended

■ With misoprostol
For **cautions, contra-indications**, and **side-effects**
of misoprostol, see section 1.3.4

Napratec® (Pharmacia) PoM

Combination pack, 56 yellow scored tablets,
naproxen 500 mg; 56 white scored tablets, misoprostol 200 micrograms. Net price = £23.76.
Label: 21
Dose: patients requiring naproxen for rheumatoid arthritis, osteoarthritis, or ankylosing spondylitis, with
prophylaxis against NSAID-induced gastroduodenal
ulceration, 1 naproxen 500-mg tablet and 1 misoprostol
200-microgram tablet taken together twice daily with
food; CHILD not recommended

PIROXICAM

Indications: pain and inflammation in rheumatic disease (including juvenile arthritis) and other musculoskeletal disorders; acute gout

Cautions: see notes above; avoid in porphyria (section 9.8.2); **interactions:** Appendix 1 (NSAIDs)

Contra-indications: see notes above

Side-effects: see notes above; pain at injection site (occasionally tissue damage); suppositories may cause rectal irritation and occasional bleeding

Dose: *by mouth*, rheumatic disease, initially 20 mg daily, maintenance 10–30 mg daily, in single or divided doses; CHILD (over 6 years), juvenile arthritis, under 15 kg, 5 mg daily; 16–25 kg, 10 mg; 26–45 kg, 15 mg; over 46 kg, 20 mg

Acute musculoskeletal disorders, 40 mg daily in single or divided doses for 2 days, then 20 mg daily for 7–14 days; CHILD not recommended

Acute gout, 40 mg initially, then 40 mg daily in single or divided doses for 4–6 days; CHILD not recommended

By deep intramuscular injection into gluteal muscle, for initial treatment of acute conditions, as dose by mouth (on short-term basis); CHILD not recommended

Piroxicam (Non-proprietary) PoM
Capsules, piroxicam 10 mg, net price 56-cap pack = £2.81; 20 mg, 28-cap pack = £3.13. Label: 21
Available from Alpharma, APS, Hillcross, IVAX, Kent
Dispersible tablets, piroxicam 10 mg, net price 56-tab pack = £9.57; 20 mg, 28-tab pack = £9.42. Label: 13, 21
Available from Generics

Feldene® (Pfizer) PoM
Capsules, piroxicam 10 mg (maroon/blue), net price 56-cap pack = £7.20; 20 mg (maroon), 28-cap pack = £7.20. Label: 21
Tablets, (Feldene Melt®)*, piroxicam 20 mg, net price 28-tab pack = £9.83. Label: 10, patient information leaflet, 21
Excipients: include aspartame equivalent to phenylalanine 140 micrograms/tablet (section 9.4.1)
NOTE. *Feldene Melt*® tablets can be taken by placing on tongue or by swallowing
Dispersible tablets, piroxicam 10 mg (scored), net price 56-tab pack = £11.70; 20 mg, 28-tab pack = £11.70. Label: 13, 21
Injection, piroxicam 20 mg/mL. Net price 1-mL amp = 84p
Gel, section 10.3.2

Brexidol® (Trinity) PoM
Tablets, yellow, scored, piroxicam (as betadex) 20 mg, net price 30-tab pack = £12.22. Label: 21
Dose: osteoarthritis, rheumatic disease and acute musculoskeletal disorders, 1 tablet daily (may be halved in elderly); CHILD not recommended

ROFECOXIB

Indications: pain and inflammation in osteoarthritis and rheumatoid arthritis; acute pain (including dysmenorrhoea and pain following dental or orthopaedic surgery)

Cautions: see notes above; history of ischaemic heart disease; **interactions**: Appendix 1 (NSAIDs)

Contra-indications: see notes above; also inflammatory bowel disease

Side-effects: see notes above; also mouth ulcers, constipation, chest pain (consider discontinuing if

ischaemic heart disease deteriorates), palpitations, weight gain, sleep disturbance, fatigue, menstrual disturbances, atopic eczema, alopecia, and muscle cramps reported; raised liver enzymes (discontinue if persistent)

Dose: osteoarthritis, 12.5 mg daily, increased if necessary to max. 25 mg once daily; CHILD not recommended

Rheumatoid arthritis, 25 mg once daily; CHILD not recommended

Acute pain, 50 mg initially then 25–50 mg once daily; CHILD not recommended

Dysmenorrhoea, 25–50 mg once daily; CHILD not recommended

Vioxx® (MSD) PoM
Tablets, rofecoxib 12.5 mg (ivory), net price 28-tab pack = £21.58; 25 mg (yellow), 28-tab pack = £21.58
Suspension, sugar-free, yellow, strawberry-flavoured, rofecoxib 12.5 mg/5 mL, net price 150 mL = £23.12; 25 mg/5 mL, 150 mL = £23.12
Vioxx® *Acute tablets*, rofecoxib 25 mg (yellow), net price 14-tab pack = £10.79; 50 mg (orange), 7-tab pack = £5.39

SULINDAC

Indications: pain and inflammation in rheumatic disease and other musculoskeletal disorders; acute gout

Cautions: see notes above; also history of renal stones and ensure adequate hydration; **interactions:** Appendix 1 (NSAIDs)

Contra-indications: see notes above

Side-effects: see notes above; also urine discoloration occasionally reported

Dose: 200 mg twice daily with food (may be reduced according to response); max. 400 mg daily; acute gout should respond within 7 days; limit treatment of peri-articular disorders to 7–10 days; CHILD not recommended

Sulindac (Non-proprietary) PoM
Tablets, sulindac 100 mg, net price 56-tab pack = £7.45; 200 mg, 56-tab pack = £13.00. Label: 21
Available from Generics

Clinoril® (MSD) PoM
Tablets, both yellow, scored, sulindac 100 mg, net price 60-tab pack = £6.73; 200 mg, 60-tab pack = £12.96. Label: 21

TENOXICAM

Indications: pain and inflammation in rheumatic disease and other musculoskeletal disorders

Cautions: see notes above; **interactions:** Appendix 1 (NSAIDs)

Contra-indications: see notes above

Side-effects: see notes above

Dose: *by mouth*, rheumatic disease, 20 mg daily; CHILD not recommended

Acute musculoskeletal disorders, 20 mg daily for 7 days; max. 14 days; CHILD not recommended

By intravenous or intramuscular injection, for initial treatment for 1–2 days, as dose by mouth; CHILD not recommended

Mobiflex® (Roche) PoM
Tablets, red-brown, f/c, tenoxicam 20 mg. Net price 28-tab pack = £13.47. Label: 21
Injection, powder for reconstitution, tenoxicam 20 mg. Net price per amp (with solvent) = 89p

TIAPROFENIC ACID

Indications: pain and inflammation in rheumatic disease and other musculoskeletal disorders

Cautions: see notes above; **interactions:** Appendix 1 (NSAIDs)

Contra-indications: see notes above; also active bladder or prostate disease (or symptoms) and history of recurrent urinary-tract disorders—if urinary symptoms develop discontinue immediately and perform urine tests and culture; see also CSM advice below

> **CSM ADVICE.** Following reports of **severe cystitis** CSM has recommended that tiaprofenic acid should not be given to patients with urinary-tract disorders and should be stopped if urinary symptoms develop. Patients should be advised to stop taking tiaprofenic acid and to report to their doctor promptly if they develop urinary-tract symptoms (such as increased frequency, nocturia, urgency, pain on urinating, or blood in urine)

Side-effects: see notes above

Dose: 600 mg daily in 2–3 divided doses; CHILD not recommended

Tiaprofenic Acid (Non-proprietary) PoM
Tablets, tiaprofenic acid 200 mg, net price 84-tab pack = £20.48; 300 mg, 56-tab pack = £20.48. Label: 21
Available from Alpharma

Surgam® (Florizel) PoM
Tablets, tiaprofenic acid 200 mg, net price 84-tab pack = £20.48; 300 mg, 56-tab pack = £20.48. Label: 21

■ Modified release

Surgam SA® (Aventis Pharma) PoM
Capsules, m/r, maroon/pink enclosing white pellets, tiaprofenic acid 300 mg. Net price 56-cap pack = £20.48. Label: 25
Dose: 2 capsules once daily; CHILD not recommended

VALDECOXIB

Indications: pain and inflammation in osteoarthritis and in rheumatoid arthritis; dysmenorrhoea

Cautions: see notes above; following coronary artery bypass graft surgery; **interactions:** Appendix 1 (NSAIDs)

Contra-indications: see notes above; sulphonamide hypersensitivity; inflammatory bowel disease

Side-effects: see notes above; dry mouth, belching; less frequently stomatitis, taste disturbance, weight gain, palpitations, syncope, coughing, hypertonia, hypoaesthesia, paraesthesia, confusion; rarely intestinal obstruction, cerebrovascular disorder, dysphonia

Dose: osteoarthritis, rheumatoid arthritis, ADULT over 18 years, 10 mg once daily, increased if necessary to max. 20 mg once daily
Dysmenorrhoea, ADULT over 18 years, 40 mg once daily (max. 40 mg twice daily on first day if necessary)

Bextra® (Pfizer) ▼ PoM
Tablets, f/c, valdecoxib 10 mg (white), net price 30-tab pack = £23.12; 20 mg (white), 30-tab pack = £23.12; 40 mg (yellow), 5-tab pack = £3.85

Aspirin and the salicylates

Aspirin was the traditional first choice anti-inflammatory analgesic but most physicians now prefer to start treatment with another NSAID which may be better tolerated and more convenient for the patient.

In regular high dosage aspirin has about the same anti-inflammatory effect as other NSAIDs. The required dose for active inflammatory joint disease is at least 3.6 g daily. There is little anti-inflammatory effect with less than 3 g daily. Gastro-intestinal side-effects such as nausea, dyspepsia, and gastro-intestinal bleeding may occur with any dosage of aspirin but anti-inflammatory doses are associated with a much higher incidence of side-effects. Anti-inflammatory doses of aspirin may also cause mild chronic salicylate intoxication (salicylism) characterised by dizziness, tinnitus, and deafness; these symptoms may be controlled by reducing the dosage.

ASPIRIN

(Acetylsalicylic Acid)

Indications: pain and inflammation in rheumatic disease and other musculoskeletal disorders (including juvenile arthritis); see also section 4.7.1; antiplatelet (section 2.9)

Cautions: asthma, allergic disease, uncontrolled hypertension, hepatic or renal impairment (avoid if severe), dehydration, pregnancy (particularly at term; see also Appendix 4), elderly; preferably avoid during fever or viral infection in adolescents (risk of Reye's syndrome, see below); G6PD-deficiency (section 9.1.5); **interactions:** Appendix 1 (aspirin)
REYE'S SYNDROME. Owing to an association with Reye's syndrome the CSM has advised that aspirin-containing preparations should not be given to children and adolescents under 16 years, unless specifically indicated, e.g. for Kawasaki syndrome

Contra-indications: previous or active peptic ulceration; children and adolescents under 16 years (unless specifically indicated e.g. for Kawasaki syndrome) and breast-feeding—risk of Reye's syndrome, see above; haemophilia and other bleeding disorders; not for treatment of gout
HYPERSENSITIVITY. Aspirin and other NSAIDs **contra-indicated** in history of hypersensitivity to aspirin or any other NSAID—which includes those in whom attacks of asthma, angioedema, urticaria or rhinitis have been precipitated by aspirin or any other NSAID

Side-effects: common with anti-inflammatory doses; gastro-intestinal discomfort or nausea, ulceration with occult bleeding (but occasionally major haemorrhage); also other haemorrhage (e.g. subconjunctival); hearing disturbances such as tinnitus (leading rarely to deafness), vertigo, confusion, hypersensitivity reactions (angioedema, bronchospasm and rashes); increased bleeding time; rarely oedema, blood disorders, particularly thrombocytopenia; **overdosage:** see Emergency Treatment of Poisoning, p. 22

Dose: 0.3–1 g every 4 hours after food; max. in acute conditions 8 g daily; CHILD, juvenile arthritis, up to 80 mg/kg daily in 5–6 divided doses after food, increased in acute exacerbations to 130 mg/kg

NOTE. High doses of aspirin are very rarely required and are now given under specialist supervision only, and with plasma monitoring (especially in children)

■ Preparations
Section 4.7.1

BENORILATE

(Benorylate)

(Aspirin-paracetamol ester; 2 g benorilate is equivalent to approximately 1.15 g aspirin and 970 mg paracetamol)

Indications: pain and inflammation in rheumatic disease and other musculoskeletal disorders; mild to moderate pain; pyrexia

Cautions: see under Aspirin (above) and Paracetamol (section 4.7.1)

Contra-indications: see under Aspirin (above) and Paracetamol (section 4.7.1)

Side-effects: see under Aspirin (above) and Paracetamol (section 4.7.1)

Dose: rheumatic disease, 4–8 g daily divided into 2–3 doses; max. 6 g daily for elderly; CHILD not recommended

Mild to moderate pain, 2 g twice daily preferably after food; CHILD not recommended

Benorilate (Non-proprietary)

Tablets, benorilate 750 mg. Net price 100-tab pack = £8.20. Label: 21, 31

Granules, benorilate 2 g /sachet. Net price 60 sachet-pack = £13.77. Label: 13, 21, 31

Suspension, sugar-free, benorilate 2 g/5 mL. Net price 300 mL = £11.23. Label: 21, 31

Available from Sanofi-Synthelabo (*Benoral*®), Sterwin

10.1.2   Corticosteroids

10.1.2.1   Systemic corticosteroids

The general actions and uses of the corticosteroids are described in section 6.3. Treatment with corticosteroids in rheumatic diseases should be reserved for specific indications, e.g. when other anti-inflammatory drugs are unsuccessful. Corticosteroids can induce osteoporosis, and prophylaxis should be considered on long-term treatment (section 6.6).

In severe, possibly life-threatening, situations a high initial dose of corticosteroid is given to induce remission and the dose is then gradually reduced to the lowest maintenance dose that will control the disease or, if possible, discontinued altogether. However, relapse may occur as the dose is reduced, particularly if the reduction is too rapid. The tendency is therefore to increase the maintenance dose and consequently the patient becomes dependent on corticosteroids. For this reason pulse doses of corticosteroids (e.g. methylprednisolone (as sodium succinate) up to 1 g intravenously on three consecutive days) are used to suppress highly active inflammatory disease while longer-term and slower-acting treatment is commenced.

Prednisolone is used for most purposes; it has the advantage over the more potent corticosteroids (see section 6.3.2) of permitting finer dosage adjustments. To minimise side-effects the maintenance

dose of prednisolone should be as low as possible, usually 7.5 mg daily. Recent evidence has suggested that prednisolone 7.5 mg daily may substantially reduce the rate of joint destruction in moderate to severe *rheumatoid arthritis* of less than 2 years duration. The reduction in joint destruction must be distinguished from mere symptomatic improvement (which lasts only 6 to 12 months at this dose) and care should be taken to avoid increasing the dosage beyond 7.5 mg daily. Current evidence supports maintenance of this anti-erosive dose for 2–4 years only after which treatment should be tapered off to reduce long-term adverse effects.

Polymyalgia rheumatica and *giant cell (temporal) arteritis* are always treated with corticosteroids. The usual initial dose of prednisolone in polymyalgia rheumatica is 10–15 mg daily and in giant cell arteritis 40–60 mg daily (the higher dose being used if visual symptoms occur). Treatment should be continued until remission of disease activity and doses are then reduced gradually to about 7.5 –10 mg daily for maintenance. Relapse is common if therapy is stopped prematurely. Many patients require treatment for at least 2 years and in some patients it may be necessary to continue long-term low-dose corticosteroid treatment.

Polyarteritis nodosa and *polymyositis* are usually treated with corticosteroids. An initial dose of 60 mg of prednisolone daily is often used and reduced to a maintenance dose of 10–15 mg daily.

Systemic lupus erythematosus is treated with corticosteroids when necessary using a similar dosage regimen to that for polyarteritis nodosa and polymyositis (above). Patients with pleurisy, pericarditis, or other systemic manifestations will respond to corticosteroids. It may then be possible to reduce the dosage; alternate-day treatment is sometimes adequate, and the drug may be gradually withdrawn. In some mild cases corticosteroid treatment may be stopped after a few months. Many mild cases of systemic lupus erythematosus do not require corticosteroid treatment. Alternative treatment with anti-inflammatory analgesics, and possibly chloroquine or hydroxychloroquine, should be considered.

Ankylosing spondylitis should not be treated with long-term corticosteroids; rarely, pulse doses may be needed and may be useful in extremely active disease that does not respond to conventional treatment.

10.1.2.2   Local corticosteroid injections

Corticosteroids are injected locally for an anti-inflammatory effect. In inflammatory conditions of the joints, particularly in rheumatoid arthritis, they are given by *intra-articular injection* to relieve pain, increase mobility, and reduce deformity in one or a few joints. Full aseptic precautions are essential; infected areas should be avoided. Occasionally an acute inflammatory reaction develops after an intra-articular or soft-tissue injection of a corticosteroid. This may be a reaction to the microcrystalline suspension of the corticosteroid used, but must be distinguished from sepsis introduced into the injection site. An almost insoluble compound such as triamcinolone hexacetonide has a long-acting (depot) effect and is preferred for intra-articular injection.

Smaller amounts of corticosteroids may also be injected directly into soft tissues for the relief of inflammation in conditions such as *tennis* or *golfer's elbow* or *compression neuropathies*. In *tendinitis*, injections should be made into the tendon sheath and not directly into the tendon (due to the absence of a true tendon sheath, the Achilles tendon should not be injected). A soluble preparation (e.g. containing betamethasone or dexamethasone sodium phosphate) is preferred for injection into the carpal tunnel.

Hydrocortisone acetate or one of the synthetic analogues such as triamcinolone hexacetonide is generally used for local injection. Flushing has been reported with intra-articular corticosteroid injections. Charcot-like arthropathies have also been reported (particularly following repeated intra-articular injections). Intra-articular injections may affect the hyaline cartilage and each joint should not usually be treated more than 3 times in one year.

Corticosteroid injections are also injected into soft tissues for the treatment of skin lesions (see section 13.4).

LOCAL CORTICOSTEROID INJECTIONS

Indications: local inflammation of joints and soft tissues (for details, consult product literature)
Cautions: see notes above and consult product literature; see also section 6.3.2
Contra-indications: see notes above and consult product literature
Side-effects: see notes above and consult product literature
Dose: see under preparations

■ Dose calculated as dexamethasone sodium phosphate

Dexamethasone (Organon) PoM

Injection, dexamethasone sodium phosphate 5 mg/mL (≡ dexamethasone 3.8 mg/mL ≡ dexamethasone phosphate 4.6 mg/mL). Net price 1-mL amp = 83p; 2-mL vial = £1.27
Dose: by intra-articular or intrasynovial injection (for details consult product literature), 0.4–4 mg (calculated as dexamethasone sodium phosphate) according to size; where appropriate may be repeated at intervals of 3–21 days according to response

■ Dose calculated as dexamethasone phosphate

Dexamethasone (Mayne) PoM

Injection, dexamethasone phosphate 4 mg/mL (as sodium phosphate) (≡ dexamethasone 3.3 mg/mL ≡ dexamethasone sodium phosphate 4.4 mg/mL), net price 1-mL amp = £1.00; 2-mL vial = £1.98
Dose: by intra-articular or intrasynovial injection (for details consult product literature), 0.4–4 mg (calculated as dexamethasone phosphate) according to size (*soft-tissue infiltration* 2–6 mg); where appropriate may be repeated at intervals of 3–21 days

■ Hydrocortisone acetate

Hydrocortistab® (Sovereign) PoM

Injection, (aqueous suspension), hydrocortisone acetate 25 mg/mL. Net price 1-mL amp = £4.77
Dose: by intra-articular or intrasynovial injection (for details consult product literature), 5–50 mg according to size; where appropriate may be repeated at intervals of 21 days; not more than 3 joints should be treated on any one day; CHILD 5–30 mg (divided)

■ Methylprednisolone acetate

Depo-Medrone® (Pharmacia) PoM

Injection (aqueous suspension), methylprednisolone acetate 40 mg/mL. Net price 1-mL vial = £2.87; 2-mL vial = £5.15; 3-mL vial = £7.47
Dose: by intra-articular or intrasynovial injection (for details consult product literature), 4–80 mg, according to size; where appropriate may be repeated at intervals of 7–35 days; also for *intralesional injection*

Depo-Medrone® with Lidocaine (Pharmacia) PoM

Injection (aqueous suspension), methylprednisolone acetate 40 mg, lidocaine hydrochloride 10 mg/mL. Net price 1-mL vial = £3.28; 2-mL vial = £5.88
Dose: by intra-articular or intrasynovial injection (for details consult product literature), 4–80 mg, according to size; where appropriate may be repeated at intervals of 7–35 days

■ Prednisolone acetate

Deltastab® (Sovereign) PoM

Injection (aqueous suspension), prednisolone acetate 25 mg/mL. Net price 1-mL amp = £4.77
Dose: by intra-articular or intrasynovial injection (for details consult product literature), 5–25 mg according to size; not more than 3 joints should be treated on any one day; where appropriate may be repeated when relapse occurs
For *intramuscular injection*, see section 6.3.2

■ Triamcinolone acetonide

Adcortyl® **Intra-articular/Intradermal** (Squibb) PoM

Injection (aqueous suspension), triamcinolone acetonide 10 mg/mL. Net price 1-mL amp = £1.02; 5-mL vial = £4.14
Dose: by intra-articular injection or intrasynovial injection (for details consult product literature), 2.5–15 mg according to size (for larger doses use *Kenalog*®); where appropriate may be repeated when relapse occurs
By intradermal injection, (for details consult product literature): 2–3 mg; max. 5 mg at any one site (total max. 30 mg); where appropriate may be repeated at intervals of 1–2 weeks
CHILD under 6 years not recommended

Kenalog® **Intra-articular/Intramuscular** (Squibb) PoM

Injection (aqueous suspension), triamcinolone acetonide 40 mg/mL, net price 1-mL vial = £1.70; 1-mL prefilled syringe = £2.11; 2-mL prefilled syringe = £3.66
NOTE. Intramuscular needle with prefilled syringe should be replaced for intra-articular injection
Dose: by intra-articular or intrasynovial injection (for details consult product literature), 5–40 mg according to size; total max. 80 mg (for doses below 5 mg use *Adcortyl*® *Intra-articular/Intradermal*); where appropriate may be repeated when relapse occurs; CHILD under 6 years not recommended
For *intramuscular injection*, see section 6.3.2

10.1.3 Drugs which suppress the rheumatic disease process

Certain drugs such as gold, penicillamine, hydroxychloroquine, chloroquine, drugs affecting the immune response, and sulfasalazine may suppress the disease process in *rheumatoid arthritis*, as may sulfasalazine, methotrexate, and possibly gold and azathioprine in *psoriatic arthritis*. They are sometimes known as second-line or disease-modifying antirheumatic drugs (DMARDs). Unlike NSAIDs they do not produce an immediate therapeutic effect but require 4 to 6 months of treatment for a full response. If one of these drugs does not lead to objective benefit within 6 months of initiating treatment or 3 months after maximum treatment, it should be discontinued and a different drug tried. Response to a disease-modifying antirheumatic drug may allow the dose of the NSAID to be reduced.

Disease-modifying antirheumatic drugs may improve not only the symptoms and signs of inflammatory joint disease but also extra-articular manifestations such as vasculitis. They reduce the erythrocyte sedimentation rate, C-reactive protein, and sometimes the titre of rheumatoid factor. Some (e.g. methotrexate and ciclosporin) are believed to retard erosive damage as judged radiologically.

Since in the first few months, the course of rheumatoid arthritis is unpredictable and the diagnosis uncertain, it is usual to start treatment with an NSAID alone. Disease-modifying antirheumatic drugs are, however, instituted by specialists as soon as diagnosis, progression, and severity of the disease have been confirmed. The choice of a disease-modifying antirheumatic drug should take into account co-morbidity and patient preference. Sulfasalazine, methotrexate, intramuscular gold and penicillamine are similar in efficacy. However, sulfasalazine or methotrexate are often used first because they may be better tolerated.

Penicillamine and drugs that affect the immune response are also sometimes used in rheumatoid arthritis where there are troublesome extra-articular features such as vasculitis, and in patients who are taking high doses of corticosteroids. Where the response is satisfactory there is often a striking reduction in requirements of both corticosteroids and other drugs. Gold and penicillamine are effective in *palindromic rheumatism*. Systemic and *discoid lupus erythematosus* are sometimes treated with chloroquine or hydroxychloroquine.

JUVENILE IDIOPATHIC ARTHRITIS. Many children with *juvenile idiopathic arthritis* (juvenile chronic arthritis) do not require disease-modifying antirheumatic drugs. Methotrexate is effective in juvenile idiopathic arthritis; sulfasalazine is an alternative but should be avoided in systemic-onset juvenile idiopathic arthritis. Gold and penicillamine are used very rarely. For the role of etanercept in polyarticular-course juvenile idiopathic arthritis, see p. 494

Gold

Gold may be given by intramuscular injection as sodium aurothiomalate or by mouth as auranofin.

Sodium aurothiomalate must be given by deep intramuscular injection and the area gently massaged. A test dose of 10 mg must be given followed by doses of 50 mg at weekly intervals until there is definite evidence of remission. Benefit is not to be expected until about 300–500 mg has been given; it should be discontinued if there is no remission after 1 g has been given. In patients who do respond, the interval between injections is then gradually increased to 4 weeks and treatment is continued for up to 5 years after complete remission. If relapse occurs the dosage frequency may be immediately increased to 50 mg weekly and only once control has been obtained again should the dosage frequency be decreased; if no response is seen within 2 months, alternative treatment should be sought. It is important to avoid complete relapse since second courses of gold are not usually effective. Children may be given 1 mg/kg weekly to a maximum of 50 mg weekly, the intervals being gradually increased to 4 weeks according to response; an initial test dose is given corresponding to one-tenth to one-fifth of the calculated dose.

Auranofin is given by mouth. If there is no response after 6 months treatment should be discontinued. Auranofin is less effective than parenteral gold.

Gold therapy should be discontinued in the presence of blood disorders or proteinuria (associated with immune complex nephritis) which is repeatedly above 300 mg/litre without other cause (such as urinary-tract infection). Urine tests and full blood counts (including total and differential white cell and platelet counts) must therefore be performed before starting treatment with gold and before each intramuscular injection; in the case of oral treatment the urine and blood tests should be carried out monthly. Rashes with pruritus often occur after 2 to 6 months of intramuscular treatment and may necessitate discontinuation of treatment; the most common side-effect of oral therapy, diarrhoea with or without nausea or abdominal pain, may respond to bulking agents (such as bran) or temporary reduction in dosage.

SODIUM AUROTHIOMALATE

Indications: active progressive rheumatoid arthritis, juvenile arthritis

Cautions: see notes above; renal and hepatic impairment, elderly, history of urticaria, eczema, colitis, drugs which cause blood disorders; annual chest X-ray; **interactions:** Appendix 1 (gold)

Contra-indications: severe renal and hepatic disease (see notes above); history of blood disorders or bone marrow aplasia, exfoliative dermatitis, systemic lupus erythematosus, necrotising enterocolitis, pulmonary fibrosis; pregnancy and breast-feeding (Appendixes 4 and 5); porphyria (section 9.8.2)

Side-effects: severe reactions (occasionally fatal) in up to 5% of patients; mouth ulcers, skin reactions (including, on prolonged parenteral treatment, irreversible pigmentation in sun-exposed areas), proteinuria, blood disorders (sometimes sudden and fatal); rarely colitis, peripheral neuritis, pulmonary fibrosis, hepatotoxicity with cholestatic jaundice, nephrotic syndrome, alopecia

Dose: *by deep intramuscular injection*, administered on expert advice, see notes above
COUNSELLING. Warn patient to tell doctor immediately if sore throat, fever, infection, non-specific illness, unexplained bleeding and bruising, purpura, mouth ulcers, metallic taste, or rashes develop; also ask patients to report immediately any breathlessness or cough

Myocrisin® (JHC) [PoM]
Injection, sodium aurothiomalate 20 mg/mL, net price 0.5-mL (10-mg) amp = £3.16; 40 mg/mL,

0.5-mL (20-mg) amp = £4.60; 100 mg/mL, 0.5-mL (50-mg) amp = £9.36. Counselling, blood disorder symptoms

AURANOFIN

Indications: active progressive rheumatoid arthritis

Cautions: see under Sodium Aurothiomalate; also caution in inflammatory bowel disease

BLOOD COUNTS. Withdraw if platelet count falls below 100 000/mm³ or if signs and symptoms suggestive of thrombocytopenia occur, see also notes above

Contra-indications: see under Sodium Aurothiomalate

Side-effects: diarrhoea most common (reduced by bulking agents such as bran); see also under Sodium Aurothiomalate

Dose: administered on expert advice, 6 mg daily (initially in 2 divided doses then if tolerated as single dose), if response inadequate after 6 months, increase to 9 mg daily (in 3 divided doses), discontinue if no response after a further 3 months; CHILD not recommended

COUNSELLING. Warn patient to tell doctor immediately if sore throat, fever, infection, non-specific illness, unexplained bleeding and bruising, purpura, mouth ulcers, metallic taste, or rashes develop; also ask patients to report immediately any breathlessness or cough

NOTE. The package insert for *Ridaura* also advises that patients must also report immediately if conjunctivitis or hair loss develops

Ridaura® (Yamanouchi) ▣**PoM**

Tablets, yellow, f/c, auranofin 3 mg. Net price 60-tab pack = £27.10. Label: 21, counselling, blood disorder symptoms (see above)

Penicillamine

Penicillamine has a similar action to gold, and more patients are able to continue treatment than with gold but side-effects occur frequently. Penicillamine should be discontinued if there is no improvement within 1 year.

Patients should be warned not to expect improvement for at least 6 to 12 weeks after treatment is initiated. If remission has been sustained for 6 months, reduction of dosage by 125 to 250 mg every 12 weeks may be attempted.

Blood counts, including platelets, and urine examinations should be carried out before starting treatment and then every 1 or 2 weeks for the first 2 months then every 4 weeks to detect blood disorders and proteinuria (they should also be carried out in the week after any dose increase). A reduction in platelet count calls for discontinuation with subsequent re-introduction at a lower dosage and then, if possible, gradual increase. Proteinuria, associated with immune complex nephritis, occurs in up to 30% of patients, but may resolve despite continuation of treatment; treatment may be continued provided that renal function tests remain normal, oedema is absent, and the 24-hour urinary excretion of protein does not exceed 2 g.

Nausea may occur but is not usually a problem provided that penicillamine is taken before food or on retiring and that low initial doses are used and only gradually increased. Loss of taste may occur about 6 weeks after treatment is started but usually returns 6 weeks later irrespective of whether or not treatment is discontinued; mineral supplements are

not recommended. Rashes are a common side-effect. Those which occur in the first few months of treatment disappear when the drug is stopped and treatment may then be re-introduced at a lower dose level and gradually increased. Late rashes are more resistant and often necessitate discontinuation of treatment.

Patients who are hypersensitive to penicillin may react rarely to penicillamine.

PENICILLAMINE

Indications: see notes above and under Dose

Cautions: see notes above; renal impairment (Appendix 3), pregnancy (Appendix 4); avoid concurrent gold, chloroquine, hydroxychloroquine, or immunosuppressive treatment; avoid oral iron within 2 hours of a dose; **interactions:** Appendix 1 (penicillamine)

BLOOD COUNTS AND URINE TESTS. See notes above. Longer intervals may be adequate in cystinuria and Wilson's disease. Consider withdrawal if platelet count falls below 120 000/mm³ or white blood cells below 2500/mm³ or if 3 successive falls within reference range (can restart at reduced dose when counts return to within reference range but permanent withdrawal necessary if recurrence of leucopenia or thrombocytopenia)

COUNSELLING. Warn patient to tell doctor immediately if sore throat, fever, infection, non-specific illness, unexplained bleeding and bruising, purpura, mouth ulcers, or rashes develop

Contra-indications: hypersensitivity (except in life-threatening situation when desensitisation may be attempted—consult product literature); lupus erythematosus

Side-effects: (see also notes above) initially nausea, anorexia, fever, and skin reactions; taste loss (mineral supplements not recommended); blood disorders including thrombocytopenia, neutropenia, agranulocytosis and aplastic anaemia; proteinuria, rarely haematuria (withdraw immediately); haemolytic anaemia, nephrotic syndrome, lupus erythematosus-like syndrome, myasthenia gravis-like syndrome, polymyositis (rarely with cardiac involvement), dermatomyositis, mouth ulcers, stomatitis, alopecia, bronchiolitis and pneumonitis, pemphigus, Goodpasture's syndrome, and Stevens-Johnson syndrome also reported; male and female breast enlargement reported; in non-rheumatoid conditions rheumatoid arthritis-like syndrome also reported; late rashes (reduce dose or withdraw treatment)

Dose: severe active rheumatoid arthritis, administered on expert advice, ADULT initially 125–250 mg daily before food for 1 month increased by similar amounts at intervals of not less than 4 weeks to usual maintenance of 500–750 mg daily in divided doses; max. 1.5 g daily; ELDERLY initially up to 125 mg daily before food for 1 month increased by similar amounts at intervals of not less than 4 weeks; max. 1 g daily; CHILD maintenance of 15–20 mg/kg daily (initial dose lower and increased at intervals of 4 weeks over a period of 3-6 months)

Wilson's disease, chronic active hepatitis, and cystinuria, section 9.8.1

Lead poisoning, see Emergency Treatment of Poisoning, p. 27

Penicillamine (Non-proprietary) PoM
Tablets, penicillamine 125 mg, net price 20 = £1.97; 250 mg, 20 = £3.41. Label: 6, 22, counselling, blood disorder symptoms (see above)
Available from Alpharma, APS, Hillcross, IVAX

Distamine* (Alliance) PoM
Tablets, all f/c, penicillamine 125 mg, net price 20 = £2.17; 250 mg, 20 = £3.74. Label: 6, 22, counselling, blood disorder symptoms (see above)

Antimalarials

The antimalarials **chloroquine** and **hydroxychloroquine** are used to treat rheumatoid arthritis of moderate inflammatory activity. These drugs are effective for mild systemic lupus erythematosus, particularly involving cutaneous and joint manifestations. Chloroquine and hydroxychloroquine should not be used for psoriatic arthritis.

Chloroquine and hydroxychloroquine are better tolerated than gold or penicillamine. Retinopathy (see below) occurs rarely provided that the recommended doses are not exceeded; in the elderly it is difficult to distinguish drug-induced retinopathy from ageing changes.

Mepacrine (section 5.4.4) is sometimes used in discoid lupus erythematosus [unlicensed].

CAUTIONS. Chloroquine and hydroxychloroquine should be used with caution in hepatic impairment and in renal impairment (Appendix 3). Manufacturers recommend regular ophthalmological examination but the evidence of practical value is unsatisfactory (see advice of Royal College of Ophthalmologists, below). It is not necessary to withdraw an antimalarial during pregnancy if the rheumatic disease is well controlled. Chloroquine and hydroxychloroquine are present in breast milk and breast-feeding should be avoided when they are used to treat rheumatic disease; chloroquine can, however, be used for malaria during pregnancy and breast-feeding (section 5.4.1). Both should be used with caution in neurological disorders (especially in those with a history of epilepsy), in severe gastro-intestinal disorders, in G6PD deficiency (section 9.1.5), in porphyria, and in the elderly (see also above). Chloroquine and hydroxychloroquine may exacerbate psoriasis and aggravate myasthenia gravis. Concurrent use of hepatotoxic drugs should be avoided; other **interactions**: Appendix 1 (chloroquine and hydroxychloroquine).

Advice of Royal College of Ophthalmologists
The Royal College of Ophthalmologists has advised that a screening protocol for chloroquine should be negotiated with local ophthalmologists; no screening is recommended for mepacrine because it is not thought to be associated with ophthalmological effects. The following recommendations relate to hydroxychloroquine.

Before treatment:
- Assess renal and liver function (adjust dose if impaired)
- Ask patient about visual impairment (not corrected by glasses). If impairment or eye disease present, assessment by an optometrist is advised and any abnormality should be referred to an ophthalmologist

- Record near visual acuity of each eye (with glasses where appropriate) using a standard reading chart
- Initiate hydroxychloroquine treatment if no abnormality detected (at a dose not exceeding hydroxychloroquine sulphate 6.5 mg/kg daily)

During treatment:
- Ask patient about visual symptoms and monitor visual acuity annually using the standard reading chart
- Refer to ophthalmologist if visual acuity changes or if vision blurred and warn patient to stop treatment and seek prescribing doctor's advice
- A child treated for juvenile arthritis should receive slit-lamp examination routinely to check for uveitis
- If long-term treatment is required (more than 5 years), individual arrangement should be agreed with the local ophthalmologist

NOTE. To avoid excessive dosage in obese patients, the dose of hydroxychloroquine and chloroquine should be calculated on the basis of lean body weight. Ocular toxicity is unlikely with chloroquine phosphate not exceeding 4 mg/kg daily (equivalent to chloroquine base approx. 2.5 mg/kg daily)

SIDE-EFFECTS. The side-effects of chloroquine and hydroxychloroquine include gastro-intestinal disturbances, headache and skin reactions (rashes, pruritus); those occurring less frequently include ECG changes, convulsions, visual changes, retinal damage (see above), keratopathy, ototoxicity, hair depigmentation, hair loss, and discoloration of skin, nails, and mucous membranes. Side-effects that occur rarely include blood disorders (including thrombocytopenia, agranulocytosis, and aplastic anaemia), mental changes (including emotional disturbances and psychosis), myopathy (including cardiomyopathy and neuromyopathy), acute generalised exanthematous pustulosis, exfoliative dermatitis, Stevens-Johnson syndrome, photosensitivity, and hepatic damage. **Important**: very toxic in overdosage—immediate advice from poisons centres essential (see also p. 24).

CHLOROQUINE

Indications: active rheumatoid arthritis (including juvenile arthritis), systemic and discoid lupus erythematosus; malaria (section 5.4.1)
Cautions: see notes above
Side-effects: see notes above
Dose: administered on expert advice, *by mouth*, chloroquine (base) 150 mg daily; max. 2.5 mg/kg daily, see recommendations above; CHILD up to 3 mg/kg daily
NOTE. Chloroquine base 150 mg ≡ chloroquine sulphate 200 mg ≡ chloroquine phosphate 250 mg (approx.).

■ Preparations
Section 5.4.1

HYDROXYCHLOROQUINE SULPHATE

Indications: active rheumatoid arthritis (including juvenile arthritis), systemic and discoid lupus erythematosus; dermatological conditions caused or aggravated by sunlight
Cautions: see notes above

Side-effects: see notes above

Dose: administered on expert advice, initially 400 mg daily in divided doses; maintenance 200–400 mg daily; max. 6.5 mg/kg daily (but not exceeding 400 mg daily), see recommendations above; CHILD, up to 6.5 mg/kg daily (max. 400 mg daily)

Plaquenil® (Sanofi-Synthelabo) [PoM]
Tablets, f/c, hydroxychloroquine sulphate 200 mg. Net price 60-tab pack = £4.55. Label: 5, 21

Drugs affecting the immune response

Methotrexate is a disease-modifying antirheumatic drug suitable for moderate to severe rheumatoid arthritis. **Azathioprine, ciclosporin, cyclophosphamide, leflunomide,** and the **cytokine inhibitors** (adalimumab, anakinra, etanercept, and infliximab) are considered more toxic and they are used in cases that have not responded to other disease-modifying drugs.

Methotrexate is usually given in an initial dose of 7.5 mg by mouth once a week, adjusted according to response to a maximum of 15 mg once a week (occasionally 20 mg once a week). Regular full blood counts (including differential white cell count and platelet count), renal and liver-function tests are required. In patients who experience mucosal or gastro-intestinal side-effects with methotrexate, folic acid 5 mg every week may help to reduce the frequency of such side-effects.

Azathioprine is usually given in a dose of 1.5 to 2.5 mg/kg daily in divided doses. Blood counts are needed to detect possible neutropenia or thrombocytopenia (usually resolved by reducing the dose). Nausea, vomiting, and diarrhoea may occur, usually starting early during the course of treatment, and may necessitate withdrawal of the drug; herpes zoster infection may also occur.

Leflunomide acts on the immune system as a disease-modifying antirheumatic drug. Its therapeutic effect starts after 4–6 weeks and improvement may continue for a further 4–6 months. Leflunomide, which is similar in efficacy to sulfasalazine and methotrexate, may be chosen when these drugs cannot be used. The active metabolite of leflunomide persists for a long period; active procedures to wash the drug out are required in case of serious adverse effects, or before starting treatment with another disease-modifying antirheumatic drug, or, in men or women, before conception. Side-effects of leflunomide include bone-marrow toxicity; its immunosuppressive effects increase the risk of infection and malignancy.

Ciclosporin (cyclosporin) is licensed for severe active rheumatoid arthritis when conventional second-line therapy is inappropriate or ineffective. There is some evidence that ciclosporin may retard the rate of erosive progression and improve symptom control in those who respond only partially to methotrexate.

Cyclophosphamide (section 8.1.1) may be used at a dose of 1 to 1.5 mg/kg daily by mouth for rheumatoid arthritis with severe systemic manifestations [unlicensed indication]; it is toxic and regular blood counts (including platelet count) should be carried out. Cyclophosphamide may also be given intravenously in a dose of 0.5 to 1 g (with prophylactic mesna) for *severe systemic rheumatoid arthritis* and for other connective tissue diseases (especially with active vasculitis), repeated initially at fortnightly then at monthly intervals (according to clinical response and haematological monitoring).

Drugs that affect the immune response are also used in the management of severe cases of *systemic lupus erythematosus* and other connective tissue disorders. They are often given in conjunction with corticosteroids for patients with severe or progressive renal disease. They may be used in cases of *polymyositis* which are resistant to corticosteroids. They are used for their corticosteroid-sparing effect in patients whose corticosteroid requirements are excessive. **Azathioprine** is usually used.

Azathioprine and methotrexate are used in the treatment of *psoriatic arthropathy* [unlicensed indication] for severe or progressive cases which are not controlled with anti-inflammatory drugs.

AZATHIOPRINE

Indications: see notes above; transplantation rejection, see section 8.2.1

Cautions: see section 8.2.1

Contra-indications: see section 8.2.1

Side-effects: see section 8.2.1

Dose: *by mouth*, initially, rarely more than 3 mg/kg daily, reduced according to response; maintenance 1–3 mg/kg daily; consider withdrawal if no improvement within 3 months

■ Preparations
Section 8.2.1

CICLOSPORIN

(Cyclosporin)

Indications: severe active rheumatoid arthritis when conventional second-line therapy inappropriate or ineffective; graft-versus-host disease (section 8.2.2); atopic dermatitis and psoriasis (section 13.5.3).

Cautions: see section 8.2.2
ADDITIONAL CAUTIONS IN RHEUMATOID ARTHRITIS. *Contra-indicated* in abnormal renal function, uncontrolled hypertension (see also below), uncontrolled infections, and malignancy. Measure serum creatinine at least twice before treatment and monitor every 2 weeks for first 3 months, then every 4 weeks (or more frequently if dose increased or concomitant NSAIDs introduced or increased (see also **interactions:** Appendix 1 (ciclosporin)), reduce dose if serum creatinine increases more than 30% above baseline in more than 1 measurement; if above 50%, reduce dose by 50% (even if within normal range) and discontinue if reduction not successful within 1 month; monitor blood pressure (discontinue if hypertension develops that cannot be controlled by antihypertensive therapy); monitor hepatic function if concomitant NSAIDs given.

Side-effects: see section 8.2.2

Dose: *by mouth*, administered in accordance with expert advice, initially 2.5 mg/kg daily in 2 divided doses, if necessary increased gradually after 6 weeks; max. 4 mg/kg daily (discontinue if response insufficient after 3 months); dose adjusted according to response for maintenance and treatment reviewed after 6 months (continue only if benefits outweigh risks); CHILD and under 18 years, not recommended

IMPORTANT. For preparations and counselling and for advice on conversion between the preparations, see section 8.2.2

■ Preparations
Section 8.2.2

LEFLUNOMIDE

Indications: moderate to severe active rheumatoid arthritis

Cautions: renal impairment (Appendix 3); impaired bone-marrow function including anaemia, leucopenia or thrombocytopenia (avoid if significant and due to causes other than rheumatoid arthritis); recent treatment with other hepatotoxic or myelotoxic disease-modifying antirheumatic drugs (avoid concomitant use); history of tuberculosis; exclude pregnancy before treatment; effective contraception **essential** during treatment and for at least 2 years after treatment in women and at least 3 months after treatment in men (plasma concentration monitoring required; waiting time before conception may be reduced with washout procedures—consult product literature and see Washout Procedure below); monitor full blood count (including differential white cell count and platelet count) before treatment and every 2 weeks for 6 months then every 8 weeks; monitor liver function—(see Hepatotoxicity below); monitor blood pressure; washout procedures recommended for serious adverse effects and before switching to other disease-modifying antirheumatic drugs (consult product literature and see below); **interactions:** Appendix 1 (leflunomide)

HEPATOTOXICITY. Potentially life-threatening hepatotoxicity reported usually in the first 6 months; monitor liver function before treatment and every 2 weeks for first 6 months then every 8 weeks. Discontinue treatment (and institute washout procedure—consult product literature and see Washout Procedure below) or reduce dose according to liver-function abnormality; if liver-function abnormality persists after dose reduction, discontinue treatment and institute washout procedure

WASHOUT PROCEDURE. To aid drug elimination in case of serious adverse effect, or before starting another disease-modifying antirheumatic drug, or before conception (see also Appendix 4), stop treatment and give *either* colestyramine 8 g 3 times daily for 11 days *or* activated charcoal 50 g 4 times daily for 11 days; the concentration of the active metabolite after washout should be less than 20 micrograms/litre (measured on 2 occasions 14 days apart) in men or women before conception—consult product literature

Contra-indications: severe immunodeficiency; serious infection; hepatic impairment; severe hypoproteinaemia; pregnancy (**important teratogenic risk:** see Cautions and Appendix 4); breast-feeding (Appendix 5)

Side-effects: diarrhoea, nausea, vomiting, anorexia, oral mucosal disorders, abdominal pain, weight loss; increase in blood pressure; headache, dizziness, asthenia, paraesthesia; tenosynovitis; alopecia, eczema, dry skin, rash, pruritus; leucopenia; rarely taste disturbances, anxiety, tendon rupture, urticaria, anaemia, thrombocytopenia, eosinophilia, hyperlipidaemia, hypokalaemia, hypophosphataemia, hepatic dysfunction (see Hepatotoxicity above); also reported, pancreatitis,

anaphylaxis, interstitial lung disease, severe infection, pancytopenia, vasculitis, Stevens-Johnson syndrome, toxic epidermal necrolysis (discontinue and initiate washout procedure—consult product literature)

Dose: initially 100 mg once daily for 3 days then maintenance, 10–20 mg once daily; CHILD under 18 years safety and efficacy not established

Arava® (Aventis Pharma) ▼ PoM
Tablets, f/c, leflunomide 10 mg, net price 30-tab pack = £46.50; 20 mg (ochre), 30-tab pack = £46.50; 100 mg, 3-tab pack = £23.25. Label: 4

METHOTREXATE

Indications: moderate to severe active rheumatoid arthritis; malignant disease (section 8.1.3); psoriasis (section 13.5.3)

Cautions: section 8.1; see CSM advice below (blood count, liver and pulmonary toxicity); extreme caution in blood disorders (avoid if severe); renal impairment (avoid in moderate or severe—Appendix 3); peptic ulceration, ulcerative colitis, diarrhoea and ulcerative stomatitis (withdraw if stomatitis develops—may be first sign of gastro-intestinal toxicity); risk of accumulation in pleural effusion or ascites—drain before treatment; porphyria (section 9.8.2); **interactions:** see below and Appendix 1 (methotrexate)

> **CSM advice.** In view of reports of blood dyscrasias (including fatalities) and liver cirrhosis with low-dose methotrexate, the CSM has advised:
>
> - full blood count and renal and liver function tests before starting treatment and repeated weekly until therapy stabilised, thereafter patients should be monitored every 2–3 months
>
> - patients should report all symptoms and signs suggestive of infection, especially sore throat
>
> Treatment with folinic acid (as calcium folinate, section 8.1) may be required in acute toxicity

BLOOD COUNT. Haematopoietic suppression may occur abruptly; factors likely to increase toxicity include advanced age, renal impairment and concomitant administration of another anti-folate drug. Any profound drop in white cell or platelet count calls for immediate withdrawal of methotrexate and introduction of supportive therapy

LIVER TOXICITY. Liver cirrhosis reported. Treatment should not be started or should be discontinued if any abnormality of liver function tests or liver biopsy is present or develops during therapy. Abnormalities may return to normal within 2 weeks after which treatment may be recommenced if judged appropriate

PULMONARY TOXICITY. Pulmonary toxicity may be a special problem in rheumatoid arthritis (patient to seek medical attention if dyspnoea, cough or fever); monitor for symptoms at each visit—discontinue if pneumonitis suspected.

ASPIRIN AND OTHER NSAIDS. If aspirin or other NSAIDs are given concurrently the dose of methotrexate should be carefully monitored. Patients should be advised to avoid self-medication with over-the-counter aspirin or ibuprofen

Contra-indications: see Cautions above, hepatic impairment (Appendix 2), pregnancy (following administration to a woman or a man, avoid conception for **at least 3 months** after stopping—Appendix 4), breast-feeding (Cytotoxic drugs, Appendix 5), active infection and immunodeficiency syndromes

Side-effects: section 8.1; also anorexia, abdominal discomfort, intestinal ulceration and bleeding, diarrhoea, toxic megacolon, hepatotoxicity (see Cautions above); ecchymosis; pulmonary oedema, pleuritic pain, pulmonary fibrosis, interstitial pneumonitis (see Pulmonary Toxicity above); anaphylactic reactions, urticaria; dizziness, drowsiness, malaise, headache, mood changes, abnormal cranial sensations; precipitation of diabetes, osteoporosis; menstrual disturbances, vaginitis, impotence, loss of libido; haematuria, dysuria, renal failure; arthralgia, myalgia, vasculitis, blurred vision; rash, pruritus, Stevens-Johnson syndrome, toxic epidermal necrolysis, photosensitivity, changes of skin pigmentation, telangiectasia

Dose: *by mouth*, 7.5 mg once weekly (as a single dose *or* divided into 3 doses of 2.5 mg given at intervals of 12 hours), adjusted according to response; max. total weekly dose 20 mg

---

Important. Note that the above dose is a **weekly** dose. The CSM has received reports of prescription and dispensing errors including fatalities. Attention should be paid to the **strength** of methotrexate tablets prescribed and the **frequency** of dosing.

Methotrexate (Non-proprietary) PoM
Tablets, yellow, methotrexate 2.5 mg, net price 28-tab pack = £3.27. Counselling, dose, NSAIDs
Available from Lederle, Mayne, Pharmacia (*Maxtrex®*)
Tablets, yellow, methotrexate 10 mg, net price 20 (Mayne) = £11.01; (Pharmacia, *Maxtrex®*) = £9.03. Counselling, dose, NSAIDs

Cytokine inhibitors

Cytokine inhibitors should be used under specialist supervision.

Adalimumab, **etanercept**, and **infliximab** inhibit the activity of tumour necrosis factor.

NICE guidance (etanercept and infliximab for rheumatoid arthritis). NICE has recommended (March 2002) the use of either etanercept or infliximab for highly active rheumatoid arthritis in adults who have failed to respond to at least 2 standard disease-modifying antirheumatic drugs, including methotrexate (unless methotrexate cannot be used because of intolerance or contra-indications). Etanercept and infliximab should be prescribed (according to the guidelines of the British Society for Rheumatology) and their use monitored by consultant rheumatologists specialising in their use. Infliximab should be given concomitantly with methotrexate.

Etanercept or infliximab should be withdrawn if severe side-effects develop or if there is no response after 3 months. There is no evidence to support treatment for longer than 4 years; a decision to continue therapy should be based on disease activity and clinical effectiveness in individual cases.

Consecutive use of etanercept and infliximab is not recommended.

Prescribers of etanercept and infliximab should register consenting patients with the Biologics Registry of the British Society for Rheumatology.

NICE guidance (etanercept for juvenile idiopathic arthritis). NICE has recommended (March 2002) the use of etanercept in children aged 4–17 years with active polyarticular-course juvenile idiopathic arthritis who have not responded adequately to methotrexate or who are intolerant of it. Etanercept should be used under specialist supervision according to the guidelines of the British Paediatric Rheumatology Group.

Etanercept should be withdrawn if severe side-effects develop or if there is no response after 6 months or if the initial response is not maintained. There is no evidence to support treatment for longer than 2 years; a decision to continue therapy should be based on disease activity and clinical effectiveness in individual cases.

Prescribers of etanercept and infliximab should register consenting patients with the Biologics Registry of the British Paediatric Rheumatology Group.

Adalimumab is licensed for moderate to severe active rheumatoid arthritis when response to other disease-modifying antirheumatic drugs (including methotrexate) has been inadequate. Adalimumab should be used in combination with methotrexate, but it may be given alone if methotrexate is inappropriate. If there is no response after 3 months, adalimumab should be discontinued.

Etanercept is also licensed for the treatment of active and progressive *psoriatic arthritis* in adults not responding adequately to other disease-modifying antirheumatic drugs, and for severe *ankylosing spondylitis* in adults not responding adequately to conventional therapy. Infliximab is also licensed for the treatment of *ankylosing spondylitis*, in patients with severe axial symptoms who have not responded adequately to conventional therapy.

Adalimumab, etanercept, and infliximab have been associated with infections, sometimes severe, including tuberculosis and septicaemia. Other side-effects include nausea, abdominal pain, worsening heart failure, hypersensitivity reactions (including angioedema, bronchospasm, urticaria, and anaphylaxis), fever, headache, depression, lupus erythematosus-like syndrome, pruritus, injection-site reactions, and blood disorders (including anaemia, leucopenia, thrombocytopenia, pancytopenia, aplastic anaemia).

Anakinra inhibits the activity of interleukin-1. Anakinra (in combination with methotrexate) is licensed for the treatment of rheumatoid arthritis which has not responded to methotrexate alone; it is not, however, recommended for routine management of rheumatoid arthritis, see NICE guidance below.

NICE guidance (anakinra for rheumatoid arthritis). NICE does not recommend (November 2003) anakinra for the treatment of rheumatoid arthritis except when used in a controlled long-term clinical study. Patients receiving anakinra for rheumatoid arthritis should continue treatment until they and their consultant consider it appropriate to stop.

ADALIMUMAB

Indications: see under Cytokine Inhibitors above
Cautions: hepatic impairment; renal impairment; monitor for infections before, during, and for 5 months after treatment (see also Tuberculosis

below); predisposition to infections; heart failure (discontinue if symptoms develop or worsen; avoid in moderate or severe heart failure); demyelinating CNS disorders (risk of exacerbation); **interactions:** Appendix 1 (adalimumab)

TUBERCULOSIS. Patients must be evaluated for active and latent tuberculosis before treatment. Tuberculosis chemoprophylaxis must be started before initiating adalimumab in latent tuberculosis (contra-indicated in active tuberculosis). Patients should be instructed to seek medical advice if they develop symptoms suggestive of tuberculosis (such as persistent cough, weight loss, fever). If active tuberculosis suspected, adalimumab should be discontinued until infection either ruled out or treated

Contra-indications: pregnancy (Appendix 4); breast-feeding (Appendix 5); severe infections (see also Cautions)

Side-effects: see under Cytokine Inhibitors and Cautions above; also diarrhoea, constipation, vomiting, oesophagitis, dyspepsia, gastritis, dysphagia, taste disturbances, mouth ulceration, hypertension, vasodilatation, chest pain, ecchymosis, cough, sore throat, asthma, dyspnoea, asthenia, insomnia, drowsiness, dizziness, agitation, tremor, paraesthesia, hypoaesthesia, neuralgia, menorrhagia, urinary frequency, haematuria, proteinuria, arthralgia, myalgia, eye disorders, rash, alopecia, sweating, hyperlipidaemia, hypokalaemia, hyperuricaemia

Dose: _by subcutaneous injection_, ADULT over 18 years, 40 mg on alternate weeks; if necessary increased to 40 mg weekly in patients receiving adalimumab alone

Humira® (Abbott) ▼ PoM
Injection, adalimumab, net price 40-mg prefilled syringe = £357.50. Counselling, tuberculosis

ANAKINRA

Indications: see under Cytokine Inhibitors above

Cautions: renal impairment (Appendix 3); predisposition to infections; history of asthma (risk of serious infection); **interactions:** Appendix 1 (anakinra)

BLOOD DISORDERS. Neutropenia reported commonly. Monitor neutrophil count before treatment, then every month for 6 months, then every 3 months—discontinue if neutropenia develops. Patients should be instructed to seek medical advice if symptoms suggestive of neutropenia (such as fever, sore throat, infection) develop

Contra-indications: pregnancy (Appendix 4); breast-feeding; neutropenia

Side-effects: injection-site reactions, headache; infections, neutropenia (see also Cautions)

Dose: _by subcutaneous injection_, ADULT over 18 years, 100 mg once daily

Kineret® (Amgen) ▼ PoM
Injection, anakinra, net price 100-mg prefilled syringe = £20.47. Counselling, blood disorder symptoms

ETANERCEPT

Indications: see under Cytokine Inhibitors above; severe, active and progressive rheumatoid arthritis in patients not previously treated with methotrexate

Cautions: predisposition to infection (avoid if predisposition to septicaemia); significant exposure to herpes zoster virus—interrupt treatment and consider varicella–zoster immunoglobulin;

heart failure (risk of exacerbation); demyelinating CNS disorders (risk of exacerbation); history of blood disorders; **interactions:** Appendix 1 (etanercept)

Contra-indications: pregnancy; breast-feeding; active infection

Side-effects: see under Cytokine Inhibitors above; also vomiting, oesophagitis, cholecystitis, pancreatitis, gastro-intestinal haemorrhage, myocardial or cerebral ischaemia, venous thromboembolism, hypotension, hypertension, dyspnoea, demyelinating disorders, seizures, bone fracture, renal impairment, polymyositis, bursitis, lymphadenopathy

Dose: _by subcutaneous injection_, rheumatoid arthritis, psoriatic arthritis, ankylosing spondylitis, ADULT over 18 years, 25 mg twice weekly

Polyarticular-course juvenile idiopathic arthritis, CHILD and ADOLESCENT 4–17 years, 400 micrograms/kg twice weekly (max. 25 mg twice weekly)

Enbrel (Wyeth) ▼ PoM
Injection, powder for reconstitution, etanercept, net price 25-mg vial = £89.38

INFLIXIMAB

Indications: see under Cytokine Inhibitors above; Crohn's disease (section 1.5)

Cautions: hepatic impairment; renal impairment; monitor for infections before, during, and for 6 months after treatment (see also Tuberculosis below); heart failure (discontinue if symptoms develop or worsen; avoid in moderate or severe heart failure); demyelinating CNS disorders (risk of exacerbation); **interactions:** Appendix 1 (infliximab)

TUBERCULOSIS. Tuberculosis (often in extrapulmonary sites) reported. Patients must be evaluated for active and latent tuberculosis before treatment. Tuberculosis chemoprophylaxis must be started before initiating infliximab in latent tuberculosis (contra-indicated in active tuberculosis). Patients should be instructed to seek medical advice if they develop symptoms suggestive of tuberculosis (such as persistent cough, weight loss, fever). If active tuberculosis suspected, infliximab should be discontinued until infection either ruled out or treated

HYPERSENSITIVITY REACTIONS. Hypersensitivity reactions (including fever, chest pain, hypotension, hypertension, dyspnoea, pruritus, urticaria, serum sickness-like reactions, angioedema, anaphylaxis) reported during or within 1–2 hours after infusion (risk greatest during first or second infusion or in patients who discontinue other immunosuppressants. All patients should be observed carefully for 1–2 hours after infusion and resuscitation equipment should be available for immediate use. Prophylactic antipyretics, antihistamines, or hydrocortisone may be administered. Readministration not recommended after infliximab-free interval of more than 16 weeks—risk of delayed hypersensitivity reactions. Patients should be advised to keep Alert card with them at all times and seek medical advice if symptoms of delayed hypersensitivity develop

Contra-indications: pregnancy (Appendix 4); breast-feeding (Appendix 5); severe infections (see also under Cautions)

Side-effects: see under Cytokine Inhibitors and Cautions above; also dyspepsia, diarrhoea, constipation, hepatitis, cholecystitis, diverticulitis, gastro-intestinal haemorrhage, flushing, bradycardia, arrhythmias, palpitation, syncope, vasospasm, peripheral ischaemia, ecchymosis, haematoma, interstitial pneumonitis or fibrosis, fatigue, anxiety, drowsiness, dizziness, insomnia, confusion, agitation, amnesia, seizures, demyelinating disorders, vaginitis, myalgia, arthralgia, endophthalmitis, rash, sweating, hyperkeratosis, skin pigmentation, alopecia

Dose: *by intravenous infusion*, rheumatoid arthritis (in combination with methotrexate), ADULT and ADOLESCENT over 17 years, 3 mg/kg, repeated at 2 weeks and 6 weeks after initial infusion, then repeated every 8 weeks

Ankylosing spondylitis, ADULT and ADOLESCENT over 17 years, 5 mg/kg, repeated at 2 weeks and 6 weeks after initial infusion, then repeated every 6–8 weeks; discontinue if no response by 6 weeks of initial infusion

Remicade® (Schering-Plough) ▼ PoM
Intravenous infusion, powder for reconstitution, infliximab, net price 100-mg vial = £451.20.
Label: 10, Alert card, counselling, tuberculosis and hypersensitivity reactions

Sulfasalazine

Sulfasalazine (sulphasalazine) has a beneficial effect in suppressing the inflammatory activity of rheumatoid arthritis. Side-effects include rashes, gastro-intestinal intolerance and, especially in patients with rheumatoid arthritis, occasional leucopenia, neutropenia, and thrombocytopenia. These haematological abnormalities occur usually in the first 3 to 6 months of treatment and are reversible on cessation of treatment. Close monitoring of full blood counts (including differential white cell count and platelet count) is necessary initially, and at monthly intervals during the first 3 months (liver-function tests also being performed at monthly intervals for the first 3 months). Although the manufacturer recommends renal function tests, evidence of practical value is unsatisfactory.

SULFASALAZINE

(Sulphasalazine)
Indications: active rheumatoid arthritis; ulcerative colitis, see section 1.5 and notes above
Cautions: see section 1.5 and notes above
The CSM has recommended that patients should be advised to report any unexplained bleeding, bruising, purpura, sore throat, fever or malaise. A blood count should be performed and the drug stopped immediately if there is suspicion of a blood dyscrasia.
Contra-indications: see section 1.5 and notes above
Side-effects: see section 1.5 and notes above
Dose: *by mouth*, administered on expert advice, as enteric-coated tablets, initially 500 mg daily, increased by 500 mg at intervals of 1 week to a max. of 2–3 g daily in divided doses

Sulfasalazine (Non-proprietary) PoM
Tablets, e/c, sulfasalazine 500 mg. Net price 112-tab pack = £8.43. Label: 5, 14, 25, counselling, blood disorder symptoms (see CSM recommendation above), contact lenses may be stained
Available from Alpharma (*Sulazine EC*®)

Salazopyrin EN-Tabs® (Pharmacia) PoM
Tablets, e/c, yellow, f/c, sulfasalazine 500 mg. Net price 112-tab pack = £8.43. Label: 5, 14, 25, counselling, blood disorder symptoms (see CSM

recommendation above), contact lenses may be stained

10.1.4 Gout and cytotoxic-induced hyperuricaemia

It is important to distinguish drugs used for the treatment of acute attacks of gout from those used in the long-term control of the disease. The latter exacerbate and prolong the acute manifestations if started during an attack.

Acute attacks of gout

Acute attacks of gout are usually treated with high doses of **NSAIDs** such as diclofenac, etoricoxib, indometacin, ketoprofen, naproxen, piroxicam, or sulindac (section 10.1.1). The use of azapropazone should be restricted to patients in whom less toxic drugs have been ineffective (**important:** see CSM restrictions on p. 480). Colchicine is an alternative. Aspirin is *not* indicated in gout. Allopurinol and uricosurics are not effective in treating an acute attack and may prolong it indefinitely if started during the acute episode.

Colchicine is probably as effective as NSAIDs. Its use is limited by the development of toxicity at higher doses, but it is of value in patients with heart failure since, unlike NSAIDs, it does not induce fluid retention; moreover it can be given to patients receiving anticoagulants.

Intra-articular injection of a **corticosteroid** may be used in acute monoarticular gout [unlicensed indication]. A corticosteroid by intramuscular injection can be effective in podagra.

COLCHICINE

Indications: acute gout, short-term prophylaxis during initial therapy with allopurinol and uricosuric drugs; prophylaxis of familial Mediterranean fever (recurrent polyserositis) [unlicensed]
Cautions: breast-feeding (Appendix 5), elderly, gastro-intestinal disease, cardiac, hepatic and renal impairment; **interactions:** Appendix 1 (colchicine)
Contra-indications: pregnancy
Side-effects: most common are nausea, vomiting, and abdominal pain; excessive doses may also cause profuse diarrhoea, gastro-intestinal haemorrhage, rashes, renal and hepatic damage. Rarely peripheral neuritis, myopathy, alopecia, inhibition of spermatogenesis, and with prolonged treatment blood disorders
Dose: treatment of gout, 1 mg initially, followed by 500 micrograms every 2–3 hours until relief of pain is obtained or vomiting or diarrhoea occurs, or until a total dose of 6 mg has been reached; the course should not be repeated within 3 days
Prevention of gout attacks during initial treatment with allopurinol or uricosuric drugs, 500 micrograms 2–3 times daily
Prophylaxis of familial Mediterranean fever [unlicensed], 0.5–2 mg daily

Colchicine (Non-proprietary) PoM
Tablets, colchicine 500 micrograms, net price 20 = £3.32
Available from Celltech, CP, IVAX

Long-term control of gout

Frequent recurrence of acute attacks of gout, the presence of tophi, or signs of chronic gouty arthritis may call for the initiation of long-term ('interval') treatment. For long-term control of gout the formation of uric acid from purines may be reduced with the xanthine-oxidase inhibitor allopurinol, or the uricosuric drug sulfinpyrazone may be used to increase the excretion of uric acid in the urine. Treatment should be continued indefinitely to prevent further attacks of gout by correcting the hyperuricaemia. These drugs should never be started during an acute attack; they are usually started 2–3 weeks after the attack has settled. The initiation of treatment may precipitate an acute attack therefore colchicine or an anti-inflammatory analgesic should be used as a prophylactic and continued for at least one month after the hyperuricaemia has been corrected (usually about 3 months of prophylaxis). However, if an acute attack develops during treatment, then the treatment should continue at the same dosage and the acute attack treated in its own right.
Allopurinol is a well tolerated drug which is widely used. It is especially useful in patients with renal impairment or urate stones where uricosuric drugs cannot be used; it is *not* indicated for the treatment of asymptomatic hyperuricaemia. It is usually given once daily, since the active metabolite of allopurinol has a long half-life, but doses over 300 mg daily should be divided. It may occasionally cause rashes.
Sulfinpyrazone (sulphinpyrazone) can be used instead of allopurinol, or in conjunction with it in cases that are resistant to treatment.
Probenecid (available on a named-patient basis) is a uricosuric drug used to prevent nephrotoxicity associated with cidofovir (section 5.3).
Crystallisation of urate in the urine may occur with the uricosuric drugs and it is important to ensure an adequate urine output especially in the first few weeks of treatment. As an additional precaution the urine may be rendered alkaline.
Aspirin and salicylates antagonise the uricosuric drugs; they do not antagonise allopurinol but are nevertheless *not* indicated in gout.

ALLOPURINOL

Indications: prophylaxis of gout and of uric acid and calcium oxalate renal stones; prophylaxis of hyperuricaemia associated with cancer chemotherapy
Cautions: administer prophylactic colchicine or NSAID (*not* aspirin or salicylates) until at least 1 month after hyperuricaemia corrected; ensure adequate fluid intake (2–3 litres/day); hepatic impairment (Appendix 2), renal impairment (monitor liver function; Appendix 3); for hyperuricaemia associated with cancer therapy, allopurinol treatment should be started before cancer therapy; pregnancy and breast-feeding; **interactions:** Appendix 1 (allopurinol)
Contra-indications: not a treatment for acute gout but continue if attack develops when already

receiving allopurinol, and treat attack separately (see notes above)
Side-effects: rashes (**withdraw** therapy; if rash mild re-introduce cautiously but **discontinue** immediately if recurrence—hypersensitivity reactions occur rarely and include exfoliation, fever, lymphadenopathy, arthralgia, and eosinophilia resembling Stevens-Johnson or Lyell's syndrome, vasculitis, hepatitis, renal impairment, and very rarely seizures); gastro-intestinal disorders; rarely malaise, headache, vertigo, drowsiness, visual and taste disturbances, hypertension, alopecia, hepatotoxicity, paraesthesia and neuropathy, gynaecomastia, blood disorders (including leucopenia, thrombocytopenia, haemolytic anaemia and aplastic anaemia)
Dose: initially 100 mg daily, preferably after food, then adjusted according to plasma or urinary uric acid concentration; usual maintenance dose in mild conditions 100–200 mg daily, in moderately severe conditions 300–600 mg daily, in severe conditions 700–900 mg daily; doses over 300 mg daily given in divided doses; CHILD under 15 years, (in neoplastic conditions, enzyme disorders) 10–20 mg/kg daily (max. 400 mg daily)

Allopurinol (Non-proprietary) PoM
Tablets, allopurinol 100 mg, net price 28-tab pack = 91p; 300 mg, 28-tab pack = £2.17. Label: 8, 21, 27
Available from Alpharma, APS, Arrow, Ashbourne (*Xanthomax*®), Berk (*Caplenal*®), CP, DDSA (*Cosuric*®), Generics, Hillcross, IVAX, Ranbaxy (*Rimapurinol*®), Sovereign

Zyloric® (GSK) PoM
Tablets, allopurinol 100 mg, net price 100-tab pack = £10.96; 300 mg, 28-tab pack = £7.86. Label: 8, 21, 27

PROBENECID

Indications: prevention of nephrotoxicity associated with cidofovir (section 5.3)
Cautions: ensure adequate fluid intake (about 2–3 litres daily) and render urine alkaline if uric acid overload is high; peptic ulceration, renal impairment (avoid if severe); transient false-positive Benedict's test; G6PD-deficiency (section 9.1.5); **interactions:** Appendix 1 (probenecid)
Contra-indications: history of blood disorders, nephrolithiasis, porphyria (section 9.8.2), acute gout attack; avoid aspirin and salicylates
Side-effects: gastro-intestinal disturbances, urinary frequency, headache, flushing, dizziness, alopecia, anaemia, haemolytic anaemia, sore gums; hypersensitivity reactions including anaphylaxis, dermatitis, pruritus, urticaria, fever and Stevens-Johnson syndrome; rarely nephrotic syndrome, hepatic necrosis, leucopenia, aplastic anaemia; toxic epidermal necrolysis reported with concurrent colchicine
Dose: used with cidofovir, see section 5.3

Probenecid (Non-proprietary) PoM
Tablets, probenecid 500 mg. Label: 12, 21, 27
Available on named-patient basis from IDIS (*Benuryl*®, *Probecid*®)

SULFINPYRAZONE
(Sulphinpyrazone)

Indications: gout prophylaxis, hyperuricaemia

Cautions: see under Probenecid; regular blood counts advisable; cardiac disease (may cause salt and water retention); **interactions:** Appendix 1 (sulfinpyrazone)

Contra-indications: see under Probenecid; avoid in hypersensitivity to NSAIDs

Side-effects: gastro-intestinal disturbances, occasionally allergic skin reactions, salt and water retention; rarely blood disorders, gastro-intestinal ulceration and bleeding, acute renal failure, raised liver enzymes, jaundice and hepatitis

Dose: initially 100–200 mg daily with food (or milk) increasing over 2–3 weeks to 600 mg daily (rarely 800 mg daily), continued until serum uric acid concentration normal then reduced for maintenance (maintenance dose may be as low as 200 mg daily)

Anturan® (Novartis) [PoM]
Tablets, both yellow, s/c, sulfinpyrazone 100 mg, net price 84-tab pack = £4.72; 200 mg, 84-tab pack = £9.38. Label: 12, 21

Hyperuricaemia associated with cytotoxic drugs

Allopurinol is used to prevent hyperuricaemia associated with cytotoxic drugs—see section 8.1 (Hyperuricaemia) and Allopurinol above.

Rasburicase is licensed for the prophylaxis and treatment of acute hyperuricaemia, before and during initiation of chemotherapy, in patients with haematological malignancy and a high tumour burden at risk of rapid lysis.

RASBURICASE

Indications: prophylaxis and treatment of acute hyperuricaemia with initial chemotherapy for haematological malignancy

Cautions: monitor closely for hypersensitivity; atopic allergies; may interfere with test for uric acid—consult product literature

Contra-indications: susceptibility to haemolytic anaemia including G6PD deficiency; pregnancy; breast-feeding

Side-effects: fever; nausea, vomiting; less frequently diarrhoea, headache, hypersensitivity reactions (including rash, bronchospasm and anaphylaxis); haemolytic anaemia, methaemoglobinaemia

Dose: *by intravenous infusion,* 200 micrograms/kg once daily for 5–7 days

Fasturtec (Sanofi-Synthelabo) ▼ [PoM]
Intravenous infusion, powder for reconstitution, rasburicase, net price 1.5-mg vial (with solvent) = £48.24; 7.5-mg vial (with solvent) = £201.00

10.2 Drugs used in neuromuscular disorders

10.2.1 Drugs which enhance neuromuscular transmission

Anticholinesterases are used as first-line treatment in *ocular myasthenia gravis* and as an adjunct to immunosuppressant therapy for *generalised myasthenia gravis.*

Corticosteroids are used when anticholinesterases do not control symptoms completely. A second-line immunosuppressant such as azathioprine is frequently used to reduce the dose of corticosteroid.

Plasmapheresis or infusion of intravenous immunoglobulin [unlicensed indication] may induce temporary remission in severe relapses, particularly where bulbar or respiratory function is compromised or before thymectomy.

Anticholinesterases

Anticholinesterase drugs enhance neuromuscular transmission in voluntary and involuntary muscle in myasthenia gravis. They prolong the action of acetylcholine by inhibiting the action of the enzyme acetylcholinesterase. Excessive dosage of these drugs may impair neuromuscular transmission and precipitate 'cholinergic crises' by causing a depolarising block. This may be difficult to distinguish from a worsening myasthenic state.

Muscarinic side-effects of anticholinesterases include increased sweating, salivary, and gastric secretion, also increased gastro-intestinal and uterine motility, and bradycardia. These parasympathomimetic effects are antagonised by atropine.

Edrophonium has a very brief action and it is therefore used mainly for the diagnosis of myasthenia gravis. However, such testing should be performed only by those experienced in its use; other means of establishing the diagnosis are available. A single test-dose usually causes substantial improvement in muscle power (lasting about 5 minutes) in patients with the disease (if respiration already impaired, *only* in conjunction with someone skilled at intubation).

Edrophonium can also be used to determine whether a patient with myasthenia is receiving inadequate or excessive treatment with cholinergic drugs. If treatment is excessive an injection of edrophonium will either have no effect or will intensify symptoms (if respiration already impaired, *only* in conjunction with someone skilled at intubation). Conversely, transient improvement may be seen if the patient is being inadequately treated. The test is best performed just before the next dose of anticholinesterase.

Neostigmine produces a therapeutic effect for up to 4 hours. Its pronounced muscarinic action is a disadvantage, and simultaneous administration of an antimuscarinic drug such as atropine or propantheline may be required to prevent colic, excessive salivation, or diarrhoea. In severe disease neostigmine may be given every 2 hours. The maximum that most patients can tolerate is 180 mg daily.

Pyridostigmine is less powerful and slower in action than neostigmine but it has a longer duration of action. It is preferable to neostigmine because of its smoother action and the need for less frequent dosage. It is particularly preferred in patients whose muscles are weak on waking. It has a comparatively mild gastro-intestinal effect but an antimuscarinic drug may still be required. It is inadvisable to exceed a total daily dose of 450 mg in order to avoid acetylcholine receptor downregulation. Immunosuppressant therapy is usually considered if the dose of pyridostigmine exceeds 360 mg daily.

Distigmine has the longest action but the danger of a 'cholinergic crisis' caused by accumulation of the drug is greater than with shorter-acting drugs; it is rarely used in the management of myasthenia gravis.

Neostigmine and edrophonium are also used to reverse the actions of the non-depolarising muscle relaxants (see section 15.1.6).

NEOSTIGMINE

Indications: myasthenia gravis; other indications (section 15.1.6)

Cautions: asthma (*extreme* caution), bradycardia, arrhythmias, recent myocardial infarction, epilepsy, hypotension, parkinsonism, vagotonia, peptic ulceration, hyperthyroidism, renal impairment, pregnancy and breast-feeding; atropine or other antidote to muscarinic effects may be necessary (particularly when neostigmine is given by injection), but not given routinely because it may mask signs of overdosage; **interactions:** Appendix 1 (parasympathomimetics)

Contra-indications: intestinal or urinary obstruction

Side-effects: nausea, vomiting, increased salivation, diarrhoea, abdominal cramps (more marked with higher doses); signs of overdosage include bronchoconstriction, increased bronchial secretions, lacrimation, excessive sweating, involuntary defaecation and micturition, miosis, nystagmus, bradycardia, heart block, arrhythmias, hypotension, agitation, excessive dreaming, and weakness eventually leading to fasciculation and paralysis

Dose: *by mouth*, neostigmine bromide 15–30 mg at suitable intervals throughout day, total daily dose 75–300 mg (but see also notes above); NEONATE 1–5 mg every 4 hours, half an hour before feeds; CHILD up to 6 years initially 7.5 mg, 6–12 years initially 15 mg, usual total daily dose 15–90 mg

By subcutaneous or intramuscular injection, neostigmine metilsulfate 1–2.5 mg at suitable intervals throughout day (usual total daily dose 5–20 mg); NEONATE 50–250 micrograms every 4 hours half an hour before feeds; CHILD 200–500 micrograms as required

Neostigmine (Non-proprietary) PoM
Tablets, scored, neostigmine bromide 15 mg. Net price 20 = £3.93
Available from Cambridge
Injection, neostigmine metilsulfate 2.5 mg/mL. Net price 1-mL amp = 58p
Available from Antigen, Phoenix

DISTIGMINE BROMIDE

Indications: myasthenia gravis (but rarely used); urinary retention and other indications (section 7.4.1)

Cautions: see under Neostigmine; also oesophagitis

Contra-indications: see under Neostigmine; also severe constipation, severe postoperative shock, serious circulatory insufficiency

Side-effects: see under Neostigmine

Dose: initially 5 mg daily half an hour before breakfast, increased at intervals of 3–4 days if necessary to a max. of 20 mg daily; CHILD up to 10 mg daily according to age

- Preparations
Section 7.4.1

EDROPHONIUM CHLORIDE

Indications: see under Dose and notes above; reversal of non-depolarising neuromuscular blockade and diagnosis of dual block (section 15.1.6)

Cautions: see under Neostigmine; have resuscitation facilities; *extreme* caution in respiratory distress (see notes above) and in asthma
NOTE. Severe cholinergic reactions can be counteracted by injection of atropine sulphate (which should always be available)

Contra-indications: see under Neostigmine

Side-effects: see under Neostigmine

Dose: diagnosis of myasthenia gravis, *by intravenous injection*, 2 mg followed after 30 seconds (if no adverse reaction has occurred) by 8 mg; in adults without suitable veins, *by intramuscular injection*, 10 mg

Detection of overdosage or underdosage of cholinergic drugs, *by intravenous injection*, 2 mg (best before next dose of anticholinesterase, see notes above)

CHILD *by intravenous injection*, 20 micrograms/kg followed after 30 seconds (if no adverse reaction has occurred) by 80 micrograms/kg

Edrophonium (Non-proprietary) PoM
Injection, edrophonium chloride 10 mg/mL. Net price 1-mL amp = £4.76
Available from Cambridge

PYRIDOSTIGMINE BROMIDE

Indications: myasthenia gravis

Cautions: see under Neostigmine; weaker muscarinic action

Contra-indications: see under Neostigmine

Side-effects: see under Neostigmine

Dose: *by mouth*, 30–120 mg at suitable intervals throughout day, total daily dose 0.3–1.2 g (but see also notes above); NEONATE 5–10 mg every 4 hours, 30–60 minutes before feeds; CHILD up to 6 years initially 30 mg, 6–12 years initially 60 mg, usual total daily dose 30–360 mg

Mestinon® (ICN) PoM
Tablets, scored, pyridostigmine bromide 60 mg. Net price 20 = £5.02

Immunosuppressant therapy

Corticosteroids (section 6.3) are established as treatment for myasthenia gravis; although they are commonly given on alternate days there is little evidence of benefit over daily administration.

Corticosteroid treatment is usually initiated under in-patient supervision and all patients should receive osteoporosis prophylaxis (section 6.6).

In *generalised myasthenia gravis* small initial doses of prednisolone (10 mg on alternate days) are increased in steps of 10 mg on alternate days to 1–1.5 mg/kg (max. 100 mg) on alternate days. When given daily, prednisolone is started at 5 mg daily and then increased in steps of 5 mg daily to usually 60–80 mg daily (0.75–1 mg/kg daily). About 10% of patients experience a transient but very serious worsening of symptoms in the first 2–3 weeks, especially if the corticosteroid is started at a high dose. However, ventilated patients may be started on 1.5 mg/kg (max. 100 mg) on alternate days. Smaller doses of corticosteroid are usually required in *ocular myasthenia*. Once clinical remission has occurred (usually after 2–6 months), the dose of prednisolone should be reduced slowly to the minimum effective dose (usually 10–40 mg on alternate days).

In generalised myasthenia gravis **azathioprine** (section 8.2.1) is usually started at the same time as the corticosteroid and it allows a lower maintenance dose of the corticosteroid to be used; azathioprine is initiated at a low dose, which is increased over 3–4 weeks to 2–2.5 mg/kg daily. **Ciclosporin** (section 8.2.2), **methotrexate** (section 8.1.3), or **mycophenolate mofetil** (section 8.2.1) may be used in patients unresponsive or intolerant to other treatments [unlicensed indications].

10.2.2 Skeletal muscle relaxants

Drugs described below are used for the relief of chronic muscle spasm or spasticity associated with multiple sclerosis or other neurological damage; they are not indicated for spasm associated with minor injuries. They act principally on the central nervous system with the exception of dantrolene which has a peripheral site of action. They differ in action from the muscle relaxants used in anaesthesia (section 15.1.5) which block transmission at the neuromuscular junction.

The underlying cause of spasticity should be treated and any aggravating factors (e.g. pressure sores, infection) remedied. Skeletal muscle relaxants are effective in most forms of spasticity except the rare alpha variety. The major disadvantage of treatment with these drugs is that reduction in muscle tone can cause a loss of splinting action of the spastic leg and trunk muscles and sometimes lead to an increase in disability.

Dantrolene acts directly on skeletal muscle and produces fewer central adverse effects making it a drug of choice. The dose should be increased slowly.

Baclofen inhibits transmission at spinal level and also depresses the central nervous system. The dose should be increased slowly to avoid the major side-effects of sedation and muscular hypotonia (other adverse events are uncommon).

Diazepam may also be used. Sedation and, occasionally, extensor hypotonus are disadvantages. Other benzodiazepines also have muscle-relaxant properties. Muscle-relaxant doses of benzodiazepines are similar to anxiolytic doses (section 4.1.2).

Tizanidine is an alpha$_2$-adrenoceptor agonist indicated for spasticity associated with multiple sclerosis or spinal cord injury.

BACLOFEN

Indications: chronic severe spasticity resulting from disorders such as multiple sclerosis or traumatic partial section of spinal cord

Cautions: renal impairment (Appendix 3); psychiatric illness, Parkinson's disease, cerebrovascular disease, elderly; respiratory impairment, epilepsy; history of peptic ulcer; diabetes; hypertonic bladder sphincter; pregnancy (Appendix 4); avoid abrupt withdrawal (risk of hyperactive state, may exacerbate spasticity, and precipitate autonomic dysfunction including hyperthermia, psychiatric reactions and convulsions, see also under Withdrawal below); porphyria (section 9.8.2); **interactions:** Appendix 1 (muscle relaxants)

WITHDRAWAL. CSM has advised that serious side-effects can occur on abrupt withdrawal; to minimise risk, discontinue by gradual dose reduction over at least 1–2 weeks (longer if symptoms occur)

DRIVING. Drowsiness may affect performance of skilled tasks (e.g. driving); effects of alcohol enhanced

Contra-indications: peptic ulceration

Side-effects: frequently sedation, drowsiness, muscular hypotonia, nausea, urinary disturbances; occasionally lassitude, confusion, speech disturbance, dizziness, ataxia, hallucinations, nightmares, headache, euphoria, insomnia, depression, anxiety, agitation, tremor, nystagmus, paraesthesias, seizures, myalgia, fever, respiratory or cardiovascular depression, hypotension, dry mouth, gastro-intestinal disturbances, sexual dysfunction, visual disorders, rash, pruritus, urticaria, hyperhidrosis, angioedema; rarely taste alterations, blood sugar changes, and paradoxical increase in spasticity

Dose: *by mouth*, 5 mg 3 times daily, preferably with or after food, gradually increased; max. 100 mg daily (discontinue if no benefit within 6 weeks); CHILD 0.75–2 mg/kg daily (over 10 years, max. 2.5 mg/kg daily) *or* 2.5 mg 4 times daily increased gradually according to age to maintenance: 1–2 years 10–20 mg daily, 2–6 years 20–30 mg daily, 6–10 years 30–60 mg daily

By intrathecal injection, see preparation below

Baclofen (Non-proprietary) ▣oM
Tablets, baclofen 10 mg, net price 28-tab pack = 76p, 84-tab pack = £2.29. Label: 2, 8
Available from Alpharma, APS, Ashbourne (*Baclospas®*), Hillcross, IVAX, Sandoz

Lioresal® (Cephalon) ▣oM
Tablets, scored, baclofen 10 mg. Net price 84-tab pack = £10.84. Label: 2, 8
Excipients: include gluten

Liquid, sugar-free, raspberry–flavoured, baclofen 5 mg/5 mL. Net price 300 mL = £8.95. Label: 2, 8

■ By intrathecal injection

Lioresal® (Novartis) ▣oM
Intrathecal injection, baclofen, 50 micrograms/mL, net price 1-mL amp (for test dose) = £2.74; 500 micrograms/mL, 20-mL amp (for use with implantable pump) = £60.77; 2 mg/mL, 5-mL amp (for use with implantable pump) = £60.77
Important: consult product literature for details on dose testing and titration—important to monitor patients closely in appropriately equipped and staffed environment during screening and immediately after pump

implantation, and to have resuscitation equipment available for immediate use

Dose: by intrathecal injection, specialist use only, severe chronic spasticity unresponsive to oral antispastic drugs (or where side-effects of oral therapy unacceptable) *or* as alternative to ablative neurosurgical procedures, initial *test dose* 25–50 micrograms over at least 1 minute via catheter or lumbar puncture, increased in 25-microgram steps (not more often than every 24 hours) to max. 100 micrograms to determine appropriate dose *then dose-titration phase,* most often using infusion pump (implanted into chest wall or abdominal wall tissues) to establish *appropriate maintenance dose* (ranging from 12 micrograms to 2 mg daily for spasticity of spinal origin *or* 22 micrograms to 1.4 mg daily for spasticity of cerebral origin) retaining some spasticity to avoid sensation of paralysis; CHILD 4–18 years (spasticity of cerebral origin only), initial *test dose* 25 micrograms then titrated as for ADULT to *appropriate maintenance dose* (ranging from 24 micrograms to 1.2 mg daily in children under 12 years)

DANTROLENE SODIUM

Indications: chronic severe spasticity of voluntary muscle; malignant hyperthermia (section 15.1.8)

Cautions: impaired cardiac and pulmonary function; test liver function before and at intervals during therapy; therapeutic effect may take a few weeks to develop but if treatment is ineffective it should be discontinued after 4–6 weeks. Avoid when spasticity is useful, for example, locomotion; **interactions:** Appendix 1 (muscle relaxants).
DRIVING. Drowsiness may affect performance of skilled tasks (e.g. driving); effects of alcohol enhanced

Contra-indications: hepatic impairment (may cause severe liver damage); acute muscle spasm

Side-effects: transient drowsiness, dizziness, weakness, malaise, fatigue, diarrhoea (withdraw if severe, discontinue treatment if recurs on re-introduction), anorexia, nausea, headache, rash; less frequently constipation, dysphagia, speech and visual disturbances, confusion, nervousness, insomnia, depression, seizures, chills, fever, increased urinary frequency; rarely, tachycardia, erratic blood pressure, dyspnoea, haematuria, possible crystalluria, urinary incontinence or retention, pleural effusion, pericarditis, dose-related hepatotoxicity (occasionally fatal) may be more common in women over 30 especially those taking oestrogens

Dose: initially 25 mg daily, may be increased at weekly intervals to max. of 100 mg 4 times daily; usual dose 75 mg 3 times daily; CHILD not recommended

Dantrium® (Procter & Gamble Pharm.) ▣PoM▣
Capsules, both orange/brown, dantrolene sodium 25 mg, net price 20 = £2.46; 100 mg, 20 = £8.61. Label: 2

DIAZEPAM

Indications: muscle spasm of varied aetiology, including tetanus; other indications (section 4.1.2, section 4.8, section 15.1.4.1)

Cautions: see section 4.1.2; special precautions for intravenous injection (section 4.8.2)

Contra-indications: see section 4.1.2

Side-effects: see section 4.1.2; also hypotonia

Dose: *by mouth,* 2–15 mg daily in divided doses, increased if necessary in spastic conditions to 60 mg daily according to response
Cerebral spasticity in selected cases, CHILD 2–40 mg daily in divided doses

By intramuscular or by slow intravenous injection (into a large vein at a rate of not more than 5 mg/minute), in acute muscle spasm, 10 mg repeated if necessary after 4 hours
NOTE. Only use intramuscular route when oral and intravenous routes not possible; special precautions for intravenous injection see section 4.8.2

Tetanus, ADULT and CHILD, *by intravenous injection,* 100–300 micrograms/kg repeated every 1–4 hours; *by intravenous infusion (or by nasoduodenal tube),* 3–10 mg/kg over 24 hours, adjusted according to response

■ **Preparations**
Section 4.1.2

TIZANIDINE

Indications: spasticity associated with multiple sclerosis or spinal cord injury or disease

Cautions: elderly, renal impairment (Appendix 3), pregnancy and breast-feeding, monitor liver function monthly for first 4 months and in those who develop unexplained nausea, anorexia or fatigue; concomitant administration of drugs that prolong QT interval; **interactions:** Appendix 1 (muscle relaxants)
DRIVING. Drowsiness may affect performance of skilled tasks (e.g. driving); effects of alcohol enhanced

Contra-indications: severe hepatic impairment

Side-effects: drowsiness, fatigue, dizziness, dry mouth, nausea, gastro-intestinal disturbances, hypotension; also reported, bradycardia, insomnia, hallucinations and altered liver enzymes (discontinue if persistently raised—consult product literature); rarely acute hepatitis

Dose: initially 2 mg daily as a single dose increased according to response at intervals of at least 3–4 days in steps of 2 mg daily (and given in divided doses) usually up to 24 mg daily in 3–4 divided doses; max. 36 mg daily; CHILD not recommended

Zanaflex® (Elan) ▣PoM▣
Tablets, scored, tizanidine (as hydrochloride) 2 mg, net price 120-tab pack = £77.50; 4 mg, 120-tab pack = £96.88. Label: 2

Other muscle relaxants

The clinical efficacy of carisoprodol, meprobamate (section 4.1.2), and methocarbamol as muscle relaxants is **not** well established although they have been included in compound analgesic preparations.

CARISOPRODOL

Indications: short-term symptomatic relief of muscle spasm (but see notes above)

Cautions: see under Meprobamate (section 4.1.2); **interactions:** Appendix 1 (muscle relaxants)

Contra-indications: see under Meprobamate (section 4.1.2); porphyria (section 9.8.2)

Side-effects: see under Meprobamate (section 4.1.2); drowsiness is common

Dose: 350 mg 3 times daily; ELDERLY half adult dose or less

Carisoma® (Forest) ▣PoM▣
Tablets, carisoprodol 125 mg, net price 100 = £7.10; 350 mg, 100 = £7.95. Label: 2

METHOCARBAMOL ◨◢

Indications: short-term symptomatic relief of muscle spasm (but see notes above)

Cautions: hepatic impairment (Appendix 2); renal impairment (Appendix 4); breast-feeding (Appendix 5); **interactions:** Appendix 1 (muscle relaxants)

DRIVING. Drowsiness may affect performance of skilled tasks (e.g. driving); effects of alcohol enhanced

Contra-indications: coma or pre-coma, brain damage, epilepsy, myasthenia gravis

Side-effects: nausea, vomiting, dyspepsia; hypersensitivity reactions (including urticaria, angioedema, anaphylaxis); fever, headache, drowsiness, dizziness, confusion, amnesia, restlessness, anxiety, tremor, seizures; blurred vision, nasal congestion; rash, pruritus; leucopenia, cholestatic jaundice

Dose: 1.5 g 4 times daily; may be reduced to 750 mg 3 times daily; ELDERLY up to 750 mg 4 times daily may be sufficient; CHILD not recommended

Robaxin® (Shire) PoM ◨◢
750 Tablets, f/c, scored, methocarbamol 750 mg, net price 20 = £2.53. Label: 2

Nocturnal leg cramps

Quinine salts (section 5.4.1) 200–300 mg at bedtime are effective in reducing the frequency of nocturnal leg cramps by about 25% in ambulatory patients. It may take up to 4 weeks for improvement to become apparent and it is then given on a continuous basis if there is benefit. Patients should be monitored closely during the early stages for adverse effects as well as for benefit. Treatment should be interrupted at intervals of approximately 3 months to assess the need for further quinine treatment. Quinine is very toxic in overdosage and accidental fatalities have occurred in children (see also below).

QUININE

Indications: see notes above; malaria (section 5.4.1)

Cautions: see section 5.4.1

Contra-indications: see section 5.4.1

Side-effects: see section 5.4.1; **important:** very toxic in **overdosage**—immediate advice from poison centres essential (see also p. 24)

Dose: see notes above

■ Preparations
Section 5.4.1

10.3 Drugs for the relief of soft-tissue inflammation

Extravasation

> Local guidelines for the management of extravasation should be followed where they exist or specialist advice sought.

Extravasation injury follows leakage of drugs or intravenous fluids from the veins or inadvertent administration into the subcutaneous or subdermal tissue. It must be dealt with **promptly** to prevent tissue necrosis.

Acidic or alkaline preparations and those with an osmolarity greater than that of plasma can cause extravasation injury and excipients including alcohol and polyethylene glycol have also been implicated. Cytotoxic drugs commonly cause extravasation injury. In addition, certain patients such as the very young and the elderly are at increased risk. Those receiving anticoagulants are more likely to lose blood into surrounding tissues if extravasation occurs whilst those receiving sedatives or analgesics may not notice the early signs or symptoms of extravasation.

PREVENTION OF EXTRAVASATION. Precautions should be taken to avoid extravasation; ideally, drugs liable to cause extravasation injury should be given through a central line and patients receiving repeated doses of hazardous drugs peripherally should have the cannula resited at regular intervals. Attention should be paid to the manufacturers' recommendations for administration. Placing a glyceryl trinitrate patch (section 2.6.1) distal to the cannula may improve the patency of the vessel in patients with small veins or in those whose veins are prone to collapse.

Patients should be asked to report any pain or burning at the site of injection immediately.

MANAGEMENT OF EXTRAVASATION. If extravasation is suspected the infusion should be stopped immediately but the cannula should not be removed until after an attempt has been made to aspirate the area (through the cannula) in order to remove as much of the drug as possible. Aspiration is sometimes possible if the extravasation presents with a raised bleb or blister at the injection site and is surrounded by hardened tissue, but it is often unsuccessful if the tissue is soft or soggy. Corticosteroids are usually given to treat inflammation, although there is little evidence to support their use in extravasation. Hydrocortisone or dexamethasone (section 6.3.2) may be given either locally by subcutaneous injection or intravenously at a site distant from the injury. Antihistamines (section 3.4.1) and analgesics (section 4.7) may be required for symptom relief.

The management of extravasation beyond these measures is not well standardised and calls for specialist advice. Treatment depends on the nature of the offending substance; one approach is to localise and neutralise the substance whereas another is to spread and dilute it. The first method may be appropriate following extravasation of vesicant drugs and involves administration of an antidote (if available) and the application of cold compresses 3–4 times a day (consult specialist literature for details of specific antidotes). Spreading and diluting the offending substance involves infiltrating the area with physiological saline, applying warm compresses, elevating the affected limb, and administering hyaluronidase (section 10.3.1). A saline flush-out technique (involving flushing the subcutaneous tissue with physiological saline) may be effective but requires specialist advice. Hyaluronidase should **not** be administered following extravasation of vesicant drugs (unless it is either specifically indicated or used in the saline flush-out technique).

10.3.1 Enzymes

Hyaluronidase is used to render the tissues more easily permeable to injected fluids, e.g. for introduction of fluids by subcutaneous infusion (termed hypodermoclysis).

HYALURONIDASE

Indications: enhance permeation of subcutaneous or intramuscular injections, local anaesthetics and subcutaneous infusions; promote resorption of excess fluids and blood

Cautions: infants or elderly (control speed and total volume and avoid overhydration especially in renal impairment)

Contra-indications: do not apply direct to cornea; avoid sites where infection or malignancy; not for anaesthesia in unexplained premature labour; not to be used to reduce swelling of bites or stings; not for intravenous administration

Side-effects: occasional severe allergy

Dose: With subcutaneous or intramuscular injection, 1500 units dissolved directly in solution to be injected (ensure compatibility)

With local anaesthetics, 1500 units mixed with local anaesthetic solution (ophthalmology, 15 units/mL)

Hypodermoclysis, 1500 units dissolved in 1 mL water for injections or 0.9% sodium chloride injection, administered before start of 500–1000 mL infusion fluid

Extravasation (see notes above) or haematoma, 1500 units dissolved in 1 mL water for injections or 0.9% sodium chloride injection, infiltrated into affected area (as soon as possible after extravasation)

Hyalase® (CP) ▐PoM▐
Injection, powder for reconstitution, hyaluronidase (ovine). Net price 1500-unit amp = £7.60

10.3.2 Rubefacients and other topical antirheumatics

Rubefacients act by counter-irritation. Pain, whether superficial or deep-seated, is relieved by any method which itself produces irritation of the skin. Counter-irritation is comforting in painful lesions of the muscles, tendons, and joints, and in non-articular rheumatism. Rubefacients probably all act through the same essential mechanism and differ mainly in intensity and duration of action.

Topical **NSAIDs** (e.g. felbinac, ibuprofen, ketoprofen and piroxicam) may provide some slight relief of pain in musculoskeletal conditions.

Topical NSAIDs and counter-irritants

CAUTIONS. Apply with gentle massage only. Avoid contact with eyes, mucous membranes, and inflamed or broken skin; discontinue if rash develops. Hands should be washed immediately after use. Not for use with occlusive dressings. Topical application of large amounts may result in systemic effects including hypersensitivity and asthma (renal disease has also been reported). Not generally suitable for children. Patient packs carry a **warning** to avoid during **pregnancy** or **breast-feeding**.

HYPERSENSITIVITY. For NSAID hypersensitivity and asthma warning, see p. 478 and p. 479

PHOTOSENSITIVITY. Patients should be advised against excessive exposure to sunlight of area treated in order to avoid possibility of photosensitivity

Ketoprofen (Non-proprietary) ▐PoM▐
Gel, ketoprofen 2.5%, net price 50 g = £3.25, 100 g = £6.25
Excipients: include fragrance
Dose: apply 2–4 times daily for up to 7 days (usual max. 15 g daily)
Available from PLIVA

Piroxicam (Non-proprietary) ▐PoM▐
Gel, piroxicam 0.5%, net price 60 g = £6.00; 112 g = £9.41
Excipients: include propylene glycol
Dose: apply 3–4 times daily
Available from Sovereign

■ Proprietary preparations

Feldene® (Pfizer) ▐PoM▐
Gel, piroxicam 0.5%. Net price 60 g = £6.00; 112 g = £9.41 (also 7.5 g starter pack, hosp. only)
Excipients: include benzyl alcohol, propylene glycol
Dose: apply 3–4 times daily; therapy should be reviewed after 4 weeks

Fenbid® Forte Gel (Goldshield) ▐PoM▐
Gel, ibuprofen 10%, net price 100 g = £6.50
Excipients: include benzyl alcohol
Dose: apply up to 4 times daily; therapy should be reviewed after 14 days

Ibugel® Forte (Dermal) ▐PoM▐
Forte gel, ibuprofen 10%, net price 100 g = £6.50
Excipients: none as listed in section 13.1.3
Dose: apply up to 3 times daily

Oruvail® (Rhône-Poulenc Rorer) ▐PoM▐
Gel, ketoprofen 2.5%. Net price 100 g = £7.12
Excipients: include fragrance
Dose: apply 2–4 times daily for up to 7 days (usual recommended dose 15 g daily)

Pennsaid® (Dimethaid) ▐PoM▐
Cutaneous solution, diclofenac sodium 1.6% in dimethyl sulfoxide, net price 60 mL = £16.00
Excipients: include propylene glycol
Dose: pain in osteoarthritis of superficial medium to large joints, apply 0.5–1 mL 4 times daily

Powergel® (Menarini) ▐PoM▐
Gel, ketoprofen 2.5%. Net price 50 g = £3.25; 100 g = £6.25
Excipients: include hydroxybenzoates (parabens), fragrance
Dose: apply 2–3 times daily for up to max. 10 days

Traxam® (Goldshield) ▐PoM▐
Foam, felbinac 3.17%. Net price 100 g = £7.00.
Label: 15
Excipients: include cetostearyl alcohol

Gel, felbinac 3%. Net price 100 g = £7.00
Excipients: none as listed in section 13.1.3
Dose: apply 2–4 times daily; max. 25 g daily; therapy should be reviewed after 14 days
NOTE. Felbinac is an active metabolite of the NSAID fenbufen

Voltarol Emulgel® (Novartis) [PoM]
Gel, diclofenac diethylammonium salt 1.16% (equivalent to diclofenac sodium 1%). Net price 20 g (hosp. only) = £1.55; 100 g = £7.00
Excipients: include propylene glycol, fragrance
Dose: apply 3–4 times daily; therapy should be reviewed after 14 days (or after 28 days for osteoarthritis)

■ Preparations on sale to the public
Topical NSAIDs and counter-irritants on sale to the public together with their significant ingredients include:

Algesal® (diethylamine salicylate), **Algipan Rub®** (capsicum oleoresin, glycol salicylate, methyl nicotinate)
Balmosa® (camphor, capsicum oleoresin, menthol, methyl salicylate), **Boots Pain Relief Balm®** (ethyl nicotinate, glycol monosalicylate, nonylic acid vanillylamide), **Boots Pain Relief Embrocation®** (camphor, turpentine oil), **Boots Pain Relief Warming Spray®** (camphor, ethyl nicotinate, methyl salicylate)
Cremalgin® (capsicin, glycol salicylate, methyl nicotinate), **Cuprofen® Ibutop® Gel** (ibuprofen)
Deep Freeze Cold Gel® (menthol), **Deep Freeze Spray®** (levomenthol), **Deep Heat Massage Liniment®**, **Deep Heat Maximum®** (menthol, methyl salicylate), **Deep Heat Rub®** (eucalyptus oil, menthol, methyl salicylate, turpentine oil), **Deep Heat Spray®** (glycol salicylate, ethyl salicylate, methyl salicylate, methyl nicotinate), **Deep Relief®** (ibuprofen, menthol), **Difflam® Cream** (benzydamine), **Difflam®-P Cream** (benzydamine), **Dubam Cream®** (methyl salicylate, menthol, cineole), **Dubam Spray®** (ethyl salicylate, methyl salicylate, glycol salicylate, methyl nicotinate)
Elliman's Universal Embrocation® (acetic acid, turpentine oil)
Feldene P® Gel (piroxicam), **Fenbid® Gel** (ibuprofen), **Fiery Jack Cream®** (capsicum oleoresin, diethylamine salicylate, glycol salicylate, methyl nicotinate), **Fiery Jack Ointment®** (capsicum oleoresin)
Goddard's White Oil Embrocation® (dilute acetic acid, dilute ammonia solution, turpentine oil)
Hansaplast® Thermo Plaster (capsaicinoids, colophony)
Ibuderm® (ibuprofen), **Ibugel®** (ibuprofen), **Ibuleve®**, **Ibuleve® Maximum Strength**, **Ibuleve Mousse®**, **Ibuleve Sports Gel®** (ibuprofen), **Ibumousse®** (ibuprofen), **Ibuspray®** (ibuprofen), **Intralgin®** (benzocaine, salicylamide)
Lloyds Cream® (diethyl salicylate)
Mentholatum® Ibuprofen Gel (ibuprofen), **Movelat® Cream** (mucopolysaccharide polysulphate, salicylic acid, thymol), **Movelat® Gel** (mucopolysaccharide polysulphate, salicylic acid), **Movelat® Relief Cream** (mucopolysaccharide polysulphate, salicylic acid, thymol), **Movelat® Relief Gel** (mucopolysaccharide polysulphate, salicylic acid)
Nasciodine® (camphor, iodine, menthol, methyl salicylate, turpentine oil), **Nella Red Oil®** (arachis oil, clove oil, mustard oil, methyl nicotinate), **Nurofen® Gel Maximum Strength** (ibuprofen), **Nurofen Muscular Pain Relief Gel®** (ibuprofen)
Oruvail® Gel (ketoprofen 30-g tube; 100-g tube prescribable on NHS ([PoM]))
PR Heat Spray® (ethyl nicotinate, methyl salicylate, camphor); **Proflex® Cream** (ibuprofen), **Proflex Pain Relief Cream®** (ibuprofen)
Radian®-B Ibuprofen Gel (ibuprofen), **Radian®-B Muscle Lotion**, **Radian®-B Heat Spray** (ammonium salicylate, camphor, menthol, salicylic acid), **Radian®-B Muscle Rub** (camphor, capsicin, menthol, methyl salicylate), **Ralgex Cream®** (capsicin, glycol monosalicylate, methyl nicotinate), **Ralgex Freeze Spray®** (dimethyl

ether, glycol monosalicylate, isopentane), **Ralgex® Ibutop® Gel** (ibuprofen), **Ralgex Low Odour Spray®** (glycol monosalicylate, methyl nicotinate), **Ralgex Spray®** (ethyl salicylate, methyl salicylate, glycol monosalicylate, methyl nicotinate), **Ralgex Stick®** (capsicin, ethyl salicylate, methyl salicylate, glycol salicylate, menthol)
Salonair® (benzyl nicotinate, camphor, glycol salicylate, menthol, methyl salicylate, squalane), **Salonpas Plasters®** (glycol salicylate, methyl salicylate), **Solpaflex®** Gel (ketoprofen)
Tiger Balm Red® (camphor, clove oil, cajuput oil, menthol), **Tiger Balm White®** (cajuput oil, camphor, clove oil, menthol), **Transvasin Cream®** (ethyl nicotinate, hexyl nicotinate, thurfyl salicylate), **Transvasin Spray®** (diethylamine salicylate, hydroxyethyl salicylate, methyl nicotinate), **Traxam Pain Relief®** (felbinac), **Voltarol Emulgel® P** (diclofenac diethylammonium)

Capsaicin

CAUTIONS. Avoid contact with eyes, and inflamed or broken skin. Hands should be washed immediately after use. Not for use under tight bandages. Avoid taking a hot shower or bath just before or after applying capsaicin—burning sensation enhanced.

SIDE–EFFECTS. Transient burning sensation may occur during initial treatment, particularly if too much cream is used, or if the frequency of administration is less than 3–4 times daily.

Axsain® (Elan) [PoM]
Cream, capsaicin 0.075%. Net price 45 g = £15.04.
Excipients: include benzyl alcohol, cetyl alcohol
Dose: for post-herpetic neuralgia (**important: after** lesions have healed), apply a small amount up to 3–4 times daily; for painful diabetic neuropathy, under supervision of hospital consultant, apply 3–4 times daily for 8 weeks then review

Zacin® (Elan) [PoM]
Cream, capsaicin 0.025%. Net price 45 g = £15.04.
Excipients: include benzyl alcohol, cetyl alcohol
Dose: symptomatic relief in osteoarthritis, apply a small amount 4 times daily

Poultices

Kaolin Poultice ◢
Poultice, heavy kaolin 52.7%, thymol 0.05%, boric acid 4.5%, peppermint oil 0.05%, methyl salicylate 0.2%, glycerol 42.5%. Net price 200 g = £2.12
Dose: warm and apply directly or between layers of muslin; avoid application of overheated poultice

Kaolin Poultice K/L Pack® (K/L) ◢
Kaolin poultice Net price 4 × 100-g pouches = £9.14

11: Eye

11.1 Administration of drugs to the eye

Drugs are most commonly administered to the eye by topical application as eye drops or eye ointments. Where a higher drug concentration is required within the eye, a local injection may be necessary.

Eye-drop dispensers are available to aid the instillation of eye drops especially amongst the elderly, visually impaired, arthritic, or otherwise physically limited patients. Eye-drop dispensers are for use with plastic eye drop bottles, for repeat use by individual patients.

EYE DROPS AND EYE OINTMENTS. Eye drops are generally instilled into the pocket formed by gently pulling down the lower eyelid and keeping the eye closed for as long as possible after application, preferably 1–2 minutes; one drop is all that is needed. A small amount of eye ointment is applied similarly; the ointment melts rapidly and blinking helps to spread it

When two different eye-drop preparations are used at the same time of day, dilution and overflow may occur when one immediately follows the other. The patient should therefore leave an interval of 5 minutes between the two.

Systemic effects may arise from absorption of drugs into the general circulation from conjunctival vessels or from the nasal mucosa after the excess preparation has drained down through the tear ducts. The extent of systemic absorption following ocular administration is highly variable; nasal drainage of drugs is associated with eye drops much more often than with eye ointments.

For warnings relating to eye drops and contact lenses, see section 11.9.

EYE LOTIONS. These are solutions for the irrigation of the conjunctival sac. They act mechanically to flush out irritants or foreign bodies as a first-aid treatment. Sterile sodium chloride 0.9% solution (section 11.8.1) is usually used. Clean water will suffice in an emergency.

OTHER PREPARATIONS. Subconjunctival injection may be used to administer anti-infective drugs, mydriatics, or corticosteroids for conditions not responding to topical therapy. The drug diffuses through the cornea and sclera to the anterior and posterior chambers and vitreous humour. However, because the dose-volume is limited (usually not more than 1 mL), this route is suitable only for drugs which are readily soluble.

Drugs such as antimicrobials and corticosteroids may be administered systemically to treat an eye condition. Implants which gradually release a drug over a prolonged period are also available (e.g. *Vitrasert*®).

PRESERVATIVES AND SENSITISERS. Information on preservatives and on substances identified as skin sensitisers (see section 13.1.3) is provided under preparation entries.

11.2 Control of microbial contamination

Preparations for the eye should be sterile when issued. Eye drops in multiple-application containers include a preservative but care should nevertheless be taken to avoid contamination of the contents during use.

Eye drops in multiple-application containers for *domiciliary use* should not be used for more than 4 weeks after first opening (unless otherwise stated).

Eye drops for use in *hospital wards* are normally discarded 1 week after first opening. Individual containers should be provided for each patient. Containers used before an operation should be discarded at the time of the operation and fresh containers supplied. A fresh supply should also be provided upon discharge from hospital; it may be acceptable in specialist ophthalmology units to issue on discharge eye drop bottles that have been in use for the patient for less than 36 hours.

In *out-patient departments* single-application packs should preferably be used; if multiple-application packs are used, they should be discarded at the end of each day. In clinics for eye diseases and in accident and emergency departments, where the dangers of infection are high, single-application packs should be used; if a multiple-application pack is used, it should be discarded after single use.

Diagnostic dyes (e.g. fluorescein) should be used only from single-application packs.

In *eye surgery* single-application containers should be used if possible; if a multiple-application pack is used, it should be discarded after single use. Preparations used during intra-ocular procedures and others that may penetrate into the anterior chamber must be isotonic and without preservatives and buffered if necessary to a neutral pH. Specially formulated fluids should be used for intra-ocular surgery; large volume intravenous infusion preparations are not suitable for this purpose. For all surgical procedures, a previously unopened container is used for each patient.

11.3 Anti-infective eye preparations

11.3.1	Antibacterials
11.3.2	Antifungals
11.3.3	Antivirals

EYE INFECTIONS. Most acute superficial eye infections can be treated topically. Blepharitis and conjunctivitis are often caused by staphylococci; keratitis and endophthalmitis may be bacterial, viral, or fungal.

Bacterial *blepharitis* is treated by application of an antibacterial eye ointment to the conjunctival sac or to the lid margins. Systemic treatment may occasionally be required and is usually undertaken after culturing organisms from the lid margin and determining their antimicrobial sensitivity; antibiotics such as the tetracyclines given for 3 months or longer may be appropriate.

Most cases of acute bacterial conjunctivitis are self-limiting; where treatment is appropriate, antibacterial eye drops or an eye ointment are used. A poor response might indicate viral or allergic conjunctivitis. *Gonococcal conjunctivitis* is treated with systemic and topical antibacterials.

Corneal ulcer and *keratitis* require specialist treatment and may call for subconjunctival or systemic administration of antimicrobials.

Endophthalmitis is a medical emergency which also calls for specialist management and often requires parenteral, subconjunctival, or intra-ocular administration of antimicrobials.

For reference to the treatment of *crab lice of the eyelashes*, see section 13.10.4

11.3.1 Antibacterials

Bacterial infections are generally treated topically with eye drops and eye ointments. Systemic administration is sometimes appropriate in blepharitis. In intra-ocular infection, a variety of routes (intracorneal, intravitreal and systemic) may be used.

Chloramphenicol has a broad spectrum of activity and is the drug of choice for *superficial eye infections*. Chloramphenicol eye drops are well tolerated and the recommendation that chloramphenicol eye drops should be avoided because of an increased risk of aplastic anaemia is not well founded.

Other antibacterials with a broad spectrum of activity include the quinolones, **ciprofloxacin** and **ofloxacin; framycetin, gentamicin,** and **neomycin** are also active against a wide variety of bacteria. Gentamicin, ciprofloxacin, and ofloxacin are effective for infections caused by *Pseudomonas aeruginosa*.

Ciprofloxacin eye drops are licensed for *corneal ulcers*; intensive application (especially in the first 2 days) is required throughout the day and night.

Trachoma which results from chronic infection with *Chlamydia trachomatis* can be treated with **azithromycin** by mouth [unlicensed indication]; alternatively a combination of an oral and a topical tetracycline can be used.

Fusidic acid is useful for staphylococcal infections.

Propamidine isetionate is of little value in bacterial infections but is specific for the rare but potentially devastating condition of *acanthamoeba keratitis* (see also section 11.9).

WITH CORTICOSTEROIDS. Many antibacterial preparations also incorporate a corticosteroid but such mixtures should **not** be used unless a patient is under close specialist supervision. In particular they should not be prescribed for undiagnosed 'red eye' which is sometimes caused by the herpes simplex virus and may be difficult to diagnose (section 11.4).

ADMINISTRATION.

Eye drops. Apply 1 drop at least every 2 hours then reduce frequency as infection is controlled and continue for 48 hours after healing.

Eye ointment. Apply *either* at night (if eye drops used during the day) *or* 3–4 times daily (if eye ointment used alone).

CHLORAMPHENICOL

Indications: see notes above
Side-effects: transient stinging; see also notes above
Dose: see notes above

Chloramphenicol (Non-proprietary) PoM
Eye drops, chloramphenicol 0.5%. Net price 10 mL = £1.23
Eye ointment, chloramphenicol 1%. Net price 4 g = £1.04

Chloromycetin® (Goldshield) PoM
Redidrops (= eye drops), chloramphenicol 0.5%. Net price 5 mL = £1.65; 10 mL = £2.01
Excipients: include phenylmercuric acetate
Ophthalmic ointment (= eye ointment), chloramphenicol 1%. Net price 4 g = £2.01

■ Single use
Minims® **Chloramphenicol** (Chauvin) PoM
Eye drops, chloramphenicol 0.5%. Net price 20 × 0.5 mL = £4.92

CIPROFLOXACIN

Indications: superficial bacterial infections, see notes above; corneal ulcers
Cautions: not recommended for children under 1 year; pregnancy and breast-feeding
Side-effects: local burning and itching; lid margin crusting; hyperaemia; taste disturbances; corneal staining, keratitis, lid oedema, lacrimation, photophobia, corneal infiltrates; nausea and visual disturbances reported
Dose: superficial bacterial infection, see notes above

Corneal ulcer, apply throughout day and night, day 1 apply every 15 minutes for 6 hours then every 30 minutes, day 2 apply every hour, days 3–14 apply every 4 hours (max. duration of treatment 21 days)

Ciloxan® (Alcon) PoM
Ophthalmic solution (= eye drops), ciprofloxacin (as hydrochloride) 0.3%. Net price 5 mL = £4.94
Excipients: include benzalkonium chloride

FRAMYCETIN SULPHATE

Indications: see notes above
Dose: see notes above

Soframycin® (Florizel) PoM
Eye drops, framycetin sulphate 0.5%. Net price 10 mL = £4.62
Excipients: include benzalkonium chloride
Eye ointment, framycetin sulphate 0.5%. Net price 5 g = £2.52

FUSIDIC ACID

Indications: see notes above
Dose: see under preparation below

Fucithalmic® (Leo) PoM
Eye drops, m/r, fusidic acid 1% in gel basis (liquifies on contact with eye). Net price 5 g = £2.09
Excipients: include benzalkonium chloride, disodium edetate
Dose: apply twice daily

GENTAMICIN

Indications: see notes above
Dose: see notes above

Garamycin® (Schering-Plough) PoM
Drops (for ear or eye), gentamicin 0.3% (as sulphate). Net price 10 mL = £1.79
Excipients: include benzalkonium chloride

Genticin® (Roche) PoM
Drops (for ear or eye), gentamicin 0.3% (as sulphate). Net price 10 mL = £1.91
Excipients: include benzalkonium chloride

■ Single use
Minims® **Gentamicin Sulphate** (Chauvin) PoM
Eye drops, gentamicin 0.3% (as sulphate). Net price 20 × 0.5 mL = £5.75

NEOMYCIN SULPHATE

Indications: see notes above
Dose: see notes above

Neomycin (Non-proprietary) PoM
Eye drops, neomycin sulphate 0.5% (3500 units/mL). Net price 10 mL = £3.11
Available from Martindale
Eye ointment, neomycin sulphate 0.5% (3500 units/g). Net price 3 g = £2.38
Available from Martindale

■ With antibacterials
Neosporin® (PLIVA) PoM
Eye drops, gramicidin 25 units, neomycin sulphate 1700 units, polymyxin B sulphate 5000 units/mL. Net price 5 mL = £5.12
Excipients: include thiomersal
Dose: apply 2–4 times daily or more frequently if required

■ With hydrocortisone
Section 12.1.1

OFLOXACIN

Indications: see notes above
Cautions: pregnancy and breast-feeding; not to be used for more than 10 days
Side-effects: local irritation including photophobia; dizziness, numbness, nausea and headache reported
Dose: see notes above

Exocin® (Allergan) PoM
Ophthalmic solution (= eye drops), ofloxacin 0.3%. Net price 5 mL = £2.17
Excipients: include benzalkonium chloride

POLYMYXIN B SULPHATE

Indications: see notes above
Dose: see notes above

■ With antibacterials
Polyfax® (PLIVA) PoM
Eye ointment, polymyxin B sulphate 10 000 units, bacitracin zinc 500 units/g. Net price 4 g = £3.26

Polytrim® (PLIVA) PoM
Eye drops, trimethoprim 0.1%, polymyxin B sulphate 10 000 units/mL. Net price 5 mL = £3.05
Excipients: include thiomersal
Eye ointment, trimethoprim 0.5%, polymyxin B sulphate 10 000 units/g. Net price 4 g = £3.05

PROPAMIDINE ISETIONATE

Indications: local treatment of infections (but see notes above)

Brolene® (Aventis Pharma)
Eye drops, propamidine isetionate 0.1%. Net price 10 mL = £2.67
Excipients: include benzalkonium chloride
Dose: apply 4 times daily
NOTE. Eye drops containing propamidine isetionate 0.1% also available from Typharm (*Golden Eye Drops*)

Eye ointment, dibromopropamidine isetionate 0.15%. Net price 5 g = £2.79

Dose: apply 1–2 times daily

NOTE. Eye ointment containing dibromopropamidine isetionate 0.15% also available from Typharm (*Golden Eye Ointment*)

11.3.2 Antifungals

Fungal infections of the cornea are rare but can occur after agricultural injuries, especially in hot and humid climates. Orbital mycosis is rarer, and when it occurs it is usually because of a direct spread of infection from the paranasal sinuses. Increasing age, debility, or immunosuppression may encourage fungal proliferation. The spread of infection through blood occasionally produces a metastatic endophthalmitis.

Many different fungi are capable of producing ocular infection; they may be identified by appropriate laboratory procedures.

Antifungal preparations for the eye are not generally available. Treatment will normally be carried out at specialist centres, but requests for information about supplies of preparations not available commercially should be addressed to the local Health Authority (or equivalent in Scotland or Northern Ireland), or to the nearest hospital ophthalmology unit, or to Moorfields Eye Hospital, City Road, London EC1V 2PD (tel. (020) 7253 3411).

11.3.3 Antivirals

Herpes simplex infections producing, for example, dendritic corneal ulcer can be treated with **aciclovir**. **Ganciclovir** eye drops are licensed for the treatment of acute herpetic keratitis.

Slow-release ocular implants containing **ganciclovir** (*Vitrasert*®, available from Bausch & Lomb) may be inserted surgically to treat immediate sight-threatening CMV retinitis. Local treatments do not protect against systemic infection or infection in the other eye. For systemic treatment of CMV retinitis, see section 5.3.

ACICLOVIR

(Acyclovir)

Indications: local treatment of herpes simplex infections

Side-effects: local irritation and inflammation reported

Dose: apply 5 times daily (continue for at least 3 days after complete healing)

Zovirax® (GSK) PoM

Eye ointment, aciclovir 3%. Net price 4.5 g = £10.67

Tablets and *injection*, see section 5.3

Cream, see section 13.10.3

GANCICLOVIR

Indications: acute herpetic keratitis

Cautions: pregnancy and breast-feeding

Side-effects: ocular irritation, visual disturbances; superficial punctate keratitis

Dose: apply 5 times daily until complete corneal re-epithelialisation, then 3 times daily for 7 days (usual duration of treatment 21 days)

Virgan® (Chauvin) ▼ PoM

Eye drops, ganciclovir 0.15 % in gel basis, net price 5 g = £10.64

Excipients: include benzalkonium chloride

11.4 Corticosteroids and other anti-inflammatory preparations

11.4.1   Corticosteroids
11.4.2   Other anti-inflammatory preparations

11.4.1 Corticosteroids

Corticosteroids administered locally (as eye drops, eye ointments or subconjunctival injection) or by mouth have an important place in treating anterior segment inflammation, including that which results from surgery.

Topical corticosteroids should normally only be used under expert supervision; three main dangers are associated with their use:

- a 'red eye', where the diagnosis is unconfirmed, may be due to herpes simplex virus, and a corticosteroid may aggravate the condition, leading to corneal ulceration, with possible damage to vision and even loss of the eye. Bacterial, fungal and amoebic infections pose a similar hazard;
- 'steroid glaucoma' may follow the use of corticosteroid eye preparations in susceptible individuals;
- a 'steroid cataract' may follow prolonged use.

Other side-effects include thinning of the cornea and sclera.

Use of a combination product containing a corticosteroid with an anti-infective is rarely justified.

Systemic corticosteroids (section 6.3.2) may be useful for ocular conditions. The risk of producing a 'steroid cataract' is very high (75%) if the equivalent of more than 15 mg prednisolone is given daily for several years.

BETAMETHASONE

Indications: local treatment of inflammation (short-term)

Cautions: see notes above

Side-effects: see notes above

Dose: apply eye drops every 1–2 hours until controlled then reduce frequency, eye ointment 2–4 times daily or at night when used with eye drops

Betnesol® (Celltech) PoM

Drops (for ear, eye, or nose), betamethasone sodium phosphate 0.1%. Net price 10 mL = £1.84

Excipients: include benzalkonium chloride, disodium edetate

Eye ointment, betamethasone sodium phosphate 0.1%. Net price 3 g = £1.12

Vista-Methasone® (Martindale) [PoM]
Drops (for ear, eye, or nose), betamethasone sodium phosphate 0.1%. Net price 5 mL = £1.10; 10 mL = £1.25
Excipients: include benzalkonium chloride

■ With neomycin
Betnesol-N® (Celltech) [PoM]
Drops (for ear, eye, or nose), see section 12.1.1
Eye ointment, betamethasone sodium phosphate 0.1%, neomycin sulphate 0.5%. Net price 3 g = £1.28
NOTE. May be difficult to obtain

Vista-Methasone N® (Martindale) [PoM]
Drops (for ear, eye, or nose), see section 12.1.1

DEXAMETHASONE

Indications: local treatment of inflammation (short-term)
Cautions: see notes above
Side-effects: see notes above
Dose: apply eye drops 4–6 times daily; severe conditions every 30–60 minutes until controlled then reduce frequency

Maxidex® (Alcon) [PoM]
Eye drops, dexamethasone 0.1%, hypromellose 0.5%. Net price 5 mL = £1.49; 10 mL = £2.95
Excipients: include benzalkonium chloride, disodium edetate, polysorbate 80

■ Single use
Minims® **Dexamethasone** (Chauvin) [PoM]
Eye drops, dexamethasone sodium phosphate 0.1%. Net price 20 × 0.5 mL = £6.95
Excipients: include disodium edetate

■ With antibacterials
Maxitrol® (Alcon) [PoM]
Eye drops, dexamethasone 0.1%, hypromellose 0.5%, neomycin 0.35% (as sulphate), polymyxin B sulphate 6000 units/mL. Net price 5 mL = £1.77
Excipients: include benzalkonium chloride, polysorbate 20
Eye ointment, dexamethasone 0.1%, neomycin 0.35% (as sulphate), polymyxin B sulphate 6000 units/g. Net price 3.5 g = £1.52
Excipients: include hydroxybenzoates (parabens), wool fat

Sofradex® (Florizel) [PoM]
Drops and ointment (for ear or eye), see section 12.1.1

Tobradex® (Alcon) [PoM]
Eye drops, dexamethasone 0.1%, tobramycin 0.3%. Net price 5 mL = £5.65
Excipients: include benzalkonium chloride, disodium edetate

FLUOROMETHOLONE

Indications: local treatment of inflammation (short-term)
Cautions: see notes above
Side-effects: see notes above
Dose: apply eye drops 2–4 times daily (initially every hour for 24–48 hours then reduce frequency)

FML® (Allergan) [PoM]
Ophthalmic suspension (= eye drops), fluoro-metholone 0.1%, polyvinyl alcohol (*Liquifilm*®) 1.4%. Net price 5 mL = £1.71; 10 mL = £2.95
Excipients: include benzalkonium chloride, disodium edetate, polysorbate 80

HYDROCORTISONE ACETATE

Indications: local treatment of inflammation (short-term)
Cautions: see notes above
Side-effects: see notes above

Hydrocortisone (Non-proprietary) [PoM]
Eye drops, hydrocortisone acetate 1%. Net price 10 mL = £3.21
Available from Martindale
Eye ointment, hydrocortisone acetate 0.5%, net price 3 g = £2.28; 1%, 3 g = £2.29; 2.5%, 3 g = £2.33
Available from Martindale

■ With neomycin
Neo-Cortef® (PLIVA) [PoM]
Drops and ointment (for ear or eye), see section 12.1.1
NOTE. May be difficult to obtain

PREDNISOLONE

Indications: local treatment of inflammation (short-term)
Cautions: see notes above
Side-effects: see notes above
Dose: apply eye drops every 1–2 hours until controlled then reduce frequency

Pred Forte® (Allergan) [PoM]
Eye drops, prednisolone acetate 1%. Net price 5 mL = £1.52; 10 mL = £3.05
Excipients: include benzalkonium chloride, disodium edetate, polysorbate 80
Dose: apply 2–4 times daily

Predsol® (Celltech) [PoM]
Drops (for ear or eye), prednisolone sodium phosphate 0.5%. Net price 10 mL = £1.83
Excipients: include benzalkonium chloride, disodium edetate

■ Single use
Minims® **Prednisolone Sodium Phosphate** (Chauvin) [PoM]
Eye drops, prednisolone sodium phosphate 0.5%. Net price 20 × 0.5 mL = £5.75
Excipients: include disodium edetate

■ With neomycin
Predsol-N® (Celltech) [PoM]
Drops (for ear or eye), see section 12.1.1

RIMEXOLONE

Indications: local treatment of inflammation (short-term)
Cautions: see notes above
Side-effects: see notes above
Dose: postoperative inflammation, apply 4 times daily for 2 weeks, beginning 24 hours after surgery
Steroid-responsive inflammation, apply at least 4 times daily for up to 4 weeks
Uveitis, apply every hour during daytime in week 1, then every 2 hours in week 2, then 4 times daily in week 3, then twice daily for first 4 days of week 4, then once daily for remaining 3 days of week 4

Vexol® (Alcon) ▼ [PoM]
Eye drops, rimexolone 1%, net price 5 mL = £5.95
Excipients: include benzalkonium chloride, disodium edetate, polysorbate 80

11.4.2 Other anti-inflammatory preparations

Other preparations used for the topical treatment of inflammation and allergic conjunctivitis include antihistamines, lodoxamide, and sodium cromoglicate.

Topical preparations of **antihistamines** such as eye drops containing **antazoline** (with xylometazoline as *Otrivine-Antistin®*), **azelastine**, **ketotifen**, **levocabastine** and **olopatadine** may be used for allergic conjunctivitis.

Sodium cromoglicate (sodium cromoglycate) and **nedocromil sodium** eye drops may be useful for vernal keratoconjunctivitis and other allergic forms of conjunctivitis.

Lodoxamide eye drops are used for allergic conjunctival conditions including seasonal allergic conjunctivitis.

Diclofenac eye drops (section 11.8.2) and **emedastine** eye drops are also licensed for seasonal allergic conjunctivitis.

ANTAZOLINE SULPHATE

Indications: allergic conjunctivitis

Otrivine-Antistin® (Novartis Consumer Health)
Eye drops, antazoline sulphate 0.5%, xylometazoline hydrochloride 0.05%. Net price 10 mL = £2.35
Excipients: include benzalkonium chloride, disodium edetate
Dose: ADULT and CHILD over 5 years apply 2–3 times daily
NOTE. Xylometazoline is a sympathomimetic; it should be avoided in angle-closure glaucoma; absorption of antazoline and xylometazoline may result in systemic side-effects and the possibility of interaction with other drugs

AZELASTINE HYDROCHLORIDE

Indications: allergic conjunctivitis
Side-effects: mild transient irritation; bitter taste reported
Dose: seasonal allergic conjunctivitis, ADULT and CHILD over 4 years, apply twice daily, increased if necessary to 4 times daily
Perennial conjunctivitis, ADULT and ADOLESCENT over 12 years, apply twice daily, increased if necessary to 4 times daily; max. duration of treatment 6 weeks

Optilast® (Viatris) PoM
Eye drops, azelastine hydrochloride 0.05%. Net price 8 mL = £6.88
Excipients: include benzalkonium chloride, disodium edetate

EMEDASTINE

Indications: seasonal allergic conjunctivitis
Side-effects: transient burning or stinging; blurred vision, local oedema, keratitis, irritation, dry eye, lacrimation, corneal infiltrates (discontinue) and staining; photophobia; headache, and rhinitis occasionally reported
Dose: ADULT and CHILD over 3 years, apply twice daily

Emadine® (Alcon) PoM
Eye drops, emedastine 0.05% (as difumarate), net price 5 mL = £7.69
Excipients: include benzalkonium chloride

KETOTIFEN

Indications: seasonal allergic conjunctivitis
Side-effects: transient burning or stinging, punctate corneal epithelial erosion; less commonly dry eye, subconjunctival haemmorhage, photophobia; headache, drowsiness, skin reactions, and dry mouth also reported
Dose: ADULT and CHILD over 3 years, apply twice daily

Zaditen® (Novartis) ▼ PoM
Eye drops, ketotifen (as fumarate) 250 micrograms/mL, net price 5 mL = £9.75
Excipients: include benzalkonium chloride

LEVOCABASTINE

Indications: seasonal allergic conjunctivitis
Side-effects: local irritation, blurred vision, local oedema, urticaria; dyspnoea, headache
Dose: ADULT and CHILD over 9 years, apply twice daily, increased if necessary to 3–4 times daily, discontinue if no improvement within 3 days

¹**Livostin®** (Novartis) PoM
Eye drops, levocabastine 0.05% (as hydrochloride). Net price 4 mL = £9.29
Excipients: include benzalkonium chloride, disodium edetate, polysorbate 80, propylene glycol

1. Levocabastine 0.05% eye drops can be sold to the public (in max. pack size of 4 mL) for treatment of seasonal allergic conjunctivitis in adults and children over 12 years; proprietary brands on sale to the public include *Livostin® Direct* eye drops

LODOXAMIDE

Indications: allergic conjunctivitis
Side-effects: mild transient burning, stinging, itching, and lacrimation; flushing and dizziness reported
Dose: ADULT and CHILD over 4 years, apply eye drops 4 times daily

Alomide® (Alcon) PoM
Ophthalmic solution (= eye drops), lodoxamide 0.1% (as trometamol). Net price 10 mL = £5.48
Excipients: include benzalkonium chloride, disodium edetate

NEDOCROMIL SODIUM

Indications: allergic conjunctivitis; vernal keratoconjunctivitis
Side-effects: transient burning and stinging; distinctive taste reported
Dose: seasonal and perennial conjunctivitis, ADULT and CHILD over 6 years, apply twice daily increased if necessary to 4 times daily; max. 12 weeks treatment for seasonal allergic conjunctivitis
Vernal keratoconjunctivitis, ADULT and CHILD over 6 years, apply 4 times daily

Rapitil® (Rhône-Poulenc Rorer) PoM
Eye drops, nedocromil sodium 2%. Net price 5 mL = £9.31
Excipients: include benzalkonium chloride, disodium edetate

OLOPATADINE

Indications: seasonal allergic conjunctivitis
Side-effects: local irritation; less commonly keratitis, dry eye, local oedema, photophobia; headache, asthenia, dizziness; dry nose also reported
Dose: ADULT and CHILD over 3 years, apply twice daily; max. duration of treatment 4 months

Opatanol® (Alcon) ▼ PoM
Eye drops, olopatadine (as hydrochloride) 1 mg/mL, net price 5 mL = £8.77
Excipients: include benzalkonium chloride

SODIUM CROMOGLICATE

(Sodium cromoglycate)
Indications: allergic conjunctivitis; vernal keratoconjunctivitis
Side-effects: transient burning and stinging
Dose: ADULT and CHILD apply eye drops 4 times daily

¹**Sodium Cromoglicate** (Non-proprietary) PoM
Eye drops, sodium cromoglicate 2%. Net price 13.5 mL = £1.97
Available from Alpharma, IVAX (*Hay-Crom® Aqueous*), Pharma-Global (*Vividrin®*), PLIVA, Rhône-Poulenc Rorer (*Opticrom® Aqueous*)

1. Sodium cromoglicate 2% eye drops can be sold to the public (in max. pack size of 10 mL) for treatment of acute seasonal and perennial allergic conjunctivitis; proprietary brands on sale to the public include *Boots Hayfever Relief*, *Clariteyes®*, *Opticrom® Allergy*, *Optrex® Allergy*, and *Vivicrom®*

11.5 Mydriatics and cycloplegics

Antimuscarinics dilate the pupil and paralyse the ciliary muscle; they vary in potency and duration of action.

Short-acting, relatively weak mydriatics, such as **tropicamide** 0.5%, facilitate the examination of the fundus of the eye. **Cyclopentolate** 1% or **atropine** are preferable for producing cycloplegia for refraction in young children. Atropine ointment 1% is sometimes preferred for children aged under 5 years because the ointment formulation reduces systemic absorption. Atropine, which has a longer duration of action, is also used for the treatment of anterior uveitis mainly to prevent posterior synechiae, often with phenylephrine 10% eye drops (2.5% in children, the elderly, and those with cardiac disease). **Homatropine** 1% is also used in the treatment of anterior segment inflammation, and may be preferred for its shorter duration of action.

CAUTIONS. Darkly pigmented iris is more resistant to pupillary dilatation and caution should be exercised to avoid overdosage. Mydriasis may precipitate acute angle-closure glaucoma in a very few patients, usually aged over 60 years and hypermetropic (long-sighted), who are predisposed to the condition because of a shallow anterior chamber. Phenylephrine may interact with systemically administered monoamine-oxidase inhibitors; other **interactions**: Appendix 1 (sympathomimetics).

DRIVING. Patients should be warned not to drive for 1–2 hours after mydriasis.

SIDE-EFFECTS. Ocular side-effects of mydriatics and cycloplegics include transient stinging and raised intra-ocular pressure; on prolonged administration, local irritation, hyperaemia, oedema and conjunctivitis may occur. Contact dermatitis (conjunctivitis) is not uncommon with the antimuscarinic mydriatic drugs, especially atropine.

Toxic systemic reactions to atropine and cyclopentolate may occur in the very young and the very old; see under Atropine Sulphate (section 1.2) for systemic side-effects of antimuscarinic drugs.

Antimuscarinics

ATROPINE SULPHATE

Indications: refraction procedures in young children; anterior uveitis—see also notes above
Cautions: risk of systemic effects with eye drops in infants under 3 months—eye ointment preferred; see also notes above
Side-effects: see notes above

Atropine (Non-proprietary) PoM
Eye drops, atropine sulphate 0.5%, net price 10 mL = £2.32; 1%, 10 mL = 89p
Available from Martindale
Eye ointment, atropine sulphate 1%. Net price 3 g = £2.78
Available from Martindale

Isopto Atropine® (Alcon) PoM
Eye drops, atropine sulphate 1%, hypromellose 0.5%. Net price 5 mL = 99p
Excipients: include benzalkonium chloride

■ Single use

Minims® Atropine Sulphate (Chauvin) PoM
Eye drops, atropine sulphate 1%. Net price 20 × 0.5 mL = £4.92

CYCLOPENTOLATE HYDROCHLORIDE

Indications: see notes above
Cautions: see notes above
Side-effects: see notes above

Mydrilate® (Intrapharm) PoM
Eye drops, cyclopentolate hydrochloride 0.5%, net price 5 mL = 73p; 1%, 5 mL = 98p
Excipients: include benzalkonium chloride

■ Single use

Minims® Cyclopentolate Hydrochloride (Chauvin) PoM
Eye drops, cyclopentolate hydrochloride 0.5 and 1%. Net price 20 × 0.5 mL (both) = £4.92

HOMATROPINE HYDROBROMIDE

Indications: see notes above
Cautions: see notes above
Side-effects: see notes above

Homatropine (Non-proprietary) PoM
Eye drops, homatropine hydrobromide 1%, net price 10 mL = £2.09; 2%, 10 mL = £2.21
Available from Martindale

TROPICAMIDE

Indications: see notes above
Cautions: see notes above

Side-effects: see notes above

Mydriacyl® (Alcon) **PoM**
Eye drops, tropicamide 0.5%, net price 5 mL =
£1.36; 1%, 5 mL = £1.68
Excipients: include benzalkonium chloride, disodium edetate

■ Single use
Minims® Tropicamide (Chauvin) **PoM**
Eye drops, tropicamide 0.5 and 1%. Net price 20 ×
0.5 mL (both) = £5.75

Sympathomimetics

PHENYLEPHRINE HYDROCHLORIDE
Indications: mydriasis; see also notes above
Cautions: children and elderly (avoid 10%
strength); cardiovascular disease (avoid or use
2.5% strength only); tachycardia; hyperthyroidism; diabetes; see also notes above
Contra-indications: angle-closure glaucoma
Side-effects: eye pain and stinging; blurred vision,
photophobia; systemic effects include arrhythmias,
hypertension, coronary artery spasm

Phenylephrine (Non-proprietary)
Eye drops, phenylephrine hydrochloride 10%. Net
price 10 mL = £3.25
Available from Martindale
See also under Hypromellose (section 11.8.1)

■ Single use
Minims® Phenylephrine Hydrochloride
(Chauvin)
Eye drops, phenylephrine hydrochloride 2.5%, net
price 20 × 0.5 mL = £5.75; 10%, 20 × 0.5 mL =
£5.75
Excipients: include disodium edetate, sodium metabisulphite

11.6 Treatment of glaucoma

Glaucoma describes a group of disorders characterised by visual field loss associated with cupping of
the optic disc and optic nerve damage. While glaucoma is generally associated with raised intra-ocular
pressure, it can occur when the intra-ocular pressure
is within the normal range.

In most parts of the world the commonest form of
glaucoma is *primary open-angle glaucoma* (chronic
simple glaucoma; wide-angle glaucoma), where the
obstruction is in the trabecular meshwork. The
condition is often asymptomatic and the patient
may present with significant visual field loss. *Acute
closed-angle glaucoma* (primary angle closure
glaucoma; closed angle glaucoma) results from
blockage of aqueous humour flow into the anterior
chamber and is a medical emergency.

Only drugs that reduce intra-ocular pressure are
available for managing glaucoma; they act by a
variety of mechanisms. A topical beta-blocker or a
prostaglandin analogue is commonly the drug of first
choice. It may be necessary to combine these drugs
or add others such as miotics, sympathomimetics and
carbonic anhydrase inhibitors to control intra-ocular
pressure.

For urgent reduction of intra-ocular pressure and
before surgery, mannitol 20% (up to max. of 500 mL)
should be given by slow intravenous infusion until
the intra-ocular pressure has been satisfactorily
reduced. Acetazolamide by intravenous injection
may also be used for the emergency management
of raised intra-ocular pressure.

Standard antiglaucoma therapy is used if supplementary treatment is required after iridotomy, iridectomy or a drainage operation in either primary
open-angle or acute closed-angle glaucoma.

Beta-blockers

Topical application of a beta-blocker to the eye
reduces intra-ocular pressure effectively in *chronic
simple glaucoma*, probably by reducing the rate of
production of aqueous humour. Administration by
mouth also reduces intra-ocular pressure but this
route is not used since side-effects may be troublesome.

Beta-blockers used as eye drops include **betaxolol,
carteolol, levobunolol, metipranolol,** and **timolol.**

CAUTIONS, CONTRA-INDICATIONS AND SIDE-
EFFECTS. Systemic absorption may follow topical
application therefore eye drops containing a beta-
blocker are contra-indicated in patients with bradycardia, heart block, or uncontrolled heart failure.
Important: for a warning to avoid in asthma see
CSM advice below. Consider also other cautions,
contra-indications and side-effects of beta-blockers
(pp. 77–8). Local side-effects of eye drops include
ocular stinging, burning, pain, itching, erythema, dry
eyes and allergic reactions including anaphylaxis and
blepharoconjunctivitis; occasionally corneal disorders have been reported.
CSM advice. The CSM has advised that beta-blockers,
even those with apparent cardioselectivity, should not be
used in patients with asthma or a history of obstructive
airways disease, unless no alternative treatment is available.
In such cases the risk of inducing bronchospasm should be
appreciated and appropriate precautions taken.

INTERACTIONS. Since systemic absorption may
follow topical application the possibility of interactions, in particular, with drugs such as verapamil
should be borne in mind. See also Appendix 1 (beta-
blockers).

BETAXOLOL HYDROCHLORIDE
Indications: see notes above
Cautions: see notes above
Contra-indications: see notes above
Side-effects: see notes above
Dose: apply twice daily

Betoptic® (Alcon) **PoM**
Ophthalmic solution (= eye drops), betaxolol (as
hydrochloride) 0.5%, net price 5 mL = £3.81
Excipients: include benzalkonium chloride, disodium edetate
Ophthalmic suspension (= eye drops), m/r, betaxolol (as hydrochloride) 0.25%, net price 5 mL =
£4.77
Excipients: include benzalkonium chloride, disodium edetate
Unit dose eye drop suspension, m/r, betaxolol (as
hydrochloride) 0.25%, net price 50 × 0.25 mL =
£14.49

CARTEOLOL HYDROCHLORIDE
Indications: see notes above
Cautions: see notes above
Contra-indications: see notes above
Side-effects: see notes above

Dose: apply twice daily

Teoptic® (Novartis) [PoM]
Eye drops, carteolol hydrochloride 1%, net price 5 mL = £4.60; 2%, 5 mL = £5.40
Excipients: include benzalkonium chloride

LEVOBUNOLOL HYDROCHLORIDE

Indications: see notes above
Cautions: see notes above
Contra-indications: see notes above
Side-effects: see notes above; anterior uveitis occasionally reported
Dose: apply once or twice daily

Levobunolol (Non-proprietary) [PoM]
Eye drops, levobunolol hydrochloride 0.5%. Net price 5 mL = £2.97
Available from Cusi

Betagan® (Allergan) [PoM]
Eye drops, levobunolol hydrochloride 0.5%, polyvinyl alcohol (*Liquifilm®*) 1.4%. Net price 5-mL= £4.66, triple pack (3 × 5 mL) = £11.89
Excipients: include benzalkonium chloride, disodium edetate, sodium metabisulphite
Unit dose eye drops, levobunolol hydrochloride 0.5%, polyvinyl alcohol (*Liquifilm®*) 1.4%. Net price 30 × 0.4 mL = £9.98
Excipients: include disodium edetate

METIPRANOLOL

Indications: see notes above but in chronic open-angle glaucoma **restricted** to patients allergic to preservatives or to those wearing soft contact lenses (in whom benzalkonium chloride should be avoided)
Cautions: see notes above
Contra-indications: see notes above
Side-effects: see notes above; granulomatous anterior uveitis reported (discontinue treatment)
Dose: apply twice daily

Minims® Metipranolol (Chauvin) [PoM]
Eye drops, metipranolol 0.1%, net price 20 × 0.5 mL = £10.19; 0.3%, 20 × 0.5 mL = £11.09

TIMOLOL MALEATE

Indications: see notes above
Cautions: see notes above
Contra-indications: see notes above
Side-effects: see notes above
Dose: apply twice daily; long-acting preparations, see under preparations below

Timolol (Non-proprietary) [PoM]
Eye drops, timolol (as maleate) 0.25%, net price 5 mL = £3.71; 0.5%, 5 mL = £3.99
Available from Alpharma, APS, Hillcross, IVAX, Martindale, Opus (*Glau-opt®*), Sandoz

Timoptol® (MSD) [PoM]
Eye drops, in Ocumeter® metered-dose unit, timolol (as maleate) 0.25%, net price 5 mL = £3.12; 0.5%, 5 mL = £3.12
Excipients: include benzalkonium chloride
Unit dose eye drops, timolol (as maleate) 0.25%, net price 30 × 0.2 mL = £8.45; 0.5%, 30 × 0.2 mL = £9.65

■ Once-daily preparations
Nyogel® (Novartis) [PoM]
Eye gel (= eye drops), timolol (as maleate) 0.1%, net price 5 mL = £2.85
Excipients: include benzalkonium chloride
Dose: apply eye drops once daily

Timoptol®-LA (MSD) [PoM]
Ophthalmic gel-forming solution (= eye drops), timolol (as maleate) 0.25%, net price 2.5 mL = £3.12; 0.5%, 2.5 mL = £3.12
Excipients: include benzododecinium bromide
Dose: apply eye drops once daily

■ With dorzolamide
See under Dorzolamide

■ With latanoprost
See under Latanoprost

Prostaglandin analogues

Latanoprost and **travoprost** are prostaglandin analogues which increase uveoscleral outflow; **bimatoprost** has been introduced, recently. They are used to reduce intra-ocular pressure in ocular hypertension or in open-angle glaucoma. Patients receiving prostaglandin analogues should be monitored for any changes in eye coloration since an increase in the brown pigment in the iris may occur; particular care is required in those with mixed coloured irides and those receiving treatment to one eye only.

BIMATOPROST

Indications: monotherapy or adjunctive therapy for raised intra-ocular pressure in open-angle glaucoma and ocular hypertension in patients intolerant or insufficiently responsive to other drugs
Cautions: see under Latanoprost and notes above
Side-effects: see under Latanoprost; also ocular pruritus, allergic conjunctivitis, cataract, conjunctival oedema, eye discharge, photophobia, superficial punctate keratitis, headache; hypertension
Dose: apply once daily, preferably in the evening; CHILD and ADOLESCENT under 18 years, not recommended

Lumigan® (Allergan) ▼ [PoM]
Eye drops, bimatoprost 300 micrograms/mL, net price 3 mL = £11.46, triple pack (3 × 3 mL) = £32.66
Excipients: include benzalkonium chloride

LATANOPROST

Indications: raised intra-ocular pressure in open-angle glaucoma and ocular hypertension
Cautions: before initiating treatment, advise patients of possible change in eye colour; monitor for eye colour change; aphakia, or pseudophakia with torn posterior lens capsule or anterior chamber lenses; risk factors for cystoid macular oedema; brittle or severe asthma; not to be used within 5 minutes of use of thiomersal-containing preparations; manufacturer advises avoid in pregnancy and in breast-feeding
Side-effects: brown pigmentation particularly in those with mixed-colour irides; blepharitis, ocular irritation and pain; darkening, thickening and lengthening of eye lashes; periorbital or lid oedema; conjunctival hyperaemia; transient punctate epithelial erosions; dyspnoea, exacerbation of

asthma; local skin reactions, macular oedema, iritis and uveitis reported rarely; darkening of palpebral skin reported very rarely
Dose: apply once daily, preferably in the evening

Xalatan® (Pharmacia) [PoM]
Eye drops, latanoprost 50 micrograms/mL, net price 2.5 mL = £11.95
Excipients: include benzalkonium chloride

■ With timolol
For cautions, contra-indications, and side-effects of timolol, see section 11.6, Beta-blockers
Xalacom® (Pharmacia) ▼ [PoM]
Eye drops, latanoprost 50 micrograms, timolol (as maleate) 5 mg/mL, net price 2.5 mL = £15.07
Excipients: include benzalkonium chloride
Dose: for raised intra-ocular pressure in patients with open-angle glaucoma and ocular hypertension when beta-blocker alone not adequate; apply once daily, in the morning

---

TRAVOPROST

Indications: raised intra-ocular pressure in open-angle glaucoma and ocular hypertension
Cautions: see under Latanoprost and notes above
Side-effects: see under Latanoprost; also headache, ocular pruritus, photophobia, and keratitis reported; rarely, hypotension, bradycardia, conjunctivitis, browache
Dose: apply once daily, preferably in the evening; CHILD and ADOLESCENT under 18 years, not recommended

Travatan® (Alcon) ▼ [PoM]
Eye drops, travoprost 40 micrograms/mL, net price 2.5 mL = £11.46
Excipients: include benzalkonium chloride

Sympathomimetics

Dipivefrine is a pro-drug of adrenaline. It is claimed to pass more rapidly than adrenaline through the cornea and is then converted to the active form.

Adrenaline (epinephrine) probably acts both by reducing the rate of production of aqueous humour and by increasing the outflow through the trabecular meshwork. It is contra-indicated in angle-closure glaucoma because it is a mydriatic, unless an iridectomy has been carried out. Side-effects include severe smarting and redness of the eye; adrenaline should be used with caution in patients with hypertension and heart disease.

Brimonidine, a selective alpha₂-adrenoceptor stimulant, is licensed for the reduction of intra-ocular pressure in open-angle glaucoma or ocular hypertension in patients for whom beta-blockers are inappropriate; it may also be used as adjunctive therapy when intra-ocular pressure is inadequately controlled by a beta-blocker alone.

Apraclonidine (section 11.8.2) is another alpha₂-adrenoceptor stimulant. Eye drops containing apraclonidine 0.5% are used for a short term to delay laser treatment or surgery for glaucoma in patients not adequately controlled by another drug; eye drops containing 1% are used for control of intra-ocular pressure after anterior segment laser surgery.

BRIMONIDINE TARTRATE

Indications: adjunct to beta-blockers or used alone in raised intra-ocular pressure in ocular hypertension or open-angle glaucoma in patients unresponsive to beta-blockers or if beta-blockers contra-indicated
Cautions: severe cardiovascular disease; cerebral or coronary insufficiency, Raynaud's syndrome, postural hypotension, depression, hepatic or renal impairment; pregnancy, breast-feeding; **interactions:** Appendix 1 (alpha₂-adrenoceptor stimulants)
DRIVING. Drowsiness may affect performance of skilled tasks (e.g. driving)
Side-effects: ocular reactions include hyperaemia, burning, stinging, blurring, pruritus, allergy, and conjunctival follicles; occasionally corneal erosion and staining, photophobia, eyelid inflammation, conjunctivitis; headache, dry mouth, taste alteration, fatigue, dizziness, drowsiness reported; rarely depression, nasal dryness, palpitations, and hypersensitivity reactions
Dose: apply twice daily

Alphagan® (Allergan) [PoM]
Eye drops, brimonidine tartrate 0.2%, net price 5 mL = £10.31
Excipients: include benzalkonium chloride

DIPIVEFRINE HYDROCHLORIDE

Indications: see notes above
Contra-indications: see notes above
Side-effects: see notes above
Dose: apply twice daily

Propine® (Allergan) [PoM]
Eye drops, dipivefrine hydrochloride 0.1%, net price 5 mL = £3.81, 10 mL = £4.77
Excipients: include benzalkonium chloride, disodium edetate

Carbonic anhydrase inhibitors and systemic drugs

The **carbonic anhydrase inhibitors**, acetazolamide and dorzolamide, reduce intra-ocular pressure by reducing aqueous humour production. Systemic use also produces weak diuresis.

Acetazolamide is given by mouth or by intravenous injection (intramuscular injections are painful because of the alkaline pH of the solution). It is used as an adjunct to other treatment for reducing intra-ocular pressure. Acetazolamide is a sulphonamide; blood disorders, rashes and other sulphonamide-related side-effects occur occasionally. It is not generally recommended for long-term use; electrolyte disturbances and metabolic acidosis that occur may be corrected by administering potassium bicarbonate (as effervescent potassium tablets, section 9.2.1.3).

Dorzolamide and **brinzolamide** are topical carbonic anhydrase inhibitors. They are licensed for use in patients resistant to beta-blockers or those in whom beta-blockers are contra-indicated. They are used alone or as an adjunct to a topical beta-blocker. Systemic absorption may rarely give rise to sulphonamide-like side-effects and may require discontinuation if severe.

The **osmotic diuretics**, intravenous hypertonic **mannitol** (section 2.2.5), or **glycerol** by mouth, are useful short-term ocular hypotensive drugs.

ACETAZOLAMIDE

Indications: reduction of intra-ocular pressure in open-angle glaucoma, secondary glaucoma, and peri-operatively in angle-closure glaucoma; diuresis (section 2.2.7); epilepsy

Cautions: not generally recommended for prolonged use but if given monitor blood count and plasma electrolyte concentration; pulmonary obstruction (risk of acidosis); elderly; pregnancy and breast-feeding; avoid extravasation at injection site (risk of necrosis); **interactions:** Appendix 1 (diuretics)

Contra-indications: hypokalaemia, hyponatraemia, hyperchloraemic acidosis; severe hepatic impairment; renal impairment; sulphonamide hypersensitivity

Side-effects: nausea, vomiting, diarrhoea, taste disturbance; loss of appetite, paraesthesia, flushing, headache, dizziness, fatigue, irritability, depression; thirst, polyuria; reduced libido; metabolic acidosis and electrolyte disturbances on long-term therapy; occasionally, drowsiness, confusion, hearing disturbances, urticaria, malaena, glycosuria, haematuria, abnormal liver function, renal calculi, blood disorders including agranulocytosis and thrombocytopenia, rashes including Stevens-Johnson syndrome and toxic epidermal necrolysis; rarely, photosensitivity, liver damage, flaccid paralysis, convulsions; transient myopia reported

Dose: *by mouth or by intravenous injection*, glaucoma, 0.25–1 g daily in divided doses

Epilepsy, 0.25–1 g daily in divided doses; CHILD 8–30 mg/kg daily, max. 750 mg daily

By intramuscular injection, as for intravenous injection but preferably avoided because of alkalinity

Diamox® (Goldshield) [PoM]
Tablets, acetazolamide 250 mg. Net price 112-tab pack = £12.68. Label: 3
Sodium Parenteral (= injection), powder for reconstitution, acetazolamide (as sodium salt). Net price 500-mg vial = £14.76
NOTE. Injection may be difficult to obtain

Diamox® SR (Goldshield) [PoM]
Capsules, m/r, two-tone orange, enclosing orange f/c pellets, acetazolamide 250 mg. Net price 28-cap pack = £11.55. Label: 3, 25
Dose: glaucoma, 1–2 capsules daily

BRINZOLAMIDE

Indications: adjunct to beta-blockers or used alone in raised intra-ocular pressure in ocular hypertension and in open-angle glaucoma if beta-blocker alone inadequate or inappropriate

Cautions: hepatic impairment; pregnancy (Appendix 4); **interactions:** Appendix 1 (brinzolamide)

Contra-indications: renal impairment (creatinine clearance less than 30 mL/minute), hyperchloraemic acidosis; breast-feeding

Side-effects: local irritation, taste disturbance; less commonly nausea, dyspepsia, dry mouth, chest pain, epistaxis, haemoptysis, dyspnoea, rhinitis, pharyngitis, bronchitis, paraesthesia, depression, dizziness, headache, dermatitis, alopecia, corneal erosion

Dose: apply twice daily increased to 3 times daily if necessary

Azopt® (Alcon) ▼ [PoM]
Eye drops, brinzolamide 10 mg/mL, net price 5 mL = £7.17
Excipients: include benzalkonium chloride, disodium edetate

DORZOLAMIDE

Indications: raised intra-ocular pressure in ocular hypertension, open-angle glaucoma, pseudo-exfoliative glaucoma *either* as adjunct to beta-blocker *or* used alone in patients unresponsive to beta-blockers or if beta-blockers contra-indicated

Cautions: hepatic impairment; systemic absorption follows topical application; history of renal calculi; chronic corneal defects, history of intra-ocular surgery; **interactions:** Appendix 1 (dorzolamide)

Contra-indications: severe renal impairment or hyperchloraemic acidosis; pregnancy and breast-feeding

Side-effects: ocular burning, stinging and itching, blurred vision, lacrimation, conjunctivitis, superficial punctate keratitis, eyelid inflammation and crusting, anterior uveitis, transient myopia, corneal oedema, iridocyclitis; headache, dizziness, paraesthesia, asthenia, sinusitis, rhinitis, nausea; hypersensitivity reactions (including urticaria, angioedema, bronchospasm); bitter taste, epistaxis, urolithiasis

Dose: used alone, apply 3 times daily; with topical beta-blocker, apply twice daily

Trusopt® (MSD) [PoM]
Ophthalmic solution (= eye drops), dorzolamide (as hydrochloride) 2%, net price 5 mL = £9.31
Excipients: include benzalkonium chloride

■ **With timolol**
For cautions, contra-indications, and side-effects of timolol, see section 11.6, Beta-blockers

Cosopt® (MSD) [PoM]
Ophthalmic solution (= eye drops), dorzolamide (as hydrochloride) 2%, timolol (as maleate) 0.5%, net price 5 mL = £13.50
Excipients: include benzalkonium chloride
Dose: for raised intra-ocular pressure in open-angle glaucoma, or pseudoexfoliative glaucoma when beta-blockers alone not adequate, apply twice daily

Miotics

The small pupil is an unfortunate side-effect of these drugs (except when pilocarpine is used temporarily before an operation for *angle-closure glaucoma*). They act by opening up the inefficient drainage channels in the trabecular meshwork resulting from contraction or spasm of the ciliary muscle.

Miotics used in the management of raised intra-ocular pressure include carbachol and pilocarpine.

CAUTIONS. A darkly pigmented iris may require higher concentration of the miotic or more frequent administration and care should be taken to avoid overdosage. Retinal detachment has occurred in susceptible individuals and those with retinal disease; therefore fundus examination is advised before starting treatment with a miotic. Care is also required in conjunctival or corneal damage. Intra-ocular pressure and visual fields should be monitored in those with chronic simple glaucoma and those receiving long-term treatment with a miotic. Miotics should be used with caution in cardiac disease, hypertension, asthma, peptic ulceration, urinary-tract obstruction, and Parkinson's disease.

COUNSELLING. Blurred vision may affect performance of skilled tasks (e.g. driving) particularly at night or in reduced lighting

CONTRA-INDICATIONS. Miotics are contra-indicated in conditions where pupillary constriction is undesirable such as acute iritis, anterior uveitis and some forms of secondary glaucoma. They should be avoided in acute inflammatory disease of the anterior segment.

SIDE-EFFECTS. Ciliary spasm leads to headache and browache which may be more severe in the initial 2–4 weeks of treatment (a particular disadvantage in patients under 40 years of age). Ocular side-effects include burning, itching, smarting, blurred vision, conjunctival vascular congestion, myopia, lens changes with chronic use, vitreous haemorrhage, and pupillary block. Systemic side-effects (see under Parasympathomimetics, section 7.4.1) are rare following application to the eye.

CARBACHOL

Indications: see notes above
Cautions: see notes above
Contra-indications: see notes above
Side-effects: see notes above
Dose: apply up to 4 times daily

Isopto Carbachol® (Alcon) PoM
Eye drops, carbachol 3%, hypromellose 1%. Net price 10 mL = £1.76
Excipients: include benzalkonium chloride

PILOCARPINE

Indications: see notes above; dry mouth (section 12.3.5)
Cautions: see notes above
Contra-indications: see notes above
Side-effects: see notes above
Dose: apply up to 4 times daily; long-acting preparations, see under preparations below

Pilocarpine Hydrochloride (Non-proprietary) PoM
Eye drops, pilocarpine hydrochloride 0.5%, net price 10 mL = £1.37; 1%, 10 mL = £1.07; 2%, 10 mL = £1.19; 3%, 10 mL = £1.44; 4%, 10 mL = £1.60
Available from Alpharma, Cusi, Hillcross, Martindale

■ Single use
Minims® Pilocarpine Nitrate (Chauvin) PoM
Eye drops, pilocarpine nitrate 2 and 4%, net price 20 × 0.5 mL (both) = £4.92

■ Long acting
Pilogel® (Alcon) PoM
Ophthalmic gel, pilocarpine hydrochloride 4%, carbomer 940 (polyacrylic acid) 3.5%, net price 5 g = £6.86
Excipients: include benzalkonium chloride, disodium edetate
Dose: apply 1–1.5 cm gel once daily at bedtime

11.7   Local anaesthetics

Oxybuprocaine and tetracaine (amethocaine) are probably the most widely used topical local anaesthetics. Proxymetacaine causes less initial stinging and is useful for children. Oxybuprocaine or a combined preparation of lidocaine (lignocaine) and fluorescein is used for tonometry. Tetracaine produces a more profound anaesthesia and is suitable for use before minor surgical procedures, such as the removal of corneal sutures. It has a temporary disruptive effect on the corneal epithelium. Lidocaine, with or without adrenaline (epinephrine), is injected into the eyelids for minor surgery, while retrobulbar or peribulbar injections are used for surgery of the globe itself. Local anaesthetics should never be used for the management of ocular symptoms.

LIDOCAINE HYDROCHLORIDE

(Lignocaine hydrochloride)
Indications: local anaesthetic

Minims® Lignocaine and Fluorescein (Chauvin) PoM
Eye drops, lidocaine hydrochloride 4%, fluorescein sodium 0.25%. Net price 20 × 0.5 mL = £6.93

OXYBUPROCAINE HYDROCHLORIDE

Indications: local anaesthetic

Minims® Benoxinate (Oxybuprocaine) Hydrochloride (Chauvin) PoM
Eye drops, oxybuprocaine hydrochloride 0.4%. Net price 20 × 0.5 mL = £4.92

PROXYMETACAINE HYDROCHLORIDE

Indications: local anaesthetic

Minims® Proxymetacaine (Chauvin) PoM
Eye drops, proxymetacaine hydrochloride 0.5%. Net price 20 × 0.5 mL = £6.95

■ With fluorescein
Minims® Proxymetacaine and Fluorescein (Chauvin) PoM
Eye drops, proxymetacaine hydrochloride 0.5%, fluorescein sodium 0.25%. Net price 20 × 0.5 mL = £7.95

TETRACAINE HYDROCHLORIDE

(Amethocaine hydrochloride)
Indications: local anaesthetic

Minims® Amethocaine Hydrochloride (Chauvin) PoM
Eye drops, tetracaine hydrochloride 0.5 and 1%. Net price 20 × 0.5 mL (both) = £5.75

11.8 Miscellaneous ophthalmic preparations

11.8.1 Tear deficiency, ocular lubricants, and astringents

11.8.2 Ocular diagnostic and peri-operative preparations and photodynamic treatment

Certain eye drops, e.g. amphotericin, ceftazidime, cefuroxime, colistin, desferrioxamine, dexamethasone, gentamicin and vancomycin may be prepared aseptically from material supplied for injection; for details on preparation of trisodium edetate eye drops see under *Limclair* section 9.5.1.2.

11.8.1 Tear deficiency, ocular lubricants, and astringents

Chronic soreness of the eyes associated with reduced or abnormal tear secretion (e.g. in Sjögren's syndrome) often responds to tear replacement therapy or pilocarpine given by mouth (section 12.3.5). The severity of the condition and patient preference will often guide the choice of preparation.

Hypromellose is the traditional choice of treatment for tear deficiency. It may need to be instilled frequently (e.g. hourly) for adequate relief. Ocular surface mucin is often abnormal in tear deficiency and the combination of hypromellose with a mucolytic such as **acetylcysteine** can be helpful.

The ability of **carbomers** to cling to the eye surface may help reduce frequency of application to 4 times daily.

Polyvinyl alcohol increases the persistence of the tear film and is useful when the ocular surface mucin is reduced.

Povidone eye drops are also used in the management of tear deficiency.

Sodium chloride 0.9% drops are sometimes useful in tear deficiency, and can be used as 'comfort drops' by contact lens wearers, and to facilitate lens removal. Special presentations of sodium chloride 0.9% and other irrigation solutions are used routinely for intra-ocular surgery.

Eye ointments containing a **paraffin** may be used to lubricate the eye surface, especially in cases of recurrent corneal epithelial erosion. They may cause temporary visual disturbance and are best suited for application before sleep. Ointments should not be used during contact lens wear.

Zinc sulphate is a traditional astringent that is now little used.

ACETYLCYSTEINE

Indications: tear deficiency, impaired or abnormal mucus production
Dose: apply eye drops 3–4 times daily

Ilube (Alcon) PoM
Eye drops, acetylcysteine 5%, hypromellose 0.35%. Net price 10 mL = £4.63
Excipients: include benzalkonium chloride, disodium edetate

CARBOMERS

(Polyacrylic acid)
Synthetic high molecular weight polymers of acrylic acid cross-linked with either allyl ethers of sucrose or allyl ethers of pentaerithrityl

Indications: dry eyes including keratoconjunctivitis sicca, unstable tear film
Dose: apply 3–4 times daily or as required

GelTears (Chauvin)
Gel (= eye drops), carbomer 980 (polyacrylic acid) 0.2%, net price 10 g = £2.80
Excipients: include benzalkonium chloride

Liposic (Bausch & Lomb)
Gel (= eye drops), carbomer 980 (polyacrylic acid) 0.2%, net price 10 g = £2.96
Excipients: include cetrimide

Viscotears (Novartis Ophthalmics)
Liquid gel (= eye drops), carbomer 980 (polyacrylic acid) 0.2%, net price 10 g = £3.12
Excipients: include cetrimide, disodium edetate
Liquid gel (= eye drops), carbomer 980 (polyacrylic acid) 0.2%, net price 30 × 0.6-mL single-dose units = £5.75

CARMELLOSE SODIUM

Indications: dry eye conditions
Dose: apply as required

Celluvisc (Allergan) ▼
Eye drops, carmellose sodium 1%, net price 30 × 0.4 mL = £5.75

HYDROXYETHYLCELLULOSE

Indications: tear deficiency

Minims Artificial Tears (Chauvin)
Eye drops, hydroxyethylcellulose 0.44%, sodium chloride 0.35%. Net price 20 × 0.5 mL = £5.75

HYPROMELLOSE

Indications: tear deficiency
NOTE. The Royal Pharmaceutical Society of Great Britain has stated that where it is not possible to ascertain the strength of hypromellose prescribed, the prescriber should be contacted to clarify the strength intended.

Hypromellose (Non-proprietary)
Eye drops, hypromellose 0.3%, net price 10 mL = 75p
Available from Alpharma, IVAX, Martindale

Isopto Alkaline (Alcon)
Eye drops, hypromellose 1%, net price 10 mL = 99p
Excipients: include benzalkonium chloride

Isopto Plain (Alcon)
Eye drops, hypromellose 0.5%, net price 10 mL = 85p
Excipients: include benzalkonium chloride

Tears Naturale (Alcon)
Eye drops, dextran '70' 0.1%, hypromellose 0.3%, net price 15 mL = £1.68
Excipients: include benzalkonium chloride, disodium edetate

■ Single use
Artelac SDU (Pharma-Global)
Eye drops, hypromellose 0.32%, net price 30 × 0.5 mL = £10.80

■ With phenylephrine

NOTE. Phenylephrine (section 11.5) acts to constrict conjunctival vessels, thus producing a whiter eye; it is not recommended for prolonged use

Isopto Frin® (Alcon) ▭

Eye drops, phenylephrine hydrochloride 0.12%, hypromellose 0.5%, net price 10 mL = £1.14
Excipients: include benzethonium chloride
Dose: temporary relief of redness due to minor irritation, apply up to 4 times daily

LIQUID PARAFFIN

Indications: dry eye conditions

Lacri-Lube® (Allergan)
Eye ointment, white soft paraffin 57.3%, liquid paraffin 42.5%, wool alcohols 0.2%. Net price 3.5 g = £1.90, 5 g = £2.47

Lubri-Tears® (Alcon)
Eye ointment, white soft paraffin 60%, liquid paraffin 30%, wool fat 10%. Net price 5 g = £2.29

PARAFFIN, YELLOW, SOFT

Indications: see notes above

Simple Eye Ointment
Ointment, liquid paraffin 10%, wool fat 10%, in yellow soft paraffin. Net price 4 g = £2.68
Available from Martindale, PLIVA

POLYVINYL ALCOHOL

Indications: tear deficiency

Hypotears® (Novartis)
Eye drops, macrogol '8000' 2%, polyvinyl alcohol 1%. Net price 15 mL = £1.09
Excipients: include benzalkonium chloride, disodium edetate

Liquifilm Tears® (Allergan)
Ophthalmic solution (= eye drops), polyvinyl alcohol 1.4%. Net price 15 mL = £1.61
Excipients: include benzalkonium chloride, disodium edetate
Ophthalmic solution (= eye drops), polyvinyl alcohol 1.4%, povidone 0.6%. Net price 30 × 0.4 mL = £5.35

Sno Tears® (Chauvin)
Eye drops, polyvinyl alcohol 1.4%. Net price 10 mL = £1.06
Excipients: include benzalkonium chloride, disodium edetate

POVIDONE

Indications: dry eye conditions
Dose: apply 4 times daily or as required

Oculotect® (Novartis)
Eye drops, povidone 5%. Net price 20 × 0.4 mL = £3.40

SODIUM CHLORIDE

Indications: irrigation, including first-aid removal of harmful substances

Sodium Chloride 0.9% Solutions
See section 13.11.1

Balanced Salt Solution
Solution (sterile), sodium chloride 0.64%, sodium acetate 0.39%, sodium citrate 0.17%, calcium chloride 0.048%, magnesium chloride 0.03%, potassium chloride 0.075%
For intra-ocular or topical irrigation during surgical procedures
Available from Alcon (15 mL, 250 mL and 500 mL) and from Novartis Ophthalmics (*Iocare®*, 15 mL and 500 mL)

■ Single use

Minims® Saline (Chauvin)
Eye drops, sodium chloride 0.9%. Net price 20 × 0.5 mL = £4.92

ZINC SULPHATE

Indications: see notes above
Cautions: see notes above

Zinc Sulphate (Non-proprietary)
Eye drops, zinc sulphate 0.25%. Net price 10 mL = £3.03
Available from Martindale

11.8.2 Ocular diagnostic and peri-operative preparations and photodynamic treatment

Ocular diagnostic preparations

Fluorescein sodium and **rose bengal** are used in diagnostic procedures and for locating damaged areas of the cornea due to injury or disease. Rose bengal is more efficient for the diagnosis of conjunctival epithelial damage but it often stings excessively unless a local anaesthetic is instilled beforehand.

FLUORESCEIN SODIUM

Indications: detection of lesions and foreign bodies

Minims® Fluorescein Sodium (Chauvin)
Eye drops, fluorescein sodium 1 or 2%. Net price 20 × 0.5 mL (both) = £4.92

■ With local anaesthetic
Section 11.7

ROSE BENGAL

Indications: detection of lesions and foreign bodies

Minims® Rose Bengal (Chauvin)
Eye drops, rose bengal 1%. Net price 20 × 0.5 mL = £5.75

Ocular peri-operative drugs

Drugs used to prepare the eye for surgery and drugs that are injected into the anterior chamber at the time of surgery are included here.

Sodium hyaluronate preparations (*Healonid®*, Pharmacia; *Ophthalin®*, Iocare) are used during surgical procedures on the eye.

Apraclonidine, an alpha$_2$-adrenoceptor stimulant, reduces intra-ocular pressure possibly by reducing the production of aqueous humour. It is used for short-term treatment only.

Special presentations of **sodium chloride 0.9%** solution are used routinely in intra-ocular surgery (section 11.8.1).

ACETYLCHOLINE CHLORIDE

Indications: cataract surgery, penetrating kerato-plasty, iridectomy, and other anterior segment surgery requiring rapid complete miosis

Miochol-E® (Novartis) PoM
Solution for intra-ocular irrigation, acetylcholine chloride 1%, mannitol 3% when reconstituted. Net price 2 mL-vial = £9.10

APRACLONIDINE

NOTE. Apraclonidine is a derivative of clonidine
Indications: control of intra-ocular pressure
Cautions: history of angina, severe coronary insuf-ficiency, recent myocardial infarction, heart fail-ure, cerebrovascular disease, vasovagal attack, chronic renal failure; depression; pregnancy and breast-feeding; monitor intra-ocular pressure and visual fields; loss of effect may occur over time; suspend treatment if reduction in vision occurs in end-stage glaucoma; monitor for excessive reduc-tion in intra-ocular pressure following peri-opera-tive use; **interactions:** Appendix 1 (alpha$_2$-adreno-ceptor stimulants)
DRIVING. Drowsiness may affect performance of skilled tasks (e.g. driving)
Contra-indications: history of severe or unstable and uncontrolled cardiovascular disease
Side-effects: dry mouth, taste disturbance; hyper-aemia, ocular pruritus, discomfort and lacrimation (withdraw if ocular intolerance including oedema of lids and conjunctiva); headache, asthenia, dry nose; lid retraction, conjunctival blanching and mydriasis reported after peri-operative use; since absorption may follow topical application systemic effects (see Clonidine Hydrochloride, section 2.5.2) may occur
Dose: see under preparations below

Iopidine® (Alcon) PoM
Ophthalmic solution (= eye drops), apraclonidine 1% (as hydrochloride). Net price 24 × 2 single use 0.25-mL units = £81.90
Dose: control or prevention of postoperative elevation of intra-ocular pressure after anterior segment laser surgery, apply 1 drop 1 hour before laser procedure then 1 drop immediately after completion of procedure; CHILD not recommended
Iopidine 0.5% ophthalmic solution (= eye drops), apraclonidine 0.5% (as hydrochloride). Net price 5 mL = £11.45
Excipients: include benzalkonium chloride
Dose: short-term adjunctive treatment of chronic glauc-oma in patients not adequately controlled by another drug (see note below), apply 1 drop 3 times daily usually for max. 1 month; CHILD not recommended
NOTE. May not provide additional benefit if patient already using two drugs that suppress the production of aqueous humour

DICLOFENAC SODIUM

Indications: inhibition of intraoperative miosis during cataract surgery (but does not possess intrinsic mydriatic properties); postoperative inflammation in cataract surgery, strabismus sur-gery or argon laser trabeculoplasty; pain in corneal epithelial defects after photorefractive keratect-omy, radial keratotomy or accidental trauma; seasonal allergic conjunctivitis (section 11.4.2)

Voltarol® **Ophtha Multidose** (Novartis) PoM
Eye drops, diclofenac sodium 0.1%, net price 5 mL = £6.68
Excipients: include benzalkonium chloride, disodium edetate, propylene glycol

▪ Single use
Voltarol® **Ophtha** (Novartis) PoM
Eye drops, diclofenac sodium 0.1%. Net price pack of 5 single-dose units = £4.00, 40 single-dose units = £32.00

FLURBIPROFEN SODIUM

Indications: inhibition of intraoperative miosis (but does not possess intrinsic mydriatic properties); anterior segment inflammation following post-operative and post-laser trabeculoplasty when corticosteroids contra-indicated

Ocufen® (Allergan) PoM
Ophthalmic solution (= eye drops), flurbiprofen sodium 0.03%, polyvinyl alcohol (Liquifilm®) 1.4%. Net price 40 × 0.4 mL = £37.15

KETOROLAC TROMETAMOL

Indications: prophylaxis and reduction of inflam-mation and associated symptoms following ocular surgery

Acular® (Allergan) PoM
Eye drops, ketorolac trometamol 0.5%. Net price 5 mL = £6.68
Excipients: include benzalkonium chloride, disodium edetate

Subfoveal choroidal neovascularisation

Verteporfin is licensed for use in the photodynamic treatment of subfoveal choroidal neovascularisation associated with age-related macular degeneration *or* with pathological myopia. It is also licensed for occult subfoveal choroidal neovascularisation with disease progression. Following intravenous infusion, verteporfin is activated by local irradiation using non-thermal red light to produce cytotoxic deriva-tives. Only specialists experienced in the manage-ment of these conditions should use it.

> **NICE guidance (photodynamic therapy for wet age-related macular degeneration).** NICE has recommended (September 2003) photodynamic therapy for wet age-related macular degeneration with a confirmed diagnosis of classic with **no** occult subfoveal choroidal neovascularisation and best-cor-rected visual acuity of 6/60 or better.
> Photodynamic therapy is **not** recommended for wet age-related macular degeneration with predominantly classic but partly occult subfoveal choroidal neovas-cularisation *except* in clinical studies.

VERTEPORFIN

Indications: see notes above—specialist use only
Cautions: photosensitivity—avoid exposure of unprotected skin and eyes to bright light during infusion and for 48 hours afterwards; hepatic impairment (avoid if severe), biliary obstruction; avoid extravasation; pregnancy (Appendix 4)
Contra-indications: porphyria; breast-feeding (Appendix 5)

Side-effects: visual disturbances (including blurred vision, flashing lights, visual-field defects), nausea, back pain, asthenia, pruritus, hypercholesterolaemia, fever; rarely lacrimation disorder, subretinal or vitreous haemorrhage, hypersensitivity reactions (including chest pain, syncope, sweating, changes in blood pressure and in heart rate); injection-site reactions including pain, oedema, inflammation, haemorrhage, discoloration

Dose: *by intravenous infusion* over 10 minutes, 6 mg/m^2
NOTE. For information on administration and light activation, consult product literature

Visudyne® (Novartis) ▼ PoM
Injection, powder for reconstitution, verteporfin, net price 15-mg vial = £850.00

11.9 Contact lenses

NOTE. Some recommendations in this section involve non-licensed indications.

For cosmetic reasons many people prefer to wear contact lenses rather than spectacles; contact lenses are also sometimes required for medical indications. Visual defects are corrected by either rigid ('hard' or gas permeable) lenses or soft (hydrogel) lenses; soft lenses are the most popular type, because they are the most comfortable, though they may not give the best vision. Lenses should usually be worn for a specified number of hours each day. Continuous (extended) wear involves much greater risks to eye health and is not recommended except where medically indicated.

Contact lenses require meticulous care. Poor compliance with directions for use, and with daily cleaning and disinfection, may result in complications which include ulcerative keratitis, conjunctival problems (such as purulent or papillary conjunctivitis). One-day disposable lenses, which are worn only once and therefore require no maintenance or storage, are becoming increasingly popular.

Acanthamoeba keratitis, a sight-threatening condition, is associated with ineffective lens cleaning and disinfection or the use of contaminated lens cases. The condition is especially associated with the use of soft lenses (including frequently replaced lenses). Acanthamoeba keratitis is treated by specialists with intensive use of polihexanide (polyhexamethylene biguanide), propamidine isetionate, chlorhexidine and neomycin drops, sometimes in combination.

CONTACT LENSES AND DRUG TREATMENT. Special care is required in prescribing eye preparations for contact lens users. Some drugs and preservatives in eye preparations can accumulate in hydrogel lenses and may induce toxic reactions. Therefore, unless medically indicated, the lenses should be removed before instillation and not worn during the period of treatment. Alternatively, unpreserved drops can be used. Eye drops may, however, be instilled over rigid corneal contact lenses. Ointment preparations should never be used in conjunction with contact lens wear; oily eye drops should also be avoided.

Many drugs given systemically can also have adverse effects on contact lens wear. These include oral contraceptives (particularly those with a higher oestrogen content), drugs which reduce blink rate (e.g. anxiolytics, hypnotics, antihistamines, and muscle relaxants), drugs which reduce lacrimation (e.g. antihistamines, antimuscarinics, phenothiazines and related drugs, some beta-blockers, diuretics, and tricyclic antidepressants), and drugs which increase lacrimation (including ephedrine and hydralazine). Other drugs that may affect contact lens wear are isotretinoin (may cause conjunctival inflammation), aspirin (salicylic acid appears in tears and may be absorbed by contact lenses—leading to irritation), and rifampicin and sulfasalazine (may discolour lenses).

12: Ear, nose, and oropharynx

12.1   Drugs acting on the ear

12.1.1   Otitis externa
12.1.2   Otitis media
12.1.3   Removal of ear wax

12.1.1   Otitis externa

Otitis externa is an inflammatory reaction of the meatal skin. It is important to exclude an underlying chronic otitis media before treatment is commenced. Many cases recover after thorough cleansing of the external ear canal by suction, dry mopping, or gentle syringing. A frequent problem in resistant cases is the difficulty in applying lotions and ointments satisfactorily to the relatively inaccessible affected skin. The most effective method is to introduce a ribbon gauze dressing soaked with **corticosteroid** ear drops or with an astringent such as **aluminium acetate** solution. When this is not practical, the ear should be gently cleansed with a probe covered in cotton wool and the patient encouraged to lie with the affected ear uppermost for ten minutes after the canal has been filled with a liberal quantity of the appropriate solution.

If infection is present, a topical anti-infective which is not used systemically (such as **neomycin** or **clioquinol**) may be used, but for only about a week as excessive use may result in fungal infections; these may be difficult to treat and require expert advice. Sensitivity to the anti-infective or solvent may occur and resistance to antibacterials is a possibility with prolonged use. **Chloramphenicol** may also be used but the ear drops contain propylene glycol and cause sensitivity in about 10% of patients (the eye ointment can be used instead [unlicensed indication]). Solutions containing an anti-infective and a corticosteroid (such as *Locorten-Vioform®*) are used for treating cases where infection is present with inflammation and eczema. In view of reports of ototoxicity in patients with a perforated tympanic membrane (eardrum), the CSM has stated that treatment with a topical aminoglycoside antibiotic is contra-indicated in those with a tympanic perforation. However, many specialists do use these drops cautiously in the presence of a perforation in patients with otitis media (section 12.1.2) and where other measures have failed for otitis externa.

A solution of **acetic acid** 2% acts as an antifungal and antibacterial in the external ear canal. It may be used to treat mild otitis externa but in severe cases an anti-inflammatory preparation with or without an anti-infective drug is required. A proprietary preparation containing acetic acid 2% (*EarCalm®* spray) is on sale to the public.

An acute infection may cause severe pain and a systemic antibacterial is required with a simple analgesic such as paracetamol. When a resistant staphylococcal infection (a boil) is present in the external auditory meatus, **flucloxacillin** is the drug of choice (section 5.1, table 1); **ciprofloxacin** (or an aminoglycoside) may be needed in pseudomonal infections which may occur if the patient has diabetes or is immunocompromised.

The skin of the pinna adjacent to the ear canal is often affected by eczema. Topical corticosteroid creams and ointments (see section 13.4) are then required, but prolonged use should be avoided.

Astringent preparations

ALUMINIUM ACETATE

Indications: inflammation in otitis externa (see notes above)

Dose: insert into meatus or apply on a gauze wick which should be kept saturated with the ear drops

Aluminium Acetate (Non-proprietary)

Ear drops 13%, aluminium sulphate 2.25 g, calcium carbonate 1 g, tartaric acid 450 mg, acetic acid (33%) 2.5 mL, purified water 7.5 mL

Available from manufacturers of 'special order' products

Ear drops 8%, dilute 8 parts aluminium acetate ear drops (13%) with 5 parts purified water. Must be freshly prepared

Anti-inflammatory preparations

BETAMETHASONE SODIUM PHOSPHATE

Indications: eczematous inflammation in otitis externa (see notes above)

Cautions: avoid prolonged use

Contra-indications: untreated infection

Side-effects: local sensitivity reactions

Betnesol® (Celltech) [PoM]

Drops (for ear, eye, or nose), betamethasone sodium phosphate 0.1%. Net price 10 mL = £1.84

Excipients: include benzalkonium chloride, disodium edetate

Dose: ear, apply 2–3 drops every 2–3 hours; reduce frequency when relief obtained; *eye*, see section 11.4.1; *nose*, see section 12.2.1

Vista-Methasone® (Martindale) [PoM]

Drops (for ear, eye, or nose), betamethasone sodium phosphate 0.1%. Net price 5 mL = £1.10; 10 mL = £1.25

Excipients: include benzalkonium chloride, disodium edetate

Dose: ear, apply 2–3 drops every 3–4 hours; reduce frequency when relief obtained; *eye*, see section 11.4.1; *nose*, see section 12.2.1

■ With antibacterial

Betnesol-N® (Celltech) [PoM]

Drops (for ear, eye, or nose), betamethasone sodium phosphate 0.1%, neomycin sulphate 0.5%.Net price 10 mL = £1.89

Excipients: include benzalkonium chloride, disodium edetate

Dose: ear, apply 2–3 drops 3–4 times daily; *eye*, see section 11.4.1; *nose*, section 12.2.3

Vista-Methasone N® (Martindale) [PoM]

Drops (for ear, eye, or nose), betamethasone sodium phosphate 0.1%, neomycin sulphate 0.5%. Net price 5 mL = £1.17; 10 mL = £1.29

Excipients: include thiomersal

Dose: ear, apply 2–3 drops every 3–4 hours; reduce frequency when relief obtained; *eye*, see section 11.4.1; *nose*, section 12.2.3

DEXAMETHASONE

Indications: eczematous inflammation in otitis externa (see notes above)

Cautions: avoid prolonged use

Contra-indications: untreated infection

Side-effects: local sensitivity reactions

■ With antibacterial

Otomize® (GSK Consumer Healthcare) [PoM]

Ear spray, dexamethasone 0.1%, neomycin sulphate 3250 units/mL, glacial acetic acid 2%. Net price 5-mL pump-action aerosol unit = £4.24

Excipients: include hydroxybenzoates (parabens)

Dose: apply 1 metered spray into the ear 3 times daily

Sofradex® (Florizel) [PoM]

Drops (for ear or eye), dexamethasone (as sodium metasulphobenzoate) 0.05%, framycetin sulphate 0.5%, gramicidin 0.005%. Net price 10 mL = £5.21

Excipients: include polysorbate 80

Dose: ear, apply 2–3 drops 3–4 times daily; *eye*, see section 11.4.1

Ointment (for ear or eye), dexamethasone 0.05%, framycetin sulphate 0.5%, gramicidin 0.005%. Net price 5 g = £3.72

Dose: ear, apply 1–2 times daily; *eye*, see section 11.4.1

FLUMETASONE PIVALATE

(Flumethasone Pivalate)

Indications: eczematous inflammation in otitis externa (see notes above)

Cautions: avoid prolonged use

Contra-indications: untreated infection

Side-effects: local sensitivity reactions

■ With antibacterial

Locorten-Vioform® (Novartis Consumer Health) [PoM]

Ear drops, flumetasone pivalate 0.02%, clioquinol 1%. Net price 7.5 mL = 97p

Dose: apply 2–3 drops into the ear twice daily for up to 7–10 days; not recommended for child under 2 years

HYDROCORTISONE

Indications: eczematous inflammation in otitis externa (see notes above)

Cautions: avoid prolonged use

Contra-indications: untreated infection

Side-effects: local sensitivity reactions

■ With antibacterial

Gentisone HC® (Roche) [PoM]

Ear drops, hydrocortisone acetate 1%, gentamicin 0.3% (as sulphate). Net price 10 mL = £3.97

Excipients: include benzalkonium chloride, disodium edetate

Dose: apply 2–4 drops into the ear 3–4 times daily and at night

Neo-Cortef® (PLIVA) [PoM]

Drops (for ear or eye), hydrocortisone acetate 1.5%, neomycin sulphate 0.5%. Net price 10 mL = £4.11

Excipients: include miripirium chloride (myristyl-gamma-picolinium chloride)

Dose: ear, apply 2–3 drops 3–4 times daily; *eye*, see section 11.4.1

NOTE. May be difficult to obtain

Ointment (for ear or eye), hydrocortisone acetate 1.5%, neomycin sulphate 0.5%. Net price 3.9 g = £1.53

Excipients: include wool fat

Dose: ear, apply 1–2 times daily; *eye*, see section 11.4.1

NOTE. May be difficult to obtain

Otosporin® (GSK) [PoM] [symbol]
Ear drops, hydrocortisone 1%, neomycin sulphate 3400 units, polymyxin B sulphate 10 000 units/mL. Net price 5 mL = £2.15; 10 mL = £4.30
Excipients: include cetostearyl alcohol, hydroxybenzoates (parabens), polysorbate 20
Dose: apply 3 drops into the ear 3–4 times daily

PREDNISOLONE SODIUM PHOSPHATE

Indications: eczematous inflammation in otitis externa (see notes above)
Cautions: avoid prolonged use
Contra-indications: untreated infection
Side-effects: local sensitivity reactions

Predsol® (Celltech) [PoM]
Drops (for ear or eye), prednisolone sodium phosphate 0.5%. Net price 10 mL = £1.83
Excipients: include benzalkonium chloride, disodium edetate
Dose: ear, apply 2–3 drops every 2–3 hours; reduce frequency when relief obtained; *eye,* see section 11.4.1

■ With antibacterial

Predsol-N® (Celltech) [PoM]
Drops (for ear or eye), prednisolone sodium phosphate 0.5%, neomycin sulphate 0.5%. Net price 10 mL = £1.95
Excipients: include benzalkonium chloride, disodium edetate
Dose: ear, apply 2–3 drops 3–4 times daily; *eye,* see section 11.4.1

TRIAMCINOLONE ACETONIDE

Indications: eczematous inflammation in otitis externa (see notes above)
Cautions: avoid prolonged use
Contra-indications: untreated infection
Side-effects: local sensitivity reactions

■ With antibacterial

Audicort® (Goldshield) [PoM]
Ear drops, triamcinolone acetonide 0.1%, neomycin (as neomycin undecenoate) 0.35%. Net price 10 mL = £5.20
Excipients: include disodium edetate, propylene glycol, sodium metabisulphite
Dose: apply 2–5 drops into the ear 3–4 times daily; CHILD not recommended

Tri-Adcortyl Otic® (Squibb) [PoM] [symbol]
Ear ointment, triamcinolone acetonide 0.1%, gramicidin 0.025%, neomycin 0.25% (as sulphate), nystatin 100 000 units/g in *Plastibase®*. Net price 10 g = £1.58
Dose: apply into the ear 2–3 times daily; CHILD under 1 year not recommended

Anti-infective preparations

CHLORAMPHENICOL [symbol]

Indications: bacterial infection in otitis externa (but see notes above)
Cautions: avoid prolonged use (see notes above)
Side-effects: high incidence of sensitivity reactions to vehicle

Chloramphenicol (Non-proprietary) [PoM] [symbol]
Ear drops, chloramphenicol in propylene glycol, net price 5%, 10 mL = £1.40; 10%, 10 mL = £1.40
Excipients: may include propylene glycol
Available from Martindale
Dose: apply 2–3 drops into the ear 2–3 times daily

CLIOQUINOL

Indications: mild bacterial or fungal infections in otitis externa (see notes above)
Cautions: avoid prolonged use (see notes above)
Contra-indications: perforated tympanic membrane
Side-effects: local sensitivity; stains skin and clothing

■ With corticosteroid
Locorten-Vioform®, [PoM] see Flumetasone

CLOTRIMAZOLE

Indications: fungal infection in otitis externa (see notes above)
Side-effects: occasional local irritation or sensitivity

Canesten® (Bayer Consumer Care)
Solution, clotrimazole 1% in polyethylene glycol 400 (macrogol 400). Net price 20 mL = £2.43
Dose: ear, apply 2–3 times daily continuing for at least 14 days after disappearance of infection; *skin,* see section 13.10.2

FRAMYCETIN SULPHATE

Indications: see under Gentamicin
Cautions: see under Gentamicin
Contra-indications: perforated tympanic membrane (see notes above)
Side-effects: local sensitivity

■ With corticosteroid
Sofradex®, [PoM] see Dexamethasone

GENTAMICIN

Indications: bacterial infection in otitis externa (see notes above)
Cautions: avoid prolonged use (see notes above)
Contra-indications: perforated tympanic membrane (but see also notes above and section 12.1.2)
Side-effects: local sensitivity

Garamycin® (Schering-Plough) [PoM]
Drops (for ear or eye), gentamicin 0.3% (as sulphate). Net price 10 mL = £1.79
Excipients: include benzalkonium chloride
Dose: ear, apply 3–4 drops 3–4 times daily; reduce frequency when relief obtained; *eye,* see section 11.3.1

Genticin® (Roche) [PoM]
Drops (for ear or eye), gentamicin 0.3% (as sulphate). Net price 10 mL = £1.91
Excipients: include benzalkonium chloride
Dose: ear, apply 2–3 drops 3–4 times daily and at night; *eye,* see section 11.3.1

■ With corticosteroid
Gentisone HC® [PoM] see Hydrocortisone

NEOMYCIN SULPHATE

Indications: bacterial infection in otitis externa (see notes above)
Cautions: avoid prolonged use (see notes above)
Contra-indications: perforated tympanic membrane (see notes above)
Side-effects: local sensitivity

- With corticosteroid

Audicort® PoM   see Triamcinolone

Betnesol-N® PoM   see Betamethasone

Neo-Cortef® PoM   see Hydrocortisone

Otomize® PoM   see Dexamethasone

Otosporin® PoM   see Hydrocortisone

Predsol-N® PoM   see Prednisolone

Tri-Adcortyl Otic® PoM   see Triamcinolone

Vista-Methasone N® PoM   see Betamethasone

Other aural preparations

Choline salicylate is a mild analgesic but it is of doubtful value when applied topically.

Audax® (SSL) NHS

Ear drops, choline salicylate 21.6%, glycerol 12.6%. Net price 10 mL = £2.62
Excipients: include propylene glycol

12.1.2   Otitis media

Acute otitis media is the commonest cause of severe pain in small children. Many infections, especially those accompanying coryza, are caused by viruses. Most uncomplicated cases resolve without antibacterial treatment and a **simple analgesic**, such as paracetamol, may be sufficient. In children without systemic features, a **systemic antibacterial** may be started after 72 hours if there is no improvement, or earlier if there is deterioration (Table 1, section 5.1). Topical treatment of acute otitis media is ineffective and there is no place for drops containing a local anaesthetic. If the tympanic membrane has perforated, culture and sensitivity testing of any discharge is helpful in selecting an appropriate systemic antibacterial (Table 1, section 5.1).

In *recurrent acute otitis media* prophylaxis with an antibacterial (e.g. amoxicillin) during the winter months can be tried in young children who live at home and do not attend day centres. A full course of a systemic antibacterial is required if otitis media recurs.

Otitis media with effusion ('glue ear') occurs in about 10% of children and in 90% of children with cleft palates. Systemic antibacterials are not usually required for otitis media with effusion. If 'glue ear' persists for more than a month or two, the child should be referred for assessment and follow up because of the risk of long-term hearing impairment which can delay language development. Untreated or resistant glue ear may be responsible for some types of *chronic otitis media*.

The organisms recovered from patients with *chronic otitis media* are often opportunists living in the debris, keratin, and necrotic bone present in the middle ear and mastoid. Thorough cleansing with an aural suction tube may completely resolve infection of many years duration. Acute exacerbations of chronic infection may require a systemic antibacterial (Table 1, section 5.1). A swab should be taken to identify the infecting organism and its antibacterial sensitivity. Presence of *Pseudomonas aeruginosa* and *Proteus* spp. requires treatment with parenteral antibacterials. Local debridement of the meatal and middle ear contents may then be followed by topical treatment with ribbon gauze dressings as for otitis

externa (section 12.1.1). This is particularly true with infections in mastoid cavities when dusting powders can also be tried.

The CSM has stated that topical treatment with ototoxic antibacterials is contra-indicated in the presence of a perforation (section 12.1.1). However, many specialists use ear drops containing **aminoglycosides** (e.g. neomycin) or **polymyxins** if the otitis media has failed to settle with systemic antibacterials; it is considered that the pus in the middle ear associated with otitis media carries a higher risk of ototoxicity than the drops themselves. Ciprofloxacin or ofloxacin ear drops [both unlicensed; available on named-patient basis from IDIS] are an effective alternative to aminoglycoside ear drops for chronic otitis media in patients with perforation of the tympanic membrane.

12.1.3   Removal of ear wax

Wax is a normal bodily secretion which provides a protective film on the meatal skin and need only be removed if it causes deafness or interferes with a proper view of the ear drum. Syringing is generally best avoided in young children, in patients with a history of recurrent otitis externa, a history of ear-drum perforation, or previous ear surgery. A person who has hearing in one ear only should not have that ear syringed because even a very slight risk of damage is unacceptable in this situation.

Wax may be removed by syringing with water (warmed to body temperature). If necessary, wax can be softened before syringing with simple remedies such as **sodium bicarbonate** ear drops, **olive oil** ear drops or **almond oil** ear drops , which are safe, effective and inexpensive. If the wax is hard and impacted the drops may be used twice daily for a few days before syringing; otherwise the wax may be softened on the day of syringing. The patient should lie with the affected ear uppermost for 5 to 10 minutes after a generous amount of the softening remedy has been introduced into the ear. Some proprietary preparations containing organic solvents can irritate the meatal skin, and in most cases the simple remedies indicated above are just as effective and less likely to cause irritation. Docusate sodium or urea–hydrogen peroxide are ingredients in a number of proprietary preparations.

Almond Oil (Non-proprietary)
Ear drops, almond oil in a suitable container
Allow to warm to room temperature before use

Olive Oil (Non-proprietary)
Ear drops, olive oil in a suitable container
Allow to warm to room temperature before use

Sodium Bicarbonate (Non-proprietary)
Ear drops, sodium bicarbonate 5%, net price 10 mL = £1.25
Available from Thornton & Ross

Cerumol® (LAB)
Ear drops, chlorobutanol 5%, paradichlorobenzene 2%, arachis (peanut) oil 57.3%. Net price 11 mL = £1.45

Exterol® (Dermal)
Ear drops, urea–hydrogen peroxide complex 5% in glycerol. Net price 8 mL = £1.97

Molcer® (Wallace Mfg) ▭
Ear drops, docusate sodium 5%. Net price 15 mL =
£1.32
Excipients: include propylene glycol

Otex® (DDD) ▭
Ear drops, urea–hydrogen peroxide 5%. Net price
8 mL = £2.64

Waxsol® (Norgine) ▭
Ear drops, docusate sodium 0.5%. Net price 10 mL
= £1.36

12.2   Drugs acting on the nose

12.2.1	Drugs used in nasal allergy
12.2.2	Topical nasal decongestants
12.2.3	Nasal preparations for infection and epistaxis

Rhinitis is often self-limiting but bacterial sinusitis
may require treatment with antibacterials (Table 1,
section 5.1). There are few indications for nasal
sprays and drops except in allergic rhinitis and
perennial rhinitis (section 12.2.1). Many nasal preparations contain sympathomimetic drugs which
may damage the nasal cilia (section 12.2.2). Some
specialists use saline sniffs for a short period after
endonasal surgery.

NASAL POLYPS. Short-term use of corticosteroid
nasal drops helps to produce significant shrinkage of
nasal polyps; to be effective, the drops must be
administered with the patient in the 'head down'
position. The reduction in swelling can be maintained by continuing treatment with a corticosteroid
nasal spray. A short course of a systemic corticosteroid may be required initially to shrink large
polyps.

12.2.1   Drugs used in nasal allergy

Mild allergic rhinitis is controlled by topical **nasal
corticosteroids** or **oral antihistamines** (section
3.4.1); systemic nasal decongestants are of doubtful
value (section 3.10).

More persistent symptoms and nasal congestion
can be relieved by topical nasal **corticosteroids** and
cromoglicate (cromoglycate); topical antihistamines
(azelastine and levocabastine) are also used in allergic rhinitis. In seasonal allergic rhinitis (e.g. hay
fever), treatment should begin 2 to 3 weeks before
the season commences and may have to be continued
for several months; treatment may be required for
years in perennial rhinitis.

In allergic rhinitis, topical preparations of corticosteroids and cromoglicate have a well-established
role; although it may be less effective, cromoglicate
is often the first choice in children. Topical antihistamines are considered less effective than topical
corticosteroids but probably more effective than
cromoglicate.

Sometimes allergic rhinitis is accompanied by
vasomotor rhinitis. In this situation, the addition of
topical nasal ipratropium bromide (section 12.2.2)
can reduce watery rhinorrhoea.

Very disabling symptoms occasionally justify the
use of **systemic corticosteroids** for short periods
(section 6.3), for example in students taking important examinations. They may also be used at the
beginning of a course of treatment with a corticosteroid spray to relieve severe mucosal oedema and
allow the spray to penetrate the nasal cavity.

Antihistamines

AZELASTINE HYDROCHLORIDE
Indications: allergic rhinitis
Side-effects: irritation of nasal mucosa; bitter taste
(if applied incorrectly)

[1]**Rhinolast**® (Viatris) PoM
Aqueous nasal spray, azelastine hydrochloride
140 micrograms (0.14 mL)/metered spray. Net
price 20 mL (with metered pump) = £11.92
Excipients: include benzalkonium chloride, sodium edetate
Dose: ADULT and CHILD over 5 years, apply 140 micrograms (1 spray) into each nostril twice daily

1. Can be sold to the public for nasal administration in
aqueous form (other than by aerosol) if supplied for the
treatment of seasonal allergic rhinitis or perennial allergic
rhinitis in adults and children over 5 years, subject to max.
single dose of 140 micrograms per nostril, max. daily dose
of 280 micrograms per nostril, and a pack size limit of 36
doses; a proprietary brand (*Aller-eze*®) is on sale to the
public

LEVOCABASTINE
Indications: treatment of allergic rhinitis
Cautions: renal impairment (see Appendix 3)
Side-effects: nasal irritation; hypersensitivity reac-
tions, headache, fatigue, drowsiness reported

[1]**Livostin**® (Novartis) PoM
Aqueous nasal spray, levocabastine (as hydrochloride) 0.05%. Net price 10-mL spray pump =
£9.74
Excipients: include disodium edetate, propylene glycol, polysorbate 80 and benzalkonium chloride
Dose: ADULT and CHILD over 9 years, apply 2 sprays into
each nostril twice daily, increased if necessary to 3–4
times daily

1. Can be sold to the public for nasal administration if
supplied for symptomatic treatment of seasonal allergic
rhinitis in adults and children over 12 years subject to max.
strength of levocabastine 0.05% and max. pack size 10 mL;
proprietary brands on sale to the public include *Livostin*®
Direct Nasal Spray

Corticosteroids

Nasal preparations containing corticosteroids (beclometasone, betamethasone, budesonide, flunisolide,
fluticasone, mometasone, and triamcinolone) have a
useful role in the prophylaxis and treatment of
allergic rhinitis (see notes above).

CAUTIONS. Corticosteroid nasal preparations
should be avoided in the presence of untreated nasal
infections, and also after nasal surgery (until healing
has occurred); they should also be avoided in pulmonary tuberculosis. Patients transferred from systemic corticosteroids may experience exacerbation
of some symptoms. Systemic absorption may follow
nasal administration particularly if high doses are
used or if treatment is prolonged; for cautions and

side-effects of systemic corticosteroids, see section 6.3.2. The risk of systemic effects may be greater with nasal drops than with nasal sprays; drops are administered incorrectly more often than sprays. The CSM recommends that the height of children receiving prolonged treatment with nasal corticosteroids is monitored; if growth is slowed, referral to a paediatrician should be considered.

SIDE-EFFECTS. Local side-effects include dryness, irritation of nose and throat, epistaxis and rarely ulceration; nasal septal perforation (usually following nasal surgery) and raised intra-ocular pressure or glaucoma may also occur rarely. Headache, smell and taste disturbances may also occur. Hypersensitivity reactions, including bronchospasm, have been reported.

BECLOMETASONE DIPROPIONATE
(Beclomethasone Dipropionate)
Indications: prophylaxis and treatment of allergic and vasomotor rhinitis
Cautions: see notes above
Side-effects: see notes above
Dose: ADULT and CHILD over 6 years, apply 100 micrograms (2 sprays) into each nostril twice daily or 50 micrograms (1 spray) into each nostril 3–4 times daily; max. total 400 micrograms (8 sprays) daily; when symptoms controlled, dose reduced to 50 micrograms (1 spray) into each nostril twice daily

¹**Beclometasone** (Non-proprietary) PoM
Nasal spray, beclometasone dipropionate 50 micrograms/metered spray. Net price 200-spray unit = £3.44
Available from Alpharma, Generics, IVAX (*Nasobec Aqueous®*)

1. Can be sold to the public for nasal administration (other than by aerosol) if supplied for the prevention and treatment of allergic rhinitis in adults over 18 years subject to max. single dose of 100 micrograms per nostril, max. daily dose of 200 micrograms per nostril for max. 3 months, and a pack size of 20 mg; proprietary brands on sale to the public include *Beclogen®, Beconase® Allergy, Boots Hayfever Relief®, Care Hayfever Relief®, Nasobec® Hayfever, Pollenase® Hayfever, Tesco Hayfever Relief®, Vivabec®*

Beconase® (A&H) PoM
Nasal spray (aqueous suspension), beclometasone dipropionate 50 micrograms/metered spray. Net price 200-spray unit with applicator = £4.01
Excipients: include benzalkonium chloride, polysorbate 80

BETAMETHASONE SODIUM PHOSPHATE
Indications: non-infected inflammatory conditions of nose
Cautions: see notes above
Side-effects: see notes above

Betnesol® (Celltech) PoM
Drops (for ear, eye, or nose), betamethasone sodium phosphate 0.1%. Net price 10 mL = £1.84
Excipients: include benzalkonium chloride, disodium edetate
Dose: nose, apply 2–3 drops into each nostril 2–3 times daily; *ear,* section 12.1.1; *eye,* see section 11.4.1

Vista-Methasone® (Martindale) PoM
Drops (for ear, eye, or nose), betamethasone sodium phosphate 0.1%. Net price 5 mL = £1.10, 10 mL = £1.25
Excipients: include benzalkonium chloride, disodium edetate
Dose: nose, apply 2–3 drops into each nostril twice daily; *ear,* section 12.1.1; *eye,* see section 11.4.1

BUDESONIDE
Indications: prophylaxis and treatment of allergic and vasomotor rhinitis; nasal polyps
Cautions: see notes above
Side-effects: see notes above
Dose: rhinitis, ADULT and CHILD over 12 years, apply 200 micrograms (2 sprays) into each nostril once daily in the morning or 100 micrograms (1 spray) into each nostril twice daily; when control achieved reduce to 100 micrograms (1 spray) into each nostril once daily
Nasal polyps, ADULT and CHILD over 12 years, 100 micrograms (1 spray) into each nostril twice daily for up to 3 months

¹**Budesonide** (Non-proprietary) PoM
Nasal spray, budesonide 100 micrograms/metered spray, net price 100-spray unit = £5.85
Available from Generics

1. Can be sold to the public for nasal administration (other than by aerosol) if supplied for the prevention and treatment of seasonal allergic rhinitis in adults over 18 years subject to max. single dose of 200 micrograms per nostril, max. daily dose of 200 micrograms per nostril for max. period of 3 months, and a pack size of 10 mg

Rhinocort Aqua® (AstraZeneca) PoM
Nasal spray, budesonide 100 micrograms/metered spray. Net price 100-spray unit = £5.85
Excipients: include disodium edetate, polysorbate 80, potassium sorbate

DEXAMETHASONE ISONICOTINATE
Indications: treatment of allergic rhinitis
Cautions: see notes above; avoid contact with eyes
Side-effects: see notes above

■ With sympathomimetic
For cautions and side-effects of sympathomimetics see Ephedrine Hydrochloride, section 12.2.2
Dexa-Rhinaspray Duo® (Boehringer Ingelheim) PoM
Nasal spray, dexamethasone isonicotinate 20 micrograms, tramazoline hydrochloride 120 micrograms/metered spray. Net price 110-dose unit = £2.15
Excipients: include benzalkonium chloride, polysorbate 80
Dose: allergic rhinitis, ADULT and CHILD over 12 years, apply 1 spray into each nostril 2–3 times daily, max. 6 times daily; max. duration 14 days; CHILD 5–12 years 1 spray into each nostril up to twice daily; under 5 years not recommended

FLUNISOLIDE
Indications: prophylaxis and treatment of allergic rhinitis
Cautions: see notes above
Side-effects: see notes above

Syntaris® (IVAX) [PoM]
Aqueous nasal spray, flunisolide 25 micrograms/
metered spray. Net price 240-spray unit with pump
and applicator = £5.05
Excipients: include benzalkonium chloride, butylated hydroxytoluene, disodium edetate, polysorbates, propylene glycol
Dose: ADULT, apply 50 micrograms (2 sprays) into each
nostril twice daily, increased if necessary to max. 3 times
daily then reduced for maintenance; CHILD 5–14 years
initially 25 micrograms (1 spray) into each nostril up to 3
times daily

FLUTICASONE PROPIONATE

Indications: see under preparations below
Cautions: see notes above
Side-effects: see notes above

¹**Flixonase**® (A&H) [PoM]
Aqueous nasal spray, fluticasone propionate
50 micrograms/metered spray. Net price 150-spray
unit with applicator = £12.57
Excipients: include benzalkonium chloride, polysorbate 80
Dose: prophylaxis and treatment of allergic rhinitis,
ADULT and CHILD over 12 years, apply 100 micrograms
(2 sprays) into each nostril once daily, preferably in the
morning, increased to max. twice daily if required; when
control achieved reduce to 50 micrograms (1 spray) into
each nostril once daily; CHILD 4–11 years, 50 micrograms
(1 spray) into each nostril once daily, increased to max.
twice daily if required

1. Can be sold to the public for nasal administration (other
than by pressurised nasal spray) if supplied for the
prevention and treatment of allergic rhinitis in adults over
18 years, subject to max. single dose of 100 micrograms per
nostril, max. daily dose of 200 micrograms per nostril for
max. 3 months, and a pack size of 3 mg; proprietary brands
on sale to the public include *Flixonase*®*Allergy*

Flixonase Nasule® (A&H) [PoM]
Nasal drops, fluticasone propionate 400 micr-
ograms/unit dose, net price 28 × 0.4-mL units =
£14.83
Excipients: include polysorbate 20
Dose: nasal polyps, apply approx. 6 drops into each
nostril once or twice daily, consider alternative treatment
if no improvement after 4–6 weeks; CHILD not recommended

MOMETASONE FUROATE

Indications: prophylaxis and treatment of allergic
rhinitis
Cautions: see notes above
Side-effects: see notes above

Nasonex® (Schering-Plough) [PoM]
Nasal spray, mometasone furoate 50 micrograms/
metered spray. Net price 140-spray unit = £10.92
Excipients: include benzalkonium chloride, polysorbate 80
Dose: ADULT and CHILD over 12 years, apply 100 micrograms (2 sprays) into each nostril once daily, increased if
necessary to max. 200 micrograms (4 sprays) into each
nostril once daily; when control achieved reduce to
50 micrograms (1 spray) into each nostril once daily;
CHILD 6–11 years, 50 micrograms (1 spray) into each
nostril once daily

TRIAMCINOLONE ACETONIDE

Indications: prophylaxis and treatment of allergic
rhinitis
Cautions: see notes above
Side-effects: see notes above

¹**Nasacort**® (Aventis Pharma) [PoM]
Aqueous nasal spray, triamcinolone acetonide
55 micrograms/metered spray. Net price 120-spray
unit = £9.60
Excipients: include benzalkonium chloride, disodium edetate,
polysorbate 80
Dose: ADULT and CHILD over 12 years apply 110 micrograms (2 sprays) into each nostril once daily; when
control achieved, reduce to 55 micrograms (1 spray) into
each nostril once daily; CHILD 6–12 years, 55 micrograms
(1 spray) into each nostril once daily

1. Can be sold to the public for nasal administration as a non-
pressurised nasal spray if supplied for the symptomatic
treatment of seasonal allergic rhinitis in adults over 18
years, subject to max. daily dose of 110 micrograms per
nostril for max. 3 months, and a pack size of 3.575 mg

Cromoglicate

SODIUM CROMOGLICATE

(Sodium Cromoglycate)
Indications: prophylaxis of allergic rhinitis
Side-effects: local irritation; rarely transient bron-
chospasm

Rynacrom® (Pantheon)
4% aqueous nasal spray, sodium cromoglicate 4%
(5.2 mg/squeeze). Net price 22 mL with pump =
£19.10
Excipients: include benzalkonium chloride, disodium edetate
Dose: ADULT and CHILD, apply 1 squeeze into each nostril
2–4 times daily

Vividrin® (Pharma-Global)
Nasal spray, sodium cromoglicate 2%. Net price
15 mL = £8.56
Excipients: include benzalkonium chloride, edetic acid, polysorbate 80
Dose: ADULT and CHILD, apply 1 spray into each nostril
4–6 times daily

■ With sympathomimetic

Rynacrom Compound® (Pantheon)
Nasal spray, sodium cromoglicate 2% (2.6 mg/
metered spray) and xylometazoline hydrochloride
0.025% (32.5 micrograms/metered spray). Net
price 26 mL with pump = £14.33
Excipients: include benzalkonium chloride, disodium edetate
Dose: apply 1 spray into each nostril 4 times daily
NOTE. A proprietary brand of sodium cromoglicate 2%
and xylometazoline hydrochloride 0.025% (*Rynacrom
Allergy*®) is on sale to the public

12.2.2 Topical nasal decongestants

The nasal mucosa is sensitive to changes in atmo-
spheric temperature and humidity and these alone
may cause slight nasal congestion. The nose and
nasal sinuses produce a litre of mucus in 24 hours
and much of this finds its way silently into the
stomach via the nasopharynx. Slight changes in the
nasal airway, accompanied by an awareness of
mucus passing along the nasopharynx causes some
patients to be inaccurately diagnosed as suffering
from chronic sinusitis. These symptoms are particularly noticeable in the later stages of the common
cold. **Sodium chloride** 0.9% given as nasal drops
may relieve nasal congestion by helping to liquefy
mucous secretions. Corticosteroid nasal drops produce shrinkage of nasal polyps (section 12.2).

Symptoms of nasal congestion associated with vasomotor rhinitis and the common cold can be relieved by the short-term use (usually not longer than 7 days) of decongestant nasal drops and sprays. These all contain sympathomimetic drugs which exert their effect by vasoconstriction of the mucosal blood vessels which in turn reduces oedema of the nasal mucosa. They are of limited value because they can give rise to a rebound congestion (rhinitis medicamentosa) on withdrawal, due to a secondary vasodilation with a subsequent temporary increase in nasal congestion. This in turn tempts the further use of the decongestant, leading to a vicious cycle of events. **Ephedrine nasal drops** is the safest sympathomimetic preparation and can give relief for several hours. The more potent sympathomimetic drugs oxymetazoline, and xylometazoline are more likely to cause a rebound effect. **All** of these preparations may cause a hypertensive crisis if used during treatment with a monoamine-oxidase inhibitor.

Non-allergic watery rhinorrhoea often responds well to treatment with the antimuscarinic **ipratropium bromide**.

Inhalation of **warm moist air** is useful in the treatment of symptoms of acute infective conditions, and the use of compounds containing volatile substances such as menthol and eucalyptus may encourage their use (section 3.8).

Systemic nasal decongestants—see section 3.10.

Sympathomimetics

EPHEDRINE HYDROCHLORIDE

Indications: nasal congestion

Cautions: avoid excessive or prolonged use; caution in infants under 3 months (no good evidence of value—if irritation occurs might narrow nasal passage); **interactions:** Appendix 1 (sympathomimetics)

Side-effects: local irritation, nausea, headache; after excessive use tolerance with diminished effect, rebound congestion; cardiovascular effects also reported

Dose: see below

Ephedrine (Non-proprietary)
Nasal drops, ephedrine hydrochloride 0.5%, net price 10 mL = £1.13; 1%, 10 mL = £1.18
NOTE. The BP directs that if no strength is specified 0.5% drops should be supplied
Dose: instil 1–2 drops into each nostril up to 3 or 4 times daily when required

XYLOMETAZOLINE HYDROCHLORIDE

Indications: nasal congestion

Cautions: see under Ephedrine Hydrochloride and notes above

Side-effects: see under Ephedrine Hydrochloride and notes above

Dose: see below

Xylometazoline (Non-proprietary)
Nasal drops, xylometazoline hydrochloride 0.1%, net price 10 mL = £1.91
Dose: instil 2–3 drops into each nostril 2–3 times daily when required; max. duration 7 days; not recommended for children under 12 years
Available from Manx (*Otradrops®*), Novartis Consumer Health (*Otrivine®* **NHS**)
Paediatric nasal drops, xylometazoline hydrochloride 0.05%, net price 10 mL = £1.59
Dose: CHILD over 3 months instil 1–2 drops into each nostril 1–2 times daily when required (not recommended for infants under 3 months of age, doctor's advice only under 2 years); max. duration 7 days
Available from Manx (*Otradrops®*), Novartis Consumer Health (*Otrivine®* **NHS**, *Tixycolds®*)
Nasal spray, xylometazoline hydrochloride 0.1%, net price 10 mL = £1.91
Dose: apply 1 spray into each nostril 2–3 times daily when required; max. duration 7 days; not recommended for children under 12 years
Available from Manx (*Otraspray®*), Novartis Consumer Health (*Otrivine®* **NHS**)

■ Preparations on Sale to the Public
Sympathomimetic nasal preparations on sale to the public (not prescribable on the NHS) include:
Afrazine® (oxymetazoline), **Dristan®** (oxymetazoline), **Fenox®** (phenylephrine), **Non Drowsy Sudafed Decongestant Nasal Spray®** (xylometazoline), **Sudafed®** nasal spray (oxymetazoline), **Vicks Sinex®** (oxymetazoline)

Antimuscarinic

IPRATROPIUM BROMIDE

Indications: rhinorrhoea associated with allergic and non-allergic rhinitis

Cautions: see section 3.1.2; avoid spraying near eyes

Side-effects: nasal dryness and epistaxis

Dose: apply 42 micrograms (2 sprays) into each nostril 2–3 times daily; CHILD under 12 years not recommended

Rinatec® (Boehringer Ingelheim) PoM
Nasal spray 0.03%, ipratropium bromide 21 micrograms/metered spray. Net price 180-dose unit = £4.55
Excipients: include benzalkonium chloride

12.2.3 Nasal preparations for infection and epistaxis

There is **no** evidence that topical anti-infective nasal preparations have any therapeutic value in rhinitis or sinusitis; for elimination of nasal staphylococci, see below.

Systemic treatment of sinusitis—see section 5.1, table 1.

Betnesol-N® (Celltech) PoM
Drops (for ear, eye, or nose), betamethasone sodium phosphate 0.1%, neomycin sulphate 0.5%. Net price 10 mL = £1.89
Excipients: include benzalkonium chloride
Dose: nose, apply 2–3 drops into nostril 2–3 times daily; *eye*, see section 11.4.1; *ear*, see section 12.1.1

¹**Locabiotal**® (Servier) PoM NHS ▭
Spray, fusafungine 500 micrograms/metered spray. Net price 50-spray unit with nasal (yellow) and oral (white) adapters = £1.55
Excipients: include alcohol
Dose: infection and inflammation of upper respiratory tract (but not recommended, see notes above), 1 spray into each nostril or into mouth every 4 hours; CHILD 1 spray into each nostril or into mouth every 6 hours; withdraw if no improvement after 7 days

1. NHS Except for treatment of infections and inflammation of the oropharynx and endorsed 'SLS'

Vista-Methasone N® (Martindale) PoM ▭
Drops (for ear, eye, or nose), betamethasone sodium phosphate 0.1%, neomycin sulphate 0.5%. Net price 5 mL = £1.17, 10 mL = £1.29
Excipients: include thiomersal
Dose: nose, apply 2–3 drops into each nostril twice daily; *eye,* see section 11.4.1; *ear,* see section 12.1.1

Nasal staphylococci

Elimination of organisms such as staphylococci from the nasal vestibule can be achieved by the use of a cream containing **chlorhexidine and neomycin** (*Naseptin*®), but re-colonisation frequently occurs. Coagulase-positive staphylococci are present in the noses of 40% of the population.

A nasal ointment containing **mupirocin** is also available; it should probably be held in reserve for resistant cases. In hospital, mupirocin nasal ointment should be reserved for the eradication (in both patients and staff) of nasal carriage of methicillin-resistant *Staphylococcus aureus* (MRSA). The ointment should be applied 3 times daily for 5 days and a sample taken 2 days after treatment to confirm eradication. The course may be repeated if the sample is positive (and the throat is not colonised). To avoid the development of resistance, the treatment course should not exceed 7 days and the course should not be repeated on more than one occasion. If the MRSA strain is mupirocin-resistant or does not respond after 2 courses, consider alternative products such as chlorhexidine and neomycin cream.

Bactroban Nasal® (GSK) PoM
Nasal ointment, mupirocin 2% (as calcium salt) in white soft paraffin basis. Net price 3 g = £6.24
Dose: for eradication of nasal carriage of staphylococci, including methicillin-resistant *Staphylococcus aureus* (MRSA), apply 2–3 times daily to the inner surface of each nostril

Naseptin® (Alliance) PoM
Cream, chlorhexidine hydrochloride 0.1%, neomycin sulphate 0.5%, net price 15 g = £1.48
Excipients: include arachis (peanut) oil, cetostearyl alcohol
Dose: for eradication of nasal carriage of staphylococci, apply to nostrils 4 times daily for 10 days; for preventing nasal carriage of staphylococci apply to nostrils twice daily

Epistaxis

Bismuth iodoform paraffin paste (BIPP) is used for packing cavities after ear, nose and oropharyngeal surgery as a mild disinfectant and astringent; it is also used to pack nasal cavities in acute epistaxis. It is available either as a paste, to be applied to ribbon gauze packing, or as BIPP-impregnated ribbon gauze.

BISMUTH SUBNITRATE AND IODOFORM

Indications: packing cavities after ear, nose or oropharyngeal surgery; epistaxis
Cautions: hyperthyroidism
Side-effects: erythematous rash (discontinue use); encephalopathy reported only with large packs or when placed directly on neural tissue

Bismuth Subnitrate and Iodoform (Non-proprietary)
Paste, 30-g sachet, net price = £9.50; 30-g tube = £9.50
Available from Aurum
Impregnated gauze, sterile, net price 1.25 cm × 100 cm, 10 = £89.70; 1.25 cm × 125 cm, 5 = £44.85; 1.25 cm × 200 cm, 5 = £62.05; 1.25 cm × 300 cm, 5 = £81.15; 2.5 cm × 100 cm, 10 = £97.20; 2.5 cm × 125 cm, 5 = £48.60; 2.5 cm × 200 cm, 5 = £70.35; 2.5 cm × 300 cm, 5 = £92.55
Available from Aurum

12.3 Drugs acting on the oropharynx

12.3.1 Drugs for oral ulceration and inflammation
12.3.2 Oropharyngeal anti-infective drugs
12.3.3 Lozenges and sprays
12.3.4 Mouthwashes, gargles, and dentifrices
12.3.5 Treatment of dry mouth

12.3.1 Drugs for oral ulceration and inflammation

Ulceration of the oral mucosa may be caused by trauma (physical or chemical), recurrent aphthae, infections, carcinoma, dermatological disorders, nutritional deficiencies, gastro-intestinal disease, haematopoietic disorders, and drug therapy. It is important to establish the diagnosis in each case as the majority of these lesions require specific management in addition to local treatment. Patients with an unexplained mouth ulcer of more than 3 weeks' duration require urgent referral to hospital to exclude oral cancer. Local treatment aims at protecting the ulcerated area, or at relieving pain or reducing inflammation.

SIMPLE MOUTHWASHES. A **saline** or **compound thymol glycerin** mouthwash (section 12.3.4) may relieve the pain of traumatic ulceration. The mouthwash is made up with warm water and used at frequent intervals until the discomfort and swelling subsides.

ANTISEPTIC MOUTHWASHES. Secondary bacterial infection may be a feature of any mucosal ulceration; it can increase discomfort and delay healing. Use of a **chlorhexidine** or **povidone–iodine** mouthwash (section 12.3.4) is often beneficial and may accelerate healing of recurrent aphthae.

MECHANICAL PROTECTION. **Carmellose gelatin paste** may relieve some discomfort arising from ulceration by protecting the ulcer site. The paste adheres to the mucosa, but is difficult to apply effectively to some parts of the mouth. *Gelclair®* is available for the management of oral lesions; it forms a film of povidone and sodium hyaluronate on the lesion.

CORTICOSTEROIDS. Topical corticosteroid therapy may be used for some forms of oral ulceration. In the case of aphthous ulcers it is most effective if applied in the 'prodromal' phase.

Thrush or other types of candidiasis are recognised complications of corticosteroid treatment.

Hydrocortisone oromucosal tablets are allowed to dissolve next to an ulcer and are useful in recurrent aphthae and erosive lichenoid lesions.

Triamcinolone dental paste is designed to keep the corticosteroid in contact with the mucosa for long enough to permit penetration of the lesion, but is difficult for patients to apply properly.

Systemic corticosteroid therapy (section 6.3.2) is reserved for severe conditions such as pemphigus vulgaris.

LOCAL ANALGESICS. Local analgesics have a limited role in the management of oral ulceration. When applied topically their action is of a relatively short duration so that analgesia cannot be maintained continuously throughout the day. The main indication for a topical local analgesic is to relieve the pain of otherwise intractable oral ulceration particularly when it is due to major aphthae. For this purpose lidocaine (lignocaine) 5% ointment or lozenges containing a local anaesthetic are applied to the ulcer. When local anaesthetics are used in the mouth care must be taken not to produce anaesthesia of the pharynx before meals as this might lead to choking.

Benzydamine mouthwash or spray may be useful in palliating the discomfort associated with a variety of ulcerative conditions. It has also been found to be effective in reducing the discomfort of post-irradiation mucositis. Some patients find the full-strength mouthwash causes some stinging and, for them, it should be diluted with an equal volume of water. **Flurbiprofen** lozenges are licensed for the relief of sore throat.

Choline salicylate dental gel has some analgesic action and may provide relief for recurrent aphthae, but excessive application or confinement under a denture irritates the mucosa and can itself cause ulceration. Benefit in teething may merely be due to pressure of application (comparable with biting a teething ring); excessive use can lead to salicylate poisoning.

OTHER PREPARATIONS. **Carbenoxolone** gel or mouthwash may be of some value for mild oral and perioral lesions. **Doxycycline** rinsed in the mouth may also be of value for severe recurrent aphthous ulceration.

PERIODONTITIS. Low-dose doxycycline (*Periostat®*) is licensed as an adjunct to scaling and root planing for the treatment of periodontitis; doxycycline reduces collagenase activity at a low dose without inhibiting bacteria associated with periodontitis. For anti-infectives used in the treatment of periodontal disease, see section 12.3.2. For

mouthwashes used for oral hygiene and plaque inhibition, see section 12.3.4.

BENZYDAMINE HYDROCHLORIDE

Indications: painful inflammatory conditions of oropharynx

Side-effects: occasional numbness or stinging; rarely hypersensitivity reactions

Difflam® (3M)

Oral rinse, green, benzydamine hydrochloride 0.15%, net price 200 mL (*Difflam® Sore Throat Rinse*) = £2.83; 300 mL = £4.31

Dose: rinse or gargle, using 15 mL (diluted with water if stinging occurs) every 1½–3 hours as required, usually for not more than 7 days; not suitable for children aged 12 years or under

Spray, benzydamine hydrochloride 0.15%. Net price 30-mL unit = £3.41

Dose: ADULT, 4–8 puffs onto affected area every 1½–3 hours; CHILD under 6 years 1 puff per 4 kg body-weight to max. 4 puffs every 1½–3 hours; 6–12 years 4 puffs every 1½–3 hours

CARBENOXOLONE SODIUM

Indications: mild oral and perioral lesions

Bioral Gel® (Merck Consumer Health)

Gel, carbenoxolone sodium 2% in adhesive basis. Net price 5 g = £2.38

Dose: apply after meals and at bedtime

Bioplex® (APS) [PoM]

Mouthwash granules, carbenoxolone sodium 1% (20 mg/sachet). Net price 24 × 2-g sachets = £8.85

Dose: for mouth ulcers, rinse with 1 sachet in 30–50 mL of warm water 3 times daily and at bedtime

CARMELLOSE SODIUM

Indications: mechanical protection of oral and perioral lesions

Orabase® (ConvaTec)

Protective paste (= oral paste), carmellose sodium 16.7%, pectin 16.7%, gelatin 16.7%, in *Plastibase®*. Net price 30 g = £1.91; 100 g = £4.24

Dose: apply a thin layer when necessary after meals

Orahesive® (ConvaTec)

Powder, carmellose sodium, pectin, gelatin, equal parts. Net price 25 g = £2.20

Dose: sprinkle on the affected area

CORTICOSTEROIDS

Indications: oral and perioral lesions

Contra-indications: untreated oral infection; manufacturer of triamcinolone contra-indicates use on tuberculous and viral lesions

Side-effects: occasional exacerbation of local infection

[1]**Adcortyl in Orabase®** (Squibb) [PoM]

Oral paste, triamcinolone acetonide 0.1% in adhesive basis. Net price 10 g = £1.27

Dose: ADULT and CHILD, apply a thin layer 2–4 times daily; do not rub in; use limited to 5 days for children and short-term use also advised for elderly

1. A 5-g tube (*Adcortyl in Orabase® for Mouth Ulcers*) is on sale to the public for the treatment of common mouth ulcers for max. 5 days

Corlan® (Celltech)
Pellets (= oromucosal tablets), hydrocortisone
2.5 mg (as sodium succinate). Net price 20 = £2.10
Dose: ADULT and CHILD, 1 lozenge 4 times daily, allowed
to dissolve slowly in the mouth in contact with the ulcer

DOXYCYCLINE

Indications: see preparations; oral herpes (section
12.3.2)
Cautions: section 5.1.3; monitor for superficial
fungal infection, particularly, if predisposition to
oral candidiasis
Contra-indications: section 5.1.3
Side-effects: section 5.1.3; fungal superinfection
Dose: see preparations

Periostat (CollaGenex) PoM
Tablets, f/c, doxycycline (as hyclate) 20 mg, net
price 56-tab pack = £16.50. Label: 6, 11, 27,
counselling, posture
Dose: periodontitis (as an adjunct to gingival scaling and
root planing), 20 mg twice daily for 3 months; CHILD
under 12 years not recommended
COUNSELLING. Tablets should be swallowed whole with
plenty of fluid, while sitting or standing

■ Local application
For severe recurrent aphthous ulceration, the contents of a 100 mg doxycycline capsule can be stirred
into a small amount of water then rinsed around the
mouth for 2–3 minutes 4 times daily usually for 3
days; it should preferably not be swallowed [unli-
censed indication].
NOTE. Doxycycline stains teeth; avoid in children under 12
years of age

FLURBIPROFEN

Indications: relief of sore throat
Cautions: see section 10.1.1
Contra-indications: see section 10.1.1
Side-effects: taste disturbance, mouth ulcers (move
lozenge around mouth); see also section 10.1.1

Strefen® (Crookes)
Lozenges, flurbiprofen 8.75 mg, net price 16 = £2.00
Dose: allow 1 lozenge to dissolve slowly in the mouth
every 3–6 hours, max. 5 lozenges in 24 hours, for max. 3
days; CHILD under 12 years not recommended

LOCAL ANAESTHETICS

Indications: relief of pain in oral lesions
Cautions: avoid prolonged use; hypersensitivity

■ Preparations
Local anaesthetics are included in some mouth ulcer
preparations, for details see below
  Local anaesthetics are also included in some throat
lozenges and sprays, see section 12.3.3

SALICYLATES

Indications: mild oral and perioral lesions
Cautions: not to be applied to dentures—leave at
least 30 minutes before re-insertion of dentures;
frequent application, especially in children, may
give rise to salicylate poisoning
NOTE. CSM warning on aspirin and Reye's syndrome
does not apply to non-aspirin salicylates or to topical
preparations such as teething gels

■ Choline salicylate
Choline Salicylate Dental Gel, BP
Oral gel, choline salicylate 8.7% in a flavoured gel
basis
Available as *Bonjela*® (R&C), net price 15 g (sugar-free) =
£1.72; *Dinnefords Teejel*® (SSL), 10 g = £1.40
Dose: apply ½-inch of gel with gentle massage not more
often than every 3 hours; CHILD over 4 months ¼-inch of
gel not more than every 3 hours; max. 6 applications
daily

■ Salicylic acid
Pyralvex® (Norgine)
Oral paint, brown, rhubarb extract (anthraquinone
glycosides 0.5%), salicylic acid 1%. Net price
10 mL with brush = £1.65
Dose: apply 3–4 times daily; CHILD under 12 years not
recommended

■ Preparations on Sale to the Public
The following list includes topical treatments for
mouth ulcers and for teething on sale to the public,
together with their active ingredients:
Anbesol Liquid® and **Anbesol Teething gel**® (cetylpyridinium, chlorocresol, lidocaine (lignocaine)), **Ban-
sor**® (cetrimide), **Bioral Gel**® (carbenoxolone),
Bonjela gel® (cetalkonium chloride, choline salicylate),
Bonjela Teething gel® (cetalkonium chloride, lidocaine
(lignocaine)), **Calgel**® (cetylpyridinium, lidocaine
(lignocaine)), **Dentinox Teething gel**® (cetylpyridinium,
lidocaine (lignocaine)), **Dinnefords Teejel**® (choline
salicylate), **Frador**® (chlorobutanol, menthol), **Medijel**®
(aminoacridine (aminacrine), lidocaine (lignocaine)),
Pyralvex® (anthraquinone glycoside, salicylic acid), **Rinstead Adult gel**® (benzocaine, chloroxylenol), **Rinstead
Contact pastilles**® (lidocaine (lignocaine)), **Rinstead
pastilles**® (cetylpyridinium, menthol), **Rinstead Teething gel**® (cetylpyridinium, lidocaine (lignocaine)),
Woodward's Teething gel® (cetylpyridinium, lidocaine
(lignocaine))

12.3.2 **Oropharyngeal anti-infective drugs**

The most common cause of a sore throat is a viral
infection which does not benefit from anti-infective
treatment. Streptococcal sore throats require systemic **penicillin** therapy (section 5.1, table 1). Acute
ulcerative gingivitis (Vincent's infection) responds to
systemic **metronidazole** 200 mg 3 times daily for 3
days (section 5.1.11).
  Preparations administered in the dental surgery for
the local treatment of periodontal disease include
gels of metronidazole (*Elyzol*®, Colgate-Palmolive)
and of minocycline (*Dentomycin*®, Blackwell).

Fungal infections

Candida albicans may cause thrush and other forms
of stomatitis which are sometimes associated with
the use of broad-spectrum antibacterials or of
cytotoxics; withdrawing the causative drug may lead
to rapid resolution. Otherwise, an antifungal drug
may be effective.
  Of the antifungal drugs used for mouth infections,
amphotericin and **nystatin** are not absorbed from

the gastro-intestinal tract and are used by local application in the mouth. **Miconazole** occupies an intermediate position since it is used by local application in the mouth but is also absorbed to the extent that potential interactions need to be considered. **Fluconazole** and **itraconazole** are absorbed when taken by mouth and are available for administration by mouth for oropharyngeal candidiasis (section 5.2). For advice on prevention of fungal infections in immunocompromised patients see p. 293.

AMPHOTERICIN

Indications: oral and perioral fungal infections
Side-effects: mild gastro-intestinal disturbances reported

Fungilin® (Squibb) PoM
Lozenges, yellow, amphotericin 10 mg. Net price 60-lozenge pack = £3.95. Label: 9, 24, counselling, after food
Dose: allow 1 lozenge to dissolve slowly in the mouth 4 times daily for 10–15 days (continued for 48 hours after lesions have resolved); increase to 8 daily if infection severe
Oral suspension, yellow, sugar-free, amphotericin 100 mg/mL. Net price 12 mL with pipette = £2.31. Label: 9, counselling, use of pipette, hold in mouth, after food
Dose: place 1 mL in the mouth after food and retain near lesions 4 times daily for 14 days (continued for 48 hours after lesions have resolved)

MICONAZOLE

Indications: see under Preparations; intestinal fungal infections (section 5.2)
Cautions: pregnancy and breast-feeding; avoid in porphyria (section 9.8.2); **interactions:** Appendix 1 (antifungals, imidazole)
Contra-indications: hepatic impairment
Side-effects: nausea and vomiting, diarrhoea (with long-term treatment); rarely allergic reactions; isolated reports of hepatitis

¹**Daktarin®** (Janssen-Cilag) PoM
Oral gel, sugar-free, orange-flavoured, miconazole 24 mg/mL (20 mg/g). Net price 15-g tube = £2.37, 80-g tube = £5.00. Label: 9, counselling, hold in mouth, after food
Dose: prevention and treatment of oral fungal infections, place 5–10 mL in the mouth after food and retain near lesions 4 times daily; CHILD under 2 years 2.5 mL twice daily, 2–6 years 5 mL twice daily, over 6 years 5 mL 4 times daily; treatment continued for 48 hours after lesions have resolved
Localised lesions, smear small amount on affected area with clean finger 4 times daily (dental prostheses should be removed at night and brushed with gel)
1. 15-g tube can be sold to the public

NYSTATIN

Indications: oral and perioral fungal infections
Side-effects: oral irritation and sensitisation, nausea reported; see also section 5.2
Dose: (as pastilles or as suspension) ADULT and CHILD, 100 000 units 4 times daily after food,

usually for 7 days (continued for 48 hours after lesions have resolved)
NOTE. Unlicensed for treating candidiasis in NEONATE under 1 month. Immunosuppressed ADULT and CHILD over 1 month may require higher doses (e.g. 500 000 units 4 times daily)
Prophylaxis, NEONATE 100 000 units once daily

Nystatin (Non-proprietary) PoM
Oral suspension, nystatin 100 000 units/mL. Net price 30 mL = £1.96. Label: 9, counselling, hold in mouth, after food
Available from Hillcross, Rosemont (*Nystamont®*, sugar-free)

Nystan® (Squibb) PoM
Pastilles, yellow/brown, nystatin 100 000 units. Net price 28-pastille pack = £3.24. Label: 9, 24, counselling, after food
Oral suspension, yellow, nystatin 100 000 units/mL. Net price 30 mL with pipette = £2.05. Label: 9, counselling, use of pipette, hold in mouth, after food

Viral infections

The management of herpes infections of the mouth is a soft diet, adequate fluid intake, analgesics as required, and the use of **chlorhexidine** mouthwash (section 12.3.4) to control plaque accumulation if toothbrushing is painful. In the case of severe herpetic stomatitis, systemic **aciclovir** is required (section 5.3). Aciclovir cream (section 13.10.3) is licensed for the treatment of labial herpes simplex infections.

Herpes infections of the mouth may also respond to **doxycycline** (section 12.3.1) rinsed in the mouth.

12.3.3 Lozenges and sprays

There is no convincing evidence that antiseptic lozenges and sprays have a beneficial action and they sometimes irritate and cause sore tongue and sore lips. Some of these preparations also contain local anaesthetics which relieve pain but may cause sensitisation.

■ Preparations on Sale to the Public
The following list includes throat lozenges and sprays on sale to the public, together with their significant ingredients.
AAA® (benzocaine), **Beechams Throat Plus®** (benzalkonium, hexylresorcinol), **Bradosol®** (benzalkonium), **Bradosol Plus®** (domiphen, lidocaine (lignocaine)), **Dequacaine®** (benzocaine, dequalinium), **Dequadin®** (dequalinium), **Dequaspray®** (lidocaine (lignocaine)), **Eludril®** spray (tetracaine (amethocaine), chlorhexidine), **Labosept®** (dequalinium), **Meggezones®** (menthol), **Mentholatum®** lozenges (amylmetacresol, menthol), **Merocaine®** (benzocaine, cetylpyridinium), **Merocets®** lozenges (cetylpyridinium), **Merocets Plus®** lozenges (cetylpyridinium, menthol), **Strepsils®** lozenges (amylmetacresol, dichlorobenzyl alcohol), **Strepsils Extra®** lozenges (hexylresorcinol), **Strepsils Pain Relief Spray®** (lidocaine (lignocaine)), **TCP®** pastilles (phenols), **Tyrozets®** (benzocaine, tyrothricin), **Vicks Ultra Chloraseptic®** (benzocaine)

12.3.4 Mouthwashes, gargles, and dentifrices

Mouthwashes have a mechanical cleansing action and freshen the mouth; warm **compound sodium chloride mouthwash** is as useful as any.

Mouthwashes containing an oxidising agent, such as **hydrogen peroxide**, may be useful in the treatment of acute ulcerative gingivitis (Vincent's infection) since the organisms involved are anaerobes. It also has a mechanical cleansing effect due to frothing when in contact with oral debris.

There is evidence that **chlorhexidine** has a specific effect in inhibiting the formation of plaque on teeth. A chlorhexidine mouthwash may be useful as an adjunct to other oral hygiene measures for oral infection or when toothbrushing is not possible.

Povidone–iodine mouthwash is useful for mucosal infections but does not inhibit plaque accumulation. It should not be used for periods longer than 14 days because a significant amount of iodine is absorbed.

There is no convincing evidence that gargles are effective.

CHLORHEXIDINE GLUCONATE

Indications: see under preparations below

Side-effects: mucosal irritation (if desquamation occurs, discontinue treatment or dilute mouthwash with an equal volume of water); reversible brown staining of teeth, and of silicate or composite restorations; tongue discoloration; parotid gland swelling reported

NOTE. Chlorhexidine gluconate may be incompatible with some ingredients in toothpaste; leave an interval of at least 30 minutes between using mouthwash and toothpaste

Chlorhexidine (Non-proprietary)
Mouthwash, chlorhexidine gluconate 0.2%, net price 300 mL = £1.83
Dose: oral hygiene and plaque inhibition, rinse mouth with 10 mL for about 1 minute twice daily
Denture stomatitis, cleanse and soak dentures in mouthwash solution for 15 minutes twice daily
Available from Blackwell (original, aniseed-, or mint-flavoured)

Chlorohex® (Colgate-Palmolive)
Chlorohex 1200® mouthwash, chlorhexidine gluconate 0.12% (mint-flavoured). Net price 300 mL = £2.20
Dose: oral hygiene and plaque inhibition, rinse mouth with 15 mL for about 30 seconds twice daily

Corsodyl® (GSK Consumer Healthcare)
Dental gel, chlorhexidine gluconate 1%. Net price 50 g = £1.21
Dose: oral hygiene and plaque inhibition and gingivitis, brush on the teeth once or twice daily
Oral candidiasis and management of aphthous ulcers, apply to affected areas once or twice daily
Mouthwash, chlorhexidine gluconate 0.2%. Net price 300 mL (original or mint) = £1.81, 600 mL (mint) = £3.62
Dose: oral hygiene and plaque inhibition, oral candidiasis, gingivitis, and management of aphthous ulcers, rinse mouth with 10 mL for about 1 minute twice daily
Denture stomatitis, cleanse and soak dentures in mouthwash solution for 15 minutes twice daily

Oral spray, chlorhexidine gluconate 0.2% (mint-flavoured). Net price 60 mL = £4.10
Dose: oral hygiene and plaque inhibition, oral candidiasis, and management of aphthous ulcers, apply as required to tooth, gingival, or ulcer surfaces using up to 12 actuations (approx. 0.14 mL/actuation) twice daily

■ With chlorobutanol

Eludril® (Ceuta)
Mouthwash or *gargle*, chlorhexidine gluconate 0.1%, chlorobutanol 0.5% (mint-flavoured), net price 90 mL = £1.22, 250 mL = £2.56, 500 mL = £4.64
Dose: oral hygiene, plaque inhibition, minor throat infections, use 10–15 mL (diluted with warm water in measuring cup provided) 2–3 times daily
Denture disinfection, soak previously cleansed dentures in mouthwash (diluted with 2 volumes of water) for 60 minutes

HEXETIDINE

Indications: oral hygiene

Oraldene® (Warner Lambert)
Mouthwash or *gargle*, red, hexetidine 0.1%. Net price 100 mL = £1.31; 200 mL = £2.02
Dose: use 15 mL undiluted 2–3 times daily

OXIDISING AGENTS

Indications: oral hygiene, see notes above

Hydrogen Peroxide Mouthwash, BP
Mouthwash, consists of Hydrogen Peroxide Solution 6% (= approx. 20 volume) BP
Dose: rinse the mouth for 2–3 minutes with 15 mL diluted in half a tumblerful of warm water 2–3 times daily

Peroxyl® (Colgate-Palmolive)
Mouthwash, hydrogen peroxide 1.5%, net price 300 mL = £2.81
Dose: rinse the mouth with 10 mL for about 1 minute up to 4 times daily (after meals and at bedtime)

POVIDONE–IODINE

Indications: oral hygiene
Cautions: pregnancy (Appendix 4); breast-feeding (Appendix 5); see also notes above
Contra-indications: avoid regular use in patients with thyroid disorders or those receiving lithium therapy
Side-effects: idiosyncratic mucosal irritation and hypersensitivity reactions; may interfere with thyroid-function tests and with tests for occult blood

Betadine® (SSL)
Mouthwash or *gargle*, amber, povidone-iodine 1%. Net price 250 mL = £1.12
Dose: adults and children over 6 years, up to 10 mL undiluted or diluted with an equal quantity of warm water for up to 30 seconds up to 4 times daily for up to 14 days

SODIUM CHLORIDE

Indications: oral hygiene, see notes above

Sodium Chloride Mouthwash, Compound, BP
Mouthwash, sodium bicarbonate 1%, sodium chloride 1.5% in a suitable vehicle with a peppermint flavour.
Dose: extemporaneous preparations should be prepared according to the following formula: sodium chloride 1.5 g, sodium bicarbonate 1 g, concentrated peppermint emulsion 2.5 mL, double-strength chloroform emulsion 50 mL, water to 100 mL
To be diluted with an equal volume of warm water

THYMOL

Indications: oral hygiene, see notes above

Mouthwash Solution-tablets
Consist of tablets which may contain antimicrobial, colouring, and flavouring agents in a suitable soluble effervescent basis to make a mouthwash suitable for dental purposes.
Dose: dissolve 1 tablet in a tumblerful of warm water

12.3.5 Treatment of dry mouth

Dry mouth (xerostomia) may be caused by drugs with antimuscarinic (anticholinergic) side-effects (e.g. antispasmodics, tricyclic antidepressants, and some antipsychotics), by irradiation of the head and neck region or by damage to or disease of the salivary glands. Patients with a persistently dry mouth may develop a burning or scalded sensation and have poor oral hygiene; they may develop increased dental caries, periodontal disease, intolerance of dentures, and oral infections (particularly candidiasis). Dry mouth may be relieved in many patients by simple measures such as frequent sips of cool drinks or sucking pieces of ice or sugar-free fruit pastilles. Sugar-free chewing gum stimulates salivation in patients with residual salivary function.

An **artificial saliva** can provide useful relief of dry mouth. A properly balanced artificial saliva should be of a neutral pH and contain electrolytes (including fluoride) to correspond approximately to the composition of saliva. Of the proprietary preparations available, *Luborant* is licensed for any condition giving rise to a dry mouth; *Biotène Oralbalance*, *BioXtra*, *Glandosane*, *Saliva Orthana*, and *Saliveze*, have ACBS approval for dry mouth associated only with radiotherapy or sicca syndrome. *Salivix* pastilles, which act locally as salivary stimulants, are also available and have similar ACBS approval. *SST* tablets may be prescribed for dry mouth in patients with salivary gland impairment (and patent salivary ducts).

Pilocarpine tablets are licensed for the treatment of xerostomia following irradiation for head and neck cancer and for dry mouth and dry eyes (xerophthalmia) in Sjögren's syndrome. They are effective only in patients who have some residual salivary gland function, and therefore should be withdrawn if there is no response.

Local treatment

AS Saliva Orthana® (AS Pharma)
Oral spray, gastric mucin 3.5%, xylitol 2%, sodium fluoride 4.2 mg/litre, with preservatives and flavouring agents. Net price 50-mL bottle = £4.25; 450-mL refill = £29.69
Lozenges, mucin 65 mg, xylitol 59 mg, in a sorbitol basis. Net price 45-lozenge pack = £3.02
Dose: ACBS: patients suffering from dry mouth as a result of having (or having undergone) radiotherapy, or sicca syndrome, spray 2–3 times onto oral and pharyngeal mucosa, when required
NOTE. *AS Saliva Orthana®* lozenges do not contain fluoride

Glandosane® (Fresenius Kabi)
Aerosol spray, carmellose sodium 500 mg, sorbitol 1.5 g, potassium chloride 60 mg, sodium chloride 42.2 mg, magnesium chloride 2.6 mg, calcium chloride 7.3 mg, and dipotassium hydrogen phosphate 17.1 mg/50 g. Net price 50-mL unit (neutral, lemon or peppermint flavoured) = £4.35
Dose: ACBS: patients suffering from dry mouth as a result of having (or having undergone) radiotherapy, or sicca syndrome, spray onto oral and pharyngeal mucosa as required

Luborant® (Antigen)
Oral spray, pink, sorbitol 1.8 g, carmellose sodium (sodium carboxymethylcellulose) 390 mg, dibasic potassium phosphate 48.23 mg, potassium chloride 37.5 mg, monobasic potassium phosphate 21.97 mg, calcium chloride 9.972 mg, magnesium chloride 3.528 mg, sodium fluoride 258 micrograms/60 mL, with preservatives and colouring agents. Net price 60-mL unit = £3.96
Dose: saliva deficiency, 2–3 sprays onto oral mucosa up to 4 times daily, or as directed
NOTE. May be difficult to obtain

Biotène Oralbalance® (Anglian)
Saliva replacement gel, lactoperoxidase, lactoferrin, lysozyme, glucose oxidase, xylitol in a gel basis, net price 50-g tube = £4.10
Dose: ACBS: patients suffering from dry mouth as a result of having (or having undergone) radiotherapy, or sicca syndrome, apply to gums and tongue as required
NOTE. Avoid use with toothpastes containing detergents (including foaming agents)

BioXtra® (Molar)
Gel, lactoperoxidase, lactoferrin, lysozyme, whey colostrum, xylitol and other ingredients, net price 40-mL tube = £2.25
Dose: ACBS: patients suffering from dry mouth as a result of having (or having undergone) radiotherapy, or sicca syndrome, apply to oral mucosa as required

Saliveze® (Wyvern)
Oral spray, carmellose sodium (sodium carboxymethylcellulose), calcium chloride, magnesium chloride, potassium chloride, sodium chloride, and dibasic sodium phosphate. Net price 50-mL bottle (mint-flavoured) = £3.50
Dose: ACBS: patients suffering from dry mouth as a result of having (or having undergone) radiotherapy, or sicca syndrome, 1 spray onto oral mucosa as required

Salivix® (Provalis)
Pastilles, sugar-free, reddish-amber, acacia, malic acid and other ingredients. Net price 50-pastille pack = £2.86
Dose: ACBS: patients suffering from dry mouth as a result of having (or having undergone) radiotherapy, or sicca syndrome, suck 1 pastille when required

SST (Sinclair)
Tablets, sugar-free, citric acid, malic acid and other ingredients in a sorbitol base, net price 100-tab pack = £4.86
Dose: symptomatic treatment of dry mouth in patients with impaired salivary gland function and patent salivary ducts, allow 1 tablet to dissolve slowly in the mouth when required

Systemic treatment

PILOCARPINE HYDROCHLORIDE

Indications: xerostomia following irradiation for head and neck cancer (see also notes above); dry mouth and dry eyes in Sjögren's syndrome

Cautions: asthma and chronic obstructive pulmonary disease (avoid if uncontrolled, see Contraindications), cardiovascular disease (avoid if uncontrolled); cholelithiasis or biliary-tract disease, peptic ulcer, hepatic impairment (Appendix 2), renal impairment; risk of increased urethral smooth muscle tone and renal colic; maintain adequate fluid intake to avoid dehydration associated with excessive sweating; cognitive or psychiatric disturbances; angle-closure glaucoma; **interactions:** Appendix 1 (parasympathomimetics)

COUNSELLING. Blurred vision or dizziness may affect performance of skilled tasks (e.g. driving) particularly at night or in reduced lighting

Contra-indications: uncontrolled asthma and chronic obstructive pulmonary disease (increased bronchial secretions and increased airways resistance); uncontrolled cardiorenal disease; acute iritis; pregnancy and breast-feeding

Side-effects: headache, influenza-like syndrome, increased urinary frequency, sweating; less frequently, nausea, vomiting, abdominal pain, dyspepsia, diarrhoea, constipation, flushing, hypertension, palpitations, rhinitis, dizziness, asthenia, lacrimation, conjunctivitis, visual disturbances, ocular pain, rash, pruritus; rarely, flatulence, urinary urgency

Dose: xerostomia following irradiation for head and neck cancer, 5 mg 3 times daily with or immediately after meals (last dose always with evening meal); if tolerated but response insufficient after 4 weeks, may be increased to max. 30 mg daily in divided doses; max. therapeutic effect normally within 4–8 weeks; discontinue if no improvement after 2–3 months; CHILD not recommended

Dry mouth and dry eyes in Sjögren's syndrome, 5 mg 4 times daily (with meals and at bedtime); if tolerated but response insufficient, may be increased to max. 30 mg daily in divided doses; discontinue if no improvement after 2–3 months; CHILD not recommended

Salagen® (Novartis) PoM
Tablets, f/c, pilocarpine hydrochloride 5 mg. Net price 84-tab pack = £51.43. Label: 21, 27, counselling, driving

13: Skin

13.1 Management of skin conditions

13.1.1 Vehicles

Both vehicle and active ingredients are important in the treatment of skin conditions; the vehicle alone may have more than a mere placebo effect. The vehicle affects the degree of hydration of the skin, has a mild anti-inflammatory effect, and aids the penetration of active drug.

Applications are usually viscous solutions, emulsions, or suspensions for application to the skin (including the scalp) or nails.

Collodions are painted on the skin and allowed to dry to leave a flexible film over the site of application.

Creams are emulsions of oil and water and are generally well absorbed into the skin. They may contain an antimicrobial preservative unless the active ingredient or basis is intrinsically bactericidal and fungicidal. Generally, creams are cosmetically more acceptable than ointments because they are less greasy and easier to apply.

Gels consist of active ingredients in suitable hydrophilic or hydrophobic bases; they generally have a high water content. Gels are particularly suitable for application to the face and scalp.

Lotions have a cooling effect and may be preferred to ointments or creams for application over a hairy area. Lotions in alcoholic basis can sting if used on broken skin. *Shake lotions* (such as calamine lotion) contain insoluble powders which leave a deposit on the skin surface.

Ointments are greasy preparations which are normally anhydrous and insoluble in water, and are more occlusive than creams. They are particularly suitable for chronic, dry lesions. The most commonly used ointment bases consist of soft paraffin or a combination of soft, liquid and hard paraffin. Some ointment bases have both *hydrophilic and lipophilic* properties; they may have occlusive properties on the skin surface, encourage hydration, and also be miscible with water; they often have a mild anti-inflammatory effect. *Water-soluble ointments* contain macrogols which are freely soluble in water and are therefore readily washed off; they have a limited but useful role where ready removal is desirable.

Pastes are stiff preparations containing a high proportion of finely powdered solids such as zinc oxide and starch suspended in an ointment. They are used for circumscribed lesions such as those which occur in lichen simplex, chronic eczema, or psoriasis. They are less occlusive than ointments and can be used to protect inflamed, lichenified, or excoriated skin.

Dusting powders are used only rarely. They reduce friction between opposing skin surfaces. Dusting powders should not be applied to moist areas because they can cake and abrade the skin. Talc is a lubricant but it does not absorb moisture whereas starch is less lubricant but absorbs water.

DILUTION. The BP directs that creams and ointments should **not** normally be diluted but that should dilution be necessary care should be taken, in particular, to prevent microbial contamination. The appropriate diluent should be used and heating should be avoided during mixing; excessive dilution may affect the stability of some creams. Diluted creams should normally be used within 2 weeks of their preparation.

13.1.2   Suitable quantities for prescribing

Suitable quantities of dermatological preparations to be prescribed for specific areas of the body are:

	Creams and Ointments	Lotions
Face	15–30 g	100 mL
Both hands	25–50 g	200 mL
Scalp	50–100 g	200 mL
Both arms or both legs	100–200 g	200 mL
Trunk	400 g	500 mL
Groins and genitalia	15–25 g	100 mL

These amounts are usually suitable for an adult for twice daily application for 1 week. The recommendations do not apply to corticosteroid preparations—for suitable quantities of corticosteroid preparations see section 13.4.

13.1.3   Excipients and sensitisation

Excipients in topical products rarely cause problems. If a patch test indicates allergy to an excipient, then products containing the substance should be avoided. The following excipients in topical preparations may rarely be associated with sensitisation; the presence of these excipients is indicated in the entries for topical products.

Beeswax	Imidurea
Benzyl alcohol	Isopropyl palmitate
Butylated hydroxyanisole	N-(3-Chloroallyl)hexami-
Butylated hydroxytoluene	nium chloride (quaternium
Cetostearyl alcohol (including	15)
cetyl and stearyl alcohol)	Polysorbates
Chlorocresol	Propylene glycol
Edetic acid (EDTA)	Sodium metabisulphite
Ethylenediamine	Sorbic acid
Fragrances	Wool fat and related sub-
Hydroxybenzoates	stances including lanolin[1]
(parabens)	

1. Purified versions of wool fat have reduced the problem

13.2   Emollient and barrier preparations

13.2.1	Emollients
13.2.2	Barrier preparations

BORDERLINE SUBSTANCES. The preparations marked 'ACBS' are regarded as drugs when prescribed in accordance with the advice of the Advisory Committee on Borderline Substances for the clinical conditions listed. Prescriptions issued in accordance with this advice and endorsed 'ACBS' will normally not be investigated. See Appendix 7 for listing by clinical condition.

13.2.1   Emollients

Emollients soothe, smooth and hydrate the skin and are indicated for all dry or scaling disorders. Their effects are short-lived and they should be applied frequently even after improvement occurs. They are useful in dry and eczematous disorders, and to a lesser extent in psoriasis (section 13.5.2). Light emollients such as **aqueous cream** are suitable for many patients with dry skin but a wide range of more greasy preparations including **white soft paraffin**, **emulsifying ointment**, and **liquid and white soft paraffin ointment** are available; the severity of the condition, patient preference and site of application will often guide the choice of emollient; emollients should be applied in the direction of hair growth. Some ingredients may rarely cause sensitisation (section 13.1.3) and this should be suspected if an eczematous reaction occurs.

Preparations such as **aqueous cream** and **emulsifying ointment** can be used as soap substitutes for hand washing and in the bath; the preparation is rubbed on the skin before rinsing off completely. The addition of a bath oil (section 13.2.1.1) may also be helpful.

Preparations containing an antibacterial should be avoided unless infection is present (section 13.10) or is a frequent complication.

Urea is employed as a hydrating agent. It is used in scaling conditions and may be useful in elderly patients. It is occasionally used with other topical agents such as corticosteroids to enhance penetration.

■ Non-proprietary emollient preparations

Aqueous Cream, BP
Cream, emulsifying ointment 30%, [1]phenoxyethanol 1% in freshly boiled and cooled purified water, net price 100 g = 21p
Excipients: include cetostearyl alcohol

1. The BP permits use of alternative antimicrobials provided their identity and concentration are stated on the label

Emulsifying Ointment, BP
Ointment, emulsifying wax 30%, white soft paraffin 50%, liquid paraffin 20%, net price 100 g = 30p
Excipients: include cetostearyl alcohol

Hydrous Ointment, BP
Ointment, (oily cream), dried magnesium sulphate 0.5%, phenoxyethanol 1%, wool alcohols ointment 50%, in freshly boiled and cooled purified water, net price 100 g = 40p

Liquid and White Soft Paraffin Ointment, NPF
Ointment, liquid paraffin 50%, white soft paraffin 50%, net price 250 g = £1.89

Paraffin, White Soft, BP
White petroleum jelly, net price 100 g = 32p

Paraffin, Yellow Soft, BP
Yellow petroleum jelly, net price 100 g = 33p

■ Proprietary emollient preparations

Aveeno® (J&J)
Cream, colloidal oatmeal in emollient basis, net price 100 mL = £3.78
Excipients: include benzyl alcohol, cetyl alcohol, isopropyl palmitate
ACBS: For endogenous and exogenous eczema, xeroderma, ichthyosis, and senile pruritus (pruritus of the elderly) associated with dry skin
Lotion, colloidal oatmeal in emollient basis, net price 400-mL pump pack = £6.42
Excipients: include benzyl alcohol, cetyl alcohol, isopropyl palmitate
ACBS: as for *Aveeno*® *Cream*

Cetraben® **Emollient Cream** (Sankyo)
Cream, white soft paraffin 13.2%, light liquid paraffin 10.5%, net price 50 g = £1.17, 125 g = £2.38, 500-g pump pack = £5.61
Excipients: include cetostearyl alcohol, hydroxybenzoates (parabens)
For inflamed, damaged, dry or chapped skin including eczema

Decubal® **Clinic** (Alpharma)
Cream, isopropyl myristate 17%, glycerol 8.5%, wool fat 6%, dimeticone 5%, net price 50 g = £1.53, 100 g = £1.98
Excipients: include cetyl alcohol, polysorbates, sorbic acid, wool fat
For dry skin conditions including ichthyosis, psoriasis, dermatitis and hyperkeratosis

Dermamist® (Yamanouchi)
Spray application, white soft paraffin 10% in a basis containing liquid paraffin, fractionated coconut oil, net price 250-mL pressurised aerosol unit = £9.91
Excipients: none as listed in section 13.1.3
For dry skin conditions including eczema, ichthyosis, pruritus of the elderly
NOTE. Flammable

Diprobase® (Schering-Plough)
Cream, cetomacrogol 2.25%, cetostearyl alcohol 7.2%, liquid paraffin 6%, white soft paraffin 15%, water-miscible basis used for *Diprosone*® cream, net price 50 g = £1.54; 500-g dispenser = £6.61
Excipients: include cetostearyl alcohol, chlorocresol
For dry skin conditions
Ointment, liquid paraffin 5%, white soft paraffin 95%, basis used for *Diprosone*® ointment, net price 50 g = £1.54
Excipients: none as listed in section 13.1.3
For dry skin conditions

Doublebase® (Dermal)
Gel, isopropyl myristate 15%, liquid paraffin 15%, net price 100 g = £2.98, 500 g = £6.55
Excipients: none as listed in section 13.1.3
For dry chapped or itchy skin conditions

Drapolene® —section 13.2.2

E45® (Crookes)
Cream, light liquid paraffin 12.6%, white soft paraffin 14.5%, hypoallergenic hydrous wool fat (hypoallergenic lanolin) 1% in self-emulsifying monostearin, net price 50 g = £1.18, 125 g = £2.39, 350 g = £4.14, 500-g pump pack = £6.20
Excipients: include cetyl alcohol, hydroxybenzoates (parabens)
For dry skin conditions

Emollient Wash Cream, soap substitute, zinc oxide 5% in an emollient basis, net price 250-mL pump pack = £2.95
Excipients: none as listed in section 13.1.3
ACBS: for endogenous and exogenous eczema, xeroderma, ichthyosis and senile pruritus (pruritus of the elderly) associated with dry skin
Lotion, light liquid paraffin 4%, cetomacrogol, white soft paraffin 10%, hypoallergenic anhydrous wool fat (hypoallergenic lanolin) 1% in glyceryl monostearate, net price 200 mL = £2.40, 500-mL pump pack = £4.50
Excipients: include isopropyl palmitate, hydroxybenzoates (parabens), benzyl alcohol
ACBS: for symptomatic relief of dry skin conditions, such as those associated with atopic eczema and contact dermatitis

Epaderm® (SSL)
Ointment, emulsifying wax 30%, yellow soft paraffin 30%, liquid paraffin 40%, net price 125 g = £3.67, 500 g = £6.21
Excipients: include cetostearyl alcohol
For use as an emollient or soap substitute

Gammaderm® (Linderma)
Cream, evening primrose oil 20%, net price 50 g = £2.83, 250 g = £8.20
Excipients: include beeswax, hydroxybenzoates (parabens), propylene glycol
Cautions: epilepsy (but hazard unlikely with topical preparations)
For dry skin conditions

Hewletts Cream® (Kestrel)
Cream, hydrous wool fat 4%, zinc oxide 8%, arachis (peanut) oil, oleic acid, white soft paraffin, net price 35 g = £1.43, 400 g = £6.69
Excipients: include fragrance
For nursing hygiene and care of skin, and chapped hands

Hydromol® (Ferndale)
Cream, sodium pidolate 2.5%, net price 50 g = £2.04, 100 g = £3.80, 500 g = £12.60
Excipients: include cetostearyl alcohol, hydroxybenzoates (parabens)
For dry skin conditions
Ointment, yellow soft paraffin 30%, emulsifying wax 30%, net price 125 g = £3.30, 500 g = £5.58
Excipients: none as listed in section 13.1.3
For use as an emollient or as a bath additive

Kamillosan® (Goldshield)
Ointment, chamomile extracts 10.5% in a basis containing wool fat, net price 50 g = £2.50, 100 g = £5.00
Excipients: include beeswax, cetostearyl alcohol, hydroxybenzoates (parabens)
For nappy rash, sore nipples and chapped hands

Keri® (Bristol-Myers Squibb)
Lotion, mineral oil 16%, with lanolin oil, net price 190-mL pump pack = £3.56, 380-mL pump pack = £5.81
Excipients: include fragrance, hydroxybenzoates (parabens), N-(3-chloroallyl)hexaminium chloride (quaternium 15), propylene glycol
For dry skin conditions and nappy rash

LactiCare® (Stiefel)
Lotion, lactic acid 5%, sodium pidolate 2.5%, net price 150 mL = £3.19
Excipients: include cetostearyl alcohol, imidurea, isopropyl palmitate, fragrance
For dry skin conditions

Lipobase (Yamanouchi)
Cream, fatty cream basis used for *Locoid Lipo-cream*, net price 50 g = £2.24
Excipients: include cetostearyl alcohol, hydroxybenzoates (parabens)
For dry skin conditions, also for use during treatment with topical corticosteroid and as diluent for *Locoid Lipo-cream*

Neutrogena **Dermatological Cream** (J&J)
Cream, glycerol 40% in an emollient basis, net price 100 g = £3.79
Excipients: include cetostearyl alcohol, hydroxybenzoates (parabens)
For dry skin conditions

Oilatum (Stiefel)
Cream, light liquid paraffin 6%, white soft paraffin 15%, net price 40 g = £1.79, 150 g = £3.38
Excipients: include benzyl alcohol, cetostearyl alcohol
For dry skin conditions
Shower emollient (gel), light liquid paraffin 70%, net price 125 g = £4.84
Excipients: include fragrance
For dry skin conditions including dermatitis

Ultrabase (Schering Health)
Cream, water-miscible, containing liquid paraffin and white soft paraffin, net price 50 g = £1.05, 500-g dispenser = £7.58
Excipients: include fragrance, hydroxybenzoates (parabens), disodium edetate, stearyl alcohol
For dry skin conditions

Unguentum M (Crookes)
Cream, cetostearyl alcohol, glyceryl monostearate, saturated neutral oil, liquid paraffin, white soft paraffin, net price 50 g = £1.59, 100 g = £3.13, 200-mL dispenser = £6.19, 500 g = £9.55
Excipients: include cetostearyl alcohol, polysorbate 40, propylene glycol, sorbic acid
For dry skin conditions and nappy rash

Vaseline Dermacare (Elida Fabergé)
Cream, dimeticone 1%, white soft paraffin 15%, net price 150 mL = £2.11
Excipients: include hydroxybenzoates (parabens)
ACBS: for endogenous and exogenous eczema, xeroderma, ichthyosis and senile pruritus (pruritus of the elderly) associated with dry skin
Lotion, dimeticone 1%, liquid paraffin 4%, white soft paraffin 5% in an emollient basis, net price 75 mL = 86p, 200 mL = £2.29
Excipients: include disodium edetate, hydroxybenzoates (parabens), wool fat
ACBS: as for *Vaseline Dermacare* *Cream*

■ Preparations containing urea

Aquadrate (Alliance)
Cream, urea 10%, net price 30 g = £1.59, 100 g = £4.79
Excipients: none as listed in section 13.1.3
Dose: for dry, scaling and itching skin, apply thinly and rub into area when required

Balneum **Plus** (Crookes)
Cream, urea 5%, lauromacrogols 3%, net price 100 g = £5.58, 175-g pump pack = £7.81, 500-g pump pack = £19.50
Excipients: include benzyl alcohol, polysorbates
Dose: for dry, scaling and itching skin, apply twice daily

Calmurid (Galderma)
Cream, urea 10%, lactic acid 5%. Diluent aqueous cream, life of diluted cream 14 days, net price 100 g = £5.70, 500-g dispenser = £21.48
Excipients: none as listed in section 13.1.3
Dose: for dry, scaling and itching skin, apply a thick layer for 3–5 minutes, massage into area, and remove excess, usually twice daily. Use half-strength cream for 1 week if stinging occurs

E45 **Itch Relief Cream** (Crookes)
Cream, urea 5%, macrogol lauryl ether 3%, net price 50 g = £2.16, 100 g = £3.47
Excipients: include benzyl alcohol, polysorbates
Dose: for dry, scaling, and itching skin, apply twice a day

Eucerin (Beiersdorf)
Cream, urea 10%, net price 50 mL = £3.69, 150 mL = £9.10
Excipients: include benzyl alcohol, isopropyl palmitate, wool fat
Dose: for dry skin conditions including eczema, ichthyosis, xeroderma, hyperkeratosis, apply thinly and rub into area twice daily
Lotion, urea 10%, net price 250 mL = £4.52
Excipients: include benzyl alcohol, isopropyl palmitate
Dose: for dry skin conditions including eczema, ichthyosis, xeroderma, hyperkeratosis, apply sparingly and rub into area twice daily

Nutraplus (Galderma)
Cream, urea 10%, net price 100 g = £4.37
Excipients: include hydroxybenzoates (parabens), propylene glycol
Dose: for dry, scaling and itching skin, apply 2–3 times daily

■ With antimicrobials

Dermol (Dermal)
Dermol *500 Lotion*, benzalkonium chloride 0.1%, chlorhexidine hydrochloride 0.1%, liquid paraffin 2.5%, isopropyl myristate 2.5%, net price 500-mL dispenser = £6.79
Excipients: include cetostearyl alcohol
Dose: for dry and pruritic skin conditions including eczema and dermatitis, apply to skin or use as soap substitute
Dermol *200 Shower Emollient*, benzalkonium chloride 0.1%, chlorhexidine hydrochloride 0.1%, liquid paraffin 2.5%, isopropyl myristate 2.5%, net price 200 mL = £3.99
Excipients: include cetostearyl alcohol
Dose: for dry and pruritic skin conditions including eczema and dermatitis, apply to skin or use as soap substitute

13.2.1.1 Emollient bath additives

Alpha Keri Bath (Bristol-Myers Squibb)
Bath oil, liquid paraffin 91.7%, oil-soluble fraction of wool fat 3%, net price 240 mL = £3.45, 480 mL = £6.43
Excipients: include fragrance
Dose: for dry skin conditions including ichthyosis and pruritus of the elderly, add 10–20 mL/bath (INFANT 5 mL)

Aveeno (J&J)
Aveeno *Bath oil*, colloidal oatmeal, white oat fraction in emollient basis, net price 250 mL = £4.28
Excipients: include beeswax, fragrance
Dose: ACBS: for endogenous and exogenous eczema, xeroderma, ichthyosis, and senile pruritus (pruritus of the elderly) associated with dry skin, add 30 mL/bath
Aveeno Colloidal *Bath additive*, oatmeal, white oat fraction in emollient basis, net price 10 × 50-g sachets = £7.33
Excipients: none as listed in section 13.1.3
Dose: ACBS: as for Aveeno Bath oil; add 1 sachet/bath (INFANT half sachet)

Balneum (Crookes)
Balneum *bath oil*, soya oil 84.75%, net price 200 mL = £2.79, 500 mL = £6.06, 1 litre = £11.70
Excipients: include butylated hydroxytoluene, propylene glycol, fragrance
Dose: for dry skin conditions including those associated with dermatitis and eczema; add 20 mL/bath (INFANT 5 mL)

Balneum Plus® *bath oil*, soya oil 82.95%, mixed lauromacrogols 15%, net price 500 mL = £7.50
Excipients: include butylated hydroxytoluene, propylene glycol, fragrance
Dose: for dry skin conditions including those associated with dermatitis and eczema where pruritus also experienced; add 20 mL/bath (INFANT 5 mL)

Cetraben® (Sankyo)
Emollient bath additive, light liquid paraffin 82.8%, net price 500 mL = £5.25
Dose: for dry skin conditions, including eczema, add 1–2 capfuls/bath (CHILD ½–1 capful)

Dermalo® (Dermal)
Bath emollient, acetylated wool alcohols 5%, liquid paraffin 65%, net price 500 mL = £3.87
Excipients: none as listed in section 13.1.3
Dose: for dermatitis, dry skin conditions including ichthyosis and pruritus of the elderly; add 15–20 mL/bath (INFANT and CHILD 5–10 mL)

Diprobath® (Schering-Plough)
Bath additive, isopropyl myristate 39%, light liquid paraffin 46%, net price 500 mL = £7.50
Excipients: none as listed in section 13.1.3
Dose: for dry skin conditions including dermatitis and eczema; add 25 mL/bath (INFANT 10 mL)

E45® (Crookes)
Emollient bath oil, cetyl dimeticone 5%, liquid paraffin 91%, net price 250 mL = £2.95, 500 mL = £4.70
Excipients: none as listed in section 13.1.3
Dose: ACBS: for endogenous and exogenous eczema, xeroderma, ichthyosis, and senile pruritus (pruritus of the elderly) associated with dry skin; add 15 mL/bath (CHILD 5–10 mL)

Emollient Medicinal Bath Oil (Ashbourne)
Emollient bath oil, liquid paraffin 65%, acetylated wool alcohols 5%, net price 250 mL = £2.75, 500 mL = £5.46
Dose: for dry skin conditions including dermatitis, pruritus of the elderly, and ichthyosis, add 15–20 mL/bath (INFANT and CHILD 5–10 mL added to a small bath or washbasin)

Hydromol Emollient® (Ferndale)
Bath additive, isopropyl myristate 13%, light liquid paraffin 37.8%, net price 150 mL = £1.87, 350 mL = £3.80, 1 litre = £9.00
Excipients: none as listed in section 13.1.3
Dose: for dry skin conditions including eczema, ichthyosis and pruritus of the elderly; add 1–3 capfuls/bath (INFANT ½–2 capfuls)

Imuderm® (Goldshield)
Bath oil, almond oil 30%, light liquid paraffin 69.6%, net price 250 mL = £3.75
Excipients: include butylated hydroxyanisole
Dose: for dry skin conditions including dermatitis, eczema, pruritus of the elderly, and ichthyosis, add 15–30 mL/bath (INFANT and CHILD 7.5–15 mL)

Oilatum® (Stiefel)
Oilatum® *Emollient bath additive* (emulsion), acetylated wool alcohols 5%, liquid paraffin 63.4%, net price 250 mL = £2.75, 500 mL = £4.57
Excipients: include isopropyl palmitate, fragrance
Dose: for dry skin conditions including dermatitis, pruritus of the elderly and ichthyosis; add 1–3 capfuls/bath (INFANT 0.5–2 capfuls)
Oilatum® *Fragrance Free bath additive*, light liquid paraffin 63.4%, net price 500 mL = £5.75
Excipients: include wool fat, isopropyl palmitate
Dose: for dry skin conditions including dermatitis, pruritus of the elderly and ichthyosis; add 1–3 capfuls/bath (INFANT 0.5–2 capfuls)

■ With antimicrobials
Dermol® (Dermal)
Dermol® *600 Bath Emollient*, benzalkonium chloride 0.5%, liquid paraffin 25%, isopropyl myristate 25%, net price 600 mL = £8.49
Excipients: include polysorbate 60
Dose: for dry and pruritic skin conditions including eczema and dermatitis, add up to 30 mL/bath (INFANT up to 15 mL)

Emulsiderm® (Dermal)
Liquid emulsion, liquid paraffin 25%, isopropyl myristate 25%, benzalkonium chloride 0.5%, net price 300 mL (with 15-mL measure) = £4.33, 1 litre (with 30-mL measure) = £13.49
Excipients: include polysorbate 60
Dose: for dry skin conditions including eczema and ichthyosis; add 7–30 mL/bath

Oilatum® (Stiefel)
Oilatum® *Plus bath additive*, benzalkonium chloride 6%, triclosan 2%, light liquid paraffin 52.5%, net price 500 mL = £7.86, 1 litre = £15.30
Excipients: include wool fat, isopropyl palmitate
Dose: for topical treatment of eczema including eczema at risk from infection; add 1–2 capfuls/bath (INFANT over 6 months 1 mL)

13.2.2 Barrier preparations

Barrier preparations often contain water-repellent substances such as **dimeticone** (dimethicone) or other silicones. They are used on the skin around stomas, bedsores, and pressure areas in the elderly where the skin is intact. Where the skin has broken down, barrier preparations have a limited role in protecting adjacent skin. They are no substitute for adequate nursing care and it is doubtful if they are any more effective than the traditional compound **zinc ointments**.

NAPPY RASH. Barrier creams and ointments are used for protection against nappy rash which is usually a local dermatitis. The first line of treatment is to ensure that nappies are changed frequently and that tightly fitting water-proof pants are avoided. The rash may clear when left exposed to the air and a barrier preparation may be helpful. If the rash is associated with a fungal infection, an antifungal cream such as clotrimazole cream (section 13.10.2) is useful. A mild corticosteroid such as hydrocortisone 1% may be useful but treatment should be limited to a week or less; the occlusive effect of nappies and water-proof pants may increase absorption (for cautions, see Hydrocortisone p. 543).

■ Non-proprietary barrier preparations
Zinc Cream, BP
Cream, zinc oxide 32%, arachis (peanut) oil 32%, calcium hydroxide 0.045%, oleic acid 0.5%, wool fat 8%, in freshly boiled and cooled purified water, net price 50 g = 39p
For nappy and urinary rash and eczematous conditions

Zinc Ointment, BP
Ointment, zinc oxide 15%, in Simple Ointment BP 1988 (which contains wool fat 5%, hard paraffin 5%, cetostearyl alcohol 5%, white soft paraffin 85%), net price 25 g = 15p
For nappy and urinary rash and eczematous conditions

Zinc and Castor Oil Ointment, BP

Ointment, zinc oxide 7.5%, castor oil 50%, arachis (peanut) oil 30.5%, white beeswax 10%, cetostearyl alcohol 2%, net price 25 g = 14p
For nappy and urinary rash

■ Proprietary barrier preparations

Conotrane® (Yamanouchi)
Cream, benzalkonium chloride 0.1%, dimeticone '350' 22%, net price 100 g = 80p, 500 g = £3.77
Excipients: include cetostearyl alcohol, fragrance
For nappy and urinary rash and pressure sores

Drapolene® (Warner Lambert)
Cream, benzalkonium chloride 0.01%, cetrimide 0.2% in a basis containing white soft paraffin, cetyl alcohol and wool fat, net price 100 g = £1.43, 200 g = £2.38, 350 g = £3.66
Excipients: include cetyl alcohol, chlorocresol, wool fat
For nappy and urinary rash; minor wounds

Medicaid® (Eastern)
Cream, cetrimide 0.5% in a basis containing light liquid paraffin, white soft paraffin, cetostearyl alcohol, glyceryl monostearate, net price 50 g = £1.69
Excipients: include cetostearyl alcohol, fragrance, hydroxybenzoates (parabens), wool fat
For nappy rash, minor burns and abrasions

Metanium® (Ransom)
Ointment, titanium dioxide 20%, titanium peroxide 5%, titanium salicylate 3% in a basis containing dimeticone, light liquid paraffin, white soft paraffin, and benzoin tincture, net price 30 g = £1.85
Excipients: none as listed in section 13.1.3
For nappy rash and related disorders

Morhulin® (Thornton & Ross)
Ointment, cod-liver oil 11.4%, zinc oxide 38%, in a basis containing liquid paraffin and yellow soft paraffin, net price 50 g = £1.56
Excipients: include wool fat derivative
For minor wounds, varicose ulcers, pressure sores, eczema and nappy rash

Siopel® (Centrapharm)
Barrier cream, dimeticone '1000' 10%, cetrimide 0.3%, arachis (peanut) oil, net price 50 g = £1.66
Excipients: include butylated hydroxytoluene, cetostearyl alcohol, hydroxybenzoates (parabens)
For protection against water-soluble irritants

Sprilon® (S&N Hlth.)
Spray application, dimeticone 1.04%, zinc oxide 12.5%, in a basis containing wool alcohols, cetostearyl alcohol, dextran, white soft paraffin, liquid paraffin, propellants, net price 115-g pressurised aerosol unit = £3.54
Excipients: include cetostearyl alcohol, hydroxybenzoates (parabens), wool fat
For urinary rash, pressure sores, leg ulcers, moist eczema, fissures, fistulae and ileostomy care
NOTE. Flammable

Sudocrem® (Forest)
Cream, benzyl alcohol 0.39%, benzyl benzoate 1.01%, benzyl cinnamate 0.15%, hydrous wool fat (hypoallergenic lanolin) 4%, zinc oxide 15.25%, net price 30 g = £1.01, 60 g = £1.07, 125 g = £1.56, 250 g = £2.66, 400 g = £3.88
Excipients: include beeswax (synthetic), polysorbates, propylene glycol, fragrance
For nappy rash and pressure sores

Vasogen® (Forest)
Barrier cream, dimeticone 20%, calamine 1.5%, zinc oxide 7.5%, net price 50 g = 80p, 100 g = £1.36
Excipients: include hydroxybenzoates (parabens), wool fat
For nappy rash, pressure sores, ileostomy and colostomy care

13.3 Topical local anaesthetics and antipruritics

Pruritus may be caused by systemic disease (such as drug hypersensitivity, obstructive jaundice, endocrine disease, and certain malignant diseases) as well as by skin disease (e.g. psoriasis, eczema, urticaria, and scabies). Where possible the underlying causes should be treated. An **emollient** (section 13.2.1) may be of value where the pruritus is associated with dry skin. Pruritus that occurs in otherwise healthy elderly people can also be treated with an emollient. For advice on the treatment of pruritus in palliative care, see, p. 15.

Preparations containing **crotamiton** are sometimes used but are of uncertain value. Preparations containing **calamine** are often ineffective.

A topical preparation containing **doxepin** 5% is licensed for the relief of pruritus in eczema; it can cause drowsiness and there may be a risk of sensitisation.

Pruritus is common in biliary obstruction, especially in primary biliary cirrhosis and drug-induced cholestasis. Oral administration of **colestyramine** (cholestyramine) is the treatment of choice (section 1.9.2).

Topical antihistamines and local anaesthetics are only marginally effective and may occasionally cause sensitisation. A short course of a topical corticosteroid is appropriate in treating *insect stings*. Insect stings should not be treated with calamine preparations.

A short treatment with a **sedating antihistamine** (section 3.4.1) may help in insect stings and in intractable pruritus where sedation is desirable.

For preparations used in *pruritus ani*, see section 1.7.1.

CALAMINE

Indications: pruritus

Calamine (Non-proprietary)
Aqueous cream, calamine 4%, zinc oxide 3%, liquid paraffin 20%, self-emulsifying glyceryl monostearate 5%, cetomacrogol emulsifying wax 5%, phenoxyethanol 0.5%, freshly boiled and cooled purified water 62.5%, net price 100 mL = 59p
Lotion (=cutaneous suspension), calamine 15%, zinc oxide 5%, glycerol 5%, bentonite 3%, sodium citrate 0.5%, liquefied phenol 0.5%, in freshly boiled and cooled purified water, net price 200 mL = 63p
Oily lotion (BP 1980), calamine 5%, arachis (peanut) oil 50%, oleic acid 0.5%, wool fat 1%, in calcium hydroxide solution, net price 200 mL = £1.08

CROTAMITON

Indications: pruritus (including pruritus after scabies—section 13.10.4); see notes above

Cautions: avoid use near eyes and broken skin; use on doctor's advice for children under 3 years
Contra-indications: acute exudative dermatoses
Dose: pruritus, apply 2–3 times daily; CHILD below 3 years, apply once daily

Eurax® (Novartis Consumer Health)
Cream, crotamiton 10%, net price 30 g = £2.27, 100 g = £3.95
Excipients: include beeswax, fragrance, hydroxybenzoates (parabens), stearyl alcohol
Lotion, crotamiton 10%, net price 100 mL = £2.99
Excipients: include cetyl alcohol, fragrance, propylene glycol, sorbic acid, stearyl alcohol

DOXEPIN HYDROCHLORIDE

Indications: pruritus in eczema; depressive illness (section 4.3.1)
Cautions: glaucoma, urinary retention, severe liver impairment, mania; avoid application to large areas; pregnancy and breast-feeding; **interactions:** Appendix 1 (antidepressants, tricyclic)
DRIVING. Drowsiness may affect performance of skilled tasks (e.g. driving); effects of alcohol enhanced
Side-effects: drowsiness; local burning, stinging, irritation, tingling and rash; dry mouth and other systemic side-effects reported (section 4.3.1)
Dose: apply thinly 3–4 times daily; usual max. 3 g per application; usual total max. 12 g daily; coverage should be less than 10% of body surface area; CHILD under 12 years not recommended

Xepin® (CHS) PoM
Cream, doxepin hydrochloride 5%, net price 30 g = £12.61. Label: 2, 10, patient information leaflet
Excipients: include benzyl alcohol

TOPICAL LOCAL ANAESTHETICS

Indications: relief of local pain, see notes above. See section 15.2 for use in surface anaesthesia
Cautions: occasionally cause hypersensitivity
NOTE. Topical local anaesthetic preparations may be absorbed, especially through mucosal surfaces, therefore excessive application should be avoided and they should preferably not be used for more than about 3 days; not generally suitable for young children

■ Preparations on sale to the public
The following is a list of topical local anaesthetic preparations on sale to the public, together with their significant ingredients:
Anethaine® (tetracaine (amethocaine)), **Anthisan® Plus** (benzocaine, mepyramine), **BurnEze®** (benzocaine), **Dermidex®** (lidocaine, alcloxa, cetrimide, chlorobutanol), **Lanacane® cream** (benzocaine, chlorothymol), **Solarcaine®** (benzocaine, triclosan), **Solarcaine® gel** (lidocaine), **Vagisil® cream** (lidocaine), **Wasp–Eze® spray** (benzocaine, mepyramine)

TOPICAL ANTIHISTAMINES

Indications: see notes above
Cautions: may cause hypersensitivity; avoid in eczema; photosensitivity (diphenhydramine); not recommended for longer than 3 days

■ Preparations on sale to the public
The following is a list of topical antihistamine preparations on sale to the public, together with their significant ingredients:
Anthisan® (mepyramine), **Anthisan® Bite and Sting** (mepyramine), **Anthisan® Plus** (mepyramine, benzocaine), **Benadryl® Skin Allergy Relief cream** (diphen-hydramine, camphor), **Benadryl® Skin Allergy Relief lotion** (diphenhydramine, camphor), **Boots Bite & Sting Relief Antihistamine cream** (mepyramine), **R.B.C.®** (antazoline, calamine, camphor, cetrimide, menthol), **Wasp–Eze® ointment** (antazoline), **Wasp–Eze® spray** (mepyramine, benzocaine)

13.4 Topical corticosteroids

Topical corticosteroids are used for the treatment of inflammatory conditions of the skin other than those due to an infection, in particular the *eczematous disorders* (for further details see section 13.5.1). Corticosteroids suppress various components of the inflammatory reaction while in use; they are in no sense curative, and when treatment is discontinued a rebound exacerbation of the condition may occur. They are indicated for the relief of symptoms and for the suppression of signs of the disorder when potentially less harmful measures are ineffective.

Topical corticosteroids are of no value in the treatment of *urticaria* and they are **contra-indicated** in *rosacea*; they may worsen ulcerated or secondarily infected lesions. They should not be used indiscriminately in *pruritus* (where they will only benefit if inflammation is causing the itch) and are **not** recommended for *acne vulgaris*.

Systemic or potent topical corticosteroids should be avoided or given only under specialist supervision *in psoriasis* because, although they may suppress the psoriasis in the short term, relapse or vigorous rebound occurs on withdrawal (sometimes precipitating severe pustular psoriasis). Topical use of potent corticosteroids on widespread psoriasis also leads to systemic as well as to local side-effects. It is reasonable, however, to prescribe a weaker corticosteroid (such as hydrocortisone) for short periods (perhaps up to 4 weeks) for *flexural* and *facial psoriasis* (**important:** not more potent than hydrocortisone 1% on the face). In the case of *scalp psoriasis* it is reasonable to use a more potent corticosteroid such as betamethasone or fluocinonide.

In general, the most potent topical corticosteroids should be reserved for recalcitrant dermatoses such as *chronic discoid lupus erythematosus, lichen simplex chronicus, hypertrophic lichen planus*, and *palmoplantar pustulosis*. Topical corticosteroids may cause skin atrophy, especially on thin skin areas such as the face or flexures, and may cause acneform pustules; on the face, they may cause a rosacea-like disorder (perioral dermatitis). Potent corticosteroids should therefore generally be avoided on the face and skin flexures, although specialists occasionally prescribe them in certain circumstances.

Intralesional corticosteroid injections (section 10.1.2.2) are more effective than the very potent topical corticosteroid preparations and they should be reserved for severe cases where there are localised lesions (such as *keloid scars, hypertrophic lichen planus*, or *localised alopecia areata*) and topical treatment has failed. Their effects may last for several weeks or even months. Particular care is needed to inject accurately into the lesion in order to avoid severe skin atrophy and loss of pigmentation.

SIDE-EFFECTS. Unlike the *potent* and *very potent* groups, the *moderate* and *mild* groups are rarely associated with side-effects. The more potent the preparation the more care is required, as absorption through the skin can cause severe pituitary-adrenal-axis suppression and Cushing's syndrome (section 6.3.2), both of which depend on the area of the body treated and the duration of the treatment. Absorption is greatest from areas of thin skin, raw surfaces, and intertriginous areas, and is increased by occlusion.

Local side-effects include:

(a) spread and worsening of untreated infection;
(b) thinning of the skin which may be restored over a period of time after stopping although the original structure may never return;
(c) irreversible striae atrophicae and telangiectasia;
(d) contact dermatitis;
(e) perioral dermatitis, an inflammatory papular disorder on the face of young women;
(f) acne at the site of application in some patients;
(g) mild depigmentation which may be reversible

CHOICE OF FORMULATION. *Water-miscible* creams are suitable for moist or weeping lesions whereas *ointments* are generally chosen for dry, lichenified or scaly lesions or where a more occlusive effect is required. *Lotions* may be useful when minimal application to a large or hair-bearing area is required or for the treatment of exudative lesions. *Occlusive polythene or hydrocolloid dressings* increase absorption, but also increase the risk of side-effects; they are therefore used only under supervision on a short-term basis for very thick areas of skin (such as the palms and soles). The *inclusion of urea* or *salicylic acid* increases the penetration of the corticosteroid.

Topical corticosteroid potencies

Potency	Examples
Mild	Hydrocortisone 1%
Moderately potent	Clobetasone butyrate 0.05%
Potent	Betamethasone 0.1% (as valerate)
	Hydrocortisone butyrate
Very potent	Clobetasol propionate 0.05%

The preparation containing the **least potent** drug at the lowest strength which is effective is the one of choice; dilution should be avoided whenever possible.

APPLICATION. Corticosteroid preparations should normally be applied once or twice daily. It is not necessary to apply them more frequently.

The length of a corticosteroid cream or ointment expelled from a tube may be used to specify the quantity to be applied to a given area of skin. This length may be measured in terms of a *fingertip unit* (the distance from the tip of the adult index finger to the first crease). One fingertip unit (approximately 500 mg) is sufficient to cover an area that is twice that of the flat adult hand.

Suitable quantities of corticosteroid preparations to be prescribed for specific areas of the body are:

	Creams and Ointments
Face and neck	15 to 30 g
Both hands	15 to 30 g
Scalp	15 to 30 g
Both arms	30 to 60 g
Both legs	100 g
Trunk	100 g
Groins and genitalia	15 to 30 g

These amounts are usually suitable for an adult for twice daily application for 1 week

CHILDREN. Children, especially babies, are particularly susceptible to side-effects. The more potent corticosteroids are **contra-indicated** in infants under 1 year, and in general they should be avoided in children or if necessary used with great care and for short periods. A mild corticosteroid such as hydrocortisone 1% ointment or cream is useful for treating nappy rash (section 13.2.2) and for atopic eczema in childhood (but see caution below). A potent or moderately potent corticosteroid may be appropriate for severe atopic eczema on the limbs, for 1–2 weeks **only**, followed by a weaker preparation as the condition improves; an emollient (section 13.2.1) should be used throughout.

COMPOUND PREPARATIONS. The advantages of including other substances (such as antibacterials or antifungals) with corticosteroids in topical preparations are debatable, but they may have a place where there is associated bacterial or fungal infection.

HYDROCORTISONE

Indications: mild inflammatory skin disorders such as eczemas (but for over-the-counter preparations, see below); nappy rash, see notes above and section 13.2.2

Cautions: see notes above; also avoid prolonged use in infants and children (extreme caution in dermatoses of infancy including nappy rash—where possible treatment should be limited to 5–7 days), avoid prolonged use on the face (and keep away from eyes); more potent corticosteroids **contra-indicated** in infants under 1 year (see also notes above)
PSORIASIS. Risks of more potent corticosteroids in psoriasis include possibility of rebound relapse, development of generalised pustular psoriasis, and local and systemic toxicity; they are specifically **contra-indicated** in widespread plaque psoriasis

Contra-indications: untreated bacterial, fungal, or viral skin lesions; rosacea (acne rosacea), perioral dermatitis; not recommended for acne vulgaris (more potent corticosteroids specifically **contra-indicated**)

Side-effects: see notes above

Dose: apply thinly 1–2 times daily

Hydrocortisone (Non-proprietary) PoM
Cream, hydrocortisone 0.5%, net price, 15 g = 35p, 30 g = 66p; 1%, 15 g = 37p. Label: 28. Potency: mild
Ointment, hydrocortisone 0.5%, net price 15 g = 36p, 30 g = 65p; 1%, 15 g = 38p. Label: 28. Potency: mild
When hydrocortisone cream or ointment is prescribed and no strength is stated, the 1% strength should be supplied

■ Over–the–counter hydrocortisone products
The following skin creams and ointments contain hydrocortisone (alone or with other ingredients) and can be sold to the public for the treatment of allergic contact dermatitis, irritant dermatitis, insect bite reactions and mild to moderate eczema

Cautions: not for children under 10 years or in pregnancy, without medical advice
Contra-indications: eyes/face, anogenital region, broken or infected skin (including cold sores, acne, and athlete's foot)

Dose: apply sparingly over small area 1–2 times daily for max. of 1 week

Dermacort® (hydrocortisone 0.1%, cream), **Eurax Hc**® (hydrocortisone 0.25%; crotamiton 10%, cream), **Hc45**® (hydrocortisone acetate 1%, cream), **Lanacort**® (hydrocortisone acetate 1%, cream and ointment), **Zenoxone**® (hydrocortisone 1%, cream)

■ Proprietary hydrocortisone preparations

NOTE. The following preparations are PoM; those on sale to the public (with restrictions) are listed above

Dioderm® (Dermal) PoM
Cream, hydrocortisone 0.1%, net price 30 g = £2.69. Label: 28. Potency: mild
Excipients: include cetostearyl alcohol, propylene glycol
NOTE. Although this contains only 0.1% hydrocortisone, the formulation is designed to provide a clinical activity comparable to that of Hydrocortisone Cream 1% BP

Efcortelan® (GSK) PoM
Cream, hydrocortisone 0.5%, net price, 30 g = 66p; 1%, 30 g = 81p; 2.5%, 30 g = £1.83. Label: 28. Potency: mild
Excipients: include cetostearyl alcohol, chlorocresol
Ointment, hydrocortisone 0.5%, net price, 30 g = 66p; 1%, 30 g = 81p; 2.5%, 30 g = £1.83. Label: 28. Potency: mild
Excipients: none as listed in section 13.1.3

Mildison® (Yamanouchi) PoM
Lipocream, hydrocortisone 1%, net price 30 g = £2.63. Label: 28. Potency: mild
Excipients: include cetostearyl alcohol, hydroxybenzoates (parabens)

■ Compound preparations

Compound preparations with coal tar see section 13.5.2

Alphaderm® (Alliance) PoM
Cream, hydrocortisone 1%, urea 10%, net price 30 g = £2.36; 100 g = £7.32. Label: 28. Potency: moderate
Excipients: none as listed in section 13.1.3

Calmurid HC® (Galderma) PoM
Cream, hydrocortisone 1%, urea 10%, lactic acid 5%, net price 30 g = £2.33, 100 g = £7.30. Label: 28. Potency: moderate
Excipients: none as listed in section 13.1.3
NOTE. Manufacturer advises dilute to half-strength with aqueous cream for 1 week if stinging occurs then transfer to undiluted preparation (but see section 13.1.1 for advice to avoid dilution where possible)

¹**Eurax-Hydrocortisone**® (Novartis Consumer Health) PoM
Cream, hydrocortisone 0.25%, crotamiton 10%, net price 30 g = 87p. Label: 28. Potency: mild
Excipients: include fragrance, hydroxybenzoates (parabens), propylene glycol, stearyl alcohol

1. A 15-g tube is on sale to the public for treatment of contact dermatitis and insect bites (*Eurax Hc*®)

■ With antimicrobials

See notes above for comment on compound preparations

¹**Canesten HC**® (Bayer Consumer Care) PoM
Cream, hydrocortisone 1%, clotrimazole 1%, net price 30 g = £2.38. Label: 28. Potency: mild
Excipients: include benzyl alcohol, cetostearyl alcohol

1. A 15-g tube is on sale to the public for the treatment of athlete's foot and fungal infection of skin folds with associated inflammation (*Canesten*® *Hydrocortisone*)

Daktacort® (Janssen-Cilag) PoM
Cream, hydrocortisone 1%, miconazole nitrate 2%, net price 30 g = £2.24. Label: 28. Potency: mild
Excipients: include butylated hydroxyanisole, disodium edetate

Ointment, hydrocortisone 1%, miconazole nitrate 2%, net price 30 g = £2.25. Label: 28. Potency: mild
Excipients: none as listed in section 13.1.3

Econacort® (Squibb) PoM
Cream, hydrocortisone 1%, econazole nitrate 1%, net price 30 g = £2.25. Label: 28. Potency: mild
Excipients: include butylated hydroxyanisole

Fucidin H® (Leo) PoM
Cream, hydrocortisone acetate 1%, fusidic acid 2%, net price 30 g = £5.30, 60 g = £10.60. Label: 28. Potency: mild
Excipients: include butylated hydroxyanisole, cetyl alcohol, potassium sorbate
Ointment, hydrocortisone acetate 1%, sodium fusidate 2%, net price 30 g = £4.35, 60 g = £8.70. Label: 28. Potency: mild
Excipients: include cetyl alcohol, wool fat

Gregoderm® (Unigreg) PoM
Ointment, hydrocortisone 1%, neomycin sulphate 0.4%, nystatin 100 000 units/g, polymyxin B sulphate 7250 units/g, net price 15 g = £2.40. Label: 28. Potency: mild
Excipients: include cetostearyl alcohol

Nystaform-HC® (Typharm) PoM
Cream, hydrocortisone 0.5%, nystatin 100 000 units/g, chlorhexidine hydrochloride 1%, net price 30 g = £2.66. Label: 28. Potency: mild
Excipients: include benzyl alcohol, cetostearyl alcohol, polysorbate '60'
Ointment, hydrocortisone 1%, nystatin 100 000 units/g, chlorhexidine acetate 1%, net price 30 g = £2.66. Label: 28. Potency: mild
Excipients: none as listed in section 13.1.3

Terra-Cortril® (Pfizer) PoM
Topical ointment, hydrocortisone 1%, oxytetracycline 3% (as hydrochloride), net price 15 g = £1.21, 30 g = £2.18. Label: 28. Potency: mild
Excipients: none as listed in section 13.1.3

Timodine® (R&C) PoM
Cream, hydrocortisone 0.5%, nystatin 100 000 units/g, benzalkonium chloride solution 0.2%, dimeticone '350' 10%, net price 30 g = £2.38. Label: 28. Potency: mild
Excipients: include butylated hydroxyanisole, cetostearyl alcohol, hydroxybenzoates (parabens), sodium metabisulphite, sorbic acid

Vioform-Hydrocortisone® (Novartis Consumer Health) PoM
Cream, hydrocortisone 1%, clioquinol 3%, net price 30 g = £1.46. Label: 28. Potency: mild
Excipients: include cetostearyl alcohol
Ointment, hydrocortisone 1%, clioquinol 3%, net price 30 g = £1.46. Label: 28. Potency: mild
Excipients: none as listed in section 13.1.3
NOTE. Stains clothing

HYDROCORTISONE BUTYRATE

Indications: severe inflammatory skin disorders such as eczemas unresponsive to less potent corticosteroids; psoriasis, see notes above

Cautions: see under Hydrocortisone and notes above

Contra-indications: see under Hydrocortisone and notes above

Side-effects: see notes above

Dose: apply thinly 1–2 times daily

Locoid® (Yamanouchi) [PoM]
Cream, hydrocortisone butyrate 0.1%, net price 30 g
= £2.46, 100 g = £7.58. Label: 28. Potency: potent
Excipients: include cetostearyl alcohol, hydroxybenzoates (parabens)
Lipocream, hydrocortisone butyrate 0.1%, net price
30 g = £2.59, 100 g = £7.94. Label: 28. Potency:
potent
Excipients: include cetostearyl alcohol, hydroxybenzoates (parabens)
NOTE. For bland cream basis see *Lipobase*®, section
13.2.1
Ointment, hydrocortisone butyrate 0.1%, net price
30 g = £2.46, 100 g = £7.58. Label: 28. Potency:
potent
Excipients: none as listed in section 13.1.3
Scalp lotion, hydrocortisone butyrate 0.1%, in an
aqueous isopropyl alcohol basis, net price 100 mL
= £10.49. Label: 15, 28. Potency: potent
Excipients: none as listed in section 13.1.3

Locoid Crelo® (Yamanouchi) [PoM]
Lotion (topical emulsion), hydrocortisone butyrate
0.1% in a water-miscible basis, net price 100 g
(with applicator nozzle) = £9.08. Label: 28.
Potency: potent
Excipients: include cetostearyl alcohol, hydroxybenzoates (parabens), propylene glycol

■ With antimicrobials
See notes above for comment on compound preparations
Locoid C® (Yamanouchi) [PoM]
Cream, hydrocortisone butyrate 0.1%, chlorquinaldol 3%, net price 30 g = £3.23. Label: 28. Potency:
potent
Excipients: include cetostearyl alcohol
NOTE. Stains clothing and can darken skin and hair
Ointment, ingredients as for cream, in a greasy
basis, net price 30 g = £3.23. Label: 28. Potency:
potent
Excipients: none as listed in section 13.1.3
NOTE. Stains clothing and can darken skin and hair

ALCLOMETASONE DIPROPIONATE

Indications: inflammatory skin disorders such as
eczemas
Cautions: see under Hydrocortisone and notes
above
Contra-indications: see under Hydrocortisone and
notes above
Side-effects: see notes above
Dose: apply thinly 1–2 times daily

Modrasone® (PLIVA) [PoM]
Cream, alclometasone dipropionate 0.05%, net
price 50 g = £2.82. Label: 28. Potency: moderate
Excipients: include cetostearyl alcohol, chlorocresol, propylene
glycol
Ointment, alclometasone dipropionate 0.05%, net
price 50 g = £2.82. Label: 28. Potency: moderate
Excipients: include beeswax, propylene glycol

BECLOMETASONE DIPROPIONATE

(Beclomethasone dipropionate)
Indications: severe inflammatory skin disorders
such as eczemas unresponsive to less potent
corticosteroids; psoriasis, see notes above
Cautions: see under Hydrocortisone and notes
above
Contra-indications: see under Hydrocortisone and
notes above
Side-effects: see notes above
Dose: apply thinly 1–2 times daily

Propaderm® (GSK) [PoM]
Cream, beclometasone dipropionate 0.025%, net
price 30 g = £1.74. Label: 28. Potency: potent
Excipients: include cetostearyl alcohol, chlorocresol
Ointment, beclometasone dipropionate 0.025%, net
price 30 g = £1.74. Label: 28. Potency: potent
Excipients: include propylene glycol

BETAMETHASONE ESTERS

Indications: severe inflammatory skin disorders
such as eczemas unresponsive to less potent
corticosteroids; psoriasis, see notes above
Cautions: see under Hydrocortisone and notes
above; use of more than 100 g per week of 0.1%
preparation likely to cause adrenal suppression
Contra-indications: see under Hydrocortisone and
notes above
Side-effects: see notes above
Dose: apply thinly 1–2 times daily

Betamethasone Valerate (Non-proprietary) [PoM]
Cream, betamethasone (as valerate) 0.1%, net price
30 g = £1.54. Label: 28. Potency: potent
Ointment, betamethasone (as valerate) 0.1%, net
price 30 g = £1.69. Label: 28. Potency: potent
Available from Dowelhurst, Futura

Betacap® (Dermal) [PoM]
Scalp application, betamethasone (as valerate)
0.1% in a water-miscible basis containing coconut
oil derivative, net price 100 mL = £4.22. Label: 15,
28. Potency: potent
Excipients: none as listed in section 13.1.3

Betnovate® (GSK) [PoM]
Cream, betamethasone (as valerate) 0.1% in a
water-miscible basis, net price 30 g = £1.54, 100 g
= £4.35. Label: 28. Potency: potent
Excipients: include cetostearyl alcohol, chlorocresol
Ointment, betamethasone (as valerate) 0.1% in an
anhydrous paraffin basis, net price 30 g = £1.54,
100 g = £4.35. Label: 28. Potency: potent
Excipients: none as listed in section 13.1.3
Lotion, betamethasone (as valerate) 0.1%, net price
100 mL = £5.23. Label: 28. Potency: potent
Excipients: include cetostearyl alcohol, hydroxybenzoates (parabens)
Scalp application, betamethasone (as valerate)
0.1% in a water-miscible basis, net price 100 mL
= £5.70. Label: 15, 28. Potency: potent
Excipients: none as listed in section 13.1.3

Betnovate-RD® (GSK) [PoM]
Cream, betamethasone (as valerate) 0.025% in a
water-miscible basis (1 in 4 dilution of *Betnovate*®
cream), net price 100 g = £3.59. Label: 28.
Potency: moderate
Excipients: include cetostearyl alcohol, chlorocresol
Ointment, betamethasone (as valerate) 0.025% in an
anhydrous paraffin basis (1 in 4 dilution of
Betnovate® ointment), net price 100 g = £3.59.
Label: 28. Potency: moderate
Excipients: none as listed in section 13.1.3

Bettamousse® (Celltech) [PoM]
Foam (= scalp application), betamethasone valerate
0.12% (≡ betamethasone 0.1%), net price 100 g =
£7.50. Label: 28. Potency: potent
Excipients: include cetyl alcohol, polysorbate 60, propylene glycol,
stearyl alcohol
NOTE. Flammable

Diprosone® (Schering-Plough) PoM
Cream, betamethasone (as dipropionate) 0.05%, net price 30 g = £2.41, 100 g = £6.84. Label: 28.
Potency: potent
Excipients: include cetostearyl alcohol, chlorocresol
Ointment, betamethasone (as dipropionate) 0.05%, net price 30 g = £2.41, 100 g = £6.84. Label: 28.
Potency: potent
Excipients: none as listed in section 13.1.3
Lotion, betamethasone (as dipropionate) 0.05%, net price 30 mL = £3.04, 100 mL = £8.71. Label: 28.
Potency: potent
Excipients: none as listed in section 13.1.3

■ With salicylic acid
See notes above for comment on compound preparations
Diprosalic® (Schering-Plough) PoM
Ointment, betamethasone (as dipropionate) 0.05%, salicylic acid 3%, net price 30 g = £3.30, 100 g = £9.50. Label: 28. Potency: potent
Excipients: none as listed in section 13.1.3
Dose: apply thinly 1–2 times daily; max. 60 g per week
Lotion, betamethasone (as dipropionate) 0.05%, salicylic acid 2%, in an alcoholic basis, net price 100 mL = £10.50. Label: 28. Potency: potent
Excipients: include disodium edetate
Dose: apply a few drops 1–2 times daily

■ With antimicrobials
See notes above for comment on compound preparations
Betnovate-C® (GSK) PoM
Cream, betamethasone (as valerate) 0.1%, clioquinol 3%, net price 30 g = £1.89. Label: 28.
Potency: potent
Excipients: include cetostearyl alcohol, chlorocresol
NOTE. Stains clothing
Ointment, betamethasone (as valerate) 0.1%, clioquinol 3%, net price 30 g = £1.89. Label: 28.
Potency: potent
Excipients: none as listed in section 13.1.3
NOTE. Stains clothing

Betnovate-N® (GSK) PoM
Cream, betamethasone (as valerate) 0.1%, neomycin sulphate 0.5%, net price 30 g = £1.89, 100 g = £5.25. Label: 28. Potency: potent
Excipients: include cetostearyl alcohol, chlorocresol
Ointment, betamethasone (as valerate) 0.1%, neomycin sulphate 0.5%, net price 30 g = £1.89, 100 g = £5.25. Label: 28. Potency: potent
Excipients: none as listed in section 13.1.3

FuciBET® (Leo) PoM
Cream, betamethasone (as valerate) 0.1%, fusidic acid 2%, net price 30 g = £6.04, 60 g = £12.07.
Label: 28. Potency: potent
Excipients: include cetostearyl alcohol, chlorocresol

Lotriderm® (PLIVA) PoM
Cream, betamethasone dipropionate 0.064% (≡ betamethasone 0.05%), clotrimazole 1%, net price 30 g = £6.34. Label: 28. Potency: potent
Excipients: include benzyl alcohol, cetostearyl alcohol, propylene glycol

CLOBETASOL PROPIONATE

Indications: short-term treatment only of severe resistant inflammatory skin disorders such as recalcitrant eczemas unresponsive to less potent corticosteroids; psoriasis, see notes above
Cautions: see under Hydrocortisone and notes above
Contra-indications: see under Hydrocortisone and notes above

Side-effects: see notes above
Dose: apply thinly 1–2 times daily for up to 4 weeks; max. 50 g of 0.05% preparation per week

Dermovate® (GSK) PoM
Cream, clobetasol propionate 0.05%, net price 30 g = £2.82, 100 g = £8.27. Label: 28. Potency: very potent
Excipients: include beeswax (or beeswax substitute), cetostearyl alcohol, chlorocresol, propylene glycol
Ointment, clobetasol propionate 0.05%, net price 30 g = £2.82, 100 g = £8.27. Label: 28. Potency: very potent
Excipients: include propylene glycol
Scalp application, clobetasol propionate 0.05%, in a thickened alcoholic basis, net price 30 mL = £3.22, 100 mL = £10.90. Label: 15, 28. Potency: very potent
Excipients: none as listed in section 13.1.3

■ With antimicrobials
See notes above for comment on compound preparations
Dermovate-NN® (GSK) PoM
Cream, clobetasol propionate 0.05%, neomycin sulphate 0.5%, nystatin 100 000 units/g, net price 30 g = £3.85. Label: 28. Potency: very potent
Excipients: include arachis (peanut) oil, beeswax substitute
Ointment, ingredients as for cream, in a paraffin basis, net price 30 g = £3.85. Label: 28. Potency: very potent
Excipients: none as listed in section 13.1.3

CLOBETASONE BUTYRATE

Indications: eczemas and dermatitis of all types; maintenance between courses of more potent corticosteroids
Cautions: see under Hydrocortisone and notes above
Contra-indications: see under Hydrocortisone and notes above
Side-effects: see notes above
Dose: apply thinly 1–2 times daily

¹**Eumovate**® (GSK) PoM
Cream, clobetasone butyrate 0.05%, net price 30 g = £1.94, 100 g = £5.68. Label: 28. Potency: moderate
Excipients: include beeswax substitute, cetostearyl alcohol, chlorocresol
Ointment, clobetasone butyrate 0.05%, net price 30 g = £1.94, 100 g = £5.68. Label: 28. Potency: moderate
Excipients: none as listed in section 13.1.3

1. Cream can be sold to the public for short-term symptomatic treatment and control of patches of eczema and dermatitis (but not seborrhoeic dermatitis) in adults and children over 12 years provided pack does not contain more than 15 g

■ With antimicrobials
See notes above for comment on compound preparations
Trimovate® (GSK) PoM
Cream, clobetasone butyrate 0.05%, oxytetracycline 3% (as calcium salt), nystatin 100 000 units/g, net price 30 g = £3.44. Label: 28.
Potency: moderate
Excipients: include cetostearyl alcohol, chlorocresol, sodium metabisulphite
NOTE. Stains clothing

DESOXIMETASONE
(Desoxymethasone)

Indications: severe acute inflammatory, allergic, and chronic skin disorders; psoriasis, see notes above

Cautions: see under Hydrocortisone and notes above

Contra-indications: see under Hydrocortisone and notes above

Side-effects: see notes above

Dose: apply thinly 1–2 times daily

Stiedex® (Stiefel) [PoM]
LP Oily cream, desoximetasone 0.05%, net price 30 g = £2.73, 100 g = £8.19. Label: 28. Potency: moderate
Excipients: include edetic acid (EDTA), wool fat
Lotion, desoximetasone 0.25%, salicylic acid 1%, net price 50 mL = £7.69. Label: 28. Potency: potent
Excipients: include disodium edetate, propylene glycol

DIFLUCORTOLONE VALERATE

Indications: severe inflammatory skin disorders such as eczemas unresponsive to less potent corticosteroids; high strength (0.3%), short-term treatment of severe exacerbations; psoriasis, see notes above

Cautions: see under Hydrocortisone and notes above

Contra-indications: see under Hydrocortisone and notes above

Side-effects: see notes above

Dose: apply thinly 1–2 times daily for up to 4 weeks (0.1% preparations) or 2 weeks (0.3% preparations), reducing strength as condition responds; max. 60 g of 0.3% per week

Nerisone® (Meadow) [PoM]
Cream, diflucortolone valerate 0.1%, net price 30 g = £1.59. Label: 28. Potency: potent
Excipients: include disodium edetate, hydroxybenzoates (parabens), stearyl alcohol
Oily cream, diflucortolone valerate 0.1%, net price 30 g = £2.56. Label: 28. Potency: potent
Excipients: include beeswax
Ointment, diflucortolone valerate 0.1%, net price 30 g = £1.59. Label: 28. Potency: potent
Excipients: none as listed in section 13.1.3

Nerisone Forte® (Meadow) [PoM]
Oily cream, diflucortolone valerate 0.3%, net price 15 g = £2.09. Label: 28. Potency: very potent
Excipients: include beeswax
Ointment, diflucortolone valerate 0.3%, net price 15 g = £2.09. Label: 28. Potency: very potent
Excipients: none as listed in section 13.1.3

FLUDROXYCORTIDE
(Flurandrenolone)

Indications: inflammatory skin disorders such as eczemas

Cautions: see under Hydrocortisone and notes above

Contra-indications: see under Hydrocortisone and notes above

Side-effects: see notes above

Dose: apply thinly 1–2 times daily, reducing strength as condition responds

Haelan® (Typharm) [PoM]
Cream, fludroxycortide 0.0125%, net price 60 g = £3.26. Label: 28. Potency: moderate
Excipients: include cetyl alcohol, propylene glycol

Ointment, fludroxycortide 0.0125%, net price 60 g = £3.26. Label: 28. Potency: moderate
Excipients: include beeswax, cetyl alcohol, polysorbate
Tape, polythene adhesive film impregnated with fludroxycortide 4 micrograms /cm^2, net price 7.5 cm × 50 cm = £9.27, 7.5 cm × 200 cm = £24.95
Dose: for chronic localised recalcitrant dermatoses (but not acute or weeping), cut tape to fit lesion, apply to clean, dry skin shorn of hair, usually for 12 of each 24 hours

FLUOCINOLONE ACETONIDE

Indications: inflammatory skin disorders such as eczemas; psoriasis, see notes above

Cautions: see under Hydrocortisone and notes above

Contra-indications: see under Hydrocortisone and notes above

Side-effects: see notes above

Dose: apply thinly 1–2 times daily, reducing strength as condition responds

Synalar® (GP Pharma) [PoM]
Cream, fluocinolone acetonide 0.025%, net price 30 g = £1.74. Label: 28. Potency: potent
Excipients: include benzyl alcohol, cetostearyl alcohol, polysorbates, propylene glycol
Gel, fluocinolone acetonide 0.025%, net price 30 g = £2.57. For use on scalp and other hairy areas. Label: 28. Potency: potent
Excipients: include hydroxybenzoates (parabens), propylene glycol
Ointment, fluocinolone acetonide 0.025%, net price 30 g = £1.74. Label: 28. Potency: potent
Excipients: include propylene glycol, wool fat

Synalar 1 in 4 Dilution® (GP Pharma) [PoM]
Cream, fluocinolone acetonide 0.00625%, net price 50 g = £2.03. Label: 28. Potency: moderate
Excipients: include benzyl alcohol, cetostearyl alcohol, polysorbates, propylene glycol
Ointment, fluocinolone acetonide 0.00625%, net price 50 g = £2.03. Label: 28. Potency: moderate
Excipients: include propylene glycol, wool fat

Synalar 1 in 10 Dilution® (GP Pharma) [PoM]
Cream, fluocinolone acetonide 0.0025%, net price 50 g = £1.92. Label: 28. Potency: mild
Excipients: include benzyl alcohol, cetostearyl alcohol, polysorbates, propylene glycol

■ With antibacterials
See notes above for comment on compound preparations
Synalar C® (GP Pharma) [PoM]
Cream, fluocinolone acetonide 0.025%, clioquinol 3%, net price 15 g = £1.12. Label: 28. Potency: potent
Excipients: include cetostearyl alcohol, disodium edetate, hydroxybenzoates (parabens), polysorbates, propylene glycol
Ointment, ingredients as for cream, net price 15 g = £1.12. Label: 28. Potency: potent.
NOTE. stains clothing
Excipients: include propylene glycol, wool fat

Synalar N® (GP Pharma) [PoM]
Cream, fluocinolone acetonide 0.025%, neomycin sulphate 0.5%, net price 30 g = £1.83. Label: 28. Potency: potent
Excipients: include cetostearyl alcohol, hydroxybenzoates (parabens), polysorbates, propylene glycol
Ointment, ingredients as for cream, in a greasy basis, net price 30 g = £1.83. Label: 28. Potency: potent
Excipients: include propylene glycol, wool fat

FLUOCINONIDE

Indications: severe inflammatory skin disorders such as eczemas unresponsive to less potent corticosteroids; psoriasis, see notes above

Cautions: see under Hydrocortisone and notes above

Contra-indications: see under Hydrocortisone and notes above

Side-effects: see notes above

Dose: apply thinly 1–2 times daily

Metosyn® (GP Pharma) PoM
FAPG cream, fluocinonide 0.05%, net price 25 g = £1.52, 100 g = £5.14. Label: 28. Potency: potent
Excipients: include propylene glycol
Ointment, fluocinonide 0.05%, net price 25 g = £1.35, 100 g = £5.07. Label: 28. Potency: potent
Excipients: include propylene glycol, wool fat

FLUOCORTOLONE

Indications: severe inflammatory skin disorders such as eczemas unresponsive to less potent corticosteroids; psoriasis, see notes above

Cautions: see under Hydrocortisone and notes above

Contra-indications: see under Hydrocortisone and notes above

Side-effects: see notes above

Dose: apply thinly 1–2 times daily, reducing strength as condition responds

Ultralanum Plain® (Meadow) PoM
Cream, fluocortolone caproate 0.25%, fluocortolone pivalate 0.25%, net price 50 g = £2.95.
Label: 28. Potency: moderate
Excipients: include disodium edetate, fragrance, hydroxybenzoates (parabens), stearyl alcohol
Ointment, fluocortolone 0.25%, fluocortolone caproate 0.25%, net price 50 g = £2.95. Label: 28.
Potency: moderate
Excipients: include wool fat, fragrance

FLUTICASONE PROPIONATE

Indications: inflammatory skin disorders such as dermatitis and eczemas unresponsive to less potent corticosteroids

Cautions: see under Hydrocortisone and notes above

Contra-indications: see under Hydrocortisone and notes above

Side-effects: see notes above

Dose: apply thinly 1–2 times daily

Cutivate® (GSK) PoM
Cream, fluticasone propionate 0.05%, net price 15 g = £2.59, 50 g = £7.65. Label: 28. Potency: potent
Excipients: include cetostearyl alcohol, imidurea, propylene glycol
Ointment, fluticasone propionate 0.005%, net price 15 g = £2.59, 50 g = £7.65. Label: 28. Potency: potent
Excipients: include propylene glycol

HALCINONIDE

Indications: short-term treatment only of severe resistant inflammatory skin disorders such as recalcitrant eczemas unresponsive to less potent corticosteroids; psoriasis, see notes above

Cautions: see under Hydrocortisone and notes above

Contra-indications: see under Hydrocortisone and notes above

Side-effects: see notes above

Dose: apply thinly 1–2 times daily

Halciderm Topical® (Squibb) PoM
Cream, halcinonide 0.1%, net price 30 g =£3.40.
Label: 28. Potency: very potent
Excipients: include propylene glycol

MOMETASONE FUROATE

Indications: severe inflammatory skin disorders such as eczemas unresponsive to less potent corticosteroids; psoriasis, see notes above

Cautions: see under Hydrocortisone and notes above

Contra-indications: see under Hydrocortisone and notes above

Side-effects: see notes above

Dose: apply thinly once daily (to scalp in case of lotion)

Elocon® (Schering-Plough) PoM
Cream, mometasone furoate 0.1%, net price 30 g = £4.88, 100 g = £14.05. Label: 28. Potency: potent
Excipients: include stearyl alcohol
Ointment, mometasone furoate 0.1%, net price 30 g =£4.88, 100 g =£14.05. Label: 28. Potency: potent
Excipients: none as listed in section 13.1.3
Scalp lotion, mometasone furoate 0.1% in an aqueous isopropyl alcohol basis, net price 30 mL = £4.88. Label: 28. Potency: potent
Excipients: include propylene glycol

TRIAMCINOLONE ACETONIDE

Indications: severe inflammatory skin disorders such as eczemas unresponsive to less potent corticosteroids; psoriasis, see notes above

Cautions: see under Hydrocortisone and notes above

Contra-indications: see under Hydrocortisone and notes above

Side-effects: see notes above

Dose: apply thinly 1–2 times daily

■ With antimicrobials
See notes above for comment on compound preparations
Aureocort® (Lederle) PoM
Ointment, triamcinolone acetonide 0.1%, chlortetracycline hydrochloride 3%, in an anhydrous greasy basis containing wool fat and white soft paraffin, net price 15 g = £2.70. Label: 28.
Potency: potent
Excipients: include wool fat
NOTE. Stains clothing

Tri-Adcortyl® (Squibb) PoM
Cream, triamcinolone acetonide 0.1%, gramicidin 0.025%, neomycin (as sulphate) 0.25%, nystatin 100 000 units/g, net price 30 g = £3.15. Label: 28.
Potency: potent
Excipients: include benzyl alcohol, ethylenediamine, propylene glycol, fragrance
Ointment, triamcinolone acetonide 0.1%, gramicidin 0.025%, neomycin (as sulphate) 0.25%, nystatin 100 000 units/g, net price 30 g = £3.15.
Label: 28. Potency: potent
Excipients: none as listed in section 13.1.3
NOTE. Not recommended owing to presence of ethylenediamine in the cream and also because combination of antibacterial with antifungal not considered useful in either the cream or ointment

13.5   Preparations for eczema and psoriasis

13.5.1	Preparations for eczema
13.5.2	Preparations for psoriasis
13.5.3	Drugs affecting the immune response

13.5.1   Preparations for eczema

Eczema (dermatitis) has several causes, which may influence treatment. The main types of eczema are irritant, allergic contact, atopic, venous and discoid; different types may co-exist. Lichenification, due to scratching and rubbing, may complicate any chronic eczema. *Atopic eczema* is the most common type and it usually involves dry skin as well as infection and lichenification.

Management of eczema involves the removal or treatment of contributory factors including occupational and domestic irritants. Known or suspected contact allergens should be avoided. Rarely, ingredients in topical medicinal products may sensitise the skin; the BNF lists active ingredients together with excipients that have been associated with skin sensitisation.

Skin dryness and the consequent irritant eczema requires **emollients** (section 13.2.1). applied regularly and liberally to the affected area; this may be supplemented with bath or shower emollients. The use of emollients should continue even if the eczema improves or if other treatment is being used.

Topical corticosteroids (section 13.4) are also required in the management of eczema; the potency of the corticosteroid should be appropriate to the severity and site of the condition. Mild corticosteroids are generally used on the face and on flexures; potent corticosteroids are generally required for use on adults with discoid or lichenified eczema or with eczema on the scalp, limbs, and trunk. Treatment should be reviewed regularly, especially if a potent corticosteroid is required. Bandages (including those containing **zinc** and **ichthammol**) are sometimes applied over topical corticosteroids to treat eczema of the limbs.

INFECTION. Bacterial infection (commonly with *Staphylococcus aureus* and occasionally with *Streptococcus pyogenes*) can exacerbate eczema and requires treatment with topical or systemic **antibacterial drugs** (section 13.10.1 and section 5.1). Antibacterial drugs should be used in short courses (typically 1 week) to reduce the risk of drug resistance or skin sensitisation. Associated eczema is treated simultaneously with a topical corticosteroid usually of moderate or high potency.

Eczema involving widespread or recurrent infection requires the use of a systemic antibacterial that is active against the infecting organism. Products that combine an antiseptic with an emollient application (section 13.2.1) and with a bath emollient (section 13.2.1.1) may also be used; antiseptic shampoos (section 13.9) may be used on the scalp.

Intertriginous eczema commonly involves candida and bacteria; it is best treated with a mild or moderately potent topical corticosteroid and a suitable antimicrobial drug.

Widespread herpes simplex infection may complicate atopic eczema and treatment with a systemic antiviral drug (section 5.3) is indicated.

The management of *seborrhoeic dermatitis* is described below.

MANAGEMENT OF OTHER FEATURES OF ECZEMA. *Lichenification*, which results from repeated scratching is treated initially with a potent corticosteroid. Bandages containing **ichthammol paste** (to reduce pruritus) and other substances such as **zinc oxide** may be applied over the corticosteroid. **Coal tar** (section 13.5.2) and **ichthammol** can be useful in some cases of *chronic eczema*.

Antihistamines (section 3.4.1) may be of some value in relieving the itch of eczema, usually because of their sedating effect.

Exudative ('*weeping*') *eczema* requires a potent corticosteroid initially; infection may also be present and require specific treatment (see above). **Potassium permanganate** solution (1 in 10 000) can be used in exudating eczema for its antiseptic and astringent effect; treatment should be stopped when exudation stops.

Severe refractory eczema is best managed under specialist supervision; it may require phototherapy, systemic corticosteroids (section 6.3.2), or other drugs acting on the immune system (section 13.5.3).

SEBORRHOEIC DERMATITIS. *Seborrhoeic dermatitis* (*seborrhoeic eczema*) is associated with species of the yeast *Malassezia* and affects the scalp, paranasal areas, and eyebrows. Shampoos active against the yeast (including those containing ketoconazole and coal tar, section 13.9) and combinations of mild corticosteroids with suitable antimicrobials (section 13.4) are used.

ICHTHAMMOL

Indications: chronic lichenified eczema
Side-effects: skin irritation
Dose: apply 1–3 times daily

Ichthammol Ointment, BP 1980
Ointment, ichthammol 10%, yellow soft paraffin 45%, wool fat 45%, net price 25 g = 53p

Zinc and Ichthammol Cream, BP
Cream, ichthammol 5%, cetostearyl alcohol 3%, wool fat 10%, in zinc cream, net price 100 g = 79p

Zinc Paste and Ichthammol Bandage, BP
(*Ichthopaste®*, *Icthaband®*), see Appendix 8 (section A8.2.9)

13.5.2   Preparations for psoriasis

Psoriasis is characterised by epidermal thickening and scaling. It commonly affects extensor surfaces and the scalp. For mild psoriasis, reassurance and treatment with an emollient may be all that is necessary.

Occasionally psoriasis is provoked or exacerbated by drugs such as lithium, chloroquine and hydroxychloroquine, beta-blockers, non-steroidal anti-inflammatory drugs, and ACE inhibitors. Psoriasis may not be seen until the drug has been taken for weeks or months.

Emollients (section 13.2.1), in addition to their effects on dryness, scaling and cracking, may have an antiproliferative effect in psoriasis. They are particularly useful in *inflammatory psoriasis* and in *plaque psoriasis of palms and soles*, in which irritant factors can perpetuate the condition. Emollients are useful adjuncts to other more specific treatment.

More specific treatment for *chronic stable plaque psoriasis* on extensor surfaces of trunk and limbs involves the use of **vitamin D analogues, coal tar, dithranol**, and the retinoid **tazarotene**. However, they can irritate the skin and they are not suitable for the more inflammatory forms of psoriasis; their use should be suspended during an inflammatory phase of psoriasis. The efficacy and the irritancy of each substance varies between patients. If a substance irritates significantly, it should be stopped or the concentration reduced; if it is tolerated, its effects should be assessed after 4 to 6 weeks and treatment continued if it is effective.

Widespread *unstable psoriasis* of erythrodermic or generalised pustular type requires urgent specialist assessment. Initial topical treatment should be limited to using emollients frequently and generously; emollients should be prescribed in quantities of 1 kg or more. More localised acute or subacute *inflammatory psoriasis* with hot, spreading or itchy lesions, should be treated topically with emollients or with a corticosteroid of medium potency.

Calcipotriol and **tacalcitol** are analogues of vitamin D that affect cell division and differentiation but have little effect on calcium metabolism. **Calcitriol**, an active form of vitamin D, has recently been introduced for topical use. Vitamin D and its analogues do not smell or stain and they may be more acceptable than tar or dithranol products. Of the vitamin D analogues, tacalcitol and calcitriol are less likely to irritate. If the efficacy of a vitamin D analogue declines after several weeks, it may be regained by suspending use for a few weeks; some patients find it helpful to alternate another treatment with a vitamin D analogue every few weeks.

Coal tar has anti-inflammatory properties that are useful in chronic plaque psoriasis; it also has antiscaling properties. Crude coal tar is the most effective form, typically in a concentration of 1 to 10% in a soft paraffin base, but few outpatients tolerate the smell and mess. Cleaner extracts of coal tar included in proprietary preparations, are more practicable for home use but they are less effective and improvement takes longer. Contact of coal tar products with normal skin is not normally harmful and they can be used for widespread small lesions; however, irritation, contact allergy, and sterile folliculitis can occur. The milder tar extracts can be used on the face and flexures. Tar baths and tar shampoos are also helpful.

Dithranol is effective for chronic plaque psoriasis. Its major disadvantages are irritation (for which individual susceptibility varies) and staining of skin and of clothing. It should be applied to chronic extensor plaques only, carefully avoiding normal skin. Dithranol is not generally suitable for widespread small lesions nor should it be used in the flexures or on the face. Treatment should be started with a low concentration such as dithranol 0.1%, and the strength increased gradually every few days up to 3%, according to tolerance. Proprietary preparations are more suitable for home use; they are usually washed off after 5 to 60 minutes ('short contact'). Specialist nurses may apply intensive treatment with dithranol paste which is covered by stockinette dressings and usually retained overnight. Dithranol should be discontinued if even a low concentration causes acute inflammation; continued use can result in the psoriasis becoming unstable. When applying dithranol, hands should be protected by gloves or they should be washed thoroughly afterwards.

Tazarotene, a retinoid, is effective in psoriasis. It is clean and odourless. Irritation is common but it is minimised by applying tazarotene sparingly to the plaques and avoiding normal skin.

A topical **corticosteroid** (section 13.4) is not generally suitable as the sole treatment of extensive chronic plaque psoriasis; any early improvement is not usually maintained and there is a risk of the condition deteriorating or of precipitating an unstable form of psoriasis (e.g. erythrodermic psoriasis or generalised pustular psoriasis). However, it may be appropriate to treat psoriasis in specific sites such as the face and flexures usually with a mild corticosteroid, and psoriasis of the scalp, hands and feet with a potent corticosteroid.

Combining the use of a corticosteroid with another specific topical treatment may be beneficial in chronic plaque psoriasis; the drugs may be used separately at different times of the day or used together in a single formulation. *Eczema* co-existing with psoriasis may be treated with a corticosteroid, or coal tar, or both.

Scalp psoriasis is usually scaly, and the scale may be thick and adherent. This requires softening with an emollient ointment, cream, or oil and usually combined with **salicylic acid** as a keratolytic.

Some preparations prescribed for psoriasis affecting the scalp combine salicylic acid with coal tar or **sulphur**. Preparations containing salicylic acid, sulphur, and coal tar are available as proprietary products. The product should be applied generously and an adequate quantity should be prescribed. It should be left on for at least an hour, often more conveniently overnight, before washing it off. If a corticosteroid lotion or gel is required (e.g. for itch), it can be used in the morning.

PHOTOTHERAPY. **Ultraviolet B** (UVB) radiation is usually effective for *chronic stable psoriasis* and for *guttate psoriasis*. It may be considered for patients with moderately severe psoriasis in whom topical treatment has failed, but it may irritate inflammatory psoriasis. Narrow-band UVB is more effective and it is less likely to burn than conventional broad-band therapy.

Photochemotherapy combining long-wave ultraviolet A radiation with a psoralen (PUVA) is available in dermatology centres. The psoralen, which enhances the effect of the irradiation, is administered either by mouth or topically. PUVA is effective in most forms of psoriasis, including the *unstable forms of psoriasis* and *localised palmoplantar pustular psoriasis*. Early adverse effects include phototoxicity and pruritus. Higher cumulative doses exaggerate signs of skin ageing, increase the risk of dysplastic and neoplastic skin lesions especially squamous cancer, and pose a theoretical risk of cataracts.

SYSTEMIC TREATMENT. **Systemic treatment** is required for severe, resistant, unstable or complicated forms of psoriasis, and it should be initiated only under specialist supervision. Systemic drugs for psoriasis include acitretin and drugs that act on the immune system (such as ciclosporin, hydroxycarbamide, and methotrexate, section 13.5.3).

Systemic corticosteroids should be used only rarely in psoriasis because rebound deterioration may occur on reducing the dose.

The main indication for **acitretin** is *psoriasis*, but it is also used in disorders of keratinisation such as severe *Darier's disease* (keratosis follicularis), and some forms of *ichthyosis*. Acitretin, a metabolite of etretinate, is a retinoid (vitamin A derivative). Although a minority of cases of psoriasis respond well to acitretin alone, it is only moderately effective in many cases and it is combined with other treatments. A therapeutic effect occurs after 2 to 4 weeks and the maximum benefit after 4 to 6 weeks or longer. Acitretin is prescribed by specialists and its availability is limited to hospital pharmacies or to a small number of specified retail pharmacies.

Apart from teratogenicity, which remains a risk for 2 years after stopping, acitretin is the least toxic systemic treatment for psoriasis; in women with a potential for child-bearing, the possibility of pregnancy must be excluded before treatment and pregnancy must be avoided during treatment and for a period of 2 years afterwards. Common side effects derive from its widespread but reversible effects on epithelia, such as dry and cracking lips, dry skin and mucosal surfaces, hair thinning, paronychia, and soft and sticky palms and soles. Liver function and blood lipid concentration should be monitored

Topical preparations for psoriasis

Vitamin D and analogues

Calcipotriol, **calcitriol**, and **tacalcitol** are used for the management of *plaque psoriasis*. They should be avoided by those with calcium metabolism disorders, and used with caution in *generalised pustular* or *erythrodermic exfoliative psoriasis* (enhanced risk of hypercalcaemia). Local skin reactions (itching, erythema, burning, paraesthesia, dermatitis) are common. Hands should be washed thoroughly after application to avoid inadvertent transfer to other body areas. Aggravation of psoriasis has also been reported.

CALCIPOTRIOL

Indications: plaque psoriasis

Cautions: see notes above; pregnancy; avoid use on face; if used with UV treatment apply at least 2 hours before UV exposure

Contra-indications: see notes above

Side-effects: see notes above; also photosensitivity; rarely facial or perioral dermatitis, skin atrophy

Dose: *cream* or *ointment* apply once or twice daily; max. 100 g weekly (less with *scalp solution*, see below); CHILD over 6 years, apply twice daily; 6–

12 years max. 50 g weekly; over 12 years max. 75 g weekly

NOTE. Patient information leaflets for *Dovonex*® cream and ointment advise liberal application (but note max. recommended weekly dose, above)

Dovonex® (Leo) [PoM]

Cream, calcipotriol 50 micrograms/g, net price 60 g = £13.66, 120 g = £27.32

Excipients: include cetostearyl alcohol, disodium edetate

Ointment, calcipotriol 50 micrograms/g, net price 60 g = £13.66, 120 g = £27.32

Excipients: include disodium edetate, propylene glycol

Scalp solution, calcipotriol 50 micrograms/mL, net price 60 mL = £20.21, 120 mL = £40.42

Excipients: include propylene glycol

Dose: scalp psoriasis, apply to scalp twice daily; max. 60 mL weekly (less with cream or ointment, see below); CHILD not recommended

NOTE. When preparations used together max. total calcipotriol 5 mg in any one week (e.g. scalp solution 60 mL with cream or ointment 30 g *or* cream or ointment 60 g with scalp solution 30 mL)

■ With betamethasone

For cautions, contra-indications, side-effects, and for comment on the limited role of corticosteroids in psoriasis, see section 13.4.

Dovobet® (Leo) ▼ [PoM]

Ointment, betamethasone 0.05% (as dipropionate), calcipotriol 50 micrograms/g, net price 60 g = £35.00. Label: 28

Excipients: none as listed in section 13.1.3

Dose: initial treatment of stable plaque psoriasis, apply once daily to max. 30% of body surface for up to 4 weeks; max. 15 g daily, max. 100 g weekly; CHILD and ADOLESCENT under 18 years not recommended

CALCITRIOL

Indications: mild to moderate plaque psoriasis

Cautions: see notes above; liver impairment (Appendix 2), renal impairment (Appendix 3); pregnancy

Contra-indications: see notes above; do not apply under occlusion

Side-effects: see notes above

Dose: apply twice daily; not more than 35% of body surface to be treated daily, max. 30 g daily; CHILD not recommended

Silkis® (Galderma) ▼ [PoM]

Ointment, calcitriol 3 micrograms/g, net price 30 g = £7.20, 100 g = £24.00

Excipients: none as listed in section 13.1.3

TACALCITOL

Indications: plaque psoriasis

Cautions: see notes above; pregnancy (Appendix 4), breast-feeding (Appendix 5); avoid eyes; monitor plasma calcium if risk of hypercalcaemia or in renal impairment; if used in conjunction with UV treatment, UV radiation should be given in the morning and tacalcitol applied at bedtime

Contra-indications: see notes above

Side-effects: see notes above

Dose: apply daily preferably at bedtime; max. 10 g daily; CHILD not recommended

Curatoderm® (Crookes) [PoM]

Ointment, tacalcitol (as monohydrate) 4 micrograms/g, net price 30 g = £15.09, 60 g = £26.06, 100 g = £34.75

Excipients: none as listed in section 13.1.3

Tazarotene

TAZAROTENE

Indications: mild to moderate plaque psoriasis affecting up to 10% of skin area

Cautions: wash hands immediately after use, avoid contact with eyes, face, intertriginous areas, hair-covered scalp, eczematous or inflamed skin; avoid excessive exposure to UV light (including sunlight, solariums, PUVA or UVB treatment); do not apply emollients or cosmetics within 1 hour of application

Contra-indications: pregnancy—advise women of child-bearing age to ensure adequate contraceptive protection; breast-feeding (Appendix 5)

Side-effects: local irritation (more common with higher concentration and may require discontinuation), pruritus, burning, erythema, desquamation, non-specific rash, contact dermatitis, and worsening of psoriasis; rarely stinging and inflamed, dry or painful skin

Dose: apply once daily in the evening usually for up to 12 weeks; CHILD under 18 years not recommended

Zorac® (Allergan) ▣PoM
Gel, tazarotene 0.05%, net price 30 g = £14.09, 60 g = £26.26; 0.1%, 30 g = £14.80, 60 g = £27.70
Excipients: include benzyl alcohol, butylated hydroxyanisole, butylated hydroxytoluene, disodium edetate, polysorbate 40

Coal tar

COAL TAR

Indications: psoriasis and occasionally chronic atopic eczema

Cautions: avoid eyes, mucosa, genital or rectal areas, and broken or inflamed skin; use suitable chemical protection gloves for extemporaneous preparation

Contra-indications: not for use in sore, acute, or pustular psoriasis or in presence of infection

Side-effects: skin irritation and acne-like eruptions, photosensitivity; stains skin, hair, and fabric

Dose: apply 1–3 times daily starting with low-strength preparations

NOTE. For shampoo preparations see section 13.9; impregnated dressings see Appendix 8 (section A8.2.9)

■ Non-proprietary preparations
May be difficult to obtain—some patients may find newer proprietary preparations more acceptable

Calamine and Coal Tar Ointment, BP
Ointment, calamine 12.5 g, strong coal tar solution 2.5 g, zinc oxide 12.5 g, hydrous wool fat 25 g, white soft paraffin 47.5 g
Excipients: include wool fat
Dose: apply 1–2 times daily

Coal Tar and Salicylic Acid Ointment, BP
Ointment, coal tar 2 g, salicylic acid 2 g, emulsifying wax 11.4 g, white soft paraffin 19 g, coconut oil 54 g, polysorbate '80' 4 g, liquid paraffin 7.6 g
Excipients: include cetostearyl alcohol
Dose: apply 1–2 times daily

Coal Tar Paste, BP
Paste, strong coal tar solution 7.5%, in compound zinc paste
Dose: apply 1–2 times daily

Zinc and Coal Tar Paste, BP
Paste, zinc oxide 6%, coal tar 6%, emulsifying wax 5%, starch 38%, yellow soft paraffin 45%
Excipients: include cetostearyl alcohol
Dose: apply 1–2 times daily

■ Proprietary preparations

Carbo-Dome® (Sandoz)
Cream, coal tar solution 10%, in a water-miscible basis, net price 30 g = £4.77, 100 g = £13.65
Excipients: include beeswax, hydroxybenzoates (parabens)
Dose: psoriasis, apply to skin 2–3 times daily

Clinitar® (CHS)
Cream, coal tar extract 1%, net price 100 g = £10.99
Excipients: include cetostearyl alcohol, isopropyl palmitate, propylene glycol
Dose: psoriasis and eczema, apply to skin 1–2 times daily

Cocois® (Celltech)
Scalp ointment, coal tar solution 12%, salicylic acid 2%, precipitated sulphur 4%, in a coconut oil emollient basis, net price 40 g (with applicator nozzle) = £5.04, 100 g = £9.46
Excipients: include cetostearyl alcohol
Dose: scaly scalp disorders including psoriasis, eczema, seborrhoeic dermatitis and dandruff, apply to scalp once weekly as necessary (if severe use daily for first 3–7 days), shampoo off after 1 hour; CHILD 6–12 years, medical supervision required (not recommended under 6 years)
NOTE. Ointment containing coal tar solution 12%, salicylic acid 2%, precipitated sulphur 4% also available from Centrapharm (*Sebco*®)

Exorex® (Forest)
Lotion, prepared coal tar 1% in an emollient basis, net price 100 mL = £8.65, 250 mL = £17.33
Excipients: include hydroxybenzoates (parabens), polysorbate 80
Dose: psoriasis, apply to skin or scalp 2–3 times daily; CHILD and ELDERLY, dilute with a few drops of water before applying

Pragmatar® (Alliance)
Cream, cetyl alcohol-coal tar distillate 4%, salicylic acid 3%, sulphur (precipitated) 3%, net price 25 g = £3.12, 100 g = £10.07
Excipients: include cetyl alcohol, fragrance
Dose: scaly skin disorders, apply thinly once daily; dandruff and other seborrhoeic conditions, apply to scalp once weekly or in severe cases daily; INFANT dilute with a few drops of water before application

Psoriderm® (Dermal)
Cream, coal tar 6%, lecithin 0.4%, net price 225 mL = £3.55
Excipients: include isopropyl palmitate, propylene glycol
Dose: psoriasis, apply to skin or scalp 1–2 times daily
Scalp lotion—section 13.9

■ Bath preparations

Coal Tar Solution, BP
Solution, coal tar 20%, polysorbate '80' 5%, in alcohol (96%), net price 100 mL = 82p
Excipients: include polysorbates
Dose: use 100 mL in a bath
NOTE. Strong Coal Tar Solution BP contains coal tar 40%

Polytar Emollient® (Stiefel)
Bath additive, coal tar solution 2.5%, arachis (peanut) oil extract of coal tar 7.5%, tar 7.5%, cade oil 7.5%, liquid paraffin 35%, net price 500 mL = £6.50
Excipients: include isopropyl palmitate
Dose: psoriasis, eczema, atopic and pruritic dermatoses, use 2–4 capfuls (15–30 mL) in bath and soak for 20 minutes

Psoriderm® (Dermal)
Bath emulsion, coal tar 40%, net price 200 mL = £3.09
Excipients: include polysorbate 20
Dose: psoriasis, use 30 mL in a bath and soak for 5 minutes

■ With corticosteroids

Alphosyl HC® (GSK Consumer Healthcare) PoM
Cream, coal tar extract 5%, hydrocortisone 0.5%, allantoin 2%, net price 100 g = £3.54. Label: 28. Potency: mild
Excipients: include beeswax, cetyl alcohol, hydroxybenzoates (parabens), isopropyl palmitate, wool fat
Dose: psoriasis, apply thinly 1–2 times daily; CHILD under 5 years not recommended

Dithranol

DITHRANOL
(Anthralin)
Indications: subacute and chronic psoriasis, see notes above
Cautions: avoid use near eyes and sensitive areas of skin; see also notes above
Contra-indications: hypersensitivity; acute and pustular psoriasis
Side-effects: local burning sensation and irritation; stains skin, hair, and fabrics
Dose: see notes above and under preparations
NOTE. Some of these dithranol preparations also contain coal tar or salicylic acid—for cautions and side-effects see under Coal Tar (above) or under Salicylic Acid

¹Dithranol Ointment, BP PoM
Ointment, dithranol, in yellow soft paraffin; usual strengths 0.1–2%. Part of basis may be replaced by hard paraffin if a stiffer preparation is required. Label: 28

1. PoM if dithranol content more than 1%, otherwise may be sold to the public

Dithranol Paste, BP
Paste, dithranol in zinc and salicylic acid (Lassar's) paste. Usual strengths 0.1–1% of dithranol. Label: 28

Dithrocream® (Dermal)
Cream, dithranol 0.1%, net price 50 g = £4.24; 0.25%, 50 g = £4.55; 0.5%, 50 g = £5.24; 1%, 50 g = £6.10; PoM 2%, 50 g = £7.64. Label: 28
Excipients: include cetostearyl alcohol, chlorocresol, salicylic acid
Dose: for application to skin or scalp; 0.1–0.5% suitable for overnight treatment, 1–2% for max. 1 hour

Micanol® (GP Pharma)
Cream, dithranol 1% in a lipid-stabilised basis, net price 50 g = £10.37; PoM 3%, 50 g = £12.92. Label: 28
Excipients: none as listed in section 13.1.3
Dose: for application to skin, for up to 30 minutes, if necessary 3% cream may be used under medical supervision; apply to scalp for up to 30 minutes
NOTE. At the end of contact time use plenty of lukewarm (not hot) water to rinse off cream; soap should not be used

Psorin® (Ayrton Saunders)
Ointment, dithranol 0.11%, crude coal tar 1%, salicylic acid 1.6%, net price 50 g = £8.20, 100 g = £16.35. Label: 28
Excipients: include beeswax, wool fat
Dose: for application to skin up to twice daily

Scalp gel, dithranol 0.25%, salicylic acid 1.6% in gel basis containing methyl salicylate, net price 50 g = £6.25. Label: 28
Excipients: none as listed in section 13.1.3
Dose: for application to scalp, initially apply on alternate days for 10–20 minutes; may be increased to daily application for max. 1 hour and then wash off

Salicylic acid

SALICYLIC ACID
For coal tar preparations containing salicylic acid, see under Coal Tar p. 552; for dithranol preparations containing salicylic acid see under Dithranol, above
Indications: hyperkeratotic skin disorders; acne (section 13.6.1); warts and calluses (section 13.7); scalp conditions (section 13.9); fungal nail infections (section 13.10.2)
Cautions: see notes above; avoid broken or inflamed skin
SALICYLATE TOXICITY. If large areas of skin are treated, salicylate toxicity may be a hazard
Side-effects: sensitivity, excessive drying, irritation, systemic effects after widespread use (see under Cautions)

Zinc and Salicylic Acid Paste, BP
Paste, (Lassar's Paste), zinc oxide 24%, salicylic acid 2%, starch 24%, white soft paraffin 50%, net price 25 g = 19p
Dose: apply twice daily

Oral retinoids for psoriasis

ACITRETIN
NOTE. Acitretin is a metabolite of etretinate
Indications: severe extensive psoriasis resistant to other forms of therapy; palmoplantar pustular psoriasis; severe congenital ichthyosis; severe Darier's disease (keratosis follicularis)
Cautions: exclude pregnancy before starting (test for pregnancy within 2 weeks before treatment and monthly thereafter; start treatment on day 2 or 3 of menstrual cycle)—women (including those with history of infertility) should avoid pregnancy for at least 1 month before, during, and for at least 2 years after treatment; patients should avoid concomitant tetracycline or methotrexate, high doses of vitamin A (more than 4000–5000 units daily) and use of keratolytics, and should not donate blood during or for at least 1 year after stopping therapy (teratogenic risk); check liver function at start, then every 1–2 weeks for 2 months, then every 3 months; monitor plasma lipids; diabetes (can alter glucose tolerance—initial frequent blood glucose checks); radiographic assessment on long-term treatment; investigate atypical musculo-skeletal symptoms; in children use only in exceptional circumstances (premature epiphyseal closure reported); avoid excessive exposure to sunlight and unsupervised use of sunlamps; **interactions:** Appendix 1 (retinoids)
Contra-indications: hepatic and renal impairment; hyperlipidaemia, pregnancy (**important teratogenic risk:** see Cautions and Appendix 4); breast-feeding
Side-effects: dryness of mucous membranes (sometimes erosion), of skin (sometimes scaling, thinning, erythema especially of face, and pruritus),

and of conjunctiva (sometimes conjunctivitis and decreased tolerance of contact lenses); sticky skin, dermatitis; other side-effects reported include palmoplantar exfoliation, epistaxis, epidermal and nail fragility, oedema, paronychia, granulomatous lesions, bullous eruptions, reversible hair thinning and alopecia, myalgia and arthralgia, occasional nausea, headache, malaise, drowsiness, rhinitis, sweating, taste disturbance, and gingivitis; benign intracranial hypertension (discontinue if severe headache, vomiting, diarrhoea, abdominal pain, and visual disturbance occur; **avoid** concomitant tetracyclines); photosensitivity, corneal ulceration, raised liver enzymes, rarely jaundice and hepatitis (**avoid** concomitant methotrexate); raised triglycerides; decreased night vision reported; skeletal hyperostosis and extraosseous calcification reported following long-term administration of etretinate (and premature epiphyseal closure in children, see Cautions)

Dose: under expert supervision, initially 25–30 mg daily (Darier's disease 10 mg daily) for 2–4 weeks, then adjusted according to response, usual range 25–50 mg daily (max. 75 mg daily) for further 6–8 weeks (in Darier's disease and ichthyosis not more than 50 mg daily for up to 6 months); CHILD (**important:** exceptional circumstances only, see Cautions), 500 micrograms/kg daily (occasionally up to 1 mg/kg daily to max. 35 mg daily for limited periods) with careful monitoring of musculo-skeletal development

Neotigason® (Roche) PoM

Capsules, acitretin 10 mg (brown/white), net price 60-cap pack = £27.15; 25 mg (brown/yellow), 60-cap pack = £63.00 (hosp. or specified retail pharmacy only—consult product literature for details, specialist dermatological supervision).
Label: 10, patient information leaflet, 21

13.5.3 Drugs affecting the immune response

Drugs affecting the immune response are used for eczema or psoriasis. Systemic drugs acting on the immune system are generally used by **specialists** in a hospital setting.

Ciclosporin (cyclosporin) by mouth can be used for *severe psoriasis* and for *severe eczema*. **Azathioprine** (section 8.2.1) or **mycophenolate mofetil** (section 8.2.1) are used for severe refractory eczema [unlicensed indication]. **Hydroxycarbamide** (hydroxyurea) (section 8.1.5) is used for severe psoriasis.

Methotrexate may be used for *severe resistant psoriasis*, the dose being adjusted according to severity of the condition and haematological and biochemical measurements; the usual dose is methotrexate 10 to 25 mg *once weekly*, by mouth. Folic acid may be given to reduce the possibility of methotrexate toxicity.

Pimecrolimus by topical application is licensed for *mild to moderate atopic eczema* for short-term use to treat signs and symptoms and for intermittent use to prevent flares. **Tacrolimus** is licensed for topical use in *moderate to severe atopic eczema*. Both are new drugs whose long-term safety and place in therapy is still being evaluated and they should not usually be considered first-line treatments unless there is a specific reason to avoid or reduce the use of topical corticosteroids. Treatment with tacrolimus should normally be initiated by a specialist. Neither drug is licensed for children aged under 2 years.

For the role of corticosteroids in eczema see section 13.5.1 and for comment on their limited role in psoriasis see section 13.4.

CICLOSPORIN

(Cyclosporin)

Indications: see under Dose; transplantation and graft-versus-host disease (section 8.2.2)

Cautions: see section 8.2.2

ADDITIONAL CAUTIONS IN ATOPIC DERMATITIS AND PSORIASIS. **Contra-indicated** in abnormal renal function, hypertension not under control (see also below), infections not under control, and malignancy (see also below). Dermatological and physical examination, including blood pressure and renal function measurements required at least twice before starting; discontinue if hypertension develops that cannot be controlled by dose reduction or antihypertensive therapy; avoid excessive exposure to sunlight and use of UVB or PUVA; *in atopic dermatitis*, also allow herpes simplex infections to clear before starting (if they occur during treatment withdraw if severe); *Staphylococcus aureus* skin infections not absolute contra-indication providing controlled (but avoid erythromycin unless no other alternative—see also **interactions**: Appendix 1 (ciclosporin)); monitor serum creatinine every 2 weeks during treatment; *in psoriasis*, also exclude malignancies (including those of skin and cervix) before starting (biopsy any lesions not typical of psoriasis) and treat patients with malignant or pre-malignant conditions of skin only after appropriate treatment (and if no other option); monitor serum creatinine every 2 weeks for first 3 months then every 2 months (monthly if dose more than 2.5 mg/kg daily), reducing dose by 25–50% if increases more than 30% above baseline (even if within normal range) and discontinuing if reduction not successful within 1 month; also discontinue if lymphoproliferative disorder develops

Side-effects: see section 8.2.2

Dose: ADULT over 16 years *by mouth*, administered in accordance with expert advice

Short-term treatment (max. 8 weeks) of severe atopic dermatitis where conventional therapy ineffective or inappropriate, initially 2.5 mg/kg daily in 2 divided doses, if good initial response not achieved within 2 weeks, increase rapidly to max. 5 mg/kg daily; initial dose of 5 mg/kg daily in 2 divided doses if very severe; CHILD under 16 years not recommended

Severe psoriasis where conventional therapy ineffective or inappropriate, initially 2.5 mg/kg daily in 2 divided doses, increased gradually to max. 5 mg/kg daily if no improvement within 1 month (discontinue if response still insufficient after 6 weeks); initial dose of 5 mg/kg daily justified if condition requires rapid improvement; CHILD under 16 years not recommended

IMPORTANT. For preparations and counselling and for advice on conversion between the preparations, see section 8.2.2

■ Preparations
Section 8.2.2

METHOTREXATE

Indications: severe uncontrolled psoriasis unresponsive to conventional therapy (specialist use only); malignant disease (section 8.1.3); rheumatoid arthritis (section 10.1.3)

Cautions: see section 10.1.3, also photosensitivity—psoriasis lesions aggravated by UV radiation (skin ulceration reported)

Contra-indications: see section 10.1.3

Side-effects: see section 10.1.3

Dose: *by mouth*, 10–25 mg once weekly, adjusted according to response; ELDERLY consider dose reduction (extreme caution); CHILD not recommended

> **Important.** Note that the above dose is a **weekly** dose. The CSM has received reports of prescription and dispensing errors including fatalities. Attention should be paid to the **strength** of methotrexate tablets prescribed and the **frequency** of dosing.

■ Preparations
Section 10.1.3

PIMECROLIMUS

Indications: acute treatment of mild to moderate atopic eczema (including flares)

Cautions: UV light (avoid excessive exposure to sunlight and sunlamps), avoid other topical treatments except emollients at treatment site

Contra-indications: contact with eyes and mucous membranes, application under occlusion; infection at treatment site; congenital epidermal barrier defects; generalised erythroderma

Side-effects: burning sensation, pruritus, erythema, skin infections (including folliculitis and rarely impetigo, herpes simplex and zoster, molluscum contagiosum); rarely papilloma; local reactions including pain, paraesthesia, peeling, dryness, oedema, and worsening of eczema

Dose: apply twice daily until symptoms resolve; CHILD under 2 years not recommended

Elidel® (Novartis) ▼ PoM
Cream, pimecrolimus 1%, net price 30 g = £19.69, 60 g = £37.41, 100 g = £59.07. Label: 28
Excipients: include benzyl alcohol, cetyl alcohol, propylene glycol, stearyl alcohol

TACROLIMUS

Indications: moderate to severe atopic eczema unresponsive to conventional therapy (specialist use only); other indications section 8.2.2

Cautions: infection at treatment site, UV light (avoid excessive exposure to sunlight and sunlamps), do not apply other topical preparations within 2 hours of application

Contra-indications: avoid contact with eyes and mucous membranes, application under occlusion; congenital epidermal barrier defects; generalised erythroderma; pregnancy and breast-feeding

Side-effects: burning or tingling sensation, pruritus, erythema, folliculitis, acne, herpes simplex infection, increased sensitivity to hot and cold, alcohol intolerance; lymphadenopathy also reported

Dose: ADULT and ADOLESCENT over 16 years initially apply 0.1% ointment thinly twice daily for up to 3 weeks then reduce to 0.03% ointment twice daily (with further reduction to once daily where appropriate) until lesion clears; CHILD 2–16 years, initially apply 0.03% ointment twice daily for up to 3 weeks then reduce to once daily until lesion clears; CHILD under 2 years not recommended

Protopic® (Fujisawa) ▼ PoM
Ointment, tacrolimus (as monohydrate) 0.03%, net price 30 g = £19.44, 60 g = £36.94; 0.1%, 30 g = £21.60, 60 g = £41.04. Label: 4, 11, 28
Excipients: include beeswax

13.6   Acne and rosacea

13.6.1   Topical preparations for acne
13.6.2   Oral preparations for acne

ACNE. Treatment of acne should be commenced early to prevent scarring. Patients should be counselled that an improvement may not be seen for at least a couple of months. The choice of treatment depends on whether the acne is predominantly inflammatory or comedonal and its severity.

Mild to moderate acne is generally treated with topical preparations (section 13.6.1). Systemic treatment (section 13.6.2) with oral antibiotics is generally used for *moderate to severe acne* or where topical preparations are not tolerated or are ineffective or where application to the site is difficult. Another oral preparation used for acne is the hormone treatment co-cyprindiol (cyproterone acetate with ethinylestradiol); it is for women only.

Severe acne, acne unresponsive to prolonged courses of oral antibiotics, scarring, or acne associated with psychological problems calls for early referral to a consultant dermatologist who may prescribe isotretinoin for administration by mouth.

ROSACEA. Rosacea is not comedonal (but may exist with acne which may be comedonal). The pustules and papules of rosacea respond to topical metronidazole (section 13.10.1.2) or to oral administration of oxytetracycline or tetracycline 500 mg twice daily (section 5.1.3) or of erythromycin 500 mg twice daily (section 5.1.5); courses usually last 6–12 weeks and are repeated intermittently. Alternatively, doxycycline (section 5.1.3) in a dose of 100 mg once daily may be used [unlicensed indication] if oxytetracycline or tetracycline is inappropriate (e.g. in renal impairment). Isotretinoin is occasionally given in refractory cases [unlicensed indication]. Camouflagers (section 13.8.2) may be required for the redness.

13.6.1   Topical preparations for acne

Significant comedonal acne responds well to topical retinoids (see p. 557), whereas both comedones and inflamed lesions respond well to benzoyl peroxide or azelaic acid (see below). Alternatively, topical application of an antibiotic such as erythromycin or clindamycin may be effective for inflammatory acne. If topical preparations prove inadequate oral preparations may be needed (section 13.6.2).

Benzoyl peroxide and azelaic acid

Benzoyl peroxide is effective in mild to moderate acne. Both comedones and inflamed lesions respond well to benzoyl peroxide. The lower concentrations seem to be as effective as higher concentrations in reducing inflammation. It is usual to start with a lower strength and to increase the concentration of benzoyl peroxide gradually. Adverse effects include local skin irritation, particularly when therapy is initiated, but the scaling and redness often subside with treatment continued at a reduced frequency of application. If the acne does not respond after 2 months then use of a topical antibacterial should be considered.

Azelaic acid has antimicrobial and anticomedonal properties. It may be an alternative to benzoyl peroxide or to a topical retinoid for treating mild to moderate comedonal acne, particularly of the face. Some patients prefer it because it is less likely to cause local irritation than benzoyl peroxide.

BENZOYL PEROXIDE

Indications: acne vulgaris
Cautions: avoid contact with eyes, mouth, and mucous membranes; may bleach fabrics and hair; avoid excessive exposure to sunlight
Side-effects: skin irritation (reduce frequency or suspend use until irritation subsides and re-introduce at reduced frequency)
Dose: apply 1–2 times daily preferably after washing with soap and water, start treatment with lower-strength preparations
NOTE. May bleach clothing

Brevoxyl® (Stiefel)
Cream, benzoyl peroxide 4% in an aqueous basis, net price 40 g = £3.30
Excipients: include cetyl alcohol, fragrance, stearyl alcohol

PanOxyl® (Stiefel)
Aquagel (= aqueous gel), benzoyl peroxide 2.5%, net price 40 g = £1.76; 5%, 40 g = £1.92; 10%, 40 g = £2.07
Excipients: include propylene glycol
Cream, benzoyl peroxide 5% in a non-greasy basis, net price 40 g = £1.51
Excipients: include isopropyl palmitate, propylene glycol
Gel, benzoyl peroxide 5% in an aqueous alcoholic basis, net price 40 g = £1.51; 10%, 40 g = £1.69
Excipients: include fragrance
Wash, benzoyl peroxide 10% in a detergent basis, net price 150 mL = £4.00
Excipients: include imidurea

■ With antimicrobials
Benzamycin® (Schwarz) PoM
Gel, pack for reconstitution, providing erythromycin 3% and benzoyl peroxide 5% in an alcoholic basis, net price per pack to provide 46.6 g = £15.27
Excipients: none as listed in section 13.1.3
Dose: apply twice daily (very fair skin, initially once daily at night)

Duac® Once Daily (Stiefel) PoM
Gel, benzoyl peroxide 5%, clindamycin 1% (as phosphate) in an aqueous basis, net price 25 g = £9.95
Excipients: include disodium edetate
Dose: apply once daily in the evening

Quinoderm® (Ferndale)
Cream, benzoyl peroxide 5%, potassium hydroxy-quinoline sulphate 0.5%, in an astringent vanishing-cream basis, net price 50 g = £2.21
Excipients: include cetostearyl alcohol, edetic acid (EDTA)
Cream, benzoyl peroxide 10%, potassium hydroxy-quinoline sulphate 0.5%, in an astringent vanish-

ing-cream basis, net price 25 g = £1.30, 50 g = £2.49
Excipients: include cetostearyl alcohol, edetic acid (EDTA)

AZELAIC ACID

Indications: acne vulgaris
Cautions: pregnancy, breast-feeding; avoid contact with eyes
Side-effects: local irritation (reduce frequency or discontinue use temporarily); rarely photosensitisation

Skinoren® (Schering Health) PoM
Cream, azelaic acid 20%, net price 30 g = £4.40
Excipients: include propylene glycol
Dose: apply twice daily (sensitive skin, once daily for first week). Extended treatment may be required but manufacturer advises period of treatment should not exceed 6 months

Topical antibacterials for acne

For many patients with mild to moderate inflammatory acne, topical antibacterials may be no more effective than topical benzoyl peroxide or tretinoin. Topical antibacterials are probably best reserved for patients who wish to avoid oral antibacterials or who cannot tolerate them. Topical preparations of **erythromycin** and **clindamycin** are effective for inflammatory acne; topical preparations of tetracycline may also be effective. Topical antibacterials can produce mild irritation of the skin, and on rare occasions cause sensitisation.

Antibacterial resistance of *Propionibacterium acnes* is increasing; there is cross-resistance between erythromycin and clindamycin. To avoid development of resistance:

- when possible use non-antibiotic antimicrobials (such as benzoyl peroxide or azelaic acid);
- avoid concomitant treatment with different oral and topical antibiotics;
- if a particular antibiotic is effective, use it for repeat courses if needed (short intervening courses of a topical antibacterial, such as benzoyl peroxide or azelaic acid, may eliminate any resistant propionibacteria);
- do not continue treatment for longer than necessary (however, treatment with a topical preparation should be continued for at least 6 months)

ANTIBIOTICS

Indications: acne vulgaris
Cautions: some manufacturers advise preparations containing alcohol are not suitable for use with benzoyl peroxide

Benzamycin® PoM see under Benzoyl Peroxide above

Dalacin T® (Pharmacia) PoM
Topical solution, clindamycin 1% (as phosphate), in an aqueous alcoholic basis, net price (both with applicator) 30 mL = £4.34, 50 mL = £7.23
Excipients: include propylene glycol
Dose: apply twice daily

Lotion, clindamycin 1% (as phosphate) in an aqueous basis, net price 30 mL = £5.08, 50 mL = £8.47
Excipients: include cetostearyl alcohol, hydroxybenzoates (parabens)
Dose: apply twice daily

Stiemycin® (Stiefel) PoM
Solution, erythromycin 2% in an alcoholic basis, net price 50 mL = £8.60
Excipients: include propylene glycol
Dose: apply twice daily

Topicycline® (Shire) PoM
Solution, powder for reconstitution, tetracycline hydrochloride, 4-epitetracycline hydrochloride, providing tetracycline hydrochloride 2.2 mg/mL when reconstituted with solvent containing *n*-decyl methyl sulphoxide and citric acid in 40% alcohol. Net price per pack of powder and solvent to provide 70 mL = £6.15
Excipients: none as listed in section 13.1.3
Dose: apply twice daily

Zindaclin® (Strakan) PoM
Gel, clindamycin 1% (as phosphate), net price 30 g = £8.66
Excipients: include propylene glycol
Dose: apply once daily

Zineryt® (Yamanouchi) PoM
Topical solution, powder for reconstitution, erythromycin 40 mg, zinc acetate 12 mg/mL when reconstituted with solvent containing ethanol, net price per pack of powder and solvent to provide 30 mL = £8.29, 90 mL = £23.91
Excipients: none as listed in section 13.1.3
Dose: apply twice daily

Topical retinoids and related preparations for acne

Tretinoin and its isomer **isotretinoin** are useful in treating comedonal acne but patients should be warned that some redness and skin peeling might occur initially but settles with time. Several months of treatment may be needed to achieve an optimal response and the treatment should be continued until no new lesions develop.

Topical **isotretinoin** is licensed to treat non-inflammatory and inflammatory lesions in patients with mild to moderate acne. Isotretinoin is also given by mouth; see section 13.6.2 for **warnings** relating to use by mouth.

Adapalene, a retinoid-like drug, is licensed for mild to moderate acne. It is less irritant than topical retinoids.

CAUTIONS. Topical retinoids should be avoided in severe acne involving large areas. Contact with eyes, nostrils, mouth and mucous membranes, eczematous, broken or sunburned skin should be avoided. These drugs should be used with caution in sensitive areas such as the neck, and accumulation in angles of the nose should be avoided. Exposure to UV light (including sunlight, solariums) should be avoided; if sun exposure is unavoidable, an appropriate sunscreen or protective clothing should be used. Use of retinoids with abrasive cleaners, comedogenic or astringent cosmetics should be avoided. Allow peeling (e.g. resulting from use of benzoyl peroxide) to subside before using a topical retinoid; alternating a preparation that causes peeling with a topical

retinoid may give rise to contact dermatitis (reduce frequency of retinoid application).

CONTRA-INDICATIONS. Topical retinoids are contra-indicated in pregnancy (Appendix 4); women of child-bearing age should take adequate contraceptive precautions. Tretinoin is contra-indicated in personal or familial history of cutaneous epithelioma.

SIDE-EFFECTS. Local reactions include burning, erythema, stinging, pruritus, dry or peeling skin (discontinue if severe). Increased sensitivity to UVB light or sunlight occurs. Temporary changes of skin pigmentation have been reported. Eye irritation and oedema, and blistering or crusting of skin have been reported rarely.

ADAPALENE
Indications: mild to moderate acne
Cautions: see notes above
Contra-indications: see notes above
Side-effects: see notes above
Dose: apply thinly once daily before retiring

Differin® (Galderma) PoM
Cream, adapalene 0.1%, net price 30 g = £8.00, 45 g = £11.40
Excipients: include disodium edetate, hydroxybenzoates (parabens)
Gel, adapalene 0.1%, net price 30 g = £8.00, 45 g = £11.40
Excipients: include disodium edetate, hydroxybenzoates (parabens), propylene glycol

TRETINOIN
NOTE. Tretinoin is the acid form of vitamin A
Indications: see under preparations below; photo-damage (section 13.8.1); malignant disease (section 8.1.5)
Cautions: see notes above
Contra-indications: see notes above
Side-effects: see notes above
Dose: see under preparations below

Retin-A® (Janssen-Cilag) PoM
Cream, tretinoin 0.025%, net price 60 g = £6.03
Excipients: include butylated hydroxytoluene, sorbic acid, stearyl alcohol
Dose: acne vulgaris, for dry or fair skin, apply thinly 1–2 times daily
Gel, tretinoin 0.01%, net price 60 g = £6.03; 0.025%, 60 g = £6.03
Excipients: include butylated hydroxytoluene
Dose: acne vulgaris and other keratotic conditions, apply thinly 1–2 times daily
Lotion, tretinoin 0.025%, net price 100 mL = £6.94
Excipients: include butylated hydroxytoluene
Dose: acne vulgaris, apply thinly 1–2 times daily

■ With antibacterial
Aknemycin® **Plus** (Crookes) PoM
Solution, tretinoin 0.025%, erythromycin 4% in an alcoholic basis, net price 25 mL = £7.94
Dose: acne, apply thinly 1–2 times daily
Excipients: none as listed in section 13.1.3

ISOTRETINOIN
NOTE. Isotretinoin is an isomer of tretinoin
IMPORTANT. For **indications, cautions, contra-indications** and **side-effects** of isotretinoin **when given by mouth,** see p. 559
Indications: see notes above; oral treatment (see section 13.6.2)

Cautions: (*topical application* **only**) see notes above

Contra-indications: (*topical application* **only**) see notes above

Dose: apply thinly 1–2 times daily

Isotrex® (Stiefel) PoM
Gel, isotretinoin 0.05%, net price 30 g = £6.65
Excipients: include butylated hydroxytoluene

■ With antibacterial
Isotrexin® (Stiefel) PoM
Gel, isotretinoin 0.05%, erythromycin 2% in ethanolic basis, net price 30 g = £8.36
Excipients: include butylated hydroxytoluene

Other topical preparations for acne

Salicylic acid is available in various preparations for sale direct to the public for the treatment of mild acne. Other products are more suitable for acne; salicylic acid is used mainly for its keratolytic effect. Preparations containing **sulphur** and **abrasive agents** are not considered beneficial in acne.

Topical **corticosteroids** should **not** be used in acne.

A topical preparation of **nicotinamide** is available for inflammatory acne.

ABRASIVE AGENTS

Indications: acne vulgaris (but see notes above)
Cautions: avoid contact with eyes; discontinue use temporarily if skin becomes irritated
Contra-indications: superficial venules, telangiectasia

Brasivol® (Stiefel)
Paste No. 1, aluminium oxide 38.09% in fine particles, in a soap-detergent basis, net price 75 g = £2.49
Excipients: include fragrance, N-(3-Chloroallyl)hexaminium chloride (quaternium 15)
Dose: use instead of soap 1–3 times daily

CORTICOSTEROIDS

Indications: use in acne not recommended (see notes above)
Cautions: see section 13.4 and notes above
Contra-indications: see section 13.4 and notes above
Side-effects: see section 13.4 and notes above

Actinac® (Peckforton) PoM
Lotion (powder for reconstitution with solvent), chloramphenicol 40 mg, hydrocortisone acetate 40 mg, allantoin 24 mg, butoxyethyl nicotinate 24 mg, precipitated sulphur 320 mg/g. Discard 21 days after reconstitution, net price 2 × 6.25-g bottles powder with 2 × 20-mL bottles solvent = £16.28. Label: 28. Potency: mild
Excipients: none as listed in section 13.1.3

NICOTINAMIDE

Indications: see under preparation
Cautions: avoid contact with eyes and mucous membranes (including nose and mouth); reduce frequency of application if excessive dryness, irritation or peeling
Side-effects: dryness of skin; also pruritus, erythema, burning and irritation

Nicam® (Dermal)
Gel, nicotinamide 4%, net price 60 g = £7.98
Excipients: none as listed in section 13.1.3
Dose: inflammatory acne vulgaris, apply twice daily; reduce to once daily or on alternate days if irritation occurs
NOTE. Formerly marketed as *Papulex®*

SALICYLIC ACID

Indications: acne; psoriasis (section 13.5.2); warts and calluses (section 13.7); fungal nail infections (section 13.10.2)
Cautions: avoid contact with mouth, eyes, mucous membranes; systemic effects after excessive use (see Aspirin and the salicylates, section 10.1.1)
Side-effects: local irritation

Acnisal® (DermaPharm)
Topical solution, salicylic acid 2% in a detergent and emollient basis, net price 177 mL = £4.13.
Excipients: include benzyl alcohol
Dose: use up to 3 times daily

SULPHUR

Cautions: avoid contact with eyes, mouth, and mucous membranes; causes skin irritation

■ With resorcinol
Prolonged application of resorcinol may interfere with thyroid function therefore not recommended
Eskamel® (Goldshield) NHS
Cream, resorcinol 2%, sulphur 8%, in a non-greasy flesh-coloured basis, net price 25 g = £3.03
Excipients: include propylene glycol, fragrance

13.6.2 Oral preparations for acne

Oral antibacterials for acne

Systemic antibacterial treatment is useful for inflammatory acne if topical treatment is not adequately effective or if it is inappropriate. Anticomedonal treatment (e.g. with topical benzoyl peroxide) may also be required.

Either **oxytetracycline** or **tetracycline** (section 5.1.3) is usually given for acne in a dose of 500 mg twice daily. If there is no improvement after the first 3 months another oral antibacterial should be used. Maximum improvement usually occurs after 4 to 6 months but in more severe cases treatment may need to be continued for 2 years or longer.

Doxycycline and **minocycline** (section 5.1.3) are alternatives to tetracycline. Doxycycline may be used in a dose of 100 mg daily. Minocycline offers less likelihood of bacterial resistance but may sometimes cause irreversible pigmentation; it is given in a dose of 100 mg daily (in one or two divided doses).

Erythromycin (section 5.1.5) in a dose of 500 mg twice daily is an alternative for the management of acne but propionibacteria strains resistant to erythromycin are becoming widespread and this may explain poor response.

Trimethoprim (section 5.1.8) in a dose of 300 mg twice daily may be used for acne resistant to other antibacterials [unlicensed indication]. Prolonged treatment with trimethoprim may depress haematopoiesis; it should generally be initiated by specialists.

Concomitant use of different topical and systemic antibacterials is undesirable owing to the increased likelihood of the development of bacterial resistance.

Hormone treatment for acne

Co-cyprindiol (cyproterone acetate with ethinylestradiol) contains an anti-androgen. It is no more effective than an oral broad-spectrum antibacterial but is useful in women who also wish to receive oral contraception.

Improvement of acne with co-cyprindiol probably occurs because of decreased sebum secretion which is under androgen control. Some women with moderately severe hirsutism may also benefit because hair growth is also androgen-dependent. Contra-indications of co-cyprindiol include pregnancy and a predisposition to thrombosis.

> **CSM advice.** Venous thromboembolism occurs more frequently in women taking co-cyprindiol than those taking a low-dose combined oral contraceptive. The CSM has reminded prescribers that co-cyprindiol is licensed for use in women with severe acne which has not responded to oral antibacterials and for moderately severe hirsutism; it should not be used solely for contraception. It is contra-indicated in those with a personal or close family history of venous thromboembolism. Women with severe acne or hirsutism may have an inherently increased risk of cardiovascular disease.

CO-CYPRINDIOL

A mixture of cyproterone acetate and ethinylestradiol in the mass proportions 2000 parts to 35 parts, respectively

Indications: severe acne in women refractory to prolonged oral antibacterial therapy (but see notes above); moderately severe hirsutism

Cautions: see under Combined Hormonal Contraceptives, section 7.3.1

Contra-indications: see under Combined Hormonal Contraceptives, section 7.3.1

Side-effects: see under Combined Hormonal Contraceptives, section 7.3.1

Dose: 1 tablet daily for 21 days starting on day 1 of menstrual cycle and repeated after a 7-day interval, usually for several months; withdraw when acne or hirsutism completely resolved (repeat courses may be given if recurrence)

Co-cyprindiol (Non-proprietary) PoM
Tablets, co-cyprindiol 2000/35 (cyproterone acetate 2 mg, ethinylestradiol 35 micrograms), net price 21-tab pack = £3.70
Available from Neolab

Dianette® (Schering Health) PoM
Tablets, beige, s/c, co-cyprindiol 2000/35 (cyproterone acetate 2 mg, ethinylestradiol 35 micrograms), net price 21-tab pack = £3.70

Oral retinoid for acne

The retinoid **isotretinoin** (*Roaccutane®*) reduces sebum secretion. It is used for the systemic treatment of nodulo-cystic and conglobate acne, severe acne, scarring, acne which has not responded to an adequate course of a systemic antibacterial, or acne which is associated with psychological problems. It is also useful in women who develop acne in the third or fourth decades of life, since late onset acne is frequently unresponsive to antibacterials.

Isotretinoin is a toxic drug that should be prescribed **only** by, or under the supervision of, a consultant dermatologist. It is given for at least 16 weeks; repeat courses are not normally required.

Side-effects of isotretinoin include severe dryness of the skin and mucous membranes, nose bleeds, and joint pains. The drug is **teratogenic** and must **not** be given to women of child-bearing age unless they practise effective contraception and then only after detailed assessment and explanation by the physician (see under Cautions below).

ISOTRETINOIN

NOTE. Isotretinoin is an isomer of tretinoin

Indications: see notes above

Cautions: exclude pregnancy before starting (perform pregnancy test 2–3 days before expected menstruation, start treatment on day 2 or 3 of menstrual cycle)—effective contraception must be practised at least 1 month before, during, and for at least 1 month after treatment; avoid blood donation during treatment and for at least 1 month after treatment; history of depression; measure hepatic function before treatment, 1 month after starting and then every 3 months (reduce dose or discontinue if transaminase raised above normal); measure serum lipids before treatment, 1 month after starting, then at end of treatment (reduce dose or discontinue if raised), discontinue if uncontrolled hypertriglyceridaemia or pancreatitis; diabetes; dry eye syndrome (associated with risk of keratitis); avoid keratolytics; **interactions:** Appendix 1 (retinoids)
WAX EPILATION AND DERMABRASION. Warn patient to avoid wax epilation during treatment and for at least 6 months after stopping (risk of epidermal stripping); avoid dermabrasion during treatment and for at least 6 months after stopping (risk of scarring)

Contra-indications: pregnancy (**important teratogenic risk:** see Cautions and Appendix 4); breast-feeding; renal or hepatic impairment; hypervitaminosis A, hyperlipidaemia

Side-effects: dryness of skin (with scaling, thinning, erythema, pruritus), epidermal fragility (trauma may cause blistering); rarely acne fulminans, facial hyperpigmentation; dryness of lips (sometimes cheilitis), dryness of nasal mucosa (with mild epistaxis), of pharyngeal mucosa (with hoarseness), of conjunctiva (sometimes conjunctivitis), decreased tolerance to contact lenses and rarely keratitis; visual disturbances (papilloedema, optic neuritis, corneal opacities, cataracts, decreased night vision, photophobia, blurred vision)—expert referral and consider withdrawal; hair thinning (reversible on withdrawal) or (rarely) hirsutism; nausea, headache, malaise, drowsiness, sweating; benign intracranial hypertension (avoid concomitant tetracyclines); myalgia and arthralgia; raised serum creatinine concentrations reported; rarely jaundice and hepatitis; raised plasma triglycerides and cholesterol (risk of pancreatitis if triglycerides above 8 g/litre); allergic vasculitis and granulomatous lesions reported, other side-effects reported include hearing deficiency, mood changes (severe depression), convulsions, menstrual irregularities, hyperuricaemia, inflammatory bowel disease, diarrhoea (discontinue if severe), paronychia and Gram-positive infections, tendinitis, bone changes (including early epiphyseal closure and skeletal hyperostosis following long-term administration), thrombocytopenia, thrombocytosis, neutropenia and anaemia, lymphadenopathy, and haematuria and proteinuria

Dose: initially 500 micrograms/kg daily (in 1–2 divided doses) with food for 4 weeks; if good response continue for further 8–12 weeks; if little response, increase to 1 mg/kg daily for 8–12 weeks; if intolerant, reduce dose to 100–200 micrograms/kg daily

Isotretinoin (Non-proprietary) PoM
Capsules, isotretinoin 5 mg, net price 56-cap pack = £18.22; 20 mg, 56-cap pack = £50.21 (hosp. only). Label: 10, patient information leaflet, 21
Available from Schering Health

Roaccutane® (Roche) PoM
Capsules, isotretinoin 5 mg (red-violet/white), net price 60-cap pack = £19.52; 20 mg (red-violet/white), 60-cap pack = £53.80 (hosp. or specified retail pharmacy only). Label: 10, patient information card, 21

13.7 Preparations for warts and calluses

Warts (verrucas) are caused by a human papillomavirus, which most frequently affects the hands, feet (plantar warts), and the anogenital region (see below); treatment usually relies on local tissue destruction. Warts may regress on their own and treatment is required only if the warts are painful, unsightly, persistent, or cause distress.

Preparations of **salicylic acid, formaldehyde, gluteraldehyde** or **silver nitrate** are available for purchase by the public; they are suitable for the removal of warts on hands and feet. **Salicylic acid** is a useful keratolytic which may be considered first; it is also suitable for the removal of *corns and calluses*. Colloidal preparations of salicylic acid are available but some patients may develop an allergy to colophony in the formulation. An ointment combining **salicylic acid** with **podophyllum resin** (*Posalfilin®*) is available for treating plantar warts.

SALICYLIC ACID

Indications: see under preparations; psoriasis (section 13.5.2); acne (section 13.6.1); fungal nail infections (section 13.10.2)
Cautions: significant peripheral neuropathy, patients with diabetes at risk of neuropathic ulcers; protect surrounding skin and avoid broken skin; not suitable for application to face, anogenital region, or large areas
Side-effects: skin irritation, see notes above
Dose: see under preparations; advise patient to apply carefully to wart and to protect surrounding skin (e.g. with soft paraffin or specially designed plaster); rub wart surface gently with file or pumice stone once weekly; treatment may need to be continued for up to 3 months

Cuplex® (S&N Hlth.)
Gel, salicylic acid 11%, lactic acid 4%, in a collodion basis, net price 5 g = £2.23. Label: 15
Dose: for plantar and mosaic warts, corns, and calluses, apply twice daily

Duofilm® (Stiefel)
Paint, salicylic acid 16.7%, lactic acid 16.7%, in flexible collodion, net price 15 mL (with applicator) = £1.95. Label: 15
Dose: for plantar and mosaic warts, apply daily

Occlusal® (DermaPharm)
Application, salicylic acid 26% in polyacrylic solution, net price 10 mL (with applicator) = £3.48. Label: 15
Dose: for common and plantar warts, apply daily

Salactol® (Dermal)
Paint, salicylic acid 16.7%, lactic acid 16.7%, in flexible collodion, net price 10 mL (with applicator) = £1.93. Label: 15
Dose: for warts, particularly plantar warts, verrucas, corns, and calluses, apply daily

Salatac® (Dermal)
Gel, salicylic acid 12%, lactic acid 4% in a collodion basis, net price 8 g (with applicator) = £3.36. Label: 15
Dose: for warts, verrucas, corns, and calluses, apply daily

Verrugon® (Pickles)
Ointment, salicylic acid 50% in a paraffin basis, net price 6 g = £2.61
Dose: for plantar warts, apply daily

■ With podophyllum

Posalfilin® (Norgine)
Ointment, podophyllum resin 20%, salicylic acid 25%, net price 10 g = £3.77
Dose: for plantar warts apply daily
NOTE. Owing to the salicylic acid content, not suitable for anogenital warts; owing to the podophyllum content also contra-indicated in pregnancy and breast-feeding

FORMALDEHYDE

Indications: see under preparations
Cautions: see under Salicylic Acid
Contra-indications: see under Salicylic Acid
Side-effects: see under Salicylic Acid

Veracur® (Typharm)
Gel, formaldehyde 0.75% in a water-miscible gel basis, net price 15 g = £2.41.
Dose: for warts, particularly plantar warts, apply twice daily

GLUTARALDEHYDE

Indications: warts, particularly plantar warts
Cautions: protect surrounding skin; not for application to face, mucosa, or anogenital areas
Side-effects: rashes, skin irritation (discontinue if severe); stains skin brown
Dose: apply twice daily (see also under Salicylic acid)

Glutarol® (Dermal)
Solution (= application), glutaraldehyde 10%, net price 10 mL (with applicator) = £2.33

SILVER NITRATE

Indications: see under preparation
Cautions: protect surrounding skin and avoid broken skin; not suitable for application to face, ano-genital region, or large areas
Side-effects: stains skin and fabric
Dose: see under preparation; instructions in proprietary packs generally incorporate advice to

remove dead skin before use by gentle filing and to cover with adhesive dressing after application

AVOCA® (Bray)

Caustic pencil, tip containing silver nitrate 95%, potassium nitrate 5%, net price, treatment pack (including emery file, 6 adhesive dressings and protector pads) = £1.78.

Dose: for common warts and verrucas, apply moistened caustic pencil tip for 1–2 minutes; repeat after 24 hours up to max. 3 applications for warts *or* max. 6 applications for verrucas

Anogenital warts

The treatment of anogenital warts (condylomata acuminata) should be accompanied by screening for other sexually transmitted diseases. **Podophyllum** and **podophyllotoxin** (the major active ingredient of podophyllum) may be used for *soft, non-keratinised* external anogenital warts; these preparations can cause considerable irritation of the treated area. They can also cause severe systemic toxicity on excessive application including gastrointestinal, renal, haematological, and CNS effects. Patients with a limited number of external warts or *keratinised* lesions may be better treated with cryotherapy or other forms of physical ablation.

Imiquimod cream is licensed for the treatment of external anogenital warts; it may be used for both keratinised and non-keratinised lesions.

Inosine pranobex (section 5.3) is licensed for adjunctive treatment of genital warts but it has been superseded by more effective drugs.

IMIQUIMOD

Indications: external genital and perianal warts

Cautions: avoid normal skin, inflamed skin and open wounds; not suitable for internal genital warts; uncircumcised males (risk of phimosis or stricture of foreskin); pregnancy

Side-effects: local reactions including itching, pain, erythema, erosion, oedema, and excoriation; less commonly local ulceration and scabbing; permanent hypopigmentation or hyperpigmentation reported

Dose: apply thinly 3 times a week at night until lesions resolve (max. 16 weeks); CHILD not recommended

IMPORTANT. Should be rubbed in and allowed to stay on the treated area for 6–10 hours then washed off with mild soap and water (uncircumcised males washing under foreskin should wash daily). The cream should be washed off before sexual contact

Aldara® (3M) [PoM]

Cream, imiquimod 5%, net price 12-sachet pack = £55.18. Label: 10, patient information leaflet

Excipients: include benzyl alcohol, cetyl alcohol, hydroxybenzoates (parabens), polysorbate 60, stearyl alcohol

Condoms: may damage latex condoms and diaphragms

PODOPHYLLUM

Indications: see under preparations

Cautions: avoid normal skin and open wounds; keep away from face; very irritant to eyes; **important:** see also warnings below

Contra-indications: pregnancy and breast-feeding; children

Side-effects: see notes above

Podophyllin Paint, Compound, BP [PoM]

(podophyllum resin 15% in compound benzoin tincture), podophyllum resin 1.5 g, compound benzoin tincture to 10 mL; 5 mL to be dispensed unless otherwise directed. Label: 15

Dose: external genital warts, applied weekly in genitourinary clinic (or at a general practitioner's surgery by trained nurses after screening for other sexually transmitted diseases)

IMPORTANT. Should be allowed to stay on the treated area for not longer than 6 hours and then washed off. Care should be taken to avoid splashing the surrounding skin during application (which must be covered with soft paraffin as a protection). Where there are a large number of warts only a few should be treated at any one time as **severe toxicity** caused by absorption of podophyllin has been reported

■ Podophyllotoxin

Condyline® (Ardern) [PoM]

Solution, podophyllotoxin 0.5% in alcoholic basis, net price 3.5 mL (with applicators) = £16.00. Label: 15

Dose: condylomata acuminata affecting the penis or the female external genitalia, apply twice daily for 3 consecutive days; treatment may be repeated at weekly intervals if necessary for a total of five 3-day treatment courses; direct medical supervision for lesions in the female and for lesions greater than 4 cm^2 in the male; max. 50 single applications ('loops') per session (consult product literature)

Warticon® (Stiefel) [PoM]

Cream, podophyllotoxin 0.15%, net price 5 g (with mirror) = £16.62

Excipients: include butylated hydroxyanisole, cetyl alcohol, hydroxybenzoates (parabens), sorbic acid, stearyl alcohol

Dose: condylomata acuminata affecting the penis or the female external genitalia, apply twice daily for 3 consecutive days; treatment may be repeated at weekly intervals if necessary for a total of four 3-day treatment courses; direct medical supervision for lesions greater than 4 cm^2

Solution, blue, podophyllotoxin 0.5% in alcoholic basis, net price 3 mL (with applicators— *Warticon*® [for men]; with applicators and mirror— *Warticon Fem*® [for women]) = £13.85. Label: 15

Dose: condylomata acuminata affecting the penis or the female external genitalia, apply twice daily for 3 consecutive days; treatment may be repeated at weekly intervals if necessary for a total of four 3-day treatment courses; direct medical supervision for lesions greater than 4 cm^2; max. 50 single applications ('loops') per session (consult product literature)

13.8   Sunscreens and camouflagers

13.8.1	Sunscreen preparations
13.8.2	Camouflagers

13.8.1   Sunscreen preparations

Solar ultraviolet irradiation can be harmful to the skin. It is responsible for disorders such as *polymorphic light eruption, solar urticaria,* and it provokes the various *cutaneous porphyrias*. It also provokes (or at least aggravates) skin lesions of *lupus erythematosus* and may aggravate *rosacea* and some other *dermatoses*. Sunlight may also cause photosensitivity in patients taking some drugs such as demeclocycline, phenothiazines, or amiodarone. All these conditions (as well as *sunburn*) may occur after relatively short periods of exposure to the sun. Solar ultraviolet irradiation may provoke attacks of recurrent herpes labialis (but it is not known whether the effect of sunlight exposure is local or systemic).

The effects of exposure over longer periods include *ageing changes* and more importantly the initiation of *skin cancer*.

Solar ultraviolet radiation is approximately 200–400 nm in wavelength. The medium wavelengths (290–320 nm, known as UVB) cause sunburn and contribute to the long-term changes responsible for skin cancer and ageing. The long wavelengths (320–400 nm, known as UVA) do not cause sunburn but are responsible for many *photosensitivity reactions* and *photodermatoses*. Both UVA and UVB contribute to long-term *photodamage* and to the pathogenesis of *skin cancer*.

Sunscreen preparations contain substances that protect the skin against UVB and hence against sunburn, but they are no substitute for covering the skin and avoiding sunlight. The sun protection factor (SPF, usually indicated in the preparation title) provides guidance on the degree of protection offered against UVB; it indicates the multiples of protection provided against burning, compared with unprotected skin; for example, an SPF of 8 should enable a person to remain 8 times longer in the sun without burning. However, in practice users do not apply sufficient sunscreen product and the protection is lower than that found in experimental studies. Sunscreen preparations, do not prevent long-term damage associated with UVA, which might not become apparent for 10 to 20 years. Preparations that also contain reflective substances, such as titanium dioxide, provide the most effective protection against UVA. Some products use a star rating system to indicate the protection against UVA relative to protection against UVB for the same product. Four stars indicate that the product offers balanced UVA and UVB protection; products with 3, 2, or 1 star rating indicate that greater protection is offered against UVB than against UVA. However, the usefulness of the star rating system remains controversial.

Some sunscreen preparations, particularly aminobenzoates, may rarely cause photosensitivity reactions.

For optimum photoprotection, sunscreen preparations should be applied **thickly** and **frequently** (approximately 2 hourly). In photodermatoses, they should be used from spring to autumn. As maximum protection from sunlight is desirable, preparations with the highest SPF should be prescribed.

BORDERLINE SUBSTANCES. The preparations marked 'ACBS' are regarded as drugs when prescribed for skin protection against ultraviolet radiation in abnormal cutaneous photosensitivity resulting from genetic disorders or photodermatoses, including vitiligo and those resulting from radiotherapy; chronic or recurrent herpes simplex labialis. Preparations with SPF less than 15 are not prescribable. See also Appendix 7.

Ambre Solaire® (Garnier)
Total Screen Sun Intolerant Skin Lotion (UVA and UVB protection; UVB-SPF 60), octocrylene 10%, titanium dioxide 5.3%, drometrizole trisiloxane 2.5%, avobenzone 2.5%, terephthalydene dicamphor sulfonic acid 0.5%, net price 200 mL = £7.98. ACBS
Excipients: include disodium edetate, hydroxybenzoates (parabens), propylene glycol

Delph® (Fenton)
Lotion, (UVA and UVB protection; UVB-SPF 15), ethylhexyl *p*-methoxycinnamate 7.5%, oxybenzone 3%, titanium dioxide 0.6%, net price 200 mL = £1.99. ACBS
Excipients: include cetostearyl alcohol, fragrance, hydroxybenzoates (parabens), imidurea
Lotion, (UVA and UVB protection; UVB-SPF 20), ethylhexyl *p*-methoxycinnamate 7.5%, oxybenzone 3%, titanium dioxide 1.6%, net price 200 mL = £1.99. ACBS
Excipients: include cetostearyl alcohol, fragrance, hydroxybenzoates (parabens), imidurea
Lotion, (UVA and UVB protection; UVB-SPF 25), avobenzone 4%, ethylhexyl *p*-methoxycinnamate 3.5%, titanium dioxide 2.1%, oxybenzone 1.3%, net price 200 mL = £2.85. ACBS
Excipients: include cetostearyl alcohol, fragrance, hydroxybenzoates (parabens), imidurea
Lotion, (UVA and UVB protection; UVB-SPF 30), ethylhexyl *p*-methoxycinnamate 4.8%, avobenzone 4%, titanium dioxide 2.5%, oxybenzone 1.5%, net price 200 mL = £2.85. ACBS
Excipients: include cetostearyl alcohol, fragrance, hydroxybenzoates (parabens), imidurea

E45 Sun® (Crookes)
Sunblock lotion (UVA and UVB protection; UVB-SPF 25), waterproof, titanium dioxide 3.6%, zinc oxide 13.9%, net price 150 mL = £6.56. ACBS
Excipients: include hydroxybenzoates (parabens), isopropyl palmitate
Sunblock lotion (UVA and UVB protection; UVB-SPF 50), waterproof, titanium dioxide 6.4%, zinc oxide 16%, net price 150 mL = £7.09. ACBS
Excipients: include hydroxybenzoates (parabens), isopropyl palmitate

RoC Total Sunblock® (J&J)
Cream (UVA and UVB protection; UVB-SPF 25), containing avobenzone 2%, ethylhexyl *p*-methoxycinnamate 7.5%, titanium dioxide 5.5%, net price 50 mL = £4.06. ACBS
Excipients: include beeswax, cetostearyl alcohol, disodium EDTA, hydroxybenzoates (parabens)

SpectraBan® (Stiefel)
Lotion (UVB protection; UVB-SPF 25), aminobenzoic acid 5%, padimate-O 3.2%, in an alcoholic basis, net price 150 mL = £3.45. ACBS
Excipients: include fragrance
NOTE. Flammable; stains clothing
Ultra lotion (UVA and UVB protection; UVB-SPF 28), water resistant, avobenzone 2%, oxybenzone 3%, padimate-O 8%, titanium dioxide 2%, net price 150 mL = £5.45. ACBS
Excipients: include benzyl alcohol, disodium edetate, sorbic acid, fragrance

Sunsense® **Ultra** (Sandoz)
Lotion (UVA and UVB protection; UVB-SPF 60), ethylhexyl *p*-methoxycinnamate 7.5% oxybenzone 3%, titanium dioxide 3.5%, net price 50-mL bottle with roll-on applicator = £3.11, 125 mL = £5.10. ACBS
Excipients: include butylated hydroxytoluene, cetyl alcohol, fragrance, hydroxybenzoates (parabens), propylene glycol

Uvistat® (Eastern)
Cream (UVA and UVB protection; UVB-SPF 22 but marketed as 'factor 20'), water-resistant, ethylhexyl *p*-methoxycinnamate 7%, avobenzone 4%, titanium dioxide 4.5%, net price 125 g = £5.10. ACBS
Excipients: include disodium edetate, fragrance, hydroxybenzoates (parabens)
Ultrablock cream (UVA and UVB protection; UVB-SPF 30), water-resistant, ethylhexyl *p*-methoxycinnamate 7.5%, avobenzone 4%, titanium dioxide 6.5%, net price 125 g = £5.10. ACBS
Excipients: include disodium edetate, fragrance, hydroxybenzoates (parabens)

Photodamage

Diclofenac gel is licensed for *actinic keratosis*. Treatment should continue for 60 to 90 days (optimal therapeutic effect may not be seen until 30 days after stopping). **Fluorouracil** cream (section 8.1.3) is also licensed for actinic keratosis. **Methyl-5-aminolevu-linate** cream (*Metvix*®, available from Galderma), followed by irradiation with red light, is licensed for treating thin non-hyperkeratotic actinic keratoses of the face and scalp when other treatments are less appropriate, or for treating superficial or nodular basal-cell carcinoma that is considered unsuitable for other therapies; it is used in specialist centres.

Application of **tretinoin** 0.05% cream is reported to be associated with gradual improvement in *photo-damaged skin* (usually within 3–4 months of starting).

DICLOFENAC SODIUM

Indications: actinic keratosis
Cautions: as for topical NSAIDs, see section 10.3.2
Contra-indications: as for topical NSAIDs, see section 10.3.2
Side-effects: as for topical NSAIDs, see section 10.3.2; also paraesthesia
Dose: apply thinly twice daily for 60–90 days; max. 8 g daily

Solaraze® (Shire) PoM
Gel, diclofenac sodium 3%, net price 25 g = £17.90
Excipients: include benzyl alcohol

TRETINOIN

NOTE. Tretinoin is the acid form of vitamin A
Indications: mottled hyperpigmentation, roughness and fine wrinkling of photodamaged skin due to chronic sun exposure; acne vulgaris (section 13.6); malignant disease (section 8.1.5)
Cautions: see section 13.6.1
Contra-indications: see section 13.6.1
Side-effects: see section 13.6.1
Dose: apply thinly at night, then reduce to 1–3 nights weekly

Retinova® (Janssen-Cilag) PoM NHS
Cream, tretinoin 0.05%, net price 20 g = £13.75.
Excipients: include fragrance

13.8.2 Camouflagers

Disfigurement of the skin can be very distressing to patients and may have a marked psychological effect. In skilled hands, or with experience, camouflage cosmetics can be very effective in concealing scars and birthmarks. The depigmented patches in vitiligo are also very disfiguring and camouflage creams are of great cosmetic value.

BORDERLINE SUBSTANCES. The preparations marked 'ACBS' are regarded as drugs when prescribed for postoperative scars and other deformities and as an adjunctive therapy in the relief of emotional disturbances due to disfiguring skin disease, such as vitiligo. See also Appendix 7.

Covermark® (Epiderm)
Classic foundation (masking cream), net price 15 mL (10 shades) = £10.75. ACBS
Excipients: include beeswax, hydroxybenzoates (parabens), fragrance

Finishing powder, net price 60 g = £10.55. ACBS
Excipients: include beeswax, hydroxybenzoates (parabens), fragrance

Dermablend® (Brodie & Stone)
Cover creme, net price 10.7 g (15 shades) = £8.19; 28.4 g (11 shades) = £12.89. ACBS
Excipients: include beeswax, hydroxybenzoates (parabens)
Leg and body cover, (9 shades), net price 64 g = £11.72. ACBS
Excipients: include beeswax, hydroxybenzoates (parabens)
Setting powder, net price 28 g = £11.13. ACBS
Excipients: include hydroxybenzoates (parabens)

Dermacolor® (Fox)
Camouflage creme, (100 shades), net price 25 g = £8.10. ACBS
Excipients: include beeswax, butylated hydroxytoluene, fragrance, propylene glycol, stearyl alcohol, wool fat
Fixing powder, (7 shades), net price 60 g = £6.55. ACBS
Excipients: include fragrance

Keromask® (Network)
Masking cream, (2 shades), net price 15 mL = £5.67. ACBS
Excipients: include butylated hydroxyanisole, hydroxybenzoates (parabens), wool fat, propylene glycol
Finishing powder, net price 20 g = £5.67. ACBS
Excipients: include butylated hydroxytoluene, hydroxybenzoates (parabens)

Veil® (Blake)
Cover cream, (20 shades), net price 19 g = £7.80, 44 g = £12.76, 70 g = £17.87. ACBS
Excipients: include hydroxybenzoates (parabens), wool fat derivative
Finishing powder, translucent, net price 35 g = £7.80. ACBS
Excipients: include butylated hydroxyanisole, hydroxybenzoates (parabens)

13.9 Shampoos and other preparations for scalp conditions

Dandruff is considered to be a mild form of seborrhoeic dermatitis (see also section 13.5.1). Shampoos containing antimicrobial agents such as **pyrithione zinc** (which are widely available) and **selenium sulphide** may have beneficial effects. Shampoos containing **tar** extracts may be useful and they are also used in *psoriasis*. **Ketoconazole** shampoo should be considered for more persistent or severe dandruff or for seborrhoeic dermatitis of the scalp.

Corticosteroid gels and lotions (section 13.4) can also be used.

Shampoos containing **coal tar** and **salicylic acid** may also be useful. A cream or an ointment containing coal tar and salicylic acid is very helpful in *psoriasis* that affects the scalp (section 13.5.2). Patients who do not respond to these treatments may need to be referred to exclude the possibility of other skin conditions.

Cradle cap in infants may be treated with **olive oil** or **arachis oil** (ground-nut oil, peanut oil) applications followed by shampooing.

See below for male-pattern baldness and also section 13.5 (psoriasis and eczema), section 13.10.4 (lice), and section 13.10.2 (ringworm).

■ Shampoos

Alphosyl 2 in 1® (GSK Consumer Healthcare)
Shampoo, alcoholic coal tar extract 5%, net price 125 mL = £1.81, 250 mL = £3.43
Excipients: include hydroxybenzoates (parabens), fragrance
Dose: dandruff, use once or twice weekly as necessary; psoriasis, seborrhoeic dermatitis, scaling and itching, use every 2–3 days

Betadine® (SSL)

Scalp and skin cleanser—section 13.11.4

Shampoo solution, povidone–iodine 4%, in a surfactant solution, net price 250 mL = £2.32

Excipients: include fragrance

Dose: seborrhoeic scalp conditions associated with excessive dandruff, pruritus, scaling, exudation and erythema, infected scalp lesions (recurrent furunculosis, infective folliculitis, impetigo), apply 1–2 times weekly; CHILD under 2 years not recommended

Cautions; Contra-indications; Side-effects: see section 13.11.4, Iodine Compounds

Capasal® (Dermal)

Shampoo, coal tar 1%, coconut oil 1%, salicylic acid 0.5%, net price 250 mL = £5.28

*Excipients: none as listed in section 13.1.3

Dose: scaly scalp disorders including psoriasis, seborrhoeic dermatitis, dandruff, and cradle cap, apply daily as necessary

Ceanel Concentrate® (Ferndale)

Shampoo, cetrimide 10%, undecenoic acid 1%, phenylethyl alcohol 7.5%, net price 150 mL = £3.40, 500 mL = £9.80

*Excipients: none as listed in section 13.1.3

Dose: scalp psoriasis, seborrhoeic dermatitis, dandruff, apply 3 times in first week then twice weekly

Clinitar® (CHS)

Shampoo solution, coal tar extract 2%, net price 100 g = £2.50

Excipients: include polysorbates, fragrance

Dose: scalp psoriasis, seborrhoeic dermatitis, and dandruff, apply up to 3 times weekly

Meted® (DermaPharm)

Shampoo, salicylic acid 3%, sulphur 5%, net price 120 mL = £3.90

Excipients: include fragrance

Dose: scaly scalp disorders including psoriasis, seborrhoeic dermatitis, and dandruff, apply at least twice weekly

Nizoral® (Janssen-Cilag) PoM

Cream—section 13.10.2

Shampoo, ketoconazole 2%, net price 120 mL = £4.09

Excipients: include imidurea

Dose: for seborrhoeic dermatitis and dandruff apply twice weekly for 2–4 weeks, for pityriasis versicolor once daily for max. 5 days

NOTE. Shampoo containing ketoconazole 2% also available from Alpharma

1. Can be sold to the public for the prevention and treatment of dandruff and seborrhoeic dermatitis of the scalp as a shampoo formulation containing ketoconazole max. 2%, in a pack containing max. 120 mL and labelled to show a max. frequency of application of once every 3 days; brands on sale to the public include *Nizoral® Dandruff Shampoo* and *Nizoral® Anti-Dandruff Shampoo*

Pentrax® (DermaPharm)

Shampoo, coal tar 4.3%, net price 120 mL = £3.90

*Excipients: none as listed in section 13.1.3

Dose: scaly scalp disorders including psoriasis, seborrhoeic dermatitis, and dandruff, apply at least twice weekly

Polytar AF® (Stiefel)

Shampoo, arachis (peanut) oil extract of coal tar 0.3%, cade oil 0.3%, coal tar solution 0.1%, pine tar 0.3%, pyrithione zinc 1%, net price 150 mL = £4.40

Excipients: include fragrance, imidurea

Dose: scaly scalp disorders including psoriasis, seborrhoeic dermatitis, and dandruff, apply 2–3 times weekly for at least 3 weeks

Psoriderm® (Dermal)

Scalp lotion (= shampoo), coal tar 2.5%, lecithin 0.3%, net price 250 mL = £5.33

Excipients: include disodium edetate

Dose: scalp psoriasis, use as necessary

Selsun® (Abbott)

Shampoo application, selenium sulphide 2.5%, net price 50 mL = £1.44, 100 mL = £1.96, 150 mL = £2.75

Excipients: include fragrance

Dose: seborrhoeic dermatitis and dandruff, apply twice weekly for 2 weeks then once weekly for 2 weeks and then as necessary; CHILD under 5 years not recommended; pityriasis versicolor, section 13.10.2 [unlicensed indication]

Cautions: avoid using 48 hours before or after applying hair colouring, straightening or waving preparations

T/Gel® (Neutrogena)

Shampoo, coal tar extract 2%, net price 125 mL = £3.18, 250 mL = £4.78

Excipients: include fragrance, hydroxybenzoates (parabens), imidurea, tetrasodium edetate

Dose: scalp psoriasis, seborrhoeic dermatitis, dandruff, apply as necessary

■ **Other scalp preparations**

Cocois®

Section 13.5.2

Polytar® (Stiefel)

Liquid, arachis (peanut) oil extract of crude coal tar 0.3%, cade oil 0.3%, coal tar solution 0.1%, oleyl alcohol 1%, tar 0.3%, net price 250 mL = £2.23

Excipients: include fragrance, imidurea, polysorbate 80

Dose: scalp disorders including psoriasis, seborrhoea, eczema, pruritus, and dandruff, apply 1–2 times weekly

Polytar Plus® (Stiefel)

Liquid, ingredients as *Polytar®* liquid with hydrolysed animal protein 3%, net price 500 mL = £4.40

Excipients: include fragrance, imidurea, polysorbate 80

Dose: scalp disorders including psoriasis, seborrhoea, eczema, pruritus, and dandruff, apply 1–2 times weekly

Pragmatar®

Section 13.5.2

Male-pattern baldness

Finasteride is licensed for the treatment of male-pattern baldness in men. Continuous use for 3–6 months is required before benefit is seen, and effects are reversed 6–12 months after treatment is discontinued.

Topical application of **minoxidil** may stimulate limited hair growth in a small proportion of adults but only for as long as it is used.

FINASTERIDE

Indications: male-pattern baldness in men

Cautions: see section 6.4.2

Side-effects: see section 6.4.2

Dose: 1 mg daily

Propecia® (MSD) ▼ PoM DHS

Tablets, f/c, beige, finasteride 1 mg, net price 28-tab pack = £26.99

MINOXIDIL

Indications: male-pattern baldness (men and women)

Cautions: see section 2.5.1 (only about 1.4–1.7% absorbed); avoid contact with eyes, mouth and mucous membranes, broken, infected, shaved, or inflamed skin; avoid inhalation of spray mist; avoid occlusive dressings and topical drugs which enhance absorption

Contra-indications: see section 2.5.1

Side-effects: see section 2.5.1; irritant dermatitis, allergic contact dermatitis, discontinue if hair loss persists for more than 2 weeks

Dose: apply 1 mL twice daily to dry hair and scalp (discontinue if no improvement after 1 year); 5% strength for use in men only

Regaine® (Pharmacia) NHS
Regaine® *Regular Strength topical solution*, minoxidil 2% in an aqueous alcoholic basis, net price 60-mL bottle with applicators = £14.16
Excipients: include propylene glycol
Regaine® *Extra Strength topical solution*, minoxidil 5% in an aqueous alcoholic basis, net price 60-mL bottle with applicators = £17.00, 3 × 60-mL bottles = £34.03
Excipients: include propylene glycol
Cautions: flammable; wash hands after application

13.10 Anti-infective skin preparations

13.10.1 Antibacterial preparations
13.10.2 Antifungal preparations
13.10.3 Antiviral preparations
13.10.4 Parasiticidal preparations
13.10.5 Preparations for minor cuts and abrasions

13.10.1 Antibacterial preparations

13.10.1.1 Antibacterial preparations only used topically
13.10.1.2 Antibacterial preparations also used systemically

For many skin infections such as *erysipelas* and *cellulitis* systemic antibacterial treatment is more appropriate because the infection is too deeply seated for adequate penetration of topical preparations. For details of suitable treatment see section 5.1, table 1.

In the community, small, localised areas of acute *impetigo* may be treated by short-term topical application of **fusidic acid**; **mupirocin** is an alternative topical treatment. If the impetigo is extensive or longstanding, an oral antibacterial such as **flucloxacillin** (or **erythromycin** in penicillin-allergy) (section 5.1, Table 1) should be used. Mild antiseptics such as **povidone–iodine** (section 13.11.4) are used to soften crusts and exudate.

Although there are a great many antibacterial drugs presented in topical preparations some are potentially hazardous and frequently their use is not necessary if adequate hygienic measures can be taken. Moreover not all skin conditions that are oozing, crusted, or characterised by pustules are actually infected. Topical antibacterials should be **avoided** on *leg ulcers* unless used in short courses for defined infections; treatment of bacterial colonisation is generally inappropriate.

To minimise the development of resistant organisms it is advisable to limit the choice of antibacterials applied topically to those not used systemically. Unfortunately some of these, for example neomycin, may cause sensitisation, and there is cross-sensitivity with other aminoglycoside antibiotics, such as gentamicin. If *large areas of skin* are being treated, ototoxicity may also be a hazard with aminoglycoside antibiotics (and also with polymyxins), particularly in children, in the elderly, and in those with renal impairment. *Resistant organisms* are more common in hospitals, and whenever possible swabs should be taken for bacteriological examination before beginning treatment.

Mupirocin is not related to any other antibacterial in use; it is effective for skin infections, particularly those due to Gram-positive organisms but it is not indicated for pseudomonal infection. Although *Staphylococcus aureus* strains with low-level resistance to mupirocin are emerging, it is generally useful in infections resistant to other antibacterials. To avoid the development of resistance, mupirocin should not be used for longer than 10 days and local microbiology advice should be sought before using it in hospital. In the presence of mupirocin-resistant MRSA infection, a polymyxin can be used, but its use should be discussed with the local microbiologist.

Silver sulfadiazine (silver sulphadiazine) is used in the treatment of infected burns.

13.10.1.1 Antibacterial preparations only used topically

MUPIROCIN

Indications: bacterial skin infections (see also notes above)

Bactroban® (GSK) PoM
Cream, mupirocin (as mupirocin calcium) 2%, net price 15 g = £4.71
Excipients: include benzyl alcohol, cetyl alcohol, stearyl alcohol
Dose: secondarily infected traumatic lesions, apply 3 times daily for up to 10 days; re-evaluate if no response after 3–5 days
Ointment, mupirocin 2%, net price 15 g = £4.71
Excipients: none as listed in section 13.1.3
NOTE. Contains macrogol and manufacturer advises caution in renal impairment; may sting
Dose: skin infections, apply up to 3 times daily for up to 10 days
Important: cream and ointment not interchangeable—prescription should specify formulation required
Nasal ointment, see section 12.2.3

NEOMYCIN SULPHATE

Indications: bacterial skin infections
Cautions: large areas, see below
LARGE AREAS. If large areas of skin are being treated ototoxicity may be a hazard, particularly in children, in the elderly, and in those with renal impairment
Contra-indications: neonates
Side-effects: sensitisation (see also notes above)

Neomycin Cream BPC PoM ▰
Cream, neomycin sulphate 0.5%, cetomacrogol emulsifying ointment 30%, chlorocresol 0.1%,

disodium edetate 0.01%, in freshly boiled and cooled purified water, net price 15 g = £1.15
Excipients: include cetostearyl alcohol, edetic acid (EDTA)
Dose: apply up to 3 times daily (short-term use)

Cicatrin® (GSK) [PoM]
Cream, neomycin sulphate 3300 units, bacitracin zinc 250 units, cysteine 2 mg, glycine 10 mg, threonine 1 mg/g, net price 15 g = 99p, 30 g = £1.98
Excipients: include wool fat derivative, polysorbates
Dose: superficial bacterial infection of skin, ADULT and CHILD over 2 years, apply up to 3 times daily (short-term use)
Dusting powder, neomycin sulphate 3300 units, bacitracin zinc 250 units, cysteine 2 mg, glycine 10 mg, threonine 1 mg/g, net price 15 g = 99p, 50 g = £3.30
Excipients: none as listed in section 13.1.3
Dose: superficial bacterial infection of skin, ADULT and CHILD over 2 years, apply up to 3 times daily (short-term use)

Graneodin® (Squibb) [PoM]
Ointment, neomycin sulphate 0.25%, gramicidin 0.025%, net price 25 g = £1.47
Excipients: none as listed in section 13.1.3
Dose: superficial bacterial infection of skin, apply 2–4 times daily (for max. 7 days—possibly longer for sycosis barbae)

POLYMYXINS

(Includes colistin sulphate and polymyxin B sulphate)
Indications: bacterial skin infections
Cautions: large areas, see below
LARGE AREAS. If large areas of skin are being treated nephrotoxicity and neurotoxicity may be a hazard, particularly in children, in the elderly, and in those with renal impairment
Side-effects: sensitisation (see also notes above)

Polyfax® (PLIVA) [PoM]
Ointment, polymyxin B sulphate 10 000 units, bacitracin zinc 500 units/g, net price 20 g = £4.62
Excipients: none as listed in section 13.1.3
Dose: apply twice daily or more frequently if required

Colomycin® (Forest) [PoM]
Powder, sterile, for making topical preparations (usually 1%), colistin sulphate, net price 1-g vial = £18.37
Excipients: none as listed in section 13.1.3

SILVER SULFADIAZINE

(Silver sulphadiazine)
Indications: prophylaxis and treatment of infection in burn wounds; as an adjunct to short-term treatment of infection in leg ulcers and pressure sores; as an adjunct to prophylaxis of infection in skin graft donor sites and extensive abrasions; for conservative management of finger-tip injuries
Cautions: hepatic and renal impairment; G6PD deficiency; pregnancy and breast-feeding (avoid in late pregnancy and in neonate—see also Appendix 4); may inactivate enzymatic debriding agents—concomitant use may be inappropriate; for large amounts see also **interactions:** Appendix 1 (sulphonamides)
LARGE AREAS. Plasma-sulphadiazine concentrations may approach therapeutic levels with *side-effects* and *interactions* as for sulphonamides (see section 5.1.8) if large areas of skin are treated. Owing to the association of sulphonamides with severe blood and skin disorders treatment should be stopped immediately if blood disorders or rashes develop—but leucopenia developing 2–3 days after starting treatment of burns patients is

reported usually to be self-limiting and silver sulfadiazine need not usually be discontinued provided blood counts are monitored carefully to ensure return to normality within a few days. Argyria may also occur if large areas of skin are treated (or if application is prolonged).
Contra-indications: pregnancy and breast-feeding; sensitivity to sulphonamides; not recommended for neonates (see also Appendix 4)
Side-effects: allergic reactions including burning, itching and rashes; argyria reported following prolonged use; leucopenia reported (monitor blood levels)

Flamazine® (S&N Hlth.) [PoM]
Cream, silver sulfadiazine 1%, net price 20 g = £3.10, 50 g = £4.11, 250 g = £11.00, 500 g = £19.48
Excipients: include cetyl alcohol, polysorbates, propylene glycol
Dose: apply with sterile applicator; burns, apply daily or more frequently if very exudative; leg ulcers or pressure sores, apply daily or on alternate days (not recommended if ulcer very exudative); finger-tip injuries, apply every 2–3 days; consult product literature for details

13.10.1.2 Antibacterial preparations also used systemically

FUSIDIC ACID

Indications: staphylococcal skin infections
Cautions: see notes above; avoid contact with eyes
Side-effects: rarely hypersensitivity reactions
Dose: apply 3–4 times daily

Fucidin® (Leo) [PoM]
Cream, fusidic acid 2%, net price 15 g = £2.74, 30 g = £4.62
Excipients: include butylated hydroxyanisole, cetyl alcohol
Ointment, sodium fusidate 2%, net price 15 g = £2.23, 30 g = £3.79
Excipients: include cetyl alcohol, wool fat

METRONIDAZOLE

Indications: see under preparations
Cautions: avoid exposure to strong sunlight or UV light
Side-effects: skin irritation
Dose: see under preparations

■ Rosacea (see also section 13.6)
Metrogel® (Novartis) [PoM]
Gel, metronidazole 0.75%, net price 40 g = £19.90. Label: 10, patient information leaflet
Excipients: include hydroxybenzoates (parabens), propylene glycol
Dose: acute inflammatory exacerbations of acne rosacea, apply thinly twice daily for 8–9 weeks

Metrosa® (Linderma) [PoM]
Gel, metronidazole 0.75%, net price 40 g = £19.90. Label: 10, patient information leaflet
Excipients: include propylene glycol
Dose: acute exacerbation of acne rosacea, apply thinly twice daily for up to 8 weeks

Noritate® (Aventis Pharma) [PoM]
Cream, metronidazole 1%, net price 30 g = £19.08. Label: 10, patient information leaflet
Excipients: include hydroxybenzoates (parabens)
Dose: acne rosacea, apply once daily for 8 weeks

Rozex® (Galderma) [PoM]
Cream, metronidazole 0.75%, net price 30 g = £13.75, 40 g = £15.28. Label: 10, patient information leaflet
Excipients: include benzyl alcohol, isopropyl palmitate

Gel, metronidazole 0.75%, net price 30 g = £13.75, 40 g = £15.28. Label: 10, patient information leaflet
Excipients: include disodium edetate, hydroxybenzoates (parabens), propylene glycol
Dose: inflammatory papules, pustules and erythema of acne rosacea, apply twice daily for 3–4 months

Zyomet® (Goldshield) PoM
Gel, metronidazole 0.75%, net price 30 g = £12.00. Label: 10, patient information leaflet
Excipients: include benzyl alcohol, disodium edetate, propylene glycol
Dose: acute inflammatory exacerbations of acne rosacea, apply thinly twice daily for 8–9 weeks

■ Malodorous tumours and skin ulcers

Anabact® (CHS) PoM
Gel, metronidazole 0.75%, net price 15 g = £4.47, 30 g = £7.89
Excipients: include hydroxybenzoates (parabens), propylene glycol
Dose: malodorous fungating tumours and malodorous gravitational and decubitus ulcers, apply to clean wound 1–2 times daily and cover with non-adherent dressing

Metrotop® (SSL) PoM
Gel, metronidazole 0.8%, net price 15 g = £4.73, 30 g = £8.36
Excipients: none as listed in section 13.1.3
Dose: malodorous fungating tumours and malodorous gravitational and decubitus ulcers, apply to clean wound 1–2 times daily and cover (flat wounds, apply liberally; cavities, smear on paraffin gauze and pack loosely)

13.10.2 Antifungal preparations

Most localised fungal infections are treated with topical preparations. Systemic therapy (section 5.2) is necessary for nail or scalp infection or if the skin infection is widespread, disseminated or intractable. Skin scrapings should be examined if systemic therapy is being considered or where there is doubt about the diagnosis.

DERMATOPHYTOSES. Ringworm infection can affect the scalp (tinea capitis), body (tinea corporis), groin (tinea cruris), hand (tinea manuum), foot (tinea pedis, athlete's foot), or nail (tinea unguium); scalp infection requires systemic treatment (section 5.2); additional topical application of an antifungal may reduce the risk of transmission. Most other local ringworm infections can be treated adequately with topical antifungal preparations (including shampoos, section 13.9). The imidazole antifungals **clotrimazole, econazole, ketoconazole, miconazole,** and **sulconazole** are all effective. **Terbinafine** cream is also effective but it is more expensive. Other topical antifungals include **amorolfine** and the **undecenoates. Compound benzoic acid ointment** (Whitfield's ointment) has been used for ringworm infections but it is cosmetically less acceptable than proprietary preparations. Topical preparations for athlete's foot containing **tolnaftate** are on sale to the public.

Antifungal dusting powders are of little therapeutic value in the treatment of fungal skin infections and may cause skin irritation; they may have some role in preventing re-infection.

Tinea infection of the nail is almost always treated systemically (section 5.2); topical application of **amorolfine** or **tioconazole** may be effective for treating early onychomycosis when involvement is limited to mild distal disease in up to 2 nails.

PITYRIASIS VERSICOLOR. Pityriasis (tinea) versicolor may be treated with **ketoconazole** shampoo (section 13.9). Alternatively, **selenium sulphide** shampoo [unlicensed indication] (section 13.9) may be used as a lotion (diluted with water to reduce irritation) and left on for at least 30 minutes or overnight; it is applied 2–7 times over a fortnight and the course repeated if necessary.

Topical imidazole antifungals **clotrimazole, econazole, ketoconazole, miconazole,** and **sulconazole** and topical **terbinafine** are alternatives but large quantities may be required.

If topical therapy fails, or if the infection is widespread, pityriasis versicolor is treated systemically with an azole antifungal (section 5.2). Relapse is common, especially in the immunocompromised.

CANDIDIASIS. Candidal skin infections may be treated with topical imidazole antifungals **clotrimazole, econazole, ketoconazole, miconazole,** and **sulconazole;** topical terbinafine is an alternative. Topical application of **nystatin** is also effective for candidiasis but it is ineffective against dermatophytosis. Refractory candidiasis requires systemic treatment (section 5.2) generally with a triazole such as fluconazole; systemic treatment with terbinafine is **not appropriate** for refractory candidiasis.

COMPOUND TOPICAL PREPARATIONS. Combination of an imidazole and a mild corticosteroid (such as hydrocortisone 1%) (section 13.4) may be of value in the treatment of eczematous intertrigo and, in the first few days only, of a severely inflamed patch of ringworm. Combination of a mild corticosteroid with either an imidazole or nystatin may be of use in the treatment of intertrigo associated with candida.

CAUTIONS. Contact with eyes and mucous membranes should be avoided.

SIDE-EFFECTS. Occasional local irritation and hypersensitivity reactions include mild burning sensation, erythema, and itching. Treatment should be discontinued if these are severe.

AMOROLFINE
Indications: see under preparations
Cautions: see notes above; also avoid contact with ears; pregnancy and breast-feeding
Side-effects: see notes above

Loceryl® (Galderma) PoM
Cream, amorolfine (as hydrochloride) 0.25%, net price 20 g = £4.83. Label: 10, patient information leaflet
Excipients: include cetostearyl alcohol, disodium edetate
Dose: fungal skin infections, apply once daily after cleansing in the evening for at least 2–3 weeks (up to 6 weeks for foot infection) continuing for 3–5 days after lesions have healed
Nail lacquer, amorolfine (as hydrochloride) 5%, net price 5-mL pack (with nail files, spatulas and cleansing swabs) = £25.00. Label: 10, patient information leaflet
Excipients: none as listed in section 13.1.3
Dose: fungal nail infections, apply to infected nails 1–2 times weekly after filing and cleansing; allow to dry (approx. 3 minutes); treat finger nails for 6 months, toe nails for 9–12 months (review at intervals of 3 months); avoid nail varnish or artificial nails during treatment

BENZOIC ACID

Indications: ringworm (tinea), but see notes above

Benzoic Acid Ointment, Compound, BP
(Whitfield's ointment)
Ointment, benzoic acid 6%, salicylic acid 3%, in emulsifying ointment
Dose: apply twice daily
Excipients: include cetostearyl alcohol

CLOTRIMAZOLE

Indications: fungal skin infections; vaginal candidiasis (section 7.2.2); otitis externa (section 12.1.1)
Cautions: see notes above
Side-effects: see notes above
Dose: apply 2–3 times daily

Clotrimazole (Non-proprietary)
Cream, clotrimazole 1%, net price 20 g = £1.77
Available from Akita (*Candiden*®), Alpharma, APS, Ashbourne (*Abtrim*®), CP, Generics, PLIVA

[1]**Canesten**® (Bayer Consumer Care)
Cream, clotrimazole 1%, net price 20 g = £2.14, 50 g = £3.80. On sale to the public as *Canesten*® *AF* cream
Excipients: include benzyl alcohol, cetostearyl alcohol, polysorbate 60
Powder, clotrimazole 1%, net price 30 g = £1.52. On sale to the public as *Canesten*® *AF* powder
Excipients: none as listed in section 13.1.3
Solution, clotrimazole 1% in macrogol 400 (polyethylene glycol 400), net price 20 mL = £2.43. For hairy areas
Excipients: none as listed in section 13.1.3
Spray, clotrimazole 1%, in 30% isopropyl alcohol, net price 40-mL atomiser = £4.99. Label: 15. For large or hairy areas. On sale to the public as *Canesten*® *AF* spray
Excipients: include propylene glycol

1. The brand name *Canesten*® *AF Once Daily* is used for bifonazole

ECONAZOLE NITRATE

Indications: fungal skin infections; vaginal candidiasis (section 7.2.2)
Cautions: see notes above
Side-effects: see notes above
Dose: skin infections apply twice daily; nail infections, apply once daily under occlusive dressing

Ecostatin® (Squibb)
Cream, econazole nitrate 1%, net price 15 g = £1.49; 30 g = £2.75
Excipients: include butylated hydroxyanisole, fragrance

Pevaryl® (Janssen-Cilag)
Cream, econazole nitrate 1%, net price 30 g = £2.65
Excipients: include butylated hydroxyanisole, fragrance

KETOCONAZOLE

Indications: fungal skin infections; systemic or resistant fungal infections (section 5.2); vulval candidiasis (section 7.2.2)
Cautions: see notes above; do **not** use within 2 weeks of a topical corticosteroid for seborrhoeic dermatitis—risk of skin sensitisation
Side-effects: see notes above
Dose: tinea pedis, apply twice daily; other fungal infections, apply 1–2 times daily

[1]**Nizoral**® (Janssen-Cilag) [PoM]
[2]*Cream*, ketoconazole 2%, net price 30 g = £3.81
Excipients: include cetyl alcohol, polysorbates, propylene glycol, stearyl alcohol
Shampoo—section 13.9

1. A 15-g tube is available for sale to the public for the treatment of tinea pedis, tinea cruris, and candidal intertrigo (*Daktarin*® *Gold*)
2. [NHS] except for seborrhoeic dermatitis and pityriasis versicolor and endorsed 'SLS'

MICONAZOLE NITRATE

Indications: fungal skin infections; intestinal fungal infections (section 5.2); oral fungal infections (section 12.3.2); vaginal candidiasis (section 7.2.2)
Cautions: see notes above
Side-effects: see notes above
Dose: apply twice daily continuing for 10 days after lesions have healed; nail infections, apply 1–2 times daily

Daktarin® (Janssen-Cilag)
Cream, miconazole nitrate 2%, net price 30 g = £2.07. Also on sale to the public as *Daktarin*® *Dual Action cream* for athlete's foot
Excipients: include butylated hydroxyanisole
NOTE. A 15-g tube [NHS] is on sale to the public.
Powder [NHS], miconazole nitrate 2%, net price 20 g = £1.81. Also on sale to the public as *Daktarin*® *Dual Action powder* for athlete's foot
Excipients: include none as listed in section 13.1.3
Dual Action Spray powder, miconazole nitrate 0.16%, in an aerosol basis, net price 100 g = £2.27
Excipients: none as listed in section 13.1.3

NYSTATIN

Indications: skin infections due to *Candida* spp.; intestinal candidiasis (section 5.2); vaginal candidiasis (section 7.2.2); oral fungal infections (section 12.3.2)
Cautions: see notes above
Side-effects: see notes above

Nystaform® (Typharm) [PoM]
Cream, nystatin 100 000 units/g, chlorhexidine hydrochloride 1%, net price 30 g = £2.62
Excipients: include benzyl alcohol, cetostearyl alcohol, polysorbate 60
Dose: apply 2–3 times daily continuing for 7 days after lesions have healed.

Nystan® (Squibb) [PoM]
Cream, nystatin 100 000 units/g, net price 30 g = £2.18
Excipients: include benzyl alcohol, propylene glycol, fragrance
Dose: apply 2–4 times daily
Ointment, nystatin 100 000 units/g, in *Plastibase*®, net price 30 g = £1.75
Excipients: none as listed in section 13.1.3
Dose: apply 2–4 times daily

Tinaderm-M® (Schering-Plough) [PoM]
Cream, nystatin 100 000 units/g, tolnaftate 1%, net price 20 g = £1.83
Excipients: include butylated hydroxytoluene, cetostearyl alcohol, hydroxybenzoates (parabens), fragrance
Dose: apply 2–3 times daily

SALICYLIC ACID

Indications: fungal nail infections, particularly tinea; hyperkeratotic skin disorders (section 13.5.2); acne vulgaris (section 13.6.1); warts and calluses (section 13.7)

Contra-indications: children under 5 years; pregnancy
Side-effects: see notes above
Dose: apply twice daily

Phytex® (Wynlit) ▭
Paint, salicylic acid 1.46% (total combined), tannic acid 4.89% and boric acid 3.12% (as borotannic complex), in a vehicle containing alcohol and ethyl acetate, net price 25 mL (with brush) = £1.56
Excipients: none as listed in section 13.1.3
NOTE. Flammable

SULCONAZOLE NITRATE
Indications: fungal skin infections
Cautions: see notes above
Side-effects: see notes above; also blistering
Dose: apply 1–2 times daily continuing for 2–3 weeks after lesions have healed

Exelderm® (Centrapharm)
Cream, sulconazole nitrate 1%, net price 30 g = £3.00
Excipients: include cetyl alcohol, polysorbates, propylene glycol, stearyl alcohol

TERBINAFINE
Indications: fungal skin infections
Cautions: pregnancy, breast-feeding; avoid contact with eyes
Side-effects: redness, itching, or stinging; rarely allergic reactions (discontinue)

[1]**Lamisil**® (Novartis) PoM
Cream, terbinafine hydrochloride 1%, net price 15 g = £4.86, 30 g = £8.76
Dose: apply thinly 1–2 times daily for up to 1 week in tinea pedis, 1–2 weeks in tinea corporis and tinea cruris, 2 weeks in cutaneous candidiasis and pityriasis versicolor; review after 2 weeks; CHILD not recommended
Excipients: include benzyl alcohol, cetyl alcohol, polysorbate 60, stearyl alcohol
Tablets, see section 5.2

1. Can be sold to the public for external use for the treatment of tinea pedis and tinea cruris as a cream containing terbinafine hydrochloride max. 1% in a pack containing max. 15 g (*Lamisil*® *AT* cream); also for the treatment of tinea pedis, tinea cruris, and tinea corporis as a spray containing terbinafine hydrochloride max. 1% in a pack containing max. 30 mL (*Lamisil*® *AT* spray)

TIOCONAZOLE
Indications: fungal nail infections
Cautions: see notes above
Contra-indications: pregnancy (Appendix 4)
Side-effects: see notes above; also local oedema, dry skin, nail discoloration, periungual inflammation, nail pain, rash, exfoliation
Dose: apply to nails and surrounding skin twice daily for up to 6 months (may be extended to 12 months)

Trosyl® (Pfizer) PoM
Cutaneous solution, tioconazole 28%, net price 12 mL (with applicator brush) = £27.38
Excipients: none as listed in section 13.1.3

UNDECENOATES
Indications: see under preparations below
Side-effects: see notes above
Dose: see under preparations below

Monphytol® (LAB) ▭
Paint, methyl undecenoate 5%, propyl undecenoate 0.7%, salicylic acid 3%, methyl salicylate 25%, propyl salicylate 5%, chlorobutanol 3%, net price 18 mL (with brush) = £1.61
Excipients: none as listed in section 13.1.3
Dose: fungal skin and nail infections, apply twice daily

Mycota® (Thornton & Ross)
Cream, zinc undecenoate 20%, undecenoic acid 5%, net price 25 g = £1.19
Excipients: include fragrance
Dose: treatment of athlete's foot, apply twice daily continuing for 7 days after lesions have healed
Prevention of athlete's foot, apply once daily
Powder, zinc undecenoate 20%, undecenoic acid 2%, net price 70 g = £1.80
Excipients: include fragrance
Dose: treatment of athlete's foot, apply twice daily continuing for 7 days after lesions have healed
Prevention of athlete's foot, apply once daily
Spray application, undecenoic acid 2.5%, dichlorophen 0.25% (pressurised aerosol pack), net price 100 mL = £1.93
Excipients: include fragrance
Dose: treatment of athlete's foot, apply twice daily continuing for 7 days after lesions have healed
Prevention of athlete's foot, apply once daily

13.10.3 Antiviral preparations

Aciclovir cream is licensed for the treatment of initial and recurrent labial and genital *herpes simplex infections*; treatment should begin as early as possible. Systemic treatment is necessary for buccal or vaginal infections or if cold sores recur frequently; *herpes zoster (shingles)* also requires systemic treatment (for details of systemic use see section 5.3). **Penciclovir** cream is licensed for the treatment of labial *herpes simplex infection*.
   Idoxuridine solution (5% in dimethyl sulfoxide) is of little value.

ACICLOVIR
(Acyclovir)
Indications: see notes above
Cautions: avoid contact with eyes and mucous membranes
Side-effects: transient stinging or burning; occasionally erythema, itching or drying of the skin
Dose: apply to lesions every 4 hours (5 times daily) for 5–10 days, starting at first sign of attack

[1]**Aciclovir** (Non-proprietary) PoM
Cream, aciclovir 5%, net price 2 g = £3.02, 10 g = £8.88
Excipients: include propylene glycol
Available from Alpharma (*excipients* also include sorbic acid), Genus, Pharmacia, Ratiopharm (*Zuvogen*®, *excipients* also include cetyl alcohol, propylene glycol)

1. A 2-g tube and a pump pack are on sale to the public for the treatment of cold sores (*Zovirax*® *Cold Sore Cream*); other brands on sale to the public include *Action*® *Cold Sore*, *Boots Avert*®, *Clearsore*®, *Herpetad*®, *Soothelip*®, *Viralief*®, and *Virasorb*®

Zovirax® (GSK) PoM
Cream, aciclovir 5%, net price 2 g = £5.29, 10 g = £15.94
Excipients: include cetostearyl alcohol, propylene glycol
Eye ointment, section 11.3.3
Tablets, section 5.3

PENCICLOVIR

Indications: see notes above

Cautions: avoid contact with eyes and mucous membranes

Side-effects: transient stinging, burning, numbness

Vectavir® (Novartis Consumer Health) PoM
Cream, penciclovir 1%, net price 2 g = £4.20
Dose: herpes labialis, apply to lesions every 2 hours during waking hours for 4 days, starting at first sign of attack; CHILD under 12 years, not recommended
Excipients: include cetostearyl alcohol, propylene glycol

IDOXURIDINE IN DIMETHYL SULFOXIDE ▱

Indications: herpes simplex and herpes zoster infection but of little value

Cautions: avoid contact with the eyes, mucous membranes, and textiles; breast-feeding (may taste unpleasant)

Contra-indications: pregnancy (Appendix 4); **not** to be used in mouth

Side-effects: stinging on application, changes in taste; overuse may cause maceration

Herpid® (Yamanouchi) PoM ▱
Application, idoxuridine 5% in dimethyl sulfoxide, net price 5 mL (with applicator) = £6.81
Dose: apply to lesions 4 times daily for 4 days, starting at first sign of attack; CHILD under 12 years, not recommended

13.10.4 Parasiticidal preparations

Suitable quantities of parasiticidal preparations

	Skin creams	Lotions	Cream rinses
Scalp (headlice)	—	50–100 mL	50–100 mL
Body (scabies)	30–60 g	100 mL	—
Body (crab lice)	30–60 g	100 mL	—

These amounts are usually suitable for an adult for single application.

Scabies

Permethrin is effective for the treatment of *scabies* (*Sarcoptes scabiei*); **malathion** can be used if permethrin is inappropriate.

Aqueous preparations are preferable to alcoholic lotions, which are not recommended owing to irritation of excoriated skin and the genitalia.

Older preparations include **benzyl benzoate**, which is an irritant and should be avoided in children; it is less effective than malathion and permethrin.

Ivermectin (*Mectizan®*, MSD, available on a named patient basis) in a single dose of 200 micrograms/kg by mouth has been used, in combination with other drugs, for the treatment of hyperkeratotic (crusted or 'Norwegian') scabies that does not respond to topical treatment alone.

APPLICATION. Although acaricides have traditionally been applied after a hot bath, this is **not** necessary and there is even evidence that a hot bath may increase absorption into the blood, removing them from their site of action on the skin.

All members of the affected household should be treated simultaneously. Treatment should be applied to the whole body including the scalp, neck, face, and ears. Particular attention should be paid to the webs of the fingers and toes and lotion brushed under the ends of nails. It is now recommended that malathion and permethrin should be applied twice, one week apart; in the case of benzyl benzoate up to 3 applications on consecutive days may be needed. It is important to warn users to reapply treatment to the hands if they are washed. Patients with hyperkeratotic scabies may require 2 or 3 applications of acaricide on consecutive days to ensure that enough penetrates the skin crusts to kill all the mites.

ITCHING. The *itch* and *eczema* of scabies persists for some weeks after the infestation has been eliminated and treatment for pruritus and eczema (section 13.5.1) may be required. Application of **crotamiton** can be used to control itching after treatment with more effective acaricides. A topical corticosteroid may help to reduce itch and inflammation after scabies has been treated successfully; however, persistent symptoms suggest that scabies eradication was not successful. Oral administration of a **sedating antihistamine** (section 3.4.1) at night may also be useful.

Head lice

Carbaryl, **malathion**, and the **pyrethroids** (permethrin and phenothrin) are effective against head lice (*Pediculus humanus capitis*) but lice in some districts have developed resistance; resistance to two or more parasiticidal preparations has also been reported. Benzyl benzoate is licensed for the treatment of head lice but it is less effective than other drugs.

Head lice infestation (pediculosis) should be treated using lotion or liquid formulations. Shampoos are diluted too much in use to be effective. Alcoholic formulations are effective but aqueous formulations are preferred in severe eczema, for patients with asthma, and small children. A contact time of 12 hours or overnight treatment is recommended for lotions and liquids; a 2-hour treatment is not sufficient to kill eggs.

In general, a course of treatment for head lice should be 2 applications of product 7 days apart to prevent lice emerging from any eggs that survive the first application.

The policy of rotating insecticides on a district-wide basis is now considered outmoded. To overcome the development of resistance, a mosaic strategy is required whereby, if a course of treatment fails to cure, a different insecticide is used for the next course. If a course of treatment with either permethrin or phenothrin fails, then a non-pyrethroid parasiticidal product should be used for the next course.

A **head lice repellent** containing piperonal 2% (*Rappell®*) is on sale to the public, but its value is uncertain.

WET COMBING METHODS. Several products are available which require the use of a plastic detection comb and hair conditioner; a head lice device (*Bug*

Buster® Kit) is prescribable on the NHS. The methods typically involve meticulous combing with the detection comb (probably for at least 30 minutes each time) over the whole scalp at 4-day intervals for a minimum of 2 weeks.

Crab lice

Carbaryl [unlicensed for crab lice], **permethrin, phenothrin**, and **malathion** are effective for *crab lice (Pthirus pubis)*. An aqueous preparation should be applied to **all** parts of the body (not merely the groins and axillae) for 12 hours or overnight; a second treatment is needed after 7 days to kill lice emerging from surviving eggs. A different insecticide should be used if a course of treatment fails. Alcoholic lotions are not recommended (owing to irritation of excoriated skin and the genitalia).

Aqueous **malathion** lotion is effective for *crab lice of the eye lashes* [unlicensed use].

Benzyl benzoate

Benzyl benzoate is effective for *scabies* but is not a first-choice for *scabies* (see notes above).

BENZYL BENZOATE

Indications: scabies (but see notes above)
Cautions: children (not recommended, see also under Dose, below), avoid contact with eyes and mucous membranes; do not use on broken or secondarily infected skin; breast-feeding (suspend feeding until product has been washed off)
Side-effects: skin irritation, burning sensation especially on genitalia and excoriations, occasionally rashes
Dose: apply over the whole body; repeat without bathing on the following day and wash off 24 hours later; a third application may be required in some cases
NOTE. Not recommended for children—dilution to reduce irritant effect also reduces efficacy. Some manufacturers recommend application to the body but to exclude the head and neck. However, application should be extended to the scalp, neck, face, and ears

Benzyl Benzoate Application, BP (Non-proprietary)
Application, benzyl benzoate 25% in an emulsion basis, net price 500 mL = £2.45
Available from Aventis Pharma (*Ascabiol®*, excipients: include triethanolamine), IVAX, Thornton & Ross

Carbaryl

Carbaryl is recommended for *head lice*; an aqueous preparation is recommended for *crab lice* (see notes above) but a suitable product is not currently licensed for this indication. In the light of experimental data in *animals* it would be prudent to consider carbaryl as a potential human carcinogen and it has been restricted to prescription only use. The Department of Health has emphasised that the risk is a theoretical one and that any risk from the intermittent use of head lice preparations is likely to be exceedingly small.

CARBARYL
(Carbaril)
Indications: see notes above and under preparations
Cautions: avoid contact with eyes; do not use on broken or secondarily infected skin; do not use more than once a week for 3 consecutive weeks; children under 6 months, medical supervision required; alcoholic lotions **not** recommended for pediculosis in asthma, in severe eczema or in small children
Side-effects: skin irritation
Dose: rub into dry hair and scalp, allow to dry naturally, shampoo after 12 hours, and comb wet hair (see also notes above)

Carylderm® (SSL) PoM
Liquid, carbaryl 1% in an aqueous basis, net price 50 mL = £2.28. For head lice
Excipients: include cetostearyl alcohol, hydroxybenzoates (parabens)
Lotion, carbaryl 0.5%, in an alcoholic basis, net price 50 mL = £2.28. Label: 15
Excipients: include fragrance
For head lice (alcoholic, see notes above)

Malathion

Malathion is recommended for *scabies, head lice* and *crab lice* (for details see notes above).

The risk of systemic effects associated with 1–2 applications of malathion is considered to be very low; however applications of lotion repeated at intervals of less than 1 week *or* application for more than 3 consecutive weeks should be **avoided** since the likelihood of eradication of lice is not increased.

MALATHION
Indications: see notes above and under preparations
Cautions: avoid contact with eyes; do not use on broken or secondarily infected skin; do not use lotion more than once a week for 3 consecutive weeks; children under 6 months, medical supervision required; alcoholic lotions **not** recommended for head lice in severe eczema, asthma or in small children, or for scabies or crab lice (see notes above)
Side-effects: skin irritation
Dose: head lice, rub 0.5% preparation into dry hair and scalp, allow to dry naturally, remove by washing after 12 hours (see also notes above) *or* apply 1% shampoo to wet hair and rinse after 5 minutes, repeat, comb wet hair, repeat twice at intervals of 3 days
Crab lice, apply 0.5% aqueous preparation over whole body, allow to dry naturally, wash off after 12 hours or overnight
Scabies, apply 0.5% preparation over whole body, and wash off after 24 hours; if hands are washed with soap within 24 hours, they should be retreated; see also notes above
NOTE. For scabies, manufacturer recommends application to the body but not necessarily to the head and neck. However, application should be extended to the scalp, neck, face, and ears

Derbac-M® (SSL)
Liquid, malathion 0.5% in an aqueous basis, net price 50 mL = £2.22, 200 mL = £5.56
Excipients: include cetostearyl alcohol, fragrance, hydroxybenzoates (parabens)
For crab lice, head lice and scabies

Prioderm® (SSL)
Lotion, malathion 0.5%, in an alcoholic basis, net price 50 mL = £2.22, 200 mL = £5.56. Label: 15
Excipients: include fragrance
For head lice (alcoholic, see notes above)
Cream shampoo ⟨NHS⟩ ◤, malathion 1%, net price 40 g = £2.77
Excipients: include cetostearyl alcohol, fragrance, hydroxybenzoates (parabens), sodium edetate, wool fat
For crab lice and head lice

Quellada M® (GSK Consumer Healthcare)
Liquid, malathion 0.5% in an aqueous basis, net price 50 mL = £1.85, 200 mL = £4.62
Excipients: include cetostearyl alcohol, fragrance, hydroxybenzoates (parabens)
For crab lice, head lice and scabies
Cream shampoo ◤, malathion 1%, net price 40 g = £2.18
Excipients: include cetostearyl alcohol, fragrance, hydroxybenzoates (parabens), sodium edetate, wool fat
For crab lice and head lice

Suleo-M® (SSL)
Lotion, malathion 0.5%, in an alcoholic basis, net price 50 mL = £2.22, 200 mL = £5.56. Label: 15
Excipients: include fragrance

For head lice (alcoholic, see notes above)

Permethrin

Permethrin is effective for *scabies, head lice*, and *crab lice* (for details see notes above).

PERMETHRIN

Indications: see notes above and under preparations
Cautions: avoid contact with eyes; do not use on broken or secondarily infected skin; children under 6 months, medical supervision required for cream rinse (head lice); children aged 2 months–2 years, medical supervision required for dermal cream (scabies)
Side-effects: pruritus, erythema, and stinging; rarely rashes and oedema
Dose: see under preparations

Lyclear® **Creme Rinse** (Warner Lambert) ◤
Cream rinse, permethrin 1% in basis containing isopropyl alcohol 20%, net price 59 mL = £2.38, 2 × 59-mL pack = £4.32
Excipients: include cetyl alcohol
Dose: head lice, apply to clean damp hair and rinse after 10 minutes
NOTE. Not affected by chlorine in swimming pools

Lyclear® **Dermal Cream** (Kestrel)
Dermal cream, permethrin 5%, net price 30 g = £5.52. Label: 10, patient information leaflet
Excipients: include butylated hydroxytoluene, wool fat derivative
Dose: scabies, apply over whole body and wash off after 8–12 hours; CHILD (see also Cautions, above) apply over whole body including face, neck, scalp and ears; if hands washed with soap within 8 hours of application, they should be treated again with cream (see notes above)
NOTE. Manufacturer recommends application to the body but to exclude head and neck. However, application should be extended to the scalp, neck, face, and ears
Larger patients may require up to two 30-g packs for adequate treatment
Crab lice, ADULT over 18 years, see notes above

Phenothrin

Phenothrin is recommended for *head lice* and *crab lice* (for details see notes above).

PHENOTHRIN

Indications: see notes above and under preparations
Cautions: avoid contact with eyes; do not use on broken or secondarily infected skin; do not use more than once a week for 3 weeks at a time; children under 6 months, medical supervision required; alcoholic preparations **not** recommended for head lice in severe eczema, in asthma, in small children, or for scabies or crab lice (see notes above)
Side-effects: skin irritation
Dose: see under preparations

Full Marks® (SSL)
Liquid, phenothrin 0.5% in an aqueous basis, net price 50 mL = £2.22, 200 mL = £5.56
Excipients: include cetostearyl alcohol, fragrance, hydroxybenzoates (parabens)
Dose: head lice, apply to dry hair, allow to dry naturally; shampoo after 12 hours or next day, comb wet hair
Lotion, phenothrin 0.2% in basis containing isopropyl alcohol 69.3%, net price 50 mL = £2.22, 200 mL = £5.56. Label: 15
Excipients: include fragrance
Dose: crab lice and head lice (alcoholic, see above), apply to dry hair, allow to dry naturally; shampoo after 12 hours [unlicensed contact duration], comb wet hair
Mousse (= foam application) ◤, phenothrin 0.5% in an alcoholic basis, net price 50 g = £2.44, 150 g = £5.95. Label: 15
Excipients: include cetostearyl alcohol
Dose: head lice (alcoholic, see above), apply to dry hair; shampoo after 30 minutes, comb wet hair

13.10.5 Preparations for minor cuts and abrasions

Some of the preparations listed are used in minor burns, and abrasions. They are applied as necessary. Preparations containing camphor and sulphonamides should be **avoided**. Preparations such as magnesium sulphate paste are also listed but are now rarely used to treat carbuncles and boils as these are best treated with antibiotics (section 5.1.1.2).

Cetrimide Cream, BP
Cream, cetrimide 0.5% in a suitable water-miscible basis such as cetostearyl alcohol 5%, liquid paraffin 50% in freshly boiled and cooled purified water, net price 50 g = 77p

Proflavine Cream, BPC
Cream, proflavine hemisulphate 0.1%, yellow beeswax 2.5%, chlorocresol 0.1%, liquid paraffin 67.3%, freshly boiled and cooled purified water 25%, wool fat 5%, net price 100 mL = 77p
NOTE. Stains clothing
Excipients: include beeswax, wool fat

▪ Preparations for boils
Magnesium Sulphate Paste, BP
Paste, dried magnesium sulphate 45 g, glycerol 55 g, phenol 500 mg, net price 25 g = 58p, 50 g = 63p
NOTE. Should be stirred before use
Dose: apply under dressing

Collodion

Flexible collodion may be used to seal minor cuts and wounds that have partially healed.

Collodion, Flexible, BP
Collodion, castor oil 2.5%, colophony 2.5% in a collodion basis, prepared by dissolving pyroxylin (10%) in a mixture of 3 volumes of ether and 1 volume of alcohol (90%), net price 10 mL = 21p. Label: 15
NOTE. Very highly flammable

Skin tissue adhesive

Tissue adhesives are used for closure of minor skin wounds and for additional suture support. They should be applied by an appropriately trained healthcare professional.

Dermabond® (Ethicon)
Topical skin adhesive, sterile, octylcyanoacrylate, net price 0.5 mL = £10.18

Epiglu® (ICN)
Tissue adhesive, sterile, ethyl-2-cyanoacrylate 954.5 mg/g, polymethylmethacrylate, net price 4 × 3-g vials = £95.00 (with dispensing pipettes and pallete)

Indermil® (Tyco)
Tissue adhesive, sterile, enbucrilate, net price 5 × 500-mg units = £32.50, 20 × 500-mg units = £130.00

Histoacryl® (Braun)
Tissue adhesive, sterile, enbucrilate, net price 5 × 200-mg unit (blue) = £32.00, 10 × 200-mg unit (blue) = £64.00, 5 × 500-mg unit (clear or blue) = £33.00, 10 × 500-mg unit (blue) = £66.00

LiquiBand® (MedLogic)
Tissue adhesive, sterile, butylcyanoacrylate, net price 0.5-g amp = £5.50

13.11 Skin cleansers and antiseptics

13.11.1 Alcohols and saline
13.11.2 Chlorhexidine salts
13.11.3 Cationic surfactants and soaps
13.11.4 Chlorine and iodine
13.11.5 Phenolics
13.11.6 Astringents, oxidisers, and dyes
13.11.7 Preparations for promotion of wound healing

Soap or detergent is used with water to cleanse intact skin; emollient preparations such as aqueous cream or emulsifying ointment (section 13.2.1) that do not irritate the skin are best used for cleansing dry skin.

An antiseptic is used for skin that is infected or that is susceptible to recurrent infection. Detergent preparations containing **chlorhexidine**, **triclosan**, or **povidone–iodine**, which should be thoroughly rinsed off, are used. Emollients may also contain antiseptics (section 13.2.1).

Antiseptics such as **chlorhexidine** or **povidone–iodine** are used on intact skin before surgical procedures; their antiseptic effect is enhanced by an alcoholic solvent. **Cetrimide** solution may be

used if a detergent effect is also required. Chlorinated solutions such as dilute sodium hypochlorite solution are too irritant and are not recommended.

For irrigating ulcers or wounds, lukewarm sterile sodium chloride 0.9% solution is used but tap water is often appropriate.

Potassium permanganate solution 1 in 10 000, a mild antiseptic with astringent properties, can be used for exudative eczematous areas; it should be stopped when the skin becomes dry. It can stain skin and nails especially with prolonged use.

13.11.1 Alcohols and saline

ALCOHOL

Indications: skin preparation before injection
Cautions: flammable; avoid broken skin; patients have suffered severe burns when diathermy has been preceded by application of alcoholic skin disinfectants

Industrial Methylated Spirit, BP
Mixture of 19 volumes of ethanol (absolute alcohol) of an appropriate strength with 1 volume of approved wood naphtha and is Industrial Methylated Spirit of the quality known either as '66 OP' or as '74 OP', net price 100 mL = 30p. Label: 15

Surgical Spirit, BP
Spirit, methyl salicylate 0.5 mL, diethyl phthalate 2%, castor oil 2.5%, in industrial methylated spirit, net price 100 mL = 20p. Label: 15

SODIUM CHLORIDE

Indications: see notes above

Sodium Chloride (Non-proprietary)
Solution (sterile), sodium chloride 0.9%, net price 10 × 10-mL unit = £3.61; 10 × 20-mL unit = £10.33; 10 × 30-mL unit = £3.00
Available from GBM, Generics (20-mL vial only)

Flowfusor® (Fresenius Kabi)
Solution (sterile), sodium chloride 0.9%, net price 120-mL Bellows Pack = £1.50

Irriclens® (ConvaTec)
Solution in aerosol can, (sterile), sodium chloride 0.9%, net price 240-mL can = £2.95

Miniversol® (Ezject)
Solution (sterile), sodium chloride 0.9%, net price 30 × 45-mL unit = £15.00

Normasol® (SSL)
Solution (sterile), sodium chloride 0.9%, net price 25 × 25-mL sachet = £5.85; 10 × 100-mL sachet = £7.16
See also section 11.8.2

Steripod® Sodium Chloride (SSL)
Steripod® sodium chloride 0.9% solution (sterile), sodium chloride 0.9%, net price 25 × 20-mL sachet = £6.83

13.11.2 Chlorhexidine salts

CHLORHEXIDINE

Indications: see under preparations; bladder irrigation and catheter patency solutions (see section 7.4.4)

Cautions: avoid contact with eyes, brain, meninges and middle ear; not for use in body cavities; alcoholic solutions not suitable before diathermy
Side-effects: occasional sensitivity

Chlorhexidine 0.05% (Baxter)
2000 Solution (sterile), pink, chlorhexidine acetate 0.05%, net price 500 mL = 72p, 1000 mL = 74p
For cleansing and disinfecting wounds and burns

Cepton® (Eastern)
Skin wash (= solution), red, chlorhexidine gluconate 1%, net price 150 mL = £1.99
For use as skin wash in acne
Lotion, blue, chlorhexidine gluconate 0.1%, net price 150 mL = £1.99
For skin disinfection in acne

CX Antiseptic Dusting Powder® (Adams Hlth.)
Dusting powder, sterile, chlorhexidine acetate 1%, net price 15 g = £1.20
For skin disinfection

Hibiscrub® (SSL)
Cleansing solution, red, chlorhexidine gluconate solution 20% (≡ 4% chlorhexidine gluconate), perfumed, in a surfactant solution, net price 250 mL = £1.10, 500 mL = £1.60, 5 litres = £12.70
Excipients: include fragrance
Use instead of soap for pre-operative hand and skin preparation and for general hand and skin disinfection

Hibisol® (SSL)
Solution, chlorhexidine gluconate solution 2.5% (≡ 0.5% chlorhexidine gluconate), in isopropyl alcohol 70% with emollients, net price 500 mL = £1.70
To be used undiluted for hand and skin disinfection

Hibitane Obstetric® (Centrapharm)
Cream, chlorhexidine gluconate solution 5% (≡ 1% chlorhexidine gluconate), in a pourable water-miscible basis, net price 250 mL = £2.22
For use in obstetrics and gynaecology as an antiseptic and lubricant (for application to skin around vulva and perineum and to hands of midwife or doctor)

Hydrex® (Adams Hlth.)
Solution, chlorhexidine gluconate solution 2.5% (≡ chlorhexidine gluconate 0.5%), in an alcoholic solution, net price 600 mL (clear) = £1.58; 600 mL (pink) = £1.58; 600 mL (blue) = £1.80
For pre-operative skin disinfection
NOTE. Flammable
Surgical scrub, chlorhexidine gluconate 4% in a surfactant solution, net price 250 mL = £1.00, 500 mL = £1.49
For pre-operative hand and skin preparation and for general hand disinfection

Unisept® (SSL)
Solution (sterile), pink, chlorhexidine gluconate 0.05%, net price 25 × 25-mL sachet = £5.59; 10 × 100-mL sachet = £6.84
For cleansing and disinfecting wounds and burns and swabbing in obstetrics

■ With cetrimide
Steripod® **Chlorhexidine/Cetrimide** (SSL)
Steripod® Chlorhexidine/Cetrimide solution, chlorhexidine gluconate solution 0.075% (≡ chlorhexidine gluconate 0.015%), cetrimide 0.15%, net price 25 × 20-mL vials = £6.52
For cleansing and disinfecting wounds and burns

Tisept® (SSL)
Solution (sterile), yellow, chlorhexidine gluconate 0.015%, cetrimide 0.15%, net price 25 × 25-mL sachet = £5.59; 10 × 100-mL sachet = £6.84
To be used undiluted for general skin disinfection and wound cleansing

Travasept 100® (Baxter)
Solution (sterile), yellow, chlorhexidine acetate 0.015%, cetrimide 0.15%, net price 500 mL = £1.80, 1 litre = £1.90
To be used undiluted in skin disinfection such as wound cleansing and obstetrics

Concentrates

Hibitane 5% Concentrate® (SSL)
Solution, red, chlorhexidine gluconate solution 25% (≡ 5% chlorhexidine gluconate), in a perfumed aqueous solution, net price 5 litres = £11.50
Dose: to be used diluted 1 in 10 (0.5%) with alcohol 70% for pre-operative skin preparation, or 1 in 100 (0.05%) with water for general skin disinfection
NOTE. Alcoholic solutions not suitable before diathermy (see Alcohol, above)

■ With cetrimide
Hibicet Hospital Concentrate® (SSL)
Solution, orange, chlorhexidine gluconate solution 7.5% (≡ chlorhexidine gluconate 1.5%), cetrimide 15%, net price 5 litres = £8.55
Dose: to be used diluted 1 in 100 (1%) to 1 in 30 with water for skin disinfection and wound cleansing, and diluted 1 in 30 in alcohol 70% for pre-operative skin preparation
NOTE. Alcoholic solutions not suitable before diathermy (see Alcohol, above)

13.11.3 Cationic surfactants and soaps

CETRIMIDE

Indications: skin disinfection
Cautions: avoid contact with eyes; avoid use in body cavities
Side-effects: skin irritation and occasionally sensitisation

■ Preparations
Ingredient of *Hibicet Hospital Concentrate*®, *Steripod*®, *Tisept*®, and *Travasept 100*, see above

13.11.4 Chlorine and iodine

CHLORINATED SOLUTIONS

Cautions: bleaches fabric; irritant (protect surrounding tissues with soft paraffin)

Chlorasol® (SSL) NHS
Solution (sterile), sodium hypochlorite, containing 0.3% available chlorine. Net price 25 × 25-mL sachets = £8.49
NOTE. Irritant, therefore no longer recommended

IODINE COMPOUNDS

Indications: skin disinfection

Cautions: pregnancy, breast-feeding; broken skin (see below); renal impairment (Appendix 3)
LARGE OPEN WOUNDS. The application of povidone–iodine to large wounds or severe burns may produce systemic adverse effects such as metabolic acidosis, hypernatraemia and impairment of renal function.

Contra-indications: avoid regular use in patients with thyroid disorders or those receiving lithium therapy

Side-effects: rarely sensitivity; may interfere with thyroid function tests

Betadine® (SSL)
Antiseptic paint, povidone–iodine 10% in an alcoholic solution, net price 8 mL (with applicator brush) = £1.01
Dose: apply undiluted to minor wounds and infections, twice daily
Alcoholic solution, povidone–iodine 10%, net price 500 mL = £1.91
Dose: apply undiluted in pre- and post-operative skin disinfection; NEONATE not recommended for regular use (and contra-indicated in very low birthweight infants)
NOTE. Flammable—caution in procedures involving hot wire cautery and diathermy
Antiseptic solution, povidone–iodine 10% in aqueous solution, net price 500 mL = £1.75
Dose: apply undiluted in pre- and post-operative skin disinfection; NEONATE not recommended for regular use (and contra-indicated in very low birthweight infants)
NOTE. Not for body cavity irrigation
Dry powder spray, povidone–iodine 2.5% in a pressurised aerosol unit, net price 150-g unit = £2.79
For skin disinfection, particularly minor wounds and infections, CHILD under 2 years not recommended
NOTE. Not for use in serous cavities
Ointment, povidone–iodine 10%, in a water-miscible basis, net price 20 g = £1.39, 80 g = £2.79
Excipients: none as listed in section 13.1.3
For skin disinfection, particularly minor wounds and infections, CHILD under 2 years not recommended
Skin cleanser solution, povidone–iodine 4%, in a surfactant basis, net price 250 mL = £2.14
Dose: for infective conditions of the skin. Retain on skin for 3–5 minutes before rinsing; repeat twice daily; CHILD under 2 years not recommended
Surgical scrub, povidone–iodine 7.5%, in a non-ionic surfactant basis, net price 500 mL = £1.58
To be used as a pre-operative scrub for hands and skin; CHILD not recommended for regular use in neonates (and contra-indicated in very low birthweight infants)

Savlon® **Dry Antiseptic** (Novartis Consumer Health)
Powder spray, povidone–iodine 1.14% in a pressurised aerosol unit, net price 50-mL unit = £2.39
For minor wounds

Videne® (Adams Hlth.)
Alcoholic tincture, povidone–iodine 10%, net price 500 mL = £1.85
To be applied undiluted in pre-operative skin disinfection
Antiseptic solution, povidone–iodine 10% in aqueous solution, net price 500 mL = £1.70
To be applied undiluted in pre-operative skin disinfection and general antisepsis
Surgical scrub, povidone–iodine 7.5% in aqueous solution, net price 500 mL = £1.52
To be used as a pre-operative scrub for hand and skin disinfection

13.11.5 Phenolics

TRICLOSAN

Indications: skin disinfection

Cautions: avoid contact with eyes

Aquasept® (SSL)
Skin cleanser, blue, triclosan 2%, net price 28.5 mL = 33p, 250 mL = £1.10, 500 mL = £1.68
Excipients: include chlorocresol, edetic acid (EDTA), propylene glycol, fragrance
For disinfection and pre-operative hand preparation

Manusept® (SSL)
Antibacterial hand rub, triclosan 0.5%, isopropyl alcohol 70%, net price 250 mL = £1.07, 500 mL = £1.56
Excipients: none as listed in section 13.1.3
For disinfection and pre-operative hand preparation
NOTE. Flammable

Ster-Zac Bath Concentrate® (SSL)
Solution, triclosan 2%, net price 28.5 mL = 40p, 500 mL = £2.24
Dose: for prevention of cross-infection use 28.5 mL/bath
Excipients: include trisodium edetate

13.11.6 Astringents, oxidisers, and dyes

HYDROGEN PEROXIDE

Indications: see under preparations below

Cautions: large or deep wounds; avoid on healthy skin and eyes; bleaches fabric; incompatible with products containing iodine or potassium permanganate

Hydrogen Peroxide Solution, BP
Solution 6% (20 vols), net price 100 mL = 16p
Solution 3% (10 vols), net price 100 mL = 19p
For skin disinfection, particularly cleansing and deodorising wounds and ulcers
NOTE. The BP directs that when hydrogen peroxide is prescribed, hydrogen peroxide solution 6% (20 vols) should be dispensed.
IMPORTANT. Strong solutions of hydrogen peroxide which contain 27% (90 vols) and 30% (100 vols) are only for the preparation of weaker solutions

Crystacide® (GP Pharma)
Cream, hydrogen peroxide 1%, net price 10 g = £3.71, 25 g = £6.21
Dose: superficial bacterial skin infection, apply 2-3 times daily for up to 3 weeks
Excipients: include edetic acid (EDTA), propylene glycol

Hioxyl®
Section 13.11.7

POTASSIUM PERMANGANATE

Indications: cleansing and deodorising suppurating eczematous reactions and wounds

Cautions: irritant to mucous membranes

Dose: wet dressings or baths, approx. 0.01% solution
NOTE. Stains skin and clothing

Potassium Permanganate Solution
Solution, potassium permanganate 0.1% (1 in 1000) in water
Dose: to be diluted 1 in 10 to provide a 0.01% (1 in 10 000) solution

Permitabs® (Centrapharm)
Solution tablets, for preparation of topical solution, potassium permanganate 400 mg, net price 30-tab pack = £5.08
NOTE. 1 tablet dissolved in 4 litres of water provides a 0.01% (1 in 10 000) solution

13.11.7 Preparations for promotion of wound healing

Desloughing agents

Desloughing agents for ulcers are second-line treatment and the underlying causes should be treated. The main beneficial effect is removal of slough and clot and the ablation of local infection. Preparations which absorb or help promote the removal of exudate may also help (Appendix 8). It should be noted that substances applied to an open area are easily absorbed and perilesional skin is easily sensitised. Gravitational dermatitis may be complicated by superimposed contact sensitivity to substances such as neomycin or lanolin. Enzyme preparations such as streptokinase-streptodornase or alternatively dextranomer (Appendix 8) are designed for applying to sloughing ulcers. Sterile larvae (maggots) (*LarvE*®, Biosurgical Research Unit) are also used for managing sloughing wounds and are prescribable on the NHS.

Aserbine® (Goldshield)
Solution, benzoic acid 0.15%, malic acid 2.25%, propylene glycol 40%, salicylic acid 0.0375%, net price 500 mL = £3.61
Excipients: include fragrance
Dose: use as wash before each application of cream (or use as wet dressing)

Hioxyl® (Ferndale)
Cream, hydrogen peroxide (stabilised) 1.5%, net price 25 g = £2.16, 100 g = £6.76
Excipients: include cetostearyl alcohol
For leg ulcers and pressure sores
Dose: apply when necessary and if necessary cover with a dressing

Varidase Topical® (Wyeth) PoM
Powder, streptokinase 100 000 units, streptodornase 25 000 units. For preparing solutions for topical use, net price with sterile physiological saline 20 mL (combi-pack) = £10.82
Excipients: none as listed in section 13.1.3
Dose: reconstitute with 20 mL sterile physiological saline (or water for injections) and apply as wet dressing 1–2 times daily; cover with semi-occlusive dressing; irrigate lesion thoroughly with physiological saline and remove loosened material before next application; also used to dissolve clots in the bladder or urinary catheters
Contra-indications: active haemorrhage, severe hypertension
Side-effects: infrequent allergic reactions (reduced by careful and frequent removal of exudate and thorough irrigation with physiological saline); fever, transient burning and hypersensitivity reactions including shock reported

Growth factor

A topical preparation of **becaplermin** (recombinant human platelet-derived growth factor) is licensed as an adjunct treatment of full-thickness, neuropathic, diabetic ulcers.

Regranex® (Janssen-Cilag) ▼ PoM
Gel, becaplermin (recombinant human platelet-derived growth factor) 0.01%, net price 15 g = £275
Excipients: include hydroxybenzoates
Dose: full-thickness, neuropathic, diabetic ulcers (no larger than 5 cm²), apply thin layer daily and cover with gauze dressing moistened with physiological saline; max. duration of treatment 20 weeks (reassess if no healing after first 10 weeks)
Cautions: malignant disease; avoid on sites with infection, malignancy, peripheral arteriopathy, or osteomyelitis
Side-effects: irritation, rarely bullous eruption, oedema

13.12 Antiperspirants

Aluminium chloride is a potent antiperspirant used in the treatment of hyperhidrosis. Aluminium salts are also incorporated in preparations used for minor fungal skin infections associated with hyperhidrosis.
In more severe cases specialists use **glycopyrronium bromide** as a 0.05% solution in the iontophoretic treatment of hyperhidrosis of plantar and palmar areas. **Botulinum A toxin-haemagglutinin complex** (section 4.9.3) is licensed for use intradermally for severe hyperhidrosis of the axillae unresponsive to topical antiperspirant or other antihidrotic treatment.

ALUMINIUM SALTS

Indications: see under Dose below
Cautions: avoid contact with eyes or mucous membranes; avoid use on broken or irritated skin; do not shave axillae or use depilatories within 12 hours of application; avoid contact with clothing
Side-effects: skin irritation
Dose: hyperhidrosis affecting axillae, hands or feet, apply liquid formulation at night to dry skin, wash off the following morning, initially daily then reduce frequency as condition improves—do not bathe immediately before use
Hyperhidrosis, bromidrosis, intertrigo, and prevention of tinea pedis and related conditions, apply powder to dry skin

Anhydrol Forte® (Dermal)
Solution (= application), aluminium chloride hexahydrate 20% in an alcoholic basis, net price 60-mL bottle with roll-on applicator = £2.82. Label: 15
Excipients: none as listed in section 13.1.3

¹**Driclor**® (Stiefel)
Application, aluminium chloride hexahydrate 20% in an alcoholic basis, net price 60-mL bottle with roll-on applicator = £2.82. Label: 15
Excipients: none as listed in section 13.1.3

1. A 30-mL pack is on sale to the public (*Driclor*® Solution)

ZeaSORB® (Stiefel)
Dusting powder, aldioxa 0.22%, chloroxylenol 0.5%, net price 50 g = £2.15
Excipients: include fragrance

GLYCOPYRRONIUM BROMIDE

Indications: iontophoretic treatment of hyperhidrosis; other indications section 15.1.3
Cautions: see section 15.1.3 (but poorly absorbed and systemic effects unlikely)

Contra-indications: see section 15.1.3 (but poorly absorbed and systemic effects unlikely), infections affecting the treatment site

Side-effects: see section 15.1.3 (but poorly absorbed and systemic effects unlikely), tingling at administration site

Dose: consult product literature; only 1 site to be treated at a time, max. 2 sites treated in any 24 hours, treatment not to be repeated within 7 days

Robinul® (Antigen) PoM
Powder, glycopyrronium bromide, net price 3 g = £110.00

13.13 Wound management products and Elastic Hosiery

■ Preparations
See Appendix 8

13.14 Topical circulatory preparations

These preparations are used to improve circulation in conditions such as bruising, superficial thrombophlebitis, chilblains and varicose veins but are of little value. Chilblains are best managed by avoidance of exposure to cold; neither systemic nor topical vasodilator therapy is established as being effective. Sclerotherapy of varicose veins is described in section 2.13.

Rubefacients are described in section 10.3.2.

Hirudoid® (Sankyo)
Cream, heparinoid 0.3% in a vanishing-cream basis, net price 50 g = £1.35
Excipients: include cetostearyl alcohol, hydroxybenzoates (parabens)
Gel, heparinoid 0.3%, net price 50 g = £1.35
Excipients: include propylene glycol, fragrance
Dose: apply up to 4 times daily in superficial soft-tissue injuries and superficial thrombophlebitis

Lasonil® (Bayer Consumer Care)
Ointment, heparinoid 0.8% in white soft paraffin, net price 40 g = £1.08
Excipients: include wool fat derivative
Dose: apply 2–3 times daily in superficial soft-tissue injuries

14: Immunological products and vaccines

> **Post-immunisation pyrexia in infants.** The parent should be advised that if pyrexia develops after childhood immunisation, the infant can be given a dose of paracetamol or ibuprofen and, if necessary, a second dose given 6 hours later. The parent should be warned to seek medical advice if the pyrexia persists after the second dose.
>
> For post-immunisation pyrexia in an infant aged 2–3 months, the dose of paracetamol is 60 mg; the dose of ibuprofen is 50 mg (on doctor's advice). An oral syringe can be obtained from any pharmacy to give the small volume required.

14.1   Active immunity

Vaccines may consist of:

1. a *live attenuated* form of a virus (e.g. rubella or measles vaccine) or bacteria (e.g. BCG vaccine)
2. *inactivated* preparations of the virus (e.g. influenza vaccine) or bacteria, or
3. *extracts of* or *detoxified exotoxins* produced by a micro-organism (e.g. tetanus vaccine).

They stimulate production of antibodies and other components of the immune mechanism.

For **live attenuated** vaccines, immunisation is generally achieved with a single dose (but 3 doses are required with oral poliomyelitis vaccine). Live attenuated vaccines usually produce a durable immunity but not always as long as that of the natural infection. When two live virus vaccines are required (and are not available as a combined preparation) they should be given either simultaneously at different sites or with an interval of at least 3 weeks.

Inactivated vaccines may require a primary series of injections of vaccine to produce adequate antibody response and in most cases booster (reinforcing) injections are required; the duration of immunity varies from months to many years. Some inactivated vaccines are adsorbed onto an adjuvant (such as aluminium hydroxide) to enhance the antibody response.

> Guidelines in this chapter reflect those in the handbook *Immunisation against Infectious Disease* (1996), which in turn reflects the advice of the Joint Committee on Vaccination and Immunisation (JCVI). Chapters from the handbook are available at www.doh.gov.uk/greenbook

SIDE-EFFECTS. Some vaccines (e.g. poliomyelitis) produce very few reactions, while others (e.g. measles and rubella) may produce a very mild form of the disease. Some vaccines may produce discomfort at the site of injection and mild fever and malaise. Occasionally there are more serious untoward reactions and these should always be reported to the CSM. Anaphylactic reactions are very rare but can be fatal (see section 3.4.3 for management). The product literature should be consulted for full details of side-effects.

CONTRA-INDICATIONS. Most vaccines have some basic contra-indication to their use, and the product literature should be consulted for details. In general, vaccination should be postponed if the individual is suffering from an *acute illness*. Minor infections without fever or systemic upset are not contra-indications. A definite severe reaction to a preceding dose is a contra-indication to further doses.

Some viral vaccines contain small quantities of antibacterials such as neomycin or polymyxin B (or both); such vaccines may need to be withheld from individuals who are *extremely sensitive to the antibacterial. Hypersensitivity to egg* contra-indicates influenza vaccine and tick-borne encephalitis vaccine (residual egg protein present) and, if evidence of previous anaphylactic reaction, also yellow fever vaccine.

Live vaccines should not be administered routinely to *pregnant women* because of possible harm to the fetus but where there is a significant risk of exposure (e.g. poliomyelitis or yellow fever), the need for vaccination outweighs any possible risk to the fetus. Live vaccines should not be given to individuals with *impaired immune response*, whether caused by disease (for special reference to *HIV infection*, see below) or as a result of radiotherapy or treatment with high doses of corticosteroids or other immunosuppressive drugs.[1,2] They should not be given to those suffering from *malignant conditions* such as leukaemia and tumours of the reticulo-endothelial system.[2]

The intramuscular route should not be used in patients with bleeding disorders such as haemophilia or thrombocytopenia.

NOTE. The Department of Health has advised *against the use of jet guns* for vaccination owing to the risk of transmitting blood-borne infections, such as HIV.

---

1. Live vaccines should be postponed until at least 3 months after stopping corticosteroids and 6 months after stopping chemotherapy.

2. Use of normal immunoglobulin should be considered after exposure to measles (see p. 595) and varicella–zoster immunoglobulin considered after exposure to chickenpox or herpes zoster (see p. 596).

VACCINES AND HIV INFECTION. HIV-positive individuals with or without symptoms can receive the following live vaccines:

MMR (but not whilst severely immunosuppressed);[1,2] and the following inactivated vaccines:

cholera, diphtheria, haemophilus influenzae type b, hepatitis A, hepatitis B, influenza, meningococcal, pertussis, pneumococcal, poliomyelitis[3], rabies, tetanus, typhoid (injection).

HIV-positive individuals should **not** receive:

BCG, yellow fever[4]

NOTE. The above advice differs from that for other immunocompromised patients.

VACCINES AND ASPLENIA. The following vaccines are recommended for asplenic patients or those with splenic dysfunction:

haemophilus influenzae type b, meningococcal group C, pneumococcal, influenza.

For antibiotic prophylaxis in asplenia see p. 256.

Immunisation schedule

Vaccines for the childhood immunisation schedule should be obtained from **local health authorities** or **direct from Farillon**—not to be prescribed on FP10 (GP10 in Scotland; WP10 in Wales) since not available to pharmacies.

During first year of life

Adsorbed Diphtheria, Tetanus and [whole-cell] Pertussis Vaccine [DTwP]

3 doses at intervals of 4 weeks; first dose at 2 months of age

Primary immunisation should continue to be with diphtheria, tetanus and *whole-cell* pertussis [DTwP] vaccine unless whole-cell pertussis is contra-indicated (because of previous reaction to the whole-cell component), in which case adsorbed diphtheria, tetanus and pertussis (acellular component) vaccine may be used

plus

Haemophilus Influenzae type b Vaccine (Hib)

3 doses at intervals of 4 weeks; first dose at 2 months of age

plus

Meningococcal Group C Conjugate Vaccine

3 doses at intervals of 4 weeks; first dose at 2 months of age

plus

Poliomyelitis Vaccine, Live (Oral)

3 doses at intervals of 4 weeks; first dose at 2 months of age

BCG Vaccine (for neonates at risk only)

See section 14.4, BCG Vaccines

During second year of life

Measles, Mumps and Rubella Vaccine, Live (MMR)

Single dose at 12–15 months of age

---

1. Use of normal immunoglobulin should be considered after exposure to measles (see p. 595) and varicella–zoster immunoglobulin considered after exposure to chickenpox or herpes zoster (see p. 596).

2. The Royal College of Paediatrics and Child Health recommends that MMR is not given to a child with HIV infection whilst severely immunosuppressed.

3. The Royal College of Paediatrics and Child Health recommends that inactivated poliomyelitis vaccine is used instead of oral poliomyelitis vaccine for routine immunisation of children with HIV infection.

4. Because insufficient evidence of safety.

Haemophilus Influenzae type b Vaccine (Hib) (if not previously immunised)

Single dose at 13 months–4 years of age (over 4 years, see section 14.4, Haemophilus Influenzae type b Vaccine)

Before school or nursery school entry

Adsorbed Diphtheria, Tetanus and Pertussis (Acellular Component) Vaccine [DTaP]

Single booster dose

Pre-school booster should comprise diphtheria, tetanus and *acellular pertussis* [DTaP] vaccine (the vaccine with whole-cell pertussis is **not** recommended because of increased reactions in older children)

Preferably allow interval of at least 3 years after completing basic course; can be given at same session as MMR Vaccine but use separate syringe and needle, and give in different limb

plus

Poliomyelitis Vaccine, Live (Oral)

Single booster dose

Preferably allow interval of at least 3 years after completing basic course

plus

Measles, Mumps and Rubella Vaccine, Live (MMR)

Single booster dose

Can be given at same session as Adsorbed Diphtheria, Tetanus and Pertussis (Acellular Component) Vaccine but use separate syringe and needle, and use different limb

Between 10–14 years of age

BCG Vaccine (for tuberculin-negative children)

Single dose

May be given simultaneously with another live vaccine; otherwise an interval of 4 weeks should be allowed between the two

Before leaving school or before employment or further education

Adsorbed Diphtheria [low dose] and Tetanus Vaccine for Adults and Adolescents

Single booster dose

Adsorbed Diphtheria and Tetanus Vaccine, DT/Vac/Ads(Child), **not** to be used for children aged over 10 years and adults

plus

Poliomyelitis Vaccine, Live (Oral)

Single booster dose

During adult life

Poliomyelitis Vaccine, Live (Oral) (if not previously immunised)

3 doses at intervals of 4 weeks

No adult should remain unimmunised; booster doses for adults are not necessary unless they are at special risk, such as healthcare workers in possible contact with poliomyelitis and travellers to areas where poliomyelitis is epidemic or endemic, see p. 591

Measles, Mumps and Rubella Vaccine, Live (MMR) (for women of child-bearing age susceptible to rubella)

Single dose

Women of child-bearing age should be tested for rubella antibodies and sero-negative women offered rubella immunisation (using the MMR vaccine)—exclude pregnancy before immunisation, but see also section 14.4, Measles, Mumps and Rubella Vaccine

Adsorbed Diphtheria [low dose] and Tetanus Vaccine for Adults and Adolescents (if not previously immunised)
3 doses at intervals of 4 weeks
Booster dose 10 years after primary course and again 10 years later maintains satisfactory level of protection

Adsorbed Diphtheria and Tetanus Vaccine, DT/Vac/ Ads(Child), **not** to be used for children aged over 10 years and adults

High-risk groups

For information on high-risk groups, see section 14.4 under individual vaccines
Hepatitis A Vaccine
Hepatitis B Vaccine
Influenza Vaccine
Pneumococcal Vaccine

14.2   Passive immunity

Immunity with immediate protection against certain infective organisms can be obtained by injecting preparations made from the plasma of immune individuals with adequate levels of antibody to the disease for which protection is sought (see under Immunoglobulin section 14.5). This passive immunity lasts only a few weeks; where necessary passive immunisation can be repeated.

Antibodies of human origin are usually termed *immunoglobulins*. The term *antiserum* is applied to material prepared in animals. Because of serum sickness and other allergic-type reactions that may follow injections of antisera, this therapy has been replaced wherever possible by the use of immuno-globulins. Reactions are theoretically possible after injection of human immunoglobulins but reports of such reactions are very rare.

14.3   Storage and use

Care must be taken to store all vaccines and other immunological products under the conditions recommended in the product literature, otherwise the preparation may become ineffective. **Refrigerated storage** is usually necessary; many vaccines need to be stored at 2–8°C and not allowed to freeze. Vaccines should be protected from light. Unused vaccine in multidose vials without preservative (most live virus vaccines) should be discarded within 1 hour of first use; those containing a preservative (including oral poliomyelitis vaccine) should be discarded within 3 hours or at the end of a session. Unused vaccines should be disposed of by incineration at a registered disposal contractor.

Particular attention must be paid to instructions on the use of diluents. Vaccines which are liquid suspensions or are reconstituted before use should be adequately mixed to ensure uniformity of the material to be injected.

14.4   Vaccines and antisera

AVAILABILITY. Anthrax and yellow fever vaccines, botulism antitoxin, diphtheria antitoxin, and snake and spider venom antitoxins are available from local designated holding centres.

For antivenom, see Emergency Treatment of Poisoning, p. 29.

Enquiries for vaccines not available commercially can also be made to:

Immunisation and Communicable Diseases Branch
Department of Health
Skipton House
80 London Road
London SE1 6LH
Tel: (020) 7972 1522

In Scotland information about availability of vaccines can be obtained from the Chief Administrative Pharmaceutical Officer of the local Health Board. In Wales enquiries should be directed to:

Welsh Office
Cathays Park
Cardiff CF1 3NQ
Tel: (029) 2082 5111, extn 4658

and in Northern Ireland:

Regional Pharmacist (procurement co-ordination)
United Hospitals TrustPharmacy Dept
Whiteabbey Hospital
Doagh Road
Newtownabbey BT37 9RH
Tel: (028) 908 65181 ext 2386)

For further details of availability, see under individual vaccines.

Anthrax vaccine

Anthrax immunisation is indicated for individuals who handle infected animals, for those exposed to imported infected animal products, and for laboratory staff who work with *Bacillus anthracis*.

In the event of possible contact with *B. anthracis*, post-exposure immunisation may be indicated, in addition to antimicrobial prophylaxis (section 5.1.12). Advice on the use of anthrax vaccine must be obtained from the Immunisation Division, Communicable Disease Surveillance Centre, Health Protection Agency, Colindale (CDSC) (tel. 020 8200 6868)

The vaccine is the alum precipitate of an antigen from *B. anthracis* and, following the primary course of injections, booster doses should be given at about yearly intervals.

Anthrax Vaccine PoM
Dose: initial course 3 doses of 0.5 mL *by intramuscular injection* at intervals of 3 weeks followed by a fourth dose after an interval of 6 months; for post-exposure prophylaxis, fifth dose recommended 1 year after exposure
Booster doses: 0.5 mL annually
NOTE. Advice on post-exposure prophylaxis must be obtained from CDSC
Available from CDSC

BCG vaccines

BCG (Bacillus Calmette-Guérin) is a live attenuated strain derived from *Mycobacterium bovis* which stimulates the development of hypersensitivity to *M. tuberculosis*. BCG vaccine should be given intradermally by operators skilled in the technique (see below).

Within 2–6 weeks a small swelling appears at the injection site which progresses to a papule or to a benign ulcer about 10 mm in diameter and heals in 6–12 weeks. A dry dressing may be used if the ulcer discharges, but air should **not** be excluded.

> The CSM has reported that serious reactions with BCG are uncommon and most often consist of prolonged ulceration or subcutaneous abscess formation due to faulty injection technique.

BCG is recommended for the following groups if BCG immunisation, as evidenced by a characteristic scar, has not previously been carried out and they are negative for tuberculoprotein hypersensitivity:

- contacts of those with active respiratory tuberculosis;
- immigrants (including infants and children) from countries with a high incidence of tuberculosis should be immunised without delay. Their infants born in the UK should also be immunised within a few days of birth, or at two months of age at the same time as the first dose of routine childhood vaccines;
- health service staff (including medical students, hospital medical staff, nurses, physiotherapists, radiographers, technical staff in pathology departments and any others considered to be at special risk because of the likelihood of contact with infective patients or their sputum; particularly important to test staff in contact with the immunocompromised, e.g. in transplant, oncology and HIV units, and staff in maternity and paediatric departments);
- children between 10 and 14 years of age (see schedule, section 14.1);
- veterinary and other staff who handle animal species known to be susceptible to tuberculosis;
- staff working in prisons, in residential homes and in hostels for refugees and the homeless;
- those intending to stay for more than 1 month in countries with a high incidence of tuberculosis (section 14.6)
- newly-born infants, children or adults where the parents or the adults request immunisation;

Apart from infants of up to 3 months, any person being considered for BCG immunisation must first be given a skin test for hypersensitivity to tuberculoprotein (see under Diagnostic agents, below).

BCG vaccine may be given simultaneously with another live vaccine (see also section 14.1), but if they are not given at the same time, an interval of 4 weeks should normally be allowed between them. However, when BCG is given to infants, there is no need to delay the primary immunisations, including poliomyelitis.

See section 14.1 for general contra-indications. BCG is also contra-indicated in subjects with generalised septic skin conditions (in the case of eczema, a vaccination site free from lesions should be chosen).

Bladder instillations of BCG are licensed for the management of bladder carcinoma (section 8.2.4).

For advice on chemoprophylaxis against tuberculosis, see section 5.1.9.

■ Intradermal

Bacillus Calmette-Guérin Vaccine ▼ PoM

BCG Vaccine, Dried Tub/Vac/BCG

A freeze-dried preparation of live bacteria of a strain derived from the bacillus of Calmette and Guérin.

Dose: by intradermal injection, 0.1 mL (INFANT under 12 months 0.05 mL)

Available from health authorities or direct from Farillon (SSI brand, multidose vial with diluent)

INTRADERMAL INJECTION TECHNIQUE. After swabbing with spirit and allowing to dry, skin is stretched between thumb and forefinger and needle (size 25G or 26G) inserted (bevel upwards) for about 2 mm into superficial layers of dermis (almost parallel with surface). Needle should be short with short bevel (can usually be seen through epidermis during insertion). Raised blanched bleb showing tips of hair follicles is sign of correct injection; 7 mm bleb ≡ 0.1 mL injection; if considerable resistance not felt, needle is removed and reinserted before giving more vaccine.

To be injected at insertion of deltoid muscle onto humerus (keloid formation more likely with sites higher on arm); tip of shoulder should be **avoided**; for cosmetic reasons, upper and lateral surface of thigh may be preferred (but in neonates, upper arm **must** be used).

■ Percutaneous

Preparations for administration by the percutaneous multiple puncture technique are not currently available

Diagnostic agents

In the *Mantoux test*, the diagnostic dose is by intradermal injection of Tuberculin Purified Protein Derivative (PPD):

Routine
10 units PPD i.e. 0.1 mL of 100 units/mL (1 in 1000)

Special (hypersensitive or TB suspected)
1 unit PPD i.e. 0.1 mL of 10 units/mL (1 in 10 000)

Special (low sensitivity)
100 units PPD i.e. 0.1 mL of 1000 units/mL (1 in 100)

In the *Heaf test* (multiple puncture) a solution containing Tuberculin Purified Protein Derivative 100 000 units/mL is used; 1 mL is sufficient for up to about 20 tests.

NOTE. Tuberculin testing should not be carried out within 4 weeks of receiving a live viral vaccine since response to tuberculin may be inhibited.

Tuberculin PPD PoM

Prepared from the heat treated products of growth and lysis of the appropriate species of mycobacterium, and containing 100 000 units/mL, net price 1-mL amp = £5.89. Also available diluted 1 in 100 (1000 units/mL), 1 in 1000 (100 units/mL), and 1 in 10 000 (10 units/mL), net price 1 mL (all) = £2.22

Available from health authorities or direct from Farillon

Botulism antitoxin

A trivalent botulism antitoxin is available for the post-exposure prophylaxis of botulism and for the treatment of persons thought to be suffering from botulism. It specifically neutralises the toxins produced by *Clostridium botulinum* types A, B, and E. It is not effective against infantile botulism as the toxin (type A) is seldom, if ever, found in the blood in this type of infection.

Hypersensitivity reactions are a problem. It is essential to read the contra-indications, warnings, and details of sensitivity tests on the package insert. Prior to treatment checks should be made regarding previous administration of any antitoxin and history of any allergic condition, e.g. asthma, hay fever, etc. All patients should be tested for sensitivity (diluting the antitoxin if history of allergy).

Botulism Antitoxin PoM

A preparation containing the specific antitoxic globulins that have the power of neutralising the toxins formed by types A, B, and E of *Clostridium botulinum*.

NOTE. The BP title Botulinum Antitoxin is not used because the preparation currently available has a higher phenol content (0.45% against 0.25%).

Dose: prophylaxis, *by intramuscular injection*, 20 mL as soon as possible after exposure; treatment, 20 mL (diluted to 100 mL with sodium chloride 0.9%) by slow intravenous infusion followed by 10 mL 2–4 hours later if necessary, and further doses at intervals of 12–24 hours.

Available from local designated centres, for details see TOXBASE (requires registration) www.spib.axl.co.uk. For supplies outside working hours apply to other designated centres and, as a last resort, to Department of Health Duty Officer (Tel (020) 7210 3000).

Cholera vaccine

Cholera vaccine contains heat-killed Inaba and Ogawa sub-types of *Vibrio cholerae*, Serovar O1. Cholera vaccine provides little protection and cannot control the spread of the disease; it is no longer available in the UK.

Cholera vaccine is no longer required for international travel. The Department of Health has advised that in the rare circumstance where an unofficial demand may be anticipated, confirmation of non-requirement of cholera vaccine may be given on official notepaper signed and stamped by the medical practitioner.

Travellers to a country where cholera exists should be warned that scrupulous attention to food and water and personal hygiene is **essential**.

Diphtheria vaccines

Protection against diphtheria is essentially due to antitoxin, the production of which is stimulated by vaccines prepared from the toxin of *Corynebacterium diphtheriae*. Adsorbed diphtheria vaccines are recommended for the routine immunisation of babies and are usually given in the form of **adsorbed diphtheria, tetanus, and [whole-cell] pertussis vaccine** (see schedule, section 14.1). Adsorbed diphtheria and tetanus vaccine is used when immunisation against pertussis is contra-indicated.

A booster dose of **adsorbed diphtheria, tetanus and pertussis (acellular component) vaccine** is recommended before school entry (3–5 years of age). This should preferably be given after an interval of at least 3 years from the last dose of the basic course. A further booster dose is recommended before leaving school; for this purpose **adsorbed diphtheria [low dose] and tetanus vaccine for adults and adolescents** is available.

For details on booster doses of diphtheria vaccine in a child over 13 years who requires treatment of a tetanus-prone wound, see under Tetanus Vaccines.

The single antigen diphtheria vaccine is no longer available; **adsorbed diphtheria [low dose] and tetanus vaccine for adults and adolescents** is a suitable replacement. The vaccine can be used if an individual has completed a full course of tetanus vaccine or has had a tetanus vaccine within the last 10 years but requires diphtheria vaccination as part of the school-leaving booster, for occupational reasons, or for foreign travel.

Staff in contact with diphtheria patients or potentially pathogenic clinical specimens or working directly with *Corynebacterium diphtheriae* should be considered for a booster or for primary immunisation following a risk assessment. **Adsorbed diphtheria [low dose] and tetanus vaccine for adults and adolescents** is used for this purpose; immunity should be checked by antibody testing at least 3 months after completion of immunisation.

Unimmunised contacts of a diphtheria case require a primary course of 3 doses of **adsorbed diphtheria and tetanus vaccine** at monthly intervals (**important:** adults and children *over 10 years* must be given a vaccine containing **low-dose** diphtheria toxoid). *Immunised* contacts require a single booster dose. Booster doses against diphtheria are not recommended as routine.

Previously immunised travellers to countries where diphtheria is endemic or epidemic require a booster dose, using a combined diphtheria and tetanus vaccine, if their primary immunisation was more than 10 years ago. *Unimmunised travellers* require a full course of 3 doses at monthly intervals (**important:** adults and children *over 10 years* requiring either a primary course or a booster should be given **adsorbed diphtheria [low-dose] and tetanus vaccine for adults and adolescents**).

See section 14.1 for general contra-indications.

Diphtheria vaccines for children

IMPORTANT. **Not** recommended for persons *aged 10 years or over* (use diphtheria vaccines for adults and adolescents instead)

■ With tetanus and pertussis (whole-cell)

Adsorbed Diphtheria, Tetanus, and [whole-cell] Pertussis Vaccine PoM

DTPer/Vac/Ads, [DTwP]

Injection, suspension of diphtheria formol toxoid, tetanus formol toxoid, and pertussis vaccine adsorbed on a mineral carrier

Dose: primary immunisation of children, *by intramuscular or deep subcutaneous injection*, 0.5 mL at 2 months followed by second dose after 4 weeks and third dose after another 4 weeks (see schedule, section 14.1)

Available from health authorities or direct from Farillon as Aventis Pasteur brand (excipients include thiomersal)

NOTE. Adsorbed diphtheria, tetanus and pertussis vaccine is available in combination with Haemophilus influenzae type b vaccine, see under Haemophilus Influenzae type b Vaccine

■ With tetanus and pertussis (acellular)

Infanrix® (GSK) ▼ PoM

Injection, suspension of diphtheria toxoid, tetanus toxoid, and acellular pertussis vaccine components adsorbed on a mineral carrier, net price 0.5-mL prefilled syringe = £11.00

Dose: primary immunisation of children, *by deep intramuscular injection* 0.5 mL at 2 months followed by a

second dose after 4 weeks and third dose after another 4 weeks (see schedule, section 14.1); booster dose for CHILD under 7 years previously immunised with 3 doses of diphtheria, tetanus, and pertussis (whole cell or acellular) vaccine, *by deep intramuscular injection*, 0.5 mL (see schedule, section 14.1)
Available as part of childhood immunisation schedule, from health authorities or Farillon

■ With tetanus
Adsorbed Diphtheria and Tetanus Vaccine PoM
DT/Vac/Ads(Child)
Injection, suspension of diphtheria formol toxoid and tetanus formol toxoid adsorbed on a mineral carrier
Dose: primary immunisation of children omitting pertussis component, *by intramuscular or deep subcutaneous injection*, 0.5 mL at 2 months followed by second dose after 4 weeks and third dose after another 4 weeks (see schedule, section 14.1); booster at school entry (if pertussis not appropriate), 0.5 mL
Available from health authorities or direct from Farillon as Chiron Vaccines Evans brand (excipients include thiomersal) or Aventis Pasteur brand (excipients include thiomersal)

Diphtheria vaccines for adolescents and adults

A low dose of diphtheria toxoid is sufficient to recall immunity in individuals previously immunised against diphtheria but whose immunity may have diminished with time; it is insufficient to cause serious reactions that may occur when a higher-dose vaccine is used in an individual who is already immune. Preparations containing low dose diphtheria must be used when immunising adults and children *over 10 years*.

■ With tetanus
Adsorbed Diphtheria [low dose] and Tetanus Vaccine for Adults and Adolescents PoM
DT/Vac/Ads(Adult)
Injection, suspension of diphtheria formol toxoid and tetanus formol toxoid adsorbed on a mineral carrier, net price 0.5-mL prefilled syringe = £2.67
Dose: primary immunisation in *patients over 10 years, by intramuscular or deep subcutaneous injection*, 3 doses each of 0.5 mL separated by intervals of 4 weeks; booster, 0.5 mL at least 10 years
Available from health authorities or direct from Farillon as Aventis Pasteur brand (*Diftavax*®; excipients include thiomersal)

■ Single antigen
No longer available in the UK. The Department of Health advises that Adsorbed Diphtheria [low dose] and Tetanus Vaccine for Adults and Adolescents be used as a replacement for all routine uses (see above).

Diphtheria antitoxin

Diphtheria antitoxin is used for passive immunisation; it is derived from horse serum, therefore reactions are common after administration.
It is now only used in suspected cases of diphtheria (without waiting for bacteriological confirmation); tests for hypersensitivity should be first carried out.
It is no longer used for prophylaxis because of the risk of hypersensitivity; unimmunised contacts should be promptly investigated and given antibacterial prophylaxis (section 5.1, table 2) and vaccine (see notes above).

Diphtheria Antitoxin PoM
Dip/Ser
Dose: prophylaxis *by intramuscular injection*, 500–2000 units (but **not** used, see notes above)
Treatment, nasal diphtheria, *by intramuscular injection*, 10 000–20 000 units; tonsillar diphtheria, *by intramuscular or intravenous injection*, 15 000–25 000 units; pharyngeal or laryngeal diphtheria, *by intramuscular or intravenous injection*, 20 000–40 000 units; combined types or delayed diagnosis, *by intravenous injection*, 40 000–60 000 units; severe diphtheria, *by intravenous injection* (or part intravenous and part intramuscular injection), 40 000–100 000 units; CHILD under 10 years half adult dose
Available from Communicable Disease Surveillance Centre (Tel (020) 8200 6868) or in Northern Ireland from Public Health Laboratory, Belfast City Hospital (Tel (028) 9032 9241).

Haemophilus influenzae type B vaccine

Children under the age of 13 months are at high risk of *Haemophilus influenzae* type b infection. **Haemophilus influenzae type b (Hib) vaccine** is a component of the primary course of childhood immunisation (see schedule, section 14.1). The course consists of 3 doses of haemophilus influenzae type b vaccine with an interval of 1 month between each dose. If primary immunisation against diphtheria, tetanus, pertussis and poliomyelitis has already been commenced or completed, children under the age of 13 months should still receive 3 doses of haemophilus influenzae type b vaccine at monthly intervals. Children over the age of 13 months are at a lower risk of infection and, if not previously immunised, need receive only 1 dose of the vaccine. The risk of infection falls sharply after the age of 4 years therefore the vaccine is not normally required for children over 4 years. However, it may be given to those over 4 years who are considered to be at increased risk of invasive *Haemophilus influenzae* type b disease (such as those with sickle cell disease and those receiving treatment for malignancy). Also, asplenic children and adults, irrespective of age or the interval from splenectomy, should receive a single dose of haemophilus influenzae type b vaccine; those under 1 year should be given 3 doses. For elective splenectomy, the vaccine should ideally be given at least 2 weeks before the operation. Side-effects reported include fever, headache, malaise, irritability, prolonged crying, loss of appetite, vomiting, diarrhoea, and rash (including urticaria); convulsions, erythema multiforme, and transient cyanosis of the lower limbs have been reported.
See section 14.1 for general contra-indications

■ Single component
Each single component product may be used to complete a course started with any other single component product listed below
ACT-HIB® (Aventis Pasteur) PoM
Injection, powder for reconstitution, capsular polysaccharide of *Haemophilus influenzae* type b (conjugated to tetanus protein), net price per vial with diluent (0.5 mL) = £8.83
Dose: *by intramuscular or deep subcutaneous injection*, 0.5 mL; for primary immunisation, 3 doses are required at intervals of 1 month (see schedule, section 14.1)
NOTE. If required, haemophilus influenzae type b vaccine is available in combination with adsorbed diphtheria, tetanus and pertussis vaccine (see below); alternatively,

ACT-HIB® may be reconstituted with 0.5 mL of Aventis Pasteur brand of adsorbed diphtheria, tetanus and pertussis vaccine

Available, as part of childhood immunisation schedule, from health authorities or Farillon

Hiberix® (GSK) ▼ PoM

Injection, powder for reconstitution, capsular polysaccharide of *Haemophilus influenzae* type b (conjugated to tetanus protein), net price single-dose vial = £9.19

> Dose: *by intramuscular injection*, 0.5 mL; for primary immunisation, 3 doses are required at intervals of 1 month (see schedule, section 14.1)
>
> NOTE. Haemophilus influenzae type b vaccine is available in combination with adsorbed diphtheria, tetanus and acellular pertussis vaccine (see below); if separate vaccines used, haemophilus influenzae vaccine type b vaccine should be injected at the same time but in a **separate limb** to the adsorbed diphtheria, tetanus and acellular pertussis vaccine

Available, as part of childhood immunisation schedule, from health authorities or Farillon

■ **With diphtheria, tetanus and pertussis vaccines**
Each combined product may be used to complete a course started with any other combined product listed here; **important** see also under Adsorbed Diphtheria, Tetanus and Pertussis Vaccine (p. 582)

ACT-HIB®DTP (Aventis Pasteur) PoM

Injection, powder for reconstitution, capsular polysaccharide of *Haemophilus influenzae* type b (conjugated to tetanus protein) with diluent containing diphtheria toxoid, tetanus toxoid and *Bordetella pertussis* cells, net price = £10.41

> Excipients: include thiomersal
>
> Dose: CHILD under 4 years, *by intramuscular or deep subcutaneous injection*, 0.5 mL; for primary immunisation, 3 doses are required at intervals of 1 month (see schedule, section 14.1)

Available, as part of childhood immunisation schedule, from health authorities or Farillon

Infanrix®-Hib (GSK) ▼ PoM

Injection, powder for reconstitution, capsular polysaccharide of *Haemophilus influenzae* type b (conjugated to tetanus protein) with diluent containing diphtheria toxoid, tetanus toxoid, and acellular pertussis vaccine adsorbed on a mineral carrier, net price 0.5-mL vial = £19.00.

> Dose: primary immunisation of children, 0.5 mL *by deep intramuscular injection* at 2 months followed by a second dose after 4 weeks and third dose after another 4 weeks (see schedule, section 14.1)

Hepatitis A vaccine

Hepatitis A vaccine is prepared from formaldehyde-inactivated hepatitis A virus grown in human diploid cells.

Immunisation is recommended for:

- laboratory staff who work directly with the virus;
- patients with haemophilia treated with Factor VIII or Factor IX concentrates or who have liver disease or who have been infected with hepatitis B or hepatitis C;
- travellers to high-risk areas (see p. 598);
- individuals who are at risk due to their sexual behaviour.

Immunisation should be considered for :

- patients with chronic liver disease;
- staff and residents of homes for those with severe learning difficulties;
- workers at risk of exposure to untreated sewage;
- prevention of secondary cases in close contacts of confirmed cases of hepatitis A, within 7 days of onset of disease in the primary case;
- parenteral drug abusers.

Patients with haemophilia and those with chronic liver disease should be checked for previous exposure before immunisation.

Side-effects of hepatitis A vaccine, usually mild, include transient soreness, erythema, and induration at the injection site. Less common effects include fever, malaise, fatigue, headache, nausea, diarrhoea, and loss of appetite; arthralgia, myalgia, and, generalised rashes are occasionally reported.

See section 14.1 for general contra-indications.

■ Single component

Avaxim® (Aventis Pasteur) PoM

Injection, suspension of formaldehyde-inactivated hepatitis A virus (GBM grown in human diploid cells) 320 antigen units/mL adsorbed onto aluminium hydroxide, net price 0.5-mL prefilled syringe = £20.63

> Dose: *by intramuscular injection* (see note below), 0.5 mL as a single dose; booster dose 0.5 mL 6–12 months after initial dose; further booster doses, 0.5 mL every 10 years; CHILD under 16 years, not recommended
>
> NOTE. The deltoid region is the preferred site of injection. The subcutaneous route may be used for patients with haemophilia

Epaxal® (MASTA) PoM

Injection, suspension of formaldehyde-inactivated hepatitis A virus (RG-SB grown in human diploid cells) at least 500 RIA units/mL, net price 0.5-mL prefilled syringe = £23.81

> Dose: *by intramuscular injection* (see note below), ADULT over 2 years, 0.5 mL as a single dose; booster dose 0.5 mL 6–12 months after initial dose (1–6 months if splenectomised)
>
> NOTE. The deltoid region is the preferred site of injection. The subcutaneous route may be used for patients with bleeding disorders
>
> IMPORTANT. *Epaxal®* contains influenza virus haem-agglutinin grown in the allantoic cavity of chick embryos, therefore contra-indicated in those hypersensitive to eggs or chicken protein.

Havrix Monodose® (GSK) PoM

Injection, suspension of formaldehyde-inactivated hepatitis A virus (HM 175 grown in human diploid cells) 1440 ELISA units/mL adsorbed onto aluminium hydroxide, net price 1-mL prefilled syringe = £23.81, 0.5-mL (720 ELISA units) prefilled syringe (*Havrix Junior Monodose®*) = £18.03

> Dose: *by intramuscular injection* (see note below), 1 mL as a single dose; booster dose, 1 mL 6–12 months after initial dose; CHILD 1–15 years 0.5 mL; booster dose, 0.5 mL 6–12 months after initial dose
>
> NOTE. Booster dose may be delayed by up to 3 years if not given after recommended interval following primary dose with *Havrix Monodose®*. The deltoid region is the preferred site of injection in adults. The subcutaneous route may be used for patients with haemophilia

Vaqta® Paediatric (Aventis Pasteur) PoM

Injection, suspension of formaldehyde-inactivated hepatitis A virus (grown in human diploid cells)

50 antigen units/mL adsorbed onto aluminium hydroxide, net price 0.5-mL vial = £15.65

Dose: by intramuscular injection (see note below) CHILD and ADOLESCENT 2–17 years, 0.5 mL as a single dose; booster dose 0.5 mL 6–18 months after initial dose; under 2 years, not recommended

NOTE. The deltoid region is the preferred site of injection

■ With hepatitis B vaccine

Twinrix® (GSK) PoM

Injection, inactivated hepatitis A virus 720 ELISA units and recombinant (DNA) hepatitis B surface antigen 20 micrograms/mL adsorbed onto aluminium hydroxide and aluminium phosphate, net price 1-mL prefilled syringe (*Twinrix® Adult*) = £29.85, 0.5-mL prefilled syringe (*Twinrix® Paediatric*) = £22.36

Dose: by intramuscular injection into deltoid muscle (see note below); primary course of 3 doses of 1 mL, the second 1 month and the third 6 months after the first dose; CHILD 1–15 years *by intramuscular injection*, 3 doses of 0.5 mL

Accelerated schedule (e.g. for travellers departing within 1 month), ADULT, second dose 7 days after first dose, third dose after further 14 days and a fourth dose after 12 months

NOTE. Primary course should be completed with *Twinrix®* (single component vaccines given at appropriate intervals may be used for booster dose); not to be injected into the buttock (vaccine efficacy reduced); subcutaneous route used for patients with haemophilia (but immune response may be reduced).

IMPORTANT. *Twinrix®* **not** recommended for post-exposure prophylaxis following percutaneous (needle-stick), ocular or mucous membrane exposure to hepatitis B virus.

■ With typhoid vaccine

Hepatyrix® (GSK) PoM

Injection, suspension of inactivated hepatitis A virus (grown in human diploid cells) 1440 ELISA units/mL adsorbed onto aluminium hydroxide, combined with typhoid vaccine containing 25 micrograms/mL virulence polysaccharide antigen of *Salmonella typhi*, net price 1-mL prefilled syringe = £34.49

Dose: by intramuscular injection (see note below), ADULT and ADOLESCENT over 15 years, 1 mL as a single dose; booster doses, see under single component hepatitis A vaccine and under polysaccharide typhoid vaccine

NOTE. The deltoid region is the preferred site of injection. The subcutaneous route may be used for patients with thrombocytopenia or haemophilia

ViATIM® (Aventis Pasteur) ▼ PoM

Injection, suspension of inactivated hepatitis A virus (grown in human diploid cells) 160 antigen units/mL adsorbed onto aluminium hydroxide, combined with typhoid vaccine containing 25 micrograms/mL virulence polysaccharide antigen of *Salmonella typhi*, net price 1-mL prefilled syringe = £32.49

Dose: by intramuscular injection (see note below), ADULT and ADOLESCENT over 16 years, 1 mL as a single dose; booster doses, see under single component hepatitis A vaccine and under polysaccharide typhoid vaccine

NOTE. The deltoid region is the preferred site of injection. The subcutaneous route may be used for patients with thrombocytopenia or haemophilia

Hepatitis B vaccine

Hepatitis B vaccine contains inactivated hepatitis B virus surface antigen (HBsAg) adsorbed on alumin-

ium hydroxide adjuvant. It is made biosynthetically using recombinant DNA technology. The vaccine is used in individuals at high risk of contracting hepatitis B.

In the UK, high-risk groups include:

- parenteral drug abusers;
- individuals who change sexual partners frequently;
- close family contacts of a case or carrier;
- infants born to mothers who *either* have had hepatitis B during pregnancy, *or* are positive for both hepatitis B surface antigen and hepatitis B e-antigen *or* are surface antigen positive without e markers (or where they have not been determined); active immunisation of the infant is started immediately after delivery and *hepatitis B immunoglobulin* (see p. 596) is given at the same time as the vaccine (but preferably at a different site). Infants born to mothers who are positive for hepatitis B surface antigen and for e-antigen antibody should receive the vaccine but not the immunoglobulin;
- haemophiliacs, those receiving regular blood transfusions or blood products, and carers responsible for the administration of such products;
- patients with chronic renal failure including those on haemodialysis. Haemodialysis patients should be monitored for antibodies annually and re-immunised if necessary. Home carers (of dialysis patients) who are negative for hepatitis B surface antigen should be vaccinated;
- healthcare personnel (including trainees) who have direct contact with blood or blood-stained body fluids or with patients' tissues;
- other occupational risk groups such as morticians and embalmers;
- staff and patients of day-care or residential accommodation for those with severe learning difficulties;
- inmates of custodial institutions;
- those travelling to areas of high prevalence who are at increased risk or who plan to remain there for lengthy periods (see p. 598);
- families adopting children from countries with a high prevalence of hepatitis B.

Immunisation takes up to 6 months to confer adequate protection; the duration of immunity is not known precisely, but a single booster 5 years after the primary course may be sufficient to maintain immunity for those who continue to be at risk.

More detailed guidance is given in the memorandum *Immunisation against Infectious Disease*. Immunisation does not eliminate the need for commonsense precautions for avoiding the risk of infection from known carriers by the routes of infection which have been clearly established, consult *Guidance for Clinical Health Care Workers: Protection against Infection with Blood-borne Viruses* and *Protecting Health Care Workers and Patients from Hepatitis B*. Accidental inoculation of hepatitis B virus-infected blood into a wound, incision, needle-prick, or abrasion may lead to infection, whereas it is unlikely that indirect exposure to a carrier will do so.

Specific **hepatitis B immunoglobulin** ('HBIG') is available for use with the vaccine in those accidentally infected and in infants (section 14.5).

A combined hepatitis A and hepatitis B vaccine is also available.

See section 14.1 for general contra-indications.

■ Single component

Engerix B® (GSK) PoM

Injection, suspension of hepatitis B surface antigen (rby, prepared from yeast cells by recombinant

DNA technique) 20 micrograms/mL adsorbed onto aluminium hydroxide, net price 0.5-mL (paediatric) vial = £9.85, 0.5-mL (paediatric) prefilled syringe = £10.40, 1-mL vial = £13.27, 1-mL prefilled syringe = £13.97

Dose: by intramuscular injection (see note below), 3 doses of 1 mL (20 micrograms), the second 1 month and the third 6 months after the first dose; CHILD birth to 15 years 3 doses of 0.5 mL (10 micrograms); if compliance likely to be low in CHILD 10–15 years increase dose to 1 mL (20 micrograms)

Accelerated schedule, third dose 2 months after first dose and a fourth dose at 12 months; exceptionally (e.g. for travellers departing within 1 month), ADULT, second dose 7 days after first dose, third dose after a further 14 days and a fourth dose after 12 months

INFANT born to hepatitis B surface antigen-positive mothers (see also notes above), 4 doses of 0.5 mL (10 micrograms), first dose at birth with hepatitis B immunoglobulin injection (separate site) the second 1 month, the third 2 months and the fourth 12 months after the first dose

Chronic haemodialysis patients, *by intramuscular injection* (see note below) 4 doses of 2 mL (40 micrograms), the second 1 month, the third 2 months and the fourth 6 months after the first dose; adjustment of immunisation schedule and booster doses may be required in those with low antibody concentration

NOTE. Deltoid muscle is preferred site of injection in adults and older children; anterolateral thigh is preferred site in neonates, infants and young children; not to be injected into the buttock (vaccine efficacy reduced); subcutaneous route used for patients with thrombocytopenia or bleeding disorders

HBvaxPRO® (Aventis Pasteur) PoM

Injection, suspension of hepatitis B surface antigen (prepared from yeast cells by recombinant DNA technique) 10 micrograms/mL adsorbed onto aluminium hydroxyphosphate sulphate, net price 0.5-mL (5-microgram) vial = £9.70, 1-mL (10-microgram) vial = £12.90; 40 micrograms/mL, 1-mL (40-microgram) vial = £31.50

Dose: by intramuscular injection (see note below), ADULT and ADOLESCENT over 16 years, 3 doses of 10 micrograms, the second 1 month and the third 6 months after the first dose; CHILD under 16 years, 3 doses of 5 micrograms

Accelerated schedule, third dose 2 months after first dose with fourth dose at 12 months

Booster doses may be required in immunocompromised patients with low antibody concentration

INFANT born to hepatitis B surface antigen-positive mothers (see also notes above), 0.5 mL (5 micrograms), first dose at birth with hepatitis B immunoglobulin injection (separate site), subsequent doses according to local policy

Chronic haemodialysis patients, *by intramuscular injection* (see note below) 3 doses of 40 micrograms, the second 1 month and the third 6 months after the first dose; booster doses may be required in those with low antibody concentration

NOTE. Deltoid muscle is preferred site of injection in adults and older children; anterolateral thigh is preferred site in infants; not to be injected into the buttock (vaccine efficacy reduced); subcutaneous route used for patients with bleeding disorders

■ With hepatitis A vaccine
See Hepatitis A Vaccine

Influenza vaccines

While most viruses are antigenically stable, the influenza viruses A and B (especially A) are constantly altering their antigenic structure as indicated by changes in the haemagglutinins (H) and neuraminidases (N) on the surface of the viruses. It is essential that influenza vaccines in use contain the H and N components of the prevalent strain or strains. Every year the World Health Organization recommends which strains should be included.

The recommended strains are grown in the allantoic cavity of chick embryos (therefore **contra-indicated** in those hypersensitive to eggs).

Since **influenza vaccines** will not control epidemics they are recommended *only for persons at high risk*. Annual immunisation is strongly recommended for individuals aged over 6 months with the following conditions:

- chronic respiratory disease, including asthma;
- chronic heart disease;
- chronic renal disease;
- diabetes mellitus;
- immunosuppression owing to disease or treatment, including asplenia or splenic dysfunction.

Influenza immunisation is also recommended for all persons aged over 65 years and for residents of nursing homes, residential homes for the elderly, and other long-stay facilities.

As part of the winter planning, NHS employers should offer vaccination to healthcare workers directly involved in patient care. Employers of social care workers should consider similar action.

Interactions: Appendix 1 (vaccines).
See section 14.1 for general contra-indications.

Inactivated Influenza Vaccine (Split Virion)
(Aventis Pasteur) PoM

Injection, suspension of formaldehyde-inactivated influenza virus (split virion) Flu/Vac/Split, net price 0.5-mL prefilled syringe = £6.29

Dose: by deep subcutaneous or by intramuscular injection, 0.5 mL as a single dose; CHILD 6–35 months 0.25–0.5 mL, 3–12 years 0.5 mL, in children dose repeated after at least 4 weeks if not previously vaccinated

Inactivated Influenza Vaccine (Surface Antigen)
(Chiron Vaccines Evans) PoM

Injection, suspension of propiolactone-inactivated influenza virus (surface antigen) Flu/Vac/SA, net price 0.5-mL prefilled syringe = £3.98

Excipients: include thiomersal

Dose: by deep subcutaneous or by intramuscular injection, 0.5 mL as a single dose; CHILD 6–35 months 0.25–0.5 mL, 3–12 years 0.5 mL, in children dose repeated after at least 4 weeks if not previously vaccinated

Agrippal® (Wyeth) PoM

Injection, suspension of formaldehyde-inactivated influenza virus (surface antigen) Flu/Vac/SA, net price 0.5-mL prefilled syringe = £6.29

Dose: by deep subcutaneous or by intramuscular injection, 0.5 mL as a single dose; CHILD 6–35 months 0.25–0.5 mL, 3–12 years 0.5 mL, in children dose repeated after at least 4 weeks if not previously vaccinated

Begrivac® (Wyeth) PoM

Injection, suspension of formaldehyde-inactivated influenza virus (split virion) Flu/Vac/Split, net price 0.5-mL prefilled syringe = £6.29

Dose: by deep subcutaneous or by intramuscular injection, 0.5 mL as a single dose; CHILD 6–35 months 0.25–0.5 mL, 3–12 years 0.5 mL, in children dose repeated after at least 4 weeks if not previously vaccinated

Fluarix® (GSK) [PoM]

Injection, suspension of formaldehyde-inactivated influenza virus (split virion) Flu/Vac/Split, net price 0.5-mL prefilled syringe = £4.39

Dose: by deep subcutaneous or by intramuscular injection, 0.5 mL as a single dose; CHILD 6–35 months 0.25–0.5 mL, 3–12 years 0.5 mL, in children dose repeated after at least 4 weeks if not previously vaccinated

Fluvirin® (Chiron Vaccines Evans) [PoM]

Injection, suspension of propiolactone-inactivated influenza virus (surface antigen) Flu/Vac/SA, net price 0.5-mL prefilled syringe = £5.97

Excipients: include thiomersal

Dose: by deep subcutaneous or by intramuscular injection, 0.5 mL as a single dose; CHILD 6–35 months 0.25–0.5 mL, 3–12 years 0.5 mL, in children dose repeated after at least 4 weeks if not previously vaccinated

Inflexal® V (Aventis Pasteur) [PoM]

Injection, suspension of inactivated influenza virus (surface antigen) Flu/Vac/SA, net price 0.5-mL prefilled syringe = £6.59

Dose: by deep subcutaneous or by intramuscular injection, 0.5 mL as a single dose; CHILD 6–35 months 0.25–0.5 mL, 3–12 years 0.5 mL, in children dose repeated after at least 4 weeks if not previously vaccinated

Influvac Sub-unit® (Solvay) [PoM]

Injection, suspension of formaldehyde-inactivated influenza virus (surface antigen) Flu/Vac/SA, net price 0.5-mL prefilled syringe = £5.49

Excipients: include thiomersal

Dose: by deep subcutaneous or by intramuscular injection, 0.5 mL as a single dose; CHILD 6–35 months 0.25–0.5 mL, 3–12 years 0.5 mL, in children dose repeated after at least 4 weeks if not previously vaccinated

Mastaflu® (MASTA) [PoM]

Injection, suspension of formaldehyde-inactivated influenza virus (surface antigen) Flu/Vac/SA, net price 0.5-mL prefilled syringe = £6.59

Excipients: include thiomersal

Dose: by deep subcutaneous or by intramuscular injection, 0.5 mL as a single dose; CHILD 6–35 months 0.25–0.5 mL, 3–12 years 0.5 mL, in children dose repeated after at least 4 weeks if not previously vaccinated

Measles vaccine

Measles vaccine has been replaced by a combined live measles, mumps and rubella vaccine (MMR vaccine) for all eligible children.

Administration of a measles-containing vaccine to children may be associated with a mild measles-like syndrome with a measles-like rash and pyrexia about a week after injection. Much less commonly, convulsions and, very rarely, encephalitis have been reported. Convulsions in infants are much less frequently associated with measles vaccines than with other conditions leading to febrile episodes.

MMR vaccine may be used in the control of outbreaks of measles (see under MMR Vaccine).

■ Single antigen vaccine
No longer available in the UK

■ Combined vaccines
See MMR vaccine

Measles, Mumps and Rubella (MMR) vaccine

A combined live **measles, mumps, and rubella vaccine** (MMR vaccine) aims to eliminate rubella (and congenital rubella syndrome), measles, and mumps. Every child should receive two doses of MMR vaccine by entry to primary school, unless there is a valid contra-indication (see below) or parental refusal. MMR vaccine should be given irrespective of previous measles, mumps or rubella infection.

The first dose of MMR vaccine is given to children aged 12–15 months. A second (booster) dose is given before starting school at 3–5 years of age (see schedule, section 14.1). Children presenting for pre-school booster who have not received the first dose of MMR vaccine should be given a dose of MMR vaccine followed 3 months later by a second dose. At school-leaving age or at entry into further education, MMR immunisation should be offered to individuals of both sexes who have not received it.

MMR vaccine should be used to protect against rubella in *seronegative women of child-bearing age* (see schedule, section 14.1), and unimmunised healthcare workers who might put pregnant women at risk of rubella. MMR vaccine may also be offered to previously *unimmunised and seronegative post-partum women*. Immunisation in susceptible post-partum women a few days after delivery is important because about 60% of congenital abnormalities from rubella infection occur in babies of women who have borne more than one child. Immigrants arriving after the age of school immunisation are particularly likely to require immunisation.

MMR vaccine may also be used in the control of outbreaks of measles and should be offered to susceptible children (including babies from 5 months of age) within 3 days of exposure to infection; these children should still receive routine MMR vaccinations. MMR vaccine is **not suitable** for prophylaxis following exposure to mumps or rubella since the antibody response to the mumps and rubella components is too slow for effective prophylaxis.

Children with partially or totally impaired immune response should not receive live vaccines (for advice on HIV see section 14.1). If they have been exposed to measles infection they should be given normal immunoglobulin (section 14.5).

Malaise, fever or a rash may occur following the first dose of MMR vaccine, most commonly about a week after vaccination and lasting about 2 to 3 days (section 14.1). Leaflets are available for parents on advice for reducing fever (including the use of paracetamol). Parotid swelling occasionally occurs, usually in the third week. Adverse reactions are considerably less common after the second dose of MMR vaccine than after the first dose.

Idiopathic thrombocytopenic purpura has occurred rarely following MMR vaccination, usually within 6 weeks of the first dose. The risk of developing idiopathic thrombocytopenic purpura after MMR vaccine is much less than the risk of developing it after infection with wild measles, mumps or rubella virus. The CSM has recommended that children who develop idiopathic thrombocytopenic purpura within 6 weeks of the first dose of MMR should undergo serological testing before the second dose is due; if the results suggest incomplete immunity against measles, mumps or rubella then a second dose of MMR is recommended. The Central Public Health Laboratory, Colindale offers free serological testing for children developing idiopathic thrombocytopenic purpura *within 6 weeks* of the first dose of MMR.

Post-vaccination meningoencephalitis was reported (rarely and with complete recovery) following vaccination with MMR vaccine containing Urabe mumps vaccine, which has now been discontinued; no cases have been confirmed in association with the currently used Jeryl Lynn mumps vaccine. Children with post-vaccination symptoms are not infectious.

> Reviews undertaken on behalf of the CSM and the Medical Research Council have not found any evidence of a link between MMR vaccination and bowel disease or autism. The Chief Medical Officers have advised that the MMR vaccine is the safest and best way to protect children against measles, mumps, and rubella. Information (including fact sheets and a list of references) may be obtained from www.immunisation.nhs.uk and www.mmrthefacts.nhs.uk

Contra-indications to MMR include:

- children with untreated malignant disease or altered immunity (for advice on vaccines and HIV see section 14.1), and those receiving immunosuppressive drugs or radiotherapy, or high-dose corticosteroids;
- children who have received another live vaccine by injection within 3 weeks;
- children with allergies to gelatin or neomycin;
- children with acute febrile illness (vaccination should be deferred);
- if given to women, pregnancy should be avoided for 1 month;
- should not be given within 3 months of an immunoglobulin injection.

The Department of Health recommends avoiding rubella vaccination during pregnancy. However, if given inadvertently during pregnancy, then termination is not recommended because extensive studies have failed to link rubella vaccination in early pregnancy with fetal damage.
NOTE. Children with a personal or close family history of convulsions should be given MMR vaccine, provided the parents understand that there may be a febrile response; doctors should seek specialist paediatric advice rather than withhold vaccination; there is increasing evidence that MMR vaccine can be given safely even when the child has had an anaphylactic reaction to food containing egg (dislike of egg or refusal to eat egg is not a contra-indication).

MMR Vaccine PoM

Live measles, mumps, and rubella vaccine
Dose: by deep subcutaneous or by intramuscular injection, 0.5 mL (see schedule, section 14.1)
Available from health authorities or direct from Farillon as *MMR II®* (Aventis Pasteur) or *Priorix®* (GSK)
NOTE. *MMR II®* is licensed for use in adults and should therefore be used for immunising seronegative women and unimmunised healthcare workers

Meningococcal vaccines

Almost all childhood meningococcal disease in the UK is caused by *Neisseria meningitidis* serogroups B and C. **Meningococcal Group C conjugate vaccine** protects only against infection by serogroup

C; it can be given from 2 months of age. After early adult life the risk of meningococcal disease declines, and immunisation is not generally recommended after the age of 25 years.

CHILDHOOD IMMUNISATION. **Meningococcal Group C conjugate vaccine** provides long-term protection against infection by serogroup C of *Neisseria meningitidis* in children from 2 months of age; it is now a component of the primary course of childhood immunisation. The recommended schedule consists of 3 doses starting at 2 months of age with an interval of 1 month between each dose (see schedule, section 14.1). Infants aged 5–12 months not previously vaccinated should receive 2 doses, with an interval of 1 month between doses. It is recommended that meningococcal group C conjugate vaccine be given to anyone aged up to 24 years who has not been vaccinated previously with this vaccine; those over 1 year receive a single dose.

Meningococcal group C conjugate vaccine is also recommended for individuals with a dysfunctional or absent spleen.

IMMUNISATION FOR TRAVELLERS. Individuals travelling to countries of risk (see below) should be immunised with a meningococcal polysaccharide vaccine that covers serotypes **A, C, W135 and Y**. The tetravalent vaccine is already required for those travelling to Saudi Arabia during the Hajj and Umrah pilgrimages (due to outbreaks of the W135 strain). Outbreaks of infection with the W135 strain of meningococcus have occured in Burkina Faso, West Africa and there have been cases in a number of other African countries. Meningococcal vaccine is no longer recommended for travellers to areas outside Africa and Saudi Arabia (during the pilgrimages) unless outbreaks occur.

Vaccination with the tetravalent (A, C, W135 and Y) vaccine should be considered particularly for those living or working with local people or visiting an area of risk during outbreaks. Countries with risk in Africa are listed below but outbreaks may also occur in countries not listed:

> Angola, Benin, Burkina Faso, Burundi, Cameroon, Central African Republic, Chad, Democratic Republic of Congo, Eritrea, Ethiopia, Gambia, Ghana, Guinea, Guinea Bissau, Ivory Coast, Kenya, Mali, Mozambique, Namibia, Niger, Nigeria, Rwanda, Senegal, Sierra Leone, Somalia, Sudan, Tanzania, Togo, Uganda, and Zambia

Proof of vaccination with the tetravalent vaccine is required for visitors arriving in Saudi Arabia for the Hajj and Umrah pilgrimages.

Travellers should be immunised with the meningococcal polysaccharide vaccine that covers serogroups A, C, W135 and Y, even if they have already received meningococcal group C conjugate vaccine. The response to serotype C in unconjugated meningococcal polysaccharide vaccines given to children aged under 18 months is not as good as in adults.

CONTACTS OF INFECTED INDIVIDUALS AND LABORATORY WORKERS. For advice on the immunisation of *close contacts* of cases of meningococcal disease in the UK and on the role of the vaccine in the control of *local outbreaks*, consult Guidelines for Public Health Management of

Meningococcal Disease in the UK in *Commun Dis Public Health* 2002; **5**: 187–204. See section 5.1 Table 2 for antibacterial prophylaxis to prevent a secondary case of meningococcal meningitis

The need for immunisation of laboratory staff who work directly with *Neisseria meningitidis* should be considered.

SIDE-EFFECTS. Side-effects of meningococcal Group C conjugate vaccine include redness, swelling, and pain at the site of the injection, mild fever, irritability, drowsiness, dizziness, nausea, vomiting, diarrhoea, headache, myalgia, rash, urticaria, pruritus, malaise, lymphadenopathy, hypotonia, paraesthesia, hypoaesthesia, and syncope. Hypersensitivity reactions (including anaphylaxis, bronchospasm, and angioedema) and seizures have been reported rarely. Symptoms of meningism have also been reported rarely, but there is no evidence that the vaccine causes meningococcal C meningitis. There have been very rare reports of Stevens-Johnson syndrome. The CSM has advised that vaccination provides benefit in terms of lives saved and disabilities prevented.

Meningococcal polysaccharide A&C and A, C, W135 and Y vaccines are associated with injection-site reactions and very rarely headache, fatigue, fever, and drowsiness. Hypersensitivity reactions including anaphylaxis have been reported.

See section 14.1 for general contra-indications.

■ Meningococcal Group C conjugate vaccine

Meningitec® (Wyeth) PoM
Injection, suspension of capsular polysaccharide antigen of *Neisseria meningitidis* group C (conjugated to *Corynebacterium diphtheriae* protein), adsorbed onto aluminium phosphate, net price 0.5-mL vial = £17.95
Dose: by intramuscular (or deep subcutaneous) injection, ADULT and CHILD over 1 year 0.5 mL as a single dose; for routine immunisation in CHILD under 1 year, 3 doses (each of 0.5 mL) are required at intervals of 1 month (see schedule, section 14.1)
Available as part of childhood immunisation schedule from Farillon
NOTE. Subcutaneous route used for patients with thrombocytopenia or haemophilia

Menjugate® (Chiron) PoM
Injection, powder for reconstitution, capsular polysaccharide antigen of *Neisseria meningitidis* group C (conjugated to *Corynebacterium diphtheriae* protein), adsorbed onto aluminium hydroxide, single-dose and 10-dose vials
Dose: by intramuscular (or deep subcutaneous) injection, ADULT and CHILD over 1 year 0.5 mL as a single dose; for routine immunisation in CHILD under 1 year, 3 doses (each of 0.5 mL) are required at intervals of 1 month (see schedule, section 14.1)
Available from Farillon
NOTE. Subcutaneous route used for patients with thrombocytopenia or haemophilia

NeisVac-C® (Baxter) PoM
Injection, suspension of polysaccharide antigen of *Neisseria meningitidis* group C (conjugated to tetanus toxoid protein), adsorbed onto aluminium hydroxide, 0.5-mL prefilled syringe
Dose: by intramuscular (or deep subcutaneous) injection, ADULT and CHILD over 1 year 0.5 mL as a single dose; for routine immunisation in CHILD under 1 year, 3 doses

(each of 0.5 mL) are required at intervals of 1 month (see schedule, section 14.1)
Available from Farillon
NOTE. Subcutaneous route used for patients with thrombocytopenia or haemophilia
The dose in the BNF may differ from that in product literature

■ Meningococcal polysaccharide A&C vaccine

Mengivac (A+C)® (Aventis Pasteur) PoM
Injection, powder for reconstitution, capsular polysaccharide antigens of *Neisseria meningitidis* (meningococcus) groups A and C, net price single-dose vial (with syringe containing diluent) = £6.39
Dose: by deep subcutaneous injection or by intramuscular injection, ADULT and CHILD over 18 months 0.5 mL
NOTE. Children aged 3–18 months respond less well to the vaccine and for these children it should be used only in epidemics; additionally, protection is of short duration. Children under 3 months respond poorly

■ Meningococcal polysaccharide A, C, W135 and Y vaccine

ACWY Vax® (GSK) PoM
Injection, powder for reconstitution, capsular polysaccharide antigens of *Neisseria meningitidis* groups A, C, W135 and Y, net price single-dose vial (with syringe containing diluent) = £17.99
Dose: by deep subcutaneous injection, ADULT and CHILD over 2 years 0.5 mL
NOTE. May be given to CHILD 2 months–2 years [unlicensed] but antibody response may be suboptimal

Mumps vaccine

■ Single antigen vaccine
No longer available in the UK

■ Combined vaccine
See MMR Vaccine

Pertussis vaccine

Pertussis vaccine is given combined with diphtheria and tetanus vaccine starting at 2 months of age (see schedule section 14.1).

With some vaccines available in the early 1960s *persistent screaming and collapse* were reported but these reactions are rarely observed with the vaccines now available. *Convulsions and encephalopathy* have been reported as rare complications, but such conditions may arise from other causes and be falsely attributed to the vaccine. Neurological complications *after whooping cough itself* are considerably more common than after the vaccine.

As with any other elective immunisation procedure it is advisable to postpone vaccination if the child is suffering from any acute illness, until fully recovered. Minor infections without fever or systemic upset are not reasons to delay immunisation. Immunisation should not be carried out in children who have a history of severe general reaction to a preceding dose; in these children immunisation should be completed with adsorbed diphtheria and tetanus vaccine. Where there has been a severe local reaction or pyrexia, acellular pertussis vaccine may be used. The following reactions should be regarded as severe:

- *Local*—an extensive area of redness and swelling which becomes indurated and involves most of the antero-lateral surface of the thigh or a major part of the circumference of the upper arm.
- *General*—temperature of 39.5°C or more within 48 hours of vaccine, anaphylaxis, bronchospasm, laryngeal oedema, generalised collapse, prolonged unresponsiveness, prolonged inconsolable screaming, and convulsions occurring within 72 hours.

A personal or family history of allergy is **not** a contra-indication to immunisation against whooping cough; nor are stable neurological conditions such as cerebral palsy or spina bifida.

CHILDREN WITH PROBLEM HISTORIES. When there is a personal or family history of *febrile* convulsions, there is an increased risk of these occurring after pertussis immunisation. In such children, immunisation is *recommended* but advice on the *prevention of fever* (see p. 578) should be given at the time of immunisation.

In a British study, children with a family history of epilepsy were immunised with pertussis vaccine without any significant adverse events.These children's developmental progress has been normal. In children with a close family history (first degree relatives) of *idiopathic epilepsy*, there may be a risk of developing a similar condition, irrespective of vaccine. Immunisation is *recommended* for these children.

Where there is a *still evolving neurological problem*, immunisation should be *deferred* until the condition is stable. Children whose epilepsy is well controlled may receive pertussis vaccine. When there has been a documented history of *cerebral damage in the neonatal period*, immunisation should be *carried out unless there is evidence of an evolving neurological abnormality*. If immunisation is to be deferred, this should be stated on the neonatal discharge summary. Where there is doubt, appropriate advice should be sought from a consultant paediatrician, local immunisation co-ordinator or consultant in communicable disease control *rather than withholding vaccine*.

OLDER CHILDREN. There is no contra-indication to administration of pertussis vaccine to unimmunised older children in order to protect the individuals and siblings under the age of immunisation; however, no suitable vaccine is available for children aged over 7 years. Guidance for immunisation against pertussis in the absence of single antigen pertussis vaccine is available at www.immunisation.nhs.uk/pertussisguide.html

■ Combined vaccine
Combined vaccine (*pertussis, tetanus,* and *diphtheria*), see under Diphtheria vaccines

Pneumococcal vaccine

A polyvalent (23-valent) unconjugated **pneumococcal polysaccharide vaccine** is used for the immunisation of persons over the age of 2 years (children under 2 years should receive the 7-valent pneumococcal conjugate vaccine, see below); it is recommended in any of the following circumstances:

- Adults over 75 years
- Homozygous sickle cell disease;
- Asplenia or severe dysfunction of the spleen;
- Chronic renal disease or nephrotic syndrome;
- Coeliac syndrome;
- Immunodeficiency or immunosuppression due to disease or treatment, including HIV infection;
- Chronic heart disease;
- Chronic lung disease;
- Chronic liver disease including cirrhosis;
- Diabetes mellitus;
- Patients with cochlear implants.

Where possible, the vaccine should be given at least 2 weeks before splenectomy, before cochlear implant surgery, and before chemotherapy; patients should be given advice about increased risk of pneumococcal infection (a patient card and information leaflet for patients with asplenia are available from the Department of Health or in Scotland from the Scottish Executive, Public Health Division 1). Prophylactic antibacterial therapy against pneumococcal infection should not be stopped after immunisation. The vaccine is effective in a single dose if the types of pneumonia in the community are reflected in the polysaccharides contained in the vaccine. It should not be given in pregnancy, or when breastfeeding, or when there is infection. Hypersensitivity reactions may occur.

A polyvalent (7-valent) **pneumococcal polysaccharide conjugated vaccine** is used for the prevention of invasive pneumococcal disease in children aged between 2 months and 2 years who are at special risk because of the conditions shown above; the number of doses required for primary immunisation varies according to age. Children aged over 2 years at high risk of pneumococcal disease who have previously received pneumococcal polysaccharide conjugated vaccine should receive the unconjugated polyvalent (23-valent) pneumococcal polysaccharide vaccine (ideally after a 2–month interval).

REVACCINATION. Revaccination with the 23–valent pneumococcal polysaccharide vaccine less than 3 years after the first injection may produce severe reactions in some subjects. Revaccination is therefore not recommended except, every 5 years, in individuals in whom the antibody concentration is likely to decline rapidly (e.g. asplenia, splenic dysfunction and nephrotic syndrome). Antibody concentration may decline more rapidly in children and revaccination after 3 years may be considered for children under 10 years. If there is doubt, the need for revaccination should be discussed with a haematologist, immunologist, or microbiologist, and measurement of antibody concentration considered.

See section 14.1 for general contra-indications.
IMPORTANT. Not for intradermal injection which may cause severe local reactions

■ Pneumococcal polysaccharide vaccines
Pneumovax® II (Aventis Pasteur) PoM
Polysaccharide from each of 23 capsular types of pneumococcus, net price 0.5-mL vial = £9.49
Dose: by subcutaneous or intramuscular injection, 0.5 mL; revaccination, see notes above; CHILD under 2 years, not recommended (suboptimal response and also safety and efficacy not established)

■ Pneumococcal polysaccharide conjugated vaccine

Prevenar® (Wyeth) ▼ [PoM]

Polysaccharide from each of 7 capsular types of pneumococcus (conjugated to diphtheria toxoid) adsorbed onto aluminium phosphate, net price 0.5-mL vial = £39.25

Dose: by intramuscular injection, INFANT 2–6 months 3 doses each of 0.5 mL separated by intervals of 1 month and a further dose in second year of life; 7–11 months 2 doses each of 0.5 mL separated by an interval of 1 month and a further dose in second year of life; CHILD 1–2 years 2 doses each of 0.5 mL separated by an interval of 2 months

NOTE. Deltoid muscle is preferred site of injection in young children; anterolateral thigh is preferred site in infants

Poliomyelitis vaccines

There are two types of poliomyelitis vaccine, poliomyelitis vaccine, live (oral) (Sabin) and poliomyelitis vaccine, inactivated (Salk). The oral vaccine, consisting of a mixture of attenuated strains of virus types 1, 2, and 3 is generally used in the UK.

A course of primary immunisation consists of 3 doses of **live (oral) poliomyelitis vaccine**, starting at 2 months of age with an interval of 1 month between each dose (see schedule, section 14.1). A course of 3 doses should also be given to all unimmunised adults; no adult should remain unimmunised against poliomyelitis.

Two booster doses of live poliomyelitis vaccine (oral), are recommended, the first before school entry and the second before leaving school (see schedule, section 14.1). Booster doses for adults are not necessary except for those at special risk such as travellers to endemic areas, or laboratory staff likely to be exposed to the viruses, or healthcare workers in possible contact with cases; booster doses should be given to such individuals every 10 years.

Vaccine-associated poliomyelitis and poliomyelitis in those coming into contact with vaccinees is rare. In England and Wales there is an annual average of 1 recipient and 1 contact case for over 2 million doses of oral vaccine. The need for strict personal hygiene must be stressed; the contacts of a recently vaccinated baby should be advised of the need to wash their hands thoroughly after changing the baby's nappies. Immunocompromised individuals should avoid close contact with children vaccinated with live (oral) poliomyelitis vaccine for 4–6 weeks.

Contra-indications to the use of oral poliomyelitis vaccine include vomiting and diarrhoea, and immunodeficiency disorders (or household contacts of patients with immunodeficiency disorders). See section 14.1 for further contra-indications.

Poliomyelitis vaccine (inactivated) may be used for those in whom poliomyelitis vaccine (oral) is contra-indicated because of immunosuppressive disorders (for advice on AIDS see section 14.1).

Either live (oral) vaccine or inactivated vaccine may be used to complete a course started with the other, except that live (oral) vaccine must **not** be used for immunosuppressed individuals or their household contacts (see above).

TRAVELLERS. Travellers to areas where poliomyelitis is epidemic or endemic should receive a full course of oral poliomyelitis vaccine if they have not been vaccinated previously. Those who have not been vaccinated in the last 10 years should receive a

booster dose of oral poliomyelitis vaccine. Details of countries in which poliomyelitis is currently epidemic or endemic can be obtained from www.travax.scot.nhs.uk or by contacting the National Travel Health Network and Centre (p. 598)

■ Live (oral) (Sabin)

Poliomyelitis Vaccine, Live (Oral) [PoM]
Pol/Vac (Oral)

¹ A suspension of suitable live attenuated strains of poliomyelitis virus, types 1, 2, and 3. Available in single-dose and 10-dose containers

Dose: 3 drops; for primary immunisation 3 doses are required (see schedule, section 14.1). May be given on a lump of sugar; not to be given with foods which contain preservatives

Available from health authorities or direct from Farillon

NOTE. Poliomyelitis vaccine loses potency once the container has been opened, therefore any vaccine remaining at the end of an immunisation session should be discarded; whenever possible sessions should be arranged to avoid undue wastage.

1. BP permits code OPV for vaccine in single doses provided it also appears on pack.

■ Inactivated (Salk)

Poliomyelitis Vaccine, Inactivated [PoM]
Pol/Vac (Inact)

An inactivated suspension of suitable strains of poliomyelitis virus, types 1, 2, and 3.

Dose: by subcutaneous injection, 0.5 mL or as stated on the label; for primary immunisation 3 doses are required at intervals of 4 weeks

Available direct from Farillon

NOTE. Should be ordered one dose at a time (on a named-patient basis) and only when required for use

Rabies vaccine

The licensed rabies vaccines, both cell-derived, are the human diploid cell vaccine (HDCV) and the purified chick embryo cell (PCEC) vaccine.

PRE-EXPOSURE PROPHYLAXIS. Pre-exposure immunisation should be offered to those at high risk—laboratory staff who handle the rabies virus, those working in quarantine stations, animal handlers, veterinary surgeons and field workers who are likely to be bitten by infected wild animals, certain port officials, and bat handlers. Human transmission of rabies has not been recorded but it is advised that those caring for patients with the disease should be vaccinated as if they have been exposed.

Pre-exposure immunisation is also recommended for those living or travelling, usually for longer than 4 weeks, in areas where rabies is endemic, especially those who will be away from medical facilities or those who may be exposed to unusual risk.

Pre-exposure prophylaxis is indicated during pregnancy if there is substantial risk of exposure to rabies.

Pre-exposure use requires 3 intramuscular doses of rabies vaccine, with further booster doses for those who remain at continued risk (see under preparations below for details of regimens). To ensure protection in persons at high risk (e.g. laboratory workers), the concentration of antirabies antibodies in plasma is used to determine the intervals between doses.

POST-EXPOSURE PROPHYLAXIS. Post-exposure prophylaxis depends on the level of risk in the country, the nature of exposure, and the individual's immune status. Specialist advice must be sought for all bat bites.

There are no specific contra-indications to the use of rabies vaccine for post-exposure prophylaxis and its use should be considered whenever a patient has been attacked by an animal in a country where rabies is endemic, even if there is no direct evidence of rabies in the attacking animal. Because of the potential consequences of untreated rabies exposure and because rabies vaccination has not been associated with fetal abnormalities, pregnancy is not considered a contra-indication to post-exposure prophylaxis.

For post-exposure prophylaxis of *fully immunised* individuals (who have previously received pre-exposure or post-exposure prophylaxis with cell-derived rabies vaccine), 2 intramuscular doses of cell-derived vaccine, separated by 3–7 days, are likely to be sufficient. Rabies immunoglobulin is not necessary in such cases.

Post-exposure treatment for *unimmunised individuals* (or those whose prophylaxis is possibly incomplete) comprises 5 intramuscular doses of rabies vaccine given over 1 month (on days 0, 3, 7, 14, and 28); depending on the level of risk (determined by factors such as the nature and country of bite and the promptness of post-exposure prophylaxis), rabies immunoglobulin is given on day 0 (section 14.5). The course may be discontinued if it is proved that the individual was not at risk.

Advice on up-to-date country-by-country information and on post-exposure immunisation and treatment of rabies is available from the Virus Reference Division, Central Public Health Laboratory, Colindale, London NW9 5HT (Tel (020) 8200 4400) or in Scotland from the Scottish Centre for Infection and Environmental Health through www.travax.scot.nhs.uk

Rabies Vaccine (Aventis Pasteur) PoM
Freeze-dried inactivated Wistar rabies virus strain PM/WI 38 1503-3M cultivated in human diploid cells, net price single-dose vial with syringe containing diluent = £22.15
Dose: prophylactic, *by deep subcutaneous or intramuscular injection* in the deltoid region, 1 mL on days 0, 7, and 28; also booster doses every 2–3 years to those at continued risk
Post-exposure, *by deep subcutaneous or intramuscular injection* in the deltoid region, 1 mL, see notes above
Also available from local designated centres (special workers and post-exposure treatment)

Rabipur® (MASTA) PoM
Freeze-dried inactivated Flury LEP rabies virus strain cultivated in chick embryo cells, net price single-dose vial = £22.15
Dose: prophylactic, *by intramuscular injection* in the deltoid muscle or anterolateral thigh in small children, 1 mL on days 0, 7 and 21 or 28; also booster doses every 2–5 years for those at continued risk
Post-exposure, *by intramuscular injection* in the deltoid muscle or anterolateral thigh in small children, 1 mL, see notes above

Rubella vaccine

A combined measles, mumps and rubella vaccine (MMR vaccine) aims to eliminate rubella (German measles) and congenital rubella syndrome. MMR vaccine is used for childhood vaccination as well as for vaccinating adults (including women of child-bearing age) who do not have immunity against rubella.

■ Single antigen vaccine
No longer available in the UK; the combined live measles, mumps and rubella vaccine is a suitable alternative (see MMR vaccine p. 587)

■ Combined vaccines
see MMR vaccine

Smallpox vaccine

Limited supplies of **smallpox vaccine** are held at the Central Public Health Laboratory, Colindale (Tel. (020) 8200 4400) for the exclusive use of workers in laboratories where pox viruses (such as vaccinia) are handled.

If a wider use of the vaccine is being considered, detailed contingency plan guidelines should be consulted at www.doh.gov.uk/epcu/cbr/cbrpdf/ smallpoxplan.pdf.

Tetanus vaccines

Tetanus vaccines stimulate the production of the protective antitoxin. In general, adsorption on aluminium hydroxide, aluminium phosphate, or calcium phosphate improves antigenicity. Adsorbed tetanus vaccine is offered routinely to babies in combination with adsorbed diphtheria vaccine (DT/ Vac/Ads(Child)) and more usually also combined with killed *Bordetella pertussis* organisms as adsorbed diphtheria, tetanus, and pertussis vaccine (DTPer/Vac/Ads), see schedule, section 14.1.

In children, adsorbed diphtheria, tetanus, and pertussis vaccine not only gives protection against tetanus in childhood but also gives the basic immunity for subsequent booster doses at school entry and at school leaving (see schedule, section 14.1) and also for a potentially tetanus-contaminated injury. The Department of Health has recommended that for the primary immunisation of adults and adolescents previously unimmunised against tetanus, and where booster doses of tetanus are indicated, following a tetanus-prone wound or for travel, adsorbed diphtheria [low dose] and tetanus vaccine for adults and adolescents is used (see p. 583).

To maintain immunity against tetanus, booster doses of adsorbed tetanus are generally given at intervals of more than 10 years to reduce the possibility of local reactions. If a child over the age of 13 years requires a tetanus booster for a wound then, provided more than 10 years have elapsed since the school-entry booster, adsorbed diphtheria [low dose] and tetanus vaccine for adults and adolescents can be given; the routine booster at school-leaving age is omitted.

Active immunisation is important for persons in older age groups who may never have had a routine or complete course of immunisation when younger. In these persons a course of adsorbed diphtheria [low dose] and tetanus vaccine for adults and adolescents may be given. Very rarely, tetanus has developed after abdominal surgery; patients awaiting elective surgery should be asked about tetanus immunisation and immunised if necessary. All laboratory staff should be offered a primary course if unimmunised.

Any adult who has received 5 doses is likely to have life-long immunity.

For travel recommendations see p. 598

WOUNDS. Wounds are considered to be tetanus-prone if they are sustained *either* more than 6 hours before surgical treatment *or* at any interval after injury and are puncture-type or show much devitalised tissue or are septic or are contaminated with soil or manure. All wounds should receive thorough surgical toilet.

- For *clean wounds*, fully immunised individuals (those who have received a total of 5 doses of tetanus vaccine at appropriate intervals) and those whose primary immunisation is complete (with boosters up to date), do not require tetanus vaccine; individuals whose primary immunisation is incomplete or whose boosters are not up to date require a reinforcing dose of an appropriate strength of combined diphtheria and tetanus vaccine (followed by further doses as required to complete the schedule); non-immunised individuals (or whose immunisation status is not known) should be given a dose of the vaccine immediately (followed by completion of the full course of the vaccine if records confirm the need).

- For *tetanus-prone wounds,* management is as for clean wounds with the addition of a dose of tetanus immunoglobulin (section 14.5) given at a different site; in fully immunised individuals and those whose primary immunisation is complete (see above) the immunoglobulin is needed only if the risk of infection is especially high (e.g. contamination with manure). Antibacterial prophylaxis (with benzylpenicillin, co-amoxiclav, or metronidazole) may also be required for tetanus-prone wounds.

See section 14.1 for general contra-indications

■ Single antigen vaccines

Adsorbed Tetanus Vaccine PoM

Tet/Vac/Ads

Injection, suspension of tetanus formol toxoid adsorbed on a mineral carrier

Dose: by deep subcutaneous or by intramuscular injection, 3 doses each of 0.5 mL separated by intervals of 1 month

NOTE. For primary immunisation in adults and adolescents and boosters, adsorbed diphtheria [low dose] and tetanus vaccine for adults and adolescents is now recommended, see notes above

Available from Chiron Vaccine Evans as Clostet®, (net price 0.5-mL single-dose syringe = £1.79)

Excipients: include thiomersal

■ Combined vaccines

See Diphtheria Vaccines

Tick-borne encephalitis vaccine

Tick-borne encephalitis vaccine is licensed for immunisation of those in high-risk areas based on official recommendations (see section 14.6). Those working, walking or camping in warm forested areas of Central and Eastern Europe and Scandinavia, particularly from April to October when ticks are most prevalent, are at greatest risk of tick-borne encephalitis. Ideally, immunisation should be completed at least one month before travel.

Fever exceeding 40°C may occur, particularly after the first dose of tick-borne encephalitis vaccine. Other side effects include arrhythmias; the vaccine should be used with caution in those with cardiovascular disease. Tick-borne encephalitis vaccine is **contra-indicated** in those with acute febrile infection and hypersensitivity to egg protein. See section 14.1 for general contra-indications and side-effects.

Tick-borne encephalitis immunoglobulin [unlicensed—available on named patient basis from Baxter BioScience] may be considered for those bitten by a tick before the second dose of tick-borne encephalitis vaccine, and rarely when immediate protection is required for those at high risk or travelling at short notice.

FSME-IMMUN® (Baxter BioScience) PoM

Injection, suspension, inactivated Neudoerfl tick-borne encephalitis virus strain, cultivated in chick embryo cells, net price 0.5-mL prefilled syringe = £32.00

Excipients: include gentamicin and neomycin

Dose: by intramuscular injection in deltoid muscle, 3 doses each of 0.5 mL (CHILD 3–15 years, first dose 0.25 mL), second dose after 3 weeks–3 months and third dose after further 9–12 months; ELDERLY over 60 years and immunocompromised (including those receiving immunosuppressants), antibody concentration may be measured 4 weeks after second dose and dose repeated if protective levels not achieved

NOTE. To achieve more rapid protection, second dose may be given 14 days after first dose

Booster doses can be given every 3 years after third dose unless antibody concentration adequate

---

Typhoid vaccines

Typhoid immunisation is advised for travellers to countries where sanitation standards may be poor, although it is not a substitute for scrupulous personal hygiene (see section 14.6). Immunisation is also advised for laboratory workers handling specimens from suspected cases.

Capsular **polysaccharide typhoid vaccine** is given by *intramuscular or deep subcutaneous injection*; further doses are needed every 3 years on continued exposure. Local reactions, including pain, swelling or erythema, may appear 48–72 hours after administration.

For general contra-indications to vaccines, see section 14.1.

■ Polysaccharide vaccine for injection

Typherix® (GSK) PoM

Injection, Vi capsular polysaccharide typhoid vaccine, 50 micrograms/mL virulence polysaccharide antigen of *Salmonella typhi*, net price 0.5-mL prefilled syringe = £10.68

Dose: by intramuscular injection, 0.5 mL; CHILD under 2 years may show suboptimal response

Typhim Vi® (Aventis Pasteur) PoM

Injection, Vi capsular polysaccharide typhoid vaccine, 50 micrograms/mL virulence polysaccharide antigen of *Salmonella typhi*, net price 0.5-mL prefilled syringe = £10.20

Dose: by deep subcutaneous or by intramuscular injection, 0.5 mL; CHILD under 18 months may show suboptimal response

■ Polysaccharide vaccine with hepatitis A vaccine

See Hepatitis A Vaccine

Varicella–zoster vaccine

Varicella–zoster vaccine (live) is licensed for immunisation against varicella in seronegative healthy adults and adolescents. It is not recommended for routine use in children but may be given to seronegative healthy children over 1 year who come into close contact with individuals at high risk of severe varicella infections. The Department of Health recommends varicella–zoster vaccine for seronegative healthcare workers who come into direct contact with patients. Those with a history of chickenpox or shingles can be considered immune, but healthcare workers with a negative or uncertain history should be tested.

Varicella–zoster vaccine is contra-indicated in pregnancy (avoid pregnancy for 3 months after vaccination) and during breast-feeding. It must not be given to individuals with primary or acquired immunodeficiency or to individuals receiving immunosuppressive therapy. For further contra-indications, see section 14.1.

Rarely, transmission of vaccine virus has occurred from the vaccinated individuals to close contacts. Therefore, after vaccination, contact with the following should be avoided if a vaccine-related cutaneous rash develops within 4–6 weeks of the first or second dose:

- varicella-susceptible pregant women;
- individuals at high risk of severe varicella, including those with immunodeficiency or those receiving immunosuppressive therapy.

Healthcare workers who develop a generalised papular or vesicular rash on vaccination should avoid contact with patients until the lesions have crusted. Those who develop a localised rash after vaccination should cover the lesions and be allowed to continue working unless in contact with patients at high risk of severe varicella.

For reference to specific **varicella–zoster immunoglobulin** see section 14.5.

Varilrix® (GSK) ▼ PoM
Injection, powder for reconstitution, live attenuated varicella–zoster virus (Oka strain) propagated in human diploid cells, net price 0.5-mL vial (with diluent) = £29.37
Excipients: include neomycin
Dose: by subcutaneous injection into upper arm, ADULT and ADOLESCENT over 13 years (see notes above), 2 doses of 0.5 mL separated by an interval of 8 weeks (minimum 6 weeks); CHILD over 1 year (but see notes above), 0.5 mL as a single dose

Yellow fever vaccine

Live yellow fever vaccine is indicated for those travelling or living in areas where infection is endemic (see p. 598) and for laboratory staff who handle the virus or who handle clinical material from suspected cases. Infants under 9 months of age should be vaccinated only if the risk of yellow fever is unavoidable since there is a small risk of encephalitis. The vaccine should not be given to those with impaired immune responsiveness, or who have had an anaphylactic reaction to egg; it should not be given during pregnancy (but where there is a significant risk of exposure the need for immuni-

sation outweighs any risk to the fetus). See section 14.1 for further contra-indications. Headache, fever, tiredness, and stiffness may occur 4–7 days after vaccination. Other side-effects include myalgia, asthenia, lymphadenopathy, rash, urticaria, and injection-site reactions.The immunity which probably lasts for life is officially accepted for 10 years starting from 10 days after primary immunisation and for a further 10 years immediately after revaccination.

Yellow Fever Vaccine, Live PoM
Yel/Vac
Injection, powder for reconstitution, preparation of 17D strain of yellow fever virus grown in fertilized hens eggs
Dose: by subcutaneous injection, 0.5 mL
Available (only to designated Yellow Fever Vaccination centres) as *Arilvax*® (Chiron Vaccine Evans) and *Stamaril*® (Aventis Pasteur)

14.5   Immunoglobulins

Human immunoglobulins have replaced immunoglobulins of animal origin (antisera) which were frequently associated with hypersensitivity. Injection of immunoglobulins produces immediate protection lasting for several weeks.

Immunoglobulins are produced from pooled human plasma or serum, and are tested and found non-reactive for hepatitis B surface antigen and for antibodies against hepatitis C virus and human immunodeficiency virus (types 1 and 2)

The two types of human immunoglobulin preparation are **normal immunoglobulin** and **specific immunoglobulins**.

Further information about immunoglobulins is included in *Immunisation against Infectious Disease* (see section 14.1).

AVAILABILITY. **Normal immunoglobulin** is available from the Immunisation Division, CDSC, Health Protection Agency, Colindale only for contacts and the control of outbreaks. It is available commercially for other purposes.

Specific immunoglobulins are available from Health Protection and microbiology laboratories with the exception of **tetanus immunoglobulin** which is distributed through BPL to hospital pharmacies or blood transfusion departments and is also available to general medical practitioners. **Rabies immunoglobulin** is available from the Specialist Reference Microbiology Division, Central Public Health Laboratory, Health Protection Agency, Colindale. The large amounts of **hepatitis B immunoglobulin** required by transplant centres should be obtained commercially.

In Scotland all immunoglobulins are available from the *Blood Transfusion Service*. **Tetanus immunoglobulin** is distributed by the *Blood Transfusion Service* to hospitals and general medical practitioners on demand.

Normal immunoglobulin

Human **normal immunoglobulin** ('HNIG') is prepared from pools of at least 1000 donations of human plasma; it contains antibody to measles, mumps, varicella, hepatitis A, and other viruses that are currently prevalent in the general population.

CAUTIONS and SIDE-EFFECTS. Side-effects of immunoglobulins include malaise, chills, fever, and rarely anaphylaxis. Normal immunoglobulin is **contra-indicated** in patients with known class specific antibody to immunoglobulin A (IgA).

Normal immunoglobulin may **interfere with the immune response to live virus vaccines** which should therefore only be given **at least 3 weeks before or 3 months after** an injection of normal immunoglobulin (this does not apply to yellow fever vaccine since normal immunoglobulin does not contain antibody to this virus). For travellers, if there is insufficient time, the recommended interval may have to be ignored.

USES. Normal immunoglobulin is administered by intramuscular injection for the protection of susceptible contacts against **hepatitis A** virus (infectious hepatitis), **measles** and, to a lesser extent, **rubella**.

Special formulations of immunoglobulins for intravenous administration are available for *replacement therapy* for patients with congenital agammaglobulinaemia and hypogammaglobulinaemia, for the treatment of idiopathic thrombocytopenic purpura and Kawasaki syndrome, and for the prophylaxis of infection following bone-marrow transplantation and in children with symptomatic HIV infection who have recurrent bacterial infections. Normal immunoglobulin may also be given intramuscularly or subcutaneously for replacement therapy, but intravenous formulations are normally preferred.

Intravenous immunoglobulin is also used in the treatment of Guillain-Barré syndrome in preference to plasma exchange.

HEPATITIS A. **Hepatitis A vaccine** is preferred for individuals at risk of infection (see p. 584) including those visiting areas where the disease is highly endemic (all countries excluding Northern and Western Europe, North America, Japan, Australia, and New Zealand). In unimmunised individuals, transmission of hepatitis A is reduced by good hygiene. Intramuscular **normal immunoglobulin** is no longer recommended for routine prophylaxis in travellers but it may be indicated for immunocompromised patients if their antibody response to vaccine is unlikely to be adequate.

Intramuscular normal immunoglobulin is of value in the prevention of infection in close contact of confirmed cases of hepatitis A where there has been a delay in identifying cases or for individuals at high risk of severe disease.

MEASLES. Intramuscular normal immunoglobulin may be given to prevent or attenuate an attack of measles in individuals who do not have adequate immunity. Children and adults with compromised immunity who have come into contact with measles should receive intramuscular normal immunoglobulin as soon as possible after exposure. It is most effective if given within 72 hours but can be effective if given within 6 days. For individuals receiving intravenous immunoglobulin, 100 mg/kg given within 3 weeks before measles exposure should prevent measles. Intramuscular normal immunoglobulin should also be considered for the following individuals if they have been in contact with a confirmed case of measles or with a person associated with a local outbreak:

- non-immune pregnant women
- infants under 9 months

Further advice should be sought from the Public Health Protection Agency Communicable Disease Surveillance Centre (tel. (020) 8200 6868).

Individuals with normal immunity who are not in the above categories and who have not been fully immunised against measles, can be given MMR vaccine (section 14.4) for prophylaxis following exposure to measles.

RUBELLA. Intramuscular immunoglobulin after exposure to rubella does **not** prevent infection in non-immune contacts and is **not** recommended for protection of pregnant women exposed to rubella. It may however reduce the likelihood of a clinical attack which may possibly reduce the risk to the fetus. It should only be used if termination of pregnancy would be unacceptable when it should be given as soon as possible after exposure. Serological follow-up of recipients is essential. For routine prophylaxis, see MMR vaccine (p. 587).

■ For intramuscular use

Normal Immunoglobulin PoM

Normal immunoglobulin injection. 250-mg vial; 750-mg vial

Dose: *by deep intramuscular injection*, to control outbreaks of hepatitis A (see notes above), 500 mg; CHILD under 10 years 250 mg

Measles prophylaxis, CHILD under 1 year 250 mg, 1–2 years 500 mg, 3 years and over 750 mg; to allow attenuated attack, CHILD under 1 year 100 mg, 1 year and over 250 mg

Rubella in pregnancy, prevention of clinical attack, 750 mg

Available from the Immunisation Division, CDSC, Health Protection Agency, Colindale (for contacts and control of outbreaks only, see above) and from SNBTS

■ For subcutaneous use

Subcuvia® (Baxter BioScience) PoM

Normal immunoglobulin injection, net price 5-mL vial = £29.60, 10-mL vial = £59.60

Dose: *by subcutaneous injection*, antibody deficiency syndromes, consult product literature

NOTE. May be administered by intramuscular injection (if subcutaneous route not possible) but **not** for patients with thrombocytopenia or other haemostatic disorders

■ For intravenous use

Normal Immunoglobulin for Intravenous Use PoM

Available as: *Flebogamma*® 5% (0.5 g, 2.5 g, 5 g, 10 g—Grifols); *Gammagard*® *S/D* (0.5 g, 2.5 g, 5 g, 10 g—Baxter BioScience); Human Immunoglobulin (3 g, 5 g, 10 g—SNBTS); *Octagam*® (2.5 g, 5 g, 10 g—Octapharma); *Sandoglobulin*® (1 g, 3 g, 6 g, 12 g—ZLB); *Vigam*®*S* (2.5 g, 5 g—BPL); *Vigam*®*Liquid* (2.5 g, 5 g, 10 g—BPL)

Dose: consult product literature

Specific immunoglobulins

Specific immunoglobulins are prepared by pooling the plasma of selected donors with high levels of the specific antibody required.

Although a hepatitis B vaccine is now available for those at high risk of infection, specific **hepatitis B immunoglobulin** ('HBIG') is available for use in association with hepatitis B vaccine for the prevention of infection in laboratory and other personnel who have been accidentally inoculated with hepatitis B virus, and in infants born to mothers who have become infected with this virus in pregnancy or who are high-risk carriers (see Hepatitis B Vaccine, p. 585).

Following exposure of an unimmunised individual to an animal in or from a high-risk country, the site of the bite should be washed with soapy water and specific **rabies immunoglobulin** of human origin should be injected at the site of the bite and also given intramuscularly. Rabies vaccine should also be given (for details see Rabies Vaccine, p. 591).

For the management of tetanus-prone wounds, **tetanus immunoglobulin** of human origin ('HTIG') should be used in addition to wound toilet and, where appropriate, antibacterial prophylaxis and adsorbed tetanus vaccine (section 14.4). Tetanus immunoglobulin, together with metronidazole (section 5.1.11) and wound toilet, should also be used for the treatment of established cases of tetanus.

Varicella–zoster immunoglobulin (VZIG) is recommended for individuals who are at increased risk of severe varicella *and* who have no antibodies to varicella–zoster virus *and* who have significant exposure to chickenpox or herpes zoster. Those at increased risk include neonates of women who develop chickenpox in the period 7 days before to 7 days after delivery, women exposed at any stage of pregnancy (but when supplies of VZIG are short, only issued to those exposed in the first 20 weeks' gestation or to those near term), and the immunosuppressed including those who have received corticosteroids in the previous 3 months at the following dose equivalents of prednisolone: *children* 2 mg/kg daily for at least 1 week or 1 mg/kg daily for 1 month; *adults* about 40 mg daily for more than 1 week. (**Important:** for full details consult *Immunisation against Infectious Disease*). **Varicella–zoster vaccine** is available—see section 14.4

Cytomegalovirus (CMV) immunoglobulin (available on a named-patient basis from SNBTS) is indicated for prophylaxis in patients receiving immunosuppressive treatment. Also batches of normal immunoglobulin with a high CMV titre are available from Grifols for treatment and prophylaxis of CMV infections [unlicensed indication].

■ Hepatitis B

Hepatitis B Immunoglobulin PoM

See notes above

Dose: by intramuscular injection (as soon as possible after exposure), ADULT 500 units; CHILD under 5 years 200 units, 5–9 years 300 units; NEONATE 200 units as soon as possible after birth; for full details consult *Immunisation against Infectious Disease*

Available from selected Health Protection Agency and NHS laboratories (except for Transplant Centres, see p. 594), also available from BPL and SNBTS

NOTE. Hepatitis B immunoglobulin for intravenous use is available from BPL and SNBTS on a named-patient basis.

■ Rabies

Rabies Immunoglobulin PoM

(Antirabies Immunoglobulin Injection)

See notes above

Dose: 20 units/kg, half *by intramuscular injection* and half *by infiltration* around wound

Available from Public Health Laboratory Service (also from BPL and SNBTS)

■ Tetanus

Tetanus Immunoglobulin PoM

(Antitetanus Immunoglobulin Injection)

See notes above

Dose: by intramuscular injection, prophylactic 250 units, increased to 500 units if more than 24 hours have elapsed or there is risk of heavy contamination or following burns

Therapeutic, 150 units/kg (multiple sites)

Available from BPL and SNBTS

Tetabulin® (Baxter BioScience) PoM

Tetanus immunoglobulin, net price 250-unit prefilled syringe = £14.80

Dose: by intramuscular injection, prophylactic, 250 units, increased to 500 units if wound older than 12 hours or if risk of heavy contamination or if patient weighs more than 90 kg; second dose of 250 units given after 3–4 weeks if patient immunosuppressed or if active immunisation with tetanus vaccine contra-indicated

Therapeutic, 30–300 units/kg

Tetanus Immunoglobulin for Intravenous Use PoM

Used for proven or suspected clinical tetanus

Dose: by intravenous infusion, 5000–10 000 units

Available from BPL and SNBTS on a named-patient basis

■ Varicella–Zoster

Varicella–Zoster Immunoglobulin PoM

(Antivaricella–zoster Immunoglobulin)

See notes above

Dose: by deep intramuscular injection, prophylaxis (as soon as possible—not later than 10 days after exposure), CHILD up to 5 years 250 mg, 6–10 years 500 mg, 11–14 years 750 mg, over 15 years 1 g; give second dose if further exposure occurs after 3 weeks of first dose

NOTE. No evidence that effective in treatment of severe disease. Normal immunoglobulin for intravenous use may be used to provide an immediate source of antibody.

Available from selected Health Protection Agency and NHS laboratories (also from BPL and SNBTS)

Anti-D (Rh₀) immunoglobulin

Anti-D (Rh_0) immunoglobulin is available to prevent a rhesus-negative mother from forming antibodies to fetal rhesus-positive cells which may pass into the maternal circulation. The objective is to protect any subsequent child from the hazard of haemolytic disease of the newborn.

Anti-D immunoglobulin should be administered following any sensitising episode (e.g. abortion, miscarriage and birth); it should be injected within 72 hours of the episode but even if a longer period has elapsed it may still give protection and should be administered. The dose of anti-D immunoglobulin is determined according to the level of exposure to rhesus-positive blood.

For routine antenatal prophylaxis (see also NICE guidance below), two doses of at least 500 units of anti-D immunoglobulin should be given, the first at 28 weeks' gestation and the second at 34 weeks.

NICE Guidance (routine antenatal anti-D prophylaxis for rhesus-negative women). NICE has recommended (May 2002) that routine antenatal anti-D prophylaxis be offered to all non-sensitised pregnant women who are rhesus negative.

Use of routine *antenatal* anti-D prophylaxis should not be affected by previous anti-D prophylaxis for a sensitising event early in the same pregnancy. Similarly, *postpartum* anti-D prophylaxis should not be affected by previous routine antenatal anti-D prophylaxis or by antenatal anti-D prophylaxis for a sensitising event.

Note. MMR vaccine may be given in the postpartum period simultaneously with anti-D (Rh$_0$) immuno-globulin injection provided that separate syringes are used and the products are administered into different limbs. If blood is transfused, the antibody response to the vaccine may be inhibited—measure rubella anti-bodies after 8 weeks and revaccinate if necessary.

Anti-D (Rh$_0$) Immunoglobulin (Non-proprietary) PoM

Injection, anti-D (Rh$_0$) immunoglobulin, net price 250-unit vial = £14.95, 500-unit vial = £19.50, 2500-unit vial = £94.40

Dose: by deep intramuscular injection, to rhesus-negative woman for prevention of Rh$_0$(D) sensitisation:

Following birth of rhesus-positive infant, 500 units immediately or within 72 hours; for transplacental bleed of over 4 mL fetal red cells, extra 100–125 units per mL fetal red cells

Following any potentially sensitising episode (e.g. still-birth, abortion, amniocentesis) up to 20 weeks' gestation 250 units per episode (after 20 weeks, 500 units) imme-diately or within 72 hours

Antenatal prophylaxis, 500 units given at weeks 28 and 34 of pregnancy; a further dose is still needed immedi-ately or within 72 hours of delivery

Following Rh$_0$(D) incompatible blood transfusion, 100–125 units per mL transfused rhesus-positive red cells

Available from Blood Centres and from BPL (*D-Gam*®) and SNBTS

Anti-D (Rh$_0$) Immunoglobulin (Baxter BioScience) PoM

Injection, anti-D (Rh$_0$) immunoglobulin 1250 units/mL (250 micrograms/mL), net price 1-mL prefilled syringe = £23.90

Dose: by intramuscular injection, to rhesus-negative woman for prevention of Rh$_0$(D) sensitisation:

Following abortion, miscarriage or birth of rhesus-positive infant, 1250 units immediately or within 72 hours; for transplacental bleed of over 25 mL fetal blood (1% of fetal erythrocytes), 5000 units (*or* 50 units per mL fetal blood)

Following any potentially sensitising episode (e.g. amniocentesis) 1250 units immediately or within 72 hours

Antenatal prophylaxis, 1250 units may be given at weeks 28 and 34 of pregnancy; a further dose is still needed immediately or within 72 hours of delivery

Following Rh$_0$(D) incompatible blood transfusion, 50–100 units per mL transfused rhesus-positive blood

NOTE. Some UK authorities recommend lower doses for antenatal prophylaxis (see notes above)

Rhophylac® (ZLB) PoM

Injection, anti-D (Rh$_0$) immunoglobulin 750 units/mL (150 micrograms/mL), net price 2-mL (1500-unit) prefilled syringe = £50.00.

Dose: by intramuscular or intravenous injection, to rhesus-negative woman for prevention of Rh$_0$(D) sensi-tisation:

Following birth of rhesus-positive infant, 1000–1500 units immediately or within 72 hours; for large

transplacental bleed, extra 100 units per mL fetal red cells (preferably by intravenous injection)

Following any potentially sensitising episode (e.g. abor-tion, amniocentesis, chorionic villous sampling) up to 12 weeks' gestation 1000 units per episode (after 12 weeks, higher doses may be required) immediately or within 72 hours

Antenatal prophylaxis, 1500 units given between weeks 28–30 of pregnancy; a further dose is still needed immediately or within 72 hours of delivery

Following Rh$_0$(D) incompatible blood transfusion, *by intravenous injection*, 50 units per mL transfused rhesus-positive blood (100 units or per mL of erythrocyte concentrate)

NOTE. Some UK authorities recommend different doses for antenatal prophylaxis (see notes above)

WinRho SDF® (Baxter BioScience) PoM

Injection, anti-D (Rh$_0$) immunoglobulin, powder for reconstitution, net price 1500-unit (300-mic-rogram) vial (with diluent) = £115.00, 5000-unit (1-mg) vial (with diluent) = £383.00

Dose: to rhesus-negative woman for prevention of Rh$_0$(D) sensitisation:

Following birth of rhesus-positive infant, *by intramus-cular injection*, 1500 units *or by intravenous injection*, 600 units immediately or within 72 hours; for transpla-cental bleed of over 25 mL fetal blood, *by intramuscular injection*, extra 50 units per mL fetal blood

Following any potentially sensitising episode (e.g. abor-tion, amniocentesis, chorionic villous sampling) up to 12 weeks' gestation, *by intramuscular injection*, 600 units per episode (after 12 weeks, 1500 units) immediately or within 72 hours

Antenatal prophylaxis, *by intramuscular or intravenous injection*, 1500 units given at week 28 of pregnancy; a further dose is still needed immediately or within 72 hours of delivery

Following Rh$_0$(D) incompatible blood transfusion, *by intramuscular injection*, at least 600 units per 10 mL transfused rhesus-positive blood, given in divided doses over several days; following Rh$_0$(D) incompatible thrombocyte transfusion in rhesus-negative woman of child-bearing age, *by intravenous injection*, 1500 units

Autoimmune (idiopathic) thrombocytopenic purpura, consult product literature

NOTE. Some UK authorities recommend different doses for antenatal prophylaxis (see notes above)

Interferons

Interferon gamma-1b is indicated for chronic granulomatous disease to reduce the frequency of serious infection.

INTERFERON GAMMA-1b

(Immune interferon)

Indications: adjunct to antibacterials to reduce frequency of serious infection in patients with chronic granulomatous disease

Cautions: severe hepatic or renal impairment; seizure disorders or compromised central nervous system function; pre-existing cardiac disease (including ischaemia, congestive heart failure, and arrhythmias); monitor before and during treatment: haematological tests (including full blood count, differential white cell count, and platelet count), blood chemistry tests (including renal and liver function tests) and urinalysis; avoid simultaneous administration of foreign proteins including immunological products (risk of exaggerated immune response); pregnancy (Appendix 4); breast-feeding (Appendix 5); **interactions:** Appendix 1 (interferons)

DRIVING. May impair ability to drive or operate machinery; effects may be enhanced by alcohol

Side-effects: fever, headache, chills, myalgia, fatigue; nausea, vomiting, arthralgia, rashes and injection-site reactions reported

Dose: see under Preparations

Immukin® (Boehringer Ingelheim) [PoM]
Injection, recombinant human interferon gamma-1b 200 micrograms/mL, net price 0.5-mL vial = £88.00
Dose: by subcutaneous injection, 50 micrograms/m^2 3 times a week; patients with body surface area of 0.5 m^2 or less, 1.5 micrograms/kg 3 times a week; not yet recommended for children under 6 months

14.6 International travel

NOTE. For advice on **malaria chemoprophylaxis**, see section 5.4.1.

No special immunisation is required for travellers to the United States, Europe, Australia, or New Zealand although all travellers should have immunity to tetanus and poliomyelitis (and childhood immunisations should be up to date). In Non-European areas surrounding the Mediterranean, in Africa, the Middle East, Asia, and South America, certain special precautions are required.

Long-term travellers to areas that have a high incidence of **poliomyelitis** or **tuberculosis** should be immunised with the appropriate vaccine; in the case of poliomyelitis previously immunised adults may be given a booster dose of oral poliomyelitis vaccine. BCG immunisation is recommended for travellers proposing to stay for longer than one month (or in close contact with the local population) in Asia, Africa, or Central and South America; it should preferably be given three months or more before departure.

Yellow fever immunisation is recommended for travel to the endemic zones of Africa and South America. Many countries require an International Certificate of Vaccination from individuals arriving from, or who have been travelling through, endemic areas, whilst other countries require a certificate from all entering travellers (consult the Department of Health Handbook, *Health Information for Overseas Travel*).

Immunisation against **meningococcal meningitis** is recommended for a number of areas of the world (for details, see p. 588).

Protection against **hepatitis A** is recommended for travellers to high-risk areas outside Northern and Western Europe, North America, Japan, Australia and New Zealand. Hepatitis A vaccine (see p. 584) is preferred and it is likely to be effective even if given shortly before departure; normal immunoglobulin is no longer given routinely but may be indicated in the immunocompromised (see p. 594).

Hepatitis B vaccine (see p. 585) is recommended for those travelling to areas of high prevalence who intend to seek employment as healthcare workers or

who plan to remain there for lengthy periods and who may therefore be at increased risk of acquiring infection as the result of medical or dental procedures carried out in those countries. Short-term tourists or business travellers are not generally at increased risk of infection but may place themselves at risk by their sexual behaviour when abroad.

Prophylactic immunisation against **rabies** (see p. 591) is recommended for travellers to enzootic areas on long journeys to areas out of reach of immediate medical attention.

Travellers who have not had a **tetanus** booster in the last 10 years and are visiting areas where medical attention may not be accessible should receive a booster dose of adsorbed diphtheria [low dose] and tetanus vaccine for adults and adolescents (see p. 583), even if they have received 5 doses of tetanus vaccine previously.

Typhoid vaccine is indicated for travellers to those countries where typhoid is endemic but the vaccine is no substitute for personal precautions. Food should be freshly prepared and hot, and uncooked vegetables (including green salads) should be avoided; only fruits which can be peeled should be eaten. Only suitable bottled water, or tap water that has been boiled, or treated with sterilising tablets should be used for drinking. This advice also applies to cholera and other diarrhoeal diseases (including travellers' diarrhoea).

Cholera vaccine has little value in preventing infections and should **not** be given for international travel (see under Cholera Vaccine). It is no longer available.

Advice on **diphtheria**, on **Japanese encephalitis** ([NHS] vaccine available on named-patient basis from Aventis Pasteur and MASTA) and on **tick-borne encephalitis** is included in *Health Information for Overseas Travel*, see below.

Information on health advice for travellers. The Department of Health booklet, *Health Advice For Travellers* (code: T6) includes information on immunisation requirements (or recommendations) around the world. The booklet can be obtained from travel agents, post-offices or by telephoning 0800 555 777 (24-hour service); also available on the Internet at: www.doh.gov.uk/hat/hatcvr.htm

The Department of Health handbook, *Health Information for Overseas Travel* (2001), which draws together essential information *for healthcare professionals* regarding health advice for travellers, can be obtained from
The Stationery Office
PO Box 29, Norwich NR3 1GN
Telephone orders, 0870 600 5522
Fax: 0870 600 5533
www.tso.co.uk

Immunisation requirements change from time to time, and information on the current requirements for any particular country may be obtained from:

National Travel Health Network and Centre
Hospital for Tropical Diseases
Mortimer Market Centre
Capper Street, off Tottenham Court Road
London WC1E 6AU
Tel: (020) 7380 9234
(09.00–12.00 weekdays for healthcare professionals **only**) www.nathnac.org

Scottish Centre for Infection and Environmental
  Health
Clifton House
Clifton Place
Glasgow G3 7LN
Tel: (0141) 300 1130
(14.00–16.00 hours weekdays)
www.travax.scot.nhs.uk (for registered users for the
  NHS website Travax only)

National Assembly for Wales
Cathays Park
Cardiff CF10 3NQ
Tel: (029) 2082 5111
Department of Health and Social Services
Castle Buildings
Stormont
Belfast BT4 3PP
Tel: (028) 9052 0000

or from the embassy or legation of the appropriate
country.

15: Anaesthesia

15.1   General anaesthesia

NOTE. The drugs in section 15.1 should be used only by experienced personnel and where adequate resuscitation equipment is available.

It is common practice to administer several drugs with different actions to produce surgical anaesthesia. An intravenous anaesthetic is usually used for induction, followed by maintenance with an inhalational anaesthetic, perhaps supplemented by other drugs administered intravenously. Specific drugs are often used to produce muscle relaxation; these drugs interfere with spontaneous respiration and intermittent positive-pressure ventilation is commonly employed.

SURGERY AND LONG-TERM MEDICATION. The risk of stopping long-term medication before surgery is often greater than the risk of continuing it during surgery; however, surgery itself may alter the need for continued drug therapy of certain conditions. It is vital that the anaesthetist knows about **all** drugs that a patient is (or has been) taking.

Patients with adrenal atrophy resulting from long-term corticosteroid use (section 6.3.2) may suffer a precipitous fall in blood pressure unless corticosteroid cover is provided during anaesthesia and in the immediate postoperative period. Anaesthetists must therefore know whether a patient is, or has been, receiving corticosteroids.

Other drugs that should normally not be stopped before surgery include antiepileptics, antiparkinsonian drugs, antipsychotics, anxiolytics, bronchodilators, cardiovascular drugs, glaucoma drugs, immunosuppressants, drugs of dependence, and thyroid or antithyroid drugs. Expert advice is required for patients receiving antivirals for HIV infection. For general advice on surgery in diabetic patients see section 6.1.1.

Patients on oral anticoagulant therapy present with increased risk for anaesthesia and surgery. In these circumstances, the anaesthetist and surgeon should assess the relative risks and decide jointly whether the anticoagulant should be stopped or replaced with heparin therapy.

Drugs that are stopped before surgery include combined oral contraceptives (see Surgery, section 7.3.1 for details); for advice on hormone replacement therapy, see section 6.4.1.1. If antidepressants need to be stopped, they should be withdrawn gradually to avoid withdrawal symptoms. In view of their hazardous interactions MAOIs should normally be stopped 2 weeks before surgery. Tricyclic antidepressants need not be stopped, but there may be an increased risk of arrhythmias and hypotension (and dangerous interaction with vasopressor drugs); therefore, the anaesthetist should be informed if they are not stopped. Lithium should be stopped 24 hours before major surgery but the normal dose can be continued for minor surgery (with careful monitoring of fluids and electrolytes). Potassium-sparing diuretics may need to be withheld on the morning of surgery because hyperkalaemia may develop if renal perfusion is impaired or if there is tissue damage.

ANAESTHESIA AND DRIVING. Patients given sedatives and analgesics during minor outpatient procedures should be very carefully warned about the risk of driving afterwards. For intravenous benzodiazepines and for a short general anaesthetic the risk extends to **at least 24 hours** after administration. Responsible persons should be available to take patients home. The dangers of taking **alcohol** should also be emphasised.

PROPHYLAXIS OF ACID ASPIRATION. Regurgitation and aspiration of gastric contents (Mendelson's syndrome) is an important complication of general anaesthesia, particularly in obstetrics and emergency surgery.

An **H₂-receptor antagonist** (section 1.3.1) or a **proton pump inhibitor** (section 1.3.5) such as omeprazole may be used before surgery to increase the pH and reduce the volume of gastric fluid. They do not affect the pH of fluid already in the stomach and this limits their value in emergency procedures; oral H₂-receptor antagonists can be given 1–2 hours before the procedure but omeprazole must be given at least 12 hours earlier. Antacids are frequently used to neutralise the acidity of the fluid already in the stomach; 'clear' (non-particulate) antacids such as sodium citrate are preferred.

Gas cylinders

Each gas cylinder bears a label with the name of the gas contained in the cylinder. The name or chemical symbol of the gas appears on the shoulder of the cylinder and is also clearly and indelibly stamped on the cylinder valve.

The colours on the valve end of the cylinder extend down to the shoulder; in the case of mixed gases the colours for the individual gases are applied in four segments, two for each colour.

Gas cylinders should be stored in a cool well-ventilated room, free from flammable materials.

No lubricant of any description should be used on the cylinder valves.

15.1.1 Intravenous anaesthetics

Intravenous anaesthetics may be used either to induce anaesthesia or for maintenance of anaesthesia throughout surgery. Intravenous anaesthetics nearly all produce their effect in one arm-brain circulation time and can cause apnoea and hypotension, and so adequate resuscitative facilities **must** be available. They are **contra-indicated** if the anaesthetist is not confident of being able to maintain the airway (e.g. in the presence of a tumour in the pharynx or larynx). Extreme care is required in surgery of the mouth, pharynx, or larynx and in patients with acute circulatory failure (shock) or fixed cardiac output.

Individual requirements vary considerably and the recommended dosage is only a guide. Smaller dosage is indicated in ill, shocked, or debilitated patients, while robust individuals may require more. To facilitate tracheal intubation, induction is followed by a neuromuscular blocking drug (section 15.1.5).

TOTAL INTRAVENOUS ANAESTHESIA. This is a technique in which major surgery is carried out with all anaesthetic drugs given intravenously. Respiration is controlled, the lungs being inflated with oxygen-enriched air. Muscle relaxants are used to provide relaxation and prevent reflex muscle movements. The main problem to be overcome is the assessment of depth of anaesthesia.

ANAESTHESIA AND DRIVING. See section 15.1.

Barbiturates

Thiopental sodium (thiopentone sodium) is used widely, but it has no analgesic properties. Induction is generally smooth and rapid, but owing to its potency, overdosage with cardiorespiratory depression may occur.

Awakening from a moderate dose of thiopental is rapid due to redistribution of the drug into other tissues. Metabolism is, however, slow and some sedative effects may persist for 24 hours. Repeated doses have a cumulative effect.

THIOPENTAL SODIUM
(Thiopentone sodium)

Indications: induction of general anaesthesia; anaesthesia of short duration; reduction of raised intracranial pressure if ventilation controlled

Cautions: see notes above; hepatic impairment (Appendix 2); reconstituted solution is highly alkaline—extravasation causes tissue necrosis and severe pain; avoid intra-arterial injection; **interactions:** Appendix 1 (anaesthetics, general)

Contra-indications: see notes above; porphyria (section 9.8.2)

Side-effects: arrhythmias, myocardial depression, laryngeal spasm, cough, sneezing, hypersensitivity reactions, rash, injection-site reactions

Dose: induction of general anaesthesia, *by intravenous injection* as a 2.5% (25 mg/mL) solution, in fit premedicated adults, initially 100–150 mg (reduced in elderly or debilitated) over 10–15 seconds (longer in elderly or debilitated), followed by further quantity if necessary according to response after 30–60 seconds; *or* up to 4 mg/kg; CHILD induction 2–7 mg/kg

Raised intracranial pressure, *by intravenous injection*, 1.5–3 mg/kg, repeated as required

Thiopental (Non-proprietary) PoM
Injection, powder for reconstitution, thiopental sodium, net price 500-mg vial = £3.06
Available from Link

Other intravenous anaesthetics

Etomidate is an induction agent associated with rapid recovery without hangover effect. It causes less hypotension than other drugs used for induction. There is a high incidence of extraneous muscle movement which can be minimised by an opioid analgesic or a short-acting benzodiazepine given just before induction. Pain on injection can be reduced by the use of a larger vein or by an opioid analgesic given just before induction. Etomidate may suppress adrenocortical function, particularly on continuous administration, and it should not be used for maintenance of anaesthesia.

Propofol is associated with rapid recovery without hangover effect and is very widely used. There is sometimes pain on intravenous injection, but significant extraneous muscle movements do not occur. Convulsions, anaphylaxis, and delayed recovery from anaesthesia have occured after propofol administration; since the onset of some convulsions can be delayed the CSM has advised special caution after day surgery. Propofol has been associated with bradycardia, occasionally profound; intravenous administration of an antimuscarinic may be necessary to prevent this.

Ketamine can be given by the intravenous or the intramuscular route and it has good analgesic properties when used in sub-anaesthetic dosage. The maximum effect occurs after more than one arm-brain circulation time. Muscle tone is increased. There is cardiovascular stimulation and arterial pressure may rise with tachycardia. The main disadvantage of ketamine is the high incidence of hallucinations and other transient psychotic sequelae, but it is believed that these are much less significant in children. The incidence of psychotic effects can be reduced when drugs such as diazepam are also used. Ketamine is **contra-indicated** in patients with hypertension and is best avoided in those prone to hallucinations. It is used mainly for paediatric anaesthesia, particularly when repeated administration is required. Recovery is relatively slow.

ETOMIDATE

Indications: induction of anaesthesia
Cautions: see notes above; avoid in porphyria (section 9.8.2); **interactions:** Appendix 1 (anaesthetics, general)
Contra-indications: see notes above
Side-effects: see notes above
Dose: see under preparations

Etomidate-Lipuro® (Braun) [PoM]
Injection (emulsion), etomidate 2 mg/mL, net price 10-mL amp = £1.53
Dose: ADULT and CHILD, *by slow intravenous injection*, 150–300 micrograms/kg; CHILD under 10 years may need up to 400 micrograms/kg; ELDERLY 150–200 micrograms/kg

Hypnomidate® (Janssen-Cilag) [PoM]
Injection, etomidate 2 mg/mL, net price 10-mL amp = £1.58
Excipients: include propylene glycol (see Excipients, p. 2)
Dose: ADULT and CHILD, *by slow intravenous injection*, 300 micrograms/kg; ELDERLY 150–200 micrograms/kg; max. total dose 60 mg

KETAMINE

Indications: induction and maintenance of anaesthesia
Cautions: see notes above; **interactions:** Appendix 1 (anaesthetics, general)
Contra-indications: see notes above
Side-effects: see notes above
Dose: *by intramuscular injection*, short procedures, initially 6.5–13 mg/kg (10 mg/kg usually produces 12–25 minutes of surgical anaesthesia)
Diagnostic manoeuvres and procedures not involving intense pain, initially 4 mg/kg
By intravenous injection over at least 60 seconds, short procedures, initially 1–4.5 mg/kg (2 mg/kg usually produces 5–10 minutes of surgical anaesthesia)
By intravenous infusion of a solution containing 1 mg/mL, longer procedures, induction, total dose of 0.5–2 mg/kg; maintenance (using microdrip infusion), 10–45 micrograms/kg/minute, rate adjusted according to response

Ketalar® (Pfizer) [PoM]
Injection, ketamine (as hydrochloride) 10 mg/mL, net price 20-mL vial = £4.22; 50 mg/mL, 10-mL vial = £8.77; 100 mg/mL, 10-mL vial = £16.10

PROPOFOL

Indications: see under dose
Cautions: see notes above; monitor blood-lipid concentration if risk of fat overload or if sedation longer than 3 days; **interactions:** Appendix 1 (anaesthetics, general)
Contra-indications: see notes above; not to be used for sedation of ventilated children and adolescents under 17 years (risk of potentially fatal effects including metabolic acidosis, cardiovascular collapse, rhabdomyolysis, hyperlipidaemia and hepatomegaly)
Side-effects: see notes above; pulmonary oedema, postoperative fever reported
Dose: *1% injection*
Induction of anaesthesia, *by intravenous injection or infusion*, 1.5–2.5 mg/kg (less in those over 55 years) at a rate of 20–40 mg every 10 seconds; CHILD over 1 month, administer slowly until response (usual dose in child over 8 years 2.5 mg/kg, may need more in younger child e.g. 2.5–4 mg/kg)
Maintenance of anaesthesia, *by intravenous injection*, 25–50 mg repeated according to response *or by intravenous infusion*, 4–12 mg/kg/hour; CHILD over 3 years, *by intravenous injection or infusion*, 9–15 mg/kg/hour
Sedation in intensive care, *by intravenous infusion*, ADULT over 17 years, 0.3–4 mg/kg/hour
Sedation for surgical and diagnostic procedures, initially *by intravenous injection* over 1–5 minutes, 0.5–1 mg/kg; maintenance, *by intravenous infusion*, 1.5–4.5 mg/kg/hour (additionally, if rapid increase in sedation required, *by intravenous injection*, 10–20 mg); those over 55 years may require lower dose; CHILD and ADOLESCENT under 17 years not recommended

2% injection
Induction of anaesthesia, *by intravenous infusion*, 1.5–2.5 mg/kg (less in those over 55 years) at a rate of 20–40 mg every 10 seconds; CHILD over 3 years,

administer slowly until response (usual dose in child over 8 years 2.5 mg/kg, may need more in younger child e.g. 2.5–4 mg/kg)

Maintenance of anaesthesia, *by intravenous infusion*, 4–12 mg/kg/hour; CHILD over 3 years, *by intravenous infusion*, 9–15 mg/kg/hour

Sedation in intensive care, *by intravenous infusion*, ADULT over 17 years, 0.3–4 mg/kg/hour

Propofol (Non-proprietary) PoM

1% injection (emulsion), propofol 10 mg/mL, net price 20-mL amp = £2.33, 50-mL bottle = £5.82, 100-mL bottle = £11.64

2% injection (emulsion), propofol 20 mg/mL, net price 50-mL vial = £11.64

Available from Baxter (1%, 2%), Braun (*Propofol-Lipuro®* 1%, 2%), Fresenius Kabi (1%, 2%), Zurich (1%, 2%)

Diprivan® (AstraZeneca) PoM

1% injection (emulsion), propofol 10 mg/mL, net price 20-mL amp = £3.88, 50-mL vial = £9.70, 50-mL prefilled syringe (for use with *Diprifusor® TCI* system) = £10.67, 100-mL vial = £19.40

2% injection (emulsion), propofol 20 mg/mL, net price 50-mL vial = £19.40, 50-mL prefilled syringe (for use with *Diprifusor® TCI* system) = £20.37

NOTE. *Diprifusor® TCI* ('target controlled infusion') system is for use **only** for induction and maintenance of general anaesthesia in adults

15.1.2 Inhalational anaesthetics

Inhalational anaesthetics may be gases or volatile liquids. They can be used both for induction and maintenance of anaesthesia and may also be used following induction with an intravenous anaesthetic (section 15.1.1).

Gaseous anaesthetics require suitable equipment for storage and administration. They may be supplied via hospital pipelines or from metal cylinders. *Volatile liquid anaesthetics* are administered using calibrated vaporisers, using air, oxygen, or nitrous oxide–oxygen mixtures as the carrier gas. It should be noted that they can all trigger malignant hyperthermia (section 15.1.8).

To prevent hypoxia inhalational anaesthetics must be given with concentrations of oxygen greater than in air.

ANAESTHESIA AND DRIVING. See section 15.1.

Volatile liquid anaesthetics

Halothane is a volatile liquid anaesthetic. Its advantages are that it is potent, induction is smooth, the vapour is non-irritant, pleasant to inhale, and seldom induces coughing or breath-holding. Despite these advantages, however, halothane is much less widely used than previously owing to its association with *severe hepatotoxicity* (**important**: see CSM advice, below).

Halothane causes cardiorespiratory depression. Respiratory depression results in elevation of arterial carbon dioxide tension and perhaps ventricular arrhythmias. Halothane also depresses the cardiac muscle fibres and may cause bradycardia. The result is diminished cardiac output and fall of arterial pressure. Adrenaline (epinephrine) infiltrations

should be avoided in patients anaesthetised with halothane as ventricular arrhythmias may result.

Halothane produces moderate muscle relaxation, but this may be inadequate for major abdominal surgery and specific muscle relaxants are then used.

CSM advice (halothane hepatotoxicity). In a publication on findings confirming that *severe hepatotoxicity* can follow halothane anaesthesia the CSM has reported that this occurs more frequently after repeated exposures to halothane and has a high mortality. The risk of severe hepatotoxicity appears to be increased by repeated exposures within a short time interval, but even after a long interval (sometimes of several years) susceptible patients have been reported to develop jaundice. Since there is no reliable way of identifying susceptible patients the CSM recommends the following precautions prior to use of halothane:

1. a careful anaesthetic history should be taken to determine previous exposure and previous reactions to halothane;

2. repeated exposure to halothane within a period of **at least 3 months should be avoided** unless there are **overriding** clinical circumstances;

3. a history of unexplained jaundice or pyrexia in a patient following exposure to halothane is an absolute **contra-indication** to its future use in that patient.

Enflurane is a volatile anaesthetic similar to halothane, but less potent, about twice the concentration being necessary for induction and maintenance.

Enflurane is a powerful cardiorespiratory depressant. Shallow respiration is likely to result in a rise of arterial carbon dioxide tension, but ventricular arrhythmias are uncommon and it is probably safe to use adrenaline (epinephrine) infiltrations. Myocardial depression may result in a fall in cardiac output and in arterial hypotension. It may cause EEG changes and should be avoided in those liable to epileptic seizures. Enflurane may cause hepatotoxicity in those sensitised to halogenated anaesthetics but the risk is smaller than with halothane.

Isoflurane is an isomer of enflurane. It has a potency intermediate between that of halothane and enflurane, and even less of an inhaled dose is metabolised than with enflurane. Heart rhythm is generally stable during isoflurane anaesthesia, but heart-rate may rise, particularly in younger patients. Systemic arterial pressure may fall, owing to a decrease in systemic vascular resistance and with less decrease in cardiac output than occurs with halothane. Respiration is depressed. Muscle relaxation is produced and muscle relaxant drugs potentiated. Isoflurane may also cause hepatotoxicity in those sensitised to halogenated anaesthetics but the risk is appreciably smaller than with halothane.

Desflurane is reported to have about one-fifth the potency of isoflurane. Owing to limited experience it is not recommended in neurosurgical patients. It is not recommended for induction in children because cough, breath-holding, apnoea, laryngospasm and increased secretions can occur. The risk of hepatotoxicity with desflurane in those sensitised to halogenated anaesthetics appears to be remote.

Sevoflurane is a rapid acting volatile liquid anaesthetic. Patients may require early postoperative pain relief as emergence and recovery are particularly rapid. Sevoflurane can interact with carbon dioxide absorbents to form compound A, a potentially nephrotoxic vinyl ether. However, in spite of extensive use, no cases of sevoflurane-induced permanent renal injury have been reported and the carbon dioxide absorbents used in the UK produce very low concentrations of compound A.

DESFLURANE

Indications: see notes above
Cautions: see notes above; **interactions:** Appendix 1 (anaesthetics, general)
Contra-indications: see notes above; susceptibility to malignant hyperthermia
Side-effects: see notes above
Dose: using a specifically calibrated vaporiser, *induction*, 4–11%; CHILD not recommended for induction
Maintenance, 2–6% in nitrous oxide; 2.5–8.5% in oxygen or oxygen-enriched air; max. 17%

Suprane® (Baxter Anaesthesia) PoM
Desflurane, net price 240 mL = £48.85

ENFLURANE

Indications: see notes above
Cautions: see notes above; epilepsy; avoid in porphyria (section 9.8.2); **interactions:** Appendix 1 (anaesthetics, general)
Contra-indications: susceptibility to malignant hyperthermia
Side-effects: see notes above
Dose: using a specifically calibrated vaporiser, *induction*, increased gradually from 0.4% to max. of 4.5% in air, oxygen, or nitrous oxide–oxygen, according to response
Maintenance, 0.5–3% in nitrous oxide–oxygen

Enflurane (Abbott)
Enflurane, net price 250 mL = £24.00

HALOTHANE

Indications: see notes above
Cautions: see notes above (**important:** CSM advice, see notes above); avoid for dental procedures in those under 18 years unless treated in hospital (high risk of arrhythmia); avoid in porphyria (section 9.8.2); **interactions:** Appendix 1 (anaesthetics, general)
Contra-indications: see notes above; susceptibility to malignant hyperthermia
Side-effects: see notes above
Dose: using a specifically calibrated vaporiser, *induction*, increased gradually to 2–4% in oxygen or nitrous oxide–oxygen; CHILD (see cautions) 1.5–2%
Maintenance, 0.5–2%

Halothane (Concord)
Halothane, net price 250 mL = £20.57

ISOFLURANE

Indications: see notes above
Cautions: see notes above; **interactions:** Appendix 1 (anaesthetics, general)
Contra-indications: susceptibility to malignant hyperthermia
Side-effects: see notes above

Dose: using a specifically calibrated vaporiser, *induction*, increased gradually from 0.5% to 3%, in oxygen or nitrous oxide–oxygen
Maintenance, 1–2.5% in nitrous oxide–oxygen; an additional 0.5–1% may be required when given with oxygen alone; caesarean section, 0.5–0.75% in nitrous oxide–oxygen

Isoflurane (Abbott)
Isoflurane, net price 250 mL = £47.50

Aerrane® (Baxter Anaesthesia)
Isoflurane, net price 100 mL = £8.21, 250 mL = £27.00

SEVOFLURANE

Indications: see notes above
Cautions: see notes above; renal impairment; **interactions:** Appendix 1 (anaesthetics, general)
Contra-indications: see notes above; susceptibility to malignant hyperthermia
Side-effects: see notes above; also agitation occurs frequently in children
Dose: using a specifically calibrated vaporiser, *induction*, up to 5% in oxygen or nitrous oxide–oxygen; CHILD up to 7%
Maintenance, 0.5–3%

Sevoflurane (Abbott) PoM
Sevoflurane, net price 250 mL = £123.00

Nitrous oxide

Nitrous oxide is used for maintenance of anaesthesia and, in sub-anaesthetic concentrations, for analgesia. For anaesthesia it is commonly used in a concentration of 50 to 70% in oxygen as part of a balanced technique in association with other inhalational or intravenous agents. Nitrous oxide is unsatisfactory as a sole anaesthetic owing to lack of potency, but is useful as part of a combination of drugs since it allows a significant reduction in dosage.

A mixture of nitrous oxide and oxygen containing 50% of each gas (*Entonox®, Equanox®*) is used to produce analgesia without loss of consciousness. Self-administration using a demand valve is popular in obstetric practice, for changing painful dressings, as an aid to postoperative physiotherapy, and in emergency ambulances.

Nitrous oxide may have a deleterious effect if used in patients with an air-containing closed space since nitrous oxide diffuses into such a space with a resulting increase in pressure. This effect may be dangerous in the presence of a pneumothorax which may enlarge to compromise respiration.

Exposure of patients to nitrous oxide for prolonged periods, either by continuous or by intermittent administration, may result in megaloblastic anaemia owing to interference with the action of vitamin B_{12}. For the same reason, exposure of theatre staff to nitrous oxide should be minimised. Depression of white cell formation may also occur.

NITROUS OXIDE

Indications: see notes above
Cautions: see notes above; **interactions:** Appendix 1 (anaesthetics, general)
Side-effects: see notes above

Dose: using suitable anaesthetic apparatus, *maintenance* of light anaesthesia, as a mixture with 25–30% oxygen

Analgesic, as a mixture with 50% oxygen, according to the patient's needs

15.1.3   Antimuscarinic drugs

Antimuscarinic drugs are used (less commonly nowadays) as premedicants to dry bronchial and salivary secretions which are increased by intubation, by surgery to the upper airways, and by some inhalational anaesthetics. They are also used before or with neostigmine (section 15.1.6) to prevent bradycardia, excessive salivation, and other muscarinic actions of neostigmine. They also prevent bradycardia and hypotension associated with drugs such as halothane, propofol, and suxamethonium.

Atropine is now rarely used for premedication but still has an emergency role in the treatment of vagotonic side-effects. For its role in acute arrhythmias after myocardial infarction, see section 2.3.1; see also cardiopulmonary resuscitation, section 2.7.3.

Hyoscine reduces secretions and also provides a degree of amnesia, sedation and anti-emesis. Unlike atropine it may produce bradycardia rather than tachycardia. In some patients, especially the elderly, hyoscine may cause the central anticholinergic syndrome (excitement, ataxia, hallucinations, behavioural abnormalities, and drowsiness).

Glycopyrronium reduces salivary secretions. When given intravenously it produces less tachycardia than atropine. It is widely used with neostigmine for reversal of non-depolarising muscle relaxants (section 15.1.5).

Phenothiazines do not effectively reduce secretions when used alone.

ATROPINE SULPHATE

Indications: drying secretions, reversal of excessive bradycardia; with neostigmine for reversal of non-depolarising neuromuscular block; antispasmodic (section 1.2); bradycardia (section 2.3.1); cardiopulmonary resuscitation (section 2.7.3); eye (section 11.5)

Cautions: cardiovascular disease; see also section 1.2; **interactions:** Appendix 1 (antimuscarinics)
DURATION OF ACTION. Since atropine has a shorter duration of action than neostigmine, late unopposed bradycardia may result; close monitoring of the patient is necessary

Contra-indications: see section 1.2

Side-effects: tachycardia; see also section 1.2

Dose: premedication, *by intravenous injection*, 300–600 micrograms immediately before induction of anaesthesia

By subcutaneous or *intramuscular injection,* 300–600 micrograms 30–60 minutes before induction; CHILD 20 micrograms/kg (max. 600 micrograms)

Intra-operative bradycardia, *by intravenous injection,* incremental doses of 100 micrograms (larger doses in emergencies)

Control of muscarinic side-effects of neostigmine in reversal of competitive neuromuscular block, *by intravenous injection,* 0.6–1.2 mg

Arrhythmias after myocardial infarction, see section 2.3.1; see also cardiopulmonary resuscitation algorithm, inside back cover

Atropine (Non-proprietary) PoM
Injection, atropine sulphate 600 micrograms/mL, net price 1-mL amp = 50p
NOTE. Other strengths also available
Injection, prefilled disposable syringe, atropine sulphate 100 micrograms/mL, net price 5 mL = £4.16, 10 mL = £4.66, 30 mL = £8.52
Available from Celltech (*Minijet*®)
Injection, prefilled disposable syringe, atropine sulphate 200 micrograms/mL, net price 5 mL = £4.45; 300 micrograms/mL, 10 mL = £4.45; 600 micrograms/mL, 1 mL = £4.45
Available from Aurum

■ With morphine
See under Morphine Salts (section 4.7.2)

GLYCOPYRRONIUM BROMIDE
(Glycopyrrolate)

Indications: see under Atropine Sulphate; hyperhidrosis (section 13.12)

Cautions: cardiovascular disease; see also Atropine sulphate (section 1.2); **interactions:** Appendix 1 (antimuscarinics)

Side-effects: see under Atropine Sulphate

Dose: premedication, *by intramuscular or intravenous injection,* 200–400 micrograms, *or* 4–5 micrograms/kg to a max. of 400 micrograms; CHILD *by intramuscular or* preferably *by intravenous injection,* 4–8 micrograms/kg to a max. of 200 micrograms

Intra-operative use, *by intravenous injection,* as for premedication, repeated if necessary

Control of muscarinic side-effects of neostigmine in reversal of non-depolarising neuromuscular block, *by intravenous injection,* 200 micrograms per 1 mg of neostigmine, *or* 10–15 micrograms/kg with neostigmine 50 micrograms/kg; CHILD 10 micrograms/kg with neostigmine 50 micrograms/kg

Robinul® (Anpharm) PoM
Injection, glycopyrronium bromide 200 micrograms/mL, net price 1-mL amp = 60p; 3-mL amp = £1.01
Available as a generic from Antigen

■ With neostigmine metilsulphate
Section 15.1.6

HYOSCINE HYDROBROMIDE
(Scopolamine hydrobromide)

Indications: drying secretions, amnesia; other indications (section 4.6)

Cautions: see under Atropine Sulphate; avoid in the elderly (see notes above)

Contra-indications: porphyria (section 9.8.2)

Side-effects: see under Atropine Sulphate; bradycardia

Dose: premedication, *by subcutaneous or intramuscular injection,* 200–600 micrograms 30–60 minutes before induction of anaesthesia, usually with papaveretum

Hyoscine (Non-proprietary) PoM
Injection, hyoscine hydrobromide 400 micrograms/mL, net price 1-mL amp = £2.71; 600 micrograms/mL, 1-mL amp = £2.81

■ With papaveretum
See under papaveretum (section 4.7.2)

15.1.4   Sedative and analgesic peri-operative drugs

15.1.4.1   Anxiolytics and neuroleptics
15.1.4.2   Non-opioid analgesics
15.1.4.3   Opioid analgesics

These drugs are given to allay the apprehension of the patient in the pre-operative period (including the night before operation), to relieve pain and discomfort when present, and to augment the action of subsequent anaesthetic agents. A number of the drugs used also provide some degree of pre-operative amnesia. The choice will vary with the individual patient, the nature of the operative procedure, the anaesthetic to be used and other prevailing circumstances such as outpatients, obstetrics, recovery facilities etc. The choice would also vary in elective and emergency operations.

PREMEDICATION IN CHILDREN. Oral administration is preferred to injections where possible but is not altogether satisfactory; the rectal route should only be used in exceptional circumstances. Oral alimemazine (trimeprazine) is still used but when given alone it may cause postoperative restlessness when pain is present.

Atropine or hyoscine is often given orally to children, but may be given intravenously immediately before induction.

The use of a suitable local anaesthetic cream (section 15.2) should be considered to avoid pain at injection site.

ANAESTHESIA AND DRIVING. See section 15.1.

15.1.4.1   Anxiolytics and neuroleptics

Anxiolytic benzodiazepines are widely used whereas neuroleptics such as **chlorpromazine** (section 4.2.1) are rarely used in the UK for premedication although chlorpromazine was used to prevent shivering in induction of hypothermia. **Alimemazine (trimeprazine)** (section 3.4.1) is still occasionally used as a premedicant for children (but see section 15.1.4).

Benzodiazepines

Benzodiazepines possess useful properties for premedication including relief of anxiety, sedation, and amnesia; short-acting benzodiazepines taken by mouth are the most common premedicants. They have no analgesic effect so an opioid analgesic may sometimes be required for pain.

Benzodiazepines can alleviate anxiety at doses that do not necessarily cause excessive sedation and they are of particular value during short procedures or during operations under local anaesthesia (including dentistry). Amnesia reduces the likelihood of any unpleasant memories of the procedure (although benzodiazepines, particularly when used for more profound sedation, can sometimes induce sexual fantasies). Benzodiazepines are also used in intensive care units for sedation, particularly in those receiving assisted ventilation.

Benzodiazepines may occasionally cause marked respiratory depression and facilities for its treatment are essential; flumazenil (section 15.1.7) is used to antagonise the effects of benzodiazepines. They are best avoided in myasthenia gravis, especially perioperatively.

Diazepam is used to produce mild sedation with amnesia. It is a long-acting drug with active metabolites and a second period of drowsiness can occur several hours after its administration. Peri-operative use of diazepam in children is not generally recommended; its effect and timing of response are unreliable and paradoxical effects may occur.

Diazepam is relatively insoluble in water and preparations formulated in organic solvents are painful on intravenous injection and give rise to a high incidence of venous thrombosis (which may not be noticed for several days after the injection). Intramuscular injection of diazepam is painful and absorption is erratic. An emulsion preparation for intravenous injection is less irritant and is followed by a negligible incidence of venous thrombosis; it is not suitable for intramuscular injection. Diazepam is also available as a rectal solution.

Temazepam is given by mouth and has a shorter duration of action and a more rapid onset than diazepam given by mouth. It has been used as a premedicant in inpatient and day-case surgery; anxiolytic and sedative effects last about 90 minutes although there may be residual drowsiness.

Lorazepam produces more prolonged sedation than temazepam and it has marked amnesic effects. It is used as a premedicant the night before major surgery; a further, smaller dose may be required the following morning if any delay in starting surgery is anticipated. Alternatively the first dose may be given early in the morning on the day of operation.

Midazolam is a water-soluble benzodiazepine which is often used in preference to intravenous diazepam; recovery is faster than from diazepam. Midazolam is associated with profound sedation when high doses are given intravenously or when used with certain other drugs.

DIAZEPAM

Indications: premedication; sedation with amnesia, and in conjunction with local anaesthesia; other indications (section 4.1.2, section 4.8.2, and section 10.2.2)

Cautions: see notes above and section 4.1.2 and section 4.8.2

Contra-indications: see notes above and section 4.1.2

Side-effects: see notes above and section 4.1.2

Dose: *by mouth*, 5 mg on night before minor or dental surgery then 5 mg 2 hours before procedure

By intravenous injection, into a large vein 10–20 mg over 2–4 minutes as sedative cover for minor surgical and medical procedures; premedication 100–200 micrograms/kg

By rectum in solution, 10 mg; ELDERLY 5 mg; CHILD not recommended (see notes above)

NOTE. Diazepam rectal solution doses in the BNF may differ from those in the product literature

■ Preparations
Section 4.1.2

LORAZEPAM

Indications: sedation with amnesia; premedication; other indications (section 4.1.2 and section 4.8.2)

Cautions: see notes above and under Diazepam (section 4.1.2 and section 4.8.2); **interactions:** Appendix 1 (anxiolytics and hypnotics)

Contra-indications: see notes above and under Diazepam (section 4.1.2)

Side-effects: see notes above and under Diazepam (section 4.1.2)

Dose: *by mouth*, 2–3 mg the night before operation; 2–4 mg 1–2 hours before operation

By slow intravenous injection, preferably diluted with an equal volume of sodium chloride intravenous infusion 0.9% or water for injections, 50 micrograms/kg 30–45 minutes before operation

By intramuscular injection, diluted as above, 50 micrograms/kg 60–90 minutes before operation

■ Preparations
Section 4.1.2

MIDAZOLAM

Indications: sedation with amnesia; sedation in intensive care; premedication, induction of anaesthesia; status epilepticus [unlicensed use], section 4.8.2

Cautions: hepatic impairment; renal impairment (Appendix 3); pregnancy (Appendix 4) and breast-feeding (Appendix 5); cardiac disease; respiratory disease; children (particularly if cardiovascular impairment); history of drug or alcohol abuse; reduce dose in elderly and debilitated; avoid prolonged use (and abrupt withdrawal thereafter); concentration of midazolam in children under 15 kg not to exceed 1 mg/mL; **interactions:** Appendix 1 (anxiolytics and hypnotics)

Contra-indications: myasthenia gravis; severe respiratory depression; acute pulmonary insufficiency

Side-effects: gastro-intestinal disturbances, increased appetite, jaundice; hypotension, cardiac arrest, heart rate changes, anaphylaxis, thrombosis; laryngospasm, bronchospasm, respiratory depression and respiratory arrest (particularly with high doses or on rapid injection); drowsiness, confusion, ataxia, amnesia, headache, euphoria, hallucinations, fatigue, dizziness, vertigo, involuntary movements, paradoxical increase in excitement and aggression; dysarthria; urinary retention, incontinence, changes in libido; blood disorders; muscle weakness; visual disturbances; salivation changes; skin reactions; on intravenous injection, pain, thrombophlebitis

Dose: conscious sedation, *by slow intravenous injection* (approx. 2 mg/minute), initially 2–2.5 mg (ELDERLY 0.5–1 mg), increased if necessary in steps of 1 mg (ELDERLY 0.5–1 mg); usual range 3.5–7.5 mg, ELDERLY max. 3.5 mg; CHILD *by intravenous injection* over 2–3 minutes, 6 months–5 years initially 50–100 micrograms/kg, dose increased if necessary in small steps (max. total dose 6 mg), 6–12 years initially 25–50 micrograms/kg, dose increased if necessary in small steps (max. total dose 10 mg)

By intramuscular injection, CHILD 1–15 years 50–150 micrograms/kg; max. 10 mg

By rectum (see note below), CHILD over 6 months 300–500 micrograms/kg

Sedative in combined anaesthesia, *by intravenous injection*, 30–100 micrograms/kg repeated as required or *by intravenous infusion*, 30–100 micrograms/kg/hour (ELDERLY lower doses needed); CHILD not recommended

Premedication, *by deep intramuscular injection*, 70–100 micrograms/kg (ELDERLY 25–50 micrograms/kg) 20–60 minutes before induction, usual dose 2–3 mg; CHILD 1–15 years 80–200 micrograms/kg

By rectum, CHILD over 6 months 300–500 micrograms/kg 15–30 minutes before induction

Induction, *by slow intravenous injection*, with premedication, 150–200 micrograms/kg (ELDERLY 100–200 micrograms/kg), without premedication, 300–350 micrograms/kg (ELDERLY 150–300 micrograms/kg); doses increased in steps not greater than 5 mg every 2 minutes; max. 600 micrograms/kg; CHILD over 7 years 150 micrograms/kg

Sedation of patients receiving intensive care, *by slow intravenous injection*, initially 30–300 micrograms/kg given in steps of 1–2.5 mg every 2 minutes, then *by slow intravenous injection or by intravenous infusion*, 30–200 micrograms/kg/hour; reduce dose (or omit initial dose) in hypovolaemia, vasoconstriction, or hypothermia; lower doses may be adequate if opioid analgesic also used; NEONATE under 32 weeks gestational age *by intravenous infusion*, 30 micrograms/kg/hour, NEONATE over 32 weeks gestational age and CHILD under 6 months 60 micrograms/kg/hour, over 6 months *by slow intravenous injection*, initially 50–200 micrograms/kg, then *by intravenous infusion*, 60–120 micrograms/kg/hour

NOTE. For rectal administration of the injection solution, attach a plastic applicator onto the end of a syringe; if the volume to be given rectally is too small, water for injection may be added to give a total volume of 10 mL

Midazolam (Non-proprietary) PoM
Injection, midazolam (as hydrochloride) 1 mg/mL, net price 50-mL vial = £6.00; 5 mg/mL, 2-mL amp = 77p, 5-mL amp = 91p, 10-mL amp = £4.86, 18-mL amp = £6.80

Available from Antigen, Aurum, CP, Phoenix

Hypnovel® (Roche) PoM
Injection, midazolam (as hydrochloride) 2 mg/mL, net price 5-mL amp = 96p; 5 mg/mL, 2-mL amp = 81p

---

TEMAZEPAM

Indications: premedication before surgery; anxiety before investigatory procedures; hypnotic (section 4.1.1)

Cautions: see notes above and under Diazepam (section 4.1.2 and section 4.8.2); **interactions:** Appendix 1 (anxiolytics and hypnotics)

Contra-indications: see notes above and under Diazepam (section 4.1.2)

Side-effects: see notes above and under Diazepam (section 4.1.2)

Dose: *by mouth*, premedication, 20–40 mg (elderly, 10–20 mg) 1 hour before operation; CHILD 1 mg/kg (max. 30 mg)

■ Preparations
Section 4.1.1

15.1.4.2 Non-opioid analgesics

Since non-steroidal anti-inflammatory drugs (NSAIDs) do not depress respiration, do not impair gastro-intestinal motility, and do not cause dependence, they may be useful alternatives (or adjuncts) to the use of opioids for the relief of postoperative pain. NSAIDs may be inadequate for the relief of severe pain.

Acemetacin, **diclofenac**, **flurbiprofen**, **ibuprofen**, **ketoprofen**, **rofecoxib** (section 10.1.1), **parecoxib**, and **ketorolac** are licensed for postoperative use. Diclofenac, ketoprofen, and ketorolac can be given by injection as well as by mouth. Intramuscular injections of diclofenac and ketoprofen are given deep into the gluteal muscle to minimise pain and tissue damage; diclofenac can also be given by intravenous infusion for the treatment or prevention of postoperative pain. Ketorolac is less irritant on intramuscular injection but pain has been reported; it can also be given by intravenous injection. Parecoxib (a selective inhibitor of cyclo-oxygenase-2) can be given by intramuscular or intravenous injection.

Suppositories of diclofenac and ketoprofen may be effective alternatives to the parenteral use of these drugs. Flurbiprofen is also available as suppositories.

KETOROLAC TROMETAMOL

Indications: short-term management of moderate to severe acute postoperative pain only

Cautions: see section 10.1.1; avoid in porphyria (section 9.8.2); **interactions:** Appendix 1 (NSAIDs)

Contra-indications: see section 10.1.1; also history of asthma, complete or partial syndrome of nasal polyps, angioedema or bronchospasm; history of peptic ulceration or gastro-intestinal bleeding; haemorrhagic diatheses (including coagulation disorders) and operations with high risk of haemorrhage or incomplete haemostasis; confirmed or suspected cerebrovascular bleeding; moderate or severe renal impairment; hypovolaemia or dehydration; pregnancy (including labour and delivery) and breast-feeding

Side-effects: see section 10.1.1; also anaphylaxis, dry mouth, excessive thirst, psychotic reactions, convulsions, myalgia, hyponatraemia, hyperkalaemia, flushing or pallor, bradycardia, hypertension, palpitations, chest pain, purpura, postoperative wound haemorrhage, haematoma, epistaxis; pain at injection site

Dose: _by mouth_, 10 mg every 4–6 hours (ELDERLY every 6–8 hours); max. 40 mg daily; max. duration of treatment 7 days; CHILD under 16 years, not recommended

By intramuscular injection or by intravenous injection over not less than 15 seconds, initially 10 mg, then 10–30 mg every 4–6 hours when required (every 2 hours in initial postoperative period); max. 90 mg daily (ELDERLY and patients weighing less than 50 kg, 60 mg daily); max. duration of treatment 2 days by either route; CHILD under 16 years, not recommended

NOTE. Pain relief may not occur for over 30 minutes after intravenous or intramuscular injection. When converting from parenteral to oral administration, total combined dose on the day of converting should not exceed 90 mg (60 mg in the elderly and patients weighing less than 50 kg) of which the oral component should not exceed

40 mg; patients should be converted to oral route as soon as possible

Toradol® (Roche) PoM
Tablets, ivory, f/c, ketorolac trometamol 10 mg, net price 20-tab pack = £6.23. Label: 17, 21
Injection, ketorolac trometamol 10 mg/mL, net price 1-mL amp = £1.02; 30 mg/mL, 1-mL amp = £1.22

PARECOXIB

NOTE. Parecoxib is a pro-drug of valdecoxib.
Indications: short-term management of acute postoperative pain
Cautions: see section 10.1.1; dehydration; following coronary artery bypass graft surgery; **interactions:** Appendix 1 (NSAIDs)
Contra-indications: see section 10.1.1; sulphonamide hypersensitivity, inflammatory bowel disease; severe congestive heart failure
Side-effects: see section 10.1.1; also flatulence, bradycardia, hypotension, hypertension, back pain, hypoaesthesia, hypokalaemia, pharyngitis, cerebrovascular disorders, rash (discontinue—risk of serious reactions including Stevens-Johnson syndrome and toxic epidermal necrolysis)
Dose: _by deep intramuscular injection or by intravenous injection_, initially 40 mg, then 20–40 mg every 6–12 hours when required; max. 80 mg daily; ELDERLY weighing less than 50 kg, initially 20 mg, then max. 40 mg daily; CHILD and ADOLESCENT under 18 years, not recommended

Dynastat® (Pharmacia) ▼ PoM
Injection, powder for reconstitution, parecoxib (as sodium salt), net price 40-mg vial = £4.96, 40-mg vial (with solvent) = £5.67

15.1.4.3 Opioid analgesics

Opioid analgesics are now rarely used as premedicants; they are more likely to be administered at induction. Pre-operative use of opioid analgesics is generally limited to those patients who require control of existing pain. The main side-effects of opioid analgesics are respiratory depression, cardiovascular depression, nausea, and vomiting; for general notes on opioid analgesics and their use in postoperative pain, see section 4.7.2.

For the management of opioid-induced respiratory depression, see section 15.1.7.

INTRA-OPERATIVE ANALGESIA. Opioid analgesics given in small doses before or with induction reduce the dose requirement of some drugs used during anaesthesia. Pethidine, morphine and papaveretum have been used for this purpose, but shorter-acting and more potent drugs such as alfentanil, fentanyl, and remifentanil are now preferred. Nalbuphine is seldom used.

Alfentanil, **fentanyl** and **remifentanil** are particularly useful because they act within 1–2 minutes. The initial doses of alfentanil or fentanyl are followed either by successive intravenous injections or by an intravenous infusion; prolonged infusions increase the duration of effect. Repeated intra-operative doses of alfentanil or fentanyl should be given with care since the respiratory depression can persist into the postoperative period and occasionally it may become apparent for the first time postoperatively when monitoring of the patient might be less intensive.

In contrast to other opioids which are metabolised in the liver, remifentanil undergoes rapid metabolism by non-specific blood and tissue esterases; its short duration of action allows prolonged administration at high dosage, without accumulation, and with little risk of residual postoperative respiratory depression. Remifentanil should not be given as a bolus injection intra-operatively, but it is well suited to continuous infusion; a supplemental analgesic will often be required after stopping the infusion.

ALFENTANIL

Indications: analgesia especially during short operative procedure and outpatient surgery; enhancement of anaesthesia; analgesia and suppression of respiratory activity in patients receiving intensive care, with assisted ventilation, for up to 4 days

Cautions: see section 4.7.2 and notes above
Contra-indications: see section 4.7.2 and notes above
Side-effects: see section 4.7.2 and notes above
Dose:

> To avoid excessive dosage in obese patients, dose may need to be calculated on the basis of ideal body-weight

By intravenous injection, spontaneous respiration, ADULT, initially up to 500 micrograms over 30 seconds; supplemental, 250 micrograms
With assisted ventilation, ADULT and CHILD, initially 30–50 micrograms/kg; supplemental, 15 micrograms/kg
By intravenous infusion, with assisted ventilation, ADULT and CHILD, initially 50–100 micrograms/kg over 10 minutes *or* as a bolus, followed by maintenance of 0.5–1 micrograms/kg/minute
Analgesia and suppression of respiratory activity during intensive care, with assisted ventilation, *by intravenous infusion*, initially 2 mg/hour subsequently adjusted according to response (usual range 0.5–10 mg/hour); more rapid initial control may be obtained with an intravenous dose of 5 mg given in divided portions over 10 minutes (slowing if hypotension or bradycardia occur); additional doses of 0.5–1 mg may be given by intravenous injection during short painful procedures

Rapifen® (Janssen-Cilag) [CD]
Injection, alfentanil (as hydrochloride) 500 micrograms/mL. Net price 2-mL amp = 72p; 10-mL amp = £3.31
Intensive care injection, alfentanil (as hydrochloride) 5 mg/mL. To be diluted before use. Net price 1-mL amp = £2.65

FENTANYL

Indications: analgesia during operation, enhancement of anaesthesia; respiratory depressant in assisted respiration; analgesia in other situations (section 4.7.2)

Cautions: see section 4.7.2 and notes above
Contra-indications: see section 4.7.2 and notes above
Side-effects: see section 4.7.2 and notes above
Dose: *by intravenous injection*, with spontaneous respiration, 50–200 micrograms, then 50 micrograms as required; CHILD 3–5 micrograms/kg, then 1 microgram/kg as required
With assisted ventilation, 0.3–3.5 mg, then 100–200 micrograms as required; CHILD 15 micrograms/kg, then 1–3 micrograms/kg as required

Fentanyl (Non-proprietary) [CD]
Injection, fentanyl (as citrate) 50 micrograms/mL, net price 2-mL amp = 24p, 10-mL amp = £1.17
Available from Antigen, Auden Mckenzie

Sublimaze® (Janssen-Cilag) [CD]
Injection, fentanyl (as citrate) 50 micrograms/mL, net price 2-mL amp = 24p, 10-mL amp = £1.17

REMIFENTANIL

Indications: supplementation of general anaesthesia during induction and analgesia during maintenance of anaesthesia (consult product literature for use in patients undergoing cardiac surgery); analgesia and sedation in ventilated, intensive care patients

Cautions: see section 4.7.2 and notes above
Contra-indications: see section 4.7.2 and notes above
Side-effects: see section 4.7.2 and notes above
Dose:

> To avoid excessive dosage in obese patients, dose should be calculated on the basis of ideal body-weight

Induction, *by intravenous infusion*, 0.5–1 microgram/kg/minute, *with or without* an initial bolus *by intravenous injection* (of a solution containing 20–250 micrograms/mL) over not less than 30 seconds, 1 microgram/kg
NOTE. If patient is to be intubated more than 8 minutes after start of intravenous infusion, initial intravenous injection dose is unnecessary
Maintenance in ventilated patients, *by intravenous infusion*, 0.05–2 micrograms/kg/minute according to anaesthetic technique and adjusted according to response; supplemental doses in light anaesthesia, *by intravenous injection* every 2–5 minutes
Maintenance in spontaneous respiration anaesthesia, *by intravenous infusion*, initially 40 nanograms/kg/minute adjusted according to response, usual range 25–100 nanograms/minute
CHILD 1–12 years, maintenance, *by intravenous infusion*, 0.05–1.3 micrograms/kg/minute (*with or without* an initial bolus *by intravenous injection* over not less than 30 seconds, 1 microgram/kg/minute) according to anaesthetic technique and adjusted according to response
Analgesia and sedation in ventilated, intensive care patients, *by intravenous infusion*, ADULT over 18 years initially 100–150 nanograms/kg/minute adjusted according to response, usual range 6–740 nanograms/kg/minute; if an infusion rate of 200 nanograms/kg/minute does not produce adequate sedation add another sedative (consult product literature for details); additional analgesia during stimulating or painful procedures, *by intravenous infusion*, ADULT over 18 years maintain infusion of at least 100 nanograms/kg/minute for at least 5 minutes before procedure and adjust every 2–5 minutes according to requirements, usual range 250–750 nanograms/kg/minute

Ultiva® (Elan) ☐CD☐

Injection, powder for reconstitution, remifentanil (as hydrochloride), net price 1-mg vial = £5.50; 2-mg vial = £11.00; 5-mg vial = £27.50

15.1.5 Muscle relaxants

Muscle relaxants used in anaesthesia are also known as **neuromuscular blocking drugs**. By specific blockade of the neuromuscular junction they enable light levels of anaesthesia to be employed with adequate relaxation of the muscles of the abdomen and diaphragm. They also relax the vocal cords and allow the passage of a tracheal tube. Their action differs from the muscle relaxants acting on the spinal cord or brain which are used in musculoskeletal disorders (section 10.2.2).

Patients who have received a muscle relaxant should **always** have their respiration assisted or controlled until the drug has been inactivated or antagonised (section 15.1.6).

Non-depolarising muscle relaxants

Non-depolarising muscle relaxants (also known as competitive muscle relaxants) compete with acetyl-choline for receptor sites at the neuromuscular junction and their action may be reversed with anticholinesterases such as neostigmine (section 15.1.6). Non-depolarising muscle relaxants may be divided into the **aminosteroid** group which includes pancuronium, rocuronium and vecuronium, and the **benzylisoquinolinium** group which includes atracurium, cisatracurium, gallamine and mivacurium.

Non-depolarising muscle relaxants have a slower onset of action than suxamethonium. These drugs can be classified by their duration of action as short-acting (15–30 minutes), intermediate-acting (30–40 minutes) and long-acting (60–120 minutes), although duration of action is dose-dependent. Drugs with a shorter or intermediate duration of action, such as atracurium and vecuronium, are more widely employed than those with a longer duration of action such as pancuronium.

Non-depolarising muscle relaxants have no sedative or analgesic effects and are not considered to be a triggering factor for malignant hyperthermia.

For patients receiving intensive care and who require tracheal intubation and mechanical ventilation, a non-depolarising muscle relaxant is chosen according to its onset of effect, duration of action and side-effects. Rocuronium, with a rapid onset of effect, may facilitate intubation. Atracurium or cisatracurium may be suitable for long-term muscle relaxation since their duration of action is not dependent on elimination by the liver or the kidneys.

CAUTIONS. Allergic cross-reactivity between neuromuscular blocking agents has been reported; caution is advised in cases of hypersensitivity to these drugs. Their activity is prolonged in patients with myasthenia gravis and in hypothermia, therefore lower doses are required. Resistance may develop in patients with burns who may require increased doses; low plasma cholinesterase activity in these patients requires dose titration for mivacurium. **Interactions:** Appendix 1 (muscle relaxants).

SIDE-EFFECTS. Benzylisoquinolinium non-depolarising muscle relaxants (except cisatracurium) are associated with histamine release which can cause skin flushing, hypotension, tachycardia, broncho-spasm and rarely, anaphylactoid reactions. Aminosteroid muscle relaxants produce minimal histamine release. Drugs possessing vagolytic activity can counteract any bradycardia that occurs during surgery.

Atracurium is a mixture of 10 isomers and is a benzylisoquinolinium muscle relaxant with an intermediate duration of action. It undergoes non-enzymatic metabolism which is independent of liver and kidney function, thus allowing its use in patients with hepatic or renal impairment. Cardiovascular effects are associated with significant histamine release.

Cisatracurium is a single isomer of atracurium. It is more potent and has a slightly longer duration of action than atracurium and provides greater cardiovascular stability because cisatracurium lacks histamine-releasing effects.

Mivacurium, a benzylisoquinolinium muscle relaxant, has a short duration of action. It is metabolised by plasma cholinesterase and muscle paralysis is prolonged in individuals deficient in this enzyme. It is not associated with vagolytic activity or ganglionic blockade although histamine release may occur, particularly with rapid injection.

Pancuronium, an aminosteroid muscle relaxant, has a long duration of action and is often used in patients receiving long-term mechanical ventilation in intensive care units. It lacks a histamine-releasing effect, but vagolytic and sympathomimetic effects can cause tachycardia and hypertension.

Rocuronium exerts an effect within 2 minutes and has the most rapid onset of any of the competitive muscle relaxants. It is an aminosteroid muscle relaxant with an intermediate duration of action. It is reported to have minimal cardiovascular effects; high doses produce mild vagolytic activity.

Vecuronium, an aminosteroid muscle relaxant, has an intermediate duration of action. It does not generally produce histamine release and lacks cardiovascular effects.

Gallamine has vagolytic and sympathomimetic properties and frequently increases pulse rate and blood pressure. It is rarely used since the other neuromuscular blocking drugs have a more predictable response and it should be avoided in patients with renal impairment.

ATRACURIUM BESILATE

(Atracurium besylate)

Indications: muscle relaxation (short to intermediate duration) for surgery or during intensive care

Cautions: see notes above

Side-effects: see notes above

Dose: surgery or intubation, ADULT and CHILD over 1 month, *by intravenous injection*, initially 300–600 micrograms/kg; maintenance, *by intravenous injection*, 100–200 micrograms/kg as required *or by intravenous infusion*, 5–10 micrograms/kg/minute (300–600 micrograms/kg/hour)

Intensive care, ADULT and CHILD over 1 month, *by intravenous injection*, initially 300–600 micrograms/kg (optional) then *by intravenous infusion* 4.5–29.5 micrograms/kg/minute (usual dose 11–13 micrograms/kg/minute)

Atracurium (Non-proprietary) [PoM]
Injection, atracurium besilate 10 mg/mL, net price
2.5-mL amp = £1.85; 5-mL amp = £3.37; 25-mL
amp = £14.45
Available from Mayne

Tracrium® (GSK) [PoM]
Injection, atracurium besilate 10 mg/mL, net price
2.5-mL amp = £1.78; 5-mL amp = £3.23; 25-mL
amp = £13.88

CISATRACURIUM

Indications: muscle relaxation (intermediate duration) for surgery or during intensive care
Cautions: see notes above
Side-effects: see notes above
Dose: intubation, *by intravenous injection*, ADULT
and CHILD over 1 month, initially 150 micrograms/
kg; maintenance, *by intravenous injection*,
30 micrograms/kg approx. every 20 minutes;
CHILD 2–12 years, 20 micrograms/kg approx.
every 9 minutes; or maintenance, *by intravenous
infusion*, ADULT and CHILD over 2 years, initially,
3 micrograms/kg/minute, *then after stabilisation*,
1–2 micrograms/kg/minute; dose reduced by up to
40% if used with enflurane or isoflurane
Intensive care, *by intravenous infusion*, ADULT 0.5–
10.2 micrograms/kg/minute (usual dose 3 micr-
ograms/kg/minute)
NOTE. Lower doses can be used for children over 2 years
when not for intubation

Nimbex® (GSK) [PoM]
Injection, cisatracurium (as besilate) 2 mg/mL, net
price 2.5-mL amp = £2.20, 5-mL amp = £4.20, 10-
mL amp = £8.12
Forte injection, cisatracurium (as besilate) 5 mg/
mL, net price 30-mL vial = £33.43

GALLAMINE TRIETHIODIDE ▰

Indications: muscle relaxation (intermediate dura-
tion) for surgery
Cautions: see notes above
Contra-indications: renal impairment
Side-effects: see notes above
Dose: *by intravenous injection*, 80–120 mg, then
20–40 mg as required; NEONATE 600 micrograms/
kg; CHILD 1.5 mg/kg

Flaxedil® (Concord) [PoM] ▰
Injection, gallamine triethiodide 40 mg/mL, net
price 2-mL amp = £4.97

MIVACURIUM

Indications: muscle relaxation (short duration) for
surgery
Cautions: see notes above; low plasma cholinesterase activity
Side-effects: see notes above
Dose: *by intravenous injection*, 70–250 micr-
ograms/kg; maintenance 100 micrograms/kg every
15 minutes; CHILD 2–6 months initially 150 micr-
ograms/kg, 7 months–12 years initially 200 micr-
ograms/kg; maintenance (CHILD 2 months–12
years) 100 micrograms/kg every 6–9 minutes
NOTE. Doses up to 150 micrograms/kg may be given over
5–15 seconds, higher doses should be given over 30
seconds. In patients with asthma, cardiovascular disease
or those who are sensitive to falls in arterial blood
pressure give over 60 seconds

By intravenous infusion, maintenance of block, 8–
10 micrograms/kg/minute, adjusted if necessary
every 3 minutes by 1 microgram/kg/minute to
usual dose of 6–7 micrograms/kg/minute; CHILD
2 months–12 years, usual dose 11–14 micrograms/
kg/minute

Mivacron® (GSK) [PoM]
Injection, mivacurium (as chloride) 2 mg/mL, net
price 5-mL amp = £3.00; 10-mL amp = £4.85

PANCURONIUM BROMIDE

Indications: muscle relaxation (long duration) for
surgery or during intensive care
Cautions: see notes above; hepatic impairment
(Appendix 2); renal impairment (Appendix 3);
pregnancy (Appendix 4) and breast-feeding
(Appendix 5)
Side-effects: see notes above
Dose: *by intravenous injection*, initially for intubation 50–100 micrograms/kg then 10–20 micr-
ograms/kg as required; CHILD initially 60–
100 micrograms/kg, then 10–20 micrograms/kg,
NEONATE 30–40 micrograms/kg initially then
10–20 micrograms/kg
Intensive care, *by intravenous injection*, 60 micr-
ograms/kg every 60–90 minutes

Pancuronium (Non-proprietary) [PoM]
Injection, pancuronium bromide 2 mg/mL, net price
2-mL amp = 65p
Available from Antigen, Mayne

ROCURONIUM BROMIDE

Indications: muscle relaxation (intermediate duration) for surgery or during intensive care
Cautions: see notes above; hepatic impairment
(Appendix 2); renal impairment (Appendix 3);
pregnancy (Appendix 4) and breast-feeding
(Appendix 5)
Side-effects: see notes above
Dose: intubation, ADULT and CHILD over 1 month,
by intravenous injection, initially 600 micrograms/
kg; maintenance *by intravenous injection*,
150 micrograms/kg (ELDERLY 75–100 micr-
ograms/kg) *or* maintenance *by intravenous infusion*, 300–600 micrograms/kg/hour (ELDERLY up to
400 micrograms/kg/hour)
Intensive care, *by intravenous injection*, ADULT
initially 600 micrograms/kg; maintenance *by intravenous infusion*, 300–600 micrograms/kg/hour for
first hour, then adjusted according to response

Esmeron® (Organon) [PoM]
Injection, rocuronium bromide 10 mg/mL, net price
5-mL vial = £3.23, 10-mL vial = £6.46

VECURONIUM BROMIDE

Indications: muscle relaxation (intermediate duration) for surgery
Cautions: see notes above
Side-effects: see notes above
Dose: *by intravenous injection*, intubation, 80–
100 micrograms/kg; maintenance 20–30 micr-
ograms/kg according to response; NEONATE and
INFANT up to 4 months, initially 10–20 micr-
ograms/kg then incremental doses to achieve
response; CHILD over 5 months, as adult dose (up
to 1 year onset more rapid and high intubation dose
may not be required)

By intravenous infusion, 0.8–1.4 micrograms/kg/minute (after initial intravenous injection of 40–100 micrograms/kg)

Norcuron® (Organon) [PoM]
Injection, powder for reconstitution, vecuronium bromide, net price 10-mg vial = £4.24 (with water for injections)

Depolarising muscle relaxants

Suxamethonium has the most rapid onset of action of any of the muscle relaxants and is ideal if fast onset and brief duration of action are required e.g. with tracheal intubation. Its duration of action is about 2 to 6 minutes following intravenous doses of about 1 mg/kg; repeated doses can be used for longer procedures.

Suxamethonium acts by mimicking acetylcholine at the neuromuscular junction but hydrolysis is much slower than for acetylcholine; depolarisation is therefore prolonged resulting in neuromuscular blockade. Unlike the non-depolarising muscle relaxants, its action cannot be reversed and recovery is spontaneous; anticholinesterases such as neostigmine potentiate the neuromuscular block.

Suxamethonium should be given after anaesthetic induction because paralysis is usually preceded by painful muscle fasciculations. While tachycardia occurs with single use, bradycardia may occur with repeated doses in adults and with the first dose in children. Premedication with atropine reduces bradycardia as well as the excessive salivation associated with suxamethonium use.

Prolonged paralysis may occur in **dual block**, which occurs with high or repeated doses of suxamethonium and is caused by the development of a non-depolarising block following the initial depolarising block; edrophonium (section 15.1.6) may be used to confirm the diagnosis of dual block. Individuals with myasthenia gravis are resistant to suxamethonium but can develop dual block resulting in delayed recovery. Prolonged paralysis may also occur in those with low or atypical plasma cholinesterase. Assisted ventilation should be continued until muscle function is restored.

SUXAMETHONIUM CHLORIDE

Indications: muscle relaxation (rapid onset, short duration)
Cautions: see notes above; pregnancy (Appendix 4); patients with cardiac, respiratory or neuromuscular disease; raised intra-ocular pressure (avoid in penetrating eye injury); severe sepsis (risk of hyperkalaemia); **interactions:** Appendix 1 (muscle relaxants)
Contra-indications: family history of malignant hyperthermia, low plasma cholinesterase activity (including severe liver disease) (Appendix 2), hyperkalaemia; major trauma, severe burns, neurological disease involving acute wasting of major muscle, prolonged immobilisation—risk of hyperkalaemia, personal or family history of congenital myotonic disease, Duchenne muscular dystrophy
Side-effects: see notes above; also postoperative muscle pain, myoglobinuria, myoglobinaemia; tachycardia, arrhythmias, cardiac arrest, hypertension, hypotension; bronchospasm, apnoea, prolonged respiratory depression, anaphylactic reactions; hyperkalaemia; hyperthermia; increased gastric pressure; rash, flushing
Dose: *by intravenous injection,* initially 1 mg/kg; maintenance, usually 0.5–1 mg/kg at 5–10 minute intervals; max. 500 mg/hour; NEONATE and INFANT, 2 mg/kg; CHILD, 1 mg/kg
By intravenous infusion of a solution containing 1–2 mg/mL (0.1–0.2%), 2.5–4 mg/minute; max. 500 mg/hour; CHILD reduce infusion rate according to body-weight
By intramuscular injection, INFANT up to 4–5 mg/kg; CHILD up to 4 mg/kg; max. 150 mg

Suxamethonium Chloride (Non-proprietary) [PoM]
Injection, suxamethonium chloride 50 mg/mL, net price 2-mL amp = 70p, 2-mL prefilled syringe = £7.00
Available from Antigen, Aurum

Anectine® (GSK) [PoM]
Injection, suxamethonium chloride 50 mg/mL, net price 2-mL amp = 77p

15.1.6 Anticholinesterases used in anaesthesia

Anticholinesterases reverse the effects of the non-depolarising (competitive) muscle relaxant drugs such as pancuronium but they prolong the action of the depolarising muscle relaxant drug suxamethonium.

Edrophonium has a transient action and may be used in the diagnosis of suspected dual block due to suxamethonium.

Neostigmine has a longer duration of action than edrophonium. It is the specific drug for reversal of non-depolarising (competitive) blockade. It acts within one minute of intravenous injection and lasts for 20 to 30 minutes; a second dose may then be necessary. Atropine or preferably glycopyrronium (section 15.1.3) should be given before or with neostigmine in order to prevent bradycardia, excessive salivation, and other muscarinic actions of neostigmine.

EDROPHONIUM CHLORIDE

Indications: see under Dose; myasthenia gravis (section 10.2.1)
Cautions: see section 10.2.1 and notes above; atropine should also be given
Contra-indications: see section 10.2.1 and notes above
Side-effects: see section 10.2.1 and notes above
Dose: brief reversal of non-depolarising neuromuscular blockade, *by intravenous injection* over several minutes, 500–700 micrograms/kg (after or with atropine sulphate 600 micrograms)
Diagnosis of dual block, *by intravenous injection,* 10 mg

Edrophonium (Non-proprietary) [PoM]
Injection, edrophonium chloride 10 mg/mL, net price 1-mL amp = £4.76
Available from Cambridge

NEOSTIGMINE METILSULFATE

(Neostigmine methylsulphate)

Indications: see under Dose

Cautions: see section 10.2.1 and notes above; atropine should also be given

Contra-indications: see section 10.2.1 and notes above

Side-effects: see section 10.2.1 and notes above

Dose: reversal of non-depolarising neuromuscular blockade, *by intravenous injection* over 1 minute, 50–70 micrograms/kg (max. 5 mg) after or with atropine sulphate 0.6–1.2 mg
Myasthenia gravis, see section 10.2.1

Neostigmine (Non-proprietary) PoM
Injection, neostigmine metilsulfate 2.5 mg/mL, net price 1-mL amp = 58p

■ With glycopyrronium
Robinul-Neostigmine® (Anpharm) PoM
Injection, neostigmine metilsulfate 2.5 mg, glyco-pyrronium bromide 500 micrograms/mL, net price 1-mL amp = £1.01
Dose: reversal of non-depolarising neuromuscular block-ade *by intravenous injection* over 10–30 seconds, 1–2 mL *or* 0.02 mL/kg, dose may be repeated if required (total max. 2 mL); CHILD 0.02 mL/kg (*or* 0.2 mL/kg of a 1 in 10 dilution using water for injections or sodium chloride injection 0.9%), dose may be repeated if required (total max. 2 mL)

15.1.7 Antagonists for central and respiratory depression

Respiratory depression is a major concern with opioid analgesics and it may be treated by artificial ventilation or be reversed by **naloxone**. Naloxone will immediately reverse opioid-induced respiratory depression but the dose may have to be repeated because of the short duration of action of naloxone; however, naloxone will also antagonise the analgesic effect.

Flumazenil is a benzodiazepine antagonist for the reversal of the central sedative effects of benzodiaz-epines after anaesthetic and similar procedures. Flumazenil has a shorter half-life than that of diazepam and midazolam (and there is a risk that patients may become resedated).

Doxapram (section 3.5.1) is a central and respir-atory stimulant but is of limited value.

FLUMAZENIL

Indications: reversal of sedative effects of benzo-diazepines in anaesthetic, intensive care, and diagnostic procedures

Cautions: short-acting (repeat doses may be neces-sary—benzodiazepine effects may persist for at least 24 hours); benzodiazepine dependence (may precipitate withdrawal symptoms); prolonged ben-zodiazepine therapy for epilepsy (risk of con-vulsions); history of panic disorders (risk of recurrence); ensure neuromuscular blockade cleared before giving; avoid rapid injection in high-risk or anxious patients and following major surgery; hepatic impairment; head injury (rapid reversal of benzodiazepine sedation may cause

convulsions); elderly, children, pregnancy and breast-feeding

Contra-indications: life-threatening condition (e.g. raised intracranial pressure, status epilepticus) controlled by benzodiazepines

Side-effects: nausea, vomiting, and flushing; if wakening too rapid, agitation, anxiety, and fear; transient increase in blood pressure and heart-rate in intensive care patients; very rarely convulsions (particularly in epileptics)

Dose: *by intravenous injection*, 200 micrograms over 15 seconds, then 100 micrograms at 60-second intervals if required; usual dose range, 300–600 micrograms; max. total dose 1 mg (2 mg in intensive care); question aetiology if no response to repeated doses
By intravenous infusion, if drowsiness recurs after injection, 100–400 micrograms/hour, adjusted according to level of arousal

Anexate® (Roche) PoM
Injection, flumazenil 100 micrograms/mL, net price 5-mL amp = £15.59

NALOXONE HYDROCHLORIDE

Indications: reversal of opioid-induced respiratory depression; overdosage with opioids (Emergency Treatment of Poisoning)

Cautions: cardiovascular disease or those receiving cardiotoxic drugs (serious adverse cardiovascular effects reported); physical dependence on opioids (precipitates withdrawal); pain (see also under Titration of Dose, below); has short duration of action (repeated doses or infusion may be neces-sary to reverse effects of opioids with longer duration of action)
TITRATION OF DOSE. In postoperative use, the dose should be titrated for each patient in order to obtain sufficient respiratory response; however, naloxone antag-onises analgesia

Side-effects: nausea and vomiting reported; tachy-cardia and fibrillation also reported

Dose: *by intravenous injection*, 100–200 micr-ograms (1.5–3 micrograms/kg); if response inade-quate, increments of 100 micrograms every 2 minutes; further doses *by intramuscular injection* after 1–2 hours if required
CHILD *by intravenous injection*, 10 micrograms/kg; subsequent dose of 100 micrograms/kg if no response; if intravenous route not possible, may be given in divided doses by *intramuscular or sub-cutaneous injection*
NEONATE *by subcutaneous, intramuscular, or intravenous injection*, 10 micrograms/kg, repeated every 2 to 3 minutes *or by intramuscular injection*, 200 micrograms (60 micrograms/kg) as a single dose at birth (onset of action slower)

Naloxone PoM —see under Emergency Treatment of Poisoning p. 24

Narcan® PoM —see under Emergency Treatment of Poisoning p. 24

Narcan Neonatal® (Bristol-Myers Squibb) PoM
Injection, naloxone hydrochloride 20 micrograms/ mL, net price 2-mL amp = £3.32

15.1.8 Drugs for malignant hyperthermia

Malignant hyperthermia is a rare but potentially lethal complication of anaesthesia. It is characterised by a rapid rise in temperature, increased muscle rigidity, tachycardia, and acidosis. The most common triggers of malignant hyperthermia are the volatile anaesthetics. Suxamethonium has also been implicated, but malignant hyperthermia is more likely if it is given following a volatile anaesthetic. Known trigger agents should be avoided during anaesthesia.

Dantrolene is used in the treatment of malignant hyperthermia. It acts on skeletal muscle cells by interfering with calcium efflux, thereby stopping the contractile process.

DANTROLENE SODIUM

Indications: malignant hyperthermia

Cautions: avoid extravasation; **interactions:** Appendix 1 (muscle relaxants)

Dose: *by rapid intravenous injection,* 1 mg/kg, repeated as required to a cumulative max. of 10 mg/kg

Dantrium Intravenous® (Procter & Gamble Pharm.) PoM

Injection, powder for reconstitution, dantrolene sodium, net price 20-mg vial = £16.22 (hosp. only)

15.2 Local anaesthesia

The use of local anaesthetics by injection or by application to mucous membranes to produce local analgesia is discussed in this section.

See also section 1.7 (colon and rectum), section 11.7 (eye), section 12.3 (oropharynx), and section 13.3 (skin).

USE OF LOCAL ANAESTHETICS. Local anaesthetic drugs act by causing a reversible block to conduction along nerve fibres. The drugs used vary widely in their potency, toxicity, duration of action, stability, solubility in water, and ability to penetrate mucous membranes. These variations determine their suitability for use by various routes, e.g. topical (surface), infiltration, plexus, epidural (extradural) or spinal block.

The cold sensation produced by **ethyl chloride** spray is used to test the onset of regional anaesthesia; it is also used as a local anaesthetic for minor skin procedures.

ADMINISTRATION. In estimating the safe dosage of these drugs it is important to take account of the rate at which they are absorbed and excreted as well as their potency. The patient's age, weight, physique, and clinical condition, the degree of vascularity of the area to which the drug is to be applied, and the duration of administration are other factors which must be taken into account.

Local anaesthetics do not rely on the circulation to transport them to their sites of action, but uptake into the systemic circulation is important in terminating their action and producing toxicity. Following most regional anaesthetic procedures, maximum arterial plasma concentrations of anaesthetic develop within about 10 to 25 minutes, so **careful surveillance** for

toxic effects is necessary during the first 30 minutes after injection. Great care must be taken to avoid accidental intravascular injection.

Epidural anaesthesia is commonly used during surgery, often combined with general anaesthesia, because of its protective effect against the stress response of surgery. It is often used when good postoperative pain relief is essential (e.g. aortic aneurysm surgery or major gut surgery).

TOXICITY. Toxic effects associated with local anaesthetics usually result from excessively high plasma concentrations; single application of topical lidocaine preparations does not generally cause systemic side-effects. Effects initially include a feeling of inebriation and lightheadedness followed by sedation, circumoral paraesthesia and twitching; convulsions can occur in severe reactions. On intravenous injection convulsions and cardiovascular collapse may occur very rapidly. Hypersensitivity reactions occur mainly with the ester-type local anaesthetics such as benzocaine, cocaine, procaine, and tetracaine (amethocaine); reactions are less frequent with the amide types such as lidocaine, (lignocaine), bupivacaine, prilocaine, and ropivacaine.

When prolonged analgesia is required, a long-acting local anaesthetic is preferred to minimise the likelihood of cumulative systemic toxicity. Local anaesthetic injections should be given slowly in order to detect inadvertent intravascular administration. Local anaesthetics should **not** be injected into inflamed or infected tissues nor should they be applied to the traumatised urethra. In such cases absorption into the blood may increase the possibility of systemic side-effects. The local anaesthetic effect may also be reduced by the altered local pH.

USE OF VASOCONSTRICTORS. Most local anaesthetics, with the exception of cocaine, cause dilation of blood vessels. The addition of a vasoconstrictor such as **adrenaline (epinephrine)** diminishes local blood flow, slows the rate of absorption of the local anaesthetic, and prolongs its local effect. Adrenaline must be used in a low concentration (e.g. 1 in 200 000) for this purpose and it should **not** be given with a local anaesthetic injection in digits and appendages; it may produce ischaemic necrosis.

When adrenaline is included the final concentration should be 1 in 200 000 (5 micrograms/mL). In dental surgery, up to 1 in 80 000 (12.5 micrograms/mL) of adrenaline is used with local anaesthetics. There is no justification for using higher concentrations.

The total dose of adrenaline should **not** exceed 500 micrograms and it is essential not to exceed a concentration of 1 in 200 000 (5 micrograms/mL) if more than 50 mL of the mixture is to be injected. For general cautions associated with the use of adrenaline, see section 2.7.3. For drug interactions, see Appendix 1 (sympathomimetics).

Lidocaine

Lidocaine (lignocaine) is effectively absorbed from mucous membranes and is a useful surface anaesthetic in concentrations of 2 to 4%. Except for surface anaesthesia, solutions should not usually exceed 1% in strength. The duration of the block (with adrenaline) is about 90 minutes.

LIDOCAINE HYDROCHLORIDE
(Lignocaine hydrochloride)

Indications: see under Dose; also dental anaesthesia (see below); ventricular arrhythmias (section 2.3.2)

Cautions: epilepsy, hepatic or respiratory impairment, impaired cardiac conduction, bradycardia; porphyria (section 9.8.2); reduce dose in elderly or debilitated; resuscitative equipment should be available; see section 2.3.2 for effects on heart; **interactions:** Appendix 1 (lidocaine)

Contra-indications: hypovolaemia, complete heart block; do not use solutions containing adrenaline for anaesthesia in appendages

Side-effects: CNS effects include confusion, respiratory depression and convulsions; hypotension and bradycardia (may lead to cardiac arrest); hypersensitivity reported; see also notes above

Dose: infiltration anaesthesia, *by injection*, according to patient's weight and nature of procedure, max. 200 mg (or 500 mg if given in solutions containing adrenaline)—see also Administration on p. 614 and see also **important** warning below
Intravenous regional anaesthesia and nerve blocks, seek expert advice
Surface anaesthesia, usual strengths 2–4%, see preparations below

> **Important.** The licensed doses stated above may not be appropriate in some settings and expert advice should be sought

■ Lidocaine hydrochloride injections

Lidocaine (Non-proprietary) PoM
Injection 0.5%, lidocaine hydrochloride 5 mg/mL, net price 10-mL amp = 35p
Injection 1%, lidocaine hydrochloride 10 mg/mL, net price 2-mL amp = 21p; 5-mL amp = 22p; 10-mL amp = 35p; 10-mL prefilled syringe = £4.53; 20-mL amp =58p
Injection 2%, lidocaine hydrochloride 20 mg/mL, net price 2-mL amp = 28p; 5-mL amp = 25p

Xylocaine® (AstraZeneca) PoM
Injection 1% with adrenaline 1 in 200 000, anhydrous lidocaine hydrochloride 10 mg/mL, adrenaline 1 in 200 000 (5 micrograms/mL), net price 20-mL vial = 76p
Injection 2% with adrenaline 1 in 200 000, anhydrous lidocaine hydrochloride 20 mg/mL, adrenaline 1 in 200 000 (5 micrograms/mL), net price 20-mL vial = 81p

■ Lidocaine injections for dental use
NOTE. Consult expert dental sources for specific advice in relation to dose of lidocaine for dental anaesthesia
A variety of lidocaine injections with adrenaline is available in dental cartridges; brand names include *Lignospan Special*®, *Lignostab*® *A*, *Rexocaine*®, *Xylocaine*®, and *Xylotox*®.

■ Lidocaine for surface anaesthesia
Important. Rapid and extensive absorption may result in systemic side-effects

Lidocaine (Non-proprietary)
Gel, lidocaine hydrochloride 1%, net price 15 mL = £1.30; 2%, 15 mL = £1.30
Dose: urethral catheterisation, into urethra at least 5 minutes before catheter insertion, MEN 10 mL followed by further 3–5 mL; WOMEN 3–5 mL; CHILD 1–5 mL

Mucocutaneous anaesthesia, 2–3 mL applied when necessary; CHILD 1–2 mL
Major aphthae in immunocompromised patients, 2–3 mL applied when necessary, max. 15 mL in 24 hours; CHILD 1–2 mL, max. 8 mL in 24 hours
Available from APS
Ointment, lidocaine hydrochloride 5%, net price 15 g = 88p
Dose: dental practice, rub gently into dry gum
Sore nipples from breast-feeding, apply using gauze and wash off immediately before feed
Pain relief (in anal fissures, haemorrhoids, pruritus ani, pruritus vulvae, herpes zoster, or herpes labialis), 1–2 mL applied when necessary; avoid long-term use
Available from APS
Solution, lidocaine hydrochloride 4%, net price 25 mL = £1.35
Dose: biopsy in mouth, 3–4 mL with suitable spray *or* swab (with adrenaline if necessary); max. 5 mL, ELDERLY lower max. dose, CHILD max. 3 mg/kg
Puncture of maxillary sinus or polypectomy, apply with swab for 2–3 minutes (with adrenaline); max. 5 mL, ELDERLY lower max. dose, CHILD max. 3 mg/kg
Bronchoscopy and bronchography, 2–3 mL with suitable spray; max. 5 mL, ELDERLY lower max. dose, CHILD max. 3 mg/kg
Available from APS

Lidocaine and chlorhexidine (Non-proprietary)
Gel, lidocaine hydrochloride 1%, chlorhexidine gluconate solution 0.25%, net price 15 mL = 70p; lidocaine hydrochloride 2%, chlorhexidine gluconate solution 0.25%, 15 mL = 70p
Dose: urethral catheterisation, into urethra at least 5 minutes before catheter insertion, MEN 10 mL followed by further 3–5 mL; WOMEN 3–5 mL; CHILD 1–5 mL
Mucocutaneous anaesthesia, 2–3 mL applied when necessary; CHILD 1–2 mL
Major aphthae in immunocompromised patients, 2–3 mL applied when necessary, max. 15 mL in 24 hours; CHILD 1–2 mL, max. 8 mL in 24 hours
Available from APS

Emla® (AstraZeneca) PoM
Drug Tariff cream, lidocaine 2.5%, prilocaine 2.5%, net price 5-g tube = £1.73
Surgical pack cream, lidocaine 2.5%, prilocaine 2.5%, net price 30-g tube = £10.25
Premedication pack cream, lidocaine 2.5%, prilocaine 2.5%, net price 5 × 5-g tube with 12 occlusive dressings = £9.75
Cautions: not for wounds, mucous membranes (except genital warts in adults), or atopic dermatitis; avoid use near eyes or middle ear; although systemic absorption low, caution in anaemia, or in congenital or acquired methaemoglobinaemia (see also Prilocaine, p. 617)
Side-effects: include transient paleness, redness, and oedema
Dose: anaesthesia before minor skin procedures including venepuncture, apply thick layer under occlusive dressing 1–5 hours before procedure (2–5 hours before procedures on large areas e.g. split skin grafting); INFANT 1–12 months [unlicensed use] single application on intact skin under specialist supervision, under 1 month not recommended (risk of methaemoglobinaemia, see Cautions below)
Removal of warts from genital mucosa in adults, apply up to 10 g 5–10 minutes before removal

Instillagel® (CliniMed)
Gel, lidocaine hydrochloride 2%, chlorhexidine gluconate solution 0.25%, in a sterile lubricant basis in disposable syringe, net price 6-mL syringe = £1.51, 11-mL syringe = £1.70
Excipients: include hydroxybenzoates (parabens)
Dose: 6–11 mL into urethra

Laryng-O-Jet ® (Celltech) [PoM]
Jet spray 4% (disposable kit for laryngotracheal anaesthesia), lidocaine hydrochloride 40 mg/mL, net price per unit (4-mL vial and disposable sterile cannula with cover and vial injector) = £5.10
Cautions: may be rapidly and almost completely absorbed from respiratory tract and systemic side-effects may occur; extreme caution if mucosa has been traumatised or if sepsis present
Dose: usually 160 mg (4 mL) as a single dose instilled as jet spray into lumen of larynx and trachea (reduce dose according to size, age and condition of patient); max. 200 mg (5 mL)

Xylocaine® (AstraZeneca)
Spray (= pump spray), lidocaine 10% (100 mg/g) supplying 10 mg lidocaine/dose; 500 spray doses per container. Net price 50-mL bottle = £3.13
Dose: dental practice, 1–5 doses
Maxillary sinus puncture, 3 doses
During delivery in obstetrics, up to 20 doses
Procedures in pharynx, larynx, and trachea, up to 20 doses
Topical 4%, anhydrous lidocaine hydrochloride 40 mg/mL, net price 30-mL bottle = £1.21
Excipients: include hydroxybenzoates (parabens)
Dose: bronchoscopy, 1–7.5 mL with suitable spray
Biopsy in mouth, 3–4 mL with suitable spray *or* swab (with adrenaline if necessary); max. 7.5 mL

▪ Lidocaine for ear, nose, and oropharyngeal use
Lidocaine with Phenylephrine (Non-proprietary)
Topical solution, lidocaine hydrochloride 5%, phenylephrine hydrochloride 0.5%, net price 2.5 mL (with nasal applicator) = £8.24. For cautions, contra-indications and side-effects of phenylephrine, see section 2.7.2
Available from Aurum

Bupivacaine

The advantage of bupivacaine over other local anaesthetics is its longer duration of action. It has a slow onset of action, taking up to 30 minutes for full effect. It is often used in lumbar epidural blockade and is particularly suitable for continuous epidural analgesia in labour. It is the principal drug for spinal anaesthesia in the UK.

BUPIVACAINE HYDROCHLORIDE

Indications: see under Dose
Cautions: see under Lidocaine Hydrochloride and notes above; myocardial depression may be more severe and more resistant to treatment; **interactions:** Appendix 1 (bupivacaine)
Contra-indications: see under Lidocaine Hydrochloride and notes above; intravenous regional anaesthesia (Bier's block)
Side-effects: see under Lidocaine Hydrochloride and notes above
Dose: adjusted according to patient's physical status and nature of procedure—**important:** see also under Administration, above
Local infiltration, 0.25% (up to 60 mL)
Peripheral nerve block, 0.25% (max. 60 mL), 0.5% (max. 30 mL)
Epidural block,
Surgery, *lumbar*, 0.5% (max. 20 mL); *caudal*, 0.5% (max. 30 mL)

Labour, *lumbar*, 0.25–0.5% (max. 12 mL); *caudal*, but rarely used, 0.25–0.5% (max. 20 mL)
Sympathetic block, 0.25% (max. 50 mL)

> **Important.** The licensed doses stated above may not be appropriate in some settings and expert advice should be sought

Bupivacaine (Non-proprietary) [PoM]
Injection, anhydrous bupivacaine hydrochloride 2.5 mg/mL (0.25%), net price 10-mL = 82p; 5 mg/mL (0.5%), 10-mL = 94p
NOTE. Bupivacaine hydrochloride injection 0.25% and 0.5% are available in glass or plastic ampoules, and sterile-wrapped glass ampoules
Infusion, anhydrous bupivacaine hydrochloride 1 mg/mL (0.1%), net price 100 mL = £8.41; 250 mL = £10.59; 1.25 mg/mL (0.125%), 250 mL = £10.80
Dose: Continuous lumbar epidural infusion during labour (once epidural block established), 10–15 mg/hour of 0.1% or 0.125% solution; max. 2 mg/kg over 4 hours and total of 400 mg in 24 hours
Continuous thoracic, upper abdominal, or lower abdominal epidural infusion for post-operative pain (once epidural block established), 4–15 mg/hour of 0.1% or 0.125% solution; max. 2 mg/kg over 4 hours and total of 400 mg in 24 hours; not recommended for use in children
Available from Antigen

Marcain® (AstraZeneca) [PoM]
Injection, anhydrous bupivacaine hydrochloride 2.5 mg/mL (*Marcain*® 0.25%), net price 10-mL *Polyamp*® = £1.06; 5 mg/mL (*Marcain*® 0.5%), 10-mL *Polyamp*® = £1.21

Marcain Heavy® (AstraZeneca) [PoM]
Injection, anhydrous bupivacaine hydrochloride 5 mg, glucose 80 mg/mL, net price 4-mL amp = 93p
Dose: spinal anaesthesia, 2–4 mL

▪ With adrenaline
Bupivacaine and Adrenaline (Non-proprietary) [PoM]
Injection, anhydrous bupivacaine hydrochloride 2.5 mg/mL (0.25%), adrenaline 1 in 200 000 (5 micrograms/mL), net price 10-mL amp = £1.23
Injection, anhydrous bupivacaine hydrochloride 5 mg/mL (0.5%), adrenaline 1 in 200 000 (5 micrograms/mL), net price 10-mL amp = £1.40
Available from Antigen

Marcain® **with Adrenaline** (AstraZeneca) [PoM]
Injection 0.25%, bupivacaine hydrochloride 2.5 mg/mL, adrenaline 1 in 200 000 (5 micrograms/mL), net price 10-mL amp = £1.18
Injection 0.5%, bupivacaine hydrochloride 5 mg/mL, adrenaline 1 in 200 000 (5 micrograms/mL), net price 10-mL amp = £1.33
NOTE. May be difficult to obtain

Levobupivacaine

Levobupivacaine, an isomer of bupivacaine, has been introduced recently. It has similar anaesthetic and analgesic properties to bupivacaine.

LEVOBUPIVACAINE HYDROCHLORIDE

NOTE. Levobupivacaine is an isomer of bupivacaine

Indications: see under Dose

Cautions: see under Lidocaine Hydrochloride and notes above; **interactions:** Appendix 1 (levobupivacaine)

Contra-indications: see under Lidocaine Hydrochloride and notes above; intravenous regional anaesthesia (Bier's block); paracervical block in obstetrics

Side-effects: see under Lidocaine Hydrochloride and notes above

Dose: adjusted according to patient's physical status and nature of procedure—**important:** see also under Administration, above

Surgical anaesthesia,

lumbar epidural, 10–20 mL (50–150 mg) of 5 or 7.5 mg/mL solution over 5 minutes; caesarean section, 15–30 mL (75–150 mg) of 5 mg/mL solution over 15–20 minutes

intrathecal, 3 mL (15 mg) of 5 mg/mL solution

peripheral nerve block, 1–40 mL of 2.5 or 5 mg/mL solution (max. 150 mg)

ilioinguinal/iliohypogastric block, CHILD 0.25–0.5 mL/kg (1.25–2.5 mg/kg) of 2.5 or 5 mg/mL solution

peribulbar block, 5–15 mL (37.5–112.5 mg) of 7.5 mg/mL solution

local infiltration, 1–60 mL (max. 150 mg) of 2.5 mg/mL solution

Acute pain,

lumbar epidural, 6–10 mL (15–25 mg) of 2.5 mg/mL solution at intervals of at least 15 minutes *or* 4–10 mL/hour (5–12.5 mg/hour) of 1.25 mg/mL solution as a continuous epidural infusion for labour pain, *or* 10–15 mL/hour (12.5–18.75 mg/hour) of 1.25 mg/mL solution or 5–7.5 mL/hour (12.5–18.75 mg/hour) of 2.5 mg/mL solution as a continuous epidural infusion for postoperative pain

NOTE. 7.5 mg/mL **contra-indicated** for use in obstetrics; for 1.25 mg/mL concentration dilute standard solutions with sodium chloride 0.9%.

Important. The licensed doses stated above may not be appropriate in some settings and expert advice should be sought

---

Chirocaine® (Abbott) ▼ PoM

Injection, levobupivacaine hydrochloride 2.5 mg/mL, net price 10-mL amp = £1.66; 5 mg/mL, 10-mL amp = £1.90; 7.5 mg/mL, 10-mL amp = £2.85

Prilocaine

Prilocaine is a local anaesthetic of low toxicity which is similar to lidocaine (lignocaine). If used in high doses, methaemoglobinaemia may occur which can be treated with intravenous injection of methylthioninium chloride (methylene blue) 1% using a dose of 1 mg/kg. Infants are particularly susceptible to methaemoglobinaemia.

PRILOCAINE HYDROCHLORIDE

Indications: infiltration anaesthesia (higher strengths for dental use only), nerve block

Cautions: see under Lidocaine Hydrochloride and notes above; renal impairment; **interactions:** Appendix 1 (prilocaine)

Contra-indications: see under Lidocaine Hydrochloride and notes above; anaemia or congenital or acquired methaemoglobinaemia

Side-effects: see under Lidocaine Hydrochloride and notes above; ocular toxicity (including blindness) reported with excessive strengths used for ophthalmic procedures

Dose: adjusted according to site of operation and response of patient, to max. 400 mg used alone, or 300 mg if used with felypressin

Citanest® (AstraZeneca) PoM

Injection 1%, prilocaine hydrochloride 10 mg/mL, net price 20-mL multidose vial = 81p

■ For dental use

Citanest® (Dentsply) PoM

Injection 4%, prilocaine hydrochloride 40 mg/mL, net price 2-mL cartridge = 16p

Citanest with Octapressin® (Dentsply) PoM

Injection 3%, prilocaine hydrochloride 30 mg/mL, felypressin 0.03 unit/mL, net price 2-mL cartridge and self-aspirating cartridge (both) = 16p

Procaine

Procaine is now seldom used. It is as potent as lidocaine (lignocaine) but has a shorter duration of action. It provides less intense analgesia because of reduced spread through the tissues. It is of no value as a surface anaesthetic.

PROCAINE HYDROCHLORIDE

Indications: local anaesthesia by infiltration and regional routes (but see notes above)

Cautions: see notes above

Side-effects: see notes above

Dose: adjusted according to site of operation and patient's response

By injection, up to 1 g (200 mL of 0.5% solution or 100 mL of 1%) with adrenaline 1 in 200 000

Procaine (Non-proprietary) PoM

Injection, procaine hydrochloride 2% (20 mg/mL) in sodium chloride intravenous infusion, net price 2-mL amp = 89p

Available from Martindale

Ropivacaine

Ropivacaine is an amide-type local anaesthetic agent.

ROPIVACAINE HYDROCHLORIDE

Indications: see under Dose

Cautions: see Lidocaine Hydrochloride and notes above; **interactions:** Appendix 1 (ropivacaine)

Contra-indications: see Lidocaine Hydrochloride and notes above; intravenous regional anaesthesia (Bier's block); paracervical block in obstetrics

Side-effects: see Lidocaine Hydrochloride and notes above

Dose: adjust according to patient's physical status and nature of procedure—see also under Administration on p. 614

Surgical anaesthesia,

lumbar epidural, 15–20 mL of 10 mg/mL solution *or* 15–25 mL of 7.5 mg/mL solution; caesarean section, 15–20 mL of 7.5 mg/mL solution

thoracic epidural (to establish block for postoperative pain), 5–15 mL of 7.5 mg/mL solution

major nerve block (brachial plexus block), 30–40 mL of 7.5 mg/mL solution

field block, up to 30 mL of 7.5 mg/mL solution

Acute pain,

lumbar epidural, 10–20 mL of 2 mg/mL solution followed by 10–15 mL of 2 mg/mL solution at intervals of at least 30 minutes *or* 6–10 mL/hour of 2 mg/mL solution as a continuous epidural infusion for labour pain *or* 6–14 mL/hour of 2 mg/mL solution as a continuous epidural infusion for postoperative pain

thoracic epidural, 6–14 mL/hour of 2 mg/mL solution as a continuous infusion

field block, up to 100 mL of 2 mg/mL solution

peripheral nerve block, 5–10 mL/hour of 2 mg/mL solution as a continuous infusion *or* by intermittent injection

CHILD over 1 year (body-weight up to 25 kg), *caudal epidural* (for pre- and post-operative pain only), 2 mg/kg of 2 mg/mL solution

Naropin® (AstraZeneca) PoM

Injection, ropivacaine hydrochloride 2 mg/mL, net price 10-mL *Polyamp*® = £1.37; 7.5 mg/mL, 10-mL *Polyamp*® = £2.65; 10 mg/mL, 10-mL *Polyamp*® = £3.20

Epidural infusion, ropivacaine hydrochloride 2 mg/mL, net price 100-mL *Polybag*® = £8.23, 200-mL *Polybag*® = £14.45

Tetracaine

Tetracaine (amethocaine) is an effective local anaesthetic for topical application; a 4% gel is indicated for anaesthesia prior to venepuncture or venous cannulation. It is rapidly absorbed from mucous membranes and should **never** be applied to inflamed, traumatised, or highly vascular surfaces. It should **never** be used to provide anaesthesia for bronchoscopy or cystoscopy, as lidocaine (lignocaine) is a safer alternative. It is used in ophthalmology (section 11.7) and in skin preparations (section 13.3). Hypersensitivity to tetracaine has been reported.

TETRACAINE

(Amethocaine)

Indications: see under preparation below

Cautions: see notes above

Contra-indications: see notes above

Side-effects: see notes above; also erythema, oedema and pruritus; very rarely blistering

Important. Rapid and extensive absorption may result in systemic side-effects (see also notes above)

Ametop® (S&N Hlth.)

Gel, tetracaine 4%, net price 1.5-g tube = £1.15

Dose: apply contents of tube to site of venepuncture or venous cannulation and cover with occlusive dressing; remove gel and dressing after 30 minutes for venepuncture and after 45 minutes for venous cannulation; PRE-

MATURE INFANT and INFANT under 1 month not recommended

Other local anaesthetics

Benzocaine is a local anaesthetic of low potency and toxicity. It is an ingredient of some proprietary topical preparations for musculoskeletal conditions (section 10.3.2), mouth-ulcer preparations (section 12.3.1), and throat lozenges (section 12.3.3).

Mepivacaine is a local anaesthetic used in dentistry; it is available in dental cartridges with or without adrenaline (epinephrine) as *Scandonest*®. **Articaine** (carticaine) is a newly introduced local anaesthetic for dental use; it is available in cartridges with adrenaline (*Septanest*®).

Cocaine readily penetrates mucous membranes and is an effective surface anaesthetic with an intense vasoconstrictor action. However, apart from its use in otolaryngology (see below), it has now been replaced by less toxic alternatives. It has marked sympathomimetic activity and should **never** be given by injection because of its toxicity. As a result of its intense stimulant effect it is a drug of addiction. In otolaryngology cocaine is applied to the nasal mucosa in concentrations of 4 to 10% (40–100 mg/mL); an oromucosal solution and nasal spray both containing cocaine hydrochloride 10% are available (Aurum). In order to avoid systemic effects, the maximum dose recommended for application to the nasal mucosa in fit adults is a total of 1.5 mg/kg, which is equivalent to a total topical dose of approximately 100 mg for an adult male; this dose relates to direct application of cocaine (application on gauze may reduce systemic absorption). It should be used only by those skilled in the precautions needed to *minimise absorption* and the *consequent risk of arrhythmias*. Although cocaine interacts with other drugs liable to induce arrhythmias, including adrenaline, some otolaryngologists consider that combined use of topical cocaine with topical adrenaline (in the form of a paste or a solution) improves the operative field and may possibly reduce absorption. Cocaine is a mydriatic as well as a local anaesthetic but owing to corneal toxicity it is now little used in ophthalmology. Cocaine should be avoided in porphyria (section 9.8.2).

Appendix 1: Interactions

Two or more drugs given at the same time may exert their effects independently or may interact. The interaction may be potentiation or antagonism of one drug by another, or occasionally some other effect. Adverse drug interactions should be reported to the CSM as for other adverse drug reactions.

Drug interactions may be **pharmacodynamic** or **pharmacokinetic**.

Pharmacodynamic interactions

These are interactions between drugs which have similar or antagonistic pharmacological effects or side-effects. They may be due to competition at receptor sites, or occur between drugs acting on the same physiological system. They are usually predictable from a knowledge of the pharmacology of the interacting drugs; in general, those demonstrated with one drug are likely to occur with related drugs. They occur to a greater or lesser extent in most patients who receive the interacting drugs.

Pharmacokinetic interactions

These occur when one drug alters the absorption, distribution, metabolism, or excretion of another, thus increasing or reducing the amount of drug available to produce its pharmacological effects. They are not easily predicted and many of them affect only a small proportion of patients taking the combination of drugs. Pharmacokinetic interactions occurring with one drug cannot be assumed to occur with related drugs unless their pharmacokinetic properties are known to be similar.

Pharmacokinetic interactions are of several types:

AFFECTING ABSORPTION. The rate of absorption or the total amount absorbed can both be altered by drug interactions. Delayed absorption is rarely of clinical importance unless high peak plasma concentrations are required (e.g. when giving an analgesic). Reduction in the total amount absorbed, however, may result in ineffective therapy.

DUE TO CHANGES IN PROTEIN BINDING. To a variable extent most drugs are loosely bound to plasma proteins. Protein-binding sites are non-specific and one drug can displace another thereby increasing its proportion free to diffuse from plasma to its site of action. This only produces a detectable increase in effect if it is an extensively bound drug (more than 90%) that is not widely distributed throughout the body. Even so displacement rarely produces more than transient potentiation because this increased concentration of free drug results in an increased rate of elimination.

Displacement from protein binding plays a part in the potentiation of warfarin by sulphonamides, and tolbutamide but the importance of these interactions is due mainly to the fact that warfarin metabolism is also inhibited.

AFFECTING METABOLISM. Many drugs are metabolised in the liver. Induction of the hepatic microsomal enzyme system by one drug can gradually increase the rate of metabolism of another, resulting in lower plasma concentrations and a reduced effect. On withdrawal of the inducer plasma concentrations increase and toxicity may occur. Barbiturates, griseofulvin, many antiepileptics, and rifampicin are the most important enzyme inducers. Drugs affected include warfarin and the oral contraceptives.

Conversely when one drug inhibits the metabolism of another higher plasma concentrations are produced, rapidly resulting in an increased effect with risk of toxicity. Some drugs which potentiate warfarin and phenytoin do so by this mechanism.

AFFECTING RENAL EXCRETION. Drugs are eliminated through the kidney both by glomerular filtration and by active tubular secretion. Competition occurs between those which share active transport mechanisms in the proximal tubule. For example, salicylates and some other NSAIDs delay the excretion of methotrexate; serious methotrexate toxicity is possible.

Relative importance of interactions

Many drug interactions are harmless and many of those which are potentially harmful only occur in a small proportion of patients; moreover, the severity of an interaction varies from one patient to another. Drugs with a small therapeutic ratio (e.g. phenytoin) and those which require careful control of dosage (e.g. anticoagulants, antihypertensives, and antidiabetics) are most often involved.

Patients at increased risk from drug interactions include the elderly and those with impaired renal or liver function.

HAZARDOUS INTERACTIONS. The symbol • has been placed against interactions that are **potentially hazardous** and where combined administration of the drugs involved should be **avoided** (or only undertaken with caution and appropriate monitoring).

Interactions that have no symbol do not usually have serious consequences.

List of drug interactions

The following is an alphabetical list of drugs and their interactions; to avoid excessive cross-referencing each drug or group is listed twice: in the alphabetical list and also against the drug or group with which it interacts; changes in the interactions lists since BNF No. 46 (September 2003) are underlined.

For explanation of symbol • see above

Abacavir
  Analgesics: abacavir possibly reduces plasma concentration of methadone
Acarbose see Antidiabetics

ACE Inhibitors

Adrenergic Neurone Blockers: enhanced hypotensive effect when ACE inhibitors given with adrenergic neurone blockers

Alcohol: enhanced hypotensive effect when ACE inhibitors given with alcohol

Aldesleukin: enhanced hypotensive effect when ACE inhibitors given with aldesleukin

Allopurinol: increased risk of toxicity when captopril given with allopurinol especially in renal impairment

Alpha-blockers: enhanced hypotensive effect when ACE inhibitors given with alpha-blockers

Alprostadil: enhanced hypotensive effect when ACE inhibitors given with alprostadil

Amifostine: possible enhanced hypotensive effect when ACE inhibitors given with amifostine

Analgesics: increased risk of renal impairment when ACE inhibitors given with NSAIDs, also hypotensive effect antagonised; increased risk of hyperkalaemia when ACE inhibitors given with ketorolac; risk of renal impairment when ACE inhibitors given with aspirin (in doses over 300 mg daily), also hypotensive effect antagonised

Angiotensin-II Receptor Antagonists: enhanced hypotensive effect when ACE inhibitors given with angiotensin-II receptor antagonists

Antacids: absorption of ACE inhibitors possibly reduced by antacids; absorption of captopril, enalapril and fosinopril reduced by antacids

Anti-arrhythmics: increased risk of toxicity when captopril given with procainamide especially in renal impairment

Antibacterials: plasma concentration of active metabolite of imidapril reduced by rifampicin (reduced antihypertensive effect); quinapril tablets reduce absorption of tetracyclines (quinapril tablets contain magnesium carbonate)

Anticoagulants: increased risk of hyperkalaemia when ACE inhibitors given with heparins

Antidepressants: hypotensive effect of ACE inhibitors possibly enhanced by MAOIs

Antidiabetics: ACE inhibitors possibly enhance hypoglycaemic effect of insulin, metformin and sulphonylureas

Antipsychotics: enhanced hypotensive effect when ACE inhibitors given with antipsychotics

Anxiolytics and Hypnotics: enhanced hypotensive effect when ACE inhibitors given with anxiolytics and hypnotics

Beta-blockers: enhanced hypotensive effect when ACE inhibitors given with beta-blockers

Calcium-channel Blockers: enhanced hypotensive effect when ACE inhibitors given with calcium-channel blockers

Cardiac Glycosides: captopril possibly increases plasma concentration of digoxin

• Ciclosporin: increased risk of hyperkalaemia when ACE inhibitors given with ●ciclosporin

Clonidine: enhanced hypotensive effect when ACE inhibitors given with clonidine; antihypertensive effect of captopril possibly delayed by previous treatment with clonidine

Corticosteroids: hypotensive effect of ACE inhibitors antagonised by corticosteroids

Cytotoxics: increased risk of leucopenia when captopril given with azathioprine

Diazoxide: enhanced hypotensive effect when ACE inhibitors given with diazoxide

• Diuretics: enhanced hypotensive effect when ACE inhibitors given with ●diuretics; increased risk of severe hyperkalaemia when ACE inhibitors given with ●potassium-sparing diuretics (monitor potas-

ACE Inhibitors

• Diuretics (continued)

sium concentration with low-dose spironolactone in heart failure)

Dopaminergics: enhanced hypotensive effect when ACE inhibitors given with levodopa

Epoetin: antagonism of hypotensive effect and increased risk of hyperkalaemia when ACE inhibitors given with epoetin

• Lithium: ACE inhibitors reduce excretion of ●lithium (increased plasma concentration)

Methyldopa: enhanced hypotensive effect when ACE inhibitors given with methyldopa

Moxisylyte (thymoxamine): enhanced hypotensive effect when ACE inhibitors given with moxisylyte

Moxonidine: enhanced hypotensive effect when ACE inhibitors given with moxonidine

Muscle Relaxants: enhanced hypotensive effect when ACE inhibitors given with baclofen or tizanidine

Nitrates: enhanced hypotensive effect when ACE inhibitors given with nitrates

Oestrogens: hypotensive effect of ACE inhibitors antagonised by oestrogens

• Potassium Salts: increased risk of severe hyperkalaemia when ACE inhibitors given with ●potassium salts

Probenecid: excretion of captopril reduced by probenecid

Progestogens: risk of hyperkalaemia when ACE inhibitors given with drospirenone (monitor serum potassium during first cycle)

Ulcer-healing Drugs: hypotensive effect of ACE inhibitors antagonised by carbenoxolone

Vasodilator Antihypertensives: enhanced hypotensive effect when ACE inhibitors given with hydralazine, minoxidil or nitroprusside

Acebutolol see Beta-blockers

Aceclofenac see NSAIDs

Acemetacin see NSAIDs

Acenocoumarol (nicoumalone) see Coumarins

Acetazolamide see Diuretics

Aciclovir

Note. Interactions do not apply to topical aciclovir preparations

Note. Valaciclovir interactions as for aciclovir

Cytotoxics: plasma concentration of aciclovir increased by mycophenolate mofetil, also plasma concentration of inactive metabolite of mycophenolate mofetil increased

Probenecid: excretion of aciclovir reduced by probenecid (increased plasma concentration)

Acitretin see Retinoids

Acrivastine see Antihistamines

Adalimumab

• Anakinra: avoid concomitant use of adalimumab with ●anakinra

• Vaccines: avoid concomitant use of adalimumab with live ●vaccines (see p. 578)

Adenosine

Note. Possibility of interaction with drugs tending to impair myocardial conduction

• Adrenergic Neurone Blockers: increased myocardial depression when anti-arrhythmics given with ●bretylium

Anaesthetics, Local: increased myocardial depression when anti-arrhythmics given with bupivacaine or levobupivacaine

• Anti-arrhythmics: increased myocardial depression when anti-arrhythmics given with other ●anti-arrhythmics

• Antihistamines: increased risk of ventricular arrhythmias when anti-arrhythmics given with ●terfenadine

Adenosine *(continued)*
- Antipsychotics: increased risk of ventricular arrhythmias when anti-arrhythmics that prolong the QT interval given with ●antipsychotics that prolong the QT interval
- Beta-blockers: increased myocardial depression when anti-arrhythmics given with ●beta-blockers
- Dipyridamole: effect of adenosine enhanced and extended by ●dipyridamole (important risk of toxicity)

Theophylline: anti-arrhythmic effect of adenosine antagonised by theophylline

Tropisetron: caution with anti-arrhythmics advised by manufacturer of tropisetron (risk of ventricular arrhythmias)

Adrenaline (epinephrine) *see* Sympathomimetics

Adrenergic Neurone Blockers

ACE Inhibitors: enhanced hypotensive effect when adrenergic neurone blockers given with ACE inhibitors

Alcohol: enhanced hypotensive effect when adrenergic neurone blockers given with alcohol

Alpha-blockers: enhanced hypotensive effect when adrenergic neurone blockers given with alpha-blockers

Alprostadil: enhanced hypotensive effect when adrenergic neurone blockers given with alprostadil

Amifostine: possible enhanced hypotensive effect when adrenergic neurone blockers given with amifostine

- Anaesthetics, General: enhanced hypotensive effect when adrenergic neurone blockers given with ●general anaesthetics

Analgesics: hypotensive effect of adrenergic neurone blockers antagonised by NSAIDs

Angiotensin-II Receptor Antagonists: enhanced hypotensive effect when adrenergic neurone blockers given with angiotensin-II receptor antagonists

- Anti-arrhythmics: increased myocardial depression when bretylium given with ●anti-arrhythmics

Antidepressants: enhanced hypotensive effect when adrenergic neurone blockers given with MAOIs; hypotensive effect of adrenergic neurone blockers antagonised by tricyclics

Antipsychotics: hypotensive effect of adrenergic neurone blockers antagonised by haloperidol; hypotensive effect of adrenergic neurone blockers antagonised by higher doses of chlorpromazine; enhanced hypotensive effect when adrenergic neurone blockers given with phenothiazines

Anxiolytics and Hypnotics: enhanced hypotensive effect when adrenergic neurone blockers given with anxiolytics and hypnotics

Beta-blockers: enhanced hypotensive effect when adrenergic neurone blockers given with beta-blockers

Calcium-channel Blockers: enhanced hypotensive effect when adrenergic neurone blockers given with calcium-channel blockers

Clonidine: enhanced hypotensive effect when adrenergic neurone blockers given with clonidine

Corticosteroids: hypotensive effect of adrenergic neurone blockers antagonised by corticosteroids

Diazoxide: enhanced hypotensive effect when adrenergic neurone blockers given with diazoxide

Diuretics: enhanced hypotensive effect when adrenergic neurone blockers given with diuretics

- Dolasetron: increased risk of ventricular arrhythmias when bretylium given with ●dolasetron—avoid concomitant use

Dopaminergics: enhanced hypotensive effect when adrenergic neurone blockers given with levodopa

Adrenergic Neurone Blockers *(continued)*

Methyldopa: enhanced hypotensive effect when adrenergic neurone blockers given with methyldopa

Moxisylyte (thymoxamine): enhanced hypotensive effect when adrenergic neurone blockers given with moxisylyte

Moxonidine: enhanced hypotensive effect when adrenergic neurone blockers given with moxonidine

Muscle Relaxants: enhanced hypotensive effect when adrenergic neurone blockers given with baclofen or tizanidine

Nitrates: enhanced hypotensive effect when adrenergic neurone blockers given with nitrates

Oestrogens: hypotensive effect of adrenergic neurone blockers antagonised by oestrogens

Pizotifen: hypotensive effect of adrenergic neurone blockers antagonised by pizotifen

- Sympathomimetics: hypotensive effect of adrenergic neurone blockers antagonised by ●ephedrine, ●isometheptene, ●metaraminol, ●methylphenidate, ●noradrenaline (norepinephrine), ●oxymetazoline, ●phenylephrine, ●phenylpropanolamine, ●pseudoephedrine and ●xylometazoline

Ulcer-healing Drugs: hypotensive effect of adrenergic neurone blockers antagonised by carbenoxolone

Vasodilator Antihypertensives: enhanced hypotensive effect when adrenergic neurone blockers given with hydralazine, minoxidil or nitroprusside

Adsorbents *see* Kaolin

Alcohol

ACE Inhibitors: enhanced hypotensive effect when alcohol given with ACE inhibitors

Adrenergic Neurone Blockers: enhanced hypotensive effect when alcohol given with adrenergic neurone blockers

Alpha-blockers: increased sedative effect when alcohol given with indoramin; enhanced hypotensive effect when alcohol given with alpha-blockers

Analgesics: enhanced hypotensive and sedative effects when alcohol given with opioid analgesics

Angiotensin-II Receptor Antagonists: enhanced hypotensive effect when alcohol given with angiotensin-II receptor antagonists

- Antibacterials: disulfiram-like reaction when alcohol given with metronidazole; possibility of disulfiram-like reaction when alcohol given with tinidazole; increased risk of convulsions when alcohol given with ●cycloserine

- Anticoagulants: major changes in consumption of alcohol may affect anticoagulant control with ●coumarins or ●phenindione

- Antidepressants: some beverages containing alcohol and some dealcoholised beverages contain tyramine which interacts with ●MAOIs (hypertensive crisis)—if no tyramine, enhanced hypotensive effect; sedative effects possibly increased when alcohol given with SSRIs; increased sedative effect when alcohol given with ●mirtazapine, ●tricyclic-related antidepressants or ●tricyclics

Antidiabetics: alcohol enhances hypoglycaemic effect of antidiabetics; increased risk of lactic acidosis when alcohol given with metformin; flushing, in susceptible subjects, when alcohol given with chlorpropamide

Antiepileptics: alcohol possibly increases CNS side-effects of carbamazepine; increased sedative effect when alcohol given with primidone

Antifungals: effects of alcohol possibly enhanced by griseofulvin

Alcohol *(continued)*

Antihistamines: increased sedative effect when alcohol given with antihistamines (possibly less effect with non-sedating antihistamines)

Antimuscarinics: increased sedative effect when alcohol given with hyoscine

Antipsychotics: increased sedative effect when alcohol given with antipsychotics

Anxiolytics and Hypnotics: increased sedative effect when alcohol given with anxiolytics and hypnotics

Barbiturates: increased sedative effect when alcohol given with barbiturates

Beta-blockers: enhanced hypotensive effect when alcohol given with beta-blockers

Calcium-channel Blockers: enhanced hypotensive effect when alcohol given with calcium-channel blockers; plasma concentration of alcohol possibly increased by verapamil

Clonidine: enhanced hypotensive effect when alcohol given with clonidine

Cytotoxics: disulfiram-like reaction when alcohol given with procarbazine

Diazoxide: enhanced hypotensive effect when alcohol given with diazoxide

Disulfiram: disulfiram reaction when alcohol given with disulfiram (see p. 247)

Diuretics: enhanced hypotensive effect when alcohol given with diuretics

Dopaminergics: alcohol reduces tolerance to bromocriptine

Lofexidine: increased sedative effect when alcohol given with lofexidine

Methyldopa: enhanced hypotensive effect when alcohol given with methyldopa

Moxonidine: enhanced hypotensive effect when alcohol given with moxonidine

Muscle Relaxants: increased sedative effect when alcohol given with baclofen, methocarbamol or tizanidine

Nabilone: increased sedative effect when alcohol given with nabilone

Nicorandil: alcohol possibly enhances hypotensive effect of nicorandil

Nitrates: enhanced hypotensive effect when alcohol given with nitrates

● Paraldehyde: increased sedative effect when alcohol given with ●paraldehyde

Retinoids: presence of alcohol causes etretinate to be formed from acitretin

Vasodilator Antihypertensives: enhanced hypotensive effect when alcohol given with hydralazine, minoxidil or nitroprusside

Aldesleukin

ACE Inhibitors: enhanced hypotensive effect when aldesleukin given with ACE inhibitors

Alpha-blockers: enhanced hypotensive effect when aldesleukin given with alpha-blockers

Angiotensin-II Receptor Antagonists: enhanced hypotensive effect when aldesleukin given with angiotensin-II receptor antagonists

Beta-blockers: enhanced hypotensive effect when aldesleukin given with beta-blockers

Calcium-channel Blockers: enhanced hypotensive effect when aldesleukin given with calcium-channel blockers

Clonidine: enhanced hypotensive effect when aldesleukin given with clonidine

Diazoxide: enhanced hypotensive effect when aldesleukin given with diazoxide

Diuretics: enhanced hypotensive effect when aldesleukin given with diuretics

Methyldopa: enhanced hypotensive effect when aldesleukin given with methyldopa

Aldesleukin *(continued)*

Moxonidine: enhanced hypotensive effect when aldesleukin given with moxonidine

Nitrates: enhanced hypotensive effect when aldesleukin given with nitrates

Vasodilator Antihypertensives: enhanced hypotensive effect when aldesleukin given with hydralazine, minoxidil or nitroprusside

Alendronic Acid *see* Bisphosphonates

Alfentanil *see* Opioid Analgesics

Alfuzosin *see* Alpha-blockers

Alimemazine (trimeprazine) *see* Antihistamines

Alkylating Drugs *see* Busulfan, Cyclophosphamide, Ifosfamide, Melphalan, and Thiotepa

Allopurinol

ACE Inhibitors: increased risk of toxicity when allopurinol given with captopril especially in renal impairment

Antibacterials: increased risk of rash when allopurinol given with amoxicillin or ampicillin

Anticoagulants: allopurinol possibly enhances anticoagulant effect of coumarins

Ciclosporin: allopurinol possibly increases plasma concentration of ciclosporin (risk of nephrotoxicity)

● Cytotoxics: allopurinol enhances effects and increases toxicity of ●azathioprine and ●mercaptopurine (reduce dose of azathioprine and mercaptopurine); avoidance of allopurinol advised by manufacturer of ●capecitabine

Theophylline: allopurinol possibly increases plasma concentration of theophylline

Almotriptan *see* 5HT₁ Agonists

Alpha₂-adrenoceptor Stimulants

Antidepressants: manufacturer of apraclonidine and brimonidine advises avoid concomitant use with MAOIs; manufacturer of apraclonidine and brimonidine advises avoid concomitant use with tricyclic-related antidepressants; manufacturer of apraclonidine and brimonidine advises avoid concomitant use with tricyclics

Alpha-blockers

ACE Inhibitors: enhanced hypotensive effect when alpha-blockers given with ACE inhibitors

Adrenergic Neurone Blockers: enhanced hypotensive effect when alpha-blockers given with adrenergic neurone blockers

Alcohol: enhanced hypotensive effect when alpha-blockers given with alcohol; increased sedative effect when indoramin given with alcohol

Aldesleukin: enhanced hypotensive effect when alpha-blockers given with aldesleukin

Alprostadil: enhanced hypotensive effect when alpha-blockers given with alprostadil

Amifostine: possible enhanced hypotensive effect when alpha-blockers given with amifostine

● Anaesthetics, General: enhanced hypotensive effect when alpha-blockers given with ●general anaesthetics

Analgesics: hypotensive effect of alpha-blockers antagonised by NSAIDs

Angiotensin-II Receptor Antagonists: enhanced hypotensive effect when alpha-blockers given with angiotensin-II receptor antagonists

● Antidepressants: enhanced hypotensive effect when alpha-blockers given with MAOIs; manufacturer of indoramin advises avoid concomitant use with ●MAOIs

Antipsychotics: enhanced hypotensive effect when alpha-blockers given with antipsychotics

Anxiolytics and Hypnotics: enhanced hypotensive and sedative effects when alpha-blockers given with anxiolytics and hypnotics

Alpha-blockers *(continued)*
- Beta-blockers: enhanced hypotensive effect when alpha-blockers given with ●beta-blockers, also increased risk of first-dose hypotension with post-synaptic alpha-blockers such as prazosin
- Calcium-channel Blockers: enhanced hypotensive effect when alpha-blockers given with ●calcium-channel blockers, also increased risk of first-dose hypotension with post-synaptic alpha-blockers such as prazosin

  Cardiac Glycosides: prazosin increases plasma concentration of digoxin

  Clonidine: enhanced hypotensive effect when alpha-blockers given with clonidine

  Corticosteroids: hypotensive effect of alpha-blockers antagonised by corticosteroids

  Diazoxide: enhanced hypotensive effect when alpha-blockers given with diazoxide
- Diuretics: enhanced hypotensive effect when alpha-blockers given with ●diuretics, also increased risk of first-dose hypotension with post-synaptic alpha-blockers such as prazosin

  Dopaminergics: enhanced hypotensive effect when alpha-blockers given with levodopa

  Methyldopa: enhanced hypotensive effect when alpha-blockers given with methyldopa
- Moxisylyte (thymoxamine): possible severe postural hypotension when alpha-blockers given with ●moxisylyte

  Moxonidine: enhanced hypotensive effect when alpha-blockers given with moxonidine

  Muscle Relaxants: enhanced hypotensive effect when alpha-blockers given with baclofen or tizanidine

  Nitrates: enhanced hypotensive effect when alpha-blockers given with nitrates

  Oestrogens: hypotensive effect of alpha-blockers antagonised by oestrogens

  Sildenafil: enhanced hypotensive effect when alpha-blockers given with sildenafil (avoid alpha-blockers for 4 hours after sildenafil)
- Tadalafil: enhanced hypotensive effect when alpha-blockers given with ●tadalafil (avoid concomitant use)

  Ulcer-healing Drugs: hypotensive effect of alpha-blockers antagonised by carbenoxolone
- Vardenafil: hypotensive effect of alpha-blockers enhanced by ●vardenafil (avoid concomitant use)

  Vasodilator Antihypertensives: enhanced hypotensive effect when alpha-blockers given with hydralazine, minoxidil or nitroprusside

Alpha-blockers (post-synaptic) *see* Alpha-blockers

Alprazolam *see* Anxiolytics and Hypnotics

Alprostadil

ACE Inhibitors: enhanced hypotensive effect when alprostadil given with ACE inhibitors

Adrenergic Neurone Blockers: enhanced hypotensive effect when alprostadil given with adrenergic neurone blockers

Alpha-blockers: enhanced hypotensive effect when alprostadil given with alpha-blockers

Angiotensin-II Receptor Antagonists: enhanced hypotensive effect when alprostadil given with angiotensin-II receptor antagonists

Beta-blockers: enhanced hypotensive effect when alprostadil given with beta-blockers

Calcium-channel Blockers: enhanced hypotensive effect when alprostadil given with calcium-channel blockers

Clonidine: enhanced hypotensive effect when alprostadil given with clonidine

Diazoxide: enhanced hypotensive effect when alprostadil given with diazoxide

Alprostadil *(continued)*

Diuretics: enhanced hypotensive effect when alprostadil given with diuretics

Methyldopa: enhanced hypotensive effect when alprostadil given with methyldopa

Moxonidine: enhanced hypotensive effect when alprostadil given with moxonidine

Nitrates: enhanced hypotensive effect when alprostadil given with nitrates

Vasodilator Antihypertensives: enhanced hypotensive effect when alprostadil given with hydralazine, minoxidil or nitroprusside

Aluminium Hydroxide *see* Antacids

Amantadine

Antimuscarinics: increased risk of antimuscarinic side-effects when amantadine given with antimuscarinics

Antipsychotics: increased risk of extrapyramidal side-effects when amantadine given with antipsychotics

Bupropion: increased risk of side-effects when amantadine given with bupropion

Domperidone: increased risk of extrapyramidal side-effects when amantadine given with domperidone
- Memantine: increased risk of CNS toxicity when amantadine given with ●memantine (manufacturer of memantine advises avoid concomitant use); effects of dopaminergics possibly enhanced by memantine

  Methyldopa: increased risk of extrapyramidal side-effects when amantadine given with methyldopa; antiparkinsonian effect of dopaminergics antagonised by methyldopa

  Metoclopramide: increased risk of extrapyramidal side-effects when amantadine given with metoclopramide

  Tetrabenazine: increased risk of extrapyramidal side-effects when amantadine given with tetrabenazine

Amifostine

Note. Limited information available—rapid clearance from plasma minimises risk of interactions; possibility of interactions with antihypertensives and other drugs which potentiate hypotension

ACE Inhibitors: possible enhanced hypotensive effect when amifostine given with ACE inhibitors

Adrenergic Neurone Blockers: possible enhanced hypotensive effect when amifostine given with adrenergic neurone blockers

Alpha-blockers: possible enhanced hypotensive effect when amifostine given with alpha-blockers

Angiotensin-II Receptor Antagonists: possible enhanced hypotensive effect when amifostine given with angiotensin-II receptor antagonists

Beta-blockers: possible enhanced hypotensive effect when amifostine given with beta-blockers

Calcium-channel Blockers: possible enhanced hypotensive effect when amifostine given with calcium-channel blockers

Clonidine: possible enhanced hypotensive effect when amifostine given with clonidine

Diazoxide: possible enhanced hypotensive effect when amifostine given with diazoxide

Diuretics: possible enhanced hypotensive effect when amifostine given with diuretics

Methyldopa: possible enhanced hypotensive effect when amifostine given with methyldopa

Moxonidine: possible enhanced hypotensive effect when amifostine given with moxonidine

Nitrates: possible enhanced hypotensive effect when amifostine given with nitrates

Vasodilator Antihypertensives: possible enhanced hypotensive effect when amifostine given with hydralazine, minoxidil or nitroprusside

Amikacin *see* Aminoglycosides

Amiloride *see* Diuretics

Aminoglutethimide

- Anticoagulants: aminoglutethimide accelerates metabolism of ●coumarins and ●phenindione (reduced anticoagulant effect)

  Antidiabetics: manufacturer of aminoglutethimide advises that metabolism of biguanides and sulphonylureas possibly accelerated

  Cardiac Glycosides: aminoglutethimide accelerates metabolism of digitoxin (reduced effect)

  Corticosteroids: aminoglutethimide accelerates metabolism of corticosteroids (reduced effect)

  Diuretics: increased risk of hyponatraemia when aminoglutethimide given with diuretics

  Hormone Antagonists: aminoglutethimide reduces plasma concentration of tamoxifen

  Progestogens: aminoglutethimide reduces plasma concentration of medroxyprogesterone

  Theophylline: aminoglutethimide accelerates metabolism of theophylline (reduced effect)

Aminoglycosides

  Analgesics: plasma concentration of amikacin and gentamicin in neonates possibly increased by indometacin

  Antibacterials: neomycin reduces absorption of phenoxymethylpenicillin; increased risk of nephrotoxicity when aminoglycosides given with colistin or polymyxins; increased risk of nephrotoxicity and ototoxicity when aminoglycosides given with capreomycin, teicoplanin or vancomycin

- Anticoagulants: experience in anticoagulant clinics suggests that INR possibly altered when neomycin (given for local action on gut) is given with ●coumarins or ●phenindione

  Antidiabetics: neomycin possibly enhances hypoglycaemic effect of acarbose, also severity of gastro-intestinal effects increased

  Antifungals: increased risk of nephrotoxicity when aminoglycosides given with amphotericin

  Bisphosphonates: increased risk of hypocalcaemia when aminoglycosides given with bisphosphonates

  Cardiac Glycosides: neomycin reduces absorption of digoxin

- Ciclosporin: increased risk of nephrotoxicity when aminoglycosides given with ●ciclosporin

- Cytotoxics: increased risk of nephrotoxicity and possibly of ototoxicity when aminoglycosides given with ●platinum compounds

- Diuretics: increased risk of ototoxicity when aminoglycosides given with ●loop diuretics

- Muscle Relaxants: aminoglycosides enhance effects of ●non-depolarising muscle relaxants and ●suxamethonium

  Oestrogens: *broad-spectrum* antibacterials possibly reduce contraceptive effect of oestrogens (risk probably small, see p. 388)

- Parasympathomimetics: aminoglycosides antagonise effects of ●neostigmine and ●pyridostigmine

Aminophylline *see* Theophylline

Aminosalicylates

  Cardiac Glycosides: sulfasalazine possibly reduces absorption of digoxin

  Cytotoxics: possible increased risk of leucopenia when aminosalicylates given with azathioprine or mercaptopurine

  Folates: sulfasalazine possibly reduces absorption of folic acid

Amiodarone

  Note. Amiodarone has a long half-life; there is a potential for drug interactions to occur for several weeks (or even months) after treatment with it has been stopped

Amiodarone *(continued)*

- Adrenergic Neurone Blockers: increased myocardial depression when anti-arrhythmics given with ●bretylium

  Anaesthetics, Local: increased myocardial depression when anti-arrhythmics given with bupivacaine or levobupivacaine

- Anti-arrhythmics: increased myocardial depression when anti-arrhythmics given with other ●anti-arrhythmics; increased risk of ventricular arrhythmias when amiodarone given with ●disopyramide—avoid concomitant use; amiodarone increases plasma concentration of ●flecainide (halve dose of flecainide); amiodarone increases plasma concentration of ●procainamide and ●quinidine (increased risk of ventricular arrhythmias—avoid concomitant use)

- Antibacterials: increased risk of ventricular arrhythmias when amiodarone given with parenteral ●erythromycin—avoid concomitant use; increased risk of ventricular arrhythmias when amiodarone given with ●moxifloxacin—avoid concomitant use; increased risk of ventricular arrhythmias when amiodarone given with ●sulfamethoxazole and ●trimethoprim (as co-trimoxazole)—avoid concomitant use of co-trimoxazole

- Anticoagulants: amiodarone inhibits metabolism of ●coumarins and ●phenindione (enhanced anticoagulant effect)

- Antidepressants: increased risk of ventricular arrhythmias when amiodarone given with ●tricyclics—avoid concomitant use

- Antiepileptics: amiodarone inhibits metabolism of ●phenytoin (increased plasma concentration)

- Antihistamines: increased risk of ventricular arrhythmias when amiodarone given with ●mizolastine or ●terfenadine—avoid concomitant use; increased risk of ventricular arrhythmias when anti-arrhythmics given with ●terfenadine

- Antimalarials: avoidance of amiodarone advised by manufacturer of ●artemether/lumefantrine (risk of ventricular arrhythmias); increased risk of ventricular arrhythmias when amiodarone given with ●chloroquine and hydroxychloroquine, ●mefloquine or ●quinine—avoid concomitant use

- Antipsychotics: increased risk of ventricular arrhythmias when anti-arrhythmics that prolong the QT interval given with ●antipsychotics that prolong the QT interval; increased risk of ventricular arrhythmias when amiodarone given with ●amisulpride, ●haloperidol, ●phenothiazines, ●pimozide, ●sertindole or ●thioridazine—avoid concomitant use

- Antivirals: increased risk of ventricular arrhythmias when amiodarone given with ●nelfinavir—avoid concomitant use; plasma concentration of amiodarone increased by ●ritonavir (increased risk of ventricular arrhythmias—avoid concomitant use)

- Beta-blockers: increased risk of bradycardia, AV block and myocardial depression when amiodarone given with ●beta-blockers; increased myocardial depression when anti-arrhythmics given with ●beta-blockers; increased risk of ventricular arrhythmias when amiodarone given with ●sotalol—avoid concomitant use

- Calcium-channel Blockers: increased risk of bradycardia, AV block and myocardial depression when amiodarone given with ●diltiazem or ●verapamil

- Cardiac Glycosides: amiodarone increases plasma concentration of ●digoxin (halve dose of digoxin)

  Ciclosporin: amiodarone possibly increases plasma concentration of ciclosporin

  Diuretics: increased cardiac toxicity with amiodarone if hypokalaemia occurs with acetazol-

Amiodarone

Diuretics *(continued)*
amide, loop diuretics or thiazides and related diuretics
- Dolasetron: increased risk of ventricular arrhythmias when amiodarone given with ●dolasetron—avoid concomitant use
- Lipid-regulating Drugs: increased risk of myopathy when amiodarone given with ●simvastatin (avoid doses of simvastatin above 20 mg daily)
Lithium: increased risk of hypothyroidism when amiodarone given with lithium
- Pentamidine Isetionate: increased risk of ventricular arrhythmias when amiodarone given with ●pentamidine isetionate—avoid concomitant use
Thyroid Hormones: for concomitant use of amiodarone and thyroid hormones see p. 73
Tropisetron: caution with anti-arrhythmics advised by manufacturer of tropisetron (risk of ventricular arrhythmias)
Ulcer-healing Drugs: plasma concentration of amiodarone increased by cimetidine

Amisulpride *see* Antipsychotics
Amitriptyline *see* Antidepressants, Tricyclic
Amlodipine *see* Calcium-channel Blockers
Amobarbital *see* Barbiturates
Amoxapine *see* Antidepressants, Tricyclic
Amoxicillin *see* Penicillins

Amphotericin

Note. Close monitoring required with concomitant administration of nephrotoxic drugs or cytotoxics
Antibacterials: increased risk of nephrotoxicity when amphotericin given with aminoglycosides or polymyxins
Antifungals: amphotericin reduces renal excretion and increases cellular uptake of flucytosine (toxicity possibly increased); effects of amphotericin possibly antagonised by imidazoles and triazoles
- Cardiac Glycosides: hypokalaemia caused by amphotericin increases cardiac toxicity with ●cardiac glycosides
- Ciclosporin: increased risk of nephrotoxicity when amphotericin given with ●ciclosporin
- Corticosteroids: increased risk of hypokalaemia when amphotericin given with ●corticosteroids—avoid concomitant use unless corticosteroids needed to control reactions
Diuretics: increased risk of hypokalaemia when amphotericin given with loop diuretics or thiazides and related diuretics
- Tacrolimus: increased risk of nephrotoxicity when amphotericin given with ●tacrolimus

Ampicillin *see* Penicillins

Amprenavir

Antacids: absorption of amprenavir possibly reduced by antacids
- Antibacterials: plasma concentration of both drugs increased when amprenavir given with erythromycin; amprenavir increases plasma concentration of ●rifabutin (halve dose of rifabutin); plasma concentration of amprenavir significantly reduced by ●rifampicin—avoid concomitant use; amprenavir possibly increases plasma concentration of dapsone
- Antidepressants: plasma concentration of amprenavir reduced by ●St John's wort—avoid concomitant use
Antiepileptics: amprenavir possibly increases plasma concentration of carbamazepine
Antifungals: amprenavir possibly increases plasma concentration of itraconazole
- Antihistamines: amprenavir possibly increases plasma concentration of loratadine; increased risk

Amprenavir

- Antihistamines *(continued)*
of ventricular arrhythmias when amprenavir given with ●terfenadine—avoid concomitant use
Antimuscarinics: avoidance of amprenavir advised by manufacturer of tolterodine
- Antipsychotics: amprenavir possibly increases plasma concentration of clozapine and thioridazine; amprenavir increases plasma concentration of ●pimozide and ●sertindole (increased risk of ventricular arrhythmias—avoid concomitant use)
Antivirals: plasma concentration of amprenavir reduced by efavirenz; plasma concentration of amprenavir possibly reduced by nevirapine; plasma concentration of both drugs increased when amprenavir given with ritonavir
- Anxiolytics and Hypnotics: increased risk of prolonged sedation and respiratory depression when amprenavir given with ●alprazolam, ●clorazepate, ●diazepam, ●flurazepam and ●midazolam
Calcium-channel Blockers: amprenavir possibly increases plasma concentration of diltiazem, nicardipine, nifedipine and nimodipine
- Cilostazol: amprenavir possibly increases plasma concentration of ●cilostazol—avoid concomitant use
- Ergot Alkaloids: increased risk of ergotism when amprenavir given with ●ergotamine and methysergide—avoid concomitant use
- Lipid-regulating Drugs: amprenavir possibly increases plasma concentration of atorvastatin; amprenavir possibly increases plasma concentration of ●simvastatin—avoid concomitant use
Oestrogens: amprenavir possibly reduces contraceptive effect of oestrogens
Progestogens: amprenavir possibly reduces contraceptive effect of progestogens
Sildenafil: amprenavir possibly increases plasma concentration of sildenafil— reduce initial dose of sildenafil
Ulcer-healing Drugs: amprenavir possibly increases plasma concentration of cimetidine

Anabolic Steroids

- Anticoagulants: anabolic steroids enhance anticoagulant effect of ●coumarins and ●phenindione
Antidiabetics: anabolic steroids possibly enhance hypoglycaemic effect of antidiabetics

Anaesthetics, General

Note. See also Surgery and Long-term Medication, p. 600
- Adrenergic Neurone Blockers: enhanced hypotensive effect when general anaesthetics given with ●adrenergic neurone blockers
- Alpha-blockers: enhanced hypotensive effect when general anaesthetics given with ●alpha-blockers
Angiotensin-II Receptor Antagonists: enhanced hypotensive effect when general anaesthetics given with angiotensin-II receptor antagonists
Antibacterials: general anaesthetics possibly potentiate hepatotoxicity of isoniazid; effects of thiopental enhanced by sulphonamides; hypersensitivity-like reactions can occur when general anaesthetics given with intravenous vancomycin
- Antidepressants: Because of hazardous interactions between general anaesthetics and ●MAOIs, MAOIs should normally be stopped 2 weeks before surgery; increased risk of arrhythmias and hypotension when general anaesthetics given with tricyclics
- Antipsychotics: enhanced hypotensive effect when general anaesthetics given with ●antipsychotics
Anxiolytics and Hypnotics: increased sedative effect when general anaesthetics given with anxiolytics and hypnotics

Anaesthetics, General *(continued)*

Beta-blockers: enhanced hypotensive effect when general anaesthetics given with beta-blockers

● Calcium-channel Blockers: enhanced hypotensive effect when general anaesthetics or isoflurane given with calcium-channel blockers; general anaesthetics enhance hypotensive effect of ●verapamil (also AV delay)

Clonidine: enhanced hypotensive effect when general anaesthetics given with clonidine

● Cytotoxics: nitrous oxide increases antifolate effect of ●methotrexate—avoid concomitant use

Diazoxide: enhanced hypotensive effect when general anaesthetics given with diazoxide

Diuretics: enhanced hypotensive effect when general anaesthetics given with diuretics

● Dopaminergics: increased risk of arrhythmias when volatile liquid general anaesthetics given with ●levodopa

Ergot Alkaloids: halothane reduces effects of ergometrine on the parturient uterus

● Memantine: increased risk of CNS toxicity when ketamine given with ●memantine (manufacturer of memantine advises avoid concomitant use)

Methyldopa: enhanced hypotensive effect when general anaesthetics given with methyldopa

Moxonidine: enhanced hypotensive effect when general anaesthetics given with moxonidine

Muscle Relaxants: volatile liquid general anaesthetics enhance effects of non-depolarising muscle relaxants and suxamethonium

Nitrates: enhanced hypotensive effect when general anaesthetics given with nitrates

Oxytocin: oxytocic effect possibly reduced, also enhanced hypotensive effect and risk of arrhythmias when volatile liquid general anaesthetics given with oxytocin

● Sympathomimetics: increased risk of arrhythmias when volatile liquid general anaesthetics given with ●adrenaline (epinephrine); increased risk of hypertension when volatile liquid general anaesthetics given with ●methylphenidate

Theophylline: increased risk of convulsions when ketamine given with theophylline; increased risk of arrhythmias when halothane given with theophylline

Vasodilator Antihypertensives: enhanced hypotensive effect when general anaesthetics given with hydralazine, minoxidil or nitroprusside

Anaesthetics, General (intravenous) *see* Anaesthetics, General

Anaesthetics, General (volatile liquids) *see* Anaesthetics, General

Anaesthetics, Local *see* Bupivacaine, Levobupivacaine, Lidocaine (lignocaine), Prilocaine, and Ropivacaine

Anakinra

● Adalimumab: avoid concomitant use of anakinra with ●adalimumab

● Etanercept: increased risk of side-effects when anakinra given with ●etanercept—avoid concomitant use

● Infliximab: avoid concomitant use of anakinra with ●infliximab

● Vaccines: avoid concomitant use of anakinra with live ●vaccines (see p. 578)

Analgesics *see* Aspirin, Nefopam, NSAIDs, Opioid Analgesics, and Paracetamol

Angiotensin-II Receptor Antagonists

ACE Inhibitors: enhanced hypotensive effect when angiotensin-II receptor antagonists given with ACE inhibitors

Angiotensin-II Receptor Antagonists *(continued)*

Adrenergic Neurone Blockers: enhanced hypotensive effect when angiotensin-II receptor antagonists given with adrenergic neurone blockers

Alcohol: enhanced hypotensive effect when angiotensin-II receptor antagonists given with alcohol

Aldesleukin: enhanced hypotensive effect when angiotensin-II receptor antagonists given with aldesleukin

Alpha-blockers: enhanced hypotensive effect when angiotensin-II receptor antagonists given with alpha-blockers

Alprostadil: enhanced hypotensive effect when angiotensin-II receptor antagonists given with alprostadil

Amifostine: possible enhanced hypotensive effect when angiotensin-II receptor antagonists given with amifostine

Anaesthetics, General: enhanced hypotensive effect when angiotensin-II receptor antagonists given with general anaesthetics

Analgesics: increased risk of renal impairment when angiotensin-II receptor antagonists given with NSAIDs, also hypotensive effect antagonised; increased risk of hyperkalaemia when angiotensin-II receptor antagonists given with ketorolac; risk of renal impairment when angiotensin-II receptor antagonists given with aspirin (in doses over 300 mg daily), also hypotensive effect antagonised

Anticoagulants: increased risk of hyperkalaemia when angiotensin-II receptor antagonists given with heparin

Antidepressants: hypotensive effect of angiotensin-II receptor antagonists possibly enhanced by MAOIs

Antipsychotics: enhanced hypotensive effect when angiotensin-II receptor antagonists given with antipsychotics

Anxiolytics and Hypnotics: enhanced hypotensive effect when angiotensin-II receptor antagonists given with anxiolytics and hypnotics

Beta-blockers: enhanced hypotensive effect when angiotensin-II receptor antagonists given with beta-blockers

Calcium-channel Blockers: enhanced hypotensive effect when angiotensin-II receptor antagonists given with calcium-channel blockers

● Cardiac Glycosides: telmisartan increases plasma concentration of ●digoxin

● Ciclosporin: increased risk of hyperkalaemia when angiotensin-II receptor antagonists given with ●ciclosporin

Clonidine: enhanced hypotensive effect when angiotensin-II receptor antagonists given with clonidine

Corticosteroids: hypotensive effect of angiotensin-II receptor antagonists antagonised by corticosteroids

Diazoxide: enhanced hypotensive effect when angiotensin-II receptor antagonists given with diazoxide

● Diuretics: enhanced hypotensive effect when angiotensin-II receptor antagonists given with ●diuretics; increased risk of hyperkalaemia when angiotensin-II receptor antagonists given with ●potassium-sparing diuretics

Dopaminergics: enhanced hypotensive effect when angiotensin-II receptor antagonists given with levodopa

Epoetin: antagonism of hypotensive effect and increased risk of hyperkalaemia when angiotensin-II receptor antagonists given with epoetin

Angiotensin-II Receptor Antagonists *(continued)*

• Lithium: angiotensin-II receptor antagonists reduce excretion of •lithium (increased plasma concentration)

Methyldopa: enhanced hypotensive effect when angiotensin-II receptor antagonists given with methyldopa

Moxisylyte (thymoxamine): enhanced hypotensive effect when angiotensin-II receptor antagonists given with moxisylyte

Moxonidine: enhanced hypotensive effect when angiotensin-II receptor antagonists given with moxonidine

Muscle Relaxants: enhanced hypotensive effect when angiotensin-II receptor antagonists given with baclofen or tizanidine

Nitrates: enhanced hypotensive effect when angiotensin-II receptor antagonists given with nitrates

Oestrogens: hypotensive effect of angiotensin-II receptor antagonists antagonised by oestrogens

• Potassium Salts: increased risk of hyperkalaemia when angiotensin-II receptor antagonists given with •potassium salts

Progestogens: risk of hyperkalaemia when angiotensin-II receptor antagonists given with drospirenone (monitor serum potassium during first cycle)

Ulcer-healing Drugs: hypotensive effect of angiotensin-II receptor antagonists antagonised by carbenoxolone

Vasodilator Antihypertensives: enhanced hypotensive effect when angiotensin-II receptor antagonists given with hydralazine, minoxidil or nitroprusside

Anion-exchange Resins *see* Colestipol and Colestyramine

Antacids

Note. Antacids should preferably not be taken at the same time as other drugs since they may impair absorption

ACE Inhibitors: antacids possibly reduce absorption of ACE inhibitors; antacids reduce absorption of captopril, enalapril and fosinopril

Analgesics: antacids reduce absorption of diflunisal; alkaline urine due to some antacids increases excretion of aspirin

Anti-arrhythmics: alkaline urine due to some antacids reduces excretion of quinidine (plasma concentration of quinidine occasionally increased)

Antibacterials: antacids reduce absorption of azithromycin, cefaclor, cefpodoxime, ciprofloxacin, isoniazid, levofloxacin, moxifloxacin, norfloxacin, ofloxacin, rifampicin and tetracyclines; oral magnesium salts (as magnesium trisilicate) reduce absorption of nitrofurantoin

Antiepileptics: antacids reduce absorption of gabapentin and phenytoin

Antifungals: antacids reduce absorption of itraconazole and ketoconazole

Antihistamines: antacids reduce absorption of fexofenadine

Antimalarials: antacids reduce absorption of chloroquine and hydroxychloroquine; oral magnesium salts (as magnesium trisilicate) reduce absorption of proguanil

Antipsychotics: antacids reduce absorption of phenothiazines and sulpiride

Antivirals: antacids possibly reduce absorption of amprenavir; antacids reduce absorption of zalcitabine

Bile Acids: antacids possibly reduce absorption of bile acids

Bisphosphonates: antacids reduce absorption of bisphosphonates

Antacids *(continued)*

Cardiac Glycosides: antacids possibly reduce absorption of digoxin

Corticosteroids: antacids reduce absorption of deflazacort

Cytotoxics: antacids reduce absorption of mycophenolate mofetil

Dipyridamole: antacids possibly reduce absorption of dipyridamole

Iron: oral magnesium salts (as magnesium trisilicate) reduce absorption of *oral* iron

Lipid-regulating Drugs: antacids reduce absorption of rosuvastatin

Lithium: sodium bicarbonate increases excretion of lithium (reduced plasma concentration)

Penicillamine: antacids reduce absorption of penicillamine

Ulcer-healing Drugs: antacids possibly reduce absorption of lansoprazole

Antazoline *see* Antihistamines

Anti-arrhythmics *see* Adenosine, Amiodarone, Bretylium, Disopyramide, Flecainide, Lidocaine (lignocaine), Mexiletine, Procainamide, Propafenone, and Quinidine

Antibacterials *see* individual drugs

Antibiotics (cytotoxic) *see* Doxorubicin

Anticoagulants *see* Coumarins, Heparins, and Phenindione

Antidepressants *see* Antidepressants, SSRI; Antidepressants, Tricyclic; Antidepressants, Tricyclic (related); MAOIs; Mirtazapine; Moclobemide; Reboxetine; St John's Wort; Tryptophan; Venlafaxine

Antidepressants, Noradrenaline Re-uptake Inhibitors *see* Reboxetine

Antidepressants, SSRI

Alcohol: sedative effects possibly increased when SSRIs given with alcohol

Anaesthetics, Local: fluvoxamine inhibits metabolism of ropivacaine—avoid prolonged administration of ropivacaine

• Analgesics: increased risk of bleeding when SSRIs given with •NSAIDs or •aspirin; fluvoxamine possibly increases plasma concentration of methadone; increased risk of CNS toxicity when SSRIs given with •tramadol

Anti-arrhythmics: fluoxetine increases plasma concentration of flecainide

• Anticoagulants: SSRIs possibly enhance anticoagulant effect of •coumarins

• Antidepressants: avoidance of fluvoxamine advised by manufacturer of •reboxetine; citalopram, escitalopram or fluvoxamine should not be started until 2 weeks after stopping •MAOIs, also MAOIs should not be started until at least 1 week after stopping citalopram, escitalopram or fluvoxamine; CNS effects of SSRIs increased by •MAOIs (risk of serious toxicity); paroxetine or sertraline should not be started until 2 weeks after stopping •MAOIs, also MAOIs should not be started until at least 2 weeks after stopping paroxetine or sertraline; fluoxetine should not be started until 2 weeks after stopping •MAOIs, also MAOIs should not be started until at least 5 weeks after stopping fluoxetine; increased risk of CNS toxicity when escitalopram given with •moclobemide, preferably avoid concomitant use; after stopping citalopram or fluvoxamine do not start •moclobemide for at least 1 week; after stopping fluoxetine do not start •moclobemide for 5 weeks; after stopping paroxetine or sertraline do not start •moclobemide for 2 weeks; increased serotonergic effects when SSRIs given with •St John's wort—avoid concomitant use; SSRIs increase plasma concentration

Antidepressants, SSRI

- Antidepressants *(continued)*
  of some ●tricyclics; agitation and nausea may
  occur when SSRIs given with ●tryptophan
- Antiepileptics: SSRIs antagonise anticonvulsant
  effect of ●antiepileptics (convulsive threshold
  lowered); plasma concentration of paroxetine
  reduced by carbamazepine, phenytoin and
  primidone; fluoxetine and fluvoxamine increase
  plasma concentration of ●carbamazepine; fluoxetine and fluvoxamine increase plasma concentration of ●phenytoin
- Antihistamines: increased risk of ventricular arrhythmias when citalopram, fluoxetine or fluvoxamine given with ●terfenadine—avoid
  concomitant use
- Antimalarials: avoidance of antidepressants advised
  by manufacturer of ●artemether/lumefantrine
  Antimuscarinics: paroxetine increases plasma concentration of procyclidine
- Antipsychotics: fluoxetine increases plasma concentration of ●clozapine, ●haloperidol, risperidone, ●sertindole and ●zotepine; paroxetine
  increases plasma concentration of ●thioridazine
  (increased risk of ventricular arrhythmias—avoid
  concomitant use); fluvoxamine, paroxetine and
  sertraline increase plasma concentration of ●cloz-
  apine; fluvoxamine increases plasma concentration of olanzapine; sertraline increases plasma
  concentration of ●pimozide (increased risk of
  ventricular arrhythmias—avoid concomitant use);
  paroxetine increases plasma concentration of
  ●sertindole
- Antivirals: plasma concentration of sertraline
  reduced by efavirenz; plasma concentration of
  SSRIs possibly increased by ●ritonavir
  Anxiolytics and Hypnotics: fluvoxamine increases
  plasma concentration of some benzodiazepines;
  sedative effects possibly increased when sertraline
  given with zolpidem
  Barbiturates: SSRIs antagonise anticonvulsant effect
  of barbiturates (convulsive threshold lowered);
  plasma concentration of paroxetine reduced by
  phenobarbital
  Beta-blockers: fluvoxamine increases plasma concentration of propranolol
- Dopaminergics: caution with paroxetine advised by
  manufacturer of entacapone; increased risk of
  hypertension and CNS excitation when paroxetine
  or sertraline given with ●selegiline (selegiline
  should not be started until 2 weeks after stopping
  paroxetine or sertraline, avoid paroxetine or
  sertraline for 2 weeks after stopping selegiline);
  increased risk of hypertension and CNS excitation
  when fluvoxamine given with ●selegiline (selegiline should not be started until 1 week after
  stopping fluvoxamine, avoid fluvoxamine for 2
  weeks after stopping selegiline); increased risk of
  hypertension and CNS excitation when fluoxetine
  given with ●selegiline (selegiline should not be
  started until 5 weeks after stopping fluoxetine,
  avoid fluoxetine for 2 weeks after stopping
  selegiline); theoretical risk of serotonin syndrome
  if citalopram given with selegiline (especially if
  dose of selegiline exceeds 10 mg daily); manufacturer of escitalopram advises caution with
  selegiline
- 5HT₁ Agonists: fluvoxamine possibly inhibits
  metabolism of frovatriptan; possible increased
  serotonergic effects when SSRIs given with
  frovatriptan; increased risk of CNS toxicity when
  citalopram, escitalopram, fluoxetine, fluvoxamine
  or paroxetine given with ●sumatriptan; increased

Antidepressants, SSRI

- 5HT₁ Agonists *(continued)*
  risk of CNS toxicity when sertraline given with
  ●sumatriptan (manufacturer of sertraline advises
  avoid concomitant use); fluvoxamine possibly
  inhibits metabolism of zolmitriptan (reduce dose
  of zolmitriptan)
- Lithium: Increased risk of CNS effects when SSRIs
  given with ●lithium (lithium toxicity reported)
  Parasympathomimetics: paroxetine increases plasma
  concentration of galantamine
- Sibutramine: increased risk of CNS toxicity when
  SSRIs given with ●sibutramine (manufacturer of
  sibutramine advises avoid concomitant use)
  Sympathomimetics: metabolism of SSRIs possibly
  inhibited by methylphenidate
- Theophylline: fluvoxamine increases plasma concentration of ●theophylline (concomitant use
  should usually be avoided, but where not possible
  halve theophylline dose and monitor plasma-
  theophylline concentration)
  Ulcer-healing Drugs: plasma concentration of sertraline increased by cimetidine

Antidepressants, SSRI (related) *see* Venlafaxine

Antidepressants, Tricyclic

Adrenergic Neurone Blockers: tricyclics antagonise
  hypotensive effect of adrenergic neurone blockers
- Alcohol: increased sedative effect when tricyclics
  given with ●alcohol
  Alpha₂-adrenoceptor Stimulants: avoidance of tricyclics advised by manufacturer of apraclonidine
  and brimonidine
  Anaesthetics, General: increased risk of arrhythmias
  and hypotension when tricyclics given with
  general anaesthetics
- Analgesics: increased risk of CNS toxicity when
  tricyclics given with ●tramadol; side-effects possibly increased when tricyclics given with
  nefopam; sedative effects possibly increased when
  tricyclics given with opioid analgesics
- Anti-arrhythmics: increased risk of ventricular
  arrhythmias when tricyclics given with ●amio-
  darone—avoid concomitant use; increased risk of
  ventricular arrhythmias when tricyclics given with
  ●disopyramide, ●flecainide, ●procainamide or
  ●quinidine; increased risk of arrhythmias when
  tricyclics given with ●propafenone
- Antibacterials: increased risk of ventricular arrhythmias when tricyclics given with ●moxifloxacin—
  avoid concomitant use; plasma concentration of
  tricyclics possibly reduced by rifampicin
- Antidepressants: increased risk of hypertension and
  CNS excitation when tricyclics given with
  ●MAOIs, tricyclics should not be started until 2
  weeks after stopping MAOIs (3 weeks if starting
  clomipramine or imipramine), also MAOIs should
  not be started for at least 1–2 weeks after stopping
  tricyclics (3 weeks in the case of clomipramine or
  imipramine); after stopping tricyclics do not start
  ●moclobemide for at least 1 week; plasma
  concentration of some tricyclics increased by
  ●SSRIs; plasma concentration of amitriptyline
  reduced by St John's wort
- Antiepileptics: tricyclics antagonise anticonvulsant
  effect of ●antiepileptics (convulsive threshold
  lowered); metabolism of tricyclics accelerated by
  ●carbamazepine (reduced plasma concentration
  and reduced effect); plasma concentration of
  tricyclics possibly reduced by ●phenytoin; tricyclics antagonise anticonvulsant effect of ●primid-
  one (convulsive threshold lowered), also
  metabolism of tricyclics possibly accelerated
  (reduced plasma concentration)

Antidepressants, Tricyclic *(continued)*

- Antihistamines: increased risk of ventricular arrhythmias when tricyclics given with ●terfenadine—avoid concomitant use; increased antimuscarinic and sedative effects when tricyclics given with antihistamines

- Antimalarials: avoidance of antidepressants advised by manufacturer of ●artemether/lumefantrine

Antimuscarinics: increased risk of antimuscarinic side-effects when tricyclics given with antimuscarinics

- Antipsychotics: plasma concentration of tricyclics increased by ●antipsychotics—possibly increased risk of ventricular arrhythmias; increased risk of ventricular arrhythmias when tricyclics given with ●pimozide or ●thioridazine—avoid concomitant use; possibly increased antimuscarinic side-effects when tricyclics given with clozapine; increased risk of antimuscarinic side-effects when tricyclics given with phenothiazines

- Antivirals: plasma concentration of tricyclics possibly increased by ●ritonavir

Anxiolytics and Hypnotics: increased sedative effect when tricyclics given with anxiolytics and hypnotics

- Barbiturates: tricyclics antagonises anticonvulsant effect of ●barbiturates (convulsive threshold lowered), also metabolism of tricyclics possibly accelerated (reduced plasma concentration)

- Beta-blockers: increased risk of ventricular arrhythmias when tricyclics given with ●sotalol

Calcium-channel Blockers: plasma concentration of imipramine increased by diltiazem and verapamil; plasma concentration of tricyclics possibly increased by diltiazem and verapamil

- Clonidine: tricyclics antagonise hypotensive effect of ●clonidine, also increased risk of hypertension on clonidine withdrawal

Disulfiram: metabolism of tricyclics inhibited by disulfiram (increased plasma concentration); concomitant amitriptyline reported to increase disulfiram reaction with alcohol

Diuretics: increased risk of postural hypotension when tricyclics given with diuretics

- Dopaminergics: caution with tricyclics advised by manufacturer of entacapone; CNS toxicity reported when tricyclics given with ●selegiline

Muscle Relaxants: tricyclics enhance muscle relaxant effect of baclofen

Nicorandil: tricyclics possibly enhance hypotensive effect of nicorandil

Nitrates: tricyclics reduce effects of sublingual tablets of nitrates (failure to dissolve under tongue owing to dry mouth)

Oestrogens: antidepressant effect of tricyclics antagonised by oestrogens (but side-effects of tricyclics possibly increased due to increased plasma concentration)

- Sibutramine: increased risk of CNS toxicity when tricyclics given with ●sibutramine (manufacturer of sibutramine advises avoid concomitant use)

- Sympathomimetics: increased risk of hypertension and arrhythmias when tricyclics given with ●adrenaline (epinephrine) (but local anaesthetics with adrenaline appear to be safe); metabolism of tricyclics possibly inhibited by methylphenidate; increased risk of hypertension and arrhythmias when tricyclics given with ●noradrenaline (norepinephrine)

Thyroid Hormones: effects of tricyclics possibly enhanced by thyroid hormones; effects of amitriptyline and imipramine enhanced by thyroid hormones

Antidepressants, Tricyclic *(continued)*

Ulcer-healing Drugs: plasma concentration of tricyclics possibly increased by cimetidine; metabolism of amitriptyline, doxepin, imipramine and nortriptyline inhibited by cimetidine (increased plasma concentration)

Antidepressants, Tricyclic (related)

- Alcohol: increased sedative effect when tricyclic-related antidepressants given with ●alcohol

Alpha₂-adrenoceptor Stimulants: avoidance of tricyclic-related antidepressants advised by manufacturer of apraclonidine and brimonidine

- Antidepressants: tricyclic-related antidepressants should not be started until 2 weeks after stopping ●MAOIs, also MAOIs should not be started until at least 1–2 weeks after stopping tricyclic-related antidepressants; after stopping tricyclic-related antidepressants do not start ●moclobemide for at least 1 week

- Antiepileptics: tricyclic-related antidepressants possibly antagonise anticonvulsant effect of ●antiepileptics (convulsive threshold lowered); plasma concentration of mianserin reduced by ●carbamazepine and ●phenytoin; metabolism of mianserin accelerated by ●primidone (reduced plasma concentration)

Antihistamines: possible increased antimuscarinic and sedative effects when tricyclic-related antidepressants given with antihistamines

- Antimalarials: avoidance of antidepressants advised by manufacturer of ●artemether/lumefantrine

Antimuscarinics: possibly increased antimuscarinic side-effects when tricyclic-related antidepressants given with antimuscarinics

- Antipsychotics: increased risk of arrhythmias when maprotiline given with ●thioridazine—avoid concomitant use; increased risk of ventricular arrhythmias when maprotiline given with ●pimozide—avoid concomitant use

Anxiolytics and Hypnotics: increased sedative effect when tricyclic-related antidepressants given with anxiolytics and hypnotics

- Barbiturates: tricyclic-related antidepressants possibly antagonise anticonvulsant effect of ●barbiturates (convulsive threshold lowered); metabolism of mianserin accelerated by ●phenobarbital (reduced plasma concentration)

Diazoxide: enhanced hypotensive effect when tricyclic-related antidepressants given with diazoxide

Dopaminergics: caution with maprotiline advised by manufacturer of entacapone

Nitrates: tricyclic-related antidepressants possibly reduce effects of sublingual tablets of nitrates (failure to dissolve under tongue owing to dry mouth)

- Sibutramine: increased risk of CNS toxicity when tricyclic-related antidepressants given with ●sibutramine (manufacturer of sibutramine advises avoid concomitant use)

Vasodilator Antihypertensives: enhanced hypotensive effect when tricyclic-related antidepressants given with hydralazine or nitroprusside

Antidiabetics

ACE Inhibitors: hypoglycaemic effect of insulin, metformin and sulphonylureas possibly enhanced by ACE inhibitors

Alcohol: hypoglycaemic effect of antidiabetics enhanced by alcohol; increased risk of lactic acidosis when metformin given with alcohol; flushing, in susceptible subjects, when chlorpropamide given with alcohol

Anabolic Steroids: hypoglycaemic effect of antidiabetics possibly enhanced by anabolic steroids

Antidiabetics *(continued)*

● Analgesics: effects of sulphonylureas possibly enhanced by ●NSAIDs; effects of sulphonylureas enhanced by ●azapropazone (avoid concomitant use)

● Antibacterials: hypoglycaemic effect of acarbose possibly enhanced by neomycin, also severity of gastro-intestinal effects increased; effects of repaglinide enhanced by clarithromycin; effects of glibenclamide possibly enhanced by ciprofloxacin; plasma concentration of nateglinide and repaglinide reduced by rifampicin; effects of sulphonylureas enhanced by ●chloramphenicol; metabolism of chlorpropamide and tolbutamide accelerated by ●rifamycins (reduced effect); metabolism of sulphonylureas possibly accelerated by ●rifamycins (reduced effect); effects of sulphonylureas rarely enhanced by sulphonamides and trimethoprim

● Anticoagulants: hypoglycaemic effect of sulphonylureas possibly enhanced by ●coumarins, also possible changes to anticoagulant effect

Antidepressants: hypoglycaemic effect of insulin, metformin and sulphonylureas enhanced by MAOIs; hypoglycaemic effect of antidiabetics possibly enhanced by MAOIs

Antiepileptics: tolbutamide transiently increases plasma concentration of phenytoin (possibility of toxicity)

● Antifungals: plasma concentration of sulphonylureas increased by ●fluconazole and ●miconazole; hypoglycaemic effect of gliclazide and glipizide enhanced by ●miconazole— avoid concomitant use; plasma concentration of sulphonylureas possibly increased by voriconazole

Antihistamines: thrombocyte count depressed when metformin given with ketotifen

Antipsychotics: hypoglycaemic effect of sulphonylureas possibly antagonised by phenothiazines

Antivirals: plasma concentration of tolbutamide possibly increased by ritonavir

Beta-blockers: warning signs of hypoglycaemia (such as tremor) with antidiabetics may be masked when given with beta-blockers; hypoglycaemic effect of insulin enhanced by beta-blockers

● Bosentan: plasma concentration of both drugs reduced when glibenclamide given with ●bosentan (avoid concomitant use)

Calcium-channel Blockers: glucose tolerance occasionally impaired when insulin given with nifedipine

Corticosteroids: hypoglycaemic effect of antidiabetics antagonised by corticosteroids

Cytotoxics: metabolism of rosiglitazone possibly inhibited by paclitaxel

Diazoxide: hypoglycaemic effect of antidiabetics antagonised by diazoxide

Diuretics: hypoglycaemic effect of antidiabetics antagonised by loop diuretics and thiazides and related diuretics; increased risk of hyponatraemia when chlorpropamide given with potassium-sparing diuretics plus thiazide

Hormone Antagonists: possible acceleration of the metabolism of biguanides and sulphonylureas advised by manufacturer of aminoglutethimide; requirements for insulin, metformin, repaglinide and sulphonylureas possibly reduced by octreotide

Leflunomide: hypoglycaemic effect of tolbutamide possibly enhanced by leflunomide

● Lipid-regulating Drugs: hypoglycaemic effect of acarbose possibly enhanced by colestyramine; increased risk of severe hypoglycaemia when repaglinide given with ●gemfibrozil—avoid concomitant use; may be improved glucose tolerance

Antidiabetics

● Lipid-regulating Drugs *(continued)*
and an additive effect when insulin or sulphonylureas given with fibrates

Oestrogens: hypoglycaemic effect of antidiabetics antagonised by oestrogens

Orlistat: avoidance of acarbose advised by manufacturer of orlistat

Pancreatin: hypoglycaemic effect of acarbose antagonised by pancreatin

Probenecid: hypoglycaemic effect of chlorpropamide possibly enhanced by probenecid

Progestogens: hypoglycaemic effect of antidiabetics antagonised by progestogens

● Sulfinpyrazone: effects of sulphonylureas enhanced by ●sulfinpyrazone

Testosterone: hypoglycaemic effect of antidiabetics possibly enhanced by testosterone

Ulcer-healing Drugs: excretion of metformin reduced by cimetidine (increased plasma concentration); hypoglycaemic effect of sulphonylureas enhanced by cimetidine

Antiepileptics see Carbamazepine, Ethosuximide, Gabapentin, Lamotrigine, Levetiracetam, Oxcarbazepine, Phenytoin, Primidone, Tiagabine, Topiramate, Valproate, and Vigabatrin

Antifungals see Amphotericin; Antifungals, Imidazole; Antifungals, Triazole; Caspofungin; Flucytosine; Griseofulvin; Terbinafine

Antifungals, Imidazole

Analgesics: ketoconazole increases plasma concentration of valdecoxib (reduce initial dose of valdecoxib); ketoconazole inhibits metabolism of alfentanil (risk of prolonged or delayed respiratory depression)

Antacids: absorption of ketoconazole reduced by antacids

● Anti-arrhythmics: miconazole increases plasma concentration of ●quinidine (increased risk of ventricular arrhythmias—avoid concomitant use)

● Antibacterials: metabolism of ketoconazole accelerated by ●rifampicin (reduced plasma concentration), also plasma concentration of rifampicin may be reduced by ketoconazole; plasma concentration of ketoconazole possibly reduced by isoniazid

● Anticoagulants: ketoconazole enhances anticoagulant effect of ●coumarins; miconazole enhances anticoagulant effect of ●coumarins (miconazole oral gel and possibly vaginal formulations absorbed)

● Antidepressants: avoidance of imidazoles advised by manufacturer of ●reboxetine; ketoconazole increases plasma concentration of mirtazapine

● Antidiabetics: miconazole enhances hypoglycaemic effect of ●gliclazide and ●glipizide— avoid concomitant use; miconazole increases plasma concentration of ●sulphonylureas

● Antiepileptics: plasma concentration of ketoconazole reduced by ●phenytoin; miconazole enhances anticonvulsant effect of ●phenytoin (plasma concentration of phenytoin increased)

Antifungals: imidazoles possibly antagonise effects of amphotericin

● Antihistamines: manufacturer of loratadine advises ketoconazole possibly increases plasma concentration of loratadine; imidazoles possibly inhibit metabolism of ●mizolastine (avoid concomitant use); ketoconazole inhibits metabolism of ●mizolastine—avoid concomitant use; imidazoles inhibit metabolism of ●terfenadine—risk of ventricular arrhythmias, avoid concomitant use of systemic or topical preparations

Antifungals, Imidazole (continued)

- Antimalarials: avoidance of imidazoles advised by manufacturer of ●artemether/lumefantrine

  Antimuscarinics: absorption of ketoconazole reduced by antimuscarinics; avoidance of ketoconazole advised by manufacturer of tolterodine

- Antipsychotics: increased risk of ventricular arrhythmias when imidazoles given with ●pimozide—avoid concomitant use; imidazoles possibly increase plasma concentration of quetiapine (reduce dose of quetiapine); increased risk of ventricular arrhythmias when ketoconazole given with ●sertindole—avoid concomitant use; possible increased risk of ventricular arrhythmias when imidazoles given with ●sertindole—avoid concomitant use

- Antivirals: ketoconazole inhibits the metabolism of indinavir; plasma concentration of ketoconazole reduced by nevirapine—avoid concomitant use; combination of ketoconazole with ●ritonavir may increase plasma concentration of either drug (or both); ketoconazole increases plasma concentration of saquinavir; imidazoles possibly increase plasma concentration of saquinavir

- Anxiolytics and Hypnotics: ketoconazole increases plasma concentration of ●midazolam (risk of prolonged sedation)

  Bosentan: ketoconazole possibly increases plasma concentration of bosentan

- Calcium-channel Blockers: ketoconazole inhibits metabolism of ●felodipine (increased plasma concentration); avoidance of ketoconazole advised by manufacturer of lercanidipine; ketoconazole possibly inhibits metabolism of dihydropyridines (increased plasma concentration)

- Ciclosporin: ketoconazole inhibits metabolism of ●ciclosporin (increased plasma concentration); miconazole possibly inhibits metabolism of ●ciclosporin (increased plasma concentration)

- Cilostazol: ketoconazole possibly increases plasma concentration of ●cilostazol—avoid concomitant use

  Corticosteroids: ketoconazole possibly inhibits metabolism of corticosteroids; ketoconazole inhibits the metabolism of methylprednisolone; ketoconazole increases plasma concentration of inhaled mometasone

  Cytotoxics: *in vitro* studies suggest a possible interaction between ketoconazole and docetaxel (consult docetaxel product literature); ketoconazole increases plasma concentration of imatinib

- Ergot Alkaloids: increased risk of ergotism when imidazoles given with ●ergotamine and methysergide—avoid concomitant use

- 5HT$_1$ Agonists: ketoconazole increases plasma concentration of ●eletriptan (risk of toxicity)—avoid concomitant use

- Lipid-regulating Drugs: possible increased risk of myopathy when imidazoles given with atorvastatin or simvastatin; increased risk of myopathy when ketoconazole given with ●simvastatin (avoid concomitant use); possible increased risk of myopathy when miconazole given with ●simvastatin—avoid concomitant use

  Oestrogens: anecdotal reports of contraceptive failure when imidazoles or ketoconazole given with oestrogens

  Parasympathomimetics: ketoconazole increases plasma concentration of galantamine

  Sildenafil: ketoconazole increases plasma concentration of sildenafil—reduce initial dose of sildenafil

- Sirolimus: ketoconazole and miconazole increase plasma concentration of ●sirolimus

Antifungals, Imidazole (continued)

- Tacrolimus: imidazoles possibly increase plasma concentration of ●tacrolimus; ketoconazole increases plasma concentration of ●tacrolimus

  Tadalafil: ketoconazole increases plasma concentration of tadalafil

- Theophylline: ketoconazole possibly increases plasma concentration of ●theophylline

  Ulcer-healing Drugs: absorption of ketoconazole reduced by histamine H$_2$-antagonists, proton pump inhibitors and sucralfate

- Vardenafil: ketoconazole increases plasma concentration of ●vardenafil—avoid concomitant use

Antifungals, Polyene *see* Amphotericin

Antifungals, Triazole

Note. In general, fluconazole interactions relate to multiple-dose treatment

Analgesics: fluconazole increases plasma concentration of celecoxib (halve dose of celecoxib); fluconazole increases plasma concentration of parecoxib (reduce dose of parecoxib); fluconazole increases plasma concentration of valdecoxib—reduce initial dose of valdecoxib

Antacids: absorption of itraconazole reduced by antacids

- Anti-arrhythmics: itraconazole and voriconazole increase plasma concentration of ●quinidine (increased risk of ventricular arrhythmias—avoid concomitant use)

- Antibacterials: plasma concentration of itraconazole increased by clarithromycin; triazoles possibly increase plasma concentration of ●rifabutin (increased risk of uveitis—reduce rifabutin dose); voriconazole increases plasma concentration of ●rifabutin, also rifabutin reduces plasma concentration of voriconazole (increase dose of voriconazole and also monitor for rifabutin toxicity); fluconazole increases plasma concentration of ●rifabutin (increased risk of uveitis—reduce rifabutin dose); plasma concentration of voriconazole reduced by ●rifampicin—avoid concomitant use; metabolism of fluconazole and itraconazole accelerated by ●rifampicin (reduced plasma concentration)

- Anticoagulants: fluconazole, itraconazole and voriconazole enhance anticoagulant effect of ●coumarins

- Antidepressants: avoidance of triazoles advised by manufacturer of ●reboxetine

- Antidiabetics: voriconazole possibly increases plasma concentration of sulphonylureas; fluconazole increases plasma concentration of ●sulphonylureas

- Antiepileptics: plasma concentration of voriconazole possibly reduced by ●carbamazepine and ●primidone—avoid concomitant use; voriconazole increases plasma concentration of ●phenytoin, also phenytoin reduces plasma concentration of voriconazole (increase dose of voriconazole and also monitor for phenytoin toxicity); plasma concentration of itraconazole reduced by ●phenytoin; fluconazole increases plasma concentration of ●phenytoin (consider reducing dose of phenytoin)

  Antifungals: triazoles possibly antagonise effects of amphotericin

- Antihistamines: itraconazole inhibits metabolism of ●mizolastine—avoid concomitant use; triazoles inhibit metabolism of ●terfenadine—risk of ventricular arrhythmias, avoid concomitant use of systemic or topical preparations

- Antimalarials: avoidance of triazoles advised by manufacturer of ●artemether/lumefantrine

Antifungals, Triazole *(continued)*

Antimuscarinics: avoidance of itraconazole advised by manufacturer of tolterodine

• Antipsychotics: increased risk of ventricular arrhythmias when triazoles given with ●pimozide—avoid concomitant use; triazoles possibly increase plasma concentration of quetiapine (reduce dose of quetiapine); possible increased risk of ventricular arrhythmias when triazoles given with ●sertindole—avoid concomitant use; increased risk of ventricular arrhythmias when itraconazole given with ●sertindole—avoid concomitant use

• Antivirals: plasma concentration of itraconazole possibly increased by amprenavir; itraconazole increases plasma concentration of ●indinavir (consider reducing dose of indinavir); itraconazole increases plasma concentration of ●nevirapine and ritonavir; combination of itraconazole with ●ritonavir may increase plasma concentration of either drug (or both); triazoles possibly increase plasma concentration of saquinavir; fluconazole increases plasma concentration of ●zidovudine (increased risk of toxicity)

• Anxiolytics and Hypnotics: fluconazole and itraconazole increase plasma concentration of ●midazolam (risk of prolonged sedation); itraconazole increases plasma concentration of buspirone (reduce dose of buspirone)

• Barbiturates: plasma concentration of voriconazole possibly reduced by ●phenobarbital—avoid concomitant use

• Bosentan: fluconazole increases plasma concentration of ●bosentan—avoid concomitant use; itraconazole possibly increases plasma concentration of bosentan

• Calcium-channel Blockers: negative inotropic effect possibly increased when itraconazole given with calcium-channel blockers; itraconazole inhibits metabolism of ●felodipine (increased plasma concentration); avoidance of itraconazole advised by manufacturer of lercanidipine; itraconazole possibly inhibits metabolism of dihydropyridines (increased plasma concentration)

• Cardiac Glycosides: itraconazole increases plasma concentration of ●digoxin

• Ciclosporin: fluconazole, itraconazole and voriconazole inhibit metabolism of ●ciclosporin (increased plasma concentration)

Corticosteroids: itraconazole possibly inhibits metabolism of methylprednisolone

Cytotoxics: itraconazole inhibits metabolism of busulfan (increased risk of toxicity); itraconazole possibly inhibits metabolism of vincristine (increased risk of neurotoxicity)

Diuretics: plasma concentration of fluconazole increased by hydrochlorothiazide

• Ergot Alkaloids: increased risk of ergotism when triazoles given with ●ergotamine and methysergide—avoid concomitant use

• 5HT₁ Agonists: itraconazole increases plasma concentration of ●eletriptan (risk of toxicity)—avoid concomitant use

• Lipid-regulating Drugs: possible increased risk of myopathy when triazoles given with atorvastatin or simvastatin; increased risk of myopathy when itraconazole given with ●atorvastatin or ●simvastatin (avoid concomitant use)

Oestrogens: anecdotal reports of contraceptive failure when fluconazole or itraconazole given with oestrogens

Sildenafil: itraconazole increases plasma concentration of sildenafil—reduce initial dose of sildenafil

• Sirolimus: voriconazole increases plasma concentration of ●sirolimus—avoid concomitant use;

Antifungals, Triazole

• Sirolimus *(continued)*
itraconazole increases plasma concentration of ●sirolimus

• Tacrolimus: triazoles possibly increase plasma concentration of ●tacrolimus; fluconazole and voriconazole increase plasma concentration of ●tacrolimus

Tadalafil: itraconazole possibly increases plasma concentration of tadalafil

• Theophylline: fluconazole possibly increases plasma concentration of ●theophylline

Ulcer-healing Drugs: voriconazole increases plasma concentration of omeprazole (reduce dose of omeprazole); absorption of itraconazole reduced by histamine H₂-antagonists and proton pump inhibitors

• Vardenafil: itraconazole possibly increases plasma concentration of ●vardenafil—avoid concomitant use

Antihistamines

Note. Sedative interactions apply to a lesser extent to the non-sedating antihistamines. Interactions do not generally apply to antihistamines used for topical action (including inhalation)

Alcohol: increased sedative effect when antihistamines given with alcohol (possibly less effect with non-sedating antihistamines)

Antacids: absorption of fexofenadine reduced by antacids

• Anti-arrhythmics: increased risk of ventricular arrhythmias when terfenadine given with ●anti-arrhythmics; increased risk of ventricular arrhythmias when mizolastine or terfenadine given with ●amiodarone—avoid concomitant use; increased risk of ventricular arrhythmias when mizolastine or terfenadine given with ●disopyramide—avoid concomitant use; increased risk of ventricular arrhythmias when mizolastine or terfenadine given with ●flecainide—avoid concomitant use; increased risk of ventricular arrhythmias when mizolastine or terfenadine given with ●mexiletine—avoid concomitant use; increased risk of ventricular arrhythmias when mizolastine or terfenadine given with ●procainamide—avoid concomitant use; increased risk of ventricular arrhythmias when mizolastine or terfenadine given with ●propafenone—avoid concomitant use; increased risk of ventricular arrhythmias when mizolastine or terfenadine given with ●quinidine—avoid concomitant use

• Antibacterials: metabolism of terfenadine inhibited by ●clarithromycin (avoid concomitant use—increased risk of ventricular arrhythmias); manufacturer of loratadine advises plasma concentration possibly increased by erythromycin; metabolism of mizolastine inhibited by ●erythromycin—avoid concomitant use; metabolism of terfenadine inhibited by ●erythromycin—risk of ventricular arrhythmias, avoid concomitant use of systemic or topical preparations; increased risk of ventricular arrhythmias when mizolastine or terfenadine given with ●moxifloxacin—avoid concomitant use; metabolism of mizolastine possibly inhibited by ●macrolides (avoid concomitant use); increased risk of ventricular arrhythmias when terfenadine given with ●quinupristin/dalfopristin or ●telithromycin—avoid concomitant use

• Antidepressants: increased risk of ventricular arrhythmias when terfenadine given with ●citalopram, ●fluoxetine, fluvoxamine or ●tricyclics—avoid concomitant use; increased antimuscarinic and sedative effects when antihistamines given with MAOIs or tricyclics; possible increased antimus-

Antihistamines

- Antidepressants *(continued)*
  carinic and sedative effects when antihistamines
  given with tricyclic-related antidepressants
  Antidiabetics: thrombocyte count depressed when
  ketotifen given with metformin
- Antifungals: manufacturer of loratadine advises
  plasma concentration possibly increased by ketoconazole; metabolism of mizolastine inhibited by
  ●itraconazole or ●ketoconazole—avoid concomitant use; metabolism of terfenadine inhibited by
  ●imidazoles and ●triazoles—risk of ventricular
  arrhythmias, avoid concomitant use of systemic or
  topical preparations; metabolism of mizolastine
  possibly inhibited by ●imidazoles (avoid concomitant use)
- Antimalarials: avoidance of terfenadine advised by
  manufacturer of ●artemether/lumefantrine (risk of
  ventricular arrhythmias); increased risk of
  ventricular arrhythmias when terfenadine given with
  ●quinine—avoid concomitant use
  Antimuscarinics: increased risk of antimuscarinic
  side-effects when antihistamines given with antimuscarinics
- Antipsychotics: increased risk of ventricular arrhythmias when terfenadine given with ●antipsy-
  chotics; increased risk of ventricular arrhythmias
  when terfenadine given with ●pimozide, ●sertin-
  dole or ●thioridazine—avoid concomitant use
- Antivirals: plasma concentration of loratadine possibly increased by amprenavir; increased risk of
  ventricular arrhythmias when terfenadine given
  with ●amprenavir, ●efavirenz, ●indinavir, ●nelfi-
  navir, ●ritonavir or ●saquinavir—avoid concomitant use; plasma concentration of non-sedating
  antihistamines possibly increased by ritonavir
  Anxiolytics and Hypnotics: increased sedative effect
  when antihistamines given with anxiolytics and
  hypnotics
- Beta-blockers: increased risk of ventricular arrhythmias when mizolastine or terfenadine given with
  ●sotalol—avoid concomitant use
  Betahistine: antihistamines theoretically antagonise
  effect of betahistine
  Cytotoxics: *in vitro* studies suggest a possible
  interaction between terfenadine and docetaxel
  (consult docetaxel product literature)
- Diuretics: risk of ventricular arrhythmias with
  terfenadine increased by hypokalaemia or other
  electrolyte imbalance caused by ●diuretics
- Grapefruit Juice: plasma concentration of terfenadine increased by ●grapefruit juice—avoid concomitant use
- Hormone Antagonists: avoidance of terfenadine
  advised by manufacturer of ●bicalutamide
  Leukotriene Antagonists: terfenadine reduces
  plasma concentration of zafirlukast
- Pentamidine Isetionate: increased risk of ventricular
  arrhythmias when terfenadine given with ●pent-
  amidine isetionate—avoid concomitant use
  Ulcer-healing Drugs: manufacturer of loratadine
  advises plasma concentration possibly increased
  by cimetidine

Antihistamines, Non-sedating *see* Antihistamines
Antihistamines, Sedating *see* Antihistamines
Antimalarials *see* Artemether with Lumefantrine,
Chloroquine and Hydroxychloroquine, Meflo-
quine, Primaquine, Proguanil, and Quinine
Antimetabolites *see* Cytarabine, Fludarabine,
Fluorouracil, Mercaptopurine, and Methotrexate
Antimuscarinics
Note. Many drugs have antimuscarinic effects; concomi-
tant use of two or more such drugs can increase side-
effects such as dry mouth, urine retention, and constipa-

tion; concomitant use can also lead to confusion in the
elderly. Interactions do not generally apply to antimuscarinics used by inhalation
Alcohol: increased sedative effect when hyoscine
given with alcohol
Analgesics: increased risk of antimuscarinic side-
effects when antimuscarinics given with nefopam
Anti-arrhythmics: increased risk of antimuscarinic
side-effects when antimuscarinics given with
disopyramide; atropine delays absorption of
mexiletine
Antibacterials: manufacturer of tolterodine advises
avoid concomitant use with clarithromycin and
erythromycin
Antidepressants: plasma concentration of procyclidine increased by paroxetine; increased risk of
antimuscarinic side-effects when antimuscarinics
given with MAOIs or tricyclics; possibly increased
antimuscarinic side-effects when antimuscarinics
given with tricyclic-related antidepressants
Antifungals: antimuscarinics reduce absorption of
ketoconazole; manufacturer of tolterodine advises
avoid concomitant use with itraconazole and
ketoconazole
Antihistamines: increased risk of antimuscarinic
side-effects when antimuscarinics given with
antihistamines
<u>Antipsychotics</u>: antimuscarinics possibly reduce
effects of haloperidol; increased risk of antimuscarinic side-effects when antimuscarinics given
with clozapine; antimuscarinics reduce plasma
concentration of phenothiazines, but risk of
antimuscarinic side-effects increased
<u>Antivirals</u>: manufacturer of tolterodine advises avoid
concomitant use with amprenavir, indinavir,
lopinavir, nelfinavir, ritonavir and saquinavir
Domperidone: antimuscarinics antagonise effects of
domperidone on gastro-intestinal activity
Dopaminergics: increased risk of antimuscarinic
side-effects when antimuscarinics given with
amantadine; antimuscarinics possibly reduce
absorption of levodopa
Memantine: effects of antimuscarinics possibly
enhanced by memantine
Metoclopramide: antimuscarinics antagonise effects
of metoclopramide on gastro-intestinal activity
Nitrates: antimuscarinics possibly reduce effects of
sublingual tablets of nitrates (failure to dissolve
under tongue owing to dry mouth)
Parasympathomimetics: antimuscarinics antagonise
effects of parasympathomimetics

Antipsychotics

Note. Increased risk of toxicity with myelosuppressive
drugs
Note. Avoid concomitant use of clozapine with drugs that
have a substantial potential for causing agranulocytosis
ACE Inhibitors: enhanced hypotensive effect when
antipsychotics given with ACE inhibitors
Adrenergic Neurone Blockers: enhanced hypotensive effect when phenothiazines given with adrenergic neurone blockers; higher doses of
chlorpromazine antagonise hypotensive effect of
adrenergic neurone blockers; haloperidol antagonises hypotensive effect of adrenergic neurone
blockers
Adsorbents: absorption of phenothiazines possibly
reduced by kaolin
Alcohol: increased sedative effect when antipsychotics given with alcohol
Alpha-blockers: enhanced hypotensive effect when
antipsychotics given with alpha-blockers
- Anaesthetics, General: enhanced hypotensive effect
  when antipsychotics given with ●general anaesthetics

Antipsychotics *(continued)*

- Analgesics: avoid concomitant use of clozapine with
  ●azapropazone (increased risk of agranulocytosis);
  possible severe drowsiness when haloperidol
  given with indometacin; increased risk of convulsions when antipsychotics given with tramadol;
  enhanced hypotensive and sedative effects when
  antipsychotics given with opioid analgesics

  Angiotensin-II Receptor Antagonists: enhanced
  hypotensive effect when antipsychotics given with
  angiotensin-II receptor antagonists

  Antacids: absorption of phenothiazines and sulpiride
  reduced by antacids

- Anti-arrhythmics: increased risk of ventricular
  arrhythmias when antipsychotics that prolong the
  QT interval given with ●anti-arrhythmics that
  prolong the QT interval; increased risk of ventricular arrhythmias when amisulpride, haloperidol,
  phenothiazines, pimozide, sertindole or thioridazine given with ●amiodarone—avoid concomitant use; increased risk of ventricular arrhythmias
  when amisulpride, pimozide, sertindole or thioridazine given with ●disopyramide—avoid concomitant use; increased risk of ventricular
  arrhythmias when phenothiazines given with
  ●disopyramide, ●procainamide or ●quinidine;
  increased risk of arrhythmias when clozapine
  given with ●flecainide; increased risk of ventricular arrhythmias when amisulpride, pimozide,
  sertindole or thioridazine given with ●procain-
  amide—avoid concomitant use; increased risk of
  ventricular arrhythmias when amisulpride,
  pimozide, sertindole or thioridazine given with
  ●quinidine—avoid concomitant use

- Antibacterials: increased risk of ventricular arrhythmias when pimozide given with ●clarithromycin,
  ●moxifloxacin or ●telithromycin—avoid concomitant use; increased risk of ventricular arrhythmias when sertindole given with ●erythromycin or
  ●moxifloxacin—avoid concomitant use; increased
  risk of ventricular arrhythmias when amisulpride
  given with parenteral ●erythromycin—avoid concomitant use; plasma concentration of clozapine
  possibly increased by ●erythromycin (possible
  increased risk of convulsions); possible increased
  risk of ventricular arrhythmias when pimozide
  given with ●erythromycin—avoid concomitant
  use; increased risk of ventricular arrhythmias when
  haloperidol or phenothiazines given with ●moxi-
  floxacin—avoid concomitant use; plasma concentration of clozapine possibly reduced by
  rifampicin; metabolism of haloperidol accelerated
  by ●rifampicin (reduced plasma concentration);
  avoid concomitant use of clozapine with ●chlor-
  amphenicol or ●sulphonamides (increased risk of
  agranulocytosis); plasma concentration of quetiapine possibly increased by macrolides (reduce
  dose of quetiapine); possible increased risk of
  ventricular arrhythmias when sertindole given
  with ●macrolides—avoid concomitant use

- Antidepressants: plasma concentration of clozapine,
  haloperidol, risperidone, sertindole and zotepine
  increased by ●fluoxetine; plasma concentration of
  clozapine and olanzapine increased by ●fluvox-
  amine; plasma concentration of clozapine and
  sertindole increased by ●paroxetine; plasma concentration of thioridazine increased by ●paroxetine
  (increased risk of ventricular arrhythmias—avoid
  concomitant use); plasma concentration of clozapine increased by ●sertraline and ●venlafaxine;
  plasma concentration of pimozide increased by
  ●sertraline (increased risk of ventricular arrhythmias—avoid concomitant use); plasma concentration of haloperidol increased by venlafaxine;

Antipsychotics

- Antidepressants *(continued)*
  increased risk of ventricular arrhythmias when
  pimozide given with ●maprotiline or ●tricyclics—
  avoid concomitant use; increased risk of arrhythmias when thioridazine given with ●maprotiline—
  avoid concomitant use; clozapine possibly
  increases CNS effects of ●MAOIs; antipsychotics
  increase plasma concentration of ●tricyclics—
  possibly increased risk of ventricular arrhythmias;
  increased risk of ventricular arrhythmias when
  thioridazine given with ●tricyclics—avoid concomitant use; increased risk of antimuscarinic
  side-effects when phenothiazines given with
  tricyclics; possibly increased antimuscarinic side-
  effects when clozapine given with tricyclics

  Antidiabetics: phenothiazines possibly antagonise
  hypoglycaemic effect of sulphonylureas

- Antiepileptics: metabolism of haloperidol, olanzapine, quetiapine, risperidone and sertindole accelerated by carbamazepine (reduced plasma
  concentration); metabolism of clozapine accelerated by ●carbamazepine (reduced plasma concentration), also avoid concomitant use of drugs with
  substantial potential for causing agranulocytosis;
  antipsychotics antagonise anticonvulsant effect of
  ●carbamazepine, ●ethosuximide, ●oxcarbazepine,
  ●phenytoin, ●primidone and ●valproate (convulsive threshold lowered); metabolism of clozapine,
  quetiapine and sertindole accelerated by phenytoin
  (reduced plasma concentration); metabolism of
  haloperidol accelerated by primidone (reduced
  plasma concentration); increased risk of neutropenia when olanzapine given with ●valproate

- Antifungals: increased risk of ventricular arrhythmias when sertindole given with ●itraconazole or
  ●ketoconazole—avoid concomitant use; possible
  increased risk of ventricular arrhythmias when
  sertindole given with ●imidazoles or ●triazoles—
  avoid concomitant use; plasma concentration of
  quetiapine possibly increased by imidazoles and
  triazoles (reduce dose of quetiapine); increased
  risk of ventricular arrhythmias when pimozide
  given with ●imidazoles or ●triazoles—avoid concomitant use

- Antihistamines: increased risk of ventricular arrhythmias when antipsychotics given with ●terfen-
  adine; increased risk of ventricular arrhythmias
  when pimozide, sertindole or thioridazine given
  with ●terfenadine—avoid concomitant use

- Antimalarials: avoidance of antipsychotics advised
  by manufacturer of ●artemether/lumefantrine;
  increased risk of ventricular arrhythmias when
  pimozide given with ●mefloquine or ●quinine—
  avoid concomitant use; increased risk of ventricular arrhythmias when thioridazine given with
  ●quinine—avoid concomitant use

  Antimuscarinics: increased risk of antimuscarinic
  side-effects when clozapine given with antimuscarinics; plasma concentration of phenothiazines reduced by antimuscarinics, but risk of
  antimuscarinic side-effects increased; effects of
  haloperidol possibly reduced by antimuscarinics

- Antipsychotics: avoid concomitant use of clozapine
  with depot formulation of ●flupentixol, ●fluphen-
  azine, ●haloperidol, ●pipotiazine or
  ●zuclopenthixol as cannot be withdrawn quickly if
  neutropenia occurs; increased risk of ventricular
  arrhythmias when amisulpride, phenothiazines,
  pimozide or sertindole given with ●thioridazine—
  avoid concomitant use; increased risk of ventricular arrhythmias when sertindole given with
  ●amisulpride—avoid concomitant use; increased

Antipsychotics

- Antipsychotics *(continued)*
  risk of ventricular arrhythmias when pimozide given with ●phenothiazines—avoid concomitant use

- Antivirals: plasma concentration of clozapine and thioridazine possibly increased by amprenavir; plasma concentration of pimozide and sertindole increased by ●amprenavir (increased risk of ventricular arrhythmias—avoid concomitant use); plasma concentration of sertindole increased by ●indinavir, ●lopinavir, ●nelfinavir, ●ritonavir and ●saquinavir (increased risk of ventricular arrhythmias—avoid concomitant use); plasma concentration of thioridazine possibly increased by indinavir, nelfinavir and saquinavir; plasma concentration of pimozide possibly increased by ●indinavir, ●nelfinavir and ●saquinavir (increased risk of ventricular arrhythmias—avoid concomitant use); plasma concentration of antipsychotics possibly increased by ●ritonavir; plasma concentration of pimozide increased by ●ritonavir (increased risk of ventricular arrhythmias—avoid concomitant use); plasma concentration of clozapine increased by ●ritonavir (increased risk of toxicity)—avoid concomitant use

  Anxiolytics and Hypnotics: increased sedative effect when antipsychotics given with anxiolytics and hypnotics; plasma concentration of zotepine increased by diazepam; plasma concentration of haloperidol increased by buspirone

- Barbiturates: antipsychotics antagonise anticonvulsant effect of ●barbiturates (convulsive threshold lowered); metabolism of haloperidol accelerated by phenobarbital (reduced plasma concentration)

- Beta-blockers: enhanced hypotensive effect when phenothiazines given with beta-blockers; plasma concentration of both drugs may increase when chlorpromazine given with ●propranolol; increased risk of ventricular arrhythmias when amisulpride, phenothiazines, pimozide or sertindole given with ●sotalol

  Calcium-channel Blockers: enhanced hypotensive effect when antipsychotics given with calcium-channel blockers

  Clonidine: enhanced hypotensive effect when phenothiazines given with clonidine

- Cytotoxics: avoid concomitant use of clozapine with ●cytotoxics (increased risk of agranulocytosis)

  Desferrioxamine: manufacturer of levomepromazine (methotrimeprazine) advises avoid concomitant use with desferrioxamine; avoidance of prochlorperazine advised by manufacturer of desferrioxamine

  Diazoxide: enhanced hypotensive effect when phenothiazines given with diazoxide

- Diuretics: risk of ventricular arrhythmias with amisulpride or sertindole increased by hypokalaemia caused by ●diuretics; risk of ventricular arrhythmias with pimozide or thioridazine increased by hypokalaemia caused by ●diuretics (avoid concomitant use); enhanced hypotensive effect when phenothiazines given with diuretics

  Dopaminergics: increased risk of extrapyramidal side-effects when antipsychotics given with amantadine; antipsychotics antagonise effects of apomorphine, levodopa, lisuride and pergolide; antipsychotics antagonise hypoprolactinaemic and antiparkinsonian effects of bromocriptine and cabergoline; manufacturer of amisulpride advises avoid concomitant use of levodopa (antagonism of effect); avoidance of antipsychotics advised by

Antipsychotics

Dopaminergics *(continued)*
  manufacturer of pramipexole and ropinirole (antagonism of effect)

- Lithium: increased risk of ventricular arrhythmias when amisulpride, sertindole or thioridazine given with ●lithium—avoid concomitant use; increased risk of extrapyramidal side-effects and possibly neurotoxicity when clozapine, haloperidol or phenothiazines given with lithium; increased risk of extrapyramidal side-effects when sulpiride given with lithium

  Memantine: effects of antipsychotics possibly reduced by memantine

  Methyldopa: enhanced hypotensive effect when antipsychotics given with methyldopa (also increased risk of extrapyramidal effects)

  Metoclopramide: increased risk of extrapyramidal side-effects when antipsychotics given with metoclopramide

  Moxonidine: enhanced hypotensive effect when phenothiazines given with moxonidine

  Muscle Relaxants: promazine possibly enhances effects of suxamethonium

  Nitrates: enhanced hypotensive effect when phenothiazines given with nitrates

- Penicillamine: avoid concomitant use of clozapine with ●penicillamine (increased risk of agranulocytosis)

- Pentamidine Isetionate: increased risk of ventricular arrhythmias when amisulpride or thioridazine given with ●pentamidine isetionate—avoid concomitant use

- Sibutramine: increased risk of CNS toxicity when antipsychotics given with ●sibutramine (manufacturer of sibutramine advises avoid concomitant use)

  Sympathomimetics: antipsychotics antagonise hypertensive effect of sympathomimetics

  Tetrabenazine: increased risk of extrapyramidal side-effects when antipsychotics given with tetrabenazine

- Ulcer-healing Drugs: effects of antipsychotics, chlorpromazine and clozapine possibly enhanced by cimetidine; increased risk of ventricular arrhythmias when sertindole given with ●cimetidine—avoid concomitant use; absorption of sulpiride reduced by sucralfate

  Vasodilator Antihypertensives: enhanced hypotensive effect when phenothiazines given with hydralazine, minoxidil or nitroprusside

Antivirals *see* Abacavir, Aciclovir, Amprenavir, Cidofovir, Didanosine, Efavirenz, Emtricitabine, Famciclovir, Foscarnet, Ganciclovir, Indinavir, Lamivudine, Lopinavir, Nelfinavir, Nevirapine, Ribavirin, Ritonavir, Saquinavir, Stavudine, Tenofovir, Valaciclovir, Zalcitabine, and Zidovudine

Anxiolytics and Hypnotics

ACE Inhibitors: enhanced hypotensive effect when anxiolytics and hypnotics given with ACE inhibitors

Adrenergic Neurone Blockers: enhanced hypotensive effect when anxiolytics and hypnotics given with adrenergic neurone blockers

Alcohol: increased sedative effect when anxiolytics and hypnotics given with alcohol

Alpha-blockers: enhanced hypotensive and sedative effects when anxiolytics and hypnotics given with alpha-blockers

Anaesthetics, General: increased sedative effect when anxiolytics and hypnotics given with general anaesthetics

Anxiolytics and Hypnotics *(continued)*

Analgesics: increased sedative effect when anxiolytics and hypnotics given with opioid analgesics

Angiotensin-II Receptor Antagonists: enhanced hypotensive effect when anxiolytics and hypnotics given with angiotensin-II receptor antagonists

- Antibacterials: metabolism of midazolam inhibited by ●clarithromycin, ●erythromycin, ●quinupristin/dalfopristin and ●telithromycin (increased plasma concentration with increased sedation); plasma concentration of buspirone increased by erythromycin (reduce dose of buspirone); metabolism of zopiclone inhibited by erythromycin and quinupristin/dalfopristin; metabolism of benzodiazepines possibly accelerated by rifampicin (possibly reduced plasma concentration); metabolism of diazepam accelerated by rifampicin (reduced plasma concentration); metabolism of buspirone and zaleplon possibly accelerated by rifampicin; metabolism of zolpidem accelerated by rifampicin (reduced plasma concentration and reduced effect); metabolism of diazepam inhibited by isoniazid

Anticoagulants: chloral and triclofos may transiently enhance anticoagulant effect of coumarins

Antidepressants: plasma concentration of some benzodiazepines increased by fluvoxamine; sedative effects possibly increased when zolpidem given with sertraline; manufacturer of buspirone advises avoid concomitant use with MAOIs; increased sedative effect when anxiolytics and hypnotics given with mirtazapine, tricyclic-related antidepressants or tricyclics

Antiepileptics: plasma concentration of clonazepam often reduced by carbamazepine, phenytoin and primidone; benzodiazepines possibly increase or decrease plasma concentration of phenytoin; diazepam increases or decreases plasma concentration of phenytoin

- Antifungals: plasma concentration of midazolam increased by ●fluconazole, ●itraconazole and ●ketoconazole (risk of prolonged sedation); plasma concentration of buspirone increased by itraconazole (reduce dose of buspirone)

Antihistamines: increased sedative effect when anxiolytics and hypnotics given with antihistamines

Antipsychotics: increased sedative effect when anxiolytics and hypnotics given with antipsychotics; buspirone increases plasma concentration of haloperidol; diazepam increases plasma concentration of zotepine

- Antivirals: increased risk of prolonged sedation and respiratory depression when alprazolam, clorazepate, diazepam, flurazepam or midazolam given with ●amprenavir; increased risk of prolonged sedation when midazolam given with ●efavirenz, ●indinavir or ●nelfinavir—avoid concomitant use; increased risk of prolonged sedation when alprazolam given with ●indinavir—avoid concomitant use; plasma concentration of anxiolytics and hypnotics possibly increased by ●ritonavir; plasma concentration of alprazolam, clorazepate, diazepam, flurazepam, midazolam and zolpidem possibly increased by ●ritonavir (risk of extreme sedation and respiratory depression —avoid concomitant use); plasma concentration of midazolam increased by ●saquinavir (risk of prolonged sedation)

Barbiturates: plasma concentration of clonazepam often reduced by phenobarbital

Beta-blockers: enhanced hypotensive effect when anxiolytics and hypnotics given with beta-blockers

Anxiolytics and Hypnotics *(continued)*

Calcium-channel Blockers: enhanced hypotensive effect when anxiolytics and hypnotics given with calcium-channel blockers; midazolam increases absorption of lercanidipine; plasma concentration of buspirone increased by diltiazem and verapamil (reduce dose of buspirone); metabolism of midazolam inhibited by diltiazem and verapamil (increased plasma concentration with increased sedation)

Clonidine: enhanced hypotensive effect when anxiolytics and hypnotics given with clonidine

Diazoxide: enhanced hypotensive effect when anxiolytics and hypnotics given with diazoxide

Disulfiram: metabolism of benzodiazepines inhibited by disulfiram (increased sedative effects); increased risk of temazepam toxicity when given with disulfiram

Diuretics: enhanced hypotensive effect when anxiolytics and hypnotics given with diuretics; administration of chloral or triclofos with parenteral furosemide (frusemide) may displace thyroid hormone from binding sites

Dopaminergics: benzodiazepines possibly antagonise effects of levodopa

Grapefruit Juice: plasma concentration of buspirone increased by grapefruit juice

Lofexidine: increased sedative effect when anxiolytics and hypnotics given with lofexidine

Methyldopa: enhanced hypotensive effect when anxiolytics and hypnotics given with methyldopa

Moxonidine: enhanced hypotensive effect when anxiolytics and hypnotics given with moxonidine; sedative effects possibly increased when benzodiazepines given with moxonidine

Muscle Relaxants: increased sedative effect when anxiolytics and hypnotics given with baclofen or tizanidine

Nabilone: increased sedative effect when anxiolytics and hypnotics given with nabilone

Nitrates: enhanced hypotensive effect when anxiolytics and hypnotics given with nitrates

Ulcer-healing Drugs: metabolism of benzodiazepines, clomethiazole and zaleplon inhibited by cimetidine (increased plasma concentration); metabolism of diazepam possibly inhibited by esomeprazole and omeprazole (increased plasma concentration)

Vasodilator Antihypertensives: enhanced hypotensive effect when anxiolytics and hypnotics given with hydralazine, minoxidil or nitroprusside

Apomorphine

Antipsychotics: effects of apomorphine antagonised by antipsychotics

Dopaminergics: effects of apomorphine possibly enhanced by entacapone

Memantine: effects of dopaminergics possibly enhanced by memantine

Methyldopa: antiparkinsonian effect of dopaminergics antagonised by methyldopa

Nitrates: sublingual apomorphine enhances hypotensive effect of nitrates

Apraclonidine *see* Alpha₂-adrenoceptor Stimulants

Artemether with Lumefantrine

- Anti-arrhythmics: manufacturer of artemether/lumefantrine advises avoid concomitant use with ●amiodarone, ●disopyramide, ●flecainide, ●procainamide or ●quinidine (risk of ventricular arrhythmias)

- Antibacterials: manufacturer of artemether/lumefantrine advises avoid concomitant use with ●macrolides and ●quinolones

Artemether with Lumefantrine *(continued)*
- Antidepressants: manufacturer of artemether/lumefantrine advises avoid concomitant use with ●antidepressants
- Antifungals: manufacturer of artemether/lumefantrine advises avoid concomitant use with ●imidazoles and ●triazoles
- Antihistamines: manufacturer of artemether/lumefantrine advises avoid concomitant use with ●terfenadine (risk of ventricular arrhythmias)
- Antimalarials: manufacturer of artemether/lumefantrine advises avoid concomitant use with ●antimalarials
- Antipsychotics: manufacturer of artemether/lumefantrine advises avoid concomitant use with ●antipsychotics
- Beta-blockers: manufacturer of artemether/lumefantrine advises avoid concomitant use with ●metoprolol and ●sotalol
- Grapefruit Juice: metabolism of artemether/lumefantrine possibly inhibited by ●grapefruit juice (avoid concomitant use)

Aspirin
ACE Inhibitors: risk of renal impairment when aspirin (in doses over 300 mg daily) given with ACE inhibitors, also hypotensive effect antagonised
Adsorbents: absorption of aspirin possibly reduced by kaolin
- Analgesics: avoid concomitant use of aspirin with ●NSAIDs (increased side-effects); antiplatelet effect of aspirin possibly reduced by ibuprofen
Angiotensin-II Receptor Antagonists: risk of renal impairment when aspirin (in doses over 300 mg daily) given with angiotensin-II receptor antagonists, also hypotensive effect antagonised
Antacids: excretion of aspirin increased by alkaline urine due to some antacids
- Anticoagulants: increased risk of bleeding when aspirin given with ●coumarins or ●phenindione (due to antiplatelet effect); aspirin enhances anticoagulant effect of ●heparins
- Antidepressants: increased risk of bleeding when aspirin given with ●SSRIs or ●venlafaxine
Antiepileptics: aspirin enhances effects of phenytoin and valproate
Cilostazol: manufacturer of cilostazol recommends dose of aspirin should not exceed 80 mg daily when given with cilostazol
Clopidogrel: increased risk of bleeding when aspirin given with clopidogrel
Corticosteroids: increased risk of gastro-intestinal bleeding and ulceration when aspirin given with corticosteroids, also corticosteroids reduce plasma concentration of salicylate
- Cytotoxics: aspirin reduces excretion of ●methotrexate (increased risk of toxicity)
Diuretics: aspirin antagonises diuretic effect of spironolactone; increased risk of toxicity when high-dose aspirin given with carbonic anhydrase inhibitors
Leukotriene Antagonists: aspirin increases plasma concentration of zafirlukast
Metoclopramide: rate of absorption of aspirin increased by metoclopramide (enhanced effect)
Mifepristone: avoidance of aspirin advised by manufacturer of mifepristone
Probenecid: aspirin antagonises effects of probenecid
Sibutramine: increased risk of bleeding when aspirin given with sibutramine
Sulfinpyrazone: aspirin antagonises effects of sulfinpyrazone
Atenolol *see* Beta-blockers

Atorvastatin *see* Statins
Atovaquone
- Antibacterials: plasma concentration of atovaquone reduced by ●rifabutin and ●rifampicin (possible therapeutic failure of atovaquone); plasma concentration of atovaquone reduced by tetracycline
Antivirals: atovaquone possibly reduces plasma concentration of indinavir
Metoclopramide: plasma concentration of atovaquone reduced by metoclopramide
Atracurium *see* Muscle Relaxants
Atropine *see* Antimuscarinics
Auranofin *see* Gold
Azapropazone *see* NSAIDs
Azathioprine
ACE Inhibitors: increased risk of leucopenia when azathioprine given with captopril
- Allopurinol: enhanced effects and increased toxicity of azathioprine when given with ●allopurinol (reduce dose of azathioprine)
Aminosalicylates: possible increased risk of leucopenia when azathioprine given with aminosalicylates
- Antibacterials: manufacturer of azathioprine reports interaction with ●rifampicin (transplants possibly rejected); increased risk of haematological toxicity when azathioprine given with ●sulfamethoxazole (as co-trimoxazole); increased risk of haematological toxicity when azathioprine given with ●trimethoprim (also with co-trimoxazole)
- Anticoagulants: azathioprine possibly reduces anticoagulant effect of ●warfarin
Antiepileptics: cytotoxics reduce absorption of phenytoin
- Antipsychotics: avoid concomitant use of cytotoxics with ●clozapine (increased risk of agranulocytosis)
Azelastine *see* Antihistamines
Azithromycin *see* Macrolides
Aztreonam
- Anticoagulants: aztreonam possibly enhances anticoagulant effect of ●coumarins
Oestrogens: *broad-spectrum* antibacterials possibly reduce contraceptive effect of oestrogens (risk probably small, see p. 388)
Baclofen *see* Muscle Relaxants
Balsalazide *see* Aminosalicylates
Bambuterol *see* Sympathomimetics, Beta$_2$
Barbiturates
Alcohol: increased sedative effect when barbiturates given with alcohol
Anti-arrhythmics: barbiturates accelerate metabolism of disopyramide and quinidine (reduced plasma concentration)
- Antibacterials: barbiturates accelerate metabolism of ●chloramphenicol, doxycycline and metronidazole (reduced plasma concentration); phenobarbital reduces plasma concentration of ●telithromycin (avoid during and for 2 weeks after phenobarbital)
- Anticoagulants: barbiturates accelerate metabolism of ●coumarins (reduced anticoagulant effect)
- Antidepressants: phenobarbital reduces plasma concentration of paroxetine; phenobarbital accelerates metabolism of ●mianserin (reduced plasma concentration); anticonvulsant effect of barbiturates possibly antagonised by MAOIs and ●tricyclic-related antidepressants (convulsive threshold lowered); anticonvulsant effect of barbiturates antagonised by SSRIs (convulsive threshold lowered); plasma concentration of phenobarbital reduced by ●St John's wort—avoid concomitant use; anticonvulsant effect of barbiturates antagonised by ●tricyclics (convulsive

Barbiturates
- Antidepressants *(continued)*
  threshold lowered), also metabolism of tricyclics possibly accelerated (reduced plasma concentration)

  Antiepileptics: phenobarbital reduces plasma concentration of carbamazepine, lamotrigine and tiagabine; phenobarbital possibly reduces plasma concentration of ethosuximide; plasma concentration of phenobarbital increased by oxcarbazepine, also plasma concentration of an active metabolite of oxcarbazepine reduced; plasma concentration of phenobarbital often increased by phenytoin, plasma concentration of phenytoin often reduced but may be increased; increased sedative effect when barbiturates given with primidone; plasma concentration of phenobarbital increased by valproate (also plasma concentration of valproate reduced); plasma concentration of phenobarbital possibly reduced by vigabatrin
- Antifungals: phenobarbital possibly reduces plasma concentration of ●voriconazole—avoid concomitant use; phenobarbital reduces absorption of griseofulvin (reduced effect)
- Antipsychotics: anticonvulsant effect of barbiturates antagonised by ●antipsychotics (convulsive threshold lowered); phenobarbital accelerates metabolism of haloperidol (reduced plasma concentration)
- Antivirals: barbiturates possibly reduce plasma concentration of ●indinavir, ●lopinavir, ●nelfinavir and ●saquinavir

  Anxiolytics and Hypnotics: phenobarbital often reduces plasma concentration of clonazepam
- Calcium-channel Blockers: barbiturates reduce effects of ●felodipine and ●isradipine; barbiturates probably reduce effects of ●dihydropyridines, ●diltiazem and ●verapamil

  Cardiac Glycosides: barbiturates accelerate metabolism of digitoxin (reduced effect)
- Ciclosporin: barbiturates accelerate metabolism of ●ciclosporin (reduced effect)
- Corticosteroids: barbiturates accelerate metabolism of ●corticosteroids (reduced effect)

  Diuretics: increased risk of osteomalacia when phenobarbital given with carbonic anhydrase inhibitors

  Folates: plasma concentration of phenobarbital possibly reduced by folates

  Hormone Antagonists: barbiturates accelerate metabolism of gestrinone (reduced plasma concentration); barbiturates possibly accelerate metabolism of toremifene (possibly reduced plasma concentration)

  Leukotriene Antagonists: phenobarbital reduces plasma concentration of montelukast

  Memantine: effects of barbiturates possibly reduced by memantine
- Oestrogens: barbiturates accelerate metabolism of ●oestrogens (reduced contraceptive effect—see p. 388)
- Progestogens: barbiturates accelerate metabolism of ●progestogens (reduced contraceptive effect—see p. 388)

  Sympathomimetics: plasma concentration of phenobarbital possibly increased by methylphenidate

  Theophylline: barbiturates accelerate metabolism of theophylline (reduced effect)

  Thyroid Hormones: barbiturates accelerate metabolism of thyroid hormones (may increase requirements for thyroid hormones in hypothyroidism)

  Tibolone: barbiturates accelerate metabolism of tibolone (reduced plasma concentration)

Barbiturates *(continued)*
  Tropisetron: phenobarbital reduces plasma concentration of tropisetron

  Vitamins: barbiturates possibly increase requirements for vitamin D

Beclometasone *see* Corticosteroids
Belladonna Alkaloids *see* Antimuscarinics
Bendroflumethiazide (bendrofluazide) *see* Diuretics
Benorilate *see* Aspirin and Paracetamol
Benperidol *see* Antipsychotics
Benzatropine (benztropine) *see* Antimuscarinics
Benzodiazepines *see* Anxiolytics and Hypnotics
Benzthiazide *see* Diuretics
Benzylpenicillin *see* Penicillins

Beta-blockers
  Note. Since systemic absorption may follow topical application of beta-blockers to the eye the possibility of interactions, in particular, with drugs such as verapamil should be borne in mind

  ACE Inhibitors: enhanced hypotensive effect when beta-blockers given with ACE inhibitors

  Adrenergic Neurone Blockers: enhanced hypotensive effect when beta-blockers given with adrenergic neurone blockers

  Alcohol: enhanced hypotensive effect when beta-blockers given with alcohol

  Aldesleukin: enhanced hypotensive effect when beta-blockers given with aldesleukin
- Alpha-blockers: enhanced hypotensive effect when beta-blockers given with ●alpha-blockers, also increased risk of first-dose hypotension with post-synaptic alpha-blockers such as prazosin

  Alprostadil: enhanced hypotensive effect when beta-blockers given with alprostadil

  Amifostine: possible enhanced hypotensive effect when beta-blockers given with amifostine

  Anaesthetics, General: enhanced hypotensive effect when beta-blockers given with general anaesthetics
- Anaesthetics, Local: propranolol increases risk of ●bupivacaine toxicity

  Analgesics: hypotensive effect of beta-blockers antagonised by NSAIDs; plasma concentration of esmolol possibly increased by morphine

  Angiotensin-II Receptor Antagonists: enhanced hypotensive effect when beta-blockers given with angiotensin-II receptor antagonists
- Anti-arrhythmics: increased myocardial depression when beta-blockers given with ●anti-arrhythmics; increased risk of bradycardia, AV block and myocardial depression when beta-blockers given with ●amiodarone; increased risk of ventricular arrhythmias when sotalol given with ●amiodarone, ●disopyramide, ●procainamide or ●quinidine—avoid concomitant use; increased risk of myocardial depression and bradycardia when beta-blockers given with ●flecainide; propranolol increases risk of ●lidocaine (lignocaine) toxicity; plasma concentration of metoprolol and propranolol increased by propafenone
- Antibacterials: increased risk of ventricular arrhythmias when sotalol given with ●moxifloxacin—avoid concomitant use; metabolism of bisoprolol and propranolol accelerated by rifampicin (plasma concentration significantly reduced)
- Antidepressants: plasma concentration of propranolol increased by fluvoxamine; enhanced hypotensive effect when beta-blockers given with MAOIs; increased risk of ventricular arrhythmias when sotalol given with ●tricyclics

  Antidiabetics: beta-blockers may mask warning signs of hypoglycaemia (such as tremor) with

Beta-blockers

Antidiabetics *(continued)*
antidiabetics; beta-blockers enhance hypoglycaemic effect of insulin

- Antihistamines: increased risk of ventricular arrhythmias when sotalol given with ●mizolastine or
●terfenadine—avoid concomitant use

- Antimalarials: avoidance of metoprolol and sotalol
advised by manufacturer of ●artemether/lumefan-
trine; increased risk of bradycardia when beta-
blockers given with mefloquine

- Antipsychotics: plasma concentration of both drugs
may increase when propranolol given with
●chlorpromazine; increased risk of ventricular
arrhythmias when sotalol given with ●amisulpride,
●phenothiazines, ●pimozide or ●sertindole;
enhanced hypotensive effect when beta-blockers
given with phenothiazines

Anxiolytics and Hypnotics: enhanced hypotensive
effect when beta-blockers given with anxiolytics
and hypnotics

- Calcium-channel Blockers: enhanced hypotensive
effect when beta-blockers given with calcium-
channel blockers; possible severe hypotension and
heart failure when beta-blockers given with
●nifedipine or ●nisoldipine; increased risk of AV
block and bradycardia when beta-blockers given
with ●diltiazem; asystole, severe hypotension and
heart failure when beta-blockers given with
●verapamil (see p. 106)

Cardiac Glycosides: increased risk of AV block and
bradycardia when beta-blockers given with cardiac
glycosides

- Ciclosporin: carvedilol increases plasma concentration of ●ciclosporin

- Clonidine: increased risk of withdrawal hypertension
when beta-blockers given with ●clonidine (withdraw beta-blockers several days before slowly
withdrawing clonidine)

Corticosteroids: hypotensive effect of beta-blockers
antagonised by corticosteroids

Diazoxide: enhanced hypotensive effect when beta-
blockers given with diazoxide

- Diuretics: enhanced hypotensive effect when beta-
blockers given with diuretics; risk of ventricular
arrhythmias with sotalol increased by hypokalaemia caused by ●loop diuretics or ●thiazides and
related diuretics

- Dolasetron: increased risk of ventricular arrhythmias
when sotalol given with ●dolasetron—avoid concomitant use

Dopaminergics: enhanced hypotensive effect when
beta-blockers given with levodopa

Ergot Alkaloids: increased peripheral vasoconstriction when beta-blockers given with ergotamine
and methysergide

$5HT_1$ Agonists: propranolol possibly increases
plasma concentration of rizatriptan (reduce dose of
rizatriptan)

Methyldopa: enhanced hypotensive effect when
beta-blockers given with methyldopa

- Moxisylyte (thymoxamine): possible severe postural
hypotension when beta-blockers given with
●moxisylyte

Moxonidine: enhanced hypotensive effect when
beta-blockers given with moxonidine

Muscle Relaxants: propranolol enhances effects of
muscle relaxants; enhanced hypotensive effect
when beta-blockers given with baclofen; possible
enhanced hypotensive effect and bradycardia
when beta-blockers given with tizanidine

Nitrates: enhanced hypotensive effect when beta-
blockers given with nitrates

Beta-blockers *(continued)*

Oestrogens: hypotensive effect of beta-blockers
antagonised by oestrogens

Parasympathomimetics: propranolol antagonises
effects of neostigmine and pyridostigmine;
increased risk of arrhythmias when beta-blockers
given with pilocarpine

- Sympathomimetics: severe hypertension when beta-
blockers given with ●adrenaline (epinephrine) or
●noradrenaline (norepinephrine) especially with
non-selective beta-blockers; possible severe
hypertension when beta-blockers given with
●dobutamine especially with non-selective beta-
blockers

Tropisetron: caution with beta-blockers advised by
manufacturer of tropisetron (risk of ventricular
arrhythmias)

Ulcer-healing Drugs: plasma concentration of
labetalol, metoprolol and propranolol increased by
cimetidine; hypotensive effect of beta-blockers
antagonised by carbenoxolone

Vasodilator Antihypertensives: enhanced hypotensive effect when beta-blockers given with hydralazine, minoxidil or nitroprusside

Betahistine

Antihistamines: effect of betahistine theoretically
antagonised by antihistamines

Betamethasone *see* Corticosteroids

Betaxolol *see* Beta-blockers

Bethanechol *see* Parasympathomimetics

Bezafibrate *see* Fibrates

Bicalutamide

Anticoagulants: bicalutamide possibly enhances
anticoagulant effect of coumarins

- Antihistamines: manufacturer of bicalutamide
advises avoid concomitant use with ●terfenadine

Biguanides *see* Antidiabetics

Bile Acids *see* Ursodeoxycholic Acid

Bisoprolol *see* Beta-blockers

Bisphosphonates

Analgesics: bioavailability of tiludronic acid
increased by indometacin

Antacids: absorption of bisphosphonates reduced by
antacids

Antibacterials: increased risk of hypocalcaemia
when bisphosphonates given with aminoglycosides

Calcium Salts: absorption of bisphosphonates
reduced by calcium salts

Iron: absorption of bisphosphonates reduced by *oral
iron*

Bosentan

Anticoagulants: manufacturer of bosentan recommends monitoring anticoagulant effect of coumarins

- Antidiabetics: plasma concentration of both drugs
reduced when bosentan given with ●glibenclamide
(avoid concomitant use)

- Antifungals: plasma concentration of bosentan
possibly increased by itraconazole and ketoconazole; plasma concentration of bosentan increased
by ●fluconazole—avoid concomitant use

Antivirals: plasma concentration of bosentan possibly increased by ritonavir

- Ciclosporin: plasma concentration of bosentan
increased by ●ciclosporin (also plasma concentration of ciclosporin reduced—avoid concomitant
use)

Lipid-regulating Drugs: bosentan reduces plasma
concentration of simvastatin

- Oestrogens: bosentan possibly causes contraceptive
failure of hormonal contraceptives containing
●oestrogens (alternative contraception recommended)

Bosentan *(continued)*
- Progestogens: bosentan possibly causes contraceptive failure of hormonal contraceptives containing ●progestogens (alternative contraception recommended)

Bretylium *see* Adrenergic Neurone Blockers
Brimonidine *see* Alpha₂-adrenoceptor Stimulants
Brinzolamide *see* Diuretics
Bromocriptine
Alcohol: tolerance of bromocriptine reduced by alcohol
Antibacterials: plasma concentration of bromocriptine increased by erythromycin (increased risk of toxicity); plasma concentration of bromocriptine possibly increased by macrolides (increased risk of toxicity)
Antipsychotics: hypoprolactinaemic and antiparkinsonian effects of bromocriptine antagonised by antipsychotics
Domperidone: hypoprolactinaemic effect of bromocriptine possibly antagonised by domperidone
Hormone Antagonists: plasma concentration of bromocriptine increased by octreotide
Memantine: effects of dopaminergics possibly enhanced by memantine
Methyldopa: antiparkinsonian effect of dopaminergics antagonised by methyldopa
Metoclopramide: hypoprolactinaemic effect of bromocriptine antagonised by metoclopramide
- Sympathomimetics: risk of toxicity when bromocriptine given with ●isometheptene or ●phenylpropanolamine

Brompheniramine *see* Antihistamines
Buclizine *see* Antihistamines
Budesonide *see* Corticosteroids
Bumetanide *see* Diuretics
Bupivacaine
Anti-arrhythmics: increased myocardial depression when bupivacaine given with anti-arrhythmics
- Beta-blockers: increased risk of bupivacaine toxicity when bupivacaine given with ●propranolol

Buprenorphine *see* Opioid Analgesics
Bupropion
Note. Bupropion should be administered with extreme caution to patients receiving other medication known to lower the seizure threshold—see CSM advice p. 248 and Cautions, Contra-indications and Side-effects of individual drugs
- Antidepressants: manufacturer of bupropion advises avoid for 2 weeks after stopping ●MAOIs; manufacturer of bupropion advises avoid concomitant use with ●moclobemide
Antiepileptics: plasma concentration of bupropion reduced by carbamazepine and phenytoin; metabolism of bupropion inhibited by valproate
- Antivirals: plasma concentration of bupropion increased by ●ritonavir (risk of toxicity)—avoid concomitant use
Dopaminergics: increased risk of side-effects when bupropion given with amantadine or levodopa

Buspirone *see* Anxiolytics and Hypnotics
Busulfan
Analgesics: metabolism of *intravenous* busulfan possibly inhibited by paracetamol (manufacturer of *intravenous* busulfan advises caution within 72 hours of paracetamol)
Antiepileptics: cytotoxics reduce absorption of phenytoin
Antifungals: metabolism of busulfan inhibited by itraconazole (increased risk of toxicity)
- Antipsychotics: avoid concomitant use of cytotoxics with ●clozapine (increased risk of agranulocytosis)

Butobarbital *see* Barbiturates
Butyrophenones *see* Antipsychotics

Cabergoline
Antibacterials: plasma concentration of cabergoline increased by erythromycin (increased risk of toxicity); plasma concentration of cabergoline possibly increased by macrolides (increased risk of toxicity)
Antipsychotics: hypoprolactinaemic and antiparkinsonian effects of cabergoline antagonised by antipsychotics
Domperidone: hypoprolactinaemic effect of cabergoline possibly antagonised by domperidone
Memantine: effects of dopaminergics possibly enhanced by memantine
Methyldopa: antiparkinsonian effect of dopaminergics antagonised by methyldopa
Metoclopramide: hypoprolactinaemic effect of cabergoline antagonised by metoclopramide

Calcium Salts
Note. see also Antacids
Antibacterials: calcium salts reduces absorption of ciprofloxacin and tetracycline
Bisphosphonates: calcium salts reduces absorption of bisphosphonates
Cardiac Glycosides: large intravenous doses of calcium salts can precipitate arrhythmias when given with cardiac glycosides
Diuretics: increased risk of hypercalcaemia when calcium salts given with thiazides and related diuretics
Thyroid Hormones: calcium salts reduces absorption of levothyroxine (thyroxine)

Calcium-channel Blockers
Note. Dihydropyridine calcium-channel blockers include amlodipine, felodipine, isradipine, lacidipine, lercanidipine, nicardipine, nifedipine, nimodipine, and nisoldipine
ACE Inhibitors: enhanced hypotensive effect when calcium-channel blockers given with ACE inhibitors
Adrenergic Neurone Blockers: enhanced hypotensive effect when calcium-channel blockers given with adrenergic neurone blockers
Alcohol: enhanced hypotensive effect when calcium-channel blockers given with alcohol; verapamil possibly increases plasma concentration of alcohol
Aldesleukin: enhanced hypotensive effect when calcium-channel blockers given with aldesleukin
- Alpha-blockers: enhanced hypotensive effect when calcium-channel blockers given with ●alpha-blockers, also increased risk of first-dose hypotension with post-synaptic alpha-blockers such as prazosin
Alprostadil: enhanced hypotensive effect when calcium-channel blockers given with alprostadil
Amifostine: possible enhanced hypotensive effect when calcium-channel blockers given with amifostine
- Anaesthetics, General: enhanced hypotensive effect when calcium-channel blockers given with general anaesthetics or isoflurane; hypotensive effect of verapamil enhanced by ●general anaesthetics (also AV delay)
Analgesics: hypotensive effect of calcium-channel blockers antagonised by NSAIDs
Angiotensin-II Receptor Antagonists: enhanced hypotensive effect when calcium-channel blockers given with angiotensin-II receptor antagonists
- Anti-arrhythmics: increased risk of bradycardia, AV block and myocardial depression when diltiazem or verapamil given with ●amiodarone; increased risk of myocardial depression and asystole when verapamil given with ●disopyramide or ●flecainide; verapamil increases plasma concentration of ●quinidine (extreme hypotension may occur);

Calcium-channel Blockers

- Anti-arrhythmics *(continued)*
nifedipine reduces plasma concentration of quinidine

- Antibacterials: metabolism of felodipine possibly inhibited by erythromycin (increased plasma concentration); manufacturer of lercanidipine advises avoid concomitant use with erythromycin; metabolism of diltiazem, nifedipine, nimodipine and verapamil accelerated by ●rifampicin (plasma concentration significantly reduced); metabolism of isradipine, nicardipine and nisoldipine possibly accelerated by ●rifampicin (possible significantly reduced plasma concentration); plasma concentration of nifedipine increased by ●quinupristin/dalfopristin

Antidepressants: diltiazem and verapamil increase plasma concentration of imipramine; enhanced hypotensive effect when calcium-channel blockers given with MAOIs; diltiazem and verapamil possibly increase plasma concentration of tricyclics

Antidiabetics: glucose tolerance occasionally impaired when nifedipine given with insulin

- Antiepileptics: effects of dihydropyridines, nicardipine and nifedipine probably reduced by carbamazepine; diltiazem and verapamil enhance effects of ●carbamazepine; effects of felodipine and isradipine reduced by carbamazepine; effects of dihydropyridines, nicardipine and nifedipine probably reduced by ●phenytoin; effects of felodipine, isradipine and verapamil reduced by phenytoin; diltiazem increases plasma concentration of ●phenytoin but also effect of diltiazem reduced; plasma concentration of nisoldipine reduced by phenytoin; effects of felodipine and isradipine reduced by ●primidone; effects of dihydropyridines, diltiazem and verapamil probably reduced by ●primidone

- Antifungals: metabolism of dihydropyridines possibly inhibited by itraconazole and ketoconazole (increased plasma concentration); metabolism of felodipine inhibited by ●itraconazole and ●ketoconazole (increased plasma concentration); manufacturer of lercanidipine advises avoid concomitant use with itraconazole and ketoconazole; negative inotropic effect possibly increased when calcium-channel blockers given with itraconazole

Antimalarials: possible increased risk of bradycardia when calcium-channel blockers given with mefloquine

Antipsychotics: enhanced hypotensive effect when calcium-channel blockers given with antipsychotics

- Antivirals: plasma concentration of diltiazem, nicardipine, nifedipine and nimodipine possibly increased by amprenavir; manufacturer of lercanidipine advises avoid concomitant use with ritonavir; plasma concentration of calcium-channel blockers possibly increased by ●ritonavir

Anxiolytics and Hypnotics: enhanced hypotensive effect when calcium-channel blockers given with anxiolytics and hypnotics; diltiazem and verapamil inhibit metabolism of midazolam (increased plasma concentration with increased sedation); absorption of lercanidipine increased by midazolam; diltiazem and verapamil increase plasma concentration of buspirone (reduce dose of buspirone)

- Barbiturates: effects of dihydropyridines, diltiazem and verapamil probably reduced by ●barbiturates;

Calcium-channel Blockers

- Barbiturates *(continued)*
effects of felodipine and isradipine reduced by ●barbiturates

- Beta-blockers: enhanced hypotensive effect when calcium-channel blockers given with beta-blockers; increased risk of AV block and bradycardia when diltiazem given with ●beta-blockers; asystole, severe hypotension and heart failure when verapamil given with ●beta-blockers (see p. 106); possible severe hypotension and heart failure when nifedipine or nisoldipine given with ●beta-blockers

Calcium-channel Blockers: plasma concentration of both drugs may increase when diltiazem given with nifedipine

- Cardiac Glycosides: nifedipine possibly increases plasma concentration of ●digoxin; diltiazem, lercanidipine and nicardipine increase plasma concentration of ●digoxin; verapamil increases plasma concentration of ●digoxin, also increased risk of AV block and bradycardia

- Ciclosporin: diltiazem, nicardipine and verapamil increase plasma concentration of ●ciclosporin; combination of lercanidipine with ●ciclosporin may increase plasma concentration of either drug (or both)—avoid concomitant use; plasma concentration of nifedipine possibly increased by ciclosporin (increased risk of toxicity including gingival hyperplasia)

- Cilostazol: diltiazem increases plasma concentration of ●cilostazol—avoid concomitant use

Clonidine: enhanced hypotensive effect when calcium-channel blockers given with clonidine

Corticosteroids: hypotensive effect of calcium-channel blockers antagonised by corticosteroids

Cytotoxics: nifedipine possibly inhibits metabolism of vincristine

Diazoxide: enhanced hypotensive effect when calcium-channel blockers given with diazoxide

Diuretics: enhanced hypotensive effect when calcium-channel blockers given with diuretics

Dopaminergics: enhanced hypotensive effect when calcium-channel blockers given with levodopa

Grapefruit Juice: plasma concentration of felodipine, isradipine, lacidipine, lercanidipine, nicardipine, nifedipine, nimodipine, nisoldipine and verapamil increased by grapefruit juice

Hormone Antagonists: diltiazem and verapamil increase plasma concentration of dutasteride

- Lipid-regulating Drugs: possible increased risk of myopathy when diltiazem given with simvastatin; increased risk of myopathy when verapamil given with ●simvastatin (avoid doses of simvastatin above 20 mg daily)

Lithium: neurotoxicity may occur when diltiazem or verapamil given with lithium without increased plasma concentration of lithium

- Magnesium (parenteral): profound hypotension reported with concomitant use of nifedipine and ●parenteral magnesium in pre-eclampsia

Methyldopa: enhanced hypotensive effect when calcium-channel blockers given with methyldopa

Moxisylyte (thymoxamine): enhanced hypotensive effect when calcium-channel blockers given with moxisylyte

Moxonidine: enhanced hypotensive effect when calcium-channel blockers given with moxonidine

Muscle Relaxants: verapamil enhances effects of non-depolarising muscle relaxants and suxamethonium; enhanced hypotensive effect when calcium-channel blockers given with baclofen or tizanidine; risk of arrhythmias when diltiazem

Calcium-channel Blockers

Muscle Relaxants *(continued)*
given with intravenous dantrolene; hypotension, myocardial depression, and hyperkalaemia when verapamil given with intravenous dantrolene; nifedipine enhances effects of non-depolarising muscle relaxants

Nitrates: enhanced hypotensive effect when calcium-channel blockers given with nitrates

Oestrogens: hypotensive effect of calcium-channel blockers antagonised by oestrogens

- Sirolimus: diltiazem increases plasma concentration of ●sirolimus
- Tacrolimus: diltiazem and nifedipine increase plasma concentration of ●tacrolimus
- Theophylline: calcium-channel blockers possibly increase plasma concentration of ●theophylline (enhanced effect); diltiazem increases plasma concentration of theophylline; verapamil increases plasma concentration of ●theophylline (enhanced effect)

Ulcer-healing Drugs: metabolism of calcium-channel blockers possibly inhibited by cimetidine (increased plasma concentration); hypotensive effect of calcium-channel blockers antagonised by carbenoxolone

Vardenafil: enhanced hypotensive effect when nifedipine given with vardenafil

Vasodilator Antihypertensives: enhanced hypotensive effect when calcium-channel blockers given with hydralazine, minoxidil or nitroprusside

Calcium-channel Blockers (dihydropyridines)

see Calcium-channel Blockers

Candesartan *see* Angiotensin-II Receptor Antagonists

Capecitabine *see* Fluorouracil

Capreomycin

Antibacterials: increased risk of nephrotoxicity when capreomycin given with colistin or polymyxins; increased risk of nephrotoxicity and ototoxicity when capreomycin given with aminoglycosides or vancomycin

Cytotoxics: increased risk of nephrotoxicity and ototoxicity when capreomycin given with platinum compounds

Oestrogens: *broad-spectrum* antibacterials possibly reduce contraceptive effect of oestrogens (risk probably small, see p. 388)

Captopril *see* ACE Inhibitors

Carbamazepine

Alcohol: CNS side-effects of carbamazepine possibly increased by alcohol

- Analgesics: effects of carbamazepine enhanced by ●dextropropoxyphene; carbamazepine reduces plasma concentration of methadone; carbamazepine reduces effects of tramadol
- Antibacterials: plasma concentration of carbamazepine increased by ●clarithromycin and ●erythromycin; plasma concentration of carbamazepine reduced by ●rifabutin; carbamazepine accelerates metabolism of doxycycline (reduced effect); plasma concentration of carbamazepine increased by ●isoniazid (also possibly increased isoniazid hepatotoxicity); carbamazepine reduces plasma concentration of ●telithromycin (avoid during and for 2 weeks after carbamazepine)
- Anticoagulants: carbamazepine accelerates metabolism of ●coumarins (reduced anticoagulant effect)
- Antidepressants: plasma concentration of carbamazepine increased by ●fluoxetine and ●fluvoxamine; carbamazepine reduces plasma concentration of ●mianserin, mirtazapine and paroxetine; manufacturer of carbamazepine

Carbamazepine

- Antidepressants *(continued)*
advises avoid for 2 weeks after stopping ●MAOIs, also antagonism of anticonvulsant effect; anticonvulsant effect of antiepileptics antagonised by MAOIs and ●tricyclic-related antidepressants (convulsive threshold lowered); anticonvulsant effect of antiepileptics antagonised by ●SSRIs and ●tricyclics (convulsive threshold lowered); plasma concentration of carbamazepine reduced by ●St John's wort—avoid concomitant use; carbamazepine accelerates metabolism of ●tricyclics (reduced plasma concentration and reduced effect)

Antiepileptics: carbamazepine possibly reduces plasma concentration of ethosuximide; carbamazepine often reduces plasma concentration of lamotrigine, also plasma concentration of an active metabolite of carbamazepine sometimes raised (but evidence is conflicting); plasma concentration of carbamazepine sometimes reduced by oxcarbazepine (but concentration of an active metabolite of carbamazepine may be increased), also plasma concentration of an active metabolite of oxcarbazepine often reduced; plasma concentration of both drugs often reduced when carbamazepine given with phenytoin, also plasma concentration of phenytoin may be increased; plasma concentration of carbamazepine often reduced by primidone, also plasma concentration of primidone sometimes reduced (but concentration of an active metabolite of primidone often increased); carbamazepine reduces plasma concentration of tiagabine; carbamazepine often reduces plasma concentration of topiramate; carbamazepine reduces plasma concentration of valproate, also plasma concentration of active metabolite of carbamazepine increased

- Antifungals: carbamazepine possibly reduces plasma concentration of ●voriconazole—avoid concomitant use; carbamazepine possibly reduces plasma concentration of ●caspofungin—consider increasing dose of caspofungin
- Antimalarials: possible increased risk of convulsions when antiepileptics given with chloroquine and hydroxychloroquine; anticonvulsant effect of antiepileptics and carbamazepine antagonised by ●mefloquine
- Antipsychotics: anticonvulsant effect of carbamazepine antagonised by ●antipsychotics (convulsive threshold lowered); carbamazepine accelerates metabolism of haloperidol, olanzapine, quetiapine, risperidone and sertindole (reduced plasma concentration); carbamazepine accelerates metabolism of ●clozapine (reduced plasma concentration), also avoid concomitant use of drugs with substantial potential for causing agranulocytosis
- Antivirals: plasma concentration of carbamazepine possibly increased by amprenavir and ●ritonavir; carbamazepine possibly reduces plasma concentration of indinavir, lopinavir, nelfinavir and saquinavir

Anxiolytics and Hypnotics: carbamazepine often reduces plasma concentration of clonazepam

Barbiturates: plasma concentration of carbamazepine reduced by phenobarbital

Bupropion: carbamazepine reduces plasma concentration of bupropion

- Calcium-channel Blockers: carbamazepine reduces effects of felodipine and isradipine; carbamazepine probably reduces effects of dihydropyridines, nicardipine and nifedipine; effects of carbamazepine enhanced by ●diltiazem and ●verapamil

Carbamazepine (continued)

Cardiac Glycosides: carbamazepine accelerates metabolism of digitoxin (reduced effect)

- Ciclosporin: carbamazepine accelerates metabolism of ●ciclosporin (reduced plasma concentration)
- Corticosteroids: carbamazepine accelerates metabolism of ●corticosteroids (reduced effect)
- Diuretics: increased risk of hyponatraemia when carbamazepine given with diuretics; plasma concentration of carbamazepine increased by ●acetazolamide
- Hormone Antagonists: metabolism of carbamazepine inhibited by ●danazol (increased risk of toxicity); carbamazepine accelerates metabolism of gestrinone (reduced plasma concentration); carbamazepine possibly accelerates metabolism of toremifene (possibly reduced plasma concentration)

Lithium: neurotoxicity may occur when carbamazepine given with lithium without increased plasma concentration of lithium

Muscle Relaxants: carbamazepine antagonises muscle relaxant effect of non-depolarising muscle relaxants (accelerated recovery from neuromuscular blockade)

- Oestrogens: carbamazepine accelerates metabolism of ●oestrogens (reduced contraceptive effect—see p. 388)
- Progestogens: carbamazepine accelerates metabolism of ●progestogens (reduced contraceptive effect—see p. 388)

Retinoids: plasma concentration of carbamazepine possibly reduced by isotretinoin

Theophylline: carbamazepine accelerates metabolism of theophylline (reduced effect)

Thyroid Hormones: carbamazepine accelerates metabolism of thyroid hormones (may increase requirements for thyroid hormones in hypothyroidism)

Tibolone: carbamazepine accelerates metabolism of tibolone (reduced plasma concentration)

- Ulcer-healing Drugs: metabolism of carbamazepine inhibited by ●cimetidine (increased plasma concentration)

Vitamins: carbamazepine possibly increases requirements for vitamin D

Carbapenems see Ertapenem, Imipenem with Cilastatin, and Meropenem

Carbenoxolone

Note. Interactions do not apply to small amounts used topically on oral mucosa

ACE Inhibitors: carbenoxolone antagonises hypotensive effect of ACE inhibitors

Adrenergic Neurone Blockers: carbenoxolone antagonises hypotensive effect of adrenergic neurone blockers

Alpha-blockers: carbenoxolone antagonises hypotensive effect of alpha-blockers

Angiotensin-II Receptor Antagonists: carbenoxolone antagonises hypotensive effect of angiotensin-II receptor antagonists

Beta-blockers: carbenoxolone antagonises hypotensive effect of beta-blockers

Calcium-channel Blockers: carbenoxolone antagonises hypotensive effect of calcium-channel blockers

Cardiac Glycosides: hypokalaemia caused by carbenoxolone increases cardiac toxicity with cardiac glycosides

Clonidine: carbenoxolone antagonises hypotensive effect of clonidine

Corticosteroids: increased risk of hypokalaemia when carbenoxolone given with corticosteroids

Carbenoxolone (continued)

Diazoxide: carbenoxolone antagonises hypotensive effect of diazoxide

Diuretics: carbenoxolone antagonises diuretic effect of diuretics; increased risk of hypokalaemia when carbenoxolone given with acetazolamide, loop diuretics or thiazides and related diuretics; ulcer-healing effect of carbenoxolone inhibited by amiloride and spironolactone

Methyldopa: carbenoxolone antagonises hypotensive effect of methyldopa

Moxonidine: carbenoxolone antagonises hypotensive effect of moxonidine

Nitrates: carbenoxolone antagonises hypotensive effect of nitrates

Vasodilator Antihypertensives: carbenoxolone antagonises hypotensive effect of hydralazine, minoxidil and nitroprusside

Carbonic Anhydrase Inhibitors see Diuretics

Carboplatin see Platinum Compounds

Carboprost see Prostaglandins

Cardiac Glycosides

ACE Inhibitors: plasma concentration of digoxin possibly increased by captopril

Alpha-blockers: plasma concentration of digoxin increased by prazosin

Aminosalicylates: absorption of digoxin possibly reduced by sulfasalazine

Analgesics: plasma concentration of cardiac glycosides possibly increased by NSAIDs, also possible exacerbation of heart failure and reduction of renal function; digoxin increases risk of tramadol toxicity

- Angiotensin-II Receptor Antagonists: plasma concentration of digoxin increased by ●telmisartan

Antacids: absorption of digoxin possibly reduced by antacids

- Anti-arrhythmics: plasma concentration of digoxin increased by ●amiodarone, ●propafenone and ●quinidine (halve dose of digoxin)

Antibacterials: absorption of digoxin reduced by neomycin; plasma concentration of digoxin possibly reduced by rifampicin; plasma concentration of digoxin increased by macrolides (increased risk of toxicity); metabolism of digitoxin accelerated by rifamycins (reduced effect); plasma concentration of digoxin possibly increased by telithromycin and trimethoprim

- Antidepressants: plasma concentration of digoxin reduced by ●St John's wort—avoid concomitant use

Antiepileptics: metabolism of digitoxin accelerated by carbamazepine, phenytoin and primidone (reduced effect); plasma concentration of digoxin possibly reduced by phenytoin

- Antifungals: increased cardiac toxicity with cardiac glycosides if hypokalaemia occurs with ●amphotericin; plasma concentration of digoxin increased by ●itraconazole
- Antimalarials: plasma concentration of digoxin possibly increased by ●chloroquine and hydroxychloroquine; possible increased risk of bradycardia when digoxin given with mefloquine; plasma concentration of digoxin increased by ●quinine

Barbiturates: metabolism of digitoxin accelerated by barbiturates (reduced effect)

Beta-blockers: increased risk of AV block and bradycardia when cardiac glycosides given with beta-blockers

Calcium Salts: arrhythmias can be precipitated when cardiac glycosides given with large intravenous doses of calcium salts

- Calcium-channel Blockers: plasma concentration of digoxin increased by ●diltiazem, ●lercanidipine

Cardiac Glycosides

- Calcium-channel Blockers *(continued)* and ●nicardipine; plasma concentration of digoxin possibly increased by ●nifedipine; plasma concentration of digoxin increased by ●verapamil, also increased risk of AV block and bradycardia
- Ciclosporin: plasma concentration of digoxin increased by ●ciclosporin (increased risk of toxicity)
  Corticosteroids: increased risk of hypokalaemia when cardiac glycosides given with corticosteroids
- Diuretics: increased cardiac toxicity with cardiac glycosides if hypokalaemia occurs with ●acetazolamide, ●loop diuretics or ●thiazides and related diuretics; plasma concentration of digitoxin possibly affected by spironolactone; plasma concentration of digoxin increased by ●spironolactone
  Hormone Antagonists: metabolism of digitoxin accelerated by aminoglutethimide (reduced effect)
  Lipid-regulating Drugs: absorption of cardiac glycosides possibly reduced by colestipol and colestyramine; plasma concentration of digoxin possibly increased by atorvastatin
  Muscle Relaxants: risk of ventricular arrhythmias when cardiac glycosides given with suxamethonium; possible increased risk of bradycardia when cardiac glycosides given with tizanidine
  Penicillamine: plasma concentration of digoxin possibly reduced by penicillamine
  Ulcer-healing Drugs: increased cardiac toxicity with cardiac glycosides if hypokalaemia occurs with carbenoxolone; plasma concentration of digoxin possibly slightly increased by proton pump inhibitors; absorption of cardiac glycosides possibly reduced by sucralfate

Carisoprodol *see* Muscle Relaxants

Carteolol *see* Beta-blockers

Carvedilol *see* Beta-blockers

Caspofungin

Antibacterials: plasma concentration of caspofungin initially increased and then reduced by rifampicin (consider increasing dose of caspofungin)
- Antiepileptics: plasma concentration of caspofungin possibly reduced by ●carbamazepine and phenytoin—consider increasing dose of caspofungin
  Antivirals: plasma concentration of caspofungin possibly reduced by efavirenz and nevirapine—consider increasing dose of caspofungin
- Ciclosporin: plasma concentration of caspofungin increased by ●ciclosporin (manufacturer of caspofungin recommends monitoring liver enzymes)
  Corticosteroids: plasma concentration of caspofungin possibly reduced by dexamethasone—consider increasing dose of caspofungin
- Tacrolimus: caspofungin reduces plasma concentration of ●tacrolimus

Cefaclor *see* Cephalosporins
Cefadroxil *see* Cephalosporins
Cefalexin *see* Cephalosporins
Cefixime *see* Cephalosporins
Cefotaxime *see* Cephalosporins
Cefoxitin *see* Cephalosporins
Cefpirome *see* Cephalosporins
Cefpodoxime *see* Cephalosporins
Cefprozil *see* Cephalosporins
Cefradine *see* Cephalosporins
Ceftazidime *see* Cephalosporins
Ceftriaxone *see* Cephalosporins
Cefuroxime *see* Cephalosporins
Celecoxib *see* NSAIDs
Celiprolol *see* Beta-blockers

Cephalosporins

Antacids: absorption of cefaclor and cefpodoxime reduced by antacids
- Anticoagulants: cephalosporins possibly enhance anticoagulant effect of ●coumarins
  Oestrogens: *broad-spectrum* antibacterials possibly reduce contraceptive effect of oestrogens (risk probably small, see p. 388)
  Probenecid: excretion of cephalosporins reduced by probenecid (increased plasma concentration)
  Ulcer-healing Drugs: absorption of cefpodoxime reduced by histamine H₂-antagonists

Cephamycins *see* Cephalosporins
Certoparin *see* Heparins
Cetirizine *see* Antihistamines
Chloral *see* Anxiolytics and Hypnotics

Chloramphenicol

Antibacterials: metabolism of chloramphenicol accelerated by rifampicin (reduced plasma concentration)
- Anticoagulants: chloramphenicol enhances anticoagulant effect of ●coumarins
- Antidiabetics: chloramphenicol enhances effects of ●sulphonylureas
- Antiepileptics: chloramphenicol increases plasma concentration of ●phenytoin (increased risk of toxicity); metabolism of chloramphenicol accelerated by ●primidone (reduced plasma concentration)
- Antipsychotics: avoid concomitant use of chloramphenicol with ●clozapine (increased risk of agranulocytosis)
- Barbiturates: metabolism of chloramphenicol accelerated by ●barbiturates (reduced plasma concentration)
- Ciclosporin: chloramphenicol possibly increases plasma concentration of ●ciclosporin
  Oestrogens: *broad-spectrum* antibacterials possibly reduce contraceptive effect of oestrogens (risk probably small, see p. 388)
- Tacrolimus: chloramphenicol possibly increases plasma concentration of ●tacrolimus

Chlordiazepoxide *see* Anxiolytics and Hypnotics
Chloroquine and Hydroxychloroquine

Adsorbents: absorption of chloroquine and hydroxychloroquine reduced by kaolin
Antacids: absorption of chloroquine and hydroxychloroquine reduced by antacids
- Anti-arrhythmics: increased risk of ventricular arrhythmias when chloroquine and hydroxychloroquine given with ●amiodarone—avoid concomitant use
- Antibacterials: increased risk of ventricular arrhythmias when chloroquine and hydroxychloroquine given with ●moxifloxacin—avoid concomitant use
  Antiepileptics: possible increased risk of convulsions when chloroquine and hydroxychloroquine given with antiepileptics
- Antimalarials: avoidance of antimalarials advised by manufacturer of ●artemether/lumefantrine; increased risk of convulsions when chloroquine and hydroxychloroquine given with ●mefloquine
- Cardiac Glycosides: chloroquine and hydroxychloroquine possibly increase plasma concentration of ●digoxin
- Ciclosporin: chloroquine and hydroxychloroquine increase plasma concentration of ●ciclosporin (increased risk of toxicity)
  Parasympathomimetics: chloroquine and hydroxychloroquine have potential to increase symptoms of myasthenia gravis and thus diminish effect of neostigmine and pyridostigmine

Chloroquine and Hydroxychloroquine *(continued)*

Ulcer-healing Drugs: metabolism of chloroquine and hydroxychloroquine inhibited by cimetidine (increased plasma concentration)

Chlorphenamine (chlorpheniramine) *see* Antihistamines

Chlorpromazine *see* Antipsychotics

Chlorpropamide *see* Antidiabetics

Chlortalidone *see* Diuretics

Chlortetracycline *see* Tetracyclines

Ciclosporin

● ACE Inhibitors: increased risk of hyperkalaemia when ciclosporin given with ●ACE inhibitors

Allopurinol: plasma concentration of ciclosporin possibly increased by allopurinol (risk of nephrotoxicity)

● Analgesics: increased risk of nephrotoxicity when ciclosporin given with ●NSAIDs; ciclosporin increases plasma concentration of ●diclofenac (halve dose of diclofenac)

● Angiotensin-II Receptor Antagonists: increased risk of hyperkalaemia when ciclosporin given with ●angiotensin-II receptor antagonists

Anti-arrhythmics: plasma concentration of ciclosporin possibly increased by amiodarone and propafenone

● Antibacterials: metabolism of ciclosporin inhibited by ●clarithromycin and ●erythromycin (increased plasma concentration); metabolism of ciclosporin accelerated by ●rifampicin (reduced plasma concentration); plasma concentration of ciclosporin possibly reduced by ●sulfadiazine; plasma concentration of ciclosporin possibly increased by ●chloramphenicol, ●doxycycline and ●telithromycin; increased risk of nephrotoxicity when ciclosporin given with ●aminoglycosides, ●polymyxins, ●quinolones, ●sulphonamides or ●vancomycin; metabolism of ciclosporin possibly inhibited by ●macrolides (increased plasma concentration); plasma concentration of ciclosporin increased by ●quinupristin/dalfopristin; increased risk of nephrotoxicity when ciclosporin given with ●trimethoprim, also plasma concentration of ciclosporin reduced by intravenous trimethoprim

● Antidepressants: plasma concentration of ciclosporin reduced by ●St John's wort—avoid concomitant use

● Antiepileptics: metabolism of ciclosporin accelerated by ●carbamazepine and ●phenytoin (reduced plasma concentration); metabolism of ciclosporin accelerated by ●primidone (reduced effect)

● Antifungals: metabolism of ciclosporin inhibited by ●fluconazole, ●itraconazole, ●ketoconazole and ●voriconazole (increased plasma concentration); metabolism of ciclosporin possibly inhibited by ●miconazole (increased plasma concentration); increased risk of nephrotoxicity when ciclosporin given with ●amphotericin; ciclosporin increases plasma concentration of ●caspofungin (manufacturer of caspofungin recommends monitoring liver enzymes); plasma concentration of ciclosporin possibly reduced by griseofulvin

● Antimalarials: plasma concentration of ciclosporin increased by ●chloroquine and hydroxychloroquine (increased risk of toxicity)

● Antivirals: plasma concentration of ciclosporin possibly increased by ●nelfinavir and ●ritonavir

● Barbiturates: metabolism of ciclosporin accelerated by ●barbiturates (reduced effect)

● Beta-blockers: plasma concentration of ciclosporin increased by ●carvedilol

● Bile Acids: absorption of ciclosporin increased by ●ursodeoxycholic acid

Ciclosporin *(continued)*

● Bosentan: ciclosporin increases plasma concentration of ●bosentan (also plasma concentration of ciclosporin reduced—avoid concomitant use)

● Calcium-channel Blockers: combination of ciclosporin with ●lercanidipine may increase plasma concentration of either drug (or both)—avoid concomitant use; plasma concentration of ciclosporin increased by ●diltiazem, ●nicardipine and ●verapamil; ciclosporin possibly increases plasma concentration of nifedipine (increased risk of toxicity including gingival hyperplasia)

● Cardiac Glycosides: ciclosporin increases plasma concentration of ●digoxin (increased risk of toxicity)

● Colchicine: possible increased risk of nephrotoxicity and myotoxicity when ciclosporin given with ●colchicine (increased plasma concentration of ciclosporin)

● Corticosteroids: plasma concentration of ciclosporin increased by high-dose ●methylprednisolone (risk of convulsions); ciclosporin increases plasma concentration of prednisolone

● Cytotoxics: increased risk of nephrotoxicity when ciclosporin given with ●melphalan; increased risk of neurotoxicity when ciclosporin given with ●doxorubicin; risk of toxicity when ciclosporin given with ●methotrexate; *in vitro* studies suggest a possible interaction between ciclosporin and docetaxel (consult docetaxel product literature)

● Diuretics: increased risk of hyperkalaemia when ciclosporin given with ●potassium-sparing diuretics

● Grapefruit Juice: plasma concentration of ciclosporin increased by ●grapefruit juice (increased risk of toxicity)

● Hormone Antagonists: metabolism of ciclosporin inhibited by danazol (increased plasma concentration); plasma concentration of ciclosporin reduced by lanreotide and ●octreotide

● Lipid-regulating Drugs: increased risk of renal impairment when ciclosporin given with fenofibrate; increased risk of myopathy when ciclosporin given with ●rosuvastatin (avoid concomitant use); ciclosporin increases plasma concentration of ezetimibe; increased risk of myopathy when ciclosporin given with ●statins

● Metoclopramide: plasma concentration of ciclosporin increased by ●metoclopramide

● Modafinil: plasma concentration of ciclosporin reduced by ●modafinil

Oestrogens: plasma concentration of ciclosporin possibly increased by oestrogens

● Orlistat: absorption of ciclosporin possibly reduced by ●orlistat

● Potassium Salts: increased risk of hyperkalaemia when ciclosporin given with ●potassium salts

● Progestogens: metabolism of ciclosporin inhibited by ●progestogens (increased plasma concentration)

Sirolimus: ciclosporin possibly increases plasma concentration of sirolimus

● Tacrolimus: plasma concentration of ciclosporin increased by ●tacrolimus (increased risk of toxicity)—avoid concomitant use

● Ulcer-healing Drugs: plasma concentration of ciclosporin possibly increased by ●cimetidine; plasma concentration of ciclosporin possibly affected by omeprazole

Cidofovir

Antivirals: combination of cidofovir with tenofovir may increase plasma concentration of either drug (or both)

Cilazapril *see* ACE Inhibitors

Cilostazol

Analgesics: manufacturer of cilostazol recommends dose of concomitant aspirin should not exceed 80 mg daily

● Antibacterials: plasma concentration of cilostazol increased by ●erythromycin (also plasma concentration of erythromycin reduced)—avoid concomitant use

● Antifungals: plasma concentration of cilostazol possibly increased by ●ketoconazole—avoid concomitant use

● Antivirals: plasma concentration of cilostazol possibly increased by ●amprenavir, ●indinavir, ●lopinavir, nelfinavir, ●ritonavir and ●saquinavir—avoid concomitant use

● Calcium-channel Blockers: plasma concentration of cilostazol increased by ●diltiazem—avoid concomitant use

● Ulcer-healing Drugs: plasma concentration of cilostazol possibly increased by ●cimetidine and ●lansoprazole—avoid concomitant use; plasma concentration of cilostazol increased by ●omeprazole (risk of toxicity)—avoid concomitant use

Cimetidine see Histamine H₂-antagonists

Cinnarizine see Antihistamines

Ciprofibrate see Fibrates

Ciprofloxacin see Quinolones

Cisatracurium see Muscle Relaxants

Cisplatin see Platinum Compounds

Citalopram see Antidepressants, SSRI

Clarithromycin see Macrolides

Clemastine see Antihistamines

Clindamycin

● Muscle Relaxants: clindamycin enhances effects of ●non-depolarising muscle relaxants and ●suxamethonium

Oestrogens: broad-spectrum antibacterials possibly reduce contraceptive effect of oestrogens (risk probably small, see p. 388)

Parasympathomimetics: clindamycin antagonises effects of neostigmine and pyridostigmine

Clobazam see Anxiolytics and Hypnotics

Clomethiazole see Anxiolytics and Hypnotics

Clomipramine see Antidepressants, Tricyclic

Clonazepam see Anxiolytics and Hypnotics

Clonidine

ACE Inhibitors: enhanced hypotensive effect when clonidine given with ACE inhibitors; previous treatment with clonidine possibly delays antihypertensive effect of captopril

Adrenergic Neurone Blockers: enhanced hypotensive effect when clonidine given with adrenergic neurone blockers

Alcohol: enhanced hypotensive effect when clonidine given with alcohol

Aldesleukin: enhanced hypotensive effect when clonidine given with aldesleukin

Alpha-blockers: enhanced hypotensive effect when clonidine given with alpha-blockers

Alprostadil: enhanced hypotensive effect when clonidine given with alprostadil

Amifostine: possible enhanced hypotensive effect when clonidine given with amifostine

Anaesthetics, General: enhanced hypotensive effect when clonidine given with general anaesthetics

Analgesics: hypotensive effect of clonidine antagonised by NSAIDs

Angiotensin-II Receptor Antagonists: enhanced hypotensive effect when clonidine given with angiotensin-II receptor antagonists

● Antidepressants: enhanced hypotensive effect when clonidine given with MAOIs; hypotensive effect of clonidine antagonised by ●tricyclics, also

Clonidine

● Antidepressants (continued)
increased risk of hypertension on clonidine withdrawal

Antipsychotics: enhanced hypotensive effect when clonidine given with phenothiazines

Anxiolytics and Hypnotics: enhanced hypotensive effect when clonidine given with anxiolytics and hypnotics

● Beta-blockers: increased risk of withdrawal hypertension when clonidine given with ●beta-blockers (withdraw beta-blockers several days before slowly withdrawing clonidine)

Calcium-channel Blockers: enhanced hypotensive effect when clonidine given with calcium-channel blockers

Corticosteroids: hypotensive effect of clonidine antagonised by corticosteroids

Diazoxide: enhanced hypotensive effect when clonidine given with diazoxide

Diuretics: enhanced hypotensive effect when clonidine given with diuretics

Dopaminergics: enhanced hypotensive effect when clonidine given with levodopa

Methyldopa: enhanced hypotensive effect when clonidine given with methyldopa

Moxisylyte (thymoxamine): enhanced hypotensive effect when clonidine given with moxisylyte

Moxonidine: enhanced hypotensive effect when clonidine given with moxonidine

Muscle Relaxants: enhanced hypotensive effect when clonidine given with baclofen or tizanidine

Nitrates: enhanced hypotensive effect when clonidine given with nitrates

Oestrogens: hypotensive effect of clonidine antagonised by oestrogens

● Sympathomimetics: possible risk of hypertension when clonidine given with adrenaline (epinephrine) or noradrenaline (norepinephrine); serious adverse events reported with concomitant use of clonidine and ●methylphenidate (causality not established)

Ulcer-healing Drugs: hypotensive effect of clonidine antagonised by carbenoxolone

Vasodilator Antihypertensives: enhanced hypotensive effect when clonidine given with hydralazine, minoxidil or nitroprusside

Clopamide see Diuretics

Clopidogrel

Analgesics: increased risk of bleeding when clopidogrel given with NSAIDs or aspirin

● Anticoagulants: manufacturer of clopidogrel advises avoid concomitant use with ●warfarin; antiplatelet action of clopidogrel enhances anticoagulant effect of ●coumarins and ●phenindione; increased risk of bleeding when clopidogrel given with heparins

Dipyridamole: increased risk of bleeding when clopidogrel given with dipyridamole

Clorazepate see Anxiolytics and Hypnotics

Clotrimazole see Antifungals, Imidazole

Clozapine see Antipsychotics

Co-amoxiclav see Penicillins

Co-beneldopa see Levodopa

Co-careldopa see Levodopa

Codeine see Opioid Analgesics

Co-fluampicil see Penicillins

Colchicine

● Ciclosporin: possible increased risk of nephrotoxicity and myotoxicity when colchicine given with ●ciclosporin (increased plasma concentration of ciclosporin)

Colestipol

Note. Other drugs should be taken at least 1 hour before or 4-6 hours after colestipol to reduce possible interference with absorption

Bile Acids: colestipol possibly reduces absorption of bile acids

Cardiac Glycosides: colestipol possibly reduces absorption of cardiac glycosides

Diuretics: colestipol reduces absorption of thiazides and related diuretics (give at least 2 hours apart)

Thyroid Hormones: colestipol reduces absorption of thyroid hormones

Colestyramine

Note. Other drugs should be taken at least 1 hour before or 4-6 hours after colestyramine to reduce possible interference with absorption

Analgesics: colestyramine reduces absorption of paracetamol

Antibacterials: colestyramine antagonises effects of oral vancomycin

* Anticoagulants: colestyramine may enhance or reduce anticoagulant effect of ●coumarins and ●phenindione

Antidiabetics: colestyramine possibly enhances hypoglycaemic effect of acarbose

Antiepileptics: colestyramine possibly reduces absorption of valproate

Bile Acids: colestyramine possibly reduces absorption of bile acids

Cardiac Glycosides: colestyramine possibly reduces absorption of cardiac glycosides

Cytotoxics: colestyramine reduces absorption of mycophenolate mofetil

Diuretics: colestyramine reduces absorption of thiazides and related diuretics (give at least 2 hours apart)

Leflunomide: colestyramine significantly decreases effect of leflunomide (enhanced elimination)—avoid unless drug elimination desired

Raloxifene: colestyramine reduces absorption of raloxifene (manufacturer of raloxifene advises avoid concomitant administration)

Thyroid Hormones: colestyramine reduces absorption of thyroid hormones

Colistin *see* Polymyxins

Contraceptives, oral *see* Oestrogens and Progestogens

Corticosteroids

Note. Interactions do not generally apply to corticosteroids used for topical action (including inhalation)

ACE Inhibitors: corticosteroids antagonise hypotensive effect of ACE inhibitors

Adrenergic Neurone Blockers: corticosteroids antagonise hypotensive effect of adrenergic neurone blockers

Alpha-blockers: corticosteroids antagonise hypotensive effect of alpha-blockers

Analgesics: increased risk of gastro-intestinal bleeding and ulceration when corticosteroids given with NSAIDs; increased risk of gastro-intestinal bleeding and ulceration when corticosteroids given with aspirin, also corticosteroids reduce plasma concentration of salicylate

Angiotensin-II Receptor Antagonists: corticosteroids antagonise hypotensive effect of angiotensin-II receptor antagonists

Antacids: absorption of deflazacort reduced by antacids

* Antibacterials: metabolism of corticosteroids possibly inhibited by erythromycin; metabolism of methylprednisolone inhibited by erythromycin; metabolism of corticosteroids accelerated by ●rifamycins (reduced effect)

Corticosteroids *(continued)*

* Anticoagulants: corticosteroids may enhance or reduce anticoagulant effect of ●coumarins (high-dose corticosteroids enhance anticoagulant effect)

Antidiabetics: corticosteroids antagonise hypoglycaemic effect of antidiabetics

* Antiepileptics: metabolism of corticosteroids accelerated by ●carbamazepine, ●phenytoin and ●primidone (reduced effect)

* Antifungals: metabolism of corticosteroids possibly inhibited by ketoconazole; plasma concentration of inhaled mometasone increased by ketoconazole; metabolism of methylprednisolone inhibited by ketoconazole; increased risk of hypokalaemia when corticosteroids given with ●amphotericin—avoid concomitant use unless amphotericin needed to control reactions; metabolism of methylprednisolone possibly inhibited by itraconazole; dexamethasone possibly reduces plasma concentration of caspofungin—consider increasing dose of caspofungin

Antivirals: dexamethasone possibly reduces plasma concentration of indinavir, lopinavir and saquinavir; plasma concentration of corticosteroids, dexamethasone and prednisolone possibly increased by ritonavir

* Barbiturates: metabolism of corticosteroids accelerated by ●barbiturates (reduced effect)

Beta-blockers: corticosteroids antagonise hypotensive effect of beta-blockers

Calcium-channel Blockers: corticosteroids antagonise hypotensive effect of calcium-channel blockers

Cardiac Glycosides: increased risk of hypokalaemia when corticosteroids given with cardiac glycosides

* Ciclosporin: high-dose methylprednisolone increases plasma concentration of ●ciclosporin (risk of convulsions); plasma concentration of prednisolone increased by ciclosporin

Clonidine: corticosteroids antagonise hypotensive effect of clonidine

* Cytotoxics: increased risk of haematological toxicity when corticosteroids given with ●methotrexate

Diazoxide: corticosteroids antagonise hypotensive effect of diazoxide

Diuretics: corticosteroids antagonise diuretic effect of diuretics; increased risk of hypokalaemia when corticosteroids given with acetazolamide, loop diuretics or thiazides and related diuretics

Hormone Antagonists: metabolism of corticosteroids accelerated by aminoglutethimide (reduced effect)

Methyldopa: corticosteroids antagonise hypotensive effect of methyldopa

Mifepristone: effect of corticosteroids (including inhaled corticosteroids) may be reduced for 3–4 days after mifepristone

Moxonidine: corticosteroids antagonise hypotensive effect of moxonidine

Nitrates: corticosteroids antagonise hypotensive effect of nitrates

Oestrogens: plasma concentration of corticosteroids increased by oral contraceptives containing oestrogens

Somatropin: corticosteroids may inhibit growth-promoting effect of somatropin

Sympathomimetics: metabolism of dexamethasone accelerated by ephedrine

Sympathomimetics, Beta$_2$: increased risk of hypokalaemia when corticosteroids given with high doses of beta$_2$ sympathomimetics—for CSM advice (hypokalaemia) see p. 135

Theophylline: increased risk of hypokalaemia when corticosteroids given with theophylline

Corticosteroids (continued)

Ulcer-healing Drugs: increased risk of hypokalaemia when corticosteroids given with carbenoxolone

- Vaccines: high doses of corticosteroids impair immune response to ●vaccines, avoid concomitant use with live vaccines (see p. 578)

Vasodilator Antihypertensives: corticosteroids antagonise hypotensive effect of hydralazine, minoxidil and nitroprusside

Cortisone see Corticosteroids

Co-trimoxazole see Trimethoprim and Sulfamethoxazole

Coumarins

Note. Change in patient's clinical condition, particularly associated with liver disease, intercurrent illness, or drug administration, necessitates more frequent testing. Major changes in diet (especially involving salads and vegetables) and in alcohol consumption may also affect anticoagulant control

- Alcohol: anticoagulant control with coumarins may be affected by major changes in consumption of ●alcohol

Allopurinol: anticoagulant effect of coumarins possibly enhanced by allopurinol

- Anabolic Steroids: anticoagulant effect of coumarins enhanced by ●anabolic steroids
- Analgesics: anticoagulant effect of coumarins possibly enhanced by ●NSAIDs, ●celecoxib, ●dextropropoxyphene, ●diflunisal, ●etodolac, ●etoricoxib, ●flurbiprofen, ●ibuprofen, ●mefenamic acid, ●meloxicam, ●piroxicam, ●rofecoxib, ●sulindac and ●valdecoxib; anticoagulant effect of coumarins enhanced by ●azapropazone (avoid concomitant use); anticoagulant effect of coumarins possibly enhanced by ●diclofenac, also increased risk of haemorrage with intravenous diclofenac (avoid concomitant use); increased risk of bleeding when coumarins given with ●ketorolac (avoid concomitant use); increased risk of bleeding when coumarins given with ●aspirin (due to antiplatelet effect); anticoagulant effect of coumarins possibly enhanced by prolonged regular use of paracetamol
- Anti-arrhythmics: metabolism of coumarins inhibited by ●amiodarone (enhanced anticoagulant effect); anticoagulant effect of coumarins enhanced by ●propafenone; anticoagulant effect of coumarins possibly enhanced by ●quinidine
- Antibacterials: experience in anticoagulant clinics suggests that INR possibly altered when coumarins are given with ●neomycin (given for local action on gut); anticoagulant effect of coumarins enhanced by ●chloramphenicol, ●ciprofloxacin, ●clarithromycin, ●erythromycin, ●metronidazole, ●nalidixic acid, ●norfloxacin and ●ofloxacin and ●sulphonamides; anticoagulant effect of coumarins possibly enhanced by ●aztreonam, ●cephalosporins, levofloxacin, ●macrolides, ●tetracyclines and trimethoprim; studies have failed to demonstrate an interaction with coumarins, but common experience in anticoagulant clinics is that INR can be altered by a course of broad-spectrum penicillins such as ampicillin; metabolism of coumarins accelerated by ●rifamycins (reduced anticoagulant effect)
- Antidepressants: anticoagulant effect of warfarin possibly enhanced by ●venlafaxine; anticoagulant effect of coumarins possibly enhanced by ●SSRIs; anticoagulant effect of warfarin reduced by ●St John's wort (avoid concomitant use); anticoagulant effect of warfarin enhanced by mirtazapine
- Antidiabetics: coumarins possibly enhance hypoglycaemic effect of ●sulphonylureas, also possible changes to anticoagulant effect

Coumarins (continued)

- Antiepileptics: metabolism of coumarins accelerated by ●carbamazepine and ●primidone (reduced anticoagulant effect); metabolism of coumarins accelerated by ●phenytoin (possibility of reduced anticoagulant effect, but enhancement also reported); anticoagulant effect of coumarins possibly enhanced by valproate
- Antifungals: anticoagulant effect of coumarins enhanced by ●fluconazole, ●itraconazole, ●ketoconazole and ●voriconazole; anticoagulant effect of coumarins enhanced by ●miconazole (miconazole oral gel and possibly vaginal formulations absorbed); anticoagulant effect of coumarins reduced by ●griseofulvin

Antimalarials: isolated reports that anticoagulant effect of warfarin may be enhanced by proguanil

- Antivirals: anticoagulant effect of warfarin may be enhanced or reduced by ●nevirapine; anticoagulant effect of coumarins possibly enhanced by ●ritonavir

Anxiolytics and Hypnotics: anticoagulant effect of coumarins may transiently be enhanced by chloral and triclofos

- Barbiturates: metabolism of coumarins accelerated by ●barbiturates (reduced anticoagulant effect)

Bosentan: monitoring anticoagulant effect of coumarins recommended by manufacturer of bosentan

- Clopidogrel: anticoagulant effect of coumarins enhanced due to antiplatelet action of ●clopidogrel; avoidance of warfarin advised by manufacturer of ●clopidogrel
- Corticosteroids: anticoagulant effect of coumarins may be enhanced or reduced by ●corticosteroids (high-dose corticosteroids enhance anticoagulant effect)
- Cranberry Juice: anticoagulant effect of warfarin possibly enhanced by ●cranberry juice—avoid concomitant use
- Cytotoxics: anticoagulant effect of coumarins possibly enhanced by ●fluorouracil and ●ifosfamide; anticoagulant effect of warfarin possibly reduced by ●azathioprine and ●mercaptopurine; replacement of warfarin with a heparin advised by manufacturer of imatinib (possibilty of enhanced warfarin effect)
- Dipyridamole: anticoagulant effect of coumarins enhanced due to antiplatelet action of ●dipyridamole
- Disulfiram: anticoagulant effect of coumarins enhanced by ●disulfiram
- Dopaminergics: anticoagulant effect of warfarin enhanced by ●entacapone
- Enteral Foods: anticoagulant effect of coumarins antagonised by vitamin K (present in some ●enteral feeds)
- Hormone Antagonists: metabolism of coumarins accelerated by ●aminoglutethimide (reduced anticoagulant effect); anticoagulant effect of coumarins possibly enhanced by bicalutamide and ●toremifene; metabolism of coumarins inhibited by ●danazol (enhanced anticoagulant effect); anticoagulant effect of coumarins enhanced by ●flutamide and ●tamoxifen

Leflunomide: anticoagulant effect of warfarin possibly enhanced by leflunomide

Leukotriene Antagonists: anticoagulant effect of warfarin enhanced by zafirlukast

- Lipid-regulating Drugs: anticoagulant effect of coumarins may be enhanced or reduced by ●colestyramine; anticoagulant effect of coumarins possibly enhanced by ●rosuvastatin; anticoagulant effect of coumarins enhanced by ●fibrates and ●simvastatin

Coumarins *(continued)*

- Oestrogens: anticoagulant effect of coumarins antagonised by ●oestrogens

  Orlistat: monitoring anticoagulant effect of coumarins recommended by manufacturer of orlistat
- Progestogens: anticoagulant effect of coumarins antagonised by ●progestogens

  Raloxifene: anticoagulant effect of coumarins antagonised by raloxifene
- Retinoids: anticoagulant effect of coumarins possibly reduced by ●acitretin

  Sibutramine: increased risk of bleeding when anticoagulants given with sibutramine
- Sulfinpyrazone: anticoagulant effect of coumarins enhanced by ●sulfinpyrazone
- Sympathomimetics: anticoagulant effect of coumarins possibly enhanced by ●methylphenidate

  Terpene Mixture: anticoagulant effect of coumarins possibly reduced by Rowachol®
- Testosterone: anticoagulant effect of coumarins enhanced by ●testosterone
- Thyroid Hormones: anticoagulant effect of coumarins enhanced by ●thyroid hormones
- Ulcer-healing Drugs: metabolism of coumarins inhibited by ●cimetidine (enhanced anticoagulant effect); anticoagulant effect of coumarins possibly enhanced by ●esomeprazole and ●omeprazole; absorption of coumarins possibly reduced by ●sucralfate (reduced anticoagulant effect)

  Vaccines: anticoagulant effect of warfarin possibly enhanced by influenza vaccine
- Vitamins: anticoagulant effect of coumarins antagonised by ●vitamin K

Cranberry Juice

- Anticoagulants: cranberry juice possibly enhances anticoagulant effect of ●warfarin—avoid concomitant use

Cyclizine *see* Antihistamines

Cyclopenthiazide *see* Diuretics

Cyclopentolate *see* Antimuscarinics

Cyclophosphamide

Antiepileptics: cytotoxics reduce absorption of phenytoin
- Antipsychotics: avoid concomitant use of cytotoxics with ●clozapine (increased risk of agranulocytosis)
- Cytotoxics: increased toxicity when high-dose cyclophosphamide given with ●pentostatin—avoid concomitant use

  Muscle Relaxants: cyclophosphamide enhances effects of suxamethonium

Cycloserine

- Alcohol: increased risk of convulsions when cycloserine given with ●alcohol

  Antibacterials: increased risk of CNS toxicity when cycloserine given with isoniazid

  Oestrogens: *broad-spectrum* antibacterials possibly reduce contraceptive effect of oestrogens (risk probably small, see p. 388)

Cyproheptadine *see* Antihistamines

Cytarabine

Antiepileptics: cytotoxics reduce absorption of phenytoin

Antifungals: cytarabine possibly reduces plasma concentration of flucytosine
- Antipsychotics: avoid concomitant use of cytotoxics with ●clozapine (increased risk of agranulocytosis)

  Cytotoxics: intracellular concentration of cytarabine increased by fludarabine

Cytotoxics *see* individual drugs

Dairy Products

Antibacterials: dairy products reduces absorption of ciprofloxacin and norfloxacin; dairy products reduces absorption of tetracyclines (except doxycycline and minocycline)

Dalteparin *see* Heparins

Danazol

- Anticoagulants: danazol inhibits metabolism of ●coumarins (enhanced anticoagulant effect)
- Antiepileptics: danazol inhibits metabolism of ●carbamazepine (increased risk of toxicity)
- Ciclosporin: danazol inhibits metabolism of ●ciclosporin (increased plasma concentration)

  Tacrolimus: danazol possibly increases plasma concentration of tacrolimus

Dantrolene *see* Muscle Relaxants

Dapsone

Antibacterials: plasma concentration of dapsone reduced by rifamycins; plasma concentration of both drugs may increase when dapsone given with trimethoprim

Antivirals: plasma concentration of dapsone possibly increased by amprenavir

Oestrogens: *broad-spectrum* antibacterials possibly reduce contraceptive effect of oestrogens (risk probably small, see p. 388)

Probenecid: excretion of dapsone reduced by probenecid (increased risk of side-effects)

Darbepoetin *see* Epoetin

Deflazacort *see* Corticosteroids

Demeclocycline *see* Tetracyclines

Desferrioxamine

Antipsychotics: avoidance of desferrioxamine advised by manufacturer of levomepromazine (methotrimeprazine); manufacturer of desferrioxamine advises avoid concomitant use with prochlorperazine

Desflurane *see* Anaesthetics, General

Desloratadine *see* Antihistamines

Desmopressin

Analgesics: effects of desmopressin enhanced by indometacin

Loperamide: plasma concentration of *oral* desmopressin increased by loperamide

Desogestrel *see* Progestogens

Dexamethasone *see* Corticosteroids

Dexamfetamine *see* Sympathomimetics

Dexketoprofen *see* NSAIDs

Dextromethorphan *see* Opioid Analgesics

Dextromoramide *see* Opioid Analgesics

Dextropropoxyphene *see* Opioid Analgesics

Diamorphine *see* Opioid Analgesics

Diazepam *see* Anxiolytics and Hypnotics

Diazoxide

ACE Inhibitors: enhanced hypotensive effect when diazoxide given with ACE inhibitors

Adrenergic Neurone Blockers: enhanced hypotensive effect when diazoxide given with adrenergic neurone blockers

Alcohol: enhanced hypotensive effect when diazoxide given with alcohol

Aldesleukin: enhanced hypotensive effect when diazoxide given with aldesleukin

Alpha-blockers: enhanced hypotensive effect when diazoxide given with alpha-blockers

Alprostadil: enhanced hypotensive effect when diazoxide given with alprostadil

Amifostine: possible enhanced hypotensive effect when diazoxide given with amifostine

Anaesthetics, General: enhanced hypotensive effect when diazoxide given with general anaesthetics

Analgesics: hypotensive effect of diazoxide antagonised by NSAIDs

Angiotensin-II Receptor Antagonists: enhanced hypotensive effect when diazoxide given with angiotensin-II receptor antagonists

Diazoxide (continued)

Antidepressants: enhanced hypotensive effect when diazoxide given with MAOIs or tricyclic-related antidepressants

Antidiabetics: diazoxide antagonises hypoglycaemic effect of antidiabetics

Antipsychotics: enhanced hypotensive effect when diazoxide given with phenothiazines

Anxiolytics and Hypnotics: enhanced hypotensive effect when diazoxide given with anxiolytics and hypnotics

Beta-blockers: enhanced hypotensive effect when diazoxide given with beta-blockers

Calcium-channel Blockers: enhanced hypotensive effect when diazoxide given with calcium-channel blockers

Clonidine: enhanced hypotensive effect when diazoxide given with clonidine

Corticosteroids: hypotensive effect of diazoxide antagonised by corticosteroids

Diuretics: enhanced hypotensive effect when diazoxide given with diuretics

Dopaminergics: enhanced hypotensive effect when diazoxide given with levodopa

Methyldopa: enhanced hypotensive effect when diazoxide given with methyldopa

Moxisylyte (thymoxamine): enhanced hypotensive effect when diazoxide given with moxisylyte

Moxonidine: enhanced hypotensive effect when diazoxide given with moxonidine

Muscle Relaxants: enhanced hypotensive effect when diazoxide given with baclofen or tizanidine

Nitrates: enhanced hypotensive effect when diazoxide given with nitrates

Oestrogens: hypotensive effect of diazoxide antagonised by oestrogens

Ulcer-healing Drugs: hypotensive effect of diazoxide antagonised by carbenoxolone

Vasodilator Antihypertensives: enhanced hypotensive effect when diazoxide given with hydralazine, minoxidil or nitroprusside

Diclofenac see NSAIDs

Dicycloverine (dicyclomine) see Antimuscarinics

Didanosine

Note. Antacids in tablet formulation may affect absorption of other drugs

Antivirals: plasma concentration of didanosine possibly increased by ganciclovir; plasma concentration of didanosine increased by tenofovir

Diflunisal see NSAIDs

Digitoxin see Cardiac Glycosides

Digoxin see Cardiac Glycosides

Dihydrocodeine see Opioid Analgesics

Diltiazem see Calcium-channel Blockers

Dimercaprol

● Iron: avoid concomitant use of dimercaprol with ●iron

Dinoprostone see Prostaglandins

Diphenhydramine see Antihistamines

Diphenoxylate see Opioid Analgesics

Diphenylpyraline see Antihistamines

Dipipanone see Opioid Analgesics

Dipivefrine see Sympathomimetics

Dipyridamole

Antacids: absorption of dipyridamole possibly reduced by antacids

● Anti-arrhythmics: dipyridamole enhances and extends the effects of ●adenosine (important risk of toxicity)

● Anticoagulants: antiplatelet action of dipyridamole enhances anticoagulant effect of ●coumarins and ●phenindione; dipyridamole enhances anticoagulant effect of heparins

Dipyridamole (continued)

Clopidogrel: increased risk of bleeding when dipyridamole given with clopidogrel

Cytotoxics: dipyridamole possibly reduces effects of fludarabine

Disodium Etidronate see Bisphosphonates

Disodium Pamidronate see Bisphosphonates

Disopyramide

● Adrenergic Neurone Blockers: increased myocardial depression when anti-arrhythmics given with ●bretylium

Anaesthetics, Local: increased myocardial depression when anti-arrhythmics given with bupivacaine or levobupivacaine

● Anti-arrhythmics: increased myocardial depression when anti-arrhythmics given with other ●anti-arrhythmics; increased risk of ventricular arrhythmias when disopyramide given with ●amiodarone—avoid concomitant use

● Antibacterials: plasma concentration of disopyramide possibly increased by ●clarithromycin (increased risk of toxicity); plasma concentration of disopyramide increased by ●erythromycin (increased risk of toxicity); increased risk of ventricular arrhythmias when disopyramide given with ●moxifloxacin or ●quinupristin/dalfopristin—avoid concomitant use; metabolism of disopyramide accelerated by ●rifamycins (reduced plasma concentration)

● Antidepressants: increased risk of ventricular arrhythmias when disopyramide given with ●tricyclics

Antiepileptics: plasma concentration of disopyramide reduced by phenytoin; metabolism of disopyramide accelerated by primidone (reduced plasma concentration)

● Antihistamines: increased risk of ventricular arrhythmias when disopyramide given with ●mizolastine or ●terfenadine—avoid concomitant use; increased risk of ventricular arrhythmias when anti-arrhythmics given with ●terfenadine

● Antimalarials: avoidance of disopyramide advised by manufacturer of ●artemether/lumefantrine (risk of ventricular arrhythmias)

Antimuscarinics: increased risk of antimuscarinic side-effects when disopyramide given with antimuscarinics

● Antipsychotics: increased risk of ventricular arrhythmias when anti-arrhythmics that prolong the QT interval given with ●antipsychotics that prolong the QT interval; increased risk of ventricular arrhythmias when disopyramide given with ●amisulpride, ●pimozide, ●sertindole or ●thioridazine—avoid concomitant use; increased risk of ventricular arrhythmias when disopyramide given with ●phenothiazines

● Antivirals: plasma concentration of disopyramide possibly increased by ●ritonavir (increased risk of toxicity)

Barbiturates: metabolism of disopyramide accelerated by barbiturates (reduced plasma concentration)

● Beta-blockers: increased myocardial depression when anti-arrhythmics given with ●beta-blockers; increased risk of ventricular arrhythmias when disopyramide given with ●sotalol—avoid concomitant use

● Calcium-channel Blockers: increased risk of myocardial depression and asystole when disopyramide given with ●verapamil

● Diuretics: increased cardiac toxicity with disopyramide if hypokalaemia occurs with ●acetazolamide, ●loop diuretics or ●thiazides and related diuretics

Disopyramide *(continued)*

- <u>Dolasetron</u>: increased risk of ventricular arrhythmias when disopyramide given with ●dolasetron—avoid concomitant use

 Nitrates: disopyramide reduces effects of sublingual tablets of nitrates (failure to dissolve under tongue owing to dry mouth)

 Tropisetron: caution with anti-arrhythmics advised by manufacturer of tropisetron (risk of ventricular arrhythmias)

Distigmine *see* Parasympathomimetics

Disulfiram

 Alcohol: disulfiram reaction when disulfiram given with alcohol (see p. 247)

 Antibacterials: psychotic reaction reported when disulfiram given with metronidazole

- <u>Anticoagulants</u>: disulfiram enhances anticoagulant effect of ●coumarins

 Antidepressants: increased disulfiram reaction with alcohol reported with concomitant amitriptyline; disulfiram inhibits metabolism of tricyclics (increased plasma concentration)

- <u>Antiepileptics</u>: disulfiram inhibits metabolism of ●phenytoin (increased risk of toxicity)

 Anxiolytics and Hypnotics: disulfiram increases risk of temazepam toxicity; disulfiram inhibits metabolism of benzodiazepines (increased sedative effects)

- Paraldehyde: risk of toxicity when disulfiram given with ●paraldehyde

 Theophylline: disulfiram inhibits metabolism of theophylline (increased risk of toxicity)

Diuretics

 Note. Since systemic absorption may follow topical application of brinzolamide to the eye, the possibility of interactions should be borne in mind

 Note. Since systemic absorption may follow topical application of dorzolamide to the eye, the possibility of interactions should be borne in mind

- <u>ACE Inhibitors</u>: enhanced hypotensive effect when diuretics given with ●ACE inhibitors; increased risk of severe hyperkalaemia when potassium-sparing diuretics given with ●ACE inhibitors (monitor potassium concentration with low-dose spironolactone in heart failure)

 Adrenergic Neurone Blockers: enhanced hypotensive effect when diuretics given with adrenergic neurone blockers

 Alcohol: enhanced hypotensive effect when diuretics given with alcohol

 Aldesleukin: enhanced hypotensive effect when diuretics given with aldesleukin

- Alpha-blockers: enhanced hypotensive effect when diuretics given with ●alpha-blockers, also increased risk of first-dose hypotension with post-synaptic alpha-blockers such as prazosin

 Alprostadil: enhanced hypotensive effect when diuretics given with alprostadil

 Amifostine: possible enhanced hypotensive effect when diuretics given with amifostine

 Anaesthetics, General: enhanced hypotensive effect when diuretics given with general anaesthetics

- <u>Analgesics</u>: possibly increased risk of hyperkalaemia when potassium-sparing diuretics given with NSAIDs; diuretics increase risk of nephrotoxicity of NSAIDs, also antagonism of diuretic effect; effects of diuretics antagonised by indometacin and ketorolac; increased risk of hyperkalaemia when potassium-sparing diuretics given with indometacin; occasional reports of reduced renal function when triamterene given with ●indometacin—avoid concomitant use; increased risk of toxicity when carbonic anhydrase inhibitors given

Diuretics

- <u>Analgesics</u> *(continued)*

 with high-dose aspirin; diuretic effect of spironolactone antagonised by aspirin

- <u>Angiotensin-II Receptor Antagonists</u>: enhanced hypotensive effect when diuretics given with ●angiotensin-II receptor antagonists; increased risk of hyperkalaemia when potassium-sparing diuretics given with ●angiotensin-II receptor antagonists

- Anti-arrhythmics: hypokalaemia caused by acetazolamide, loop diuretics or thiazides and related diuretics increases cardiac toxicity with amiodarone; hypokalaemia caused by acetazolamide, loop diuretics or thiazides and related diuretics increases cardiac toxicity with ●disopyramide; hypokalaemia caused by acetazolamide, loop diuretics or thiazides and related diuretics increases cardiac toxicity with ●flecainide; hypokalaemia caused by acetazolamide, loop diuretics or thiazides and related diuretics antagonises action of ●lidocaine (lignocaine); hypokalaemia caused by acetazolamide, loop diuretics or thiazides and related diuretics antagonises action of ●mexiletine; hypokalaemia caused by loop diuretics or thiazides and related diuretics increases cardiac toxicity with ●quinidine; acetazolamide reduces excretion of ●quinidine (occasionally increased plasma concentration), also cardiac toxicity of quinidine increased if hypokalaemia occurs

- <u>Antibacterials</u>: avoidance of diuretics advised by manufacturer of lymecycline; increased risk of ototoxicity when loop diuretics given with ●aminoglycosides, ●polymyxins or ●vancomycin; acetazolamide antagonises effects of ●methenamine

 Antidepressants: possible increased risk of hypokalaemia when loop diuretics or thiazides and related diuretics given with reboxetine; enhanced hypotensive effect when diuretics given with MAOIs; increased risk of postural hypotension when diuretics given with tricyclics

 Antidiabetics: loop diuretics and thiazides and related diuretics antagonise hypoglycaemic effect of antidiabetics; increased risk of hyponatraemia when thiazides and related diuretics plus potassium-sparing diuretic given with chlorpropamide

- <u>Antiepileptics</u>: increased risk of hyponatraemia when diuretics given with carbamazepine; acetazolamide increases plasma concentration of ●carbamazepine; increased risk of osteomalacia when carbonic anhydrase inhibitors given with phenytoin or primidone; acetazolamide possibly reduces plasma concentration of primidone

 Antifungals: increased risk of hypokalaemia when loop diuretics or thiazides and related diuretics given with amphotericin; hydrochlorothiazide increases plasma concentration of fluconazole

- Antihistamines: hypokalaemia or other electrolyte imbalance with diuretics increases risk of ventricular arrhythmias with ●terfenadine

- Antipsychotics: hypokalaemia caused by diuretics increases risk of ventricular arrhythmias with ●pimozide or ●thioridazine (avoid concomitant use); hypokalaemia caused by diuretics increases risk of ventricular arrhythmias with ●amisulpride or ●sertindole; enhanced hypotensive effect when diuretics given with phenothiazines

 Anxiolytics and Hypnotics: enhanced hypotensive effect when diuretics given with anxiolytics and hypnotics; administration of parenteral furosemide (frusemide) with chloral or triclofos may displace thyroid hormone from binding sites

Diuretics *(continued)*

Barbiturates: increased risk of osteomalacia when carbonic anhydrase inhibitors given with phenobarbital

● Beta-blockers: enhanced hypotensive effect when diuretics given with beta-blockers; hypokalaemia caused by loop diuretics or thiazides and related diuretics increases risk of ventricular arrhythmias with ●sotalol

Calcium Salts: increased risk of hypercalcaemia when thiazides and related diuretics given with calcium salts

Calcium-channel Blockers: enhanced hypotensive effect when diuretics given with calcium-channel blockers

● Cardiac Glycosides: hypokalaemia caused by acetazolamide, loop diuretics or thiazides and related diuretics increases cardiac toxicity with ●cardiac glycosides; spironolactone possibly affects plasma concentration of digitoxin; spironolactone increases plasma concentration of ●digoxin

● Ciclosporin: increased risk of hyperkalaemia when potassium-sparing diuretics given with ●ciclosporin

Clonidine: enhanced hypotensive effect when diuretics given with clonidine

Corticosteroids: diuretic effect of diuretics antagonised by corticosteroids; increased risk of hypokalaemia when acetazolamide, loop diuretics or thiazides and related diuretics given with corticosteroids

Cytotoxics: increased risk of nephrotoxicity and ototoxicity when diuretics given with platinum compounds

Diazoxide: enhanced hypotensive effect when diuretics given with diazoxide

Diuretics: increased risk of hypokalaemia when loop diuretics or thiazides and related diuretics given with acetazolamide; profound diuresis possible when metolazone given with furosemide (frusemide); increased risk of hypokalaemia when thiazides and related diuretics given with loop diuretics

Dopaminergics: enhanced hypotensive effect when diuretics given with levodopa

Hormone Antagonists: increased risk of hyponatraemia when diuretics given with aminoglutethimide; increased risk of hypercalcaemia when thiazides and related diuretics given with toremifene; increased risk of hyperkalaemia when potassium-sparing diuretics given with trilostane

Lipid-regulating Drugs: absorption of thiazides and related diuretics reduced by colestipol and colestyramine (give at least 2 hours apart)

● Lithium: loop diuretics and thiazides and related diuretics reduce excretion of ●lithium (increased plasma concentration and risk of toxicity)—loop diuretics safer than thiazides; potassium-sparing diuretics reduce excretion of ●lithium (increased plasma concentration and risk of toxicity); acetazolamide increases the excretion of ●lithium

Methyldopa: enhanced hypotensive effect when diuretics given with methyldopa

Moxisylyte (thymoxamine): enhanced hypotensive effect when diuretics given with moxisylyte

Moxonidine: enhanced hypotensive effect when diuretics given with moxonidine

Muscle Relaxants: enhanced hypotensive effect when diuretics given with baclofen or tizanidine

Nitrates: enhanced hypotensive effect when diuretics given with nitrates

Oestrogens: diuretic effect of diuretics antagonised by oestrogens

Diuretics *(continued)*

● Potassium Salts: increased risk of hyperkalaemia when potassium-sparing diuretics given with ●potassium salts

Progestogens: risk of hyperkalaemia when potassium-sparing diuretics given with drospirenone (monitor serum potassium during first cycle)

Sympathomimetics, Beta₂: increased risk of hypokalaemia when acetazolamide, loop diuretics or thiazides and related diuretics given with high doses of beta₂ sympathomimetics—for CSM advice (hypokalaemia) see p. 135

● Tacrolimus: increased risk of hyperkalaemia when potassium-sparing diuretics given with ●tacrolimus

Theophylline: increased risk of hypokalaemia when acetazolamide, loop diuretics or thiazides and related diuretics given with theophylline

Ulcer-healing Drugs: diuretic effect of diuretics antagonised by carbenoxolone; increased risk of hypokalaemia when acetazolamide, loop diuretics or thiazides and related diuretics given with carbenoxolone; amiloride and spironolactone inhibit ulcer-healing effect of carbenoxolone

Vasodilator Antihypertensives: enhanced hypotensive effect when diuretics given with hydralazine, minoxidil or nitroprusside

Vitamins: increased risk of hypercalcaemia when thiazides and related diuretics given with vitamin D

Diuretics, Loop *see* Diuretics
Diuretics, Potassium-sparing *see* Diuretics
Diuretics, Thiazide and related *see* Diuretics
Dobutamine *see* Sympathomimetics
Docetaxel

Antibacterials: *in vitro* studies suggest a possible interaction between docetaxel and erythromycin (consult docetaxel product literature)

Antiepileptics: cytotoxics reduce absorption of phenytoin

Antifungals: *in vitro* studies suggest a possible interaction between docetaxel and ketoconazole (consult docetaxel product literature)

Antihistamines: *in vitro* studies suggest a possible interaction between docetaxel and terfenadine (consult docetaxel product literature)

● Antipsychotics: avoid concomitant use of cytotoxics with ●clozapine (increased risk of agranulocytosis)

Ciclosporin: *in vitro* studies suggest a possible interaction between docetaxel and ciclosporin (consult docetaxel product literature)

Dolasetron

● Adrenergic Neurone Blockers: increased risk of ventricular arrhythmias when dolasetron given with ●bretylium—avoid concomitant use

● Anti-arrhythmics: increased risk of ventricular arrhythmias when dolasetron given with ●amiodarone, ●disopyramide, ●flecainide, ●lidocaine (lignocaine), ●mexiletine, ●procainamide or ●propafenone—avoid concomitant use

● Beta-blockers: increased risk of ventricular arrhythmias when dolasetron given with ●sotalol—avoid concomitant use

Domperidone

Analgesics: effects of domperidone on gastro-intestinal activity antagonised by opioid analgesics; domperidone increases absorption of paracetamol (enhanced effect)

Antimuscarinics: effects of domperidone on gastro-intestinal activity antagonised by antimuscarinics

Dopaminergics: increased risk of extrapyramidal side-effects when domperidone given with amantadine; domperidone possibly antagonises hypo-

Domperidone
Dopaminergics *(continued)*
prolactinaemic effects of bromocriptine and cabergoline
Donepezil *see* Parasympathomimetics
Dopamine *see* Sympathomimetics
Dopaminergics *see* Amantadine, Apomorphine, Bromocriptine, Cabergoline, Entacapone, Levodopa, Lisuride, Pergolide, Pramipexole, Quinagolide, Ropinirole, and Selegiline
Dopexamine *see* Sympathomimetics
Dorzolamide *see* Diuretics
Dosulepin (dothiepin) *see* Antidepressants, Tricyclic
Doxapram
Antidepressants: effects of doxapram enhanced by MAOIs
Sympathomimetics: increased risk of hypertension when doxapram given with sympathomimetics
Theophylline: increased CNS stimulation when doxapram given with theophylline
Doxazosin *see* Alpha-blockers
Doxepin *see* Antidepressants, Tricyclic
Doxorubicin
Antiepileptics: cytotoxics reduce absorption of phenytoin
• Antipsychotics: avoid concomitant use of cytotoxics with ●clozapine (increased risk of agranulocytosis)
Antivirals: doxorubicin possibly inhibits effects of stavudine
• Ciclosporin: increased risk of neurotoxicity when doxorubicin given with ●ciclosporin
Doxycycline *see* Tetracyclines
Doxylamine *see* Antihistamines
Drospirenone *see* Progestogens
Drotrecogin Alfa
• Anticoagulants: manufacturer of drotrecogin alfa advises avoid concomitant use with high doses of ●heparin—consult product literature
Dutasteride
Calcium-channel Blockers: plasma concentration of dutasteride increased by diltiazem and verapamil
Dydrogesterone *see* Progestogens
Edrophonium *see* Parasympathomimetics
Efavirenz
Analgesics: efavirenz reduces plasma concentration of methadone
Antibacterials: increased risk of rash when efavirenz given with clarithromycin; efavirenz reduces plasma concentration of rifabutin—increase dose of rifabutin; plasma concentration of efavirenz reduced by rifampicin—increase dose of efavirenz
• Antidepressants: efavirenz reduces plasma concentration of sertraline; plasma concentration of efavirenz reduced by ●St John's wort—avoid concomitant use
Antifungals: efavirenz possibly reduces plasma concentration of caspofungin—consider increasing dose of caspofungin
• Antihistamines: increased risk of ventricular arrhythmias when efavirenz given with ●terfenadine—avoid concomitant use
Antivirals: efavirenz reduces plasma concentration of amprenavir, indinavir and lopinavir; plasma concentration of efavirenz reduced by nevirapine; toxicity of efavirenz increased by ritonavir; monitor liver function tests; efavirenz significantly reduces plasma concentration of saquinavir
• Anxiolytics and Hypnotics: increased risk of prolonged sedation when efavirenz given with ●midazolam—avoid concomitant use
Grapefruit Juice: plasma concentration of efavirenz possibly increased by grapefruit juice

Efavirenz *(continued)*
Oestrogens: efavirenz possibly reduces contraceptive effect of oestrogens
Eletriptan *see* 5HT$_1$ Agonists
Emtricitabine
Antivirals: manufacturer of emtricitabine advises avoid concomitant use with lamivudine and zalcitabine
Enalapril *see* ACE Inhibitors
Enflurane *see* Anaesthetics, General
Enoxaparin *see* Heparins
Entacapone
• Anticoagulants: entacapone enhances anticoagulant effect of ●warfarin
Antidepressants: manufacturer of entacapone advises caution with maprotiline, moclobemide, paroxetine, tricyclics and venlafaxine; avoid concomitant use of entacapone with non-selective MAOIs
Dopaminergics: entacapone possibly enhances effects of apomorphine; manufacturer of entacapone advises max. dose of 10 mg selegiline if used concomitantly
Iron: absorption of entacapone reduced by oral iron
Memantine: effects of dopaminergics possibly enhanced by memantine
Methyldopa: entacapone possibly enhances effects of methyldopa; antiparkinsonian effect of dopaminergics antagonised by methyldopa
Sympathomimetics: entacapone possibly enhances effects of adrenaline (epinephrine), dobutamine, dopamine and noradrenaline (norepinephrine)
Enteral Foods
• Anticoagulants: the presence of vitamin K in some enteral feeds can antagonise the anticoagulant effect of ●coumarins and ●phenindione
Antiepileptics: enteral feeds possibly reduce absorption of phenytoin
Ephedrine *see* Sympathomimetics
Epinephrine (adrenaline) *see* Sympathomimetics
Epoetin
ACE Inhibitors: antagonism of hypotensive effect and increased risk of hyperkalaemia when epoetin given with ACE inhibitors
Angiotensin-II Receptor Antagonists: antagonism of hypotensive effect and increased risk of hyperkalaemia when epoetin given with angiotensin-II receptor antagonists
Eprosartan *see* Angiotensin-II Receptor Antagonists
Ergometrine *see* Ergot Alkaloids
Ergot Alkaloids
Anaesthetics, General: effects of ergometrine on the parturient uterus reduced by halothane
• Antibacterials: increased risk of ergotism when ergotamine and methysergide given with ●macrolides or ●telithromycin—avoid concomitant use; avoidance of ergotamine and methysergide advised by manufacturer of ●quinupristin/dalfopristin; increased risk of ergotism when ergotamine and methysergide given with tetracyclines
Antidepressants: possible risk of hypertension when ergotamine and methysergide given with reboxetine
• Antifungals: increased risk of ergotism when ergotamine and methysergide given with ●imidazoles or ●triazoles—avoid concomitant use
• Antivirals: increased risk of ergotism when ergotamine and methysergide given with ●amprenavir, ●indinavir, ●nelfinavir, ●ritonavir or ●saquinavir—avoid concomitant use
Beta-blockers: increased peripheral vasoconstriction when ergotamine and methysergide given with beta-blockers

Ergot Alkaloids *(continued)*
- 5HT$_1$ Agonists: increased risk of vasospasm when ergotamine and methysergide given with ●almotriptan, ●rizatriptan, ●sumatriptan or ●zolmitriptan (avoid ergotamine and methysergide for 6 hours after almotriptan, rizatriptan, sumatriptan or zolmitriptan, avoid almotriptan, rizatriptan, sumatriptan or zolmitriptan for 24 hours after ergotamine and methysergide); increased risk of vasospasm when ergotamine and methysergide given with ●eletriptan or ●frovatriptan (avoid ergotamine and methysergide for 24 hours after eletriptan or frovatriptan, avoid eletriptan or frovatriptan for 24 hours after ergotamine and methysergide)

  Sympathomimetics: increased risk of ergotism when ergotamine and methysergide given with sympathomimetics
- Ulcer-healing Drugs: increased risk of ergotism when ergotamine and methysergide given with ●cimetidine—avoid concomitant use

Ergotamine and Methysergide *see* Ergot Alkaloids

Ertapenem
  Antiepileptics: ertapenem possibly reduces plasma concentration of valproate

  Oestrogens: *broad-spectrum* antibacterials possibly reduce contraceptive effect of oestrogens (risk probably small, see p. 388)

Erythromycin *see* Macrolides

Erythropoetin *see* Epoetin

Escitalopram *see* Antidepressants, SSRI

Esmolol *see* Beta-blockers

Esomeprazole *see* Proton Pump Inhibitors

Estradiol *see* Oestrogens

Estriol *see* Oestrogens

Estrone *see* Oestrogens

Estropipate *see* Oestrogens

Etanercept
- Anakinra: increased risk of side-effects when etanercept given with ●anakinra—avoid concomitant use
- Vaccines: avoid concomitant use of etanercept with live ●vaccines (see p. 578)

Ethinylestradiol *see* Oestrogens

Ethosuximide
- Antibacterials: metabolism of ethosuximide inhibited by ●isoniazid (increased plasma concentration and risk of toxicity)
- Antidepressants: anticonvulsant effect of antiepileptics possibly antagonised by MAOIs and ●tricyclic-related antidepressants (convulsive threshold lowered); anticonvulsant effect of antiepileptics antagonised by ●SSRIs and ●tricyclics (convulsive threshold lowered)
- Antiepileptics: plasma concentration of ethosuximide possibly reduced by carbamazepine and primidone; plasma concentration of ethosuximide possibly reduced by ●phenytoin, also plasma concentration of phenytoin possibly increased; plasma concentration of ethosuximide possibly increased by valproate
- Antimalarials: possible increased risk of convulsions when antiepileptics given with chloroquine and hydroxychloroquine; anticonvulsant effect of antiepileptics antagonised by ●mefloquine
- Antipsychotics: anticonvulsant effect of ethosuximide antagonised by ●antipsychotics (convulsive threshold lowered)

  Barbiturates: plasma concentration of ethosuximide possibly reduced by phenobarbital

Etodolac *see* NSAIDs

Etomidate *see* Anaesthetics, General

Etonogestrel *see* Progestogens

Etoricoxib *see* NSAIDs

Etynodiol *see* Progestogens

Ezetimibe
  Ciclosporin: plasma concentration of ezetimibe increased by ciclosporin
- Lipid-regulating Drugs: manufacturer of ezetimibe advises avoid concomitant use with ●fibrates

Famciclovir
  Probenecid: excretion of famciclovir possibly reduced by probenecid (increased plasma concentration)

Famotidine *see* Histamine H$_2$-antagonists

Felodipine *see* Calcium-channel Blockers

Fenbufen *see* NSAIDs

Fenofibrate *see* Fibrates

Fenoprofen *see* NSAIDs

Fenoterol *see* Sympathomimetics, Beta$_2$

Fentanyl *see* Opioid Analgesics

Ferrous Salts *see* Iron

Fexofenadine *see* Antihistamines

Fibrates
- Anticoagulants: fibrates enhance anticoagulant effect of ●coumarins and ●phenindione
- Antidiabetics: fibrates may improve glucose tolerance and have an additive effect with insulin or sulphonylureas; increased risk of severe hypoglycaemia when gemfibrozil given with ●repaglinide

  Ciclosporin: increased risk of renal impairment when fenofibrate given with ciclosporin
- Lipid-regulating Drugs: avoidance of fibrates advised by manufacturer of ●ezetimibe; increased risk of myopathy when gemfibrozil given with ●statins (preferably avoid concomitant use); increased risk of myopathy when fibrates given with ●statins

Filgrastim
  Note. Pegfilgrastim interactions as for filgrastim
  Cytotoxics: neutropenia possibly exacerbated when filgrastim given with fluorouracil

Flavoxate *see* Antimuscarinics

Flecainide
- Adrenergic Neurone Blockers: increased myocardial depression when anti-arrhythmics given with ●bretylium

  Anaesthetics, Local: increased myocardial depression when anti-arrhythmics given with bupivacaine or levobupivacaine
- Anti-arrhythmics: increased myocardial depression when anti-arrhythmics given with other ●anti-arrhythmics; plasma concentration of flecainide increased by ●amiodarone (halve dose of flecainide)
- Antidepressants: plasma concentration of flecainide increased by fluoxetine; increased risk of ventricular arrhythmias when flecainide given with ●tricyclics
- Antihistamines: increased risk of ventricular arrhythmias when flecainide given with ●mizolastine or ●terfenadine—avoid concomitant use; increased risk of ventricular arrhythmias when anti-arrhythmics given with ●terfenadine
- Antimalarials: avoidance of flecainide advised by manufacturer of ●artemether/lumefantrine (risk of ventricular arrhythmias); plasma concentration of flecainide increased by ●quinine
- Antipsychotics: increased risk of ventricular arrhythmias when anti-arrhythmics that prolong the QT interval given with ●antipsychotics that prolong the QT interval; increased risk of arrhythmias when flecainide given with ●clozapine
- Antivirals: plasma concentration of flecainide increased by ●ritonavir (increased risk of ventricular arrhythmias—avoid concomitant use)

Flecainide *(continued)*
- Beta-blockers: increased risk of myocardial depression and bradycardia when flecainide given with •beta-blockers; increased myocardial depression when anti-arrhythmics given with •beta-blockers
- Calcium-channel Blockers: increased risk of myocardial depression and asystole when flecainide given with •verapamil
- Diuretics: increased cardiac toxicity with flecainide if hypokalaemia occurs with •acetazolamide, •loop diuretics or •thiazides and related diuretics
- Dolasetron: increased risk of ventricular arrhythmias when flecainide given with •dolasetron—avoid concomitant use

    Tropisetron: caution with anti-arrhythmics advised by manufacturer of tropisetron (risk of ventricular arrhythmias)

    Ulcer-healing Drugs: metabolism of flecainide inhibited by cimetidine (increased plasma concentration)

Flucloxacillin *see* Penicillins
Fluconazole *see* Antifungals, Triazole
Flucytosine

    Antifungals: renal excretion of flucytosine decreased and cellular uptake increased by amphotericin (toxicity possibly increased)

    Cytotoxics: plasma concentration of flucytosine possibly reduced by cytarabine

Fludarabine

    Antiepileptics: cytotoxics reduce absorption of phenytoin

- Antipsychotics: avoid concomitant use of cytotoxics with •clozapine (increased risk of agranulocytosis)
- Cytotoxics: fludarabine increases intracellular concentration of cytarabine; increased pulmonary toxicity when fludarabine given with •pentostatin (unacceptably high incidence of fatalities)

    Dipyridamole: effects of fludarabine possibly reduced by dipyridamole

Fludrocortisone *see* Corticosteroids
Flunisolide *see* Corticosteroids
Flunitrazepam *see* Anxiolytics and Hypnotics
Fluorouracil

    Note. Capecitabine is a prodrug of fluorouracil
    Note. Tegafur is a prodrug of fluorouracil

- Allopurinol: manufacturer of capecitabine advises avoid concomitant use with •allopurinol

    Antibacterials: metabolism of fluorouracil inhibited by metronidazole (increased toxicity)

- Anticoagulants: fluorouracil possibly enhances anticoagulant effect of •coumarins

    Antiepileptics: cytotoxics reduce absorption of phenytoin

- Antipsychotics: avoid concomitant use of cytotoxics with •clozapine (increased risk of agranulocytosis)

    Filgrastim: neutropenia possibly exacerbated when fluorouracil given with filgrastim

- Temoporfin: increased skin photosensitivity when topical fluorouracil used with •temoporfin

    Ulcer-healing Drugs: metabolism of fluorouracil inhibited by cimetidine (increased plasma concentration)

Fluoxetine *see* Antidepressants, SSRI
Flupentixol *see* Antipsychotics
Fluphenazine *see* Antipsychotics
Flurazepam *see* Anxiolytics and Hypnotics
Flurbiprofen *see* NSAIDs
Flutamide
- Anticoagulants: flutamide enhances anticoagulant effect of •coumarins

Fluticasone *see* Corticosteroids
Fluvastatin *see* Statins
Fluvoxamine *see* Antidepressants, SSRI

Folates

    Aminosalicylates: absorption of folic acid possibly reduced by sulfasalazine

    Antiepileptics: folates possibly reduce plasma concentration of phenytoin and primidone

    Barbiturates: folates possibly reduce plasma concentration of phenobarbital

Folic Acid *see* Folates
Folinic Acid *see* Folates
Formoterol (eformoterol) *see* Sympathomimetics, Beta₂
Foscarnet

    Antivirals: avoidance of foscarnet advised by manufacturer of lamivudine

Fosinopril *see* ACE Inhibitors
Fosphenytoin *see* Phenytoin
Framycetin *see* Aminoglycosides
Frovatriptan *see* 5HT₁ Agonists
Furosemide (frusemide) *see* Diuretics
Fusidic Acid

    Oestrogens: *broad-spectrum* antibacterials possibly reduce contraceptive effect of oestrogens (risk probably small, see p. 388)

Gabapentin

    Antacids: absorption of gabapentin reduced by antacids

- Antidepressants: anticonvulsant effect of antiepileptics possibly antagonised by MAOIs and •tricyclic-related antidepressants (convulsive threshold lowered); anticonvulsant effect of antiepileptics antagonised by •SSRIs and •tricyclics (convulsive threshold lowered)
- Antimalarials: possible increased risk of convulsions when antiepileptics given with chloroquine and hydroxychloroquine; anticonvulsant effect of antiepileptics antagonised by •mefloquine

Galantamine *see* Parasympathomimetics
Gallamine *see* Muscle Relaxants
Ganciclovir

    Note. Increased risk of myelosuppression with other myelosuppressive drugs—consult product literature
    Note. Valganciclovir interactions as for ganciclovir

- Antibacterials: increased risk of convulsions when ganciclovir given with •imipenem with cilastatin
- Antivirals: ganciclovir possibly increases plasma concentration of didanosine; avoidance of intravenous ganciclovir advised by manufacturer of lamivudine; profound myelosuppression when ganciclovir given with •zidovudine (if possible avoid concomitant administration, particularly during initial ganciclovir therapy)

    Cytotoxics: plasma concentration of ganciclovir possibly increased by mycophenolate mofetil, also plasma concentration of inactive metabolite of mycophenolate mofetil possibly increased

    Probenecid: excretion of ganciclovir reduced by probenecid (increased plasma concentration and risk of toxicity)

Gemeprost *see* Prostaglandins
Gemfibrozil *see* Fibrates
Gentamicin *see* Aminoglycosides
Gestodene *see* Progestogens
Gestonorone *see* Progestogens
Gestrinone

    Antibacterials: metabolism of gestrinone accelerated by rifampicin (reduced plasma concentration)

    Antiepileptics: metabolism of gestrinone accelerated by carbamazepine, phenytoin and primidone (reduced plasma concentration)

    Barbiturates: metabolism of gestrinone accelerated by barbiturates (reduced plasma concentration)

Glibenclamide *see* Antidiabetics
Gliclazide *see* Antidiabetics
Glimepiride *see* Antidiabetics

Glipizide *see* Antidiabetics
Gliquidone *see* Antidiabetics
Glyceryl Trinitrate *see* Nitrates
Glycopyrronium *see* Antimuscarinics
Gold
  Note. Increased risk of toxicity with other nephrotoxic and myelosuppressive drugs
Grapefruit Juice
- Antihistamines: grapefruit juice increases plasma concentration of ●terfenadine—avoid concomitant use
- Antimalarials: grapefruit juice possibly inhibits metabolism of ●artemether/lumefantrine (avoid concomitant use)
  Antivirals: grapefruit juice possibly increases plasma concentration of efavirenz
  Anxiolytics and Hypnotics: grapefruit juice increases plasma concentration of buspirone
  Calcium-channel Blockers: grapefruit juice increases plasma concentration of felodipine, isradipine, lacidipine, lercanidipine, nicardipine, nifedipine, nimodipine, nisoldipine and verapamil
- Ciclosporin: grapefruit juice increases plasma concentration of ●ciclosporin (increased risk of toxicity)
  Lipid-regulating Drugs: grapefruit juice increases plasma concentration of simvastatin
  Sildenafil: grapefruit juice possibly increases plasma concentration of sildenafil
- Sirolimus: grapefruit juice increases plasma concentration of ●sirolimus—avoid concomitant use
- Tacrolimus: grapefruit juice increases plasma concentration of ●tacrolimus
  Tadalafil: grapefruit juice possibly increases plasma concentration of tadalafil
- Vardenafil: grapefruit juice possibly increases plasma concentration of ●vardenafil—avoid concomitant use
Griseofulvin
  Alcohol: griseofulvin possibly enhances effects of alcohol
- Anticoagulants: griseofulvin reduces anticoagulant effect of ●coumarins
  Antiepileptics: absorption of griseofulvin reduced by primidone (reduced effect)
  Barbiturates: absorption of griseofulvin reduced by phenobarbital (reduced effect)
  Ciclosporin: griseofulvin possibly reduces plasma concentration of ciclosporin
- Oestrogens: griseofulvin accelerates metabolism of ●oestrogens (reduced contraceptive effect—see p. 388)
- Progestogens: griseofulvin accelerates metabolism of ●progestogens (reduced contraceptive effect—see p. 388)
Guanethidine *see* Adrenergic Neurone Blockers
Haloperidol *see* Antipsychotics
Halothane *see* Anaesthetics, General
Heparin *see* Heparins
Heparins
  ACE Inhibitors: increased risk of hyperkalaemia when heparins given with ACE inhibitors
- Analgesics: possible increased risk of bleeding when heparins given with NSAIDs; increased risk of haemorrhage when heparins given with intravenous ●diclofenac (avoid concomitant use, including low-dose heparin); increased risk of haemorrhage when heparins given with ●ketorolac (avoid concomitant use, including low-dose heparin); anticoagulant effect of heparins enhanced by ●aspirin
  Angiotensin-II Receptor Antagonists: increased risk of hyperkalaemia when heparin given with angiotensin-II receptor antagonists

Heparins *(continued)*
  Clopidogrel: increased risk of bleeding when heparins given with clopidogrel
  Dipyridamole: anticoagulant effect of heparins enhanced by dipyridamole
- Drotrecogin Alfa: avoidance of concomitant use of high doses of heparin with drotrecogin alfa advised by manufacturer of ●drotrecogin alfa—consult product literature
- Nitrates: anticoagulant effect of heparins reduced by infusion of ●glyceryl trinitrate
  Sibutramine: increased risk of bleeding when anticoagulants given with sibutramine
Histamine H$_2$-antagonists
  Analgesics: cimetidine possibly increases plasma concentration of azapropazone; cimetidine inhibits metabolism of opioid analgesics (increased plasma concentration)
- Anti-arrhythmics: cimetidine increases plasma concentration of amiodarone, ●procainamide, ●propafenone and ●quinidine; cimetidine inhibits metabolism of flecainide (increased plasma concentration); cimetidine increases plasma concentration of ●lidocaine (lignocaine) (increased risk of toxicity)
  Antibacterials: histamine H$_2$-antagonists reduce absorption of cefpodoxime; cimetidine increases plasma concentration of erythromycin (increased risk of toxicity, including deafness); cimetidine inhibits metabolism of metronidazole (increased plasma concentration); metabolism of cimetidine accelerated by rifampicin (reduced plasma concentration); ranitidine bismuth citrate reduces absorption of tetracyclines
- Anticoagulants: cimetidine inhibits metabolism of ●coumarins (enhanced anticoagulant effect)
  Antidepressants: cimetidine increases plasma concentration of mirtazapine and sertraline; cimetidine inhibits metabolism of amitriptyline, doxepin, imipramine and nortriptyline (increased plasma concentration); cimetidine increases plasma concentration of moclobemide (halve dose of moclobemide); cimetidine possibly increases plasma concentration of tricyclics
  Antidiabetics: cimetidine reduces excretion of metformin (increased plasma concentration); cimetidine enhances hypoglycaemic effect of sulphonylureas
- Antiepileptics: cimetidine inhibits metabolism of ●carbamazepine, ●phenytoin and ●valproate (increased plasma concentration)
  Antifungals: histamine H$_2$-antagonists reduce absorption of itraconazole and ketoconazole; cimetidine increases plasma concentration of terbinafine
  Antihistamines: manufacturer of loratadine advises cimetidine possibly increases plasma concentration of loratadine
  Antimalarials: cimetidine inhibits metabolism of chloroquine and hydroxychloroquine and quinine (increased plasma concentration)
- Antipsychotics: cimetidine possibly enhances effects of antipsychotics, chlorpromazine and clozapine; increased risk of ventricular arrhythmias when cimetidine given with ●sertindole—avoid concomitant use
  Antivirals: plasma concentration of cimetidine possibly increased by amprenavir; ranitidine increases plasma concentration of saquinavir; cimetidine possibly increases plasma concentration of zalcitabine
  Anxiolytics and Hypnotics: cimetidine inhibits metabolism of benzodiazepines, clomethiazole and zaleplon (increased plasma concentration)

Histamine H$_2$-antagonists *(continued)*

Beta-blockers: cimetidine increases plasma concentration of labetalol, metoprolol and propranolol

Calcium-channel Blockers: cimetidine possibly inhibits metabolism of calcium-channel blockers (increased plasma concentration)

● Ciclosporin: cimetidine possibly increases plasma concentration of ●ciclosporin

● Cilostazol: cimetidine possibly increases plasma concentration of ●cilostazol—avoid concomitant use

Cytotoxics: cimetidine inhibits metabolism of fluorouracil (increased plasma concentration)

Dopaminergics: cimetidine reduces excretion of pramipexole (increased plasma concentration)

● Ergot Alkaloids: increased risk of ergotism when cimetidine given with ●ergotamine and methysergide—avoid concomitant use

Hormone Antagonists: absorption of cimetidine possibly delayed by octreotide

5HT$_1$ Agonists: cimetidine inhibits metabolism of zolmitriptan (reduce dose of zolmitriptan)

Mebendazole: cimetidine possibly inhibits metabolism of mebendazole (increased plasma concentration)

Sildenafil: cimetidine increases plasma concentration of sildenafil (reduce initial dose of sildenafil)

● Theophylline: cimetidine inhibits metabolism of ●theophylline (increased plasma concentration)

Thyroid Hormones: cimetidine reduces absorption of levothyroxine (thyroxine)

Homatropine *see* Antimuscarinics

Hormone Antagonists *see* Aminoglutethimide, Bicalutamide, Danazol, Dutasteride, Flutamide, Gestrinone, Lanreotide, Octreotide, Tamoxifen, Toremifene, and Trilostane

5HT$_1$ Agonists

● Antibacterials: plasma concentration of eletriptan increased by ●clarithromycin and ●erythromycin (risk of toxicity)—avoid concomitant use; metabolism of zolmitriptan possibly inhibited by quinolones (reduce dose of zolmitriptan)

● Antidepressants: increased risk of CNS toxicity when sumatriptan given with ●citalopram, ●escitalopram, ●fluoxetine, ●fluvoxamine or ●paroxetine; metabolism of frovatriptan possibly inhibited by fluvoxamine; metabolism of zolmitriptan possibly inhibited by fluvoxamine (reduce dose of zolmitriptan); increased risk of CNS toxicity when sumatriptan given with ●sertraline (manufacturer of sertraline advises avoid concomitant use); risk of CNS toxicity when rizatriptan or sumatriptan given with ●MAOIs (avoid rizatriptan or sumatriptan for 2 weeks after MAOIs); increased risk of CNS toxicity when zolmitriptan given with ●MAOIs; risk of CNS toxicity when rizatriptan or sumatriptan given with ●moclobemide (avoid rizatriptan or sumatriptan for 2 weeks after moclobemide); risk of CNS toxicity when zolmitriptan given with ●moclobemide (reduce dose of zolmitriptan); possible increased serotonergic effects when frovatriptan given with SSRIs; increased serotonergic effects when 5HT$_1$ agonists given with ●St John's wort—avoid concomitant use

● Antifungals: plasma concentration of eletriptan increased by ●itraconazole and ●ketoconazole (risk of toxicity)—avoid concomitant use

● Antivirals: plasma concentration of eletriptan increased by ●indinavir, ●nelfinavir and ●ritonavir (risk of toxicity)—avoid concomitant use

Beta-blockers: plasma concentration of rizatriptan possibly increased by propranolol (reduce dose of rizatriptan)

5HT$_1$ Agonists *(continued)*

● Ergot Alkaloids: increased risk of vasospasm when almotriptan, rizatriptan, sumatriptan or zolmitriptan given with ●ergotamine and methysergide (avoid ergotamine and methysergide for 6 hours after almotriptan, rizatriptan, sumatriptan or zolmitriptan, avoid almotriptan, rizatriptan, sumatriptan or zolmitriptan for 24 hours after ergotamine and methysergide); increased risk of vasospasm when eletriptan or frovatriptan given with ●ergotamine and methysergide (avoid ergotamine and methysergide for 24 hours after eletriptan or frovatriptan, avoid eletriptan or frovatriptan for 24 hours after ergotamine and methysergide)

Ulcer-healing Drugs: metabolism of zolmitriptan inhibited by cimetidine (reduce dose of zolmitriptan)

Hydralazine *see* Vasodilator Antihypertensives
Hydrochlorothiazide *see* Diuretics
Hydrocortisone *see* Corticosteroids
Hydroflumethiazide *see* Diuretics
Hydromorphone *see* Opioid Analgesics
Hydrotalcite *see* Antacids
Hydroxychloroquine *see* Chloroquine and Hydroxychloroquine
Hydroxyzine *see* Antihistamines
Hyoscine *see* Antimuscarinics
Ibandronic Acid *see* Bisphosphonates
Ibuprofen *see* NSAIDs
Ifosfamide

● Anticoagulants: ifosfamide possibly enhances anticoagulant effect of ●coumarins

Antiepileptics: cytotoxics reduce absorption of phenytoin

● Antipsychotics: avoid concomitant use of cytotoxics with ●clozapine (increased risk of agranulocytosis)

Imatinib

● Antibacterials: plasma concentration of imatinib reduced by ●rifampicin—avoid concomitant use

Anticoagulants: manufacturer of imatinib advises replacement of warfarin with a heparin (possibilty of enhanced warfarin effect)

● Antiepileptics: plasma concentration of imatinib reduced by ●phenytoin—avoid concomitant use; cytotoxics reduce absorption of phenytoin

Antifungals: plasma concentration of imatinib increased by ketoconazole

● Antipsychotics: avoid concomitant use of cytotoxics with ●clozapine (increased risk of agranulocytosis)

Lipid-regulating Drugs: imatinib increases plasma concentration of simvastatin

Imidapril *see* ACE Inhibitors

Imipenem with Cilastatin

● Antivirals: increased risk of convulsions when imipenem with cilastatin given with ●ganciclovir

Oestrogens: *broad-spectrum* antibacterials possibly reduce contraceptive effect of oestrogens (risk probably small, see p. 388)

Imipramine *see* Antidepressants, Tricyclic
Immunoglobulins

Note. For advice on immunoglobulins and live virus vaccines, see under Normal Immunoglobulin, p. 595

Immunosuppressants (antiproliferative) *see* Azathioprine and Mycophenolate Mofetil

Indapamide *see* Diuretics

Indinavir

● Antibacterials: plasma concentration of indinavir decreases (increase dose) and plasma concentration of rifabutin increases (reduce dose) when given together; metabolism of indinavir accelerated by ●rifampicin (reduced plasma concentration—avoid concomitant use)

Indinavir *(continued)*

- Antidepressants: plasma concentration of indinavir reduced by ●St John's wort—avoid concomitant use
- Antiepileptics: plasma concentration of indinavir possibly reduced by carbamazepine, phenytoin and ●primidone
- Antifungals: metabolism of indinavir inhibited by ketoconazole; plasma concentration of indinavir increased by ●itraconazole (consider reducing dose of indinavir)
- Antihistamines: increased risk of ventricular arrhythmias when indinavir given with ●terfenadine—avoid concomitant use

  Antimuscarinics: avoidance of indinavir advised by manufacturer of tolterodine
- Antipsychotics: indinavir possibly increases plasma concentration of thioridazine; indinavir possibly increases plasma concentration of ●pimozide (increased risk of ventricular arrhythmias—avoid concomitant use); indinavir increases plasma concentration of ●sertindole (increased risk of ventricular arrhythmias—avoid concomitant use)

  Antivirals: plasma concentration of indinavir reduced by efavirenz and nevirapine; combination of indinavir with nelfinavir may increase plasma concentration of either drug (or both); plasma concentration of indinavir increased by ritonavir; indinavir increases plasma concentration of saquinavir
- Anxiolytics and Hypnotics: increased risk of prolonged sedation when indinavir given with ●alprazolam or ●midazolam—avoid concomitant use

  Atovaquone: plasma concentration of indinavir possibly reduced by atovaquone
- Barbiturates: plasma concentration of indinavir possibly reduced by ●barbiturates
- Cilostazol: indinavir possibly increases plasma concentration of ●cilostazol—avoid concomitant use

  Corticosteroids: plasma concentration of indinavir possibly reduced by dexamethasone
- Ergot Alkaloids: increased risk of ergotism when indinavir given with ●ergotamine and methysergide—avoid concomitant use
- 5HT$_1$ Agonists: indinavir increases plasma concentration of ●eletriptan (risk of toxicity)—avoid concomitant use
- Lipid-regulating Drugs: possible increased risk of myopathy when indinavir given with atorvastatin; increased risk of myopathy when indinavir given with ●simvastatin (avoid concomitant use)

  Sildenafil: indinavir increases plasma concentration of sildenafil—reduce initial dose of sildenafil
- Vardenafil: indinavir increases plasma concentration of ●vardenafil—avoid concomitant use

Indometacin *see* NSAIDs
Indoramin *see* Alpha-blockers
Infliximab

- Anakinra: avoid concomitant use of infliximab with ●anakinra
- Vaccines: avoid concomitant use of infliximab with live ●vaccines (see p. 578)

Influenza Vaccine *see* Vaccines
Insulin *see* Antidiabetics
Interferon Alfa *see* Interferons
Interferon Gamma *see* Interferons
Interferons

  Note. Peginterferon alfa interactions as for interferon alfa

  Theophylline: interferon alfa inhibits metabolism of theophylline (increased plasma concentration)

  Vaccines: manufacturer of interferon gamma advises avoid concomitant use with vaccines

Ipratropium *see* Antimuscarinics
Irbesartan *see* Angiotensin-II Receptor Antagonists
Iron

  Antacids: absorption of *oral* iron reduced by oral magnesium salts (as magnesium trisilicate)

  Antibacterials: *oral* iron reduces absorption of ciprofloxacin, levofloxacin, moxifloxacin, norfloxacin and ofloxacin; *oral* iron reduces absorption of tetracyclines, also absorption of *oral* iron reduced by tetracyclines

  Bisphosphonates: *oral* iron reduces absorption of bisphosphonates
- Dimercaprol: avoid concomitant use of iron with ●dimercaprol

  Dopaminergics: *oral* iron reduces absorption of entacapone; *oral* iron possibly reduces absorption of levodopa

  Methyldopa: *oral* iron antagonises hypotensive effect of methyldopa

  Penicillamine: *oral* iron reduces absorption of penicillamine

  Thyroid Hormones: *oral* iron reduces absorption of levothyroxine (thyroxine) (give at least 2 hours apart)

  Trientine: absorption of *oral* iron reduced by trientine

  Zinc: *oral* iron reduces absorption of zinc, also absorption of *oral* iron reduced by zinc

Isocarboxazid *see* MAOIs
Isoflurane *see* Anaesthetics, General
Isometheptene *see* Sympathomimetics
Isoniazid

  Anaesthetics, General: hepatotoxicity of isoniazid possibly potentiated by general anaesthetics

  Antacids: absorption of isoniazid reduced by antacids

  Antibacterials: increased risk of CNS toxicity when isoniazid given with cycloserine
- Antiepileptics: isoniazid increases plasma concentration of ●carbamazepine (also possibly increased isoniazid hepatotoxicity); isoniazid inhibits metabolism of ●ethosuximide (increased plasma concentration and risk of toxicity); isoniazid inhibits metabolism of ●phenytoin (increased plasma concentration)

  Antifungals: isoniazid possibly reduces plasma concentration of ketoconazole

  Anxiolytics and Hypnotics: isoniazid inhibits the metabolism of diazepam

  Oestrogens: *broad-spectrum* antibacterials possibly reduce contraceptive effect of oestrogens (risk probably small, see p. 388)

  Theophylline: isoniazid possibly increases plasma concentration of theophylline

Isosorbide Dinitrate *see* Nitrates
Isosorbide Mononitrate *see* Nitrates
Isotretinoin *see* Retinoids
Isradipine *see* Calcium-channel Blockers
Itraconazole *see* Antifungals, Triazole
Kaolin

  Analgesics: kaolin possibly reduces absorption of aspirin

  Anti-arrhythmics: kaolin possibly reduces absorption of quinidine

  Antibacterials: kaolin possibly reduces absorption of tetracyclines

  Antimalarials: kaolin reduces absorption of chloroquine and hydroxychloroquine

  Antipsychotics: kaolin possibly reduces absorption of phenothiazines

Ketamine *see* Anaesthetics, General
Ketoconazole *see* Antifungals, Imidazole
Ketoprofen *see* NSAIDs

Ketorolac see NSAIDs
Ketotifen see Antihistamines
Labetalol see Beta-blockers
Lacidipine see Calcium-channel Blockers
Lamivudine
 Antibacterials: plasma concentration of lamivudine increased by trimethoprim (as co-trimoxazole)—avoid concomitant use of high-dose co-trimoxazole
 Antivirals: avoidance of lamivudine advised by manufacturer of emtricitabine; manufacturer of lamivudine advises avoid concomitant use with foscarnet; manufacturer of lamivudine advises avoid concomitant use of intravenous ganciclovir; lamivudine possibly inhibits effects of zalcitabine (manufacturers advise avoid concomitant use)
Lamotrigine
• Antidepressants: anticonvulsant effect of antiepileptics possibly antagonised by MAOIs and ●tricyclic-related antidepressants (convulsive threshold lowered); anticonvulsant effect of antiepileptics antagonised by ●SSRIs and ●tricyclics (convulsive threshold lowered)
 Antiepileptics: plasma concentration of lamotrigine often reduced by carbamazepine, also plasma concentration of an active metabolite of carbamazepine sometimes raised (but evidence is conflicting); plasma concentration of lamotrigine reduced by phenytoin and primidone; plasma concentration of lamotrigine increased by valproate
• Antimalarials: possible increased risk of convulsions when antiepileptics given with chloroquine and hydroxychloroquine; anticonvulsant effect of antiepileptics antagonised by ●mefloquine
 Barbiturates: plasma concentration of lamotrigine reduced by phenobarbital
Lanreotide
 Ciclosporin: lanreotide reduces plasma concentration of ciclosporin
Lansoprazole see Proton Pump Inhibitors
Leflunomide
 Note. Increased risk of toxicity with other haematotoxic and hepatotoxic drugs
 Anticoagulants: leflunomide possibly enhances anticoagulant effect of warfarin
 Antidiabetics: leflunomide possibly enhances hypoglycaemic effect of tolbutamide
 Antiepileptics: leflunomide possibly increases plasma concentration of phenytoin
 Lipid-regulating Drugs: the effect of leflunomide is significantly reduced by colestyramine (enhanced elimination)—avoid unless drug elimination desired
• Vaccines: avoid concomitant use of leflunomide with live ●vaccines (see p. 578)
Lercanidipine see Calcium-channel Blockers
Leukotriene Antagonists
 Analgesics: plasma concentration of zafirlukast increased by aspirin
 Antibacterials: plasma concentration of zafirlukast reduced by erythromycin
 Anticoagulants: zafirlukast enhances anticoagulant effect of warfarin
 Antiepileptics: plasma concentration of montelukast reduced by primidone
 Antihistamines: plasma concentration of zafirlukast reduced by terfenadine
 Barbiturates: plasma concentration of montelukast reduced by phenobarbital
 Theophylline: zafirlukast possibly increases plasma concentration of theophylline, also plasma concentration of zafirlukast reduced

Levetiracetam
• Antidepressants: anticonvulsant effect of antiepileptics possibly antagonised by MAOIs and ●tricyclic-related antidepressants (convulsive threshold lowered); anticonvulsant effect of antiepileptics antagonised by ●SSRIs and ●tricyclics (convulsive threshold lowered)
• Antimalarials: possible increased risk of convulsions when antiepileptics given with chloroquine and hydroxychloroquine; anticonvulsant effect of antiepileptics antagonised by ●mefloquine
Levobunolol see Beta-blockers
Levobupivacaine
 Anti-arrhythmics: increased myocardial depression when levobupivacaine given with anti-arrhythmics
Levocabastine see Antihistamines
Levocetirizine see Antihistamines
Levodopa
 ACE Inhibitors: enhanced hypotensive effect when levodopa given with ACE inhibitors
 Adrenergic Neurone Blockers: enhanced hypotensive effect when levodopa given with adrenergic neurone blockers
 Alpha-blockers: enhanced hypotensive effect when levodopa given with alpha-blockers
• Anaesthetics, General: increased risk of arrhythmias when levodopa given with ●volatile liquid general anaesthetics
 Angiotensin-II Receptor Antagonists: enhanced hypotensive effect when levodopa given with angiotensin-II receptor antagonists
• Antidepressants: risk of hypertensive crisis when levodopa given with ●MAOIs, avoid levodopa for at least two weeks after stopping MAOIs; increased risk of side-effects when levodopa given with moclobemide
 Antiepileptics: effects of levodopa possibly reduced by phenytoin
 Antimuscarinics: absorption of levodopa possibly reduced by antimuscarinics
 Antipsychotics: effects of levodopa antagonised by antipsychotics; avoidance of levodopa advised by manufacturer of amisulpride (antagonism of effect)
 Anxiolytics and Hypnotics: effects of levodopa possibly antagonised by benzodiazepines
 Beta-blockers: enhanced hypotensive effect when levodopa given with beta-blockers
 Bupropion: increased risk of side-effects when levodopa given with bupropion
 Calcium-channel Blockers: enhanced hypotensive effect when levodopa given with calcium-channel blockers
 Clonidine: enhanced hypotensive effect when levodopa given with clonidine
 Diazoxide: enhanced hypotensive effect when levodopa given with diazoxide
 Diuretics: enhanced hypotensive effect when levodopa given with diuretics
 Dopaminergics: enhanced effects and increased toxicity of levodopa when given with selegiline (reduce dose of levodopa)
 Iron: absorption of levodopa possibly reduced by *oral* iron
 Memantine: effects of dopaminergics possibly enhanced by memantine
 Methyldopa: enhanced hypotensive effect when levodopa given with methyldopa; antiparkinsonian effect of dopaminergics antagonised by methyldopa
 Moxonidine: enhanced hypotensive effect when levodopa given with moxonidine

Levodopa *(continued)*

Muscle Relaxants: possible agitation, confusion and hallucinations when levodopa given with baclofen

Nitrates: enhanced hypotensive effect when levodopa given with nitrates

Vasodilator Antihypertensives: enhanced hypotensive effect when levodopa given with hydralazine, minoxidil or nitroprusside

Vitamins: effects of levodopa reduced by pyridoxine when given without dopa-decarboxylase inhibitor

Levofloxacin *see* Quinolones

Levomepromazine (methotrimeprazine) *see* Antipsychotics

Levonorgestrel *see* Progestogens

Levothyroxine (thyroxine) *see* Thyroid Hormones

Lidocaine (lignocaine)

Note. Interactions less likely when lidocaine used topically

- Adrenergic Neurone Blockers: increased myocardial depression when anti-arrhythmics given with ●bretylium

  Anaesthetics, Local: increased myocardial depression when anti-arrhythmics given with bupivacaine or levobupivacaine

- Anti-arrhythmics: increased myocardial depression when anti-arrhythmics given with other ●anti-arrhythmics

- Antibacterials: increased risk of ventricular arrhythmias when lidocaine (lignocaine) given with ●quinupristin/dalfopristin—avoid concomitant use

- Antihistamines: increased risk of ventricular arrhythmias when anti-arrhythmics given with ●terfenadine

- Antipsychotics: increased risk of ventricular arrhythmias when anti-arrhythmics that prolong the QT interval given with ●antipsychotics that prolong the QT interval

- Beta-blockers: increased myocardial depression when anti-arrhythmics given with ●beta-blockers; increased risk of lidocaine (lignocaine) toxicity when given with ●propranolol

- Diuretics: action of lidocaine (lignocaine) antagonised by hypokalaemia caused by ●acetazolamide, ●loop diuretics or ●thiazides and related diuretics

- Dolasetron: increased risk of ventricular arrhythmias when lidocaine (lignocaine) given with ●dolasetron—avoid concomitant use

  Muscle Relaxants: neuromuscular blockade enhanced and prolonged when lidocaine (lignocaine) given with suxamethonium

  Tropisetron: caution with anti-arrhythmics advised by manufacturer of tropisetron (risk of ventricular arrhythmias)

- Ulcer-healing Drugs: plasma concentration of lidocaine (lignocaine) increased by ●cimetidine (increased risk of toxicity)

Linezolid

Note. Linezolid is a reversible, non-selective MAO inhibitor—see interactions of MAOIs

Oestrogens: *broad-spectrum* antibacterials possibly reduce contraceptive effect of oestrogens (risk probably small, see p. 388)

Liothyronine *see* Thyroid Hormones

Lipid-regulating Drugs *see* Colestipol, Colestyramine, Ezetimibe, Fibrates, Nicotinic Acid, and Statins

Lisinopril *see* ACE Inhibitors

Lisuride

Antipsychotics: effects of lisuride antagonised by antipsychotics

Memantine: effects of dopaminergics possibly enhanced by memantine

Lisuride *(continued)*

Methyldopa: antiparkinsonian effect of dopaminergics antagonised by methyldopa

Lithium

- ACE Inhibitors: excretion of lithium reduced by ●ACE inhibitors (increased plasma concentration)

- Analgesics: excretion of lithium probably reduced by ●NSAIDs (increased risk of toxicity); excretion of lithium reduced by ●azapropazone, ●diclofenac, ●ibuprofen, ●indometacin, ●mefenamic acid, ●naproxen, ●parecoxib, ●piroxicam, ●rofecoxib and ●valdecoxib (increased risk of toxicity); excretion of lithium reduced by ●ketorolac (increased risk of toxicity)—avoid concomitant use

- Angiotensin-II Receptor Antagonists: excretion of lithium reduced by ●angiotensin-II receptor antagonists (increased plasma concentration)

  Antacids: excretion of lithium increased by sodium bicarbonate (reduced plasma concentration)

  Anti-arrhythmics: increased risk of hypothyroidism when lithium given with amiodarone

  Antibacterials: increased risk of lithium toxicity when given with metronidazole

- Antidepressants: increased risk of CNS effects when lithium given with ●SSRIs (lithium toxicity reported)

  Antiepileptics: neurotoxicity may occur when lithium given with carbamazepine or phenytoin without increased plasma concentration of lithium

- Antipsychotics: increased risk of extrapyramidal side-effects and possibly neurotoxicity when lithium given with clozapine, haloperidol or phenothiazines; increased risk of ventricular arrhythmias when lithium given with ●amisulpride, ●sertindole or ●thioridazine—avoid concomitant use; increased risk of extrapyramidal side-effects when lithium given with sulpiride

  Calcium-channel Blockers: neurotoxicity may occur when lithium given with diltiazem or verapamil without increased plasma concentration of lithium

- Diuretics: excretion of lithium increased by ●acetazolamide; excretion of lithium reduced by ●loop diuretics and ●thiazides and related diuretics (increased plasma concentration and risk of toxicity)—loop diuretics safer than thiazides; excretion of lithium reduced by ●potassium-sparing diuretics (increased plasma concentration and risk of toxicity)

- Methyldopa: neurotoxicity may occur when lithium given with ●methyldopa without increased plasma concentration of lithium

  Muscle Relaxants: lithium enhances effects of muscle relaxants; hyperkinesis caused by lithium possibly aggravated by baclofen

  Parasympathomimetics: lithium antagonises effects of neostigmine and pyridostigmine

  Theophylline: excretion of lithium increased by theophylline (reduced plasma concentration)

Lofepramine *see* Antidepressants, Tricyclic

Lofexidine

Alcohol: increased sedative effect when lofexidine given with alcohol

Anxiolytics and Hypnotics: increased sedative effect when lofexidine given with anxiolytics and hypnotics

Loperamide

Desmopressin: loperamide increases plasma concentration of *oral* desmopressin

Lopinavir

Note. In combination with ritonavir as Kaletra® (ritonavir is present to inhibit lopinavir metabolism and increase plasma-lopinavir concentration)—see also Ritonavir

Lopinavir *(continued)*
- Antibacterials: plasma concentration of lopinavir reduced by ●rifampicin—avoid concomitant use
- Antiepileptics: plasma concentration of lopinavir possibly reduced by carbamazepine, phenytoin and ●primidone
  Antimuscarinics: avoidance of lopinavir advised by manufacturer of tolterodine
- Antipsychotics: lopinavir increases plasma concentration of ●sertindole (increased risk of ventricular arrhythmias—avoid concomitant use)
  Antivirals: plasma concentration of lopinavir reduced by efavirenz; plasma concentration of lopinavir possibly reduced by nevirapine; lopinavir increases plasma concentration of tenofovir (also plasma concentration of lopinavir reduced)
- Barbiturates: plasma concentration of lopinavir possibly reduced by ●barbiturates
- Cilostazol: lopinavir possibly increases plasma concentration of ●cilostazol—avoid concomitant use
  Corticosteroids: plasma concentration of lopinavir possibly reduced by dexamethasone

Loprazolam *see* Anxiolytics and Hypnotics
Loratadine *see* Antihistamines
Lorazepam *see* Anxiolytics and Hypnotics
Lormetazepam *see* Anxiolytics and Hypnotics
Losartan *see* Angiotensin-II Receptor Antagonists
Lumefantrine *see* Artemether with Lumefantrine
Lymecycline *see* Tetracyclines
Macrolides
Note. See also Telithromycin
Note. Interactions do not apply to small amounts of erythromycin used topically
  Analgesics: erythromycin increases plasma concentration of alfentanil
  Antacids: absorption of azithromycin reduced by antacids
- Anti-arrhythmics: increased risk of ventricular arrhythmias when parenteral erythromycin given with ●amiodarone—avoid concomitant use; erythromycin increases plasma concentration of ●disopyramide (increased risk of toxicity); clarithromycin possibly increases plasma concentration of ●disopyramide (increased risk of toxicity)
- Antibacterials: increased risk of ventricular arrhythmias when parenteral erythromycin given with ●moxifloxacin—avoid concomitant use; macrolides possibly increase plasma concentration of ●rifabutin (increased risk of uveitis—reduce rifabutin dose); clarithromycin increases plasma concentration of ●rifabutin (increased risk of uveitis—reduce rifabutin dose)
- Anticoagulants: macrolides possibly enhance anticoagulant effect of ●coumarins; clarithromycin and erythromycin enhance anticoagulant effect of ●coumarins
- Antidepressants: avoidance of macrolides advised by manufacturer of ●reboxetine
  Antidiabetics: clarithromycin enhances effects of repaglinide
- Antiepileptics: clarithromycin and erythromycin increase plasma concentration of ●carbamazepine; clarithromycin inhibits metabolism of phenytoin (increased plasma concentration); erythromycin possibly inhibits metabolism of valproate (increased plasma concentration)
  Antifungals: clarithromycin increases plasma concentration of itraconazole
- Antihistamines: manufacturer of loratadine advises erythromycin possibly increases plasma concentration of loratadine; macrolides possibly inhibit metabolism of ●mizolastine (avoid concomitant

Macrolides
- Antihistamines *(continued)*
  use); erythromycin inhibits metabolism of ●mizolastine—avoid concomitant use; clarithromycin inhibits metabolism of ●terfenadine (avoid concomitant use—increased risk of ventricular arrhythmias); erythromycin inhibits metabolism of ●terfenadine—risk of ventricular arrhythmias, avoid concomitant use of systemic or topical preparations
- Antimalarials: avoidance of macrolides advised by manufacturer of ●artemether/lumefantrine
  Antimuscarinics: avoidance of clarithromycin and erythromycin advised by manufacturer of tolterodine
- Antipsychotics: increased risk of ventricular arrhythmias when parenteral erythromycin given with ●amisulpride—avoid concomitant use; erythromycin possibly increases plasma concentration of ●clozapine (possible increased risk of convulsions); increased risk of ventricular arrhythmias when clarithromycin given with ●pimozide—avoid concomitant use; possible increased risk of ventricular arrhythmias when erythromycin given with ●pimozide—avoid concomitant use; macrolides possibly increase plasma concentration of quetiapine (reduce dose of quetiapine); increased risk of ventricular arrhythmias when erythromycin given with ●sertindole—avoid concomitant use; possible increased risk of ventricular arrhythmias when macrolides given with ●sertindole—avoid concomitant use
- Antivirals: plasma concentration of both drugs increased when erythromycin given with amprenavir; increased risk of rash when clarithromycin given with efavirenz; plasma concentration of clarithromycin increased by ●ritonavir (reduce dose of clarithromycin in renal impairment); plasma concentration of azithromycin and erythromycin possibly increased by ritonavir; clarithromycin tablets reduce absorption of zidovudine
- Anxiolytics and Hypnotics: clarithromycin and erythromycin inhibit metabolism of ●midazolam (increased plasma concentration with increased sedation); erythromycin increases plasma concentration of buspirone (reduce dose of buspirone); erythromycin inhibits the metabolism of zopiclone
  Calcium-channel Blockers: erythromycin possibly inhibits metabolism of felodipine (increased plasma concentration); avoidance of erythromycin advised by manufacturer of lercanidipine
  Cardiac Glycosides: macrolides increase plasma concentration of digoxin (increased risk of toxicity)
- Ciclosporin: macrolides possibly inhibit metabolism of ●ciclosporin (increased plasma concentration); clarithromycin and erythromycin inhibit metabolism of ●ciclosporin (increased plasma concentration)
- Cilostazol: erythromycin increases plasma concentration of ●cilostazol (also plasma concentration of erythromycin reduced)—avoid concomitant use
  Corticosteroids: erythromycin possibly inhibits metabolism of corticosteroids; erythromycin inhibits the metabolism of methylprednisolone
- Cytotoxics: *in vitro* studies suggest a possible interaction between erythromycin and docetaxel (consult docetaxel product literature); erythromycin increases toxicity of ●vinblastine—avoid concomitant use
  Dopaminergics: erythromycin increases plasma concentration of bromocriptine and cabergoline

Macrolides

Dopaminergics *(continued)*
(increased risk of toxicity); macrolides possibly increase plasma concentration of bromocriptine and cabergoline (increased risk of toxicity)

● Ergot Alkaloids: increased risk of ergotism when macrolides given with ●ergotamine and methysergide—avoid concomitant use

● 5HT₁ Agonists: clarithromycin and erythromycin increase plasma concentration of ●eletriptan (risk of toxicity)—avoid concomitant use

Leukotriene Antagonists: erythromycin reduces plasma concentration of zafirlukast

● Lipid-regulating Drugs: clarithromycin increases plasma concentration of atorvastatin; possible increased risk of myopathy when erythromycin given with atorvastatin; erythromycin reduces plasma concentration of rosuvastatin; increased risk of myopathy when clarithromycin or erythromycin given with ●simvastatin (avoid concomitant use)

Oestrogens: *broad-spectrum* antibacterials possibly reduce contraceptive effect of oestrogens (risk probably small, see p. 388)

Parasympathomimetics: erythromycin increases plasma concentration of galantamine

Sildenafil: erythromycin increases plasma concentration of sildenafil—reduce initial dose of sildenafil

● Tacrolimus: clarithromycin and erythromycin increase plasma concentration of ●tacrolimus

Tadalafil: clarithromycin and erythromycin possibly increase plasma concentration of tadalafil

● Theophylline: clarithromycin inhibits metabolism of ●theophylline (increased plasma concentration); erythromycin inhibits metabolism of ●theophylline (increased plasma concentration), if erythromycin given by mouth, also decreased plasma-erythromycin concentration

Ulcer-healing Drugs: plasma concentration of erythromycin increased by cimetidine (increased risk of toxicity, including deafness); plasma concentration of both drugs increased when clarithromycin given with omeprazole

Vardenafil: erythromycin increases plasma concentration of vardenafil (reduce dose of vardenafil)

Magnesium (parenteral)

● Calcium-channel Blockers: profound hypotension reported with concomitant use of parenteral magnesium and ●nifedipine in pre-eclampsia

Muscle Relaxants: parenteral magnesium enhances effects of non-depolarising muscle relaxants and suxamethonium

Magnesium Salts (oral) *see* Antacids

MAOIs

Note. For interactions of reversible MAO-A inhibitors (RIMAs) see Moclobemide, and for interactions of MAO-B inhibitors see Selegiline; the antibacterial linezolid is a reversible, non-selective MAO inhibitor

ACE Inhibitors: MAOIs possibly enhance hypotensive effect of ACE inhibitors

Adrenergic Neurone Blockers: enhanced hypotensive effect when MAOIs given with adrenergic neurone blockers

● Alcohol: MAOIs interact with tyramine found in some beverages containing ●alcohol and some dealcoholised beverages (hypertensive crisis)—if no tyramine, enhanced hypotensive effect

Alpha₂-adrenoceptor Stimulants: avoidance of MAOIs advised by manufacturer of apraclonidine and brimonidine

● Alpha-blockers: avoidance of MAOIs advised by manufacturer of ●indoramin; enhanced hypotensive effect when MAOIs given with alpha-blockers

MAOIs *(continued)*

● Anaesthetics, General: Because of hazardous interactions between MAOIs and ●general anaesthetics, MAOIs should normally be stopped 2 weeks before surgery

● Analgesics: CNS excitation or depression (hypertension or hypotension) when MAOIs given with ●pethidine—avoid concomitant use and for 2 weeks after stopping MAOIs; avoidance of MAOIs advised by manufacturer of ●nefopam; possible CNS excitation or depression (hypertension or hypotension) when MAOIs given with ●opioid analgesics—avoid concomitant use and for 2 weeks after stopping MAOIs

Angiotensin-II Receptor Antagonists: MAOIs possibly enhance hypotensive effect of angiotensin-II receptor antagonists

● Antidepressants: increased risk of hypertension and CNS excitation when MAOIs given with ●reboxetine (MAOIs should not be started until 1 week after stopping reboxetine, avoid reboxetine for 2 weeks after stopping MAOIs); after stopping MAOIs do not start ●citalopram, ●escitalopram or ●fluvoxamine for 2 weeks, also MAOIs should not be started until at least 1 week after stopping citalopram, escitalopram or fluvoxamine; after stopping MAOIs do not start ●fluoxetine for 2 weeks, also MAOIs should not be started until at least 5 weeks after stopping fluoxetine; after stopping MAOIs do not start ●mirtazapine, ●paroxetine or ●sertraline for 2 weeks, also MAOIs should not be started until at least 2 weeks after stopping mirtazapine, paroxetine or sertraline; enhanced CNS effects and toxicity when MAOIs given with ●venlafaxine (venlafaxine should not be started until 2 weeks after stopping MAOIs, avoid MAOIs for 1 week after stopping venlafaxine); MAOIs can cause increased risk of hypertension and CNS excitation when given with other ●MAOIs (avoid for at least 2 weeks after stopping previous MAOIs and then start at a reduced dose); after stopping MAOIs do not start ●moclobemide for at least 1 week; MAOIs increase CNS effects of ●SSRIs (risk of serious toxicity); after stopping MAOIs do not start ●tricyclic-related antidepressants for 2 weeks, also MAOIs should not be started until at least 1–2 weeks after stopping tricyclic-related antidepressants; increased risk of hypertension and CNS excitation when MAOIs given with ●tricyclics, tricyclics should not be started until 2 weeks after stopping MAOIs (3 weeks if starting clomipramine or imipramine), also MAOIs should not be started for at least 1–2 weeks after stopping tricyclics (3 weeks in the case of clomipramine or imipramine); CNS excitation and confusion when MAOIs given with ●tryptophan (reduce dose of tryptophan)

Antidiabetics: MAOIs possibly enhance hypoglycaemic effect of antidiabetics; MAOIs enhance hypoglycaemic effect of insulin, metformin and sulphonylureas

● Antiepileptics: MAOIs possibly antagonise anticonvulsant effect of antiepileptics (convulsive threshold lowered); avoidance for 2 weeks after stopping MAOIs advised by manufacturer of ●carbamazepine, also antagonism of anticonvulsant effect; avoidance of MAOIs advised by manufacturer of ●oxcarbazepine

Antihistamines: increased antimuscarinic and sedative effects when MAOIs given with antihistamines

● Antimalarials: avoidance of antidepressants advised by manufacturer of ●artemether/lumefantrine

MAOIs *(continued)*

Antimuscarinics: increased risk of antimuscarinic side-effects when MAOIs given with antimuscarinics

● Antipsychotics: CNS effects of MAOIs possibly increased by ●clozapine

Anxiolytics and Hypnotics: avoidance of MAOIs advised by manufacturer of buspirone

Barbiturates: MAOIs possibly antagonise anticonvulsant effect of barbiturates (convulsive threshold lowered)

Beta-blockers: enhanced hypotensive effect when MAOIs given with beta-blockers

● Bupropion: avoidance of bupropion for 2 weeks after stopping MAOIs advised by manufacturer of ●bupropion

Calcium-channel Blockers: enhanced hypotensive effect when MAOIs given with calcium-channel blockers

Clonidine: enhanced hypotensive effect when MAOIs given with clonidine

Diazoxide: enhanced hypotensive effect when MAOIs given with diazoxide

Diuretics: enhanced hypotensive effect when MAOIs given with diuretics

● Dopaminergics: avoid concomitant use of nonselective MAOIs with entacapone; risk of hypertensive crisis when MAOIs given with ●levodopa, avoid levodopa for at least two weeks after stopping MAOIs; enhanced hypotensive effect when MAOIs given with selegiline

Doxapram: MAOIs enhance effects of doxapram

● 5HT₁ Agonists: risk of CNS toxicity when MAOIs given with ●rizatriptan or ●sumatriptan (avoid rizatriptan or sumatriptan for 2 weeks after MAOIs); increased risk of CNS toxicity when MAOIs given with ●zolmitriptan

● Methyldopa: avoidance of MAOIs advised by manufacturer of ●methyldopa

Moxonidine: enhanced hypotensive effect when MAOIs given with moxonidine

<u>Muscle Relaxants</u>: phenelzine enhances effects of suxamethonium

Nicorandil: enhanced hypotensive effect when MAOIs given with nicorandil

Nitrates: enhanced hypotensive effect when MAOIs given with nitrates

● Sibutramine: increased CNS toxicity when MAOIs given with ●sibutramine (manufacturer of sibutramine advises avoid concomitant use), also avoid sibutramine for 2 weeks after stopping MAOIs

● Sympathomimetics: risk of hypertensive crisis when MAOIs given with ●dexamfetamine, ●dopamine, ●dopexamine, ●ephedrine, ●isometheptene, ●methylphenidate, ●phenylephrine, ●phenylpropanolamine, ●pseudoephedrine or ●sympathomimetics

● Tetrabenazine: risk of CNS excitation and hypertension when MAOIs given with ●tetrabenazine

Vasodilator Antihypertensives: enhanced hypotensive effect when MAOIs given with hydralazine, minoxidil or nitroprusside

MAOIs, reversible *see* Moclobemide

Maprotiline *see* Antidepressants, Tricyclic (related)

Mebendazole

Ulcer-healing Drugs: metabolism of mebendazole possibly inhibited by cimetidine (increased plasma concentration)

Meclozine *see* Antihistamines

Medroxyprogesterone *see* Progestogens

Mefenamic Acid *see* NSAIDs

Mefloquine

● Anti-arrhythmics: increased risk of ventricular arrhythmias when mefloquine given with ●amio-

Mefloquine

● Anti-arrhythmics *(continued)*
darone—avoid concomitant use; increased risk of ventricular arrhythmias when mefloquine given with ●quinidine

● Antibacterials: increased risk of ventricular arrhythmias when mefloquine given with ●moxifloxacin—avoid concomitant use

● Antiepileptics: mefloquine antagonises anticonvulsant effect of ●antiepileptics, ●carbamazepine and ●valproate

● Antimalarials: avoidance of antimalarials advised by manufacturer of ●artemether/lumefantrine; increased risk of convulsions when mefloquine given with ●chloroquine and hydroxychloroquine; increased risk of convulsions when mefloquine given with ●quinine (but should not prevent the use of intravenous quinine in severe cases)

● Antipsychotics: increased risk of ventricular arrhythmias when mefloquine given with ●pimozide—avoid concomitant use

Beta-blockers: increased risk of bradycardia when mefloquine given with beta-blockers

Calcium-channel Blockers: possible increased risk of bradycardia when mefloquine given with calcium-channel blockers

Cardiac Glycosides: possible increased risk of bradycardia when mefloquine given with digoxin

Megestrol *see* Progestogens

Meloxicam *see* NSAIDs

Melphalan

Antibacterials: increased risk of melphalan toxicity when given with nalidixic acid

Antiepileptics: cytotoxics reduce absorption of phenytoin

● Antipsychotics: avoid concomitant use of cytotoxics with ●clozapine (increased risk of agranulocytosis)

● Ciclosporin: increased risk of nephrotoxicity when melphalan given with ●ciclosporin

Memantine

● Anaesthetics, General: increased risk of CNS toxicity when memantine given with ●ketamine (manufacturer of memantine advises avoid concomitant use)

● Analgesics: increased risk of CNS toxicity when memantine given with ●dextromethorphan (manufacturer of memantine advises avoid concomitant use)

<u>Antiepileptics</u>: memantine possibly reduces effects of primidone

Antimuscarinics: memantine possibly enhances effects of antimuscarinics

Antipsychotics: memantine possibly reduces effects of antipsychotics

Barbiturates: memantine possibly reduces effects of barbiturates

● Dopaminergics: memantine possibly enhances effects of dopaminergics and selegiline; increased risk of CNS toxicity when memantine given with ●amantadine (manufacturer of memantine advises avoid concomitant use)

Muscle Relaxants: memantine possibly modifies effects of baclofen and dantrolene

Mepacrine

Antimalarials: mepacrine increases plasma concentration of primaquine (increased risk of toxicity)

Meprobamate *see* Anxiolytics and Hypnotics

Meptazinol *see* Opioid Analgesics

Mercaptopurine

● Allopurinol: enhanced effects and increased toxicity of mercaptopurine when given with ●allopurinol (reduce dose of mercaptopurine)

Mercaptopurine *(continued)*

Aminosalicylates: possible increased risk of leucopenia when mercaptopurine given with aminosalicylates

- Antibacterials: increased risk of haematological toxicity when mercaptopurine given with •sulfamethoxazole (as co-trimoxazole); increased risk of haematological toxicity when mercaptopurine given with •trimethoprim (also with co-trimoxazole)
- Anticoagulants: mercaptopurine possibly reduces anticoagulant effect of •warfarin

Antiepileptics: cytotoxics reduce absorption of phenytoin

- Antipsychotics: avoid concomitant use of cytotoxics with •clozapine (increased risk of agranulocytosis)

Meropenem

Antiepileptics: meropenem reduces plasma concentration of valproate

Oestrogens: *broad-spectrum* antibacterials possibly reduce contraceptive effect of oestrogens (risk probably small, see p. 388)

Probenecid: excretion of meropenem reduced by probenecid (manufacturers of meropenem advise avoid concomitant use)

Mesalazine *see* Aminosalicylates

Mestranol *see* Oestrogens

Metaraminol *see* Sympathomimetics

Metformin *see* Antidiabetics

Methadone *see* Opioid Analgesics

Methenamine

- Antibacterials: increased risk of crystalluria when methenamine given with •sulphonamides
- Diuretics: effects of methenamine antagonised by •acetazolamide

Oestrogens: *broad-spectrum* antibacterials possibly reduce contraceptive effect of oestrogens (risk probably small, see p. 388)

Potassium Salts: avoid concomitant use of methenamine with potassium citrate

Methocarbamol *see* Muscle Relaxants

Methotrexate

- Anaesthetics, General: antifolate effect of methotrexate increased by •nitrous oxide—avoid concomitant use
- Analgesics: excretion of methotrexate probably reduced by •NSAIDs (increased risk of toxicity); excretion of methotrexate reduced by •azapropazone (avoid concomitant use); excretion of methotrexate reduced by •aspirin, •diclofenac, •ibuprofen, •indometacin, •ketoprofen, •meloxicam and •naproxen (increased risk of toxicity)
- Antibacterials: excretion of methotrexate possibly reduced by ciprofloxacin (possibly increased risk of toxicity); antifolate effect of methotrexate increased by •sulfamethoxazole (as co-trimoxazole)—avoid concomitant use; increased risk of methotrexate toxicity when given with doxycycline, sulphonamides or tetracycline; excretion of methotrexate reduced by penicillins (increased risk of toxicity); antifolate effect of methotrexate increased by •trimethoprim—avoid concomitant use

Antiepileptics: antifolate effect of methotrexate increased by phenytoin; cytotoxics reduce absorption of phenytoin

- Antimalarials: antifolate effect of methotrexate increased by •pyrimethamine
- Antipsychotics: avoid concomitant use of cytotoxics with •clozapine (increased risk of agranulocytosis)
- Ciclosporin: risk of toxicity when methotrexate given with •ciclosporin

Methotrexate *(continued)*

- Corticosteroids: increased risk of haematological toxicity when methotrexate given with •corticosteroids
- Probenecid: excretion of methotrexate reduced by •probenecid (increased risk of toxicity)
- Retinoids: plasma concentration of methotrexate increased by •acitretin (also increased risk of hepatotoxicity)—avoid concomitant use

Ulcer-healing Drugs: excretion of methotrexate possibly reduced by omeprazole (possibly increased risk of toxicity)

Methoxamine *see* Sympathomimetics

Methyldopa

ACE Inhibitors: enhanced hypotensive effect when methyldopa given with ACE inhibitors

Adrenergic Neurone Blockers: enhanced hypotensive effect when methyldopa given with adrenergic neurone blockers

Alcohol: enhanced hypotensive effect when methyldopa given with alcohol

Aldesleukin: enhanced hypotensive effect when methyldopa given with aldesleukin

Alpha-blockers: enhanced hypotensive effect when methyldopa given with alpha-blockers

Alprostadil: enhanced hypotensive effect when methyldopa given with alprostadil

Amifostine: possible enhanced hypotensive effect when methyldopa given with amifostine

Anaesthetics, General: enhanced hypotensive effect when methyldopa given with general anaesthetics

Analgesics: hypotensive effect of methyldopa antagonised by NSAIDs

Angiotensin-II Receptor Antagonists: enhanced hypotensive effect when methyldopa given with angiotensin-II receptor antagonists

- Antidepressants: manufacturer of methyldopa advises avoid concomitant use with •MAOIs

Antipsychotics: enhanced hypotensive effect when methyldopa given with antipsychotics (also increased risk of extrapyramidal effects)

Anxiolytics and Hypnotics: enhanced hypotensive effect when methyldopa given with anxiolytics and hypnotics

Beta-blockers: enhanced hypotensive effect when methyldopa given with beta-blockers

Calcium-channel Blockers: enhanced hypotensive effect when methyldopa given with calcium-channel blockers

Clonidine: enhanced hypotensive effect when methyldopa given with clonidine

Corticosteroids: hypotensive effect of methyldopa antagonised by corticosteroids

Diazoxide: enhanced hypotensive effect when methyldopa given with diazoxide

Diuretics: enhanced hypotensive effect when methyldopa given with diuretics

Dopaminergics: methyldopa antagonises antiparkinsonian effect of dopaminergics; increased risk of extrapyramidal side-effects when methyldopa given with amantadine; effects of methyldopa possibly enhanced by entacapone; enhanced hypotensive effect when methyldopa given with levodopa

Iron: hypotensive effect of methyldopa antagonised by *oral* iron

- Lithium: neurotoxicity may occur when methyldopa given with •lithium without increased plasma concentration of lithium

Moxisylyte (thymoxamine): enhanced hypotensive effect when methyldopa given with moxisylyte

Moxonidine: enhanced hypotensive effect when methyldopa given with moxonidine

Methyldopa *(continued)*

Muscle Relaxants: enhanced hypotensive effect when methyldopa given with baclofen or tizanidine

Nitrates: enhanced hypotensive effect when methyldopa given with nitrates

Oestrogens: hypotensive effect of methyldopa antagonised by oestrogens

● Sympathomimetics, Beta₂: acute hypotension reported when methyldopa given with infusion of ●salbutamol

Ulcer-healing Drugs: hypotensive effect of methyldopa antagonised by carbenoxolone

Vasodilator Antihypertensives: enhanced hypotensive effect when methyldopa given with hydralazine, minoxidil or nitroprusside

Methylphenidate *see* Sympathomimetics
Methylprednisolone *see* Corticosteroids
Methysergide *see* Ergot Alkaloids
Metipranolol *see* Beta-blockers
Metoclopramide

Analgesics: metoclopramide increases rate of absorption of aspirin (enhanced effect); effects of metoclopramide on gastro-intestinal activity antagonised by opioid analgesics; metoclopramide increases absorption of paracetamol (enhanced effect)

Antimuscarinics: effects of metoclopramide on gastro-intestinal activity antagonised by antimuscarinics

Antipsychotics: increased risk of extrapyramidal side-effects when metoclopramide given with antipsychotics

Atovaquone: metoclopramide reduces plasma concentration of atovaquone

● Ciclosporin: metoclopramide increases plasma concentration of ●ciclosporin

Dopaminergics: increased risk of extrapyramidal side-effects when metoclopramide given with amantadine; metoclopramide antagonises hypoprolactinaemic effects of bromocriptine and cabergoline; metoclopramide antagonises antiparkinsonian effect of pergolide; metoclopramide antagonises antiparkinsonian effect of ropinirole (manufacturers of ropinirole advise avoid concomitant use)

Muscle Relaxants: metoclopramide enhances effects of suxamethonium

Tetrabenazine: increased risk of extrapyramidal side-effects when metoclopramide given with tetrabenazine

Metolazone *see* Diuretics
Metoprolol *see* Beta-blockers
Metronidazole

Alcohol: disulfiram-like reaction when metronidazole given with alcohol

● Anticoagulants: metronidazole enhances anticoagulant effect of ●coumarins

● Antiepileptics: metronidazole inhibits metabolism of ●phenytoin (increased plasma concentration); metabolism of metronidazole accelerated by primidone (reduced plasma concentration)

Barbiturates: metabolism of metronidazole accelerated by barbiturates (reduced plasma concentration)

Cytotoxics: metronidazole inhibits metabolism of fluorouracil (increased toxicity)

Disulfiram: psychotic reaction reported when metronidazole given with disulfiram

Lithium: metronidazole increases risk of lithium toxicity

Oestrogens: *broad-spectrum* antibacterials possibly reduce contraceptive effect of oestrogens (risk probably small, see p. 388)

Metronidazole *(continued)*

Ulcer-healing Drugs: metabolism of metronidazole inhibited by cimetidine (increased plasma concentration)

Mexiletine

● Adrenergic Neurone Blockers: increased myocardial depression when anti-arrhythmics given with ●bretylium

Anaesthetics, Local: increased myocardial depression when anti-arrhythmics given with bupivacaine or levobupivacaine

Analgesics: absorption of mexiletine delayed by opioid analgesics

● Anti-arrhythmics: increased myocardial depression when anti-arrhythmics given with other ●anti-arrhythmics

Antibacterials: metabolism of mexiletine accelerated by rifampicin (reduced plasma concentration)

Antiepileptics: metabolism of mexiletine accelerated by phenytoin (reduced plasma concentration)

● Antihistamines: increased risk of ventricular arrhythmias when mexiletine given with ●mizolastine or ●terfenadine—avoid concomitant use; increased risk of ventricular arrhythmias when anti-arrhythmics given with ●terfenadine

Antimuscarinics: absorption of mexiletine delayed by atropine

● Antipsychotics: increased risk of ventricular arrhythmias when anti-arrhythmics that prolong the QT interval given with ●antipsychotics that prolong the QT interval

● Antivirals: plasma concentration of mexiletine possibly increased by ●ritonavir (increased risk of toxicity)

● Beta-blockers: increased myocardial depression when anti-arrhythmics given with ●beta-blockers

● Diuretics: action of mexiletine antagonised by hypokalaemia caused by ●acetazolamide, ●loop diuretics or ●thiazides and related diuretics

● Dolasetron: increased risk of ventricular arrhythmias when mexiletine given with ●dolasetron—avoid concomitant use

Theophylline: mexiletine increases plasma concentration of theophylline

Tropisetron: caution with anti-arrhythmics advised by manufacturer of tropisetron (risk of ventricular arrhythmias)

Mianserin *see* Antidepressants, Tricyclic (related)
Miconazole *see* Antifungals, Imidazole
Midazolam *see* Anxiolytics and Hypnotics
Mifepristone

Analgesics: manufacturer of mifepristone advises avoid concomitant use with NSAIDs and aspirin

Corticosteroids: mifepristone may reduce effect of corticosteroids (including inhaled corticosteroids) for 3–4 days

Minocycline *see* Tetracyclines
Minoxidil *see* Vasodilator Antihypertensives
Mirtazapine

● Alcohol: increased sedative effect when mirtazapine given with ●alcohol

Anticoagulants: mirtazapine enhances anticoagulant effect of warfarin

● Antidepressants: mirtazapine should not be started until 2 weeks after stopping ●MAOIs, also MAOIs should not be started until at least 2 weeks after stopping mirtazapine; after stopping mirtazapine do not start ●moclobemide for at least 1 week

Antiepileptics: plasma concentration of mirtazapine reduced by carbamazepine and phenytoin

Antifungals: plasma concentration of mirtazapine increased by ketoconazole

● Antimalarials: avoidance of antidepressants advised by manufacturer of ●artemether/lumefantrine

Mirtazapine *(continued)*

Anxiolytics and Hypnotics: increased sedative effect when mirtazapine given with anxiolytics and hypnotics

- Sibutramine: increased risk of CNS toxicity when mirtazapine given with ●sibutramine (manufacturer of sibutramine advises avoid concomitant use)

Ulcer-healing Drugs: plasma concentration of mirtazapine increased by cimetidine

Mivacurium *see* Muscle Relaxants

Mizolastine *see* Antihistamines

Moclobemide

- Analgesics: possible CNS excitation or depression (hypertension or hypotension) when moclobemide given with ●dextromethorphan or ●pethidine—avoid concomitant use; possible CNS excitation or depression (hypertension or hypotension) when moclobemide given with ●opioid analgesics
- Antidepressants: moclobemide should not be started for at least 1 week after stopping ●MAOIs, ●SSRI-related antidepressants, ●citalopram, ●fluvoxamine, ●mirtazapine, ●tricyclic-related antidepressants or ●tricyclics; increased risk of CNS toxicity when moclobemide given with ●escitalopram, preferably avoid concomitant use; moclobemide should not be started until 5 weeks after stopping ●fluoxetine; moclobemide should not be started until 2 weeks after stopping ●paroxetine or ●sertraline
- Antimalarials: avoidance of antidepressants advised by manufacturer of ●artemether/lumefantrine
- Bupropion: avoidance of moclobemide advised by manufacturer of ●bupropion
- Dopaminergics: caution with moclobemide advised by manufacturer of entacapone; increased risk of side-effects when moclobemide given with levodopa; avoid concomitant use of moclobemide with ●selegiline
- 5HT$_1$ Agonists: risk of CNS toxicity when moclobemide given with ●rizatriptan or ●sumatriptan (avoid rizatriptan or sumatriptan for 2 weeks after moclobemide); risk of CNS toxicity when moclobemide given with ●zolmitriptan (reduce dose of zolmitriptan)
- Sibutramine: increased CNS toxicity when moclobemide given with ●sibutramine (manufacturer of sibutramine advises avoid concomitant use), also avoid sibutramine for 2 weeks after stopping moclobemide
- Sympathomimetics: risk of hypertensive crisis when moclobemide given with ●dexamfetamine, ●dopamine, ●dopexamine, ●ephedrine, ●isometheptene, ●methylphenidate, ●phenylephrine, ●phenylpropanolamine, ●pseudoephedrine or ●sympathomimetics

Ulcer-healing Drugs: plasma concentration of moclobemide increased by cimetidine (halve dose of moclobemide)

Modafinil

Antiepileptics: modafinil possibly increases plasma concentration of phenytoin

- Ciclosporin: modafinil reduces plasma concentration of ●ciclosporin
- Oestrogens: modafinil accelerates metabolism of ●oestrogens (reduced contraceptive effect—see p. 388)

Moexipril *see* ACE Inhibitors

Mometasone *see* Corticosteroids

Monobactams *see* Aztreonam

Montelukast *see* Leukotriene Antagonists

Morphine *see* Opioid Analgesics

Moxifloxacin *see* Quinolones

Moxisylyte (thymoxamine)

ACE Inhibitors: enhanced hypotensive effect when moxisylyte given with ACE inhibitors

Adrenergic Neurone Blockers: enhanced hypotensive effect when moxisylyte given with adrenergic neurone blockers

- Alpha-blockers: possible severe postural hypotension when moxisylyte given with ●alpha-blockers

Angiotensin-II Receptor Antagonists: enhanced hypotensive effect when moxisylyte given with angiotensin-II receptor antagonists

- Beta-blockers: possible severe postural hypotension when moxisylyte given with ●beta-blockers

Calcium-channel Blockers: enhanced hypotensive effect when moxisylyte given with calcium-channel blockers

Clonidine: enhanced hypotensive effect when moxisylyte given with clonidine

Diazoxide: enhanced hypotensive effect when moxisylyte given with diazoxide

Diuretics: enhanced hypotensive effect when moxisylyte given with diuretics

Methyldopa: enhanced hypotensive effect when moxisylyte given with methyldopa

Moxonidine: enhanced hypotensive effect when moxisylyte given with moxonidine

Nitrates: enhanced hypotensive effect when moxisylyte given with nitrates

Vasodilator Antihypertensives: enhanced hypotensive effect when moxisylyte given with hydralazine, minoxidil or nitroprusside

Moxonidine

ACE Inhibitors: enhanced hypotensive effect when moxonidine given with ACE inhibitors

Adrenergic Neurone Blockers: enhanced hypotensive effect when moxonidine given with adrenergic neurone blockers

Alcohol: enhanced hypotensive effect when moxonidine given with alcohol

Aldesleukin: enhanced hypotensive effect when moxonidine given with aldesleukin

Alpha-blockers: enhanced hypotensive effect when moxonidine given with alpha-blockers

Alprostadil: enhanced hypotensive effect when moxonidine given with alprostadil

Amifostine: possible enhanced hypotensive effect when moxonidine given with amifostine

Anaesthetics, General: enhanced hypotensive effect when moxonidine given with general anaesthetics

Analgesics: hypotensive effect of moxonidine antagonised by NSAIDs

Angiotensin-II Receptor Antagonists: enhanced hypotensive effect when moxonidine given with angiotensin-II receptor antagonists

Antidepressants: enhanced hypotensive effect when moxonidine given with MAOIs

Antipsychotics: enhanced hypotensive effect when moxonidine given with phenothiazines

Anxiolytics and Hypnotics: enhanced hypotensive effect when moxonidine given with anxiolytics and hypnotics; sedative effects possibly increased when moxonidine given with benzodiazepines

Beta-blockers: enhanced hypotensive effect when moxonidine given with beta-blockers

Calcium-channel Blockers: enhanced hypotensive effect when moxonidine given with calcium-channel blockers

Clonidine: enhanced hypotensive effect when moxonidine given with clonidine

Corticosteroids: hypotensive effect of moxonidine antagonised by corticosteroids

Moxonidine *(continued)*

Diazoxide: enhanced hypotensive effect when moxonidine given with diazoxide

Diuretics: enhanced hypotensive effect when moxonidine given with diuretics

Dopaminergics: enhanced hypotensive effect when moxonidine given with levodopa

Methyldopa: enhanced hypotensive effect when moxonidine given with methyldopa

Moxisylyte (thymoxamine): enhanced hypotensive effect when moxonidine given with moxisylyte

Muscle Relaxants: enhanced hypotensive effect when moxonidine given with baclofen or tizanidine

Nitrates: enhanced hypotensive effect when moxonidine given with nitrates

Oestrogens: hypotensive effect of moxonidine antagonised by oestrogens

Ulcer-healing Drugs: hypotensive effect of moxonidine antagonised by carbenoxolone

Vasodilator Antihypertensives: enhanced hypotensive effect when moxonidine given with hydralazine, minoxidil or nitroprusside

Muscle Relaxants

ACE Inhibitors: enhanced hypotensive effect when baclofen or tizanidine given with ACE inhibitors

Adrenergic Neurone Blockers: enhanced hypotensive effect when baclofen or tizanidine given with adrenergic neurone blockers

Alcohol: increased sedative effect when baclofen, methocarbamol or tizanidine given with alcohol

Alpha-blockers: enhanced hypotensive effect when baclofen or tizanidine given with alpha-blockers

Anaesthetics, General: effects of non-depolarising muscle relaxants and suxamethonium enhanced by volatile liquid general anaesthetics

Analgesics: excretion of baclofen possibly reduced by NSAIDs (possibly increased risk of toxicity); excretion of baclofen reduced by ibuprofen (increased risk of toxicity)

Angiotensin-II Receptor Antagonists: enhanced hypotensive effect when baclofen or tizanidine given with angiotensin-II receptor antagonists

- Anti-arrhythmics: neuromuscular blockade enhanced and prolonged when suxamethonium given with lidocaine (lignocaine); effects of muscle relaxants enhanced by ●procainamide and ●quinidine

- Antibacterials: effects of non-depolarising muscle relaxants and suxamethonium enhanced by piperacillin; effects of non-depolarising muscle relaxants and suxamethonium enhanced by ●aminoglycosides; effects of non-depolarising muscle relaxants and suxamethonium enhanced by ●clindamycin; effects of non-depolarising muscle relaxants and suxamethonium enhanced by ●polymyxins; effects of suxamethonium enhanced by ●vancomycin

Antidepressants: effects of suxamethonium enhanced by phenelzine; muscle relaxant effect of baclofen enhanced by tricyclics

Antiepileptics: muscle relaxant effect of non-depolarising muscle relaxants antagonised by carbamazepine and phenytoin (accelerated recovery from neuromuscular blockade)

Antimalarials: effects of suxamethonium possibly enhanced by quinine

Antipsychotics: effects of suxamethonium possibly enhanced by promazine

Anxiolytics and Hypnotics: increased sedative effect when baclofen or tizanidine given with anxiolytics and hypnotics

Beta-blockers: enhanced hypotensive effect when baclofen given with beta-blockers; possible

Muscle Relaxants

Beta-blockers *(continued)*

enhanced hypotensive effect and bradycardia when tizanidine given with beta-blockers; effects of muscle relaxants enhanced by propranolol

Calcium-channel Blockers: enhanced hypotensive effect when baclofen or tizanidine given with calcium-channel blockers; effects of non-depolarising muscle relaxants enhanced by nifedipine and verapamil; risk of arrhythmias when intravenous dantrolene given with diltiazem; hypotension, myocardial depression, and hyperkalaemia when intravenous dantrolene given with verapamil; effects of suxamethonium enhanced by verapamil

Cardiac Glycosides: possible increased risk of bradycardia when tizanidine given with cardiac glycosides; risk of ventricular arrhythmias when suxamethonium given with cardiac glycosides

Clonidine: enhanced hypotensive effect when baclofen or tizanidine given with clonidine

Cytotoxics: effects of suxamethonium enhanced by cyclophosphamide and thiotepa

Diazoxide: enhanced hypotensive effect when baclofen or tizanidine given with diazoxide

Diuretics: enhanced hypotensive effect when baclofen or tizanidine given with diuretics

Dopaminergics: possible agitation, confusion and hallucinations when baclofen given with levodopa

Lithium: effects of muscle relaxants enhanced by lithium; baclofen possibly aggravates hyperkinesis caused by lithium

Magnesium (parenteral): effects of non-depolarising muscle relaxants and suxamethonium enhanced by parenteral magnesium

Memantine: effects of baclofen and dantrolene possibly modified by memantine

Methyldopa: enhanced hypotensive effect when baclofen or tizanidine given with methyldopa

Metoclopramide: effects of suxamethonium enhanced by metoclopramide

Moxonidine: enhanced hypotensive effect when baclofen or tizanidine given with moxonidine

Nitrates: enhanced hypotensive effect when baclofen or tizanidine given with nitrates

Parasympathomimetics: effects of non-depolarising muscle relaxants possibly antagonised by donepezil; effects of suxamethonium possibly enhanced by donepezil; effects of non-depolarising muscle relaxants antagonised by edrophonium, neostigmine, pyridostigmine and rivastigmine; effects of suxamethonium enhanced by edrophonium, galantamine, neostigmine, pyridostigmine and rivastigmine

Sympathomimetics, Beta$_2$: effects of suxamethonium enhanced by bambuterol

Trimetaphan: effects of suxamethonium enhanced by trimetaphan

Vasodilator Antihypertensives: enhanced hypotensive effect when baclofen or tizanidine given with hydralazine; enhanced hypotensive effect when baclofen or tizanidine given with minoxidil; enhanced hypotensive effect when baclofen or tizanidine given with nitroprusside

Muscle Relaxants, depolarising *see* Muscle Relaxants

Muscle Relaxants, non-depolarising *see* Muscle Relaxants

Mycophenolate Mofetil

Antacids: absorption of mycophenolate mofetil reduced by antacids

Antiepileptics: cytotoxics reduce absorption of phenytoin

Mycophenolate Mofetil (continued)
- Antipsychotics: avoid concomitant use of cytotoxics with ●clozapine (increased risk of agranulocytosis)
  Antivirals: mycophenolate mofetil increases plasma concentration of aciclovir, also plasma concentration of inactive metabolite of mycophenolate mofetil increased; mycophenolate mofetil possibly increases plasma concentration of ganciclovir, also plasma concentration of inactive metabolite of mycophenolate mofetil possibly increased
  Lipid-regulating Drugs: absorption of mycophenolate mofetil reduced by colestyramine

Nabilone
  Alcohol: increased sedative effect when nabilone given with alcohol
  Anxiolytics and Hypnotics: increased sedative effect when nabilone given with anxiolytics and hypnotics

Nabumetone see NSAIDs
Nadolol see Beta-blockers
Nalbuphine see Opioid Analgesics
Nalidixic Acid see Quinolones
Nandrolone see Anabolic Steroids
Naproxen see NSAIDs
Naratriptan see 5HT₁ Agonists
Nateglinide see Antidiabetics
Nebivolol see Beta-blockers

Nefopam
- Antidepressants: manufacturer of nefopam advises avoid concomitant use with ●MAOIs; side-effects possibly increased when nefopam given with tricyclics
  Antimuscarinics: increased risk of antimuscarinic side-effects when nefopam given with antimuscarinics

Nelfinavir
  Analgesics: nelfinavir reduces plasma concentration of methadone
- Anti-arrhythmics: increased risk of ventricular arrhythmias when nelfinavir given with ●amiodarone or ●quinidine—avoid concomitant use
- Antibacterials: nelfinavir increases plasma concentration of ●rifabutin (halve dose of rifabutin); plasma concentration of nelfinavir significantly reduced by ●rifampicin—avoid concomitant use
- Antidepressants: plasma concentration of nelfinavir reduced by ●St John's wort—avoid concomitant use
- Antiepileptics: plasma concentration of nelfinavir possibly reduced by carbamazepine and ●primidone; nelfinavir reduces plasma concentration of phenytoin
- Antihistamines: increased risk of ventricular arrhythmias when nelfinavir given with ●terfenadine—avoid concomitant use
  Antimuscarinics: avoidance of nelfinavir advised by manufacturer of tolterodine
- Antipsychotics: nelfinavir possibly increases plasma concentration of thioridazine; nelfinavir possibly increases plasma concentration of ●pimozide (increased risk of ventricular arrhythmias—avoid concomitant use); nelfinavir increases plasma concentration of ●sertindole (increased risk of ventricular arrhythmias—avoid concomitant use)
  Antivirals: combination of nelfinavir with indinavir, ritonavir or saquinavir may increase plasma concentration of either drug (or both)
- Anxiolytics and Hypnotics: increased risk of prolonged sedation when nelfinavir given with ●midazolam—avoid concomitant use
- Barbiturates: plasma concentration of nelfinavir possibly reduced by ●barbiturates
- Ciclosporin: nelfinavir possibly increases plasma concentration of ●ciclosporin

Nelfinavir (continued)
  Cilostazol: nelfinavir possibly increases plasma concentration of cilostazol—avoid concomitant use
- Ergot Alkaloids: increased risk of ergotism when nelfinavir given with ●ergotamine and methysergide—avoid concomitant use
- 5HT₁ Agonists: nelfinavir increases plasma concentration of ●eletriptan (risk of toxicity)—avoid concomitant use
- Lipid-regulating Drugs: possible increased risk of myopathy when nelfinavir given with atorvastatin; increased risk of myopathy when nelfinavir given with ●simvastatin (avoid concomitant use)
- Oestrogens: nelfinavir accelerates metabolism of ●oestrogens (reduced contraceptive effect—see p. 388)
  Sildenafil: nelfinavir possibly increases plasma concentration of sildenafil— reduce initial dose of sildenafil
- Tacrolimus: nelfinavir possibly increases plasma concentration of ●tacrolimus

Neomycin see Aminoglycosides
Neostigmine see Parasympathomimetics
Netilmicin see Aminoglycosides

Nevirapine
  Analgesics: nevirapine possibly reduces plasma concentration of methadone
- Antibacterials: plasma concentration of nevirapine reduced by ●rifampicin—avoid concomitant use
- Anticoagulants: nevirapine may enhance or reduce anticoagulant effect of ●warfarin
- Antidepressants: plasma concentration of nevirapine reduced by ●St John's wort—avoid concomitant use
- Antifungals: nevirapine reduces plasma concentration of ●ketoconazole—avoid concomitant use; plasma concentration of nevirapine increased by ●fluconazole; nevirapine possibly reduces plasma concentration of caspofungin—consider increasing dose of caspofungin
- Antivirals: nevirapine possibly reduces plasma concentration of amprenavir and lopinavir; nevirapine reduces plasma concentration of efavirenz and indinavir; nevirapine reduces plasma concentration of ●saquinavir—avoid concomitant use
- Oestrogens: nevirapine accelerates metabolism of ●oestrogens (reduced contraceptive effect—see p. 388)
- Progestogens: nevirapine accelerates metabolism of ●progestogens (reduced contraceptive effect—see p. 388)

Nicardipine see Calcium-channel Blockers

Nicorandil
  Alcohol: hypotensive effect of nicorandil possibly enhanced by alcohol
  Antidepressants: enhanced hypotensive effect when nicorandil given with MAOIs; hypotensive effect of nicorandil possibly enhanced by tricyclics
- Sildenafil: hypotensive effect of nicorandil significantly enhanced by ●sildenafil (avoid concomitant use)
- Tadalafil: hypotensive effect of nicorandil significantly enhanced by ●tadalafil (avoid concomitant use)
- Vardenafil: hypotensive effect of nicorandil possibly enhanced by ●vardenafil—avoid concomitant use
  Vasodilator Antihypertensives: possible enhanced hypotensive effect when nicorandil given with hydralazine, minoxidil or nitroprusside

Nicotinic Acid
  Note. Interactions apply to lipid-regulating doses of nicotinic acid

Nicotinic Acid *(continued)*
- Lipid-regulating Drugs: increased risk of myopathy when nicotinic acid given with ●statins (applies to lipid regulating doses of nicotinic acid)

Nifedipine *see* Calcium-channel Blockers
Nimodipine *see* Calcium-channel Blockers
Nisoldipine *see* Calcium-channel Blockers
Nitrates

ACE Inhibitors: enhanced hypotensive effect when nitrates given with ACE inhibitors

Adrenergic Neurone Blockers: enhanced hypotensive effect when nitrates given with adrenergic neurone blockers

Alcohol: enhanced hypotensive effect when nitrates given with alcohol

Aldesleukin: enhanced hypotensive effect when nitrates given with aldesleukin

Alpha-blockers: enhanced hypotensive effect when nitrates given with alpha-blockers

Alprostadil: enhanced hypotensive effect when nitrates given with alprostadil

Amifostine: possible enhanced hypotensive effect when nitrates given with amifostine

Anaesthetics, General: enhanced hypotensive effect when nitrates given with general anaesthetics

Analgesics: hypotensive effect of nitrates antagonised by NSAIDs

Angiotensin-II Receptor Antagonists: enhanced hypotensive effect when nitrates given with angiotensin-II receptor antagonists

Anti-arrhythmics: effects of sublingual tablets of nitrates reduced by disopyramide (failure to dissolve under tongue owing to dry mouth)

- Anticoagulants: infusion of glyceryl trinitrate reduces anticoagulant effect of ●heparins

Antidepressants: enhanced hypotensive effect when nitrates given with MAOIs; effects of sublingual tablets of nitrates possibly reduced by tricyclic-related antidepressants (failure to dissolve under tongue owing to dry mouth); effects of sublingual tablets of nitrates reduced by tricyclics (failure to dissolve under tongue owing to dry mouth)

Antimuscarinics: effects of sublingual tablets of nitrates possibly reduced by antimuscarinics (failure to dissolve under tongue owing to dry mouth)

Antipsychotics: enhanced hypotensive effect when nitrates given with phenothiazines

Anxiolytics and Hypnotics: enhanced hypotensive effect when nitrates given with anxiolytics and hypnotics

Beta-blockers: enhanced hypotensive effect when nitrates given with beta-blockers

Calcium-channel Blockers: enhanced hypotensive effect when nitrates given with calcium-channel blockers

Clonidine: enhanced hypotensive effect when nitrates given with clonidine

Corticosteroids: hypotensive effect of nitrates antagonised by corticosteroids

Diazoxide: enhanced hypotensive effect when nitrates given with diazoxide

Diuretics: enhanced hypotensive effect when nitrates given with diuretics

Dopaminergics: hypotensive effect of nitrates enhanced by sublingual apomorphine; enhanced hypotensive effect when nitrates given with levodopa

Methyldopa: enhanced hypotensive effect when nitrates given with methyldopa

Moxisylyte (thymoxamine): enhanced hypotensive effect when nitrates given with moxisylyte

Moxonidine: enhanced hypotensive effect when nitrates given with moxonidine

Nitrates *(continued)*

Muscle Relaxants: enhanced hypotensive effect when nitrates given with baclofen or tizanidine

Oestrogens: hypotensive effect of nitrates antagonised by oestrogens

- Sildenafil: hypotensive effect of nitrates significantly enhanced by ●sildenafil (avoid concomitant use)
- Tadalafil: hypotensive effect of nitrates significantly enhanced by ●tadalafil (avoid concomitant use)

Ulcer-healing Drugs: hypotensive effect of nitrates antagonised by carbenoxolone

- Vardenafil: hypotensive effect of nitrates possibly enhanced by ●vardenafil—avoid concomitant use

Vasodilator Antihypertensives: enhanced hypotensive effect when nitrates given with hydralazine, minoxidil or nitroprusside

Nitrazepam *see* Anxiolytics and Hypnotics
Nitrofurantoin

Antacids: absorption of nitrofurantoin reduced by oral magnesium salts (as magnesium trisilicate)

Oestrogens: *broad-spectrum* antibacterials possibly reduce contraceptive effect of oestrogens (risk probably small, see p. 388)

Probenecid: excretion of nitrofurantoin reduced by probenecid (increased risk of side-effects)

Sulfinpyrazone: excretion of nitrofurantoin reduced by sulfinpyrazone (increased risk of toxicity)

Nitroimidazoles *see* Metronidazole and Tinidazole
Nitroprusside *see* Vasodilator Antihypertensives
Nitrous Oxide *see* Anaesthetics, General
Nizatidine *see* Histamine H_2-antagonists
Noradrenaline (norepinephrine) *see* Sympathomimetics
Norelgestromin *see* Progestogens
Norepinephrine (noradrenaline) *see* Sympathomimetics
Norethisterone *see* Progestogens
Norfloxacin *see* Quinolones
Norgestimate *see* Progestogens
Norgestrel *see* Progestogens
Nortriptyline *see* Antidepressants, Tricyclic
NSAIDs

Note. See also Aspirin. Interactions do not generally apply to topical NSAIDs

ACE Inhibitors: increased risk of renal impairment when NSAIDs given with ACE inhibitors, also hypotensive effect antagonised; increased risk of hyperkalaemia when ketorolac given with ACE inhibitors

Adrenergic Neurone Blockers: NSAIDs antagonise hypotensive effect of adrenergic neurone blockers

Alpha-blockers: NSAIDs antagonise hypotensive effect of alpha-blockers

- Analgesics: avoid concomitant use of NSAIDs with ●NSAIDs or ●aspirin (increased side-effects); avoid concomitant use of NSAIDs with ●ketorolac (increased side-effects and haemorrhage); ibuprofen possibly reduces antiplatelet effect of aspirin

Angiotensin-II Receptor Antagonists: increased risk of renal impairment when NSAIDs given with angiotensin-II receptor antagonists, also hypotensive effect antagonised; increased risk of hyperkalaemia when ketorolac given with angiotensin-II receptor antagonists

Antacids: absorption of diflunisal reduced by antacids

- Antibacterials: indometacin possibly increases plasma concentration of amikacin and gentamicin in neonates; plasma concentration of etoricoxib and rofecoxib reduced by rifampicin; possible increased risk of convulsions when NSAIDs given with quinolones

- Anticoagulants: celecoxib, diflunisal, etodolac, etoricoxib, flurbiprofen, ibuprofen, mefenamic

NSAIDs

- Anticoagulants *(continued)*
  acid, meloxicam, piroxicam, rofecoxib, sulindac and valdecoxib possibly enhance anticoagulant effect of ●coumarins; azapropazone enhances anticoagulant effect of ●coumarins (avoid concomitant use); NSAIDs possibly enhance anticoagulant effect of ●coumarins and ●phenindione; increased risk of bleeding when ketorolac given with ●coumarins (avoid concomitant use); diclofenac possibly enhances anticoagulant effect of ●coumarins, also increased risk of haemorrage with intravenous diclofenac (avoid concomitant use); increased risk of haemorrhage when intravenous diclofenac given with ●heparins (avoid concomitant use, including low-dose heparin); possible increased risk of bleeding when NSAIDs given with heparins; increased risk of haemorrhage when ketorolac given with ●heparins (avoid concomitant use, including low-dose heparin); diclofenac enhances anticoagulant effect of ●phenindione, also increased risk of haemorrhage with intravenous diclofenac (avoid concomitant use); ketorolac enhances anticoagulant effect of ●phenindione (increased risk of haemorrhage—avoid concomitant use)

- Antidepressants: increased risk of bleeding when NSAIDs given with ●SSRIs or ●venlafaxine

- Antidiabetics: azapropazone enhances effects of ●sulphonylureas (avoid concomitant use); NSAIDs possibly enhance effects of ●sulphonylureas

- Antiepileptics: NSAIDs possibly enhance effects of ●phenytoin; azapropazone enhances effects of ●phenytoin (avoid concomitant use)

  Antifungals: plasma concentration of valdecoxib increased by ketoconazole (reduce initial dose of valdecoxib); plasma concentration of valdecoxib increased by fluconazole—reduce initial dose of valdecoxib; plasma concentration of parecoxib increased by fluconazole (reduce dose of parecoxib); plasma concentration of celecoxib increased by fluconazole (halve dose of celecoxib)

- Antipsychotics: possible severe drowsiness when indometacin given with haloperidol; avoid concomitant use of azapropazone with ●clozapine (increased risk of agranulocytosis)

- Antivirals: plasma concentration of piroxicam increased by ●ritonavir (risk of toxicity)—avoid concomitant use; plasma concentration of NSAIDs possibly increased by ritonavir; increased risk of haematological toxicity when NSAIDs given with zidovudine

  Beta-blockers: NSAIDs antagonise hypotensive effect of beta-blockers

  Bisphosphonates: indometacin increases bioavailability of tiludronic acid

  Calcium-channel Blockers: NSAIDs antagonise hypotensive effect of calcium-channel blockers

  Cardiac Glycosides: NSAIDs possibly increase plasma concentration of cardiac glycosides, also possible exacerbation of heart failure and reduction of renal function

- Ciclosporin: increased risk of nephrotoxicity when NSAIDs given with ●ciclosporin; plasma concentration of diclofenac increased by ●ciclosporin (halve dose of diclofenac)

  Clonidine: NSAIDs antagonise hypotensive effect of clonidine

  Clopidogrel: increased risk of bleeding when NSAIDs given with clopidogrel

NSAIDs *(continued)*

  Corticosteroids: increased risk of gastro-intestinal bleeding and ulceration when NSAIDs given with corticosteroids

- Cytotoxics: NSAIDs probably reduce excretion of ●methotrexate (increased risk of toxicity); azapropazone reduces excretion of ●methotrexate (avoid concomitant use); diclofenac, ibuprofen, indometacin, ketoprofen, meloxicam and naproxen reduce excretion of ●methotrexate (increased risk of toxicity)

  Desmopressin: indometacin enhances effects of desmopressin

  Diazoxide: NSAIDs antagonise hypotensive effect of diazoxide

- Diuretics: risk of nephrotoxicity of NSAIDs increased by diuretics, also antagonism of diuretic effect; indometacin and ketorolac antagonise effects of diuretics; occasional reports of reduced renal function when indometacin given with ●triamterene—avoid concomitant use; possibly increased risk of hyperkalaemia when NSAIDs given with potassium-sparing diuretics; increased risk of hyperkalaemia when indometacin given with potassium-sparing diuretics

- Lithium: NSAIDs probably reduce excretion of ●lithium (increased risk of toxicity); azapropazone, diclofenac, ibuprofen, indometacin, mefenamic acid, naproxen, parecoxib, piroxicam, rofecoxib and valdecoxib reduce excretion of ●lithium (increased risk of toxicity); ketorolac reduces excretion of ●lithium (increased risk of toxicity)—avoid concomitant use

  Methyldopa: NSAIDs antagonise hypotensive effect of methyldopa

  Mifepristone: avoidance of NSAIDs advised by manufacturer of mifepristone

  Moxonidine: NSAIDs antagonise hypotensive effect of moxonidine

  Muscle Relaxants: ibuprofen reduces excretion of baclofen (increased risk of toxicity); NSAIDs possibly reduce excretion of baclofen (possibly increased risk of toxicity)

  Nitrates: NSAIDs antagonise hypotensive effect of nitrates

  Oestrogens: etoricoxib and valdecoxib increase plasma concentration of ethinylestradiol

- Pentoxifylline (oxpentifylline): possible increased risk of bleeding when NSAIDs given with pentoxifylline (oxpentifylline); increased risk of bleeding when ketorolac given with ●pentoxifylline (oxpentifylline) (avoid concomitant use)

- Probenecid: excretion of indometacin, ketoprofen and naproxen reduced by ●probenecid (increased plasma concentration); excretion of ketorolac reduced by ●probenecid (increased plasma concentration)—avoid concomitant use

  Progestogens: risk of hyperkalaemia when NSAIDs given with drospirenone (monitor serum potassium during first cycle)

  Sibutramine: increased risk of bleeding when NSAIDs given with sibutramine

- Tacrolimus: possible increased risk of nephrotoxicity when NSAIDs given with tacrolimus; increased risk of nephrotoxicity when ibuprofen given with ●tacrolimus

  Theophylline: rofecoxib increases plasma concentration of theophylline

  Ulcer-healing Drugs: plasma concentration of azapropazone possibly increased by cimetidine; valdecoxib increases plasma concentration of omeprazole

NSAIDs *(continued)*

Vasodilator Antihypertensives: NSAIDs antagonise hypotensive effect of hydralazine, minoxidil and nitroprusside

Octreotide

Antidiabetics: octreotide possibly reduces requirements for insulin, metformin, repaglinide and sulphonylureas

● Ciclosporin: octreotide reduces plasma concentration of ●ciclosporin

Dopaminergics: octreotide increases plasma concentration of bromocriptine

Ulcer-healing Drugs: octreotide possibly delays absorption of cimetidine

Oestrogens

Note. Interactions of combined oral contraceptives may also apply to combined contraceptive patches; in case of hormone replacement therapy low dose unlikely to induce interactions

ACE Inhibitors: oestrogens antagonise hypotensive effect of ACE inhibitors

Adrenergic Neurone Blockers: oestrogens antagonise hypotensive effect of adrenergic neurone blockers

Alpha-blockers: oestrogens antagonise hypotensive effect of alpha-blockers

Analgesics: plasma concentration of ethinylestradiol increased by etoricoxib and valdecoxib

Angiotensin-II Receptor Antagonists: oestrogens antagonise hypotensive effect of angiotensin-II receptor antagonists

● Antibacterials: contraceptive effect of oestrogens possibly reduced by broad-spectrum antibacterials and ●penicillins (risk probably small, see p. 388); metabolism of oestrogens accelerated by ●rifamycins (reduced contraceptive effect—see p. 388); contraceptive effect of oestrogens possibly reduced by ●tetracyclines (risk probably small, see p. 388)

● Anticoagulants: oestrogens antagonise anticoagulant effect of ●coumarins and ●phenindione

● Antidepressants: contraceptive effect of oestrogens reduced by ●St John's wort (avoid concomitant use); oestrogens antagonise antidepressant effect of tricyclics (but side-effects of tricyclics possibly increased due to increased plasma concentration)

Antidiabetics: oestrogens antagonise hypoglycaemic effect of antidiabetics

● Antiepileptics: metabolism of oestrogens accelerated by ●carbamazepine, ●oxcarbazepine, ●phenytoin, ●primidone and ●topiramate (reduced contraceptive effect—see p. 388)

● Antifungals: anecdotal reports of contraceptive failure when oestrogens given with fluconazole, imidazoles, itraconazole or ketoconazole; metabolism of oestrogens accelerated by ●griseofulvin (reduced contraceptive effect—see p. 388); occasional reports of breakthrough bleeding when oestrogens (used for contraception) given with terbinafine

● Antivirals: contraceptive effect of oestrogens possibly reduced by amprenavir and efavirenz; metabolism of oestrogens accelerated by ●nelfinavir, ●nevirapine and ●ritonavir (reduced contraceptive effect—see p. 388)

● Barbiturates: metabolism of oestrogens accelerated by ●barbiturates (reduced contraceptive effect—see p. 388)

Beta-blockers: oestrogens antagonise hypotensive effect of beta-blockers

Bile Acids: elimination of cholesterol in bile increased when oestrogens given with bile acids

● Bosentan: possible contraceptive failure of hormonal contraceptives containing oestrogens when given

Oestrogens

● Bosentan *(continued)*

with ●bosentan (alternative contraception recommended)

Calcium-channel Blockers: oestrogens antagonise hypotensive effect of calcium-channel blockers

Ciclosporin: oestrogens possibly increase plasma concentration of ciclosporin

Clonidine: oestrogens antagonise hypotensive effect of clonidine

Corticosteroids: oral contraceptives containing oestrogens increase plasma concentration of corticosteroids

Diazoxide: oestrogens antagonise hypotensive effect of diazoxide

Diuretics: oestrogens antagonise diuretic effect of diuretics

Dopaminergics: oestrogens increase plasma concentration of ropinirole

Lipid-regulating Drugs: plasma concentration of ethinylestradiol increased by rosuvastatin

Methyldopa: oestrogens antagonise hypotensive effect of methyldopa

● Modafinil: metabolism of oestrogens accelerated by ●modafinil (reduced contraceptive effect—see p. 388)

Moxonidine: oestrogens antagonise hypotensive effect of moxonidine

Nitrates: oestrogens antagonise hypotensive effect of nitrates

Somatropin: oestrogens (when used as oral replacement therapy) may increase dose requirements of somatropin

Tacrolimus: contraceptive effect of oestrogens possibly reduced by tacrolimus

Theophylline: oestrogens reduce excretion of theophylline (increased plasma concentration)

Vasodilator Antihypertensives: oestrogens antagonise hypotensive effect of hydralazine, minoxidil and nitroprusside

Oestrogens, conjugated *see* Oestrogens

Ofloxacin *see* Quinolones

Olanzapine *see* Antipsychotics

Olmesartan *see* Angiotensin-II Receptor Antagonists

Olsalazine *see* Aminosalicylates

Omeprazole *see* Proton Pump Inhibitors

Opioid Analgesics

Alcohol: enhanced hypotensive and sedative effects when opioid analgesics given with alcohol

Anti-arrhythmics: opioid analgesics delay absorption of mexiletine

Antibacterials: plasma concentration of alfentanil increased by erythromycin; avoidance of pre-medication with opioid analgesics advised by manufacturer of ciprofloxacin (reduced plasma concentration of ciprofloxacin) when ciprofloxacin used for surgical prophylaxis; metabolism of methadone accelerated by rifampicin (reduced effect)

● Anticoagulants: dextropropoxyphene possibly enhances anticoagulant effect of ●coumarins

● Antidepressants: plasma concentration of methadone possibly increased by fluvoxamine; CNS excitation or depression (hypertension or hypotension) when pethidine given with ●MAOIs—avoid concomitant use and for 2 weeks after stopping MAOIs; possible CNS excitation or depression (hypertension or hypotension) when opioid analgesics given with ●MAOIs—avoid concomitant use and for 2 weeks after stopping MAOIs; possible CNS excitation or depression (hypertension or hypotension) when opioid analgesics

Opioid Analgesics

- Antidepressants *(continued)*

  given with ●moclobemide; possible CNS excitation or depression (hypertension or hypotension) when dextromethorphan or pethidine given with ●moclobemide—avoid concomitant use; increased risk of CNS toxicity when tramadol given with ●SSRIs or ●tricyclics; sedative effects possibly increased when opioid analgesics given with tricyclics

- Antiepileptics: dextropropoxyphene enhances effects of ●carbamazepine; effects of tramadol reduced by carbamazepine; plasma concentration of methadone reduced by carbamazepine; metabolism of methadone accelerated by phenytoin (reduced effect and risk of withdrawal effects)

  Antifungals: metabolism of alfentanil inhibited by ketoconazole (risk of prolonged or delayed respiratory depression)

  Antipsychotics: enhanced hypotensive and sedative effects when opioid analgesics given with antipsychotics; increased risk of convulsions when tramadol given with antipsychotics

- Antivirals: plasma concentration of methadone possibly reduced by abacavir and nevirapine; plasma concentration of methadone reduced by efavirenz, nelfinavir and ritonavir; plasma concentration of fentanyl increased by ●ritonavir; plasma concentration of dextropropoxyphene and pethidine increased by ●ritonavir (risk of toxicity)—avoid concomitant use; plasma concentration of opioid analgesics (except methadone) possibly increased by ●ritonavir; methadone possibly increases plasma concentration of zidovudine

  Anxiolytics and Hypnotics: increased sedative effect when opioid analgesics given with anxiolytics and hypnotics

  Beta-blockers: morphine possibly increases plasma concentration of esmolol

  Cardiac Glycosides: increased risk of tramadol toxicity when given with digoxin

  Domperidone: opioid analgesics antagonise effects of domperidone on gastro-intestinal activity

- Dopaminergics: caution in antidepressant advised by manufacturer of selegiline; hyperpyrexia and CNS toxicity reported when pethidine given with ●selegiline (avoid concomitant use)

- Memantine: increased risk of CNS toxicity when dextromethorphan given with ●memantine (manufacturer of memantine advises avoid concomitant use)

  Metoclopramide: opioid analgesics antagonise effects of metoclopramide on gastro-intestinal activity

  Ulcer-healing Drugs: metabolism of opioid analgesics inhibited by cimetidine (increased plasma concentration)

Orciprenaline *see* Sympathomimetics

Orlistat

  Anticoagulants: manufacturer of orlistat recommends monitoring anticoagulant effect of coumarins

  Antidiabetics: manufacturer of orlistat advises avoid concomitant use with acarbose

- Ciclosporin: orlistat possibly reduces absorption of ●ciclosporin

Orphenadrine *see* Antimuscarinics

Oxaliplatin *see* Platinum Compounds

Oxazepam *see* Anxiolytics and Hypnotics

Oxcarbazepine

- Antidepressants: manufacturer of oxcarbazepine advises avoid concomitant use with ●MAOIs;

Oxcarbazepine

- Antidepressants *(continued)*

  anticonvulsant effect of antiepileptics possibly antagonised by MAOIs and ●tricyclic-related antidepressants (convulsive threshold lowered); anticonvulsant effect of antiepileptics antagonised by ●SSRIs and tricyclics (convulsive threshold lowered)

  Antiepileptics: oxcarbazepine sometimes reduces plasma concentration of carbamazepine (but concentration of an active metabolite of carbamazepine may be increased), also plasma concentration of an active metabolite of oxcarbazepine often reduced; oxcarbazepine increases plasma concentration of phenytoin, also plasma concentration of an active metabolite of oxcarbazepine reduced; oxcarbazepine increases plasma concentration of an active metabolite of primidone, also plasma concentration of an active metabolite of oxcarbazepine reduced; plasma concentration of an active metabolite of oxcarbazepine sometimes reduced by valproate

- Antimalarials: possible increased risk of convulsions when antiepileptics given with chloroquine and hydroxychloroquine; anticonvulsant effect of antiepileptics antagonised by ●mefloquine

- Antipsychotics: anticonvulsant effect of oxcarbazepine antagonised by ●antipsychotics (convulsive threshold lowered)

  Barbiturates: oxcarbazepine increases plasma concentration of phenobarbital, also plasma concentration of an active metabolite of oxcarbazepine reduced

- Oestrogens: oxcarbazepine accelerates metabolism of ●oestrogens (reduced contraceptive effect—see p. 388)

- Progestogens: oxcarbazepine accelerates metabolism of ●progestogens (reduced contraceptive effect—see p. 388)

Oxprenolol *see* Beta-blockers

Oxybutynin *see* Antimuscarinics

Oxycodone *see* Opioid Analgesics

Oxymetazoline *see* Sympathomimetics

Oxytetracycline *see* Tetracyclines

Oxytocin

  Anaesthetics, General: oxytocic effect possibly reduced, also enhanced hypotensive effect and risk of arrhythmias when oxytocin given with volatile liquid general anaesthetics

  Prostaglandins: uterotonic effect of oxytocin potentiated by prostaglandins

  Sympathomimetics: risk of hypertension when oxytocin given with vasoconstrictor sympathomimetics (due to enhanced vasopressor effect)

Paclitaxel

  Antidiabetics: paclitaxel possibly inhibits metabolism of rosiglitazone

  Antiepileptics: cytotoxics reduce absorption of phenytoin

- Antipsychotics: avoid concomitant use of cytotoxics with ●clozapine (increased risk of agranulocytosis)

Pancreatin

  Antidiabetics: pancreatin antagonises hypoglycaemic effect of acarbose

Pancuronium *see* Muscle Relaxants

Pantoprazole *see* Proton Pump Inhibitors

Papaveretum *see* Opioid Analgesics

Paracetamol

  Anticoagulants: prolonged regular use of paracetamol possibly enhances anticoagulant effect of coumarins

  Cytotoxics: paracetamol possibly inhibits metabolism of *intravenous* busulfan (manufacturer of

Paracetamol

Cytotoxics (continued)

intravenous busulfan advises caution within 72 hours of paracetamol)

Domperidone: absorption of paracetamol increased by domperidone (enhanced effect)

Lipid-regulating Drugs: absorption of paracetamol reduced by colestyramine

Metoclopramide: absorption of paracetamol increased by metoclopramide (enhanced effect)

Paraldehyde

• Alcohol: increased sedative effect when paraldehyde given with ●alcohol

• Disulfiram: risk of toxicity when paraldehyde given with ●disulfiram

Parasympathomimetics

Anti-arrhythmics: effects of neostigmine and pyridostigmine antagonised by procainamide; effects of neostigmine and pyridostigmine possibly antagonised by propafenone; effects of neostigmine and pyridostigmine antagonised by quinidine

• Antibacterials: plasma concentration of galantamine increased by erythromycin; effects of neostigmine and pyridostigmine antagonised by ●aminoglycosides; effects of neostigmine and pyridostigmine antagonised by clindamycin; effects of neostigmine and pyridostigmine antagonised by ●polymyxins

Antidepressants: plasma concentration of galantamine increased by paroxetine

Antifungals: plasma concentration of galantamine increased by ketoconazole

Antimalarials: effects of neostigmine and pyridostigmine may be diminished because of potential for chloroquine and hydroxychloroquine to increase symptoms of myasthenia gravis

Antimuscarinics: effects of parasympathomimetics antagonised by antimuscarinics

Beta-blockers: increased risk of arrhythmias when pilocarpine given with beta-blockers; effects of neostigmine and pyridostigmine antagonised by propranolol

Lithium: effects of neostigmine and pyridostigmine antagonised by lithium

Muscle Relaxants: donepezil possibly enhances effects of suxamethonium; edrophonium, galantamine, neostigmine, pyridostigmine and rivastigmine enhance effects of suxamethonium; donepezil possibly antagonises effects of non-depolarising muscle relaxants; edrophonium, neostigmine, pyridostigmine and rivastigmine antagonise effects of non-depolarising muscle relaxants

Parecoxib see NSAIDs

Paroxetine see Antidepressants, SSRI

Pegfilgrastim see Filgrastim

Peginterferon Alfa see Interferons

Penicillamine

Antacids: absorption of penicillamine reduced by antacids

• Antipsychotics: avoid concomitant use of penicillamine with ●clozapine (increased risk of agranulocytosis)

Cardiac Glycosides: penicillamine possibly reduces plasma concentration of digoxin

Iron: absorption of penicillamine reduced by oral iron

Zinc: absorption of penicillamine reduced by zinc

Penicillins

Allopurinol: increased risk of rash when amoxicillin or ampicillin given with allopurinol

Penicillins (continued)

Antibacterials: absorption of phenoxymethylpenicillin reduced by neomycin

Anticoagulants: common experience in anticoagulant clinics is that INR can be altered by a course of broad-spectrum penicillins such as ampicillin, although studies have failed to demonstrate an interaction with coumarins or phenindione

Cytotoxics: penicillins reduce excretion of methotrexate (increased risk of toxicity)

Muscle Relaxants: piperacillin enhances effects of non-depolarising muscle relaxants and suxamethonium

• Oestrogens: broad-spectrum antibacterials and penicillins possibly reduce contraceptive effect of ●oestrogens (risk probably small, see p. 388)

Probenecid: excretion of penicillins reduced by probenecid (increased plasma concentration)

Pentamidine Isetionate

• Anti-arrhythmics: increased risk of ventricular arrhythmias when pentamidine isetionate given with ●amiodarone—avoid concomitant use

• Antibacterials: increased risk of ventricular arrhythmias when pentamidine isetionate given with ●moxifloxacin—avoid concomitant use

• Antihistamines: increased risk of ventricular arrhythmias when pentamidine isetionate given with ●terfenadine—avoid concomitant use

• Antipsychotics: increased risk of ventricular arrhythmias when pentamidine isetionate given with ●amisulpride or ●thioridazine—avoid concomitant use

Pentazocine see Opioid Analgesics

Pentostatin

Antiepileptics: cytotoxics reduce absorption of phenytoin

• Antipsychotics: avoid concomitant use of cytotoxics with ●clozapine (increased risk of agranulocytosis)

• Cytotoxics: increased toxicity when pentostatin given with high-dose ●cyclophosphamide—avoid concomitant use; increased pulmonary toxicity when pentostatin given with ●fludarabine (unacceptably high incidence of fatalities)

Pentoxifylline (oxpentifylline)

• Analgesics: possible increased risk of bleeding when pentoxifylline (oxpentifylline) given with NSAIDs; increased risk of bleeding when pentoxifylline (oxpentifylline) given with ●ketorolac (avoid concomitant use)

Theophylline: pentoxifylline (oxpentifylline) increases plasma concentration of theophylline

Pergolide

Antipsychotics: effects of pergolide antagonised by antipsychotics

Memantine: effects of dopaminergics possibly enhanced by memantine

Methyldopa: antiparkinsonian effect of dopaminergics antagonised by methyldopa

Metoclopramide: antiparkinsonian effect of pergolide antagonised by metoclopramide

Pericyazine see Antipsychotics

Perindopril see ACE Inhibitors

Perphenazine see Antipsychotics

Pethidine see Opioid Analgesics

Phenazocine see Opioid Analgesics

Phenelzine see MAOIs

Phenindione

Note. Change in patient's clinical condition particularly associated with liver disease, intercurrent illness, or drug administration, necessitates more frequent testing. Major changes in diet (especially involving salads and vegetables) and in alcohol consumption may also affect anticoagulant control

Phenindione (continued)

- Alcohol: anticoagulant control with phenindione may be affected by major changes in consumption of ●alcohol
- Anabolic Steroids: anticoagulant effect of phenindione enhanced by ●anabolic steroids
- Analgesics: anticoagulant effect of phenindione possibly enhanced by ●NSAIDs; anticoagulant effect of phenindione enhanced by ●diclofenac, also increased risk of haemorrhage with intravenous diclofenac (avoid concomitant use); anticoagulant effect of phenindione enhanced by ●ketorolac (increased risk of haemorrhage—avoid concomitant use); increased risk of bleeding when phenindione given with ●aspirin (due to antiplatelet effect)
- Anti-arrhythmics: metabolism of phenindione inhibited by ●amiodarone (enhanced anticoagulant effect)
- Antibacterials: experience in anticoagulant clinics suggests that INR possibly altered when phenindione is given with ●neomycin (given for local action on gut); anticoagulant effect of phenindione possibly enhanced by levofloxacin and ●tetracyclines; studies have failed to demonstrate an interaction with phenindione, but common experience in anticoagulant clinics is that INR can be altered by a course of broad-spectrum penicillins such as ampicillin
- Antivirals: anticoagulant effect of phenindione possibly enhanced by ●ritonavir
- Clopidogrel: anticoagulant effect of phenindione enhanced due to antiplatelet action of ●clopidogrel
- Dipyridamole: anticoagulant effect of phenindione enhanced due to antiplatelet action of ●dipyridamole
- Enteral Foods: anticoagulant effect of phenindione antagonised by vitamin K (present in some ●enteral feeds)
- Hormone Antagonists: metabolism of phenindione accelerated by ●aminoglutethimide (reduced anticoagulant effect)
- Lipid-regulating Drugs: anticoagulant effect of phenindione may be enhanced or reduced by ●colestyramine; anticoagulant effect of phenindione possibly enhanced by ●rosuvastatin; anticoagulant effect of phenindione enhanced by ●fibrates
- Oestrogens: anticoagulant effect of phenindione antagonised by ●oestrogens
- Progestogens: anticoagulant effect of phenindione antagonised by ●progestogens
- Sibutramine: increased risk of bleeding when anticoagulants given with sibutramine
- Testosterone: anticoagulant effect of phenindione enhanced by ●testosterone
- Thyroid Hormones: anticoagulant effect of phenindione enhanced by ●thyroid hormones
- Vitamins: anticoagulant effect of phenindione antagonised by ●vitamin K

Phenobarbital see Barbiturates
Phenoperidine see Opioid Analgesics
Phenothiazines see Antipsychotics
Phenoxybenzamine see Alpha-blockers
Phenoxymethylpenicillin see Penicillins
Phentolamine see Alpha-blockers
Phenylephrine see Sympathomimetics
Phenylpropanolamine see Sympathomimetics
Phenytoin

- Analgesics: effects of phenytoin possibly enhanced by ●NSAIDs; effects of phenytoin enhanced by ●azapropazone (avoid concomitant use); phenytoin accelerates metabolism of methadone

Phenytoin

- Analgesics (continued)
(reduced effect and risk of withdrawal effects); effects of phenytoin enhanced by aspirin
- Antacids: absorption of phenytoin reduced by antacids
- Anti-arrhythmics: metabolism of phenytoin inhibited by ●amiodarone (increased plasma concentration); phenytoin reduces plasma concentration of disopyramide; phenytoin accelerates metabolism of mexiletine and ●quinidine (reduced plasma concentration)
- Antibacterials: metabolism of phenytoin inhibited by clarithromycin, ●isoniazid and ●metronidazole (increased plasma concentration); plasma concentration of phenytoin increased or decreased by ciprofloxacin; phenytoin accelerates metabolism of doxycycline (reduced plasma concentration); plasma concentration of phenytoin increased by ●chloramphenicol (increased risk of toxicity); metabolism of phenytoin accelerated by ●rifamycins (reduced plasma concentration); plasma concentration of phenytoin possibly increased by sulphonamides; phenytoin reduces plasma concentration of ●telithromycin (avoid during and for 2 weeks after phenytoin); plasma concentration of phenytoin increased by ●trimethoprim (also increased antifolate effect)
- Anticoagulants: phenytoin accelerates metabolism of ●coumarins (possibility of reduced anticoagulant effect, but enhancement also reported)
- Antidepressants: plasma concentration of phenytoin increased by ●fluoxetine and ●fluvoxamine; phenytoin reduces plasma concentration of mianserin, mirtazapine and paroxetine; anticonvulsant effect of antiepileptics possibly antagonised by MAOIs and ●tricyclic-related antidepressants (convulsive threshold lowered); anticonvulsant effect of antiepileptics antagonised by ●SSRIs and ●tricyclics (convulsive threshold lowered); plasma concentration of phenytoin reduced by ●St John's wort—avoid concomitant use; phenytoin possibly reduces plasma concentration of ●tricyclics
- Antidiabetics: plasma concentration of phenytoin transiently increased by tolbutamide (possibility of toxicity)
- Antiepileptics: plasma concentration of both drugs often reduced when phenytoin given with carbamazepine, also plasma concentration of phenytoin may be increased; plasma concentration of phenytoin possibly increased by ●ethosuximide, also plasma concentration of ethosuximide possibly reduced; phenytoin reduces plasma concentration of lamotrigine and tiagabine; plasma concentration of phenytoin increased by oxcarbazepine, also plasma concentration of an active metabolite of oxcarbazepine reduced; phenytoin possibly reduces plasma concentration of primidone (but concentration of an active metabolite increased), plasma concentration of phenytoin often reduced but may be increased; plasma concentration of phenytoin increased by ●topiramate (also plasma concentration of topiramate reduced); plasma concentration of phenytoin increased or possibly reduced when given with valproate, also plasma concentration of valproate reduced; plasma concentration of phenytoin reduced by vigabatrin
- Antifungals: phenytoin reduces plasma concentration of ●itraconazole and ●ketoconazole; anticonvulsant effect of phenytoin enhanced by ●miconazole (plasma concentration of phenytoin

Phenytoin
- Antifungals *(continued)*
  increased); plasma concentration of phenytoin
  increased by ●fluconazole (consider reducing dose
  of phenytoin); plasma concentration of phenytoin
  increased by ●voriconazole, also phenytoin
  reduces plasma concentration of voriconazole
  (increase dose of voriconazole and also monitor
  for phenytoin toxicity); phenytoin reduces plasma
  concentration of caspofungin—
  consider increasing dose of caspofungin
- Antimalarials: possible increased risk of convulsions
  when antiepileptics given with chloroquine and
  hydroxychloroquine; anticonvulsant effect of
  antiepileptics antagonised by ●mefloquine; anticonvulsant effect of phenytoin antagonised by
  ●pyrimethamine, also increased antifolate effect
- Antipsychotics: anticonvulsant effect of phenytoin
  antagonised by ●antipsychotics (convulsive
  threshold lowered); phenytoin accelerates metabolism of clozapine, quetiapine and sertindole
  (reduced plasma concentration)

  Antivirals: phenytoin possibly reduces plasma concentration of indinavir, lopinavir and saquinavir;
  plasma concentration of phenytoin reduced by
  nelfinavir; plasma concentration of phenytoin
  increased or decreased by zidovudine

  Anxiolytics and Hypnotics: phenytoin often reduces
  plasma concentration of clonazepam; plasma
  concentration of phenytoin increased or decreased
  by diazepam; plasma concentration of phenytoin
  possibly increased or decreased by benzodiazepines

  Barbiturates: phenytoin often increases plasma
  concentration of phenobarbital, plasma concentration of phenytoin often reduced but may be
  increased

  Bupropion: phenytoin reduces plasma concentration
  of bupropion
- Calcium-channel Blockers: phenytoin reduces
  effects of felodipine, isradipine and verapamil;
  phenytoin probably reduces effects of dihydropyridines, nicardipine and ●nifedipine; phenytoin
  reduces plasma concentration of nisoldipine;
  plasma concentration of phenytoin increased by
  ●diltiazem but also effect of diltiazem reduced

  Cardiac Glycosides: phenytoin accelerates metabolism of digitoxin (reduced effect); phenytoin
  possibly reduces plasma concentration of digoxin
- Ciclosporin: phenytoin accelerates metabolism of
  ●ciclosporin (reduced plasma concentration)
- Corticosteroids: phenytoin accelerates metabolism
  of corticosteroids (reduced effect)
- Cytotoxics: phenytoin increases antifolate effect of
  methotrexate; absorption of phenytoin reduced by
  cytotoxics; phenytoin reduces plasma concentration of ●imatinib—avoid concomitant use
- Disulfiram: metabolism of phenytoin inhibited by
  ●disulfiram (increased risk of toxicity)

  Diuretics: increased risk of osteomalacia when
  phenytoin given with carbonic anhydrase inhibitors

  Dopaminergics: phenytoin possibly reduces effects
  of levodopa

  Enteral Foods: absorption of phenytoin possibly
  reduced by enteral feeds

  Folates: plasma concentration of phenytoin possibly
  reduced by folates

  Hormone Antagonists: phenytoin accelerates
  metabolism of gestrinone (reduced plasma concentration); phenytoin possibly accelerates
  metabolism of toremifene

Phenytoin *(continued)*
  Leflunomide: plasma concentration of phenytoin
  possibly increased by leflunomide

  Lithium: neurotoxicity may occur when phenytoin
  given with lithium without increased plasma
  concentration of lithium

  Modafinil: plasma concentration of phenytoin possibly increased by modafinil

  Muscle Relaxants: phenytoin antagonises muscle
  relaxant effect of non-depolarising muscle
  relaxants (accelerated recovery from neuromuscular blockade)
- Oestrogens: phenytoin accelerates metabolism of
  ●oestrogens (reduced contraceptive effect—see
  p. 388)
- Progestogens: phenytoin accelerates metabolism of
  ●progestogens (reduced contraceptive effect—see
  p. 388)
- Sulfinpyrazone: plasma concentration of phenytoin
  increased by ●sulfinpyrazone

  Sympathomimetics: plasma concentration of
  phenytoin increased by methylphenidate

  Thyroid Hormones: phenytoin accelerates metabolism of thyroid hormones (may increase requirements in hypothyroidism), also plasma
  concentration of phenytoin possibly increased

  Tibolone: phenytoin accelerates metabolism of
  tibolone
- Ulcer-healing Drugs: metabolism of phenytoin
  inhibited by ●cimetidine (increased plasma concentration); effects of phenytoin enhanced by
  ●esomeprazole; effects of phenytoin possibly
  enhanced by omeprazole; absorption of phenytoin
  reduced by ●sucralfate

  Vaccines: effects of phenytoin enhanced by influenza vaccine

  Vitamins: phenytoin possibly increases requirements
  for vitamin D

Physostigmine *see* Parasympathomimetics
Pilocarpine *see* Parasympathomimetics
Pimozide *see* Antipsychotics
Pindolol *see* Beta-blockers
Pioglitazone *see* Antidiabetics
Piperacillin *see* Penicillins
Pipotiazine *see* Antipsychotics
Piroxicam *see* NSAIDs
Pivmecillinam *see* Penicillins
Pizotifen
  Adrenergic Neurone Blockers: pizotifen antagonises
  hypotensive effect of adrenergic neurone blockers
Platinum Compounds
- Antibacterials: increased risk of nephrotoxicity and
  possibly of ototoxicity when platinum compounds
  given with ●aminoglycosides or ●polymyxins;
  increased risk of nephrotoxicity and ototoxicity
  when platinum compounds given with capreomycin; increased risk of nephrotoxicity and possibly
  of ototoxicity when cisplatin given with vancomycin

  Antiepileptics: cytotoxics reduce absorption of
  phenytoin
- Antipsychotics: avoid concomitant use of cytotoxics
  with ●clozapine (increased risk of agranulocytosis)

  Diuretics: increased risk of nephrotoxicity and
  ototoxicity when platinum compounds given with
  diuretics

Polymyxin B *see* Polymyxins
Polymyxins
  Antibacterials: increased risk of nephrotoxicity when
  colistin or polymyxins given with aminoglycosides; increased risk of nephrotoxicity when
  colistin or polymyxins given with capreomycin;
  increased risk of nephrotoxicity and ototoxicity
  when colistin given with teicoplanin or vanco-

Polymyxins

Antibacterials *(continued)*
mycin; increased risk of nephrotoxicity when polymyxins given with vancomycin
Antifungals: increased risk of nephrotoxicity when polymyxins given with amphotericin
- Ciclosporin: increased risk of nephrotoxicity when polymyxins given with ●ciclosporin
- Cytotoxics: increased risk of nephrotoxicity and possibly of ototoxicity when polymyxins given with ●platinum compounds
- Diuretics: increased risk of otoxicity when polymyxins given with ●loop diuretics
- Muscle Relaxants: polymyxins enhance effects of ●non-depolarising muscle relaxants and ●suxamethonium
Oestrogens: *broad-spectrum* antibacterials possibly reduce contraceptive effect of oestrogens (risk probably small, see p. 388)
- Parasympathomimetics: polymyxins antagonise effects of ●neostigmine and ●pyridostigmine

Potassium Aminobenzoate

Antibacterials: potassium aminobenzoate inhibits effects of sulphonamides

Potassium Bicarbonate *see* Potassium Salts
Potassium Chloride *see* Potassium Salts
Potassium Citrate *see* Potassium Salts

Potassium Salts

Note. Includes salt substitutes
- ACE Inhibitors: increased risk of severe hyperkalaemia when potassium salts given with ●ACE inhibitors
- Angiotensin-II Receptor Antagonists: increased risk of hyperkalaemia when potassium salts given with ●angiotensin-II receptor antagonists
Antibacterials: avoid concomitant use of potassium citrate with methenamine
- Ciclosporin: increased risk of hyperkalaemia when potassium salts given with ●ciclosporin
- Diuretics: increased risk of hyperkalaemia when potassium salts given with ●potassium-sparing diuretics
- Tacrolimus: increased risk of hyperkalaemia when potassium salts given with ●tacrolimus

Pramipexole

Antipsychotics: manufacturer of pramipexole advises avoid concomitant use of antipsychotics (antagonism of effect)
Memantine: effects of dopaminergics possibly enhanced by memantine
Methyldopa: antiparkinsonian effect of dopaminergics antagonised by methyldopa
Ulcer-healing Drugs: excretion of pramipexole reduced by cimetidine (increased plasma concentration)

Pravastatin *see* Statins
Prazosin *see* Alpha-blockers
Prednisolone *see* Corticosteroids

Prilocaine

Antibacterials: increased risk of methaemoglobinaemia when prilocaine given with sulphonamides

Primidone

Alcohol: increased sedative effect when primidone given with alcohol
Anti-arrhythmics: primidone accelerates metabolism of disopyramide and quinidine (reduced plasma concentration)
- Antibacterials: primidone accelerates metabolism of ●chloramphenicol, doxycycline and metronid-

Primidone

- Antibacterials *(continued)*
azole (reduced plasma concentration); primidone reduces plasma concentration of ●telithromycin (avoid during and for 2 weeks after primidone)
- Anticoagulants: primidone accelerates metabolism of ●coumarins (reduced anticoagulant effect)
- Antidepressants: primidone reduces plasma concentration of paroxetine; primidone accelerates metabolism of ●mianserin (reduced plasma concentration); anticonvulsant effect of antiepileptics possibly antagonised by MAOIs and ●tricyclic-related antidepressants (convulsive threshold lowered); anticonvulsant effect of antiepileptics antagonised by ●SSRIs and ●tricyclics (convulsive threshold lowered); plasma concentration of active metabolite of primidone reduced by ●St John's wort—avoid concomitant use; anticonvulsant effect of primidone antagonised by ●tricyclics (convulsive threshold lowered), also metabolism of tricyclics possibly accelerated (reduced plasma concentration)
- Antiepileptics: primidone often reduces plasma concentration of carbamazepine, also plasma concentration of primidone sometimes reduced (but concentration of an active metabolite of primidone often increased); primidone possibly reduces plasma concentration of ethosuximide; primidone reduces plasma concentration of lamotrigine and tiagabine; plasma concentration of an active metabolite of primidone increased by oxcarbazepine, also plasma concentration of an active metabolite of oxcarbazepine reduced; plasma concentration of primidone possibly reduced by phenytoin (but concentration of an active metabolite increased), plasma concentration of phenytoin often reduced but may be increased; plasma concentration of primidone possibly increased by ●valproate (plasma concentration of active metabolite of primidone increased), also plasma concentration of valproate reduced; plasma concentration of primidone possibly reduced by vigabatrin
- Antifungals: primidone possibly reduces plasma concentration of ●voriconazole—avoid concomitant use; primidone reduces absorption of griseofulvin (reduced effect)
- Antimalarials: possible increased risk of convulsions when antiepileptics given with chloroquine and hydroxychloroquine; anticonvulsant effect of antiepileptics antagonised by ●mefloquine
- Antipsychotics: anticonvulsant effect of primidone antagonised by ●antipsychotics (convulsive threshold lowered); primidone accelerates metabolism of haloperidol (reduced plasma concentration)
- Antivirals: primidone possibly reduces plasma concentration of ●indinavir, ●lopinavir, ●nelfinavir and ●saquinavir
Anxiolytics and Hypnotics: primidone often reduces plasma concentration of clonazepam
Barbiturates: increased sedative effect when primidone given with barbiturates
- Calcium-channel Blockers: primidone reduces effects of ●felodipine and ●isradipine; primidone probably reduces effects of ●dihydropyridines, ●diltiazem and ●verapamil
Cardiac Glycosides: primidone accelerates metabolism of digitoxin (reduced effect)
- Ciclosporin: primidone accelerates metabolism of ●ciclosporin (reduced effect)
- Corticosteroids: primidone accelerates metabolism of ●corticosteroids (reduced effect)

Primidone *(continued)*

Diuretics: plasma concentration of primidone possibly reduced by acetazolamide; increased risk of osteomalacia when primidone given with carbonic anhydrase inhibitors

Folates: plasma concentration of primidone possibly reduced by folates

Hormone Antagonists: primidone accelerates metabolism of gestrinone and toremifene (reduced plasma concentration)

Leukotriene Antagonists: primidone reduces plasma concentration of montelukast

Memantine: effects of primidone possibly reduced by memantine

● Oestrogens: primidone accelerates metabolism of ●oestrogens (reduced contraceptive effect—see p. 388)

● Progestogens: primidone accelerates metabolism of ●progestogens (reduced contraceptive effect—see p. 388)

Sympathomimetics: plasma concentration of primidone possibly increased by methylphenidate

Theophylline: primidone accelerates metabolism of theophylline (reduced effect)

Thyroid Hormones: primidone accelerates metabolism of thyroid hormones (may increase requirements for thyroid hormones in hypothyroidism)

Tibolone: primidone accelerates metabolism of tibolone (reduced plasma concentration)

Tropisetron: primidone reduces plasma concentration of tropisetron

Vitamins: primidone possibly increases requirements for vitamin D

Probenecid

ACE Inhibitors: probenecid reduces excretion of captopril

● Analgesics: probenecid reduces excretion of ●indometacin, ●ketoprofen and ●naproxen (increased plasma concentration); probenecid reduces excretion of ●ketorolac (increased plasma concentration)—avoid concomitant use; effects of probenecid antagonised by aspirin

Antibacterials: probenecid reduces excretion of meropenem (manufacturers of meropenem advise avoid concomitant use); probenecid reduces excretion of cephalosporins, ciprofloxacin, nalidixic acid, norfloxacin and penicillins (increased plasma concentration); probenecid reduces excretion of dapsone and nitrofurantoin (increased risk of side-effects); effects of probenecid antagonised by pyrazinamide

Antidiabetics: probenecid possibly enhances hypoglycaemic effect of chlorpropamide

Antivirals: probenecid reduces excretion of aciclovir (increased plasma concentration); probenecid possibly reduces excretion of famciclovir and zalcitabine (increased plasma concentration); probenecid reduces excretion of ganciclovir and zidovudine (increased plasma concentration and risk of toxicity)

● Cytotoxics: probenecid reduces excretion of ●methotrexate (increased risk of toxicity)

Procainamide

ACE Inhibitors: increased risk of toxicity when procainamide given with captopril especially in renal impairment

● Adrenergic Neurone Blockers: increased myocardial depression when anti-arrhythmics given with ●bretylium

Anaesthetics, Local: increased myocardial depression when anti-arrhythmics given with bupivacaine or levobupivacaine

● Anti-arrhythmics: increased myocardial depression when anti-arrhythmics given with other ●anti-

Procainamide

● Anti-arrhythmics *(continued)*
arrhythmics; plasma concentration of procainamide increased by ●amiodarone (increased risk of ventricular arrhythmias—avoid concomitant use)

● Antibacterials: increased risk of ventricular arrhythmias when procainamide given with ●moxifloxacin—avoid concomitant use; plasma concentration of procainamide increased by trimethoprim

● Antidepressants: increased risk of ventricular arrhythmias when procainamide given with ●tricyclics

● Antihistamines: increased risk of ventricular arrhythmias when procainamide given with ●mizolastine or ●terfenadine—avoid concomitant use; increased risk of ventricular arrhythmias when anti-arrhythmics given with ●terfenadine

● Antimalarials: avoidance of procainamide advised by manufacturer of ●artemether/lumefantrine (risk of ventricular arrhythmias)

● Antipsychotics: increased risk of ventricular arrhythmias when anti-arrhythmics that prolong the QT interval given with ●antipsychotics that prolong the QT interval; increased risk of ventricular arrhythmias when procainamide given with ●amisulpride, ●pimozide, ●sertindole or ●thioridazine—avoid concomitant use; increased risk of ventricular arrhythmias when procainamide given with ●phenothiazines

● Beta-blockers: increased myocardial depression when anti-arrhythmics given with ●beta-blockers; increased risk of ventricular arrhythmias when procainamide given with ●sotalol—avoid concomitant use

● Dolasetron: increased risk of ventricular arrhythmias when procainamide given with ●dolasetron—avoid concomitant use

● Muscle Relaxants: procainamide enhances effects of ●muscle relaxants

Parasympathomimetics: procainamide antagonises effects of neostigmine and pyridostigmine

Tropisetron: caution with anti-arrhythmics advised by manufacturer of tropisetron (risk of ventricular arrhythmias)

● Ulcer-healing Drugs: plasma concentration of procainamide increased by ●cimetidine

Procarbazine

Alcohol: disulfiram-like reaction when procarbazine given with alcohol

Antiepileptics: cytotoxics reduce absorption of phenytoin

● Antipsychotics: avoid concomitant use of cytotoxics with ●clozapine (increased risk of agranulocytosis)

Prochlorperazine *see* Antipsychotics

Procyclidine *see* Antimuscarinics

Progesterone *see* Progestogens

Progestogens

Note. Interactions of combined oral contraceptives may also apply to combined contraceptive patches

ACE Inhibitors: risk of hyperkalaemia when drospirenone given with ACE inhibitors (monitor serum potassium during first cycle)

Analgesics: risk of hyperkalaemia when drospirenone given with NSAIDs (monitor serum potassium during first cycle)

Angiotensin-II Receptor Antagonists: risk of hyperkalaemia when drospirenone given with angiotensin-II receptor antagonists (monitor serum potassium during first cycle)

● Antibacterials: metabolism of progestogens accelerated by ●rifamycins (reduced contraceptive effect—see p. 388)

● Anticoagulants: progestogens antagonise anticoagulant effect of ●coumarins and ●phenindione

Progestogens *(continued)*

- Antidepressants: contraceptive effect of progestogens reduced by ●St John's wort (avoid concomitant use)

  Antidiabetics: progestogens antagonise hypoglycaemic effect of antidiabetics

- Antiepileptics: metabolism of progestogens accelerated by ●carbamazepine, ●oxcarbazepine, ●phenytoin, ●primidone and ●topiramate (reduced contraceptive effect—see p. 388)

- Antifungals: metabolism of progestogens accelerated by ●griseofulvin (reduced contraceptive effect—see p. 388); occasional reports of breakthrough bleeding when progestogens (used for contraception) given with terbinafine

- Antivirals: contraceptive effect of progestogens possibly reduced by amprenavir; metabolism of progestogens accelerated by ●nevirapine (reduced contraceptive effect—see p. 388)

- Barbiturates: metabolism of progestogens accelerated by ●barbiturates (reduced contraceptive effect—see p. 388)

- Bosentan: possible contraceptive failure of hormonal contraceptives containing progestogens when given with ●bosentan (alternative contraception recommended)

- Ciclosporin: progestogens inhibit metabolism of ●ciclosporin (increased plasma concentration)

  Diuretics: risk of hyperkalaemia when drospirenone given with potassium-sparing diuretics (monitor serum potassium during first cycle)

  Hormone Antagonists: plasma concentration of medroxyprogesterone reduced by aminoglutethimide

  Lipid-regulating Drugs: plasma concentration of norgestrel increased by rosuvastatin

- Retinoids: efficacy of low dose progestogens may be reduced by ●tretinoin but need not affect prescribing of combined oral contraceptives, there is no compelling evidence of interaction between isotretinoin and combined oral contraceptives

  Tacrolimus: contraceptive effect of progestogens possibly reduced by tacrolimus

Proguanil

  Antacids: absorption of proguanil reduced by oral magnesium salts (as magnesium trisilicate)

  Anticoagulants: isolated reports that proguanil may enhance anticoagulant effect of warfarin

- Antimalarials: avoidance of antimalarials advised by manufacturer of ●artemether/lumefantrine; increased antifolate effect when proguanil given with pyrimethamine

Promazine *see* Antipsychotics

Promethazine *see* Antihistamines

Propafenone

- Adrenergic Neurone Blockers: increased myocardial depression when anti-arrhythmics given with ●bretylium

  Anaesthetics, Local: increased myocardial depression when anti-arrhythmics given with bupivacaine or levobupivacaine

- Anti-arrhythmics: increased myocardial depression when anti-arrhythmics given with other ●anti-arrhythmics; plasma concentration of propafenone increased by quinidine

- Antibacterials: metabolism of propafenone accelerated by ●rifampicin (reduced effect)

- Anticoagulants: propafenone enhances anticoagulant effect of ●coumarins

- Antidepressants: increased risk of arrhythmias when propafenone given with ●tricyclics

- Antihistamines: increased risk of ventricular arrhythmias when propafenone given with ●mizolastine or ●terfenadine—avoid concomitant use;

Propafenone

- Antihistamines *(continued)*
  increased risk of ventricular arrhythmias when anti-arrhythmics given with ●terfenadine

- Antipsychotics: increased risk of ventricular arrhythmias when anti-arrhythmics that prolong the QT interval given with ●antipsychotics that prolong the QT interval

- Antivirals: plasma concentration of propafenone increased by ●ritonavir (increased risk of ventricular arrhythmias—avoid concomitant use)

- Beta-blockers: increased myocardial depression when anti-arrhythmics given with ●beta-blockers; propafenone increases plasma concentration of metoprolol and propranolol

- Cardiac Glycosides: propafenone increases plasma concentration of ●digoxin (halve dose of digoxin)

  Ciclosporin: propafenone possibly increases plasma concentration of ciclosporin

- Dolasetron: increased risk of ventricular arrhythmias when propafenone given with ●dolasetron—avoid concomitant use

  Parasympathomimetics: propafenone possibly antagonises effects of neostigmine and pyridostigmine

  Theophylline: propafenone increases plasma concentration of theophylline

  Tropisetron: caution with anti-arrhythmics advised by manufacturer of tropisetron (risk of ventricular arrhythmias)

- Ulcer-healing Drugs: plasma concentration of propafenone increased by ●cimetidine

Propantheline *see* Antimuscarinics

Propiverine *see* Antimuscarinics

Propofol *see* Anaesthetics, General

Propranolol *see* Beta-blockers

Prostaglandins

  Oxytocin: prostaglandins potentiate uterotonic effect of oxytocin

Proton Pump Inhibitors

  Analgesics: plasma concentration of omeprazole increased by valdecoxib

  Antacids: absorption of lansoprazole possibly reduced by antacids

  Antibacterials: plasma concentration of both drugs increased when omeprazole given with clarithromycin

- Anticoagulants: esomeprazole and omeprazole possibly enhance anticoagulant effect of ●coumarins

- Antiepileptics: omeprazole possibly enhances effects of phenytoin; esomeprazole enhances effects of ●phenytoin

  Antifungals: proton pump inhibitors reduce absorption of itraconazole and ketoconazole; plasma concentration of omeprazole increased by voriconazole (reduce dose of omeprazole)

  Anxiolytics and Hypnotics: esomeprazole and omeprazole possibly inhibit metabolism of diazepam (increased plasma concentration)

  Cardiac Glycosides: proton pump inhibitors possibly slightly increase plasma concentration of digoxin

  Ciclosporin: omeprazole possibly affects plasma concentration of ciclosporin

- Cilostazol: omeprazole increases plasma concentration of ●cilostazol (risk of toxicity)—avoid concomitant use; lansoprazole possibly increases plasma concentration of ●cilostazol—avoid concomitant use

  Cytotoxics: omeprazole possibly reduces excretion of methotrexate (possibly increased risk of toxicity)

  Tacrolimus: omeprazole possibly increases plasma concentration of tacrolimus

Proton Pump Inhibitors *(continued)*
Ulcer-healing Drugs: absorption of lansoprazole possibly reduced by sucralfate
Pseudoephedrine *see* Sympathomimetics
Pyrazinamide
Oestrogens: *broad-spectrum* antibacterials possibly reduce contraceptive effect of oestrogens (risk probably small, see p. 388)
Probenecid: pyrazinamide antagonises effects of probenecid
Sulfinpyrazone: pyrazinamide antagonises effects of sulfinpyrazone
Pyridostigmine *see* Parasympathomimetics
Pyridoxine *see* Vitamins
Pyrimethamine
● Antibacterials: increased antifolate effect when pyrimethamine (includes Fansidar®) given with ●sulphonamides; increased antifolate effect when pyrimethamine given with ●trimethoprim
● Antiepileptics: pyrimethamine antagonises anticonvulsant effect of ●phenytoin, also increased antifolate effect
● Antimalarials: avoidance of antimalarials advised by manufacturer of ●artemether/lumefantrine; increased antifolate effect when pyrimethamine given with proguanil
Antivirals: increased antifolate effect when pyrimethamine given with zidovudine
● Cytotoxics: pyrimethamine increases antifolate effect of ●methotrexate
Quetiapine *see* Antipsychotics
Quinagolide
Memantine: effects of dopaminergics possibly enhanced by memantine
Methyldopa: antiparkinsonian effect of dopaminergics antagonised by methyldopa
Quinapril *see* ACE Inhibitors
Quinidine
● Adrenergic Neurone Blockers: increased myocardial depression when anti-arrhythmics given with ●bretylium
Adsorbents: absorption of quinidine possibly reduced by kaolin
Anaesthetics, Local: increased myocardial depression when anti-arrhythmics given with bupivacaine or levobupivacaine
Antacids: excretion of quinidine reduced by alkaline urine due to some antacids (plasma concentration of quinidine occasionally increased)
● Anti-arrhythmics: increased myocardial depression when anti-arrhythmics given with other ●anti-arrhythmics; plasma concentration of quinidine increased by ●amiodarone (increased risk of ventricular arrhythmias—avoid concomitant use); quinidine increases plasma concentration of propafenone
● Antibacterials: increased risk of ventricular arrhythmias when quinidine given with ●moxifloxacin or ●quinupristin/dalfopristin—avoid concomitant use; metabolism of quinidine accelerated by ●rifamycins (reduced plasma concentration)
● Anticoagulants: quinidine possibly enhances anticoagulant effect of ●coumarins
● Antidepressants: increased risk of ventricular arrhythmias when quinidine given with ●tricyclics
● Antiepileptics: metabolism of quinidine accelerated by ●phenytoin and primidone (reduced plasma concentration)
● Antifungals: plasma concentration of quinidine increased by ●itraconazole, ●miconazole and ●voriconazole (increased risk of ventricular arrhythmias—avoid concomitant use)
● Antihistamines: increased risk of ventricular arrhythmias when quinidine given with ●mizolastine or

Quinidine
● Antihistamines *(continued)*
●terfenadine—avoid concomitant use; increased risk of ventricular arrhythmias when anti-arrhythmics given with ●terfenadine
● Antimalarials: avoidance of quinidine advised by manufacturer of ●artemether/lumefantrine (risk of ventricular arrhythmias); increased risk of ventricular arrhythmias when quinidine given with ●mefloquine
● Antipsychotics: increased risk of ventricular arrhythmias when anti-arrhythmics that prolong the QT interval given with ●antipsychotics that prolong the QT interval; increased risk of ventricular arrhythmias when quinidine given with ●amisulpride, ●pimozide, ●sertindole or ●thioridazine—avoid concomitant use; increased risk of ventricular arrhythmias when quinidine given with ●phenothiazines
● Antivirals: increased risk of ventricular arrhythmias when quinidine given with ●nelfinavir—avoid concomitant use; plasma concentration of quinidine increased by ●ritonavir (increased risk of ventricular arrhythmias—avoid concomitant use)
Barbiturates: metabolism of quinidine accelerated by barbiturates (reduced plasma concentration)
● Beta-blockers: increased myocardial depression when anti-arrhythmics given with ●beta-blockers; increased risk of ventricular arrhythmias when quinidine given with ●sotalol—avoid concomitant use
● Calcium-channel Blockers: plasma concentration of quinidine reduced by nifedipine; plasma concentration of quinidine increased by ●verapamil (extreme hypotension may occur)
● Cardiac Glycosides: quinidine increases plasma concentration of ●digoxin (halve dose of digoxin)
● Diuretics: excretion of quinidine reduced by ●acetazolamide (occasionally increased plasma concentration), also cardiac toxicity of quinidine increased if hypokalaemia occurs; increased cardiac toxicity with quinidine if hypokalaemia occurs with ●loop diuretics or ●thiazides and related diuretics
● Muscle Relaxants: quinidine enhances effects of ●muscle relaxants
Parasympathomimetics: quinidine antagonises effects of neostigmine and pyridostigmine
Tropisetron: caution with anti-arrhythmics advised by manufacturer of tropisetron (risk of ventricular arrhythmias)
● Ulcer-healing Drugs: plasma concentration of quinidine increased by ●cimetidine

Quinine
● Anti-arrhythmics: increased risk of ventricular arrhythmias when quinine given with ●amiodarone—avoid concomitant use; quinine increases plasma concentration of ●flecainide
● Antibacterials: increased risk of ventricular arrhythmias when quinine given with ●moxifloxacin—avoid concomitant use
● Antihistamines: increased risk of ventricular arrhythmias when quinine given with ●terfenadine—avoid concomitant use
● Antimalarials: avoidance of antimalarials advised by manufacturer of ●artemether/lumefantrine; increased risk of convulsions when quinine given with ●mefloquine (but should not prevent the use of intravenous quinine in severe cases)
● Antipsychotics: increased risk of ventricular arrhythmias when quinine given with ●pimozide or ●thioridazine—avoid concomitant use

Quinine *(continued)*
- Cardiac Glycosides: quinine increases plasma concentration of ●digoxin
- Muscle Relaxants: quinine possibly enhances effects of suxamethonium
- Ulcer-healing Drugs: metabolism of quinine inhibited by cimetidine (increased plasma concentration)

Quinolones
- Analgesics: possible increased risk of convulsions when quinolones given with ●NSAIDs; manufacturer of ciprofloxacin advises avoid premedication with opioid analgesics (reduced plasma concentration of ciprofloxacin) when ciprofloxacin used for surgical prophylaxis
- Antacids: absorption of ciprofloxacin, levofloxacin, moxifloxacin, norfloxacin and ofloxacin reduced by antacids
- Anti-arrhythmics: increased risk of ventricular arrhythmias when moxifloxacin given with ●amiodarone, ●disopyramide, ●procainamide or ●quinidine—avoid concomitant use
- Antibacterials: increased risk of ventricular arrhythmias when moxifloxacin given with parenteral ●erythromycin—avoid concomitant use
- Anticoagulants: levofloxacin possibly enhances anticoagulant effect of coumarins and phenindione; ciprofloxacin, nalidixic acid, norfloxacin and ofloxacin enhance anticoagulant effect of ●coumarins
- Antidepressants: increased risk of ventricular arrhythmias when moxifloxacin given with ●tricyclics—avoid concomitant use
- Antidiabetics: ciprofloxacin possibly enhances effects of glibenclamide
- Antiepileptics: ciprofloxacin increases or decreases plasma concentration of phenytoin
- Antihistamines: increased risk of ventricular arrhythmias when moxifloxacin given with ●mizolastine or ●terfenadine—avoid concomitant use
- Antimalarials: avoidance of quinolones advised by manufacturer of ●artemether/lumefantrine; increased risk of ventricular arrhythmias when moxifloxacin given with ●chloroquine and hydroxychloroquine, ●mefloquine or ●quinine—avoid concomitant use
- Antipsychotics: increased risk of ventricular arrhythmias when moxifloxacin given with ●haloperidol, ●phenothiazines, ●pimozide or ●sertindole—avoid concomitant use
- Beta-blockers: increased risk of ventricular arrhythmias when moxifloxacin given with ●sotalol—avoid concomitant use
- Calcium Salts: absorption of ciprofloxacin reduced by calcium salts
- Ciclosporin: increased risk of nephrotoxicity when quinolones given with ●ciclosporin
- Cytotoxics: nalidixic acid increases risk of melphalan toxicity; ciprofloxacin possibly reduces excretion of methotrexate (possibly increased risk of toxicity)
- Dairy Products: absorption of ciprofloxacin and norfloxacin reduced by dairy products
- 5HT$_1$ Agonists: quinolones possibly inhibit metabolism of zolmitriptan (reduce dose of zolmitriptan)
- Iron: absorption of ciprofloxacin, levofloxacin, moxifloxacin, norfloxacin and ofloxacin reduced by *oral* iron
- Oestrogens: *broad-spectrum* antibacterials possibly reduce contraceptive effect of oestrogens (risk probably small, see p. 388)
- Pentamidine Isetionate: increased risk of ventricular arrhythmias when moxifloxacin given with ●pentamidine isetionate—avoid concomitant use

Quinolones *(continued)*
- Probenecid: excretion of ciprofloxacin, nalidixic acid and norfloxacin reduced by probenecid (increased plasma concentration)
- Theophylline: possible increased risk of convulsions when quinolones given with ●theophylline; ciprofloxacin and norfloxacin increase plasma concentration of ●theophylline
- Ulcer-healing Drugs: absorption of ciprofloxacin, levofloxacin, moxifloxacin, norfloxacin and ofloxacin reduced by sucralfate
- Zinc: absorption of ciprofloxacin, levofloxacin, moxifloxacin, norfloxacin and ofloxacin reduced by zinc

Quinupristin with Dalfopristin
- Anti-arrhythmics: increased risk of ventricular arrhythmias when quinupristin/dalfopristin given with ●disopyramide, ●lidocaine (lignocaine) or ●quinidine—avoid concomitant use
- Antibacterials: manufacturer of quinupristin/dalfopristin recommends monitoring liver function when given with rifampicin
- Antihistamines: increased risk of ventricular arrhythmias when quinupristin/dalfopristin given with ●terfenadine—avoid concomitant use
- Antivirals: quinupristin/dalfopristin possibly increases plasma concentration of saquinavir
- Anxiolytics and Hypnotics: quinupristin/dalfopristin inhibits metabolism of ●midazolam (increased plasma concentration with increased sedation); quinupristin/dalfopristin inhibits the metabolism of zopiclone
- Calcium-channel Blockers: quinupristin/dalfopristin increases plasma concentration of ●nifedipine
- Ciclosporin: quinupristin/dalfopristin increases plasma concentration of ●ciclosporin
- Ergot Alkaloids: manufacturer of quinupristin/dalfopristin advises avoid concomitant use with ●ergotamine and methysergide
- Oestrogens: *broad-spectrum* antibacterials possibly reduce contraceptive effect of oestrogens (risk probably small, see p. 388)
- Tacrolimus: quinupristin/dalfopristin increases plasma concentration of ●tacrolimus

Rabeprazole *see* Proton Pump Inhibitors

Raloxifene
- Anticoagulants: raloxifene antagonises anticoagulant effect of coumarins
- Lipid-regulating Drugs: absorption of raloxifene reduced by colestyramine (manufacturer of raloxifene advises avoid concomitant administration)

Ramipril *see* ACE Inhibitors

Ranitidine *see* Histamine H$_2$-antagonists

Ranitidine Bismuth Citrate *see* Histamine H$_2$-antagonists

Reboxetine
- Antibacterials: manufacturer of reboxetine advises avoid concomitant use with ●macrolides
- Antidepressants: manufacturer of reboxetine advises avoid concomitant use with ●fluvoxamine; increased risk of hypertension and CNS excitation when reboxetine given with ●MAOIs (MAOIs should not be started until 1 week after stopping reboxetine, avoid reboxetine for 2 weeks after stopping MAOIs)
- Antifungals: manufacturer of reboxetine advises avoid concomitant use with ●imidazoles and ●triazoles
- Antimalarials: avoidance of antidepressants advised by manufacturer of ●artemether/lumefantrine
- Diuretics: possible increased risk of hypokalaemia when reboxetine given with loop diuretics or thiazides and related diuretics

Reboxetine *(continued)*

Ergot Alkaloids: possible risk of hypertension when reboxetine given with ergotamine and methysergide

- Sibutramine: increased risk of CNS toxicity when noradrenaline re-uptake inhibitors given with ●sibutramine (manufacturer of sibutramine advises avoid concomitant use)

Remifentanil *see* Opioid Analgesics

Repaglinide *see* Antidiabetics

Retinoids

Alcohol: etretinate formed from acitretin in presence of alcohol

- Antibacterials: possible increased risk of benign intracranial hypertension when retinoids given with ●tetracyclines (avoid concomitant use)
- Anticoagulants: acitretin possibly reduces anticoagulant effect of ●coumarins

Antiepileptics: isotretinoin possibly reduces plasma concentration of carbamazepine

- Cytotoxics: acitretin increases plasma concentration of ●methotrexate (also increased risk of hepatotoxicity)—avoid concomitant use
- Progestogens: oral tretinoin may reduce contraceptive efficacy of low dose ●progestogens but need not affect prescribing of combined oral contraceptives, there is no compelling evidence of interaction between isotretinoin and combined oral contraceptives

Vitamins: risk of hypervitaminosis A when retinoids given with vitamin A

Reviparin *see* Heparins

Ribavirin

- Antivirals: ribavirin possibly inhibits effects of ●stavudine; ribavirin possibly inhibits effects of ●zidovudine (manufacturer of zidovudine advises avoid concomitant use)

Rifabutin *see* Rifamycins

Rifampicin *see* Rifamycins

Rifamycins

ACE Inhibitors: rifampicin reduces plasma concentration of active metabolite of imidapril (reduced antihypertensive effect)

Analgesics: rifampicin reduces plasma concentration of etoricoxib and rofecoxib; rifampicin accelerates metabolism of methadone (reduced effect)

Antacids: absorption of rifampicin reduced by antacids

- Anti-arrhythmics: rifamycins accelerate metabolism of ●disopyramide and ●quinidine (reduced plasma concentration); rifampicin accelerates metabolism of mexiletine (reduced plasma concentration); rifampicin accelerates metabolism of ●propafenone (reduced effect)
- Antibacterials: plasma concentration of rifabutin increased by ●clarithromycin (increased risk of uveitis—reduce rifabutin dose); rifampicin accelerates metabolism of chloramphenicol (reduced plasma concentration); rifamycins reduce plasma concentration of dapsone; plasma concentration of rifabutin possibly increased by ●macrolides (increased risk of uveitis—reduce rifabutin dose); monitoring of liver function with rifampicin recommended by manufacturer of quinupristin/dalfopristin; rifampicin reduces plasma concentration of ●telithromycin (avoid during and for 2 weeks after rifampicin)
- Anticoagulants: rifamycins accelerate metabolism of ●coumarins (reduced anticoagulant effect)

Antidepressants: rifampicin possibly reduces plasma concentration of tricyclics

- Antidiabetics: rifamycins accelerate metabolism of ●chlorpropamide and ●tolbutamide (reduced effect); rifampicin reduces plasma concentration of

Rifamycins

- Antidiabetics *(continued)*

nateglinide and repaglinide; rifamycins possibly accelerate metabolism of ●sulphonylureas (reduced effect)

- Antiepileptics: rifabutin reduces plasma concentration of ●carbamazepine; rifamycins accelerate metabolism of ●phenytoin (reduced plasma concentration)
- Antifungals: rifampicin accelerates metabolism of ●ketoconazole (reduced plasma concentration), also plasma concentration of rifampicin may be reduced by ketoconazole; plasma concentration of rifabutin increased by ●fluconazole (increased risk of uveitis—reduce rifabutin dose); rifampicin accelerates metabolism of ●fluconazole and ●itraconazole (reduced plasma concentration); plasma concentration of rifabutin increased by ●voriconazole, also rifabutin reduces plasma concentration of voriconazole (increase dose of voriconazole and also monitor for rifabutin toxicity); rifampicin reduces plasma concentration of ●voriconazole—avoid concomitant use; rifampicin initially increases and then reduces plasma concentration of caspofungin (consider increasing dose of caspofungin); rifampicin reduces plasma concentration of terbinafine; plasma concentration of rifabutin possibly increased by ●triazoles (increased risk of uveitis—reduce rifabutin dose)
- Antipsychotics: rifampicin accelerates metabolism of ●haloperidol (reduced plasma concentration); rifampicin possibly reduces plasma concentration of clozapine
- Antivirals: rifampicin significantly reduces plasma concentration of ●amprenavir and ●nelfinavir—avoid concomitant use; plasma concentration of rifabutin increased by ●amprenavir and ●nelfinavir (halve dose of rifabutin); plasma concentration of rifabutin reduced by efavirenz—increase dose of rifabutin; rifampicin reduces plasma concentration of efavirenz—increase dose of efavirenz; rifampicin accelerates metabolism of ●indinavir (reduced plasma concentration—avoid concomitant use); plasma concentration of rifabutin increases (reduce dose) and plasma concentration of ●indinavir decreases (increase dose) when given together; rifampicin reduces plasma concentration of ●lopinavir and ●nevirapine—avoid concomitant use; plasma concentration of rifabutin increased by ●ritonavir (risk of uveitis—avoid concomitant use); rifamycins significantly reduce plasma concentration of ●saquinavir—avoid concomitant use unless another protease inhibitor also given e.g. ritonavir; avoidance of rifampicin advised by manufacturer of zidovudine

Anxiolytics and Hypnotics: rifampicin accelerates metabolism of diazepam (reduced plasma concentration); rifampicin possibly accelerates metabolism of benzodiazepines (possibly reduced plasma concentration); rifampicin possibly accelerates metabolism of buspirone and zaleplon; rifampicin accelerates metabolism of zolpidem (reduced plasma concentration and reduced effect)

- Atovaquone: rifabutin and rifampicin reduce plasma concentration of ●atovaquone (possible therapeutic failure of atovaquone)

Beta-blockers: rifampicin accelerates metabolism of bisoprolol and propranolol (plasma concentration significantly reduced)

- Calcium-channel Blockers: rifampicin possibly accelerates metabolism of ●isradipine, ●nicardipine and ●nisoldipine (possible significantly reduced plasma concentration); rifampicin accel-

Rifamycins

- Calcium-channel Blockers *(continued)* erates metabolism of ●diltiazem, ●nifedipine, ●nimodipine and ●verapamil (plasma concentration significantly reduced)

  Cardiac Glycosides: rifamycins accelerate metabolism of digitoxin (reduced effect); rifampicin possibly reduces plasma concentration of digoxin
- Ciclosporin: rifampicin accelerates metabolism of ●ciclosporin (reduced plasma concentration)
- Corticosteroids: rifamycins accelerate metabolism of ●corticosteroids (reduced effect)
- Cytotoxics: interaction with rifampicin reported by manufacturer of ●azathioprine (transplants possibly rejected); rifampicin reduces plasma concentration of ●imatinib—avoid concomitant use

  Hormone Antagonists: rifampicin accelerates metabolism of gestrinone (reduced plasma concentration)

  Lipid-regulating Drugs: rifampicin accelerates metabolism of fluvastatin (reduced effect)
- Oestrogens: rifamycins accelerate metabolism of ●oestrogens (reduced contraceptive effect—see p. 388); *broad-spectrum* antibacterials possibly reduce contraceptive effect of oestrogens (risk probably small, see p. 388)
- Progestogens: rifamycins accelerate metabolism of ●progestogens (reduced contraceptive effect—see p. 388)
- Sirolimus: rifampicin reduces plasma concentration of ●sirolimus
- Tacrolimus: rifampicin reduces plasma concentration of ●tacrolimus

  Tadalafil: rifampicin reduces plasma concentration of tadalafil

  Theophylline: rifampicin accelerates metabolism of theophylline (reduced plasma concentration)

  Thyroid Hormones: rifampicin accelerates metabolism of levothyroxine (thyroxine) (may increase requirements for levothyroxine (thyroxine) in hypothyroidism)

  Tibolone: rifampicin accelerates metabolism of tibolone (reduced plasma concentration)

  Tropisetron: rifampicin reduces plasma concentration of tropisetron

  Ulcer-healing Drugs: rifampicin accelerates metabolism of cimetidine (reduced plasma concentration)

Riluzole

Note. No clinical data available but since riluzole extensively metabolised by the liver, possibility of interactions with a number of drugs—consult product literature

Risedronate Sodium *see* Bisphosphonates

Risperidone *see* Antipsychotics

Ritodrine *see* Sympathomimetics, Beta$_2$

Ritonavir

- Analgesics: ritonavir possibly increases plasma concentration of NSAIDs; ritonavir increases plasma concentration of ●dextropropoxyphene, ●pethidine and ●piroxicam (risk of toxicity)—avoid concomitant use; ritonavir increases plasma concentration of ●fentanyl; ritonavir reduces plasma concentration of methadone; ritonavir possibly increases plasma concentration of ●opioid analgesics (except methadone)
- Anti-arrhythmics: ritonavir increases plasma concentration of ●amiodarone, ●flecainide, ●propafenone and ●quinidine (increased risk of ventricular arrhythmias—avoid concomitant use); ritonavir possibly increases plasma concentration of ●disopyramide and ●mexiletine (increased risk of toxicity)

Ritonavir *(continued)*

- Antibacterials: ritonavir possibly increases plasma concentration of azithromycin and erythromycin; ritonavir increases plasma concentration of ●clarithromycin (reduce dose of clarithromycin in renal impairment); ritonavir increases plasma concentration of ●rifabutin (risk of uveitis—avoid concomitant use)
- Anticoagulants: ritonavir possibly enhances anticoagulant effect of ●coumarins and ●phenindione
- Antidepressants: ritonavir possibly increases plasma concentration of ●SSRIs and ●tricyclics; plasma concentration of ritonavir reduced by ●St John's wort—avoid concomitant use

  Antidiabetics: ritonavir possibly increases plasma concentration of tolbutamide
- Antiepileptics: ritonavir possibly increases plasma concentration of ●carbamazepine
- Antifungals: combination of ritonavir with ●itraconazole or ●ketoconazole may increase plasma concentration of either drug (or both); plasma concentration of ritonavir increased by fluconazole
- Antihistamines: increased risk of ventricular arrhythmias when ritonavir given with ●terfenadine—avoid concomitant use; ritonavir possibly increases plasma concentration of non-sedating antihistamines

  Antimuscarinics: avoidance of ritonavir advised by manufacturer of tolterodine
- Antipsychotics: ritonavir possibly increases plasma concentration of ●antipsychotics; ritonavir increases plasma concentration of ●clozapine (increased risk of toxicity)—avoid concomitant use; ritonavir increases plasma concentration of ●pimozide and ●sertindole (increased risk of ventricular arrhythmias—avoid concomitant use)
- Antivirals: plasma concentration of both drugs increased when ritonavir given with amprenavir; ritonavir increases toxicity of efavirenz, monitor liver function tests; ritonavir increases plasma concentration of indinavir and ●saquinavir; combination of ritonavir with nelfinavir may increase plasma concentration of either drug (or both)
- Anxiolytics and Hypnotics: ritonavir possibly increases plasma concentration of ●anxiolytics and hypnotics; ritonavir possibly increases plasma concentration of ●alprazolam, ●clorazepate, ●diazepam, ●flurazepam, ●midazolam and ●zolpidem (risk of extreme sedation and respiratory depression —avoid concomitant use)

  Bosentan: ritonavir possibly increases plasma concentration of bosentan
- Bupropion: ritonavir increases plasma concentration of ●bupropion (risk of toxicity)—avoid concomitant use
- Calcium-channel Blockers: ritonavir possibly increases plasma concentration of ●calcium-channel blockers; avoidance of ritonavir advised by manufacturer of lercanidipine
- Ciclosporin: ritonavir possibly increases plasma concentration of ●ciclosporin
- Cilostazol: ritonavir possibly increases plasma concentration of ●cilostazol—avoid concomitant use

  Corticosteroids: ritonavir possibly increases plasma concentration of corticosteroids, dexamethasone and prednisolone
- Ergot Alkaloids: increased risk of ergotism when ritonavir given with ●ergotamine and methysergide—avoid concomitant use
- 5HT$_1$ Agonists: ritonavir increases plasma concentration of ●eletriptan (risk of toxicity)—avoid concomitant use

Ritonavir *(continued)*
- Lipid-regulating Drugs: increased risk of myopathy when ritonavir given with ●simvastatin (avoid concomitant use)
- Oestrogens: ritonavir accelerates metabolism of ●●oestrogens (reduced contraceptive effect—see p. 388)
- Sildenafil: ritonavir significantly increases plasma concentration of ●sildenafil—avoid concomitant use
- Tacrolimus: ritonavir possibly increases plasma concentration of ●tacrolimus
- Tadalafil: ritonavir increases plasma concentration of tadalafil
- Theophylline: ritonavir accelerates metabolism of ●theophylline (reduced plasma concentration)
- Vardenafil: ritonavir possibly increases plasma concentration of ●vardenafil—avoid concomitant use

Rivastigmine *see* Parasympathomimetics
Rizatriptan *see* 5HT$_1$ Agonists
Rocuronium *see* Muscle Relaxants
Rofecoxib *see* NSAIDs
Ropinirole
Antipsychotics: manufacturer of ropinirole advises avoid concomitant use of antipsychotics (antagonism of effect)
Memantine: effects of dopaminergics possibly enhanced by memantine
Methyldopa: antiparkinsonian effect of dopaminergics antagonised by methyldopa
Metoclopramide: antiparkinsonian effect of ropinirole antagonised by metoclopramide (manufacturers of ropinirole advise avoid concomitant use)
Oestrogens: plasma concentration of ropinirole increased by oestrogens
Ropivacaine
Antidepressants: metabolism of ropivacaine inhibited by fluvoxamine—avoid prolonged administration of ropivacaine
Rosiglitazone *see* Antidiabetics
Rosuvastatin *see* Statins
Rowachol®
Anticoagulants: Rowachol® possibly reduces anticoagulant effect of coumarins
St John's Wort
- Antibacterials: St John's wort reduces plasma concentration of ●telithromycin (avoid during and for 2 weeks after St John's wort)
- Anticoagulants: St John's wort reduces anticoagulant effect of ●warfarin (avoid concomitant use)
- Antidepressants: St John's wort reduces plasma concentration of amitriptyline; increased serotonergic effects when St John's wort given with ●SSRIs—avoid concomitant use
- Antiepileptics: St John's wort reduces plasma concentration of ●carbamazepine and ●phenytoin—avoid concomitant use; St John's wort reduces plasma concentration of active metabolite of ●primidone—avoid concomitant use
- Antimalarials: avoidance of antidepressants advised by manufacturer of ●artemether/lumefantrine
- Antivirals: St John's wort reduces plasma concentration of ●amprenavir, ●efavirenz, ●indinavir, ●nelfinavir, ●nevirapine, ●ritonavir and ●saquinavir—avoid concomitant use
- Barbiturates: St John's wort reduces plasma concentration of ●phenobarbital—avoid concomitant use
- Cardiac Glycosides: St John's wort reduces plasma concentration of ●digoxin—avoid concomitant use
- Ciclosporin: St John's wort reduces plasma concentration of ●ciclosporin—avoid concomitant use

St John's Wort *(continued)*
- 5HT$_1$ Agonists: increased serotonergic effects when St John's wort given with ●5HT$_1$ agonists—avoid concomitant use
- Lipid-regulating Drugs: St John's wort reduces plasma concentration of simvastatin
- Oestrogens: St John's wort reduces contraceptive effect of ●oestrogens (avoid concomitant use)
- Progestogens: St John's wort reduces contraceptive effect of ●progestogens (avoid concomitant use)
- Tacrolimus: St John's wort reduces plasma concentration of ●tacrolimus—avoid concomitant use
- Theophylline: St John's wort reduces plasma concentration of ●theophylline—avoid concomitant use

Salbutamol *see* Sympathomimetics, Beta$_2$
Salmeterol *see* Sympathomimetics, Beta$_2$
Saquinavir
- Antibacterials: plasma concentration of saquinavir possibly increased by quinupristin/dalfopristin; plasma concentration of saquinavir significantly reduced by ●rifamycins—avoid concomitant use unless another protease inhibitor also given e.g. ritonavir
- Antidepressants: plasma concentration of saquinavir reduced by ●St John's wort—avoid concomitant use
- Antiepileptics: plasma concentration of saquinavir possibly reduced by carbamazepine, phenytoin and ●primidone
- Antifungals: plasma concentration of saquinavir increased by ketoconazole; plasma concentration of saquinavir possibly increased by imidazoles and triazoles
- Antihistamines: increased risk of ventricular arrhythmias when saquinavir given with ●terfenadine—avoid concomitant use
- Antimuscarinics: avoidance of saquinavir advised by manufacturer of tolterodine
- Antipsychotics: saquinavir possibly increases plasma concentration of thioridazine; saquinavir possibly increases plasma concentration of ●pimozide (increased risk of ventricular arrhythmias—avoid concomitant use); saquinavir increases plasma concentration of ●sertindole (increased risk of ventricular arrhythmias—avoid concomitant use)
- Antivirals: plasma concentration of saquinavir significantly reduced by efavirenz; plasma concentration of saquinavir increased by indinavir and ●ritonavir; combination of saquinavir with nelfinavir may increase plasma concentration of either drug (or both); plasma concentration of saquinavir reduced by ●nevirapine—avoid concomitant use
- Anxiolytics and Hypnotics: saquinavir increases plasma concentration of ●midazolam (risk of prolonged sedation)
- Barbiturates: plasma concentration of saquinavir possibly reduced by ●barbiturates
- Cilostazol: saquinavir possibly increases plasma concentration of ●cilostazol—avoid concomitant use
- Corticosteroids: plasma concentration of saquinavir possibly reduced by dexamethasone
- Ergot Alkaloids: increased risk of ergotism when saquinavir given with ●ergotamine and methysergide—avoid concomitant use
- Lipid-regulating Drugs: possible increased risk of myopathy when saquinavir given with atorvastatin; increased risk of myopathy when saquinavir given with ●simvastatin (avoid concomitant use)
- Sildenafil: saquinavir possibly increases plasma concentration of sildenafil— reduce initial dose of sildenafil

Saquinavir *(continued)*

Tadalafil: saquinavir possibly increases plasma concentration of tadalafil

Ulcer-healing Drugs: plasma concentration of saquinavir increased by ranitidine

Secobarbital *see* Barbiturates

Selegiline

Note. Selegiline is a MAO-B inhibitor

- Analgesics: hyperpyrexia and CNS toxicity reported when selegiline given with ●pethidine (avoid concomitant use); manufacturer of selegiline advises caution with tramadol

- Antidepressants: theoretical risk of serotonin syndrome if selegiline given with citalopram (especially if dose of selegiline exceeds 10 mg daily); caution with selegiline advised by manufacturer of escitalopram; increased risk of hypertension and CNS excitation when selegiline given with ●fluoxetine (selegiline should not be started until 5 weeks after stopping fluoxetine, avoid fluoxetine for 2 weeks after stopping selegiline); increased risk of hypertension and CNS excitation when selegiline given with ●fluvoxamine or ●venlafaxine (selegiline should not be started until 1 week after stopping fluvoxamine or venlafaxine, avoid fluvoxamine or venlafaxine for 2 weeks after stopping selegiline); increased risk of hypertension and CNS excitation when selegiline given with ●paroxetine or ●sertraline (selegiline should not be started until 2 weeks after stopping paroxetine or sertraline, avoid paroxetine or sertraline for 2 weeks after stopping selegiline); enhanced hypotensive effect when selegiline given with MAOIs; avoid concomitant use of selegiline with ●moclobemide; CNS toxicity reported when selegiline given with ●tricyclics

Dopaminergics: max. dose of 10 mg selegiline advised by manufacturer of entacapone if used concomitantly; selegiline enhances effects and increases toxicity of levodopa (reduce dose of levodopa)

Memantine: effects of dopaminergics and selegiline possibly enhanced by memantine

Methyldopa: antiparkinsonian effect of dopaminergics antagonised by methyldopa

Sermorelin

Note. Avoid preparations which affect release of growth hormone

Sertindole *see* Antipsychotics

Sertraline *see* Antidepressants, SSRI

Sevoflurane *see* Anaesthetics, General

Sibutramine

Analgesics: increased risk of bleeding when sibutramine given with NSAIDs or aspirin

Anticoagulants: increased risk of bleeding when sibutramine given with anticoagulants

- Antidepressants: increased CNS toxicity when sibutramine given with ●MAOIs or ●moclobemide (manufacturer of sibutramine advises avoid concomitant use), also avoid sibutramine for 2 weeks after stopping MAOIs or moclobemide; increased risk of CNS toxicity when sibutramine given with ●SSRI-related antidepressants, ●SSRIs, ●mirtazapine, ●noradrenaline re-uptake inhibitors, ●tricyclic-related antidepressants, ●tricyclics or ●tryptophan (manufacturer of sibutramine advises avoid concomitant use)

- Antipsychotics: increased risk of CNS toxicity when sibutramine given with ●antipsychotics (manufacturer of sibutramine advises avoid concomitant use)

Sildenafil

Alpha-blockers: enhanced hypotensive effect when sildenafil given with alpha-blockers (avoid alpha-blockers for 4 hours after sildenafil)

Antibacterials: plasma concentration of sildenafil increased by erythromycin—reduce initial dose of sildenafil

Antifungals: plasma concentration of sildenafil increased by itraconazole and ketoconazole—reduce initial dose of sildenafil

- Antivirals: plasma concentration of sildenafil possibly increased by amprenavir, nelfinavir and saquinavir— reduce initial dose of sildenafil; plasma concentration of sildenafil increased by indinavir—reduce initial dose of sildenafil; plasma concentration of sildenafil significantly increased by ●ritonavir—avoid concomitant use

Grapefruit Juice: plasma concentration of sildenafil possibly increased by grapefruit juice

- Nicorandil: sildenafil significantly enhances hypotensive effect of ●nicorandil (avoid concomitant use)

- Nitrates: sildenafil significantly enhances hypotensive effect of ●nitrates (avoid concomitant use)

Ulcer-healing Drugs: plasma concentration of sildenafil increased by cimetidine (reduce initial dose of sildenafil)

Simvastatin *see* Statins

Sirolimus

- Antibacterials: plasma concentration of sirolimus reduced by rifampicin; plasma concentration of sirolimus possibly increased by ●telithromycin

- Antifungals: plasma concentration of sirolimus increased by ●itraconazole, ●ketoconazole and ●miconazole; plasma concentration of sirolimus increased by ●voriconazole—avoid concomitant use

- Calcium-channel Blockers: plasma concentration of sirolimus increased by ●diltiazem

Ciclosporin: plasma concentration of sirolimus possibly increased by ciclosporin

- Grapefruit Juice: plasma concentration of sirolimus increased by ●grapefruit juice—avoid concomitant use

Sodium Aurothiomalate *see* Gold

Sodium Bicarbonate *see* Antacids

Sodium Clodronate *see* Bisphosphonates

Sodium Polystyrene Sulphonate

Thyroid Hormones: sodium polystyrene sulphonate reduces absorption of levothyroxine (thyroxine)

Sodium Valproate *see* Valproate

Somatropin

Corticosteroids: growth-promoting effect of somatropin may be inhibited by corticosteroids

Oestrogens: increased doses of somatropin may be needed when given with oestrogens (when used as oral replacement therapy)

Sotalol *see* Beta-blockers

Spironolactone *see* Diuretics

Statins

Antacids: absorption of rosuvastatin reduced by antacids

- Anti-arrhythmics: increased risk of myopathy when simvastatin given with ●amiodarone (avoid doses of simvastatin above 20 mg daily)

- Antibacterials: plasma concentration of atorvastatin increased by clarithromycin; increased risk of myopathy when simvastatin given with ●clarithromycin, ●erythromycin or ●telithromycin (avoid concomitant use); plasma concentration of rosuvastatin reduced by erythromycin; possible increased risk of myopathy when atorvastatin given with erythromycin; metabolism of fluvasta-

Statins

- Antibacterials *(continued)*
tin accelerated by rifampicin (reduced effect);
increased risk of myopathy when atorvastatin
given with ●telithromycin (avoid concomitant use)
- Anticoagulants: simvastatin enhances anticoagulant
effect of ●coumarins; rosuvastatin possibly
enhances anticoagulant effect of ●coumarins and
●phenindione
Antidepressants: plasma concentration of simvastatin reduced by St John's wort
- Antifungals: increased risk of myopathy when
simvastatin given with ●itraconazole or ●keto-
conazole (avoid concomitant use); possible
increased risk of myopathy when simvastatin
given with ●miconazole—avoid concomitant use;
increased risk of myopathy when atorvastatin
given with ●itraconazole (avoid concomitant use);
possible increased risk of myopathy when atorvastatin or simvastatin given with imidazoles;
possible increased risk of myopathy when atorvastatin or simvastatin given with triazoles
- Antivirals: plasma concentration of simvastatin
possibly increased by ●amprenavir—avoid concomitant use; plasma concentration of atorvastatin
possibly increased by amprenavir; possible
increased risk of myopathy when atorvastatin
given with indinavir, nelfinavir or saquinavir;
increased risk of myopathy when simvastatin
given with ●indinavir, ●nelfinavir, ●ritonavir or
●saquinavir (avoid concomitant use)
Bosentan: plasma concentration of simvastatin
reduced by bosentan
- Calcium-channel Blockers: possible increased risk
of myopathy when simvastatin given with diltiazem; increased risk of myopathy when simvastatin given with ●verapamil (avoid doses of
simvastatin above 20 mg daily)
Cardiac Glycosides: atorvastatin possibly increases
plasma concentration of digoxin
- Ciclosporin: increased risk of myopathy when statins
given with ●ciclosporin; increased risk of myopathy when rosuvastatin given with ●ciclosporin
(avoid concomitant use)
Cytotoxics: plasma concentration of simvastatin
increased by imatinib
Grapefruit Juice: plasma concentration of simvastatin increased by grapefruit juice
- Lipid-regulating Drugs: increased risk of myopathy
when statins given with ●gemfibrozil (preferably
avoid concomitant use); increased risk of myopathy when statins given with ●fibrates; increased
risk of myopathy when statins given with ●nico-
tinic acid (applies to lipid regulating doses of
nicotinic acid)
Oestrogens: rosuvastatin increases plasma concentration of ethinylestradiol
Progestogens: rosuvastatin increases plasma concentration of norgestrel

Stavudine

- Antivirals: effects of stavudine possibly inhibited by
●ribavirin; effects of stavudine possibly inhibited
by ●zidovudine (manufacturers advise avoid
concomitant use)
Cytotoxics: effects of stavudine possibly inhibited
by doxorubicin

Streptomycin *see* Aminoglycosides

Sucralfate

- Antibacterials: sucralfate reduces absorption of
ciprofloxacin, levofloxacin, moxifloxacin, norfloxacin, ofloxacin and tetracyclines
- Anticoagulants: sucralfate possibly reduces absorption of ●coumarins (reduced anticoagulant effect)

Sucralfate *(continued)*

- Antiepileptics: sucralfate reduces absorption of
●phenytoin
Antifungals: sucralfate reduces absorption of ketoconazole
Antipsychotics: sucralfate reduces absorption of
sulpiride
Cardiac Glycosides: sucralfate possibly reduces
absorption of cardiac glycosides
Thyroid Hormones: sucralfate reduces absorption of
levothyroxine (thyroxine)
Ulcer-healing Drugs: sucralfate possibly reduces
absorption of lansoprazole

Sulfadiazine *see* Sulphonamides
Sulfadoxine *see* Sulphonamides
Sulfamethoxazole *see* Sulphonamides
Sulfasalazine *see* Aminosalicylates

Sulfinpyrazone

Analgesics: effects of sulfinpyrazone antagonised by
aspirin
Antibacterials: sulfinpyrazone reduces excretion of
nitrofurantoin (increased risk of toxicity); effects
of sulfinpyrazone antagonised by pyrazinamide
- Anticoagulants: sulfinpyrazone enhances anticoagulant effect of ●coumarins
- Antidiabetics: sulfinpyrazone enhances effects of
●sulphonylureas
- Antiepileptics: sulfinpyrazone increases plasma
concentration of ●phenytoin
Theophylline: sulfinpyrazone reduces plasma concentration of theophylline

Sulindac *see* NSAIDs

Sulphonamides

Anaesthetics, General: sulphonamides enhance
effects of thiopental
Anaesthetics, Local: increased risk of methaemoglobinaemia when sulphonamides given with
prilocaine
- Anti-arrhythmics: increased risk of ventricular
arrhythmias when sulfamethoxazole (as co-trimoxazole) given with ●amiodarone—avoid concomitant use of co-trimoxazole
- Antibacterials: increased risk of crystalluria when
sulphonamides given with ●methenamine
- Anticoagulants: sulphonamides enhance anticoagulant effect of ●coumarins
Antidiabetics: sulphonamides rarely enhance the
effects of sulphonylureas
Antiepileptics: sulphonamides possibly increase
plasma concentration of phenytoin
- Antimalarials: increased antifolate effect when
sulphonamides given with ●pyrimethamine
(includes Fansidar®)
- Antipsychotics: avoid concomitant use of sulphonamides with ●clozapine (increased risk of
agranulocytosis)
- Ciclosporin: increased risk of nephrotoxicity when
sulphonamides given with ●ciclosporin; sulfadiazine possibly reduces plasma concentration of
●ciclosporin
- Cytotoxics: increased risk of haematological toxicity
when sulfamethoxazole (as co-trimoxazole) given
with ●azathioprine or ●mercaptopurine; sulphonamides increase risk of methotrexate toxicity;
sulfamethoxazole (as co-trimoxazole) increases
antifolate effect of ●methotrexate—avoid concomitant use
Oestrogens: *broad-spectrum* antibacterials possibly
reduce contraceptive effect of oestrogens (risk
probably small, see p. 388)
Potassium Aminobenzoate: effects of sulphonamides inhibited by potassium aminobenzoate

Sulphonylureas *see* Antidiabetics
Sulpiride *see* Antipsychotics

Sumatriptan *see* 5HT$_1$ Agonists
Suxamethonium *see* Muscle Relaxants
Sympathomimetics
- Adrenergic Neurone Blockers: ephedrine, isometheptene, metaraminol, methylphenidate, noradrenaline (norepinephrine), oxymetazoline, phenylephrine, phenylpropanolamine, pseudoephedrine and xylometazoline antagonise hypotensive effect of ●adrenergic neurone blockers
- Anaesthetics, General: increased risk of arrhythmias when adrenaline (epinephrine) given with ●volatile liquid general anaesthetics; increased risk of hypertension when methylphenidate given with ●volatile liquid general anaesthetics
- Anticoagulants: methylphenidate possibly enhances anticoagulant effect of ●coumarins
- Antidepressants: risk of hypertensive crisis when dexamfetamine, dopamine, dopexamine, ephedrine, isometheptene, methylphenidate, phenylephrine, phenylpropanolamine, pseudoephedrine or sympathomimetics given with ●MAOIs; risk of hypertensive crisis when dexamfetamine, dopamine, dopexamine, ephedrine, isometheptene, methylphenidate, phenylephrine, phenylpropanolamine, pseudoephedrine or sympathomimetics given with ●moclobemide; methylphenidate possibly inhibits metabolism of SSRIs and tricyclics; increased risk of hypertension and arrhythmias when noradrenaline (norepinephrine) given with ●tricyclics; increased risk of hypertension and arrhythmias when adrenaline (epinephrine) given with ●tricyclics (but local anaesthetics with adrenaline appear to be safe)
  Antiepileptics: methylphenidate increases plasma concentration of phenytoin; methylphenidate possibly increases plasma concentration of primidone
  Antipsychotics: hypertensive effect of sympathomimetics antagonised by antipsychotics
  Barbiturates: methylphenidate possibly increases plasma concentration of phenobarbital
- Beta-blockers: severe hypertension when adrenaline (epinephrine) or noradrenaline (norepinephrine) given with ●beta-blockers especially with non-selective beta-blockers; possible severe hypertension when dobutamine given with ●beta-blockers especially with non-selective beta-blockers
- Clonidine: possible risk of hypertension when adrenaline (epinephrine) or noradrenaline (norepinephrine) given with clonidine; serious adverse events reported with concomitant use of methylphenidate and ●clonidine (causality not established)
  Corticosteroids: ephedrine accelerates metabolism of dexamethasone
- Dopaminergics: risk of toxicity when isometheptene or phenylpropanolamine given with ●bromocriptine; effects of adrenaline (epinephrine), dobutamine, dopamine and noradrenaline (norepinephrine) possibly enhanced by entacapone
  Doxapram: increased risk of hypertension when sympathomimetics given with doxapram
  Ergot Alkaloids: increased risk of ergotism when sympathomimetics given with ergotamine and methysergide
  Oxytocin: risk of hypertension when vasoconstrictor sympathomimetics given with oxytocin (due to enhanced vasopressor effect)
- Sympathomimetics: effects of adrenaline (epinephrine) possibly enhanced by ●dopexamine; dopexamine possibly enhances effects of ●noradrenaline (norepinephrine)

Sympathomimetics, Beta$_2$
  Corticosteroids: increased risk of hypokalaemia when high doses of beta$_2$ sympathomimetics given with corticosteroids—for CSM advice (hypokalaemia) see p. 135
  Diuretics: increased risk of hypokalaemia when high doses of beta$_2$ sympathomimetics given with acetazolamide, loop diuretics or thiazides and related diuretics—for CSM advice (hypokalaemia) see p. 135
- Methyldopa: acute hypotension reported when infusion of salbutamol given with ●methyldopa
  Muscle Relaxants: bambuterol enhances effects of suxamethonium
  Theophylline: increased risk of hypokalaemia when high doses of beta$_2$ sympathomimetics given with theophylline—for CSM advice (hypokalaemia) see p. 135

Tacrolimus
- Analgesics: possible increased risk of nephrotoxicity when tacrolimus given with NSAIDs; increased risk of nephrotoxicity when tacrolimus given with ●ibuprofen
- Antibacterials: plasma concentration of tacrolimus increased by ●clarithromycin, ●erythromycin and ●quinupristin/dalfopristin; plasma concentration of tacrolimus reduced by ●rifampicin; plasma concentration of tacrolimus possibly increased by ●chloramphenicol and ●telithromycin
- Antidepressants: plasma concentration of tacrolimus reduced by ●St John's wort—avoid concomitant use
- Antifungals: plasma concentration of tacrolimus increased by ●fluconazole, ●ketoconazole and ●voriconazole; increased risk of nephrotoxicity when tacrolimus given with ●amphotericin; plasma concentration of tacrolimus reduced by ●caspofungin; plasma concentration of tacrolimus possibly increased by ●imidazoles and ●triazoles
- Antivirals: plasma concentration of tacrolimus possibly increased by ●nelfinavir and ●ritonavir
- Calcium-channel Blockers: plasma concentration of tacrolimus increased by ●diltiazem and ●nifedipine
- Ciclosporin: tacrolimus increases plasma concentration of ●ciclosporin (increased risk of toxicity)—avoid concomitant use
- Diuretics: increased risk of hyperkalaemia when tacrolimus given with ●potassium-sparing diuretics
- Grapefruit Juice: plasma concentration of tacrolimus increased by ●grapefruit juice
  Hormone Antagonists: plasma concentration of tacrolimus possibly increased by danazol
  Oestrogens: tacrolimus possibly reduces contraceptive effect of oestrogens
- Potassium Salts: increased risk of hyperkalaemia when tacrolimus given with ●potassium salts
  Progestogens: tacrolimus possibly reduces contraceptive effect of progestogens
  Ulcer-healing Drugs: plasma concentration of tacrolimus possibly increased by omeprazole

Tadalafil
- Alpha-blockers: enhanced hypotensive effect when tadalafil given with ●alpha-blockers (avoid concomitant use)
  Antibacterials: plasma concentration of tadalafil possibly increased by clarithromycin and erythromycin; plasma concentration of tadalafil reduced by rifampicin
  Antifungals: plasma concentration of tadalafil increased by ketoconazole; plasma concentration of tadalafil possibly increased by itraconazole

Tadalafil *(continued)*

Antivirals: plasma concentration of tadalafil increased by ritonavir; plasma concentration of tadalafil possibly increased by saquinavir

Grapefruit Juice: plasma concentration of tadalafil possibly increased by grapefruit juice

● Nicorandil: tadalafil significantly enhances hypotensive effect of ●nicorandil (avoid concomitant use)

● Nitrates: tadalafil significantly enhances hypotensive effect of ●nitrates (avoid concomitant use)

Tamoxifen

● Anticoagulants: tamoxifen enhances anticoagulant effect of ●coumarins

Hormone Antagonists: plasma concentration of tamoxifen reduced by aminoglutethimide

Tamsulosin *see* Alpha-blockers

Taxanes *see* Docetaxel and Paclitaxel

Tegafur with uracil *see* Fluorouracil

Teicoplanin

Antibacterials: increased risk of nephrotoxicity and ototoxicity when teicoplanin given with aminoglycosides or colistin

Oestrogens: *broad-spectrum* antibacterials possibly reduce contraceptive effect of oestrogens (risk probably small, see p. 388)

Telithromycin

● Antibacterials: plasma concentration of telithromycin reduced by ●rifampicin (avoid during and for 2 weeks after rifampicin)

● Antidepressants: plasma concentration of telithromycin reduced by ●St John's wort (avoid during and for 2 weeks after St John's wort)

● Antiepileptics: plasma concentration of telithromycin reduced by ●carbamazepine, ●phenytoin and ●primidone (avoid during and for 2 weeks after carbamazepine, phenytoin and primidone)

● Antihistamines: increased risk of ventricular arrhythmias when telithromycin given with ●terfenadine—avoid concomitant use

● Antipsychotics: increased risk of ventricular arrhythmias when telithromycin given with ●pimozide—avoid concomitant use

● Anxiolytics and Hypnotics: telithromycin inhibits metabolism of ●midazolam (increased plasma concentration with increased sedation)

● Barbiturates: plasma concentration of telithromycin reduced by ●phenobarbital (avoid during and for 2 weeks after phenobarbital)

Cardiac Glycosides: telithromycin possibly increases plasma concentration of digoxin

● Ciclosporin: telithromycin possibly increases plasma concentration of ●ciclosporin

● Ergot Alkaloids: increased risk of ergotism when telithromycin given with ●ergotamine and methysergide—avoid concomitant use

● Lipid-regulating Drugs: increased risk of myopathy when telithromycin given with ●atorvastatin or ●simvastatin (avoid concomitant use)

Oestrogens: *broad-spectrum* antibacterials possibly reduce contraceptive effect of oestrogens (risk probably small, see p. 388)

● Sirolimus: telithromycin possibly increases plasma concentration of ●sirolimus

● Tacrolimus: telithromycin possibly increases plasma concentration of ●tacrolimus

Telmisartan *see* Angiotensin-II Receptor Antagonists

Temazepam *see* Anxiolytics and Hypnotics

Temoporfin

● Cytotoxics: increased skin photosensitivity when temoporfin given with topical ●fluorouracil

Temozolomide

Antiepileptics: cytotoxics reduce absorption of phenytoin; plasma concentration of temozolomide increased by valproate

● Antipsychotics: avoid concomitant use of cytotoxics with ●clozapine (increased risk of agranulocytosis)

Tenofovir

Antivirals: combination of tenofovir with cidofovir may increase plasma concentration of either drug (or both); tenofovir increases plasma concentration of didanosine; plasma concentration of tenofovir increased by lopinavir (also plasma concentration of lopinavir reduced)

Tenoxicam *see* NSAIDs

Terazosin *see* Alpha-blockers

Terbinafine

Antibacterials: plasma concentration of terbinafine reduced by rifampicin

Oestrogens: occasional reports of breakthrough bleeding when terbinafine given with oestrogens (when used for contraception)

Progestogens: occasional reports of breakthrough bleeding when terbinafine given with progestogens (when used for contraception)

Ulcer-healing Drugs: plasma concentration of terbinafine increased by cimetidine

Terbutaline *see* Sympathomimetics, Beta$_2$

Terfenadine *see* Antihistamines

Terpene Mixture *see* Rowachol®

Testosterone

● Anticoagulants: testosterone enhances anticoagulant effect of ●coumarins and ●phenindione

Antidiabetics: testosterone possibly enhances hypoglycaemic effect of antidiabetics

Tetrabenazine

● Antidepressants: risk of CNS excitation and hypertension when tetrabenazine given with ●MAOIs

Antipsychotics: increased risk of extrapyramidal side-effects when tetrabenazine given with antipsychotics

Dopaminergics: increased risk of extrapyramidal side-effects when tetrabenazine given with amantadine

Metoclopramide: increased risk of extrapyramidal side-effects when tetrabenazine given with metoclopramide

Tetracosactide *see* Corticosteroids

Tetracycline *see* Tetracyclines

Tetracyclines

ACE Inhibitors: absorption of tetracyclines reduced by quinapril tablets (quinapril tablets contain magnesium carbonate)

Adsorbents: absorption of tetracyclines possibly reduced by kaolin

Antacids: absorption of tetracyclines reduced by antacids

● Anticoagulants: tetracyclines possibly enhance anticoagulant effect of ●coumarins and ●phenindione

Antiepileptics: metabolism of doxycycline accelerated by carbamazepine (reduced effect); metabolism of doxycycline accelerated by phenytoin and primidone (reduced plasma concentration)

Atovaquone: tetracycline reduces plasma concentration of atovaquone

Barbiturates: metabolism of doxycycline accelerated by barbiturates (reduced plasma concentration)

Calcium Salts: absorption of tetracycline reduced by calcium salts

● Ciclosporin: doxycycline possibly increases plasma concentration of ●ciclosporin

Cytotoxics: doxycycline or tetracycline increase risk of methotrexate toxicity

Tetracyclines *(continued)*

Dairy Products: absorption of tetracyclines (except doxycycline and minocycline) reduced by dairy products

Diuretics: manufacturer of lymecycline advises avoid concomitant use with diuretics

Ergot Alkaloids: increased risk of ergotism when tetracyclines given with ergotamine and methysergide

Iron: absorption of tetracyclines reduced by *oral* iron, also absorption of *oral* iron reduced by tetracyclines

● Oestrogens: tetracyclines possibly reduce contraceptive effect of ●oestrogens (risk probably small, see p. 388); *broad-spectrum* antibacterials possibly reduce contraceptive effect of oestrogens (risk probably small, see p. 388)

● Retinoids: possible increased risk of benign intracranial hypertension when tetracyclines given with ●retinoids (avoid concomitant use)

Ulcer-healing Drugs: absorption of tetracyclines reduced by ranitidine bismuth citrate, sucralfate and tripotassium dicitratobismuthate

Zinc: absorption of tetracyclines reduced by zinc, also absorption of zinc reduced by tetracyclines

Theophylline

Allopurinol: plasma concentration of theophylline possibly increased by allopurinol

Anaesthetics, General: increased risk of convulsions when theophylline given with ketamine; increased risk of arrhythmias when theophylline given with halothane

Analgesics: plasma concentration of theophylline increased by rofecoxib

Anti-arrhythmics: theophylline antagonises antiarrhythmic effect of adenosine; plasma concentration of theophylline increased by mexiletine and propafenone

● Antibacterials: metabolism of theophylline inhibited by ●clarithromycin (increased plasma concentration); metabolism of theophylline inhibited by ●erythromycin (increased plasma concentration), if erythromycin given by mouth, also decreased plasma-erythromycin concentration; plasma concentration of theophylline increased by ●ciprofloxacin and ●norfloxacin; metabolism of theophylline accelerated by rifampicin (reduced plasma concentration); plasma concentration of theophylline possibly increased by isoniazid; possible increased risk of convulsions when theophylline given with ●quinolones

● Antidepressants: plasma concentration of theophylline increased by ●fluvoxamine (concomitant use should usually be avoided, but where not possible halve theophylline dose and monitor plasma-theophylline concentration); plasma concentration of theophylline reduced by ●St John's wort—avoid concomitant use

Antiepileptics: metabolism of theophylline accelerated by carbamazepine and primidone (reduced effect)

● Antifungals: plasma concentration of theophylline possibly increased by ●fluconazole and ●ketoconazole

● Antivirals: metabolism of theophylline accelerated by ●ritonavir (reduced plasma concentration)

Barbiturates: metabolism of theophylline accelerated by barbiturates (reduced effect)

● Calcium-channel Blockers: plasma concentration of theophylline possibly increased by ●calcium-channel blockers (enhanced effect); plasma concentration of theophylline increased by diltiazem; plasma concentration of theophylline increased by ●verapamil (enhanced effect)

Theophylline *(continued)*

Corticosteroids: increased risk of hypokalaemia when theophylline given with corticosteroids

Disulfiram: metabolism of theophylline inhibited by disulfiram (increased risk of toxicity)

Diuretics: increased risk of hypokalaemia when theophylline given with acetazolamide, loop diuretics or thiazides and related diuretics

Doxapram: increased CNS stimulation when theophylline given with doxapram

Hormone Antagonists: metabolism of theophylline accelerated by aminoglutethimide (reduced effect)

Interferons: metabolism of theophylline inhibited by interferon alfa (increased plasma concentration)

Leukotriene Antagonists: plasma concentration of theophylline possibly increased by zafirlukast, also plasma concentration of zafirlukast reduced

Lithium: theophylline increases excretion of lithium (reduced plasma concentration)

Oestrogens: excretion of theophylline reduced by oestrogens (increased plasma concentration)

Pentoxifylline (oxpentifylline): plasma concentration of theophylline increased by pentoxifylline (oxpentifylline)

Sulfinpyrazone: plasma concentration of theophylline reduced by sulfinpyrazone

Sympathomimetics, Beta$_2$: increased risk of hypokalaemia when theophylline given with high doses of beta$_2$ sympathomimetics—for CSM advice (hypokalaemia) see p. 135

Tobacco: metabolism of theophylline increased by tobacco smoking (reduced plasma concentration)

● Ulcer-healing Drugs: metabolism of theophylline inhibited by ●cimetidine (increased plasma concentration)

Vaccines: plasma concentration of theophylline possibly increased by influenza vaccine

Thiazolidinediones *see* Antidiabetics

Thiopental *see* Anaesthetics, General

Thioridazine *see* Antipsychotics

Thiotepa

Antiepileptics: cytotoxics reduce absorption of phenytoin

● Antipsychotics: avoid concomitant use of cytotoxics with ●clozapine (increased risk of agranulocytosis)

Muscle Relaxants: thiotepa enhances effects of suxamethonium

Thioxanthenes *see* Antipsychotics

Thyroid Hormones

Anti-arrhythmics: for concomitant use of thyroid hormones and amiodarone see p. 73

Antibacterials: metabolism of levothyroxine (thyroxine) accelerated by rifampicin (may increase requirements for levothyroxine (thyroxine) in hypothyroidism)

● Anticoagulants: thyroid hormones enhance anticoagulant effect of ●coumarins and ●phenindione

Antidepressants: thyroid hormones enhance effects of amitriptyline and imipramine; thyroid hormones possibly enhance effects of tricyclics

Antiepileptics: metabolism of thyroid hormones accelerated by carbamazepine and primidone (may increase requirements for thyroid hormones in hypothyroidism); metabolism of thyroid hormones accelerated by phenytoin (may increase requirements in hypothyroidism), also plasma concentration of phenytoin possibly increased

Barbiturates: metabolism of thyroid hormones accelerated by barbiturates (may increase requirements for thyroid hormones in hypothyroidism)

Calcium Salts: absorption of levothyroxine (thyroxine) reduced by calcium salts

Iron: absorption of levothyroxine (thyroxine) reduced by *oral* iron (give at least 2 hours apart)

Thyroid Hormones *(continued)*
  Lipid-regulating Drugs: absorption of thyroid hormones reduced by colestipol and colestyramine
  Sodium Polystyrene Sulphonate: absorption of levothyroxine (thyroxine) reduced by sodium polystyrene sulphonate
  Ulcer-healing Drugs: absorption of levothyroxine (thyroxine) reduced by cimetidine and sucralfate

Tiagabine
• Antidepressants: anticonvulsant effect of antiepileptics possibly antagonised by MAOIs and •tricyclic-related antidepressants (convulsive threshold lowered); anticonvulsant effect of antiepileptics antagonised by •SSRIs and •tricyclics (convulsive threshold lowered)
  Antiepileptics: plasma concentration of tiagabine reduced by carbamazepine, phenytoin and primidone
• Antimalarials: possible increased risk of convulsions when antiepileptics given with chloroquine and hydroxychloroquine; anticonvulsant effect of antiepileptics antagonised by •mefloquine
  Barbiturates: plasma concentration of tiagabine reduced by phenobarbital

Tiaprofenic Acid *see* NSAIDs

Tibolone
  Antibacterials: metabolism of tibolone accelerated by rifampicin (reduced plasma concentration)
  Antiepileptics: metabolism of tibolone accelerated by carbamazepine and primidone (reduced plasma concentration); metabolism of tibolone accelerated by phenytoin
  Barbiturates: metabolism of tibolone accelerated by barbiturates (reduced plasma concentration)

Ticarcillin *see* Penicillins

Tiludronic Acid *see* Bisphosphonates

Timolol *see* Beta-blockers

Tinidazole
  Alcohol: possibility of disulfiram-like reaction when tinidazole given with alcohol
  Oestrogens: *broad-spectrum* antibacterials possibly reduce contraceptive effect of oestrogens (risk probably small, see p. 388)

Tinzaparin *see* Heparins

Tiotropium *see* Antimuscarinics

Tizanidine *see* Muscle Relaxants

Tobacco
  Theophylline: tobacco smoking increases theophylline metabolism (reduced plasma concentration)

Tobramycin *see* Aminoglycosides

Tolbutamide *see* Antidiabetics

Tolfenamic Acid *see* NSAIDs

Tolterodine *see* Antimuscarinics

Topiramate
• Antidepressants: anticonvulsant effect of antiepileptics possibly antagonised by MAOIs and •tricyclic-related antidepressants (convulsive threshold lowered); anticonvulsant effect of antiepileptics antagonised by •SSRIs and •tricyclics (convulsive threshold lowered)
• Antiepileptics: plasma concentration of topiramate often reduced by carbamazepine; topiramate increases plasma concentration of •phenytoin (also plasma concentration of topiramate reduced)
• Antimalarials: possible increased risk of convulsions when antiepileptics given with chloroquine and hydroxychloroquine; anticonvulsant effect of antiepileptics antagonised by •mefloquine
• Oestrogens: topiramate accelerates metabolism of •oestrogens (reduced contraceptive effect—see p. 388)

Topiramate *(continued)*
• Progestogens: topiramate accelerates metabolism of •progestogens (reduced contraceptive effect—see p. 388)

Torasemide *see* Diuretics

Toremifene
• Anticoagulants: toremifene possibly enhances anticoagulant effect of •coumarins
  Antiepileptics: metabolism of toremifene possibly accelerated by carbamazepine (possibly reduced plasma concentration); metabolism of toremifene possibly accelerated by phenytoin; metabolism of toremifene accelerated by primidone (reduced plasma concentration)
  Barbiturates: metabolism of toremifene possibly accelerated by barbiturates (possibly reduced plasma concentration)
  Diuretics: increased risk of hypercalcaemia when toremifene given with thiazides and related diuretics

Tramadol *see* Opioid Analgesics

Trandolapril *see* ACE Inhibitors

Tranylcypromine *see* MAOIs

Trazodone *see* Antidepressants, Tricyclic (related)

Tretinoin *see* Retinoids

Triamcinolone *see* Corticosteroids

Triamterene *see* Diuretics

Triclofos *see* Anxiolytics and Hypnotics

Trientine
  Iron: trientine reduces absorption of *oral* iron

Trifluoperazine *see* Antipsychotics

Trihexyphenidyl (benzhexol) *see* Antimuscarinics

Trilostane
  Diuretics: increased risk of hyperkalaemia when trilostane given with potassium-sparing diuretics

Trimetaphan
  Muscle Relaxants: trimetaphan enhances effects of suxamethonium

Trimethoprim
• Anti-arrhythmics: increased risk of ventricular arrhythmias when trimethoprim (as co-trimoxazole) given with •amiodarone—avoid concomitant use of co-trimoxazole; trimethoprim increases plasma concentration of procainamide
  Antibacterials: plasma concentration of both drugs may increase when trimethoprim given with dapsone
  Anticoagulants: trimethoprim possibly enhances anticoagulant effect of coumarins
  Antidiabetics: trimethoprim rarely enhances the effects of sulphonylureas
• Antiepileptics: trimethoprim increases plasma concentration of •phenytoin (also increased antifolate effect)
• Antimalarials: increased antifolate effect when trimethoprim given with •pyrimethamine
  Antivirals: trimethoprim (as co-trimoxazole) increases plasma concentration of lamivudine—avoid concomitant use of high-dose co-trimoxazole; trimethoprim possibly increases plasma concentration of zalcitabine
  Cardiac Glycosides: trimethoprim possibly increases plasma concentration of digoxin
• Ciclosporin: increased risk of nephrotoxicity when trimethoprim given with •ciclosporin, also plasma concentration of ciclosporin reduced by intravenous trimethoprim
• Cytotoxics: increased risk of haematological toxicity when trimethoprim (also with co-trimoxazole) given with •azathioprine or •mercaptopurine; trimethoprim increases antifolate effect of •methotrexate—avoid concomitant use

Trimethoprim *(continued)*

Oestrogens: *broad-spectrum* antibacterials possibly reduce contraceptive effect of oestrogens (risk probably small, see p. 388)

Trimipramine *see* Antidepressants, Tricyclic

Tripotassium Dicitratobismuthate

Antibacterials: tripotassium dicitratobismuthate reduces absorption of tetracyclines

Triprolidine *see* Antihistamines

Tropicamide *see* Antimuscarinics

Tropisetron

Anti-arrhythmics: manufacturer of tropisetron advises caution with anti-arrhythmics (risk of ventricular arrhythmias)

Antibacterials: plasma concentration of tropisetron reduced by rifampicin

Antiepileptics: plasma concentration of tropisetron reduced by primidone

Barbiturates: plasma concentration of tropisetron reduced by phenobarbital

Beta-blockers: manufacturer of tropisetron advises caution with beta-blockers (risk of ventricular arrhythmias)

Trospium *see* Antimuscarinics

Tryptophan

● Antidepressants: CNS excitation and confusion when tryptophan given with ●MAOIs (reduce dose of tryptophan); agitation and nausea may occur when tryptophan given with ●SSRIs

● Antimalarials: avoidance of antidepressants advised by manufacturer of ●artemether/lumefantrine

● Sibutramine: increased risk of CNS toxicity when tryptophan given with ●sibutramine (manufacturer of sibutramine advises avoid concomitant use)

Ulcer-healing Drugs *see* Carbenoxolone, Histamine H₂-antagonists, Proton Pump Inhibitors, Sucralfate, and Tripotassium Dicitratobismuthate

Ursodeoxycholic Acid

Antacids: absorption of bile acids possibly reduced by antacids

● Ciclosporin: ursodeoxycholic acid increases absorption of ●ciclosporin

Lipid-regulating Drugs: absorption of bile acids possibly reduced by colestipol and colestyramine

Oestrogens: elimination of cholesterol is increased when bile acids given with oestrogens

Vaccines

Note. For a general warning on live vaccines and high doses of corticosteroids or other immunosuppressive drugs, see p. 578; for advice on live vaccines and immunoglobulins, see under Normal Immunoglobulin, p. 595

● Adalimumab: avoid concomitant use of live vaccines with ●adalimumab (see p. 578)

● Anakinra: avoid concomitant use of live vaccines with ●anakinra (see p. 578)

Anticoagulants: influenza vaccine possibly enhances anticoagulant effect of warfarin

Antiepileptics: influenza vaccine enhances effects of phenytoin

● Corticosteroids: immune response to vaccines impaired by high doses of ●corticosteroids, avoid concomitant use with live vaccines (see p. 578)

● Etanercept: avoid concomitant use of live vaccines with ●etanercept (see p. 578)

● Infliximab: avoid concomitant use of live vaccines with ●infliximab (see p. 578)

Interferons: avoidance of vaccines advised by manufacturer of interferon gamma

● Leflunomide: avoid concomitant use of live vaccines with ●leflunomide (see p. 578)

Theophylline: influenza vaccine possibly increases plasma concentration of theophylline

Valaciclovir *see* Aciclovir

Valdecoxib *see* NSAIDs

Valganciclovir *see* Ganciclovir

Valproate

Analgesics: effects of valproate enhanced by aspirin

Antibacterials: plasma concentration of valproate possibly reduced by ertapenem; plasma concentration of valproate reduced by meropenem; metabolism of valproate possibly inhibited by erythromycin (increased plasma concentration)

Anticoagulants: valproate possibly enhances anticoagulant effect of coumarins

● Antidepressants: anticonvulsant effect of antiepileptics possibly antagonised by MAOIs and ●tricyclic-related antidepressants (convulsive threshold lowered); anticonvulsant effect of antiepileptics antagonised by ●SSRIs and ●tricyclics (convulsive threshold lowered)

● Antiepileptics: plasma concentration of valproate reduced by carbamazepine, also plasma concentration of active metabolite of carbamazepine increased; valproate possibly increases plasma concentration of ethosuximide; valproate increases plasma concentration of lamotrigine; valproate sometimes reduces plasma concentration of an active metabolite of oxcarbazepine; valproate increases or possibly decreases plasma concentration of phenytoin, also plasma concentration of valproate reduced; valproate possibly increases plasma concentration of ●primidone (plasma concentration of active metabolite of primidone increased), also plasma concentration of valproate reduced

● Antimalarials: possible increased risk of convulsions when antiepileptics given with chloroquine and hydroxychloroquine; anticonvulsant effect of antiepileptics and valproate antagonised by ●mefloquine

● Antipsychotics: anticonvulsant effect of valproate antagonised by ●antipsychotics (convulsive threshold lowered); increased risk of neutropenia when valproate given with ●olanzapine

Antivirals: valproate possibly increases plasma concentration of zidovudine (increased risk of toxicity)

Barbiturates: valproate increases plasma concentration of phenobarbital (also plasma concentration of valproate reduced)

Bupropion: valproate inhibits the metabolism of bupropion

Cytotoxics: valproate increases plasma concentration of temozolomide

Lipid-regulating Drugs: absorption of valproate possibly reduced by colestyramine

● Ulcer-healing Drugs: metabolism of valproate inhibited by ●cimetidine (increased plasma concentration)

Valsartan *see* Angiotensin-II Receptor Antagonists

Vancomycin

Anaesthetics, General: hypersensitivity-like reactions can occur when intravenous vancomycin given with general anaesthetics

Antibacterials: increased risk of nephrotoxicity and ototoxicity when vancomycin given with aminoglycosides, capreomycin or colistin; increased risk of nephrotoxicity when vancomycin given with polymyxins

● Ciclosporin: increased risk of nephrotoxicity when vancomycin given with ●ciclosporin

Cytotoxics: increased risk of nephrotoxicity and possibly of ototoxicity when vancomycin given with cisplatin

● Diuretics: increased risk of otoxicity when vancomycin given with ●loop diuretics

Vancomycin *(continued)*
 Lipid-regulating Drugs: effects of oral vancomycin antagonised by colestyramine
- Muscle Relaxants: vancomycin enhances effects of ●suxamethonium
 Oestrogens: *broad-spectrum* antibacterials possibly reduce contraceptive effect of oestrogens (risk probably small, see p. 388)

Vardenafil
- Alpha-blockers: vardenafil enhances hypotensive effect of ●alpha-blockers (avoid concomitant use)
 Antibacterials: plasma concentration of vardenafil increased by erythromycin (reduce dose of vardenafil)
- Antifungals: plasma concentration of vardenafil increased by ●ketoconazole—avoid concomitant use; plasma concentration of vardenafil possibly increased by ●itraconazole—avoid concomitant use
- Antivirals: plasma concentration of vardenafil increased by ●indinavir—avoid concomitant use; plasma concentration of vardenafil possibly increased by ●ritonavir—avoid concomitant use
 Calcium-channel Blockers: enhanced hypotensive effect when vardenafil given with nifedipine
- Grapefruit Juice: plasma concentration of vardenafil possibly increased by ●grapefruit juice—avoid concomitant use
- Nicorandil: vardenafil possibly enhances hypotensive effect of ●nicorandil—avoid concomitant use
- Nitrates: vardenafil possibly enhances hypotensive effect of ●nitrates—avoid concomitant use

Vasodilator Antihypertensives
 ACE Inhibitors: enhanced hypotensive effect when hydralazine, minoxidil or nitroprusside given with ACE inhibitors
 Adrenergic Neurone Blockers: enhanced hypotensive effect when hydralazine, minoxidil or nitroprusside given with adrenergic neurone blockers
 Alcohol: enhanced hypotensive effect when hydralazine, minoxidil or nitroprusside given with alcohol
 Aldesleukin: enhanced hypotensive effect when hydralazine, minoxidil or nitroprusside given with aldesleukin
 Alpha-blockers: enhanced hypotensive effect when hydralazine, minoxidil or nitroprusside given with alpha-blockers
 Alprostadil: enhanced hypotensive effect when hydralazine, minoxidil or nitroprusside given with alprostadil
 Amifostine: possible enhanced hypotensive effect when hydralazine, minoxidil or nitroprusside given with amifostine
 Anaesthetics, General: enhanced hypotensive effect when hydralazine, minoxidil or nitroprusside given with general anaesthetics
 Analgesics: hypotensive effect of hydralazine, minoxidil and nitroprusside antagonised by NSAIDs
 Angiotensin-II Receptor Antagonists: enhanced hypotensive effect when hydralazine, minoxidil or nitroprusside given with angiotensin-II receptor antagonists
 Antidepressants: enhanced hypotensive effect when hydralazine, minoxidil or nitroprusside given with MAOIs; enhanced hypotensive effect when hydralazine or nitroprusside given with tricyclic-related antidepressants
 Antipsychotics: enhanced hypotensive effect when hydralazine, minoxidil or nitroprusside given with phenothiazines

Vasodilator Antihypertensives *(continued)*
 Anxiolytics and Hypnotics: enhanced hypotensive effect when hydralazine, minoxidil or nitroprusside given with anxiolytics and hypnotics
 Beta-blockers: enhanced hypotensive effect when hydralazine, minoxidil or nitroprusside given with beta-blockers
 Calcium-channel Blockers: enhanced hypotensive effect when hydralazine, minoxidil or nitroprusside given with calcium-channel blockers
 Clonidine: enhanced hypotensive effect when hydralazine, minoxidil or nitroprusside given with clonidine
 Corticosteroids: hypotensive effect of hydralazine, minoxidil and nitroprusside antagonised by corticosteroids
 Diazoxide: enhanced hypotensive effect when hydralazine, minoxidil or nitroprusside given with diazoxide
 Diuretics: enhanced hypotensive effect when hydralazine, minoxidil or nitroprusside given with diuretics
 Dopaminergics: enhanced hypotensive effect when hydralazine, minoxidil or nitroprusside given with levodopa
 Methyldopa: enhanced hypotensive effect when hydralazine, minoxidil or nitroprusside given with methyldopa
 Moxisylyte (thymoxamine): enhanced hypotensive effect when hydralazine, minoxidil or nitroprusside given with moxisylyte
 Moxonidine: enhanced hypotensive effect when hydralazine, minoxidil or nitroprusside given with moxonidine
 Muscle Relaxants: enhanced hypotensive effect when hydralazine, minoxidil or nitroprusside given with baclofen; enhanced hypotensive effect when hydralazine, minoxidil or nitroprusside given with tizanidine
 Nicorandil: possible enhanced hypotensive effect when hydralazine, minoxidil or nitroprusside given with nicorandil
 Nitrates: enhanced hypotensive effect when hydralazine, minoxidil or nitroprusside given with nitrates
 Oestrogens: hypotensive effect of hydralazine, minoxidil and nitroprusside antagonised by oestrogens
 Ulcer-healing Drugs: hypotensive effect of hydralazine, minoxidil and nitroprusside antagonised by carbenoxolone
 Vasodilator Antihypertensives: enhanced hypotensive effect when hydralazine given with minoxidil or nitroprusside; enhanced hypotensive effect when minoxidil given with nitroprusside

Vecuronium *see* Muscle Relaxants

Venlafaxine
- Analgesics: increased risk of bleeding when venlafaxine given with ●NSAIDs or ●aspirin
- Anticoagulants: venlafaxine possibly enhances anticoagulant effect of ●warfarin
- Antidepressants: enhanced CNS effects and toxicity when venlafaxine given with ●MAOIs (venlafaxine should not be started until 2 weeks after stopping MAOIs, avoid MAOIs for 1 week after stopping venlafaxine); after stopping SSRI-related antidepressants do not start ●moclobemide for at least 1 week
- Antimalarials: avoidance of antidepressants advised by manufacturer of ●artemether/lumefantrine
- Antipsychotics: venlafaxine increases plasma concentration of ●clozapine and haloperidol
- Dopaminergics: caution with venlafaxine advised by manufacturer of entacapone; increased risk of

Venlafaxine

- Dopaminergics *(continued)*
  hypertension and CNS excitation when venlafaxine given with ●selegiline (selegiline should not be started until 1 week after stopping venlafaxine, avoid venlafaxine for 2 weeks after stopping selegiline)
- Sibutramine: increased risk of CNS toxicity when SSRI-related antidepressants given with ●sibutramine (manufacturer of sibutramine advises avoid concomitant use)

Verapamil *see* Calcium-channel Blockers

Vigabatrin

- Antidepressants: anticonvulsant effect of antiepileptics possibly antagonised by MAOIs and ●tricyclic-related antidepressants (convulsive threshold lowered); anticonvulsant effect of antiepileptics antagonised by ●SSRIs and ●tricyclics (convulsive threshold lowered)
  Antiepileptics: vigabatrin reduces plasma concentration of phenytoin; vigabatrin possibly reduces plasma concentration of primidone
- Antimalarials: possible increased risk of convulsions when antiepileptics given with chloroquine and hydroxychloroquine; anticonvulsant effect of antiepileptics antagonised by ●mefloquine
  Barbiturates: vigabatrin possibly reduces plasma concentration of phenobarbital

Vinblastine

- Antibacterials: toxicity of vinblastine increased by ●erythromycin—avoid concomitant use
  Antiepileptics: cytotoxics reduce absorption of phenytoin
- Antipsychotics: avoid concomitant use of cytotoxics with ●clozapine (increased risk of agranulocytosis)

Vincristine

Antiepileptics: cytotoxics reduce absorption of phenytoin
Antifungals: metabolism of vincristine possibly inhibited by itraconazole (increased risk of neurotoxicity)
- Antipsychotics: avoid concomitant use of cytotoxics with ●clozapine (increased risk of agranulocytosis)
Calcium-channel Blockers: metabolism of vincristine possibly inhibited by nifedipine

Vitamin A *see* Vitamins
Vitamin D *see* Vitamins
Vitamin K (Phytomenadione) *see* Vitamins
Vitamins

- Anticoagulants: vitamin K antagonises anticoagulant effect of ●coumarins and ●phenindione
  Antiepileptics: vitamin D requirements possibly increased when given with carbamazepine, phenytoin or primidone
  Barbiturates: vitamin D requirements possibly increased when given with barbiturates
  Diuretics: increased risk of hypercalcaemia when vitamin D given with thiazides and related diuretics
  Dopaminergics: pyridoxine reduces effects of levodopa when given without dopa-decarboxylase inhibitor
  Retinoids: risk of hypervitaminosis A when vitamin A given with retinoids

Voriconazole *see* Antifungals, Triazole
Warfarin *see* Coumarins
Xipamide *see* Diuretics
Xylometazoline *see* Sympathomimetics
Zafirlukast *see* Leukotriene Antagonists
Zalcitabine
  Note. Clinical data limited. Avoid use with other drugs which have a potential to cause peripheral neuropathy or pancreatitis—for further details consult product literature

Zalcitabine *(continued)*
  Antacids: absorption of zalcitabine reduced by antacids
  Antibacterials: plasma concentration of zalcitabine possibly increased by trimethoprim
  Antivirals: avoidance of zalcitabine advised by manufacturer of emtricitabine; effects of zalcitabine possibly inhibited by lamivudine (manufacturers advise avoid concomitant use)
  Probenecid: excretion of zalcitabine possibly reduced by probenecid (increased plasma concentration)
  Ulcer-healing Drugs: plasma concentration of zalcitabine possibly increased by cimetidine

Zaleplon *see* Anxiolytics and Hypnotics
Zidovudine
  Note. Increased risk of toxicity with nephrotoxic and myelosuppressive drugs - for further details consult product literature
  Analgesics: increased risk of haematological toxicity when zidovudine given with NSAIDs; plasma concentration of zidovudine possibly increased by methadone
  Antibacterials: absorption of zidovudine reduced by clarithromycin tablets; manufacturer of zidovudine advises avoid concomitant use with rifampicin
  Antiepileptics: zidovudine increases or decreases plasma concentration of phenytoin; plasma concentration of zidovudine possibly increased by valproate (increased risk of toxicity)
- Antifungals: plasma concentration of zidovudine increased by ●fluconazole (increased risk of toxicity)
  Antimalarials: increased antifolate effect when zidovudine given with pyrimethamine
- Antivirals: profound myelosuppression when zidovudine given with ●ganciclovir (if possible avoid concomitant administration, particularly during initial ganciclovir therapy); effects of zidovudine possibly inhibited by ●ribavirin (manufacturer of zidovudine advises avoid concomitant use); zidovudine possibly inhibits effects of ●stavudine (manufacturers advise avoid concomitant use)
  Probenecid: excretion of zidovudine reduced by probenecid (increased plasma concentration and risk of toxicity)

Zinc
  Antibacterials: zinc reduces absorption of ciprofloxacin, levofloxacin, moxifloxacin, norfloxacin and ofloxacin; zinc reduces absorption of tetracyclines, also absorption of zinc reduced by tetracyclines
  Iron: absorption of zinc reduced by *oral* iron, also absorption of *oral* iron reduced by zinc
  Penicillamine: zinc reduces absorption of penicillamine

Zoledronic Acid *see* Bisphosphonates
Zolmitriptan *see* 5HT$_1$ Agonists
Zolpidem *see* Anxiolytics and Hypnotics
Zopiclone *see* Anxiolytics and Hypnotics
Zotepine *see* Antipsychotics
Zuclopenthixol *see* Antipsychotics

Appendix 2: Liver disease

Liver disease may alter the response to drugs in several ways as indicated below, and drug prescribing should be kept to a minimum in all patients with severe liver disease. The main problems occur in patients with jaundice, ascites, or evidence of encephalopathy.

IMPAIRED DRUG METABOLISM. Metabolism by the liver is the main route of elimination for many drugs, but the hepatic reserve appears to be large and liver disease has to be severe before important changes in drug metabolism occur. Routine liver-function tests are a poor guide to the capacity of the liver to metabolise drugs, and in the individual patient it is not possible to predict the extent to which the metabolism of a particular drug may be impaired.

A few drugs, e.g. rifampicin and fusidic acid, are excreted in the bile unchanged and may accumulate in patients with intrahepatic or extrahepatic obstructive jaundice.

HYPOPROTEINAEMIA. The hypoalbuminaemia in severe liver disease is associated with reduced protein binding and increased toxicity of some highly protein-bound drugs such as phenytoin and prednisolone.

REDUCED CLOTTING. Reduced hepatic synthesis of blood-clotting factors, indicated by a prolonged prothrombin time, increases the sensitivity to oral anticoagulants such as warfarin and phenindione.

HEPATIC ENCEPHALOPATHY. In severe liver disease many drugs can further impair cerebral function and may precipitate hepatic encephalopathy. These include all sedative drugs, opioid analgesics, those diuretics that produce hypokalaemia, and drugs that cause constipation.

FLUID OVERLOAD. Oedema and ascites in chronic liver disease may be exacerbated by drugs that give rise to fluid retention, e.g. NSAIDs, corticosteroids, and carbenoxolone.

HEPATOTOXIC DRUGS. Hepatotoxicity is either dose-related or unpredictable (idiosyncratic). Drugs causing dose-related toxicity may do so at lower doses than in patients with normal liver function, and some drugs producing reactions of the idiosyncratic kind do so more frequently in patients with liver disease. These drugs should be avoided or used very carefully.

Table of drugs to be avoided or used with caution in liver disease

The list of drugs given below is not comprehensive and is based on current information concerning the use of these drugs in therapeutic dosage. Products introduced or amended since publication of BNF No. 46 (September 2003) are underlined.

Drug	Comment
Abacavir	Avoid in moderate hepatic impairment unless essential; avoid in severe hepatic impairment
Abciximab	Avoid in severe liver disease—increased risk of bleeding
Acamprosate	Avoid in severe liver disease
Acarbose	Avoid
ACE inhibitors	Use of prodrugs such as cilazapril, enalapril, fosinopril, imidapril, moexipril, perindopril, quinapril, ramipril, and trandolapril requires close monitoring in patients with impaired liver function
Aceclofenac	*see* NSAIDs
Acemetacin	*see* NSAIDs
Acenocoumarol (nicoumalone)	*see* Anticoagulants, Oral
Acitretin	Avoid—further impairment of liver function may occur
Aclarubicin	Manufacturer advises caution
Alfentanil	*see* Opioid Analgesics
Alfuzosin	Reduce dose in mild to moderate liver disease; avoid if severe
Alimemazine (trimeprazine)	Avoid—may precipitate coma in severe liver disease; hepatotoxic
Allopurinol	Reduce dose
Almotriptan	Manufacturer advises caution in mild to moderate liver disease; avoid in severe liver disease
Alprazolam	*see* Anxiolytics and Hypnotics
Amfebutamone	*see* Bupropion
Amifostine	Manufacturer advises avoid
Aminophylline	*see* Theophylline
Amitriptyline	*see* Antidepressants, Tricyclic (and related)
Amlodipine	Half-life prolonged—may need dose reduction
Amoxapine	*see* Antidepressants, Tricyclic (and related)
Amprenavir	Avoid oral solution due to high propylene glycol content; reduce dose of capsules to 450 mg every 12 hours in moderate hepatic impairment and reduce dose to 300 mg every 12 hours in severe impairment
Amsacrine	Reduce dose
Anabolic steroids	Preferably avoid—dose-related toxicity
Analgesics	*see* Aspirin, NSAIDs, Opioid Analgesics and Paracetamol

Drug	Comment
Anastrozole	Avoid in moderate to severe liver disease
Androgens	Preferably avoid—dose-related toxicity with some, and produce fluid retention
Antacids	In patients with fluid retention, avoid those containing large amounts of sodium, e.g. magnesium trisilicate mixture, *Gaviscon*® Avoid those causing constipation—can precipitate coma
Anticoagulants, oral	Avoid in severe liver disease, especially if prothrombin time already prolonged
Antidepressants, MAOI	May cause idiosyncratic hepatotoxicity; see also Moclobemide
Antidepressants, SSRI	Reduce dose or avoid in severe liver disease
Antidepressants, tricyclic (and related)	Tricyclics preferable to MAOIs but sedative effects increased (avoid in severe liver disease)
Antihistamines	*see* individual entries
Antipsychotics	All can precipitate coma; phenothiazines are hepatotoxic; *see also* Clozapine, Olanzapine, Quetiapine, Risperidone and Sertindole
Anxiolytics and hypnotics	All can precipitate coma; avoid chloral hydrate; small dose of oxazepam or temazepam probably safest; reduce oral dose of clomethiazole; reduce dose of zaleplon to 5 mg (avoid if severe); reduce dose of zolpidem to 5 mg (avoid if severe); reduce dose of zopiclone (avoid if severe)
Apomorphine	Low sublingual doses may be used with caution for erectile dysfunction
Artemether [ingredient]	*see Riamet*®
Aspirin	Avoid—increased risk of gastro-intestinal bleeding
Atorvastatin	*see* Statins
Atosiban	No information available
Atovaquone	Manufacturer advises caution—monitor more closely
Auranofin	Caution in mild to moderate liver disease; avoid in severe liver disease
Azapropazone	*see* NSAIDs
Azathioprine	May need dose reduction
Azithromycin	Avoid; jaundice reported
Bambuterol	Avoid in severe liver disease
Bemiparin	Manufacturer advises avoid in severe liver disease
Bendrofluazide	*see* Thiazides and Related Diuretics
Bendroflumethiazide (bendrofluazide)	*see* Thiazides and Related Diuretics
Benorilate [aspirin-paracetamol ester]	*see* Aspirin and Paracetamol
Benperidol	*see* Antipsychotics
Benzthiazide	*see* Thiazides and Related Diuretics
Bexarotene	Avoid
Bezafibrate	Avoid in severe liver disease

Drug	Comment
Bicalutamide	Increased accumulation possible in moderate to severe hepatic impairment
Bisoprolol	Max. 10 mg daily in severe liver impairment
Bosentan	Avoid in moderate and severe hepatic impairment
Brompheniramine	Sedation inappropriate in severe liver disease—avoid
Buclizine	Sedation inappropriate in severe liver disease—avoid
Budesonide	Plasma-budesonide concentration may increase on oral administration
Bumetanide	*see* Loop Diuretics
Bupivacaine	*see* Lidocaine
Buprenorphine	*see* Opioid Analgesics
Bupropion	Manufacturer recommends 150 mg daily; avoid in severe hepatic cirrhosis
Buspirone	Reduce dose in mild to moderate liver disease; avoid in severe liver disease
Cabergoline	Reduce dose in severe hepatic impairment
Calcitriol	Manufacturer of topical calcitriol advises avoid in severe liver disease
Candesartan	Halve initial dose in mild or moderate liver disease; avoid if severe
Capecitabine	Manufacturer advises avoid in severe hepatic impairment
Carbamazepine	Metabolism impaired in advanced liver disease
Carbenoxolone	Produces sodium and water retention and hypokalaemia
Carvedilol	Avoid
Caspofungin	70 mg on first day then 35 mg once daily in moderate hepatic impairment; no information available for severe hepatic impairment
Ceftriaxone	Reduce dose and monitor plasma concentration if both hepatic and severe renal impairment
Celecoxib	*see* NSAIDs
Certoparin	*see* Heparin
Cetrorelix	Manufacturer advises avoid in moderate liver impairment
Chloral hydrate	*see* Anxiolytics and Hypnotics
Chloramphenicol	Avoid if possible—increased risk of bone-marrow depression; reduce dose and monitor plasma-chloramphenicol concentration
Chlordiazepoxide	*see* Anxiolytics and Hypnotics
Chlorphenamine (chlorpheniramine)	Sedation inappropriate in severe liver disease—avoid
Chlorpheniramine	*see* Chlorphenamine
Chlorpromazine	*see* Antipsychotics
Chlorpropamide	*see* Sulphonylureas
Chlortalidone	*see* Thiazides and Related Diuretics
Chlortetracycline	*see* Tetracyclines
Ciclosporin	May need dose adjustment
Cilazapril	*see* ACE Inhibitors
Cilostazol	Avoid in moderate or severe liver disease

Drug	Comment
Cimetidine	Increased risk of confusion; reduce dose
Cinnarizine	Sedation inappropriate in severe liver disease—avoid
Ciprofibrate	Avoid in severe liver disease
Citalopram	Use doses at lower end of range
Cladribine	Regular monitoring recommended
Clarithromycin	Hepatic dysfunction including jaundice reported
Clavulanic acid [ingredient]	see Co-amoxiclav, p. 693 and Timentin®, p. 693
Clemastine	Sedation inappropriate in severe liver disease—avoid
Clindamycin	Reduce dose
Clobazam	see Anxiolytics and Hypnotics
Clomethiazole	see Anxiolytics and Hypnotics
Clomifene	Avoid in severe liver disease
Clomipramine	see Antidepressants, Tricyclic (and related)
Clopamide	see Thiazides and Related Diuretics
Clopidogrel	Manufacturer advises caution (risk of bleeding); avoid in severe hepatic impairment
Clorazepate	see Anxiolytics and Hypnotics
Clozapine	Initial dose 12.5 mg daily increased slowly with regular monitoring of liver function; avoid in symptomatic or progressive liver disease or hepatic failure
Co-amoxiclav	Monitor liver function in liver disease. Cholestatic jaundice, see p. 262
Codeine	see Opioid Analgesics
Colestyramine	Interferes with absorption of fat-soluble vitamins and may aggravate malabsorption in primary biliary cirrhosis; likely to be ineffective in complete biliary obstruction
Contraceptives, oral	Avoid in active liver disease and if history of pruritus or cholestasis during pregnancy
Co-trimoxazole	Manufacturer advises avoid in severe liver disease
Cyclizine	Sedation inappropriate in severe liver disease—avoid
Cyclopenthiazide	see Thiazides and Related Diuretics
Cyclophosphamide	Reduce dose
Cyclosporin	see Ciclosporin
Cyproheptadine	Sedation inappropriate in severe liver disease—avoid
Cyproterone acetate	Dose-related toxicity; see also side-effects of cyproterone, section 8.3.4.2
Cytarabine	Reduce dose
Dacarbazine	Dose reduction may be required in mild to moderate liver disease; avoid if severe
Dalfopristin [ingredient]	see Synercid®
Dalteparin	see Heparin
Dantrolene	Avoid—may cause severe liver damage
Darbepoetin	Manufacturer advises caution
Daunorubicin	Reduce dose

Drug	Comment
Debrisoquine	May need dose reduction
Demeclocycline	see Tetracyclines
Desflurane	Reduce dose
Desogestrel	Avoid; see also Contraceptives, Oral
Dexketoprofen	see NSAIDs
Dextromethorphan	see Opioid Analgesics
Dextropropoxyphene	see Opioid Analgesics
Diamorphine	see Opioid Analgesics
Diazepam	see Anxiolytics and Hypnotics
Diclofenac	see NSAIDs
Didanosine	Insufficient information but consider dose reduction
Diethylstilbestrol	Avoid; see also Contraceptives, Oral
Diflunisal	see NSAIDs
Dihydrocodeine	see Opioid Analgesics
Diltiazem	Reduce dose
Diphenhydramine	Caution in mild to moderate liver disease; avoid in severe disease if sedation is inappropriate
Diphenoxylate	see Opioid Analgesics
Diphenylpyraline	Caution in mild to moderate liver disease; avoid in severe disease if sedation is inappropriate
Dipipanone	see Opioid Analgesics
Disopyramide	Half-life prolonged—may need dose reduction
Docetaxel	Monitor liver function—reduce dose according to liver enzymes; avoid in severe hepatic impairment
Dosulepin (dothiepin)	see Antidepressants, Tricyclic (and related)
Dothiepin	see Antidepressants, Tricyclic (and related)
Doxazosin	No information—manufacturer advises caution
Doxepin	see Antidepressants, Tricyclic (and related)
Doxorubicin	Reduce dose according to bilirubin concentration
Doxycycline	see Tetracyclines
Doxylamine	Caution in mild to moderate liver disease; avoid in severe disease if sedation is inappropriate
Drotrecogin alfa (activated)	Avoid in chronic severe liver disease
Dutasteride	Manufacturer advises avoid in severe liver impairment—no information available
Dydrogesterone	Avoid; see also Contraceptives, Oral
Efavirenz	In mild to moderate liver disease, monitor liver function; avoid in severe hepatic impairment
Eformoterol	see Formoterol
Eletriptan	Manufacturer advises avoid in severe hepatic impairment
Enalapril	see ACE Inhibitors
Enfuvirtide	Manufacturer advises caution—no information available
Enoxaparin	see Heparin
Entacapone	Avoid
Epirubicin	Reduce dose according to bilirubin concentration

Drug	Comment
Epoetin	Manufacturers advise caution in chronic hepatic failure
Eprosartan	Halve initial dose in mild or moderate liver disease; avoid if severe
Eptifibatide	Avoid in severe liver disease—increased risk of bleeding
Ergometrine	Avoid in severe liver disease
Ergotamine	Avoid in severe liver disease—risk of toxicity increased
Erythromycin	May cause idiosyncratic hepatotoxicity
Escitalopram	Initial dose 5 mg daily (for 2 weeks), increased to 10 mg daily according to response
Esomeprazole	In severe liver disease dose should not exceed 20 mg daily
Estradiol	Avoid; see also Contraceptives, Oral
Estramustine	Manufacturer advises caution and regular liver function tests; avoid in severe liver disease
Estriol	Avoid; see also Contraceptives, Oral
Estrone	Avoid; see also Contraceptives, Oral
Estropipate	Avoid; see also Contraceptives, Oral
Ethinylestradiol	Avoid; see also Contraceptives, Oral
Etodolac	see NSAIDs
Etoposide	Avoid in severe hepatic impairment
Etynodiol diacetate	Avoid; see also Contraceptives, Oral
Exemestane	Manufacturer advises caution
Ezetimibe	Avoid in moderate and severe hepatic impairment—may accumulate
Famciclovir	Usual dose in well compensated liver disease (information not available on decompensated)
Felodipine	Reduce dose
Fenbufen	see NSAIDs
Fenofibrate	Avoid in severe liver disease
Fenoprofen	see NSAIDs
Fentanyl	see Opioid Analgesics
Flecainide	Avoid (or reduce dose) in severe liver disease
Flucloxacillin	Cholestatic jaundice, see p. 260
Fluconazole	Toxicity with related drugs
Flunitrazepam	see Anxiolytics and Hypnotics
Fluorouracil	Manufacturer advises caution
Fluoxetine	see Antidepressants, SSRI
Flupentixol	see Antipsychotics
Fluphenazine	see Antipsychotics
Flurazepam	see Anxiolytics and Hypnotics
Flurbiprofen	see NSAIDs
Flutamide	Use with caution (hepatotoxic)
Fluvastatin	see Statins
Fluvoxamine	see Antidepressants, SSRI
Formoterol (eformoterol)	Metabolism possibly reduced in severe cirrhosis
Fosinopril	see ACE Inhibitors
Fosphenytoin	Consider 10–25% reduction in dose or infusion rate (except initial dose for status epilepticus)

Drug	Comment
Frovatriptan	Avoid in severe hepatic impairment
Frusemide	see Loop Diuretics
Furosemide (frusemide)	see Loop Diuretics
Fusidic acid	see Sodium Fusidate
Galantamine	Reduce dose in moderate hepatic impairment; avoid in severe impairment
Ganirelix	Manufacturer advises avoid in moderate or severe hepatic impairment
Gemcitabine	Manufacturer advises caution
Gemfibrozil	Avoid in liver disease
Gestodene	Avoid; see also Contraceptives, Oral
Gestonorone	Avoid; see also Contraceptives, Oral
Gestrinone	Avoid in severe liver disease
Glibenclamide	see Sulphonylureas
Gliclazide	see Sulphonylureas
Glimepiride	Manufacturer advises avoid in severe hepatic impairment
Glipizide	see Sulphonylureas
Gliquidone	see Sulphonylureas
Griseofulvin	Avoid in severe liver disease
Haloperidol	see Antipsychotics
Halothane	Avoid if history of unexplained pyrexia or jaundice following previous exposure to halothane
Heparin	Reduce dose in severe liver disease
Hydralazine	Reduce dose
Hydrochlorothiazide	see Thiazides and Related Diuretics
Hydroflumethiazide	see Thiazides and Related Diuretics
Hydromorphone	see Opioid Analgesics
Hydroxyzine	Sedation inappropriate in severe liver disease—avoid
Hypnotics	see Anxiolytics and Hypnotics
Ibandronic acid	Manufacturer advises caution in severe hepatic impairment—limited information available
Ibuprofen	see NSAIDs
Idarubicin	Reduce dose according to bilirubin concentration
Ifosfamide	Avoid
Imidapril	see ACE Inhibitors
Imipramine	see Antidepressants, Tricyclic (and related)
Indapamide	see Thiazides and Related Diuretics
Indinavir	Reduce dose to 600 mg every 8 hours in mild to moderate hepatic impairment; not studied in severe impairment
Indometacin	see NSAIDs
Indoramin	Manufacturer advises caution
Interferon alfa	Close monitoring in mild to moderate hepatic impairment; avoid if severe
Interferon beta	Avoid in decompensated liver disease

Drug	Comment
Irinotecan	Monitor closely for neutropenia if plasma-bilirubin concentration up to 1.5 times upper limit of normal range; avoid if plasma-bilirubin concentration greater than 1.5 times upper limit of normal range
Iron dextran	Avoid in severe hepatic impairment
Iron sorbital	Avoid
Iron sucrose	Avoid
Isocarboxazid	*see* Antidepressants, MAOI
Isoniazid	Use with caution; monitor liver function regularly and particularly frequently in the first 2 months; *see also* p. 284
Isotretinoin	Avoid—further impairment of liver function may occur
Isradipine	Reduce dose
Itraconazole	Half-life prolonged—dose reduction may be necessary
Kaletra®	Avoid oral solution because of propylene glycol content; use capsules with caution in mild to moderate hepatic impairment and avoid in severe impairment
Ketoconazole	Avoid
Ketoprofen	*see* NSAIDs
Ketorolac	*see* NSAIDs
Ketotifen	Sedation inappropriate in severe liver disease—avoid
Labetalol	Avoid—severe hepatocellular injury reported
Lacidipine	Antihypertensive effect possibly increased
Lamotrigine	Halve dose in moderate liver disease; quarter dose in severe liver disease
Lansoprazole	In severe liver disease dose should not exceed 30 mg daily
Leflunomide	Avoid—active metabolite may accumulate
Lepirudin	No information—manufacturer advises that cirrhosis may affect renal excretion
Lercanidipine	Avoid in severe liver disease
Levetiracetam	Halve dose in severe hepatic impairment (due to concomitant renal impairment)
Levobupivacaine	Manufacturer advises caution in liver disease
Levomepromazine (methotrimeprazine)	*see* Antipsychotics
Levonorgestrel	Avoid; *see also* Contraceptives, Oral
Lidocaine (lignocaine)	Avoid (or reduce dose) in severe liver disease
Lignocaine	*see* Lidocaine
Linezolid	In severe hepatic impairment manufacturer advises use only if potential benefit outweighs risk
Lofepramine	*see* Antidepressants, Tricyclic (and related)
Loop diuretics	Hypokalaemia may precipitate coma (use potassium-sparing diuretic to prevent this); increased risk of hypomagnesaemia in alcoholic cirrhosis
Lopinavir [ingredient]	*see* Kaletra®

Drug	Comment
Loprazolam	*see* Anxiolytics and Hypnotics
Lorazepam	*see* Anxiolytics and Hypnotics
Lormetazepam	*see* Anxiolytics and Hypnotics
Losartan	Consider lower dose
Lumefantrine [ingredient]	*see* Riamet®
Lymecycline	*see* Tetracyclines
Magnesium salts	Avoid in hepatic coma if risk of renal failure
Maprotiline	*see* Antidepressants, Tricyclic (and related)
Meclozine	Sedation inappropriate in severe liver disease—avoid
Medroxyprogesterone	Avoid; *see also* Contraceptives, Oral
Mefenamic acid	*see* NSAIDs
Mefloquine	Avoid for prophylaxis in severe liver disease
Megestrol	Avoid; *see also* Contraceptives, Oral
Meloxicam	*see* NSAIDs
Meprobamate	*see* Anxiolytics and Hypnotics
Meptazinol	*see* Opioid Analgesics
Mercaptopurine	May need dose reduction
Meropenem	Monitor transaminase and bilirubin concentrations
Mesterolone	*see* Androgens
Mestranol	Avoid; *see also* Contraceptives, Oral
Metformin	Withdraw if tissue hypoxia likely—manufacturers advise avoid
Methadone	*see* Opioid Analgesics
Methenamine	Avoid
Methionine	May precipitate coma
Methocarbamol	Manufacturer advises caution; half-life may be prolonged
Methotrexate	Dose-related toxicity—avoid in non-malignant conditions (e.g. psoriasis)
Methotrimeprazine	*see* Antipsychotics
Methoxsalen	Avoid or reduce dose
Methyldopa	Manufacturer advises caution in history of liver disease; avoid in active liver disease
Methysergide	Avoid
Metoclopramide	Reduce dose
Metolazone	*see* Thiazides and Related Diuretics
Metoprolol	Reduce oral dose
Metronidazole	In severe liver disease reduce total daily dose to one-third, and give once daily
Mexiletine	Avoid (or reduce dose) in severe liver disease
Mianserin	*see* Antidepressants, Tricyclic (and related)
Miconazole	Avoid
Midazolam	*see* Anxiolytics and Hypnotics
Minocycline	*see* Tetracyclines
Mirtazapine	Manufacturer advises caution
Mitoxantrone	Manufacturer advises caution in severe hepatic impairment
Mivacurium	Reduce dose
Mizolastine	Manufacturer recommends avoid in significant hepatic impairment

Drug	Comment
Moclobemide	Reduce dose in severe liver disease
Modafinil	Halve dose in severe liver disease
Moexipril	see ACE Inhibitors
Morphine	see Opioid Analgesics
Moxifloxacin	Manufacturer advises avoid in severe hepatic impairment
Moxonidine	Avoid in severe liver disease
Nabumetone	see NSAIDs
Nalbuphine	see Opioid Analgesics
Nalidixic acid	Manufacturer advises caution in liver disease
Nandrolone	see Anabolic Steroids
Naproxen	see NSAIDs
Naratriptan	Max. 2.5 mg in 24 hours in moderate hepatic impairment; avoid if severe
Nateglinide	Manufacturer advises caution in moderate hepatic impairment; avoid in severe impairment—no information available
Nebivolol	No information available—manufacturer advises avoid
Nelfinavir	No information available—manufacturer advises caution
Neomycin	Absorbed from gastro-intestinal tract in liver disease—increased risk of ototoxicity
Nevirapine	Manufacturer advises caution in moderate hepatic impairment; avoid in severe hepatic impairment; see also p. 306
Nicardipine	Reduce dose
Nicoumalone	see Anticoagulants, Oral
Nifedipine	Reduce dose
Nimodipine	Elimination reduced in cirrhosis—monitor blood pressure
Nisoldipine	Formulation not suitable in hepatic impairment
Nitrazepam	see Anxiolytics and Hypnotics
Nitrofurantoin	Cholestatic jaundice and chronic active hepatitis reported
Nitroprusside	see Sodium Nitroprusside
Nizatidine	Manufacturer advises caution
Norethisterone	Avoid; see also Contraceptives, Oral
Norgestimate	Avoid; see also Contraceptives, Oral
Norgestrel	Avoid; see also Contraceptives, Oral
Nortriptyline	see Antidepressants, Tricyclic (and related)

Drug	Comment
NSAIDs	Increased risk of gastro-intestinal bleeding and can cause fluid retention; avoid in severe liver disease; aceclofenac, initially 100 mg daily; celecoxib, halve initial dose in moderate liver disease; etoricoxib, max. 60 mg daily in mild hepatic impairment (max. 60 mg on alternate days in moderate hepatic impairment); parecoxib, halve dose in moderate hepatic impairment (max. 40 mg daily); rofecoxib max. 12.5 mg daily in moderate hepatic impairment; valdecoxib max. 10 mg daily for osteoarthritis and rheumatoid arthritis (max. 20 mg daily for dysmenorrhoea) in moderate hepatic impairment
Oestrogens	Avoid; see also Contraceptives, Oral
Ofloxacin	Elimination may be reduced in severe hepatic impairment
Olanzapine	Consider initial dose of 5 mg daily
Olmesartan	No information available—manufacturer advises avoid
Omeprazole	In liver disease not more than 20 mg daily should be needed
Ondansetron	Reduce dose; not more than 8 mg daily in severe liver disease
Opioid analgesics	Avoid or reduce dose—may precipitate coma
Oral contraceptives	see Contraceptives, Oral
Oxazepam	see Anxiolytics and Hypnotics
Oxcarbazepine	No dosage adjustment required in mild to moderate hepatic impairment; no information in severe impairment
Oxprenolol	Reduce dose
Oxybutynin	Manufacturer advises caution
Oxycodone	see Opioid Analgesics
Oxytetracycline	see Tetracyclines
Paclitaxel	Avoid in severe liver disease
Pancuronium	Possibly slower onset, higher dose requirement and prolonged recovery time
Pantoprazole	Max. 20 mg daily in severe hepatic impairment and cirrhosis—monitor liver function (discontinue if deterioration)
Papaveretum	see Opioid Analgesics
Paracetamol	Dose-related toxicity—avoid large doses
Parecoxib	see NSAIDs
Paroxetine	see Antidepressants, SSRI
Peginterferon alfa	Avoid in severe hepatic impairment
Pentazocine	see Opioid Analgesics
Pericyazine	see Antipsychotics
Perindopril	see ACE Inhibitors
Perphenazine	see Antipsychotics
Pethidine	see Opioid Analgesics
Phenazocine	see Opioid Analgesics
Phenelzine	see Antidepressants, MAOI
Phenindione	see Anticoagulants, Oral
Phenobarbital	May precipitate coma
Phenoperidine	see Opioid Analgesics

Drug	Comment
Phenothiazines	*see* Antipsychotics
Phenytoin	Reduce dose to avoid toxicity
Pholcodine	*see* Opioid Analgesics
Pilocarpine	Reduce initial oral dose in moderate or severe cirrhosis
Pimozide	*see* Antipsychotics
Pioglitazone	Avoid
Piperazine	Manufacturer advises avoid
Pipotiazine	*see* Antipsychotics
Piracetam	Avoid
Piroxicam	*see* NSAIDs
Pravastatin	*see* Statins
Prazosin	Initially 500 micrograms daily; increased with caution
Prednisolone	Side-effects more common
Primidone	Reduce dose; may precipitate coma
Procainamide	Avoid or reduce dose
Procarbazine	Avoid in severe hepatic impairment
Prochlorperazine	*see* Antipsychotics
Progesterone	Avoid; *see also* Contraceptives, Oral
Progestogens	Avoid; *see also* Contraceptives, Oral
Promazine	*see* Antipsychotics
Promethazine	Avoid—may precipitate coma in severe liver disease; hepatotoxic
Propafenone	Reduce dose
Propantheline	Manufacturer advises caution
Propiverine	Avoid
Propranolol	Reduce oral dose
Propylthiouracil	Reduce dose
Pyrazinamide	Avoid—idiosyncratic hepatotoxicity more common; *see also* p. 285
Pyrimethamine	Manufacturer advises caution
Quetiapine	Manufacturer advises initial dose of 25 mg daily, increased daily in steps of 25–50 mg
Quinagolide	Manufacturer advises avoid—no information available
Quinapril	*see* ACE Inhibitors
Quinupristin [ingredient]	*see* Synercid®
Rabeprazole	Manufacturer advises caution in severe hepatic dysfunction
Raloxifene	Manufacturer advises avoid
Raltitrexed	Caution in mild or moderate disease; avoid if severe
Ramipril	*see* ACE Inhibitors
Reboxetine	Initial dose 2 mg twice daily, increased according to tolerance
Remifentanil	*see* Opioid Analgesics
Repaglinide	Manufacturer advises avoid in severe liver disease
Reviparin	Manufacturer advises avoid in severe hepatic impairment
Riamet®	Manufacturer advises caution in severe hepatic impairment—monitor ECG and plasma potassium concentration
Ribavirin	No dosage adjustment required; avoid oral administration in severe hepatic dysfunction or decompensated cirrhosis
Rifabutin	Reduce dose in severe hepatic impairment

Drug	Comment
Rifampicin	Impaired elimination; monitor liver function; avoid or do not exceed 8 mg/kg daily; *see also* p. 285
Riluzole	Avoid
Risperidone	Manufacturer advises initial oral dose of 500 micrograms twice daily increased in steps of 500 micrograms twice daily to 1–2 mg twice daily; if an oral dose of at least 2 mg daily tolerated, 25 mg as a depot injection can be given every 2 weeks
Ritonavir	Avoid in severe hepatic impairment
Rivastigmine	No information available—manufacturer advises avoid in severe liver disease
Rizatriptan	Reduce dose to 5 mg in mild to moderate liver disease; avoid in severe liver disease
Rocuronium	Reduce dose
Rofecoxib	*see* NSAIDs
Ropinirole	Avoid in severe hepatic impairment
Ropivacaine	Manufacturer advises caution in severe liver disease
Rosiglitazone	Avoid
Saquinavir	Plasma concentration possibly increased; manufacturer advises caution with *Fortovase®* in moderate hepatic impairment and with *Invirase®* in severe impairment; avoid *Fortovase®* in severe impairment
Sertindole	Slower titration and lower maintenance dose in mild to moderate hepatic impairment; avoid in severe hepatic impairment; *see also* Antipsychotics
Sertraline	*see* Antidepressants, SSRI
Sibutramine	Increased plasma-sibutramine concentration; manufacturer advises caution in mild to moderate hepatic impairment; avoid if severe impairment
Sildenafil	Initial dose 25 mg; manufacturer advises avoid in severe hepatic impairment
Simvastatin	*see* Statins
Sirolimus	Monitor blood-sirolimus trough concentration
Sodium aurothiomalate	Caution in mild to moderate liver disease; avoid in severe liver disease
Sodium bicarbonate	*see* Antacids
Sodium fusidate	Impaired biliary excretion; possibly increased risk of hepatotoxicity; avoid or reduce dose
Sodium nitroprusside	Avoid in severe liver disease
Sodium phenylbutyrate	Manufacturer advises caution
Sodium valproate	*see* Valproate
Statins	Avoid in active liver disease or unexplained persistent elevations in serum transaminases
Stilboestrol (diethylstilbestrol)	Avoid; *see also* Contraceptives, Oral
Sulindac	*see* NSAIDs

Drug	Comment
Sulphonylureas	Increased risk of hypoglycaemia in severe liver disease; avoid or use small dose; can produce jaundice; *see also* Glimepiride
Sulpiride	*see* Antipsychotics
Sumatriptan	Manufacturer advises 50 mg oral dose in hepatic impairment; avoid in severe hepatic impairment
Suxamethonium	Prolonged apnoea may occur in severe liver disease due to reduced hepatic synthesis of pseudocholinesterase
Synercid®	Consider reducing dose to 5 mg/kg every 8 hours in moderate hepatic impairment, adjusted according to clinical response; avoid in severe hepatic impairment or if plasma-bilirubin concentration greater than 3 times upper limit of reference range
Tacrolimus	Reduce dose
Tadalafil	Max. dose 10 mg
Tamsulosin	Avoid in severe hepatic impairment
Tegafur with uracil	*see Uftoral®*
Telmisartan	20–40 mg once daily in mild or moderate impairment; avoid in severe hepatic impairment or biliary obstruction
Temazepam	*see* Anxiolytics and Hypnotics
Tenoxicam	*see* NSAIDs
Terbinafine	Manufacturer advises avoid—elimination reduced
Terfenadine	Avoid—risk of arrhythmias
Testosterone and esters	*see* Androgens
Tetracyclines	Avoid (or use with caution); tetracycline and demeclocycline max. 1 g daily in divided doses
Theophylline	Reduce dose
Thiazides and related diuretics	Avoid in severe liver disease; hypokalaemia may precipitate coma (potassium-sparing diuretic can prevent); increased risk of hypomagnesaemia in alcoholic cirrhosis
Thiopental	Reduce dose for induction in severe liver disease
Thioridazine	*see* Antipsychotics
Tiagabine	Maintenance dose 5–10 mg 1–2 times daily initially in mild to moderate hepatic impairment; avoid in severe impairment
Tiaprofenic acid	*see* NSAIDs
Tibolone	Avoid in severe liver disease
Ticarcillin [ingredient]	*see* Timentin®
Timentin®	Cholestatic jaundice, *see* under Co-amoxiclav p. 262
Tinzaparin	*see* Heparin
Tirofiban	Caution in mild to moderate liver disease; avoid in severe liver disease—increased risk of bleeding
Tizanidine	Avoid in severe liver disease
Tolbutamide	*see* Sulphonylureas
Tolfenamic acid	*see* NSAIDs
Tolterodine	Reduce dose to 1 mg twice daily

Drug	Comment
Topiramate	Use with caution in hepatic impairment—clearance may be decreased
Topotecan	Avoid in severe hepatic impairment
Torasemide	*see* Loop Diuretics
Toremifene	Elimination decreased in hepatic impairment—avoid if severe
Tramadol	*see* Opioid Analgesics
Trandolapril	*see* ACE Inhibitors
Tranylcypromine	*see* Antidepressants, MAOI
Trazodone	*see* Antidepressants, Tricyclic (and related)
Tretinoin (oral)	Reduce dose
Tribavirin	*see* Ribavirin
Triclofos	*see* Anxiolytics and Hypnotics
Trifluoperazine	*see* Antipsychotics
Trimeprazine	*see* Alimemazine
Trimetrexate	Manufacturer advises caution; interrupt treatment if severe abnormalities in liver function tests (consult product literature)
Trimipramine	*see* Antidepressants, Tricyclic (and related)
Triprolidine	Sedation inappropriate in severe liver disease—avoid
Trospium	Manufacturer advises avoid—no information available
Uftoral®	Manufacturer advises monitor liver function in mild to moderate hepatic impairment and avoid in severe impairment
Ursodeoxycholic acid	Avoid in chronic liver disease (but used in primary biliary cirrhosis)
Valaciclovir	Manufacturer advises caution with high doses used for preventing cytomegalovirus disease—no information available
Valproate	Avoid if possible—hepatotoxicity and hepatic failure may occasionally occur (usually in first 6 months); *see also* p. 233
Valproic acid	*see* Valproate
Valsartan	Halve dose in mild to moderate hepatic impairment; avoid if severe
Vardenafil	Initial dose 5 mg; manufacturer advises avoid in severe hepatic impairment
Venlafaxine	Halve dose in moderate hepatic impairment; avoid if severe
Verapamil	Reduce oral dose
Verteporfin	Avoid in severe hepatic impairment
Vinblastine	Dose reduction may be necessary
Vincristine	Dose reduction may be necessary
Vindesine	Dose reduction may be necessary
Vinorelbine	Dose reduction may be required in significant hepatic impairment

Drug	Comment
Voriconazole	In mild to moderate hepatic cirrhosis use normal loading dose then halve normal maintenance dose; no information available for severe hepatic cirrhosis—manufacturer advises use only if potential benefit outweighs risk
Warfarin	*see* Anticoagulants, Oral
Xipamide	*see* Thiazides and Related Diuretics
Zafirlukast	Manufacturer advises avoid
Zalcitabine	Further impairment of liver function may occur
Zaleplon	*see* Anxiolytics and Hypnotics
Zidovudine	Accumulation may occur
Zoledronic acid	Manufacturer advises caution in severe hepatic impairment—limited information available
Zolmitriptan	Max. 5 mg in 24 hours in moderate or severe hepatic impairment
Zolpidem	*see* Anxiolytics and Hypnotics
Zopiclone	*see* Anxiolytics and Hypnotics
Zotepine	Initial dose 25 mg twice daily, increased gradually according to response (max. 75 mg twice daily); monitor liver function at weekly intervals for first 3 months
Zuclopenthixol	*see* Antipsychotics

Appendix 3: Renal impairment

The use of drugs in patients with reduced renal function can give rise to problems for several reasons:

- failure to excrete a drug or its metabolites may produce toxicity;
- sensitivity to some drugs is increased even if elimination is unimpaired;
- many side-effects are tolerated poorly by patients in renal failure;
- some drugs cease to be effective when renal function is reduced.

Many of these problems can be avoided by reducing the dose or by using alternative drugs.

Principles of dose adjustment in renal impairment

The level of renal function below which the dose of a drug must be reduced depends on whether the drug is eliminated entirely by renal excretion or is partly metabolised, and on how toxic it is.

For many drugs with only minor or no dose-related side-effects very precise modification of the dose regimen is unnecessary and a simple scheme for dose reduction is sufficient.

For more toxic drugs with a small safety margin dose regimens based on glomerular filtration rate should be used. For those where both efficacy and toxicity are closely related to plasma concentrations recommended regimens should be seen only as a guide to initial treatment; subsequent treatment must be adjusted according to clinical response and plasma concentration.

The total daily maintenance dose of a drug can be reduced either by reducing the size of the individual doses or by increasing the interval between doses. For some drugs, if the size of the maintenance dose is reduced it will be important to give a loading dose if an immediate effect is required. This is because when a patient is given a regular dose of any drug it takes more than five times the half-life to achieve steady-state plasma concentrations. As the plasma half-life of drugs excreted by the kidney is prolonged in renal failure it may take many days for the reduced dosage to achieve a therapeutic plasma concentration. The loading dose should usually be the same size as the initial dose for a patient with normal renal function.

Nephrotoxic drugs should, if possible, be avoided in patients with renal disease because the consequences of nephrotoxicity are likely to be more serious when the renal reserve is already reduced.

Use of dosage table

Dose recommendations are based on the severity of renal impairment. This is expressed in terms of glomerular filtration rate (GFR), usually measured by the **creatinine clearance** (best calculated from a 24-hour urine collection). The serum-creatinine concentration is sometimes used instead as a measure of renal function but is only a **rough guide** even when corrected for age, weight, and sex. Nomograms are available for making the correction and should be used where accuracy is important.

For *prescribing purposes* renal impairment is arbitrarily divided into 3 grades (definitions vary for grades of renal impairment; therefore, where the product literature does not correspond with this grading, values for creatinine clearance or another measure of renal function are included):

Grade	GFR	Serum creatinine (approx.) (but see above)
Mild	20–50 mL/minute	150–300 micromol/litre
Moderate	10–20 mL/minute	300–700 micromol/litre
Severe	< 10 mL/minute	> 700 micromol/litre

NOTE. Conversion factors are:
Litres/24 hours = mL/minute × 1.44
mL/minute = Litres/24 hours × 0.69

Dialysis. For prescribing in patients on continuous ambulatory peritoneal dialysis (CAPD) or haemodialysis, consult specialist literature.

Renal function declines with age; many elderly patients have a glomerular filtration rate below 50 mL/minute which, because of reduced muscle mass, may not be indicated by a raised serum creatinine. It is wise to assume at least mild impairment of renal function when prescribing for the elderly.

The following table may be used as a guide to drugs which are known to require a reduction in dose in renal impairment, and to those which are potentially harmful or are ineffective. Drug prescribing should be kept to the minimum in all patients with severe renal disease.

If even mild renal impairment is considered likely on clinical grounds, renal function should be checked before prescribing **any** drug which requires dose modification.

Table of drugs to be avoided or used with caution in renal impairment

Products introduced or amended since publication of BNF No. 46 (September 2003) are underlined.

Drug and degree of impairment	Comment
Abacavir	
Severe	Avoid
Abciximab	
Severe	Avoid—increased risk of bleeding
Acamprosate	
Mild	Avoid; excreted in urine
Acarbose	
Moderate to severe	Manufacturer advises avoid—no information available

Drug and degree of impairment	Comment

ACE inhibitors
Mild to moderate — Use with caution and monitor response (see also p. 90). Hyperkalaemia and other side-effects more common. Initial doses: captopril 12.5 mg twice daily, cilazapril 500 micrograms once daily, enalapril 2.5 mg once daily, imidapril 2.5 mg once daily (avoid if creatinine clearance less than 30 mL/minute), moexipril 3.75 mg once daily, perindopril 2 mg once daily (2 mg once daily on alternate days in moderate impairment), quinapril 2.5 mg once daily, ramipril 1.25 mg once daily, trandolapril 500 micrograms once daily

Acebutolol — *see* Beta-blockers

Aceclofenac — *see* NSAIDs

Acemetacin — *see* NSAIDs

Acenocoumarol (nicoumalone) — *see* Anticoagulants, Oral

Acetazolamide
Mild — Avoid; metabolic acidosis

Aciclovir
Mild — Reduce intravenous dose
Moderate to severe — Reduce dose

Acipimox
Mild — Reduce dose; avoid if creatinine clearance less than 30 mL/minute

Acitretin
Mild — Avoid; increased risk of toxicity

Aclarubicin — Manufacturer advises caution

Acrivastine
Moderate — Avoid; excreted by kidney

Adefovir dipivoxil
Mild — 10 mg every 48 hours
Moderate — 10 mg every 72 hours
Severe — No information available

Adrenergic neurone blockers
Moderate to severe — Avoid; increased postural hypotension; decrease in renal blood flow

Alendronic acid
Mild — Manufacturer advises avoid if creatinine clearance less than 35 mL/minute

Alfentanil — *see* Opioid Analgesics

Alfuzosin — Start at 2.5 mg twice daily and adjust according to response

Alimemazine (trimeprazine)
Severe — Avoid

Allopurinol
Moderate — 100–200 mg daily; increased toxicity; rashes
Severe — 100 mg on alternate days (max. 100 mg daily)

Almotriptan
Severe — Max. 12.5 mg in 24 hours

Alprazolam — *see* Anxiolytics and Hypnotics

Alteplase
Moderate — Risk of hyperkalaemia

Aluminium salts
Severe — Aluminium is absorbed and may accumulate

NOTE. Absorption of aluminium from aluminium salts is increased by citrates, which are contained in many effervescent preparations (such as effervescent analgesics)

Amantadine
Mild to moderate — Reduce dose; avoid in elderly if creatinine clearance less than 60 mL/minute
Severe — Avoid

Amfebutamone — *see* Bupropion

Amifostine — Manufacturer advises avoid

Amikacin — *see* Aminoglycosides

Amiloride — *see* Potassium-sparing Diuretics

Aminoglycosides
Mild — Reduce dose; monitor serum concentrations; *see also* section 5.1.4

Amisulpride
Mild — Manufacturer advises use half normal dose
Moderate — Manufacturer advises use one-third of normal dose
Severe — Manufacturer advises dose reduction and intermittent treatment

Amobarbital
Severe — Reduce dose; active metabolite accumulates

Amoxicillin
Severe — Reduce dose; rashes more common

Amphotericin
Mild — Use only if no alternative; nephrotoxicity may be reduced with use of complexes

Ampicillin
Severe — Reduce dose; rashes more common

Amprenavir
Mild to moderate — Use oral solution with caution due to high propylene glycol content
Severe — Avoid oral solution

Amsacrine — Reduce dose

Anakinra
Mild — Manufacturer advises caution if creatinine clearance 30–50 mL/minute; avoid if creatinine clearance less than 30 mL/minute

Analgesics — *see* Opioid Analgesics and NSAIDs

Anastrozole
Moderate to severe — Avoid—no information available

Anticoagulants, oral
Severe — Avoid

Antipsychotics
Severe — Start with small doses; increased cerebral sensitivity; *see also* Amisulpride, Clozapine, Olanzapine, Quetiapine, Risperidone and Sulpiride

Anxiolytics and hypnotics
Severe — Start with small doses; increased cerebral sensitivity; *see also* chloral hydrate

Drug and degree of impairment	Comment
Apomorphine	
Severe	Use with caution; max. sublingual dose 2 mg
Artemether [ingredient]	*see* Riamet®
Aspirin	
Severe	Avoid; sodium and water retention; deterioration in renal function; increased risk of gastrointestinal bleeding
Atenolol	*see* Beta-blockers
Atosiban	No information available
Atovaquone	Manufacturer advises caution—monitor more closely
Auranofin	*see* Sodium Aurothiomalate
Azapropazone	
Mild to moderate	Max. 300 mg twice daily in rheumatoid arthritis and ankylosing spondylitis; avoid in gout if creatinine clearance less than 60 mL/minute
Severe	Avoid
Azathioprine	
Severe	Reduce dose
Azithromycin	
Moderate to severe	No information available
Aztreonam	
Moderate	Reduce dose
Baclofen	
Mild	Use smaller doses (e.g. 5 mg daily); excreted by kidney
Balsalazide	
Moderate to severe	Manufacturer advises avoid
Bambuterol	
Mild	Reduce dose
Bemiparin	*see* Heparin
Bendrofluazide	*see* Thiazides and Related Diuretics
Bendroflumethiazide (bendrofluazide)	*see* Thiazides and Related Diuretics
Benorilate [aspirin–paracetamol ester]	*see* Aspirin and Paracetamol
Benperidol	*see* Antipsychotics
Benzodiazepines	*see* Anxiolytics and Hypnotics
Benzylpenicillin	
Severe	Max. 6 g daily; neurotoxicity—high doses may cause convulsions
Beta-blockers	
Mild	Start with 2.5 mg of nebivolol; reduce dose of celiprolol if creatinine clearance less than 40 mL/minute
Moderate	Start with small dose of acebutolol (active metabolite accumulates); reduce dose of atenolol, bisoprolol, nadolol, pindolol, sotalol (all excreted unchanged); avoid celiprolol if creatinine clearance less than 15 mL/minute
Severe	Start with small dose; higher plasma concentrations after oral administration; may reduce renal blood flow and adversely affect renal function in severe impairment; manufacturer advises avoid celiprolol and sotalol

Drug and degree of impairment	Comment
Bezafibrate	
Mild to moderate	Reduce dose; avoid if creatinine clearance less than 15 mL/minute
Bisoprolol	*see* Beta-blockers
Bleomycin	
Moderate	Reduce dose
Bumetanide	
Moderate	May need high doses
Buprenorphine	*see* Opioid Analgesics
Bupropion	Manufacturer recommends 150 mg daily
Buspirone	
Mild	Reduce dose
Moderate to severe	Avoid
Calcitriol	
Severe	Manufacturer of topical calcitriol advises avoid—no information available
Candesartan	
Moderate	Halve initial dose
Severe	Avoid
Capecitabine	
Mild	Use three-quarters of starting dose if creatinine clearance 30–50 mL/minute; avoid if creatinine clearance less than 30 mL/minute
Capreomycin	
Mild	Reduce dose; nephrotoxic; ototoxic
Captopril	*see* ACE Inhibitors
Carbamazepine	Manufacturer advises caution
Carbenoxolone	
Moderate	Avoid; fluid retention
Carboplatin	
Mild	Reduce dose and monitor haematological parameters and renal function
Moderate to severe	Avoid
Cefaclor	No dose adjustment required—manufacturer advises caution
Cefadroxil	
Moderate	Reduce dose
Cefalexin	
Mild to moderate	Max. 3 g daily if creatinine clearance 40–50 mL/minute; max. 1.5 g daily if creatinine clearance 10–40 mL/minute
Severe	Max. 750 mg daily
Cefixime	
Moderate	Reduce dose
Cefotaxime	
Severe	Loading dose of 1 g then use half normal dose
Cefoxitin	
Mild	Reduce dose
Cefpirome	
Mild	Usual initial dose, then use half normal dose
Moderate to severe	Usual initial dose, then use one-quarter normal dose
Cefpodoxime	
Mild	Reduce dose
Cefprozil	Usual initial dose, then use half normal dose
Cefradine	
Moderate to severe	Reduce dose

Drug and degree of impairment	Comment
Ceftazidime	
Mild	Reduce dose
Ceftriaxone	
Severe	Max. 2 g daily; also monitor plasma concentration if both hepatic and severe renal impairment
Cefuroxime	
Moderate to severe	Reduce parenteral dose
Celecoxib	*see* NSAIDs
Celiprolol	*see* Beta-blockers
Certoparin	*see* Heparin
Cetirizine	
Moderate	Use half normal dose
Cetrorelix	
Moderate	Manufacturer advises avoid
Chloral hydrate	Avoid
Chloramphenicol	
Severe	Avoid unless no alternative; dose-related depression of haematopoiesis
Chlordiazepoxide	*see* Anxiolytics and Hypnotics
Chloroquine	
Mild to moderate	Reduce dose (but for malaria prophylaxis see section 5.4.1)
Severe	Avoid (but for malaria prophylaxis see section 5.4.1)
Chlorpromazine	*see* Antipsychotics
Chlorpropamide	Avoid
Chlortalidone	*see* Thiazides and Related Diuretics
Chlortetracycline	*see* Tetracyclines
Ciclosporin	*see* p. 425 (*see also* p. 554 if used in atopic dermatitis or psoriasis and p. 492 if used in rheumatoid arthritis)
Cidofovir	
Mild	Avoid; nephrotoxic
Cilastatin [ingredient]	*see Primaxin®*
Cilazapril	*see* ACE Inhibitors
Cilostazol	
Mild	Avoid if creatinine clearance less than 25 mL/minute
Cimetidine	
Mild to moderate	600–800 mg daily; occasional risk of confusion
Severe	400 mg daily
Ciprofibrate	
Moderate	100 mg on alternate days
Severe	Avoid
Ciprofloxacin	
Moderate	Use half normal dose
Cisplatin	
Mild	Avoid if possible; nephrotoxic and neurotoxic
Citalopram	
Moderate to severe	No information available
Citramag®	
Severe	Avoid—risk of hypermagnesaemia
Citrates	Absorption of aluminium from aluminium salts is increased by citrates, which are contained in many effervescent preparations (such as effervescent analgesics)
Cladribine	Regular monitoring recommended

Drug and degree of impairment	Comment
Clarithromycin	
Mild	Use half normal dose if creatinine clearance less than 30 mL/minute; avoid *Klaricid XL®* if creatinine clearance less than 30 mL/minute
Clavulanic acid [ingredient]	*see* Co-amoxiclav and *Timentin®*
Clobazam	*see* Anxiolytics and Hypnotics
Clodronate sodium	*see* Sodium Clodronate
Clomethiazole	*see* Anxiolytics and Hypnotics
Clopamide	*see* Thiazides and Related Diuretics
Clopidogrel	Manufacturer advises caution
Clorazepate	*see* Anxiolytics and Hypnotics
Clozapine	
Mild to moderate	Initial dose 12.5 mg daily increased slowly
Severe	Avoid
Co-amoxiclav	
Moderate to severe	Reduce dose
Codeine	*see* Opioid Analgesics
Colchicine	
Moderate	Reduce dose
Severe	Avoid or reduce dose if no alternative
Colistin	
Mild	Reduce dose; nephrotoxic; neurotoxic
Co-trimoxazole	
Mild	Use half normal dose if creatinine clearance 15–30 mL/minute; avoid if creatinine clearance less than 15 mL/minute and if plasma-sulfamethoxazole concentration cannot be monitored
Cyclopenthiazide	*see* Thiazides and Related Diuretics
Cyclophosphamide	Reduce dose
Cycloserine	
Mild to moderate	Reduce dose
Severe	Avoid
Cyclosporin	*see* Ciclosporin
Dacarbazine	
Mild to moderate	Dose reduction may be required
Severe	Avoid
Dalteparin	*see* Heparin
Daunorubicin	
Mild to moderate	Reduce dose
Debrisoquine	*see* Adrenergic Neurone Blockers
Demeclocycline	*see* Tetracyclines
Desflurane	
Moderate	Reduce dose
Desloratadine	
Severe	Manufacturer advises caution
Desmopressin	Antidiuretic effect may be reduced
Dexketoprofen	*see* NSAIDs
Dextromethorphan	*see* Opioid Analgesics
Dextropropoxyphene	*see* Opioid Analgesics
Diamorphine	*see* Opioid Analgesics
Diazepam	*see* Anxiolytics and Hypnotics
Diazoxide	
Severe	75–150 mg i/v; increased sensitivity to hypotensive effect

Drug and degree of impairment	Comment
Diclofenac	*see* NSAIDs
Didanosine	
Mild	Reduce dose; consult product literature
Diflunisal	*see* NSAIDs (excreted by kidney)
Digitoxin	
Severe	Max. 100 micrograms daily
Digoxin	
Mild	Reduce dose; toxicity increased by electrolyte disturbances
Dihydrocodeine	*see* Opioid Analgesics
Diltiazem	Start with smaller dose
Diphenoxylate	*see* Opioid Analgesics
Dipipanone	*see* Opioid Analgesics
Disodium etidronate	
Mild	Reduce dose
Moderate to severe	Avoid
Disodium pamidronate	Max. infusion rate 20 mg/hour
Moderate to severe	
Disopyramide	
Mild	100 mg every 8 hours *or* 150 mg every 12 hours
Moderate	100 mg every 12 hours
Severe	150 mg every 24 hours
NOTE. Sustained release preparations may be unsuitable; monitor plasma-disopyramide concentrations	
Diuretics, potassium-sparing	*see* Potassium-sparing Diuretics
Doxycycline	*see* Tetracyclines
Drospirenone [ingredient]	*see* Yasmin®
Efavirenz	
Severe	Manufacturer advises caution—no information available
Eletriptan	
Mild	Reduce initial dose to 20 mg; max. 40 mg in 24 hours; avoid if creatinine clearance less than 30 mL/minute
Emtricitabine	
Mild	Reduce dose
Enalapril	*see* ACE Inhibitors
Enflurane	
Severe	Avoid
Enfuvirtide	Manufacturer advises caution if creatinine clearance less than 35 mL/minute—no information available
Enoxaparin	*see* Heparin
Enoximone	Consider dose reduction
Ephedrine	
Severe	Avoid; increased CNS toxicity
Eprosartan	
Mild	Halve initial dose
Eptifibatide	
Mild	Avoid if creatinine clearance less than 30 mL/minute
Ergometrine	
Severe	Manufacturer advises avoid
Ergotamine	
Moderate	Avoid; nausea and vomiting; risk of renal vasoconstriction
Ertapenem	
Mild	Manufacturer advises avoid if creatinine clearance less than 30 mL/minute

Drug and degree of impairment	Comment
Erythromycin	
Severe	Max. 1.5 g daily (ototoxicity)
Escitalopram	
Mild	Manufacturer advises caution
Esmolol	*see* Beta-blockers
Esomeprazole	
Severe	Manufacturer advises caution
Estramustine	Manufacturer advises caution
Ethambutol	
Mild	Reduce dose; if creatinine clearance less than 30 mL/minute monitor plasma-ethambutol concentration; optic nerve damage
Etidronate disodium	*see* Disodium Etidronate
Etodolac	*see* NSAIDs
Etoricoxib	*see* NSAIDs
Exemestane	Manufacturer advises caution
Famciclovir	
Mild to moderate	Reduce dose
Famotidine	
Severe	Max. 20 mg at night
Fenbufen	*see* NSAIDs
Fenofibrate	
Mild	134 mg daily
Moderate	67 mg daily
Severe	Avoid
Fenoprofen	*see* NSAIDs
Fentanyl	*see* Opioid Analgesics
Flecainide	
Mild	Max. initial dose 100 mg daily
Fleet Phospho-soda®	
Severe	Avoid
Flucloxacillin	
Severe	Reduce dose
Fluconazole	
Mild to moderate	Usual initial dose then halve subsequent doses
Flucytosine	Reduce dose and monitor plasma-flucytosine concentration—consult product literature
Fludarabine	
Mild	Reduce dose; avoid if creatinine clearance less than 30 mL/minute
Flunitrazepam	*see* Anxiolytics and Hypnotics
Fluoxetine	
Mild to moderate	Reduce dose (give on alternate days)
Severe	Avoid
Flupentixol	*see* Antipsychotics
Fluphenazine	*see* Antipsychotics
Flurazepam	*see* Anxiolytics and Hypnotics
Flurbiprofen	*see* NSAIDs
Fluvastatin	
Severe	Avoid
Fluvoxamine	
Moderate	Start with smaller dose
Fondaparinux	Increased risk of bleeding; avoid if creatinine clearance less than 30 mL/minute
Foscarnet	
Mild	Reduce dose; consult product literature
Fosinopril	*see* ACE Inhibitors
Fosphenytoin	Consider 10–25% reduction in dose or infusion rate (except initial dose for status epilepticus)

Drug and degree of impairment	Comment
Frusemide	*see* Furosemide
Furosemide (frusemide)	
Moderate	May need high doses; deafness may follow rapid i/v injection
Fybogel Mebeverine®	
Severe	Avoid; contains 7 mmol potassium per sachet
Gabapentin	
Mild	Reduce dose; consult product literature
Galantamine	
Severe	Avoid
Gallamine	
Moderate	Avoid; prolonged paralysis
Ganciclovir	
Mild	Reduce dose; consult product literature
Ganirelix	
Moderate to severe	Manufacturer advises avoid
Gaviscon®	
Severe	Avoid; high sodium content
Gemcitabine	Manufacturer advises caution
Gemeprost	Manufacturer advises avoid
Gemfibrozil	
Severe	Start with 900 mg daily
Gentamicin	*see* Aminoglycosides
Gestrinone	
Severe	Avoid
Glatiramer	No information available—manufacturer advises caution
Glibenclamide	
Severe	Avoid
Gliclazide	
Mild to moderate	Reduce dose
Severe	Avoid if possible; if no alternative reduce dose and monitor closely
Glimepiride	
Severe	Avoid
Glipizide	
Mild to moderate	Increased risk of hypoglycaemia; avoid if hepatic impairment also present
Severe	Avoid
Gliquidone	Avoid in renal failure
Guanethidine	*see* Adrenergic Neurone Blockers
Haloperidol	*see* Antipsychotics
Heparin	
Severe	Risk of bleeding increased
Hetastarch	
Severe	Avoid; excreted by kidney
Hydralazine	
Mild	Reduce dose if creatinine clearance less than 30 mL/minute
Hydrochlorothiazide	*see* Thiazides and Related Diuretics
Hydroflumethiazide	*see* Thiazides and Related Diuretics
Hydromorphone	*see* Opioid Analgesics
Hydroxychloroquine	
Mild to moderate	Reduce dose; only on prolonged use
Severe	Avoid
Hydroxyzine	Use half normal dose
Hypnotics	*see* Anxiolytics and Hypnotics
Ibandronic acid	Avoid if serum creatinine above 442 micromol/litre

Drug and degree of impairment	Comment
Ibuprofen	*see* NSAIDs
Idarubicin	
Mild	Reduce dose
Ifosfamide	
Mild	Avoid if serum creatinine concentration greater than 120 micromol/litre
Imidapril	*see* ACE Inhibitors
Imipenem [ingredient]	*see Primaxin*®
Indapamide	*see* Thiazides and Related Diuretics
Indometacin	*see* NSAIDs
Indoramin	Manufacturer advises caution
Inosine pranobex	
Mild	Avoid; metabolised to uric acid
Insulin	
Severe	May need dose reduction; insulin requirements fall; compensatory response to hypoglycaemia is impaired
Interferon alfa	
Mild to moderate	Close monitoring required
Severe	Avoid
Interferon beta	No information available—monitoring advised
Irinotecan	No information available
Isoniazid	
Severe	Max. 200 mg daily; peripheral neuropathy
Isotretinoin	
Mild	Avoid; increased risk of toxicity
Itraconazole	Bioavailability of oral formulations possibly reduced; avoid intravenous infusion if creatinine clearance less than 30 mL/minute
Kaletra®	Avoid oral solution due to propylene glycol content; use capsules with caution in severe impairment
Ketoprofen	*see* NSAIDs
Ketorolac	*see* NSAIDs
Lamivudine	
Mild	Reduce dose; consult product literature
Lamotrigine	
Moderate to severe	Metabolite may accumulate
Leflunomide	
Moderate to severe	Manufacturer advises avoid—no information available
Lepirudin	
Mild to moderate	Manufacturer advises reducing initial dose by 50% and subsequent doses by 50–85%
Severe	Avoid or stop infusion (unless APTT is below therapeutic levels when alternate day administration may be considered)
Lercanidipine	
Severe	Avoid

Drug and degree of impairment	Comment
Levetiracetam	
Mild to moderate	Max. 2 g daily if creatinine clearance 50–80 mL/minute; max. 1.5 g daily if creatinine clearance 30–50 mL/minute; max. 1 g daily if creatinine clearance less than 30 mL/minute
Severe	0.5–1 g daily (as a single dose) in end-stage disease
Levocabastine	
Severe	Manufacturer advises avoid
Levocetirizine	
Mild to moderate	5 mg on alternate days if creatinine clearance 30–50 mL/minute; 5 mg every 3 days if creatinine clearance less than 30 mL/minute
Severe	Avoid
Levofloxacin	
Mild	Usual initial dose, then use half normal dose
Moderate to severe	Reduce dose; consult product literature
Levomepromazine (methotrimeprazine)	see Antipsychotics
Linezolid	Manufacturer advises metabolites may accumulate if creatinine clearance less than 30 mL/minute
Lisinopril	see ACE Inhibitors
Lithium salts	
Mild	Avoid if possible or reduce dose and monitor plasma concentration carefully
Moderate	Avoid
Lopinavir [ingredient]	see Kaletra®
Loprazolam	see Anxiolytics and Hypnotics
Lorazepam	see Anxiolytics and Hypnotics
Lormetazepam	see Anxiolytics and Hypnotics
Losartan	
Moderate to severe	Start with 25 mg once daily
Lumefantrine [ingredient]	see Riamet®
Lymecycline	see Tetracyclines
Magnesium salts	
Moderate	Avoid or reduce dose; increased risk of toxicity; magnesium carbonate mixture and magnesium trisilicate mixture also have high sodium content
Malarone®	
Mild	Avoid for malaria prophylaxis (and if possible for malaria treatment) if creatinine clearance less than 30 mL/minute
Mefenamic acid	see NSAIDs
Meloxicam	see NSAIDs
Melphalan	Reduce dose initially; avoid high doses in moderate to severe impairment
Memantine	
Mild	Reduce dose to 10 mg daily if creatinine clearance 40–60 mL/minute
Moderate to severe	Manufacturer advises avoid—no information available
Meprobamate	see Anxiolytics and Hypnotics

Drug and degree of impairment	Comment
Meptazinol	see Opioid Analgesics
Mercaptopurine	
Moderate	Reduce dose
Meropenem	
Mild	Increase dose interval to every 12 hours
Moderate	Use half normal dose every 12 hours
Severe	Use half normal dose every 24 hours
Mesalazine	
Moderate	Use with caution
Severe	Manufacturers advise avoid
Metformin	
Mild	Avoid; increased risk of lactic acidosis
Methadone	see Opioid Analgesics
Methenamine	
Severe	Avoid
Methocarbamol	Manufacturer advises caution
Methotrexate	
Mild	Reduce dose; accumulates; nephrotoxic
Moderate	Avoid
Methotrimeprazine	see Antipsychotics
Methyldopa	
Moderate	Start with small dose; increased sensitivity to hypotensive and sedative effect
Methysergide	Avoid
Metoclopramide	
Severe	Avoid or use small dose; increased risk of extrapyramidal reactions
Metolazone	see Thiazides and Related Diuretics
Metoprolol	see Beta-blockers
Midazolam	see Anxiolytics and Hypnotics
Milrinone	
Mild	Reduce dose and monitor response
Minocycline	see Tetracyclines
Mirtazapine	Manufacturer advises caution
Mivacurium	
Severe	Reduce dose; prolonged paralysis
Modafinil	
Severe	Use half normal dose
Moexipril	see ACE Inhibitors
Morphine	see Opioid Analgesics
Moxifloxacin	Manufacturer advises avoid if creatinine clearance less than 30 mL/minute—no information available
Moxonidine	
Mild	Max. single dose 200 micrograms and max. daily dose 400 micrograms
Moderate to severe	Avoid
Nabumetone	see NSAIDs
Nadolol	see Beta-blockers
Nalbuphine	see Opioid Analgesics
Nalidixic acid	
Moderate to severe	Use half normal dose; ineffective in renal failure because concentration in urine is inadequate
Naproxen	see NSAIDs

Drug and degree of impairment	Comment
Naratriptan	
Moderate	Max. 2.5 mg in 24 hours
Severe	Avoid
Narcotic analgesics	*see* Opioid Analgesics
Nebivolol	*see* Beta-blockers
Nelfinavir	No information available—manufacturer advises caution
Neomycin	
Mild	Avoid; ototoxic; nephrotoxic
Neostigmine	
Moderate	May need dose reduction
Netilmicin	*see* Aminoglycosides
Nicardipine	
Moderate	Start with small dose
Nicotine	
Severe	May affect clearance of nicotine or its metabolites
Nicoumalone	*see* Anticoagulants, Oral
Nimodipine	Manufacturer advises caution with intravenous administration
Nitrazepam	*see* Anxiolytics and Hypnotics
Nitrofurantoin	
Mild	Avoid; peripheral neuropathy; ineffective because of inadequate urine concentrations
Nitroprusside	*see* Sodium Nitroprusside
Nizatidine	
Mild	Use half normal dose
Moderate	Use one-quarter normal dose
Norfloxacin	
Mild to moderate	Use half normal dose if creatinine clearance less than 30 mL/minute
NSAIDs	
Mild	Use lowest effective dose and monitor renal function; sodium and water retention; deterioration in renal function possibly leading to renal failure; deterioration also reported after topical use; *see also* Azapropazone
Moderate to severe	Avoid if possible; *see also* Azapropazone
Ofloxacin	
Mild	Usual initial dose, then use half normal dose
Moderate	Usual initial dose, then 100 mg every 24 hours
Olanzapine	Consider initial dose of 5 mg daily
Olmesartan	Max. 20 mg daily if creatinine clearance 20–60 mL/minute; avoid if creatinine clearance less than 20 mL/minute
Olsalazine	
Moderate	Use with caution
Severe	Manufacturer advises avoid
Opioid analgesics	
Moderate to severe	Reduce doses or avoid; increased and prolonged effect; increased cerebral sensitivity
Oseltamivir	
Mild to moderate	Reduce dose if creatinine clearance less than 30 mL/minute
Severe	Avoid

Drug and degree of impairment	Comment
Oxaliplatin	
Mild	Manufacturer advises avoid if creatinine clearance less than 30 mL/minute
Oxazepam	*see* Anxiolytics and Hypnotics
Oxcarbazepine	
Mild	Initial dose 300 mg daily if creatinine clearance less than 30 mL/minute; increase according to response at intervals of at least 1 week
Oxpentifylline	*see* Pentoxifylline
Oxprenolol	*see* Beta-blockers
Oxybutynin	Manufacturer advises caution
Oxycodone	*see* Opioid Analgesics
Oxytetracycline	*see* Tetracyclines
Pamidronate disodium	*see* Disodium Pamidronate
Pancuronium	
Severe	Prolonged duration of block
Pantoprazole	Max. 40 mg daily
Papaveretum	*see* Opioid Analgesics
Paroxetine	
Mild	Usual initial dose; small increments if necessary
Peginterferon alfa	Close monitoring required—reduce dose if necessary
Penicillamine	
Mild	Avoid if possible or reduce dose; nephrotoxic
Pentamidine	
Mild	Reduce dose; consult product literature
Pentazocine	*see* Opioid Analgesics
Pentoxifylline (oxpentifylline)	
Mild	Reduce dose by 30–50% if creatinine clearance less than 30 mL/minute
Pericyazine	*see* Antipsychotics
Perindopril	*see* ACE Inhibitors
Perphenazine	*see* Antipsychotics
Pethidine	*see* Opioid Analgesics
Phenazocine	*see* Opioid Analgesics
Phenindione	*see* Anticoagulants, Oral
Phenobarbital	
Severe	Avoid large doses
Phenoperidine	*see* Opioid Analgesics
Phenothiazines	*see* Antipsychotics
Pholcodine	*see* Opioid Analgesics
Picolax®	
Severe	Avoid—risk of hypermagnesaemia
Pilocarpine	Manufacturer advises caution with tablets
Pimozide	*see* Antipsychotics
Pindolol	*see* Beta-blockers
Piperacillin [ingredient]	*see Tazocin®*
Piperazine	
Severe	Avoid—neurotoxic
Pipotiazine	*see* Antipsychotics
Piracetam	
Mild	Use half normal dose
Moderate	Use one-quarter normal dose
Severe	Avoid
Piroxicam	*see* NSAIDs

Drug and degree of impairment	Comment
Potassium salts	
Moderate	Avoid routine use; high risk of hyperkalaemia
Potassium-sparing diuretics	Monitor plasma K$^+$; high risk of
Mild	hyperkalaemia in renal impairment; amiloride excreted by kidney unchanged
Moderate	Avoid
Povidone–iodine	
Severe	Avoid regular application to inflamed or broken mucosa
Pramipexole	
Mild	Initially 88 micrograms twice daily; if renal function declines, reduce dose further
Moderate to severe	Initially 88 micrograms daily; if renal function declines, reduce dose further
Pravastatin	
Moderate to severe	Start at lower end of dosage range
Prazosin	
Moderate to severe	Initially 500 micrograms daily; increased with caution
Primaxin®	
Mild	Reduce dose
Primidone	*see* Phenobarbital
Probenecid	
Moderate	Avoid; ineffective and toxicity increased
Procainamide	
Mild	Avoid or reduce dose
Procarbazine	
Severe	Avoid
Prochlorperazine	*see* Antipsychotics
Proguanil	
Mild	100 mg once daily
Moderate	50 mg on alternate days
Severe	50 mg once weekly; increased risk of haematological toxicity
Promazine	*see* Antipsychotics
Propantheline	Manufacturer advises caution
Propiverine	
Severe	Avoid
Propranolol	*see* Beta-blockers
Propylthiouracil	
Mild to moderate	Use three-quarters normal dose
Severe	Use half normal dose
Pseudoephedrine	
Severe	Avoid; increased CNS toxicity
Pyridostigmine	
Moderate	Reduce dose; excreted by kidney
Pyrimethamine	Manufacturer advises caution
Quetiapine	Manufacturer advises initial dose of 25 mg daily, increased daily in steps of 25–50 mg
Quinagolide	Manufacturer advises avoid—no information available
Quinapril	*see* ACE Inhibitors
Quinine	Reduce parenteral maintenance dose for malaria treatment, *see* section 5.4.1
Raloxifene	
Severe	Avoid

Drug and degree of impairment	Comment
Raltitrexed	
Mild	Reduce dose and increase dosing interval
Moderate to severe	Avoid
Ramipril	*see* ACE Inhibitors
Ranitidine	
Severe	Use half normal dose; occasional risk of confusion
Ranitidine bismuth citrate	
Severe	Avoid
Reboxetine	Initial dose 2 mg twice daily, increased according to tolerance
Regulan®	
Severe	Avoid; contains 6.4 mmol potassium per sachet
Reviparin	
Severe	Manufacturer advises avoid
Riamet®	Manufacturer advises caution in severe renal impairment—monitor ECG and plasma potassium concentration
Ribavirin	
Mild	Plasma-ribavirin concentration increased; manufacturer advises avoid oral ribavirin unless essential—monitor haemoglobin concentration closely
Rifabutin	
Mild	Use half normal dose if creatinine clearance less than 30 mL/minute
Riluzole	No information available—manufacturer advises avoid
Risedronate sodium	
Mild	Manufacturer advises avoid if creatinine clearance less than 30 mL/minute
Risperidone	Manufacturer advises initial oral dose of 500 micrograms twice daily increased in steps of 500 micrograms twice daily to 1–2 mg twice daily; if an oral dose of at least 2 mg daily tolerated, 25 mg as a depot injection can be given every 2 weeks
Ritonavir [ingredient]	*see Kaletra*®
Rivastigmine	Manufacturer advises caution
Rizatriptan	
Mild to moderate	Reduce dose to 5 mg
Severe	Avoid
Rocuronium	
Moderate	Reduce dose; prolonged paralysis
Rofecoxib	*see* NSAIDs
Ropinirole	
Severe	Avoid
Rosiglitazone	
Mild	Manufacturer advises caution, if creatinine clearance less than 30 mL/minute
Rosuvastatin	
Mild	Avoid if creatinine clearance less than 30 mL/minute
Saquinavir	
Severe	Dose adjustment possibly required
Sertraline	Manufacturer advises caution

Drug and degree of impairment	Comment
Sevoflurane	Manufacturer advises caution
Sibutramine	
Mild to moderate	Manufacturer advises caution
Severe	Avoid
Sildenafil	
Mild	Initial dose 25 mg if creatinine clearance less than 30 mL/minute
Simvastatin	
Moderate to severe	Doses above 10 mg daily should be used with caution
Sirolimus	Adjust immunosuppressant regimen in patients with raised serum creatinine
Sodium aurothiomalate	Avoid; nephrotoxic
Mild	
Sodium bicarbonate	
Severe	Avoid; specialised role in some forms of renal disease
Sodium clodronate	
Mild to moderate	Use half normal dose and monitor serum creatinine
Severe	Avoid
Sodium nitroprusside	
Moderate	Avoid prolonged use
Sodium valproate	*see* Valproate
Solpadeine®	
Severe	Avoid; contains 18.5 mmol sodium per tablet
Solpadol®	
Severe	Avoid; contains 18.6 mmol sodium per tablet
Sotalol	*see* Beta-blockers
Spironolactone	*see* Potassium-sparing Diuretics
Stavudine	
Mild	20 mg twice daily (15 mg if < 60 kg)
Moderate to severe	20 mg once daily (15 mg if < 60 kg)
Streptomycin	*see* Aminoglycosides
Sucralfate	
Severe	Avoid; aluminium is absorbed and may accumulate
Sulfadiazine	
Severe	Avoid; high risk of crystalluria
Sulfasalazine	
Moderate	Risk of toxicity including crystalluria—ensure high fluid intake
Severe	Avoid
Sulfinpyrazone	
Moderate	Avoid; ineffective as uricosuric
Sulindac	*see* NSAIDs
Sulphonamides	
Moderate	Ensure high fluid intake; rashes and blood disorders; crystalluria a risk
Sulphonylureas	*see under* individual drugs
Sulpiride	
Moderate	Avoid if possible, or reduce dose
Tacalcitol	Monitor serum calcium concentration
Tadalafil	
Mild	Max. dose 10 mg
Tamsulosin	
Severe	Manufacturer advises caution

Drug and degree of impairment	Comment
Tazobactam [ingredient]	*see Tazocin®*
Tazocin®	
Mild	Adult: Max. 4.5 g every 8 hours if creatinine clearance 20–80 mL/minute
Moderate to severe	Adult: Max. 4.5 g every 12 hours; Child under 12 years: Consult product literature
Teicoplanin	
Mild	On day 4 use half normal dose if creatinine clearance is 40–60 mL/minute and use one-third normal dose if creatinine clearance is less than 40 mL/minute
Telithromycin	
Mild	Use half normal dose if creatinine clearance less than 30 mL/minute
Telmisartan	
Severe	Avoid
Temazepam	*see* Anxiolytics and Hypnotics
Tenofovir	
Mild to moderate	Monitor renal function weekly—interrupt treatment if further deterioration; 245 mg every 2 days if creatinine clearance 30–50 mL/minute; 245 mg every 3–4 days if creatinine clearance 10–30 mL/minute
Severe	No information available
Tenoxicam	*see* NSAIDs
Terbinafine	
Mild	Use half normal dose
Terfenadine	
Mild	Use half normal dose if creatinine clearance less than 40 mL/minute
Tetracyclines	
Mild	Avoid tetracyclines except doxycycline or minocycline which may be used cautiously (avoid excessive doses)
Thiazides and related diuretics	
Moderate	Avoid; ineffective (metolazone remains effective but risk of excessive diuresis)
Thioridazine	*see* Antipsychotics
Tiaprofenic acid	*see* NSAIDs
Ticarcillin [ingredient]	*see Timentin®*
Tiludronic acid	
Moderate to severe	Avoid
Timentin®	
Mild	Reduce dose
Timolol	*see* Beta-blockers
Tinzaparin	
Severe	May need dose reduction
Tioguanine	
Moderate	Reduce dose
Tiotropium	Plasma-tiotropium concentration raised; manufacturer advises caution
Tirofiban	
Mild	Use half normal dose if creatinine clearance less than 30 mL/minute

Drug and degree of impairment	Comment
Tizanidine	
Mild	Initially 2 mg once daily if creatinine clearance less than 25 mL/minute; increase once-daily dose gradually according to response before increasing frequency
Tobramycin	*see* Aminoglycosides
Tolbutamide	
Mild to moderate	Reduce dose
Severe	Avoid if possible; if no alternative reduce dose and monitor closely
Tolfenamic acid	*see* NSAIDs
Tolterodine	Reduce dose to 1 mg twice daily if creatinine clearance less than 30 mL/minute
Topiramate	
Moderate to severe	Longer time to steady-state plasma concentrations
Topotecan	
Moderate	Reduce dose
Severe	Avoid
Torasemide	
Moderate	May need high doses
Tramadol	*see* Opioid Analgesics
Trandolapril	*see* ACE Inhibitors
Tranexamic acid	
Mild to moderate	Reduce dose
Severe	Avoid
Tretinoin (oral)	
Mild	Reduce dose
Triamterene	*see* Potassium-sparing Diuretics
Tribavirin	*see* Ribavirin
Triclofos	*see* Anxiolytics and Hypnotics
Trifluoperazine	*see* Antipsychotics
Trimeprazine	*see* Alimemazine
Trimethoprim	
Mild	Use half normal dose after 3 days if creatinine clearance 15–30 mL/minute
Moderate to severe	Use half normal dose if creatinine clearance less than 15 mL/minute—avoid if creatinine clearance less than 10 mL/minute (unless plasma-trimethoprim concentration monitored)
Tripotassium dicitratobismuthate Severe	Avoid
Trisodium edetate	
Mild	Avoid
Trospium	
Mild to moderate	Reduce dose to 20 mg once daily or 20 mg on alternate days if creatinine clearance 10–30 mL/minute
Severe	Avoid
Tylex®	
Moderate to severe	Avoid effervescent tablets; contain 13.6 mmol sodium per tablet
Valaciclovir	
Mild	Reduce treatment dose for herpes zoster; reduce dose according to creatinine clearance for cytomegalovirus prophylaxis following renal transplantation
Moderate to severe	Reduce dose for all indications
Valdecoxib	*see* NSAIDS

Drug and degree of impairment	Comment
Valganciclovir	Reduce dose; consult product literature
Valproate	
Mild to moderate	Reduce dose
Severe	Alter dosage according to free serum valproic acid concentration
Valproic acid	*see* Valproate
Valsartan	
Moderate to severe	Start with 40 mg once daily
Vancomycin	
Mild	Reduce dose—monitor plasma-vancomycin concentration and renal function regularly
Vardenafil	
Mild	Initial dose 5 mg if creatinine clearance less than 30 mL/minute; avoid in endstage renal disease requiring dialysis
Venlafaxine	
Mild to moderate	Use half normal dose if creatinine clearance 10–30 mL/minute
Severe	Avoid
Vigabatrin	
Mild	Excreted by kidney—lower maintenance dose may be required
Voriconazole	
Mild	Intravenous vehicle may accumulate—manufacturer advises use intravenous infusion only if potential benefit outweighs risk, and monitor renal function; alternatively, use tablets (no dose adjustment required)
Warfarin	*see* Anticoagulants, Oral
Xipamide	*see* Thiazides and Related Diuretics
Yasmin®	
Severe	Manufacturer advises avoid
Zafirlukast	
Moderate to severe	Manufacturer advises caution
Zalcitabine	
Mild to moderate	750 micrograms every 12 hours
Severe	750 micrograms daily
Zidovudine	
Severe	Reduce dose; manufacturer advises oral dose of 300–400 mg daily in divided doses or intravenous dose of 1 mg/kg 3–4 times daily
Zoledronic acid	Manufacturer advises avoid if serum creatinine above 400 micromol/litre in tumor-induced hypercalcaemia or if above 265 micromol/litre in cancer and bone metastases; if renal function deteriorates in patients with bone metastases, withold dose until serum creatinine returns to within 10% of baseline value
Zopiclone	*see* Anxiolytics and Hypnotics
Zotepine	Initial dose 25 mg twice daily, increased gradually according to response (max. 75 mg twice daily)
Zuclopenthixol	*see* Antipsychotics

Appendix 4: Pregnancy

Drugs can have harmful effects on the fetus at any time during pregnancy. It is important to bear this in mind when prescribing for a woman of *childbearing age*.

During the *first trimester* drugs may produce congenital malformations (teratogenesis), and the period of greatest risk is from the third to the eleventh week of pregnancy.

During the *second* and *third trimesters* drugs may affect the growth and functional development of the fetus or have toxic effects on fetal tissues; and drugs given shortly before term or during labour may have adverse effects on labour or on the neonate after delivery.

The following list includes drugs which:

- may have harmful effects in pregnancy and indicates the trimester of risk
- are not known to be harmful in pregnancy

The list is based on human data but information on *animal* studies has been included for some drugs when its omission might be misleading.

Drugs should be prescribed in pregnancy only if the expected benefit to the mother is thought to be greater than the risk to the fetus, and all drugs should be avoided if possible during the first trimester. Drugs which have been extensively used in pregnancy and appear to be usually safe should be prescribed in preference to new or untried drugs; and the smallest effective dose should be used.

Few drugs have been shown conclusively to be teratogenic in man but no drug is safe beyond all doubt in early pregnancy. Screening procedures are available where there is a known risk of certain defects.

Absence of a drug from the list does not imply safety. It should be noted that the BNF provides independent advice and may not always agree with the product literature.

Information on drugs and pregnancy is also available from the National Teratology Information Service Telephone: (0191) 232 1525
(0191) 223 1307 (out of hours emergency only)
www.nyrdtc.nhs.uk/services/teratology/
teratology.html

Table of drugs to be avoided or used with caution in pregnancy

Products introduced or amended since publication of BNF No. 46 (September 2003) are underlined.

Drug (trimester of risk)	Comment
Abacavir	Manufacturer advises avoid (toxicity in *animal* studies)
Abciximab	Manufacturer advises use only if potential benefit outweighs risk—no information available
Acamprosate	Manufacturer advises avoid

Drug (trimester of risk)	Comment
Acarbose	Manufacturer advises avoid; insulin is normally substituted in all diabetics
ACE inhibitors (1, 2, 3)	Avoid; may adversely affect fetal and neonatal blood pressure control and renal function; also possible skull defects and oligo-hydramnios; toxicity in *animal* studies
Acebutolol	*see* Beta-blockers
Aceclofenac	*see* NSAIDs
Acemetacin	*see* NSAIDs
Acenocoumarol (nicoumalone)	*see* Anticoagulants, Oral
Acetazolamide	*see* Diuretics
Aciclovir	Not known to be harmful—manufacturers advise use only when potential benefit outweighs risk; limited absorption from topical aciclovir preparations
Acipimox	Manufacturer advises avoid
Acitretin (1, 2, 3)	Teratogenic; effective contraception must be used for at least 1 month before treatment, during treatment, and for at least 2 years after stopping
Aclarubicin	Avoid (toxicity in *animal* studies); *see also* section 8.1
Acrivastine	*see* Antihistamines
Adalimumab	Avoid; manufacturer advises adequate contraception during and for at least 5 months after last dose
Adapalene	Manufacturer advises terato-genicity in *animal* studies and recommends effective contra-ception during treatment
Adefovir dipivoxil	Toxicity in *animal* studies—manufacturer advises use only if potential benefit outweighs risk; effective contraception required during treatment
Alclometasone	*see* Corticosteroids
Alcohol (1, 2)	Regular daily drinking is terato-genic (fetal alcohol syndrome) and may cause growth retarda-tion; occasional single drinks are probably safe
(3)	Withdrawal syndrome may occur in babies of alcoholic mothers
Alendronic acid	*see* Bisphosphonates
Alfentanil	*see* Opioid Analgesics
Alimemazine (tri-meprazine)	*see* Antihistamines
Allopurinol	Toxicity not reported; manufac-turer advises avoid; use only if no safer alternative and disease carries risk for mother or child

Drug (trimester of risk)	Comment
Almotriptan	*see* 5HT$_1$ Agonists
Alpha-blockers, post-synaptic	No evidence of teratogenicity; manufacturers advise use only when potential benefit outweighs risk
Alprazolam	*see* Benzodiazepines
Alprostadil (urethral application only)	Manufacturer advises barrier contraception if partner pregnant
Alteplase	*see* Streptokinase
Amantadine	Avoid; toxicity in *animal* studies
Amfebutamone	*see* Bupropion
Amifostine	Manufacturer advises avoid—no information available
Amikacin	*see* Aminoglycosides
Amiloride	*see* Diuretics
Aminoglutethimide	Avoid; toxicity in *animal* studies and may affect fetal sexual development
Aminoglycosides (2, 3)	Auditory or vestibular nerve damage; risk greatest with streptomycin; probably very small with gentamicin and tobramycin, but avoid unless essential (if given, serum-aminoglycoside concentration monitoring essential)
Aminophylline	*see* Theophylline
Amiodarone (2, 3)	Possible risk of neonatal goitre; use only if no alternative
Amisulpride	Manufacturer advises avoid
Amitriptyline	*see* Antidepressants, Tricyclic (and related)
Amlodipine	*see* Calcium-channel Blockers
Amobarbital	*see* Barbiturates
Amorolfine	Systemic absorption very low, but manufacturer advises avoid—no information available
Amoxapine	*see* Antidepressants, Tricyclic (and related)
Amoxicillin	*see* Penicillins
Amphotericin	Not known to be harmful but manufacturers advise avoid unless potential benefit outweighs risk
Ampicillin	*see* Penicillins
Amprenavir	Avoid oral solution due to high propylene glycol content; manufacturer advises use capsules only if potential benefit outweighs risk
Amsacrine	Avoid (teratogenic and toxic in *animal* studies); may reduce fertility; *see also* section 8.1
Anabolic steroids (1, 2, 3)	Masculinisation of female fetus
Anaesthetics, general (3)	Depress neonatal respiration
Anaesthetics, local (3)	With large doses, neonatal respiratory depression, hypotonia, and bradycardia after paracervical or epidural block; neonatal methaemoglobinaemia with prilocaine and procaine

Drug (trimester of risk)	Comment
Anakinra	Manufacturer advises avoid; effective contraception must be used during treatment
Analgesics	*see* Opioid Analgesics, Nefopam, NSAIDs, and Paracetamol
Androgens (1, 2, 3)	Masculinisation of female fetus
Anticoagulants, oral (1, 2, 3)	Congenital malformations; fetal and neonatal haemorrhage; *see also* section 2.8.2
Antidepressants, MAOI (1, 2, 3)	No evidence of harm but manufacturers advise avoid unless compelling reasons
Antidepressants, SSRI	Manufacturers advise use only if potential benefit outweighs risk (no evidence of teratogenicity); toxicity in *animal* studies with escitalopram
Antidepressants, tricyclic (and related) (3)	Tachycardia, irritability, and muscle spasms in neonate reported with imipramine
Antiepileptics	Benefit of treatment outweighs risk to fetus; risk of teratogenicity greater if more than one drug used; **important:** *see also* Carbamazepine, Ethosuximide, Phenobarbital, Phenytoin, Valproate, Vigabatrin, and p. 227
Antihistamines	No evidence of teratogenicity; embryotoxicity in *animal* studies with high doses of hydroxyzine and loratadine; manufacturers of cetirizine, desloratadine, hydroxyzine, loratadine, mizolastine and terfenadine advise avoid
Antimalarials (1, 3)	Benefit of prophylaxis and treatment in malaria outweighs risk; **important:** *see also* individual drugs, p. 313 and p. 314
Antipsychotics	*See also* Amisulpride, Clozapine, Olanzapine, Quetiapine, Risperidone, Sertindole, Zotepine
(3)	Extrapyramidal effects in neonate occasionally reported
Apomorphine	Avoid
Artemether [ingredient]	*see* Riamet®
Aspirin (3)	Impaired platelet function and risk of haemorrhage; delayed onset and increased duration of labour with increased blood loss; avoid analgesic doses if possible in last few weeks (low doses probably not harmful); with high doses, closure of fetal ductus arteriosus *in utero* and possibly persistent pulmonary hypertension of newborn; kernicterus in jaundiced neonates
Atenolol	*see* Beta-blockers
Atorvastatin	*see* Statins

Drug (trimester of risk)	Comment
Atosiban	For use in premature labour *see* section 7.1.3
Atovaquone	Manufacturer advises avoid unless potential benefit outweighs risk—no information available
Atracurium	Does not cross placenta in significant amounts but manufacturer advises use only if potential benefit outweighs risk
Atropine	Not known to be harmful; manufacturer advises caution
Auranofin	Manufacturer advises teratogenicity in *animal* studies; effective contraception should be used during and for at least 6 months after treatment
Azapropazone	*see* NSAIDs
Azathioprine	*see* p. 423
Azelastine	*see* Antihistamines
Azithromycin	Manufacturer advises use only if adequate alternatives not available
Aztreonam	Manufacturer advises avoid—no information available
Baclofen	Manufacturer advises use only if potential benefit outweighs risk (toxicity in *animal* studies)
Balsalazide	Manufacturer advises avoid
Bambuterol	*see* section 3.1
Barbiturates (3)	Withdrawal effects in neonate; *see also* Phenobarbital
Basiliximab	Avoid; adequate contraception must be used during treatment and for 8 weeks after last dose
Beclometasone	*see* Corticosteroids
Bemiparin	Manufacturer advises avoid unless essential—no information available
Bendrofluazide	*see* Diuretics
Bendroflumethiazide (bendrofluazide)	*see* Diuretics
Benorilate [aspirin–paracetamol ester]	*see* Aspirin and Paracetamol
Benperidol	*see* Antipsychotics
Benzodiazepines	Avoid regular use (risk of neonatal withdrawal symptoms); use only if clear indication such as seizure control (high doses during late pregnancy or labour may cause neonatal hypothermia, hypotonia and respiratory depression)
Benzylpenicillin	*see* Penicillins
Beta-blockers	May cause intra-uterine growth restriction, neonatal hypoglycaemia, and bradycardia; risk greater in severe hypertension; *see also* section 2.5
Betamethasone	*see* Corticosteroids
Bethanechol	Manufacturer advises avoid—no information available
Bexarotene	Avoid; manufacturer advises effective contraception during and for at least 1 month after administration to men or women; *see also* section 8.1

Drug (trimester of risk)	Comment
Bezafibrate	*see* Fibrates
Bimatoprost	Manufacturer advises use only if potential benefit outweighs risk
Bisoprolol	*see* Beta-blockers
Bisphosphonates	Manufacturers advise avoid
Bleomycin	Avoid (teratogenic and carcinogenic in *animal* studies); *see also* section 8.1
Bosentan	Avoid (teratogenic in *animal* studies); effective contraception required during and for at least 3 months after administration
Botulinum toxin	Manufacturers advise avoid; toxicity in *animal* studies
Brinzolamide	Manufacturer advises avoid unless essential
Brompheniramine	*see* Antihistamines
Buclizine	*see* Antihistamines
Budesonide	*see* Corticosteroids
Bumetanide	*see* Diuretics
Bupivacaine	*see* Anaesthetics, Local
Buprenorphine	*see* Opioid Analgesics
Bupropion	Manufacturer advises avoid—no information available
Buserelin	Avoid
Buspirone	Manufacturer advises avoid
Busulfan	Avoid (teratogenic in *animals*); manufacturer advises effective contraception during administration to men or women; *see also* section 8.1
Cabergoline	No evidence of harm; manufacturer advises discontinuation one month before intended conception and avoidance during pregnancy; *see also* section 6.7.1
Calcipotriol	Manufacturer advises avoid if possible
Calcitonin (salmon) (salcatonin)	Manufacturer advises avoid unless potential benefit outweighs risk (toxicity in *animal* studies)
Calcitriol	*see* Vitamin D
Calcium folinate	Manufacturer advises use only if potential benefit outweighs risk
Calcium levofolinate	*see* Calcium Folinate
Calcium-channel blockers	May inhibit labour and manufacturers advise that diltiazem and some dihydropyridines are teratogenic in *animals*, but risk to fetus should be balanced against risk of uncontrolled maternal hypertension
Candesartan	*As for* ACE Inhibitors
Capecitabine	Avoid (teratogenic in animal studies); *see also* section 8.1
Capreomycin	Manufacturer advises use only if potential benefit outweighs risk—teratogenic in *animal* studies
Captopril	*see* ACE Inhibitors

Drug (trimester of risk)	Comment
Carbamazepine (1)	Risk of teratogenesis including increased risk of neural tube defects (counselling and screening and adequate folate supplements advised, e.g. 5 mg daily); *see also* Antiepileptics and p. 227
(3)	May possibly cause vitamin K deficiency and risk of neonatal bleeding; if vitamin K not given at birth, neonate should be monitored closely for signs of bleeding
Carbenoxolone (3)	Avoid; causes sodium retention with oedema
Carbimazole (2, 3)	Neonatal goitre and hypothyroidism; has been associated with aplasia cutis of the neonate
Carbocisteine (1)	Manufacturer advises avoid
Carboplatin	Avoid (teratogenic and embryotoxic in *animal* studies); *see also* section 8.1
Carglumic acid	Manufacturer advises avoid unless essential—no information available
Carmustine	Avoid (teratogenic and embryotoxic in *animals*); manufacturer advises effective contraception during administration to men or women; *see also* section 8.1
Carnitine	No evidence of teratogenicity in *animal* studies; consider serious consequence of discontinuing treatment
Carvedilol	*see* Beta-blockers
Caspofungin	Manufacturer advises avoid unless essential—toxicity in *animal* studies
Cefaclor	Not known to be harmful
Cefadroxil	Not known to be harmful
Cefalexin	Not known to be harmful
Cefixime	Not known to be harmful
Cefotaxime	Not known to be harmful
Cefoxitin	Not known to be harmful
Cefpirome	Manufacturer advises avoid
Cefpodoxime	Not known to be harmful
Cefprozil	Not known to be harmful
Cefradine	Not known to be harmful
Ceftazidime	Not known to be harmful
Ceftriaxone	Not known to be harmful
Cefuroxime	Not known to be harmful
Celecoxib	Manufacturer advises avoid (teratogenic in *animal* studies); *see also* NSAIDs
Celiprolol	*see* Beta-blockers
Certoparin	*see* Heparin
Cetirizine	*see* Antihistamines
Chloral hydrate	Avoid
Chlorambucil	Avoid; manufacturer advises effective contraception during administration to men or women; *see also* section 8.1

Drug (trimester of risk)	Comment
Chloramphenicol (3)	Neonatal 'grey' syndrome
Chlordiazepoxide	*see* Benzodiazepines
Chlormethine (mustine)	Avoid; *see also* section 8.1
Chloroquine	*see* Antimalarials
Chlorphenamine (chlorpheniramine)	*see* Antihistamines
Chlorpheniramine	*see* Antihistamines
Chlorpromazine	*see* Antipsychotics
Chlorpropamide	*see* Sulphonylureas
Chlortalidone	*see* Diuretics
Chlortetracycline	*see* Tetracyclines
Ciclosporin	*see* p. 423
Cidofovir	Avoid (toxicity in *animal* studies); effective contraception required during and for 1 month after treatment; also men should avoid fathering a child during and for 3 months after treatment
Cilastatin [ingredient]	*see Primaxin®*
Cilazapril	*see* ACE Inhibitors
Cilostazol	Avoid—toxicity in *animal* studies
Cimetidine	Manufacturer advises avoid unless essential
Cinnarizine	*see* Antihistamines
Ciprofibrate	*see* Fibrates
Ciprofloxacin	*see* Quinolones
Cisatracurium	Manufacturer advises avoid—no information available
Cisplatin	Avoid (teratogenic and toxic in *animal* studies); *see also* section 8.1
Citalopram	*see* Antidepressants, SSRI
Cladribine	Avoid (teratogenic in *animal* studies); *see also* section 8.1
Clarithromycin	Manufacturer advises avoid unless potential benefit outweighs risk
Clavulanic acid [ingredient]	*see* Co-amoxiclav, *Timentin®*
Clemastine	*see* Antihistamines
Clindamycin	Not known to be harmful
Clobazam	*see* Benzodiazepines
Clobetasol	*see* Corticosteroids
Clobetasone	*see* Corticosteroids
Clodronate sodium	*see* Bisphosphonates
Clomethiazole	Avoid if possible—especially during first and third trimesters
Clomifene	Possible effects on fetal development
Clomipramine	*see* Antidepressants, Tricyclic (and related)
Clonazepam	*see* Benzodiazepines
Clopidogrel	Manufacturer advises avoid—no information available
Clorazepate	*see* Benzodiazepines
Clozapine	Manufacturer advises avoid
Co-amoxiclav	*see* Penicillins
Co-beneldopa	*see* Levodopa
Co-careldopa	*see* Levodopa
Co-cyprindiol (1, 2, 3)	Feminisation of male fetus (due to cyproterone)
Codeine	*see* Opioid Analgesics

Drug (trimester of risk)	Comment
Co-fluampicil	*see* Penicillins
Colchicine	Avoid—teratogenicity in animal studies
Colistin (2, 3)	Avoid—possible risk of fetal toxicity
Contraceptives, oral	Epidemiological evidence suggests no harmful effects on fetus
Corticosteroids	Benefit of treatment, e.g. in asthma, outweighs risk (*see also* CSM advice, section 6.3.2); risk of intra-uterine growth retardation on prolonged or repeated systemic treatment; corticosteroid cover required by mother during labour; monitor closely if fluid retention
Co-trimoxazole (1)	Teratogenic risk (trimethoprim a folate antagonist)
(3)	Neonatal haemolysis and methaemoglobinaemia; fear of increased risk of kernicterus in neonates appears to be unfounded
Crisantaspase	Avoid; *see also* section 8.1
Cromoglicate	*see* Sodium Cromoglicate
Cyclizine	*see* Antihistamines
Cyclopenthiazide	*see* Diuretics
Cyclophosphamide	Avoid (manufacturer advises effective contraception during and for at least 3 months after administration to men or women); *see also* section 8.1
Cycloserine	Manufacturer advises use only if potential benefit outweighs risk—crosses the placenta
Cyclosporin	*see* p. 423
Cyproheptadine	*see* Antihistamines
Cyproterone [ingredient]	*see* Co-cyprindiol
Cytarabine	Avoid (teratogenic in *animal* studies); *see also* section 8.1
Dacarbazine	Avoid (carcinogenic and teratogenic in *animal* studies); ensure effective contraception during and for at least 6 months after administration to men or women; *see also* section 8.1
Daclizumab	Avoid
Dactinomycin	Avoid (teratogenic in *animal* studies); *see also* section 8.1
Dalfopristin [ingredient]	*see* Synercid®
Dalteparin	*see* Heparin
Danazol (1, 2, 3)	Avoid; has weak androgenic effects and virilisation of female fetus reported
Dantron (danthron)	Manufacturer advises avoid—no information available
Dapsone (3)	Neonatal haemolysis and methaemoglobinaemia; folic acid 5 mg daily should be given to mother

Drug (trimester of risk)	Comment
Darbepoetin	No evidence of harm in *animal* studies—manufacturer advises caution
Daunorubicin	Avoid (teratogenic and carcinogenic in *animal* studies); *see also* section 8.1
Debrisoquine	*see* Guanethidine
Deferiprone	Manufacturer advises avoid—teratogenic and embryotoxic in *animal* studies
Deflazacort	*see* Corticosteroids
Demeclocycline	*see* Tetracyclines
Desferrioxamine	Teratogenic in *animal* studies; manufacturer advises use only if potential benefit outweighs risk
Desflurane	*see* Anaesthetics, General
Desmopressin (3)	Small oxytocic effect in third trimester; increased risk of pre-eclampsia
Desogestrel	*see* Contraceptives, Oral
Desoximetasone	*see* Corticosteroids
Dexamethasone	*see* Corticosteroids
Dexamfetamine	Manufacturer advises avoid (retrospective evidence of uncertain significance suggesting possible embryotoxicity)
Dexketoprofen	*see* NSAIDs
Dextran	Avoid—reports of anaphylaxis in mother causing fetal anoxia, neurological damage and death
Dextromethorphan	*see* Opioid Analgesics
Dextropropoxyphene	*see* Opioid Analgesics
Diamorphine	*see* Opioid Analgesics
Diazepam	*see* Benzodiazepines
Diazoxide (2, 3)	Prolonged use may produce alopecia and impaired glucose tolerance in neonate; inhibits uterine activity during labour
Diclofenac	*see* NSAIDs
Didanosine	Manufacturer advises use only if potential benefit outweighs risk—no information available
Diethylstilbestrol (1)	High doses associated with vaginal carcinoma, urogenital abnormalities, and reduced fertility in female offspring; increased risk of hypospadias in male offspring
Diflucortolone	*see* Corticosteroids
Diflunisal	*see* NSAIDs
Digoxin	May need dosage adjustment
Dihydrocodeine	*see* Opioid Analgesics
Diloxanide	Manufacturer advises avoid—no information available
Diltiazem	*see* Calcium-channel Blockers
Diphenhydramine	*see* Antihistamines
Diphenoxylate	*see* Opioid Analgesics
Diphenylpyraline	*see* Antihistamines
Dipipanone	*see* Opioid Analgesics
Dipyridamole	Not known to be harmful
Disodium etidronate	*see* Bisphosphonates
Disodium pamidronate	*see* Bisphosphonates

Drug (trimester of risk)	Comment
Disopyramide (3)	May induce labour
Distigmine	Manufacturer advises avoid (may stimulate uterine contractions)
Disulfiram (1)	High concentrations of acetaldehyde which occur in presence of alcohol may be teratogenic
Diuretics	Not used to treat hypertension in pregnancy
(1)	Manufacturers advise avoid acetazolamide and torasemide (toxicity in *animal* studies)
(3)	Thiazides may cause neonatal thrombocytopenia
Docetaxel	Avoid (toxicity and reduced fertility in *animal* studies); manufacturer advises effective contraception during and for at least 3 months after administration; *see also* section 8.1
Docusate sodium	Not known to be harmful—manufacturer advises caution
Dolasetron	Manufacturer advises avoid unless potential benefit outweighs risk—no information available
Domperidone	Manufacturer advises avoid
Dornase alfa	No evidence of teratogenicity; manufacturer advises use only if potential benefit outweighs risk
Dosulepin (dothiepin)	*see* Antidepressants, Tricyclic (and related)
Dothiepin	*see* Antidepressants, Tricyclic (and related)
Doxazosin	*see* Alpha-blockers, Post-synaptic
Doxepin	*see* Antidepressants, Tricyclic (and related)
Doxorubicin	Avoid (teratogenic and toxic in *animal* studies); manufacturer of liposomal product advises effective contraception during and for at least 6 months after administration to men or women; *see also* section 8.1
Doxycycline	*see* Tetracyclines
Doxylamine	*see* Antihistamines
Drotrecogin alfa (activated)	Manufacturer advises avoid unless benefit outweighs risk—no information available
Dutasteride (1, 2, 3)	Avoid unprotected intercourse (*see* section 6.4.2). May cause feminisation of male fetus
Dydrogesterone	Not known to be harmful
Econazole	Not known to be harmful
Edrophonium	Manufacturer advises use only if potential benefit outweighs risk
Efavirenz	Toxicity in *animal* studies; manufacturer advises use only if potential benefit outweighs risk and no alternative options available
Eformoterol	*see* Formoterol
Eletriptan	*see* 5HT$_1$ Agonists

Drug (trimester of risk)	Comment
Emtricitabine	No information available—manufacturer advises use only if essential
Enalapril	*see* ACE Inhibitors
Enflurane	*see* Anaesthetics, General
Enfuvirtide	Manufacturer advises use only if potential benefit outweighs risk
Enoxaparin	Manufacturer advises avoid unless no safer alternative
Enoximone	Manufacturer advises use only if potential benefit outweighs risk
Entacapone	Manufacturer advises avoid—no information available
Epoetin	No evidence of harm; benefits probably outweigh risk of anaemia and of transfusion in pregnancy
Eprosartan	*As for* ACE Inhibitors
Eptifibatide	Manufacturer advises use only if potential benefit outweighs risk—no information available
Ergotamine (1, 2, 3)	Oxytocic effects on the pregnant uterus
Ertapenem	Manufacturer advises avoid unless potential benefit outweighs risk
Erythromycin	Not known to be harmful
Escitalopram	*see* Antidepressants, SSRI
Esmolol	*see* Beta-blockers
Esomeprazole	Manufacturer advises caution—no information available
Etanercept	Manufacturer advises avoid—no information available
Ethambutol	Not known to be harmful; *see also* p. 282
Ethinylestradiol	*see* Contraceptives, Oral
Ethionamide (1)	May be teratogenic
Ethosuximide (1)	May possibly be teratogenic; *see* Antiepileptics
Etidronate disodium	*see* Bisphosphonates
Etodolac	*see* NSAIDs
Etomidate	*see* Anaesthetics, General
Etoposide	Avoid (teratogenic in *animal* studies); *see also* section 8.1
Etoricoxib	*see* NSAIDs
Etynodiol	*see* Contraceptives, Oral
Ezetimibe	Manufacturer advises use only if potential benefit outweighs risk—no information available
Famciclovir	*see* Aciclovir
Famotidine	Manufacturer advises avoid unless potential benefit outweighs risk

Drug (trimester of risk)	Comment
Fansidar®	
(1)	Possible teratogenic risk (pyrimethamine a folate antagonist)
(3)	Neonatal haemolysis and methaemoglobinaemia; fear of increased risk of kernicterus in neonates appears to be unfounded
	see also Antimalarials
Felodipine	*see* Calcium-channel Blockers
Fenbufen	*see* NSAIDs
Fenofibrate	*see* Fibrates
Fenoprofen	*see* NSAIDs
Fenoterol	*see* section 3.1
Fentanyl	*see* Opioid Analgesics
Fenticonazole	Manufacturer advises avoid unless essential
Fexofenadine	*see* Antihistamines
Fibrates	Embryotoxicity in *animal* studies—manufacturers advise avoid
Filgrastim	Toxicity in *animal* studies; manufacturer advises use only if potential benefit outweighs risk
Finasteride	
(1, 2, 3)	Avoid unprotected intercourse (*see* section 6.4.2). May cause feminisation of male fetus
Flavoxate	Manufacturer advises avoid unless no safer alternative
Flecainide	Manufacturer advises toxicity in *animal* studies
Flucloxacillin	*see* Penicillins
Fluconazole	Manufacturer advises avoid—multiple congenital abnormalities reported with long-term high doses
Flucytosine	Teratogenic in *animal* studies; manufacturer advises use only if potential benefit outweighs risk
Fludarabine	Avoid (embryotoxic and teratogenic in *animal* studies); manufacturer advises effective contraception during and for at least 6 months after administration to men or women; *see also* section 8.1
Fludrocortisone	*see* Corticosteroids
Fludroxycortide (flurandrenolone)	*see* Corticosteroids
Flumazenil	Manufacturer advises avoid unless potential benefit outweighs risk
Flunisolide	*see* Corticosteroids
Flunitrazepam	*see* Benzodiazepines
Fluocinolone	*see* Corticosteroids
Fluocinonide	*see* Corticosteroids
Fluocortolone	*see* Corticosteroids
Fluorouracil	Avoid (teratogenic); *see also* section 8.1
Fluoxetine	*see* Antidepressants, SSRI
Flupentixol	*see* Antipsychotics
Fluphenazine	*see* Antipsychotics
Flurandrenolone	*see* Corticosteroids
Flurazepam	*see* Benzodiazepines
Flurbiprofen	*see* NSAIDs
Fluticasone	*see* Corticosteroids

Drug (trimester of risk)	Comment
Fluvastatin	*see* Statins
Fluvoxamine	*see* Antidepressants, SSRI
Follitropin alfa and beta	Avoid
Fondaparinux	Manufacturer advises avoid unless potential benefit outweighs possible risk—no information available
Formoterol (eformoterol)	Manufacturers advise use only if potential benefit outweighs risk; *see also* section 3.1
Foscarnet	Manufacturer advises avoid
Fosinopril	*see* ACE Inhibitors
Fosphenytoin	*see* Phenytoin
Framycetin	*see* Aminoglycosides
Frovatriptan	*see* 5HT$_1$ Agonists
Frusemide	*see* Diuretics
Furosemide (frusemide)	*see* Diuretics
Fusidic acid	*see* Sodium Fusidate
Gabapentin	*see* Antiepileptics
Galantamine	No information available
Ganciclovir	Avoid—teratogenic risk; *see also* p. 308
Gemcitabine	Avoid (teratogenic in *animal* studies); *see also* section 8.1
Gemfibrozil	*see* Fibrates
Gentamicin	*see* Aminoglycosides
Gestodene	*see* Contraceptives, Oral
Gestrinone	
(1, 2, 3)	Avoid
Glatiramer	Manufacturer advises avoid unless potential benefit outweighs risk
Glibenclamide	*see* Sulphonylureas
Gliclazide	*see* Sulphonylureas
Glimepiride	*see* Sulphonylureas
Glipizide	*see* Sulphonylureas
Gliquidone	*see* Sulphonylureas
Goserelin	Manufacturer advises avoid in pregnancy—exclude pregnancy before treatment and use non-hormonal contraceptives during treatment
Granisetron	Manufacturer advises use only when compelling reasons—no information available
Griseofulvin	Avoid (fetotoxicity and teratogenicity in *animals*); effective contraception required during and for at least 1 month after administration (**important:** effectiveness of oral contraceptives reduced, see p. 388); also men should avoid fathering a child during and for at least 6 months after administration
Guanethidine	
(3)	Postural hypotension and reduced uteroplacental perfusion; should not be used to treat hypertension in pregnancy
Haem arginate	Manufacturer advises avoid unless essential
Halcinonide	*see* Corticosteroids
Haloperidol	*see* Antipsychotics
Halothane	*see* Anaesthetics, General

Drug (trimester of risk)	Comment
Heparin (1, 2, 3)	Osteoporosis has been reported after prolonged use (*see also* Enoxaparin, Lepirudin, Reviparin and Tinzaparin); multidose vials may contain benzyl alcohol—some manufacturers advise avoid
5HT₁ agonists	Limited experience—manufacturers advise avoid unless potential benefit outweighs risk
Human menopausal gonadotrophins	Avoid
Hydralazine (1, 2)	Manufacturer advises avoid before third trimester; no reports of serious harm following use in third trimester
Hydrochlorothiazide	*see* Diuretics
Hydrocortisone	*see* Corticosteroids
Hydroflumethiazide	*see* Diuretics
Hydromorphone	*see* Opioid Analgesics
Hydroxycarbamide (hydroxyurea)	Avoid (teratogenic in *animal* studies); manufacturer advises effective contraception before and during administration; *see also* section 8.1
Hydroxychloroquine	Manufacturer advises avoid but see p. 491
Hydroxyurea	*see* Hydroxycarbamide
Hydroxyzine	*see* Antihistamines
Hyoscine butylbromide	Manufacturer advises use only if potential benefit outweighs risk
Ibandronic acid	*see* Bisphosphonates
Ibuprofen	*see* NSAIDs
Idarubicin	Avoid (teratogenic and toxic in *animal* studies); *see also* section 8.1
Idoxuridine	Teratogenic in *animal* studies
Ifosfamide	Avoid (teratogenic and carcinogenic in *animals*); manufacturer advises adequate contraception during and for at least 6 months after administration to men or women; *see also* section 8.1
Imatinib	Manufacturer advises avoid unless potential benefit outweighs risk; *see also* section 8.1
Imidapril	*see* ACE Inhibitors
Imiglucerase	Manufacturer advises use only if potential benefit outweighs risk—no information available
Imipenem [ingredient]	*see Primaxin*®
Imipramine	*see* Antidepressants, Tricyclic (and related)
Imiquimod	No evidence of teratogenicity or toxicity in *animal* studies; manufacturer advises caution
Indapamide	*see* Diuretics
Indinavir	Toxicity in *animal* studies; manufacturer advises use only if potential benefit outweighs risk; theoretical risk of hyperbilirubinaemia and renal stones in neonate if used at term
Indometacin	*see* NSAIDs

Drug (trimester of risk)	Comment
Infliximab	Avoid; manufacturer advises adequate contraception during and for at least 6 months after last dose
Inosine	Manufacturer advises avoid
Insulin (1, 2, 3)	Insulin requirements should be assessed frequently by an experienced diabetic physician
Interferons	Manufacturers recommend avoid unless compelling reasons; effective contraception to be used by men and women receiving treatment
Iodine and iodides (2, 3)	Neonatal goitre and hypothyroidism
Iodine, radioactive (1, 2, 3)	Permanent hypothyroidism—avoid
Iodoform	*see* Povidone–iodine
Ipratropium	Not known to be harmful; *see* section 3.1
Irbesartan	*As for* ACE Inhibitors
Irinotecan	Avoid (teratogenic and toxic in *animal* studies); manufacturer advises effective contraception during and for at least 3 months after administration; *see also* section 8.1
Iron (parenteral)	Avoid in early pregnancy
Isocarboxazid	*see* Antidepressants, MAOI
Isoflurane	*see* Anaesthetics, General
Isoniazid	Not known to be harmful; *see also* p. 282
Isotretinoin (1, 2, 3)	Teratogenic; effective contraception must be used for at least 1 month before oral treatment, during treatment and for at least 1 month after stopping; also avoid topical treatment
Isradipine	*see* Calcium-channel Blockers
Itraconazole	Manufacturer advises use only in life-threatening situations (toxicity at high doses in *animal* studies); ensure effective contraception during treatment and until the next menstrual period following end of treatment
Kaletra®	Avoid oral solution due to high propylene glycol content; manufacturer advises use capsules only if potential benefit outweighs risk (toxicity in *animal* studies)
Ketamine	*see* Anaesthetics, General
Ketoconazole	Manufacturer advises teratogenicity in *animal* studies; packs carry a warning to avoid in pregnancy
Ketoprofen	*see* NSAIDs
Ketorolac	*see* NSAIDs
Ketotifen	*see* Antihistamines
Labetalol	*see* Beta-blockers
Lacidipine	*see* Calcium-channel Blockers
Lactulose	Not known to be harmful

Drug (trimester of risk)	Comment
Lamivudine (1)	Manufacturer advises avoid during first trimester—no information available
Lamotrigine	*see* Antiepileptics
Lanreotide	Manufacturer advises use only if potential benefit outweighs risk
Lansoprazole	Manufacturer advises avoid
Latanoprost	Manufacturer advises avoid
Leflunomide	Avoid—active metabolite teratogenic in *animal* studies; effective contraception essential during treatment and for at least 2 years after treatment in women and at least 3 months after treatment in men (*see also* Leflunomide section 10.1.3)
Lenograstim	Toxicity in *animal* studies; manufacturer advises use only if potential benefit outweighs risk
Lepirudin	Avoid
Lercanidipine	*see* Calcium-channel Blockers
Leuprorelin	Avoid—teratogenic in *animal* studies
Levetiracetam	Toxicity in *animal* studies—manufacturer advises use only if potential benefit outweighs risk; *see also* Antiepileptics
Levobupivacaine (1)	Manufacturer advises avoid if possible—toxicity in *animal* studies; *see also* Anaesthetics, Local
Levocabastine	*see* Antihistamines
Levocetirizine	*see* Antihistamines
Levodopa	Manufacturers advise toxicity in *animal* studies
Levofloxacin	*see* Quinolones
Levomepromazine (methotrimeprazine)	*see* Antipsychotics
Levonorgestrel	*see* Contraceptives, Oral
Levothyroxine (thyroxine)	Monitor maternal serum-thyrotrophin concentration—dosage adjustment may be necessary
Lidocaine (lignocaine)	*see* Anaesthetics, Local
Lignocaine	*see* Anaesthetics, Local
Linezolid	Manufacturer advises use only if potential benefit outweighs risk—no information available
Liothyronine	Does not cross the placenta in significant amounts; monitor maternal thyroid function tests—dosage adjustment may be necessary
Lisinopril	*see* ACE Inhibitors
Lithium salts (1)	Avoid if possible (risk of teratogenicity, including cardiac abnormalities)
(2, 3)	Dose requirements increased (but on delivery return to normal abruptly); close monitoring of serum-lithium concentration advised (risk of toxicity in neonate)

Drug (trimester of risk)	Comment
Lofepramine	*see* Antidepressants, Tricyclic (and related)
Loperamide	Manufacturers advise avoid—no information available
Lopinavir [ingredient]	*see* Kaletra®
Loprazolam	*see* Benzodiazepines
Loratadine	Embryotoxic in *animal* studies; *see also* Antihistamines
Lorazepam	*see* Benzodiazepines
Lormetazepam	*see* Benzodiazepines
Losartan	*As for* ACE Inhibitors
Lumefantrine [ingredient]	*see* Riamet®
Lymecycline	*see* Tetracyclines
Magnesium sulphate (3)	Not known to be harmful for short-term intravenous administration in eclampsia but excessive doses cause neonatal respiratory depression
Malarone®	Manufacturer advises avoid unless essential
Maprotiline	*see* Antidepressants, Tricyclic (and related)
Mebendazole	Manufacturer advises toxicity in *animal* studies
Mebeverine	Not known to be harmful; manufacturers advise caution
Medroxyprogesterone	Avoid—genital malformations and cardiac defects reported in male and female fetuses
Mefenamic acid	*see* NSAIDs
Mefloquine (1)	Manufacturer advises teratogenicity in *animal* studies, but *see* p. 313 and p. 314
Meloxicam	*see* NSAIDs
Melphalan	Avoid (manufacturer advises adequate contraception during administration to men or women); *see also* section 8.1
Menadiol (3)	Neonatal haemolytic anaemia, hyperbilirubinaemia and increased risk of kernicterus in jaundiced infants
Menotrophin	Avoid
Meprobamate	Manufacturer advises avoid if possible
Meptazinol	*see* Opioid Analgesics
Mercaptamine	Manufacturer advises avoid
Mercaptopurine	Avoid (teratogenic); *see also* section 8.1
Meropenem	Manufacturer advises use only if potential benefit outweighs risk—no information available
Mesalazine	Negligible quantities cross placenta
Mesna	Not known to be harmful; *see also* section 8.1
Mesterolone	*see* Androgens
Mestranol	*see* Contraceptives, Oral
Metaraminol	May reduce placental perfusion—manufacturer advises use only if potential benefit outweighs risk

Drug (trimester of risk)	Comment
Metformin (1, 2, 3)	Avoid; insulin is normally substituted in all diabetics
Methadone	see Opioid Analgesics
Methocarbamol	Manufacturer advises avoid unless potential benefit outweighs risk
Methotrexate	Avoid (teratogenic; fertility may be reduced during therapy but this may be reversible); manufacturer advises effective contraception during and for at least 3 months after administration to men or women; see also section 8.1
Methotrimeprazine	see Antipsychotics
Methyldopa	Not known to be harmful
Methylphenidate	Limited experience—manufacturer advises avoid unless potential benefit outweighs risk; toxicity in animals
Methylprednisolone	see Corticosteroids
Methysergide	Manufacturer advises avoid
Metoclopramide	Not known to be harmful but manufacturer advises use only when compelling reasons
Metolazone	see Diuretics
Metoprolol	see Beta-blockers
Metronidazole	Manufacturer advises avoidance of high-dose regimens
Metyrapone	Avoid (may impair biosynthesis of fetal-placental steroids)
Mianserin	see Antidepressants, Tricyclic (and related)
Miconazole	Manufacturer advises avoid unless essential
Midazolam	see Benzodiazepines
Mifepristone	Manufacturer advises that if treatment fails, essential that pregnancy be terminated by another method
Milrinone	Manufacturer advises use only if potential benefit outweighs risk
Minocycline	see Tetracyclines
Minoxidil (3)	Neonatal hirsutism reported
Misoprostol (1, 2, 3)	Avoid—potent uterine stimulant (has been used to induce abortion) and may be teratogenic
Mitomycin	Avoid (teratogenic in animal studies); see also section 8.1
Mitoxantrone (mitozantrone)	Avoid; manufacturer advises effective contraception during and for at least 6 months after administration to men or women; see also section 8.1
Mitozantrone	see Mitoxantrone
Mivacurium	Manufacturer advises avoid—no information available
Mizolastine	Manufacturer advises avoid; see also Antihistamines
Moclobemide	see Antidepressants, MAOI
Modafinil	Manufacturer advises avoid
Moexipril	see ACE Inhibitors

Drug (trimester of risk)	Comment
Molgramostim	Toxicity in animal studies—manufacturer advises avoid unless potential benefit outweighs risk
Montelukast	Manufacturer advises avoid unless essential
Morphine	see Opioid Analgesics
Movicol®	Manufacturer advises use only if essential—no information available
Moxifloxacin	see Quinolones
Moxisylyte (thymoxamine)	Manufacturer advises avoid
Moxonidine	Manufacturer advises avoid—no information available
Mupirocin	Manufacturer advises avoid unless potential benefit outweighs risk—no information available
Mustine	see Chlormethine
Mycophenolate mofetil	Manufacturer advises avoid—toxicity in animal studies; effective contraception required during and for 6 weeks after discontinuation of treatment
Nabumetone	see NSAIDs
Nadolol	see Beta-blockers
Nafarelin	Avoid
Nalbuphine	see Opioid Analgesics
Nalidixic acid	see Quinolones
Naloxone	Manufacturer advises use only if potential benefit outweighs risk
Nandrolone	see Anabolic Steroids
Naproxen	see NSAIDs
Naratriptan	see 5HT$_1$ Agonists
Narcotic analgesics	see Opioid Analgesics
Nateglinide	Manufacturer advises avoid—toxicity in animal studies; insulin is normally substituted in all diabetics
Nebivolol	see Beta-blockers
Nedocromil	see section 3.1
Nefopam	No information available—manufacturer advises avoid unless no safer treatment
Nelfinavir	No information available—manufacturer advises use only if potential benefit outweighs risk
Neomycin	see Aminoglycosides
Neostigmine	Manufacturer advises use only if potential benefit outweighs risk
Netilmicin	see Aminoglycosides
Nevirapine	Although manufacturers advise avoid, may be appropriate to use if clearly indicated; see also p. 300
Nicardipine	see Calcium-channel Blockers
Nicorandil	Manufacturer advises use only if potential benefit outweighs risk—no information available
Nicotine	Use only if smoking cessation without nicotine replacement fails; avoid liquorice-flavoured nicotine products; patient information for some products contraindicates use
Nicoumalone	see Anticoagulants, Oral

Drug (trimester of risk)	Comment
Nifedipine	*see* Calcium-channel Blockers
Nimodipine	*see* Calcium-channel Blockers
Nisoldipine	*see* Calcium-channel Blockers
Nitrazepam	*see* Benzodiazepines
Nitrofurantoin (3)	May produce neonatal haemolysis if used at term
Nitrous oxide	*see* Anaesthetics, General
Nizatidine	Manufacturer advises avoid unless essential
Noradrenaline (norepinephrine) (1, 2, 3)	Avoid—may reduce placental perfusion
Norethisterone	Masculinisation of female fetuses and other defects reported; *see also* Contraceptives, Oral
Norfloxacin	*see* Quinolones
Norgestimate	*see* Contraceptives, Oral
Norgestrel	*see* Contraceptives, Oral
Nortriptyline	*see* Antidepressants, Tricyclic (and related)
NSAIDs	Most manufacturers advise avoid (or avoid unless potential benefit outweighs risk); ketorolac contra-indicated during pregnancy, labour and delivery
(3)	With regular use closure of fetal ductus arteriosus *in utero* and possibly persistent pulmonary hypertension of the newborn. Delayed onset and increased duration of labour
Nystatin	No information available, but absorption from gastro-intestinal tract negligible
Octreotide (1, 2, 3)	Possible effect on fetal growth; manufacturer advises use only if potential benefit outweighs risk
Oestrogens	*see* Contraceptives, Oral
Ofloxacin	*see* Quinolones
Olanzapine (3)	Manufacturer advises use only if potential benefit outweighs risk; neonatal lethargy, tremor, and hypertonia reported
Olmesartan	*As for* ACE inhibitors
Olsalazine	Manufacturer advises avoid unless potential benefit outweighs risk
Omeprazole	Manufacturer advises toxicity in *animal* studies
Ondansetron	No information available; manufacturer advises avoid unless potential benefit outweighs risk
Opioid analgesics (3)	Depress neonatal respiration; withdrawal effects in neonates of dependent mothers; gastric stasis and risk of inhalation pneumonia in mother during labour
Oral contraceptives	*see* Contraceptives, Oral
Orlistat	Manufacturer advises avoid—no information available
Orphenadrine	Manufacturer advises caution

Drug (trimester of risk)	Comment
Oseltamivir	Manufacturer advises avoid unless potential benefit outweighs risk
Oxaliplatin	Manufacturer advises avoid—no information available; *see also* section 8.1
Oxazepam	*see* Benzodiazepines
Oxcarbazepine (1)	Risk of teratogenesis including increased risk of neural tube defects (counselling and screening and adequate folate supplements advised, e.g. 5 mg daily); *see also* Antiepileptics and p. 227
(3)	Because of neonatal bleeding tendency associated with some antiepileptics, manufacturer advises prophylactic vitamin K_1 for mother before delivery (as well as for neonate)
Oxprenolol	*see* Beta-blockers
Oxybutynin	Manufacturer advises avoid unless potential benefit outweighs risk—toxicity in *animal* studies
Oxycodone	*see* Opioid Analgesics
Oxytetracycline	*see* Tetracyclines
Paclitaxel	Avoid (toxicity in *animal* studies); *see also* section 8.1
Pamidronate disodium	*see* Bisphosphonates
Pancreatin	Not known to be harmful
Pancuronium	Manufacturer advises avoid unless potential benefit outweighs risk—no information available
Pantoprazole	Manufacturer advises avoid unless potential benefit outweighs risk—fetotoxic in *animals*
Papaveretum	*see* Opioid Analgesics
Paracetamol	Not known to be harmful
Paraldehyde	Manufacturer advises avoid unless essential—crosses the placenta
Parecoxib	*see* NSAIDS
Paroxetine	*see* Antidepressants, SSRI
Pegfilgrastim	Toxicity in *animal* studies; manufacturer advises use only if potential benefit ouweighs risk
Penicillamine (1, 2, 3)	Fetal abnormalities reported rarely; avoid if possible
Penicillins	Not known to be harmful
Pentamidine isetionate	Manufacturer advises avoid unless essential
Pentazocine	*see* Opioid Analgesics
Pentostatin	Avoid (teratogenic in *animal* studies); manufacturer advises that men should not father children and for 6 months after administration; *see also* section 8.1
Pergolide	Manufacturer advises use only if potential benefit outweighs risk
Pericyazine	*see* Antipsychotics
Perindopril	*see* ACE Inhibitors

Drug (trimester of risk)	Comment
Perphenazine	*see* Antipsychotics
Pethidine	*see* Opioid Analgesics
Phenelzine	*see* Antidepressants, MAOI
Phenindione	*see* Anticoagulants, Oral
Phenobarbital (1, 3)	Congenital malformations. May possibly cause vitamin K deficiency and risk of neonatal bleeding; if vitamin K not given at birth, neonate should be monitored closely for signs of bleeding; *see also* Antiepileptics
Phenothiazines	*see* Antipsychotics
Phenoxymethylpenicillin	*see* Penicillins
Phentolamine	No information available
Phenytoin (1, 3)	Congenital malformations (screening advised); adequate folate supplements should be given to mother (e.g. folic acid 5 mg daily). May possibly cause vitamin K deficiency and risk of neonatal bleeding; if vitamin K not given at birth, neonate should be monitored closely for signs of bleeding. Caution in interpreting plasma concentrations—bound may be reduced but free (i.e. effective) unchanged; *see also* Antiepileptics
Pholcodine	*see* Opioid Analgesics
Phytomenadione	Manufacturer advises use only if potential benefit outweighs risk—no specific information available
Pilocarpine	Avoid—smooth muscle stimulant; toxicity in *animal* studies
Pimozide	*see* Antipsychotics
Pindolol	*see* Beta-blockers
Pioglitazone	Manufacturer advises avoid—toxicity in *animal* studies; insulin is normally substituted in all diabetics
Piperacillin [ingredient]	*see* Tazocin®
Piperazine	Not known to be harmful but manufacturer advises avoid in first trimester
Pipotiazine	*see* Antipsychotics
Piracetam	Manufacturer advises avoid
Piroxicam	*see* NSAIDs
Pivmecillinam	*see* Penicillins
Podophyllum	Avoid—neonatal death and teratogenesis have been reported
Polystyrene sulphonate resins	Manufacturers advise use only if potential benefit outweighs risk—no information available
Porfimer	Manufacturer advises avoid unless essential
Povidone–iodine (2, 3)	Sufficient iodine may be absorbed to affect the fetal thyroid
Pramipexole	Manufacturer advises use only if potential benefit outweighs risk—no information available

Drug (trimester of risk)	Comment
Pravastatin	*see* Statins
Prazosin	*see* Alpha-blockers, Post-synaptic
Prednisolone	*see* Corticosteroids
Prilocaine (3)	Neonatal methaemoglobinaemia reported after paracervical block or pudendal block; *see also* Anaesthetics, Local
Primaquine (3)	Neonatal haemolysis and methaemoglobinaemia; *see also* Antimalarials
Primaxin®	Manufacturer advises avoid unless potential benefit outweighs risk (toxicity in *animal* studies)
Primidone	*see* Phenobarbital
Procaine (3)	Neonatal methaemoglobinaemia; *see also* Anaesthetics, Local
Procarbazine	Avoid (teratogenic in *animal* studies and isolated reports in humans); *see also* section 8.1
Prochlorperazine	*see* Antipsychotics
Progesterone	Not known to be harmful
Proguanil	Adequate folate supplements should be given to mother; *see also* Antimalarials
Promazine	*see* Antipsychotics
Promethazine	*see* Antihistamines
Propafenone	Manufacturer advises avoid—no information available
Propantheline	Manufacturer advises avoid—no information available
Propiverine	Manufacturer advises avoid (retardation of skeletal development in *animals*)
Propofol	*see* Anaesthetics, General
Propranolol	*see* Beta-blockers
Propylthiouracil (2, 3)	Neonatal goitre and hypothyroidism
Protionamide (1)	May be teratogenic
Pseudoephedrine	Not known to be harmful
Pyrazinamide	Manufacturer advises use only if potential benefit outweighs risk; see also p. 282
Pyridostigmine	Manufacturer advises use only if potential benefit outweighs risk
Pyrimethamine (1)	Theoretical teratogenic risk (folate antagonist); adequate folate supplements should be given to mother; *see also* Antimalarials
Quetiapine	Manufacturer advises use only if potential benefit outweighs risk
Quinagolide	Manufacturer advises discontinue when pregnancy confirmed unless medical reason for continuing
Quinapril	*see* ACE Inhibitors

Drug (trimester of risk)	Comment
Quinine (1)	High doses are teratogenic; but in malaria benefit of treatment outweighs risk
Quinolones (1, 2, 3)	Avoid—arthropathy in *animal* studies; safer alternatives available
Quinupristin [ingredient]	*see Synercid®*
Rabeprazole	Manufacturer advises avoid—no information available
Raltitrexed	Pregnancy must be excluded before treatment; ensure effective contraception during and for at least 6 months after administration to men or women; *see also* section 8.1
Ramipril	*see ACE Inhibitors*
Ranitidine	Manufacturer advises avoid unless essential, but not known to be harmful
Ranitidine bismuth citrate	Safety not established
Rasburicase	Manufacturer advises avoid—no information available
Razoxane	Avoid (teratogenic in *animal* studies); *see also* section 8.1
Reboxetine	Manufacturer advises avoid (and discontinue if pregnancy occurs)—no information available
Remifentanil	No information available; *see also* Opioid Analgesics
Repaglinide	Manufacturer advises avoid; insulin is normally substituted in all diabetics
Reteplase	*see Streptokinase*
Reviparin	Manufacturer advises avoid—no information available
Riamet®	Toxicity in *animal* studies with artemether; manufacturer advises use only if potential benefit outweighs risk
Ribavirin	Avoid; teratogenicity in *animal* studies; ensure effective contraception during oral administration and for 6 months after treatment in women and in men; *see also* Ribavirin section 5.3
Rifabutin	Manufacturer advises avoid—no information available
Rifampicin (1)	Manufacturers advise very high doses teratogenic in *animal* studies; *see also* p. 282
(3)	Risk of neonatal bleeding may be increased
Riluzole	No information available; manufacturer advises avoid
Risedronate sodium	*see Bisphosphonates*
Risperidone	Manufacturer advises use only if potential benefit outweighs risk
Ritodrine	For use in premature labour *see* section 7.1.3
Ritonavir	Manufacturer advises use only if potential benefit outweighs risk—no information available

Drug (trimester of risk)	Comment
Rituximab	Avoid unless potential benefit to mother outweighs risk of B-lymphocyte depletion in fetus—effective contraception required during and for 12 months after treatment
Rivastigmine	Manufacturer advises use only if potential benefit outweighs risk
Rizatriptan	*see 5HT₁ Agonists*
Rocuronium	Manufacturer advises avoid unless potential benefit outweighs risk
Rofecoxib	*see NSAIDs*
Ropivacaine	Safety not established but not known to be harmful
Rosiglitazone	Manufacturer advises avoid—toxicity in *animal* studies; insulin is normally substituted in all diabetics
Rosuvastatin	*see Statins*
Salbutamol (3)	For use in asthma *see* section 3.1
	For use in premature labour *see* section 7.1.3
Salcatonin	*see Calcitonin (salmon)*
Salmeterol	*see* section 3.1
Saquinavir	Manufacturer advises use only if potential benefit outweighs risk
Selegiline	Manufacturer advises avoid—no information available
Sertindole	Manufacturer advises avoid
Sertraline	*see Antidepressants, SSRI*
Sevelamer	Manufacturer advises use only if potential benefit outweighs risk
Sevoflurane	*see Anaesthetics, General*
Sibutramine	Manufacturer advises avoid—toxicity in *animal* studies
Silver sulfadiazine	*see Sulphonamides*
Simvastatin	*see Statins*
Sirolimus	Manufacturer advises avoid (toxicity in *animal* studies); effective contraception must be used during treatment and for 12 weeks after stopping
Sodium aurothiomalate	Manufacturer advises avoid
Sodium clodronate	*see Bisphosphonates*
Sodium cromoglicate	Not known to be harmful; *see also* section 3.1
Sodium fusidate	Not known to be harmful; manufacturer advises use only if potential benefit outweighs risk
Sodium phenylbutyrate	Avoid (toxicity in *animal* studies); manufacturer advises adequate contraception during administration
Sodium valproate	*see Valproate*
Somatropin	Discontinue if pregnancy occurs—no information available but theoretical risk
Sotalol	*see Beta-blockers*
Spironolactone	Manufacturers advise toxicity in *animal* studies
Statins	Avoid—congenital anomalies reported; decreased synthesis of cholesterol possibly affects fetal development

Drug (trimester of risk)	Comment
Stavudine	Manufacturer advises use only if potential benefit outweighs risk
Streptokinase (1, 2, 3)	Possibility of premature separation of placenta in first 18 weeks; theoretical possibility of fetal haemorrhage throughout pregnancy; risk of maternal haemorrhage on post-partum use
Streptomycin	*see* Aminoglycosides
Sulfadiazine	*see* Sulphonamides
Sulfadoxine	*see* Sulphonamides
Sulfasalazine (3)	Theoretical risk of neonatal haemolysis; adequate folate supplements should be given to mother
Sulindac	*see* NSAIDs
Sulphonamides (3)	Neonatal haemolysis and methaemoglobinaemia; fear of increased risk of kernicterus in neonates appears to be unfounded
Sulphonylureas (3)	Neonatal hypoglycaemia; insulin is normally substituted in all diabetics; if oral drugs are used therapy should be stopped at least 2 days before delivery
Sulpiride	*see* Antipsychotics
Sumatriptan	*see* 5HT$_1$ Agonists
Suxamethonium	Mildly prolonged maternal paralysis may occur
Synercid®	Manufacturer advises avoid unless potential benefit outweighs risk—no information available
Tacalcitol	Manufacturer advises avoid unless no safer alternative—no information available
Tacrolimus	Avoid; manufacturer advises toxicity in *animal* studies following systemic administration
Tamoxifen	Avoid—possible effects on fetal development; effective contraception must be used during treatment and for 2 months after stopping
Tazarotene	Avoid; effective contraception required
Tazobactam [ingredient]	*see* Tazocin®
Tazocin®	Manufacturer advises use only if potential benefit outweighs risk
Tegafur with uracil	*see* Uftoral®
Teicoplanin	Manufacturer advises use only if potential benefit outweighs risk
Telithromycin	Toxicity in animal studies—manufacturer advises use only if potential benefit outweighs risk
Telmisartan	*As for* ACE Inhibitors
Temazepam	*see* Benzodiazepines

Drug (trimester of risk)	Comment
Temozolomide	Avoid (teratogenic and embryotoxic in *animal* studies); manufacturer advises adequate contraception during administration; *see also* section 8.1; also men should avoid fathering a child during and for at least 6 months after treatment
Tenecteplase	*see* Streptokinase
Tenofovir	No information available—manufacturer advises use only if potential benefit outweighs risk
Tenoxicam	*see* NSAIDs
Terazosin	*see* Alpha-blockers, Post-synaptic
Terbinafine	Manufacturer advises use only if potential benefit outweighs risk—no information available
Terbutaline (3)	For use in asthma *see* section 3.1 For use in premature labour *see* section 7.1.3
Terfenadine	*see* Antihistamines
Testosterone	*see* Androgens
Tetrabenazine	Inadequate information but no evidence of harm
Tetracyclines (1)	Effects on skeletal development in *animal* studies
(2, 3)	Dental discoloration; maternal hepatotoxicity with large parenteral doses
Theophylline (3)	Neonatal irritability and apnoea have been reported
Thiazides and related diuretics	*see* Diuretics
Thiopental	*see* Anaesthetics, General
Thioridazine	*see* Antipsychotics
Thiotepa	Avoid (teratogenic and embryotoxic in *animals*); *see also* section 8.1
Thymoxamine	*see* Moxisylyte
Thyroxine	*see* Levothyroxine
Tiagabine	Manufacturer advises avoid unless potential benefit outweighs risk
Tiaprofenic acid	*see* NSAIDs
Ticarcillin [ingredient]	*see* Penicillins
Tiludronic acid	*see* Bisphosphonates
Timentin®	*see* Penicillins
Timolol	*see* Beta-blockers
Tinidazole	Manufacturer advises avoid in first trimester
Tinzaparin	Manufacturer advises avoid unless no safer alternative
Tioconazole	Manufacturer advises avoid
Tioguanine	Avoid (teratogenicity reported when men receiving tioguanine have fathered children); ensure effective contraception during administration to men or women; *see also* section 8.1
Tiotropium	Toxicity in *animal* studies—manufacturer advises use only if potential benefit outweighs risk

Drug (trimester of risk)	Comment
Tirofiban	Manufacturer advises use only if potential benefit outweighs risk—no information available
Tizanidine	Manufacturer advises use only if potential benefit outweighs risk—no information available
Tobramycin	*see* Aminoglycosides
Tocopheryl acetate (1, 2, 3)	No evidence of safety of high doses
Tolbutamide	*see* Sulphonylureas
Tolfenamic acid	*see* NSAIDs
Tolterodine	Manufacturer advises avoid—toxicity in *animal* studies
Topiramate	Manufacturer advises avoid unless potential benefit outweighs potential risk; *see also* Antiepileptics
Topotecan	Avoid (teratogenicity and fetal loss in *animal* studies); *see also* section 8.1
Torasemide	*see* Diuretics
Tramadol	Embryotoxic in animal studies—manufacturers advise avoid; *see also* Opioid Analgesics
Trandolapril	*see* ACE Inhibitors
Tranexamic acid	No evidence of teratogenicity in *animal* studies; manufacturer advises use only if potential benefit outweighs risk—crosses the placenta
Tranylcypromine	*see* Antidepressants, MAOI
Trastuzumab	Avoid unless potential benefit outweighs risk
Travoprost	Manufacturer advises use only if potential benefit outweighs risk
Trazodone	*see* Antidepressants, Tricyclic (and related)
Treosulfan	Avoid; *see also* section 8.1
Tretinoin (1, 2, 3)	Teratogenic; effective contraception must be used for at least 1 month before oral treatment, during treatment and for at least 1 month after stopping; also avoid topical treatment
Triamcinolone	*see* Corticosteroids
Triamterene	*see* Diuretics
Tribavirin	*see* Ribavirin
Triclofos	Avoid
Trientine	Manufacturer advises use only if potential benefit outweighs risk; monitor maternal and neonatal serum-copper concentration; teratogenic in *animal* studies
Trifluoperazine	*see* Antipsychotics
Trilostane (1, 2, 3)	Interferes with placental sex hormone production
Trimeprazine	*see* Antihistamines
Trimetaphan (3)	Avoid; risk of paralytic ileus in newborn
Trimethoprim (1)	Teratogenic risk (folate antagonist); manufacturers advise avoid
Trimipramine	*see* Antidepressants, Tricyclic (and related)
Tripotassium dicitratobismuthate	Manufacturer advises avoid on theoretical grounds
Triprolidine	*see* Antihistamines
Tropisetron	Manufacturer advises toxicity in *animal* studies
Trospium	Manufacturer advises caution—no information available
Uftoral®	Avoid; manufacturer advises effective contraception during and for 3 months after administration to men or women
Ursodeoxycholic acid	No evidence of harm but manufacturer advises avoid
Vaccines (live) (1)	Theoretical risk of congenital malformations, but need for vaccination may outweigh possible risk to fetus (*see also* p. 578); avoid MMR and Rubella vaccines but *see* p. 592
Valaciclovir	*see* Aciclovir
Valdecoxib	*see* NSAIDS
Valganciclovir	*see* Ganciclovir
Valproate (1, 3)	Increased risk of congenital malformations and developmental delay (counselling and screening advised—**important:** *see also* p. 227); neonatal bleeding (related to hypofibrinaemia) and neonatal hepatotoxicity also reported
Valproic acid	*see* Valproate
Valsartan	*As for* ACE Inhibitors
Vancomycin	Manufacturer advises use only if potential benefit outweighs risk—plasma-vancomycin concentration monitoring essential to reduce risk of fetal toxicity
Vasopressin	Oxytocic effect in third trimester
Vecuronium	Manufacturer advises avoid unless potential benefit outweighs risk—no information available
Venlafaxine	Manufacturer advises avoid—no information available
Verapamil	*see* Calcium-channel Blockers
Verteporfin	Manufacturer advises use only if potential benefit outweighs risk (teratogenic in *animal* studies)
Vigabatrin	Congenital anomalies reported—manufacturer advises avoid unless potential benefit outweighs risk; *see also* Antiepileptics
Vinblastine	Avoid (limited experience suggests fetal harm; teratogenic in *animal* studies); *see also* section 8.1
Vincristine	Avoid (teratogenicity and fetal loss in *animal* studies); *see also* section 8.1
Vindesine	Avoid (teratogenic in *animal* studies); *see also* section 8.1

Drug (trimester of risk)	Comment
Vinorelbine	Avoid (teratogenicity and fetal loss in *animal* studies); *see also* section 8.1
Vitamin A (1)	Excessive doses may be teratogenic; *see also* p. 466
Vitamin D	High systemic doses teratogenic in *animals* but therapeutic doses unlikely to be harmful; manufacturer of *topical* calcitriol advises avoid; *see also* Calcipotriol and Tacalcitol
Voriconazole	Toxicity in *animal* studies—manufacturer advises avoid unless potential benefit outweighs risk; effective contraception required during treatment
Warfarin	*see* Anticoagulants, Oral
Xipamide	*see* Diuretics
Zafirlukast	Manufacturer advises use only if potential benefit outweighs risk
Zalcitabine	Limited information available; use only if potential benefit outweighs risk
Zaleplon	Manufacturer advises avoid in early pregnancy—no information available; risk of neonatal withdrawal symptoms if used in late pregnancy
Zanamivir	Manufacturer advises use only if potential benefit outweighs risk—no information available
Zidovudine	Limited information available; manufacturer advises use only if clearly indicated; *see also* p. 300
Zinc sulphate	Safety not established—crosses placenta
Zoledronic acid	Manufacturer advises avoid—toxicity in *animal* studies
Zolmitriptan	*see* $5HT_1$ Agonists
Zolpidem	*see* Benzodiazepines
Zopiclone	*see* Benzodiazepines
Zotepine	Manufacturer advises avoid unless potential benefit outweighs risk
Zuclopenthixol	*see* Antipsychotics

Appendix 5: Breast-feeding

Administration of some drugs (e.g. ergotamine) to nursing mothers may harm the infant, whereas administration of others (e.g. digoxin) has little effect. Some drugs inhibit lactation (e.g. bromocriptine).

Toxicity to the infant can occur if the drug enters the milk in pharmacologically significant quantities. The concentration in milk of some drugs (e.g. iodides) may exceed the concentration in maternal plasma so that therapeutic doses in the mother may cause toxicity to the infant. Some drugs inhibit the infant's sucking reflex (e.g. phenobarbital). Drugs in breast milk may, at least theoretically, cause hypersensitivity in the infant even when concentration is too low for a pharmacological effect. The following table lists drugs:

- which should be used with caution or which are contra-indicated in breast-feeding for the reasons given above;
- which, on present evidence, may be given to the mother during breast-feeding, because they appear in milk in amounts which are too small to be harmful to the infant;
- which are not known to be harmful to the infant although they are present in milk in significant amounts.

For many drugs insufficient evidence is available to provide guidance and it is advisable to administer only essential drugs to a mother during breast-feeding. Because of the inadequacy of information on drugs in breast milk the following table should be used only as a guide; absence from the table does not imply safety.

Table of drugs present in breast milk

Products introduced or amended since publication of BNF No. 46 (September 2003) are underlined.

Drug	Comment
Abacavir	Breast-feeding not advised in HIV infection
Abciximab	Manufacturer advises avoid—no information available
Acamprosate	Manufacturer advises avoid
Acarbose	Manufacturer advises avoid
Acebutolol	*see* Beta-blockers
Aceclofenac	Manufacturer advises avoid—no information available
Acemetacin	Manufacturer advises avoid
Acenocoumarol (nicoumalone)	*see* Anticoagulants, Oral
Acetazolamide	Amount too small to be harmful
Aciclovir	Significant amount in milk after systemic administration—not known to be harmful but manufacturer advises caution
Acipimox	Manufacturer advises avoid
Acitretin	Avoid
Aclarubicin	*see* Cytotoxic Drugs
Acrivastine	*see* Antihistamines

Drug	Comment
Adalimumab	Avoid; manufacturer advises avoid for at least 5 months after last dose
Adapalene	Manufacturer advises avoid (if used, avoid application to chest)—no information available
Adefovir dipivoxil	Manufacturer advises avoid—no information available
Alcohol	Large amounts may affect infant and reduce milk consumption
Alendronic acid	No information available
Alfacalcidol	*see* Vitamin D
Alimemazine (trimeprazine)	*see* Antihistamines
Allopurinol	Present in milk
Almotriptan	Present in milk in *animal* studies—withhold breast-feeding for 24 hours
Alprazolam	*see* Benzodiazepines
Alverine	Manufacturer advises avoid—little information available
Amantadine	Avoid; present in milk; toxicity in infant reported
Amethocaine	*see* Tetracaine
Amfebutamone	*see* Bupropion
Amifostine	No information available
Amiloride	Manufacturer advises avoid—no information available
Aminoglutethimide	Avoid
Aminophylline	*see* Theophylline
Amiodarone	Avoid; present in milk in significant amounts; theoretical risk from release of iodine; *see also* Iodine
Amisulpride	Manufacturer advises avoid—no information available
Amitriptyline	*see* Antidepressants, Tricyclic (and related)
Amlodipine	Manufacturer advises avoid—no information available
Amobarbital	*see* Barbiturates
Amorolfine	Manufacturer advises avoid—no information available
Amoxapine	*see* Antidepressants, Tricyclic (and related)
Amoxicillin	*see* Penicillins
Amphetamines	Significant amount in milk. Avoid
Amphotericin	No information available
Ampicillin	*see* Penicillins
Amprenavir	Breast-feeding not advised in HIV infection
Amsacrine	*see* Cytotoxic Drugs
Anakinra	Manufacturer advises avoid—no information available
Analgesics	*see* Aspirin, NSAIDs, Opioid Analgesics and Paracetamol
Androgens	Avoid; may cause masculinisation in the female infant or precocious development in the male infant; high doses suppress lactation

Drug	Comment
Anthraquinones	Avoid; large doses may cause increased gastric motility and diarrhoea (particularly cascara and dantron)
Anticoagulants, oral	Risk of haemorrhage; increased by vitamin-K deficiency; warfarin appears safe but phenindione should be avoided; manufacturer of acenocoumarol (nicoumalone) recommends prophylactic vitamin K for the infant (consult product literature)
Antidepressants, SSRI	*see* individual entries
Antidepressants, tricyclic (and related)	Amount of tricyclic antidepressants (including related drugs such as mianserin and trazodone) too small to be harmful but most manufacturers advise avoid; accumulation of doxepin metabolite may cause sedation and respiratory depression
Antihistamines	Significant amount of some antihistamines present in milk; although not known to be harmful manufacturers of alimemazine, cetirizine, cyproheptadine, desloratadine, fexofenadine, hydroxyzine, loratadine, mizolastine and terfenadine advise avoid; adverse effects in infant reported with clemastine
Antipsychotics	Although amount excreted in milk probably too small to be harmful, *animal* studies indicate possible adverse effects of these drugs on developing nervous system therefore avoid unless absolutely necessary; *see also* Amisulpride, Chlorpromazine, Clozapine, Olanzapine, Quetiapine, Risperidone, Sertindole, Sulpiride, Zotepine
Apomorphine	Manufacturer advises avoid—no information available
Artemether [ingredient]	*see* Riamet®
Aspirin	Avoid—possible risk of Reye's syndrome; regular use of high doses could impair platelet function and produce hypoprothrombinaemia in infant if neonatal vitamin K stores low
Atenolol	*see* Beta-blockers
Atorvastatin	Manufacturer advises avoid—no information available
Atosiban	Small amounts present in milk
Atovaquone	Manufacturer advises avoid—no information available
Atracurium	Breast-feeding unlikely to be harmful following recovery from neuromuscular block; some manufacturers advise avoiding breast-feeding for 24 hours after administration
Atropine	Small amount present in milk—manufacturer advises caution
Auranofin	Present in milk; manufacturer advises avoid
Azapropazone	Avoid—small amounts in milk
Azathioprine	*see* Cytotoxic Drugs

Drug	Comment
Azithromycin	Manufacturer advises use only if no suitable alternative—no information available
Aztreonam	Amount probably too small to be harmful—manufacturer advises avoid
Baclofen	Amount too small to be harmful
Balsalazide	Manufacturer advises avoid
Barbiturates	Avoid if possible (*see also* Phenobarbital); large doses may produce drowsiness
Basiliximab	Avoid
Beclometasone	*see* Corticosteroids
Bemiparin	Manufacturer advises avoid—no information available
Bendrofluazide	*see* Thiazides and Related Diuretics
Bendroflumethiazide (bendrofluazide)	*see* Thiazides and Related Diuretics
Benorilate	*see* Aspirin and Paracetamol
Benperidol	*see* Antipsychotics
Benzodiazepines	Present in milk—avoid if possible
Benzylpenicillin	*see* Penicillins
Beta-blockers	Monitor infant; possible toxicity due to beta-blockade but amount of most beta-blockers excreted in milk too small to affect infant; acebutolol, atenolol, nadolol, and sotalol are present in greater amounts than other beta-blockers; manufacturers advise avoid celiprolol and nebivolol
Betamethasone	*see* Corticosteroids
Bethanechol	Manufacturer advises avoid
Bexarotene	*see* Cytotoxic Drugs
Bezafibrate	Manufacturer advises avoid—no information available
Bimatoprost	Manufacturer advises avoid
Bisoprolol	*see* Beta-blockers
Bleomycin	*see* Cytotoxic Drugs
Bosentan	Manufacturer advises avoid—no information available
Botulinum toxin	Manufacturers advise avoid—no information available
Bromocriptine	Suppresses lactation
Brompheniramine	*see* Antihistamines
Buclizine	*see* Antihistamines
Budesonide	*see* Corticosteroids
Bumetanide	Manufacturer advises avoid if possible—no information available
Bupivacaine	Amount too small to be harmful
Buprenorphine	Amount too small to be harmful; manufacturer advises contraindicated in the treatment of opioid dependence
Bupropion	Present in milk—manufacturer advises avoid
Buserelin	Small amount present in milk—manufacturer advises avoid
Buspirone	Manufacturer advises avoid
Busulfan	*see* Cytotoxic Drugs
Butobarbital	*see* Barbiturates
Cabergoline	Suppresses lactation
Caffeine	Regular intake of large amounts can affect infant
Calciferol	*see* Vitamin D

Drug	Comment
Calcipotriol	No information available
Calcitonin (salmon) (salcatonin)	Avoid; inhibits lactation in *animals*
Calcitriol	*see* Vitamin D
Calcium folinate	Manufacturer advises caution—no information available
Calcium levofolinate	*see* Calcium Folinate
Candesartan	Manufacturer advises avoid—no information available
Capecitabine	Discontinue breast-feeding
Capreomycin	Manufacturer advises caution—no information available
Captopril	Excreted in milk— manufacturers advise avoid
Carbamazepine	Amount probably too small to be harmful but severe skin reaction reported in 1 infant
Carbenoxolone	Manufacturer advises avoid—no information available
Carbimazole	Amounts in milk may be sufficient to affect neonatal thyroid function therefore lowest effective dose should be used (*see also* section 6.2.2)
Carbocisteine	No information available
Carboplatin	*see* Cytotoxic Drugs
Carglumic acid	Manufacturer advises avoid unless essential—no information available
Carisoprodol	Concentrated in milk; no adverse effects reported but best avoided
Carmustine	*see* Cytotoxic Drugs
Carvedilol	*see* Beta-blockers
Cascara	*see* Anthraquinones
Caspofungin	Present in milk in *animal* studies—manufacturer advises avoid
Cefaclor	Present in milk in low concentration
Cefadroxil	Present in milk in low concentration
Cefalexin	Present in milk in low concentration
Cefixime	Manufacturer advises avoid—no information available
Cefotaxime	Present in milk in low concentration
Cefoxitin	Present in milk in low concentration
Cefpirome	Present in milk—manufacturer advises avoid
Cefpodoxime	Present in milk in low concentration
Cefprozil	Present in milk in low concentration
Cefradine	Present in milk in low concentration
Ceftazidime	Present in milk in low concentration
Ceftriaxone	Present in milk in low concentration
Cefuroxime	Present in milk in low concentration
Celecoxib	Manufacturer advises avoid—no information available
Celiprolol	*see* Beta-blockers
Cetirizine	*see* Antihistamines
Cetrorelix	Manufacturer advises avoid

Drug	Comment
Chloral hydrate	Sedation in infant—manufacturer advises avoid
Chlorambucil	*see* Cytotoxic Drugs
Chloramphenicol	Use another antibiotic; may cause bone-marrow toxicity in infant; concentration in milk usually insufficient to cause 'grey syndrome'
Chlordiazepoxide	*see* Benzodiazepines
Chlormethine (mustine)	*see* Cytotoxic Drugs
Chloroquine	Amount probably too small to be harmful when used for malaria prophylaxis; inadequate for reliable protection against malaria, *see* section 5.4.1; avoid breast-feeding when used for rheumatic diseases
Chlorphenamine (chlorpheniramine)	*see* Antihistamines
Chlorpheniramine	*see* Antihistamines
Chlorpromazine	Drowsiness in infant reported; *see* Antipsychotics
Chlorpropamide	*see* Sulphonylureas
Chlortalidone	*see* Thiazides and Related Diuretics
Chlortetracycline	*see* Tetracyclines
Ciclosporin	Present in milk—manufacturer advises avoid
Cidofovir	Manufacturer advises avoid
Cilastatin [ingredient]	*see Primaxin*®
Cilazapril	No information available—manufacturer advises avoid
Cilostazol	Present in milk in *animal* studies—manufacturer advises avoid
Cimetidine	Significant amount—not known to be harmful but manufacturer advises avoid
Ciprofibrate	Manufacturer advises avoid—present in milk in *animal* studies
Ciprofloxacin	Avoid—high concentrations in breast milk
Cisatracurium	No information available
Cisplatin	*see* Cytotoxic Drugs
Citalopram	Present in milk—manufacturer advises avoid
Cladribine	*see* Cytotoxic Drugs
Clarithromycin	Manufacturer advises avoid unless potential benefit outweighs risk—present in milk
Clavulanic acid [ingredient]	see Co-amoxiclav, *Timentin*®
Clemastine	*see* Antihistamines
Clindamycin	Amount probably too small to be harmful but bloody diarrhoea reported in 1 infant
Clobazam	*see* Benzodiazepines
Clodronate sodium	*see* Sodium Clodronate
Clomethiazole	Amount too small to be harmful
Clomifene	May inhibit lactation
Clomipramine	*see* Antidepressants, Tricyclic (and related)
Clopidogrel	Manufacturer advises avoid
Clorazepate	*see* Benzodiazepines
Clozapine	Manufacturer advises avoid
Co-amoxiclav	*see* Penicillins
Co-beneldopa	*see* Levodopa
Co-careldopa	*see* Levodopa

Drug	Comment
Codeine	Amount too small to be harmful
Co-fluampicil	*see* Penicillins
Colchicine	Present in milk but no adverse effects reported; manufacturers advise avoid because of risk of cytotoxicity
Colecalciferol	*see* Vitamin D
Colistin	Present in milk—manufacturer advises use only if potential benefit outweighs risk
Contraceptives, oral	Avoid combined oral contraceptives until weaning or for 6 months after birth (adverse effects on lactation); progestogen-only contraceptives do not affect lactation (start 3 weeks after birth or later)
Corticosteroids	Systemic effects in infant unlikely with maternal dose of prednisolone up to 40 mg daily; monitor infant's adrenal function with higher doses—the amount of inhaled drugs in breast milk is probably too small to be harmful
Cortisone acetate	*see* Corticosteroids
Co-trimoxazole	Small risk of kernicterus in jaundiced infants and of haemolysis in G6PD-deficient infants (due to sulfamethoxazole)
Crisantaspase	*see* Cytotoxic Drugs
Cromoglicate	*see* Sodium Cromoglicate
Cyclopenthiazide	*see* Thiazides and Related Diuretics
Cyclophosphamide	Discontinue breast-feeding during and for 36 hours after stopping treatment
Cycloserine	Amount too small to be harmful
Cyclosporin	*see* Ciclosporin
Cyproheptadine	*see* Antihistamines
Cyproterone	Caution; possibility of anti-androgen effects in neonate
Cytarabine	*see* Cytotoxic Drugs
Cytotoxic drugs	Discontinue breast-feeding
Daclizumab	Avoid
Dactinomycin	*see* Cytotoxic Drugs
Dalfopristin [ingredient]	*see* Synercid®
Dalteparin	No information available
Danazol	No data available but avoid because of possible androgenic effects in infant
Dantron	*see* Anthraquinones
Dapsone	Haemolytic anaemia; although significant amount in milk, risk to infant very small unless infant is G6PD deficient
Darbepoetin	Manufacturer advises avoid—no information available
Daunorubicin	*see* Cytotoxic Drugs
Deferiprone	Manufacturer advises avoid—no information available
Deflazacort	*see* Corticosteroids
Demeclocycline	*see* Tetracyclines
Desferrioxamine	Manufacturer advises use only if potential benefit outweighs risk—no information available
Desmopressin	Not known to be harmful
Desogestrel	*see* Contraceptives, Oral
Dexamethasone	*see* Corticosteroids

Drug	Comment
Dexamfetamine	*see* Amphetamines
Dexketoprofen	Manufacturer advises avoid—no information available
Dextromoramide	No information available—manufacturer advises avoid
Dextropropoxyphene	Amount too small to be harmful
Diamorphine	Therapeutic doses unlikely to affect infant; withdrawal symptoms in infants of dependent mothers; breast-feeding no longer considered best method of treating dependence in offspring of dependent mothers and should be stopped
Diazepam	*see* Benzodiazepines
Diclofenac	Amount too small to be harmful
Didanosine	Breast-feeding not advised in HIV infection
Diflunisal	Manufacturer advises avoid
Digoxin	Amount too small to be harmful
Dihydrocodeine	Manufacturer advises use only if potential benefit outweighs risk
Dihydrotachysterol	*see* Vitamin D
Diloxanide	Manufacturer advises avoid
Diltiazem	Significant amount—no evidence of harm but avoid unless no safer alternative
Diphenhydramine	*see* Antihistamines
Diphenylpyraline	*see* Antihistamines
Dipyridamole	Small amount present in milk—manufacturer advises caution
Disodium etidronate	No information available
Disodium pamidronate	Manufacturer advises avoid
Disopyramide	Present in milk—use only if essential and monitor infant for antimuscarinic effects
Distigmine	No information available
Docetaxel	*see* Cytotoxic Drugs
Docusate sodium	Present in milk following oral administration—manufacturer advises caution; rectal administration not known to be harmful
Dolasetron	Manufacturer advises avoid—no information available
Domperidone	Amount probably too small to be harmful
Dornase alfa	Amount probably too small to be harmful—manufacturer advises caution
Dosulepin (dothiepin)	*see* Antidepressants, Tricyclic (and related)
Dothiepin	*see* Antidepressants, Tricyclic (and related)
Doxazosin	Accumulates in milk—manufacturer advises avoid
Doxepin	*see* Antidepressants, Tricyclic (and related)
Doxorubicin	*see* Cytotoxic Drugs
Doxycycline	*see* Tetracyclines
Doxylamine	*see* Antihistamines
Drotrecogin alfa (activated)	Manufacturer advises avoid—no information available
Dydrogesterone	Present in milk—no adverse effects reported
Edrophonium	Amount probably too small to be harmful

Drug	Comment
Efavirenz	Breast-feeding not advised in HIV infection
Eformoterol	see Formoterol
Eletriptan	Present in milk—avoid breast-feeding for 24 hours
Emtricitabine	Breast-feeding not advised in HIV infection
Enalapril	Amount probably too small to be harmful
Enfuvirtide	Breast-feeding not advised in HIV infection
Enoxaparin	Manufacturer advises avoid—no information available
Enoximone	Manufacturer advises caution—no information available
Entacapone	Manufacturer advises avoid—present in milk in *animal* studies
Ephedrine	Irritability and disturbed sleep reported
Epirubicin	see Cytotoxic Drugs
Epoetin	Manufacturers advise avoid—no information available
Eprosartan	Manufacturer advises avoid unless potential benefit outweighs risk
Ergocalciferol	see Vitamin D
Ergotamine	Avoid; ergotism may occur in infant; repeated doses may inhibit lactation
Ertapenem	Present in milk—manufacturer advises avoid
Erythromycin	Only small amounts in milk
Escitalopram	Manufacturer advises avoid—no information available
Esmolol	see Beta-blockers
Esomeprazole	Manufacturer advises avoid—no information available
Etamsylate	Significant amount but not known to be harmful
Etanercept	Manufacturer advises avoid—no information available
Ethambutol	Amount too small to be harmful
Ethinylestradiol	see Oestrogens
Ethosuximide	Present in milk but unlikely to be harmful; manufacturer advises avoid
Etidronate disodium	see Disodium Etidronate
Etodolac	Manufacturer advises avoid
Etomidate	Avoid breast-feeding for 24 hours after administration
Etoposide	see Cytotoxic Drugs
Etoricoxib	Manufacturer advises avoid—present in milk in *animal* studies
Etynodiol	see Contraceptives, Oral
Ezetimibe	Present in milk in *animal* studies—manufacturer advises avoid
Famciclovir	Manufacturer advises avoid unless potential benefit outweighs risk—present in milk in *animal* studies
Famotidine	Present in milk—not known to be harmful but manufacturer advises avoid
Fansidar®	Small risk of kernicterus in jaundiced infants and of haemolysis in G6PD-deficient infants (due to sulfadoxine)
Felodipine	Appears in milk

Drug	Comment
Fenbufen	Small amount present in milk—manufacturer advises avoid
Fenofibrate	Manufacturer advises avoid—no information available
Fenoprofen	Amount too small to be harmful
Fentanyl	Manufacturer advises avoid
Fenticonazole	Manufacturer advises avoid unless essential—present in milk in *animal* studies
Fexofenadine	see Antihistamines
Filgrastim	No information available—manufacturer advises avoid
Flavoxate	Manufacturer advises caution—no information available
Flecainide	Significant amount but not known to be harmful
Flucloxacillin	see Penicillins
Fluconazole	Manufacturer advises avoid—present in milk
Flucytosine	Manufacturer advises avoid
Fludarabine	see Cytotoxic Drugs
Flunitrazepam	see Benzodiazepines
Fluorouracil	see Cytotoxic Drugs
Fluoxetine	Present in milk—manufacturer advises avoid
Flupentixol	see Antipsychotics
Fluphenazine	see Antipsychotics
Flurazepam	see Benzodiazepines
Flurbiprofen	Amount too small to be harmful
Fluticasone	see Corticosteroids
Fluvastatin	Manufacturer advises avoid
Fluvoxamine	Present in milk—manufacturer advises avoid
Follitropin alfa and beta	Avoid
Fomepizole	Manufacturer advises caution—no information available
Fondaparinux	Present in milk in *animal* studies—manufacturer advises avoid
Formoterol (eformoterol)	Amount in milk probably too small to be harmful but manufacturers advise avoid
Fosinopril	Present in milk—manufacturer advises avoid
Fosphenytoin	see Phenytoin
Frovatriptan	Present in milk in *animal* studies—withhold breast-feeding for 24 hours
Frusemide	see Furosemide
Furosemide (frusemide)	Amount too small to be harmful
Fusidic acid	see Sodium Fusidate
Gabapentin	Present in milk—manufacturer advises avoid
Galantamine	Manufacturer advises avoid—no information available
Ganciclovir	Avoid
Gemcitabine	see Cytotoxic Drugs
Gemfibrozil	Manufacturer advises avoid—no information available
Gestodene	see Contraceptives, Oral
Gestrinone	Manufacturer advises avoid
Glatiramer	Manufacturer advises caution—no information available
Glibenclamide	see Sulphonylureas
Gliclazide	see Sulphonylureas
Glimepiride	see Sulphonylureas

Drug	Comment
Glipizide	*see* Sulphonylureas
Gliquidone	*see* Sulphonylureas
Goserelin	Manufacturer advises avoid
Granisetron	Manufacturer advises avoid—no information available
Griseofulvin	Avoid—no information available
Haem arginate	Manufacturer advises avoid unless essential—no information available
Haloperidol	*see* Antipsychotics
Halothane	Excreted in milk
Hepatitis A vaccine	No information available
Human menopausal gonadotrophins	Avoid
Hydralazine	Present in milk but not known to be harmful; monitor infant
Hydrochlorothiazide	*see* Thiazides and Related Diuretics
Hydrocortisone	*see* Corticosteroids
Hydroflumethiazide	*see* Thiazides and Related Diuretics
Hydromorphone	Manufacturer advises avoid—no information available
Hydroxycarbamide (hydroxyurea)	*see* Cytotoxic Drugs
Hydroxychloroquine	Avoid—risk of toxicity in infant
Hydroxyurea	*see* Cytotoxic Drugs
Hydroxyzine	*see* Antihistamines
Hyoscine	Amount too small to be harmful
Ibandronic acid	Manufacturer advises avoid
Ibuprofen	Amount too small to be harmful but some manufacturers advise avoid (including topical use)
Idarubicin	*see* Cytotoxic Drugs
Idoxuridine	May make milk taste unpleasant
Ifosfamide	*see* Cytotoxic Drugs
Imatinib	*see* Cytotoxic Drugs
Imidapril	Manufacturer advises avoid—no information available
Imiglucerase	No information available
Imipenem [ingredient]	*see Primaxin®*
Imipramine	*see* Antidepressants, Tricyclic (and related)
Imiquimod	Manufacturer advises no information available
Indapamide	No information available—manufacturer advises avoid
Indinavir	Breast-feeding not advised in HIV infection
Indometacin	Amount probably too small to be harmful but convulsions reported in one infant—manufacturers advise avoid
Infliximab	Avoid; manufacturer advises avoid for at least 6 months after last dose
Insulin	Amount too small to be harmful
Interferons	Manufacturers advise avoid—no information available
Iodine and iodides	Stop breast-feeding; danger of neonatal hypothyroidism or goitre; appears to be concentrated in milk

Drug	Comment
Iodine, radioactive	Breast-feeding contra-indicated after therapeutic doses. With diagnostic doses withhold breast-feeding for at least 24 hours
Ipratropium	Amount probably too small to be harmful
Irbesartan	Manufacturer advises avoid—no information available
Irinotecan	*see* Cytotoxic Drugs
Isoniazid	Monitor infant for possible toxicity; theoretical risk of convulsions and neuropathy; prophylactic pyridoxine advisable in mother and infant
Isotretinoin	Avoid
Itraconazole	Small amounts present in milk—may accumulate; manufacturer advises unless potential benefit outweighs risk
Kaletra®	Breast-feeding not advised in HIV infection
Ketoconazole	Manufacturer advises avoid
Ketoprofen	Amount probably too small to be harmful but manufacturer advises avoid unless essential
Ketorolac	Avoid
Ketotifen	*see* Antihistamines
Labetalol	*see* Beta-blockers
Lacidipine	Manufacturer advises avoid—no information available
Lamivudine	Present in milk—manufacturer advises avoid; breast-feeding not advised in HIV infection
Lamotrigine	Present in milk but limited data suggest no harmful effects on infants
Lanreotide	Manufacturer advises avoid unless potential benefit outweighs risk—no information available
Lansoprazole	Manufacturer advises avoid unless essential—present in milk in *animal* studies
Latanoprost	May be present in milk—manufacturer advises avoid
Leflunomide	Present in milk—manufacturer advises avoid
Lenograstim	Manufacturer advises avoid—no information available
Lepirudin	Avoid
Lercanidipine	Manufacturer advises avoid
Levetiracetam	Manufacturer advises avoid—present in milk in *animal* studies
Levobupivacaine	Likely to be present in milk but risk to infant minimal
Levocabastine	Amount too small to be harmful
Levocetirizine	*see* Antihistamines
Levodopa	May suppress lactation; present in milk—manufacturers advise avoid
Levofloxacin	Manufacturer advises avoid
Levomepromazine (methotrimeprazine)	*see* Antipsychotics
Levonorgestrel	*see* Contraceptives, Oral
Levothyroxine (thyroxine)	Amount too small to affect tests for neonatal hypothyroidism

Drug	Comment
Lidocaine (lignocaine)	Amount too small to be harmful
Lignocaine	*see* Lidocaine
Linezolid	Manufacturer advises avoid—present in milk in *animal* studies
Liothyronine	Amount too small to affect tests for neonatal hypothyroidism
Lisinopril	No information available—manufacturer advises caution
Lisuride	May suppress lactation
Lithium salts	Present in milk and risk of toxicity in infant—manufacturers advise avoid
Lofepramine	*see* Antidepressants, Tricyclic (and related)
Loperamide	Amount probably too small to be harmful
Lopinavir [ingredient]	*see* Kaletra®
Loprazolam	*see* Benzodiazepines
Loratadine	*see* Antihistamines
Lorazepam	*see* Benzodiazepines
Lormetazepam	*see* Benzodiazepines
Losartan	Manufacturer advises avoid—no information available
Lumefantrine [ingredient]	*see* Riamet®
Lymecycline	*see* Tetracyclines
Macrogols	Manufacturers advise use only if essential—no information available
Malarone®	Manufacturer advises avoid; *see* also Atovaquone and Proguanil
Maprotiline	*see* Antidepressants, Tricyclic (and related)
Mebendazole	No information available
Mebeverine	Amount too small to be harmful
Medroxyprogesterone	Present in milk—no adverse effects reported
Mefenamic acid	Amount too small to be harmful but manufacturer advises avoid
Mefloquine	Present in milk but risk to infant minimal
Meloxicam	No information available—manufacturer advises avoid
Melphalan	*see* Cytotoxic Drugs
Menotrophin	Avoid
Meprobamate	Avoid; concentration in milk may exceed maternal plasma concentrations fourfold and may cause drowsiness in infant
Meptazinol	Manufacturer advises use only if potential benefit outweighs risk
Mercaptamine	Manufacturer advises avoid
Mercaptopurine	*see* Cytotoxic Drugs
Meropenem	Manufacturer advises avoid unless potential benefit justifies potential risk
Mesalazine	Diarrhoea reported but manufacturers advise negligible amounts detected in breast milk
Mesterolone	*see* Androgens
Mestranol	*see* Oestrogens
Metaraminol	Manufacturer advises caution—no information available
Metformin	Manufacturer advises avoid; present in milk

Drug	Comment
Methadone	Withdrawal symptoms in infant; breast-feeding permissible during maintenance but dose should be as low as possible and infant monitored to avoid sedation
Methenamine	Amount too small to be harmful
Methocarbamol	Present in milk in *animal* studies—manufacturer advises caution
Methotrexate	*see* Cytotoxic Drugs
Methotrimeprazine	*see* Antipsychotics
Methyldopa	Amount too small to be harmful
Methylphenidate	No information available—manufacturer advises avoid
Methylprednisolone	*see* Corticosteroids
Methysergide	Manufacturer advises avoid
Metoclopramide	Small amount present in milk; manufacturer advises avoid
Metolazone	*see* Thiazides and Related Diuretics
Metoprolol	*see* Beta-blockers
Metronidazole	Significant amount in milk; manufacturer advises avoid large single doses
Metyrapone	Manufacturer advises avoid—no information available
Mexiletine	Amount too small to be harmful
Mianserin	*see* Antidepressants, Tricyclic (and related)
Miconazole	Manufacturer advises caution—no information available
Midazolam	*see* Benzodiazepines
Mifepristone	No information available—manufacturer advises stop breast-feeding for 14 days after administration
Milrinone	Manufacturer advises caution—no information available
Minocycline	*see* Tetracyclines
Minoxidil	Present in milk but not known to be harmful
Mirtazapine	Manufacturer advises avoid—present in milk in *animal* studies
Misoprostol	No information available—manufacturer advises avoid
Mitomycin	*see* Cytotoxic Drugs
Mitoxantrone (mitozantrone)	*see* Cytotoxic Drugs
Mitozantrone	*see* Cytotoxic Drugs
Mizolastine	*see* Antihistamines
Moclobemide	Amount too small to be harmful, but patient leaflet advises avoid
Modafinil	Manufacturer advises avoid—no information available
Moexipril	Manufacturer advises avoid—no information available
Molgramostim	Manufacturer advises avoid (potential for adverse effects in infant)—no information available
Montelukast	Manufacturer advises avoid unless essential

Drug	Comment
Morphine	Therapeutic doses unlikely to affect infant; withdrawal symptoms in infants of dependent mothers; breast-feeding not best method of treating dependence in offspring and should be stopped
Moxifloxacin	Manufacturer advises avoid—present in milk in *animal* studies
Moxonidine	Present in milk—manufacturer advises avoid
Mupirocin	Manufacturer advises avoid unless potential benefit outweighs risk—no information available
Mustine	*see* Cytotoxic Drugs
Mycophenolate mofetil	No information available—manufacturer advises avoid
Nabumetone	No information available—manufacturer advises avoid
Nadolol	*see* Beta-blockers
Nafarelin	Manufacturer advises avoid—no information available
Nalbuphine	Manufacturer advises caution—no information available
Nalidixic acid	Risk to infant very small but one case of haemolytic anaemia reported
Naloxone	No information available
Naproxen	Amount too small to be harmful but manufacturer advises avoid
Naratriptan	Manufacturer advises caution—no information available
Nateglinide	Manufacturer advises avoid—present in milk in *animal* studies
Nebivolol	*see* Beta-blockers
Nedocromil	Unlikely to be present in milk
Nelfinavir	Breast-feeding not advised in HIV infection
Neostigmine	Amount probably too small to be harmful; monitor infant
Nevirapine	Breast-feeding not advised in HIV infection
Nicardipine	Manufacturer advises avoid
Nicorandil	No information available—manufacturer advises avoid
Nicotine	Present in milk; use only if smoking cessation without nicotine replacement fails; patient information for some products contra-indicates use
Nicoumalone	*see* Anticoagulants, Oral
Nifedipine	Amount too small to be harmful but manufacturers advise avoid
Nimodipine	No information available
Nisoldipine	Manufacturer advises avoid—no information available
Nitrazepam	*see* Benzodiazepines
Nitrofurantoin	Only small amounts in milk but could be enough to produce haemolysis in G6PD-deficient infants
Nizatidine	Amount too small to be harmful
Nonoxynol-9	Present in milk in *animal* studies
Norethisterone	Higher doses may suppress lactation and alter milk composition—use lowest effective dose; *see also* Contraceptives, Oral

Drug	Comment
Norfloxacin	No information available—manufacturer advises avoid
Norgestimate	*see* Contraceptives, Oral
Norgestrel	*see* Contraceptives, Oral
Nortriptyline	*see* Antidepressants, Tricyclic (and related)
NSAIDs	*see* individual entries
Nystatin	No information available, but absorption from gastro-intestinal tract negligible
Octreotide	Manufacturer advises avoid unless essential—no information available
Oestrogens	Avoid; adverse effects on lactation; *see also* Contraceptives, Oral
Ofloxacin	Manufacturer advises avoid
Olanzapine	Manufacturer advises avoid—no information available
Olmesartan	Manufacturer advises avoid—present in milk in *animal* studies
Olsalazine	Manufacturer advises avoid
Omeprazole	Manufacturers advise avoid—no information available
Ondansetron	Manufacturer advises avoid—no information available
Opioid analgesics	*see* individual entries
Oral contraceptives	*see* Contraceptives, Oral
Orlistat	Manufacturer advises avoid—no information available
Orphenadrine	Present in milk—manufacturer advises avoid
Oseltamivir	Manufacturer advises use only if potential benefit outweighs risk—present in milk in *animal* studies
Oxaliplatin	*see* Cytotoxic Drugs
Oxazepam	*see* Benzodiazepines
Oxcarbazepine	Present in milk—manufacturer advises avoid
Oxprenolol	*see* Beta-blockers
Oxybutynin	Present in milk—manufacturers advise avoid
Oxycodone	Present in milk—manufacturer advises avoid
Oxytetracycline	*see* Tetracyclines
Paclitaxel	*see* Cytotoxic Drugs
Pamidronate disodium	*see* Disodium Pamidronate
Pancuronium	Manufacturer advises avoid unless potential benefit outweighs risk—no information available
Pantoprazole	Manufacturer advises avoid unless potential benefit outweighs risk—small amount present in milk in *animal* studies
Papaveretum	*see* Morphine
Paracetamol	Amount too small to be harmful
Paraldehyde	Manufacturer advises avoid unless essential—present in milk
Parecoxib	Manufacturer advises avoid—present in milk in animal studies
Paroxetine	Present in milk—manufacturer advises discontinuation of breast-feeding should be considered
Pegfilgrastim	No information available—manufacturer advises avoid

Drug	Comment
Peginterferon alfa	*see* Interferons
Penicillins	Trace amounts in milk
Pentamidine isetion-ate	Manufacturer advises avoid unless essential
Pentazocine	Small amount present in milk—manufacturer advises caution
Pentostatin	*see* Cytotoxic Drugs
Pergolide	May suppress lactation
Pericyazine	*see* Antipsychotics
Perindopril	Manufacturer advises avoid—no information available
Perphenazine	*see* Antipsychotics
Phenindione	*see* Anticoagulants, Oral
Phenobarbital	Avoid when possible; drowsiness may occur but risk probably small; one report of methaemoglobinaemia with phenobarbital and phenytoin
Phenoxymethylpeni-cillin	*see* Penicillins
Phentolamine	No information available
Phenytoin	Small amount present in milk; manufacturer advises avoid—but *see* section 4.8.1
Phytomenadione	Present in milk
Pilocarpine	Manufacturer advises avoid—no information available
Pimozide	*see* Antipsychotics
Pindolol	*see* Beta-blockers
Pioglitazone	Manufacturer advises avoid—present in milk in *animal* studies
Piperacillin [ingredient]	*see* Tazocin®
Piperazine	Present in milk—manufacturer advises avoid breast-feeding for 8 hours after dose (express and discard milk during this time)
Piracetam	Manufacturer advises avoid
Piroxicam	Amount too small to be harmful
Pizotifen	Amount probably too small to be harmful, but patient information leaflet advises avoid
Podophyllum	Avoid
Porfimer	No information available—manufacturer advises avoid
Povidone–iodine	Avoid; iodine absorbed from vaginal preparations is concentrated in milk
Pramipexole	May suppress lactation; manufacturer advises avoid—present in milk in *animal* studies
Pravastatin	Small amount excreted in milk—manufacturer advises avoid
Prazosin	Amount probably too small to be harmful
Prednisolone	*see* Corticosteroids
Primaxin®	Present in milk—manufacturer advises avoid
Primidone	*see* Phenobarbital
Probenecid	No information available
Procainamide	Present in milk—manufacturer advises avoid
Procarbazine	*see* Cytotoxic Drugs
Prochlorperazine	*see* Antipsychotics
Progesterone	Manufacturers advise avoid—present in milk
Proguanil	*see* Chloroquine
Promazine	*see* Antipsychotics

Drug	Comment
Promethazine	*see* Antihistamines
Propafenone	Manufacturer advises avoid—no information available
Propantheline	May suppress lactation
Propiverine	Manufacturer advises avoid—present in milk in *animal* studies
Propofol	Manufacturer advises avoid—no information available
Propranolol	*see* Beta-blockers
Propylthiouracil	Monitor infant's thyroid status but amounts in milk probably too small to affect infant; high doses might affect neonatal thyroid function
Protirelin	Breast enlargement and leaking of milk reported
Pseudoephedrine	Amount too small to be harmful
Pyrazinamide	Amount too small to be harmful
Pyridostigmine	Amount probably too small to be harmful
Pyrimethamine	Significant amount—avoid administration of other folate antagonists to infant; avoid breast-feeding during toxoplasmosis treatment
Quetiapine	Manufacturer advises avoid—no information available
Quinagolide	Suppresses lactation
Quinapril	No information available—manufacturer advises caution
Quinidine	Significant amount but not known to be harmful
Quinupristin [ingredient]	*see* Synercid®
Rabeprazole	Manufacturer advises avoid—no information available
Raltitrexed	*see* Cytotoxic Drugs
Ramipril	Manufacturer advises avoid—no information available
Ranitidine	Significant amount but not known to be harmful
Ranitidine bismuth citrate	Manufacturer advises avoid—no information available
Rasburicase	Manufacturer advises avoid—no information available
Razoxane	*see* Cytotoxic Drugs
Reboxetine	Manufacturer advises avoid—no information available
Remifentanil	Manufacturer advises caution—present in milk in *animal* studies
Repaglinide	Manufacturer advises avoid—present in milk in *animal* studies
Reteplase	Manufacturer advises avoid breast-feeding for 24 hours after dose (express and discard milk during this time)
Reviparin	No information available
Riamet®	Manufacturer advises avoid breast-feeding for at least 1 week after last dose; present in milk in *animal* studies
Ribavirin	Avoid—no information available
Rifabutin	Manufacturer advises avoid—no information available
Rifampicin	Amount too small to be harmful
Riluzole	Manufacturer advises avoid—no information available
Risedronate sodium	Manufacturer advises avoid

Drug	Comment
Risperidone	Present in milk—manufacturer advises avoid
Ritonavir	Breast-feeding not advised in HIV infection
Rituximab	Avoid
Rivastigmine	Present in milk in *animal* studies—manufacturer advises avoid
Rizatriptan	Present in milk in *animal* studies—withhold breast-feeding for 24 hours
Rocuronium	Manufacturer advises avoid unless potential benefit outweighs risk—present in milk in *animal* studies
Rofecoxib	Manufacturer advises avoid—present in milk in *animal* studies
Rosiglitazone	Manufacturer advises avoid—present in milk in *animal* studies
Rosuvastatin	Manufacturer advises avoid—no information available
Salbutamol	Probably present in milk; manufacturer advises avoid unless potential benefit outweighs risk—the amount of inhaled drugs in breast milk is probably too small to be harmful
Salcatonin	*see* Calcitonin (salmon)
Saquinavir	Breast-feeding not advised in HIV infection
Secobarbital	*see* Barbiturates
Selegiline	Manufacturer advises avoid—no information available
Senna	*see* Anthraquinones
Sertindole	Manufacturer advises avoid—no information available
Sertraline	Present in milk but not known to be harmful in short-term use
Sevelamer	Manufacturer advises use only if potential benefit outweighs risk
Sibutramine	Manufacturer advises avoid—no information available
Silver sulfadiazine	*see* Sulphonamides
Simvastatin	Manufacturer advises avoid—no information available
Sirolimus	Discontinue breast-feeding
Sodium aurothiomalate	Caution—present in milk; theoretical possibility of rashes and idiosyncratic reactions
Sodium clodronate	No information available
Sodium cromoglicate	Unlikely to be present in milk
Sodium fusidate	Present in milk—manufacturer advises caution
Sodium phenylbutyrate	Manufacturer advises avoid—no information available
Sodium valproate	*see* Valproate
Somatropin	No information available
Sotalol	*see* Beta-blockers
Stavudine	Breast-feeding not advised in HIV infection
Sulfadiazine	*see* Sulphonamides
Sulfasalazine	Small amounts in milk (1 report of bloody diarrhoea and rashes); theoretical risk of neonatal haemolysis especially in G6PD-deficient infants
Sulfinpyrazone	No information available
Sulindac	No information available

Drug	Comment
Sulphonamides	Small risk of kernicterus in jaundiced infants particularly with long-acting sulphonamides, and of haemolysis in G6PD-deficient infants
Sulphonylureas	Theoretical possibility of hypoglycaemia in infant
Sulpiride	Best avoided; present in milk; *see also* Antipsychotics
Sumatriptan	Present in milk—withhold breast-feeding for 24 hours
Suxamethonium	No information available
Synercid®	Manufacturer advises avoid—no information available
Tacalcitol	Manufacturer advises avoid application to breast area—no information available
Tacrolimus	Avoid—present in milk following systemic administration
Tamoxifen	Supresses lactation; manufacturer advises avoid unless potential benefit outweighs risk
Tazarotene	Manufacturer advises avoid—present in milk in *animal* studies
Tazobactam [ingredient]	*see* Tazocin®
Tazocin®	Present in milk—manufacturer advises use only if potential benefit outweighs risk
Tegafur with uracil	*see* Cytotoxic Drugs
Teicoplanin	No information available
Telithromycin	Manufacturer advises avoid—present in milk in *animal* studies
Telmisartan	Manufacturer advises avoid—no information available
Temazepam	*see* Benzodiazepines
Temozolomide	*see* Cytotoxic Drugs
Tenecteplase	Manufacturer advises avoid breast-feeding for 24 hours after dose (express and discard milk during this time)
Tenofovir	Breast-feeding not advised in HIV infection
Tenoxicam	No information available
Terazosin	No information available
Terbinafine	Present in milk—manufacturer advises avoid
Terbutaline	Amount too small to be harmful
Terfenadine	*see* Antihistamines
Terlipressin	Not known to be harmful
Testosterone	*see* Androgens
Tetrabenazine	Manufacturer advises avoid
Tetracaine (amethocaine)	No information available
Tetracyclines	Avoid (although absorption and therefore discoloration of teeth in infant probably usually prevented by chelation with calcium in milk)
Theophylline	Present in milk—irritability in infant reported; modified-release preparations preferable
Thiamine	Severely thiamine-deficient mothers should avoid breast-feeding as toxic methyl-glyoxal excreted in milk
Thiazides and related diuretics	Amount too small to be harmful; large doses may suppress lactation

Drug	Comment
Thioridazine	*see* Antipsychotics
Thiotepa	*see* Cytotoxic Drugs
Thyroxine	*see* Levothyroxine
Tiagabine	Manufacturer advises avoid unless potential benefit outweighs risk
Tiaprofenic acid	Amount too small to be harmful
Ticarcillin [ingredient]	*see* Penicillins
Tiludronic acid	Manufacturer advises avoid—no information available
Timentin®	*see* Penicillins
Timolol	*see* Beta-blockers
Tinidazole	Present in milk—manufacturer advises avoid breast-feeding during and for 3 days after stopping treatment
Tinzaparin	Manufacturer advises avoid—no information available
Tioguanine	*see* Cytotoxic Drugs
Tiotropium	Amount in milk probably too small to be harmful (present in milk in *animal* studies)—manufacturer advises use only if potential benefit outweighs risk
Tirofiban	Manufacturer advises avoid—no information available
Tizanidine	Manufacturer advises use only if potential benefit outweighs risk—no information available
Tolbutamide	*see* Sulphonylureas
Tolfenamic acid	Amount too small to be harmful
Tolterodine	Manufacturer advises avoid—no information available
Topiramate	Manufacturer advises avoid
Topotecan	*see* Cytotoxic Drugs
Torasemide	No information available
Tramadol	Amount probably too small to be harmful, but manufacturer advises avoid
Trandolapril	Manufacturers advise avoid
Tranexamic acid	Small amount present in milk—antifibrinolytic effect in infant unlikely
Trastuzumab	Avoid breast-feeding during treatment and for six months after
Travoprost	Present in milk in animal studies; manufacturer advises avoid
Trazodone	*see* Antidepressants, Tricyclic (and related)
Treosulfan	*see* Cytotoxic Drugs
Tretinoin	Avoid
Triamcinolone	*see* Corticosteroids
Tribavirin	*see* Ribavirin
Trifluoperazine	*see* Antipsychotics
Trimeprazine	*see* Antihistamines
Trimethoprim	Present in milk—short-term use not known to be harmful
Trimipramine	*see* Antidepressants, Tricyclic (and related)
Triprolidine	*see* Antihistamines
Tropisetron	No information available
Trospium	Manufacturer advises caution—no information available
Ursodeoxycholic acid	Not known to be harmful but manufacturer advises avoid

Drug	Comment
Valaciclovir	No information available; *see also* Aciclovir
Valdecoxib	Manufacturer advises avoid—present in milk in *animal* studies
Valganciclovir	*see* Ganciclovir
Valproate	Amount too small to be harmful
Valproic acid	*see* Valproate
Valsartan	Manufacturer advises avoid—no information available
Vancomycin	Present in milk—significant absorption following oral administration unlikely
Vasopressin	Not known to be harmful
Vecuronium	No information available
Venlafaxine	Present in milk—manufacturer advises avoid
Verapamil	Amount too small to be harmful
Verteporfin	No information available—manufacturer advises avoid breast-feeding for 48 hours after administration
Vigabatrin	Present in milk—manufacturer advises avoid
Vinblastine	*see* Cytotoxic Drugs
Vincristine	*see* Cytotoxic Drugs
Vindesine	*see* Cytotoxic Drugs
Vinorelbine	*see* Cytotoxic Drugs
Vitamin A	Theoretical risk of toxicity in infants of mothers taking large doses
Vitamin D	Caution with high systemic doses; may cause hypercalcaemia in infant; manufacturer of *topical* calcitriol advises avoid; *see also* Calcipotriol and Tacalcitol
Voriconazole	Manufacturer advises avoid—no information available
Warfarin	*see* Anticoagulants, Oral
Xipamide	No information available
Zafirlukast	Present in milk—manufacturer advises avoid
Zalcitabine	Breast-feeding not advised in HIV infection
Zaleplon	Present in milk—manufacturer advises avoid
Zanamivir	Manufacturer advises avoid—present in milk in *animal* studies
Zidovudine	Breast-feeding not advised in HIV infection
Zoledronic acid	Manufacturer advises avoid—no information available
Zolmitriptan	Manufacturer advises caution—present in milk in *animal* studies
Zolpidem	Small amounts present in milk—manufacturer advises avoid
Zopiclone	Present in milk—manufacturer advises avoid
Zotepine	Manufacturer advises avoid
Zuclopenthixol	*see* Antipsychotics

Appendix 6: Intravenous Additives

INTRAVENOUS ADDITIVES POLICIES. A local policy on the addition of drugs to intravenous fluids should be drawn up by a multi-disciplinary team in each Health Authority and issued as a document to the members of staff concerned.

Centralised additive services are provided in a number of hospital pharmacy departments and should be used in preference to making additions on wards.

The information that follows should be read in conjunction with local policy documents.

Guidelines

1. Drugs should only be added to infusion containers when constant plasma concentrations are needed or when the administration of a more concentrated solution would be harmful.
2. In general, only one drug should be added to any infusion container and the components should be compatible. Ready-prepared solutions should be used whenever possible. Drugs should not normally be added to blood products, mannitol, or sodium bicarbonate. Only specially formulated additives should be used with fat emulsions or amino-acid solutions (section 9.3).
3. Solutions should be thoroughly mixed by shaking and checked for absence of particulate matter before use.
4. Strict asepsis should be maintained throughout and in general the giving set should not be used for more than 24 hours (for drug admixtures).
5. The infusion container should be labelled with the patient's name, the name and quantity of additives, and the date and time of addition (and the new expiry date or time). Such additional labelling should not interfere with information on the manufacturer's label that is still valid. When possible, containers should be retained for a period after use in case they are needed for investigation.
6. It is good practice to examine intravenous infusions from time to time while they are running. If cloudiness, crystallisation, change of colour, or any other sign of interaction or contamination is observed the infusion should be discontinued.

Problems

MICROBIAL CONTAMINATION. The accidental entry and subsequent growth of micro-organisms converts the infusion fluid pathway into a potential vehicle for infection with micro-organisms, particularly species of Candida, Enterobacter, and Klebsiella. Ready-prepared infusions containing the additional drugs, or infusions prepared by an additive service (when available) should therefore be used in preference to making extemporaneous additions to infusion containers on wards etc. However, when this is necessary strict aseptic procedure should be followed.

INCOMPATIBILITY. Physical and chemical incompatibilities may occur with loss of potency, increase in toxicity, or other adverse effect. The solutions may become opalescent or precipitation may occur, but in many instances there is no visual indication of incompatibility. Interaction may take place at any point in the infusion fluid pathway, and the potential for incompatibility is increased when more than one substance is added to the infusion fluid.

Common incompatibilities. Precipitation reactions are numerous and varied and may occur as a result of pH, concentration changes, 'salting-out' effects, complexation or other chemical changes. Precipitation or other particle formation must be avoided since, apart from lack of control of dosage on administration, it may initiate or exacerbate adverse effects. This is particularly important in the case of drugs which have been implicated in either thrombophlebitis (e.g. diazepam) or in skin sloughing or necrosis caused by extravasation (e.g. sodium bicarbonate and certain cytotoxic drugs). It is also especially important to effect solution of colloidal drugs and to prevent their subsequent precipitation in order to avoid a pyrogenic reaction (e.g. amphotericin).

It is considered undesirable to mix beta-lactam antibiotics, such as semi-synthetic penicillins and cephalosporins, with proteinaceous materials on the grounds that immunogenic and allergenic conjugates could be formed.

A number of preparations undergo significant loss of potency when added singly or in combination to large volume infusions. Examples include ampicillin in infusions that contain glucose or lactates, and chlormethine hydrochloride (mustine hydrochloride) in physiological saline. The breakdown products of dacarbazine have been implicated in adverse effects.

Blood. Because of the large number of incompatibilities, drugs should not normally be added to blood and blood products for infusion purposes. Examples of incompatibility with blood include hypertonic mannitol solutions (irreversible crenation of red cells), dextrans (rouleaux formation and interference with cross-matching), glucose (clumping of red cells), and oxytocin (inactivated).

If the giving set is not changed after the administration of blood, but used for other infusion fluids, a fibrin clot may form which, apart from blocking the set, increases the likelihood of microbial growth.

Intravenous fat emulsions may break down with coalescence of fat globules and separation of phases when additions such as antibacterials or electrolytes are made, thus increasing the possibility of embolism. Only specially formulated products such as *Vitlipid N®* (section 9.3) may be added to appropriate intravenous fat emulsions.

Other infusions that frequently give rise to incompatibility include amino acids, mannitol, and sodium bicarbonate.

Bactericides such as chlorocresol 0.1% or phenylmercuric nitrate 0.001% are present in some injection solutions. The total volume of such solutions added to a container for infusion on one occasion should not exceed 15 mL.

Method

Ready-prepared infusions should be used whenever available. **Potassium chloride** is usually available in concentrations of 20, 27, and 40 mmol/litre in sodium chloride intravenous infusion (0.9%), glucose intravenous infusion (5%) or sodium chloride and glucose intravenous infusion. **Lidocaine hydrochloride** (lignocaine hydrochloride) is usually available in concentrations of 0.1 or 0.2% in glucose intravenous infusion (5%).

When addition is required to be made extemporaneously, any product reconstitution instructions such as those relating to concentration, vehicle, mixing, and handling precautions should be strictly followed using an aseptic technique throughout. Once the product has been reconstituted, addition to the infusion fluid should be made immediately in order to minimise microbial contamination and, with certain products, to prevent degradation or other formulation change which may occur; e.g. reconstituted ampicillin injection degrades rapidly on standing, and also may form polymers which could cause sensitivity reactions.

It is also important in certain instances that an infusion fluid of specific pH be used (e.g. **furosemide** (frusemide) injection requires dilution in infusions of pH greater than 5.5).

When drug additions are made it is important to mix thoroughly; additions should not be made to an infusion container that has been connected to a giving set, as mixing is hampered. If the solutions are not thoroughly mixed a concentrated layer of the additive may form owing to differences in density. **Potassium chloride** is particularly prone to this 'layering' effect when added without adequate mixing to infusions packed in non-rigid infusion containers; if such a mixture is administered it may have a serious effect on the heart.

A time limit between addition and completion of administration must be imposed for certain admixtures to guarantee satisfactory drug potency and compatibility. For admixtures in which degradation occurs without the formation of toxic substances, an acceptable limit is the time taken for 10% decomposition of the drug. When toxic substances are produced stricter limits may be imposed. Because of the risk of microbial contamination a maximum time limit of 12 hours may be appropriate for additions made elsewhere than in hospital pharmacies offering central additive service.

Certain injections must be protected from light during continuous infusion to minimise oxidation, e.g. amphotericin, dacarbazine, and sodium nitroprusside.

Dilution with a small volume of an appropriate vehicle and administration using a motorised infusion pump is advocated for preparations such as heparin where strict control over administration is required. In this case the appropriate dose may be dissolved in a convenient volume (e.g. 24 to 48 mL) of sodium chloride intravenous infusion (0.9%).

Use of table

The table lists preparations given by three methods:

continuous infusion,
intermittent infusion, and
addition via the drip tubing.

Drugs for **continuous infusion** must be diluted in a large volume infusion. Penicillins and cephalosporins are not usually given by continuous infusion because of stability problems and because adequate plasma and tissue concentrations are best obtained by intermittent infusion. Where it is necessary to administer them by continuous infusion, detailed literature should be consulted.

Drugs that are both compatible and clinically suitable may be given by **intermittent infusion** in a relatively small volume of infusion over a short period of time, e.g. 100 mL in 30 minutes. The method is used if the product is incompatible or unstable over the period necessary for continuous infusion; the limited stability of ampicillin or amoxicillin in large volume glucose or lactate infusions may be overcome in this way.

Intermittent infusion is also used if adequate plasma and tissue concentrations are not produced by continuous infusion as in the case of drugs such as carbenicillin, dacarbazine, gentamicin, and ticarcillin.

An in-line burette may be used for intermittent infusion techniques in order to achieve strict control over the time and rate of administration, especially for infants and children and in intensive care units. Intermittent infusion may also make use of the 'piggy-back' technique provided that no additions are made to the primary infusion. In this method the drug is added to a small secondary container connected to a Y-type injection site on the primary infusion giving set; the secondary solution is usually infused within 30 minutes.

Addition *via* the drip tubing is indicated for a number of cytotoxic drugs in order to minimise extravasation. The preparation is added aseptically *via* the rubber septum of the injection site of a fast-running infusion. In general, drug preparations intended for a bolus effect should be given directly into a separate vein where possible. Failing this, administration may be made *via* the drip tubing provided that the preparation is compatible with the infusion fluid when given in this manner.

Table of drugs given by intravenous infusion

Covers addition to *Glucose intravenous infusion* 5 and 10%, *Sodium chloride intravenous infusion* 0.9%, *Compound sodium chloride intravenous infusion* (Ringer's solution), and *Compound sodium lactate intravenous infusion* (Hartmann's solution). Compatibility with glucose 5% and with sodium chloride 0.9% indicates compatibility with *Sodium chloride and glucose intravenous infusion*. Infusion of a large volume of hypotonic solution should be avoided therefore care should be taken if water for injections is used. The information in the Table relates to the proprietary preparations indicated; for other preparations suitability should be checked with the manufacturer

Abciximab (*ReoPro®*)
Continuous *in* Glucose 5% *or* Sodium chloride
0.9%
Withdraw from vial, dilute in infusion fluid and give *via* infusion pump through a non-pyrogenic low protein-binding 0.2 or 0.22 micron filter

Acetylcysteine (*Parvolex®*)
Continuous *in* Glucose 5% or Sodium chloride
0.9%
Glucose 5% is preferable—see Emergency Treatment of Poisoning

Aciclovir (as sodium salt) (*Zovirax IV®; Aciclovir IV*, Mayne; *Aciclovir IV*, Genus; *Aciclovir Sodium*, Zurich)
Intermittent *in* Sodium chloride 0.9% *or* Sodium chloride and glucose *or* Compound sodium lactate
For *Zovirax IV®, Aciclovir IV* (Genus) and *Aciclovir Sodium* (Zurich) initially reconstitute to 25 mg/mL in water for injections or sodium chloride 0.9% then dilute to not more than 5 mg/mL with the infusion fluid; to be given over 1 hour; alternatively, may be administered in a concentration of 25 mg/mL using a suitable infusion pump and given over 1 hour; for *Aciclovir IV* (Mayne) dilute to not more than 5 mg/mL with infusion fluid; give over 1 hour

Aclarubicin (as hydrochloride) (*Aclacin®*)
Intermittent *in* Glucose 5% *or* Sodium chloride
0.9%
Dissolve initially in 10 mL water for injections or sodium chloride 0.9% then dilute with 200–500 mL infusion fluid to a concentration of 200–500 micrograms/mL; give over 30–60 minutes and protect from light during administration; pH of glucose infusion should be between 5 and 6

Alemtuzumab (*MabCampath®*)
Intermittent *in* Glucose 5% or Sodium chloride
0.9%
Add requisite dose through a low protein binding 5-micron filter to 100 mL infusion fluid; infuse over 2 hours

Alfentanil (as hydrochloride) (*Rapifen® preparations*)
Continuous *or* intermittent *in* Glucose 5% *or* Sodium chloride 0.9% *or* Compound sodium lactate

Alprostadil (*Prostin VR®*)
Continuous *in* Glucose 5% *or* Sodium chloride
0.9%
Add directly to the infusion solution avoiding contact with the walls of plastic containers

Alteplase (*Actilyse®*)
Continuous *or* intermittent *in* Sodium chloride
0.9%
Dissolve in water for injections to a concentration of 1 mg/mL and infuse intravenously; alternatively dilute the solution further in the infusion fluid to a concentration of not less than 200 micrograms/mL; not to be infused in glucose solution

Amifostine (*Ethyol®*)
Intermittent *in* Sodium chloride 0.9%

Amikacin sulphate (*Amikin®*)
Intermittent *in* Glucose 5% *or* Sodium chloride 0.9% *or* Compound sodium lactate
To be given over 30 minutes

Aminophylline
Continuous *in* Glucose 5% *or* Sodium chloride 0.9% *or* Compound sodium lactate

Amiodarone hydrochloride (*Cordarone X®*)
Continuous *or* intermittent *in* Glucose 5%
Suggested initial infusion volume 250 mL given over 20–120 minutes; for repeat infusions up to 1.2 g in max. 500 mL; infusion in extreme emergency see section 2.3.2; should not be diluted to less than 600 micrograms/mL; incompatible with sodium chloride infusion; avoid equipment containing the plasticizer di-2-ethylhexyphthalate (DEHP)

Amoxicillin (as sodium salt) (*Amoxil®*)
Intermittent *in* Glucose 5% *or* Sodium chloride
0.9%
Reconstituted solutions diluted and given without delay; suggested volume 100 mL given over 30–60 minutes
via drip tubing *in* Glucose 5% *or* Sodium chloride
0.9%
Continuous infusion not usually recommended

Amphotericin (colloidal) (*Amphocil®*)
Intermittent *in* Glucose 5%
Initially reconstitute with water for injections (50 mg in 10 mL, 100 mg in 20 mL), shaking gently to dissolve (fluid may be opalescent) then dilute to a concentration of 625 micrograms/mL (1 volume of reconstituted solution with 7 volumes of infusion fluid); give at a rate of 1–2 mg/kg/hour or slower if not tolerated (initial test dose 2 mg of a 100 microgram/mL solution over 10 minutes); incompatible with sodium chloride or other electrolyte solutions, flush existing intravenous line with glucose 5% or use separate line

Amphotericin (lipid complex) (*Abelcet®*)
Intermittent *in* Glucose 5%
Allow suspension to reach room temperature, shake gently to ensure no yellow settlement, withdraw requisite dose (using 17–19 gauge needle) into one or more 20-mL syringes; replace needle on syringe with a 5-micron filter needle provided (fresh needle for each syringe) and dilute to a concentration of 1 mg/mL (2 mg/mL in fluid restriction); preferably give *via* an infusion pump at a rate of 2.5 mg/kg/hour (initial test dose of 1 mg given over 15 minutes); an in-line filter (pore size no less than 15 micron) may be used; do not use sodium chloride or other electrolyte solutions, flush existing intravenous line with glucose 5% or use separate line

Amphotericin (liposomal) (*AmBisome®*)
Intermittent *in* Glucose 5%
Reconstitute each vial with 12 mL water for injections and shake vigorously to produce a preparation containing 4 mg/mL; withdraw requisite dose from vial and introduce into infusion fluid through the 5 micron filter provided to produce a final concentration of 0.2–2 mg/mL; infuse over 30–60 minutes (initial test dose 1 mg over 10 minutes); incompatible with sodium chloride solutions, flush existing intravenous line with glucose 5% or use separate line

Amphotericin (as sodium deoxycholate complex) (*Fungizone®*)
Intermittent *in* Glucose 5%
Reconstitute each vial with 10 mL water for injections and shake immediately to produce a 5 mg/mL colloidal solution; dilute further in infusion fluid to a concentration of 100 micrograms/mL; pH of the glucose must not be below 4.2 (check each container—see product literature for details of buffer); infuse over 2–4 hours, or longer if not tolerated (initial test dose 1 mg over 20–30 minutes); begin infusion immediately after dilution and protect from light; incompatible with sodium chloride solutions, flush existing intravenous line with glucose 5% or use separate line

Ampicillin sodium (*Penbritin®*)
Intermittent *in* Glucose 5% *or* Sodium chloride
0.9%
Reconstituted solutions diluted and given without delay; suggested volume 100 mL given over 30–60 minutes
via drip tubing *in* Glucose 5% *or* Sodium chloride
0.9% *or* Ringer's solution *or* Compound sodium lactate
Continuous infusion not usually recommended

Amsacrine (*Amsidine*®)
Intermittent in Glucose 5%
Reconstitute with diluent provided and dilute to suggested volume 500 mL; give over 60–90 minutes; use glass syringes; incompatible with sodium chloride infusion

Atenolol (*Tenormin*®)
Intermittent *in* Glucose 5% *or* Sodium chloride 0.9%
Suggested infusion time 20 minutes

Atosiban (*Tractocile*®)
Continuous *in* Glucose 5% *or* Sodium chloride 0.9% *or* Compound sodium lactate
Withdraw 10 mL infusion fluid from 100-mL bag and replace with 10 mL atosiban concentrate (7.5 mg/mL) to produce a final concentration of 750 micrograms/mL

Atracurium besilate (*Tracrium*®; *Atracurium besilate injection*, Mayne; *Atracurium injection/infusion*, Genus)
Continuous *in* Glucose 5% *or* Sodium chloride 0.9% *or* Compound sodium lactate
Stability varies with diluent; dilute requisite dose with infusion infusion fluid to a concentration of 0.5–5 mg/mL

Azathioprine (as sodium salt) (*Imuran*®)
Intermittent *in* Sodium chloride 0.9% *or* Sodium chloride and glucose
Reconstitute 50 mg with 5–15 mL water for injections; dilute with 20–200 mL infusion fluid

Aztreonam (*Azactam*®)
Intermittent *in* Glucose 5% *or* Sodium chloride 0.9% *or* Ringer's solution *or* Compound sodium lactate
Dissolve initially in water for injections (1 g per 3 mL) then dilute to a concentration of less than 20 mg/mL; to be given over 20–60 minutes

Basiliximab (*Simulect*®)
Intermittent in Glucose 5% or Sodium chloride 0.9%
Reconstitute 10 mg with 5 mL water for injections then dilute to at least 25 mL with infusion fluid; reconstitute 20 mg with 10 mL water for injections then dilute to at least 50 mL with infusion fluid; give over 20–30 minutes

Benzylpenicillin sodium (*Crystapen*®)
Intermittent *in* Glucose 5% *or* Sodium chloride 0.9%
Suggested volume 100 mL given over 30–60 minutes
Continuous infusion not usually recommended

Betamethasone (as sodium phosphate) (*Betnesol*®)
Continuous *or* intermittent *or via* drip tubing *in* Glucose 5% *or* Sodium chloride 0.9%

Bleomycin sulphate
Intermittent *in* Sodium chloride 0.9%
To be given slowly; suggested volume 200 mL

Bumetanide (*Burinex*®)
Intermittent *in* Glucose 5% *or* Sodium chloride 0.9%
Suggested volume 500 mL given over 30–60 minutes

Busulfan (*Busilvex*®)
Intermittent in Glucose 5% or Sodium chloride 0.9%
Dilute to a concentration of 500 micrograms/mL; give through a central venous catheter over 2 hours

Calcitonin (salmon)/Salcatonin (*Forcaltonin*®, *Miacalcic*®)
Intermittent *in* Sodium chloride 0.9%
Diluted solution given without delay; dilute in 500 mL and give over at least 6 hours; glass or hard plastic containers should not be used; approx. 20% loss of potency on dilution (take into account when calculating dose)

Calcium folinate (*Calcium Leucovorin*®, *Refolinon*®)
Intermittent *in* Sodium chloride 0.9%
Calcium Leucovorin® can also be infused in Glucose 5 and 10% or Compound sodium lactate
Protect from light

Calcium gluconate
Continuous *in* Glucose 5% *or* Sodium chloride 0.9%
Avoid bicarbonates, phosphates, or sulphates

Calcium levofolinate (*Isovorin*®)
Intermittent *in* Glucose 5 and 10% *or* Sodium chloride 0.9% *or* Compound sodium lactate
Protect from light

Carboplatin (*Paraplatin*®)
Intermittent *in* Glucose 5% *or* Sodium chloride 0.9%
Final concentration as low as 500 micrograms/mL; give over 15–60 minutes

Carmustine (*BiCNU*®)
Intermittent *in* Glucose 5% *or* Sodium chloride 0.9%
Reconstitute with solvent provided; give over 1–2 hours

Caspofungin
Intermittent *in* Sodium chloride 0.9% *or* Compound sodium lactate
Allow vial to reach room temperature; initially reconstitute each vial with 10.5 mL water for injections, mixing gently to dissolve then dilute requisite dose in 250 mL infusion fluid (35- or 50-mg doses may be diluted in 100 mL infusion fluid if necessary); give over 60 minutes; incompatible with glucose solutions

Cefotaxime (as sodium salt) (*Claforan*®; *Cefotaxime Injection*, Genus)
Intermittent *in* Glucose 5% *or* Sodium chloride 0.9% *or* Compound sodium lactate *or* Water for injections
Suggested volume 40–100 mL given over 20–60 minutes

Cefoxitin (as sodium salt) (*Mefoxin*®)
Intermittent *or via* drip tubing in Glucose 5 and 10% *or* Sodium chloride 0.9%
Reconstitute initially with water for injections

Cefradine (*Velosef*®)
Continuous *or* intermittent *in* Glucose 5 and 10% or Sodium chloride 0.9% *or* Ringer's solution *or* Compound sodium lactate
Reconstitute 500 mg with 5 mL water for injections or glucose 5% or sodium chloride 0.9% then dilute with infusion fluid

Ceftazidime (as pentahydrate) (*Fortum*®, *Kefadim*®)
Intermittent *or via* drip tubing *in* Glucose 5 and 10% *or* Sodium chloride 0.9% *or* Compound sodium lactate
Dissolve 2 g initially in 10 mL (3 g in 15 mL) infusion fluid; for *Fortum*® dilute further to a concentration of 40 mg/mL; for *Kefadim*® dilute further to a concentration of 20 mg/mL; give over up to 30 minutes

Ceftriaxone (as sodium salt) (*Rocephin®*;
Ceftriaxone Injection, Genus)
Intermittent *or via* drip tubing *in* Glucose 5 and
10% *or* Sodium chloride 0.9%
Reconstitute 2-g vial with 40 mL infusion fluid; give
intermittent infusion over at least 30 minutes (60 minutes
in neonates); not to be given with infusion fluids
containing calcium

Cefuroxime (as sodium salt) (*Zinacef®*;
Cefuroxime Injection, Lilly)
Intermittent *or via* drip tubing *in* Glucose 5% *or*
Sodium chloride 0.9% *or* Compound sodium
lactate
Dissolve initially in water for injections (at least 2 mL for
each 250 mg, 15 mL for 1.5 g); suggested volume 50–
100 mL given over 30 minutes

Chloramphenicol (as sodium succinate)
(*Kemicetine®*)
Intermittent *or via* drip tubing *in* Glucose 5% *or*
Sodium chloride 0.9%

**Chlormethine hydrochloride/Mustine
hydrochloride** (Abbott)
via drip tubing *in* Glucose 5% *or* Sodium chloride
0.9%

Chloroquine sulphate (*Nivaquine®*)
Continuous *in* Sodium chloride 0.9%
See also section 5.4.1

Ciclosporin (*Sandimmun®*)
Continuous *in* Glucose 5% *or* Sodium chloride
0.9%
Dilute to a concentration of 50 mg in 20–100 mL; give
over 2–6 hours; not to be used with PVC equipment

Cidofovir (*Vistide®*)
Intermittent *in* Sodium chloride 0.9%
Dilute requisite dose with 100 mL infusion fluid; infuse
over 1 hour

Cimetidine (*Tagamet®*)
Continuous *or* intermittent *in* Glucose 5% *or*
Sodium chloride 0.9%
For intermittent infusion suggested volume 100 mL given
over 30–60 minutes

Cisatracurium (*Nimbex®, Nimbex Forte®*)
Continuous *in* Glucose 5% *or* Sodium chloride
0.9%
Solutions of 2 mg/mL and 5 mg/mL may be infused
undiluted; alternatively dilute with infusion fluid to a
concentration of 0.1–2 mg/mL

Cisplatin (*Cisplatin*, Pharmacia; *Cisplatin
injection solution*, Mayne)
Intermittent *in* Sodium chloride 0.9% *or* Sodium
chloride and glucose
Reconstitute initially with water for injections to produce
1 mg/mL solution then dilute in 2 litres infusion fluid;
give over 6–8 hours

Cladribine (*Leustat®*)
Continuous *in* Sodium chloride 0.9%
Dilute with 100–500 mL; glucose solutions are unsuitable

Clarithromycin (*Klaricid® I.V.*)
Intermittent *in* Glucose 5% *or* Sodium chloride
0.9% *or* Ringer's solution *or* Compound sodium
lactate
Dissolve initially in water for injections (500 mg in
10 mL) then dilute to a concentration of 2 mg/mL; give
over 60 minutes

Clindamycin (as phosphate) (*Dalacin® C
Phosphate*)
Continuous *or* intermittent *in* Glucose 5% *or*
Sodium chloride 0.9%
Give over at least 10–60 minutes (1.2 g over at least 60
minutes; higher doses by continuous infusion)

Clonazepam (*Rivotril®*)
Intermittent *in* Glucose 5 and 10% *or* Sodium
chloride 0.9%
Suggested volume 250 mL

Co-amoxiclav (*Augmentin®*)
Intermittent *in* Sodium chloride 0.9% *or* Water for
injections; see also package leaflet
Suggested volume 50–100 mL given over 30–40 minutes
and completed within 4 hours of reconstitution
via drip tubing *in* Glucose 5% *or* Sodium chloride
0.9%

Co-fluampicil (as sodium salts) (*Magnapen®*)
Intermittent *in* Glucose 5% *or* Sodium chloride
0.9%
Reconstituted solutions diluted and given without delay;
suggested volume 100 mL given over 30–60 minutes
via drip tubing *in* Glucose 5% *or* Sodium chloride
0.9% *or* Ringer's solution *or* Compound sodium
lactate

Colistimethate sodium (*Colomycin®*)
Intermittent *in* Sodium chloride 0.9% *or* Water for
injections
Dilute with 50 mL infusion fluid and give over 30 minutes

Co-trimoxazole (*Septrin® for infusion*)
Intermittent *in* Glucose 5 and 10% *or* Sodium
chloride 0.9% *or* Ringer's solution
Dilute contents of 1 ampoule (5 mL) to 125 mL, 2
ampoules (10 mL) to 250 mL or 3 ampoules (15 mL) to
500 mL; suggested duration of infusion 60–90 minutes
(but may be adjusted according to fluid requirements); if
fluid restriction necessary, 1 ampoule (5 mL) may be
diluted with 75 mL glucose 5% and infused over max. 60
minutes

Cyclophosphamide (*Endoxana®*)
via drip tubing *in* Glucose 5% *or* Sodium chloride
0.9%
Reconstitute with sodium chloride 0.9%

Cyclosporin *see* Ciclosporin

Cytarabine (*Cytosar®*)
Continuous *or* intermittent *or via* drip tubing *in*
Glucose 5% *or* Sodium chloride 0.9%
Reconstitute *Cytosar®* with water for injections or with
infusion fluid; check container for haze or precipitate
during administration

Dacarbazine (*DTIC-Dome®*; *Dacarbazine*,
Medac)
Intermittent *in* Glucose 5% *or* Sodium chloride
0.9%
Reconstitute initially with water for injections then for
DTIC-Dome® dilute in 125–250 mL infusion fluid; for
Dacarbazine (Medac) dilute in 200–300 mL infusion
fluid; give over 15–30 minutes; protect infusion from
light

Daclizumab (*Zenapax®*)
Intermittent *in* Sodium chloride 0.9%
Dilute requisite dose in 50 mL infusion fluid; infuse over
15 minutes

Dactinomycin (*Cosmegen Lyovac®*)
Intermittent *or via* drip tubing *in* Glucose 5% *or*
Sodium chloride 0.9%
Reconstitute with water for injections

Daunorubicin (as hydrochloride)   (*Cerubidin*®)
via drip tubing *in* Sodium chloride 0.9%
Reconstitute vial with 4 mL water for injections to give
5 mg/mL solution; dilute requisite dose with infusion
fluid to a concentration of 1 mg/mL; give over 20 minutes

Daunorubicin (liposomal)   (*DaunoXome*®)
Intermittent *in* Glucose 5%
Dilute to a concentration of 0.2–1 mg/mL; give over 30–
60 minutes; incompatible with sodium chloride solutions;
in-line filter not recommended (if used, pore size should
be no less than 5 micron)

Desferrioxamine mesilate   (*Desferal*®)
Continuous *or* intermittent *in* Glucose 5% *or*
Sodium chloride 0.9%
Dissolve initially in water for injections (500 mg in 5 mL)
then dilute with infusion fluid

Desmopressin   (*DDAVP*®)
Intermittent *in* Sodium chloride 0.9%
Dilute with 50 mL and give over 20 minutes

Dexamethasone sodium phosphate
(*Decadron*®; *Dexamethasone*, Mayne;
Dexamethasone, Organon)
Continuous *or* intermittent *or via* drip tubing *in*
Glucose 5% *or* Sodium chloride 0.9%
Dexamethasone (Organon) can also be infused in Ring-
er's solution *or* Compound sodium lactate

Diamorphine hydrochloride   (*Diamorphine
Injection*, CP)
Continuous *in* Glucose 5% *or* Sodium chloride
0.9%
Glucose is preferred as infusion fluid

Diazepam (solution)   (*Diazepam*, CP)
Continuous *in* Glucose 5% *or* Sodium chloride
0.9%
Dilute to a concentration of not more than 10 mg in
200 mL; max. 6 hours between addition and completion
of administration; adsorbed to some extent by the plastics
of the infusion set

Diazepam (emulsion)   (*Diazemuls*®)
Continuous *in* Glucose 5 and 10%
May be diluted to a max. concentration of 200 mg in
500 mL; max. 6 hours between addition and completion
of administration; adsorbed to some extent by the plastics
of the infusion set
via drip tubing *in* Glucose 5 and 10% *or* Sodium
chloride 0.9%
Adsorbed to some extent by the plastics of the infusion set

Diclofenac sodium   (*Voltarol*®)
Continuous *or* intermittent *in* Glucose 5% *or*
Sodium chloride 0.9%
Dilute 75 mg with 100–500 mL infusion fluid (previously
buffered with 0.5 mL sodium bicarbonate 8.4% solution
or with 1 mL sodium bicarbonate 4.2% solution); for
intermittent infusion give 25–50 mg over 15–60 minutes
or 75 mg over 30–120 minutes; for continuous infusion
give at a rate of 5 mg/hour

Digoxin   (*Lanoxin*®)
Intermittent *in* Glucose 5% *or* Sodium chloride
0.9%
To be given over at least 2 hours

Digoxin-specific antibody fragments
(*Digibind*®)
Intermittent *in* Sodium chloride 0.9%
Dissolve initially in water for injections (4 mL/vial) then
dilute with the sodium chloride 0.9% and give through a
0.22 micron sterile, disposable filter over 30 minutes

Dinoprostone   (*Prostin E2*®)
Continuous *or* intermittent *in* Glucose 5% *or*
Sodium chloride 0.9%

Disodium folinate   (*Sodiofolin*®)
Intermittent *in* Sodium chloride 0.9%
Protect from light
Avoid bicarbonate containing infusions

Disodium pamidronate   (*Aredia*®; *Disodium
pamidronate*, Mayne)
Intermittent *in* Sodium chloride 0.9%
For *Aredia*® reconstitute initially with water for injections
(15 mg in 5 mL, 30 mg or 90 mg in 10 mL); for *Aredia*®
and *Disodium pamidronate* (Mayne), dilute with infusion
fluid to a concentration of not more than 60 mg in
250 mL; give at a rate not exceeding 1 mg/minute; not
to be given with infusion fluids containing calcium

Disopyramide (as phosphate)   (*Rythmodan*®)
Continuous *or* intermittent *in* Glucose 5% *or*
Sodium chloride 0.9% *or* Ringer's solution *or*
Compound sodium lactate
Max. rate by continuous infusion 20–30 mg/hour (or
400 micrograms/kg/hour)

Dobutamine (as hydrochloride)   (*Dobutrex*®,
Posiject®)
Continuous *in* Glucose 5% *or* Sodium chloride
0.9%
Dilute to a concentration of 0.5–1 mg/mL and give *via* a
controlled infusion device; give higher concentration
(max. 5 mg/mL) with infusion pump; incompatible with
bicarbonate

Docetaxel   (*Taxotere*®)
Intermittent *in* Glucose 5% *or* Sodium chloride
0.9%
Stand docetaxel vials and diluent at room temperature for
5 minutes; add diluent to produce a concentrate containing 10 mg/mL and allow to stand for a further 5 minutes;
dilute the requisite dose with at least 250 mL infusion
fluid to a final concentration not exceeding 740 micr-
ograms/mL; infuse over 1 hour

Dolasetron mesilate   (*Anzemet*®)
Intermittent *in* Glucose 5% *or* Sodium chloride
0.9% *or* Compound sodium lactate
Suggested volume 50 mL given over 30 seconds–15
minutes

Dopamine hydrochloride   (*Intropin*®)
Continuous *in* Glucose 5% *or* Sodium chloride
0.9% *or* Compound sodium lactate
Dilute to a concentration of 1.6 mg/mL; incompatible
with bicarbonate

Dopexamine hydrochloride   (*Dopacard*®)
Continuous *in* Glucose 5% *or* Sodium chloride
0.9%
Dilute to a concentration of 400 or 800 micrograms/mL;
max. concentration *via* large peripheral vein 1 mg/mL,
concentrations up to 4 mg/mL may be infused *via* central
vein; give *via* infusion pump or other device which
provides accurate control of rate; contact with metal
should be minimised; incompatible with bicarbonate

Doxorubicin hydrochloride   (*Doxorubicin Rapid
Dissolution*, *Doxorubicin Solution*) (both
Pharmacia)
via drip tubing *in* Glucose 5% *or* Sodium chloride
0.9%
Reconstitute *Doxorubicin Rapid Dissolution* with water
for injections or sodium chloride 0.9% (10 mg in 5 mL,
50 mg in 25 mL); give over 2–3 minutes

Doxorubicin hydrochloride (liposomal)
(*Caelyx®*)
via drip tubing *in* Glucose 5%
Dilute up to 90 mg in 250 mL infusion fluid and over
90 mg in 500 mL infusion fluid

Enoximone (*Perfan®*)
Continuous *or* intermittent *in* Sodium chloride
0.9% *or* Water for injections
Dilute to a concentration of 2.5 mg/mL; incompatible
with glucose solutions; use only plastic containers or
syringes

Epirubicin hydrochloride (*Pharmorubicin®*
Rapid Dissolution, *Pharmorubicin® Solution*)
via drip tubing *in* Sodium chloride 0.9%
Reconstitute *Pharmorubicin® Rapid Dissolution* with
sodium chloride 0.9% or with water for injections
(10 mg in 5 mL, 20 mg in 10 mL, 50 mg in 25 mL); give
over 3–5 minutes

Epoprostenol (*Flolan®*)
Continuous *in* Sodium chloride 0.9%
Reconstitute with the solvent provided (pH 10.5) to make
a concentrate; use this concentrate within 12 hours and
store at 2–8°C; dilute with not more than 6 times the
volume of sodium chloride 0.9% before use

Ertapenem (*Invanz®*)
Intermittent *in* Sodium chloride 0.9%
Reconstitute 1 g with 10 mL water for injections or
sodium chloride 0.9% then dilute in 50 mL infusion fluid;
give over 30 minutes; incompatible with glucose solutions

Erythromycin (as lactobionate)
Continuous *or* intermittent *in* Glucose 5% (neu-
tralised with sodium bicarbonate) *or* Sodium
chloride 0.9%
Dissolve initially in water for injections (1 g in 20 mL)
then dilute to a concentration of 1 mg/mL for continuous
infusion and 1–5 mg/mL for intermittent infusion; give
intermittent infusion over 20–60 minutes

Esmolol hydrochloride (*Brevibloc®*)
Continuous *or* intermittent *in* Glucose 5% *or*
Sodium chloride 0.9%
Dilute to a concentration of 10 mg/mL; for continuous
infusion use a suitable infusion control device; incompa-
tible with bicarbonate

Ethanol
Continuous *in* Glucose 5% *or* Sodium chloride
0.9% *or* Ringer's solution *or* Compound sodium
lactate
Dilute to a concentration of 5–10%

Etoposide (*Eposin®*; *Vepesid®*; *Etoposide*, APS
and Mayne)
Intermittent *in* Sodium chloride 0.9%
For *Vepesid®* dilute to a concentration of not more than
250 micrograms/mL and give over not less than 30
minutes; for *Etoposide* (APS) dilute with either sodium
chloride 0.9% or glucose 5% to a concentration of
200 micrograms/mL and give over 30–60 minutes; for
Etoposide (Mayne) dilute with either sodium chloride
0.9% or glucose 5% to a concentration of not more than
250 micrograms/mL and give over not less than 30
minutes; for *Eposin®* dilute with either sodium chloride
0.9% or glucose 5% to a concentration of 200–400 micr-
ograms/mL and give over at least 30 minutes; check
container for haze or precipitate during infusion

Etoposide (as phosphate) (*Etopophos®*)
Intermittent *in* Glucose 5% *or* Sodium chloride
0.9%
Reconstitute with 5–10 mL of either water for injections
or with infusion fluid then dilute further with infusion
fluid to a concentration as low as 100 micrograms/mL and
give over 5 minutes to 3.5 hours

Filgrastim (*Neupogen®*)
Continuous *or* intermittent *in* Glucose 5%
For a filgrastim concentration of less than 1 500 000 units/
mL (15 micrograms/mL) albumin solution (human serum
albumin) is added to produce a final albumin concentration of 2 mg/mL; should not be diluted to a filgrastim
concentration of less than 200 000 units/mL (2 micr-
ograms/mL) and should not be diluted with sodium
chloride solution

Flecainide acetate (*Tambocor®*)
Continuous *or* intermittent *in* Glucose 5% *or*
Sodium chloride 0.9% *or* Compound sodium
lactate
Minimum volume in infusion fluids containing chlorides
500 mL

Flucloxacillin (as sodium salt) (*Floxapen®*)
Intermittent *in* Glucose 5% *or* Sodium chloride
0.9%
Suggested volume 100 mL given over 30–60 minutes
via drip tubing *in* Glucose 5% *or* Sodium chloride
0.9% *or* Ringer's solution *or* Compound sodium
lactate
Continuous infusion not usually recommended

Fludarabine phosphate (*Fludara®*)
Intermittent *in* Sodium chloride 0.9%
Reconstitute each 50 mg with 2 mL water for injections
and dilute requisite dose in 100 mL; give over 30 minutes

Flumazenil (*Anexate®*)
Continuous *in* Glucose 5% *or* Sodium chloride
0.9%

Fluorouracil (as sodium salt)
Continuous *or* intermittent *or* *via* drip tubing *in*
Glucose 5% *or* Sodium chloride 0.9%
Give intermittent infusion over 30–60 minutes or over 4
hours

Foscarnet sodium (*Foscavir®*)
Intermittent *in* Glucose 5% *or* Sodium chloride
0.9%
Dilute to a concentration of 12 mg/mL for infusion into
peripheral vein (undiluted solution *via* central venous line
only); infuse over at least 1 hour

Fosphenytoin Sodium (*Pro-Epanutin®*)
Intermittent *in* Glucose 5% *or* Sodium chloride
0.9%
Dilute to a concentration of 1.5–25 mg (phenytoin sodium
equivalent)/mL

Furosemide/Frusemide (as sodium salt)
(*Lasix®*)
Continuous *in* Sodium chloride 0.9% *or* Ringer's
solution
Infusion pH must be above 5.5 and rate should not exceed
4 mg/minute; glucose solutions are unsuitable

Fusidic acid (as sodium salt) (*Fucidin®*)
Continuous *in* Glucose 5% (but see below) *or*
Sodium chloride 0.9%
Reconstitute with the buffer solution provided and dilute
to 500 mL; give through central venous line over 2 hours
(or over 6 hours if superficial vein used); incompatible in
solution of pH less than 7.4

Ganciclovir (as sodium salt) (*Cymevene®*)
Intermittent *in* Glucose 5% *or* Sodium chloride
0.9% *or* Ringer's solution *or* Compound sodium
lactate
Reconstitute initially in water for injections (500 mg/
10 mL) then dilute to not more than 10 mg/mL with
infusion fluid (usually 100 mL); give over 1 hour

Gemcitabine (*Gemzar*®)
Intermittent *in* Sodium chloride 0.9%
Reconstitute initially with sodium chloride 0.9% (200 mg in at least 5 mL, 1 g in at least 25 mL); may be diluted further with infusion fluid; give over 30 minutes

Gentamicin (as sulphate) (*Cidomycin*®)
Intermittent *or via* drip tubing *in* Glucose 5% *or* Sodium chloride 0.9%
Suggested volume for intermittent infusion 50–100 mL given over 20 minutes

Glyceryl trinitrate (*Nitrocine*®, *Nitronal*®, *Tridil*®)
Continuous *in* Glucose 5% *or* Sodium chloride 0.9%
For *Tridil*® dilute to a concentration of not more than 400 micrograms/mL; for *Nitrocine*® suggested infusion concentration 100 micrograms/mL; incompatible with polyvinyl chloride infusion containers such as *Viaflex*® or *Steriflex*®; use glass or polyethylene containers or give *via* a syringe pump

Granisetron (as hydrochloride) (*Kytril*®)
Intermittent *in* Glucose 5% *or* Sodium chloride 0.9% *or* Compound sodium lactate
Dilute 3 mL in 20–50 mL infusion fluid (up to 3 mL in 10–30 mL for children); give over 5 minutes

Haem arginate (*Normosang*®)
Intermittent *in* Sodium chloride 0.9%
Dilute requisite dose in 100 mL infusion fluid in glass bottle and give over at least 30 minutes *via* large antebrachial vein; administer within 1 hour after dilution

Heparin sodium
Continuous *in* Glucose 5% *or* Sodium chloride 0.9%
Administration with a motorised pump advisable

Hydralazine hydrochloride (*Apresoline*®)
Continuous *in* Sodium chloride 0.9% *or* Ringer's solution
Suggested infusion volume 500 mL

Hydrocortisone (as sodium phosphate) (*Efcortesol*®)
Continuous *or* intermittent *or via* drip tubing *in* Glucose 5% *or* Sodium chloride 0.9%

Hydrocortisone (as sodium succinate) (*SoluCortef*®)
Continuous *or* intermittent *or via* drip tubing *in* Glucose 5% *or* Sodium chloride 0.9%

Ibandronic acid (*Bondronat*®)
Intermittent *in* Glucose 5% *or* Sodium chloride 0.9%
Dilute requisite dose in 500 mL infusion fluid and give over 2 hours

Idarubicin hydrochloride (*Zavedos*®)
via drip tubing *in* Sodium chloride 0.9%
Reconstitute with water for injections; give over 5–10 minutes

Ifosfamide (*Mitoxana*®)
Continuous *or* intermittent *or via* drip tubing *in* Glucose 5% *or* Sodium chloride 0.9%
For continuous infusion, suggested volume 3 litres given over 24 hours; for intermittent infusion, give over 30–120 minutes

Imiglucerase (*Cerezyme*®)
Intermittent *in* Sodium chloride 0.9%
Initially reconstitute with 5.1 mL water for injections to give 40 units/mL solution; dilute requisite dose in 100–200 mL infusion fluid and give over 1–2 hours *or* at a rate not exceeding 1 unit/kg/minute; administer within 3 hours after reconstitution

Imipenem with cilastatin (as sodium salt) (*Primaxin*®)
Intermittent *in* Sodium chloride 0.9% *or* Sodium chloride and Glucose
Dilute to a concentration of 5 mg (as imipenem)/mL; infuse 250–500 mg (as imipenem) over 20–30 minutes, 1 g over 40–60 minutes
Continuous infusion not usually recommended

Infliximab (*Remicade*®)
Intermittent *in* Sodium chloride 0.9%
Reconstitute each 100-mg vial with 10 mL water for injections; gently swirl vial without shaking to dissolve; allow to stand for 5 minutes; dilute requisite dose with infusion fluid to a final volume of 250 mL and give through a low protein-binding filter (1.2 micron or less) over at least 2 hours; start infusion within 3 hours of reconstitution

Insulin (soluble)
Continuous *in* Sodium chloride 0.9% *or* Compound sodium lactate
Adsorbed to some extent by plastics of infusion set; see also section 6.1.3; ensure insulin is not injected into 'dead space' of injection port of the infusion bag

Insulin aspart
Continuous *in* Sodium chloride 0.9% *or* Glucose 5%
Dilute to 0.05–1 unit/mL with infusion fluid; adsorbed to some extent by plastics of infusion set

Insulin lispro
Continuous *in* Sodium chloride 0.9% *or* Glucose 5%

Interferon alfa-2b (*IntronA*®)
Intermittent *in* Sodium chloride 0.9%
For *IntronA*® solution, dilute requisite dose in 50 mL infusion fluid and administer over 20 minutes; not to be diluted to less than 300 000 units/mL
For *IntronA*® powder, reconstitute with 1 mL water for injections; dilute requisite dose in 100 mL infusion fluid and administer over 20 minutes; not to be diluted to less than 100 000 units/mL

Irinotecan hydrochloride (*Campto*®)
Intermittent *in* Glucose 5% *or* Sodium chloride 0.9%
Dilute requisite dose in 250 mL infusion fluid; give over 30–90 minutes

Isosorbide dinitrate (*Isoket 0.05%*®, *Isoket 0.1%*®)
Continuous *in* Glucose 5% *or* Sodium chloride 0.9%
Adsorbed to some extent by polyvinyl chloride infusion containers; preferably use glass or polyethylene containers or give *via* a syringe pump; *Isoket 0.05%*® can alternatively be administered undiluted using a syringe pump with a glass or rigid plastic syringe

Itraconazole (*Sporanox*®)
Intermittent *in* Sodium chloride 0.9%
Dilute 250 mg in 50 mL infusion fluid and infuse only **60 mL** through an in-line filter (0.2 micron) over 60 minutes

Ketamine (as hydrochloride) (*Ketalar*®)
Continuous *in* Glucose 5% *or* Sodium chloride 0.9%
Dilute to 1 mg/mL; microdrip infusion for maintenance of anaesthesia

Labetalol hydrochloride (*Trandate*®)
Intermittent *in* Glucose 5% *or* Sodium chloride and glucose
Dilute to a concentration of 1 mg/mL; suggested volume 200 mL; adjust rate with in-line burette

Lenograstim (*Granocyte®*)
Intermittent *in* Sodium chloride 0.9%
Initially reconstitute with 1 mL water for injection provided (do not shake vigorously) then dilute with up to 50 mL infusion fluid for each vial of *Granocyte-13* or up to 100 mL infusion fluid for *Granocyte-34*; give over 30 minutes

Lepirudin (*Refludan®*)
Continuous *in* Glucose 5% *or* Sodium chloride 0.9%
Reconstitute initially with water for injections *or* sodium chloride 0.9% then dilute to a concentration of 2 mg/mL with infusion fluid

Magnesium sulphate
Continuous *in* Glucose 5% *or* Sodium chloride 0.9%
Suggested concentration up to 200 mg/mL

Melphalan (*Alkeran®*)
Intermittent *or via* drip tubing *in* Sodium chloride 0.9%
Reconstitute with the solvent provided then dilute with infusion fluid; max. 90 minutes between addition and completion of administration; incompatible with glucose infusion

Meropenem (*Meronem®*)
Intermittent *in* Glucose 5 and 10% *or* Sodium chloride 0.9%
Dilute in 50–200 mL infusion fluid and give over 15–30 minutes

Mesna (*Uromitexan®*)
Continuous *or via* drip tubing *in* Glucose 5% *or* Sodium chloride 0.9%

Metaraminol (as tartrate) (*Aramine®*)
Continuous *or via* drip tubing *in* Glucose 5% *or* Sodium chloride 0.9%
Suggested volume 500 mL

Methotrexate (as sodium salt) (*Methotrexate*, *Lederle*)
Continuous *or via* drip tubing *in* Glucose 5% *or* Sodium chloride 0.9% *or* Compound sodium lactate *or* Ringer's solution
Dilute in a large-volume infusion; max. 24 hours between addition and completion of administration

Methylprednisolone (as sodium succinate) (*Solu-Medrone®*)
Continuous *or* intermittent *or via* drip tubing *in* Glucose 5% *or* Sodium chloride 0.9%
Reconstitute initially with water for injections; doses up to 250 mg should be given over at least 5 minutes, high doses over at least 30 minutes

Metoclopramide hydrochloride (*Maxolon High Dose®*)
Continuous *or* intermittent *in* Glucose 5% *or* Sodium chloride 0.9% *or* Compound sodium lactate
Continuous infusion recommended; loading dose, dilute with 50–100 mL and give over 15–20 minutes; maintenance dose, dilute with 500 mL and give over 8–12 hours; for intermittent infusion dilute with at least 50 mL and give over at least 15 minutes

Mexiletine hydrochloride (*Mexitil®*)
Continuous *in* Glucose 5% *or* Sodium chloride 0.9%

Milrinone (*Primacor®*)
Continuous *in* Glucose 5% *or* Sodium chloride 0.9%
Dilute to a suggested concentration of 200 micrograms/mL

Mitoxantrone/Mitozantrone (as hydrochloride) (*Novantrone®*, *Onkotrone®*)
Intermittent *or via* drip tubing *in* Glucose 5% *or* Sodium chloride 0.9%
For administration *via* drip tubing suggested volume at least 50 mL given over at least 3–5 minutes; for intermittent infusion (*Onkotrone®* only), dilute with 50–100 mL and give over 15–30 minutes

Mivacurium (as chloride) (*Mivacron®*)
Continuous *in* Glucose 5% *or* Sodium chloride 0.9%
Dilute to a concentration of 500 micrograms/mL; may also be given undiluted

Molgramostim (*Leucomax®*)
Intermittent *in* Glucose 5% *or* Sodium chloride 0.9%
Reconstitute each vial with 1 mL water for injections; dilute with 25–100 mL infusion fluid to a concentration of not less than 80 000 units/mL; give over 4–6 hours; infusion through low protein binding 0.2 or 0.22 micron filter recommended; some infusion sets (e.g. *Port-A-Cath®*) adsorb molgramostim and should not be used

Mycophenolate mofetil (as hydrochloride) (*CellCept®*)
Intermittent *in* Glucose 5%
Reconstitute each 500-mg vial with 14 mL glucose 5% and dilute the contents of 2 vials in 140 mL infusion fluid; give over 2 hours

Naloxone (*Min-I-Jet® Naloxone Hydrochloride*, *Narcan®*)
Continuous *in* Glucose 5% *or* Sodium chloride 0.9%
Reversal of opioid-induced respiratory depression, dilute to a concentration of 4 micrograms/mL; opioid overdose only, dilute 10 mg in 50 mL glucose 5%, see Emergency Treatment of Poisoning

Netilmicin (as sulphate) (*Netillin®*)
Intermittent *or via* drip tubing *in* Glucose 5 and 10% *or* Sodium chloride 0.9%
For intermittent infusion suggested volume 50–200 mL given over 30–120 minutes

Nimodipine (*Nimotop®*)
via drip tubing *in* Glucose 5% *or* Sodium chloride 0.9% *or* Ringer's solution
Not to be added to infusion container; administer *via* an infusion pump through a Y-piece into a central catheter; incompatible with polyvinyl chloride giving sets or containers; protect infusion from light

Nizatidine (*Axid®*)
Continuous *or* intermittent *in* Glucose 5% *or* Sodium chloride 0.9% *or* Compound sodium lactate
For continuous infusion, dilute 300 mg in 150 mL and give at a rate of 10 mg/hour; for intermittent infusion, dilute 100 mg in 50 mL and give over 15 minutes

Noradrenaline acid tartrate/Norepinephrine bitartrate
Continuous *in* Glucose 5% *or* Sodium chloride and glucose
Give *via* controlled infusion device; for administration *via* syringe pump, dilute 4 mg noradrenaline acid tartrate (2 mL solution) with 48 mL; for administration *via* drip counter dilute 40 mg (20 mL solution) with 480 mL; give through a central venous catheter; incompatible with alkalis

Omeprazole (as sodium salt) (*Losec®*)
Intermittent *in* Glucose 5% *or* Sodium chloride 0.9%
Reconstitute with infusion fluid and dilute to 100 mL; give over 20–30 minutes

Ondansetron (as hydrochloride) (*Zofran®*)
Continuous *or* intermittent *in* Glucose 5% *or* Sodium chloride 0.9% *or* Ringer's solution
For intermittent infusion, dilute 32 mg in 50–100 mL and give over at least 15 minutes

Oxaliplatin (*Eloxatin®*)
Continuous *in* Glucose 5%
Reconstitute with water for injections or glucose 5% to a concentration of 5 mg/mL; dilute with 250–500 mL infusion fluid and give over 2–6 hours

Oxycodone hydrochloride (*OxyNorm®*)
Continuous *or* intermittent *in* Glucose 5% *or* Sodium chloride 0.9%
Dilute to a concentration of 1 mg/mL

Oxytocin (*Syntocinon®*)
Continuous *in* Glucose 5% *or* Sodium chloride 0.9% or Compound sodium lactate *or* Ringer's solution
Preferably given *via* a variable-speed infusion pump in a concentration appropriate to the pump; if given by drip infusion for *induction or enhancement of labour*, dilute 5 units in 500 mL infusion fluid; for *postpartum uterine haemorrhage* dilute 5–30 units in 500 mL; if high doses given for prolonged period (e.g. for inevitable or missed abortion or for postpartum haemorrhage), use low volume of an electrolyte-containing infusion fluid (not Glucose 5%) given at higher concentration than for induction or enhancement of labour; close attention to patient's fluid and electrolyte status essential

Paclitaxel (*Taxol®*)
Continuous *in* Glucose 5% *or* Sodium chloride 0.9%
Dilute to a concentration of 0.3–1.2 mg/mL and give through an in-line filter (0.22 micron or less) over 3 hours; not to be used with PVC equipment (short PVC inlet or outlet on filter may be acceptable)

Pantoprazole (as sodium sesquihydrate) (*Protium®*)
Intermittent *in* Glucose 5 and 10% *or* Sodium chloride 0.9%
Reconstitute 40 mg with 10 mL sodium chloride 0.9% and dilute to 100 mL with infusion fluid

Pentamidine isetionate (*Pentacarinat®*)
Intermittent *in* Glucose 5% *or* Sodium chloride 0.9%
Dissolve initially in water for injections (300 mg in 3–5 mL) then dilute in 50–250 mL; give over at least 60 minutes

Pentostatin (*Nipent®*)
Intermittent *in* Glucose 5% *or* Sodium chloride 0.9%
Reconstitute initially with 5 mL water for injections to produce a 2 mg/mL solution; dilute requisite dose in 25–50 mL infusion fluid (final concentration 180–330 micrograms/mL) and give over 20–30 minutes

Phenoxybenzamine hydrochloride
Intermittent *in* Sodium chloride 0.9%
Dilute in 200–500 mL infusion; give over at least 2 hours; max. 4 hours between dilution and completion of administration

Phentolamine mesilate (*Rogitine®*)
Intermittent *in* Glucose 5% *or* Sodium chloride 0.9%

Phenylephrine hydrochloride
Intermittent *in* Glucose 5% *or* Sodium chloride 0.9%
Dilute 10 mg in 500 mL infusion fluid

Phenytoin sodium (*Epanutin®*)
Intermittent *in* Sodium chloride 0.9%
Flush intravenous line with Sodium chloride 0.9% before and after infusion; dilute in 50–100 mL infusion fluid (final concentration not to exceed 10 mg/mL) and give through an in-line filter (0.22–0.50 micron) at a rate not exceeding 50 mg/minute (neonates, give at a rate of 1–3 mg/kg/minute); complete administration within 1 hour of preparation

Phytomenadione (in mixed micelles vehicle) (*Konakion® MM*)
Intermittent *in* Glucose 5%
Dilute with 55 mL; may be injected into lower part of infusion apparatus

Piperacillin with tazobactam (as sodium salts) (*Tazocin®*)
Intermittent *in* Glucose 5% *or* Sodium chloride 0.9% *or* Water for injections
Reconstitute initially with water for injections or sodium chloride infusion 0.9% (2.25 g in 10 mL, 4.5 g in 20 mL) then dilute to at least 50 mL with infusion fluid; give over 20–30 minutes

Potassium chloride
Continuous *in* Glucose 5% *or* Sodium chloride 0.9%
Dilute in a large-volume infusion; mix thoroughly to avoid 'layering', especially in non-rigid infusion containers; use ready-prepared solutions when possible

Procainamide hydrochloride (*Pronestyl®*)
Continuous *or* intermittent *in* Glucose 5%
For maintenance, dilute to a concentration of *either* 2 mg/mL and give at a rate of 1–3 mL/minute *or* 4 mg/mL and give at a rate of 0.5–1.5 mL/minute

Propofol (emulsion) (*Diprivan®*; Abbott; Baxter; *Propofol-Lipuro®*, Braun; Mayne; Fresenius Kabi; Zurich)
1% or 2% emulsion
via drip tubing *in* Glucose 5% *or* Sodium chloride 0.9%
To be administered *via* a Y-piece close to injection site
1% emulsion only
Continuous *in* Glucose 5% (*or* Sodium chloride 0.9% for *Propofol-Lipuro®*, Braun, Fresenius Kabi, and Zurich brands only)
Dilute to a concentration not less than 2 mg/mL; administer using suitable device to control infusion rate; use glass or PVC containers (if PVC bag used it should be full—withdraw volume of infusion fluid equal to that of propofol to be added); give within 6 hours of preparation; propofol may alternatively be infused undiluted using a suitable infusion pump

Quinine dihydrochloride
Continuous *in* Sodium chloride 0.9%
To be given over 4 hours; see also section 5.4.1

Quinupristin with dalfopristin (*Synercid®*)
Intermittent *in* Glucose 5%
Reconstitute 500 mg with 5 mL water for injections or glucose 5%; gently swirl vial without shaking to dissolve; allow to stand for at least 2 minutes until foam disappears; dilute requisite dose in 100 mL infusion fluid and give over 60 minutes *via* central venous catheter (in an emergency, first dose may be diluted in 250 mL infusion fluid and given over 60 minutes *via* peripheral line); flush line with glucose 5% before and after infusion; incompatible with sodium chloride solutions

Raltitrexed (*Tomudex®*)
Intermittent *in* Glucose 5% *or* Sodium chloride 0.9%
Reconstitute with water for injections; dilute requisite dose in 50–250 mL infusion fluid and give over 15 minutes

Ranitidine (as hydrochloride) (*Zantac*®)
Intermittent *in* Glucose 5% *or* Sodium chloride 0.9% *or* Compound sodium lactate

Rasburicase (*Fasturtec*®)
Intermittent *in* Sodium chloride 0.9%
Reconstitute with solvent provided; gently swirl vial without shaking to dissolve; dilute requisite dose to 50 mL with infusion fluid and give over 30 minutes

Remifentanil (*Ultiva*®)
Intermittent *or via* drip tubing *in* Glucose 5% *or* Sodium chloride 0.9% *or* Water for injections
Reconstitute with infusion fluid to a concentration of 1 mg/mL then dilute further to a concentration of 20–250 micrograms/mL (50 micrograms/mL recommended for general anaesthesia)

Rifampicin (*Rifadin*®, *Rimactane*®)
Intermittent *in* Glucose 5 and 10% *or* Sodium chloride 0.9% *or* Ringer's solution
Reconstitute with solvent provided then dilute with 250 mL (*Rimactane*®) or 500 mL (*Rifadin*®) infusion fluid; give over 2–3 hours

Ritodrine hydrochloride (*Yutopar*®)
Continuous *in* Glucose 5%
Give *via* controlled infusion device, preferably a syringe pump; if syringe pump available dilute to a concentration of 3 mg/mL; if syringe pump not available dilute to a concentration of 300 micrograms/mL; close attention to patient's fluid and electrolyte status essential

Rituximab (*MabThera*®)
Intermittent *in* Glucose 5% *or* Sodium chloride 0.9%
Dilute to 1–4 mg/mL and gently invert bag to avoid foaming

Rocuronium bromide (*Esmeron*®)
Continuous *or via* drip tubing *in* Glucose 5% *or* Sodium chloride 0.9%

Salbutamol (as sulphate) (*Ventolin*® *For Intravenous Infusion*)
Continuous *in* Glucose 5%
For *bronchodilatation* dilute 5 mg with 500 mL glucose 5% or sodium chloride 0.9%; for *premature labour* dilute with glucose 5% to a concentration of 200 micrograms/mL for use in a syringe pump *or* for other infusion methods (preferably *via* controlled infusion device), dilute to a concentration of 20 micrograms/mL; close attention to patient's fluid and electrolyte status essential

Sodium calcium edetate (*Ledclair*®)
Continuous *in* Glucose 5% *or* Sodium chloride 0.9%
Dilute to a concentration of not more than 3%; suggested volume 250–500 mL given over at least 1 hour

Sodium clodronate (*Bonefos*® *Concentrate*, *Loron*®)
Continuous *in* Sodium chloride 0.9%
Dilute 300 mg in 500 mL and give over at least 2 hours or 1.5 g in 500 mL and give over at least 4 hours; *Bonefos*® *Concentrate* can also be diluted in Glucose 5%

Sodium nitroprusside (Mayne)
Continuous *in* Glucose 5%
Reconstitute 50 mg with 2–3 mL glucose 5% then dilute immediately with 250–1000 mL infusion fluid; preferably infuse *via* infusion device to allow precise control; protect infusion from light

Sodium valproate (*Epilim*®)
Continuous *or* intermittent *in* Glucose 5% *or* Sodium chloride 0.9%
Reconstitute with solvent provided then dilute with infusion fluid

Sotalol hydrochloride (*Sotacor*®)
Continuous *or* intermittent *in* Glucose 5% *or* Sodium chloride 0.9%
Dilute to a concentration of between 0.01–2 mg/mL

Streptokinase (*Streptase*®; *Streptokinase*, Braun)
Continuous *or* intermittent *in* Glucose 5% *or* Sodium chloride 0.9%
Reconstitute *Streptase*® with sodium chloride 0.9%, and *Streptokinase* (Braun) with either water for injections or sodium chloride 0.9% then dilute further with infusion fluid

Sulfadiazine sodium
Continuous *in* Sodium chloride 0.9%
Suggested volume 500 mL; ampoule solution has a pH of over 10

Suxamethonium chloride (*Anectine*®)
Continuous *in* Glucose 5% *or* Sodium chloride 0.9%

Tacrolimus (*Prograf*®)
Continuous *in* Glucose 5% *or* Sodium chloride 0.9%
Dilute concentrate in infusion fluid to a final concentration of 4–100 micrograms/mL; give over 24 hours; incompatible with PVC

Teicoplanin (*Targocid*®)
Intermittent *in* Glucose 5% *or* Sodium chloride 0.9% *or* Compound sodium lactate
Reconstitute initially with water for injections provided; infuse over 30 minutes
Continuous infusion not usually recommended

Terbutaline sulphate (*Bricanyl*®)
Continuous *in* Glucose 5%
For *bronchodilatation* dilute 1.5–2.5 mg with 500 mL glucose 5% or sodium chloride 0.9% and give over 8–10 hours; for *premature labour* dilute in glucose 5% and give *via* controlled infusion device preferably a syringe pump; if syringe pump available dilute to a concentration of 100 micrograms/mL; if syringe pump not available dilute to a concentration of 10 micrograms/mL; close attention to patient's fluid and electrolyte status essential

Ticarcillin sodium with clavulanic acid (*Timentin*®)
Intermittent *in* Glucose 5% *or* Water for injections
Suggested volume (depending on dose) glucose 5% 100–150 mL or water for injections 50–100 mL; given over 30–40 minutes

Tirofiban (*Aggrastat*®)
Continuous *in* Glucose 5% *or* Sodium chloride 0.9%
Withdraw 50 mL infusion fluid from 250-mL bag and replace with 50 mL tirofiban concentrate (250 micrograms/mL) to give a final concentration of 50 micrograms/mL

Tobramycin (as sulphate) (*Nebcin*®)
Intermittent *or via* drip tubing *in* Glucose 5% *or* Sodium chloride 0.9%
For adult intermittent infusion suggested volume 50–100 mL (children proportionately smaller volume) given over 20–60 minutes

Topotecan (as hydrochloride) (*Hycamtin*®)
Intermittent *in* Glucose 5% *or* Sodium chloride 0.9%
Reconstitute 4 mg with 4 mL water for injections then dilute to a final concentration of 25–50 micrograms/mL; give over 30 minutes

Tramadol hydrochloride (*Zydol*®)
Continuous *or* intermittent *in* Glucose 5% *or* Sodium chloride 0.9% *or* Ringer's solution *or* Compound sodium lactate

Tranexamic acid (*Cyklokapron*®)
Continuous *in* Glucose 5% *or* Sodium chloride 0.9% *or* Ringer's solution

Trastuzumab (*Herceptin* ®)
Intermittent *in* Sodium chloride 0.9%
Reconstitute each 150-mg vial with 7.2 mL water for injections to produce 21 mg/mL solution, swirl vial gently to avoid excessive foaming and allow to stand for approximately 5 minutes; dilute requisite dose in 250 mL infusion fluid

Treosulfan (*Treosulfan*) (Medac)
Intermittent *in* Water for injections
Infusion suggested for doses above 5 g; dilute to a concentration of 5 g in 100 mL

Trimetaphan camsilate (Cambridge)
Intermittent *in* Sodium chloride 0.9% *or* Sodium chloride and glucose
Dilute to a concentration of 0.05–0.1% (0.25% if fluid restriction necessary)

Trisodium edetate (*Limclair*®)
Continuous *in* Glucose 5% *or* Sodium chloride 0.9%
Dilute to a concentration of 10 mg/mL; give over 2–3 hours

Tropisetron (as hydrochloride) (*Navoban*®)
Intermittent *or via* drip tubing *in* Glucose 5% *or* Sodium chloride 0.9% *or* Ringer's solution
Suggested concentration for infusion 50 micrograms/mL

Vancomycin (as hydrochloride) (*Vancocin*®)
Intermittent *in* Glucose 5% *or* Sodium chloride 0.9%
Reconstitute each 500 mg with 10 mL water for injections and dilute with infusion fluid to a concentration of up to 5 mg/mL (10 mg/mL in fluid restriction but increased risk of infusion-related effects); give over at least 60 minutes (rate not to exceed 10 mg/minute for doses over 500 mg); use continuous infusion only if intermittent not feasible

Vasopressin, synthetic (*Pitressin*®)
Intermittent *in* Glucose 5%
Suggested concentration 20 units/100 mL given over 15 minutes

Vecuronium bromide (*Norcuron*®)
Continuous *in* Glucose 5% *or* Sodium chloride 0.9% *or* Ringer's solution
Reconstitute with the solvent provided

Verteporfin (*Visudyne*®)
Intermittent *in* Glucose 5%
Reconstitute each 15 mg with 7 mL water for injections to produce a 2 mg/mL solution then dilute requisite dose with infusion fluid to a final volume of 30 mL and give over 10 minutes; protect from light and administer within 4 hours of reconstitution. Incompatible with sodium chloride infusion

Vinblastine sulphate (*Velbe*®)
via drip tubing *in* Sodium chloride 0.9%
Reconstitute with sodium chloride 0.9%; give over approx. 1 minute

Vincristine sulphate (*Oncovin*®)
via drip tubing *in* Glucose 5% *or* Sodium chloride 0.9%

Vindesine sulphate (*Eldisine*®)
via drip tubing *in* Glucose 5% *or* Sodium chloride 0.9%
Reconstitute with sodium chloride 0.9%; give over 1–3 minutes

Vinorelbine (*Navelbine*®)
Intermittent *in* Glucose 5% *or* Sodium chloride 0.9%
Dilute in 125 mL infusion fluid; give over 20–30 minutes

Vitamins B & C (*Pabrinex*® *I/V High potency*)
Intermittent *or via* drip tubing *in* Glucose 5% *or* Sodium chloride 0.9%
Ampoule contents should be mixed, diluted, and administered without delay; give over 10 minutes (see CSM advice, section 9.6.2)

Vitamins, multiple
(*Cernevit*®)
Intermittent *in* Glucose 5% *or* Sodium chloride 0.9%
Dissolve initially in 5 mL water for injections (or infusion fluid)
(*Solivito N*®)
Intermittent *in* Glucose 5 and 10%
Suggested volume 500–1000 mL given over 2–3 hours; see also section 9.3

Voriconazole (*Vfend*®)
Intermittent *in* Glucose 5% *or* Sodium chloride 0.9% *or* Compound sodium lactate
Reconstitute each 200 mg with 19 mL water for injections to produce a 10 mg/mL solution; dilute dose in infusion fluid to concentration of 0.5–5 mg/mL; give at a rate not exceeding 3 mg/kg/hour

Zidovudine (*Retrovir*®)
Intermittent *in* Glucose 5%
Dilute to a concentration of 2 mg/mL or 4 mg/mL and give over 1 hour

Zoledronic acid (*Zometa*®)
Intermittent *in* Glucose 5% *or* Sodium chloride 0.9%
Reconstitute 4 mg vial with 5 mL water for injections, then dilute with 100 mL infusion fluid; infuse over at least 15 minutes

Appendix 7: Borderline substances

In certain conditions some foods (and toilet preparations) have characteristics of drugs and the Advisory Committee on Borderline Substances advises as to the circumstances in which such substances may be regarded as drugs. Prescriptions issued in accordance with the Committee's advice and endorsed 'ACBS' will normally not be investigated.

> General Practitioners are reminded that the ACBS recommends products on the basis that they may be regarded as drugs for the management of specified conditions. Doctors should satisfy themselves that the products can safely be prescribed, that patients are adequately monitored and that, where necessary, expert hospital supervision is available.

Foods which may be prescribed on FP10, GP10 (Scotland), or when available WP10 (Wales)

NOTE. This is a list of food products which the ACBS has approved. The clinical condition for which the product has approval follows each entry.

Foods included in this Appendix may contain cariogenic sugars and patients should be advised to take appropriate oral hygiene measures.

Alcoholic Beverages see under Rectified Spirit

Alembicol D® (Alembic Products)
Fractionated coconut oil. Net price 5 kg = £125.55.
For steatorrhoea associated with cystic fibrosis of the pancreas, intestinal lymphangiectasia, surgery of the intestine, chronic liver disease, liver cirrhosis, other proven malabsorption syndromes; in a ketogenic diet in the management of epilepsy; type 1 hyperlipoproteinaemia

Aminex® (Gluten Free Foods Ltd)
Low-protein. Biscuits, net price 200 g = £3.75. Cookies, 150 g = £3.75. Rusks, 200 g = £3.75.
For inherited metabolic disorders, renal or liver failure requiring a low-protein diet

Amino Acid Modules (SHS)
XLEU Faladon, powder, essential and non-essential amino acids 93%, except leucine. Net price 200 g = £49.59.
For isovaleric acidaemia
XMET Homidon, powder, essential and non-essential amino acids 93%, except methionine. Net price 200 g = £49.59.
For homocystinuria or hypermethioninaemia
XMTVI Asadon, powder, essential and non-essential amino acids 93%, except methionine, threonine, and valine, with trace amounts of isoleucine. Net price 200 g = £49.59.
For methylmalonic acidaemia or propionic acidaemia
XPTM Tyrosidon, powder, essential and non-essential amino acids 93%, except methionine, phenylalanine, and tyrosine. Net price 500 g = £123.98.
For tyrosinaemia type I where plasma concentrations are above normal

XPHEN TYR Tyrosidon, powder, essential and non-essential amino acids 93%, except phenylalanine and tyrosine. Net price 500 g = £130.18
For tyrosinaemia where plasma methionine concentrations are normal

Aminogran® (UCB Pharma)
Food Supplement, powder, containing all essential amino acids except phenylalanine, for use with mineral mixture (see below), net price 500 g = £42.77. Aminogran PKU tablet (≡ 1 g powder), net price 150-tab pack = £30.00.
For the dietary management of phenylketonuria. Tablets not to be prescribed for any child under 8 years
Mineral Mixture, powder, containing all appropriate minerals for use with the above food supplement and other synthetic diets. Net price 250 g = £7.24.
For phenylketonuria and as a mineral supplement in synthetic diets

Analog® (SHS)
NOTE. Analog products are generally intended for use in children up to 1 year, see also Flavour Sachets, for use with unflavoured amino acid and peptide products from SHS
MSUD Analog, powder, essential and non-essential amino acids 15.5% except isoleucine, leucine and valine, with carbohydrate, fat, vitamins, minerals, and trace elements. Net price 400 g = £24.00.
For maple syrup urine disease
XLeu Analog, powder, essential and non-essential amino acids 15.5% except leucine, with carbohydrate, fat, vitamins, minerals, and trace elements. Net price 400 g = £24.00.
For isovaleric acidaemia
Ingredients: include arachis oil (peanut oil)
XLys Analog, powder, essential and non-essential amino acids 15.5% except lysine, with carbohydrate, fat, vitamins, minerals, and trace elements. Net price 400 g = £24.00.
For hyperlysinaemia
XLys, Try Low Analog, powder, essential and non-essential amino acids 15.5% except lysine, and low tryptophan, with carbohydrate, fat, vitamins, minerals, and trace elements. Net price 400 g = £24.00.
For type 1 glutaric aciduria
XMet Analog, powder, essential and non-essential amino acids 15.5% except methionine, with carbohydrate, fat, vitamins, minerals, and trace elements. Net price 400 g = £24.00.
For hypermethioninaemia; homocystinuria
XMTVI Analog, powder, essential and non-essential amino acids 15.5% except methionine, threonine, valine and low isoleucine, with carbohydrate, fat, vitamins, minerals, and trace elements. Net price 400 g = £24.00.
For methylmalonic acidaemia or propionic acidaemia
XP Analog, powder, essential and non-essential amino acids 15.5% except phenylalanine, with carbohydrate, fat, vitamins, minerals, and trace elements. Net price 400 g = £19.18.
For phenylketonuria
XP LCPAnalog, powder, essential and non-essential amino acids except phenylalanine 15.5%, with carbohydrate, fat, vitamins, minerals and trace

elements. Gluten- and lactose-free. Net price 400 g = £21.82.

For phenylketonuria in infants and children under 2 years of age

XPhen, Tyr Analog, powder, essential and non-essential amino acids 15.5% except phenylalanine and tyrosine, with carbohydrate, fat, vitamins, minerals and trace elements. Net price 400 g = £24.00.

For tyrosinaemia

XPTM Analog, powder, essential and non-essential amino acids 15.5% except phenylalanine, tyrosine and methionine, with carbohydrate, fat, vitamins, minerals and trace elements. Net price 400 g = £24.00.

For tyrosinaemia

Aproten® (Ultrapharm)

Gluten-free. Flour. Net price 500 g = £4.99.

For gluten-sensitive enteropathies including steatorrhoea due to gluten sensitivity, coeliac disease, and dermatitis herpetiformis

Low protein. Low Na^+ and K^+. Net prices: biscuits 180 g (36) = £2.88; bread mix 250 g = £2.17; cake mix 300 g = £2.10; crispbread 260 g = £4.06; pasta (anellini, ditalini, rigatini, spaghetti) 500 g = £4.06; tagliatelle 250 g = £2.16.

For inherited metabolic disorders, renal or liver failure requiring a low-protein diet

L-Arginine (SHS)

Powder, net price 100 g = £8.39.

For use as a supplement in urea cycle disorders other than arginase deficiency, such as hyperammonaemia types I and II, citrullaemia, arginosuccinic aciduria, and deficiency of N-acetyl glutamate synthetase

Arnott® (Ultrapharm)

Rice Cookies, gluten-free. Net price 200 g = £2.06.

For gluten-sensitive enteropathies including steatorrhoea due to gluten sensitivity, coeliac disease, and dermatitis herpetiformis

Baker's Delight®

Gluten-free. Bread, net price 100 g = 80p.

For established gluten enteropathy

Barkat® (Gluten Free Foods Ltd)

Gluten-free. Bread mix, net price 500 g = £4.12. Multi Grain Bread, 450 g = £2.79. Rice bread (sliced), brown or white, 450 g = £2.79. Rice pizza crust, brown or white, 150 g = £2.21.

For gluten-sensitive enteropathies including steatorrhoea due to gluten sensitivity, coeliac disease, and dermatitis herpetiformis

Bi-Aglut® (Novartis Consumer Health)

Gluten-free. Biscuits, net price 180 g = £2.89. Crackers, 150 g = £2.36. Cracker toast, 240 g = £4.18. Pasta (fusilli, macaroni, penne, spaghetti), 500 g = £5.23; Lasagne, 250 g = £2.95.

For gluten-sensitive enteropathies including steatorrhoea due to gluten sensitivity, coeliac disease, and dermatitis herpetiformis

Calogen® (SHS)

Emulsion, arachis oil (peanut oil) 50% in water, net price, 250 mL = £4.21 (banana or natural flavour), £4.21 (strawberry flavour); 1 litre = £16.16 (natural flavour), £16.16 (banana or butterscotch flavour).

For disease-related malnutrition, malabsorption states or other conditions requiring fortification with a high-fat supplement with or without fluid and electrolyte restrictions

Caloreen® (Nestlé Clinical)

Powder, water-soluble dextrins, 390 kcal/100 g, with less than 1.8 mmol of Na^+ and 0.3 mmol of

K^+/100 g. Gluten-, lactose-, and fructose-free. Net price 500 g = £3.02.

For disease-related malnutrition, malabsorption states or other conditions requiring fortification with a high or readily available carbohydrate supplement

Calshake® (Fresenius Kabi)

Powder, protein 4 g, carbohydrate 58 g, fat 20.4 g, energy 1809 kJ (432 kcal)/87 g. Gluten-free. Strawberry, vanilla, neutral, and banana flavours, net price 87-g sachet = £1.77; also available chocolate flavour (protein 4 g, carbohydrate 58 g, fat 20.4 g, fibre 1.6 g, energy 1809 kJ (432 kcal)/ 90 g = £1.77.

For disease-related malnutrition, malabsorption states or other conditions requiring fortification with a fat/ carbohydrate supplement

Caprilon® (SHS)

Powder, protein 11.8%, carbohydrate 55.1%, fat 28.3% (medium chain triglycerides 21.3%). Low in lactose, gluten- and sucrose-free. Used as a 12.7% solution. Net price 420 g = £12.15.

For disorders in which a high intake of MCT is beneficial

Carobel, Instant® (Cow & Gate)

Powder, carob seed flour. Net price 135 g = £2.63.

For thickening feeds in the treatment of vomiting

Casilan 90® (Heinz)

Powder, whole protein, containing all essential amino acids, 90% with less than 0.1% Na^+. Net price 250 g = £5.13.

For biochemically proven hypoproteinaemia

Clinutren® (Nestlé Clinical)

Clinutren Dessert, protein 12 g, carbohydrate 19 g, fat 3.3 g, energy 650 kJ (160 kcal)/ 125 g with vitamins and minerals. Gluten-free. Flavours: caramel, chocolate, peach or vanilla, net price 4 × 125-g pot = £4.20.

For use as a nutritional supplement prescribed on medical grounds for: short bowel syndrome, intractable malabsorption, pre-operative preparation of undernourished patients, proven inflammatory bowel disease, following total gastrectomy, dysphagia, bowel fistulas, disease-related malnutrition, continuous ambulatory peritoneal dialysis (CAPD), haemodialysis. Not suitable for any child under 3 years; maximum of 3 units daily for children aged 3 to 6 years

Clinutren Fruit, protein 8 g, carbohydrate 54 g, fat less than 0.4 g, energy 1040 kJ (250 kcal)/200 mL with vitamins and minerals. Gluten-free. Low-lactose. Flavours: grapefruit, orange, pear-cherry, or raspberry-blackcurrant, net price 4 × 200-mL cup = £6.00.

For use as a nutritional supplement prescribed on medical grounds for: short-bowel syndrome, intractable malabsorption, pre-operative preparation of undernourished patients, proven inflammatory bowel disease, following total gastrectomy, dysphagia, bowel fistulas, disease-related malnutrition. Not suitable for any child under 3 years; maximum of 3 units daily for children aged 3 to 6 years

Clinutren ISO, protein 7.6 g, carbohydrate 28 g, fat 6.6 g, energy 840 kJ (200 kcal)/200 mL with vitamins and minerals. Gluten-free. Flavours: chocolate or vanilla, net price 4 × 200-mL pot = £4.72.

For indications see *Clinutren Fruit*

Clinutren 1.5, protein 11 g, carbohydrate 42 g, fat 10 g, energy 1260 kJ (300 kcal)/200 mL with vitamins and minerals. Gluten-free; clinically lactose-free. Flavours: apricot, banana, chocolate, coffee, strawberry-raspberry or vanilla, net price 4 × 200-mL pot = £5.60.

For indications see *Clinutren Fruit*

Clinutren Thickener, powder, modified maize starch, gluten-free, net price 300 g = £4.53.
Thickening of foods and fluids in dysphagia. Not to be used for children under 3 years

Clinutren Thickened Drinks, liquid, modified maize starch, gluten-free. Flavours: orange, peppermint, and tea, net price 4 × 125 g = £1.96.
Thickening of foods and fluids in dysphagia. Not to be used for children under 3 years

Comminuted Chicken Meat (SHS)
Suspension (aqueous). Net price 150 g = £2.50.
For carbohydrate intolerance in association with possible or proven intolerance of milk; glucose and galactose intolerance

Corn flour and corn starch
For hypoglycaemia associated with glycogen-storage disease

Dextrose *see* Glucose

Dialamine® (SHS)
Powder, essential amino acids 30%, with carbohydrate 62%, energy 1500 kJ (360 kcal)/100 g, with ascorbic acid, minerals, and trace elements. Flavour: orange. Net price 200 g = £24.48.
For oral feeding where essential amino acid supplements are required; e.g. chronic renal failure, hypoproteinaemia, wound fistula leakage with excessive protein loss, conditions requiring a controlled nitrogen intake, and haemodialysis

DS Dietary Specials (Nutrition Point)
Gluten-free. Bread. Loaf, sliced (brown, white or multigrain) 400 g = £2.50; bread rolls, long (white) 3 = £1.55. Bread mix (brown or white), net price 500 g = £4.75; cake mix (white), 750 g = £4.75; white or fibre mix, 500 g = £4.75; pastry mix, 600 g = £4.75; digestive biscuits, 150 g = £1.70.
For gluten-sensitive enteropathies, coeliac disease, and dermatitis herpetiformis

Duobar® (SHS)
Bar, protein-free (phenylalanine nil added), carbohydrate 49.9 g, fat 49.9 g, energy 2692 kJ (648 kcal)/100 g. Low sodium and potassium. Strawberry, toffee, or neutral flavours. Net price 45-g bar = £1.31.
For disease-related malnutrition, malabsorption states or other conditions requiring fortification with fat/carbohydrate supplement

Duocal® (SHS)
Liquid, emulsion providing carbohydrate 23.4 g, fat 7.1 g, energy 661 kJ (158 kcal)/100 mL. Low-electrolyte, gluten-, lactose-, and protein-free. Net price 250 mL = £2.68; 1 litre = £9.53
MCT Powder, carbohydrate 74 g, fat 23.2 g (of which MCT 83%), energy 2042 kJ (486 kcal)/100 g. Low electrolyte, gluten-, protein- and lactose-free. Net price 400 g = £14.32
Super Soluble Powder, carbohydrate 72.7 g, fat 22.3 g, energy 2061 kJ (492 kcal)/100 g. Low electrolyte, gluten-, protein-, and lactose-free. Net price 400 g = £12.05
All for disease-related malnutrition, malabsorption states or other conditions requiring fortification with fat/carbohydrate supplement

Elemental 028® (SHS)
NOTE. see also Flavour Sachets, for use with unflavoured amino acid and peptide products from SHS
028 Powder, amino acids 12%, carbohydrate 70.5–72%, fat 6.64%, energy 1544–1568 kJ (364–370 kcal)/100 g with vitamins and minerals. For preparation with water before use. Net price 100-g box (orange flavoured or plain) = £3.93
028 Extra powder, amino acids 15%, carbohydrate 59%, fat 17.45%, energy 1860 kJ (443 kcal)/100 g, with vitamins, minerals, and trace elements. For

preparation with water before use. Net price 100 g (plain) = £4.67; also available orange-flavoured (carbohydrate 55%, energy 1793 kJ (427 kcal)/100 g), 100 g = £4.76
028 Extra liquid, amino acids 7.5 g, carbohydrate 27.5 g, fat 8.7 g, energy 896 kJ (215 kcal)/250 mL, with vitamins, minerals, and trace elements. Flavours: grapefruit, orange and pineapple, summer fruits. Net price 250-mL carton = £2.45
All for use as the sole source of nutrition or as a nutritional supplement prescribed on medical grounds for: short-bowel syndrome, intractable malabsorption, proven inflammatory bowel disease, bowel fistulas. Not to be prescribed for any child under 1 year; use with caution for children up to 5 years

Emsogen® (SHS)
Powder, amino acids 15%, carbohydrate 60%, fat 16.4%, energy 1839 kJ (438 kcal)/100 g, with vitamins, minerals, and trace elements. For preparation with water before use. Net price 100 g = £4.91; also available orange-flavoured (carbohydrate 55%, energy 1754 kJ (418 kcal)/100 g), 100 g = £4.91.
For use as the sole source of nutrition or as a nutritional supplement prescribed on medical grounds for short-bowel syndrome, intractable malabsorption, proven inflammatory bowel disease, bowel fistulas. Not to be prescribed for any child under 1 year; use with caution for children up to 5 years

Ener-G® (General Dietary)
Gluten-free. Cookies (vanilla flavour), net price 435 g = £4.88. Rice bread (sliced), brown, 474 g = £4.28; white, 456 g = £4.28. Rice loaf (sliced), 612 g = £4.28. Seattle brown loaf, 600 g = £4.93. Tapioca bread (sliced), 480 g = £4.28. Rice pasta (macaroni, shells, small shells, and lasagne), 454 g = £3.98; spaghetti, 447 g = £3.98; tagliatelle, 400 g = £3.98; vermicelli, 300 g = £3.98; cannelloni, 335 g = £3.98. Brown rice pasta: lasagne, 454 g = £3.98; macaroni, 454 g = £3.98; spaghetti, 447 g = £3.98. Xanthan gum, 170 g = £6.76.
For gluten-sensitive enteropathies including steatorrhoea due to gluten sensitivity, coeliac disease, and dermatitis herpetiformis
Gluten-free. Pizza bases, 372 g = £3.75. Six flour bread loaf, 576 g = £3.60. Seattle brown rolls (round or long), 4 x 119 g = £3.00
For established gluten enteropathy with coexisting established wheat sensitivity only
Low protein egg replacer, carbohydrate 94 g, energy 1574 kJ (376 kcal)/100 g. Egg-, gluten-and lactose-free, net price 454 g = £4.05.
For phenylketonuria, similar amino acid abnormalities, renal failure, liver failure and liver cirrhosis.
Low protein pasta (lasagne, macaroni, large shells, small shells, spaghetti), net price 454 g = £5.05.
For phenylketonuria, similar amino acid abnormalities, renal failure, liver failure requiring a low-protein diet
Low protein rice bread, net price 600 g = £4.39.
For inherited metabolic disorders, renal or liver failure requiring a low-protein diet

Energivit® (SHS)
Powder, protein-free, carbohydrate 66.7 g, fat 25 g, energy 2059 kJ, (492 kcal)/100 g with vitamins, minerals and trace elements, net price 400 g = £14.66.
For infants requiring additional enegy, vitamins, minerals and trace elements following a protein restricted diet

Enfamil® (Mead Johnson)
AR (Anti-Reflux), powder, protein 13 g, fat 26 g, carbohydrate 56 g, energy 2124 kJ (508 kcal)/100 g

with vitamins, minerals and trace elements, net price 400 g = £2.55.

For significant reflux disease. For use not in excess of a 6-month period. Not to be used in conjunction with any other thickener or antacid product.

Lactofree, powder, protein 11.9 g, fat 28 g, carbohydrate 56 g, energy 2176 kJ (520 kcal)/100 g with vitamins, minerals and trace elements. Lactose- and sucrose-free, net price 400 g = £3.51.

For proven lactose intolerance

Enlive® (Abbott)

Liquid, protein 9.6 g, carbohydrate 65.4 g, energy 1274 kJ (300 kcal)/240 mL, with vitamins, minerals and trace elements. Fat- and gluten-free; clinically lactose-free. Flavours: apple, fruit punch, grapefruit, lemon and lime, orange, peach, pineapple, strawberry. Net price 240-mL Tetrapak® = £1.66.

For use as a nutritional supplement prescribed on medical grounds: for short-bowel syndrome, intractable malabsorption, pre-operative preparation of patients who are undernourished, proven inflammatory bowel disease, following total gastrectomy, dysphagia, bowel fistulas, disease-related malnutrition. Not to be prescribed for any child under 1 year; use with caution for children up to 5 years

Enrich® (Abbott)

Liquid with dietary fibre, providing protein 9.4 g, carbohydrate 34.9 g, fat 8.8 g, fibre 3.4 g, energy 1079 kJ (256 kcal)/250 mL with vitamins and minerals. Lactose- and gluten-free. Vanilla and chocolate flavours. Net price 250-mL can = £2.24.

For use as the sole source of nutrition or as a nutritional supplement prescribed on medical grounds for: short-bowel syndrome, intractable malabsorption, pre-operative preparation of patients who are undernourished, proven inflammatory bowel disease, following total gastrectomy, dysphagia, disease-related malnutrition. Not to be prescribed for any child under 1 year; use with caution for children up to 5 years

Enrich Plus® (Abbott)

Liquid with dietary fibre, providing protein 6.25 g, carbohydrate 21.5 g, fat 4.92 g, fibre 1.25 g, energy 642.5 kJ (152.5 kcal)/100 mL with vitamins and minerals. Lactose- and gluten-free. Vanilla, chocolate, raspberry and banana flavours. Net price 220-mL tetrapak = £1.71; 500-mL ready-to-hang = £4.10.

For use as a nutritional supplement for patients with disease-related malnutrition, continuous ambulatory peritoneal dialysis (CAPD), short-bowel syndrome, intractable malabsorption, dysphagia, proven inflammatory bowel disease, bowel fistulas, gastrectomy, and pre-operative preparation of undernourished patients. Not to be prescribed for any child under 1 year; use with caution for children up to 5 years

Ensure® (Abbott)

Liquid, protein 10.0 g, fat 8.4 g, carbohydrate 33.9 g, energy 1057 kJ (251 kcal)/250 mL with minerals and vitamins, lactose- and gluten-free. Vanilla, chocolate, coffee, eggnog, nut, chicken, mushroom, and asparagus flavours. Net price 250-mL can = £1.92; 500-mL ready-to-hang (vanilla) = £3.74

Powder, same composition as Ensure liquid when reconstituted. Vanilla flavour. Net price 400 g = £11.39

Both for use as the sole source of nutrition or as a nutritional supplement prescribed on medical grounds for: short-bowel syndrome, intractable malabsorption, pre-operative preparation of patients who are undernourished, proven inflammatory bowel disease, following total gastrectomy, dysphagia, bowel fistulas, disease-related malnutrition. Neither to be prescribed

for any child under 1 year; use with caution for children up to 5 years

Ensure Plus® (Abbott)

Liquid, protein 13.8 g, fat 10.8 g, carbohydrate 44.4 g, with vitamins and minerals, lactose- and gluten-free, energy 1390 kJ (330 kcal)/220 mL. Vanilla flavour, (formulations may vary slightly). Net price 220-mL Tetrapak® = £1.59; 250-mL can = £2.10; 500-mL ready-to-hang (unflavoured) = £3.91; 1-litre ready-to-hang (unflavoured) = £7.63; 1.5-litre ready-to-hang (unflavoured) = £11.44. Caramel, chocolate, strawberry, banana, fruit of the forest, raspberry, orange, coffee, black currant, peach, vanilla or neutral flavours. Net price 220-mL Tetrapak® = £1.59.

Yoghurt Style, protein 13.8 g, fat 10.8 g, carbohydrate 44.4 g, with vitamins, minerals and trace elements, gluten-free, clinically lactose-free, energy 1390 kJ (330 kcal)/220 mL. Peach, pineapple, or strawberry flavour, net price 220-mL Tetrapak® = £1.59.

Both as nutritional supplements prescribed on medical grounds for: short-bowel syndrome, intractable malabsorption, pre-operative preparation of patients who are undernourished, proven inflammatory bowel disease, following total gastrectomy, dysphagia, bowel fistulas, disease-related malnutrition, continuous ambulatory peritoneal dialysis (CAPD), and haemodialysis. Not to be prescribed for any child under 1 year; use with caution for children up to 5 years

Entera® see Fresubin® Energy

Farley's Soya Formula (Heinz)

Powder, providing protein 2%, carbohydrate 7%, fat 3.8% with vitamins and minerals when reconstituted. Gluten-, sucrose-, and lactose-free. Net price 450 g = £3.79.

For proven lactose and associated sucrose intolerance in pre-school children, galactokinase deficiency, galactosaemia, and cow's milk protein intolerance

Fate® (Fate)

Low protein. All-purpose mix, net price 500 g = £5.50; Cake mix, 2 × 250 g = £5.50; Chocolate-flavour cake mix, 2 × 250 g = £5.50.

For inherited metabolic disorders, renal or liver failure requiring a low-protein diet

FlavourPac® (Vitaflo)

Powder, flavours: blackcurrant, lemon, orange, and raspberry, net price 4 × 30 × 4-g sachets = £40.00.

For use in conjuntion with Vitaflo's Inborn Error range of protein substitutes

Flavour Sachets (SHS)

Powder, flavours: cherry-vanilla, grapefruit, harvest fruits, lemon-lime, net price 20 × 5-g sachets = £8.11.

For use with SHS unflavoured amino acid and peptide products

Foodlink Complete (Foodlink)

Powder, protein 21.9 g, carbohydrate 57.3 g, fat 13.3 g, energy 1838 kJ (436.5 kcal)/100 g with vitamins and minerals, Flavours: banana, chocolate, natural, or strawberry, net price 450-g carton = £3.19; also available, vanilla with fibre, protein 19.5 g, carbohydrate 60.2 g, fat 12.3 g, fibre 8 g, energy 1804 kJ (428 kcal)/100 g = £3.75.

As a nutritional supplement prescribed on medical grounds for: short-bowel syndrome, intractable malabsorption, pre-operative preparation of undernourished patients, proven inflammatory bowel disease, following total gastrectomy, dysphagia, bowel fistulas, disease-related malnutrition. Not to be prescribed for any child under 1 year; use with caution for children up to 5 years

Formance® (Abbott)

Semi-solid, protein 4 g, carbohydrate 27 g, fat 5 g, energy 703 kJ (167 kcal)/113 g with vitamins and minerals. Gluten-free. Vanilla and butterscotch flavours. Net price 113-g pot = £1.40.

As a nutritional supplement prescribed on medical grounds for: short-bowel syndrome, intractable malabsorption, pre-operative preparation of patients who are undernourished, proven inflammatory bowel disease, following total gastrectomy, dysphagia, bowel fistulas, disease-related malnutrition, continuous ambulatory peritoneal dialysis (CAPD), and haemodialysis. Not to be prescribed for any child under 1 year; use with caution for children up to 5 years

Forticreme® (Nutricia Clinical)

Semi-solid, protein 10 g, carbohydrate 19 g, fat 5 g, energy 680 kJ (161 kcal)/100 g with vitamins and minerals. Gluten-free. Vanilla, chocolate, coffee, banana, and forest fruit flavours, net price 4 × 125-g pot = £5.99.

As a nutritional supplement prescribed on medical grounds for: short-bowel syndrome, intractable malabsorption, pre-operative preparation of patients who are undernourished, proven inflammatory bowel disease, following total gastrectomy, dysphagia, bowel fistulas, disease-related malnutrition, continuous ambulatory peritoneal dialysis (CAPD) and haemodialysis. Not to be prescribed for any child under 3 years; use with caution for children aged 3 to 5 years

Fortifresh® (Nutricia Clinical)

Liquid, protein 12 g, carbohydrate 37.4 g, fat 11.6 g, energy 1260 kJ (300 kcal)/200 mL with vitamins, minerals and trace elements. Gluten-free. Flavours: black currant, peach and orange, pineapple, raspberry, and vanilla and lemon, net price 200 mL carton = £1.54.

For use as a nutritional supplement prescribed on medical grounds for: intractable malabsorption, preoperative preparation of patients who are undernourished, inflammatory bowel disease, dysphagia, disease-related malnutrition. Not to be prescribed for any child under 3 years; use with caution for children aged 3 to 5 years

Fortijuce® (Nutricia Clinical)

Liquid, protein 8 g, carbohydrate 67 g, energy 1270 kJ (300 kcal)/200 mL, with vitamins, minerals and trace elements. Fat-free. Flavours: apricot, blackcurrant, lemon and lime, peach and orange, pineapple, apple and pear, forest fruits. Net price 200-mL carton = £1.54.

As a nutritional supplement prescribed on medical grounds for: short-bowel syndrome, intractable malabsorption, pre-operative preparation of patients who are undernourished, proven inflammatory bowel disease, following total gastrectomy, dysphagia, bowel fistulas, disease-related malnutrition. Not to be prescribed for any child under 3 years; use with caution for children up to 5 years

Fortimel® (Nutricia Clinical)

Liquid, protein 20 g, carbohydrate 20.8 g, fat 4.2 g, energy 840 kJ (200 kcal)/200 mL with vitamins and minerals. Gluten-free. Vanilla, strawberry, coffee, chocolate, and forest fruits flavours. Net price 200-mL carton = £1.31.

As a nutritional supplement prescribed on medical grounds for: short-bowel syndrome, intractable malabsorption, pre-operative preparation of patients who are undernourished, proven inflammatory bowel disease, following total gastrectomy, dysphagia, bowel fistulas, disease-related malnutrition. Not to be prescribed for any child under 3 years; use with caution for children up to 5 years

Fortini® (Nutricia Clinical)

Liquid, protein 3.4 g, carbohydrate 18.8 g, fat 6.8 g, energy 630 kJ (150 kcal)/100 mL with vitamins, minerals, and trace elements. Gluten- and lactose-free. Flavours: strawberry or vanilla, net price 200-mL tetrapak® = £2.31.

For use as a nutritional supplement prescribed on medical grounds for: disease-related malnutrition, and growth failure. Not to be prescribed for any child under 1 year

Fortini Multifibre® (Nutricia Clinical)

Liquid, protein 3.4 g, carbohydrate 18.8 g, fat 6.8 g, fibre 1.5 g, energy 630 kJ (150 kcal)/100 mL with vitamins, minerals, and trace elements. Gluten- and lactose-free. Flavours: banana, chocolate, strawberry, and vanilla, net price 200-mL tetrapak® = £2.42.

For indications see Fortini liquid

Fortisip® (Nutricia Clinical)

Liquid, protein 12 g, carbohydrate 36.8 g, fat 11.6 g, energy 1260 kJ (300 kcal)/200 mL, with vitamins, minerals and trace elements. Gluten-free; clinically lactose-free. Vanilla, banana, chocolate, orange, strawberry, tropical fruits, toffee, and neutral flavours, net price 200 mL = £1.54.

As a nutritional supplement prescribed on medical grounds for: short-bowel syndrome, intractable malabsorption, pre-operative preparation of patients who are undernourished, proven inflammatory bowel disease, following total gastrectomy, dysphagia, bowel fistulas, disease-related malnutrition. Not to be prescribed for any child under 3 years; use with caution for children aged 3 to 5 years

Fortisip® **Multi Fibre** (Nutricia Clinical)

Liquid, protein 12 g, carbohydrate 36.8 g, fat 11.6 g, fibre 4.5 g, energy 1260 kJ (300 kcal)/200 mL, with vitamins, minerals and trace elements. Gluten-free, clinically lactose-free. Banana, chicken, orange, strawberry, vanilla flavours; also available chocolate flavour (protein 10 g, carbohydrate 36 g, fat 13 g, fibre 4.5 g, energy 1260 kJ (300 kcal)/ 200 mL, net price 200 mL = £1.59.

As a nutritional supplement prescribed on medical grounds for: short-bowel syndrome, intractable malabsorption, pre-operative preparation of undernourished patients, proven inflammatory bowel disease, following total gastrectomy, dysphagia, disease-related malnutrition. Not to be prescribed for any child under 3 years; use with caution for children aged 3 to 5 years

Fortisip® **Protein** (Nutricia Clinical)

Liquid, protein 10 g, carbohydrate 14.7 g, fat 3.5 g, energy 550 kJ (130 kcal)/100 mL, with vitamins, minerals and trace elements. Gluten-free. Chocolate, forest fruits, strawberry, and vanilla flavour, net price 200 mL = £1.54.

As a nutritional supplement prescribed on medical grounds for: short-bowel syndrome, intractable malabsorption, pre-operative preparation of undernourished patients, proven inflammatory bowel disease, following total gastrectomy, dysphagia, bowel fistulas, disease-related malnutrition. Not to be prescribed for any child under 6 years

Frebini® **Energy Fibre** (Fresenius Kabi)

Liquid, tube feed, protein 18.75 g, carbohydrate 93.75 g, fat 33.5 g, fibre 5.65 g, energy 3150 kJ (750 kcal)/500 mL, with vitamins, minerals and trace elements. Gluten-free, clinically lactose-free. Flavour: neutral, net price 500-mL EasyBag® = £6.10.

Sole source of nutrition or as a nutritional supplement for children aged 1 to 10 years or 8 to 30 kg with disease-related malnutrition and/or growth failure, proven inflammatory bowel disease, following total gastrectomy, short-bowel syndrome, intractable malabsorption, dysphagia, bowel fistulas, pre-operative preparation of undernourished patients. Not to be prescribed for any child under 1 year

Frebini® Original (Fresenius Kabi)

Liquid, protein 12.5 g, carbohydrate 67.5 g, fat 20 g, energy 2100 kJ (500 kcal)/500 mL, with vitamins, minerals and trace elements. Flavour: neutral, net price 200-mL bottle = £1.89.

For use as the sole source of nutrition or as a nutritional supplement for children aged 1–6 years with short-bowel syndrome, intractable malabsorption, pre-operative preparation of patients who are undernourished, proven inflammatory bowel disease, following total gastrectomy, dysphagia, bowel fistulas, disease-related malnutrition and/or growth failure. Not to be prescribed for any child under 1 year

Fresubin HP Energy® (Fresenius Kabi)

Liquid, protein 37.5 g, carbohydrate 85 g, fat 30 g, energy 3150 kJ (750 kcal)/500 mL with vitamins, minerals, and trace elements. Gluten-free and low lactose. Vanilla flavour. Net price 500-mL bottle = £3.67; 500-mL EasyBag® = £3.72; 1-litre Easy-Bag® = £7.44.

As a nutritional supplement prescribed on medical grounds for: short-bowel syndrome, intractable malabsorption, pre-operative preparation of patients who are undernourished, proven inflammatory bowel disease, following total gastrectomy, dysphagia, bowel fistulas, disease-related malnutrition, continuous ambulatory peritoneal dialysis (CAPD), and haemodialysis. Not to be prescribed for any child under 1 year; use with caution for children up to 5 years

Fresubin® 1000 Complete (Fresenius Kabi)

Liquid, tube feed, protein 5.5 g, carbohydrate 12.5 g, fat 3.1 g, energy 420 kJ (100 kcal)/100mL with vitamins, minerals and trace elements. Gluten-free, clinically lactose-free, net price 1-litre EasyBag® = £8.20.

For use as the sole source of nutrition or as a nutritional supplement prescribed on medical grounds for: short-bowel syndrome, intractable malabsorption, pre-operative preparation of undernourished patients, proven inflammatory bowel disease, following total gastrectomy, dysphagia, bowel fistulas, disease-related malnutrition. Not to be prescribed for any child under 1 year; use with caution for children up to 5 years

Fresubin® 1200 Complete (Fresenius Kabi)

Liquid, tube feed, protein 4 g, carbohydrate 10 g, fat 2.7 g, fibre 2 g, energy 336 kJ (80 kcal)/100 mL with vitamins, minerals and trace elements. Gluten-free, clinically lactose-free, net price 1.5-litre EasyBag® = £10.20.

For use as the sole source of nutrition or as a nutritional supplement prescribed on medical grounds for: short-bowel syndrome, intractable malabsorption, pre-operative preparation of undernourished patients, proven inflammatory bowel disease, following total gastrectomy, bowel fistulas, disease-related malnutrition. Not to be prescribed for any child under 5 years

Fresubin® Original (Fresenius Kabi)

Energy, liquid, protein 11.3 g, carbohydrate 37.6 g, fat 11.66 g, energy 1260 kJ (300 kcal)/200 mL, with vitamins and minerals. Net price 200-mL carton = £1.55 (flavours: vanilla, strawberry, butterscotch, blackcurrant, banana, orange, pineapple, chocolate-mint, vegetable cream, and neutral); 500-mL bottle = £3.69 (flavour: neutral); 500-mL EasyBag® = £3.77; 1-litre EasyBag® = £7.48.

For use as sole source of nutrition or as a nutritional supplement prescribed on medical grounds for: short-bowel syndrome, intractable malabsorption, pre-

operative preparation of undernourished patients, proven inflammatory bowel disease, following total gastrectomy, dysphagia, bowel fistulas, disease-related malnutrition. Not to be prescribed for any child under 1 year; use with caution for children under 5 years

Energy Fibre, sip feed, protein 11.3 g, carbohydrate 37.6 g, fat 11.6 g, fibre 5 g, energy 1260 kJ (300 kcal)/ 200 mL, with vitamins, minerals and trace elements. Gluten-free; clinically lactose-free. Flavours: banana, cappucino, chocolate, lemon, strawberry, vanilla. Net price 200-mL carton = £1.65.

For indications see *Fresubin® Energy*

Energy Fibre, tube feed, protein 28 g, carbohydrate 94 g, fat 29 g, fibre 10 g, energy 3150 kJ (750 kcal)/ 500 mL, with vitamins, minerals and trace elements. Gluten-free; clinically lactose-free. Unflavoured, net price 500-mL EasyBag® = £3.88; 1-litre EasyBag® = £7.76.

For indications see *Fresubin® Energy*

Liquid, protein 7.6 g, carbohydrate 27.6 g, fat 6.8 g, energy 840 kJ (200 kcal)/200 mL with vitamins and minerals. Gluten-free, low lactose and cholesterol. Net price 200-mL carton (nut, peach, blackcurrant, chocolate, mocha, and vanilla flavours) = £1.55; 500-mL bottle (neutral flavour) = £2.99; 500-mL EasyBag® = £2.90; 1-litre Easy-Bag® = £5.80.

For use as the sole source of nutrition or as a nutritional supplement prescribed on medical grounds for: short-bowel syndrome, intractable malabsorption, pre-operative preparation of patients who are undernourished, proven inflammatory bowel disease, following total gastrectomy, dysphagia, bowel fistulas, disease-related malnutrition, and Refsum's disease. Not to be prescribed for any child under 1 year; use with caution for children up to 5 years

Fresubin® Original Fibre (Fresenius Kabi)

Liquid with dietary fibre, protein 19 g, carbohydrate 69 g, fat 17 g, energy 2100 kJ (500 kcal)/500 mL, with vitamins and minerals. Flavour: neutral. Net price 500-mL bottle = £3.38; 500-mL EasyBag® = £3.51; 1-litre EasyBag® = £7.03.

For use as sole source of nutrition or as a nutritional supplement prescribed on medical grounds for: short-bowel syndrome, intractable malabsorption, pre-operative preparation of patients who are undernourished, proven inflammatory bowel disease, following total gastrectomy, dysphagia, disease-related malnutrition. Not to be prescribed for any child under 2 years; use with caution for children up to 5 years

Fructose

(Laevulose)

For proven glucose/galactose intolerance

Gadsby's

Gluten-free. White bread flour, net price 1 kg = £4.99. White sliced bread, 400 g = £2.50. White bread rolls, 4 × 75 g = £2.00

For established gluten enteropathy

Galactomin® (SHS)

Formula 17, powder, protein 14.5 g, fat 25.9 g, carbohydrate 56.9 g, mineral salts 3.4 g/100 g. Used as a 13.1% solution with additional vitamins in place of milk. Net price 400 g = £11.19.

For proven lactose intolerance in preschool children, galactosaemia and galactokinase deficiency

Formula 19, powder, protein 14.6 g, fat 30.8 g, carbohydrate 49.7 g (fructose as carbohydrate source), mineral salts 2.1 g/100 g, with vitamins. Used as a 12.9% solution in place of milk. Net price 400 g = £29.48.

For glucose plus galactose intolerance

Generaid® (SHS)

Powder, whey protein and additional branched-chain amino acids (protein equivalent 81%). Net price 200 g (unflavoured) = £20.39. See also Flavour Sachets.

For patients with chronic liver disease and/or porto-hepatic encephalopathy

Plus Powder, whey protein and additional branched-chain amino acids (protein equivalent 11%) carbohydrate 62%, fat 19% with vitamins, minerals and trace elements. Net price 400 g = £14.58.

For children over 1 year with hepatic disorders

Glucose

(Dextrose monohydrate)
Net price 100 g = 21p.

For glycogen storage disease and sucrose/isomaltose intolerance

Glutafin® (Nutricia Dietary)

Gluten-free. Biscuits, savoury, 125 g = £1.60; 150 g = £2.19. Biscuits, digestive, sweet or tea, 150 g = £1.60. Biscuits, 200 g = £3.21. Cake mix, 500 g = £5.00. Crackers, 200 g = £2.60. High fibre crackers, 200 g = £2.18. Pasta (penne, shells, spirals, spaghetti), 500 g = £5.05; (lasagne, tagliatelle), 250 g = £2.65. Pizza bases, 2 × 110 g = £3.60.

Select Gluten-free. Fibre loaf (sliced or unsliced), 400 g = £2.57; part-baked, 400 g = £2.88. Fresh Bread, white loaf, (sliced), 400 g = £2.85. White loaf (sliced or unsliced), 400 g = £2.57; part-baked, 400 g = £2.88. Fibre rolls (part-baked), 4 = £2.88; long, 2 = £2.88. White rolls (part-baked), 4 = £2.88; long, 2 = £2.88. Mixes (bread, cake, fibre, fibre bread, pastry, and white), 500 g = £5.00

For gluten-sensitive enteropathies including steatorrhoea due to gluten sensitivity, coeliac disease, and dermatitis herpetiformis

Gluten-free, wheat-free, crisp bread, 2 × 125 g = £3.50; crisp roll, 220 g = £3.50. Fibre loaf (sliced or unsliced), 400 g = £2.88. Fibre rolls, 4 = £2.88. White loaf (sliced or unsliced), 400 g = £2.88. White rolls, 4 = £2.88. Mixes (fibre bread, bread, white or fibre), 500 g = £5.00; cake or pastry mix, 500 g = £5.15.

For gluten-sensitive enteropathy with co-existing established wheat sensitivity

Glutano® (Gluten Free Foods Ltd)

Gluten-free. Biscuits, net price 125 g = £1.58; wheat-free digestive biscuit, 125 g = £1.58. Short-cake rings, 100 g = £1.12. Crispbread, 125 g = £1.58. Crackers, 150 g = £1.58. Flour mix, 750 g = £4.12. Pasta (animal shapes, spaghetti, spirals, tagliatelle), 250 g = £1.58; macaroni, 500 g = £3.16. White sliced bread (par-baked), 300 g = £1.86. Wholemeal bread (sliced), 500 g = £2.24. Baguette or rolls (par-baked), 200 g = £1.49.

For gluten-sensitive enteropathies including steatorrhoea due to gluten sensitivity, coeliac disease, and dermatitis herpetiformis

HCU-gel® (Vitaflo)

Powder, protein (essential and non-essential amino acids except methionine) 10.1 g, carbohydrate 8.6 g, fat 0.03 g, energy 285.5 kJ (68 kcal)/20 g with vitamins, minerals and trace elements. Unflavoured, net price 30 × 20-g sachets = £125.50

For the dietary management of homocystinuria in children between 12 months and 10 years of age

InfaSoy® (Cow & Gate)

Powder, carbohydrate 7.1%, fat 3.6%, and protein 1.8% with vitamins and minerals when used as a

12.7% solution. Net price 450 g = £3.77; 900 g = £7.23.

For proven lactose and associated sucrose intolerance in preschool children, galactokinase deficiency, galactosaemia, and proven whole cow's milk sensitivity

Infatrini® (Nutricia Clinical)

Liquid, protein 2.6 g, carbohydrate 10.3 g, fat 5.4 g, energy 420 kJ (100 kcal)/100 mL with vitamins, minerals and trace elements. Gluten-free. Net price 100 mL = 88p, 200-mL Tetrapak® = £1.75

For use as a sole source of nutrition or as a nutritional supplement prescribed on medical grounds for: failure to thrive, disease-related malnutrition and malabsorption. Manufacturer advises suitable for infants up to 1 year or 8 kg body weight

Instant Carobel®

see **Carobel, Instant®**

Isomil® (Abbott)

Powder, protein 1.8%, carbohydrate 6.9%, fat 3.7% with vitamins and minerals when reconstituted. Lactose-free. Net price 400 g = £3.38.

For proven lactose intolerance in preschool children, galactokinase deficiency, galactosaemia, and proven whole cow's milk sensitivity

Isosource® (Novartis Consumer Health)

Energy, liquid, protein 28.5 g, carbohydrate 100 g, fat 31 g, energy 3300 kJ (800 kcal)/500 mL with vitamins, minerals and trace elements. Gluten-free; clinically lactose-free. Net price 500-mL bottle = £3.13, 500-mL flexible pouch = £3.55, 1–litre flexible pouch = £7.10.

For indications see *Isosource Standard*

Fibre, liquid, protein 19 g, carbohydrate 68 g, fat 17 g, fibre 7 g, energy 2110 kJ (500 kcal)/500 mL with vitamins, minerals and trace elements. Gluten-free; clinically lactose-free. Net price 500-mL bottle = £2.90, 500-mL flexible pouch = £3.29, 1-litre flexible pouch = £6.58.

For indications see *Isosource Standard*

Junior, liquid, protein 13.5 g, carbohydrate 85 g, fat 23.5 g, energy 2560 kJ (610 kcal)/500 mL with vitamins, minerals and trace elements. Gluten-free; clinically lactose-free. Net price 500-mL flexible pouch = £4.70.

Nutritionally complete feed for disease-related malnutrition, short-bowel syndrome, intractable malabsorption, pre-operative preparation of undernourished patients, following total gastrectomy, dysphagia, bowel fistulas, growth failure, for children aged 1 to 6 years or 8 to 20 kg

Standard, liquid, protein 20.5 g, carbohydrate 71 g, fat 17.5 g, energy 2205 kJ (525 kcal)/500 mL with vitamins, minerals and trace elements. Gluten-free; clinically lactose-free. Net price 500-mL bottle = £2.60, 500-mL flexible pouch = £2.89, 1-litre flexible pouch = £5.78.

For use as a sole source of nutrition or as a nutritional supplement prescribed on medical grounds for: short-bowel syndrome, intractable malabsorption, pre-operative preparation of undernourished patients, proven inflammatory bowel disease, following total gastrectomy, dysphagia, bowel fistulas, disease-related malnutrition. Not to be prescribed for any child under 1 year; use with caution for children up to 5 years

Jevity® (Abbott)

Liquid, protein 4 g, fat 3.5 g, carbohydrate 14.8 g, dietary fibre 1.1 g, energy 441 kJ (106 kcal)/100 mL, with vitamins and minerals. Gluten-, lactose-, and sucrose-free. Net price 500-mL ready-to-hang = £3.53, 1-litre ready-to-hang = £6.82, 1.5-litre ready-to-hang = £10.23.

For use as the sole source of nutrition or as a nutritional supplement prescribed on medical grounds for: short-bowel syndrome, intractable malabsorption, pre-operative preparation of patients who are undernourished, proven inflammatory bowel disease, bowel fistulas, following total gastrectomy, dysphagia, disease-related malnutrition. Not to be prescribed for any child under 2 years; use with caution for children up to 5 years

Plus liquid, protein 5.6 g, carbohydrate 16.1 g, fat 3.9 g, dietary fibre 1.2 g, energy 504 kJ (120 kcal)/100 mL, with vitamins and minerals. Gluten- and lactose-free. Net price 500-mL ready-to-hang = £4.00, 1-litre ready-to-hang = £8.18, 1.5-litre ready-to-hang = £12.28.

For indications see under *Jevity*®.

Jevity 1.5 kcal® (Abbott)

Liquid, tube feed, protein 6.38 g, carbohydrate 21.1 g, fat 4.9 g, energy 640 kJ (152 kcal)/100 mL, with vitamins, minerals and trace elements. Gluten- and lactose-free. Net price 500-mL ready-to-hang = £4.42, 1-litre ready-to-hang = £8.20, 1.5-litre ready-to-hang = £12.80.

For use as the sole source of nutrition or as a nutritional supplement prescribed on medical grounds for: short-bowel syndrome, intractable malabsorption, pre-operative preparation of undernourished patients, proven inflammatory bowel disease, bowel fistulas, following total gastrectomy, dysphagia, disease-related malnutrition. Not to be prescribed for any child under 2 years; use with caution for children up to 10 years

Juvela® (SHS)

Gluten-free. Harvest mix, fibre mix, and flour mix, net price 500 g = £5.34. Bread (whole or sliced), 400-g loaf = £2.58; part-baked loaf (with or without fibre), 400 g = £2.88. Fibre bread (sliced and unsliced), 400-g loaf = £2.52. Bread rolls, 5 × 85 g = £3.47, fibre bread rolls, 5 × 85 g = £3.47, part-baked rolls (with or without fibre), 5 × 75 g = £3.58. Crispbread, 210 g = £3.37. Pasta (fusilli, macaroni, spaghetti), 500 g = £5.23. Pizza bases, 2 × 180 g = £6.37. Savoury biscuits, 110 g = £1.97. Digestive biscuits, 160 g = £2.22. Tea biscuits, 160 g = £2.22.

For gluten-sensitive enteropathies including steatorrhoea due to gluten sensitivity, coeliac disease, and dermatitis herpetiformis

Low Protein. Mix, net price 500 g = £5.67. Bread (whole or sliced), 400-g loaf = £2.58. Bread rolls, 5 × 70 g = £3.30. Biscuits, orange and cinnamon flavour, 125 g = £5.54; chocolate chip, 130 g = £5.54.

For inherited metabolic disorders, renal or liver failure requiring a low-protein diet

Kindergen® (SHS)

Powder, protein 7.5 g, carbohydrate 60.5 g, fat 26.1 g, energy 2060 kJ (492 kcal)/100 g with vitamins and minerals. Net price 400 g = £19.36.

For complete nutritional support or supplementary feeding for infants and children with chronic renal failure who are receiving peritoneal rapid overnight dialysis

Leucine-Free Amino Acid Mix

see Amino Acid Modules, Xleu Faladon

Lifestyle® (Ultrapharm)

Gluten-free. Brown bread (sliced and unsliced), net price 400 g = £2.63. White bread (sliced and unsliced), 400 g = £2.63. High fibre bread (unsliced), 400 g = £2.63. Bread rolls, 400 g = £2.63.

For gluten-sensitive enteropathies including steatorrhoea due to gluten sensitivity, coeliac disease, and dermatitis herpetiformis

Liquigen® (SHS)

Emulsion, medium chain triglycerides 52%. Net price 250 mL = £6.18; 1 litre = £25.93.

For steatorrhoea associated with cystic fibrosis of the pancreas; intestinal lymphangiectasia, surgery of the intestine; chronic liver disease and liver cirrhosis; other proven malabsorption syndromes; ketogenic diet in the management of epilepsy; type I hyperlipoproteinaemia

Locasol® (SHS)

Powder, protein 14.6 g, carbohydrate 56.5 g, fat 26.1 g, mineral salts 1.9 g, not more than 55 mg of Ca^{2+}/100 g and vitamins. Used as a 13.1% solution in place of milk. Net price 400 g = £15.56.

For calcium intolerance

Loprofin® (SHS)

Low protein. Sweet biscuits, net price 150 g = £1.78; chocolate cream-filled biscuits, 125 g = £1.78; cookies (chocolate chip or cinnamon), 100 g = £4.70; wafers (orange, vanilla, or chocolate), 100 g = £1.72. Breakfast cereal, 375 g = £5.51. Egg replacer, 500 g = £10.03. Egg-white replacer, 100 g = £6.65. Bread (sliced or whole), 400-g loaf = £2.65. Rolls (part-baked) 4 × 65 g = £2.79. Mix, 500 g = £5.64. Crackers, 150 g = £2.42. Herb crackers, 150 g = £2.42. Pasta (lasagne, macaroni, pasta spirals, spaghetti), 500 g = £5.88. Pasta (vermicelli), 250 g = £2.93.

For inherited metabolic disorders, renal or liver failure requiring a low-protein diet

PKU Drink, protein 0.4 g (phenylalanine 10 mg), lactose 9.4 g, fat 2 g, energy 165 kJ (40 kcal)/100 mL. Net price 200-mL Tetrapak® = 51p.

For phenylketonuria

Low protein drink (Milupa)

Powder, protein 0.4%, carbohydrate 5.1%, fat 2% when reconstituted. Net price 400 g = £7.23.

For inherited disorders of amino acid metabolism in childhood

NOTE. Termed *Milupa*® *lpd* by manufacturer

[1]**Maxamaid**® (SHS)

MSUD Maxamaid, powder, essential and non-essential amino acids 30% except isoleucine, leucine, and valine, with carbohydrate, fat less than 0.5%, vitamins, minerals, and trace elements. Net price 500 g = £65.45.

For maple syrup urine disease

XLeu Maxamaid, powder, essential and non-essential amino acids 28.6% except leucine, with carbohydrate, fat less than 0.5%, vitamins, minerals, and trace elements. Net price 500 g = £65.45.

For isovaleric acidaemia

XLys Maxamaid, powder, essential and non-essential amino acids 30% except lysine, with carbohydrate, fat less than 0.5%, vitamins, minerals, and trace elements. Net price 500 g = £65.45.

For hyperlysinaemia

XLys, Low Try, Maxamaid, powder, essential and non-essential amino acids 30% except lysine, with carbohydrate, fat less than 0.5%, vitamins, minerals, and trace elements. Net price 500 g = £65.45.

For type 1 glutaric aciduria

XMet Maxamaid, powder, essential and non-essential amino acids 30% except methionine, with carbohydrate, fat less than 0.5%, vitamins, minerals, and trace elements. Net price 500 g = £65.45

For hypermethioninaemia, homocystinuria

XMTVI Maxamaid, powder, essential and non-essential amino acids 30% except methionine, threonine, valine and low isoleucine, with carbo-

---

1. Maxamaid products are generally intended for use in children aged 1 to 8 years, see also Flavour Sachets, for use with unflavoured amino acid and peptide products from SHS

hydrate, fat less than 0.5%, vitamins, minerals, and trace elements. Net price 500 g = £65.45.

For methylmalonic acidaemia or propionic acidaemia

XP Maxamaid, essential and non-essential amino acids 30% except phenylalanine, with carbohydrate, vitamins, minerals, and trace elements. Net price powder (unflavoured), 500 g = £38.73; (orange-flavoured), 500 g = £38.73.

For phenylketonuria. Not to be prescribed for children under 2 years

XP Maxamaid Concentrate, powder, essential and non-essential amino acids 65% except phenylalanine, with carbohydrate, fat less than 0.5%, vitamins, minerals, and trace elements. Unflavoured. Net price 500 g = £99.15.

For phenylketonuria. Not to be prescribed for children under 2 years

XPhen, Tyr Maxamaid, powder, essential and non-essential amino acids 30% except phenylalanine and tyrosine, with carbohydrate, fat less than 0.5%, vitamins, minerals, and trace elements. Unflavoured. Net price 500 g = £65.45.

For tyrosinaemia

[1]**Maxamum**® (SHS)

MSUD Maxamum, powder, essential and non-essential amino acids 47% except isoleucine, leucine, and valine, with carbohydrate, fat less than 0.5%, vitamins, minerals, and trace elements. Flavours: orange, unflavoured, see also Flavour Sachets. Net price 500 g = £104.93.

For maple syrup urine disease

XMet Maxamum, powder, essential and non-essential amino acids 47% except methionine, with carbohydrate, fat less than 0.5%, vitamins, minerals, and trace elements. Unflavoured, see also Flavour Sachets. Net price 500 g = £104.93.

For hypermethioninaemia, homocystinuria

XMTVI Maxamum, powder, essential and non-essential amino acids 47% except methionine, threonine, valine, and low isoleucine, with carbohydrate, fat less than 0.5%, vitamins, minerals, and trace elements. Unflavoured, see also Flavour Sachets. Net price 500 g = £104.93.

For methylmalonic acidaemia or propionic acidaemia

XP Maxamum, powder, essential and non-essential amino acids 47% except phenylalanine, with carbohydrates, vitamins, minerals, and trace elements. Flavours: orange, unflavoured, see also Flavour Sachets. Net price 500 g = £59.87.

For phenylketonuria. Not to be prescribed for children under 8 years

Maxijul® (SHS)

Liquid, carbohydrate 50%, with potassium 0.004%, sodium 0.023%. Gluten-, lactose-, and fructose-free. Flavours: black currant, lemon and lime, orange, and natural. Net price 200 mL = £1.09

LE Powder, modification of *Maxijul*® with lower concentrations of sodium and potassium. Net price 200 g = £3.72, 2 kg = £25.95

Super Soluble Powder, glucose polymer, potassium 0.004%, sodium 0.046%. Gluten-, lactose-, and fructose-free. Net price 4 × 132-g sachet pack = £4.18, 200 g = £1.74, 2.5 kg = £15.27, 25 kg = £103.66

All for disease-related malnutrition; malabsorption states or other conditions requiring fortification with high or readily available carbohydrate supplement

Maxipro Super Soluble® (SHS)

Powder, whey protein and additional amino acids (protein equivalent 80%). Net price 200 g = £8.43; 1 kg = £33.79.

For biochemically proven hypoproteinaemia. Not to be prescribed for any child under 1 year; unsuitable as a sole source of nutrition

Maxisorb® (SHS)

Powder, protein 12 g, carbohydrate 9 g, fat 6 g, energy 579 kJ (138 kcal)/30 g with minerals. Vanilla, strawberry and chocolate flavours. Net price 5 × 30-g sachets = £3.54.

For biochemically proven hypoproteinaemia. Not to be prescribed for any child under 1 year; use with caution for children up to 5 years

MCT Oil

Triglycerides from medium chain fatty acids. For steatorrhoea associated with cystic fibrosis of the pancreas; intestinal lymphangiectasia; surgery of the intestine; chronic liver disease and liver cirrhosis; other proven malabsorption syndromes; in a ketogenic diet in the management of epilepsy; in type I hyperlipoproteinaemia

Available from Mead Johnson (net price 950 mL = £12.18); SHS (net price 500 mL = £9.79)

MCT Pepdite® (SHS)

Powder, essential and non-essential amino acids, peptides, medium chain triglycerides, monoglyceride of sunflower oil, with carbohydrate, fat, vitamins, minerals, and trace elements. Flavour Sachets available.

MCT Pepdite 0–2. Net price 400 g = £13.61

MCT Pepdite 1+. Net price 400 g = £13.61

Both for disorders in which a high intake of medium chain triglyceride is beneficial

Metabolic Mineral Mixture® (SHS)

Powder, essential mineral salts. Net price 100 g = £8.46.

For mineral supplementation in synthetic diets

Methionine-Free Amino Acid Mix *see* Amino Acid Modules, XMET Homidon

Methionine, Threonine, Valine-Free and Isoleucine-Low Amino Acid Mix *see* Amino Acid Modules, XMTVI Asadon

Milupa® **lpd** *see under* Low Protein Drink

Milupa® **PKU2 and PKU3** *see under* PKU2 and PKU3

Modulen IBD® (Nestlé)

Powder, protein 18 g, carbohydrate 54 g, fat 23 g, energy 2040 kJ (500 kcal)/100 g with vitamins, minerals and trace elements. Net price 400 g = £9.72.

For use as the sole source of nutrition during the active phase of Crohn's disease and for nutritional support during the remission phase in patients who are malnourished. Not to be prescribed for any child under one year; use with caution for children up to 5 years

May be flavoured with Nestlé Clinical Nutrition Flavour Sachets (see under *Peptamen*)

Monogen® (SHS)

Powder, protein 11.4 g, carbohydrate 68 g, fat 11.4 g (of which MCT 93%), energy 1772 kJ (420 kcal)/100 g, with vitamins, minerals and trace elements. Net price 400 g = £13.54.

For long-chain acyl-CoA dehydrogenase deficiency (LCAD), carnitine palmitoyl transferase deficiency (CPTD), primary and secondary lipoprotin lipase deficiency

---

1. Maxamum products are generally intended for use in children aged over 8 years

MSUD Aid III® (SHS)

Powder, containing full range of amino acids except isoleucine, leucine, and valine, with vitamins, minerals, and trace elements. Net price 500 g = £123.98.

For maple syrup urine disease and related conditions where it is necessary to limit the intake of branched chain amino acids

Neocate® (SHS)

Advance, powder, essential and non-essential amino acids, carbohydrate, fat, vitamins, minerals and trace elements. Milk protein-, soy- and lactose-free. Net price 100 g = £4.10; banana-vanilla flavour 15 x 50 g = £32.40.

For proven whole protein intolerance, short-bowel syndrome, intractable malabsorption, and other gastro-intestinal disorders where an elemental diet is specifically indicated

Powder, essential and non-essential amino acids, maltodextrin, fat, vitamins, minerals, and trace elements. Net price 400 g = £19.48.

For proven whole protein intolerance, short-bowel syndrome, intractable malabsorption, and other gastro-intestinal disorders where an elemental diet is specifically indicated

Nepro® (Abbott)

Liquid, protein 7 g, carbohydrate 20.6 g, fat 9.6 g, energy 840 kJ (200 kcal)/100 mL with vitamins and minerals. Net price 237-mL can = £2.28; 500–mL ready-to-hang = £4.81.

For patients with chronic renal failure who are on haemodialysis or continuous ambulatory peritoneal dialysis (CAPD), or patients with cirrhosis or other conditions requiring a high energy, low fluid, low electrolyte diet

Nestargel® (Nestlé)

Powder, carob seed flour 96.5%, calcium lactate 3.5%. Net price 125 g = £2.62.

For thickening feeds in the treatment of vomiting

Novasource® **Forte** (Novartis Consumer Health)

Liquid, protein 30 g, carbohydrate 91.5 g, fat 29.5 g, fibre 11 g, energy 3155 kJ (750 kcal)/ 500 mL with vitamins, minerals and trace elements. Gluten-free; low-lactose, net price 500-mL flexible pouch = £4.36.

For use as a sole source of nutrition or as a nutritional supplement prescribed on medical grounds for: short-bowel syndrome, intractable malabsorption, pre-operative preparation of undernourished patients, proven inflammatory bowel disease, following total gastrectomy, dysphagia, bowel fistulas, disease-related malnutrition, neoplasia-related cachexia. Not to be prescribed for any child under 1 year; use with caution for children up to 5 years

Novasource GI Control® (Novartis Consumer Health)

Liquid, protein 4.1 g, carbohydrate 14.2 g, fat 3.5 g, fibre 2.2 g, energy 440 kJ (100 kcal)/100 mL with vitamins minerals and trace elements. Gluten-free; clinically lactose-free, net price 500-mL bottle = £4.10, 500-mL flexible pouch = £4.39.

For use as a sole source of nutrition or as a nutritional supplement prescribed on medical grounds for: short-bowel syndrome, intractable malabsorption, pre-operative preparation of undernourished patients, proven inflammatory bowel disease, following total gastrectomy, dysphagia, bowel fistulas, disease-related malnutrition. Not to be prescribed for any child under 1 year; use with caution for children up to 5 years

Nutilis® (Nutricia Clinical)

Powder, modified maize starch, gluten- and lactose-free. Net price 225 g = £3.66.

For thickening of foods in dysphagia. Not to be prescribed for children under 3 years

Nutramigen® (Mead Johnson)

Powder, protein 1.9 g, carbohydrate 7.5 g, fat 3.4 g, energy 280 kJ (68 kcal)/100 mL with vitamins and minerals. Gluten-, sucrose-, and lactose-free. Net price 400 g = £7.81.

For disaccharide and/or whole protein intolerance where additional medium chain triglyceride is not indicated

Nutramigen® **2** (Mead Johnson)

Powder, protein 2.3 g, carbohydrate 7.8 g, fat 3.5 g with vitamins, minerals and trace elements. Gluten-, sucrose-, and lactose-free, net price 425 g = £7.81.

For disaccharide and/or whole protein intolerance where additional medium chain triglyceride is not indicated. Not suitable for infants under 6 months

Nutrini® (Nutricia Clinical)

Liquid, protein 5.5 g, carbohydrate 24.6 g, fat 8.8 g, energy 840 kJ (200 kcal)/200 mL. Gluten- and sucrose-free; clinically lactose-free. Net price 200-mL bottle = £1.87, 500-mL flexible pack = £4.69, 1000-mL flexible pack = £9.38.

For use as the sole source of nutrition or as a nutritional supplement prescribed on medical grounds for: short-bowel syndrome, intractable malabsorption, pre-operative preparation of undernourished patients, dysphagia, bowel fistulas, disease-related malnutrition and/or growth failure. Not to be prescribed for any child under 1 year

Energy, liquid, protein 8.2 g, carbohydrate 37 g, fat 13.4 g, energy 1260 kJ (300 kcal)/200 mL. Gluten- and sucrose-free; clinically lactose-free. Net price 200-mL bottle = £2.31, 500-mL collapsible pack = £5.87.

For use as the sole source of nutrition or as a nutritional supplement prescribed on medical grounds for: disease-related malnutrition and growth failure

Energy Multi Fibre, liquid, tube feed, protein 4.1 g, carbohydrate 18.5 g, fat 6.7 g, fibre 0.75 g, energy 630 kJ (150 kcal)/100 mL with vitamins, minerals and trace elements. Gluten- and lactose-free, net price 200-mL bottle = £2.50, 500-mL pack = £6.25.

For short-bowel syndrome, intractable malabsorption, pre-operative preparation of undernourished patients, total gastrectomy, dysphagia, disease-related malnutrition, and growth failure. Not to be prescribed for any child under 1 year

Low Energy Multi Fibre, liquid, tube feed, protein 1.7 g, carbohydrate 10.4 g, fat 3 g, fibre 0.75 g, energy 315 kJ (75 kcal)/100mL with vitamins, minerals and trace elements. Gluten- and lactose-free, net price 200-mL bottle = £1.77, 500-mL pack = £4.43

For indications see *Nutrini Energy Multi Fibre*

Multi Fibre, liquid, protein 5.5 g, carbohydrate 24.6 g, fat 8.8 g, fibre 1.5 g, energy 840 kJ (200 kcal)/200 mL. Gluten- and sucrose-free; clinically lactose-free. Net price 200-mL bottle = £2.08, 500-mL collapsible pack = £5.20.

For indications see *Nutrini Liquid*

Nutriprem 2® (Cow & Gate)

Powder, protein 2 g, carbohydrate 7.4 g, fat 4.1 g, energy 310 kJ (75 kcal) per 100 mL when reconstituted, with vitamins and minerals. Net price 900 g = £8.80.

For catch-up growth in pre-term infants (less than 35 weeks at birth), and small-for-gestational-age infants, until 6 months corrected age

Nutrison® (Nutricia Clinical)

Energy, liquid, protein 30 g, carbohydrate 92 g, fat 29 g, energy 3200 kJ (750 kcal)/500 mL with vitamins, minerals and trace elements. Gluten- and sucrose-free; clinically lactose-free. Net price 500-

mL bottle = £3.66; 500-mL pack = £4.04; 1-litre pack = £7.32; 1.5-litre pack = £10.98.

As a nutritional supplement prescribed on medical grounds for: short-bowel syndrome, intractable malabsorption, pre-operative preparation of undernourished patients, proven inflammatory bowel disease, following total gastrectomy, dysphagia, bowel fistulas, disease-related malnutrition. Not to be prescribed for any child under 1 year; use with caution for children up to 5 years

Energy Multi Fibre, liquid, protein 30 g, carbohydrate 92.5 g, fat 29 g, fibre 7.5 g, energy 3150 kJ (750 kcal)/500 mL with vitamins, minerals, and trace elements. Gluten-free and clinically lactose-free. Net price 500-mL bottle = £4.07; 500-mL pack = £4.48; 1-litre pack = £8.14; 1.5-litre pack = £13.05.

For use as the sole source of nutrition or as a nutritional supplement prescribed on medical grounds for: short-bowel syndrome, intractable malabsorption, pre-operative preparation of undernourished patients, proven inflammatory bowel disease, following total gastrectomy, dysphagia, disease-related malnutrition. Not to be prescribed for any child under 1 year; use with caution for children up to 6 years

Multi Fibre, liquid, protein 20 g, carbohydrate 61.5 g, fat 19.5 g, fibre 7.5 g, energy 2100 kJ (500 kcal)/500 mL with vitamins, minerals and trace elements. Gluten- and sucrose-free; clinically lactose-free. Net price 500-mL bottle = £3.30; 500-mL pack = £3.63; 1-litre pack = £6.59; 1.5-litre pack = £9.89.

For indications see *Nutrison Standard* excluding bowel fistulas. Not to be prescribed for any child under 1 year; use with caution for children up to 5 years

Soya, liquid, protein 20 g, carbohydrate 61.5 g, fat 19.5 g, energy 2100 kJ (500 kcal)/500 mL, with vitamins, minerals and trace elements. Gluten- and sucrose-free; clinically lactose-free. Net price 500-mL bottle = £3.53; 1-litre pack = £7.06.

For indications see *Nutrison Standard*

Standard, liquid, protein 20 g, carbohydrate 61.5 g, fat 19.5 g, energy 2125 kJ (500 kcal)/500 mL, with vitamins, minerals and trace elements. Gluten- and sucrose-free; clinically lactose-free. Net price 500-mL bottle = £3.03; 500-mL pack = £3.36; 1-litre pack = £5.91; 1.5-litre pack = £8.87.

For use as the sole source of nutrition or as a nutritional supplement prescribed on medical grounds for: short-bowel syndrome, intractable malabsorption, pre-operative preparation of undernourished patients, proven inflammatory bowel disease, following total gastrectomy, dysphagia, bowel fistulas, disease-related malnutrition. Not to be prescribed for any child under 1 year; use with caution for children up to 5 years

Nutrison MCT® (Nutricia Clinical)

Liquid, protein 25 g, carbohydrate 61.5 g, fat 16.5 g, energy 2095 kJ (500 kcal)/500 mL with vitamins, minerals and trace elements. Gluten- and fructose-free, clinically lactose-free. Vanilla flavour. Net price 500-mL bottle = £3.32; 1-litre pack = £6.63.

For indications see *Nutrison Energy*. Not to be prescribed for any child under 1 year; use with caution for children up to 5 years

Nutrison® **Vitaplus Multi Fibre** (Nutricia Clinical)

Liquid, protein 5.5 g, carbohydrate 15 g, fat 4.3 g, energy 505 kJ (120 kcal)/100 mL, with vitamins, minerals and trace elements. Gluten- and lactose-free, net price 500-mL bottle = £4.03; 1-litre pack = £8.05; 1.5-litre pack = £12.08.

As a nutritional supplement prescribed on medical grounds for: short-bowel syndrome, intractable malabsorption, pre-operative preparation of undernourished patients, proven inflammatory bowel disease, following total gastrectomy, dysphagia, disease-

related malnutrition. Not to be prescribed for any child under 1 year; use with caution for children up to 5 years

Orgran® (Community)

Gluten-free. Pasta: lasagne (corn, rice and maize), 150 g = £2.89; shells (split pea and soya), 200 g = £2.25; spaghetti (corn, rice, rice and maize), 250 g = £2.25; spirals (buckwheat, corn, rice, rice and millet, rice and maize), 250 g = £2.25, spirals (organic brown rice), 250 g = £2.60. Crispbread (corn or rice), 200 g = £2.39. Pizza and pastry mix, 375 g = £3.33.

For gluten-sensitive enteropathies including steatorrhoea due to gluten sensitivity, coeliac disease, and dermatitis herpetiformis

Osmolite® (Abbott)

Liquid, protein 10.0 g, carbohydrate 33.9 g, fat 8.5 g, energy 1060 kJ (252 kcal)/250 mL with vitamins and minerals. Gluten- and lactose-free. Net price 250-mL can = £1.69; 500-mL bottle = £3.10, 1-litre bottle = £5.99, 1.5-litre bottle = £8.99.

For use as the sole source of nutrition or as a nutritional supplement prescribed on medical grounds for: short-bowel syndrome, intractable malabsorption, pre-operative preparation of undernourished patients, proven inflammatory bowel disease, following total gastrectomy, bowel fistulas, disease-related malnutrition, dysphagia. Not to be prescribed for any child under 1 year; use with caution for children up to 5 years

Plus, liquid, protein 5.6 g, carbohydrate 15.8 g, fat 3.9 g, energy 508 kJ (121 kcal)/100 mL with vitamins, minerals and trace elements. Gluten-free and clinically lactose-free. Net price 500-mL ready-to-hang = £3.73, 1-litre ready-to-hang = £7.20, 1.5-litre ready-to-hang = £10.79.

For indications see *Osmolite Liquid*

Paediasure® (Abbott)

Liquid, protein 7 g, carbohydrate 27.9 g, fat 12.5 g, energy 1054 kJ (252 kcal)/250 mL with vitamins and minerals. Gluten-free, clinically lactose-free. Flavours: vanilla (can, ready-to-hang and tetrapaks), strawberry, chocolate and banana (tetrapaks). Net price 250-mL can = £2.34, 500-mL ready-to-hang = £4.69, 200-mL tetrapaks = £1.88.

For use as the sole source of nutrition or as a nutritional supplement prescribed on medical grounds for children aged 1 to 10 years for short-bowel syndrome, intractable malabsorption, pre-operative preparation of undernourished patients, dysphagia, bowel fistulas, and disease-related malnutrition and/or growth failure. Not to be prescribed for any child under 1 year

Liquid with fibre, protein 7 g, carbohydrate 27.9 g, fat 12.5 g, fibre 1.3 g, energy 1054 kJ (252 kcal)/250 mL with vitamins and minerals. Gluten-free, clinically lactose-free. Flavours: vanilla (can, ready-to-hang and tetrapak), banana (tetrapak) strawberry (tetrapak). Net price 250-mL can = £2.60, 500-mL ready-to-hang = £5.20, 200-mL tetrapak = £2.08.

For indications see *Paediasure Liquid*

Paediasure® **Plus** (Abbott)

Liquid, protein 4.2 g, carbohydrate 16.7 g, fat 7.5 g, energy 632 kJ (151 kcal)/100 mL with vitamins and minerals. Gluten-free, clinically lactose-free. Flavours: vanilla (ready-to-hang and tetrapak), strawberry (tetrapak). Net price 200-mL tetrapak = £2.30, 500-mL ready-to-hang = £5.87.

For indications see *Paediasure liquid*

Liquid with fibre, tube feed, protein 4.2 g, carbohydrate 16.7 g, fat 7.5 g, energy 629 kJ (150 kcal)/100 mL with vitamins and minerals. Gluten-free, clinically lactose-free, net price 500-mL ready-to-hang = £6.25.

As a sole source of nutrition, or as a nutritional supplement for children aged 1 to 10 years with disease-related malnutrition and/or growth failure, short-bowel syndrome, intractable malabsorption, dysphagia, bowel fistulas, pre-operative preparation of undernourished patients. Not to be prescribed for any child under 1 year.

Paediatric Seravit® (SHS)

Powder, vitamins, minerals, low sodium and potassium, and trace elements. Net price 200 g (unflavoured) = £11.93; pineapple flavour, 200 g = £12.71.

For vitamin and mineral supplementation in restrictive therapeutic diets in infants and children

Pepdite® (SHS)

Powder, peptides, essential and non-essential amino acids, with carbohydrate, fat, vitamins, minerals, and trace elements. Flavour Sachets available.
Pepdite. Providing 1925 kJ (472 kcal)/100 g. Net price 400 g = £12.51
Pepdite 1+. Providing 1787 kJ (439 kcal)/100 g. Net price 400 g = £13.61; 15 x 57 g (banana flavour) = £31.88

Both for disaccharide and/or whole protein intolerance, or where amino acids or peptides are indicated in conjunction with medium chain triglycerides

Peptamen® (Nestlé Clinical)

Liquid, protein 4 g, carbohydrate 12.7 g, fat 3.7 g, energy 420 kJ (100 kcal)/100 mL, with vitamins, minerals and trace elements. Lactose- and gluten-free. Flavours: unflavoured (can), vanilla (cup, see also *Flavour Sachets*). Net price 375-mL can = £3.69, 200-mL cup = £2.25; 500-mL (Dripac-Flex) = £4.57, 1-litre = £8.23.

For use as the sole source of nutrition or as a nutritional supplement prescribed on medical grounds for: short-bowel syndrome, intractable malabsorption, proven inflammatory bowel disease, bowel fistulas. Not to be prescribed for any child under 1 year; use with caution for children up to 5 years

Nestlé Clinical Nutrition Flavour Sachets for use with *Peptamen Liquid* 200-mL cup and *Modulen IBD*. Flavours: banana, chocolate, coffee, lemon and lime, strawberry. Net price 18-sachet pack = £5.62

Pepti-Junior® (Cow & Gate)

Powder, protein 15.3 g, fat 28.3 g, carbohydrate 55.1 g, energy 2140 kJ (507 kcal)/100 g with vitamins and minerals. Used as a 13.1% solution in place of milk. Net price 450 g = £8.22.

For disaccharide and/or whole protein intolerance or where amino acids and peptides are indicated in conjunction with medium chain triglycerides

Peptisorb® (Nutricia Clinical)

Liquid, protein 20 g, carbohydrate 88 g, fat 8.5 g, energy 2100 kJ (500 kcal)/500 mL with vitamins, minerals and trace elements. Gluten-free. Net price 500-mL bottle = £4.71; 500-mL pack = £5.18; 1-litre pack = £9.36.

For use as the sole source of nutrition or as a nutritional supplement prescribed on medical grounds for: short-bowel syndrome, intractable malabsorption, proven inflammatory bowel disease, bowel fistulas. Not to be prescribed for any child under 1 year; use with caution for children up to 5 years

Perative® (Abbott)

Liquid, providing protein 15.8 g, carbohydrate 42 g, fat 8.8 g, energy 1308 kJ (310 kcal)/237 mL, with vitamins and minerals. Gluten-free, unflavoured.

Net price 237-mL can = £2.68, 500-mL ready-to-hang = £5.36, 1-litre ready-to-hang = £10.72.

For use as a nutritional supplement prescribed on medical grounds for: short-bowel syndrome, intractable malabsorption, pre-operative preparation of patients who are undernourished, proven inflammatory bowel disease, following total gastrectomy, bowel fistulas, disease-related malnutrition. Not to be prescribed for any child under 5 years

Phenylalanine, Tyrosine and Methionine-Free Amino Acid Mix *see* Amino Acid Modules, XPTM Tyrosidon

Phlexy-10® **Exchange System** (SHS)

Bar, essential and non-essential amino acids except phenylalanine 8.33 g, carbohydrate 20.5 g, fat 4.5 g/42-g bar. Citrus fruit flavour. Net price per bar = £4.06
Capsules, essential and non-essential amino acids except phenylalanine 500 mg/capsule. Net price 200-cap pack = £28.36
Tablets, essential and non-essential amino acids except phenylalanine, 1 g tablet. Net price 75-tab pack = £18.38
Drink Mix, powder, containing essential and non-essential amino acids except phenylalanine 10 g, carbohydrate 8.8 g/20-g sachet. Apple and blackcurrant, citrus, or tropical flavour. Net price 20-g sachet = £2.85

All for phenylketonuria

Phlexyvits® (SHS)

Powder, vitamins, minerals and trace elements, net price 30 × 7-g sachets = £47.70.

For use as a vitamin and mineral component of restricted therapeutic diets in older children from the age of around 11 years and over and adults with phenylketonuria and similar amino acid abnormalities

PK Aid 4® (SHS)

Powder, containing essential and non-essential amino acids except phenylalanine. Net price 500 g = £95.31.

For phenylketonuria

PK Foods (Gluten Free Foods Ltd)

Bread, white (sliced), 550 g = £4.00. Crispbread, 75 g = £2.00. Pasta (spirals), 250 g = £2.00.

For phenylketonuria and similar amino acid abnormalities

Cookies (chocolate chip, orange, or cinnamon), 150 g = £3.75. Egg replacer, 350 g = £3.75. Flour mix, 750 g = £6.99. Jelly (orange or cherry flavour), 4 × 80 g = £5.76.

For phenylketonuria

PKU 2® (Milupa)

Granules, containing essential and non-essential amino acids except phenylalanine; with vitamins, minerals, trace elements, 7.1% sucrose. Flavour: vanilla. Net price 500 g = £44.75.

For phenylketonuria

PKU 3® (Milupa)

Granules, containing essential and non-essential amino acids except phenylalanine, vitamins, minerals, and trace elements, with 3.4% sucrose. Flavour: vanilla. Net price 500 g = £44.75.

For phenylketonuria, not recommended for child under 8 years

PKU-Express® (Vitaflo)

Powder, protein (containing essential and non-essential amino acids, phenylalanine-free) 72 g, carbohydrate 15.1 g, energy 1260 kJ (301.5 kcal)/100 g with vitamins, minerals, and trace elements. Lemon, orange, or unflavoured, net price 30 x 25 g sachets = £132.00.

For phenylketonuria, not recommended for children under 8 years

PKU-gel® (Vitaflo)
Powder, protein (containing essential and non-essential amino acids, phenylalanine-free) 10.1 g, carbohydrate 8.6 g, fat 0.03 g, energy 285.5 kJ (68 kcal)/20 g with vitamins, minerals and trace elements. Orange or unflavoured, net price 30 × 20-g sachets = £76.12.
For use as part of the low-protein dietary management of phenylketonuria in children aged 1 to 10 years. Not recommended for children under 1 year

Pleniday® (TOL)
Gluten-free. Bread: loaf (sliced) net price 350 g = £1.79; country loaf (sliced), 500 g = £2.84; rustic loaf (par-baked baguette), 400 g =£2.09; petit pain, 2 × 150 g =£2.01. Pasta (penne), 250 g =£1.27; (rigate), 250 g =£1.50
For gluten-sensitive enteropathies including steatorrhoea due to gluten sensitivity, coeliac disease, and dermatitis herpetiformis

Polial® (Ultrapharm)
Biscuits. Gluten- and lactose-free. Net price 200-g pack = £2.85.
For gluten-sensitive enteropathies including steatorrhea due to gluten sensitivity, coeliac disease, and dermatitis herpetiformis

Polycal® (Nutricia Clinical)
Powder, glucose, maltose, and polysaccharides, providing 1615 kJ (380 kcal)/100 g. Net price 400 g = £3.06
Liquid, glucose polymers providing carbohydrate 61.9 g/100 mL. Low-electrolyte, protein-free. Flavours: orange and neutral. Net price 200 mL = £1.21
Both for disease-related malnutrition; malabsorption states or other conditions requiring fortification with a high or readily available carbohydrate supplement

Polycose® (Abbott)
Powder, glucose polymers, providing carbohydrate 94 g, energy 1598 kJ (376 kcal)/100 g. Net price 350-g can = £3.30.
For disease-related malnutrition; malabsorption states or other conditions requiring fortification with a high or readily available carbohydrate supplement

Pregestimil® (Mead Johnson)
Powder, protein 12.8%, carbohydrate 61.6%, fat 18.3% with vitamins and minerals. Gluten-, sucrose-, and lactose-free. Net price 400 g = £8.91.
For disaccharide and/or whole protein intolerance or where amino acids or peptides are indicated in conjunction with medium chain triglycerides

Prejomin® (Milupa)
Granules, protein 13.5 g, carbohydrate 57 g, fat 24 g, energy 2085 kJ (497 kcal)/100 g, with vitamins and minerals. Gluten-free. For preparation with water before use. Net price 400 g = £9.44.
For disaccharide and/or whole protein intolerance where additional medium chain triglyceride is not indicated

PremCare® (Heinz)
Powder, protein 1.85 g, carbohydrate 7.24 g, fat 3.96 g, energy 301 kJ (72 kcal) per 100 mL when reconstituted, with vitamins and minerals. Gluten-, sucrose-, and lactose-free. Net price 450 g = £3.58.
For catch-up growth in pre-term infants (less than 35 weeks at birth), and small-for-gestational-age infants, until 6 months post-natal age

Pro-Cal® (Vitaflo)
Powder, protein 13.5 g, carbohydrate 26.8 g, fat 56.2 g, energy 2788 kJ (667 kcal)/100 g, net price 25 x 15 g sachets =£11.04, 510 g =£10.16, 1.5 kg = £20.86, 12.5 kg = £140, 25 kg = £250.
For disease-related malnutrition, malabsorption states or other conditions requiring fortification with a fat/ carbohydrate supplement. Not to be prescribed for any child under 1 year; use with caution for young children up to 5 years

Promin® (Firstplay Dietary)
Low protein. Cous Cous, 500 g = £5.40. Pasta (alphabets, macaroni, shells, shortcut spaghetti, spirals); Pasta tricolour (alphabets, shells, spirals), net price 500 g = £5.40; Lasagne sheets, 200 g = £2.20. Pasta shells in tomato, pepper and herb sauce, 4 x 72-g sachets = £6.00; Pasta elbows in cheese and broccoli sauce, 4 x 66- g sachets = £6.00. Pasta meal, 500 g = £5.40. Pasta imitation rice, 500 g = £5.40.
For inherited metabolic disorders, renal or liver failure requiring a low-protein diet

ProMod® (Abbott)
Powder, protein 75 g, carbohydrate 7.5 g, fat 6.9 g/100 g. Gluten-free. Net price 275-g can = £8.82.
For biochemically proven hypoproteinaemia

Prosobee® (Mead Johnson)
Powder, protein 15.6%, carbohydrate 51.4%, fat 27.9% with vitamins and minerals. Gluten-, sucrose-, and lactose-free. Net price 400 g = £3.51.
For proven lactose and associated sucrose intolerance in pre-school children, galactokinase deficiency, galactosaemia, and proven whole cow's milk sensitivity

ProSure® (Abbott)
Liquid, protein 6.65 g, carbohydrate 19.4 g, fat 2.56 g, fibre 0.97 g, energy 528 kJ (125 kcal)/ 100 mL with vitamins, minerals, and trace elements. Gluten-free, clinically lactose-free. Vanilla, orange, or banana flavour, net price, 240-mL Tetrapak® = £2.70; 500-mL ready-to-hang = £5.63 (vanilla only).
As a nutritional supplement for patients with cancer cachexia. Not to be prescribed for children under 1 year; use with caution in children under 4 years

Protenplus® (Fresenius Kabi)
Liquid, protein 20 g, carbohydrate 19 g, fat 5.2 g, energy 840 kJ (200 kcal)/200 mL, with vitamins, minerals, and trace elements. Gluten-free. Vanilla, strawberry, and chocolate flavours. Net price 200-mL carton = £1.31.
As a nutritional supplement prescribed on medical grounds for: short-bowel syndrome, intractable malabsorption, pre-operative preparation of patients who are undernourished, proven inflammatory bowel disease, following total gastrectomy, dysphagia, bowel fistulas, disease-related malnutrition, continuous ambulatory peritoneal dialysis (CAPD) and haemodialysis. Not to be prescribed for any child under 1 year; use with caution for young children up to 5 years

Protifar® (Nutricia Clinical)
Powder, protein 88.5%. Low lactose, gluten- and sucrose-free. Net price 225 g = £6.20.
For biochemically proven hypoproteinaemia

Provide® (Fresenius Kabi)
Xtra Liquid, protein 3.75 g, carbohydrate 27.5 g, energy 525 kJ (125 kcal)/100 mL with vitamins, minerals and trace elements. Gluten-free. Apple, blackcurrant, carrott-apple, cherry, citrus cola, lemon & lime, melon, orange & pineapple, or tomato flavour. Net price 200-mL carton = £1.58.
As a nutritional supplement prescribed on medical grounds for: short-bowel syndrome, intractable malabsorption, pre-operative preparation of patients who are undernourished, proven inflammatory bowel disease, following total gastrectomy, dysphagia, bowel fistulas, disease-related malnutrition. Not to be prescribed for any child under 1 year; use with caution for children up to 5 years

QuickCal® (Vitaflo)

Powder, protein 4.6 g, carbohydrate 17 g, fat 77 g, energy 3260 kJ (780 kcal)/100 g, net price 25 × 13-g sachets = £9.90, 1.5 kg = £16.65.

For disease-related malnutrition, malabsorption states or other conditions requiring fortification with a fat/carbohydrate supplement. Not to be prescribed for any child under 1 year; use with caution for young children up to 5 years

Rectified Spirit Where the therapeutic qualities of alcohol are required rectified spirit (suitably flavoured and diluted) should be prescribed

Renamil® (KoRa)

Powder, protein 4.7 g, carbohydrate 70.2 g, fat 18.7 g, 1984 kJ (468 kcal)/100 g, with vitamins and minerals. Net price 1 kg = £25.40.

For chronic renal failure. Not suitable for infants and children under 1 year

Renapro® (KoRa)

Powder, whey protein providing protein 92 g, carbohydrate less than 300 mg, fat 500 mg, 1562 kJ (367 kcal)/100 g. Net price 20-g sachet = £2.32.

For dialysis and hypoproteinaemia. Not suitable for infants and children under 1 year

Resource® **Benefiber**® (Novartis Consumer Health)

Powder, soluble dietary fibre, carbohydrate 47.5 g, fibre 195 g, energy 808 kJ (190 kcal)/250 g with minerals. Gluten-free; low lactose, net price 250 g pack = £8.76, 16 x 8-g sachets = £5.72.

As a nutritional supplement prescribed on medical grounds for: short-bowel syndrome, intractable malabsorption, pre-operative preparation of undernourished patients, proven inflammatory bowel disease, following total gastrectomy, bowel fistulas, disease-related malnutrition. Not to be prescribed for children under 5 years

Resource® **Energy Dessert** (Novartis Consumer Health)

Semi-solid, protein 6 g, carbohydrate 26.5 g, fat 7.8 g, energy 839 kJ (200 kcal)/125 g with vitamins, minerals, and trace elements. Gluten-free; low lactose. Flavours: caramel, chocolate, or vanilla, net price 125-g cup = £1.35.

For use as a nutritional supplement prescribed on medical grounds for: disease-related malnutrition, short-bowel syndrome, intractable malabsorption, proven inflammatory bowel disease, bowel fistulas, dysphagia, pre-operative preparation of undernourished patients, after total gastrectomy, continuous ambulatory peritoneal dialysis (CAPD), haemodialysis. Not to be prescribed for any child under 1 year; use with caution for children up to 5 years

Resource® **Fruit Flavour Drink** (Novartis Consumer Health)

Liquid, protein 8 g, carbohydrate 67 g, energy 1276 kJ (300 kcal)/200 mL with vitamins, minerals, and trace elements. Fat- and gluten-free; low lactose. Flavours: apple, orange, or pineapple, net price 125-g carton = £1.49.

For use as a nutritional supplement prescribed on medical grounds for: disease-related malnutrition, short-bowel syndrome, intractable malabsorption, proven inflammatory bowel disease, bowel fistulas, dysphagia, pre-operative preparation of undernourished patients, after total gastrectomy. Not to be prescribed for any child under 3 years; use with caution for children up to 5 years

Resource® **Protein Extra** (Novartis Consumer Health)

Liquid, protein 18.8 g, carbohydrate 31.2 g, fat 5.6 g, energy 1057 kJ (250 kcal)/200 mL with vitamins, minerals and trace elements. Gluten-free;

low lactose. Flavours: apricot, chocolate, summer fruits, or vanilla. Net price 200-mL carton = £1.29.

For use as a nutritional supplement prescribed on medical grounds for: disease-related malnutrition, short-bowel syndrome, intractable malabsorption, proven inflammatory bowel disease, bowel fistulas, dysphagia, pre-operative preparation of undernourished patients, after total gastrectomy. Not to be prescribed for any child under 1 year; use with caution for children up to 5 years

Resource® **Shake** (Novartis Consumer Health)

Liquid, protein 8.9 g, carbohydrate 39.6 g, fat 12.3 g, energy 1280 kJ (305 kcal)/175 mL with vitamins, minerals and trace elements. Gluten-free; low lactose. Flavours: banana, chocolate, lemon, strawberry, summer fruits, toffee, or vanilla. Net price 175-mL carton = £1.46.

For use as a nutritional supplement prescribed on medical grounds for: disease-related malnutrition, short-bowel syndrome, intractable malabsorption, proven inflammatory bowel disease, bowel fistulas, dysphagia, pre-operative preparation of undernourished patients, after total gastrectomy. Not to be prescribed for any child under 1 year; use with caution for children up to 5 years

Resource® **Thickened Drink** (Novartis Consumer Health)

Liquid, carbohydrate 25 g, energy: orange 437 kJ (102 kcal); apple 428 kJ (101 kcal)/114 mL. Syrup and custard consistencies. Gluten-free; clinically lactose free, net price 12 × 114-mL cups = £7.08.

For dysphagia. Not suitable for children under 1 year

Resource® **Thickened Squash** (Novartis Consumer Health)

Liquid, syrup consistency: carbohydrate 16.9 g, energy 287 kJ (68 kcal)/100 mL; custard consistency: carbohydrate 17.8 g, energy 303 kJ (71 kcal)/100 mL. Gluten-free; clinically lactose-free. Orange and lemon flavour, net price 1.89-litre bottle = £3.99.

For dysphagia. Not suitable for children under 1 year

Resource® **ThickenUp**® (Novartis Consumer Health)

Powder, modified maize starch. Gluten- and lactose-free, net price 225 g = £3.99.

For thickening of foods in dysphagia. Not to be prescribed for children under 1 year

Rite-Diet® **Gluten-free** (Nutricia Dietary)

Gluten-free. White bread (sliced or unsliced), 400 g = £2.59. White loaf (part-baked), 400 g = £2.91. Fibre bread (sliced or unsliced), 400 g = £2.59. Fibre loaf (part-baked), 400 g = £2.91. White rolls, 4 = £2.64; (part-baked) long, 2 = £2.88. Fibre rolls, 4 = £2.64; (part-baked) long, 2 = £2.88. Flour mix (white or fibre), 500 g = £5.00.

For gluten-sensitive enteropathies including steatorrhoea due to gluten sensitivity, coeliac disease, and dermatitis herpetiformis

Rite-Diet® **Low-protein** (SHS)

Low protein. Baking mix. Net price 500 g = £5.64. Flour mix. 400 g = £4.83.

For inherited metabolic disorders, renal or liver failure requiring a low-protein diet

Scandishake® **Mix** (SHS)

Powder, protein 11.7 g, carbohydrate 66.8 g, fat 30.4 g, energy 2457 kJ (588 kcal)/serving (serving = 1 sachet reconstituted with 240 mL whole milk). Flavours: banana, caramel, chocolate, strawberry, vanilla, and unflavoured. Net price 85-g sachet = £1.85.

For disease-related malnutrition; malabsorption states or other conditions requiring fortification with a fat/carbohydrate supplement

Schar® (Nutrition Point)

Gluten-free. Bread.(white, sliced), net price 2 x 200 g = £2.50. Baguette (french bread), 400 g = £2.90. Bread rolls, 150 g = £1.50. Lunch rolls, 150 g = £1.50. White bread buns, 200 g = £2.00. Bread mix, 1 kg = £4.50. Ertha brown bread, 2 x 250 g = £3.00. Cake mix, 500 g = £4.25. Flour mix, 1 kg = £4.50. Breadsticks (Grissini), 150 g = £1.22. Cracker toast, 150 g = £1.80. Crackers, 200 g = £2.15. Crispbread, 250 g = £3.00. Pasta (fusilli, penne), 500 g = £2.80; lasagne, 250 g = £2.80; macaroni pipette, 500 g = £2.80; spaghetti, 500 g = £2.80. Pizza bases, 300 g (2 × 150 g) = £4.50. Biscuits, 200 g = £2.00. Savoy biscuits, 200 g = £2.00.

For gluten-sensitive enteropathies including steatorrhoea due to gluten sensitivity, coeliac disease, and dermatitis herpetiformis

SHS Modjul® Flavour System (SHS)

Powder, black currant, orange, pineapple, and savoury tomato flavours. Net price 100 g = £8.11.

For use with any unflavoured products based on peptides or amino acids

SMA High Energy® (SMA Nutrition)

Liquid, protein 2 g, carbohydrate 9.8 g, fat 4.9 g, energy 382 kJ (91 kcal)/100mL, with vitamins and minerals. Net price 250 mL = £1.75.

For disease-related malnutrition, malabsorption, and growth failure

SMA LF® (SMA Nutrition)

Powder, protein 1.5 g, carbohydrate 7.2 g, fat 3.6 g, energy 282 kJ (67 kcal)/100 mL, with vitamins and minerals. Net price 430 g = £3.99.

For proven lactose intolerance

Sno-Pro® (SHS)

Drink, protein 220 mg (phenylalanine 12.5 mg), carbohydrate 8 g, fat 3.8 g, energy 280 kJ (67 kcal)/100 mL. Net price 200 mL = 83p.

For phenylketonuria, chronic renal failure, and other inborn errors of metabolism

Sondalis® (Nestlé Clinical)

Sondalis Junior, powder, protein 13.9 g, carbohydrate 62.2 g, fat 18.3 g, energy 1950 kJ (467 kcal)/100 g with vitamins, minerals and trace elements. Gluten-free; clinically lactose-free. Flavour: vanilla, net price 400 g = £9.72.

For use as a sole source of nutrition or as a nutritional supplement prescribed on medical grounds for: short bowel syndrome, intractable malabsorption, pre-operative preparation of undernourished patients, proven inflammatory bowel disease, following gastrectomy, dysphagia, bowel fistulas, disease-related malnutrition, and growth failure in children aged 1-6 years. Not to be prescribed for any child under 1 year

Sunnyvale® (Everfresh)

Mixed grain bread, gluten-free. Net price 400 g = £1.79.

For gluten-sensitive enteropathies including steatorrhoea due to gluten sensitivity, coeliac disease and dermatitis herpetiformis

Suplena® (Abbott)

Liquid, protein 7.1 g, carbohydrate 60.4 g, fat 22.7 g, energy 1994 kJ (476 kcal)/237 mL. Flavour: vanilla. Net price 237-mL can = £2.28.

For patients with chronic or acute renal failure who are not undergoing dialysis; chronic or acute liver disease with fluid restriction; other conditions requiring a high-energy, low-protein, low-electrolyte, low-volume enteral feed

Survimed OPD® (Fresenius Kabi)

Liquid, protein 22.5 g, carbohydrate 75 g, fat 13 g, energy 2100 kJ (500 kcal)/500 mL, with vitamins, minerals, and trace elements. Gluten-free, and low lactose. Net price 500-mL EasyBag® = £4.85.

As a nutritional supplement prescribed on medical grounds for: short-bowel syndrome, intractable malabsorption, pre-operative preparation of patients who are undernourished, proven inflammatory bowel disease, following total gastrectomy, dysphagia, bowel fistulas, disease-related malnutrition. Not to be prescribed for any child under 1 year; use with caution for children up to 5 years

Tentrini® (Nutricia Clinical)

Liquid, tube feed, protein 3.3 g, carbohydrate 12.3 g, fat 4.2 g, energy 420 kJ (100 kcal)/100 mL, with vitamins, minerals and trace elements. Gluten- and lactose-free. Unflavoured, net price 500-mL bottle or pack = £4.00

For short-bowel syndrome, intractable malabsorption, pre-operative preparation of undernourished patients, inflammatory bowel disease, total gastrectomy, dysphagia, bowel fistulas, disease-related malnutrition, and growth failure. Not to be prescribed for any child under 1 year; use with caution for children under 7 years or 21 kg

Tentrini® Energy (Nutricia Clinical)

Liquid, tube feed, protein 4.9 g, carbohydrate 18.5 g, fat 6.3 g, energy 630 kJ (150 kcal)/100 mL, with vitamins, minerals and trace elements. Gluten- and lactose-free. Unflavoured, net price 500-mL bottle or pack = £4.95

For indications see *Tentrini*

Tentrini® Energy Multi Fibre (Nutricia Clinical)

Liquid, tube feed, protein 4.9 g, carbohydrate 18.5 g, fat 6.3 g, fibre 1.12 g, energy 630 kJ (150 kcal)/100 mL, with vitamins, minerals and trace elements. Gluten- and lactose-free. Unflavoured, net price 500-mL bottle or pack = £5.45

For indications see *Tentrini Multi Fibre*

Tentrini® Multi Fibre (Nutricia Clinical)

Liquid, tube feed, protein 3.3 g, carbohydrate 12.3 g, fat 4.2 g, fibre 1.12 g, energy 420 kJ (100 kcal)/100 mL, with vitamins, minerals and trace elements. Gluten- and lactose-free. Unflavoured, net price 500-mL bottle or pack = £4.38

For short-bowel syndrome, intractable malabsorption, pre-operative preparation of undernourished patients, inflammatory bowel disease, total gastrectomy, dysphagia, disease-related malnutrition, and growth failure. Not to be prescribed for any child under 1 year; use with caution for children under 7 years or 21 kg

Thick and Easy® (Fresenius Kabi)

Powder. Modified maize starch, net price 225-g can = £3.99; 100 × 9-g sachets = £25.58; 4.54 kg = £68.48.

Dairy. Pre-thickened milk, net price 250 mL = £1.34

Thickened Juices, liquid, modified food starch. Flavours: apple, blackcurrant, cranberry, kiwi-strawberry, and orange, net price 118-mL pot = 50p; 1.42-litre bottle = £3.50.

For thickening of foods in dysphagia. Not to be prescribed for children under 1 year except in cases of failure to thrive

Thixo-D® (Sutherland)

Powder, modified maize starch, gluten-free. Net price 375-g tub = £5.79.

For thickening of foods in dysphagia. Not to be prescribed for children under 1 year except in cases of failure to thrive

Tinkyada® (General Dietary)
Gluten-free. Brown rice pasta (elbows, fettucini, fusilli, penne, shells, spaghetti, spirals). Net price 454 g = £3.00.
For gluten-sensitive enteropathies including steatorrhoea due to gluten-sensitivity, coeliac disease and dermatitis herpetiformis

Tritamyl® (Gluten Free Foods Ltd)
Gluten-free. Flour, net price 1 kg = £5.60. Brown bread mix, 1 kg = £5.60. White bread mix, 1 kg = £5.60.
For gluten-sensitive enteropathies including steatorrhoea due to gluten sensitivity, coeliac disease and dermatitis herpetiformis

L-Tyrosine (SHS)
Powder, net price 100 g = £12.53.
For use as a supplement in maternal phenylketonurics who have low plasma tyrosine concentrations

Ultra® (Ultrapharm)
Gluten-free. Baguette, net price 400 g = £2.46. Bread, net price 400 g = £2.46. High-fibre bread, 500 g = £3.35. Crackerbread, 100 g = £1.77. Pizza base, net price 400 g = £2.65.
For gluten-sensitive enteropathies including steatorrhoea due to gluten sensitivity, coeliac disease and dermatitis herpetiformis
Low protein. PKU bread, 400 g = £2.16. PKU flour, 500 g = £3.07. PKU biscuits, 200 g = £2.21. PKU cookies, 250 g = £2.31. PKU pizza base, 400 g = £2.21. PKU savoy biscuits, 150 g = £2.06.
For inherited metabolic disorders, renal or liver failure requiring a low-protein diet

Vita-Bite® (Vitaflo)
Bar, protein 30 mg (less than 2.5 mg phenylalanine), carbohydrate 15.35 g, fat 8.4 g, energy 572 kJ (137 kcal)/25 g. Chocolate flavoured, net price 25 g = 85p.
For inherited metabolic disorders, renal or liver failure requiring a low-protein diet. Not recommended for any child under 1 year

Vitajoule® (Vitaflo)
Powder, glucose polymers, providing carbohydrate 96 g, energy 1610 kJ (380 kcal)/100 g. Net price 125 g = 99p, 200 g = £1.65, 500 g = £3.04, 2.5 kg = £15.00, 25 kg = £98.00.
For disease-related malnutrition; malabsorption states or other conditions requiring fortification with a high or readily available carbohydrate supplement

Vitamins and Minerals
Only for use in the management of actual or potential vitamin or mineral deficiency; not to be prescribed as dietary supplements or 'pick-me-ups'

Vitapro® (Vitaflo)
Powder, whole milk proteins, containing all essential amino acids, 75%. Net price 250 g = £6.10, 2 kg = £47.90.
For biochemically proven hypoproteinaemia

Vitaquick® (Vitaflo)
Powder. Modified maize starch. Net price 100 g = £2.38, 300 g = £5.67; 2 kg = £28.92; 6 kg = £73.86.
For thickening of foods in dysphagia. Not to be prescribed for children under 1 year except in cases of failure to thrive

Vitasavoury® (Vitaflo)
Powder, protein 12 g, carbohydrate 24 g, fat 54 g, energy 2610 kJ (630 kcal)/100 g, net price 10 x 50-g sachets = £13.75, 12 x 33-g ready cups = £11.62. Flavours: chicken, leek and potato, mushroom.
As a nutritional supplement for disease-related malnutrition, malabsorption states or other conditions requiring fortification with a fat/carbohydrate supple-

ment. Not to be prescribed for any child under 1 year; use with caution for young children up to 5 years

Wysoy® (Wyeth)
Powder, carbohydrate 6.9%, fat 3.6%, and protein 2.1% with vitamins and minerals when reconstituted. Net price 430 g = £3.98; 860 g = £7.58.
For proven lactose and associated sucrose intolerance in preschool children, galactokinase deficiency, galactosaemia and proven whole cow's milk sensitivity

---

Conditions for which foods may be prescribed on FP10, GP10 (Scotland), or when available WP10 (Wales)

NOTE. This is a list of clinical conditions for which the ACBS has approved food products. It is essential to check the list of products (above) for availability.

Amino acid metabolic disorders and similar protein disorders
See histidinaemia; homocystinuria; maple syrup urine disease; phenylketonuria; low-protein products; synthetic diets; tyrosinaemia.

Bowel fistulas
Complete foods: Complan Ready-to-Drink; Elemental 028 and 028 Extra; Emsogen; Enrich and Enrich Plus; Ensure; Ensure Powder; Foodlink Complete; Frebini, Frebini Energy, Frebini Energy Fibre; Fresubin Energy, Fresubin Original Liquid and Sip feeds, Fresubin 1000, and Fresubin 1200 Complete; Isosource Energy, Standard; Jevity; Novasource Forte and GI Control; Nutrini, Nutrini Energy and Fibre; Nutrison Standard and Multifibre; Osmolite Liquid and Plus; Paediasure Liquid and Plus; Peptamen; Peptisorb; Sondalis; Tentrini and Energy.
Nutritional supplements: Clinutren Dessert, Fruit, ISO and 1.5; Enlive; Ensure Plus; Formance; Forticreme; Fortifresh; Fortijuce; Fortimel; Fortisip; Fortisip Multi Fibre, Protein; Fresubin HP Energy; Modulen IBD; Nutrison Energy, and MCT; Perative; Protenplus; Provide Xtra; Resource Benefiber, Energy, Dessert, Protein Extra, Shake; Survimed OPD.

Calcium intolerance
Locasol.

Carbohydrate malabsorption
See also synthetic diets; malabsorption states.

(a) *Disaccharide intolerance*: Caloreen; Calsip; Duocal Super Soluble and Duocal Liquid; Maxijul LE, Liquid, Super Soluble; Nutramigen; Nutrison Soya; Pepdite; Pepti-Junior; Polycal liquid and powder; Polycose powder; Pregestimil; Prejomin; Pro-Cal; QuickCal; Vitajoule; Vitasavoury. See also lactose intolerance; lactose with associated sucrose intolerance.

(b) *Isomaltose intolerance*: Glucose (dextrose).

(c) *Glucose and galactose intolerance*: Comminuted Chicken Meat (Cow & Gate); Fructose; Galactomin 19 (fructose formula).

(d) *Lactose intolerance*: Colief; Comminuted Chicken Meat (SHS); Enfamil Lactofree; Farley's Soya Formula; Galactomin 17; InfaSoy; Isomil powder; Nutramigen; Nutrison Soya; Pepdite; Pregestimil; Prejomin; Prosobee; SMA LF; Wysoy.

(e) *Lactose with associated sucrose intolerance*: Comminuted Chicken Meat (SHS); Farley's Soya Formula; Galactomin 17; InfaSoy; Nutramigen; Nutrison Soya; Pepti-Junior; Pregestimil; Prejomin; Prosobee; Wysoy.

(f) *Sucrose intolerance*: Glucose (dextrose) and see also synthetic diets; malabsorption states; lactose with associated sucrose intolerance.

NOTE. Lactose or sucrose intolerance is defined as a condition of intolerance to an intake of the relevant disaccharide confirmed by demonstrated clinical benefit of the effectiveness of the disaccharide-free diet, and presence of reducing substances and/or excessive acid in the stools, a low concentration of the corresponding disaccharidase enzyme on intestinal biopsy, or by breath tests or lactose tolerance tests

Carnitine palmitoyl transferase deficiency (CPTD)
Monogen

Coeliac disease
See gluten-sensitive enteropathies.

Continuous Ambulatory Peritoneal Dialysis (CAPD)
See dialysis.

Cystic fibrosis
See malabsorption states.

Dermatitis Herpetiformis
See gluten-sensitive enteropathies.

Dialysis
Nutritional supplements for haemodialysis or continuous ambulatory peritoneal dialysis (CAPD) patients: Clinutren Dessert; Enrich Plus; Ensure Plus; Formance; Forticreme; Fresubin HP Energy; Kindergen; Nepro; Protenplus; Renapro; Resource Energy Dessert; Suplena.

Disaccharide intolerance
See carbohydrate malabsorption.

Dysphagia
Complete foods: Enfamil AR; Enrich and Enrich Plus; Ensure; Ensure Powder; Foodlink Complete; Frebini Original, Energy Fibre and Energy; Fresubin Energy, Fresubin Energy Fibre (sip and tube feed), Fresubin Original Fibre, Fresubin Original Liquid and Sip Feeds, Fresubin 1000, and Fresubin 1200 Complete; Isosource Energy, Fibre Junior and Standard; Jevity; Novasource GI Control and Forte; Nutrini Fibre and Standard; Nutrison Multi Fibre, Energy Multi Fibre, Soya, Standard and Vitaplus Multifibre; Osmolite Liquid and Plus; Paediasure Liquid, Liquid with fibre and Plus; Sondalis; Tentrini, Energy, Energy Multi Fibre, Multi Fibre.
Nutritional supplements: Clinutren Dessert, Fruit, ISO, and 1.5; Clinutren Thickened Drinks, Enlive; Ensure Plus and Yoghurt style; Formance; Forticreme; Fortifresh; Fortijuce; Fortimel; Fortisip, Multi Fibre, Protein; Fresubin HP Energy; Nutrison Energy and MCT; Protenplus; Provide Xtra; Resource Energy Dessert, Resource Benefiber, Protein Extra, ThickenUp, Thickened Squash, and Shake; Survimed OPD.
Thickeners: Clinutren Thickener, Nutilis; Thick & Easy powder and thickened juices; Thixo-D; Vitaquick.
NOTE. Dysphagia is defined as that associated with intrinsic disease of the oesophagus, e.g. oesophagitis; neuromuscular disorders, e.g. multiple sclerosis and motor neurone disease; major surgery and/or radiotherapy for cancer of the upper digestive tract; protracted severe inflammatory disease of the upper digestive tract, e.g. Stevens-Johnson syndrome and epidermolysis bullosa

Epilepsy (ketogenic diet in)
Alembicol D; Liquigen; Medium-Chain Triglyceride Oil (MCT).

Flavouring
For use with any unflavoured SHS product based on peptides or amino acids: SHS Flavour Modjul; Flavour Sachets

Galactokinase deficiency and galactosaemia
Farley's Soya Formula; Galactomin 17; InfaSoy; Isomil powder; Prosobee; Wysoy

Gastrectomy (total)
Complete foods: Enrich; Enrich Plus; Ensure; Ensure Powder; Foodlink Complete; Frebini Original; Fresubin Energy, Fresubin Energy Fibre (sip and tube feed), Fresubin Original Fibre, Fresubin Original Liquid and Sip Feeds, Fresubin 1000, and Fresubin 1200 Complete; Isosource Energy, Fibre and Standard; Jevity and Plus; Novasource GI Control, and Forte; Nutrison Multi Fibre, Energy Multi Fibre, Soya and Standard; Osmolite Liquid and Plus; Sondalis Junior; Tentrini, Energy, Energy Multi Fibre, Multi Fibre.
Nutritional supplements: Clinutren Dessert, Fruit, ISO and 1.5; Enlive; Ensure Plus; Formance; Fortijuce; Fortimel; Fortipudding; Fortisip, Multi Fibre, Protein; Fresubin HP Energy; Nutrison Energy and MCT; Perative; Provide Xtra; Resource Benefiber, Resource Energy Dessert, Protein Extra, and Shake; Survimed OPD.

Glucose/galactose intolerance
See carbohydrate malabsorption.

Glutaric aciduria
XLys, Low Try Maxamaid

Gluten-sensitive enteropathies
Aproten flour; Arnott gluten-free rice cookies; Baker's Delight wheat-, gluten- and dairy-free bread; Barkat gluten-free bread mix, brown or white rice bread (unsliced), Brown or white rice pizza crust; Bi-Aglut biscuits, crackers, cracker toast, lasagne, pasta (fusilli, macaroni, penne, spaghetti); DS Dietary Specials Mixes: brown or white bread, white cake, white or fibre; Ener-G brown and white rice bread, gluten-free tapioca bread, rice loaf, Seattle brown loaf, cookies (vanilla), xanthum gum, gluten-free rice pasta (cannelloni, lasagna, macaroni, shells, small shells, spaghetti, tagliatelli, vermicelli); brown rice pasta (lasagna, macaroni, spaghetti); Gadsby's white bread (sliced or unsliced), white bread flour, white bread rolls; Glutafin bread, multigrain white loaf (sliced or unsliced, white or part-baked), rolls (white or part-baked), fibre bread, mixes (white, multigrain white, fibre, multigrain fibre), biscuits (digestive, savoury, sweet (without chocolate or sultanas), tea), crackers, high fibre crackers and pasta (lasagne, penne, spirals, spaghetti), pizza bases; Glutano gluten-free biscuits, crackers, crisp-bread, flour mix, pastas (animal shapes, macaroni, spaghetti, spirals, tagliatelle), wholemeal bread (sliced or par-baked), baguette or rolls (par-baked), white sliced bread (par-baked); Juvela gluten-free harvest mix, loaf and high-fibre loaf (sliced and unsliced), bread rolls, fibre bread rolls, part-baked

rolls with or without fibre, crispbread, mix and fibre mix; digestive biscuits, savoury biscuits and tea biscuits, pizza bases; Lifestyle gluten-free bread rolls, brown and white bread, high-fibre bread or rolls; Pleniday bread and pastas; Polial gluten-free biscuits; Rite-Diet gluten-free fibre rolls, high-fibre bread (sliced and unsliced), white bread (sliced and unsliced), white rolls, part-baked fibre loaf and long rolls; Schar gluten-free bread, bread mix, ertha brown bread, bread rolls and buns, crackers, cake mix, cracker toast, crispbread, flour mix, french bread (baguette), pasta (fusilli, lasagne, macaroni pipette penne, rigati, rings, shells, spaghetti), pizza base, biscuits, savoy biscuits, white bread buns, wholemeal flour mix; Sunnyvale gluten-free bread; Tinkyada gluten-free brown rice pasta (elbows, fettucini, fusilli, penne, shells, spaghetti, spirals); Tritamyl flour, brown bread mix and white bread mix; Ultra gluten-free baguette, bread, bread rolls, high-fibre bread, crackerbread, pizza base; Valpiform bread mix, country loaf, pastry mix, petites baguettes

Gluten-sensitive enteropathies with coexisting established wheat sensitivity
Ener-G pizza bases, Seattle brown rolls (round or long), Six flour loaf; Glutafin Crisp Bread, Crisp Roll

Glycogen storage disease
Caloreen; Corn Flour or Corn Starch; Glucose (dextrose); Maxijul LE, Liquid (orange flavour), and Super Soluble; Polycal; Polycal Liquid and powder; Polycose; Pro-Cal; QuickCal; Vitajoule; Vitasavoury.

Growth Failure (disease related)
Enrich Plus ready-to-hang; Fortini, Fortini Multifibre; Frebini Original; Infatrini; Nutrini Extra, Multifibre and Standard; Paediasure Liquid and Liquid with fibre and Plus; SMA High Energy; Sondalis Junior; Survimed OPD; Tentrini, Energy, Energy Multi Fibre, Multi Fibre.

Haemodialysis
See dialysis.

Histidinaemia
See low-protein products; synthetic diets.

Homocystinuria
Analog XMet; Methionine-Free Amino Acid Mix; Vitaflo Flavour Pac, HCU gel; XMet Maxamaid; XMet Maxamum, and see also low-protein products; synthetic diets.

Hyperlipoproteinaemia type I
Alembicol D; Liquigen; Medium Chain Triglyceride Oil.

Hyperlysinaemia
Analog XLys; XLys Maxamaid

Hypermethioninaemia
Analog XMet; Methionine-Free Amino Acid Mix; XMet Maxamaid; XMet Maxamum.

Hypoglycaemia
Corn Flour or Corn Starch; and see also glycogen storage disease.

Hypoproteinaemia
Casilan 90; Dialamine; Maxipro Super Soluble; Maxisorb; ProMod; Protifar; Renapro; Vitapro.

Inflammatory Bowel Disease
Complete foods: Elemental 028; Elemental 028 Extra; Emsogen; Enrich; Ensure; Ensure Powder; Foodlink Complete; Frebini Original; Fresubin

Energy, Fresubin Energy Fibre (sip and tube feed) Fresubin Original Liquid and Sip Feeds, Fresubin 1000, and Fresubin 1200 Complete; Isosource Energy, Fibre and Standard; Jevity and Plus; Novasource GI Control, and Forte; Nutini Extra, and Fibre; Nutrison Multi Fibre, Energy Multi Fibre, Soya and Standard; Osmolite Liquid and Plus; Peptamen, Sondalis Junior; Tentrini, Energy, Energy Multi Fibre, Multi Fibre.
Nutritional supplements: Clinutren Dessert, ISO, Fruit and 1.5; Enlive; Ensure Plus; Formance; Forticreme; Fortifresh; Fortijuce; Fortimel; Fortipudding; Fortisip, Multi Fibre, Protein; Fresubin HP Energy; Nutrison Energy, MCT and Pepti Powder; Perative; Provide Xtra; Resource Benefiber, Dessert Energy, Protein Extra, and Shake; Survimed OPD.

Intestinal lymphangiectasia
See malabsorption states.

Intestinal surgery
See malabsorption states

Isomaltose intolerance
See carbohydrate malabsorption.

Isovaleric acidaemia
Leucine-Free Amino Acid Mix; XLeu Analog; XLeu Maxamaid.

Lactose intolerance
See carbohydrate malabsorption.

Lipoprotein lipase deficiency (primary and secondary)
Monogen

Liver failure
Alembicol D; Aminex low-protein biscuits, cookies and rusks; Aproten products (anellini, biscuits, bread mix, cake mix, crispbread, ditalini, rigatini, spaghetti, tagliatelle); Ener-G low protein egg replacer, rice bread; Generaid; Generaid Plus; Juvela low-protein (chocolate chip, orange, and cinnamon flavour) cookies, loaf (sliced and unsliced), bread rolls, mix; Liquigen; Loprofin egg replacer, egg white replacer; Loprofin low-protein bread (sliced and unsliced), bread rolls (part-baked), white rolls, fibre bread (sliced and unsliced), mix, breakfast cereal, pasta (macaroni, penne, spaghetti long, pasta spirals, vermicelli), sweet biscuits, chocolate cream-filled biscuits, crackers, cookies (chocolate chip, cinnamon), wafers (orange, chocolate, vanilla); Medium Chain Triglyceride Oil; Nepro; Promin low-protein pasta (alphabets, macaroni, shells, shortcut spaghetti, spirals), pasta tricolour (alphabets, shells, spirals), pasta meal, Rite-Diet low-protein baking mix, flour mix; Suplena; Ultra low-protein, canned bread (brown and white); Ultra PKU biscuits, bread, cookies, flour, pizza base and savoy biscuits; Valpiform cookies with chocolate nuggets, shortbread biscuits; Vita-Bite.

Long chain acyl-CoA dehydrogenase deficiency (LCAD)
Monogen

Low-protein products
Aminex low-protein biscuits, cookies and rusks; Aproten products (anellini, biscuits, bread mix, cake mix, crispbread, ditalini, rigatini, spaghetti, tagliatelle); Ener-G low protein egg replacer, rice bread; Juvela low-protein (chocolate chip, orange, and cinnamon flavour) cookies, loaf (sliced and unsliced), mix, bread rolls; Loprofin egg replacer,

egg white replacer; Loprofin low-protein bread (sliced and unsliced), mix, rolls (part-baked), fibre bread (sliced or unsliced), herb crackers, pasta (macaroni, spaghetti long, pasta spirals, vermicelli); sweet biscuits, chocolate cream-filled biscuits, crackers, cookies (chocolate chip, cinnamon), wafers (orange, chocolate, vanilla), breakfast cereal; PK Foods bread (sliced), crispbread, pasta (spirals); PKU-Gel; Promin low-protein pasta (alphabets, macaroni, shells, shortcut spaghetti, spirals), pasta tricolour (alphabets, shells, spirals), pasta meal, pasta imitation rice; Rite-Diet low-protein flour mix, baking mix; Ultra low-protein, canned bread (brown and white); Ultra PKU biscuits, bread, cookies, flour, pizza base and savoy biscuits; Valpiform cookies with chocolate nuggets, shortbread biscuits; Vita-Bite.

Malabsorption states
(see also gluten-sensitive enteropathies; liver failure; carbohydrate malabsorption; intestinal lymphangiectasia; milk intolerance and synthetic diets); includes short-bowel syndrome. It should be noted that hyperosmolar feeds should be **avoided** if the short bowel ends in a stoma or the short bowel is anastomosed to the colon.

(a) *Protein sources*: Caprilon Formula; Comminuted Chicken Meat (Cow & Gate); Duocal Super Soluble and Liquid; Maxipro Super Soluble; Maxisorb; MCT Pepdite; Neocate; Neocate Advance; Pepdite.

(b) *Fat sources*: Alembicol D; Calogen; Caprilon Formula; Liquigen; MCT Pepdite; Medium Chain Triglyceride Oil; Pro-Cal; QuickCal; Vitasavoury.

(c) *Carbohydrate*: Caloreen; Maxijul LE, Liquid, and Super Soluble; Novasource GI Control, and Forte; Nutini Extra and Multifibre, Polycal Liquid and Powder; Polycose; Pro-Cal; QuickCal; Resource Benefiber; Vitajoule; Vitasavoury.

(d) *Fat/carbohydrate sources*: Calshake; Duobar; Duocal Liquid, MCT and Super Soluble; Scandishake; SPS Energy Bar.

(e) *Complete Feeds*: For use as the sole source of nutrition or as a nutritional supplement prescribed on medical grounds: Caprilon Formula; Elemental 028; Elemental 028 Extra; Emsogen; Enrich; Ensure; Ensure Powder; Foodlink Complete; Frebini Original; Fresubin Energy, Fresubin Energy Fibre (sip and tube feed), Fresubin Original Liquid and Sip Feeds, Fresubin 1000, and Fresubin 1200 Complete; Isosource Energy, Fibre and Standard; Jevity, and Plus; MCT Pepdite; Novasource GI Control, and Forte; Nutrini, Extra and Fibre; Nutrison Multi Fibre, Energy Multi Fibre, Soya, Standard, Vitaplus Multi Fibre; Osmolite Liquid and Plus; Paediasure Liquid, Liquid with fibre and Plus; Pepdite; Peptamen; Pepti-Junior; Pregestimil; SMA High Energy; Sondalis Junior; Tentrini, Energy, Energy Multi Fibre, Multi Fibre.

(f) *Nutritional supplements*: Nutritional supplements prescribed on medical grounds: Clinutren Dessert, Fruit, ISO, Junior, and 1.5; Enlive; Enrich Plus; Ensure Bar and Plus; Formance; Forticreme; Fortifresh; Fortijuce; Fortimel; Fortisip, Multi Fibre, Protein; Fresubin HP Energy; Nutrison Energy, MCT, and Pepti Powder; Perative; Protenplus; Provide Xtra; Resource Shake and Benefiber; Survimed OPD.

(g) *Minerals*: Aminogran Mineral Mixture; Metabolic Mineral Mixture.

(h) *Vitamins*: As appropriate, and see synthetic diets.

(i) *Vitamins and Minerals*: Energivit; Paediatric Seravit

Malnutrition (disease-related)
Complete foods: Calogen; Caloreen; Calshake; Duobar; Duocal Liquid, MCT, and Super Soluble; Enrich and Plus; Ensure; Ensure Powder; Foodlink Compete; Frebini Original; Fresubin Energy, Fresubin Energy Fibre (sip and tube feed), Fresubin Original Liquid and Sip Feeds, Fresubin 1000, and Fresubin 1200 Complete; Infatrini; Isosource Energy, Fibre and Standard; Jevity and Plus; Maxijul LE, Liquid and Super Soluble; Novasource GI Control and Forte; Nutrini Extra, Fibre and Standard; Nutrison Multi Fibre, Energy Multi Fibre, Soya, Standard, Vitaplus Multi Fibre; Osmolite Liquid and Plus; Paediasure Liquid, Liquid with fibre and Plus; Polycal Liquid and Powder; Polycose; Scandishake; SMA High Energy; Tentrini, Energy, Energy Multi Fibre, Multi Fibre; Vitajoule.
Nutritional supplements: Clinutren Dessert, Fruit, ISO and 1.5; Enlive; Ensure Plus; Formance; Forticreme; Fortifresh; Fortijuce; Fortimel; Fortini, Fortini Multifibre, Fortipudding; Fortisip, Multi Fibre, Protein; Fresubin HP Energy; Nutrison Energy and MCT; Perative; ProSure, Provide Xtra; Pro-Cal; Quickcal; Resource Benefiber, Dessert Energy, Protein Xtra, and Shake; Sondalis Junior; Survimed OPD; Vitasavoury.

Maple syrup urine disease
Analog MSUD; MSUD Maxamaid; MSUD Maxamum; MSUD Aid III, and see also low-protein products; synthetic diets.

Methylmalonic acidaemia
Analog XMet, Thre, Val, Isoleu; XMet, Thre, Val, Isoleu Maxamaid; XMet, Thre, Val, Isoleu Maxamum; Methionine, Threonine, Valine-Free and Isoleucine-Low Amino Acid Mix.

Milk protein sensitivity
Comminuted Chicken Meat (SHS); Farley's Soya Formula; InfaSoy; Isomil powder; Nutramigen; Prosobee; Wysoy; and see also synthetic diets.

Nutritional support for adults
(a) **Nutritionally complete feeds.** For use as the sole source of nutrition or as a necessary nutritional supplement prescribed on medical grounds:
   (i) Gluten-Free: Foodlink Complete; Fortifresh; Fresubin Liquid and Sip Feeds; Nutrison Multi Fibre, Energy Multi Fibre and Standard; Sondalis Junior.
   (ii) Lactose- and Gluten-Free: Enrich; Ensure, Ensure Powder; Fresubin Original Fibre; Nutrison Soya; Osmolite Liquid and Plus; Sondalis 1.5.
   (iii) Containing fibre: Enrich; Fresubin Energy Fibre (tube and sip feed), Fresubin Original Fibre; Isosource Fibre; Jevity; Novasource GI Control, and Forte; Nutrini Extra, and Fibre; Nutrison Multi Fibre, Energy Multi Fibre; Paediasure with Fibre.
   (iv) Elemental Feeds: Elemental 028; Elemental 028 Extra; Emsogen; Peptamen; Peptisorb.

(b) **Nutritional source supplements**: see synthetic diets; malabsorption states.
   (i) General supplements. Necessary nutritional supplements prescribed on medical grounds: Clinutren

range; Enlive; Enrich Plus; Ensure Plus; Foodlink Complete; Formance; Forticreme; Fortijuce; Fortimel; Fortini, Fortini MultiFibre; Fortisip; Fortisip Multi Fibre; Fresubin HP Energy; Fresubin 1000, and 1200 Complete; Maxisorb; Nutrison Energy and MCT; Perative; Provide Xtra; Resource Shake; Survimed OPD.

(ii) Carbohydrates; lactose-free and gluten-free; [1]Caloreen; [1]Maxijul LE Liquid, and Super Soluble; [1]Polycal; [1]Polycal Liquid; Polycose; Pro-Cal; QuickCal; Resource Benefiber; Vitajoule; Vita-savoury.

(iii) Fat: Alembicol D; Calogen; Liquigen; MCT Oil.

(iv) Fat/carbohydrate sources: Calshake; Duobar; Duocal Liquid, MCT Powder and Super Soluble (low-electrolyte content); Scandishake, SPS Energy Bar.

(v) Nitrogen sources: Casilan 90 (whole protein based, low-sodium); Maxipro Super Soluble (whey protein based, low-sodium); Maxisorb; Pro-Mod (whey protein based, low-sodium).

(vi) Minerals: Aminogran Mineral Mixture; Metabolic Mineral Mixture.

Phenylketonuria Aminex low-protein biscuits, cookies and rusks; Aminogran Food Supplement (powder and tablets) and Mineral Mixture; Analog LCP; Analog XP; Aproten products (annellini, biscuits, bread mix, cake mix, crispbread, ditalini, rigatini, spaghetti, tagliatelle); Ener-G low protein egg replacer; Juvela low-protein loaf (sliced and unsliced), bread rolls, cookies (chocolate chip, orange, and cinnamon flavour), mix; Lofenalac; Loprofin egg replacer; Loprofin low-protein bread (sliced and unsliced), breakfast cereal, rolls (part-baked), rolls (white), fibre bread (sliced and unsliced), mix and pasta (macaroni, penne, spaghetti long, pasta spirals, vermicelli), sweet biscuits, chocolate cream-filled biscuits, crackers, cookies (chocolate chip, cinnamon), wafers (orange, chocolate, vanilla); Loprofin PKU drink; Metabolic Mineral Mixture; Milupa PKU2 and PKU3; Phlexy-10 exchange system; Phlexyvits; PK Aid 4; PK Foods bread (sliced), crispbread, pasta (spirals), cookies (chocolate chip, orange, cinnamon), egg replacer, flour mix, jelly (orange, cherry); PKU-Gel; Promin low-protein pasta (alphabets, macaroni, shells, shortcut spaghetti, spirals), pasta tricolour (alphabets, shells, spirals), pasta meal; Rite-Diet low-protein baking mix, flour mix; Sno-Pro; L-Tyrosine supplement; Ultra low-protein, canned white bread; Ultra PKU biscuits, bread, cookies, flour, pizza base, savoy biscuits; Valpiform cookies, shortbread biscuits; XP Maxamaid XP Concentrate Maxamaid; XP Maxamum; and see low-protein products and synthetic diets

Propionic acidaemia
Analog XMet, Thre, Val, Isoleu; XMet, Thre, Val, Isoleu Maxamaid; XMet Thre, Val, Isoleu Maxamum; Methionine, Threonine, Valine-Free and Isoleucine-Low Amino Acid Mix.

Protein intolerance
See amino acid metabolic disorders, low-protein products, milk protein sensitivity, synthetic diets, and whole protein sensitivity.

---

1. Have low electrolyte content

Refsum's Disease
Fresubin Original Liquid and Sip Feeds.

Renal dialysis
See Dialysis.

Renal failure
Aminex low-protein biscuits, cookies and rusks; Aproten products (annellini, biscuits, bread mix, cake mix, crispbread, ditalini, rigatini, spaghetti, tagliatelle); Dialamine; Ener-G low protein egg replacer, rice bread; Juvela low-protein (chocolate chip, orange, and cinnamon flavour) cookies, loaf (sliced and unsliced), bread rolls and flour mix; Kindergen; Loprofin egg replacer, egg white replacer, Loprofin bread (sliced and unsliced), breakfast cereal, rolls (part-baked), rolls (white), fibre bread (sliced and unsliced), mix and pasta (macaroni, penne, spaghetti long, pasta spirals, vermicelli), sweet biscuits, chocolate cream-filled biscuits, crackers, cookies (chocolate chip, cinnamon), wafers (orange, chocolate, vanilla); Nepro; Promin low-protein pasta (alphabets, macaroni, shells, shortcut spaghetti, spirals), pasta tricolour (alphabets, shells, spirals), pasta meal; Renamil; Rite-Diet low-protein flour mix, baking mix, Sno-Pro Drink; Suplena; Ultra low-protein, canned bread (brown and white); Ultra PKU bread, biscuits, cookies, flour, pizza base and savoy biscuits; Valpiform cookies with chocolate nuggets, shortbread biscuits, Vita-Bite

Short-bowel syndrome
See Malabsorption states.

Sicca Syndrome
Bioxtra Moisturising Gel; Glandosane; Luborant; Oralbalance; Saliva Orthana; Salivace; Saliveze; Salivix.

Sucrose intolerance
See Carbohydrate malabsorption.

Synthetic diets
(a) *Fat*: Alembicol D; Calogen; Liquigen; Medium Chain Triglyceride Oil; Pro-Cal; QuickCal; Vitasavoury.
(b) *Carbohydrate*: Caloreen; Maxijul LE, Liquid, Super Soluble; Polycal; Polycal Liquid; Polycose powder; Pro-Cal; QuickCal; Vitasavoury.
(c) *Fat/carbohydrate sources*: Calshake; Duobar; Duocal Liquid, MCT Powder and Super Soluble (low-electrolyte content); Scandishake.
(d) *Minerals*: Aminogran Mineral Mixture; Metabolic Mineral Mixture.
(e) *Protein sources*: see malabsorption states, complete feeds.
(f) *Vitamins*: as appropriate and see malabsorption states, nutritional support for adults.
(g) *Vitamins and Minerals*: Paediatric Seravit; Phlexyvits.

Tyrosinaemia
Analog XPhen, Tyr; Analog XPhen, Tyr, Met; XPhen, Tyr Maxamaid; XPTM Tyrosidon; XPT Tyrosidon.

Urea cycle disorders
L-Arginine supplement

Vomiting in infancy
Instant Carobel, Nestargel.

Whole protein sensitivity
Caprilon Formula; MCT Pepdite; Neocate; Neocate Advance; Nutramigen; Pepdite; Pepti-Junior; Pregestimil; Prejomin.
NOTE. Defined as intolerance to whole protein, proven by at least two withdrawal and challenge tests, as suggested by an accurate dietary history

Xerostomia
Bioxtra Moisturising Gel; Glandosane; Luborant;
Biotene Oralbalance Dry Mouth Saliva Replacement
Gel; Saliva Orthana; Saliveze; Salivix.

Conditions for which toilet preparations may be prescribed on FP10, GP10 (Scotland), WP10 (Wales)

NOTE. This is a list of clinical conditions for which the
ACBS has approved toilet preparations. For details of the
preparations see Chapter 13.

Birthmarks
See disfiguring skin lesions.

Dermatitis
Aveeno Bath Oil; Aveeno Cream; Aveeno Colloidal;
Aveeno Baby Colloidal ; E45 Emollient Bath Oil;
E45 Emollient Wash Cream; E45 Lotion; Vaseline
Dermacare Cream and Lotion

Dermatitis herpetiformis
See gluten-sensitive enteropathies.

**Disfiguring skin lesions (birthmarks, mutilating
lesions, scars, vitiligo)**
Covermark classic foundation and finishing powder;
Dermablend Cover Creme, Leg and Body Cover, and
Setting Powder; Dermacolor Camouflage cream and
fixing powder; Keromask masking cream and
finishing powder; Veil Cover cream and Finishing
Powder. (Cleansing Creams, Cleansing Milks, and
Cleansing Lotions are excluded)

Disinfectants (antiseptics)
May be prescribed on an FP10 only when ordered in
such quantities and with such directions as are
appropriate for the treatment of patients, but not for
general hygenic purposes.

Eczema
See dermatitis.

Photodermatoses (skin protection in)
Ambre Solaire Total Screen for Sun Intolerant skin
SPF 60; Coppertone Ultrashade 23; Delph Sun
Lotion SPF 15, SPF 20, SPF 25, and SPF 30; E45
Sun Block SPF 25, and 50; RoC Total Sunblock
Cream SPF 25; Spectraban 25, and Ultra; Sunsense
Ultra; Uvistat Sun Block Cream Factor 20, and
Ultrablock Suncream Factor 30.

Pruritus
See dermatitis.

Appendix 8: Wound management products and elastic hosiery

A8.1　Wound dressings

An overview of the management of *chronic wounds* (including venous ulcers and pressure sores) and the role of different dressings is given below as is the NICE guidance on difficult-to-heal surgical wounds; the notes do not deal with the management of clean surgical wounds which usually heal very rapidly. The correct dressing for wound management depends not only on the type of wound but also on the stage of the healing process. The principal stages of healing are:

- cleansing, removal of debris;
- granulation, vascularisation;
- epithelialisation.

Greater understanding of the requirements of a surgical dressing, including recognition of the benefits of maintaining a moist environment for wound healing, has improved the management of chronic wounds.

The ideal dressing needs to ensure that the wound remains:

- moist with exudate, but not macerated;
- free of clinical infection and excessive slough;
- free of toxic chemicals, particles or fibres;
- at the optimum temperature for healing;
- undisturbed by the need for frequent changes;
- at the optimum pH value.

As wound healing passes through its different stages, variations in dressing type may be required to satisfy better one or other of these requirements. Depending on the type of wound or the stage of the healing process, the functions of dressings may be summarised as follows:

Type of wound	Role of dressing
Dry, necrotic, black Yellow, sloughy	Moisture retention or rehydration If dry, moisture retention or rehydration If moist, fluid absorption Possibly odour absorption Possibly antimicrobial activity
Clean, exuding (granulating)	Fluid absorption Thermal insulation Possibly odour absorption Possibly antimicrobial activity
Dry, low exudate (epithelialising)	Moisture retention or rehydration Low adherence Thermal insulation

A decrease in pain and reduction in healing time is achieved to a marked extent with **alginate**, **foam**, **hydrogel** and **hydrocolloid** dressings and also to an important extent with **vapour-permeable films** and **membranes**; dressings such as dry gauze have little place. Practices such as the use of irritant cleansers may be harmful and are largely obsolete; removal of debris and dressing remnants should need minimal irrigation with physiological saline.

Alginate, **foam**, **hydrogel** and **hydrocolloid** dressings are designed to absorb wound exudate and thus to control the state of hydration of a wound. All are claimed to be effective, but as yet there have been few trials able to establish a clear advantage for any particular product. The choice between different dressings may therefore often depend not only on the type and stage of the wound, but also on personal experience, availability of the dressing, patient preference or tolerance and site of the wound.

***

NICE guidance (debriding agents for difficult-to-heal surgical wounds). The National Institute for Clinical Excellence has stated that alginate, foam, hydrocolloid, hydrogel, and polysaccharide (as beads or paste) dressings as well as maggots may reduce pain from difficult-to-heal surgical wounds. There is insufficient evidence to support one debriding agent over another and choice should be based on patient acceptability (including factors such as comfort and odour control), type and location of the wound, and total cost (including time for changing the dressings).

***

A8.1.1   Alginate dressings

The gelling characteristics of alginate dressings vary according to the product used. Some products only gel to a limited extent to form a partially gelled sheet that can be lifted off; others form an amorphous gel that can be rinsed off with water or physiological saline. A secondary covering is needed. They are highly absorbent and are therefore suitable for moderately or heavily exuding wounds, but not for eschars or for dry wounds.

Algisite® M (S&N Hlth.)
Calcium alginate fibre, sterile, flat non-woven dressing, net price 5 cm × 5 cm = 79p, 10 cm × 10 cm = £1.63, 15 cm × 20 cm = £4.37
Uses: moderately to heavily exuding wounds
Algisite® M Rope, net price 2 cm × 30 cm = £2.89
Uses: moderately to heavily exuding cavity wounds

Algosteril® (Beiersdorf)
Calcium alginate dressing. Net price 5 cm × 5 cm = 78p, 10 cm × 10 cm = £1.78, 10 cm × 20 cm = £3.02
Uses: moderately to heavily exuding wounds
Algosteril® Rope, net price 2 g, 30 cm = £3.16
Uses: moderately to heavily exuding cavity wounds

Curasorb® (Tyco)
Calcium alginate dressing, net price 5 cm × 5 cm = 69p, 10 cm × 10 cm = £1.46, 10 cm × 14 cm = £2.36, 10 cm × 20 cm = £2.87, 15 cm × 25 cm = £5.05, 30 cm × 61 cm = £26.50 (other sizes **NHS**)
Curasorb® Plus, calcium alginate dressing, 10 cm × 10 cm = £2.00
Curasorb® Zn, calcium alginate and zinc dressing, 5 cm × 5 cm = 78p, 10 cm × 10 cm = £1.65, 10 cm × 20 cm = £3.24 (other sizes **NHS**)

Kaltostat® (ConvaTec)
(Alginate Dressing, BP 1993, type C). Calcium alginate fibre, flat non-woven pads, 5 cm × 5 cm, net price = 80p, 7.5 cm × 12 cm = £1.73, 10 cm × 20 cm = £3.43, 15 cm × 25 cm = £5.90, (**NHS**) 30 cm × 60 cm = £24.68
Uses: moderately to heavily exuding wounds
Kaltostat® Wound Packing, net price 2 g = £3.22
Uses: moderately to heavily exuding cavity wounds

Melgisorb® (Mölnlycke)
Calcium sodium alginate fibre, sterile, highly absorbent, gelling dressing, flat non-woven pads, net price 5 cm × 5 cm = 78p, 10 cm × 10 cm = £1.62, 10 cm × 20 cm = £3.03
Uses: moderately to heavily exuding wounds including leg ulcers, dermal lesions and traumatic wounds
Melgisorb® Cavity, calcium sodium alginate fibre, sterile, highly absorbent, gelling filler ribbon, net price 32 cm × 2.2 cm, 3 pieces (2 g) = £3.06
Uses: moderately to heavily exuding cavity wounds, fistulas, sinuses, pressure sores and deep leg ulcers

SeaSorb® (Coloplast)
SeaSorb® Soft, alginate containing hydrocolloid dressing, sterile, highly absorbent, gelling dressing, 5 cm × 5 cm = 82p, 10 cm × 10 cm = £1.95, 15 cm × 15 cm = £3.70
Uses: heavily exuding wounds including leg ulcers and pressure sores
SeaSorb® Soft Filler, calcium sodium alginate fibre, highly absorbent, gelling filler, 44 cm = £2.30
Uses: moderately to heavily exuding cavity wounds, fistulas, sinus drainage, decubitus and deep leg ulcers

Sorbalgon® (Hartmann)
Calcium alginate dressing, net price 5 cm × 5 cm = 70p, 10 cm × 10 cm = £1.47
Uses: for medium to heavily exuding wounds
Sorbalgon T®, calcium alginate cavity dressing, net price 2 g, 32 cm = £3.00
Uses: for medium to heavily exuding wounds

Sorbsan® (Unomedical)
(Alginate Dressing, BP 1993, type A). Calcium alginate fibre, highly absorbent, flat non-woven pads, 5 cm × 5 cm, net price = 72p, 10 cm × 10 cm = £1.52, 10 cm × 20 cm = £2.85
Uses: moderately to heavily exuding wounds
Sorbsan® Plus, alginate dressing bonded to a secondary absorbent viscose pad, net price 7.5 cm × 10 cm = £1.54, 10 cm × 15 cm = £2.72, 10 cm × 20 cm = £3.47, 15 cm × 20 cm = £4.81
Uses: moderately to heavily exuding shallow wounds and ulcers
Sorbsan® Surgical Packing, 30 cm (2 g) = £3.16
Sorbsan® Ribbon, 40 cm (with 12.5-cm probe) = £1.84
Uses: moderately to heavily exuding cavity wounds
Sorbsan® SA **NHS** calcium alginate fibre, highly absorbent flat non-woven pads for wound contact bonded to adhesive semi-permeable polyurethane foam. Net price 9 cm × 11 cm = £2.24
Uses: moderately to lightly exuding shallow wounds

Tegagen® (3M)
(Alginate Dressing, BP 1993, type B). Net price 5 cm × 5 cm = 74p, 10 cm × 10 cm = £1.53
Uses: for leg ulcers, pressure sores, second degree burns, post-operative wounds, fungating carcinomas
Tegagen® Rope, net price 2 cm × 30 cm = £2.59
Uses: moderately to heavily exudating cavity wounds

Urgosorb® (Parema)
Alginate containing hydrocolloid dressing without adhesive border, sterile, net price 10 cm × 10 cm = £1.80, 10 cm × 20 cm = £3.30
Urgosorb Rope cavity dressing, net price 30 cm = £2.40

A8.1.2   Foam dressings

Foam dressings vary from products that are suitable for lightly exuding wounds to highly absorbent structures for heavily exuding wounds. They may also be used as secondary dressings. In hypergranulating (or overgranulating) tissue (which may arise from the use of occlusive dressings such as hydro-colloids), changing to a more permeable product such as a foam dressing may be beneficial.

Polyurethane Foam Dressing, BP 1993

Absorbent foam dressing of low adherence, sterile
Lyofoam®, net price 7.5 cm × 7.5 cm = 95p, 10 cm × 10 cm = £1.12, 10 cm × 17.5 cm = £1.75, 15 cm × 20 cm = £2.36, other sizes (NHS) 10 cm × 25 cm = £4.71 (hosp. only), 25 cm × 30 cm = £11.35 (SSL)
Uses: treatment of burns, decubitus ulcers, donor sites, granulating wounds

Polyurethane Foam Film Dressing, Sterile, with Adhesive Border

(Drug Tariff specification 47)
Allevyn® *Lite Island*, net price 9.75 cm × 16.5 cm = £1.68; 13.5 cm × 13.5 cm = £2.19; 16 cm × 16 cm = £2.60; 13.5 cm × 23.5 cm = £3.35 (S & N Hlth)
Lyofoam® *Extra Adhesive*, net price 9 cm × 9 cm = £1.18; 15 cm × 15 cm = £2.21; 22 cm × 22 cm = £4.36; 30 cm × 30 cm = £6.34; sacral, 15 cm × 13 cm = £1.81; 22 cm × 26 cm = £3.43 (SSL)
Lyofoam® *K*, net price 9 cm × 9 cm = £1.26 (SSL)
Tielle®, net price 11 cm × 11 cm = £2.17; 15 cm × 15 cm = £3.54; 18 cm × 18 cm = £4.51; 7 cm × 9 cm = £1.17; 15 cm × 20 cm = £4.43; *Tielle*® *Sacrum* 18 cm × 18 cm = £3.28 (J&J)
Trufoam®, net price 7 cm × 9 cm = £1.05; 11 cm × 11 cm = £2.00 (Unomedical)
Uses: light to moderately exuding wounds, not recommended for dry superficial wounds

Polyurethane Foam Film Dressing, Sterile, without Adhesive Border

(Drug Tariff specification 47)
Allevyn® *Lite*, net price 5 cm × 5 cm = 96p; 10 cm × 10 cm = £1.74; 10 cm × 20 cm = £2.98; 15 cm × 20 cm = £3.72 (S&N Hlth)
Allevyn® *Thin* (with adhesive border) 5 cm × 6 cm = 89p, 10 cm × 10 cm = £1.80, 15 cm × 15 cm = £2.97, 15 cm × 20 cm = £3.60
FlexiPore®, net price 10 cm × 10 cm = £1.73; 10 cm × 30 cm = £3.60 (TSL)
Lyofoam® *Extra*, net price 10 cm × 10 cm = £1.88; 17.5 cm × 10 cm = £3.18; 20 cm × 15 cm = £4.12; 25 cm × 10 cm = £3.84; (NHS) 30 cm × 25 cm = £14.35 (SSL)
Transorbent®, net price 5 cm × 7 cm = 93p; 10 cm × 10 cm = £1.75; 15 cm × 15 cm = £3.22; 20 cm × 20 cm = £5.14 (Unomedical)
Uses: light to moderately exuding wounds, not recommended for dry superficial wounds

Polyurethane Foam Film Dressing, Sterile, with Adhesive Border

Tielle® *Lite*, net price 11 cm × 11 cm = £2.08; 7 cm × 9 cm = £1.10; 8 cm × 15 cm = £2.56; 8 cm × 20 cm = £2.71 (J&J)
Uses: light to non-exuding wounds
Allevyn® *Adhesive*, 7.5 cm × 7.5 cm = £1.27, 10 cm × 10 cm = £1.86, 12.5 cm × 12.5 cm = £2.28, 17.5 cm × 17.5 cm = £4.50, 12.5 cm × 22.5 cm = £3.50, 22.5 cm × 22.5 cm = £6.56 (S&N Hlth)
Allevyn® *Plus Adhesive* (with adhesive border) 12.5 cm × 12.5 cm = £2.80; 17.5 cm × 17.5 cm = £5.40; 12.5 cm × 22.5 cm = £4.96
Allevyn® *Sacrum* (with adhesive border), shaped, 17 cm × 17 cm = £3.36, 22 cm × 22 cm = £4.93
Uses: light to moderately exuding sacral wounds
Biatain® *Adhesive*, net price 12 cm × 12 cm = £2.21; 18 cm × 18 cm = £4.42; 23 cm × 23 cm (sacral) = £3.78, 19 cm × 20 cm (heel) = £4.41; 6 cm diameter = £1.48 (Coloplast)
Uses: moderate to heavily exuding wounds

Curafoam® *Island*, net price 10 cm × 10 cm = £1.21, 15 cm × 15 cm = £2.19, 20 cm × 20 cm = £4.34 (Tyco)
Uses: moderate to heavily exuding wounds
Tielle® *Plus*, net price 11 cm × 11 cm = £2.40; 15 cm × 15 cm = £3.91; 15 cm × 20 cm = £4.91; 15 cm × 15 cm (sacrum) = £2.85 (J&J)
Uses: moderate to heavily exuding wounds
Trufoam®, net price 15 cm × 15 cm = £3.35, 15 cm × 20 cm = £4.20 (Unomedical)
Uses: moderate to heavily exuding wounds

Polyurethane Foam Film Dressing, Sterile, without Adhesive Border

Advazorb®, net price 5 cm × 7.5 cm = 45p, 10 cm × 10 cm = 80p (Advancis)
Allevyn®, net price 5 cm × 5 cm = £1.08, 9 cm × 9 cm = £3.00 (NHS), 10 cm × 10 cm = £2.13, 10 cm × 20 cm = £3.43, 20 cm × 20 cm = £5.72 10.5 cm × 13.5 cm (heel) = £4.28 (S&N Hlth)
Allevyn® *Compression*, net price 5 cm × 6 cm = £1.06; 10 cm × 10 cm = £2.19; 15 cm × 15 cm = £3.65, 15 cm × 20 cm = £4.16 (S&N Hlth)
Uses: moderately exuding wounds, burns, decubitus ulcers, and leg ulcers
Biatain® *Non-Adhesive*, net price 10 cm × 10 cm = £2.00; 15 cm × 15 cm = £3.69; 20 cm × 20 cm = £5.60; circular, 5 cm diameter = £1.05; 8 cm diameter = £1.48 (Coloplast)
Curafoam® *Plus*, net price 6 cm × 6 cm = £1.06, 10 cm × 10 cm = £1.65, 10 cm × 13 cm = £2.05, 10 cm × 20 cm = £3.20, 20 cm × 20 cm = £5.04 (Tyco)
Hydrafoam®, net price 10 cm × 10 cm = £1.73, 10 cm × 20 cm = £3.10, 15 cm × 15 cm = £3.32, 20 cm × 20 cm = £5.15 (Tyco)
3M®, net price 8.9 cm × 8.9 cm (fenestrated) = £2.09, 10 cm × 10 cm = £2.05, 10 cm × 20 cm = £3.48, 20 cm × 20 cm = £5.55, 10 cm × 60 cm = £11.75 (3M)
Tielle® *Plus Borderless*, net price 11 cm × 11 cm = £2.88; 15 cm × 20 cm = £5.40 (J&J)
Trufoam® *NA*, net price 5 cm × 5 cm = £1.00, 10 cm × 10 cm = £1.90, 15 cm × 15 cm = £3.50 (Unomedical)
Uses: moderate to heavily exuding wounds

Allevyn® (S&N Hlth.)

Hydrophilic polyurethane dressing, foam sheets with trilaminate structure, non-adherent wound contact layer, foam based central layer, bacteria-and water-proof outer layer
Allevyn® *Plus Cavity* Sterile, highly absorbent polyurethane dressing consisting of a vapour-permeable foam matrix, net price 1.5 cm × 20 cm = £1.58, 5 cm × 6 cm = £1.58; 10 cm × 10 cm = £2.63; 15 cm × 20 cm = £5.27
Uses: heavily exuding deep wounds, including deep leg ulcers, decubitus ulcers, abscesses; management of post-operative wounds including pilonidal sinus excision
Allevyn® *Cavity*, circular, 5 cm diameter = £3.52, 10 cm = £8.38, tubular 9 cm × 2.5 cm = £3.41, 12 cm × 4 cm = £6.00
Uses: moderately to heavily exuding cavity wounds including deep pressure sores and leg ulcers, surgical incisions and excisions such as pilonidal sinus excisions

Avance® (SSL)

Silver impregnated polyurethane foam film dressing
Avance® (without adhesive border), 10 cm × 10 cm = £2.55, 10 cm × 17 cm = £4.06, 15 cm × 20 cm = £5.61
Avance®*A* (with adhesive border), 9 cm × 9 cm = £2.14, 12 cm × 12 cm = £3.55, 15 cm × 15 cm = £4.35, 15 cm × 13 cm (sacral) = £3.20
Uses: for exudating wounds

Cavi-Care® (S&N Hlth.)

Soft, conforming cavity wound dressing prepared by mixing thoroughly for 15 seconds immediately before use and allowing to expand its volume within the cavity. Net price 20 g = £16.55

Uses: in the management of open post-operative granulating cavity wounds (with no underlying tracts or sinuses) such as pilonidal sinus excision, dehisced surgical wounds, hydradenitis suppurativa wounds, peri-anal wounds, perineal wounds, pressure sores

A8.1.3 Hydrogel dressings

Hydrogel dressings are most commonly supplied as an amorphous, cohesive material that can take up the shape of a wound. A secondary covering is needed. These dressings are generally used to donate liquid to dry sloughy wounds and facilitate autolytic debridement but they may also have the ability to absorb limited amounts of exudate. Hydrogel sheets are also available which have a fixed structure; such products have limited fluid handling capacity. Hydrogel sheets are best avoided in the presence of infection.

Aquaform® (Unomedical)

(Drug Tariff specification 50) Hydrogel containing modified starch copolymer. Net price 15 g = £1.77

Uses: for dry, sloughy or necrotic wounds, lightly exuding wounds, granulating wounds

Aquaflo® (Tyco)

Net price 4 cm diameter = £2.41, 7.5 cm = £2.50, 12 cm = £5.16

Curagel® (Tyco)

Net price 5 cm × 7.5 cm = £1.74, 10 cm × 10 cm = £2.71

Curagel Island (with adhesive border), net price 7.5 cm × 10 cm = £2.47, 12.5 cm × 12.5 cm = £3.58

Debrisan® (Pharmacia)

Beads, dextranomer. Net price 60-g castor = £29.01

Uses: for exudative and infected wounds, decubital ulcers, leg ulcers, hand burns, surgical wounds, post-traumatic wounds, sprinkle onto wound to a thickness of at least 3 mm and cover with appropriate dressing, renew before saturation occurs (usually once or twice daily)

Paste, dextranomer in a soft paste basis. Net price 10-g pouch = £4.99

Uses: for exudative and infected wounds, decubital ulcers, leg ulcers, surgical wounds, post-traumatic wounds, apply to a thickness of at least 3 mm and cover with appropriate dressing, renew before saturation occurs (usually once or twice daily)

Geliperm® (Geistlich)

Gel sheets in wet form, 10 cm × 10 cm = £2.19, 12 cm × 13 cm = £4.88 ([NHS]); 12 cm × 26 cm = £8.73 ([NHS])

Uses: wound and ulcer dressing, burns, donor sites

GranuGel® (ConvaTec)

(Drug Tariff Specification 50). Net price 15 g = £1.94

Uses: dry, sloughy or necrotic wounds, lightly exuding wounds, granulating wounds

Hydrosorb® (Hartmann)

Absorbent, transparent, hydrogel sheets containing polyurethane polymers covered with a semi-permeable film

Hydrosorb®, 5 cm × 7.5 cm = £1.74; 10 cm × 10 cm = £2.74; 20 cm × 20 cm = £6.60

Hydrosorb® comfort (with adhesive border, water-proof), 4.5 cm × 6.5 cm = £1.60; 7.5 cm × 10 cm = £2.50; 12.5 cm × 12.5 cm = £3.60

Uses: second degree burns, donor sites; chronic wounds where granulation is unsatisfactory, including leg ulcers, pressure sores

Intrasite Conformable® (S&N Hlth.)

(Drug Tariff specification 50). Soft and easily moulded non-woven dressing impregnated with Intrasite gel, net price 10 cm × 10 cm = £1.51; 10 cm × 20 cm = £2.03; 10 cm × 40 cm = £3.63

Uses: for dry, sloughy or necrotic wounds, lightly exuding wounds; granulating wounds

Intrasite® Gel (S&N Hlth.)

(Drug Tariff specification 50). A ready-mixed hydrogel containing modified carmellose polymer applied directly into the wound. Net price 8-g sachet = £1.51, 15-g sachet = £2.02, 25-g sachet = £3.05

Uses: for dry, sloughy or necrotic wounds; lightly exuding wounds; granulating wounds

Iodoflex® (S&N Hlth.)

Paste, iodine 0.9% as cadexomer–iodine in a paste basis with gauze backing, net price 5-g unit = £3.90; 10 g = £7.80; 17 g = £12.34

Uses: for treatment of chronic exuding wounds, such as leg ulcers, apply to wound surface, remove gauze backing and cover; renew when saturated (usually 2–3 times weekly, daily for heavily exuding wounds); max. single application 50 g, max. weekly application 150 g; max. duration up to 3 months in any single course of treatment

Cautions: caution in patients with severe renal impairment or history of thyroid disorders; iodine may be absorbed particularly if large wounds treated

Contra-indications: avoid in thyroid disorders, in those receiving lithium, in pregnancy and breast-feeding and use in children

Iodosorb® (S&N Hlth.)

Ointment, iodine 0.9% as cadexomer–iodine in an ointment basis, net price 10 g = £4.31; 20 g = £8.62

Powder, iodine 0.9% as cadexomer–iodine microbeads, net price 3-g sachet = £1.84

Uses: for treatment of chronic exuding wounds, such as leg ulcers, apply to wound surface to depth of approx. 3 mm and cover; renew when saturated (usually 2–3 times weekly, daily for heavily exuding wounds); max. single application 50 g, max. weekly application 150 g; max. duration up to 3 months in any single course of treatment

Cautions: caution in patients with severe renal impairment or history of thyroid disorders; iodine may be absorbed particularly if large wounds treated

Contra-indications: avoid in thyroid disorders, in those receiving lithium, in pregnancy and breast-feeding, and use in children

Novogel® (Ford)

Sterile, glycerol-based hydrogel sheets, net price 10 cm × 10 cm = £2.90; 30 cm × 30 cm, standard = £12.28, thin = £11.60; 5 cm × 7.5 cm = £1.78; 15 cm × 20 cm = £5.54; 20 cm × 40 cm = £10.54; 7.5 cm diameter = £2.64

Uses: diabetic wounds, burns, leg ulcers, decubitus ulcers, donor sites

Nu-Gel® (J&J)

(Drug Tariff Specification 50). A ready-mixed hydrogel containing alginate, applied directly into wound and covered with secondary dressing. Net price 15 g = £1.91

Uses: dry, sloughy or necrotic, lightly exuding or granulating wounds

Purilon® Gel (Coloplast)

(Drug Tariff specification 50). Net price 8 g = £1.47, 15 g = £1.95

Uses: for dry, sloughy or necrotic wounds; lightly exuding wounds; granulating wounds

■ Protease modulating matrix

Promogran® (J&J)

Sterile, collagen and oxidised regenerated cellulose matrix, applied directly to wound and covered with secondary dressing, net price 28 cm^2 (hexagonal) = £4.63, 123 cm^2 (hexagonal) = £14.23

Uses: chronic wounds free of necrotic tissue and infection, e.g. leg ulcers, pressure sores, diabetic foot ulcers

---

A8.1.4   Hydrocolloid dressings

Hydrocolloid dressings are usually presented as an absorbent layer on a vapour-permeable film or foam. Because of their impermeable nature, hydrocolloid dressings facilitate rehydration and autolytic debridement of dry, sloughy, or necrotic wounds; they are also suitable for promoting granulation. Fibrous dressings made from modified carmellose fibres resemble alginate dressings (e.g. *Aquacel*®); these are not occlusive.

Alione® (Coloplast)

Sterile, semi-permeable hydrocolloid dressing with adhesive border, net price 10 cm × 10 cm = £2.69, 12.5 cm × 12.5 cm = £3.70, 15 cm × 15 cm = £4.68, 20 cm × 20 cm = £7.01; without adhesive border 10 cm × 10 cm = £2.69, 12.5 cm × 12.5 cm = £3.70, 15 cm × 15 cm = £4.68, 20 cm × 20 cm = £7.01

Uses: chronic and exudating wounds

Aquacel® (ConvaTec)

Soft sterile non-woven pad containing hydrocolloid fibres, net price 5 cm × 5 cm = 97p; 10 cm × 10 cm = £2.31; 15 cm × 15 cm = £4.35

Uses: moderately to heavily exuding wounds

Aquacel® *Ribbon*, 2 cm × 45 cm = £2.36

Uses: moderately to heavily exuding cavity wounds

Aquacel® *Ag* (silver impregnated), net price 5 cm × 5 cm = £1.65, 10 cm × 10 cm = £3.93, 15 cm × 15 cm = £7.40, 20 cm × 30 cm = £18.36

Uses: moderately to heavily exuding wounds

Aquacel® *Ag Ribbon* (silver impregnated), net price 2 cm × 45 cm = £3.95

Uses: moderately to heavily exuding cavity wounds

Askina® **Biofilm Transparent** (Braun)

Sterile, semi-permeable, polyurethane film dressing with hydrocolloid adhesive, net price, 10 cm × 10 cm = 98p, 15 cm × 15 cm = £2.23, 20 cm × 20 cm = £2.91

Biofilm S® (Braun) [NHS]

Hydrocolloid dressing with polyurethane-polyester backing; also in powder form for direct application into wound, 10 cm × 10 cm, net price = £1.65; 20 cm × 20 cm = £5.70; *Biofilm*® powder, 1 sachet = £1.82

CombiDERM® (ConvaTec)

Dressing with hydrocolloid adhesive border and absorbent wound contact pad, net price 10 cm × 10 cm = £1.39; 14 cm × 14 cm = £1.93; 15 cm × 18 cm (triangular) = £3.34; 20 cm × 20 cm = £3.64; 20 cm × 23 cm (triangular) = £4.39

Uses: chronic exuding wounds such as leg ulcers, pressure sores; postoperative wounds

CombiDERM N® Hydrocolloid absorbent dressing, net price 7.5 cm × 7.5 cm = £1.09; 14 cm × 14 cm = £1.94; 15 cm × 25 cm = £3.95

Uses: chronic wounds (e.g. leg ulcers and diabetic ulcers) and exuding wounds (e.g. biopsies), and surgical wounds

Comfeel® (Coloplast)

Soft elastic pad consisting of carmellose sodium particles embedded in adhesive mass; smooth outer layer and polyurethane film backing; available as sheets, powder in plastic blister units and paste for

direct application into the wound: Ulcer dressing, net price 10 cm × 10 cm = £2.33; 15 cm × 15 cm = £4.66; 20 cm × 20 cm = £7.13; other sizes ([NHS]): 4 cm × 6 cm = £1.17; powder 6 g = £3.97; paste 12-g sachet = £1.53; 50 g = £5.89

Comfeel® **Plus** (Coloplast)

Hydrocolloid dressings containing carmellose sodium and calcium alginate. Contour dressing 6 cm × 8 cm = £1.86; 9 cm × 11 cm = £3.22; Ulcer Dressing, 4 cm × 6 cm = 82p; 10 cm × 10 cm = £2.09; 15 cm × 15 cm = £4.48; 18 cm × 20 cm (triangular) = £4.79; 20 cm × 20 cm = £6.45; Transparent Dressing, 5 cm × 7 cm = 56p; 9 cm × 14 cm = £2.04; 15 cm × 20 cm = £2.83; Pressure Relieving Dressing, 7 cm diameter = £2.95; 10 cm = £3.95; 15 cm = £5.95

Cutinova® (Beiersdorf)

Cutinova® *Hydro Border* Sterile, highly absorbent semi-transparent two-layered polyurethane dressing with vapour-permeable foam matrix on a semi-permeable film backing, net price 5 cm × 6 cm = £1.06; 10 cm × 10 cm = £2.12; 15 cm × 20 cm = £4.49

Uses: moderately to heavily exuding wounds including burns and decubitus ulcers

Cutinova® *Thin* [NHS] Sterile, highly absorbent, semi-transparent two-layered polyurethane dressing on a semi-permeable film backing, net price 5 cm × 6 cm = £1.16; 10 cm × 10 cm = £1.87; 15 cm × 20 cm = £5.13

Uses: lightly exuding wounds including abrasions, burns, decubitus ulcers, donor sites, skin protection and postoperative wounds

DuoDERM® (ConvaTec)

Extra Thin (formerly *Granuflex*® *Extra Thin*), net price 5 cm × 10 cm = 64p; 7.5 cm × 7.5 cm = 67p; 10 cm × 10 cm = £1.10; 15 cm × 15 cm = £2.38; [NHS] 5 cm × 20 cm = £1.38

Uses: minimally exuding wounds, such as abrasions, minor burns or minor surgery

Signal, hydrocolloid dressing with 'Time to change' indicator net price 10 cm × 10 cm = £1.79, 14 cm × 14 cm = £3.14, 20 cm × 20 cm = £6.24, 18.5 cm × 19.5 cm (heel) = £4.39, 22.5 cm × 20 cm (sacral) = £5.13

Uses: leg ulcers, pressure sores, diabetic ulcers, burns, postoperative wounds

Granuflex® (ConvaTec)

Hydrocolloid wound contact layer bonded to plastic foam layer, with outer semi-permeable polyurethane film, net price 10 cm × 10 cm = £2.33; 15 cm × 15 cm = £4.43; 15 cm × 20 cm = £4.80; 20 cm × 20 cm = £6.66; [NHS] 20 cm × 30 cm = £11.15

Granuflex® *Paste* ([NHS]), net price 30 g = £2.68

Granuflex® *Bordered Dressing*, 6 cm × 6 cm = £1.48; 10 cm × 10 cm = £2.78; 15 cm × 15 cm = £5.35; triangular dressing, 10 cm × 13 cm = £3.28; 15 cm × 18 cm = £5.11

Uses: chronic ulcers, pressure sores, open wounds, debridement of wounds; powders, gel, and pastes used with sheet dressings to fill deep or heavily exuding wounds

Hydrocoll® (Hartmann)

Hydrocolloid dressing with adhesive border and absorbent wound contact pad, net price 5 cm × 5 cm = 87p; 7.5 cm × 7.5 cm = £1.43; 10 cm × 10 cm = £2.08; 15 cm × 15 cm = £3.91; Concave dressing, 8 cm × 12 cm = £1.83; Sacral dressing, 12 cm × 18 cm = £3.11; Basic dressing without adhesive border, 10 cm × 10 cm = £2.11; Thin film dressing, 7.5 cm × 7.5 cm = 60p; 10 cm × 10 cm = 99p, 15 cm × 15 cm = £2.24

Uses: light to medium exuding wounds

Replicare Ultra® (S&N Hlth.)
Sterile, adhesive hydrocolloid dressing with outer semi-permeable polyurethane film backing, net price 10 cm × 10 cm = £2.21, 15 cm × 15 cm = £4.40, 20 cm × 20 cm = £6.49; Sacral dressing, 15 cm × 18 cm = £4.16
Uses: lightly to moderately exuding wounds such as leg ulcers, pressure sores; postoperative wounds; superficial burns

Tegasorb® (3M)
Hydrocolloid dressing with adhesive border, net price 10 cm × 12 cm (oval) = £2.16; 13 cm × 15 cm (oval) = £4.04; without adhesive border 10 cm × 10 cm = £2.21; 15 cm × 15 cm = £4.27
Uses: chronic wounds such as leg ulcers and pressure sores

Tegasorb® Thin Sterile, semi-permeable, clear film dressing with hydrocolloid and adhesive border, net price 10 cm × 12 cm (oval) = £1.44; 13 cm × 15 cm (oval) = £2.69; without adhesive border 10 cm × 10 cm = £1.44
Uses: low to moderately exuding wounds including leg ulcers, abrasions, burns, and donor sites

Ultec Pro® (Tyco)
Sterile, semi-permeable hydrocolloid dressing with adhesive border, net price 10.5 cm × 10.5 cm = £1.39, 14 cm × 14 cm = £2.24, 21 cm × 21 cm = £4.49, 15 cm × 18 cm (sacral) = £3.17, 19.5 cm × 23 cm (sacral) = £4.88; without adhesive border 10 cm × 10 cm = £2.19, 15 cm × 15 cm = £4.27, 20 cm × 20 cm = £6.43
Uses: lightly to moderately exuding wounds

Versiva® (ConvaTec)
Sterile, semi-permeable hydrocolloid dressing with adhesive border, net price 9 cm × 9 cm = £2.22, 14 cm × 14 cm = £4.14, 19 cm × 19 cm = £6.45, 19 cm × 24 cm = £7.79, 19 cm × 17.7 cm (sacral) = £5.49, 21 cm × 22.5 cm (sacral) = £7.79, 19.5 cm × 18.5 cm (heel) = £6.62
Uses: chronic and acute exudating wounds

■ Keloid dressings
Silicone gel sheets are used to reduce and prevent hypertrophic and keloid scarring. They should not be used on open wounds. Application times should be increased gradually. Silicone sheets can be washed and reused.

Cica-Care® (S&N Hlth.)
Soft, self-adhesive, semi-occlusive silicone gel sheet with backing. Net price, 6 cm × 12 cm = £12.44; 15 cm × 12 cm = £24.25

Mepiform® (Mölnlycke)
Self-adhesive silicone gel sheet with polyurethane film backing, net price 5 cm × 7.5 cm = £3.13; 10 cm × 18 cm = £12.70; 4 cm × 30 cm = £8.94

Silgel® (Nagor)
Silicone gel sheet, net price 10 cm × 10 cm = £13.50; 20 cm × 20 cm = £40.00; 40 cm × 40 cm = £144.00; 10 cm × 5 cm = £7.50; 15 cm × 10 cm = £19.50; 30 cm × 5 cm = £19.50; 10 cm × 30 cm = £31.50; 25 cm × 15 cm (submammary) = £21.12; 46 cm × 8.5 cm (abdominal) = £39.46; 5 cm diameter (circular) = £4.00
Silgel® STC-SE silicone gel, net price, 20-mL tube = £19.00

■ Hyaluronic acid
Hyalofill® (ConvaTec)
Hyalofill-F, [NHS] flat, non-woven, absorbent fibrous fleece of *Hyaff* (an ester of hyaluronic

acid), net price 5 cm × 5 cm = £9.80, 10 cm × 10 cm = £27.18
Uses: for treatment of chronic or acute wounds, place on surface of lesion and cover with sterile dressing, renew daily or when saturated (at least every 2–3 days)
Hyalofill-R, [NHS] absorbent fibrous rope of *Hyaff* (an ester of hyaluronic acid), net price, 500 mg = £27.18
Uses: for treatment of chronic or acute wounds, position gently inside cavity and cover with sterile dressing, renew daily or when saturated (at least every 2–3 days)

A8.1.5   Vapour-permeable films and membranes

Vapour-permeable films and membranes allow the passage of water vapour and oxygen but not of water or micro-organisms, and are suitable for mildly exuding wounds. They are highly conformable, convenient to use, provide a moist healing environment, and some may permit constant observation of the wound. However, water vapour loss may occur at a slower rate than exudate is generated, so that fluid accumulates under the dressing, which can lead to tissue maceration and to wrinkling at the adhesive contact site (with risk of bacterial entry). Newer versions have increased moisture vapour permeability; some also contain water-soluble antimicrobials. Despite these advances vapour-permeable films and membranes remain less suitable for large heavily exuding wounds and are probably not suitable for chronic leg ulcers. They are most commonly used as secondary dressings over alginates or gels; they are also sometimes used to protect fragile skin of patients at risk of developing minor skin damage.

Vapour-permeable Adhesive Film Dressing, BP 1993
(Semi-permeable Adhesive Dressing)
Sterile, extensible, waterproof, water vapour-permeable polyurethane film coated with synthetic adhesive mass; transparent. Supplied in single-use pieces.
Alldress®, net price 10 cm × 10 cm = 81p, 15 cm × 15 cm = £1.76, 15 cm × 20 cm = £2.17 (Mölnlycke)
Bioclusive®, 10.2 cm × 12.7 cm = £1.36 (J&J)
Blisterfilm®, net price 5 cm × 8 cm = 40p, 9 cm × 10 cm = 70p, 10 cm × 13 cm = 90p, 14 cm × 15 cm = £1.23 (Tyco)
C-View®, 6 cm × 7 cm = 36p, 10 cm × 12 cm = £1.00, 15 cm × 20 cm = £2.29, 20 cm × 30 cm = £3.53 ([NHS]) (Unomedical)
Hydrofilm®, 6 cm × 9 cm = 48p, 10 cm × 15 cm = £1.27, 12 cm × 25 cm = £2.29 (Hartmann)
Mefilm®, 6 cm × 7 cm = 40p, 10 cm × 12.7 cm = £1.06, 10 cm × 25 cm = £2.07, 15 cm × 21.5 cm = £2.63 (Mölnlycke)
Mepore® Ultra, 6 cm × 7 cm = 26p, 9 cm × 10 cm = 57p, 9 cm × 15 cm = 85p, 9 cm × 20 cm = £1.29, 9 cm × 25 cm = £1.42, 9 cm × 30 cm = £2.35 (Mölnlycke)
OpSite® Flexigrid, 6 cm × 7 cm = 33p, 12 cm × 12 cm = 94p, 15 cm × 20 cm = £2.38, 12 cm × 25 cm = £3.10 ([NHS]), 10 cm × 12 cm = £2.00 ([NHS]), *OpSite® Plus*, 5 cm × 5 cm = 26p, 9.5 cm × 8.5 cm = 74p, 10 cm × 12 cm = £1.00, 10 cm × 20 cm = £1.69, 35 cm × 10 cm = £2.79 (S&N Hlth)
Polyskin® II, net price 4 cm × 4 cm = 35p, 5 cm × 7 cm = 38p, 10 cm × 12 cm = 99p, 10 cm × 20 cm = £1.96, 15 cm × 20 cm = £2.26, 20 cm × 25 cm = £3.95 (Tyco)
Polyskin® MR, net price 5 cm × 7 cm = 40p, 10 cm × 12 cm = £1.08, 15 cm × 20 cm = £2.53 (Tyco)

Tegaderm®, 6 cm × 7 cm = 38p, 12 cm × 12 cm = £1.23, 15 cm × 20 cm = £2.34 (3M)

Uses: postoperative dressing, donor sites, i/v sites, superficial decubitus ulcers, amputation stumps, stoma care; protective cover to prevent skin breakdown

Omiderm® (Chemical Search) [NHS]

Sterile, water-vapour permeable polyurethane film (plain and meshed versions). Net price 5 cm × 7 cm = £2.00; 8 cm × 10 cm = £3.50, meshed = £4.75; 18 cm × 10 cm = £6.40, meshed = £9.50; 60 cm × 10 cm = £23.50; 21 cm × 31 cm = £24.00, meshed = £32.00; meshed 23 cm × 39 cm = £48.75

Uses: ulcers; donor sites; superficial and partial thickness burns; meshed: donor sites, skin grafts

---

A8.1.6 Low adherence dressing and wound contact materials

Low adherence dressings and wound contact materials are used as interface layers under secondary absorbent dressings.

Tulle dressings are manufactured from cotton or viscose fibres which are impregnated with white or yellow soft paraffin to prevent the fibres from sticking, but this is only partly successful and it may be necessary to change the dressings frequently. The paraffin reduces absorbency of the dressing. Dressings with a reduced content of soft paraffin (i.e. *Paratulle*® and *Unitulle*®) are less liable to interfere with absorption; those containing the traditional amount (such as *Jelonet*®) have been considered more suitable for skin graft transfer.

Medicated tulle dressings are not generally recommended for wound care. Although hypersensitivity is unlikely with **chlorhexidine gauze dressing**, its antibacterial efficacy has not been established.

Povidone–iodine fabric dressing is a knitted viscose dressing with povidone–iodine incorporated in a hydrophilic polyethylene glycol basis; this facilitates diffusion of the iodine into the wound and permits removal of the dressing by irrigation. The iodine has a wide spectrum of antimicrobial activity but it is rapidly deactivated by wound exudate; systemic absorption of iodine may occur.

Perforated film absorbent dressings partially overcome the problems of adherence but they are suitable only for wounds with mild to moderate amounts of exudate; they are **not** appropriate for leg ulcers or for other lesions that produce large quantities of viscous exudate.

Knitted viscose primary dressing is an alternative to tulle dressings for exuding wounds; it is sometimes used as the initial layer of multi-layer compression bandaging.

Absorbent Cellulose Dressing with Fluid Repellent Backing

Exu-Dry®, net price 10 cm × 15 cm = 94p, 15 cm × 23 cm = £1.92, 23 cm × 38 cm = £4.46 (S&N Hlth)

Uses: primary or secondary dressing for medium to heavily exuding wounds

Mesorb® cellulose wadding pad with gauze wound contact layer and non-woven repellent backing, net price 10 cm × 10 cm = 54p, 10 cm × 15 cm = 70p, 10 cm × 20 cm = 86p, 15 cm × 20 cm = £1.22, 20 cm × 25 cm = £1.93, 20 cm × 30 cm = £2.19 (Mölnlycke)

Uses: post-operative use for heavily exuding wounds

Absorbent Perforated Dressing with Adhesive Border

Low adherence dressing consisting of viscose and rayon absorbent pad with adhesive border.

Cosmopor E®, net price 5 cm × 7.2 cm, = 7p; 6 cm × 10 cm = 13p; 8 cm × 10 cm = 15p; 6 cm × 15 cm = 17p; 8 cm × 15 cm = 24p; 8 cm × 20 cm = 32p; 10 cm × 20 cm = 39p; 10 cm × 25 cm = 48p; 10 cm × 35 cm = 67p (Hartmann)

Medipore® + *Pad*, net price 5 cm × 7.2 cm = 7p, 10 cm × 10 cm = 14p, 10 cm × 15 cm = 23p, 10 cm × 20 cm = 35p, 10 cm × 25 cm = 43p, 10 cm × 35 cm = 60p (3M)

Mepore®, net price 7 cm × 8 cm = 9p, 10 cm × 11 cm = 19p, 11 cm × 15 cm = 31p, 9 cm × 20 cm = 38p, 9 cm × 25 cm = 52p, 9 cm × 30 cm = 60p, 9 cm × 35 cm = 65p (Mölnlycke)

Neosafe® , net price 9 cm × 10 cm = 16p, 9 cm × 20 cm = 34p (Neomedic)

Primapore®, net price 6 cm × 8.3 cm = 15p, 8 cm × 10 cm = 16p, 8 cm × 15 cm = 28p, 10 cm × 20 cm = 36p, 10 cm × 25 cm = 42p, 10 cm × 30 cm = 52p, 12 cm × 35 cm = 87p (S&N Hlth)

Sterifix®, net price 5 cm × 7 cm = 17p, 7 cm × 10 cm = 28p, 10 cm × 14 cm = 50p (Hartmann)

Telfa® *Island*, net price 5 cm × 10 cm = 8p, 10 cm × 20 cm = 34p (Tyco)

Uses: lightly exuding and post-operative wounds

Absorbent Perforated Plastic Film Faced Dressing

(Drug Tariff specification 9). Low-adherence dressing consisting of 3 layers.

Cutilin®, net price 5 cm × 5 cm = 12p, 10 cm × 10 cm = 21p, 10 cm × 20 cm = 39p (Beiersdorf)

Interpose®, net price 5 cm × 5 cm = 9p, 10 cm × 10 cm = 15p, 10 cm × 20 cm = 32p (Frontier)

Melolin®, net price 5 cm × 5 cm = 14p, 10 cm × 10 cm = 23p, 20 cm × 10 cm = 45p (S&N Hlth)

Release®, net price 5 cm × 5 cm = 13p, 10 cm × 10 cm = 21p, 20 cm × 10 cm = 40p (J&J)

Skintact®, net price 5 cm × 5 cm = 10p, 10 cm × 10 cm = 17p, 20 cm × 10 cm = 34p (Robinson)

Solvaline N®, net price 5 cm × 5 cm = 9p, 10 cm × 10 cm = 16p, 10 cm × 20 cm = 32p (Vernon-Carus)

Telfa®, net price 5 cm × 7.5 cm = 12p, 10 cm × 7.5 cm = 15p, 15 cm × 7.5 cm = 17p, 20 cm × 7.5 cm = 28p (Tyco)

Where no size specified by the prescriber, the 5 cm × 5 cm size to be supplied

Uses: dressing for post-operative and low exudate wounds; low adherence property and low absorption capacity

Knitted Viscose Primary Dressing, BP 1993

Warp knitted fabric manufactured from a bright viscose monofilament.

N-A Dressing®, net price 9.5 cm × 9.5 cm = 32p, 9.5 cm × 19 cm = 61p (J&J)

N-A Ultra® (silicone-coated), net price 9.5 cm × 9.5 cm = 30p, 9.5 cm × 19 cm = 58p (J&J)

Paratex® net price 9.5 cm × 9.5 cm = 25p (Parema)

Robinson Primary®, net price 12.5 cm × 14.5 cm = 39p (Robinsons)

Setoprime®, net price 9.5 cm × 9.5 cm = 28p (SSL)

Tricotex®, net price 9.5 cm × 9.5 cm = 27p (S&N Hlth)

Uses: low adherence wound contact layer for use on ulcerative and other granulating wounds with superimposed absorbent pad

Paraffin Gauze Dressing, BP 1993

(Tulle Gras). Fabric of leno weave, weft and warp threads of cotton and/or viscose yarn, impregnated with white or yellow soft paraffin, sterile, 10 cm × 10 cm, net price (light loading) = 25p; (normal loading) = 34p (most suppliers including Vernon-

Carus—*Paranet*® (light loading); SSL—
Paratulle® (light loading); Aventis Pharma—
Unitulle® (light loading); S&N Hlth—*Jelonet*®
(normal loading))
Uses: treatment of abrasions, burns, and other injuries of
skin, and ulcerative conditions; postoperatively as penile
and vaginal dressing and for sinus packing; heavier
loading for skin graft transfer

Chlorhexidine Gauze Dressing, BP 1993 ⬛
Fabric of leno weave, weft and warp threads of
cotton and/or viscose yarn, impregnated with
ointment containing chlorhexidine acetate, sterile,
5 cm × 5 cm, net price = 24p; 10 cm × 10 cm = 51p
(S&N Hlth—*Bactigras*®)

Povidone–iodine Fabric Dressing
(Drug Tariff specification 43). Knitted viscose
primary dressing impregnated with povidone–
iodine ointment 10%, net price 5 cm × 5 cm = 29p;
9.5 cm × 9.5 cm = 44p (J&J—*Inadine*®); 5 cm ×
5 cm = 26p, 9.5 cm × 9.5 cm = 37p (SSL—
Poviderm®)
Uses: wound contact layer for abrasions and superficial
burns

Atrauman® (Hartmann)
Non-adherent knitted polyester primary dressing
impregnated with neutral triglycerides, 5 cm ×
5 cm = 23p, 7.5 cm × 10 cm = 24p, 10 cm × 10 cm
= 54p
Uses: abrasions, burns, and other injuries of skin, and
ulcerative conditions; postoperatively for granulating
wounds

Mepilex® (Mölnlycke)
Low adherence, absorbent, silicone dressing with
polyurethane foam film backing, net price 10 cm ×
10 cm = £2.25, 10 cm × 20 cm = £3.71, 15 cm ×
15 cm = £4.18, 20 cm × 20 cm = £6.19; with
silicone adhesive border (*Mepilex*® *Border*) 7.5 cm
× 7.5 cm = £1.33, 10 cm × 10 cm = £2.40, 15 cm ×
15 cm = £3.93, 15 cm × 20 cm = £4.92; 15 cm ×
20 cm = £9.17, 20 cm × 50 cm = £23.42 (*Mepilex*®
Transfer)
Uses: pressure sores, venous ulcers, diabetic ulcers, donor
sites, dermal lesions, traumatic wounds; should be
covered with simple absorbent secondary dressing

Mepitel® (Mölnlycke)
Non-adherent silicone dressing. Net price 5 cm ×
7.5 cm = £1.54, 7.5 cm × 10 cm = £2.70, 10 cm ×
18 cm = £5.83, 20 cm × 30 cm = £14.73
Uses: leg ulcers, decubitus ulcers, burns, fixation of skin
grafts; should be covered with simple absorbent secondary dressing

Physiotulle® (Coloplast)
Non-adherent soft polymer wound contact dressing, net price 10 cm × 10 cm = £1.95, 15 cm ×
20 cm = £5.93
Uses: leg ulcers, pressure sores, burns, postoperative
wounds, donor sites, skin abrasions

¹**Surgipad**® (J&J) ⬛
Absorbent pad of absorbent cotton and viscose in
sleeve of non-woven viscose fabric, sterile, net
price pouch 12 cm × 10 cm = 18p, 20 cm × 10 cm
= 25p, 20 cm × 20 cm = 30p, 40 cm × 20 cm = 41p;
non-sterile, net price pack 12 cm × 10 cm = 5p,
20 cm × 10 cm = 10p, 20 cm × 20 cm = 17p, 40 cm
× 20 cm = 28p
Uses: for heavily exuding wounds requiring frequent
dressing changes

1. ⬛ Except in Sterile Dressing Pack with Non-woven
Pads

Tegapore® (3M)
Non-adherent soft polymer wound contact dressing, net price 7.5 cm × 10 cm = £2.09, 7.5 cm ×
20 cm = £4.10, 20 cm × 25 cm = £9.98

Urgotul® (Parema)
Non-adherent soft polymer wound contact dressing, net price 10 cm × 10 cm = £2.34, 10 cm ×
40 cm = £9.20, 15 cm × 20 cm = £7.11
Urgotul® *SSD* (silver impregnated), net price 10 cm
× 12 cm = £2.80, 15 cm × 20 cm = £7.05

A8.1.7 Odour absorbent dressings

These dressings have an important role in absorbing
the odour of infected wounds. Some dressings may
also benefit wound healing by binding bacteria, but
this effect awaits confirmation.

Actisorb® **Silver 200** (J&J)
(formerly Actisorb® Plus) Knitted fabric of activated charcoal, with one-way stretch, with silver
residues, within spun-bonded nylon sleeve. Net
price 6.5 cm × 9.5 cm = £1.50, 10.5 cm × 10.5 cm
= £2.35, 10.5 cm × 19 cm = £4.28

CarboFLEX® (ConvaTec)
Dressing in 5 layers: wound-facing absorbent layer
containing alginate and hydrocolloid; water-resistant second layer; third layer containing activated
charcoal; non-woven absorbent fourth layer;
water-resistant backing layer. Net price 10 cm ×
10 cm = £2.69, 8 cm × 15 cm = £3.23, 15 cm ×
20 cm = £6.12

Carbonet® (S&N Hlth.) ⬛
Activated charcoal dressing, net price 10 cm ×
10 cm = £3.04, 10 cm × 20 cm = £5.92

Carbopad® **VC** (Vernon-Carus)
Activated charcoal non-absorbent dressing, net
price 10 cm × 10 cm = £1.59, 10 cm × 20 cm =
£2.15

CliniSorb® **Odour Control Dressings** (CliniMed)
Layer of activated charcoal cloth between viscose
rayon with outer polyamide coating. Net price
10 cm × 10 cm = £1.62, 10 cm × 20 cm = £2.16,
15 cm × 25 cm = £3.48

Lyofoam C® (SSL)
Lyofoam sheet with layer of activated charcoal
cloth and additional outer envelope of polyurethane foam. Net price 10 cm × 10 cm = £2.64,
15 cm × 20 cm = £6.00, 25 cm × 10 cm = £5.39

A8.1.8 Dressing packs

The role of dressing packs is very limited. They are
used to provide a clean or sterile working surface;
packs shown below include cotton wool balls, but
they are not recommended for use on wounds.

Sterile Dressing Pack
(Drug Tariff specification 10). Contains gauze and
cotton tissue pad, gauze swabs, absorbent cotton
wool balls, absorbent paper towel, water repellent
inner wrapper. Net price per pack = 77p (Vernon-
Carus—*Vernaid*®)

Sterile Dressing Pack with Non-woven Pads
(Drug Tariff specification 35). Contains non-
woven fabric covered dressing pad, non-woven
fabric swabs, absorbent cotton wool balls, absorbent paper towel, water repellent inner wrapper.
Net price per pack = 75p (Vernon-Carus—
Vernaid®)

A8.1.9 Surgical absorbents

Surgical absorbent dressings, applied directly to the wound, have many disadvantages, since they adhere to the wound, shed fibres into it, and dehydrate it; they also permit leakage of exudate ('strike through') with an associated risk of infection. Surgical absorbents may be used as secondary absorbent layers in the management of heavily exuding wounds.

Absorbent Cotton, BP
Carded cotton fibres of not less than 10 mm average staple length, available in rolls and balls, 25 g, net price = 63p; 100 g = £1.44; 500 g = £4.84 (most suppliers). 25-g pack to be supplied when weight not stated
Uses: general purpose cleansing and swabbing, pre-operative skin preparation, application of medicaments; supplementary absorbent pad to absorb excess wound exudate

Absorbent Cotton, Hospital Quality
As for absorbent cotton but lower quality materials, shorter staple length etc. 100 g, net price = £1.00; 500 g = £3.15 (most suppliers)
Drug Tariff specifies to be supplied only where specifically ordered
Uses: suitable only as general purpose absorbent, for swabbing, and routine cleansing of incontinent patients; not for wound cleansing

Gauze and Cotton Tissue, BP 1988
Consists of absorbent cotton enclosed in absorbent cotton gauze type 12 or absorbent cotton and viscose gauze type 2. 500 g, net price = £6.14 (most suppliers, including Robinsons—*Gamgee Tissue®* (blue label))
Uses: absorbent and protective pad, as burns dressing on non-adherent layer

Gauze and Cotton Tissue
(Drug Tariff specification 14). Similar to above. 500 g, net price = £4.48 (most suppliers, including Robinsons—*Gamgee Tissue®* (pink label))
Drug Tariff specifies to be supplied only where specifically ordered
Uses: absorbent and protective pad, as burns dressing on non-adherent layer

Absorbent Lint, BPC
Cotton cloth of plain weave with nap raised on one side from warp yarns. 25 g, net price = 78p; 100 g = £2.40; 500 g = £10.09 (most suppliers). 25-g pack supplied where no quantity stated
NOTE. Not recommended for wound management

Absorbent Cotton Gauze, BP 1988
Cotton fabric of plain weave, in rolls and as swabs (see below), usually Type 13 light, sterile. 90 cm (all) × 1 m, net price = 95p; 3 m = £1.98; 5 m = £3.08; 10 m = £5.90 (most suppliers). 1-m packet supplied when no size stated
Uses: pre-operative preparation, for cleansing and swabbing
NOTE. Drug Tariff also includes unsterilised absorbent cotton gauze, 25 m roll, net price = £13.50

Absorbent Muslin, BP 1988 [NHS]
Fabric of plain weave, warp threads of cotton, weft threads of cotton and/or viscose
Uses: wet dressing, soaked in 0.9% sterile sodium chloride solution

Absorbent Cotton Ribbon Gauze, BP 1993 [NHS]
Cotton fabric of plain weave in ribbon form with fast selvedge edges
Uses: post-surgery cavity packing for sinus, dental, throat cavities etc.

Absorbent Cotton and Viscose Ribbon Gauze, BP 1993
Woven fabric in ribbon form with fast selvedge edges, warp threads of cotton, weft threads of viscose or combined cotton and viscose yarn, sterile. 5 m (both) × 1.25 cm, net price = 71p; 2.5 cm = 79p
Uses: post-surgery cavity packing for sinus, dental, throat cavities etc.

Gauze Swab, BP 1988
Consists of absorbent cotton gauze type 13 light or absorbent cotton and viscose gauze type 1 folded into squares or rectangles of 8-ply with no cut edges exposed, sterile, 7.5 cm × 7.5 cm, net price 5-pad packet = 34p; non-sterile, 10 cm × 10 cm 100-pad packet = £5.54 (most suppliers)

Filmated Gauze Swab, BP 1988
As for Gauze Swab, but with thin layer of Absorbent Cotton enclosed within, non-sterile, 10 cm × 10 cm, net price 100-pad packet = £6.99 (Vernon-Carus—*Cotfil®*)
Uses: general swabbing and cleansing

Non-woven Fabric Swab
(Drug Tariff specification 28). Consists of non-woven fabric folded 4-ply; alternative to gauze swabs, type 13 light, sterile, 7.5 cm × 7.5 cm, net price 5-pad packet = 22p; non-sterile, 10 cm × 10 cm, 100-pad packet = £2.51 (J & J—*Topper 8®*); 100-pad pack = £2.74 (CliniMed)
Uses: general purpose swabbing and cleansing; absorbs more quickly than gauze

Filmated Non-woven Fabric Swab
(Drug Tariff specification 29). Film of viscose fibres enclosed within non-woven viscose fabric folded 8-ply, non-sterile, 10 cm × 10 cm, net price 100-pad packet = £5.63 (J & J—*Regal®*)
Uses: general purpose swabbing and cleansing

A8.2 Bandages and adhesives

According to their structure and performance bandages are used for dressing retention, for support, and for compression.

A8.2.1 Non-extensible bandages

Bandages made from non-extensible woven fabrics have generally been replaced by more conformable products, therefore their role is now extremely limited. Triangular calico bandage has a role as a sling.

Open-wove Bandage, BP 1988
Cotton cloth, plain weave, warp of cotton, weft of cotton, viscose, or combination, one continuous length. Type 1, 5 m (all): 2.5 cm, net price = 31p; 5 cm = 51p; 7.5 cm = 72p; 10 cm = 94p (most suppliers) 5 m × 5 cm supplied when size not stated
Uses: protection and retention of absorbent dressings; support for minor strains, sprains; securing splints

Triangular Calico Bandage, BP 1980
Unbleached calico rt. angle triangle. 90 cm × 90 cm × 1.27 m, net price = £1.13 (most suppliers)
Uses: sling

Domette Bandage, BP 1988 [NHS]
Fabric, plain weave, cotton warp and wool weft (hospital quality also available, all cotton). 5 m

(all): 5 cm, net price = 54p; 7.5 cm = 81p; 10 cm = £1.08; 15 cm = £1.61 (Bailey, Robert)
Uses: protection and support where warmth required

Multiple Pack Dressing No. 1
(Drug Tariff). Contains absorbent cotton, absorbent cotton gauze type 13 light (sterile), open-wove bandages (banded). Net price per pack = £3.58

A8.2.2 Light-weight conforming bandages

Lightweight conforming bandages are used for dressing retention, with the aim of keeping the dressing close to the wound without inhibiting movement or restricting blood flow. The elasticity of **conforming-stretch bandages** (also termed contour bandages) is greater than that of **cotton conforming bandages**.

Cotton Conforming Bandage, BP 1988
Cotton fabric, plain weave, treated to impart some elasticity to warp and weft. 3.5 m (all): type A, 5 cm, net price = 64p, 7.5 cm = 80p, 10 cm = 98p, 15 cm = £1.34 (S&N Hlth— *Crinx*®)

Knitted Polyamide and Cellulose Contour Bandage, BP 1988
Fabric, knitted warp of polyamide filament, weft of cotton or viscose, fast edges, one continuous length. 4 m stretched (all):
K-Band®, net price 5 cm = 18p, 7 cm = 23p, 10 cm = 25p, 15 cm = 45p (Parema)
Knit Fix®, net price 5 cm = 13p, 7 cm = 18p, 10 cm = 19p, 15 cm = 35p (Bailey, Robert)

Polyamide and Cellulose Contour Bandage, BP 1988
(formerly Nylon and Viscose Stretch Bandage)
Fabric, plain weave, warp of polyamide filament, weft of cotton or viscose, fast edges, one continuous length. 4 m stretched (all):
Acti-Wrap®, cohesive, net price 6 cm = 39p, 8 cm = 57p, 10 cm = 68p; latex-free 6 cm = 45p, 8 cm = 65p, 10 cm = 77p (Activa)
Stayform®, net price 5 cm = 31p, 7.5 cm = 39p, 10 cm = 44p, 15 cm = 74p (Robinsons)
Slinky®, net price 5 cm = 39p, 7.5 cm = 57p, 10 cm = 68p, 15 cm = 97p (SSL)
Easifix®, net price 5 cm = 34p, 7.5 cm = 42p, 10 cm = 48p, 15 cm = 82p (S&N Hlth)

Conforming Bandage (Synthetic)
Fabric, plain weave, warp of polyamide, weft of viscose. 4 m stretched (all):
Hospiform® (formerly *Peha Crepp*® *E*), net price 6 cm = 13p, 8 cm = 15p, 10 cm = 18p, 12 cm = 22p (Hartmann)

A8.2.3 Tubular bandages

Tubular bandages are available in different forms, according to the function required of them. Some are used under orthopaedic casts and some are suitable for protecting areas to which creams or ointments (other than those containing potent corticosteroids) have been applied. The conformability of the elasticated versions makes them particularly suitable for retaining dressings on difficult parts of the body or for soft tissue injury, but their use as the only means of applying pressure to an oedematous limb or to a varicose ulcer is not appropriate, since the pressure they exert is inadequate. Compression

hosiery (section A8.3.1) reduces the recurrence of venous leg ulcers and should be considered after wound healing.

Cotton Stockinette, Bleached, BP 1988
Knitted fabric, cotton yarn, tubular, 1 m × 2.5 cm, net price = 30p; 5 cm = 47p; 7.5 cm = 57p; 6 m × 10 cm = £3.85 (J&J, SSL)
Uses: 1 m lengths, basis (with wadding) for Plaster of Paris bandages etc.; 6 m length, compression bandage

Elasticated Tubular Bandage, BP 1993
(formerly Elasticated Surgical Tubular Stockinette). Knitted fabric, elasticated threads of rubber-cored polyamide or polyester with cotton or cotton and viscose yarn, tubular. Lengths 50 cm and 1 m, widths 6.25 cm, 6.75 cm, 7.5 cm, 8.75 cm, 10 cm, 12 cm (other sizes ᴺᴴˢ); Shiloh—*Comfigrip*®; Easigrip—*EasiGRIP*®; Sallis—Esiban®; Sigma—*Sigma ETB*®; S&N Hlth—*Tensogrip*® ᴺᴴˢ]; JLB—*Textube*®; SSL—*Tubigrip*®. Where no size stated by prescriber the 50 cm length should be supplied and width endorsed
Uses: retention of dressings on limbs, abdomen, trunk

Elasticated Surgical Tubular Stockinette, Foam padded
(Drug Tariff specification 25). Fabric as for Elasticated Tubular Bandage with polyurethane foam lining. Heel, elbow, knee, small, net price = £2.58, medium = £2.79, large = £2.98; sacral, small, medium, and large (all) = £13.32 (SSL—*Tubipad*®)
Uses: relief of pressure and elimination of friction in relevant area; porosity of foam lining allows normal water loss from skin surface

Elasticated Viscose Stockinette
(Drug Tariff specification 46). Lightweight plain-knitted elasticated tubular bandage.
Acti-Fast®, net price 3.5 cm red line (small limb), length 1 m = 74p; 5 cm green line (medium limb), length 1 m = 80p, 3 m = £2.27, 5 cm = £3.85 blue line (large limb), length 1 m = £1.06, 3 m = £2.99, 5 m = £5.22; 10.75 cm yellow line (child trunk), length 1 m = £1.70, 3 m = £4.86, 5 m = £8.36; 17.5 cm beige line (adult trunk), length 1 m = £2.15 (Activa)
Comfifast®, net price 3.5 cm red line (small limb), length 1 m = 63p; 5 cm green line (medium limb), length 1 m = 67p, 3 m = £1.91, 5 m = £3.27; 7.5 cm blue line (large limb), length 1 m = 90p, 3 m = £2.52, 5 m = £ 4.39; 10.75 cm yellow line (child trunk), length 1 m = £1.43, 3 m = £4.10, 5 m = £7.04; 17.5 cm beige line (adult trunk), length 1 m = £1.81 (Shiloh)
Coverflex®, net price 3.5 cm red line (small limb), length 1 m = 72p; 5 cm green line (medium limb), length 1 m = 75p, 3 m = £2.20, 5 m = £3.80; 7.5 cm blue line (large limb), length 1 m = £1.05, 3 m = £2.50, 5 m = £ 4.95; 10.75 cm yellow line (child trunk), length 1 m = £1.65, 3 m = £4.75, 5 m = £8.35; 17.5 cm beige line (adult trunk), length 1 m = £2.20 (Hartmann)
Tubifast®, net price 3.5 cm red line (small limb), length 1 m = 79p; 5 cm green line (medium limb), length 1 m = 85p, 3 m = £2.43, 5 m = £4.16; 7.5 cm blue line (large limb), length 1 m = £1.14, 3 m = £3.20, 5 m = £5.58; 10.75 cm yellow line (child trunk), length 1 m = £1.82, 3 m = £5.21, 5 m = £8.95; 17.5 cm beige line (adult trunk), length 1 m = £2.30; vest, 6–24 months = £9.90, 2–5 years = £13.20, 5–8 years = £14.85, 8–11 years = £16.20, 11–14 years = £16.50; tights (pair) 6–24 months = £9.90; leggings (pair) 2–5 years = £12.30, 5–8 years = £14.85, 8–11 years = £16.50, 11–14 years = £16.50; socks (pair) = £4.13 (SSL)
Uses: retention of dressings

Elastic Net Surgical Tubular Stockinette
(Drug Tariff Specification 26). Lightweight elastic open-work net tubular fabric.

type A : arm/leg, 40 cm × 1.8 cm (size C), net price = 38p; thigh/head, 60 cm × 2.5 cm (size E) = 68p; trunk (adult), 60 cm × 4.5 cm (size F) = 99p; trunk (OS adult) 60 cm × 5.4 cm (size G) = £1.33 (SSL—*Netelast*®)

Ribbed Cotton and Viscose Surgical Tubular Stockinette, BP 1988
Knitted fabric of 1:1 ribbed structure, singles yarn spun from blend of two-thirds cotton and one-third viscose fibres. Length 5 m (all):

type A (lightweight): arm/leg (child), arm (adult) 5 cm, net price = £2.19; arm (OS adult), leg (adult) 7.5 cm = £2.87; leg (OS adult) 10 cm = £3.81; trunk (child) 15 cm = £5.48; trunk (adult) 20 cm = £6.33; trunk (OS adult) 25 cm = £7.57 (SSL)

type B (heavyweight): sizes as for type A, net price £2.19–£7.57 (Sallis—*Eesiban*®)

Drug Tariff specifies various combinations of sizes to provide sufficient material for part or full body coverage

Uses: protective dressings with tar-based and other nonsteroid ointments

Tubular Gauze Bandage, Seamless ⟦NHS⟧
Unbleached cotton yarn, positioned with applicators. 20 m roll (all): 00, net price = £2.95; 01 = £3.55; 12 = £4.60; 34 = £6.75; 56 = £9.35; 78 = £10.75; T1 = £14.75; T2 = £19.00 (SSL—*Tubegauz*®)

Uses: retention of dressings on limbs, abdomen, trunk

A8.2.4 Support bandages

Light support bandages, which include the various forms of crepe bandage, are used in the prevention of oedema; they are also used to provide support for mild sprains and joints but their effectiveness has not been proven for this purpose. Since they have limited extensibility, they are able to provide light support without exerting undue pressure. For a warning against injudicious compression see section A8.2.5.

Crepe Bandage, BP 1988
Fabric, plain weave, warp of wool threads and crepe-twisted cotton threads, weft of cotton threads; stretch bandage. 4.5 m stretched (all): 5 cm, net price = 90p; 7.5 cm = £1.26; 10 cm = £1.66; 15 cm = £2.40 (most suppliers)

Uses: light support system for strains, sprains, compression over paste bandages for varicose veins

Cotton Crepe Bandage
light support bandage, 4.5 m stretched (all): 5 cm, net price = 48p; 7.5 cm = 67p; 10 cm = 87p; 15 cm = £1.27 (Bailey, Robert– *Hospicrepe 239*)

Cotton Crepe Bandage, BP 1988
Fabric, plain weave, warp of crepe-twisted cotton threads, weft of cotton and/or viscose threads; stretch bandage. 4.5 m stretched (both): 7.5 cm, net price = £2.83; 10 cm = £3.64; other sizes ⟦NHS⟧ (most suppliers)

Uses: light support system for strains, sprains, compression over paste bandages for varicose ulcers

Cotton, Polyamide and Elastane Bandage
Fabric, cotton, polyamide, and elastane; light support bandage (Type 2). 4.5 m stretched (all): 5 cm, net price = 59p; 7.5 cm = 79p, 10 cm = 99p (Neomedic—*Neosport*®); 5 cm, net price = 67p, 7.5 cm = 95p, 10 cm = £1.22, 15 cm = £1.78 (S&N Hlth —*Softcrepe*®); 10 cm, net price = £1.16 (SSL—*Setocrepe*®)

Uses: light support for sprains and strains; retention of dressings

Cotton Stretch Bandage, BP 1988
Fabric, plain weave, warp of crepe-twisted cotton threads, weft of cotton threads; stretch bandage, lighter than cotton crepe. 4.5 m stretched (all): 5 cm, net price = 56p; 7.5 cm = 78p; 10 cm = £1.04; 15 cm = £1.48 (Bailey, Robert—*Hospicrepe 233*)

Uses: light support system for strains, sprains, compression over paste bandages for varicose veins

Cotton Suspensory Bandage
(Drug Tariff). Type 1: cotton net bag with draw tapes and webbing waistband; net price small, medium, and large (all) = £1.57, extra large = £1.66. Type 2: cotton net bag with elastic edge and webbing waistband; small = £1.73, medium = £1.78, large = £1.85, extra large = £1.93. Type 3: cotton net bag with elastic edge and webbing waistband with elastic insertion; small, medium, and large (all) = £1.87; extra large = £1.94. Type supplied to be endorsed

Uses: support of scrotum

Knitted Elastomer and Viscose Bandage
Knitted fabric, viscose and elastomer yarn. Type 2 (light support bandage) 4.5 m stretched (all):

Knit-Firm®, net price 5 cm = 39p, 7 cm = 55p, 10 cm = 72p, 15 cm = £1.04 (Bailey, Robert)

Ultra-Lite®, net price 5 cm = 49p, 7 cm = 69p, 10 cm = 91p, 15 cm = £1.30 (Parema)

Uses: light support for sprains and strains

Type 3a (light compression bandage):

Elset®, 6 m stretched, net price 10 cm = £2.50, 15 cm = £2.71; 8 m stretched, 10 cm = £3.21 (SSL)

Elset® S, 12 m stretched, net price 15 cm = £5.29 (SSL)

Mill Plus®, 6 m stretched, net price 10 cm = £1.32; 8.7 m stretched, 10 cm = £1.78 (Bailey, Robert)

Ultra-Plus®, 6 m stretched, net price 10 cm = £1.34; 8.7 m stretched, 10 cm = £1.81 (Parema)

A8.2.5 High compression bandages

High compression products are used to provide the high compression needed for the management of gross varices, post-thrombotic venous insufficiency, venous leg ulcers, and gross oedema in average-sized limbs. Their use calls for an expert knowledge of the elastic properties of the products and experience in the technique of providing careful graduated compression. Inappropriate application can lead to uneven and inadequate pressures or to hazardous levels of pressure. In particular, injudicious use of compression in limbs with arterial disease has been reported to cause severe skin and tissue necrosis (in some instances calling for amputation). Doppler testing is required before treatment with compression. Pentoxifylline (section 2.6.4.1) may be of benefit if a chronic venous leg ulcer does not respond to compression bandaging (unlicensed indication)

■ High compression bandages (Drug Tariff specification 52)

PEC High Compression Bandage
(Drug Tariff). Polyamide, elastane, and cotton compression (high) extensible bandage, 3.5 m unstretched (both): 7.5 cm, net price = £2.63; 10 cm = £3.40 (SSL—*Setopress*®)

VEC High Compression Bandage
(Drug Tariff). Viscose, elastane, and cotton compression (high) extensible bandage, 3 m unstretched (both); 7.5 cm, net price = £2.61; 10 cm = £3.35 (S&N—*Tensopress*®)

High Compression Bandage
  (Drug Tariff). Cotton, viscose, nylon, and Lycra®
  extensible bandage, 3 m (unstretted), 10 cm =
  £3.29 (ConvaTec—*SurePress*®)

■ Short Stretch Compression Bandage
Short stretch bandages help to reduce oedema and
promote healing of venous leg ulcers. They are also
used to reduce swelling associated with lymphoedema. They are applied at full stretch over padding
(*see* Sub-compression Wadding Bandage below)
which protects areas of high pressure and sites at
high risk of pressure damage.

Actiban® (Activa)
  Net price (all 5 m), 8 cm = £3.11; 10 cm = £3.33;
  12 cm = £4.06

Actico® (Activa)
  Cohesive, net price 6 m × 10 cm = £3.10

Comprilan® (Beiersdorf)
  Net price (all 5 m) 6 cm = £2.58; 8 cm = £3.04;
  10 cm = £3.27; 12 cm = £3.98

Rosidal K® (Vernon-Carus)
  Net price (all 5 m) 8 cm = £3.08; 10 cm = £3.36;
  12 cm = £4.08; N̶H̶S̶ 6 cm = £2.95

Silkolan® (Parema)
  Net price (all 5 m) 8 cm = £3.15; 10 cm = £3.56

Varex® **short stretch** (SSL)
  Net price 5 m × 10 cm = £3.33

■ Sub-compression Wadding Bandage
Advasoft® (Advancis)
  Net price 3.5 m unstreched, 10 cm = 39p

Cellona® **Undercast Padding** (Vernon-Carus)
  Net price 2.75 m unstretched (all): 7.5 cm = 37p;
  10 cm = 46p; 15 cm = 59p

Flexi-Ban® (Activa)
  Padding, net price 3.5 m unstretched, 10cm = 47p

K-Soft® (Parema)
  Net price 3.5 m unstretched, 10 cm = 42p

Ortho-Band Plus® (Bailey, Robert)
  Net price 10 cm × 3.5 cm unstretched = 40p

Profore® **#1** (S&N Hlth.)
  Natural fleece, net price 3.5 m unstretched, 10 cm =
  63p
  (Formerly *Soffban*® *Natural*)

Softexe® (SSL)
  Net price 3.5 m unstretched, 10 cm = 61p

SurePress® (ConvaTec)
  Absorbent padding, net price 3 m unstretched,
  10 cm = 50p

Ultra Soft® (Robinsons)
  Soft absorbent bandage, net price 3.5 m
  unstretched, 10 cm = 42p

Velband® (J&J)
  Absorbent padding, net price 4.5 m unstretched,
  10 cm = 72p

A8.2.6   Extra-high performance compression bandages

These bandages are capable of applying pressures
even higher than those of high compression bandages, therefore the same stringent warnings apply.
Their use is reserved for the largest and most

oedematous limbs. Extra-high performance compression bandages are poorly tolerated by patients.

Elastic Web Bandage, BP 1993
  (Also termed Blue Line Webbing). Characteristic
  fabric woven ribbon fashion, warp threads of
  cotton and rubber with mid-line threads coloured
  blue, weft threads of cotton or combined cotton and
  viscose; may be dyed skin colour; with or without
  foot loop. Per m (both) 7.5 cm, net price = 78p;
  10 cm = £1.11; with foot loop (Drug Tariff
  specification 2a) 7.5 cm = £4.46 (SSL)
  Uses: provision of support and high compression over
  large surface

Elastic Web Bandage without Foot Loop
  (Also termed Red Line Webbing) (Drug Tariff
  specification 2b) (Scott-Curwen). Characteristic
  fabric woven ribbon fashion, warp threads of
  cotton and rubber with mid-line threads coloured
  red, weft threads of cotton or combined cotton and
  viscose. 7.5 cm × 2.75 m (2.5 m unstretched), net
  price = £3.53; 7.5 cm × 3.75 m (3.5 m unstretched)
  = £4.26
  Uses: provision of support and high compression over
  large surfaces

Heavy Cotton and Rubber Elastic Bandage, BP 1993
  Heavy version of above with one end folded as foot
  loop; fastener also supplied. 1.8 m unstretched ×
  7.5 cm, net price = £11.97 (SSL, S&N Hlth—
  Elastoweb®).
  Uses: provision of high even compression over large
  surface

A8.2.7   Adhesive bandages

Elastic adhesive bandages are used to provide
compression in the treatment of varicose veins and
for the support of injured joints; they should no
longer be used for the support of fractured ribs and
clavicles. They have also been used with **zinc paste
bandage** in the treatment of venous ulcers, but they
can cause skin reactions in susceptible patients and
may not produce sufficient pressures for healing
(significantly lower than those provided by other
compression bandages).

Elastic Adhesive Bandage, BP 1993
  Woven fabric, elastic in warp (crepe-twisted cotton
  threads), weft of cotton and/or viscose threads
  spread with adhesive mass containing zinc oxide.
  4.5 m stretched (all): 5 cm, net price = £3.34;
  7.5 cm = £4.83; 10 cm = £6.43 (Robinsons—
  Flexoplast®; S&N Hlth—*Elastoplast*® Bandage).
  7.5 cm width supplied when size not stated
  Uses: compression for chronic leg ulcers; compression
  and support for swollen or sprained joints

A8.2.8   Cohesive bandages

Cohesive bandages adhere to themselves, but not to
the skin, and are useful for providing support for
sports use where ordinary stretch bandages might
become displaced and adhesive bandages are inappropriate. Care is needed in their application, however, since the loss of ability for movement between
turns of the bandage to equalise local areas of high
tension carries the potential for creating a tourniquet
effect. They should not be used if arterial disease is
suspected.

■ Cohesive extensible bandages

These elastic bandages adhere to themselves and not to skin; this prevents slipping during use.

Uses: support of sprained joints; outer layer of multi-layer compression bandaging

Coban® (3M)

Net price 6 m stretched, 10 cm = £2.82; other sizes NHS 4.5 m stretched (all): 2.5 cm = £1.25; 5 cm = £1.76; 7.5 cm = £2.64; 10 cm = £3.50; 15 cm = £5.17

Ultra Fast® (Robinsons)

Latex-free, net price 6.3 m stretched, 10 cm = £2.82

A8.2.9 Medicated bandages

Zinc Paste Bandage remains one of the standard treatments for leg ulcers and can be left on undisturbed for up to a week; it is often used in association with compression for treatment of venous ulcers.

Zinc paste bandages are also used with **coal tar** or **ichthammol** in chronic lichenified skin conditions such as chronic eczema (ichthammol often being preferred since its action is considered to be milder). They are also used with **calamine** in milder eczematous skin conditions (but the inclusion of **clioquinol** may lead to irritation in susceptible subjects).

Zinc Paste Bandage, BP 1993

Cotton fabric, plain weave, impregnated with suitable paste containing zinc oxide; requires additional bandaging. Net price 6 m × 7.5 cm = £3.28 (SSL—*Steripaste*® (15%), *excipients: include* polysorbate 80); £3.23 (SSL—*Zincaband*® (15%), *excipients: include* hydroxybenzoates); £3.31 (S&N Hlth—*Viscopaste PB7*® (10%), *excipients: include* hydroxybenzoates)

Zinc Paste and Calamine Bandage

(Drug Tariff specification 5). Cotton fabric, plain weave, impregnated with suitable paste containing calamine and zinc oxide; requires additional bandaging. Net price 6 m × 7.5 cm = £3.33 (SSL—*Calaband*®)

Zinc Paste, Calamine, and Clioquinol Bandage, BP 1993

Cotton fabric, plain weave, impregnated with suitable paste containing calamine, clioquinol, and zinc oxide; requires additional bandaging. Net price 6 m × 7.5 cm = £3.33 (SSL—*Quinaband*®, *excipients: include* hydroxybenzoates)

Zinc Paste and Ichthammol Bandage, BP 1993

Cotton fabric, plain weave, impregnated with suitable paste containing zinc oxide and ichthammol; requires additional bandaging. Net price 6 m × 7.5 cm = £3.24 (SSL—*Icthaband*®(15/2%), *excipients: include* hydroxybenzoates; S&N Hlth—*Ichthopaste*®(6/2%)

Excipients: none as listed in section 13.1.3

Uses: see section 13.5

■ Medicated stocking

Zipzoc® (S&N Hlth.)

Sterile rayon stocking impregnated with ointment containing zinc oxide 20%. Net price 4-pouch carton = £13.33; 10-pouch carton = £33.33

Uses: chronic leg ulcers; can be used under appropriate compression bandages or hosiery in chronic venous insufficiency

A8.2.10 Multi-layer compression bandaging

Multi-layer compression bandaging systems are an alternative to High Compression Bandages (section A8.2.5) for the treatment of venous leg ulcers. Compression is achieved by the combined effects of two or three extensible bandages applied over a layer of orthopaedic wadding.

Hospifour® (Bailey, Robert)

Hospifour® # 1 (Ortho-Band Plus®—see Sub-compression Wadding Bandage); *Hospifour*® # 2 (*Hospicrepe 239*®—see Cotton Crepe Bandage); *Hospifour*® # 3 (*Mill Plus*® —see Knitted Elastomer and Viscose Bandage); *Hospifour*® # 4 (*AAA-Flex*®), net price 10 cm × 6.3 m (stretched) = £1.93

K-Four® (Parema)

K-Four® # 1 (*K-Soft*®—see Sub-compression Wadding Bandage); *K-Four*® # 2 (*Ultra-Lite*®— see Knitted Elastomer and Viscose Bandage); *K-Four*® # 3 (*Ultra-Plus*®—see Knitted Elastomer and Viscose Bandage); *K-Four*® # 4 (*Ko-Flex*®), net price 10 cm × 6 m (unstretched) = £2.85

Multi-layer compression bandaging kit, four layer system, for ankle circumference 18–25 cm, net price = £6.55

Profore® (S&N Hlth.)

Profore® wound contact layer (*Tricotex*®—see Knitted Viscose Primary Dressing); *Profore*® #1 (see Sub-compression Wadding bandage); *Profore*® #2 (*Soffcrepe*®—see Cotton, Polyamide and Elastane Bandage); *Profore*® #3 (*Litepress*®—see Knitted Elastomer and Viscose Bandage); *Profore*® #4 (*Co-Plus*®—see Cohesive bandages); *Profore*® *Plus* = £3.35

Multi-layer compression bandaging kit, four layer system, for ankle circumference up to 18 cm, net price = £9.25, 18–25 cm = £8.62, 25–30 cm = £7.15, above 30 cm = £10.71

Proguide® (S&N Hlth.)

Multi-layer compression bandaging kit, two layer system, for ankle circumference 18–22 cm (red), net price = £8.92, 22–28 cm (yellow) = £9.41, 28–32 cm (green) = £9.89

System 4® (SSL)

System 4® wound contact layer (*Setoprime*®—see Knitted Viscose Primary Dressing); *System 4*® #1 (*Softexe*®—see Sub-compression Wadding Bandage), *System 4*® #2 (*Setocrepe*®—see Cotton, Polyamide and Elastane Bandage); *System 4*® #3 (*Elset*®—see Knitted Elastomer and Viscose Bandage); *System 4*® #4 (*Coban*®—see Cohesive bandages)

Multi-layer compression bandaging kit, four layer system, for ankle circumference 18–25 cm, net price = £8.15

Ultra Four® (Robinsons)

Ultra Four® wound dressing 14.5 cm × 12.5 cm; *Ultra Four*® #1 (Robinsons—*Ultra Soft*®—see Sub-compression Wadding Bandage); *Ultra Four*® #2 (Parema—*Ultra Lite*®—see Knitted Elastomer and Viscose Bandage); *Ultra Four*® #3 (Parema—*Ultra Plus*®—see Knitted Elastomer and Viscose Bandage); *Ultra Four*® #4 (Robinsons—*Ultra Fast*®—see Cohesive bandages)

Multi-layer compression bandaging kit, four layer system, for ankle circumference 18–25 cm, net price = £6.16

Surgical adhesive tapes

Adhesive tapes are useful for retaining dressings on joints or awkward body parts. These tapes, particularly those containing rubber, can cause irritant and allergic reactions in susceptible patients; synthetic adhesives have been developed to overcome this problem, but they, too, may sometimes be associated with reactions. Adhesive tapes that are occlusive may cause skin maceration. Care is needed not to apply these tapes under tension, to avoid creating a tourniquet effect. If applied over joints they need to be orientated so that the area of maximum extensibility of the fabric is in the direction of movement of the limb.

Permeable adhesive tapes

Zinc Oxide Adhesive Tape, BP 1988
(Zinc Oxide Plaster). Fabric, plain weave, warp and weft of cotton and/or viscose, spread with an adhesive containing zinc oxide. 5 m (all): 1.25 cm, net price = 85p; 2.5 cm = £1.23; 5 cm = £2.08; 7.5 cm = £3.12 (most suppliers)
Uses: securing dressings and immobilising small areas

Strappal (BSN Medical)
Zinc oxide adhesive tape. 5 m (all): 1.25 cm, net price = 83p, 2.5 cm = £1.20, 5 cm = £2.02, 7.5 cm = £3.05; other sizes [NHS]

Permeable Woven Synthetic Adhesive Tape, BP 1988
Non-extensible closely woven fabric, spread with a polymeric adhesive. 5 m (all): 1.25 cm, net price = 70p; 2.5 cm = £1.02; 5 cm = £1.78 (Beiersdorf—*Leukosilk®*)
Uses: securing dressings for patients with skin reactions to other plasters and strapping, which require use for long periods

Elastic Adhesive Tape, BP 1988
(Elastic Adhesive Plaster). Woven fabric, elastic in warp (crepe-twisted cotton threads), weft of cotton and/or viscose, spread with adhesive mass containing zinc oxide. 4.5 m stretched × 2.5 cm, net price= £1.50 (Robinsons—*Flexoplast®*; S&N—*Elastoplast®*)
Uses: securing dressings
For 5 cm width, see Elastic Adhesive Bandage

Permeable Non-woven Synthetic Adhesive Tape, BP 1988
Backing of paper-based or non-woven textile material spread with a polymeric adhesive mass. 5 m (all):
Clinipore®, net price 1.25 cm = 35p, 2.5 cm = 59p, 5 cm = 99p (Clinisupplies)
Leukofix®, net price 1.25 cm = 50p, 2.5 cm = 80p, 5 cm = £1.40 (BSN Medical)
Leukopor®, net price 1.25 cm = 45p, 2.5 cm = 70p, 5 cm = £1.23 (Beiersdorf)
Mediplast®, net price 1.25 cm = 49p, 2.5 cm = 73p (Neomedic)
Micropore®, net price 1.25 cm = 59p, 2.5 cm = 88p, 5 cm = £1.55 (3M)
Scanpor®, net price 1.25 cm = 39p, 2.5 cm = 63p, 5 cm = £1.09 (BioDiagnostics)
Where no brand stated by prescriber, net price of tape supplied not to exceed 35p (1.25 cm), 59p (2.5 cm), 99p (5 cm)
Uses: securing dressings; skin closures for small incisions for patients with skin reactions to other plasters and strapping, which require use for long periods

Permeable, Apertured Non-Woven Synthetic Adhesive Tape, BP 1988
Non-woven fabric with a polyacrylate adhesive.
Hypafix® 10 m (all): 2.5 cm, net price = £1.46, 5 cm = £2.31, 10 cm = £4.04, 15 cm = £5.98, 20 cm = £7.93, 30 cm = £11.46 (BSN Medical)
Mefix® 5 m (all): 2.5 cm, net price = 88p, 5 cm = £1.56; 10 cm = £2.49, 15 cm = £3.39, 20 cm = £4.34, 30 cm = £6.23 (Mölnlycke)
Omnifix® 10 m (all): 5 cm, net price = £2.07, 10 cm = £3.49, 15 cm = £5.15 (Hartmann)
Uses: securing dressings

Occlusive adhesive tapes

Impermeable Plastic Adhesive Tape, BP 1988
Extensible water-impermeable plastic film spread with an adhesive mass. 2.5 cm × 3 m, net price = £1.19; 2.5 cm × 5 m = £1.78; 5 cm × 5 m = £2.25; 7.5 cm × 5 m = £3.27 (Robinsons; SSL; S&N Hlth)
Uses: securing dressings; covering site of infection where exclusion of air, water, and water vapour is required

Impermeable Plastic Synthetic Adhesive Tape, BP 1988
Extensible water-impermeable plastic film spread with a polymeric adhesive mass. 5 m (both): net price, 2.5 cm = £1.69; 5 cm = £3.22 (3M—*Blenderm®*)
Uses: isolating wounds from external environment; covering sites where total exclusion of water and water vapour required; securing dressings and appliances

Adhesive dressings

Adhesive dressings (also termed 'island dressings') have a limited role for minor wounds only. The inclusion of an antiseptic is not particularly useful and may cause skin irritation in susceptible subjects.

Permeable adhesive dressings

Elastic Adhesive Dressing, BP 1993 [NHS]
Wound dressing or dressing strip, pad attached to piece of extension plaster, leaving suitable adhesive margin; both pad and margin covered with suitable protector; pad may be dyed yellow and may be impregnated with suitable antiseptic (see below); extension plaster may be perforated or ventilated
Uses: general purpose wound dressing
NOTE. Permitted antiseptics are aminoacridine hydrochloride (aminacrine hydrochloride), chlorhexidine hydrochloride (both 0.07–0.13%), chlorhexidine gluconate (0.11–0.20%); domiphen bromide (0.05–0.25%)

Permeable Plastic Wound Dressing, BP 1993 [NHS]
Consisting of an absorbent pad, which may be dyed and impregnated with a suitable antiseptic (see under Elastic Adhesive Dressing), attached to a piece of permeable plastic surgical adhesive tape, to leave a suitable adhesive margin; both pad and margin covered with suitable protector (most suppliers)
Uses: general purpose wound dressing, permeable to air and water

Vapour permeable adhesive dressings

Vapour-permeable Waterproof Plastic Wound Dressing, BP 1993

(former Drug Tariff title: Semipermeable Waterproof Plastic Wound Dressing). Consists of absorbent pad, may be dyed and impregnated with suitable antiseptic (see under Elastic Adhesive Dressing), attached to piece of semi-permeable waterproof surgical adhesive tape, to leave suitable adhesive margin; both pad and margin covered with suitable protector. 8.5 cm × 6 cm, net price = 33p (S&N Hlth—*Elastoplast Airstrip®*)
Uses: general purpose waterproof wound dressing, permeable to air and water vapour

Occlusive adhesive dressings

Impermeable Plastic Wound Dressing, BP 1993
NHS

Consists of absorbent pad, may be dyed and impregnated with suitable antiseptic (see under Elastic Adhesive Dressing), attached to piece of impermeable plastic surgical adhesive tape, to leave suitable adhesive margin; both pad and margin covered with suitable protector (most suppliers)
Uses: protective covering for wounds requiring an occlusive dressing

A8.2.13 Skin closure dressings

Skin closure strips are used as an alternative to sutures for minor cuts and lacerations.

Skin closure strips, sterile

Leukostrip®, 6.4 mm × 76 mm, 3 strips per envelope. Net price 10 envelopes = £5.37 (Beiersdorf)
Steri-strip®, 6 mm × 75 mm, 3 strips per envelope. Net price 12 envelopes = £8.52; NHS 3 mm × 75 mm, 12 envelopes = £8.32; 12 mm × 100 mm, 12 envelopes = £10.89 (3M)
Drug Tariff specifies that these are specifically for personal administration by the prescriber

A8.3 Elastic hosiery

Before elastic hosiery can be dispensed, the quantity (single or pair), article (including accessories), and compression class (I, II or III) must be specified by the prescriber; all dispensed articles must state on the packaging that they conform with Drug Tariff technical specification No. 40, for further details see Drug Tariff.
NOTE. Graduated compression tights are NHS.

A8.3.1 Graduated compression hosiery

Class 1 Light Support

Hosiery, compression at ankle 14–17 mm Hg, thigh length or below knee with knitted in heel. Net price per pair, circular knit (standard), thigh length = £6.78, below knee = £6.19; light weight elastic net (made-to-measure), thigh length = £18.15, below knee = £14.17
Uses: superficial or early varices, varicosis during pregnancy

Class 2 Medium Support

Hosiery, compression at ankle 18–24 mm Hg, thigh length or below knee with knitted in heel. Net price per pair, circular knit (standard), thigh length = £10.08, below knee = £9.06, (made-to-measure), thigh length = £33.67, below knee = £21.06; net (made-to-measure), thigh length = £18.15, below knee = £14.17; flat bed (made-to-measure, only with closed heel and open toe), thigh length = £33.67, below knee = £21.06
Uses: varices of medium severity, ulcer treatment and prophylaxis, mild oedema, varicosis during pregnancy

Class 3 Strong Support

Hosiery, compression at ankle 25–35 mm Hg, thigh length or below knee with knitted in heel. Net price per pair, circular knit (standard), thigh length = £11.94, below knee = £10.26, (made-to-measure) thigh length = £33.67, below knee = £21.06; flat bed (made-to-measure, only with open heel and open toe), thigh length = £33.67, below knee = £21.06
Uses: gross varices, post thrombotic venous insufficiency, gross oedema, ulcer treatment and prophylaxis

A8.3.2 Accessories

Suspender

Suspender, for thigh stockings, net price = 59p, belt (specification 13), = £4.52, fitted (additional price) = 59p

A8.3.3 Anklets

Class 2 Medium Support

Anklets, compression 18–24 mm Hg, circular knit (standard and made-to-measure), net price per pair = £5.93; flat bed (standard and made-to-measure) = £12.38; made-to-measure = £12.33
Uses: soft tissue support

Class 3 Strong Support

Anklets, compression 25–35 mm Hg, circular knit (standard and made-to-measure), net price per pair = £8.28; flat bed (standard) = £8.28; made-to-measure = £12.33
Uses: soft tissue support

A8.3.4 Knee caps

Class 2 Medium Support

Kneecaps, compression 18–24 mm Hg, circular knit (standard and made-to-measure), net price per pair = £5.93; flat bed (standard and made-to-measure) = £12.33; net made-to-measure = £9.69
Uses: soft tissue support

Class 3 Strong Support

Kneecaps, compression 25–35 mm Hg, circular knit (standard and made-to-measure), net price per pair = £7.91; flat bed (standard) = £7.91; made-to-measure = £12.33
Uses: soft tissue support

Appendix 9: Cautionary and advisory labels for dispensed medicines

Numbers following the preparation entries in the BNF correspond to the code numbers of the cautionary labels that pharmacists are recommended to add when dispensing. It is also expected that pharmacists will counsel patients when necessary.

Counselling needs to be related to the age, experience, background, and understanding of the individual patient. The pharmacist should ensure that the patient understands how to take or use the medicine and how to follow the correct dosage schedule. Any effects of the medicine on driving or work, any foods or medicines to be avoided, and what to do if a dose is missed should also be explained. Other matters, such as the possibility of staining of the clothes or skin by a medicine should also be mentioned.

For some preparations there is a special need for counselling, such as an unusual method or time of administration or a potential interaction with a common food or domestic remedy, and this is indicated where necessary.

ORIGINAL PACKS. Most preparations are now dispensed in unbroken original packs (see Patient Packs, p. vii) that include further advice for the patient in the form of patient information leaflets. Label 10 may be of value where appropriate. More general leaflets advising on the administration of preparations such as eye drops, eye ointments, inhalers, and suppositories are also available.

SCOPE OF LABELS. In general no label recommendations have been made for injections on the assumption that they will be administered by a healthcare professional or a well-instructed patient. The labelling is not exhaustive and pharmacists are recommended to use their professional discretion in labelling new preparations and those for which no labels are shown.

Individual labelling advice is not given on the administration of the large variety of antacids. In the absence of instructions from the prescriber, and if on enquiry the patient has had no verbal instructions, the directions given under 'Dose' should be used on the label.

It is recognised that there may be occasions when pharmacists will use their knowledge and professional discretion and decide to omit one or more of the recommended labels for a particular patient. In this case counselling is of the utmost importance. There may also be an occasion when a prescriber does not wish additional cautionary labels to be used, in which case the prescription should be endorsed 'NCL' (no cautionary labels). The exact wording that is required instead should then be specified on the prescription.

Pharmacists label medicines with various wordings in addition to those directions specified on the prescription. Such labels include 'Shake the bottle', 'For external use only', and 'Store in a cool place', as well as 'Discard . . . . days after opening' and 'Do not use after . . . .', which apply particularly to antibiotic mixtures, diluted liquid and topical preparations, and to eye-drops. Although not listed in the BNF these labels should continue to be used when appropriate; indeed, 'For external use only' is a legal requirement on external liquid preparations, while 'Keep out of the reach of children' is a legal requirement on all dispensed medicines. Care should be taken not to obscure other relevant information with adhesive labelling.

It is the usual practice for patients to take standard tablets with water or other liquid and for this reason no separate label has been recommended.

The label wordings recommended by the BNF apply to medicines dispensed against a prescription. Patients should be aware that a dispensed medicine should never be taken by, or shared with, anyone other than for whom the prescriber intended it. Therefore, the BNF does not include warnings against the use of a dispensed medicine by persons other than for whom it was specifically prescribed.

The label or labels for each preparation are recommended after careful consideration of the information available. However, it is recognised that in some cases this information may be either incomplete or open to a different interpretation. The Executive Editor will therefore be grateful to receive any constructive comments on the labelling suggested for any preparation.

Recommended label wordings

Wordings which can be given as separate warnings are labels 1-19 and labels 29-33. Wordings which can be incorporated in an appropriate position in the directions for dosage or administration are labels 21-28. A label has been omitted for number 20.

If separate labels are used it is recommended that the wordings be used without modification. If changes are made to suit computer requirements, care should be taken to retain the sense of the original.

1 **Warning. May cause drowsiness**
To be used on *preparations for children* containing antihistamines, or other preparations given to children where the warnings of label 2 on driving or alcohol would not be appropriate.

2 **Warning. May cause drowsiness. If affected do not drive or operate machinery. Avoid alcoholic drink**
To be used on *preparations for adults that can cause drowsiness*, thereby affecting the ability to drive and operate hazardous machinery; label 1 is more appropriate for children. *It is an offence to drive while under the influence of drink or drugs.*
Some of these preparations may only cause drowsiness in the first few days of treatment and some only cause drowsiness in higher doses.
In such cases the patient should be told that the advice applies until the effects have worn off. However, many of

these preparations can produce a slowing of reaction time and a loss of mental concentration that can have the same effects as drowsiness.

Avoidance of alcoholic drink is recommended because the effects of CNS depressants are enhanced by alcohol. Strict prohibition however could lead to some patients not taking the medicine. Pharmacists should therefore explain the risk and encourage compliance, particularly in patients who may think they already tolerate the effects of alcohol (see also label 3). Queries from patients with epilepsy regarding fitness to drive should be referred back to the patient's doctor.

Side-effects unrelated to drowsiness that may affect a patient's ability to drive or operate machinery safely include *blurred vision, dizziness, or nausea*. In general, no label has been recommended to cover these cases, but the patient should be suitably counselled.

3   **Warning. May cause drowsiness. If affected do not drive or operate machinery**

To be used on *preparations containing monoamine-oxidase inhibitors*; the warning to avoid alcohol and dealcoholised (low alcohol) drink is covered by the patient information leaflet.

Also to be used as for label 2 but where alcohol is not an issue.

4   **Warning. Avoid alcoholic drink**

To be used on *preparations where a reaction such as flushing may occur if alcohol is taken* (e.g. metronidazole and chlorpropamide). Alcohol may also enhance the hypoglycaemia produced by some oral antidiabetic drugs but routine application of a warning label is not considered necessary.

5   **Do not take indigestion remedies at the same time of day as this medicine**

To be used with label 25 on *preparations coated to resist gastric acid* (e.g. enteric-coated tablets). This is to avoid the possibility of premature dissolution of the coating in the presence of an alkaline pH.

Label 5 also applies to drugs such as ketoconazole *where the absorption is significantly affected by antacids*; the usual period of avoidance recommended is 2 to 4 hours.

6   **Do not take indigestion remedies or medicines containing iron or zinc at the same time of day as this medicine**

To be used on *preparations containing ciprofloxacin and some other quinolones, doxycycline, lymecycline, minocycline, and penicillamine*. These drugs chelate calcium, iron and zinc and are less well absorbed when taken with calcium-containing antacids or preparations containing iron or zinc. These incompatible preparations should be taken 2-3 hours apart.

7   **Do not take milk, indigestion remedies, or medicines containing iron or zinc at the same time of day as this medicine**

To be used on *preparations containing norfloxacin or tetracyclines that chelate, calcium, iron, magnesium, and zinc* and are thus less available for absorption; these incompatible preparations should be taken 2-3 hours apart. Doxycycline, lymecycline and minocycline are less liable to form chelates and therefore only require label 6 (see above).

8   **Do not stop taking this medicine except on your doctor's advice**

To be used on *preparations that contain a drug which is required to be taken over long periods without the patient necessarily perceiving any benefit* (e.g. antituberculous drugs).

Also to be used on *preparations that contain a drug whose withdrawal is likely to be a particular hazard* (e.g. clonidine for hypertension). Label 10 (see below) is more appropriate for corticosteroids.

9   **Take at regular intervals. Complete the prescribed course unless otherwise directed**

To be used on *preparations where a course of treatment should be completed* to reduce the incidence of relapse or failure of treatment.

The preparations are antimicrobial drugs given by mouth. Very occasionally, some may have severe side-effects (e.g. diarrhoea in patients receiving clindamycin) and in such cases the patient may need to be advised of reasons for stopping treatment quickly and returning to the doctor.

10   **Warning. Follow the printed instructions you have been given with this medicine**

To be used particularly on *preparations containing anticoagulants, lithium and oral corticosteroids*. The appropriate treatment card should be given to the patient and any necessary explanations given.

This label may also be used on other preparations to remind the patient of the instructions that have been given.

11   **Avoid exposure of skin to direct sunlight or sun lamps**

To be used on *preparations that may cause phototoxic or photoallergic reactions* if the patient is exposed to ultraviolet radiation. Many drugs other than those listed (e.g. phenothiazines and sulphonamides) may on rare occasions cause reactions in susceptible patients. Exposure to high intensity ultraviolet radiation from sunray lamps and sunbeds is particularly likely to cause reactions.

12   **Do not take anything containing aspirin while taking this medicine**

To be used on *preparations containing probenecid and sulfinpyrazone* whose activity is reduced by aspirin. Label 12 should not be used for anticoagulants since label 10 is more appropriate.

13   **Dissolve or *mix with water* before taking**

To be used on *preparations that are intended to be dissolved in water* (e.g. soluble tablets) or *mixed with water* (e.g. powders, granules) before use. In a few cases other liquids such as fruit juice or milk may be used.

14   **This medicine may colour the urine**

To be used on *preparations that may cause the patient's urine to turn an unusual colour*. These include phenolphthalein (alkaline urine pink), triamterene (blue under some lights), levodopa (dark reddish), and rifampicin (red).

15   **Caution flammable: keep away from fire or flames**

To be used on *preparations containing sufficient flammable solvent to render them flammable if exposed to a naked flame*.

16   **Allow to dissolve under the tongue. Do not transfer from this container. Keep tightly closed. Discard eight weeks after opening**

To be used on *glyceryl trinitrate tablets* to remind the patient not to transfer the tablets to plastic or less suitable containers.

17   **Do not take more than . . . in 24 hours**

To be used on *preparations for the treatment of acute migraine* except those containing ergotamine, for which label 18 is used. The dose form should be specified, e.g. tablets or capsules.

It may also be used on preparations for which no dose has been specified by the prescriber.

18   **Do not take more than . . . in 24 hours or . . . in any one week**

To be used on preparations containing ergotamine. The dose form should be specified, e.g. tablets or suppositories.

19   **Warning. Causes drowsiness which may continue the next day. If affected do not drive or operate machinery. Avoid alcoholic drink**

To be used on *preparations containing hypnotics (or some other drugs with sedative effects) prescribed to be taken at night*. On the rare occasions (e.g. nitrazepam in epilepsy) when hypnotics are prescribed for daytime administration this label would clearly not be appropriate. Also to be used as an *alternative to the label 2 wording* (the choice being at the discretion of the pharmacist) *for anxiolytics prescribed to be taken at night*.

It is hoped that this wording will convey adequately the problem of residual morning sedation after taking 'sleeping tablets'.

21   **. . . with or after food**

To be used on *preparations that are liable to cause gastric irritation, or those that are better absorbed with food*.

Patients should be advised that a *small amount of food is sufficient*.

22   **. . . half to one hour before food**

To be used on some preparations *whose absorption is thereby improved*.

Most oral antibacterials require label 23 instead (see below).

23 **. . . an hour before food or on an empty stomach**
To be used on *oral antibacterials whose absorption may
be reduced by the presence of food and acid in the
stomach.*

24 **. . . sucked or chewed**
To be used on *preparations that should be sucked or
chewed.*
The pharmacist should use discretion as to which of these
words is appropriate.

25 **. . . swallowed whole, not chewed**
To be used on *preparations that are enteric-coated or
designed for modified-release.*
Also to be used on *preparations that taste very
unpleasant or may damage the mouth* if not swallowed
whole.

26 **. . . dissolved under the tongue**
To be used on *preparations designed for sublingual use.*
Patients should be advised to hold under the tongue and
avoid swallowing until dissolved. The buccal mucosa
between the gum and cheek is occasionally specified by
the prescriber.

27 **. . . with plenty of water**
To be used on *preparations that should be well diluted*
(e.g. chloral hydrate), *where a high fluid intake is
required* (e.g. sulphonamides), or *where water is
required to aid the action* (e.g. methylcellulose). The
patient should be advised that 'plenty' means at least
150 mL (about a tumblerful). In most cases fruit juice,
tea, or coffee may be used.

28 **To be spread thinly . . .**
To be used on *external preparations* that should be
applied sparingly (e.g. corticosteroids, dithranol).

29 **Do not take more than 2 at any one time. Do not take
more than 8 in 24 hours**
To be used on containers of dispensed *solid dose
preparations containing paracetamol for adults* when
the instruction on the label indicates that the dose can be
taken on an 'as required' basis. The dose form should be
specified, e.g. tablets or capsules.
This label has been introduced because of the serious
consequences of overdosage with paracetamol.

30 **Do not take with any other paracetamol products**
To be used on all containers of dispensed *preparations
containing paracetamol.*

31 **Contains aspirin and paracetamol. Do not take with
any other paracetamol products**
To be used on all containers of dispensed *preparations
containing aspirin and paracetamol* (e.g. benorilate).

32 **Contains aspirin**
To be used on containers of dispensed *preparations
containing aspirin* when the name on the label does not
include the word 'aspirin'.

33 **Contains an aspirin-like medicine**
To be used on containers of dispensed *preparations
containing aspirin derivatives.*

Products and their labels

Products introduced or amended since publication of BNF No. 46 (September 2003) are underlined.
Proprietary names are in *italic*.
C = counselling advised; see BNF = consult product entry in BNF

Abacavir, C, hypersensitivity reactions, see BNF
Acamprosate, 21, 25
Acarbose, C, administration, see BNF
Accolate, 23
Acebutolol, 8
Aceclofenac, 21
Acemetacin, 21, C, driving
Acenocoumarol, 10, anticoagulant card
Acetazolamide, 3
Acetazolamide m/r, 3, 25
Aciclovir susp and tabs, 9
Acipimox, 21
Acitretin, 10, patient information leaflet, 21
Acrivastine, C, driving, alcohol, see BNF
Actinac, 28
Actiq, 2
Actonel, C, administration, food and calcium, see BNF
Acupan, 2, 14, (urine pink)
Adalat LA, 25
Adalat Retard, 25
Adalimumab, C, tuberculosis
Adcal, 24
Adcal-D₃, 24
Adcortyl with Graneodin, 28
Adipine MR, 21, 25
Adizem preps, 25
AeroBec, 8, C, dose
AeroBec Forte, 8, 10, steroid card, C, dose

Aerocrom, 8
Agenerase caps, 5
Agenerase oral solution, 4, 5
Airomir, C, dose, change to CFC-free inhaler, see BNF
Albendazole, 9
Alclometasone external preps, 28
Aldara, 10, patient information leaflet
Aldomet, 3, 8
Alendronic acid, C, administration, see BNF
Alfuzosin, 3, C, dose, see BNF
Alfuzosin m/r, 3, 21, 25, C, dose, see BNF
Alimemazine, 2
Allegron, 2
Allopurinol, 8, 21, 27
Almogran, 3
Almotriptan, 3
Alphosyl HC, 28
Alphaderm, 28
Alprazolam, 2
Alvedon, 30
Alvercol, 25, 27, C, administration, see BNF
Amantadine, C, driving
Aminophylline m/r, see preps
Amiodarone, 11
Amisulpride, 2
Amitriptyline, 2
Amitriptyline m/r, 2, 25
Amobarbital, 19
Amorolfine, 10, patient information leaflet

Amoxapine, 2
Amoxicillin, 9
Amoxicillin chewable tabs, 9, 10, patient information leaflet
Amoxicillin dispersible sachets, 9, 13
Amoxil, 9
Amoxil dispersible sachets, 9, 13
Amoxil paed susp, 9, C, use of pipette
Amphotericin loz, 9, 24, C, after food
Amphotericin mixt (g.i.), 9, C, use of pipette
Amphotericin mixt (mouth), 9, C, use of pipette, hold in mouth, after food
Amphotericin tabs, 9
Ampicillin, 9, 23
Amprenavir caps, 5
Amprenavir oral solution, 4, 5
Amytal, 19
Anafranil, 2
Anafranil m/r, 2, 25
Anakinra, C, blood disorder symptoms
Androcur, 21
Andropatch, C, administration, see BNF
Angettes-75, 32
Angiopine 40 LA, 21, 25
Angitil SR, 25
Angitil XL, 25
Anhydrol Forte, 15

Dantrium, 2
Dantrolene, 2
Dapsone, 8
DDAVP tabs and intranasal, C, fluid intake, see BNF
Decadron tabs, 10, steroid card, 21
Deferiprone, 14, C, blood disorders
Deflazacort, 5, 10, steroid card
Deltacortril e/c, 5, 10, steroid card, 25
Deltastab inj, 10, steroid card
Demeclocycline, 7, 9, 11, 23
De-Noltab, C, administration, see BNF
Depakote, 25
Depixol, 2
Depo-Medrone (systemic), 10, steroid card
Dermestril, C, administration, see BNF
Dermovate cream and oint, 28
Dermovate scalp application, 15, 28
Dermovate-NN, 28
Deseril, 2, 21
Desmopressin tabs and intranasal, C, fluid intake, see BNF
Desmospray, C, fluid intake, see BNF
Desmotabs, C, fluid intake, see BNF
Desoximetasone external preps, 28
Destolit, 21
Detecho, 7, 9, 11, 23, C, posture
Detrunorm, 3
Detrusitol m/r, 25
Dexamethasone inj, 10, steroid card
Dexamethasone tabs, 10, steroid card, 21
Dexamfetamine, C, driving
Dexedrine, C, driving
Dexketoprofen, 22
Dextropropoxyphene, 2
DF118 Forte, 2, 21
DHC Continus, 2, 25
Diamorphine preps, 2
Diamox tabs, 3
Diamox SR, 3, 25
Diazepam, 2 or 19
Diclofenac dispersible tabs, 13, 21
Diclofenac e/c, 5, 25
Diclofenac m/r, 21, 25
Dicloflex Retard, 21, 25
Diclomax 75 mg SR and Retard, 21, 25
Diconal, 2
Didanosine e/c caps, 25, C, administration
Didanosine tabs, 23, C, administration
Didronel, C, food and calcium, see BNF
Didronel PMO, 10, patient leaflet, C, food and calcium, see BNF
Diflucan 50 and 200mg, 9
Diflucan susp, 9
Diflucortolone external preps, 28

Diflunisal, 21, 25, C, avoid aluminium hydroxide
Digoxin elixir, C, use of pipette
Dihydrocodeine, 2, 21
Dihydrocodeine m/r, 2, 25
Dihydroergotamine, nasal spray, 18, C, dosage
Dilcardia SR, 25
Diloxanide, 9
Diltiazem, 25
Dilzem preps, 25
Dimotane, 2
Dimotane LA, 2, 25
Dimotane Plus, 2
Dimotane Plus, Paediatric, 1
Dindevan, 10, anticoagulant card, 14, (urine pink or orange)
Dioderm, 28
Dipentum, 21, C, blood disorder symptoms, see BNF
Diphenhydramine, 2
Diphenylpyraline m/r, 2, 25
Diprosalic, 28
Diprosone, 28
Dipyridamole, 22
Dipyridamole m/r, 21, 25
Disipal, C, driving
Disodium etidronate, C, food and calcium, see BNF
Disopyramide m/r, 25
Disprin CV, 25, 32
Disprol, 30
Distaclor, 9
Distaclor MR, 9, 21, 25
Distalgesic, 2, 10, patient information leaflet, 29, 30
Distamine, 6, 22, C, blood disorder symptoms, see BNF
Distigmine, 22
Disulfiram, 2, C, alcohol reaction, see BNF
Dithranol preps, 28
Dithrocream preps, 28
Dithrolan, 28
Ditropan, 3
Dolmatil, 2
Dolobid, 21, 25, C, avoid aluminium hydroxide
Doloxene, 2
Doloxene Compound, 2, 21, 32
Domperamol, 17, 30
Doralese, 2
Dostinex, 21, C, hypotensive reactions, see BNF
Dosulepin, 2
Dovobet, 28
Doxazosin m/r, 25
Doxepin, 2
Doxepin topical, 2, 10, patient information leaflet
Doxycycline caps, 6, 9, 11, 27, C, posture, see BNF
Doxycycline dispersible tabs, 6, 9, 11, 13
Doxycycline tabs, 6, 11, 27, C, posture, see BNF
Dozic, 2
Driclor, 15
Droleptan, 2

Dromadol XL, 2, 25
Droperidol, 2
Dulcolax tabs, 5, 25
Dumicoat, 10, patient information leaflet
Duofilm, 15
Duovent inhalations, C, dose
Duraphat toothpaste, C, administration
Durogesic, 2
Dutasteride, 25
Dutonin, 3
Dyazide, 14, (urine blue in some lights), 21
Dyspamet tabs, C, administration, see BNF
Dytac, 14, (urine blue in some lights), 21
Dytide, 14, (urine blue in some lights), 21

Econacort, 28
Edronax, C, driving
Efcortelan external preps, 28
Efcortesol, 10, steroid card
Efexor, 21, C, driving, skin reactions, see BNF
Efexor XL, 21, 25, C, driving, skin reactions, see BNF
Elantan preps, 25
Elleste Solo MX patches, C, administration, see BNF
Elocon, 28
Emcor preps, 8
Emeside, 8, C, blood disorder symptoms (see BNF), driving (see BNF)
Emflex, 21, C, driving
En-De-Kay mouthwash, C, food and drink, see BNF
Endoxana, 27
Enfuvirtide, C, hypersensitivity reactions, see BNF
Entacapone, 14, (urine reddish-brown), C, driving
Entocort CR, 5, 10, steroid card, 22, 25
Epanutin caps, 8, 27, C, administration, blood or skin disorder symptoms (see BNF), driving (see BNF)
Epanutin Infatabs, 8, 24, C, blood or skin disorder symptoms (see BNF), driving (see BNF)
Epanutin susp, 8, C, administration, blood or skin disorder symptoms (see BNF), driving (see BNF)
Epilim Chrono, 8, 25, C, blood or hepatic disorder symptoms (see BNF), driving (see BNF)
Epilim e/c tabs, 5, 8, 25, C, blood or hepatic disorder symptoms (see BNF), driving (see BNF)
Epilim crushable tabs, liquid and syrup, 8, C, blood or hepatic disorder symptoms (see BNF), driving (see BNF)
Eprosartan, 21

Equanil, 2
Ergotamine, 18, C, dosage
Erymax, 5, 9, 25
Erythrocin, 9
Erythromycin caps, 5, 9, 25
Erythromycin ethyl succinate, 9
Erythromycin ethyl succinate gran, 9, 13
Erythromycin stearate tabs, 9
Erythromycin tabs, 5, 9, 25
Erythroped, 9
Erythroped A tabs, 9
Escitalopram, C, driving
Esomeprazole, C, administration, see BNF
Estracombi, C, administration, see BNF
Estracyt, 23, C, dairy products, see BNF
Estraderm MX, C, administration, see BNF
Estraderm TTS, C, administration, see BNF
Estradiol vaginal ring, 10, patient information leaflet
Estrapak-50, C, administration, see BNF
Estramustine, 23, C, dairy products, see BNF
Estring, 10, patient information leaflet
Estriol, 25
Ethambutol, 8
Ethosuximide, 8, C, blood disorder symptoms (see BNF), driving (see BNF)
Etidronate, C, food and calcium, see BNF
Etodolac m/r, 25
Etonogestrel implant, C, see patient information leaflet
Etoposide caps, 23
Eucardic, 8
Eumovate external preps, 28
Eurax-Hydrocortisone, 28
Evorel preps, C, administration, see BNF
Exelon caps, 21, 25
Exelon solution, 21
Exemestane, 21

Famciclovir, 9
Famvir, 9
Farlutal 500-mg tabs, 27
Fasigyn, 4, 9, 21, 25
Faverin, C, driving, see BNF
Fefol, 25
Fefol-Vit, 25
Felbinac foam, 15
Feldene caps, 21
Feldene dispersible tabs, 13, 21
Feldene Melt, 10, patient information leaflet, 21
Felodipine m/r, 25
Fematrix, C, administration, see BNF
Femapak, C, administration, see BNF

FemSeven, C, administration, see BNF
Fenbid, 25
Fenbufen, 21
Fenofibrate, 21
Fenofibrate m/r, 21, 25
Fenogal, 21
Fenoprofen, 21
Fenopron, 21
Fentanyl patches and lozenges, 2
Fentazin, 2
Feospan, 25
Ferriprox, 14, C, blood disorders
Ferrograd, 25
Ferrograd C, 25
Ferrograd Folic, 25
Ferrous salts m/r, see preps
Ferrous sulphate paed mixt, 27
Fexofenadine, C, driving, see BNF
Flagyl S, 4, 9, 23
Flagyl supps, 4, 9
Flagyl tabs, 4, 9, 21, 25, 27
Fleet Phospho-soda, 10, patient information leaflet, C, administration
Flixotide, 8, 10, steroid card (high-dose preparations only), C, dose
Flixotide Evohaler, 8, C, dose, change to CFC-free inhaler (see BNF), 10, steroid card (250-*Evohaler* only)
Flomax MR, 25
Florinef, 10, steroid card
Floxapen, 9, 23
Fluanxol, 2, C, administration, driving, see BNF
Flucloxacillin, 9, 23
Fluconazole 50 and 200mg, 9
Fluconazole susp, 9
Fludrocortisone, 10, steroid card
Fludroxycortide external preps, 28
Flunitrazepam, 19
Fluocinolone external preps, 28
Fluocinonide external preps, 28
Fluocinonide scalp lotion, 15, 28
Fluocortolone external preps, 28
Fluorigard mouthwash, C, food and drink, see BNF
Fluoxetine, C, driving, see BNF
Flupentixol, see preps
Fluphenazine, 2
Flurazepam, 19
Flurbiprofen, 21
Flurbiprofen m/r, 21, 25
Fluticasone inhalations, 8, 10, steroid card (high-dose preparations only), C, dose
Fluticasone inhalations (CFC-free), 8, C, dose, change to CFC-free inhaler (see BNF), 10, steroid card (high-dose preparations only)
Fluvastatin, C, muscle effects, see BNF
Fluvastatin m/r, 25, C, muscle effects, see BNF
Fluvoxamine, C, driving, see BNF
Foradil, C, dose, see BNF

Formoterol fumarate, C, dose, see BNF
Fortagesic, 2, 21, 29, 30
Fortipine LA 40, 21, 25
Fortovase, 21
Fortral caps and tabs, 2, 21
Fortral supps, 2
Fosamax, C, administration, see BNF
Franol, 21
Franol Plus, 21
Frisium, 2 or 19, 8, C, driving (see BNF)
Froben, 21
Froben SR, 21, 25
Frovatriptan, 3
Frusene, 14, (urine blue in some lights), 21
Fucibet, 28
Fucidin susp, 9, 21
Fucidin tabs, 9
Fucidin H, 28
Full Marks lotion, mousse, 15
Fungilin loz, 9, 24, C, after food
Fungilin susp (g.i.), 9, C, use of pipette
Fungilin susp (mouth), 9, C, use of pipette, hold in mouth, after food
Fungilin tabs, 9
Furadantin, 9, 14, (urine yellow or brown), 21
Furamide, 9
Fuzeon, C, hypersensitivity reactions, see BNF
Fybogel, 13, C, administration, see BNF
Fybogel Mebeverine, 13, 22, C, administration, see BNF

Gabapentin, 3, 5, 8, C, driving (see BNF)
Gabitril, 21
Galake, 21, 29, 30
Galantamine, 21
Gamanil, 2
Ganciclovir, 21
Gastrobid Continus, 25
Glucobay, C, administration, see BNF
Glucophage, 21
Glyceryl trinitrate patch, see preps
Glyceryl trinitrate m/r, 25
Glyceryl trinitrate tabs, 16
Gregoderm, 28
Griseofulvin, 9, 21, C, driving
Grisovin, 9, 21, C, driving
GTN 300 mcg, 16

Haelan, 28
Halciderm Topical, 28
Halcinonide external preps, 28
Haldol, 2
Half-Inderal LA, 8, 25
Half-Securon SR, 25
Half-Sinemet CR, 14, (urine reddish), 25
Haloperidol, 2
HeliClear, 5, 9, 25

Lithium citrate m/r, 10, lithium card, 25, C, fluid and salt intake, see BNF

Lithonate, 10, lithium card, 25, C, fluid and salt intake, see BNF

Loceryl, 10, patient information leaflet

Locoid cream, oint, and topical emulsion, 28

Locoid scalp lotion, 15, 28

Locoid C, 28

Lofepramine, 2

Lofexidine, 2

Loprazolam, 19

Lopresor, 8

Lopresor SR, 8, 25

Loratadine, C, driving, alcohol, see BNF

Lorazepam, 2 or 19

Lormetazepam, 19

Loron caps and tabs, 10, patient information leaflet, C, food and calcium, see BNF

Losec, C, administration, see BNF

Lotriderm, 28

Ludiomil, 2

Lugol's solution, 27

Lustral, C, driving, see BNF

Lyclear Dermal cream, 10, patient information leaflet

Lymecycline, 6, 9

Lysovir, C, driving

Macrobid, 9, 14, (urine yellow or brown), 21, 25

Macrodantin, 9, 14, (urine yellow or brown), 21

Madopar, 14, (urine reddish), 21, C, driving

Madopar dispersible tabs, 14, (urine reddish), 21, C, administration, driving, see BNF

Madopar CR, 5, 14, (urine reddish), 25, C, driving

Magnapen, 9, 22

Magnesium citrate effervescent pdr, 10, patient information leaflet, 13, C, administration

Magnesium sulphate, 13, 23

Malarone, 21

Manerix, 10, patient information leaflet, 21

Manevac, 25, 27

Maprotiline, 2

Marevan, 10, anticoagulant card

Maxalt, 3

Maxalt Melt, 3, C, administration

Maxepa, 21

Maxolon paed liquid, C, use of pipette

Maxolon SR, 25

Maxtrex (methotrexate), C, NSAIDs (see BNF)

Mebeverine, C, administration, see BNF

Mecysteine, 5, 22, 25

Medrone tabs, 10, steroid card, 21

Mefenamic acid caps, paed susp, and tabs, 21

Mefloquine, 21, 25, 27, C, driving, malaria prophylaxis, see BNF

Melleril, 2

Meloxicam tabs, 21

Menorest, C, administration, see BNF

Menoring 50, 10, patient information leaflet

Mepacrine, 4, 9, 14, 21

Meprobamate, 2

Meptazinol, 2

Meptid, 2

Mesalazine e/c, see preps

Mesalazine m/r, see preps

Mesalazine enema and supps, C, blood disorder symptoms, see BNF

Mesalazine gran, see preps

Mesren MR, 5, 25, C, blood disorder symptoms, see BNF

Metformin, 21

Methadone, 2

Methadose, 2

Methenamine, 9

Methocarbamol, 2

Methotrexate tabs, C, NSAIDs (see BNF)

Methylcellulose (constipation or diarrhoea), C, administration, see BNF

Methylcellulose tabs (anorectic), C, administration, see BNF

Methyldopa, 3, 8

Methylphenidate m/r, 25

Methylprednisolone external preps, 28

Methylprednisolone inj, 10, steroid card

Methylprednisolone tabs, 10, steroid card, 21

Methysergide, 2, 21

Metirosine, 2

Metoclopramide paed liquid, C, use of pipette

Metoclopramide m/r, see preps

Metopirone, 21, C, driving

Metoprolol, 8

Metoprolol m/r, see preps

Metosyn cream and oint, 28

Metosyn scalp lotion, 15, 28

Metrogel, 10, patient information leaflet

Metrolyl supps, 4, 9

Metronidazole gel, see preps

Metronidazole mixt, 4, 9, 23

Metronidazole supps, 4, 9

Metronidazole tabs, 4, 9, 21, 25, 27

Metyrapone, 21, C, driving

Mianserin, 2, 25

Micanol, 28

Miconazole denture lacquer, 10, patient information leaflet

Miconazole oral gel, 9, C, hold in mouth, after food

Miconazole tabs, 9, 21

Mictral, 9, 11, 13

Midrid, 30, C, dosage

Mifegyne, 10, patient information leaflet

Mifepristone, 10, patient information leaflet

Migard, 3

Migraleve, 2, (pink tablets), 17, 30

Migranal, 18, C, dosage

Migravess, 13, 17, 32

Migravess Forte, 13, 17, 32

Migril, 2, 18, C, dosage

Mildison, 28

Minocin, 6, 9, C, posture, see BNF

Minocin MR, 6, 25

Minocycline, 6, 9, C, posture, see BNF

Minocycline m/r, 6, 25

Mintec, 5, 22, 25

Mintezol, 3, 21, 24

Mirapexin, C, hypotensive reactions, driving, see BNF

Mirtazapine, 2, 25

Mizolline, 25, C, driving

Mizollen, 25, C, driving

Mobic tabs, 21

Mobiflex, 21

Moclobemide, 10, patient information leaflet, 21

Modisal XL, 25

Moditen, 2

Modrasone, 28

Modrenal, 21

Moducren, 8

Mogadon, 19

Molipaxin, 2, 21

Mometasone cream, 28

Mometasone inhaler, 8, 10, steroid card, C, dose

Mometasone ointment, 28

Mometasone scalp lotion, 28

Monit preps, 25

Mono-Cedocard, 25

Monocor, 8

Monomax SR, 25

Monomax XL, 25

Monosorb XL, 25

Monotrim, 9

Montelukast chewable tabs, 23, 24

Morcap SR, 2, C, administration, see BNF

Morphine preps, 2

Morphine m/r susp, 2, 13

Morphine m/r caps and tabs, see preps

Motifene, 25

Motival, 2

Movicol, 13

Movicol-Half, 13

Moxifloxacin, 6, 9, C, driving

Moxisylate, 21

Moxonidine, 3

MST Continus susp, 2, 13

MST Continus tabs, 2, 25

MXL, 2, C, administration, see BNF

Myambutol, 8

Mycobutin, 8, 14, (urine orange-red), C, soft lenses

Mynah, 8, 23

Myocrisin inj, C, blood disorder symptoms, see BNF

Dental Practitioners' Formulary

The following list has been approved by the appropriate Secretaries of State, and the preparations therein may be prescribed by dental practitioners on form FP10D (GP14 in Scotland).

Sugar-free versions, where available, are preferred.

Aciclovir Cream, BP
Aciclovir Oral Suspension, BP, 200 mg/5 mL
Aciclovir Tablets, BP, 200 mg
Amoxicillin Capsules, BP
Amoxicillin Oral Powder, DPF[1]
Amoxicillin Oral Suspension, BP
Amphotericin Lozenges, BP
Amphotericin Oral Suspension, BP
Ampicillin Capsules, BP
Ampicillin Oral Suspension, BP
Artificial Saliva, DPF[2]
Artificial Saliva Substitutes as listed below (to be prescribed only for indications approved by ACBS[3]):
　　AS Saliva Orthana®
　　Glandosane®
　　Biotene Oralbalance®
　　BioXtra®
　　Saliveze®
　　Salivix®

Ascorbic Acid Tablets, BP
Aspirin Tablets, Dispersible, BP[4]
Azithromycin Oral Suspension, 200 mg/5 mL, DPF
Benzydamine Mouthwash, BP 0.15%
Benzydamine Oromucosal Spray, BP 0.15%
Carbamazepine Tablets, BP
Carmellose Gelatin Paste, DPF
Cefalexin Capsules, BP
Cefalexin Oral Suspension, BP
Cefalexin Tablets, BP
Cefradine Capsules, BP
Cefradine Oral Solution, DPF
Chlorhexidine Gluconate 1% Gel, DPF
Chlorhexidine Mouthwash, BP
Chlorhexidine Oral Spray, DPF
Chlorphenamine Tablets/Chlorpheniramine Tablets, BP
Choline Salicylate Dental Gel, BP
Clindamycin Capsules, BP
Diazepam Oral Solution, BP, 2 mg/5 mL
Diazepam Tablets, BP
Diflunisal Tablets, BP
Dihydrocodeine Tablets, BP, 30 mg
Doxycycline Capsules, BP, 100 mg

Doxycycline Tablets, 20 mg, DPF
Ephedrine Nasal Drops, BP
Erythromycin Ethyl Succinate Oral Suspension, BP
Erythromycin Ethyl Succinate Tablets, BP
Erythromycin Stearate Tablets, BP
Erythromycin Tablets, BP
Fluconazole Capsules, 50 mg, DPF
Fluconazole Oral Suspension, 50 mg/5 mL, DPF
Hydrocortisone Cream, BP, 1%
Hydrocortisone Oromucosal Tablets, BP
Hydrocortisone and Miconazole Cream, DPF
Hydrocortisone and Miconazole Ointment, DPF
Hydrogen Peroxide Mouthwash, BP
Ibuprofen Oral Suspension, BP, sugar-free
Ibuprofen Tablets, BP
Lidocaine 5% Ointment/Lignocaine 5% Ointment, DPF
Menthol and Eucalyptus Inhalation, BP 1980[5]
Metronidazole Oral Suspension, DPF
Metronidazole Tablets, BP
Miconazole Oromucosal Gel, BP
Mouthwash Solution-tablets, DPF
Nitrazepam Tablets, BP
Nystatin Ointment, BP
Nystatin Oral Suspension, BP
Nystatin Pastilles, BP
Oxytetracycline Tablets, BP
Paracetamol Oral Suspension, BP[6]
Paracetamol Tablets, BP
Paracetamol Tablets, Soluble, BP
Penciclovir Cream, DPF
Pethidine Tablets, BP
Phenoxymethylpenicillin Oral Solution, BP
Phenoxymethylpenicillin Tablets, BP
Povidone–Iodine Mouthwash, BP, 1%
Promethazine Hydrochloride Tablets, BP
Promethazine Oral Solution, BP
Rofecoxib Tablets, DPF
Sodium Chloride Mouthwash, Compound, BP
Sodium Fluoride Oral Drops, BP
Sodium Fluoride Tablets, BP
Sodium Fusidate Ointment, BP
Temazepam Oral Solution, BP
Temazepam Tablets, BP
Tetracycline Tablets, BP
Triamcinolone Dental Paste, BP
Vitamin B Tablets, Compound, Strong, BPC
Zinc Sulphate Mouthwash, DPF

> Preparations in this list which are not included in the BP or BPC are described on p. 803

---

1. Amoxicillin Dispersible Tablets are no longer available

2. Supplies may be difficult to obtain

3. Indications approved by the ACBS are: patients suffering from dry mouth as a result of having (or having undergone) radiotherapy or sicca syndrome

4. The BP directs that when soluble aspirin tablets are prescribed, dispersible aspirin tablets should be dispensed

5. This preparation does not appear in subsequent editions of the BP

6. The BP directs that when Paediatric Paracetamol Oral Suspension or Paediatric Paracetamol Mixture is prescribed and no strength stated Paracetamol Oral Suspension 120 mg/5 mL should be dispensed

Details of DPF preparations

Preparations on the List of Dental Preparations which are specified as DPF are described as follows in the DPF.

Although brand names have sometimes been included for identification purposes preparations on the list should be prescribed by non-proprietary name.

Amoxicillin Oral Powder PoM (proprietary product: *Amoxil Sachets SF*), amoxicillin (as trihydrate) 750 mg[1] and 3 g sachet

1. 750-mg sachets are no longer available

Artificial Saliva, (proprietary product: *Luborant*) consists of sorbitol 1.8 g, carmellose sodium (sodium carboxymethylcellulose) 390 mg, dibasic potassium phosphate 48.23 mg, potassium chloride 37.5 mg, monobasic potassium phosphate 21.97 mg, calcium chloride 9.972 mg, magnesium chloride 3.528 mg, sodium fluoride 258 micrograms/60 mL, with preservatives and colouring agents

Azithromycin Oral Suspension 200 mg/5 mL PoM (proprietary product: *Zithromax*); azithromycin (as dihydrate) 200 mg/5 mL when reconstituted with water

Carmellose Gelatin Paste (proprietary product: *Orabase Oral Paste*), gelatin, pectin, carmellose sodium, 16.58% of each in a suitable basis

Cefradine Oral Solution PoM (proprietary product: *Velosef Syrup*), cefradine 250 mg/5mL when reconstituted with water

Chlorhexidine Gluconate 1% Gel (proprietary product: *Corsodyl Dental Gel*), chlorhexidine gluconate 1%

Chlorhexidine Oral Spray (proprietary product: *Corsodyl Oral Spray*), chlorhexidine gluconate 0.2%

Doxycycline Tablets 20 mg PoM (proprietary product: *Periostat*), doxycycline (as hyclate) 20 mg

Fluconazole Capsules 50 mg PoM (proprietary product: *Diflucan*), fluconazole 50 mg

Fluconazole Oral Suspension 50 mg/5 mL PoM (proprietary product: *Diflucan*), fluconazole 50 mg/5 mL when reconstituted with water

Hydrocortisone and Miconazole Cream PoM (proprietary product: *Daktacort Cream*), hydrocortisone 1%, miconazole nitrate 2%

Hydrocortisone and Miconazole Ointment PoM (proprietary product: *Daktacort Ointment*), hydrocortisone 1%, miconazole nitrate 2%

Lidocaine 5% Ointment/Lignocaine 5% Ointment lidocaine 5% in a suitable basis

Metronidazole Oral Suspension PoM (proprietary product: *Flagyl S*), metronidazole (as benzoate) 200 mg/5mL

Mouthwash Solution-tablets consist of tablets which may contain antimicrobial, colouring and flavouring agents in a suitable soluble effervescent basis to make a mouthwash suitable for dental purposes

Penciclovir Cream PoM (proprietary product: *Vectavir Cream*), penciclovir 1%

Rofecoxib Tablets PoM (proprietary product: *VioxxAcute*), rofecoxib 25 mg and 50 mg

Zinc Sulphate Mouthwash consists of zinc sulphate lotion, BP. Directions for use: dilute 1 part with 4 parts of warm water
NOTE. May be difficult to obtain

Nurse Prescribers' Formulary

Nurse Prescribers Formulary for District Nurses and Health Visitors

Nurse Prescribers' Formulary Appendix (Appendix NPF). List of preparations approved by the Secretary of State which may be prescribed on form FP10P (form HS21(N) in Northern Ireland, form GP10(N) in Scotland, forms FP10(CN) and FP10(PN) in Wales or when available WP10P in Wales (ordered as WP10CN and WP10PN)) by Nurses for National Health Service patients

Medicinal Preparations

> *Preparations* on this list which are not included in the BP or BPC are described on p. 807

Almond Oil Ear Drops, BP
Arachis Oil Enema, NPF
[1]Aspirin Tablets, Dispersible, 300 mg, BP
Bisacodyl Suppositories, BP (includes 5-mg and 10-mg strengths)
Bisacodyl Tablets, BP
Cadexomer-Iodine Ointment, NPF
Cadexomer-Iodine Paste, NPF
Cadexomer-Iodine Powder, NPF
Catheter Maintenance Solution, Chlorhexidine, NPF
Catheter Maintenance Solution, Mandelic Acid, NPF
Catheter Maintenance Solution, Sodium Chloride, NPF
Catheter Maintenance Solution, 'Solution G', NPF
Catheter Maintenance Solution, 'Solution R', NPF
Choline Salicylate Dental Gel, BP
Clotrimazole Cream 1%, BP
Co-danthramer Capsules, NPF
Co-danthramer Capsules, Strong, NPF
Co-danthramer Oral Suspension, NPF
Co-danthramer Oral Suspension, Strong, NPF
Co-danthrusate Capsules, BP
Co-danthrusate Oral Suspension, NPF
Crotamiton Cream, BP
Crotamiton Lotion, BP
Dextranomer Beads, NPF
Dextranomer Paste, NPF
Dimeticone barrier creams containing at least 10%
Docusate Capsules, BP
Docusate Enema, NPF
Docusate Enema, Compound, BP
Docusate Oral Solution, BP
Docusate Oral Solution, Paediatric, BP
Econazole Cream 1%, BP
Emollients as listed below:
    Aqueous Cream, BP
    Arachis Oil, BP
    Cetraben® Emollient Cream
    Decubal® Clinic
    Dermamist®
    Diprobase® Cream

Diprobase® Ointment
Doublebase®
E45® Cream
Emulsifying Ointment, BP
Epaderm®
Gammaderm® Cream
Hydromol® Cream
Hydromol® Ointment
Hydrous Ointment, BP
Keri® Therapeutic Lotion
LactiCare® Lotion
Lipobase®
Liquid and White Soft Paraffin Ointment, NPF
Neutrogena® Dermatological Cream
Oilatum® Cream
Paraffin, White Soft, BP
Paraffin, Yellow Soft, BP
Ultrabase®
Unguentum M®
Emollient Bath Additives as listed below:
    Alpha Keri® Bath Oil
    Ashbourne Emollient Medicinal Bath Oil
    [2]Balneum®
    Cetraben®
    Dermalo® Bath Emollient
    Diprobath®
    Hydromol® Emollient
    Imuderm® Bath Oil
    Oilatum® Emollient
    Oilatum® Fragrance Free
    Oilatum® Gel
Folic Acid 400 micrograms/5 mL Oral Solution, NPF
Folic Acid Tablets 400 micrograms, BP
Glycerol Suppositories, BP
[3]Ibuprofen Oral Suspension, BP
[3]Ibuprofen Tablets, BP
Ispaghula Husk Granules, BP
Ispaghula Husk Granules, Effervescent, BP
Ispaghula Husk Oral Powder, BP
Lactulose Solution, BP
Lidocaine Gel/Lignocaine Gel, BP
Lidocaine Ointment/Lignocaine Ointment, BP
Lidocaine and Chlorhexidine Gel/Lignocaine and Chlorhexidine Gel, BP
Macrogol Oral Powder, NPF
Macrogol Oral Powder, Compound, NPF
Magnesium Hydroxide Mixture, BP
Magnesium Sulphate Paste, BP
Malathion alcoholic lotions containing at least 0.5%
Malathion aqueous lotions containing at least 0.5%
Mebendazole Oral Suspension, NPF
Mebendazole Tablets, NPF
Methylcellulose Tablets, BP
Miconazole Cream 2%, BP
Miconazole Oromucosal Gel, BP
Mouthwash Solution-tablets, NPF

---

1. Max. 96 tablets; max. pack size 32 tablets

2. Except pack sizes that are not to be prescribed under the NHS (see Part XVIIIA of the Drug Tariff, Part XI of the Northern Ireland Drug Tariff)

3. Except for indications and doses that are PoM

Nicotine Inhalation Cartridge for Oromucosal Use, NPF
Nicotine Lozenge, NPF
Nicotine Medicated Chewing Gum, NPF
Nicotine Nasal Spray, NPF
Nicotine Sublingual Tablets, NPF
Nicotine Transdermal Patches, NPF
Nystatin Oral Suspension, BP
Nystatin Pastilles, BP
Olive Oil Ear Drops, BP
Paracetamol Oral Suspension, BP (includes 120 mg/5 mL and 250 mg/5 mL strengths—both of which are available as sugar-free formulations)
[1]Paracetamol Tablets, BP
[1]Paracetamol Tablets, Soluble, BP (includes 120-mg and 500-mg tablets)
Permethrin Cream, NPF
Phenothrin Alcoholic Lotion, NPF
Phenothrin Aqueous Lotion, NPF
Phosphates Enema, BP
Piperazine and Senna Powder, NPF
Povidone–Iodine Solution, BP
Senna Granules, Standardised, BP
Senna Oral Solution, NPF
Senna Tablets, BP
Senna and Ispaghula Granules, NPF
[2]Sodium Bicarbonate Ear Drops, BP
Sodium Chloride Solution, Sterile, BP
Sodium Citrate Compound Enema, NPF
Sodium Picosulfate Capsules, NPF
Sodium Picosulfate Elixir, NPF
Spermicidal contraceptives as listed below:
    Delfen® Foam
    Duragel® Gel
    Gynol II® Jelly
    Ortho-Creme® Cream
    Orthoforms® Pessaries
Sterculia Granules, NPF
Sterculia and Frangula Granules, NPF
Streptokinase and Streptodornase Topical Powder, NPF
Thymol Glycerin, Compound, BP 1988
Titanium Ointment, BP
Water for Injections, BP
Zinc and Castor Oil Ointment, BP
Zinc Cream, BP
Zinc Ointment, BP
Zinc Oxide and Dimeticone Spray, NPF
Zinc Oxide Impregnated Medicated Stocking, NPF

Appliances and Reagents (including Wound Management Products)

> *In* the Drug Tariff Appliances and Reagents which may **not** be prescribed by Nurses are annotated Ⓝ (N**x** in the Scottish Drug Tariff and Ⓝ in the Northern Ireland Drug Tariff)

Applicators, Vaginal as listed in Part IXA of the Drug Tariff (Part 3 of the Scottish Drug Tariff, not prescribable by nurses in Northern Ireland)
Atomizers, Hand Operated as listed in Part IXA of the Drug Tariff (Part 3 of the Scottish Drug

Tariff, not prescribable by nurses in Northern Ireland)
Auto Inflation Device (for treatment of glue ear) as listed in Part IXA of the Drug Tariff (Part 3 of the Scottish Drug Tariff, Part III of the Northern Ireland Drug Tariff)
Breast Reliever as listed in Part IXA of the Drug Tariff (Part 3 of the Scottish Drug Tariff, not prescribable by nurses in Northern Ireland)
Breast Shields as listed in Part IXA of the Drug Tariff (not prescribable by nurses in Scotland or Northern Ireland)
Chemical Reagents
The following as listed in Part IXR of the Drug Tariff (Part 9 of the Scottish Drug Tariff, Part II of the Northern Ireland Drug Tariff):
    Detection Tablets for Glycosuria
    Detection Tablets for Ketonuria
    Detection Strips for Glycosuria
    Detection Strips for Ketonuria
    Detection Strips for Proteinuria
    Detection Strips for Blood Glucose
    Reagent solutions (Gerhardt's Reagent and Ammonia Solution, Strong, BP) (not prescribable by nurses in Northern Ireland)
Catheter Accessories as listed in Part IXA of the Drug Tariff (Part 3 of the Scottish Drug Tariff, Part III of the Northern Ireland Drug Tariff)
Catheter Maintenance Solutions as listed in Part IXA of the Drug Tariff (Part 3 of the Scottish Drug Tariff, Part III of the Northern Ireland Drug Tariff)
Catheters, Urethral Sterile as listed under Catheters in Part IXA of the Drug Tariff (Part 3 of the Scottish Drug Tariff, Part III of the Northern Ireland Drug Tariff)
Cervical Collar, Soft Foam as listed in Part IXA of the Drug Tariff (Part 3 of the Scottish Drug Tariff, not prescribable by nurses in Northern Ireland)
Chiropody Appliances as listed in Part IXA of the Drug Tariff (Part 2 of the Scottish Drug Tariff (except for Corn Plasters), not prescribable by nurses in Northern Ireland)
Contraceptive Devices as listed in Part IXA of the Drug Tariff (Part 3 of the Scottish Drug Tariff, Part III of the Northern Ireland Drug Tariff (fertility (ovulation) thermometers only))
Douches (with vaginal and rectal fittings) as listed in Part IXA of the Drug Tariff (Part 3 of the Scottish Drug Tariff, not prescribable by nurses in Northern Ireland)
Droppers as listed in Part IXA of the Drug Tariff (Part 3 of the Scottish Drug Tariff, not prescribable by nurses in Northern Ireland)
Ear Wax Softening Medical Devices as listed in Part IXA of the Drug Tariff (Part 3 of the Scottish Drug Tariff, Part III of the Northern Ireland Drug Tariff)
Elastic Hosiery including accessories as listed in Part IXA of the Drug Tariff (Part 4 of the Scottish Drug Tariff, Part III of the Northern Ireland Drug Tariff)
Eye Baths as listed in Part IXA of the Drug Tariff (Part 3 of the Scottish Drug Tariff, not prescribable by nurses in Northern Ireland)
Eye-drop Dispensers as listed in Part IXA of the Drug Tariff (Part 3 of the Scottish Drug Tariff, Part III of the Northern Ireland Drug Tariff)

---

1. Max. 96 tablets; max. pack size 32 tablets

2. Included in the Drug Tariff, Scottish Drug Tariff, and Northern Ireland Drug Tariff

Eye Shades as listed in Part IXA of the Drug Tariff (Part 3 of the Scottish Drug Tariff, not prescribable by nurses in Northern Ireland)

Finger Cots as listed in Part IXA of the Drug Tariff (Part 3 of the Scottish Drug Tariff, not prescribable by nurses in Northern Ireland)

Finger Stalls as listed in Part IXA of the Drug Tariff (Part 3 of the Scottish Drug Tariff, not prescribable by nurses in Northern Ireland)

Head Lice Device as listed in Part IXA of the Drug Tariff (Part 3 of the Scottish Drug Tariff, Part III of the Northern Ireland Drug Tariff)

Hypodermic Equipment as listed in Part IXA of the Drug Tariff (Part 3 of the Scottish Drug Tariff, Part III of the Northern Ireland Drug Tariff (with some exceptions))

Incontinence Appliances as listed in Part IXB of the Drug Tariff (Part 5 of the Scottish Drug Tariff, Part III of the Northern Ireland Drug Tariff)

Inhaler, Spare Tops as listed in Part IXA of the Drug Tariff (Part 3 of the Scottish Drug Tariff, not prescribable by nurses in Northern Ireland)

Insufflators as listed in Part IXA of the Drug Tariff (Part 3 of the Scottish Drug Tariff, not prescribable by nurses in Northern Ireland)

Irrigation Fluids as listed in Part IXA of the Drug Tariff (Part 2 of the Scottish Drug Tariff, Part III of the Northern Ireland Drug Tariff)

Latex Foam, Adhesive as listed in Part IXA of the Drug Tariff (not prescribable by nurses in Scotland or Northern Ireland)

Lubricating Jelly as listed in Part IXA of the Drug Tariff (Part 2 of the Scottish Drug Tariff, not prescribable by nurses in Northern Ireland)

Nasal Device (nasal dilator) as listed in Part IXA of the Drug Tariff (Part 3 of the Scottish Drug Tariff, Part III of the Northern Ireland Drug Tariff)

Nipple Shields, Plastic as listed in Part IXA of the Drug Tariff (Part 3 of the Scottish Drug Tariff, not prescribable by nurses in Northern Ireland)

Peak Flow Meters as listed in Part IXA of the Drug Tariff (Part 3 of the Scottish Drug Tariff, not prescribable by nurses in Northern Ireland)

Pessaries as listed in Part IXA of the Drug Tariff (Part 3 of the Scottish Drug Tariff, Part III of the Northern Ireland Drug Tariff (with some exceptions))

Protectives as listed in Part IXA of the Drug Tariff (Part 2 of the Scottish Drug Tariff, Part III of the Northern Ireland Drug Tariff (EMA Disposable Film Gloves only))

Saliva Stimulating Tablets as listed in Part IXA of the Drug Tariff (Part 3 of the Scottish Drug Tariff, not prescribable by nurses in Northern Ireland)

Stoma Appliances and Associated Products as listed in Part IXC of the Drug Tariff (Part 6 of the Scottish Drug Tariff, Part III of the Northern Ireland Drug Tariff)

Suprapubic Belts (replacements only) as listed in Part IXA of the Drug Tariff (Part 3 of the Scottish Drug Tariff, not prescribable by nurses in Northern Ireland)

Suprapubic Catheters as listed in Part IXA of the Drug Tariff (Part 3 of the Scottish Drug Tariff, not prescribable by nurses in Northern Ireland)

Synovial Fluid as listed in Part IXA of the Drug Tariff (Part 3 of the Scottish Drug Tariff, not prescribable by nurses in Northern Ireland)

Syringes (Bladder/Irrigating, Ear, Enema, Spare Vaginal Pipes) as listed in Part IXA of the Drug Tariff (Part 3 of the Scottish Drug Tariff, not prescribable by nurses in Northern Ireland)

Test Tubes as listed in Part IXA of the Drug Tariff (Part 3 of the Scottish Drug Tariff, not prescribable by nurses in Northern Ireland)

Tracheostomy and Laryngectomy Appliances as listed in Part IXA of the Drug Tariff (Part 2 of the Scottish Drug Tariff, not prescribable by nurses in Northern Ireland)

Trusses as listed in Part IXA of the Drug Tariff (Part 3 of the Scottish Drug Tariff, not prescribable by nurses in Northern Ireland)

Urine Sugar Analysis Equipment as listed in Part IXA of the Drug Tariff (Parts 3 and 9 of the Scottish Drug Tariff, Part III of the Northern Ireland Drug Tariff)

Vacuum Pumps and Constrictor Rings for Erectile Dysfunction as listed in Part IXA of the Drug Tariff (Part 3 of the Scottish Drug Tariff, Part III of the Northern Ireland Drug Tariff)—prescribing restrictions may apply (see Drug Tariff)

Wound Management and Related Products (including bandages, dressings, gauzes, lint, stockinette, etc)

The following as listed in Part IXA of the Drug Tariff (Part 2 of the Scottish Drug Tariff, Part III of the Northern Ireland Drug Tariff):

  Absorbent Cellulose Dressing with Fluid Repellent Backing

  Absorbent Cottons

  Absorbent Cotton Gauzes

  Absorbent Cotton and Viscose Ribbon Gauze, BP 1988

  Absorbent Dressing Pads, Sterile

  Absorbent Lint, BPC

  Absorbent Perforated Dressing with Adhesive Border

  Absorbent Perforated Plastic Film Faced Dressing

  Arm Slings

  Belladonna Adhesive Plaster BP 1980

  Boil Dressing Pack

  Cellulose Wadding, BP 1988

  Chlorhexidine Gauze Dressing, BP

  Conforming Bandage (Synthetic)

  Cotton Conforming Bandage, BP 1988

  Cotton Crêpe Bandage, BP 1988

  Cotton Crêpe Bandage, Hospicrepe 239

  Cotton, Polyamide and Elastane Bandage

  Cotton Stretch Bandage, BP 1988

  Crêpe Bandage, BP 1988

  Elastic Adhesive Bandage, BP

  Elastic Diachylon Bandage, Ventilated BPC

  Elastic Web Bandages

  Elastomer and Viscose Bandage, Knitted

  Gauze and Cotton Tissues

  Heavy Cotton and Rubber Elastic Bandage, BP

  High Compression Bandages (Extensible)

  Knitted Polyamide and Cellulose Contour Bandage, BP 1988

  Knitted Viscose Primary Dressing, BP, Type 1

  Multi-layer Compression Bandaging

  Multiple Pack Dressing No. 1

  Open-wove Bandage, BP 1988, Type 1

  Paraffin Gauze Dressing, BP

  Plaster of Paris Bandage BP 1988

Polyamide and Cellulose Contour Bandage, BP 1988

Polyester Primary Dressing with Neutral Triglycerides, Knitted

Povidone–Iodine Fabric Dressing, Sterile

Short Stretch Compression Bandage

Skin Adhesive, Sterile

Skin Closure Strips, Sterile

Standard Dressings

Sterile Dressing Packs

Stockinettes

Sub-compression Wadding Bandage

Surgical Adhesive Tapes

Surgical Sutures (absorbable and non-absorbable)

Suspensory Bandages, Cotton

Swabs

Triangular Calico Bandage, BP 1980

Vapour-permeable Adhesive Film Dressing, BP (including with absorbent pad)

Vapour-permeable Waterproof Plastic Wound Dressing, BP, Sterile

Wound Drainage Pouch

Wound Management Dressings (including activated charcoal, alginate, capillary-action, cavity, hydrocolloid, hydrogel, foam, polyurethane matrix, protease modulating matrix, silicone, silver-coated and silver-impregnated, and soft polymer dressings)

Zinc Paste Bandages (including both plain and with additional ingredients)

In the Drug Tariff Appliances and Reagents which may **not** be prescribed by Nurses are annotated Ⓝ (**Nx** in the Scottish Drug Tariff and **Ⅎ** in the Northern Ireland Drug Tariff)

Details of NPF preparations

Preparations on the Nurse Prescribers' Formulary which are not included in the BP or BPC are described as follows in the Nurse Prescribers' Formulary.

Although brand names have sometimes been included for identification purposes, it is recommended that non-proprietary names should be used for prescribing medicinal preparations in the NPF except where a non-proprietary name is not available.

Arachis Oil Enema
(proprietary product: *Fletchers' Arachis Oil Retention Enema*), arachis oil

Cadexomer–Iodine Ointment
(proprietary product: *Iodosorb Ointment*), cadexomer–iodine containing iodine 0.9% in an ointment basis

Cadexomer–Iodine Paste PoM
(proprietary product: *Iodoflex*), cadexomer–iodine containing iodine 0.9% in a paste basis

Cadexomer–Iodine Powder PoM
(proprietary product: *Iodosorb Powder*), cadexomer–iodine containing iodine 0.9%

Catheter Maintenance Solution, Chlorhexidine
(proprietary products: *Uro-Tainer Chlorhexidine*; *Uriflex C*), chlorhexidine 0.02%

Catheter Maintenance Solution, Mandelic Acid
(proprietary product: *Uro-Tainer Mandelic Acid*), mandelic acid 1%

Catheter Maintenance Solution, Sodium Chloride
(proprietary products: *Uro-Tainer Sodium Chloride*; *Uriflex-S*), sodium chloride 0.9%

Catheter Maintenance Solution, 'Solution G'
(proprietary products: *Uro-Tainer Suby G, Uriflex G*), citric acid 3.23%, magnesium oxide 0.38%, sodium bicarbonate 0.7%, disodium edetate 0.01%

Catheter Maintenance Solution, 'Solution R'
(proprietary products: *Uro-Tainer Solution R, Uriflex R*), citric acid 6%, gluconolactone 0.6%, magnesium carbonate 2.8%, disodium edetate 0.01%

Co-danthramer Capsules PoM
co-danthramer 25/200 (dantron 25 mg, poloxamer '188' 200 mg)

Co-danthramer Capsules, Strong PoM
co-danthramer 37.5/500 (dantron 37.5 mg, poloxamer '188' 500 mg)

Co-danthramer Oral Suspension PoM
(proprietary product: *Codalax*), co-danthramer 25/200 in 5 mL (dantron 25 mg, poloxamer '188' 200 mg/5 mL)

Co-danthramer Oral Suspension, Strong PoM
(proprietary product: *Codalax Forte*), co-danthramer 75/1000 in 5 mL (dantron 75 mg, poloxamer '188' 1 g/5 mL)

Co-danthrusate Oral Suspension PoM
(proprietary product: *Normax*), co-danthrusate 50/60 (dantron 50 mg, docusate sodium 60 mg/5 mL)

Dextranomer Beads
(proprietary product: *Debrisan Beads*), dextranomer

Dextranomer Paste
(proprietary product: *Debrisan Paste*), dextranomer in a soft paste basis

Dimeticone barrier creams
(proprietary products: *Conotrane Cream*, dimeticone '350' 22%; *Siopel Barrier Cream*, dimeticone '1000' 10%; *Vasogen Barrier Cream*, dimeticone 20%), dimeticone 10–22%

Docusate Enema
(proprietary product: *Norgalax Micro-enema*) docusate sodium 120 mg in 10 g

Folic Acid Oral Solution 400 micrograms/5 mL
(proprietary product: *Folicare*), folic acid 400 micrograms/5 mL

Liquid and White Soft Paraffin Ointment
liquid paraffin 50%, white soft paraffin 50%

Macrogol Oral Powder
(proprietary product: *Idrolax*), macrogol '4000' (polyethylene glycol '4000') 10 g/sachet

Macrogol Oral Powder, Compound
(proprietary products: *Movicol*), macrogol '3350' (polyethylene glycol '3350') 13.125 g, sodium bicarbonate 178.5 mg, sodium chloride 350.7 mg, potassium chloride 46.6 mg/sachet; *Movicol-Half*, macrogol '3350' (polyethylene glycol '3350') 6.563 g, sodium bicarbonate 89.3 g, sodium chloride 175.4 mg, potassium chloride 23.3 mg/sachet

Malathion alcoholic lotions
(proprietary products: *Prioderm Lotion*; *Suleo-M Lotion*), malathion 0.5% in an alcoholic basis

Malathion aqueous lotions
(proprietary products: *Derbac-M Liquid*; *Quellada M Liquid*), malathion 0.5% in an aqueous basis

Mebendazole Oral Suspension PoM
(proprietary product: *Vermox*), mebendazole 100 mg/5 mL

[1]**Mebendazole Tablets** PoM
(proprietary products: *Ovex, Vermox*), mebendazole 100 mg

Mouthwash Solution-tablets
consist of tablets which may contain antimicrobial, colouring and flavouring agents in a suitable soluble effervescent basis to make a mouthwash

[2]**Nicotine Inhalation Cartridge for Oromucosal Use**
(proprietary products: *Nicorette Inhalator, Boots Nicotine Inhalator*), nicotine 10 mg

Nicotine Lozenge
nicotine (as bitartrate) 1 mg (proprietary product: *Nicotinell Mint Lozenge*) or nicotine (as polacrilex) 2 mg or 4 mg (proprietary product: *NiQuitin CQ Lozenges*)

Nicotine Medicated Chewing Gum
(proprietary products: *Nicorette Gum, Nicorette Plus Gum, Nicotinell Gum, Nicotinell Plus Gum, NiQuitin CQ Gum, Boots Nicotine Gum*), nicotine 2 mg or 4 mg

Nicotine Nasal Spray
(proprietary product: *Nicorette Nasal Spray*), nicotine 500 micrograms/metered spray

[3]**Nicotine Sublingual Tablets**
(proprietary product: *Nicorette Microtab*), nicotine (as a cyclodextrin complex) 2 mg

[4]**Nicotine Transdermal Patches**
releasing in each 16 hours, nicotine approx. 5 mg, 10 mg, or 15 mg (proprietary product: *Nicorette Patch*) or releasing in each 24 hours nicotine approx. 7 mg, 14 mg, or 21 mg (proprietary products: *Nicotinell TTS, NiQuitin CQ, Boots NRT Patch*)

Permethrin Cream
(proprietary product: *Lyclear Dermal Cream*), permethrin 5%

Phenothrin Alcoholic Lotion
(proprietary product: *Full Marks Lotion*), phenothrin 0.2% in a basis containing isopropyl alcohol

Phenothrin Aqueous Lotion
(proprietary product: *Full Marks Liquid*), phenothrin 0.5% in an aqueous basis

Piperazine and Senna Powder
(proprietary product: *Pripsen Oral Powder*), piperazine phosphate 4 g, sennosides 15.3 mg/sachet

Senna Oral Solution
(proprietary product: *Senokot Syrup*), sennosides 7.5 mg/5 mL

Senna and Ispaghula Granules
(proprietary product: *Manevac Granules*), senna fruit 12.4%, ispaghula 54.2%

Sodium Citrate Compound Enema
(proprietary products: *Micolette Micro-enema; Micralax Micro-enema; Relaxit Micro-enema*), sodium citrate 450 mg with glycerol, sorbitol and an anionic surfactant

Sodium Picosulfate Capsules
(proprietary products: *Dulco-lax Perles*), sodium picosulfate 2.5 mg

---

1. For PoM exemption, see p. 323

2. For use with inhalation mouthpiece; to be prescribed as either a starter pack (6 cartridges with inhalator device and holder) or refill pack (42 cartridges with inhalator device)

3. To be prescribed as either a starter pack (2 x 15-tablet discs with dispenser) or refill pack (7 x 15-tablet discs)

4. Prescriber should specify the brand to be dispensed

Sodium Picosulfate Elixir
(proprietary products: *Dulco-lax Liquid, Laxoberal* NHS), sodium picosulfate 5 mg/5 mL

Sterculia Granules
(proprietary product: *Normacol Granules*), sterculia 62%

Sterculia and Frangula Granules
(proprietary product: *Normacol Plus Granules*), sterculia 62%, frangula (standardised) 8%

Streptokinase and Streptodornase Topical Powder PoM
(proprietary product: *Varidase Topical*), streptokinase 100 000 units, streptodornase 25 000 units

Zinc Oxide and Dimeticone Spray
(proprietary product: *Sprilon*), dimeticone 1.04%, zinc oxide 12.5% in a pressurised aerosol unit

Zinc Oxide Impregnated Medicated Stocking
(proprietary product: *Zipzoc*), sterile rayon stocking impregnated with ointment containing zinc oxide 20%

Nurse Prescribers' Extended Formulary

List of preparations which may be prescribed by Extended Formulary Nurse Prescribers on Form FP10P, for NHS patients in England (Form HS21(N) in Northern Ireland, Form GP10(N2) in Scotland).

Independent nurse prescribers who have completed the necessary training and are authorised to prescribe from the Nurse Prescribers' Extended Formulary list may prescribe all General Sales List and Pharmacy medicines currently prescribable by GPs, together with specified Prescription Only Medicines. In addition they may prescribe all items in the nurse prescribing list for District Nurses and Health Visitors on p. 804. The Committee on Safety of Medicines and the Medicines Commission advise that Extended Formulary Nurse Prescribers should prescribe medicines (including pharmacy-only and general sales list medicines) **only** for the medical conditions specified below. This advice is reinforced in the Department of Health Guide to Implementation of Independent Nurse Prescribing (available at www.doh.gov.uk/nurseprescribing). Nurses should **not** prescribe independently for conditions other than those on the list.

Medical Conditions

	BNF section[5]
Circulatory	
Haemorrhoids	1.7.1, 1.7.2
Phlebitis, superficial	-
Ear	
Furuncle	-
Otitis externa	12.1.1
Otitis media	12.1.2
Wax in ear	12.1.3

5. BNF sections appropriate to the listed conditions are shown. However, not all drugs in these sections are prescribable by nurses. Also, in some cases preparations (including General Sales List and Pharmacy medicines) in other BNF sections may be suitable. Before choosing a Prescription Only Medicine, nurses need to check the Nurse Prescribers' Extended Formulary list and to satisfy themselves that the product is licensed for the condition they wish to prescribe for and that the condition falls within the remit of the Nurse Prescribers' Extended Formulary.

Endocrine
Hypoglycaemia   6.1.4

Eye
Blepharitis   11.3.1
Conjunctivitis, allergic   11.4.2
Conjunctivitis, infective   11.3.1
Local anaesthetic for ophthalmic   11.7
    conditions

Gastro-intestinal conditions
Constipation   1.6
Gastro-enteritis   1.4
Heartburn   1.1
Infantile colic   1.1.1
Worms—threadworms   5.5.1

Immunisations
Routine childhood and specific   14.1, 14.4
    vaccinations

Musculoskeletal
Back pain, acute uncomplicated   4.7.1, 10.1.1
Neck pain, acute uncomplicated   4.7.1, 10.1.1
Soft tissue injury   4.7.1, 10.1.1,
                                        10.3.2
Sprains   4.7.1, 10.1.1,
                                        10.3.2

Oral conditions
Aphthous ulcer   12.3.1
Candidiasis, oral   12.3.2
Dental abscess   4.7.1, 10.1.1
Gingivitis   12.3.4
Stomatitis   -

Respiratory
Acute attacks of asthma   3.1
Acute nasopharyngitis (coryza)   12.2.2
Laryngitis   12.3.1
Pharyngitis   12.3.1
Rhinitis, allergic   3.4.1, 12.2.1,
                                        12.2.2
Sinusitis, acute   3.4.1
Tonsillitis   12.2.2, 12.3.1

Skin
Abrasions   13.10.5
Acne   13.6
Animal and human bites   5.1 (table 1)
Boil/carbuncle   13.10.5
Burn/scald   13.11, App. 8
Candidiasis, skin   13.10.2
Chronic skin ulcer   13.11.7,
                                        13.10.1
Dermatitis, atopic   13.5.1
Dermatitis, contact   13.5.1
Dermatitis, seborrhoeic   13.5.1
Dermatophytosis of the skin   13.10.2
    (ringworm)
Herpes labialis   13.10.3
Impetigo   5.1 (table 1),
                                        13.10.1
Insect bite/sting   13.3
Lacerations   13.11, App. 8
Local anaesthetic for occasions when proce- 15.2
    dure requires it
Local anaesthetic for suturing of lacerations 15.2
Nappy rash   13.2.2
Pediculosis (head lice)   13.10.4
Pruritus in chicken pox   13.3
Scabies   13.10.4
Urticaria   3.4.1
Warts (including verrucas)   13.7

Substance Dependence
Smoking cessation   4.10

Urinary system
Urinary tract infection (women)   5.1 (table 1),
—lower, uncomplicated   7.4.3

Female genital system
Bacterial vaginosis   5.1.11, 7.2.2
Candidiasis, vulvovaginal   7.2.2
Contraception   7.3
Dysmenorrhoea   4.7.1, 10.1.1
Emergency contraception   7.3
Laboratory-confirmed uncomplicated genital 5.1 (table 1)
    chlamydia infection (and the sexual part-
    ners of these patients)
Menopausal vaginal atrophy   7.2.1
Preconceptual counselling   9.1.2
Trichomonas vaginalis infection (and the 5.4.3
    sexual partners of these patients)

Male genital system
Balanitis   13.10.2

Palliative Care
Bowel colic   Prescribing in
                                        palliative care
Candidiasis, oral   12.3.2
Constipation   Prescribing in
                                        palliative care
Cough   Prescribing in
                                        palliative care
Dry mouth   Prescribing in
                                        palliative care
Excessive respiratory secretions   Prescribing in
                                        palliative care
Fungating malodorous tumours   13.10.1.2
Nausea and vomiting   Prescribing in
                                        palliative care
Neuropathic pain in palliative care   Prescribing in
                                        palliative care
Pain control   Prescribing in
                                        palliative care

Nurse Prescribers' Extended Formulary

1. All licensed P and GSL Medicines prescribable
   on the NHS
2. Prescription Only Medicines from the list below
   by the route or form specified
3. See above for the list of those medical conditions for which nurses may prescribe independently

**List of prescription only medicines for prescribing
by extended formulary nurse prescribers**

Oral antibacterials marked *—see separate list below for
indications

Drug	Route of adminis-tration, use or pharmaceutical form
Aciclovir	External
Acrivastine	Oral
Adapalene	External
Alclometasone dipropionate	External
Alimemazine tartrate (trimeprazine tartrate)	Oral
Amitriptyline hydrochloride	Oral
Amorolfine hydrochloride	External
Amoxicillin trihydrate*	Oral
Aspirin	Oral

Azelaic acid	External
Azelastine hydrochloride	Ophthalmic, nasal
Azithromycin dihydrate*	Oral
Baclofen	Palliative care—oral
Beclometasone dipropionate	External, nasal
Betamethasone sodium phosphate	Aural, nasal
Betamethasone valerate	External, rectal
Budesonide	Nasal
Carbamazepine	Oral, rectal
Carbaryl	External
Carbenoxolone sodium	Mouthwash
Cetirizine hydrochloride	Oral
Chloramphenicol	Ophthalmic
Cimetidine	Oral
Cinchocaine hydrochloride	Rectal
[1]Clavulanic acid	Oral
Clindamycin phosphate	External, vaginal
Clobetasone butyrate	External
Clotrimazole	External
Codeine phosphate	Oral
Conjugated oestrogens (equine)	External
Co-phenotrope	Oral
Cyclizine	Palliative care—parenteral
Dantrolene sodium	Palliative care—oral
Dantron	Oral
[2]Desogestrel	Oral
Desoximetasone	External
Dexamethasone	Aural
Dexamethasone isonicotinate	Nasal
Diazepam	Palliative care—oral, parenteral and rectal
Diclofenac diethylammonium	External
Diclofenac potassium	Oral
Diclofenac sodium	Oral, rectal
Dihydrocodeine tartrate	Oral
Domperidone	Palliative care—oral and rectal
Domperidone maleate	Palliative care—oral
Doxycycline*	Oral
Doxycycline hyclate*	Oral
Econazole nitrate	External, vaginal
Emedastine	Ophthalmic
Erythromycin*	External, oral
Erythromycin ethyl succinate*	Oral
Erythromycin stearate*	Oral
Estradiol	External
Estriol	External
[2]Ethinylestradiol	Oral
Etonogestrel	Implant
[2]Etynodiol diacetate	Oral
Famotidine	Oral
Felbinac	External
Fenticonazole nitrate	Vaginal
Fexofenadine hydrochloride	Oral
Flucloxacillin magnesium*	Oral
Flucloxacillin sodium*	Oral
Fluconazole	Oral
Fludroxycortide (flurandrenolone)	External
Flumazenil	Parenteral
Flumetasone pivalate	Aural
Flunisolide	Nasal
Fluocinolone acetonide	External
Fluocinonide	External
Fluocortolone hexanoate	External, rectal
Fluocortolone pivalate	External, rectal
Flurbiprofen	Lozenges
Fluticasone propionate	External, nasal
Fusidic acid	External
Gabapentin	Oral
Gentamicin sulphate	Aural

[2]Gestodene	Oral
Glucagon hydrochloride	Parenteral
Glucose	Parenteral
Hydrocortisone	External including rectal
Hydrocortisone acetate	External including rectal
Hydrocortisone butyrate	External
Hydrocortisone sodium succinate	Lozenges
Hyoscine butylbromide	Palliative care—parenteral
Hyoscine hydrobromide	Palliative care—oral, parenteral
Ibuprofen	External, oral
Ibuprofen lysine	Oral
Imipramine hydrochloride	Oral
Ipratropium bromide	Nasal
Isotretinoin	External
Ketoconazole	External
Ketoprofen	External
Levocabastine hydrochloride	Nasal and ophthalmic
Levomepromazine (methotrimeprazine) maleate	Palliative care—oral
Levomepromazine (methotrimeprazine) hydrochloride	Palliative care—parenteral
[2]Levonorgestrel	Oral
Lidocaine hydrochloride	External, parenteral
Lithium succinate	External
Lodoxamide trometamol	Ophthalmic
Loperamide hydrochloride	Oral
Loratadine	Oral
Lorazepam	Palliative care—oral, parenteral
Lymecycline*	Oral
Mebendazole	Oral
[2]Medroxyprogesterone acetate	Injection
[2]Mestranol	Oral
Metoclopramide hydrochloride	Palliative care—oral and parenteral
Metronidazole*	Oral, external, vaginal, rectal
Metronidazole benzoate*	Oral
Miconazole	Dental lacquer
Miconazole nitrate	External, vaginal
Midazolam	Palliative care—parenteral
Minocycline hydrochloride*	Oral
Mizolastine	Oral
Mometasone furoate	External, nasal
Nedocromil sodium	Ophthalmic
Nefopam hydrochloride	Oral
Neomycin sulphate	Aural
Neomycin undecanoate	Aural
Nitrofurantoin*	Oral
Nizatidine	Oral
[2]Norethisterone	Oral
[2]Norethisterone acetate	Oral
[2]Norethisterone enanthate	Parenteral
[2]Norgestimate	Oral
[2]Norgestrel	Oral
Nortriptyline hydrochloride	Oral
Nystatin	External, local mouth treatment, vaginal
Oxytetracycline dihydrate*	Oral
Paracetamol	Oral
Penciclovir	External
Piroxicam	External
Prednisolone	Oral
Prednisolone hexanoate	Rectal
Prednisolone sodium phosphate	Aural, oral
Ranitidine hydrochloride	Oral
Salbutamol sulphate	Inhalation
Silver sulfadiazine	External

Footnotes—see next page

Sodium cromoglicate	Ophthalmic
Sodium fusidate	External
Streptodornase	External
Streptokinase	External
Sulconazole nitrate	External
Terbinafine hydrochloride	External
Terbutaline sulphate	Inhalation
Tetracycline hydrochloride*	External, oral
Tretinoin	External
Triamcinolone acetonide	Aural, external, nasal, oral paste
Trimethoprim*	Oral
[3]Tuberculin PPD	Injection
[3]Vaccine, Adsorbed Diphtheria	Injection
[3]Vaccine, Adsorbed Diphtheria and Tetanus	Injection
[3]Vaccine, Adsorbed Diphtheria and Tetanus for Adults and Adolescents	Injection
[3]Vaccine, Adsorbed Diphtheria for Adults and Adolescents	Injection
[3]Vaccine, Adsorbed Diphtheria, Tetanus and Pertussis	Injection
[3]Vaccine, Adsorbed Diphtheria, Tetanus Toxoid and Pertussis (Acellular Component)	Injection
[3]Vaccine, BCG	Injection
[3]Vaccine, BCG Percutaneous	Injection
[3]Vaccine, Haemophilus Influenzae Type B (Hib)	Injection
[3]Vaccine, Haemophilus Influenzae Type B (Hib) with Diphtheria, Tetanus and Pertussis	Injection
[3]Vaccine, Haemophilus Influenzae Type B, (Hib) with Diphtheria, Tetanus and Acellular Pertussis	Injection
[4]Vaccine, Hepatitis A	Injection
[4]Vaccine, Hepatitis A with Typhoid	Injection
[4]Vaccine, Hepatitis A, Inactivated, with recombinant (DNA) Hepatitis B	Injection
[4]Vaccine, Hepatitis B	Injection
[4]Vaccine, Influenza	Injection
[3]Vaccine, Live Measles, Mumps and Rubella (MMR)	Injection
[3]Vaccine, Meningococcal Group C Conjugate	Injection
[3] or [4]Vaccine, Meningococcal Polysaccharide A and C	Injection
[4]Vaccine, Pneumococcal	Injection
[3]Vaccine, Poliomyelitis, Live (Oral)	Oral
[3]Vaccine, Rubella, Live	Injection
[4]Vaccine, Tetanus, Adsorbed	Injection
Vaccine, Typhoid, Live Attenuated (Oral)	Oral
[4]Vaccine, Typhoid, Polysaccharide	Injection
Water for Injections	Parenteral

* Oral antibacterials and indications considered suitable for nurse prescribing

Drug	Indication
[5]Amoxicillin trihydrate	Lower urinary-tract infection (women), animal and human bites
Azithromycin dihydrate	Laboratory-confirmed uncomplicated genital chlamydial infection, plus sexual partners of these patients
Doxycycline hyclate	Acne, animal and human bites, laboratory-confirmed uncomplicated genital chlamydial infection, plus sexual partners of these patients
Doxycycline monohydrate	Acne, animal and human bites, laboratory-confirmed uncomplicated genital chlamydial infection, plus sexual partners of these patients
Erythromycin	Impetigo, animal and human bites, laboratory-confirmed uncomplicated genital chlamydial infection, plus sexual partners of these patients
Erythromycin ethyl succinate	Impetigo, animal and human bites, laboratory-confirmed uncomplicated genital chlamydial infection, plus sexual partners of these patients
Erythromycin stearate	Impetigo, animal and human bites, laboratory-confirmed uncomplicated genital chlamydial infection, plus sexual partners of these patients
Flucloxacillin magnesium	Impetigo
Flucloxacillin sodium	Impetigo
Lymecycline	Acne
Metronidazole	Animal and human bites; fungating malodorous tumours; bacterial vaginosis; *trichomonas vaginalis* infection plus sexual partners of these patients
Metronidazole benzoate	Animal and human bites
Minocycline hydrochloride	Acne
Nitrofurantoin	Lower urinary-tract infection (women)
Oxytetracycline dihydrate	Acne, animal and human bites
Tetracycline hydrochloride	Acne
Trimethoprim	Lower urinary-tract infection (women)

1. Present as potassium clavulanate in co-amoxiclav
2. Nurse Prescribers in Family Planning Clinics—where it is not appropriate for nurse prescribers in family planning clinics to prescribe contraceptive drugs using form FP10(P) (forms FP10(CN) and FP10(PN) in Wales), they may prescribe using the same system as doctors in the clinic.
3. Centrally supplied vaccine excluded from reimbursement via prescription route
4. High Volume Personally Administered Vaccine. Claims for these vaccines should be ordered on form FP34D
5. With Clavulanic acid (as co-amoxiclav) for animal and human bites

Index of manufacturers

Ashbourne
Ashbourne Pharmaceuticals Ltd
Victors Barns
Northampton Rd, Brixworth
Northampton, NN6 9DQ.
Tel: (01604) 883 100
Fax: (01604) 881 640

AstraZeneca
AstraZeneca UK Ltd
Horizon Place
600 Capability Green, Luton
Beds, LU1 3LU.
Tel: 0800 7830 033
Fax: (01582) 838 003
medical.informationgb@astrazeneca.
com

Athena
Athena Neurosciences
See Elan.

Auden Mckenzie
Auden Mckenzie (Pharma Division)
Ltd
30 Stadium Business Centre
North End Rd, Wembley
Middx, HA9 0AT.
Tel: (020) 8900 2122
Fax: (020) 8903 9620

Aurum
Aurum Pharmaceuticals Ltd
Hubert Rd
Brentwood, Essex, CM14 4LZ.
Tel: (01277) 266600
Fax: (01277) 848 976
info@martindalepharma.co.uk

Aventis Behring
Aventis Behring Ltd
Aventis House
Market Place, Haywards Heath
West Sussex, RH16 1DB.
Tel: (01444) 447 400
Fax: (01444) 447 401
medinfo@aventis.com

Aventis Pasteur
Aventis Pasteur MSD Ltd
Mallards Reach
Bridge Ave, Maidenhead
Berks, SL6 1QP.
Tel: (01628) 785 291
Fax: (01628) 671 722

Aventis Pharma
Aventis Pharma Ltd
Aventis House
50 Kings Hill Ave, Kings Hill
West Malling, Kent, ME19 4AH.
Tel: (01732) 584 000
Fax: (01732) 584 080

Ayrton Saunders
Ayrton Saunders Ltd
Ayrton House
Commerce Way,
Parliament Business Park
Liverpool, Merseyside, L8 7BA.
Tel: (0151) 709 2074
Fax: (0151) 709 7336
info@ayrtons.com

Bailey, Robert
Robert Bailey Healthcare Ltd
Unit 6
Heapham Rd Industrial Estate,
Gainsborough
Lincs, DN21 1RZ.
Tel: (01427) 677 559
Fax: (01427) 677 654
marketing@cottonwool.uk.com

Bard
Bard Ltd
Forest House
Brighton Rd, Crawley
West Sussex, RH11 9BP.
Tel: (01293) 527 888
Fax: (01293) 552 428

Bausch & Lomb
Bausch & Lomb UK Ltd
106 London Rd
Kingston-upon-Thames, Surrey
KT2 6TN.
Tel: (020) 8781 2900
Fax: (01344) 8781 2901

Baxter
Baxter Healthcare Ltd
Caxton Way
Thetford
Norfolk, IP24 3SE.
Tel: (01842) 767 189
Fax: (01842) 767 099

Baxter Anaesthesia
Baxter Anaesthesia
Unit 31 Wellington Business Park
Dukes Ride, Crowthorne
Berks, RG45 6LS.
Tel: (01344) 759 300
Fax: (01344) 759 330

Baxter BioScience
Baxter BioScience
Wallingford Rd
Compton, Newbury
Berks, RG20 7QW.
Tel: (01635) 206 345
Fax: (01635) 206 373

Baxter Oncology
Baxter Healthcare Ltd
Wallingford Rd
Compton, Newbury
Berks, RG20 7QW.
Tel: (01635) 206 161
Fax: (01635) 206 103

Bayer
Bayer plc
Pharmaceutical Division
Bayer House, Strawberry Hill,
Newbury
Berks, RG14 1JA.
Tel: (01635) 563 000
Fax: (01635) 563 393
medical.science@bayer.co.uk

Bayer Consumer Care
See Bayer.

Bayer Diagnostics
Bayer plc
Diagnostics Division
Bayer House, Strawberry Hill,
Newbury
Berks, RG14 1JA.
Tel: (01635) 563 000
Fax: (01635) 563 393

BCM Specials
BCM Specials Manufacturing
D10 First 114
Nottingham, NG90 2PR.
Tel: 0800 952 1010
Fax: 0800 085 0673
bcm-specials@bcm-ltd.co.uk

Beacon
Beacon Pharmaceuticals Ltd
85 High St
Tunbridge Wells, TN1 1YG.
Tel: (01892) 506 958
Fax: (01892) 610 397
info@beaconpharma.co.uk

Becton Dickinson
Becton Dickinson UK Ltd
Between Towns Rd
Cowley, Oxford
Oxon, OX4 3LY.
Tel: (01865) 748 844
Fax: (01865) 717 313

Beiersdorf
Beiersdorf UK Ltd
Yeomans Drive, Blakelands
Milton Keynes
Bucks, MK14 5LS.
Tel: (01908) 211 444
Fax: (01908) 211 555

Bell and Croyden
John Bell and Croyden
54 Wigmore St
London, W1H 0AU.
Tel: (020) 7935 5555
Fax: (020) 7935 9605

Berk
Berk Pharmaceuticals
See APS.

BHR
BHR Pharmaceuticals Ltd
41 Centenary Business Centre
Hammond Close, Attleborough
Fields, Nuneaton
Warwickshire, CV11 6RY.
Tel: (024) 7635 3742
Fax: (024) 7632 7812
info@bhr.co.uk

Bio Diagnostics
Bio Diagnostics Ltd
Upton Industrial Estate
Rectory Rd, Upton-upon-Severn
Worcs, WR8 0XL.
Tel: (01684) 592 262
Fax: (01684) 592 501

Biogen
Biogen Ltd
5d Roxborough Way
Foundation Park, Maidenhead
Berks, SL6 3UD.
Tel: (01628) 501 000
Fax: (01628) 501 010

Biolitec
Biolitec Pharma Ltd
Block 5.3
Research Avenue South, Heriot Watt
Research Park
Edinburgh, EH14 4AP.
Tel: (0131) 451 1970
Fax: (0131) 449 7218
medical.info@biolitec.com

Biomatrix
Biomatrix UK Ltd
Lamb House
Church Street, Chiswick
London, W4 2PD.
Tel: (020) 8987 8830
Fax: (020) 8994 7083

Biomet Merck
Biomet Merck Ltd
Waterton Industrial Estate
Bridgend, South Wales, CF31 3XA.
Tel: (01656) 655 221
Fax: (01656) 645 454

Biosurgical Research
Biosurgical Research Unit
Surgical Materials Testing
Laboratory
Princess of Wales Hospital,
Coity Rd, Bridgend,
Mid Glamorgan
South Wales, CF31 1RQ.
Tel: (01656) 752 820
Fax: (01656) 752 830
maggots@smtl.co.uk

Blackwell
Blackwell Supplies Ltd
Medcare House
Centurion Close, Gillingham
Business Park, Gillingham
Kent, ME8 0SB.
Tel: (01634) 877 620
Fax: (01634) 877 621

Blake
Thomas Blake & Co
The Byre House
Fearby, Nr. Masham
North Yorks, HG4 4NF.
Tel: (01765) 689 042
Fax: (01765) 689 042
sales@veilcover.com

BOC
BOC Medical
The Priestley Centre,
10 Priestley Rd, Surrey Research Park
Guildford, Surrey, GU2 7XY.
Tel: 0800 111 333
Fax: 0800 111 555

Boehringer Ingelheim
Boehringer Ingelheim Ltd
Ellesfield Ave
Bracknell
Berks, RG12 8YS.
Tel: (01344) 424 600
Fax: (01344) 741 444

Boots
Boots The Chemists
Medical Services
Thane Rd, D90 East S10
Nottingham, NG90 1BS.
Tel: (0115) 959 5168
Fax: (0115) 959 2565

Borg
Borg Medicare
PO Box 99
Hitchin
Herts, SG5 2GF.
Tel: (01462) 442 993
Fax: (01462) 441 293

BPL
Bio Products Laboratory
Dagger Lane
Elstree
Herts, WD6 3BX.
Tel: (020) 8258 2200
Fax: (020) 8258 2601

BR
BR Pharmaceuticals Ltd
Clayton Wood Close
West Park Ring Road, Leeds
LS16 6QE.
Tel: (0113) 275 0000
Fax: (0113) 275 0055

Braun
B Braun (Medical) Ltd
Brookdale Rd
Thorncliffe Park Estate, Chapel-
town, Sheffield S35 2PW.
Tel: (0114) 225 9000
Fax: (0114) 225 9111
enquiry@bbmuk.demon.co.uk

Braun Biotrol
See Braun.

Bray
Bray Health & Leisure
1 Regal Way
Faringdon
Oxon, SN7 7BX.
Tel: (01367) 240 736
Fax: (01367) 242 625
solportLtd@btinternet.com

Bristol
Bristol Laboratories Ltd
Suite 3, 2nd Floor, Congress House
14 Lyon Rd, Harrow
Middlesex, HA1 2EN.
Tel: (020) 8863 8855
bristlab@btinternet.com

Bristol-Myers Squibb
Bristol-Myers Squibb
Pharmaceuticals Ltd
141-149 Staines Rd, Hounslow
Middx, TW3 3JA.
Tel: (020) 8572 7422
Fax: (020) 8754 3789
medical.information@bms.com

Britannia
Britannia Pharmaceuticals Ltd
41-51 Brighton Rd, Redhill
Surrey, RH1 6YS.
Tel: (01737) 773 741
Fax: (01737) 762 672
medicalservices@forumgroup.co.uk

Brodie & Stone
Brodie and Stone International plc
51 Calthorpe St
London, WC1X 0HH.
Tel: (020) 7278 9597
Fax: (020) 7278 2458
mailbox@brodieandstone.com

BSIA
See Torbet.

BSN Medical
BSN Medical Ltd
Healthcare House
Goulton St, Hull
North Humberside, HU3 4DJ.
Tel: (01482) 222 200
Fax: (01482) 222 211

Cambridge
Cambridge Laboratories
Deltic House, Kingfisher Way
Silverlink Business Park, Wallsend,
Tyne & Wear, NE28 9NX.
Tel: (0191) 296 9369
Fax: (0191) 296 9368
enquries@camb-labs.com

Castlemead
Castlemead Healthcare Ltd
PO Box 57
Ware, SG10 6LL.
Tel: (01462) 454 452
Fax: (01462) 435 684

Celltech
Celltech Pharmaceuticals Ltd
208 Bath Rd
Slough
Berks, SL1 3WE.
Tel: (01753) 534 655
Fax: (01753) 536 632
medicalinformationuk@
celltechgroup.com

CeNeS
CeNeS Pharmaceuticals
Compass House
Vision Park, Chivers Way, Histon
Cambs, CB4 9ZR.
Tel: (0870) 241 3674
Fax: (01223) 266 467
medinfo@cenes.co.uk

Centrapharm
Centrapharm Ltd
Dale House
Suckley Rd, Knightwick
Worcs, WR6 5QE.
Tel: (01886) 822 116
Fax: (01886) 822 125
info@centrapharm.co.uk

Cephalon
Cephalon UK Ltd
11-13 Frederick Sanger Rd
Surrey Research Park, Guildford
Surrey, GU2 7YD.
Tel: 0800 783 4869
Fax: (01483) 453 324
ukmedinfo@cephalon.com

Ceuta
Ceuta Healthcare Ltd
Hill House
41 Richmond Hill, Bournemouth
Dorset, BH2 6HS.
Tel: (01202) 780 558
Fax: (01202) 780 559

Chauvin
Chauvin Pharmaceuticals Ltd
106 London Rd
Kingston-Upon-Thames, Surrey
KT2 6TN.
Tel: (020) 8781 2900
Fax: (020) 8781 2901

Chemical Search
Chemical Search International Ltd
29th floor
1 Canada Square, Canary Wharf
London, E14 5DY.
Tel: (020) 7712 1758
Fax: (020) 7712 1759
info@chemicalsearch.co.uk

Chemidex
Chemidex Pharma Ltd
Chemidex House
Egham Business Village, Crabtree
Rd, Egham
Surrey, TW20 8RB.
Tel: (01784) 477 167
Fax: (01784) 471 776
info@chemidex.co.uk

Chiron
Chiron UK Ltd
PathoGenesis House
Park Lane, Cranford
Hounslow, TW5 9RR.
Tel: (020) 8580 4000
Fax: (020) 8580 4001

Chiron Vaccines Evans
Chiron Vaccines Evans Ltd
Gaskill Rd
Speke, Liverpool, L24 9GR.
Tel: (08457) 451 500
Fax: (0151) 7055 669
service@evans.com

CHS
Cambridge Healthcare Supplies Ltd
14D Wendover Rd
Rackheath Industrial Estate,
Rackheath
Norwich, NR13 6LH.
Tel: (01603) 735 200
Fax: (01603) 735 217

Chugai
Chugai Pharma UK Ltd
Mulliner House, Flanders Rd
Turnham Green, London, W4 1NN.
Tel: (020) 8987 5680
Fax: (020) 8987 5661

Clement Clarke
Clement Clarke International Ltd
Edinburgh Way
Harlow
Essex, CM20 2TT.
Tel: (01279) 414 969
Fax: (01279) 456 304
resp@clement-clarke.com

CliniMed
CliniMed Ltd
Cavell House, Knaves Beech Way
Loudwater, High Wycombe
Bucks, HP10 9QY.
Tel: (01628) 850 100
Fax: (01628) 850 331
enquires@clinimed.co.uk

Clinisupplies
Clinisupplies Ltd
9 Crystal Way
Elmgrove Rd, Harrow
Middx, HA1 2HP.
Tel: (020) 8863 4168
Fax: (020) 8426 0768
info@clinisupplies.co.uk

Clonmel
Clonmel Healthcare Ltd
Waterford Rd
Clonmel, Co. Tipperary
Ireland.
Tel: (00353) 52 77777
Fax: (00353) 52 77799
info@clonmelhealthcare.com

Co-Pharma
Co-Pharma Ltd
Unit 4
Metro Centre, Tolpits Lane, Watford
Herts, WD1 8SS.
Tel: (01923) 255 580
Fax: (01923) 255 581
sales@co-pharma.co.uk

Codan
Codan Ltd
Eastheath Ave
Wokingham
Berks, RH41 2PR.
Tel: (0118) 978 3663
Fax: (0118) 877 6274
babk@codanmed.co.uk

Colgate-Palmolive
Colgate-Palmolive Ltd
Guildford Business Park
Middleton Rd, Guildford
Surrey, GU2 5LZ.
Tel: (01483) 302 222
Fax: (01483) 303 003

CollaGenex
CollaGenex International Ltd
The Old Stable Block
7 Buttermarket, Thame
Oxon, OX9 3EW.
Tel: (01844) 218 989
Fax: (01844) 218 795
david@cgpi.co.uk

Coloplast
Coloplast Ltd
Peterborough Business Park
Peterborough, PE2 6FX.
Tel: (01733) 392 000
Fax: (01733) 233 348
gbcareteam@coloplast.com

Community
Community Foods Ltd
Micross, Brent Terrace
London, NW2 1LT.
Tel: (020) 8450 9411
Fax: (020) 8208 1803
email@communityfoods.co.uk

Concord
Concord Pharmaceuticals Ltd
PO Box 5970
Dunmow
Essex, CM6 1FY.
Tel: (0845) 602 0137
Fax: 0870 241 2335
enquires@concord-pharma.com

ConvaTec
ConvaTec Ltd
Harrington House, Milton Rd
Ickenham, Uxbridge
Middx, UB10 8PU.
Tel: (01895) 628 400
Fax: (01895) 628 456

Cow & Gate
See Nutricia Clinical.
Tel: (01225) 768 381
Fax: (01225) 768 847

CP
CP Pharmaceuticals Ltd
Ash Rd North
Wrexham Industrial Estate,
Wrexham, LL13 9UF.
Tel: (01978) 661 261
Fax: (01978) 660 130
mail@cppharma.co.uk

Crawford
Crawford Pharmaceuticals
Furtho House
20 Towcester Rd, Milton Keynes
MK19 6AQ.
Tel: (01908) 262 346
Fax: (01908) 567 730

Crookes
Crookes Healthcare Ltd
D80 Building
Nottingham, NG90 1LP.
Tel: (0115) 953 9922
Fax: (0115) 968 8722
dawn.kennard@crookes.co.uk

Cupal
Cupal Ltd
See SSL.

Cusi
Cusi Ophthalmic Generics
Pentagon Park
Boundary Way, Hemel Hempstead
Herts, HP2 7UD.
Tel: (01442) 341 326
Fax: (01442) 341 281

DDD
DDD Ltd
94 Rickmansworth Rd
Watford, Herts, WD18 7JJ.
Tel: (01923) 229 251
Fax: (01923) 220 728

DDSA
DDSA Pharmaceuticals Ltd
310 Old Brompton Rd
London, SW5 9JQ.
Tel: (020) 7373 7884
Fax: (020) 7370 4321

De Vilbiss
De Vilbiss Health Care UK Ltd
High Street
Wollaston, West Midlands, DY8 4PS.
Tel: (01384) 446 688
Fax: (01384) 446 699

De Witt
E C De Witt & Co Ltd
Tudor Rd
Manor Park, Runcorn
Cheshire, WA7 1SZ.
Tel: (01928) 579 029
Fax: (01928) 579 712
ecdewitt@ecdewitt.com

Denfleet
Denfleet Pharmaceuticals Ltd
260 Centennial Park
Elstree Hill South, Elstree
Herts, WD6 3SR.
Tel: (020) 8236 0000
Fax: (020) 8236 3501

Dental Health
Dental Health Products Ltd
60 Boughton Lane
Maidstone
Kent, ME15 9QS.
Tel: (01622) 749 222
Fax: (01622) 744 672

Dentsply
Dentsply Ltd
Hamm Moor Lane
Addlestone, Weybridge
Surrey, KT15 2SE.
Tel: (01932) 837 279
Fax: (01932) 858 970

Deproco
Deproco UK Ltd
Units R & S
Orchard Business Centre,
St. Barnabas Close, Allington
Maidstone, Kent, ME16 0JZ.
Tel: (01622) 695 520
Fax: (01622) 695 521
information@septodont.co.uk

Dermal
Dermal Laboratories Ltd
Tatmore Place
Gosmore, Hitchin
Herts, SG4 7QR.
Tel: (01462) 458 866
Fax: (01462) 420 565

DermaPharm
DermaPharm Ltd
Penrhyn House
10 St Mark's Hill, Surbiton
Surrey, KT6 4PW.
Tel: (020) 8399 3040
Fax: (020) 8399 0808
info@dermapharm.co.uk

Dexcel
Dexcel-Pharma Ltd
1 Cottesbrooke Park
Heartlands Business Park, Daventry
Northamptonshire, NN11 5YL.
Tel: (01327) 312 266
Fax: (01327) 312 262
office@dexcelpharma.co.uk

DiagnoSys
DiagnoSys Medical
Cams Hall
Fareham, Hants, PO16 8AB.
Tel: 0800 085 8808
Fax: (01329) 227 599

Dimethaid
Dimethaid International
PO Box 2963
Cookham, Maidenhead
Berks, SL6 9ZL.
Tel: (0800) 781 3642
Fax: (01628) 488 607

Discovery
Discovery Pharmaceuticals Ltd
Milton Heath House
Westcott Rd, Dorking
Surrey, RH4 3NB.
Tel: (01306) 886 715
Fax: (01306) 877 777
admin@discoverypharma.co.uk

Disetronic
Disetronic Medical Systems Ltd
Stoneleigh Deer Park
Stareton
Nr Kenilworth, CV8 2LY.
Tel: (02476) 531 338
Fax: (02476) 531 345
info@disetronic.co.uk

Dista
Dista Products Ltd
See Lilly.

Dowelhurst
Dowelhurst Ltd
1 Hawkes Drive
Heathcote Industrial Estate,
Warwick, CV34 6LX.
Tel: (01926) 461 600
Fax: (01926) 461 626

DuPont
See Bristol-Myers Squibb.

Durbin
Durbin plc
180 Northolt Rd
South Harrow
Middx, HA2 8TL.
Tel: (020) 8869 6500
Fax: (020) 8869 6565
info@durbin.co.uk

Easigrip
Easigrip Ltd
Unit 13, Scar Bank
Millers Rd, Warwick
Warwickshire, CV34 5DB.
Tel: (01926) 497 108
Fax: (01926) 497 109
enquiry@easigrip.co.uk

Eastern
Eastern Pharmaceuticals Ltd
Coomb House
7 St Johns Rd, Isleworth
Middx, TW7 6NA.
Tel: (020) 8569 8174
Fax: (020) 8569 8175

Eisai
Eisai Ltd
3 Shortlands
Hammersmith, London, W6 8EE.
Tel: (020) 8600 1400
Fax: (020) 8600 1401
Lmedinfo@eisai.net

Elan
Elan Pharma Ltd
Abel Smith House
Gunnels Wood Rd, Stevenage
Herts, SG1 2FG.
Tel: (01438) 765 100
Fax: (01438) 765 008
medinfo.uk@elan.com

Elida Fabergé
Elida Fabergé Ltd
Coal Rd, Seacroft
Leeds, LS14 2AR.
Tel: (0113) 222 5000
Fax: (0113) 222 5362

Entaco
Entaco Ltd
Royal Victoria Works
Birmingham Rd, Studley
Warwickshire, B80 7AP.
Tel: (01527) 852 306
Fax: (01527) 857 447
sales@entaco.com

Epiderm
Epiderm Ltd
Wass Lane
Sotby, Market Rasen, LN8 5LR.
Tel: (01507) 343 091
Fax: (01507) 343 092
djjcovermarkcryo@aol.com

Espire
Espire Healthcare Ltd
The Search Offices
Main Gate Road,
The Historic Dockyard
Chatham, ME4 4TE.
Tel: (01634) 812 144
Fax: (01634) 813 601
info@espirehealth.com

Ethicon
Ethicon Ltd
P.O. Box 408
Bankhead Avenue, Edinburgh
EH11 4HE.
Tel: (0131) 453 5555
Fax: (0131) 442 5114

Everfresh
Everfresh Natural Foods
Gatehouse Close
Aylesbury
Bucks, HP19 3DE.
Tel: (01296) 425 333
Fax: (01296) 422 545

Exelgyn
Exelgyn Laboratories
PO Box 4511
Henley-on-Thames,
Oxon, RG9 5ZQ.
Tel: (01491) 642 137
Fax: (0800) 731 6120

Ezject
Ezject Ltd
Bishops House
Bishops Rd, Claverham
Somerset, BS49 4NF.
Tel: (01934) 835 694
Fax: (01934) 876 790
info@ezject.co.uk

Fabre
Pierre Fabre Ltd
Hyde Abbey House
23 Hyde St, Winchester
Hampshire, SO23 7DR.
Tel: (01962) 856 956
Fax: (01962) 844 014
PFabreUK@aol.com

Farillon
Farillon Ltd
Ashton Rd
Harold Hill, Romford
Essex, RM3 8UE.
Tel: (01708) 379 000
Fax: (01708) 376 554

Fate
Fate Special Foods
Unit E2
Brook Street Business Centre,
Brook St, Tipton
West Midlands, DY4 9DD.
Tel: (01215) 224 433
Fax: (01215) 224 433

Fenton
Fenton Pharmaceuticals Ltd
4J Portman Mansions
Chiltern St, London, W1U 6NS.
Tel: (020) 7224 1388
Fax: (020) 7486 7258
mail@Fent-Pharm.co.uk

Ferndale
Ferndale Pharmaceuticals Ltd
Unit 605, Thorp Arch Estate
Wetherby, West Yorks
LS23 7BJ.
Tel: (01937) 541 122
Fax: (01937) 849 682
info@ferndale.co.uk

Ferraris
Ferraris Medical Ltd
4 Harforde Court
John Tate Rd, Hertford
Herts, SG13 7NW.
Tel: (01992) 526 300
Fax: (01992) 526 320
ferraris@globalnet.co.uk

Ferring
Ferring Pharmaceuticals (UK)
The Courtyard
Waterside Drive, Langley
Berks, SL3 6EZ.
Tel: (01753) 214 800
Fax: (01753) 214 801

Firstplay Dietary
Firstplay Dietary Foods Ltd
338 Turncroft Lane
Offerton, Stockport
Cheshire, SK1 4BP.
Tel: (0161) 474 7576
Fax: (0161) 474 7576

Florizel
Florizel Ltd
PO Box 138
Stevenage, SG2 8YN.
Tel: (01462) 436 156
Fax: (01462) 457 402

Flynn
Flynn Pharma Ltd
7 Serlby Court
Addison Rd, London W14 8EE.
Tel: (01462) 458 974
Fax: (01462) 450 755

Foodlink
Foodlink (UK) Ltd
2B Plymouth Rd
Plympton, Plymouth, PL7 4JR.
Tel: (01752) 344 544
Fax: (01752) 342 412
info@foodlinkltd.co.uk

Ford
Ford Medical Associates Ltd
2 Bridport Way
Braintree
Essex, CM7 9FJ.
Tel: (01376) 343 061
Fax: (01376) 339 014
tmf@globalnet.co.uk

Forest
Forest Laboratories UK Ltd
Bourne Rd
Bexley, Kent, DA5 1NX.
Tel: (01322) 550 550
Fax: (01322) 555 469
medinfo@forest-labs.co.uk

Fournier
Fournier Pharmaceuticals Ltd
19-20 Progress Business Centre
Whittle Parkway
Slough, SL1 6DQ.
Tel: (01753) 740 400
Fax: (01753) 740 444

Fox
C. H. Fox Ltd
22 Tavistock St
London, WC2E 7PY.
Tel: (020) 7240 3111
Fax: (020) 7379 3410

FP
Family Planning Sales Ltd
28 Kelburne Rd
Cowley, Oxford, OX4 3SZ.
Tel: (01865) 772 486
Fax: (01865) 748 746

Fresenius Kabi
Fresenius Kabi Ltd
Hampton Court
Tudor Rd, Manor Park, Runcorn
Cheshire, WA7 1UF.
Tel: (01928) 594 200
Fax: (01928) 594 314
med.info-uk@fresenius-kabi.com

Frontier
Frontier Multigate
Newbridge Rd Industrial Estate
Blackwood
South Wales, NP12 2YL.
Tel: (01495) 233 050
Fax: (01495) 233 055
multigate@frontier-group.co.uk

Fujisawa
Fujisawa Ltd
Fujisawa House
62 London Rd, Staines, TW18 4HB.
Tel: (01784) 227 500
Fax: (01784) 227 501
medinfo@fujisawa.co.uk

Futuna
Futuna Ltd
229 Preston Rd
Clayton-le-Woods,
Preston, PR6 7PT.
Tel: (0870) 601 2037
Fax: (0870) 601 2036

Galderma
Galderma (UK) Ltd
Galderma House
Church lane, Kings Langley
Herts, WD4 8JP.
Tel: (01923) 291 033
Fax: (01923) 291 060

Galen
Galen Ltd
Seagoe Industrial Estate
Craigavon, Northern Ireland
BT63 5UA.
Tel: (028) 3833 4974
Fax: (028) 3835 0206

Garnier
Laboratoires Garnier
PO Box 5
Pontyclun, Glamorgan, CF7 8XW.
Tel: (01443) 233 724
Fax: (01443) 233 726

GBM
GBM Healthcare Ltd
Beechlawn House
Hurtmore Rd, Godalming
Surrey, GU7 2RA.
Tel: (01483) 860 881
Fax: (01483) 425 715
mba_gbm@compuserve.com

Geistlich
Geistlich Pharma
Newton Bank
Long Lane, Chester, CH2 2PF.
Tel: (01244) 347 534
Fax: (01244) 319 327

General Dietary
General Dietary Ltd
PO Box 38
Kingston upon Thames
Surrey, KT2 7YP.
Tel: (020) 8336 2323
Fax: (020) 8942 8274

Generics
Generics (UK) Ltd
Albany Gate
Darkes Lane, Potters Bar
Herts, EN6 1AG.
Tel: (01707) 853 000
Fax: (01707) 643 148

Genus
Genus Pharmaceuticals
Benham ValenceNewbury
Berks, RG20 8LU.
Tel: (01635) 568 400
Fax: (01635) 568 401
enquires@genuspharma.com

Genzyme
Genzyme Biosurgery
4620 Kingsgate
Cascade Way, Oxford Business Park
South, Oxford, OX4 2SU.
Tel: (01865) 405 200
Fax: (01865) 774 172

Gilead
Gilead Sciences
The Flowers Building
Granta Park, Great Abington
Cambs, CB1 6GT.
Tel: (01223) 897 300
Fax: (01223) 897 282

GlaxoSmithKline
See GSK.

Glenwood
Glenwood Laboratories Ltd
Jenkins Dale
Chatham
Kent, ME4 5RD.
Tel: (01634) 830 535
Fax: (01634) 831 345
g.wooduk@virgin.net

Gluten Free Foods Ltd
Gluten Free Foods Ltd
Unit 270 Centennial Park
Centennial Ave, Elstree,
Borehamwood
Herts, WD6 3SS.
Tel: (020) 8953 4444
Fax: (020) 8953 8285
info@glutenfree-foods.co.uk

Goldshield
Goldshield Pharmaceuticals Ltd
NLA Tower
12-16 Addiscombe Rd, Croydon
CR0 0XT.
Tel: (020) 8649 8500
Fax: (020) 8686 0807

GP Pharma
GP Pharma
ARC Progress
Beckerings Park Rd, Lidlington
Beds, MK43 0RD.
Tel: (01525) 288 588
Fax: (01525) 289 339
info@gppharma.co.uk

Grifols
Grifols UK Ltd
72 St Andrew's Rd
Cambs, CB4 1GS.
Tel: (01223) 446 900
Fax: (01223) 446 911

GSK
GlaxoSmithKline
Stockley Park West
Uxbridge
Middx, UB11 1BT.
Tel: 0800 221 441
Fax: (020) 8990 4328
customercontactuk@gsk.com

GSK Consumer Healthcare
GlaxoSmithKline Consumer
Healthcare
GSK House
980 Great West Rd, Brentford
Middx, TW8 9GS.
Tel: (0500) 888 878
Fax: (020) 8047 6860
customer.relations@gsk.com

Hansam
Hansam Healthcare Ltd
PO Box 23876
London, SE15 4WT.
Tel: (0870) 241 3019
Fax: (020) 7207 6850

Hartmann
Paul Hartmann Ltd
Unit P2, Parklands
Heywood Distribution Park,
Pilsworth Rd, Heywood
Lancs, OL10 2TT.
Tel: (01706) 363 200
Fax: (01706) 363 201
info@uk.hartmann.info

Hawgreen
Hawgreen Ltd
The Maltings, 2nd Floor
Bridge St, Hitchin
Herts, SG5 2DE.
Tel: (01462) 441 831
Fax: (01462) 435 868

Healthcare Logistics
Healthcare Logistics Ltd
The Ridgeway
Iver, Bucks, SL0 9JW.
Tel: (01753) 650 099
Fax: (01753) 654 455
Ray.Ferris@Healthcarelogistics.co.uk

Heinz
H. J. Heinz Company Ltd
South Building
Hayes Park, Hayes, UB4 8AL.
Tel: (020) 8573 7757
Fax: (020) 8848 2325
Farleys_Heinz@Heinz.co.uk

Helios
Helios Healthcare Ltd
PO Box 203
Hitchin, SG5 2ZQ.
Tel: (01462) 441 834
Fax: (01462) 435 417

Henleys
Henleys Medical Supplies Ltd
Brownfields
Welwyn Garden City
Herts, AL7 1AN.
Tel: (01707) 333 164
Fax: (01707) 334 795

Hillcross
AAH Pharmaceuticals Ltd
Sapphire Court
Walsgrave Triangle, Coventry,
CV2 2TX.
Tel: (024) 7643 2000
Fax: (024) 7643 2001

HK Pharma
HK Pharma Ltd
PO Box 105
Hitchin
Herts, SG5 2GG.
Tel: (01462) 433 993
Fax: (01462) 450 755

Hoechst Marion Roussel
See Aventis Pharma.

Hypoguard
Hypoguard Ltd
Dock Lane
Melton, Woodbridge
Suffolk, IP12 1PE.
Tel: (01394) 387 333
Fax: (01394) 380 152
enquiries@hypoguard.com

ICN
ICN Pharmaceuticals Ltd
Cedarwood
Chineham Business Park, Crockford
Lane, Basingstoke
Hants, RG24 8WD.
Tel: (01256) 374 607
Fax: (01256) 707 334
icnuk@icnpharm.com

IDIS
IDIS World Medicines
171-185 Ewell Rd
Millbank House, Surbiton
Surrey, KT6 6AX.
Tel: (020) 8410 0700
Fax: (020) 8410 0800
idis@idis.co.uk

Infai
Infai UK Ltd
Innovation Centre
University of York Science Park,
University Rd
Heslington, York, YO10 5DG.
Tel: (01904) 435 228
Fax: (01904) 435 112
infai@infaiuk.ymn.co.uk

Intrapharm
Intrapharm Laboratories Ltd
60 Boughton Lane
Maidstone
Kent, ME15 9QS.
Tel: (01622) 749 222
Fax: (01622) 744 672
sales@intraphamlabs.com

Invicta
See Pfizer.

Ipsen
Ipsen Ltd
190 Bath Rd
Slough, Berks, SL1 3XE.
Tel: (01753) 627 777
Fax: (01753) 627 778
medical.information@ipsen.ltd.uk

IVAX
IVAX Pharmaceuticals UK Ltd
IVAX Quay, Albert Basin
Royal Docks, London, E16 2QJ.
Tel: (08705) 020 304
Fax: (08705) 323 334

Janssen-Cilag
Janssen-Cilag Ltd
PO Box 79
Saunderton, High Wycombe
Bucks, HP14 4HJ.
Tel: (01494) 567 567
Fax: (01494) 567 568

JHC
JHC Healthcare Ltd
The Maltings, 2nd Floor
Bridge St, Hitchin
Herts, SG5 2DE.
Tel: (01462) 432 533
Fax: (01462) 432 535

J&J
Johnson & Johnson Ltd
Foundation Park
Roxborough Way, Maidenhead
Berks, SL6 3UG.
Tel: (01628) 822 222
Fax: (01628) 821 222

J&J Medical
Johnson & Johnson Medical
Coronation Rd
Ascot, Berks, SL5 9EY.
Tel: (01344) 871 000
Fax: (01344) 872 599

J&J MSD
Johnson & Johnson MSD
Enterprise House, Station Rd
Loudwater, High Wycombe
Bucks, HP10 9UF.
Tel: (01494) 450 778
Fax: (01494) 450 487

JLB
B. Braun JLB Ltd
Unit 2A
St Columb Industrial Estate,
St Columb Major
Cornwall, TR9 6SF.
Tel: (01637) 880 065
Fax: (01637) 881 549

Kent
Kent Pharmaceuticals Ltd
Wotton Rd
Ashford
Kent, TN23 6LL.
Tel: (01233) 638 614
Fax: (01233) 646 899

Kestrel
Kestrel Ltd
Network House
Basing View, Basingstoke
RG21 4HG.
Tel: (01256) 307 580
Fax: (01256) 307 590
kestrel@ventiv.co.uk

King
King Pharmaceuticals Ltd
3 Ash Street
Leicester, LE5 0DA.
Tel: (01462) 434 366
Fax: (01462) 450 755

KoRa
KoRa Healthcare Ltd
Frans Maas House
Swords Business Park, Swords,
Co. Dublin
Ireland.
Tel: (00353) 1890 0406
Fax: (00353) 1890 3016
Kora@ireland.com

Kyowa Hakko
Kyowa Hakko UK Ltd
258 Bath Rd
Slough, Berks, SL1 4DX.
Tel: (01753) 566 020
Fax: (01753) 566 030

LAB
Laboratories for Applied Biology
91 Amhurst Park
London, N16 5DR.
Tel: (020) 8800 2252
Fax: (020) 8809 6884

Lamberts
Lamberts (Dalston) Ltd
PO Box 883
Oxford, OX4 3RR.
Tel: (01865) 717 300
Fax: (01865) 748 746

Lederle
See Wyeth.

Leo
Leo Pharma
Longwick Rd
Princes Risborough
Bucks, HP27 9RR.
Tel: (01844) 347 333
Fax: (01844) 342 278
medical-info.uk@leo-pharma.com

Lexon
Lexon UK Ltd
18 Oxleasow Rd
East Moons Moat, Redditch
Worcestershire, B98 0RE.
Tel: (0800) 614 242
Fax: (0800) 731 2901
sales@lexonuk.com

LifeScan
LifeScan
50-100 Holmers Farm Way
High Wycombe, Bucks, HP12 4DP.
Tel: (01494) 658 750
Fax: (01494) 658 751

Lilly
Eli Lilly & Co Ltd
Lilly House
Priestley Rd, Basingstoke
Hampshire, RG24 9NL.
Tel: (01256) 315 999
Fax: (01256) 775 858

Linderma
Linderma Ltd
Canon Bridge House
Canon Bridge, Madley
Hereford, HR2 9JF.
Tel: (01981) 250 124
Fax: (01981) 251 412
linderma@virgin.net

Link
Link Pharmaceuticals Ltd
Bishops Weald House
Albion Way, Horsham
West Sussex, RH12 1AH.
Tel: (01403) 272 451
Fax: (01403) 272 455
medical.information@linkpharm.
co.uk

Lundbeck
Lundbeck Ltd
Lundbeck House
Caldecotte Lake Business Park,
Caldecotte, Milton Keynes
Bucks, MK7 8LF.
Tel: (01908) 649 966
Fax: (01908) 647 888
ukmedicalinformation@lundbeck.
com

3M
3M Health Care Ltd
3M House
Morley St, Loughborough
Leics, LE11 1EP.
Tel: (01509) 611611
Fax: (01509) 237288

Mandeville
Mandeville Medicines
Stoke Mandeville Hospital
Aylesbury
Bucks, HP21 8AL.
Tel: (01296) 394 142
Fax: (01296) 397 223

Manx
Manx Healthcare
1 Hawkes Drive
Heathcote Industrial Estate,
Warwick
Warickshire, CV34 6LX.
Tel: (01926) 461 628
Fax: (01926) 461 621
info@manxhealthcare.com

Martindale
Martindale Pharmaceuticals Ltd
Hubert Rd
Brentwood, Essex, CM14 4LZ.
Tel: (01277) 266 600
Fax: (01277) 848 976
info@martindalepharma.co.uk

MASTA
MASTA
Moorfield Rd
Yeadon
Leeds, LS19 7BN.
Tel: (0113) 238 7500
Fax: (0113) 238 7501
medical@masta.org

Mayne
Mayne Pharma plc
Queensway
Royal Leamington Spa,
Warwickshire, CV31 3RW.
Tel: (01926) 820 820
Fax: (01926) 821 041
medinfouk@uk.maynepharma.com

MDE
MDE Diagnostics Europe Ltd
The Surrey Technology Centre
40 Occam Rd, Surrey Research
Park, Guildford
Surrey, GU2 7YG.
Tel: (01483) 688 400
info@mdediagnostic.co.uk

Mead Johnson
Mead Johnson Nutritional
See Bristol-Myers Squibb.

Meadow
Meadow Laboratories Ltd
18 Avenue Rd
Chadwell Heath, Romford
Essex, RM6 4JF.
Tel: (020) 8597 1203
enquiries@meadowlabs.fsnet.co.uk

Meda
Meda Pharmaceuticals Ltd
Regus House, Herald Way
Pegasus Business Park
Castle Donnington
Derbyshire, DE74 2TZ.
Tel: (01332) 638 033
Fax: (01332) 638 192
information@uk.meda.se

Medac
Medac (UK)
13 Lynedoch Crescent
Glasgow, G3 6EQ.
Tel: (0141) 332 8464
Fax: (0141) 332 8619
info@medac-uk.co.uk

Medical House
The Medical House plc
199 Newhall Rd
Sheffield, S9 2QJ.
Tel: (0114) 261 9011
Fax: (0114) 243 1597
info@themedicalhouse.com

Medigas
Medigas Ltd
Enterprise Drive
Four Ashes, Wolverhampton
WV10 7DF.
Tel: (01902) 791 944
Fax: (01902) 791 125

MediSense
MediSense
Abbott Laboratories Ltd
Mallory House,
Vanwall Business Park
Maidenhead, Berks, SL6 4UD.
Tel: (01628) 678 900
Fax: (01628) 678 805

Medix
See Clement Clarke.

MedLogic
MedLogic Global Ltd
Western Wood Way
Langage Science Park, Plympton
Plymouth, Devon, PL7 5BG.
Tel: (01752) 209 955
Fax: (01752) 209 956
enquiries@mlgl.co.uk

Menarini
A. Menarini Pharmaceuticals UK
Ltd
Menarini House
Mercury Park, Wycombe Lane,
Wooburn Green
Bucks, HP10 0HH.
Tel: (01628) 856 400
Fax: (01628) 856 402

Menarini Diagnostics
A. Menarini Diagnostics
Wharfedale Rd
Winnersh, Wokingham
Berks, RG41 5RA.
Tel: (0118) 944 4100
Fax: (0118) 944 4111

Merck
Merck Pharmaceuticals
Harrier House
High St, West Drayton
Middx, UB7 7QG.
Tel: (01895) 452 307
Fax: (01895) 452 296
medinfo@merckpharma.co.uk

Merck Consumer Health
See Seven Seas.

Merck Sharp & Dohme
See MSD.

Milupa
Milupa Ltd
White Horse Business Park
Trowbridge, Wilts, BA14 0XQ.
Tel: (01225) 711 511
Fax: (01225) 711 970

Molar
Molar Ltd
The Borough Yard
The Borough, Wedmore
Somerset, BS28 4EB.
Tel: (01934) 710 022
Fax: (01934) 710 033
info@molar.ltd.uk

Mölnlycke
Mölnlycke Health Care Ltd
The Arenson Centre
Arenson Way, Dunstable
Beds, LU5 5UL.
Tel: (0870) 606 0766
Fax: (0870) 608 1888
info.uk@molnlycke.net

MSD
Merck Sharp & Dohme Ltd
Hertford Rd, Hoddesdon
Herts, EN11 9BU.
Tel: (01992) 467 272
Fax: (01992) 451 066

Myogen
Myogen GmbH
PO Box 122
Richmond, North Yorks, DL10 5YA.
Tel: (01748) 828 812
Fax: (01748) 828 801
info@myogen.de

Nagor
Nagor Ltd
PO Box 21, Global House
Isle of Man Business Park, Douglas
Isle of Man, IM99 1AX.
Tel: (01624) 625 556
Fax: (01624) 661 656
enquiries@nagor.com

Napp
Napp Pharmaceuticals Ltd
Cambridge Science Park
Milton Rd, Cambs, CB4 0GW.
Tel: (01223) 424 444
Fax: (01223) 424 441

Neolab
Neolab Ltd
57 High St
Odiham, Hampshire, RG29 1LF.
Tel: (01256) 704 110
Fax: (01256) 701 144
info@neolab.co.uk

Neomedic
Neomedic Ltd
2a Crofters Rd
Northwood, Middx, HA6 3ED.
Tel: (01923) 836 379
Fax: (01923) 840 160
marketing@neomedic.co.uk

Nestlé
Nestlé UK Ltd
St. George's House
Park Lane, Croydon
Surrey, CR9 1NR.
Tel: (020) 8686 3333
Fax: (020) 8686 6072

Nestlé Clinical
Nestlé Clinical Nutrition
St George's House
Park Lane, Croydon
Surrey, CR9 1NR.
Tel: (020) 8667 5130
Fax: (020) 8667 6061

Network
Network Health & Beauty
Network House
41 Invincible Rd, Farnborough
Hants, GU14 7QU.
Tel: (01252) 533 333
Fax: (01252) 533 344
networkm@globalnet.co.uk

Neutrogena
See J&J.

Niche
Niche Generics Ltd
1 The Cam Centre
Wilbury Way, Hitchin
Herts, SG4 0TW.
Tel: (01462) 633 800
Fax: (01462) 438 279

Nordic
Nordic Pharma UK Ltd
Abbey House
1650 Arlington Business Park,
Theale, Reading, RG7 4SA.
Tel: (0118) 929 8233
Fax: (0118) 929 8234
info@nordicpharma.co.uk

Norgine
Norgine Ltd
Chaplin House
Moorhall Rd, Harefield
Middx, UB9 6NS.
Tel: (01895) 826 600
Fax: (01895) 825 865

Novartis
Novartis Pharmaceuticals UK Ltd
Frimley Business Park
Frimley, Camberley
Surrey, GU16 7SR.
Tel: (01276) 692 255
Fax: (01276) 692 508

Novartis Consumer Health
Novartis Consumer Health
Wimblehurst Rd
Horsham
West Sussex, RH12 5AB.
Tel: (01403) 210 211
Fax: (01403) 323 939
medicalaffairs.uk@ch.novartis.com

Novartis Ophthalmics
See Novartis.
Tel: (01276) 692 255

Novo Nordisk
Novo Nordisk Ltd
Broadfield Park
Brighton Rd, Crawley
West Sussex, RH11 9RT.
Tel: (01293) 613 555
Fax: (01293) 613 535
customercareuk@novonordisk.com

Nutricia Clinical
Nutricia Clinical Care
Nutricia Ltd
White Horse Business Park,
Trowbridge
Wilts, BA14 0XQ.
Tel: (01225) 711 688
Fax: (01225) 711 798
cndirect@nutricia.co.uk

Nutricia Dietary
Nutricia Dietary Care
see Nutricia Clinical.
Tel: (01225) 711 801
Fax: (01225) 711 567

Nutrition Point
Nutrition Point Ltd
13 Taurus Park
Westbrook, Warrington
Cheshire, WA5 7ZT.
Tel: (07041) 544 044
Fax: (07041) 544 055
info@nutritionpoint.co.uk

Octapharma
Octapharma Ltd
6 Elm Court
Copse Drive, Meriden Green,
Coventry, CV5 9RG.
Tel: (01676) 521 000
Fax: (01676) 521 200
octapharma@octapharma.co.uk

Omron
Omron Healthcare (UK) Ltd
Opal Drive
Fox Milne, Milton Keynes
MK15 0DG.
Tel: (01908) 258 285
Fax: (01908) 258 286
information@eu.omron.com

Opus
See Trinity.

Oral B Labs
Oral B Laboratories Ltd
Gillette Corner
Great West Rd, Isleworth
Middx, TW7 5NP.
Tel: (020) 8847 7800
Fax: (020) 8847 7828

Orbis
Orbis Consumer Products Ltd
Unit 31
Northfields Industrial Estate,
Beresford Ave
Wembley, HA0 1NW.
Tel: (020) 8902 3736
Fax: (020) 8902 4723

Organon
Organon Laboratories Ltd
Cambridge Science Park
Milton Rd, Cambs, CB4 0FL.
Tel: (01223) 432 700
Fax: (01223) 424 368

Orion
Orion Pharma (UK) Ltd
Leat House, Overbridge Square
Hambridge Lane, Newbury
Berks, RG14 5UX.
Tel: (01635) 520 300
Fax: (01635) 520 319
medicalinformation@orionpharma.
com

Orphan Europe
Orphan Europe (UK) Ltd
Isis House
43 Station Rd, Henley-on-Thames
Oxon, RG9 1AT.
Tel: (01491) 414 333
Fax: (01491) 414 443
info.uk@orphan-europe.com

Otsuka
Otsuka Pharmaceutical (UK) Ltd
Commonwealth House
2 Chalkhill Rd, Hammersmith
London, W6 8DW.
Tel: (020) 8600 6770
Fax: (020) 8600 6794
medinfo@otsuka-europe.com

Owen Mumford
Owen Mumford Ltd
Brook Hill
Woodstock, Oxford, OX20 1TU.
Tel: (01993) 812 021
Fax: (01993) 813 466

Oxygen Therapy Co Ltd
The Oxygen Therapy Co Ltd
Dumballs Rd
Cardiff, CF1 6JE.
Tel: (0800) 373 580

Paines & Byrne
Paines & Byrne Ltd
Yamanouchi House
Pyrford Rd, West Byfleet
Surrey, KT14 6RA.
Tel: (01932) 355 405
Fax: (01932) 353 458

Pantheon
Pantheon Healthcare Ltd
Studio 8
48 Tierney Rd, London, SW2 4QS.
Tel: (0845) 602 0137

Parema
Parema Ltd
Sullington Rd
Shepshed, Loughborough
Leics, LE12 9JJ.
Tel: (01509) 502 051
Fax: (01509) 650 898

Pari
PARI Medical Ltd
Enterprise House
Station Approach, West Byfleet
Surrey, KT14 6NE.
Tel: (01932) 341 122
Fax: (01932) 341 134
parimedical@compuserve.com

Parke-Davis
See Pfizer.

Parkside
Parkside Healthcare
12 Parkside Ave
Salford, M7 4HB.
Tel: (0161) 795 2792
Fax: (0161) 795 4076

Peckforton
Peckforton Pharmaceuticals Ltd
Crewe Hall
Crewe
Cheshire, CW1 6UL.
Tel: (01270) 582 255
Fax: (01270) 582 299

Penn
Penn Pharmaceuticals Services Ltd
Unit 23 & 24, Tafarnaubach
Industrial Estate
Tredegar
Gwent, NP22 3AA.
Tel: (01495) 711 222
Fax: (01495) 711 225
penn@pennpharm.co.uk

Pfizer
Pfizer Ltd
Walton Oaks
Dorking Rd, Walton-on-the-Hill
Surrey, KT20 7NS.
Tel: (01304) 616 161
Fax: (01304) 656 221

Pfizer Consumer
Pfizer Consumer Healthcare
Walton Oaks
Dorking Rd, Walton-on-the-Hill
Surrey, KT20 7NS.
Tel: (01304) 616 161
Fax: (01304) 656 221

Pharma-Global
Pharma-Global Ltd
SEQ Ltd, Nerin House
26 Ridgeway St, Douglas, Isle of
Man, IM1 1EL.
Tel: (01624) 613 997
Fax: (01624) 613 998

Pharmacia
see Pfizer.
Tel: (01304) 616 161
Fax: (01304) 656 221

Pharmion
Pharmion Ltd
The McClintock Building
Granta Park, Gt Abington
CB1 6GX.
Tel: (01223) 897 040
Fax: (01223) 897 041
info-UK@pharmion.com

Phoenix
Phoenix Pharma
Glevum Works
Upton St
Gloucester, GL1 4LA.
Tel: (01452) 522 255
Fax: (01452) 306 051
enquiries@phoenixpharma.com

Pickles
J. Pickles Healthcare
Beech House
62 High St, Knaresborough
N. Yorks, HG5 0EA.
Tel: (01423) 867 314
Fax: (01423) 869 177

Pinewood
Pinewood Healthcare
Ballymacabry
Clonmel, Co Tipperary
Eire.
Tel: (00353) 523 6253
Fax: (00353) 523 6311

PLIVA
PLIVA Pharma Ltd
Vision House
Bedford Rd, Petersfield
Hampshire, GU32 3QB.
Tel: (01730) 710900
Fax: (01730) 710901
medinfo@pliva-pharma.co.uk

Procter & Gamble
Procter & Gamble UK
The Heights
Brooklands, Weybridge
Surrey, KT13 0XP.
Tel: (01932) 896 000
Fax: (01932) 896 200

Procter & Gamble Pharm.
Procter & Gamble Technical Centres
Medical Dept
Rusham Park, Whitehall Lane
Egham, Surrey, TW20 9NW.
Tel: (01784) 474 900
Fax: (01784) 474 705

Profile
Profile Pharma Ltd
Heath Place
Bognor Regis, West Sussex
PO22 9SL.
Tel: (0870) 770 2025
Fax: (0870) 770 2224
info@profilepharma.com

Profile Respiratory
Profile Respiratory Systems Ltd
Heath Place
Bognor Regis, West Sussex, PO22 9SL.
Tel: (0870) 770 3434
Fax: (0870) 770 3433
info@profilehs.com

Provalis
Provalis Healthcare Ltd
Newtech Square
Deeside Industrial Park, Deeside
Flintshire, CH5 2NT.
Tel: (01244) 288 888
Fax: (01244) 280 342
enquiries@provalis.plc.uk

Q-Med
Q-Med (UK) Ltd
Castle Court
41 London Rd, Reigate
Surrey, RH2 9RJ.
Tel: (01737) 735 503
Fax: (01737) 735 203

Ranbaxy
Ranbaxy (UK) Ltd
6th Floor, CP House
97-107 Uxbridge Rd, Ealing
London, W5 5TL.
Tel: (020) 8280 1600
Fax: (020) 8280 1616

Rand Rocket
Rand Rocket Ltd
ABCare House
Hownsgill Industrial Park, Consett
County Durham, DH8 7NU.
Tel: (01207) 591 099
Fax: (01207) 591 098

Ransom
Ransom Consumer Healthcare
104 Bancroft
Hitchin, Herts, SG5 1LY.
Tel: (01462) 437 615
Fax: (01462) 443 512
info@williamransom.com

Ratiopharm
Ratiopharm UK Ltd
5 Jackson Close
Grove Road, Cosham
Portsmouth, Hants, PO6 1UP.
Tel: (023) 9238 6199
Fax: (023) 9238 6208
info@ratiopharm.co.uk

R&C
See Reckitt Benckiser.

Reckitt Benckiser
Reckitt Benckiser Healthcare
Dansom Lane
Hull, HU8 7DS.
Tel: (01482) 326 151
Fax: (01482) 582 526
miu@reckittbenckiser.com

Regent
Regent-GM Laboratories Ltd
861 Coronation Rd
Park Royal
London, NW10 7PT.
Tel: (020) 8961 6868
Fax: (020) 8961 9311
info@regent-gm.com

Rhône-Poulenc Rorer
See Aventis Pharma.

Richmond
Richmond Pharmaceuticals Ltd
Coomb House
7 St John's Rd, Isleworth
Middx, TW7 6NA.
Tel: (020) 8569 8174
Fax: (020) 8569 8175

Robinsons
Robinson Healthcare Ltd
Waterside
Walton, Chesterfield
Derbyshire, S40 1YF.
Tel: (01246) 220 022
Fax: (01246) 505 115
enquiries@robinsoncare.com

Roche
Roche Products Ltd
P.O. Box 8
40 Broadwater Rd,
Welwyn Garden City
Herts, AL7 3AY.
Tel: (0800) 328 1629
Fax: (01707) 390 378
medinfo.uk@roche.com

Roche Consumer Health
See Roche.
Tel: (01707) 366 000
Fax: (0800) 394 353
welwyn.rch@roche.com

Roche Diagnostics
Roche Diagnostics Ltd
Bell Lane, Lewes
East Sussex, BN7 1LG.
Tel: (01273) 480 444
Fax: (01273) 480 266

Rosemont
Rosemont Pharmaceuticals Ltd
Rosemont House
Yorkdale Industrial Park,
Braithwaite St
Leeds, LS11 9XE.
Tel: (0113) 244 1999
Fax: (0113) 246 0738

Rowa
Rowa Pharmaceuticals Ltd
Bantry
Co Cork, Ireland
Tel: (00 353 27) 50077
Fax: (00 353 27) 50417
rowa@rowa-pharma.ie

Rybar
See Shire.

Sallis
E. Sallis Ltd
Vernon Works
Waterford St, Basford
Nottingham, NG6 0DH.
Tel: (0115) 978 7841
Fax: (0115) 942 2272

Sandoz
Sandoz Ltd
37 Woolmer Way
Bordon, Hants, GU35 9QE.
Tel: (01420) 478 301
Fax: (01420) 474 427

Sankyo
Sankyo Pharma UK Ltd
Sankyo House
Repton Place, White Lion Rd,
Amersham
Bucks, HP7 9LP.
Tel: (01494) 766 866
Fax: (01494) 766 557
medinfo@sankyo.co.uk

Sanochemia
Sanochemia Diagnostics UK Ltd
Argentum
510 Bristol Business Park,
Coldharbour Lane
Bristol, BS16 1EJ.
Tel: (0117) 906 3562
Fax: (0117) 906 3709

Sanofi-Synthelabo
Sanofi-Synthelabo
1 Onslow St
Guildford
Surrey, GU1 4YS.
Tel: (01483) 505 515
Fax: (01483) 535 432

Schering Health
Schering Health Care Ltd
The Brow
Burgess Hill
West Sussex, RH15 9NE.
Tel: (0845) 609 6767
Fax: (01444) 465 878
customer.care@schering.co.uk

Schering-Plough
Schering-Plough Ltd
Shire Park
Welwyn Garden City
Herts, AL7 1TW.
Tel: (01707) 363 636
Fax: (01707) 363 763
medical.info@spcorp.com

Schwarz
Schwarz Pharma Ltd
Schwarz House
East St, Chesham
Bucks, HP5 1DG.
Tel: (01494) 797 500
Fax: (01494) 774 960

Searle
See Pfizer.

Serono
Serono Pharmaceuticals Ltd
Bedfont Cross
Stanwell Rd, Feltham
Middx, TW14 8NX.
Tel: (020) 8818 7200
Fax: (020) 8818 7222
serono_uk@serono.com

Servier
Servier Laboratories Ltd
Gallions
Wexham Springs, Framewood Rd
Wexham, SL3 6RL.
Tel: (01753) 662 744
Fax: (01753) 663 456

Seven Seas
Seven Seas Ltd
Hedon Rd
Marfleet, Hull, HU9 5NJ.
Tel: (01482) 375 234
Fax: (01482) 374 345

Shiloh
Shiloh Healthcare Ltd
Lion Mill
Fitton St, Royton
Oldham, OL2 5JX.
Tel: (0161) 624 5641
Fax: (0161) 627 0902
enquiry@shiloh.co.uk

Shire
Shire Pharmaceuticals Ltd
Hampshire International Business
Park, Chineham, Basingstoke
Hants, RG24 8EP.
Tel: (01256) 894 000
Fax: (01256) 894 708

SHS
SHS International Ltd
100 Wavertree Boulevard
Wavertree Technology Park
Liverpool, L7 9PT.
Tel: (0151) 228 8161
Fax: (0151) 230 5365
seve@shsint.co.uk

Sigma
Sigma Pharmaceuticals plc
PO Box 233
Unit 1-7 Colonial Way, Watford
Herts, WD24 4YR.
Tel: (01923) 444 999
Fax: (01923) 444 998
info@sigpharm.co.uk

Sinclair
Sinclair Pharmaceuticals Ltd
Borough Rd
Godalming
Surrey, GU7 2AB.
Tel: (01483) 426 644
Fax: (01483) 860 927

SMA Nutrition
See Wyeth.

S&N Hlth.
Smith & Nephew Healthcare Ltd
Healthcare House
Goulton St, Hull, HU3 4DJ.
Tel: (01482) 222 200
Fax: (01482) 222 211
advice@smith-nephew.com

SNBTS
Scottish National Blood Transfusion
Service
Protein Fractionation Centre
Ellen's Glen Rd, Edinburgh
EH17 7QT.
Tel: (0131) 536 5700
Fax: (0131) 536 5781

Solvay
Solvay Healthcare Ltd
Mansbridge RdWest End
Southampton, SO18 3JD.
Tel: (023) 8046 7000
Fax: (023) 8046 5350
medinfo.shl@solvay.com

Sovereign
Sovereign Medical
Sovereign House
Miles Gray Rd, Basildon
Essex, SS14 3FR.
Tel: (01268) 535 200
Fax: (01268) 535 299

Special Products
Special Products Ltd
Orion House
49 High Street, Addlestone
Surrey, KT15 1TU.
Tel: (01932) 820 666
Fax: (01932) 850 444
graham.march@specprod.co.uk

Specials Laboratory
The Specials Laboratory Ltd
Unit 1, Regents Drive
Lower Prudhoe Industrial Estate,
Northumberland, NE42 6PX.
Tel: (0800) 028 4925
Fax: (0800) 083 4222

Squibb
See Bristol-Myers Squibb.

SSL
SSL International plc
Canute Court
Toft Rd, Knutsford, WA16 0NL.
Tel: (01565) 625 000
Fax: (01565) 625 050
medical.infomation@
ssl-international.com

STD Pharmaceutical
STD Pharmaceutical Products Ltd
Plough Lane
Hereford, HR4 0EL.
Tel: (01432) 373 555
Fax: (01432) 373 314
enquiries@stdpharm.co.uk

Sterling Health
See GSK Consumer Healthcare.

Sterwin
Sterwin Medicines Ltd
PO Box 611
Guildford, Surrey, GU1 4YS.
Tel: (01483) 554 101
Fax: (01483) 554 810
sales@sterwin.com

Stiefel
Stiefel Laboratories (UK) Ltd
Holtspur Lane
Wooburn Green, High Wycombe
Bucks, HP10 0AU.
Tel: (01628) 524 966
Fax: (01628) 810 021
general@stiefel.co.uk

Strakan
Strakan Ltd
Buckholm Mill
Galashiels, TD1 2HB.
Tel: (01896) 668 060
Fax: (01896) 668 061
medinfo@strakan.com

Sussex
Sussex Pharmaceuticals Ltd
Charlswoods Rd
East Grinstead
Sussex, RH19 2HL.
Tel: (01342) 311 311
Fax: (01342) 313 078

Sutherland
Sutherland Health Ltd
Unit 1, Rivermead
Pipers Way, Thatcham
Berks, RG19 4EP.
Tel: (01635) 874 488
Fax: (01635) 877 622

Swedish Orphan
Swedish Orphan International (UK)
Ltd
The White House
Wilderspool Park, Greenalls Ave,
Stockton Heath, Warrington
Cheshire, WA4 6HL.
Tel: (01925) 438 028
Fax: (01925) 438 001

Syner-Med
Syner-Med (Pharmaceutical Pro-
ducts) Ltd
Airport House
Purley Way, Croydon
Surrey, CR0 0XZ.
Tel: (020) 8410 6400
Fax: (020) 8410 6409
mail@syner-med.com

Takeda
Takeda UK Ltd
Takeda House, Mercury Park
Wycombe Lane, Wooburn Green
High Wycombe, Bucks, HP10 0HH.
Tel: (01628) 537 900
Fax: (01628) 526 615

Taro
Taro Pharmaceuticals (UK) Ltd
1st Floor, Prince of Wales House
3 Bluecoats Ave, Hertford, SG14 1PB.
Tel: (01992) 557 440
Fax: (01992) 557 447
customerservice@taropharma.co.uk

Tarus
See Chemidex.

Teva
Teva Pharmaceuticals Ltd
Barclays House
1 Gatehouse Way, Aylesbury
Bucks, HP19 8DB.
Tel: (01296) 719 768
Fax: (01296) 719 769
info@tevapharma.co.uk

TheraSense
TheraSense UK
Centaur House
Ancells Business Park, Ancells Rd,
Fleet, Hants, GU51 2UJ.
Tel: (01252) 761 392
Fax: (01252) 761 393

Thornton & Ross
Thornton & Ross Ltd
Linthwaite Laboratories
Huddersfield, HD7 5QH.
Tel: (01484) 842 217
Fax: (01484) 847 301
mail@thorntonross.com

Tillomed
Tillomed Laboratories Ltd
3 Howard Rd
Eaton Socon, St Neots
Cambs, PE19 3ET.
Tel: (01480) 402 400
Fax: (01480) 402 402

TOL
Tree of Life
Coaldale Rd
Lymedale Business Park,
Newcastle Under Lyme
Staff, ST5 9QX.
Tel: (01782) 567 100
Fax: (01782) 567 199
health@tol-europe.com

Torbet
Torbet Laboratories Ltd
14D Wendover Rd
Rackheath Industrial Estate,
Rackheath
Norwich, NR13 6LH.
Tel: (01603) 735 200
Fax: (01603) 735 217
torbet@typharm.com

Transdermal
Transdermal Ltd
35 Grimwade Ave
Croydon
Surrey, CR0 5DJ.
Tel: (020) 8654 2251
Fax: (020) 8654 2252

TRB Chemedica
TRB Chemedica (UK) Ltd
14 Brindley Court
Lymedale Business Quarter,
Newcastle under Lyme, ST5 9QA.
Tel: (0845) 330 7556
Fax: (0845) 330 7557
info@trbchemedica.co.uk

Trinity
Trinity Pharmaceuticals Ltd
The Old Exchange
12 Compton Rd, Wimbledon
London, SW19 7QD.
Tel: (020) 8944 9443
Fax: (020) 8947 9325

TSL
Tissue Science Laboratories plc
Victoria House
Victoria Rd, Aldershot
Hants, GU11 1EJ.
Tel: (01252) 333 002
Fax: (01252) 333 010
enquiries@tissuescience.com

Tyco
Tyco Healthcare
154 Fareham Rd
Gosport, Hants, PO13 0AS.
Tel: (01329) 224 000

Typharm
Typharm Ltd
14D Wendover Rd
Rackheath Industrial Estate,
Rackheath
Norwich, NR13 6LH.
Tel: (01603) 735 200
Fax: (01603) 735 217
customerservices@typharm.com

UCB Pharma
UCB Pharma Ltd
3 George St, Watford
Herts, WD1 8UH.
Tel: (01923) 211 811
Fax: (01923) 229 002

Ultrapharm
Ultrapharm Ltd
Centenary Business Park
Henley-on-Thames
Oxon, RG9 1DS.
Tel: (01491) 578 016
Fax: (01491) 570 001
orders@glutenfree.co.uk

UniChem
UniChem Ltd
UniChem House
Cox Lane, Chessington
Surrey, KT9 1SN.
Tel: (020) 8391 2323
Fax: (020) 8974 1707

Unigreg
Unigreg Ltd
Enterprise House
181-189 Garth Rd, Morden
Surrey, SM4 4LL.
Tel: (020) 8330 1421
Fax: (020) 8330 6812
admin@unigreg.co.uk

Univar
Univar Ltd
International House
Zenith, Paycocke Rd, Basildon
Essex, SS14 3DW.
Tel: (01268) 594 400
Fax: (01268) 594 481
trientine@univareurope.com

Unomedical
Unomedical Ltd
Thornhill Rd
Redditch, B98 7NL.
Tel: (01527) 587 700
Fax: (01527) 592 111

Vernon-Carus
Vernon-Carus Ltd
Penwortham Mills
Preston, Lancs, PR1 9SN.
Tel: (01772) 744 493
Fax: (01772) 748 754
mail@vernon-carus.co.uk

Viatris
Viatris Pharmaceuticals Ltd
Building 2000
Beach Drive,
Cambridge Research Park
Waterbeach, Cambs, CB5 9PD.
Tel: (01223) 205 999
Fax: (01223) 205 998

Vitaflo
Vitaflo Ltd
11 Century Building
Brunswick Business Park,
Liverpool, L3 4BL.
Tel: (0151) 709 9020
Fax: (0151) 709 9727
vitaflo@vitaflo.co.uk

Vitaline
Vitaline Pharmaceuticals UK Ltd
8 Ridge Way
Drakes Drive,
Crendon Business Park
Long Crendon, Bucks, HP18 9BF.
Tel: (01844) 202 044
Fax: (01844) 202 077

Vitalograph
Vitalograph Ltd
Maids Moreton
Buckingham, MK18 1SW.
Tel: (01280) 827 110
Fax: (01280) 823 302
sales@vitalograph.co.uk

Wallace Mfg
Wallace Manufacturing Chemists Ltd
Wallace House
New Abbey Court, 51-53 Stert St,
Abingdon
Oxon, OX14 3JF.
Tel: (01235) 538 700
Fax: (01235) 538 800
wallace@alinter.co.uk

Wanskerne
Wanskerne Ltd
31 High Cross St
St. Austell
Cornwall, PL25 4AN.
Tel: (01726) 69500
Fax: (01726) 69135

Warner Lambert
See Pfizer.

W-L
Warner Lambert UK Ltd
See Pfizer.

Wyeth
Wyeth Pharmaceuticals
Huntercombe Lane South
Taplow, Maidenhead
Berks, SL6 0PH.
Tel: (01628) 604 377
Fax: (01628) 666 368

Wynlit
Wynlit Laboratories
153 Furzehill Rd
Borehamwood, Herts, WD6 2DR.
Tel: (07903) 370 130
Fax: (020) 8292 6117

Wyvern
Wyvern Medical Ltd
PO Box 17
Ledbury
Herefordshire, HR8 2ES.
Tel: (01531) 631 105
Fax: (01531) 634 844

Yamanouchi
Yamanouchi Pharma Ltd
Yamanouchi House
Pyrford Rd, West Byfleet
Surrey, KT14 6RA.
Tel: (01932) 342 291
Fax: (01932) 353 458

Zeal
G. H. Zeal Ltd
Deer Park Rd
London, SW19 3UU.
Tel: (020) 8542 2283
Fax: (020) 8543 7840
scientific@zeal.co.uk

ZLB
ZLB Bioplasma UK Ltd
Brackland House
St. Nicholas St, Thetford
Norfolk, IP24 1BT.
Tel: (01842) 755 025
Fax: (01842) 755 174
info-uk@zlb.com

Zurich
See Trinity.

Special-order Manufacturers

The following **companies** manufacture 'special-order' products: BCM Specials, Eldon Laboratories, Mandeville, Martindale, Oxford Pharmaceuticals, Phoenix, Rosemont, Special Products, The Specials Laboratory (see Index of Manufacturers for contact details).

Hospital manufacturing units also manufacture 'special-order' products, details may be obtained from any of the centres listed below.

> It should be noted that when a product has a licence the *Department of Health recommends that the licensed product should be ordered* unless a specific formulation is required

England

East Anglian and Oxford
Mr G. Hanson,
Production Manager
Pharmacy Manufacturing Unit
The Ipswich Hospital NHS Trust
Heath Rd
Ipswich, IP4 5PD.
Tel: (01473) 703 603
Fax: (01473) 703 609
con.hanson@ipsh-tr.anglox.nhs.uk

London
Mr M. Lillywhite,
Regional Technical Pharmacist
St. Bartholomew's Hospital
West Smithfield
London, EC1A 7BE.
Tel: (020) 7601 7475/7491
Fax: (020) 7601 7486
mike.lillywhite@
bartsandthelondon.nhs.uk

Mr P. Forsey,
Production Manager
Guy's and St. Thomas' Hospital
Trust
St. Thomas' Hospital,
Lambeth Palace Rd
London, SE1 7EH.
Tel: (020) 7118 4992
Fax: (020) 7118 5013
paul.forsey@gstt.sthames.nhs.uk

Mr C. Evans,
Production Manager
Pharmacy Department
St. George's Hospital
Blackshaw Rd
Tooting, London, SW17 0QT.
Tel: (020) 8725 1770
Fax: (020) 8725 3690
chris.evans@stgeorges.nhs.uk

Mr A. Krol,
Director of Commercial Services
Pharmacy Manufacturing Unit
Moorfields Eye Hospital NHS Trust
City Rd
London, EC1V 2PD.
Tel: (020) 7566 2363
Fax: 0800 328 8191 or
(020) 7566 2367
alan.krol@moorfields.nhs.uk

North West
Mr M.D. Booth,
Production & Aseptic Services Manager
Stockport Pharmaceuticals
Stepping Hill Hospital
Poplar Grove
Stockport, Cheshire SK2 7JE.
Tel: (0161) 419 5657
Fax: (0161) 419 5664
mike.booth@stockport-tr.nwest.
nhs.uk

Northern
Mr C. Adams,
Principal Pharmacist
Pharmacy Manufacturing Unit
Newcastle General Hospital
Westgate Rd
Newcastle-upon-Tyne, NE4 6BE.
Tel: (0191) 273 8811 ext 22689
Fax: (0191) 226 0620
pharmacyNGH@nuth.northy.nhs.
uk

South East
Ms G. Middlehurst,
Production Manager
Pharmacy Manufacturing Unit
Queen Alexandra Hospital
Cosham
Portsmouth, Hants, PO6 3LY.
Tel: (02392) 286 335
Fax: (02392) 378 288
gillian.middlehurst@porthosp.nhs.
uk

South Western
Mr P. S. Bendell,
Principal Pharmacist
Unit Manager, Torbay PMU
South Devon Healthcare
Long Rd
Paignton, Devon TQ4 7TW.
Tel: (01803) 664 707
Fax: (01803) 664 354
phil.bendell@sdevonhc-tr.swest.
nhs.uk

Trent
Mr R.W. Brookes,
Production Pharmacist
Royal Hallamshire Hospital
Glossop Rd
Sheffield, S10 2JF.
Tel: (0114) 271 3104
Fax: (0114) 271 2783
roger.brookes@sth.nhs.uk

West Midlands
Mr A. Broad,
Principal Pharmacist
Sterile Fluids Manufacturing Unit
Queen Elizabeth Medical Centre
Edgbaston
Birmingham, B15 2TH.
Tel: (0121) 627 2326
Fax: (0121) 627 2168
alan.broad@uhb.nhs.uk

Mr P.G. Williams,
Principal Pharmacist
Pharmacy Manufacturing Unit
Queens Hospital
Burton Hospitals NHS Trust,
Belvedere Rd
Burton-on-Trent, DE13 0RB.
Tel: (01283) 566 333/511 511
Extn 5138
Fax: (01283) 593 036
paul.williams@
queens.burtonh-tr.wmids.nhs.uk

Yorkshire
Dr J. Harwood,
Production Manager
Pharmacy Manufacturing Unit
Huddersfield Royal Infirmary
Lindley
Huddersfield
West Yorks, HD3 3EA.
Tel: (01484) 342 421
Fax: (01484) 342 074
john.harwood@cht.nhs.uk

Northern Ireland
Mrs S.M. Millership,
Principal Pharmacist
Victoria Pharmaceuticals
The Royal Hospitals
77 Boucher Cres
Belfast, BT12 6HU.
Tel: (028) 9055 3407
Fax: (028) 9055 3498
vicpharm@aol.com

Scotland
Mr J.A. Cook,
Principal Pharmacist—Production
Tayside Pharmaceuticals
Ninewells Hospital
Dundee, DD1 9SY.
Tel: (01382) 632 273
Fax: (01382) 632 060
jon.a.cook@tuht.scot.nhs.uk

Wales
Mr P. Spark,
Principal Pharmacist
Pharmacy Department
Cardiff and Vale NHS Trust
Heath Park
Cardiff, CF14 4XW.
Tel: (029) 2074 4828
Fax: (029) 2074 3114
paul.spark@cardiffandvale.wales.
nhs.uk

Index

Principal page references are printed in **bold** type. Proprietary (trade) names are printed in *italic* type.

In Confidence

MHRA
Medicines and Healthcare products
Regulatory Agency

SUSPECTED ADVERSE DRUG REACTIONS

If you are suspicious that an adverse reaction may be related to a drug or combination of drugs please complete this Yellow Card. Please report all adverse reactions for black triangle (▼) drugs and only serious adverse reactions for established drugs. Suspected ADRs can also be reported electronically. For additional reporting advice please see page 10 of the BNF or the MHRA website medicines.mhra.gov.uk. Do not be put off reporting because some details are not known.

PATIENT DETAILS	Patient Initials: _____	Sex: M / F	Weight if known (kg): _____
Age (at time of reaction): _____	Identification (Your Practice / Hospital Ref.)*: _____		

SUSPECTED DRUG(S)

Give brand name of drug and batch number if known	Route	Dosage	Date started	Date stopped	Prescribed for

SUSPECTED REACTION(S)

Please describe the reaction(s) and any treatment given:

Date reaction(s) started: _____   Date reaction(s) stopped: _____

Do you consider the reaction to be serious? Yes / No

If *yes*, please indicate why the reaction is considered to be serious (please tick all that apply):

☐ Patient died due to reaction   ☐ Involved or prolonged inpatient hospitalisation
☐ Life threatening   ☐ Involved persistent or significant disability or incapacity
☐ Congenital abnormality   ☐ Medically significant; please give details:

Outcome

☐ Recovered
☐ Recovering
☐ Continuing
☐ Other

* This is to enable you to identify the patient in any future correspondence concerning this report
Please attach additional pages if necessary

OTHER DRUGS (including self-medication & herbal remedies)

Did the patient take any other drugs in the last 3 months prior to the reaction?   Yes / No

If yes, please give the following information if known:

Drug (Brand, if known)	Route	Dosage	Date started	Date stopped	Prescribed for

Additional relevant information e.g. medical history, test results, known allergies, rechallenge (if performed), suspected drug interactions. For congenital abnormalities please state all other drugs taken during pregnancy and the date of the last menstrual period.

REPORTER DETAILS
Name and Professional Address:

Post code: _____ Tel No: _____

Speciality:

Signature: Date:

CLINICIAN (if not the reporter)
Name and Professional Address:

Post code:

Tel No: _____ Speciality: _____

If you would like information about other adverse reactions associated with the suspected drug, please tick this box   ☐

Send to **MHRA, CSM FREEPOST, LONDON SW8 5BR** or if you are in one of the following NHS regions:

to **CSM Mersey, FREEPOST, Liverpool L3 3AB**   or **CSM Scotland, CARDS, FREEPOST NAT3271, Edinburgh EH3 0BR**

or **CSM Northern & Yorkshire, FREEPOST 1085, Newcastle upon Tyne NE1 1BR**   or **CSM Wales, FREEPOST, Cardiff CF4 1ZZ**

or **CSM West Midlands, FREEPOST SW2991, Birmingham B18 7BR**

COMMITTEE ON SAFETY OF MEDICINES

In Confidence

MHRA
Medicines and Healthcare products
Regulatory Agency

SUSPECTED ADVERSE DRUG REACTIONS

If you are suspicious that an adverse reaction may be related to a drug or combination of drugs please complete this Yellow Card. Please report all adverse reactions for black triangle (▼) drugs and only serious adverse reactions for established drugs. Suspected ADRs can also be reported electronically. For additional reporting advice please see page 10 of the BNF or the MHRA website medicines.mhra.gov.uk. Do not be put off reporting because some details are not known.

PATIENT DETAILS   Patient Initials: _____   Sex: M / F   Weight if known (kg): _____

Age (at time of reaction): _____   Identification (Your Practice / Hospital Ref.)*: _____

SUSPECTED DRUG(S)

Give brand name of drug and batch number if known	Route	Dosage	Date started	Date stopped	Prescribed for

SUSPECTED REACTION(S)
Please describe the reaction(s) and any treatment given:

Date reaction(s) started: _____   Date reaction(s) stopped: _____

Do you consider the reaction to be serious?   Yes / No

If *yes*, please indicate why the reaction is considered to be serious (please tick all that apply):

Patient died due to reaction ☐   Involved or prolonged inpatient hospitalisation ☐

Life threatening ☐   Involved persistent or significant disability or incapacity ☐

Congenital abnormality ☐   Medically significant; please give details: ☐

Outcome

Recovered ☐
Recovering ☐
Continuing ☐
Other ☐

* This is to enable you to identify the patient in any future correspondence concerning this report
Please attach additional pages if necessary

OTHER DRUGS (including self-medication & herbal remedies)

Did the patient take any other drugs in the last 3 months prior to the reaction? Yes / No

If *yes*, please give the following information if known:

Drug (Brand, if known)	Route	Dosage	Date started	Date stopped	Prescribed for

Additional relevant information e.g. medical history, test results, known allergies, rechallenge (if performed), suspected drug interactions. For congenital abnormalities please state all other drugs taken during pregnancy and the date of the last menstrual period.

REPORTER DETAILS
Name and Professional Address:

Post code: _____ Tel No: _____

Speciality: _____

Signature: _____ Date: _____

CLINICIAN (if not the reporter)
Name and Professional Address:

Post code: _____

Tel No: _____ Speciality: _____

If you would like information about other adverse reactions associated with the suspected drug, please tick this box ☐

Send to **MHRA, CSM FREEPOST, LONDON SW8 5BR** or if you are in one of the following NHS regions:

to **CSM Mersey, FREEPOST, Liverpool L3 3AB** or **CSM Scotland, CARDS, FREEPOST NAT3271, Edinburgh EH3 0BR**

or **CSM Northern & Yorkshire, FREEPOST 1085, Newcastle upon Tyne NE1 1BR** or **CSM Wales, FREEPOST, Cardiff CF4 1ZZ**

or **CSM West Midlands, FREEPOST SW2991, Birmingham B18 7BR**

COMMITTEE ON SAFETY OF MEDICINES

In Confidence

SUSPECTED ADVERSE DRUG REACTIONS

MHRA
Medicines and Healthcare products
Regulatory Agency

If you are suspicious that an adverse reaction may be related to a drug or combination of drugs please complete this Yellow Card. Please report all adverse reactions for black triangle (▼) drugs and only serious adverse reactions for established drugs. Suspected ADRs can also be reported electronically. For additional reporting advice please see page 10 of the BNF or the MHRA website medicines.mhra.gov.uk. Do not be put off reporting because some details are not known.

PATIENT DETAILS	Patient Initials:		Sex: M / F	Weight if known (kg):
Age (at time of reaction):		Identification (Your Practice / Hospital Ref.)*:		

SUSPECTED DRUG(S)

Give brand name of drug and batch number if known	Route	Dosage	Date started	Date stopped	Prescribed for

SUSPECTED REACTION(S)

Please describe the reaction(s) and any treatment given:

Date reaction(s) started: _____ Date reaction(s) stopped: _____

Do you consider the reaction to be serious? Yes / No

If *yes*, please indicate why the reaction is considered to be serious (please tick all that apply):

☐ Patient died due to reaction
☐ Life threatening
☐ Congenital abnormality

☐ Involved or prolonged inpatient hospitalisation
☐ Involved persistent or significant disability or incapacity
☐ Medically significant; please give details:

Outcome

☐ Recovered
☐ Recovering
☐ Continuing
☐ Other

* This is to enable you to identify the patient in any future correspondence concerning this report
Please attach additional pages if necessary

OTHER DRUGS (including self-medication & herbal remedies)

Did the patient take any other drugs in the last 3 months prior to the reaction? Yes / No

If *yes*, please give the following information if known:

Drug (Brand, if known)	Route	Dosage	Date started	Date stopped	Prescribed for

Additional relevant information e.g. medical history, test results, known allergies, rechallenge (if performed), suspected drug interactions. For congenital abnormalities please state all other drugs taken during pregnancy and the date of the last menstrual period.

REPORTER DETAILS Name and Professional Address:	**CLINICIAN (if not the reporter)** Name and Professional Address:
Post code:	Post code:
Speciality: _____ Tel No: _____	Tel No: _____ Speciality: _____
Signature:	If you would like information about other adverse reactions associated with the suspected drug, please tick this box ☐
Date:	

Send to **MHRA, CSM FREEPOST, LONDON SW8 5BR** or if you are in one of the following NHS regions:

to **CSM Mersey, FREEPOST, Liverpool L3 3AB**   or **CSM Scotland, CARDS, FREEPOST NAT3271, Edinburgh EH3 0BR**

or **CSM Northern & Yorkshire, FREEPOST 1085, Newcastle upon Tyne NE1 1BR**   or **CSM Wales, FREEPOST, Cardiff CF4 1ZZ**

or **CSM West Midlands, FREEPOST SW2991, Birmingham B18 7BR**

COMMITTEE ON SAFETY OF MEDICINES

In Confidence

SUSPECTED ADVERSE DRUG REACTIONS

MHRA

Medicines and Healthcare products
Regulatory Agency

If you are suspicious that an adverse reaction may be related to a drug or combination of drugs please complete this Yellow Card. Please report all adverse reactions for black triangle (▼) drugs and only serious adverse reactions for established drugs. Suspected ADRs can also be reported electronically. For additional reporting advice please see page 10 of the BNF or the MHRA website medicines.mhra.gov.uk. Do not be put off reporting because some details are not known.

PATIENT DETAILS   Patient Initials: _____   Sex: M / F   Weight if known (kg): _____

Age (at time of reaction): _____   Identification (Your Practice / Hospital Ref.)*: _____

SUSPECTED DRUG(S)

Give brand name of drug and batch number if known	Route	Dosage	Date started	Date stopped	Prescribed for

SUSPECTED REACTION(S)
Please describe the reaction(s) and any treatment given:

Date reaction(s) started: _____   Date reaction(s) stopped: _____

Do you consider the reaction to be serious? Yes / No

If *yes*, please indicate why the reaction is considered to be serious (please tick all that apply):

Patient died due to reaction ☐   Involved or prolonged inpatient hospitalisation ☐

Life threatening ☐   Involved persistent or significant disability or incapacity ☐

Congenital abnormality ☐   Medically significant; please give details:

Outcome

Recovered ☐
Recovering ☐
Continuing ☐
Other ☐

* This is to enable you to identify the patient in any future correspondence concerning this report
Please attach additional pages if necessary

OTHER DRUGS (including self-medication & herbal remedies)

Did the patient take any other drugs in the last 3 months prior to the reaction?   Yes / No

If *yes*, please give the following information if known:

Drug (Brand, if known)	Route	Dosage	Date started	Date stopped	Prescribed for

Additional relevant information e.g. medical history, test results, known allergies, rechallenge (if performed), suspected drug interactions. For congenital abnormalities please state all other drugs taken during pregnancy and the date of the last menstrual period.

REPORTER DETAILS Name and Professional Address:	**CLINICIAN (if not the reporter)** Name and Professional Address:
Post code: _____ Tel No: _____	Tel No: _____ Post code: _____
Speciality: _____	Speciality: _____
Signature: _____ Date: _____	If you would like information about other adverse reactions associated with the suspected drug, please tick this box ☐

Send to **MHRA, CSM FREEPOST, LONDON SW8 5BR** or if you are in one of the following NHS regions:

to **CSM Mersey, FREEPOST, Liverpool L3 3AB** or **CSM Scotland, CARDS, FREEPOST NAT3271, Edinburgh EH3 0BR**

or **CSM Northern & Yorkshire, FREEPOST 1085, Newcastle upon Tyne NE1 1BR** or **CSM Wales, FREEPOST, Cardiff CF4 1ZZ**

or **CSM West Midlands, FREEPOST SW2991, Birmingham B18 7BR**

Joint British Societies Coronary Risk Prediction Chart

British Cardiac Society - British Hypertension Society - British Hyperlipidaemia Association - Diabetes UK

NO DIABETES

MEN

CHD risk <15% over next 10 years
CHD risk 15-30% over next 10 years
CHD risk >30% over next 10 years

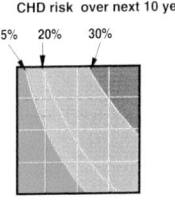

CHD risk over next 10 years

15%   20%   30%

SBP = systolic blood pressure mmHg
TC : HDL = serum total cholesterol to
HDL cholesterol ratio.

How to use the Coronary Risk Prediction Charts for Primary Prevention

These charts are for estimating coronary heart disease (CHD) risk (non-fatal MI, coronary death and new angina pectoris) for individuals who have **not** already developed CHD or other major atherosclerotic disease. They are an aid to making clincial decisions about how intensively to intervene on lifestyle and whether to use antihypertensive and lipid lowering medication, but should **not replace clinical judgement**.

- The use of these charts is **not appropriate** for patients who have existing diseases which already put them at high risk. Such diseases are:

  - CHD or other major atherosclerotic disease

  - Familial hypercholesterolaemia or other inherited dyslipidaemias

  - Renal dysfunction including diabetic nephropathy

(Continued over)

WOMEN

AGE **35 - 44** YEARS

CHD risk <15% over next 10 years
CHD risk 15-30% over next 10 years
CHD risk >30% over next 10 years

CHD risk over next 10 years

SBP = systolic blood pressure mmHg
TC : HDL = serum total cholesterol to
HDL cholesterol ratio.

- The charts should not be used to decide whether to introduce antihypertensive medication when blood pressure is persistently at or above 160/100 or when target organ damage due to hypertension is present. In both cases antihypertensive medication is recommended regardless of CHD risk.

- To estimate an individual's absolute 10 year risk of developing CHD choose the table for his or her gender, diabetes (yes/no), smoking status (smoker/non-smoker) and age. Within this square define the level of risk according to the point where the coordinates for systolic blood pressure and the ratio of total cholesterol to high density lipoprotein (HDL) cholesterol meet. If no HDL cholesterol result is available, then assume this is 1.00mmol/l and the lipid scale can be used for total serum cholesterol alone. Diabetes refers to type 2 diabetes. See later notes, if patient has type 1 diabetes or impaired fasting glucose.

- Higher risk individuals are defined as those whose 10 year CHD risk exceeds 15% which is equivalent to a combined risk of CHD and stroke (cardiovascular risk) of >20% over the same period. As a minimum those at highest CHD risk (>30% red) should be targeted and treated now. When resources allow others with a CHD risk of >15% (orange) should be progressively targeted.

- Smoking status should reflect lifetime exposure to tobacco and not simply tobacco use at the

(Continued over)

MEN

AGE **35 - 44** YEARS

NON-SMOKER SMOKER

AGE **45 - 54** YEARS

NON-SMOKER SMOKER

AGE **55 - 64** YEARS

NON-SMOKER SMOKER

AGE **65 - 74** YEARS

NON-SMOKER SMOKER

SBP — 180 160 140 120

TC: HDL — 4 6 8 10

CHD risk <15% over next 10 years
CHD risk 15-30% over next 10 years
CHD risk >30% over next 10 years

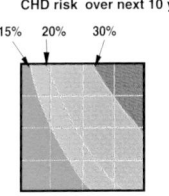

CHD risk over next 10 years

15%   20%   30%

SBP = systolic blood pressure mmHg
TC : HDL = serum total cholesterol to
HDL cholesterol ratio.

time of assessment. For example, those who have given up smoking within 5 years should be regarded as current smokers for the purposes of the charts.

- The initial blood pressure and the first random (non-fasting) total cholesterol and HDL cholesterol are used to estimate an individual's risk. However, the decision on using drug therapy should generally be based on repeat risk factor measurements over a period of time.

- These charts (and all other currently available methods of CHD risk prediction) are based on groups of people with **untreated** levels of blood pressure, total cholesterol and HDL cholesterol. In patients already receiving antihypertensive therapy in whom the decision is to be made about whether to introduce lipid-lowering medication or vice versa the charts can act as a guide, but unless recent pre-treatment risk factor values are available it is generally safest to assume that CHD risk is higher than that predicted by current levels of blood pressure or lipids on treatment.

- CHD risk is also higher than indicated in the charts for:-
  - Those with a family history of premature CHD (male first degree relatives aged <55 years and female first degree relatives aged <65 years) which increases the risk by a factor of approximately 1.5
  - Those with raised triglyceride levels
  - Women with premature menopause

(Continued over)

DIABETES

WOMEN

AGE **35 - 44** YEARS

NON-SMOKER | SMOKER

AGE **45 - 54** YEARS

NON-SMOKER | SMOKER

AGE **55 - 64** YEARS

NON-SMOKER | SMOKER

AGE **65 - 74** YEARS

NON-SMOKER | SMOKER

SBP: 180, 160, 140, 120
TC: HDL: 4, 6, 8, 10

CHD risk <15% over next 10 years
CHD risk 15-30% over next 10 years
CHD risk >30% over next 10 years

CHD risk over next 10 years

15%   20%   30%

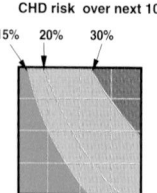

SBP = systolic blood pressure mmHg
TC : HDL = serum total cholesterol to
HDL cholesterol ratio.

- Those who are not yet diabetic but have impaired fasting glucose (6.1-6.9mmol/l
- Patients with Type 1 diabetes in whom the risk is often greater than predicted by the total cholesterol to HDL cholesterol ratio. It may be more accurate to ignore HDL cholesterol in them and use the lipid scale for total serum cholesterol alone, but direct evidence for this is currently lacking.
- As the person approaches the next age category. Risk increases exponentially with age so the risk will be closer to the higher decennium for the last four years of each decade.

• In some ethnic minorities the risk charts underestimate CHD risk because they have not been validated in these populations. For example, in people originating from the Indian subcontinent it is safest to assume that the CHD risk is higher than predicted from the charts (1.4-1.5 times).

• An individual can be shown on the chart the direction in which his or her risk of CHD can be reduced by changing smoking status, blood pressure or cholesterol, but it should be borne in mind that the estimate of risk is for a group of people with similar risk factors and that within that group there will be considerable variation in risk. The charts are primarily to assist in directing intervention to those who typically stand to benefit most.

ADULT ADVANCED LIFE SUPPORT

Precordial thump
if appropriate

Basic Life Support
if appropriate

| Check responsiveness | Open airway Check breathing | Give 2 effective breaths | Check for signs of a circulation | 15:2 Compress chest Continue CPR |

Attach defibrillator-monitor

Assess rhythm

± Check pulse

VF / VT

Non VF / VT

Defibrillate x 3 as necessary

CPR 1 min

During CPR
Correct reversible causes*

If not already
Check — electrode/paddle positions & contact

Attempt/verify — airway & O₂ i.v. access

Give — epinephrine (adrenaline) every 3 min

Consider — amiodarone atropine/pacing buffers

CPR 3 min
1 min if immediately after defibrillation

---

*Potentially reversible causes

Hypoxia	Tension pneumothorax
Hypovolaemia	Tamponade
Hyper/hypokalaemia & metabolic disorders	Toxic/therapeutic disorders
Hypothermia	Thrombo-embolic & mechanical obstruction

Precordial thump if appropriate

Call for help
Fill in local emergency No.

☏ - - - - - - - - - - - - - - - - - - -

Fetch
1. Defibrillator
2. Oxygen
3. Resuscitation equipment

Place electrodes/paddles correctly

If flat trace, check switches, connections and gain

Give oxygen

Secure airway

Secure IV access

© ERC 2001
Illustrations courtesy of Laerdal
HE 0045 ERC rev D

Available from:
LAERDAL MEDICAL LTD.
Laerdal House, Orpington,
Kent BR6 0HX,
Tel. 01689 876634, Fax. 01689 873800

European Resuscitation Council   In co-operation with   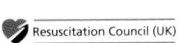 Resuscitation Council (UK)

Approximate conversions and units

lb	kg	stones	kg	mL	fl oz
1	0.45	1	6.35	50	1.8
2	0.91	2	12.70	100	3.5
3	1.36	3	19.05	150	5.3
4	1.81	4	25.40	200	7.0
5	2.27	5	31.75	500	17.6
6	2.72	6	38.10	1000	35.2
7	3.18	7	44.45		
8	3.63	8	50.80		
9	4.08	9	57.15		
10	4.54	10	63.50		
11	4.99	11	69.85		
12	5.44	12	76.20		
13	5.90	13	82.55		
14	6.35	14	88.90		
		15	95.25		

Prescribing in children

Age	Ideal body-weight		Height		Body-surface
	kg	lb	cm	inch	m²
Newborn*	3.5	7.7	50	20	0.23
1 month*	4.2	9	55	22	0.26
3 months*	5.6	12	59	23	0.32
6 months	7.7	17	67	26	0.40
1 year	10	22	76	30	0.47
3 years	15	33	94	37	0.62
5 years	18	40	108	42	0.73
7 years	23	51	120	47	0.88
12 years	39	86	148	58	1.25
Adult					
Male	68	150	173	68	1.80
Female	56	123	163	64	1.60

* The figures relate to full term and not preterm infants who may need reduced dosage according to their clinical condition.

Length

1 metre (m)		= 1000 millimetres (mm)
1 centimetre (cm)		= 10 mm
1 inch (in)		= 25.4 mm
1 foot (ft)	= 12 inches	= 304.8 mm

Mass

1 kilogram (kg)	= 1000 grams (g)
1 gram (g)	= 1000 milligrams (mg)
1 milligram (mg)	= 1000 micrograms
1 microgram	= 1000 nanograms
1 nanogram	= 1000 picograms

Volume

1 litre	= 1000 millilitres (mL)
1 millilitre (1 mL)	= 1000 microlitres
1 pint	≈ 568 mL

Other units

1 kilocalorie (kcal)	= 4186.8 joules (J)
1000 kilocalories (kcal)	= 4.1868 megajoules (MJ)
1 megajoule (MJ)	= 238.8 kilocalories (kcal)
1 millimetre of mercury (mmHg)	= 133.3 pascals (Pa)
1 kilopascal (kPa)	= 7.5 mmHg (pressure)

Plasma-drug concentrations in the BNF are expressed in mass units per litre (e.g. mg/litre). The approximate equivalent in terms of amount of substance units (e.g. micromol/litre) is given in brackets.

Recommended wording of cautionary and advisory labels

For details see Appendix 9

1   Warning. May cause drowsiness

2   Warning. May cause drowsiness. If affected do not drive or operate machinery. Avoid alcoholic drink

3   Warning. May cause drowsiness. If affected do not drive or operate machinery

4   Warning. Avoid alcoholic drink

5   Do not take indigestion remedies at the same time of day as this medicine

6   Do not take indigestion remedies or medicines containing iron or zinc at the same time of day as this medicine

7   Do not take milk, indigestion remedies, or medicines containing iron or zinc at the same time of day as this medicine

8   Do not stop taking this medicine except on your doctor's advice

9   Take at regular intervals. Complete the prescribed course unless otherwise directed

10 Warning. Follow the printed instructions you have been given with this medicine

11 Avoid exposure of skin to direct sunlight or sun lamps

12 Do not take anything containing aspirin while taking this medicine

13 Dissolve or mix with water before taking

14 This medicine may colour the urine

15 Caution flammable: keep away from fire or flames

16 Allow to dissolve under the tongue. Do not transfer from this container. Keep tightly closed. Discard 8 weeks after opening

17 Do not take more than ... in 24 hours

18 Do not take more than ... in 24 hours or ... in any one week

19 Warning. Causes drowsiness which may continue the next day. If affected do not drive or operate machinery. Avoid alcoholic drink

21 ... with or after food

22 ... half to one hour before food

23 ... an hour before food or on an empty stomach

24 ... sucked or chewed

25 ... swallowed whole, not chewed

26 ... dissolved under the tongue

27 ... with plenty of water

28 To be spread thinly ...

29 Do not take more than 2 at any one time. Do not take more than 8 in 24 hours

30 Do not take with any other paracetamol products

31 Contains aspirin and paracetamol. Do not take with any other paracetamol products

32 Contains aspirin

33 Contains an aspirin-like medicine